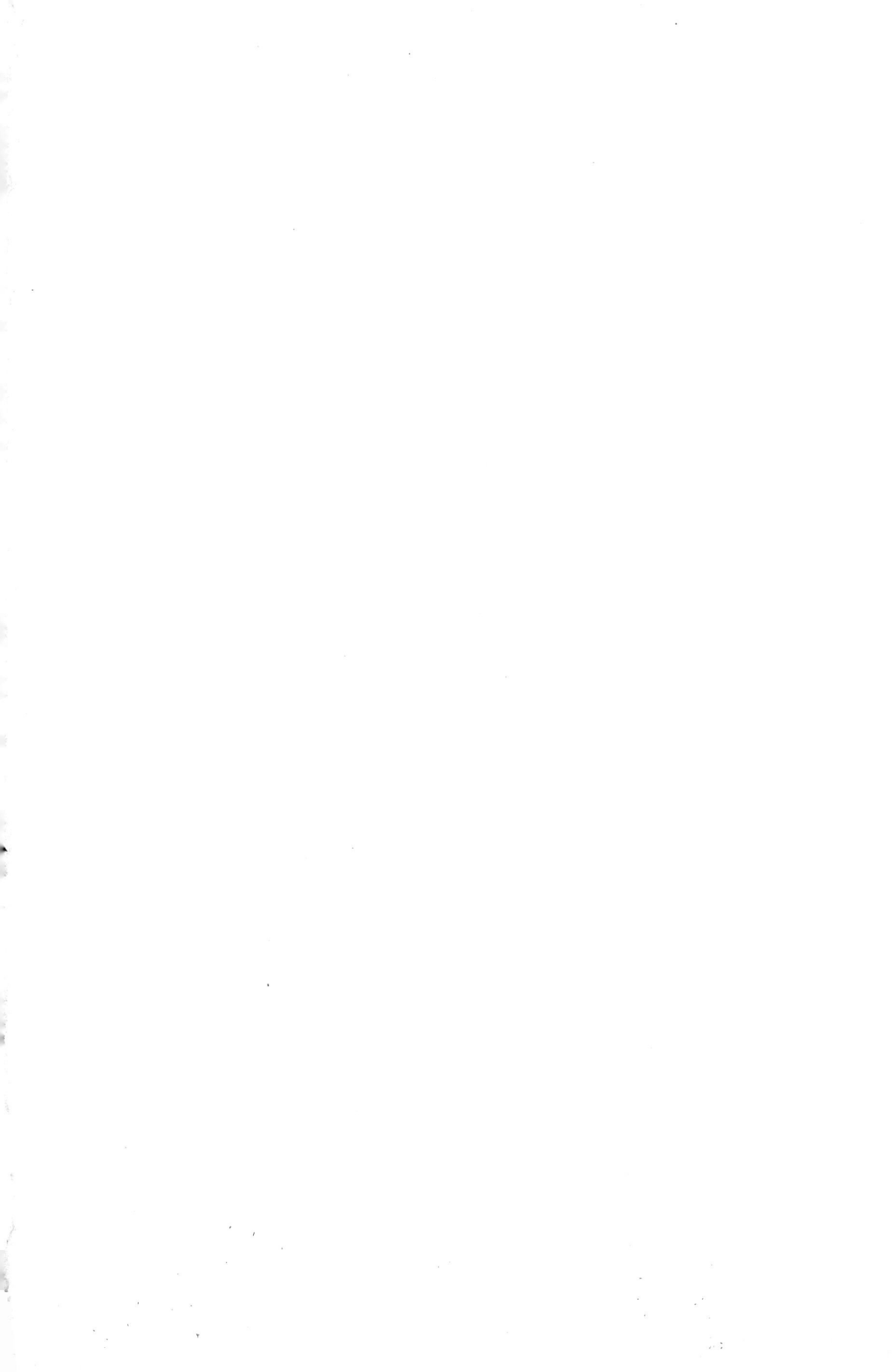

PSYCHIATRIE DER GEGENWART

FORSCHUNG UND PRAXIS

Herausgegeben von

K. P. Kisker, J. E. Meyer, C. Müller,
E. Strömgren

Band I

Zweite Auflage

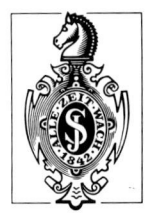

Springer-Verlag Berlin Heidelberg New York 1980

GRUNDLAGEN UND METHODEN DER PSYCHIATRIE

Teil 2

Bearbeitet von

J. Angst, A. Carlsson, J. Gross, R. Jung, P. Kempe, H. Künkel,
L. Laitinen, N. Matussek, J.-O. Ottosson, D. Ploog, D. Richter, B. Woggon,
E. Zerbin-Rüdin, D. von Zerssen

Mit 184 Abbildungen

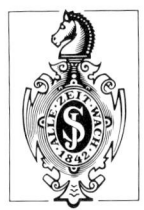

Springer-Verlag Berlin Heidelberg NewYork 1980

Professor Dr. Dr. K.P. KISKER, Medizinische Hochschule, Psychiatrische Klinik, Karl-Wiechert-Allee 9, D-3000 Hannover 61
Professor Dr. J.E. MEYER, Psychiatrische Universitätsklinik, von-Siebold-Str. 5, D-3400 Göttingen
Professor Dr. C. MÜLLER, Hôpital de Cery, Clinique Psychiatrique Universitaire, Canton de Vaud, CH-1008 Prilly
Professor Dr. E. STRÖMGREN, Psychiatrisches Krankenhaus, DK-8240 Risskov

ISBN 3-540-09619-1 Springer-Verlag Berlin Heidelberg New York
ISBN 0-387-09619-1 Springer-Verlag New York Heidelberg Berlin

CIP-Kurztitelaufnahme der Deutschen Bibliothek
Psychiatrie der Gegenwart: Forschung u. Praxis / hrsg. von K.P. Kisker ... – Berlin, Heidelberg, New York: Springer.
NE: Kisker, Karl Peter (Hrsg.) Bd. 1. – Grundlagen und Methoden der Psychiatrie Teil. 2 / Bearb. von J. Angst ... – 2. Aufl. – 1979. (Psychiatrie der Gegenwart; Bd. 1)
ISBN 3-540-09619-1 (Berlin, Heidelberg, New York)
ISBN 0-387-09619-1 (New York, Heidelberg, Berlin)
NE: Angst, Jules (Bearb.)

Das Werk ist urheberrechtlich geschützt. Die dadurch begründeten Rechte, insbesondere die der Übersetzung, des Nachdruckes, der Entnahme von Abbildungen, der Funksendung, der Wiedergabe auf photomechanischem oder ähnlichem Wege und der Speicherung in Datenverarbeitungsanlagen bleiben, auch bei nur auszugsweiser Verwertung, vorbehalten. Bei Vervielfältigung für gewerbliche Zwecke ist gemäß § 54 UrhG eine Vergütung an den Verlag zu zahlen, deren Höhe mit dem Verlag zu vereinbaren ist.
© by Springer-Verlag Berlin Heidelberg 1980.
Printed in Germany
Die Wiedergabe von Gebrauchsnamen, Handelsnamen, Warenbezeichnungen usw. in diesem Werk berechtigt auch ohne besondere Kennzeichnung nicht zu der Annahme, daß solche Namen im Sinne der Warenzeichen- und Markenschutz-Gesetzgebung als frei zu betrachten wären und daher von jedermann benutzt werden dürften.
Satz, Druck und Bindearbeiten: Universitätsdruckerei H. Stürtz AG, Würzburg 2122/3130-543210

Inhaltsverzeichnis

D. Biologische Grundlagen

Neurochemistry. By D. RICHTER. With 4 Figures	1
Stoffwechselpathologie der Zyklothymie und Schizophrenie. Von N. MATUSSEK. Mit 15 Abbildungen	65
Elektroenzephalographie und Psychiatrie. Von H. KÜNKEL. Mit 36 Abbildungen	115
Psychopharmacology: Basic Aspects. By A. CARLSSON. With 3 Figures	197
Psychopharmakotherapie. Von J. ANGST und B. WOGGON	243
Convulsive Therapy. By J.-O. OTTOSSON. With 1 Figure	315
Psychosurgery. By L. LAITINEN. With 5 Figures	351
Soziobiologie der Primaten. Von D. PLOOG. Mit 62 Abbildungen	379
Psychiatrische Genetik. Von E. ZERBIN-RÜDIN	545
Konstitution. Von D. VON ZERSSEN. Mit 12 Abbildungen	619
Deprivationsforschung und Psychiatrie. Von P. KEMPE und J. GROSS	707
Neurophysiologie und Psychiatrie. Von R. JUNG. Mit 46 Abbildungen	753
Namenverzeichnis – Author Index	1105
Sachverzeichnis – Subject Index	1187

Inhaltsverzeichnis Band I/1

A. Klinische und psychopathologische Grundlagen

Psychopathologie. Von H. Heimann. Mit 2 Abbildungen
Psychodynamik als Grundlagenforschung der Psychiatrie. Von G. Benedetti
Psychophysiologie. Von J. Fahrenberg. Mit 1 Abbildung
Neuropsychologie. Von G. Assal und H. Hecaen
Endokrinologische Psychiatrie. Von M. Bleuler
Zum Problem der psychiatrischen Primärprävention. Von L. Ciompi
Psychiatric Therapy of Mentally Abnormal Offenders. Is it Possible? By B.B. Svendsen†

B. Psychologische Grundlagen

Theoretische Grundlagen psychologischer Forschungsmethoden in der Psychiatrie. Von H. Legewie. Mit 5 Abbildungen
Lerntheoretische Grundlagen für Theorie und Praxis der Psychiatrie. Von J. Bergold. Mit 3 Abbildungen
Grundlagen und Probleme der Einstellungsforschung. Von H. Feldmann. Mit 5 Abbildungen
Sprache, Persönlichkeitsstruktur und psychoanalytisches Verfahren. Von A. Lorenzer

C. Sozial- und geisteswissenschaftliche Grundlagen

Kommunikation und Interaktion in psychiatrischer Sicht. Von P. Watzlawick. Mit 1 Abbildung
Longitudinal Methods in the Study of Normal and Pathological Development. By L.N. Robins
Demographic and Epidemiological Methods in Psychiatric Research. By B. Cooper. With 1 Figure
Crosscultural Psychiatry. Von N. Sartorius
Ethnopsychiatrie. Von G. Hofer
Psychiatrie und Gesellschaftstheorien. Von K. Dörner
Antipsychiatrie. Von K.P. Kisker
Psychiatrie und Philosophie. Von W. Blankenburg
Psychiatrie und Kunst. Von A. Bader und L. Navratil. Mit 10 Abbildungen

Namenverzeichnis

Sachverzeichnis

Mitarbeiterverzeichnis

Angst, J., Prof. Dr., Psychiatrische Universitätsklinik, Forschungsdirektion, CH-8029 Zürich 8

Carlsson, A., Dr., Göteborgs Universitet, Farmakologiska Institutionen, Fack, S-400 33 Göteborg

Gross, J., Prof. Dr., Universitäts-Krankenhaus Eppendorf, Psychiatrische und Nervenklinik, Martinistraße 52, D-2000 Hamburg 20

Jung, R., Prof. Dr., Klinikum der Albert-Ludwigs-Universität, Abt. Klinische Neurologie und Neurophysiologie, Hansastr. 9, D-7800 Freiburg

Kempe, P., Dr., Universitäts-Krankenhaus Eppendorf, Psychiatrische und Nervenklinik, Martinistraße 52, D-2000 Hamburg 20

Künkel, H., Prof. Dr., Medizinische Hochschule, Abt. für Klinische Neurophysiologie und Experimentelle Neurologie, Karl-Wiechert-Allee 9, D-3000 Hannover 61

Laitinen, L., Dr., Department of Neurosurgery, 5016 Haukeland Sykehus, N-Bergen

Matussek, N., Prof. Dr., Nervenklinik der Universität, Psychiatrische Klinik und Poliklinik, Nußbaumstraße 7, D-8000 München 2

Ottosson, J.-O., Prof. Dr., Göteborgs Universitet, Psykiatriska Kliniken I, Sahlgrenska Sjukhuset, S-413 45 Göteborg

Ploog, D., Prof. Dr., Max-Planck-Institut für Psychiatrie, Deutsche Forschungsanstalt für Psychiatrie, Kraepelinstraße 2 und 10, D-8000 München 40

Richter, D., Prof. Dr., International Brain Research Organisation, Walton-on-the-Hill, GB-Tadworth, Surrey KT20 7TT

Woggon, B., Dr., Psychiatrische Universitätsklinik, Forschungsdirektion, CH-8029 Zürich 8

Zerbin-Rüdin, E., Prof. Dr., Max-Planck-Institut für Psychiatrie, Kraepelinstraße 2 und 10, D-8000 München 40

Zerssen, D. von, Prof. Dr., Max-Planck-Institut für Psychiatrie, Klinik, Kraepelinstraße 10, D-8000 München 40

Neurochemistry

By

D. Richter

Contents

A. Introduction 2
   I. Development of Neurochemistry 2
   II. Present Review 3

B. Experimental Approaches 4
   I. Mammalian Brain in Vivo 4
   II. Brain Metabolism in Vivo 6
   III. Brain Perfusion Techniques 7
   IV. Incorporation of Labelled Metabolites in Vivo 7
   V. Tissue Slice Techniques in Vitro 8
   VI. Tissue Culture Methods 9
   VII. Separation of Neurons and Glial Cells 10
   VIII. Subcellular Fractionation 11
       1. Myelin 11
       2. Cell Nuclei 12
       3. Mitochondria 12
       4. Synaptosomes 13
       5. Synaptic Membranes 13
       6. Synaptic Vesicles 14
       7. Microtubules 14
       8. Microsomal Fraction 14
   IX. Histochemical Methods 14

C. Chemical Composition of Neural Tissues 15
   I. Distribution of Components 15
   II. Lipids 17
       1. Extraction of Lipids 17
       2. Composition of Brain Lipids 18
   III. Proteins 20
       1. Soluble Brain Proteins 20
       2. Membrane Proteins 21
       3. Neuroreceptor Proteins 24
   IV. Neurotransmitters 26
       1. Chemical Transmission 26
       2. Acetylcholine 28
       3. Dopamine 28
       4. Noradrenalin (Norepinephrine) 31
       5. Adrenaline (Epinephrine) 32
       6. 5-Hydroxytryptamine (Serotonin) 34

       7. Amino Acids 35
       8. Histamine 37
       9. Neural Modulators 38
    V. Peptide Neuroeffectors 39
       1. Metabolism 39
       2. Substance P 39
       3. Somatostatin 40
       4. Encephalins 40
       5. Oxytocin and Vasopressin 41
       6. Hypothalamic Regulatory Factors 41
D. Barrier Systems and Compartmentation 44
    I. Blood-Brain Barrier 44
   II. Blood-CSF Barrier 45
  III. Metabolic Compartmentation 46
E. Metabolism and Function 47
    I. Metabolism of Growth 47
   II. Protein Metabolism 49
  III. Lipid Metabolism 51
   IV. Energy Metabolism and Function 52
    V. Pathological Deviations 53
References 55

A. Introduction

I. Development of Neurochemistry

Neurochemistry is the branch of neurobiology that is concerned with the structure and functions of the nervous system at a molecular level. It attempts to relate the neurological mechanisms involved in behaviour to the metabolic processes occurring in brain and nerve and aims to give an adequate and acceptable description of molecular dynamics in the living cells and tissues.

Neurochemistry is one of the younger of the neurosciences, and the study in depth of the biochemical characteristics of neural tissues has developed only in recent years. The earliest approach was that of determining the chemical composition of tissue samples taken from different parts of the brain and from peripheral nerves. In that way, a general idea was obtained of the main classes of lipids, proteins and carbohydrates that are present. Grey matter was separated from the white matter of the brain, and some differences were noted in the composition of different anatomical areas. The analytical methods at first available could be applied only to relatively large samples of tissue obtained by manual dissection, and it took many years before micromethods were developed that made it possible to determine metabolites in microgram quantities of tissue and even in single isolated nerve cells. The development of tracer techniques and of sensitive new methods for the microassay of enzymes then brought information about the dynamics of the metabolic processes in different regions of the brain. Attention was at first directed mainly towards the energy metabolism, but gradually the field was enlarged to include the metabolism of the proteins, lipids and transmitter compounds in neural tissues. New techniques for the isolation of specific cell types and subcellular organelles then greatly extended our understanding of the localization of metabolic function. In this way, it became possible to study the metabolic characteristics, not only of different types of neuronal and glial cells, but also of specific nerve ending and membrane structures, so laying the foundations for our current concepts on the mechanisms of synaptic transmission.

The recent rapid growth of neurochemistry is in part a reflection of the natural interest of scientists in the basic mechanisms of the brain. Besides being the organ that is the most complex and least understood, it is now recognised to be one of the most metabolically active organs in the body. Interest has also derived from the appreciation of the relevance of neurochemical data to problems in the related fields of neurophysiology, neuroendocrinology, neuropathology and pharmacology. The early work of GARROD (1923) in showing an association between mental deficiency and inborn errors of metabolism drew attention to the relevance of neurochemical mechanisms to the operation of genetic factors that influence thinking and behaviour. Another important influence was the work of GJESSING (1947) who demonstrated for the first time in periodic catatonia a form of psychosis associated with specific changes in the protein metabolism of the brain. The increasing awareness of the many applications of neurochemistry to problems in other fields helped to make what had started as no more than a minor branch of biochemistry develop into one of the most active of the neurosciences. Present indications suggest that this is still only a beginning and that neurochemistry will continue to develop.

The growth of interest in neurochemistry brought a corresponding increase in the literature. Before the 1950s, PAGE's *Chemistry of the Brain* (1937) was the only general textbook on the subject and there was no neurochemical journal. In 1952 an international group of neurochemists agreed to organize a series of symposia arranged for the primary purpose of collecting information on important aspects of neurochemistry, and the first volume of the series, *Biochemistry of the Developing Nervous System*, edited by WAELSCH, appeared in 1955. Subsequent volumes on *Metabolism of the Nervous System* (RICHTER, 1957), *Chemical Pathology of the Nervous System* (FOLCH-PI, 1961), *Regional Neurochemistry* (KETY and ELKES, 1961), and *Comparative Neurochemistry* (RICHTER, 1964) helped to establish the modern literature of neurochemistry. The textbook *Neurochemistry* (ELLIOTT, PAGE and QUASTEL) appeared in 1955 and the *Journal of Neurochemistry* (1956–) then provided an international journal. More recently several excellent textbooks have been produced on different aspects of the subject, and special mention must be made of the comprehensive *Handbook of Neurochemistry*, in seven volumes, edited by LAJTHA (1969).

II. Present Review

The present review gives a selection of those aspects of neurochemistry that appear to be most relevant to the problems of psychiatry. Emphasis has been laid on biochemical factors in which neural tissues differ from other organs and especially on studies of the mammalian brain. Attention has been given to the neurotransmitter and receptor systems in the brain and to biochemical mechanisms that may be concerned in the therapeutic actions of drugs.

The validity of neurochemical data of various kinds depends very much on the reliability of the methods by which they were obtained. Their proper appreciation requires an understanding of the experimental methods employed, and in the following section, an outline is therefore given of some of the main techniques that have been used in neurochemical research.

Most of the older neurochemical work has now been recorded in the text-books, where reference to original sources can be found. In the present review, the general policy has been to give references to recent review articles and to quote later papers in a series, rather than attempting to cite all the relevant literature including the earlier investigations that are already well-documented elsewhere.

B. Experimental Approaches

I. Mammalian Brain in Vivo

If the living brain is observed with a microscope through a small hole in the skull, it is seen to be constantly pulsating as the walls of the arterioles dilate with each beat of the heart, and arterial blood is forced in bursts into the deeper structures of the brain. The blue tint of the blood reappearing at the surface in the veins reveals a rapid gaseous exchange due mainly to the combustion of glucose in the dendrites of the nerve cells, where the metabolic rate is especially high. Rapid changes in blood flow are seen to occur in response to the ever-changing pattern of neuronal activity, which can be recorded through electrodes applied to the surface of the brain or inserted in the deeper layers. By the use of windows in the skull, it is possible to study the circulatory changes induced by metabolic factors or by drugs, and those occurring during seizures and in other pathologic states.

The neurons and glial cells normally live and function in the fluid environment of the extracellular space, which occupies some 15%–20% of the total volume of the brain. This is far from a static environment for, besides the pulsation of the arterioles, there is a constant local disturbance as the red blood corpuscles, around 7 μ in diameter, push their way through the narrowed lumen of the capillaries that intertwine among the processes of the neurons and glial cells. There is evidence of movement also in the oligodendrocytes, which are the most numerous cells in the mammalian brain; when grown in tissue culture, the cell body of the oligodendrocyte shows a characteristic rhythmic contraction similar to that of a muscle cell (LUMSDEN and POMERAT, 1951). It is thought that in this way the oligodendrocytes may aid the flow of axoplasm in the neuronal axons to which they are attached. The oligodendrocytes account for most of the metabolic activity of the white matter of the brain and their relatively high metabolic activity and content of mitochondria would be consistent with a physiological function of this kind.

The nerve cells are structurally designed for the propagation of signals that are carried in waves of depolarization that travel at speed along their extended polarized surface membranes. The different types of neurons differ greatly in size and shape, but all have a cell body (soma or perikaryon), receiving processes (or dendrites) and a transmitting process (or axon). Some neurons also transmit information from their dendrites at junctions of a dendrodendritic type (SCHMITT et al., 1976). In having relatively large nuclei, the nerve cells resemble the cells of secretory organs active in protein synthesis, but the various types of neurons differ again in the chemical nature of the neurotransmitters, peptides or proteins they synthesize and secrete or liberate at the nerve endings. Characteristic of the nerve cells are the spindle-shaped granules of liponucleoprotein (Nissl granules) containing RNA, in the cell body, and they also have thread-like fibres (neurofibrils) and long tubular structures (neurotubules) running through the dendrites and axons. Associated with these structures is an active flow of axoplasm in which particles are carried through from the cell body to the periphery. The movements of particles in the rapid "carrier stream" in the axons can be observed directly in live neurons grown in tissue culture. The rate of flow varies in neurons of different types, but in some it is as high as 600 μm per minute (EDSTRÖM and MATTSSON, 1972; SCHUBERT and KREUTZBERG, 1975). There is also evidence of a flow in the reverse direction and of cytoplasmic flow in the dendrites. The smaller particles in the cytoplasm are in a state of constant agitation due to Brownian movement.

The nerve cells are commonly arranged in clusters round the capillaries, where they are enmeshed in the processes of the astrocytes that are attached to the capillaries by long 'sucker feet.' The constant movement in vivo of the extracellular fluid helps to account for the rapid rate of diffusion of glucose and other metabolites through the fluid lying between the capillaries and the cells. The brain has no lymphatic system, and the extracellular fluid serves as a common pathway for all metabolites entering and leaving the cells. Waste products are eliminated mainly through the capillaries, but there is also some exchange of metabolites between the extracellular fluid and the cerebrospinal fluid (CSF) at the surface of the brain and through the ependymal linings of the ventricles. The composition of the CSF at the surface of the brain therefore reflects to some extent the composition of the extracellular fluid of the brain.

The cerebral blood flow is normally controlled by the CO_2 content of the arterial blood. A rise in the CO_2 concentration dilates the arterioles and decreases the cerebrovascular resistance, so increasing the cerebral blood flow. The cerebral vascular response to CO_2 is mediated mainly by changes of pH in the extracellular fluid of the brain. Hyperventilation causes a rise in interstitial pH and decreases the blood flow: the pH then falls and the normal blood flow is restored (RAICHLE et al., 1971).

The brain is commonly said to function as a whole, but many of its functions are localized, and it is an oversimplification to regard it as a single organ. It is in fact a system of interrelated organs that differ in metabolic characteristics as well as in physiological role, which develop and mature at different times. The controlling mechanisms of the hypothalamus are active early in life, long before the mechanisms for the processing of sensory data, for the coordination of motor activity and for higher intellectual functions. In the human species, we must differentiate further between the characteristics of the right and left hemispheres, which differ appreciably in anatomy, development and functional capacities. In order to extend our understanding of the mechanisms operating in the brain, it is clearly necessary to obtain information about the different neurotransmitters and other specific metabolites and their distribution in different parts of the brain. This is discussed in Section C.

II. Brain Metabolism in Vivo

Information about the metabolism of the brain as a whole in vivo can be obtained by determining differences in the composition of the blood entering and leaving the brain. Samples of venous blood taken from the internal jugular vein have a lower content of glucose and O_2 and a higher content of CO_2 than arterial blood. By measuring also the rate of cerebral blood flow, we can determine the overall rate of metabolism in vivo of the brain. Such measurements have been made, not only in conscious animals but also in man.

Evidence of the rate of blood flow through the brain can be obtained with a thermoelectric blood-flow recorder that records the cooling effect of the blood flow on a heated needle inserted in the brain. In this way, a continuous record showing *changes* in the rate of blood flow can be obtained; but this procedure does not give an exact measure of the rate of flow expressed as millilitres blood per 100 g brain per minute.

The rate of blood flow can also be recorded by measuring the radiation emitted from any region of the brain or from the whole head after administering a radioactive gas. The labelled gas can be introduced in the respired air or by injecting a solution containing the gas into the carotid artery. The cerebral blood flow is then calculated from the slope of the curve showing the disappearance of radioactivity from the head over a period of time (INGVAR and LASSEN, 1965).

A more laborious but more exact method of measuring the cerebral blood flow is that of administering an inert or radioactive gas and determining the content of gas simultaneously in samples of arterial blood and also in venous blood taken from the internal jugular vein (KETY, 1951). This technique was used by KETY and SCHMIDT (1949) in a series of investigations of the metabolism of the brain in normal healthy human volunteers and also in patients with mental disorders of various kinds (KETY, 1957). Studies of arteriovenous differences in the levels of various metabolites showed that the brain is metabolically one of the most active organs in the body, and although the brain represents only about 2% of the total body weight, it accounts for about 20% of the total oxygen consumption of the body in the normal resting state. The oxygen is used mainly for the oxidation of glucose, but other compounds are also utilized at a lower rate. The normal rate of utilization of oxygen by the whole brain is about 3.5 ml O_2 per 100 g brain per minute.

Studies of regional and whole brain blood flow have given evidence of two compartments in the brain with different rates of blood flow. From animal experiments in which the grey matter was separated from the white, it appeared that the compartment with faster blood flow is the grey matter, in which the flow is some four times faster than in the white (INGVAR and LASSEN, 1965). This agrees with other evidence indicating that the grey matter has a higher metabolic rate than the white. It is also confirmed by measurements of the local concentrations of oxygen, carbon dioxide and hydrogen ions (pO_2, pCO_2 and pH) in different regions of the brain in vivo, which can be determined by the use of selective electrodes inserted in the tissue.

III. Brain Perfusion Techniques

It is estimated that in primates and in man no more than 3% of the blood in the internal jugular vein comes from tissues other than the brain, but in most other animals the proportion is larger, since there is more extensive communication between the cerebral and extracerebral venous beds. Errors due to contamination of blood from the brain by extracerebral blood can be avoided in studies with the isolated perfused brain. In the methods developed by GEIGER (1958) and his colleagues, a perfusion fluid of "simplified blood" containing washed erythrocytes, serum albumin, glucose, cytidine and uridine was able to maintain the electric activity of the cat brain for more than 4 h. In perfusion experiments with [^{14}C]glucose, ALLWEIS and MAGNES (1958) showed that the perfused cat brain utilizes glucose at a high rate, oxidizing about one-quarter to CO_2 and converting most of the remainder into lactic acid: but there is also a significant utilization of other noncarbohydrate compounds in the brain and a considerable labelling of amino acids, lipids and proteins with ^{14}C. WOODS et al. (1976) have described a method for perfusing the isolated rat brain, in which there was good preservation for more than 2 h of the metabolic characteristics and tissue structure as shown by electron microscopy.

IV. Incorporation of Labelled Metabolites in Vivo

A technique that has proved of considerable value for studying many different metabolic processes in experimental animals in vivo is that of introducing a metabolite labelled with a radioisotope such as ^{3}H or ^{14}C and determining the rate at which the label is incorporated into specific components of the tissues. Thus, in animals killed at different times after injecting [^{14}C]glucose, the ^{14}C is found to be incorporated to varying extents in the different carbohydrates, amino acids and lipids in the brain. The rate of incorporation of a precursor of known specific radioactivity into a brain constituent provides an index of its *turnover* in vivo. The *turnover*, which may be expressed in micromoles resynthesized per gram tissue per hour or in similar terms, provides a valuable index of the metabolic activity of any compound that remains at a constant concentration but is continuously being broken down and resynthesized.

The interpretation of the experimental findings generally depends on knowing the specific radioactivity of the precursor metabolite incorporated into a brain constituent, but difficulties can arise in view of the fact that the brain is not a homogeneous system. Apart from the different anatomical compartments represented for example by the nerve cell bodies, axons, glial cells, and vascular tissue cells, the work with labelled metabolites has shown that metabolites such as amino acids and carbohydrates are not uniformly distributed, but generally contained in separates *metabolic compartments* in which they are metabolized at different rates (BALÁZS and CREMER, 1973). The 'size' of any particular metabolic compartment depends on the metabolic pathway concerned and the route of entry, which determines the rate at which the molecules under consideration pass through the various plasma and intracellular membranes of the cells in the brain to reach the sites at which they are metabolized. It must be understood that what appears to be a 'large' metabolic compartment, representing a main metabolic pathway in terms of molecules metabolized per gram brain tissue per minute, may in fact involve only a small *anatomical* volume and vice versa. The metabolic compartments are not the same for all reactions but depend on the type of metabolism that is involved, and the same metabolite may have different specific radioactivities in the different compartments under consideration.

When a sample of brain tissue is taken from an animal for analysis, the blood supply is interrupted and the tissue becomes anoxic, since the supply of oxygen is cut off. The glucose in the tissue quickly disappears, as also other labile metabolites such as glycogen, phosphocreatine and α-ketoglutarate. Within a few minutes, irreversible changes will have occurred. Changes of this kind in biologically labile metabolites can be reduced by the rapid freezing of the brain tissue. With small animals, this may be done by dropping the head or even the whole animal into liquid nitrogen, which boils at $-196°C$, or by blowing cold nitrogen over the brain (VEECH and HAWKINS, 1974). With larger animals, a sample taken from the exposed brain may be quickly frozen or the brain tissue may be frozen in situ by applying to the surface of the brain a metal vessel containing liquid nitrogen (ALLWEIS and MAGNES, 1958). The frozen brains or brain samples may be kept in the frozen state at a temperature such as $-70°C$ until analysis is carried out. The frozen tissue is then broken up, ground in a previously cooled mortar, and treated with an appropriate solvent such as cooled perchloric acid solution, which precipitates the proteins and extracts metabolites stable at acid pH. For compounds unstable under acid conditions, an alkaline extractant may be used. While it is possible to make a rough separation of the fragments from different regions of the frozen brain, it is difficult to make an accurate dissection of small brain areas. An alternative method for stopping postmortem changes is the use of microwave irradiation, which preserves the brain morphology so that accurate dissection is then possible (GUIDOTTI et al., 1974).

V. Tissue Slice Techniques in Vitro

Much of our present knowledge of the metabolism of the nervous system has been obtained from studies with thin slices of freshly dissected tissue suspended in buffered saline solution in an atmosphere of oxygen. Tissues studied in this way include peripheral nerve and invertebrate giant axons as well as sympathetic ganglia and brain. With brain tissue, which has a relatively high metabolic rate, it is necessary to use thin slices (about 0.3 mm thick) to ensure that there is an adequate rate of diffusion of oxygen to the cells within the slice. Gas containing 95%–100% oxygen may be bubbled through the medium, or the slices may be shaken in an air apparatus of the type developed by WARBURG (1930) and his colleagues in which manometers attached to the containing vessels permit the respiration of the slices to be measured at 37° or other desired temperatures (QUASTEL, 1957).

While many of the cells are inevitably damaged in the process of preparing a tissue slice and the suspending medium differs significantly from the surrounding interstitial fluid in which the cells normally exist in vivo, the cell membranes remain to a large extent functionally intact. Isolated tissue slices therefore reproduce the metabolism of the intact organ in vivo much more closely than breis or homogenates in which the normal membrane relationships are destroyed, so that autolysis quickly proceeds. The approach towards more physiological conditions may be increased by electrical stimulation of the slices in vessels provided with grid electrodes through which electrical impulses can be applied (MCILWAIN and BACHELARD, 1971; LAJTHA, 1969). Electrical stimulation increases the rate of respiration of isolated brain slices by as much as 100% and brings it close to that normal for the brain in vivo. The metabolism of tissue slices respiring in a bath of saline is quickly affected by the washing out of coenzymes and inorganic ions from the tissue, and to correct this it is necessary to add such cofactors to the suspending medium (QUASTEL, 1957).

VI. Tissue Culture Methods

Cells grown in tissue culture retain sufficient properties of the original cells in vivo to make their study of value in helping to define the metabolic characteristics of specific cell types. Pure cultures of neurons from the superior cervical ganglion of the rat maintained in culture for a few weeks increase in size and form a complex network of processes (BRAY, 1970). Detailed biochemical and physiological studies of these cells have shown that they have the ultrastructural characteristics of adrenergic neurons and function as would be expected for such neurons in vivo in synthesizing noradrenaline, maintaining resting potentials and generating action potentials. It is of interest that these adrenergic neurons in tissue culture have been reported to make *cholinergic* synapses with one another, suggesting that such neurons are able to synthesize acetylcholine as well as noradrenaline in response to appropriate environmental clues (BUNGE, 1975). Sensory neurons from dorsal root ganglia have also been grown in complete isolation (OKUN, 1972), and relatively pure cultures of neurons from the central nervous system have been obtained (NELSON and PEACOCK, 1973; LASHER, 1974). The behaviour of clonal lines of neuroblastoma and glioma cells has been studied with a view to using them as model systems for the study of neuronal and glial function.

The earlier studies with mixed cultures of neurons and supporting cells made it possible to study in vitro the way in which the myelin sheath is formed around the axons of individual neurons. They made it possible to study the process of axon elongation by the development of the 'growth cone' at the tip of the growing nerve fibre and demonstrated the active uptake of medium components by pinocytosis (MURRAY, 1965). More recent studies have included observations on the development of synapses of various different types and the conditions controlling neurotransmitter release (BUNGE, 1975). Of special interest is the work on the properties and mechanism of action of the nerve growth factor, which was shown by LEVI-MONTALCINI and her colleagues to act specifically in stimulating the growth of certain classes of neurons (LEVI-MONTALCINI and ANGELETTI, 1971). Humoral and cellular factors influencing neuronal development have been reviewed by VARON (1975).

VII. Separation of Neurons and Glial Cells

Brain tissue contains several different types of neurons that differ in their chemical characteristics (cholinergic, adrenergic, dopaminergic, etc.) as well as in shape and size. It also contains a relatively larger number of glial cells of various types and cells of the blood vessels that permeate the tissue. Within a given cell, there are differences again in the chemical composition and metabolic properties of different regions, as in the cell body and dendritic, axonal and synaptic regions of the neuron. In trying to extend our knowledge of the metabolic characteristics of the different cell types in the brain, attempts have been made to fractionate brain tissue by separating it into its constituent classes of cells and especially to separate nerve cells from glia (ROSE, 1969; LAJTHA, 1969; BOCK and HAMBERGER, 1976). Since neurons and glia have very different functions, it was to be expected that metabolic differences would also be found. This was indicated by earlier work in which comparison was made between the respiratory rate of cerebral cortex, in which about 50% of the cells are small neurons, and corpus callosum, in which there are no neuronal cell bodies and most of the cells are glial (oligodendroglia and astrocytes). Calculations based on estimates of the cell number (from the DNA content) and on differential cell counts led to the conclusion that the neurons of the cerebral cortex are metabolically much more active than the glia, so that about 85% of the respiration of the tissue is due to the neurons. The neurons of the cerebral cortex are also metabolically more active than those of the cerebellum (ELLIOTT and HELLER, 1957).

For the bulk separation of neurons and glia, the first step is the disruption of the tissue so as to obtain a cellular suspension. This can be achieved by incubating brain slices in buffered saline at 37° C for 45 min and then pressing through nylon meshes of successively smaller sizes with pore sizes down to 50 µm (BOCK and HAMBERGER, 1976). For some purposes prior disruption of the tissue by digestion with trypsin or by treatment with acetone and glycerol has been used (APPEL et al., 1972). The isolation of various cell types from the suspension may be done by zonal centrifugation using sucrose or Ficoll sucrose solutions of graded concentrations, so that cells of different density float into different layers. Thus, using the method described by NORTON and PODUSLO (1970), the main neuronal fraction collects at the interface between $1.55\,M$ and $2.0\,M$ sucrose whereas on the $1.55\,M$ layer is a mixture of glia, neurons and capillaries. Above $1.35\,M$ sucrose is the main glial fraction and above the $0.9\,M$ layer are myelin and small debris. By repeated zonal centrifugation, the different fractions can be further purified, but this also involves a loss of material so that the ultimate yield is reduced.

In assessing the purity of the isolated cell fractions obtained by various procedures, some contaminants can be recognised by light microscopy or electron microscopy and use has been made of enzymes as markers. However, the cells in these separated fractions are for the most part severely damaged cells, since the neurons generally retain little more than the stumps of dendrites and axons. The glial cell processes are also not left intact. It has been claimed that cell fractions isolated by such procedures can be more than 90% pure, but until more satisfactory methods have been devised for assessing their purity, it would appear safer to regard them simply as fractions *enriched* to a variable extent by neuronal or glial cells (MORGAN, 1976).

VIII. Subcellular Fractionation

If brain tissue is disrupted in saline to the extent that the individual cell membranes are broken down, a suspension is obtained containing cell nuclei, mitochondria, lysosomes, ribosomes, nerve ending structures (synaptosomes), membrane fragments (microsomes) and myelin together with pieces of capillary network and other fragments. These can be separated by differential and zonal centrifugation into fractions with a relatively high content of any one of the constituents. The methods available for disrupting the cells include swelling, osmotic shock and sonication after homogenizing the tissue in a buffered saline or sucrose solution (APPEL et al. 1972). The yield of any fraction depends on the degree of purity that is required: an increase in purity involves a smaller yield. By careful choice of the starting material and of the optimum conditions for homogenization, cell disruption and centrifugation, the degree of contamination of any particular fraction by material of other types can be greatly reduced, but it must be remembered that the preparations of nuclei, mitochondria, etc. so obtained are heterogeneous in that they come from glial cells as well as from neuronal cells of different types.

1. Myelin

Myelin is the layered membrane structure that results from the growth of glial cell membranes in concentric layers around axons; it may be regarded as a greatly extended and modified plasma membrane. Myelin fragments can be isolated in high yield and relatively high purity by the usual methods of subcellular fractionation. Starting with a homogenate of brain or spinal cord, the myelin is separated from the other subcellular fractions by differential and density gradient centrifugation (APPEL et al., 1972; SPOHN and DAVISON, 1972; NORTON, 1975; TOEWS et al., 1976). The myelin prepared by the usual fractionation procedures commonly contains fragments of axon membranes and traces of axoplasm and cytoplasm from the generating cell. Because of the close binding of the glial cell membranes to the axonal membranes, such contamination is difficult to avoid and it may account for some of the enzymatic activity found in some samples of myelin. Further purification by subjecting the myelin fragments to hypo-osmotic shock in distilled water helps to release trapped materials and enables a purer sample of myelin to be obtained (NORTON, 1975).

Myelin is present in most parts of the nervous system: it accounts for up to 35% of the dry weight of the human brain and 50%–60% of the dry weight of the white matter. In composition myelin is characterized by its high content of lipids, which account for 70%–85% of the dry weight. The chief lipids of the myelin in the mammalian brain are phospholipids (40%–45%), galactosphingolipids (27%–30%) and cholesterol (25%–28%), but the lipid composition changes appreciably with age. Thus, at maturity the molar ratio of galactolipid to phosphatidylcholine is more than twice that at 15 days (NORTON and PODUSLO, 1973). The myelin obtained from the spinal cord has a higher lipid content than that isolated from the brain; the myelin of the peripheral nervous system differs again in having a considerably higher sphingomyelin content. The myelins obtained from different parts of the nervous system differ also in their protein composition (NORTON, 1975). The water content of myelin, which is relatively low, is estimated to be about 40%.

In keeping with its physiological function as an insulating sleeve required for saltatory conduction in the axon, myelin is more stable and less metabolically active than other neural membranes, but there is evidence of a slow turnover of some of the lipid and protein components. It also contains a few enzymes including a protein kinase, a cholesterol ester hydrolase and a nucleotide phosphohydrolase of which the functions are unknown (NORTON, 1975).

2. Cell Nuclei

The isolation of cell nuclei from brain homogenates is aided by their relatively high density due to their high content of DNA. Under suitable conditions, as after homogenizing in 2.2 M sucrose containing 1 mM MgCl$_2$, and 10 mM potassium succinate, the nuclei may be centrifuged down at 78,000 g to form a pellet while all the other cellular material floats. By further fractionation on discontinuous sucrose gradients of 2.2, 2.4, 2.6 and 2.8 M sucrose, a partial separation of the larger nuclei of the neurons from the smaller nuclei of the glial cells can be achieved (MANDEL et al., 1967; LØVTRUP-REIN and McEWEN, 1966). The nuclei of rat brain have been shown to contain an enzyme, poly-C synthetase, which catalyzes the polymerization of cytidine triphosphate (CTP).

3. Mitochondria

Mitochondria are abundant in brain tissue, where they account for as much as 15% of the total brain protein content (ABOOD, 1969). They are relatively concentrated in the neurons and especially in the synaptic regions. A proportion occur also in the oligodendroglia, but the astrocytes and microglia contain relatively few. Mitochondria isolated from brain homogenates are thus mainly of neuronal origin, with a smaller proportion from glial cells. The isolation procedures are facilitated by the fact that the outer membrane of the mitochondria is relatively tough and not as easily disrupted as the plasma membranes of the neurons and glial cells. Differential centrifugation and step gradients may both be used, and the purification is aided by the use of Ficoll, which enables the density to be increased without unduly increasing the osmotic pressure (ABDEL-LATIF and ABOOD, 1964; APPEL et al., 1972).

4. Synaptosomes

At many synaptic junctions, the membranes of the nerve endings are distended to form pockets of axoplasm containing mitochondria, endoplasmic reticulum, neurotubules and synaptic vesicles. When brain tissue is homogenized, these nerve ending structures are broken off from their axons and they reseal to form enclosed structures to which a portion of the postsynaptic membrane and the material of the intersynaptic cleft are generally attached. In the usual subcellular fractionation procedures, the nerve ending structures, or 'synaptosomes,' are found mainly in the crude mitochondrial fraction, and a variety of techniques have been used to obtain preparations of synaptosomes in reasonable yield and as free as possible from other contaminants. The methods currently used generally employ gradient centrifugation on sucrose or Ficoll gradients (COTMAN, 1974; MORGAN, 1976; APPEL et al., 1972). By selecting the denser fractions, contamination with membrane fragments can be reduced, but mitochondrial contamination tends to be increased. The purity of the preparation can be assessed by electron microscopy and by determining choline acetyltransferase, in which the synaptosomes from mammalian brain are enriched. Other types of nerve endings besides the cholinergic are present as well in such preparations since they are derived from the whole synaptic population of the brain. The isolation of nerve ending structures by these methods from the brain made possible a series of investigations by DE ROBERTIS, WHITTAKER and others on synaptic mechanisms in the brain.

5. Synaptic Membranes

If synaptosomes are allowed to swell in hypotonic buffer at slightly alkaline pH, they release their contents, consisting mainly of mitochondria, synaptic vesicles and cytoplasm, leaving the outer synaptic membranes as 'ghosts.' The resulting mixture of synaptic components can again be fractionated on sucrose or Ficoll gradients to give preparations of synaptic membranes which are 70%–90% pure (MOORE, 1975; MORGAN, 1976; APPEL et al., 1972; McBRIDE and VAN TASSEL, 1972). Some laboratories use the crude mitochondrial fraction instead of isolated synaptosomes as the starting point for applying osmotic shock, as in the original procedure developed by WHITTAKER et al. (1964). The resulting preparations of synaptic membranes are of value for studying the properties of neuronal membranes relatively free from glial cell membranes.

By further treatment of the synaptic membrane preparations with agents such as triton X-100 or sodium N-lauryl sarcosinate, it is possible to strip off most of the neuronal plasma membrane from the 'synaptic junctions,' which consist of pieces of presynaptic and postsynaptic membrane with the densely staining material in the synaptic cleft. In this way a fraction enriched in synaptic junctions can be obtained.

6. Synaptic Vesicles

The synaptic vesicles obtained from ruptured brain synaptosomes are small membrane-bound organelles of around 500 Å diameter containing acetylcholine or catecholamines and proteins (WHITTAKER et al., 1964; MORGAN, 1976). The synaptosomal fraction contains significant amounts of the putative transmitter amino acids that are released by electrical stimulation or electric shock, but they are not known to be stored in synaptic vesicles (RASSIN, 1972). The vesicles are apparently formed from smooth tubular endoplasmic reticulum, which reforms into vesicles near the presynaptic ending, but since this process can be induced by the fixatives used to reveal them by electron microscopy, it is not known to what extent the synaptic vesicles exist as such in vivo (GRAY, 1975).

7. Microtubules

The microtubules, which run through the axons of the neurons forming a relatively rigid skeletal structure, are of special interest in view of their apparent role in connection with axonal transport (GROSS, 1975; DROZ, 1975). According to the 'microstream hypothesis,' the microtubules generate a local carrier stream through the axoplasm in which macromolecules and discrete particles are transported towards the nerve ending. The involvement of the microtubules in axonal transport is suggested by the observation that transport is interrupted by the alkaloids colchicine and vinblastine, which bind specifically to the protein tubulin of which the microtubules are mainly composed (OCHS, 1975). It is known that axonal transport is ATP dependent, which indicates ATP as the primary energy source, and ATPase activity has been reported to be associated with the microtubules isolated from mammalian brain. The methods of isolation of microtubules from brain homogenates include discontinuous gradient centrifugation at low temperature on gradients consisting of sucrose dissolved in hexylene glycol (KIRKPATRICK et al., 1970).

8. Microsomal Fraction

This fraction containing mainly fragments of plasma membranes and endothelial reticulum from neurons and glial cells is clearly heterogeneous. It may also contain myelin fragments and lysosomes, which vary considerably in size and may therefore contaminate any of the subcellular fractions (APPEL et al., 1972). The microsomal fraction can be used in studies of membrane-attached enzymes. The purification of the microsomal fraction from rat spinal cord was reported by TOEWS et al. (1976).

IX. Histochemical Methods

The development of microchemical techniques of high sensitivity made it possible to study directly the relationships between the individual cells that make up the structural complexity of the brain. The value of this approach has been shown in the laboratories of CARLSSON, GLICK, HYDÉN, LOWRY, POPE and others. The application of specific staining methods for lipids, proteins,

RNA, and other substances was extended to include studies of the localization of enzymes in different regions, using sections cut from freeze-dried samples of neural tissues (DAVID, 1964; KOELLE, 1961). In this way the roles of enzymes such as acetylcholine esterase and the monoamine oxidase (MAO) were more clearly defined. Of special value is the application of fluorescence techniques to demonstrate the localization of the catecholamines as markers of monoamine-carrying neuronal pathways (DAHLSTRÖM and FUXE, 1965; ANDÉN et al., 1969). The distribution of proteins and polypeptides has been studied by immuno-fluorescence techniques (HÖKFELT et al., 1976). The introduction of radioautographic methods made it possible to obtain information about the metabolic activity as well as the localization of tissue components, by showing the extent of incorporation of labelled metabolites: in this way evidence was obtained of the localization of protein synthesis in the brain, by administering [^{35}S]-methionine in vivo and taking autoradiograms after allowing time for incorporation of the amino acid into the tissue proteins (RICHTER et al., 1960).

A different approach is the *quantitative* microchemical analysis of samples as small as 10 µg (2 µg dry weight) obtained by microdissection from freeze-dried sections at specific sites in the nervous system (LOWRY, 1975). While the general principles of quantitative histochemistry are similar to those of general analytical biochemistry, special techniques have been developed to deal with samples of the smallest size. The sample may be obtained from a frozen section by warming to room temperature and dissecting freehand under a dissecting microscope. In that way it is possible to reduce the sample size to that of a single neuron (HYDÉN and LANGE, 1961). Cell bodies of 15 µ diameter or more and even Purkinje cells, which readily shell out of the surrounding tissue, can be handled in this way. After weighing the samples on a quartz fibre 'fish-pole' balance, the assays for enzymes or metabolites are carried out. Many different colorimetric, fluorometric and manometric methods have been used, but the method of widest applicability is probably that developed by LOWRY, which depends on generating a nicotinamide adenine dinucleotide (as NADPH) that can be determined fluorometrically (LOWRY, 1975). The reactions are commonly carried out in droplets pipetted into minute 'oil wells' containing a mixture of hexadecane and light mineral oil, which reduce loss by evaporation. In an enzymatic reaction that produces only a very small amount of NADPH, the NADPH formed can be used to catalyze further reactions so that the amount is increased several thousand times and brought into the range suitable for fluorometric estimation. By the use of this process of amplification, known as 'cycling,' quantities far too small for direct estimation can be conveniently measured.

C. Chemical Composition of Neural Tissues

I. Distribution of Components

The tissues of the nervous system are characterized by a relatively high lipid content. This is due mainly to the lipid-rich membranes of which neural tissues are to a large extent composed. About 50% of the dry weight of the white matter of the brain and spinal cord is myelin, which is a modified membrane sheath. The grey matter contains less myelin, but has a high content of membranous structures in the dendrites, axon terminals, synaptic structures and processes of the glial cells, which are known collectively as the 'neuropil.' It could in fact be said that neurochemistry is concerned to a large extent with the study of the properties of complex lipoprotein membranes and of the neurotransmitters and other metabolites that influence their behaviour.

The brain has a high water content. The water content of the grey matter is 82% and of the white matter 72% in the human adult. It is higher still in the fetal and infant brain and decreases throughout life. A considerable decrease in water content (or increase in dry weight) results from the laying down of lipids during myelination. In the human brain myelination proceeds at a maximum rate in the period immediately after birth, but it is still continuing at some sites even up to the age of 20. In the rat brain myelination becomes active shortly after birth and myelin is still being deposited up to the age of 425 days. However, the myelin in the adult differs significantly from that deposited at an earlier age in that it contains 50% more galactolipids and differs in protein composition as well (NORTON, 1975). In view of the changes that occur during development, it is clearly necessary to consider the age in expressing the chemical composition of brain tissue as a percentage of the wet or dry weight.

The distribution of the water in the brain cannot be inferred from electron micrographs of the usual type prepared from samples of dehydrated tissue. The appearance they present, showing little or no extracellular space between the cells, has led some investigators to conclude that the water in the brain is almost entirely intracellular. However, by the use of special techniques that enable electron micrographs to be obtained without dehydrating the tissue, the pictures so obtained show appreciable gaps between the cells, representing an extracellular fluid space estimated to be 15%–20% of the total volume (VAN HARREVELD et al., 1965). This agrees with estimates made by measuring the distribution in brain slices of substances such as inulin, which enter the extracellular fluid space but are not taken up into the cells (BAKAY, 1957). It would therefore appear that the extracellular fluid is one of the main components of brain tissue.

The extracellular fluid is a dilute saline solution of similar composition to the cerebrospinal fluid. It contains sodium chloride and some other electrolytes at about the same concentration as in the blood, but the concentrations of K^+, Ca^{2+}, and Mg^{2+} ions are maintained at a generally lower and more constant level (KATZMAN, 1975). The K^+ concentration in the extracellular fluid is important in determining the neuronal and glial plasma membrane potentials. If the cortical tissue is damaged so that K^+ ions from injured cells enter the extracellular fluid, the resulting depolarization of the neighbouring cells causes a liberation of K^+ ions from the stimulated neurons, and the local disturbance can spread out over the cerebral cortex, constituting the phenomenon known as 'spreading depression' (ROITBAK and BOBROV, 1975). The same effect can be evoked by local application of KCl solution to the cerebral cortex.

Apart from electrolytes and the metabolites transferring to and from the blood, the extracellular fluid has a small content of mucoids and mucopolysaccharides. The hydrogen ion concentration is influenced by the HCO_3^- and H^+ ions formed from CO_2 in the presence of carbonic anhydrase: it therefore depends on the metabolic activity of the tissue and hence on the extent of neuronal activity.

The neurons in different parts of the brain are similar in their basic mechanism of energy metabolism, but they differ in the transmitters they synthesize and release. In the cerebral cortex most of the neurons respond to acetylcholine, and cholinergic transmission is dominant, but in the cerebellum the concentration of acetylcholine is less than one-tenth of that in the cerebral cortex and here as elsewhere other mechanisms are apparently operative. The distribution of cholinergic transmission is reflected in the distribution of the enzyme choline acetyl transferase that synthesizes acetylcholine. It was noted by FELDBERG and VOGT (1948) that cholinergic pathways with high choline acetyl transferase content tend to alternate with noncholinergic pathways in different parts of the brain and spinal cord. The distribution of some other neurotransmitters such as noradrenalin and dopamine is much more limited than that of acetylcholine. Noradrenalin is found in highest concentration (about 1 µg/g fresh tissue) in the hypothalamus and area postrema of the fourth ventricle; dopamine occurs in the thalamus, hypothalamus, caudate nucleus, putamen and mesolimbic region. Localized again are the systems responsible for the synthesis and secretion of the polypeptide hormones, ACTH, prolactin, etc. of the hypophysis.

II. Lipids

1. Extraction of Lipids

In brain sections examined after staining for lipids with Sudan II, it can be seen that lipids are present in the myelin sheath of the nerve fibres and also in significant amounts in the plasma membranes, nuclei, mitochondria and cytoplasm of the cells. In order to study the nature and functions of the lipids in the brain, we can extract them directly from the whole tissue or we can first separate the myelin and other tissue fractions before extracting with lipid solvents. If freshly minced brain is shaken with ether, some of the lipids pass quickly into the ether layer, but the rate of extraction soon falls off and even after 24 h it is far from complete. This is partly because of the high water content of fresh brain tissue and partly because some of the lipids, such as the lecithins, are normally present in hydrated forms that are sparingly soluble in lipid solvents. Some lipids normally occur in close association with the tissue proteins with which they form loose molecular complexes, and some are bound to proteins by covalent bonds forming lipoproteins or proteolipids, which liberate the free lipid only when decomposed by procedures such as heating or drying, to denature the protein part of the molecule. Solvents that may be used include ethanol, ether, acetone, petroleum ether and chloroform, but the tissue lipids vary widely in their solubility in different solvents, and it is therefore advantageous to use two or more different solvents if a complete extraction of all the lipids is desired. For many purposes a mixture of chloroform and methanol (2:1, vol/vol) is the solvent of choice (FOLCH-PI et al., 1957). This extracts the proteolipids and phosphatidylpeptides as well as most of the free lipids, but further extraction procedures are needed to obtain complete extraction of the gangliosides and polyphosphoinositides (SUZUKI, 1972).

2. Composition of Brain Lipids

The lipids of the brain can be fractionated by making use of their different solubilities in solvents, by column chromatography, and by using precipitation procedures. For analytical purposes thin layer chromatography permits the rapid separation of seven main fractions – cholesterol, cerebrosides, ethanolamine phospholipids (cephalins), sulphatides, lecithins, sphingomyelins and serine phospholipids. Gas liquid chromatography may be used in addition to a variety of colorimetric methods for the determination of individual lipids.

Table 1 gives a survey of the complex lipids extracted from the grey matter of the adult human brain. While desmosterol, the precursor of cholesterol, is present in measurable amounts in the developing brain, relatively little is found in the adult brain. For categories such as 'lecithins,' etc., the plural is used since in all the complex lipids of the brain the fatty acid parts of the molecules vary; they include unsaturated derivatives as well as the saturated fatty acids, and in the galactolipids α-hydroxy fatty acids have also been found. Free fatty acids are not present in significant amounts in the brain in vivo, but they may be found post mortem. It may be noted that fresh brain tissue contains an active cephalinase that can cause a rapid postmortem breakdown of lipids of the cephalin fraction (phosphatidylethanolamine and phosphatidylserine). The plasmalogens are also relatively labile and quickly decomposed by formalin. In the classification used in Table 1, the sphingomyelins are grouped with the sphingolipids, but they could also be included in the phospholipids in view of their phosphorus content. The triglycerides, which are present in very small amounts, probably come mainly from the vascular tissue in the brain.

The white matter contains a range of complex lipids comparable to that in the grey matter, but the total lipid content is higher because of the higher myelin content. The typical myelin lipids, cholesterol, cerebrosides and sulphatides are present in relatively large amounts. On the other hand, the ganglioside content of white matter is much lower than in the grey matter of the brain. HESS et al. (1976) have determined the ganglioside content by histochemical methods in different layers of the cerebral cortex and have shown that the ganglioside sialic acid content corresponds to the density of neuronal plasma membranes and synapses in the region.

The presence of prostaglandins in central and peripheral nervous tissues is a comparatively recent discovery (SAMUELSSON, 1964), and the study of their metabolism and functions is actively proceeding at the present time. It is known that the prostaglandins are formed from essential fatty acids and that a common precursor is arachidonic acid. An important characteristic of the prostaglandins is the 'prostanoate' structure, which is that of a 20 C monocarboxylic acid with a cyclopentane ring. The enzymes required for the biosynthesis of prosta-

Table 1. Lipid extraction by chloroform-methanol mixtures from grey matter of human brain

Total lipids (100%)	Steroids (22%)	Cholesterol Desmosterol	
	Phospholipids (62%)	Lecithins (27%) (phosphatidylcholine) Ethanolamine phospholipids (23%) (phosphatidylethanolamine) Serine phospholipids (phosphatidylserine) Plasmalogens (acetylphosphatides) Phosphoinositides (phosphatidylinositol)	
	Sphingolipids (14%)	Sphingomyelins (ceramide phosphoryl choline)	
		Galactolipids (galactosyl (ceramides)	Cerebrosides { Kerasin, Nervone, Oxynervon, Cerebron } Sulphatides
		Gangliosides (sialogalactose-ceramides) Strandins	
	Triglycerides	Saturated glycerol esters Unsaturated glycerol esters	
	Prostaglandins	PGE_2, PGF_2, PGD_2	
	Lipid derivatives	Fatty acids (arachidonic acid)	

glandins have been shown to be present in mammalian brain, and it has been reported that the synthesis of prostaglandin E_2 is stimulated by pyrogens and by the neurotransmitters noradrenalin and serotonin. Conversely, antipyretics including aspirin are inhibitors of prostaglandin synthesis. These observations have led to the hypothesis that prostaglandins are involved in the mechanisms of temperature regulation and in the pathogenesis of fever (COCEANI, 1976). The prostaglandins in the brain are believed to be associated especially with the neuronal plasma membrane, but there is evidence that they occur in low concentration in the extracellular fluid and cerebrospinal fluid (HARVEY and MILTON, 1975). This is in keeping with the role assigned to them as 'messengers' or modulators of cellular response to stimuli.

This section can provide no more than a brief introduction to the biochemistry of the brain lipids, and it is not possible to deal here with their metabolism. For further information on the lipids of neural tissues, the reader is referred to the following books and review articles: ANSELL and HAWTHORNE, 1964; COCEANI, 1976; DAVISON, 1968; DAWSON, 1966; EICHBERG et al., 1969; FOLCH-PI and STOFFYN, 1972; LAJTHA, 1970; SUZUKI, 1972, 1975.

III. Proteins

1. Soluble Brain Proteins

If brain tissue is homogenized in neutral buffer solution, a number of proteins pass into solution and remain in the supernatant after centrifugation. These water-soluble proteins, coming mainly from the cytoplasm of the neurons and glial cells, can be separated by polyacrylamide gel disk electrophoresis into 23 or more fractions of varying electrophoretic mobility (KAWAKITA, 1972). Besides several albumins and globulins, some of which have enzymatic activity, the fractions contain fibrous proteins, lipoproteins, glycoproteins, a liponucleoprotein, a copper-containing protein (cerebrocuprein), and also serum albumin and hemoglobin from the blood vessels in the brain (ROSSITER, 1962). The enzymes include a number concerned in intermediary metabolism that are apparently similar to those found in other organs.

a) Neurostenin

The fibrous proteins, neurin and stenin, extracted from brain are similar in amino acid composition and general properties to the actin and myosin of muscle, but they are not identical (WELLINGTON et al., 1976). Thus, they differ in the conditions under which they polymerize. The ATPase activity of neurostenin (corresponding to the actomyosin contractile system) and its presence in the sciatic nerve have suggested that it may be concerned in axoplasmic transport (BERL et al., 1973; OCHS, 1975). The fibrous proteins are present in relatively high concentration in growing structures such as the neurites that grow out of the nerve cells in tissue culture, and they may be involved in the active movements of the growth cones. The amount of actin extracted from neural tissue is increased by sonication (PARDEE and BAMBURG, 1976). Brain actin (neurin) constitutes 8%–10% of the soluble proteins of the developing chick brain at 15 days and about 6% in the adult. Since the part of this coming from the brain arteries is estimated to be less than 0.6%, it is present mainly in the neurons and glial cells.

b) Tubulin

When brain tissue is homogenized in neutral phosphate buffer, the microtubules contained in the nerve axons pass into solution as the soluble protein tubulin. Being an acidic protein, tubulin reacts with alkaloids such as colchicine and vinblastine; it can be separated from other proteins and purified by precipitation with vinblastine (TWOMEY et al., 1976). Tubulin accounts for about 15% of the total soluble proteins of the adult mammalian brain and an even higher proportion in the developing brain (BARONDES and DUTTON, 1972). The microtubules extend through the axons and migrate with the slow component of axoplasmic transport to the nerve endings, where the concentration of tubulin is relatively high. Since axoplasmic transport is blocked by colchicine, it has been suggested that the tubules are an essential part of the mechanism of axonal transport (GROSS, 1975).

c) Brain-Specific Soluble Proteins

Special interest attaches to certain proteins that are found exclusively in nervous tissues and are therefore believed to be closely concerned with neural function. Among the soluble brain proteins is an acidic protein that is not precipitated by ammonium sulphate and, because of its exceptional solubility in 100% saturated ammonium sulphate solution, is known as the "S-100" protein (MOORE and McGREGOR, 1965). The acidic nature of this protein, which facilitates its purification on ion exchange columns or by electrophoresis, is due to its high content of glutamic and aspartic acids. By immunizing rabbits with the purified S-100 protein, it has been possible to obtain antibody preparations that have been used to test for the presence of the protein in other tissues. In that way it was shown that the S-100 protein is present in the nervous system in many different animal species but not in any other organ (LEVINE, 1967). In the mammalian brain the S-100 protein accounts for about 1% of the soluble proteins; it is present in higher concentration in the white matter than in the grey. Studies of the localization of the S-100 protein by fluorescent antibody and other techniques have shown it to be present mainly in the oligodendroglia but also in the astroglia and on the plasma membrane of the nerve cells (HANSSON et al., 1975). It is found, possibly as an artefact (MATUS and MUGHAL, 1975), in isolated synaptosomes (BOCK and HAMBERGER, 1976). At the present time the functions of the S-100 protein are still unknown. One hypothesis is that it is concerned in the binding of calcium, which is concerned in the release of transmitters at the synapses.

Several other brain-specific soluble proteins have been described. These include a protein "14.3.2" investigated by MOORE (1972), which is apparently of neuronal origin; a similar protein "NSP-R" has been shown by immunochemical techniques to be specific for certain neurons in the brain (PICKEL et al., 1976; KAWAKITA, 1972). A glial fibrillary acidic protein (GFA) that is present in a relatively large amount is a specific marker for the astroglia (BOCK and HAMBERGER, 1976). The enzyme dopamine β-hydroxylase has been demonstrated as a major component of the soluble proteins of adrenal chromatin granules and of noradrenergic vesicles isolated from the ox splenic nerve (BARTLETT et al., 1976). By subjecting the water-soluble proteins of the rat brain to chromatography on a DNA cellulose column, MIANI et al. (1976) have isolated a brain-specific acidic protein that has a selective affinity for single-stranded DNA. This protein, which they designated DNA-110, has a molecular weight of 68,000 and isoelectric point 5.9; it accounts for nearly 2% of the total soluble proteins of the rat brain.

A brain-specific ribonucleoprotein has been isolated from the soluble proteins of goat brain by SHARMA and TALWAR (1973). This protein is not found in other organs but is present in the brain of monkey, rat, chick and many other species. It was shown to be synthesized in vitro by cultured astrocytoma cells and is therefore believed to be derived from the astroglia.

2. Membrane Proteins

The plasma membrane of the neurons and glial cells is believed to consist basically of a lipid core two molecules thick, with monomolecular layers of glycoprotein on the inner and outer surface (WOODBURY, 1970). In the central lipid layer, the lipid molecules are packed tightly enough to prevent the penetration of hydrated ions, but there is evidence that certain membrane proteins, such as those of the transport and receptor systems, extend through the lipid layer and so can form a channel between the extracellular fluid and the cytoplasm inside the cell.

Homogenization of neural tissues with surface-active detergents such as triton X-100 or sodium dodecylsulphate breaks up the membranes and brings into solution a proportion of the membrane proteins. By the combined use of detergents and sonication, 65% or more of the total brain proteins can so be "solubilized." The membrane proteins can then be fractionated by electrophoresis and in this way a number of brain-specific membrane proteins have been obtained. Special interest attaches to the specific brain proteins separated from the synaptic membranes, which have been determined by crossed immunoelectrophoresis using antisera from immunized rabbits (BOCK and HAMBERGER, 1976). It has been shown that the membrane proteins obtained from noradrenergic vesicles are similar in electrophoretic mobility to those obtained from adrenal chromaffin granules (BARTLETT et al., 1976) and the properties of a number of other membrane proteins have been studied.

a) Proteolipids

Treatment of brain tissue with certain nonpolar lipid solvents such as chloroform acetone (2:1 vol/vol) dissolves the myelin and extracts a proportion of the other membrane proteins together with phosphatidy/peptides and a variety of lipids. The main protein extracted in this way is the proteolipid, in which inositol-containing phospholipids, mainly diphosphoinositide, are associated with an apoprotein containing 3% of fatty acid radicals bound by ester linkages to the polypeptide chain (FOLCH-PI, 1975; FOLCH-PI et al., 1957; FOLCH-PI and STOFFYN, 1972). The proteolipid apoprotein appears to exist in different states of molecular aggregation (minimum 12,000 daltons) and associated with different lipids, so that proteolipids of varying molecular weight and properties have been described. The apoprotein has a relatively high content of the sulphur-containing amino acids cysteine and methionine, and it also contains tryptophan. A proteolipid extractable from brain tissue by chloroform methanol under acid conditions ('proteolipid 2') was shown to differ from the original proteolipids in being trypsin-digestible (GAITONDE, 1961; WOLFGRAM, 1966).

b) Myelin Basic Protein

About 30% of the total myelin proteins are accounted for by a strongly basic protein that can be extracted from myelin by dilute acid solutions. This protein has been shown to be responsible for a form of encephalitis that is induced when myelin proteins are injected into an experimental animal. The condition induced in this way, which is known as experimental allergic encephalitis (EAE), is a cellular antibody response to the basic protein, involving focal inflammation and demyelination in areas of the brain, such as occur in multiple sclerosis (EYLAR, 1972).

The myelin basic protein, unlike the proteolipids, contains no cysteine. The complete amino acid sequences have now been determined for the basic proteins of human and bovine myelin and it has been shown that a relatively small peptide sequence containing one molecule of tryptophan is the essential requirement for producing EAE in the guinea pig, but some other sequences are apparently active in other animals (NORTON, 1975; MORELL, 1976). It may be noted that the myelin proteins differ significantly in different animal species; rats and mice have an additional basic myelin protein of smaller molecular weight than the encephalitogenic brain protein.

The proteins of myelin from the peripheral nervous system are different from those in brain myelin; proteolipids are reported to be absent and the three major proteins are two basic proteins (P0 and P1) and a glycoprotein (BROSTOFF et al., 1975; WOOD and DAWSON, 1973). It has been reported that in multiple sclerosis and EAE there is increased activity in affected brain areas of lysosomal enzymes including cathepsins A and D, which break down the myelin basic protein into polypeptides, some of which are encephalitogenic (MARKS et al., 1976).

c) Glycoproteins

Histochemical staining techniques have shown that the surfaces of cells of many different types contain oligosaccharides bound to the proteins of the plasma membranes. The glycoproteins, which have a carbohydrate residue bound to a protein moiety, are not easily detached from the membranes to which they belong, but by the use of detergents, sonication and other procedures some of them can be brought into solution for investigation while others remain attached as insoluble membrane proteins. The solutions obtained in this way contain a heterogeneous mixture of glycoproteins, and it is difficult to obtain individual components for characterization and analysis. In view of the difficulty in stripping the glycoproteins cleanly from the membranes, BRUNNGRABER (1969) used proteolytic enzymes to break down the membrane proteins and convert the glycoproteins into water-soluble glycopeptides that could be more easily fractionated and studied. In this way it was possible to show that the oligosaccharide moieties of the brain glycoproteins are comparable to those in other tissues in that they are made up of the sugars galactose, mannose and fucose, and may also contain N-acetylglucosamine, N-acetylgalactosamine, sialic acid and sulphate.

Studies on separated cells and subcellular fractions have shown that the glycoproteins are present in high concentration in the microsomal and synaptosomal fractions. In the rat brain the proportion of glycoproteins increases considerably during development: large increases in glycoprotein mannose, galactose and glucosamine are accompanied by smaller increases in fucose and sialic acid (MARGOLIS et al., 1976). In the immature bovine brain, 85% of the glycoproteins are sulphated, and in 12 glycopeptide fractions separated by anion exchange chromatography the ester sulphate content ranged from 5.6%–21.9%. The sulphate is present in the glycoproteins as galactose 6-O-sulphate and N-acetylglucosamine 6-O-sulphate (ALLEN et al., 1976).

The glycoprotein content of CNS myelin, which is a relatively inactive modified type of membrane, is small, but when the myelin proteins solubilized with sodium dodecyl sulphate are separated by electrophoresis on polyacrylamide gels, a band is obtained that stains positively for carbohydrate with periodic acid-Schiff reagent. This CNS myelin glycoprotein that is labelled in rats injected with [^{14}C]fucose may come from the membrane structures of the oligodendroglial-axonal junction (QUARLES, 1975); it is different from the glycoprotein that is a major component of the myelin of peripheral nerve (WOOD and DAWSON, 1973).

The soluble proteins obtained when a brain homogenate in neutral buffer is extracted with ethanol contain two glycoproteins that have been shown to be arylsulphatases A and B from the lysosomes (BALASUBRAMANIAN and BACHHAWAT, 1976). They can be separated and purified by fractional precipitation with zinc acetate and purified by fractional precipitation with zinc acetate and chromatography on a medium containing concanavalin A, which binds with the α-glucosyl or α-mannosyl residue of glycoproteins. Several other brain glycoproteins have been described (MIANI et al., 1976). The glycoproteins in nervous tissues have been reviewed by QUARLES (1975).

3. Neuroreceptor Proteins

Nerve cells are influenced by several different types of endogenous metabolites, including growth factors, steroids, inorganic ions, plasmalogens, cyclic nucleotides, amino acids and biogenic amines; they are also influenced by a variety of exogenous dietary factors, toxins and drugs. The specificity of the response generally depends on a specific receptor protein built into the plasma membrane at a site on the cell surface or at a synapse. The receptor proteins are comparable to the active centres of an enzyme in that they have the property of binding molecules of a particular type and thereby triggering a specific biochemical response. This may result in the depolarization or hyperpolarization of the adjacent membrane or the activation of an enzyme concerned in one of the functions of the cell. Our present knowledge of the receptor proteins and of the neurochemical processes involved in the actions of the different types of neurotransmitters is still very limited and this is a field of active investigation at the present time.

a) Amino Acid Receptors

L-Glutamic acid has a strong excitatory action on neurons of the mammalian brain and has therefore been considered as a possible neurotransmitter or a modulator of synaptic activity. Conversely, GABA has an inhibitory action. The excitatory action of L-glutamic acid is stereospecific in that it is not produced by the D-isomer and is not produced when injected intracellularly but only when applied to the neuronal surface. This suggests that glutamic acid acts on a specific receptor at the cell membrane. Studies of the binding of L-glutamic acid by different subcellular fractions of the rat brain have identified a binding site of high affinity, strongly stereoselective for the L-isomer, localized mainly in the membranes of the nerve endings. The binding is inhibited specifically by glutamic acid diethyl ester, which does not affect the uptake of glutamic acid into the synaptosomes (ROBERTS, 1974). DE ROBERTIS and his colleagues (1976) have reported the presence in the rat brain of two proteolipids that can be separated on Sephadex LH20 columns, which have the property of binding selectively L-glutamic acid or GABA. These proteins that come from the hydrophobic part of the neuronal plasma membrane have some properties in common with receptor proteins for glutamic acid previously reported in insect and crustacean muscle, but they differ in showing a greater affinity of the binding sites for L-aspartic acid, which also has an excitatory action on neurons (CURTIS and WATKINS, 1960).

Evidence of a receptor protein for glycine in the spinal cord was obtained by YOUNG and SNYDER (1973) who showed that labelled strychnine, which blocks the inhibitory action of glycine at spinal synapses, binds to synaptic membrane fractions from spinal cord. The bound strychnine is displaced by glycine.

b) Acetylcholine Receptors

A rich source of the nicotinic type of acetylcholine receptors is the electric organ of the electric eel, and this has been used in several attempts to isolate and characterize the receptor protein. By homogenizing in $0.2\,M$ sucrose solution, membrane fragments are obtained that respond to acetylcholine by increased efflux of Na^+ ions from associated microsacs, whereas the efflux is inhibited by the antagonist d-tubocurarine, thereby indicating the presence of an acetylcholine receptor in the membrane fragments. The further purification and characterization of the receptor protein was aided by the observation that certain venom toxins, such as α-bungarotoxin, bind tightly to the acetylcholine receptor (CHANGEUX et al., 1970). The molecular weight of the polypeptide part of the receptor protein was estimated to be about 40,000–45,000 daltons. Toxin binding has been used also in studies of the properties of the acetylcholine receptor protein of mammalian brain (MOORE, 1975). The nicotinic acetylcholine receptor protein can be separated from acetylcholinesterase, which is a different type of acetylcholine receptor protein. The properties of membrane-bound and solubilized preparations of the nicotinic acetylcholine receptor protein have been reviewed by KARLIN and COWBURN (1974).

Acetycholine receptors of a different type, which are stimulated by muscarinic agents (pilocarpine and oxotremorine) and blocked by atropine, are present in the hypothalamus. The muscarinic receptors as well as receptors of the nicotinic type are both concerned in the mechanisms of thermoregulation (TANGRI et al., 1976).

c) Catecholamine Receptors

The neuroreceptors for dopamine, noradrenalin, and adrenaline are closely associated with nucleotide cyclase enzymes. The adenylate cyclase catalyzes the formation of cyclic adenosine $3^1 5^1$-monophosphate (cAMP) from ATP, while the guanylate cyclase similarly catalyzes the formation of cyclic guanosine $3^1 5^1$-monophosphate (cGMP) from GTP. The adenylate and guanylate cyclases are believed to be built into the neuronal plasma membranes, so that the cAMP or cGMP are formed intracellularly, to mediate the actions of the catecholamine transmitters within the cells (ROBISON et al., 1971). The sensitivity of the cyclase activity to catecholamine transmitters depends apparently on receptor proteins, which in some cases can be separated from the cyclase enzymes. Thus, homogenization of brain tissue appears to uncouple the adenylate cyclase from the β-adrenergic receptor localized in the synaptosomes, and protein fractions rich in adenylate cyclase or in β-adrenergic receptors can be separated on a linear sucrose density gradient (DAVIS and LEFKOWITZ, 1976).

d) Other Receptors

The presence in synaptosomes, and associated with serotonergic tracts, of a soluble protein with a high affinity for binding serotonin has been reported by TAMIR et al. (1976). Partial purification of the protein resulted in loss of binding capacity, but this loss could be restored by addition of 10^{-4} M Fe^{2+} ions. The binding of serotonin was inhibited by reserpine and vinblastine. They suggest that this protein may be concerned in the storage of serotonin. Since serotonin binds to gangliosides, these have been proposed as the serotonin receptors of the plasma membrane, but the mechanism of action of serotonin on cells remains obscure (OCHOA and BANGHAM, 1976).

Steroid hormones, being lipid soluble, pass through the lipid barrier of the plasma membrane and bind to specific receptor proteins in the cytoplasm. The steroid-receptor complex then moves to the cell nucleus and produces physiological changes by influencing RNA formation so that an enzyme is induced or genetic expression is modified in some way. Receptor systems for oestrogens and androgens have been identified in the hypothalamus and amygdala; receptor proteins for glucocorticoids are present in the hippocampus. The oestrogen receptor protein in the cerebral cortex of the newborn animal, which effects the permanent sexual differentiation of the developing brain, is different from that of the adult brain; it can be purified by ammonium sulphate fractionation and analyzed on linear sucrose density gradients using bound [^{3}H]oestradiol as a marker (WESTLEY et al., 1976). Studies of the distribution in the brain and properties of corticoid-receptor proteins have also been reported (McEWEN et al., 1976; NELSON et al., 1976).

It is now established that the mammalian brain contains opiate receptors that bind encephalins as well as morphine and other opiate drugs. The opiate receptors appear to be concentrated in the regions of the caudate nucleus, globus pallidus and anterior hypothalamus as also in the periaqueductal grey, but the nature of the receptor protein is not yet clear (ELDE et al., 1976; JAQUET and LAJTHA, 1976). The methods used for the labelling and isolation of neuroreceptors have been reviewed by FEWTRELL (1976). Interactions of hormone receptors in the brain and evidence for the presence of thyroid receptors have been discussed by EBERHARDT et al. (1976).

IV. Neurotransmitters

1. Chemical Transmission

The transmission of signals from one neuron to another is the function of the neurotransmitters. When the depolarization wave on a neuronal plasma membrane reaches the nerve ending, it causes the release of neurotransmitter molecules into the synaptic cleft. The binding of the neurotransmitter with the receptor protein then triggers a response in the postsynaptic neuron. The nerve endings are generally enlarged at the synapses to make room for the storage of a supply of neurotransmitters that may be contained in small storage vesicles. The stock of neurotransmitter at the synapse may be replenished 1) by local synthesis in the nerve ending, 2) by carriage in vesicles down the axon from a site of synthesis in the cell body, or 3) by the re-uptake of excess neurotransmitter released into the synaptic cleft. Some of the excess of neurotransmitter may be taken up by the glia or may diffuse away in the extracellular fluid, and some may be inactivated enzymatically in the synaptic cleft. For every type of synapse there are six processes to be considered – neurotransmitter synthesis, storage, release, reception, re-uptake and inactivation.

Similar mechanisms operate at neuromuscular and other junctions in which a neuroeffector produces a response by binding to a receptor protein. The coupling of the nerve action potential with the release of neurotransmitter at a nerve ending requires the presence of Ca^{2+} ions in the extracellular fluid; conversely Mg^{2+} ions have an inhibitory effect (KOELLE, 1975). Besides acetylcholine and the catecholamines, which are now well-established as neurotransmitters, there are a number of other compounds such as 5-HT, GABA and glutamic acid that apparently have this function but are commonly described as 'putative transmitters' to indicate that the evidence for their transmitter function is not accepted by all as sufficient. Other compounds to which transmitter functions have been ascribed include glycine, aspartic acid, histamine, β-alanine, taurine (HUXTABLE and BARBEAU, 1976), and certain peptides (BURNSTOCK, 1976). It may be noted that the study of chemical transmission in the mammalian brain has been helped by the study of neuroeffector systems operative in invertebrates. Thus, evidence for the inhibitory function of GABA at vertebrate synapses came from earlier studies of the properties of GABA in the stretch receptor system of the crayfish.

The chief criteria for the acceptance of a compound as a neurotransmitter are:
1. It must occur in relatively high concentration at nerve endings, preferably concentrated in synaptic vesicles.
2. It must be released selectively when the nerve is stimulated.
3. There must be a mechanism for ending the synaptic action of the compound released, by enzymatic inactivation or by reuptake.
4. The compound must resemble the natural transmitter in its behavior with respect to specific agonists and antagonists.

It is generally assumed that each neuron makes and releases only one neurotransmitter, in keeping with Dale's Principle, but there is evidence that adrenergic nerves can store and release, besides noradrenalin, amines such as octopamine (β-hydroxytyramine), which have been described as 'cotransmitters' (BURNSTOCK, 1976). It is also known that some neurons are able to take up other amines such as phenylethylamine, which may then be released as 'false transmitters' when the nerve is stimulated. Compounds such as prostaglandins, which are synthesized as a result of nerve stimulation and which influence postsynaptic activity, are known as 'modulators' of neurotransmission (DUBCOVICH and LANGER, 1975). Tissue culture techniques are now being used to study the response of neurons of different types to putative transmitters and drugs (BONKOWSKI and DRYDEN, 1976).

2. Acetylcholine

Acetylcholine, which is quaternary ammonium base, is normally present in aqueous solution at neutral pH as the cation $(CH_3)_3N^+-CH_2CH_2O.COCH_3$. Acetylcholine is synthesized by the transfer of an acetyl group to choline from acetyl CoA in the presence of the enzyme choline acetyltransferase (ChAc), which is found in cholinergic neurons, mainly in the cytoplasm of the nerve endings. Choline taken up from the extracellular fluid is acetylated in the cytoplasm, and the acetylcholine formed is incorporated into the synaptic vesicles, together with a specific protein, vesiculin (WHITTAKER and DOWDALL, 1975).

In most areas of the brain, iontophoretic application of acetylcholine to the neurons produces predominantly excitatory responses, but in some areas such as the medulla and hypothalamus up to 50% of the cholinoceptive neurons give inhibitory responses (BRADLEY, 1968). The receptors mediating inhibitory responses are thought to be exclusively muscarinic (i.e., responding also to muscarine and blocked by atropine), whereas excitatory responses are mediated either by muscarinic or by nicotinic receptors.

The quanta of acetylcholine released when an impulse reaches a cholinergic synapse are thought to be generally greater that the amount required to bind the receptor protein on the postsynaptic neuron. The excess of acetylcholine is then quickly hydrolyzed in the synaptic cleft by acetylcholinesterase to form acetate and choline, which is returned to the extracellular fluid. It has been shown by electron-microscopic histochemical techniques that acetylcholinesterase is present in high concentration at the surfaces of the presynaptic and postsynaptic membranes (KOELLE, 1975). There are several different isoenzymes of acetylcholinesterase with varying properties. There are also a number of other esterases (described as 'pseudo-cholinesterase,' butyrylcholinesterase, etc.) that hydrolyze acetylcholine but at a relatively slow rate.

3. Dopamine

Dopaminergic neurons with cell bodies in the *substantia nigra* provide some 10% of the nerve terminals in the striatum, where much of the dopamine in the brain is found. Dopaminergic neurons also extend through a second mesolimbic system, which includes the olfactory tubercle, nucleus accumbens, amygdala and certain parts of the paleocortex (CARLSSON, 1976). A third dopaminergic system in the hypothalamus mediates the release of hormones from the hypophysis (SNYDER, 1972). Dopamine is formed in the brain from tyrosine, which is first oxidized to dihydroxyphenylalanine (DOPA) through the action of the tyrosine hydroxylase. The DOPA is then decarboxylated by the dopa decarboxylase to give dopamine (Fig. 1). Dopamine is an intermediate in the pathway from tyrosine to noradrenalin (norepinephrine) and adrenaline

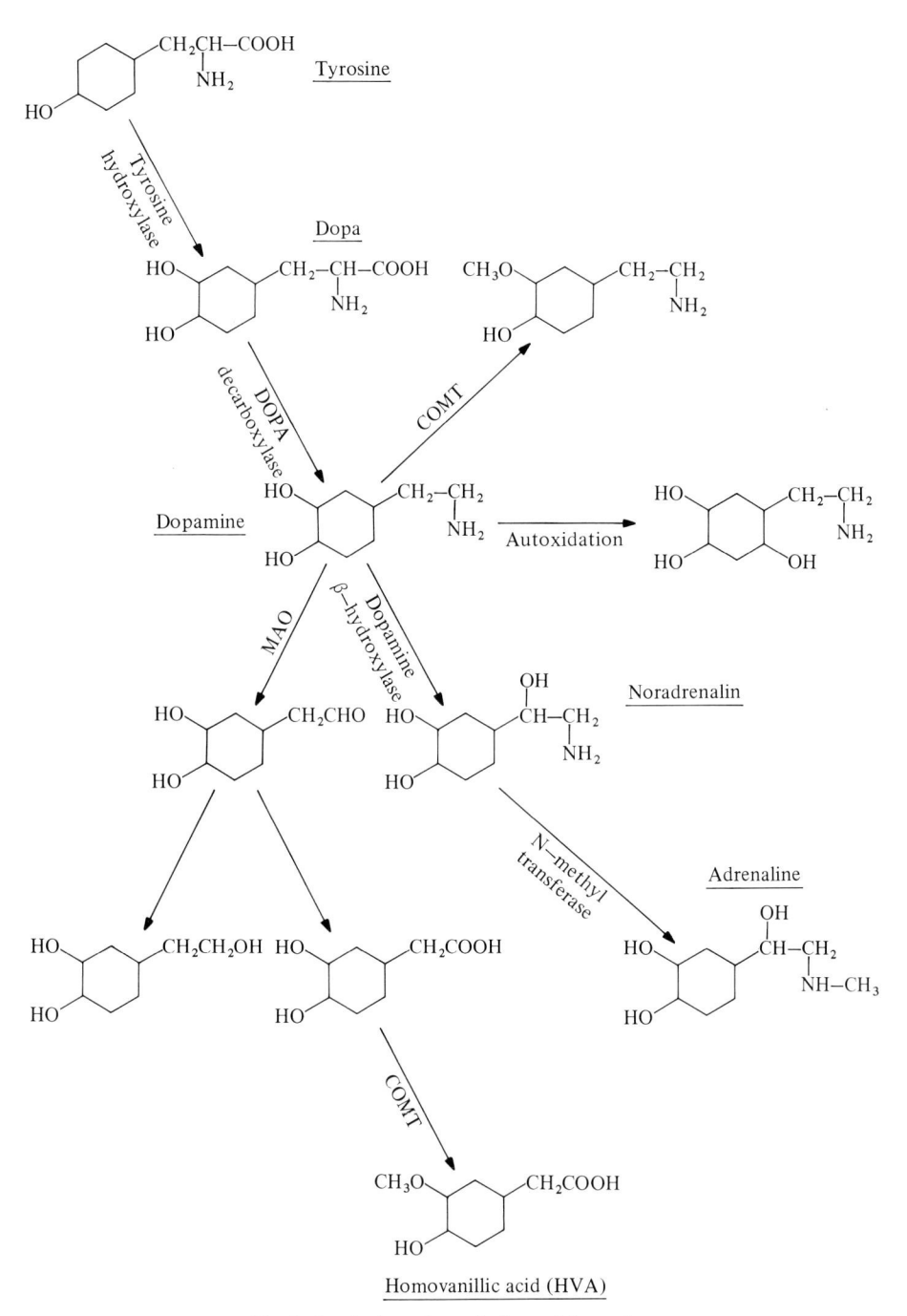

Fig. 1. Synthesis and metabolism of dopamine

(epinephrine). The rate-limiting step in the biosynthesis of the catecholamines is the hydroxylation of tyrosine by the tyrosine hydroxylase, an enzyme that requires tetrahydrobiopterin as a cofactor (GUROFF, 1975).

Dopamine has been shown to exert an inhibitory action on neurons in many parts of the CNS, this effect being most pronounced in the forebrain and thalamus and weakest in the spinal cord. The inhibitory action is attributed to a hyperpolarization of the plasma membranes due to an increase in K^+ conductance or a reduction in Na^+ conductance (KRNJEVIC, 1975). The hypothesis that dopamine activates an adenylate cyclase, which converts ATP in the neurons into cyclic adenosine monophosphate (cAMP), derives from the work of ROBISON et al. (1971), who concluded that the actions of the catecholamines are mediated by cAMP, which thus acts as a 'second messenger' within the postsynaptic neurons. This idea has been developed by GREENGARD (1975) and his collaborators who have obtained evidence that the cAMP formed in this way alters the plasma membrane permeability by phosphorylating a protein kinase, which is one of the factors determining membrane permeability (UEDA et al., 1973). They conclude that the dopamine receptor is a dopamine-binding component of a specific dopamine-sensitive adenylate cyclase and that the cAMP formed acts by modulating nicotinic cholinergic transmission. Support for this view has come from the observation that the properties of the dopamine receptors in vivo in being blocked by phenothiazines and other antipsychotic drugs are matched to a large extent by the properties of the dopamine-sensitive adenylate cyclase present in homogenates of the caudate nucleus studied in vitro (KEBABIAN et al., 1975). Recent reports that the adenylate cyclase can be separated from the β-adrenergic receptors indicate that, although closely associated, the cyclase enzyme and the receptors are not identical (DAVIS and LEFKOWITZ, 1976). That there is a link between the dopaminergic and cholinergic systems is suggested by the observation that agents that increase dopaminergic activity in vivo, such as L-DOPA, amphetamine and piribedil, also increase the level of striatal acetylcholine, whereas agents such as chlorpromazine that block dopamine receptors decrease striatal acetylcholine, apparently by increasing the rate of release of acetylcholine in the striatum (STADLER et al., 1973). There are several different ways in which dopamine can be metabolized.

1. *Dopamine β-hydroxylase* catalyzes the oxidation of the side chain, so converting dopamine into noradrenalin (norepinephrine).

2. *Autoxidation* of dopamine leads to the formation of the toxic compound 6-hydroxydopamine, but it is not established that this actually occurs to an appreciable extent in the tissues (STEIN and WISE, 1971).

3. *Catechol-O-methyl transferase (COMT)* catalyzes the transfer of a methyl group from S-adenosylmethionine to the metahydroxyl group to give 3-O-methyldopamine.

4. *Monoamine oxidase (MAO)* occurs in the tissues as different isoenzymes some of which are more specific for the oxidation of dopamine. The MAO isoenzymes oxidize dopamine to dihydroxyphenylacetaldehyde, which may either be reduced in the tissues to the corresponding alcohol or oxidized further to the carboxylic acid.

The removal of excess dopamine released at the nerve endings under normal physiological conditions is believed to be predominantly by re-uptake into the nerve endings and then into the synaptic vesicles, since dopaminergic neurons have a specific, high-affinity uptake mechanism in the plasma membrane (COYLE and SNYDER, 1969). A part of the dopamine formed in the striatum is oxidized to homovanillic acid (HVA or 4-hydroxy-3-methoxy-phenylacetic acid), which appears in the cerebrospinal fluid and is excreted in the urine. The formation of HVA from dopamine requires oxidation by MAO and methylation by COMT, either of which could happen first. What actually happens is suggested by histochemical studies that have shown that these two enzymes are located separately at different points; MAO is closely associated with the mitochondria within the nerve terminals, whereas COMT is situated outside the catecholamine nerve terminals. It is concluded that the dopamine released into the synaptic cleft and not taken up again into the neurons is indicated by the amount of the methylated derivative, 3-O-methyl dopamine produced, whereas HVA reflects dopamine that leaks from the vesicles and is oxidized by the MAO within the nerve terminals before being methylated to give HVA (SNYDER, 1972). The HVA level in the cerebrospinal fluid is reduced in patients with parkinsonism, and the HVA level has been used as an indication of the activity of dopaminergic neurons in the brain.

4. Noradrenalin (Norepinephrine)

Noradrenalin is the main transmitter of the sympathetic nerves. In the brain, noradrenergic neurons are found in high concentration in the locus coeruleus and in clusters in the reticular formation. Some of the nerve fibres pass down in the lateral sympathetic columns of the spinal cord and others ascend to the hypothalamus, the limbic forebrain and other regions including the cerebral cortex. The noradrenalin in the sympathetic nerves is stored in vesicles and released at the nerve endings, probably by exocytosis, from the vesicles directly into the extracellular space (LAGERCRANTZ, 1976). The vesicles also contain the proteins chromogranin A, chromomembrin B and dopamine β-hydroxylase, which are released together with the noradrenalin; the sympathetic neuron is thus a protein-secreting cell. The vesicles are formed in the cell body of the neurons and transported along the axons to the nerve endings at a relatively rapid rate, estimated to be up to 10 mm/h in the cat sciatic nerve (OESCH et al., 1973). The tyrosine hydroxylase and DOPA-decarboxylase travel along the axons on separate particles at a slower rate. Noradrenergic neurons show a considerable degree of plasticity in their response to stressful conditions. Prolonged stimulation of sympathetic activity by procedures such as cold stress increase the level of dopamine β-hydroxylase and tyrosine hydroxylase in the cell bodies and terminal networks. The increase depends on neuronal activity, since it is prevented by cutting the preganglionic cholinergic nerves; the phenomenon is known as trans-synaptic induction. The plasma level of dopamine β-hydroxylase in man reflects the extent of sympathetic nervous activity (USDIN and SNYDER, 1973). The sympathetic nervous system is involved in the regulation of body temperature. Exposure to cold increases the synthesis and excretion of noradrenalin, and nonshivering heat production is accompanied by the release of noradrenalin from sympathetic nerve endings. Acclimatization to cold increases the release of noradrenalin and increases the efficiency of noradrenergic transmission (PRESTON and SCHÖNBAUM, 1976).

Dopamine β-hydroxylase, which effects the oxidation of dopamine to noradrenalin, is a copper-containing glycoprotein. It requires ascorbic acid for maximum activity, which is increased by fumarate; it is inhibited by compounds that chelate with copper. The formation of dopamine β-hydroxylase and tyrosine hydroxylase in sympathetic neurons is increased by injection of nerve growth factor (GUROFF, 1975). The characteristics and functional roles of the vesicles in sympathetic neurons have been reviewed by LAGERCRANTZ (1976).

Application of noradrenalin by iontophoresis to central neurons with β-adrenergic receptors, such as Purkinje cells, produces an inhibitory response associated with hyperpolarization and either no change or an increase in membrane resistance. The response is apparently mediated by cAMP produced intracellularly through stimulation of adenylate cyclase associated with noradrenalin-sensitive receptors (BLOOM, 1975). Some neurons give an excitatory response to noradrenalin, and it is believed that excitatory responses are mediated by intracellular synthesis of cyclic guanosine monophosphate (cGMP). The part played by cyclic nucleotides as intracellular mediators of the actions of neurotransmitters in the nervous system and in other organs is still under active investigation. The present state of our knowledge has been reviewed by GREENGARD (1975). The apparent role of prostaglandins as 'messengers' or modulators of responses to noradrenalin has been discussed by COCEANI (1976).

Noradrenalin released at the nerve endings is removed to a large extent by re-uptake into the storage vesicles, but a part is O-methylated through the action of COMT to give normetanephrine (Fig. 2). MAO acts on normetanephrine to form the aldehyde, which is further oxidized to vanillylmandelic acid (VMA) or reduced to the glycol, 3-methoxy-4-hydroxy-phenylglycol (MHPG). The main product from noradrenalin in the peripheral organs is VMA, which is excreted in the urine; the VMA level in the urine has been used as an index of sympathetic nervous function. In the brain the aldehyde is mainly reduced to the glycol MHPG, which is then conjugated with sulphate to form the sulphate ester, and is excreted in the urine in that form. Some 20% of the MHPG sulphate ester excreted in the urine is derived from noradrenalin released in the brain (SNYDER, 1972).

5. Adrenaline (Epinephrine)

The adrenal medulla, which is related ontogenetically to the sympathetic nerves, contains adrenaline as the main hormone together with a smaller amount of noradrenalin. The catecholamines are contained in 'chromaffin granules' that resemble the vesicles of sympathetic nerves in containing also dopamine β-hydroxylase, chromogranin A, and other proteins. The isolation and properties of the chromaffin granules have been reviewed by WINKLER (1976). Adrenaline is also present in small amounts in sympathetic nerves and in the brain, where it occurs in the hypothalamus and in other parts of the diencephalon and

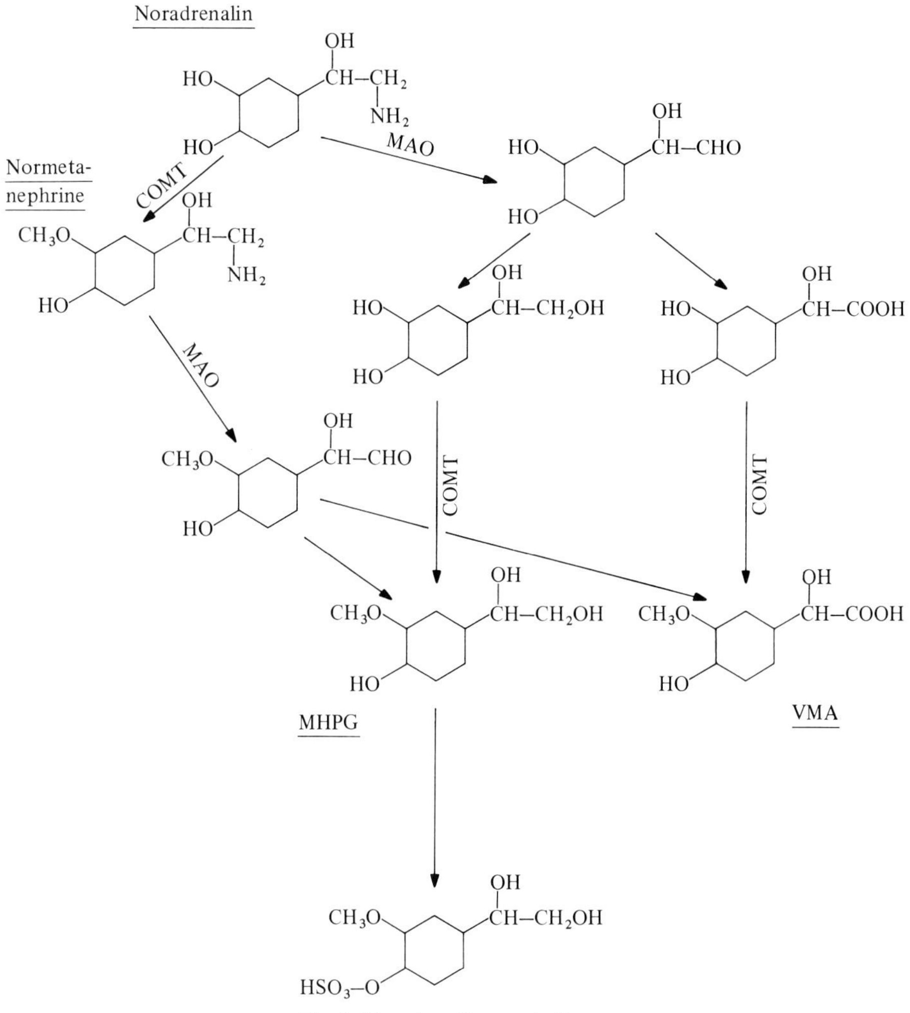

Fig. 2. Noradrenalin metabolism

brain stem (VOGT, 1957). While noradrenalin release from sympathetic nerves appears to be the primary mechanism of chemical thermoregulation, exposure to cold induces the release of adrenaline from the adrenal medulla, and it is thought that adrenaline release constitutes a second line of defence (PRESTON and SCHÖNBAUM, 1976).

Adrenaline is catabolized by COMT and MAO to form vanillomandelic acid (VMA) as a major end-metabolite. After infusion of adrenaline in man, the urine contains VMA and the sulphate esters of adrenaline and metanephrine as well as some unchanged adrenaline (GOODALL, 1959). Adrenalectomy in man greatly reduces the excretion of adrenaline metabolites, but about 20% of the normal level remains.

6. 5-Hydroxytryptamine (Serotonin)

5-Hydroxytryptamine (5-HT) is present in the neuronal cell bodies of the raphe nuclei situated dorsally in the midline of the brain stem. The nerve terminals extend through the hypothalamus and other parts of the brain and spinal cord. Destruction of the raphe nuclei greatly reduces the 5-HT content of the brain. The insomnia that results gives evidence of one of the main physiological functions of the tryptaminergic (serotonergic) system in regulating sleep. 5-HT also plays a part in the hypothalamic mechanisms of thermoregulation (PRESTON and SCHÖNBAUM, 1976), and there is evidence that central 5-HT neurons are concerned in sexual behaviour and in the action of hallucinogenic drugs such as LSD, which act on the presynaptic 5-HT receptors (FUXE et al., 1976).

5-HT is synthesized from plasma L-tryptophan, which is oxidized through the action of tryptophan hydroxylase to 5-hydroxytryptophan. Decarboxylation by the aromatic amino acid decarboxylase then results in the formation of 5-HT. The rate of synthesis of 5-HT is determined mainly by the availability of L-tryptophan in the brain, and this depends on the level of free L-tryptophan in the blood plasma. Most of the plasma L-tryptophan is bound to plasma proteins and is therefore not immediately available for transport into the brain and synthesis of 5-HT.

Tryptaminergic neurons in the mammalian brain have a specific mechanism for the re-uptake of 5-HT, and it is likely that this is the main process for terminating the action of 5-HT released at the nerve endings (SNYDER, 1972). 5-HT is oxidized by the action of MAO to the aldehyde, which on further oxidation forms 5-hydroxyindole-acetic acid (5-HIAA). 5-HIAA is the main metabolite of 5-HT found in the cerebrospinal fluid and excreted in the urine. 5-HT can also be inactivated by conjugation with sulphate through the action of an O-sulphotransferase (IVERSEN, 1973).

a) Melatonin

5-HT has a special role in the pineal gland where it occurs in high concentrations that fluctuate in phase with a regular diurnal rhythm. Thus, the 5-HT level in the pineal gland of the rat is ten times higher at midday than at midnight. The metabolism of 5-HT in the pineal gland is unique in that it leads to the formation of two metabolites, 5-methoxytryptophol and melatonin, which are not formed in any other organ (Fig. 3). N-Acetylation of 5-HT by the N-acetyl transferase is followed by O-methylation by an enzyme hydroxyindole-O-methyl transferase (HIOMT), which occurs only in the pineal gland, to give melatonin. 5-Hydroxytryptophol is formed by reduction of the aldehyde produced when 5-HT is oxidized by MAO. Methylation by the enzyme HIOMT results in the formation of 5-methoxytryptophol.

The melatonin content of the rat pineal gland is influenced by the lighting conditions; it is higher in rats kept in darkness than in those kept in the light. The diurnal changes in melatonin content and the effects of light are determined by sympathetic nerves that liberate noradrenalin, which stimulates β-adrenergic receptors on the pineal gland cells. Stimulation of the β-adrenergic receptors causes the formation of cAMP, which mediates the synthesis of the

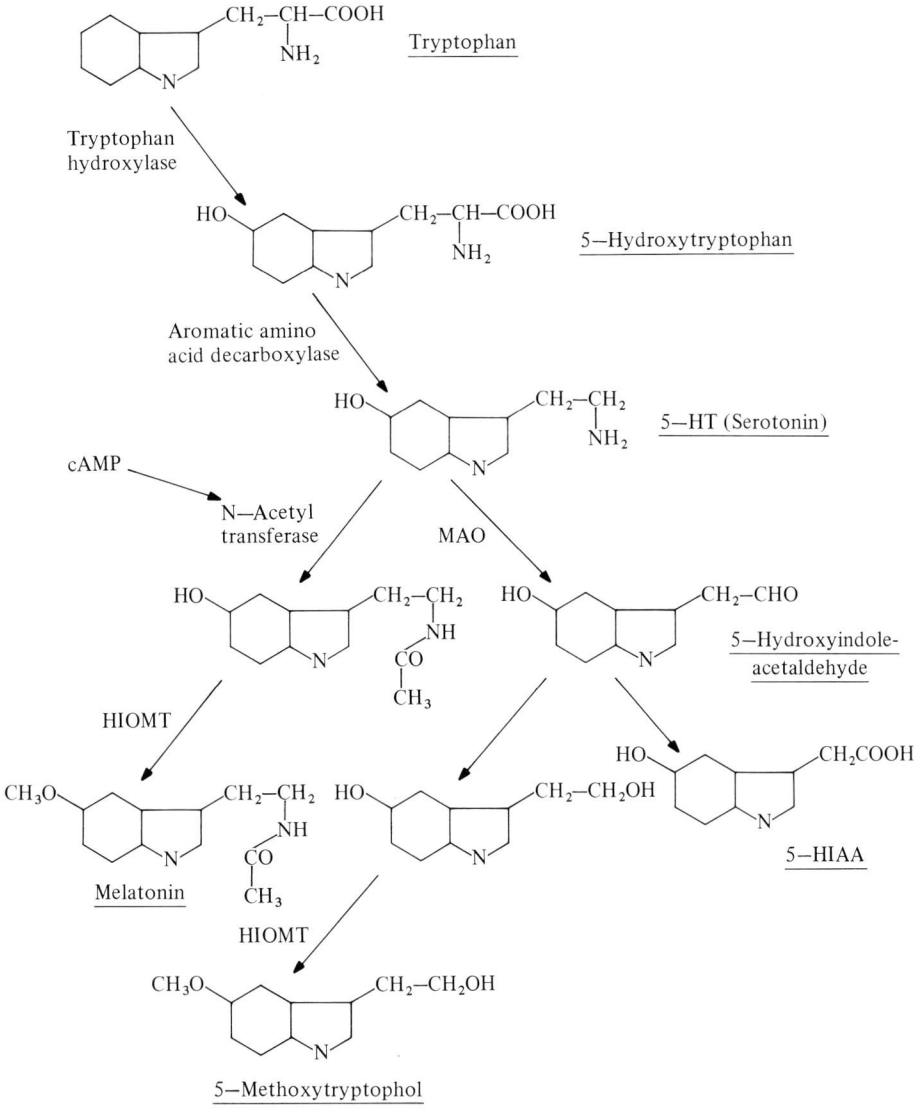

Fig. 3. Synthesis and metabolism of 5-HT

rate-limiting enzyme N-acetyltransferase. In that way the synthesis of melatonin is increased (AXELROD, 1975). Melatonin influences gonadal function in the rat and is concerned in the pigmentation of the skin in amphibians and in fish.

7. Amino Acids

a) γ-Aminobutyric Acid (GABA)

GABA, glutamate and glycine are found in high concentration in tissues of the central nervous system and are capable of exerting powerful effects

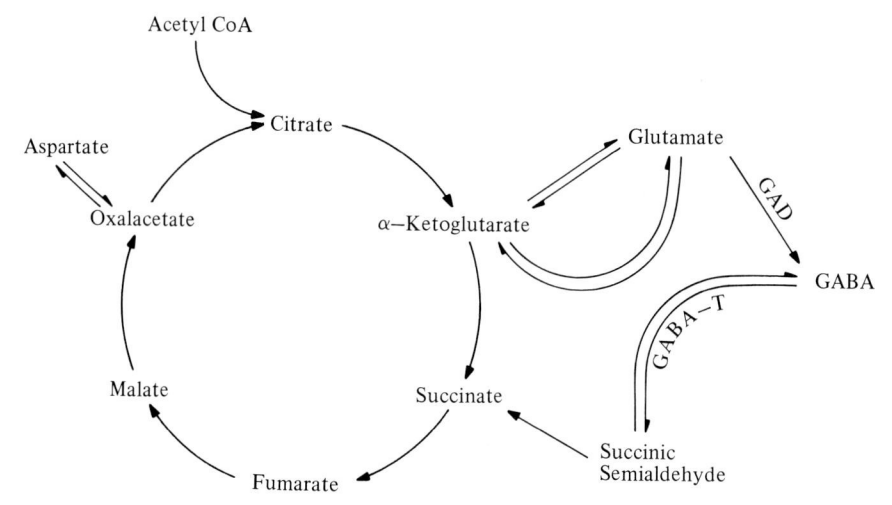

Fig. 4. Derivation of glutamate, GABA, and aspartate from metabolites in the tricarboxylic acid cycle

on neuronal activity. It is now widely believed that they act physiologically as neurotransmitters. When applied iontophoretically to neurons of the mammalian central nervous system, GABA causes hyperpolarization and depresses the firing rate. The distribution of GABA and of the glutamic acid decarboxylase (GAD) that forms GABA suggest that GABA acts as an inhibitory transmitter in the cerebral cortex, cerebellum hippocampus, and other areas in the brain. This is supported by studies of the action of bicuculline, which is a fairly specific GABA antagonist. The evidence for the transmitter function of GABA and other amino acids has been reviewed by KRNJEVIĆ (1974), CURTIS and JOHNSTON (1974), and SNYDER (1975). GABA is formed by the decarboxylation of glutamic acid in the presence of the glutamic acid decarboxylase (GAD), an enzyme that is found in the mammalia almost exclusively in the central nervous system, mainly concentrated at nerve endings in the grey matter of the brain (Fig. 4). The pathway from α-ketoglutarate via glutamate, GABA, and succinic semialdehyde to succinate is thus a route of oxidation alternative to the tricarboxylic acid cycle. This pathway, known as the 'GABA shunt,' was estimated to account for about 8% of the total flux in the tricarboxylic acid cycle in the cerebral cortex (BALÁZS et al., 1970; PATEL et al., 1974). The enzymes GAD and GABA-T both require pyridoxal phosphate as a cofactor. The GAD is located mainly in the presynaptic nerve endings and GABA-T is found in the mitochondria.

When brain tissue is subjected to subcellular fractionation, the endogenous GABA is found in the synaptosomes, where it is apparently not confined in synaptic vesicles. GABA is accumulated in the nerve endings by a high-affinity Na^+-dependent uptake system and is taken up by the synaptosomes in brain homogenates (IVERSEN and BLOOM, 1972). GABA is also taken up into the glia by a second low-affinity system (LEVI and RAITERI, 1973). There is a selective release of GABA when brain tissue is depolarized by raising the K^+ concentration in the surrounding medium (BALÁZS et al., 1970). The evidence indicates that glial uptake is the primary process for the rapid removal of GABA released at the synapses (CURTIS et al., 1976).

b) Glutamic Acid

Glutamic acid, which is the most abundant amino acid in the mammalian brain, is found in highest concentration in the cerebral cortex, where it is probably the principal excitatory transmitter. Electrical stimulation of the ascending reticular activating system produces a marked release of glutamate and reduced release of GABA in the cerebral cortex (JASPER and KOYAMA, 1969). Glutamate and aspartate are both powerful excitants of almost all neurons in the brain, and in view of their close structural similarity, it is difficult to distinguish between them and to know which is normally involved. Glutamate and aspartate are both taken up into the synaptosomes by a high-affinity Na^+-dependent uptake system and released together with GABA by potassium depolarization, whereas other amino acids are not released (SNYDER, 1975). The depolarization increases the permeability to Na^+ and K^+ ions.

c) Glycine

Glycine is present in relatively high concentration in the brain stem and spinal cord, where it is a potent inhibitor of the motor neurons. It resembles the natural transmitter of the interneurons in that its hyperpolarizing action is antagonized by strychnine. High-affinity Na^+-dependent uptake of glycine has been found to occur in synaptosomal preparations from the spinal cord but not in those from the cerebral cortex. Autoradiographic studies of the distribution of synapses with high-affinity uptake of [^{3}H]glycine have shown that about 25% of the nerve terminals in the spinal cord take up glycine in this way (IVERSEN and BLOOM, 1972). Glycine can be formed in nervous tissues from glucose by a pathway with 3-phosphoglycerate and 3-phosphoserine as intermediates. There are also other possible biosynthetic pathways (ROBERTS and HAMMERSCHLAG, 1972).

8. Histamine

Histamine is found in sensory nerves, in postganglionic fibres of the sympathetic nervous system, in the optic nerves, hypothalamus and other areas of the brain. In the cerebral cortex, histamine depresses the activity of more than 65% of the neurons, but excitatory responses are also observed. While it acts as a neuroeffector in the periphery, it is at present uncertain whether it also serves as a transmitter at synapses in the central nervous system. In many tissues the histamine is contained largely in the mast cells, but these are almost absent from the brain, which has histamine concentrations of the order of 50 mg per gram. Histamine can be formed by the decarboxylation of histidine by the histidine decarboxylase, which is present in the brain (PALACIOS et al., 1976). It can be metabolized in the tissues in a number of different ways. In the presence of histaminase (or diamine oxidase), histamine is oxidized and deaminated to give imidazole acetaldehyde. Methylation by the imidazole N-methyltransferase yields 1-methylhistamine and N-dimethylhistamine. Evidence for the existence of specific histamine receptors linked to an adenylate cyclase system has been reviewed by SATTIN et al. (1975).

9. Neural Modulators

Synaptic transmission involves not only the neurotransmitters released into the synaptic clefts but also other chemical factors that can influence the properties of the membranes of the presynaptic and postsynaptic neurons, so affecting transmitter release and the events that follow the binding of the transmitter. Such factors, described as 'modulators,' include adenosine, ATP, 5^1-AMP and cAMP, which are pharmacologically active and appear to play a part in synaptic transmission (SATTIN et al., 1975). When ATP and other adenine derivatives are applied to neurons in different parts of the brain, they affect the rate of firing and produce a variety of responses. Adenosine is readily taken up by the neurons and partly converted into cAMP; it is then transported by axonal flow to the synapses, where adenosine is released on stimulation. The amount released is sufficient to affect cell firing and to regenerate active concentrations of cAMP. The observed cytoplasmic transport of a neural modulator thus constitutes a form of signal transmission complementary to that of the action potential, but persisting for a longer time and travelling at much slower speed (MCILWAIN, 1976). The role of cAMP as a 'messenger' between extracellular and intracellular events has been considered above in discussing the mechanism of action of the catecholamines.

That prostaglandins (PGs) may play a part in mediating neural responses was suggested by the observation that small quantities of prostaglandins of the E series (PGEs) injected into the ventricles or the anterior hypothalamic region of the cat produce a rapid rise in body temperature (MILTON and WENDLANDT, 1971). Further investigation showed that pyrogens cause the release of prostaglandins into the cerebrospinal fluid, whereas antipyretic drugs, which abolish the fever, cause the PGE content to fall (FELDBERG and GUPTA, 1973). Antipyretics also inhibit the synthesis of prostaglandins by the prostaglandin synthetase in vitro (FLOWER and VANE, 1972). The evidence indicates that prostaglandin receptors in the anterior hypothalamic-preoptic area mediate the fever induced by pyrogens. It has been postulated further that prostaglandins are concerned in the normal mechanisms of thermoregulation, and various hypotheses of their mode of action at central noradrenergic synapses have been proposed, but the evidence supporting this view is insufficient to warrant further discussion here (COCEANI, 1976; HARVEY and MILTON, 1975). The possibility that prostaglandins and catecholamines interact in the central control of ovulation is also under consideration at the present time (LINTON et al., 1977). The part played by modulators in neural transmission has been reviewed by IVERSEN et al. (1975).

V. Peptide Neuroeffectors

1. Metabolism

Besides peptides such as glutathione (γ-glutamylcysteinylglycine), which are found in most tissues of the body, there are a number that are present predominantly or uniquely in the brain. This applies to homocarnosine (γ-aminobutyryl histidine), of which the human brain contains 8 mg per 100 g fresh tissue, and homoanserine (β-alanyl-1-methyl histidine). N-Acetyl-α-aspartyglutamic acid is again found only in the brain, at concentrations up to 30 mg per 100 g fresh tissue. The functions of these three peptides are unknown. Two 'dynein-like' polypeptides found in the brain and splenic nerve are of interest because they are closely associated with the intra-axonal microtubule transport system (BANKS, 1976). Several peptides have been proposed as putative neurotransmitters in invertebrate and in vertebrate nervous systems. The peptides of the hypothalamus, which regulate the release of substances from the anterior pituitary, are described as 'releasing factors' or as 'regulatory hormones' (BESSER, 1974).

Measurements of the rate of incorporation of labelled amino acids have shown that there is an active turnover of the peptides in the brain, but little information is available as to the enzyme systems involved in their biosynthesis and breakdown. Peptides can be formed either by 1) biosynthesis de novo from free precursor amino acids or by 2) breakdown of preexisting polypeptides, so as to release segments with the required amino acid sequence. There is evidence that vasopressin, growth hormone, and some other hormonal peptides are formed by the breakdown of precursors (SACHS, 1970). On the other hand, it has been reported that the thyrotropin-releasing hormone (TRH) is formed when rat hypothalamus slices are incubated in vitro in the presence of proline, glutamate and histidine together with Mg^{2+} and ATP. A nonribosomal "TRH synthetase" system is apparently responsible (MARKS and STERN, 1974a). The brain, like other tissues, contains a number of specific proteinases and peptidases, for several of which the hormonal peptides are good substrates. It appears likely that these enzymes are responsible for the degradation of the peptide hormones in vivo (MARKS and STERN, 1974b).

The determination of the chemical constitution of the different peptides and their synthesis has been of value in making the pure substances available for the physiological investigation of their properties. Their investigation has also been helped by the development of sensitive new techniques, such as radioimmunoassay, for the accurate determination of the small traces of hormones that are present in the blood and in the tissues (YALOW and BERSON, 1960).

2. Substance P

The structure of substance P as a peptide was determined by CHANG et al. (1971). It has now been synthesized and the amino acid sequence is (TREGEAR et al., 1971):

$$\text{Arg-Pro-Lys-Pro-Gln-Gln-Phe-Gly-Leu-Met-NH}_2$$

Substance P is present in sensory nerves and in the central nervous system. Studies of the localization of substance P by immunohistochemical and other techniques have shown that it occurs in small neuronal cell bodies in the spinal ganglia, in fibres in the dorsal horn of the spinal cord and in fibres in the intestinal wall (HÖKFELT et al., 1976). In the brain, concentrations are high in the basal ganglia and highest in the substantia nigra, where it is localized in the synaptosomal fraction; it has therefore been suggested that substance P may act as an excitatory neurotransmitter in this nucleus (KANAZAWA and JESSELL, 1976). Substance P is about 250 times more potent than glutamate in exciting neurons in the dorsal grey matter of the spinal cord, where it appears to act as an afferent transmitter (SNYDER, 1975). There is some evidence from electrophysiological studies that substance P may be specially concerned in the perception of pain (HENRY, 1975). In the periphery, substance P acts as a hypotensive agent by relaxing the smooth muscle of the arterioles. It also causes salivation and stimulates the smooth muscle of the intestine.

3. Somatostatin

This tetradecapeptide was first identified as a factor inhibiting the release of growth hormone in the hypothalamus, but it is also found in other brain areas as well as in primary sensory neurons and in fibres in the intestinal wall (VALE et al., 1975). The responses of neurons in the brain to somatostatin are mainly inhibitory, and it is possible that it acts as an inhibitory neurotransmitter at central synapses. HÖKFELT et al. (1976), who have studied the distribution of somatostatin in sensory neurons by immunohistochemical techniques, have found that it is present in different cells from those containing substance P. They conclude that there are two types of primary sensory neurons containing either somatostatin or substance P.

4. Encephalins

Following the identification of specific opiate receptors associated with neuronal membranes in the brain by PERT et al. (1975), two pentapeptides that act as agonists on opiate receptor sites were isolated, characterized and synthesized by HUGHES et al. (1975). The two peptides, which were named methionine encephalin and leucine encephalin, are present in the caudate nucleus, globus pallidus, nucleus accumbens and anterior hypothalamus. Immunohistochemical studies using antibodies to leucine encephalin have indicated that encephalins are contained in nerve terminals close to the opiate receptors (ELDE et al., 1976). The depressant action of morphine on neurons in the nucleus accumbens is closely mimicked by the encephalins (McCARTHY et al., 1977). Encephalin binding in the brain is influenced by Na^+, Mg^{2+} and other agents in the same way as observed for opiate agonists. Encephalins have not been found in invertebrates, but they are present in all vertebrates hitherto examined. Changes in encephalin levels in the brains of rats treated with morphine parallel the development of tolerance and withdrawal symptoms. It is concluded that the encephalins are concerned in the central mediation of pain perception in vertebrate species (SIMANTOV et al., 1976). Methionine encephalin has the structure H-Tyr-Gly-

Gly-Phe-Met-OH. The same amino acid sequence occurs in the pituitary prohormone β-lipotropin, of which some of the peptide fragments (endorphins) exhibit strong morphine-like action (KOSTERLITZ and HUGHES, 1977). The properties of the opioid peptides have been reviewed by SNYDER and SIMANTOV (1977), and GUILLEMIN (1976) has discussed their clinical significance and functions in the brain.

5. Oxytocin and Vasopressin

The two peptides oxytocin and vasopressin are synthesized in neurons of secretory type in the paraventricular and supraoptic nuclei of the hypothalamus. In association with carrier glycoproteins (neurophysins) with which they form granules, they are transported by axonal flow to the terminals in the posterior lobe of the pituitary gland (the neurohypophysis) where they are stored until finally secreted into the blood stream. The secretion is determined by the depolarization waves propagated down the axons in the supraoptico-neurohypophyseal tract. The depolarization of the nerve ending permits the uptake of Ca^{2+} ions into the neurons, and the peptides are then released together with the neurophysin, apparently by exocytosis (SACHS, 1970). The structures of these nonpeptides were established by DU VIGNAUD (1956), who showed that oxytocin has the amino acid sequence:

$$\overline{Cys\text{-}Tyr\text{-}Ile\text{-}Gln\text{-}Asn\text{-}Cys}\text{-}Pro\text{-}Leu\text{-}Gly\text{-}NH_2$$

Vasopressin is found in two forms as lysine vasopressin in the pig family and arginine vasopressin in other animals including man. Arginine vasopressin has the amino acid sequence:

$$\overline{Cys\text{-}Tyr\text{-}Phe\text{-}Gln\text{-}Asn\text{-}Cys}\text{-}Pro\text{-}Arg\text{-}Gly\text{-}NH_2$$

The ring structure of these peptides results from the formation of S-S bonds between the cystein residues. Their synthesis made the pure compounds available for the investigation of their physiological actions. Oxytocin was shown to cause contraction of the uterus and smooth muscle of the mammary glands. Vasopressin is active as an antidiuretic.

6. Hypothalamic Regulatory Factors

The secretion of the trophic hormones of the adenohypophysis is regulated by a series of peptides (releasing factors) synthesized in specialized neurons in the hypothalamus and carried in the hypophyseal portal circulation to the anterior lobe of the pituitary gland. The axons of these hypothalamic neurons end and discharge the regulatory factors in the median eminence and infundibulum close to the capillary network of the portal system where there is no blood-brain barrier, so that substances released from the axon terminals can diffuse into the portal blood stream. In this way, the controlling mechanisms of the hypothalamus influence the function of the adrenal, thyroid and mammary glands, as well as the gonads and the tissues influenced by growth hormone, including those producing insulin, glucagon and gastrin (Table 2).

Table 2. Actions of hypothalamic regulatory factors (BESSER, 1974)

Hypothalamic regulatory factors	Anterior pituitary hormones	Target organs
CRF (corticotrophin-releasing factor) releases	ACTH (adrenocorticotrophic hormone)	Adrenal cortex
TRF (thyrotrophin-releasing factor) releases	TSH (thyroid-stim. hormone, Thyrotrophin)	Thyroid gland
	Prolactin	Mammary gland
	FSH (follicle-stim. hormone) in men	Testis
	LH (luteinizing hormone) in women at luteal peak	Ovaries
	GH (growth hormone) in acromegaly	Many tissues
LH/FSH-RF or LRF (luteinizing and follicle-stim. hormone releasing factor) releases	LH (luteinizing hormone)	Ovaries
	FSH (follicle-stim. hormone)	Gonads
	GH (growth hormone) in acromegaly	Many tissues
GRF (growth hormone-releasing factor) releases	GH (growth hormone)	Many tissues
GH-RIF (growth hormone release-inhib. factor) inhibits release of	GH (growth hormone)	Many tissues
	TSH } after TRF	Thyroid gland
	FSH	Gonads
PIF (prolactin inhib. factor) inhibits release of	Prolactin	Mammary gland

It might be expected that there would be one releasing factor for each of the hormones of the anterior pituitary gland, but it is found that the regulatory factors are to some extent unspecific and that each can affect the secretion of more than one pituitary hormone. There is also evidence that one regulatory factor can influence the releasing action of another. Thus, it has been shown that the growth hormone release-inhibiting factor (GH-RIF) interferes with the action of TRF on the pituitary, since it impairs the release of TSH and FSH produced by TRF (BESSER, 1974). A growth hormone releasing factor is believed to exist, but it has not hitherto been isolated and characterized (FRANZ and ZIMMERMAN, 1975). The melanocyte-stimulating hormone (MSH), which redistributes melanin in the skin of amphibians and fish, is also present in the vertebrates including man, where its normal function is not clear. MSH is released in the pars intermedia, which is associated anatomically with the posterior lobe but belongs to the adenohypophysis in origin and function. The release of MSH is controlled in the hypothalamus by the releasing and release-inhibiting factors MRF and MIF.

The regulatory factors of the hypothalamus are all peptides of relatively low molecular weight. TRF is the tripeptide (p)Glu-His-Pro(NH_2), in which the glutamate is cyclized and the proline is in the amide form. MIF is believed to be the tripeptide Pro-Lau-Gly-NH_2, which is the terminal part of oxytocin (SIEGEL and EISENMAN, 1972), and the releasing factor MRF is apparently the pentapeptide Cys-Tyr-Ile-Glu-Asn-OH, which has the same sequence as in the ring of oxytocin. The luteinizing hormone release factor (LRF) is the decapeptide:

$$(p)Glu\text{-}His\text{-}Trp\text{-}Ser\text{-}Tyr\text{-}Gly\text{-}Leu\text{-}Arg\text{-}Pro\text{-}Gly\text{-}NH_2$$

The neurons that liberate regulatory factors in the hypothalamus are controlled by other neurons with cell bodies in other areas of the central nervous system, including the limbic and reticular activating systems. These neurons have axon terminals in the hypothalamus, which have been shown by fluorescence techniques to contain dopamine, noradrenalin or 5-HT. Cholinergic terminals are also present, and the high histamine content of the hypothalamus has suggested that histaminergic terminals may be present as well. Infusion of dopamine into the third ventricle raises the content of LH/FSH-RF and PIF in the hypophyseal portal blood and results in an increase in the plasma LH and FSH levels and decrease in plasma prolactin. The action of 5-HT is inhibitory and drugs, such as chlorpromazine, which block dopaminergic transmission raise the plasma prolactin level. Such observations have led to the identification of a dopaminergic system arising in the arcuate nucleus and terminating at the hypophyseal portal plexus, concerned in controlling the secretion of the regulatory factors of the hypothalamus (SIEGEL and EISENMAN, 1972).

As with other endocrine glands, the secretory activity of the anterior pituitary changes to suit the body's needs. This is achieved by negative feedback mechanisms with receptors sensitive to the hormone levels in the general circulation. Thus, systemic administration of thyroxin activates receptors that reduce the release of TRF and the secretion of thyrotropin; hence, the secretion of thyroxin by the thyroid gland falls as well. There are feedback mechanisms operating at several different levels; it has been shown that there are receptors sensitive not only to the hormone secreted by the target organ but also to the trophic hormones secreted by the pituitary gland.

In the case of the gonadotrophic hormones (LH-FSH), there is evidence of a further type of positive feedback that operates so as to produce a rapid rise in the plasma oestrogen level at a critical point in the oestrus cycle, thereby inducing ovulation. Under these conditions, a low dose of estrogen activates receptors that stimulate the secretion of the hypothalamic releasing factor LH-RF, leading to increased output of LH and a further increase in the plasma estrogen level (RUF et al., 1976).

D. Barrier Systems and Compartmentation

I. Blood-Brain Barrier

It has long been known that dyes that stain other tissues of the body when injected into a vein may leave the brain unstained. This could be because the dye is prevented from entering the brain, or because when it gets there it is quickly metabolized. The existence of barriers to prevent foreign substances entering from the blood is consistent with the need to maintain a constant environment for the delicate mechanisms operating in the brain. The blood-brain barrier acts selectively in permitting the free entry of certain substances such as glucose, while retarding or preventing the entry of others. Thus, fructose is not taken up or utilized appreciably by the brain in vivo, although it is readily metabolized by brain slices in vitro.

The anatomical basis of the blood-brain barrier lies in the structure of the brain capillaries, which differ from those of other organs in that the endothelial cells in the walls of the brain capillaries are fused tightly together, leaving no gaps between them. Except in certain limited areas, they also have no fenestrae through which proteins could pass, and pinocytosis is almost absent. Molecules entering the brain from the blood must therefore pass through the plasma membranes of the endothelial cells. These are permeable to small molecules such as those of O_2, CO_2 and water, but they retard the passage of larger molecules and are practically impermeable to proteins.

There is a rapid exchange between blood and brain of lipid-soluble substances that can diffuse through the lipoprotein layers in the plasma membranes of the endothelial cells. The rate of penetration of the blood-brain barrier is determined largely by their oil-water partition coefficient, which indicates their readiness to enter the membrane lipid from water (OLDENDORF, 1975). Thus, ethanol and many drugs quickly enter the brain because of their lipid solubility, whereas polar molecules and ions, which are not lipid-soluble, are excluded, unless present to an appreciable extent in undissociated form. It may be noted that there is a DC potential across the blood-brain barrier, positive on the side of the brain.

The presence of special carrier systems for the transport of glucose, amino acids, and other metabolites is indicated by the observation that the blood-brain barrier discriminates between the D- and L-stereoisomers. It also shows saturation kinetics and competitive interaction for a number of metabolites. Carrier systems have also been demonstrated for certain nucleosides, purines, and short-chain carboxylic acids. An active (uphill) transport system from brain to blood exists for K^+ ions, which are present at about 40% lower concentration in brain extracellular fluid and CSF than in the blood. The fact that the endothelial cells of the brain capillaries have about five times as many mitochondria as muscle capillaries agrees with other evidence that energy-dependent transport systems are operative there.

The distribution of metabolites between blood and brain depends not only on the anatomical characteristics and transport systems of the brain capillaries but also on metabolic factors determining the fate of molecules entering the brain. Thus, the concentration of amines in the brain is quickly reduced by the amine oxidases that are present in the capillaries, neurons and glial cells. Conversely, the relatively high amino acid concentration in the brain depends on the active uptake mechanisms in the neurons and glial cells. The uneven distribution of metabolites in different parts of the brain is due partly to such factors, but in certain regions the capillary endothelium is fenestrated, so permitting a freer exchange of substances including proteins between blood and brain. Such areas include the median eminence of the hypothalamus, the area postrema and the pineal gland. Studies of the blood-brain barrier have been reviewed by RAPOPORT (1976) and by PARTRIDGE and OLDENDORF (1977).

II. Blood-CSF Barrier

The capillaries of the choroid plexus act like those in the brain in keeping the composition of the cerebrospinal fluid (CSF) similar to that of the extracellular fluid of the brain. The CSF is a dilute saline solution containing very little protein (about 20 mg per 100 ml) and comparable in composition to a dialysate of serum. That the CSF is in fact secreted by the choroid plexus is indicated by the observation that the rate of formation is largely independent of the CSF pressure. In man about a tenth of the CSF is changed every hour. The concentrations of certain ions such as K^+, Cl^-, Ca^{2+} and Mg^{2+} in the CSF are also different from those in the serum and are maintained at a more constant level. The CSF changes appreciably in composition in its passage from the choroid plexus to the cisterna magna and to the sites of removal at the nerve root sheaths in the spinal column. This is due in part to the diffusion into the CSF of metabolites from the brain. The membranes at the surface of the brain are porous enough to permit the passage in both directions, not only of ions and organic substances but also of macromolecules. The CSF therefore contains appreciable amounts of all the metabolites that are present in the extracellular fluid of the brain. These include those that relate to transmitter function such as HVA, VMA, MHPG, 5-HIAA, choline, acetylcholine and an isoenzyme of acetylcholinesterase (GREENFIELD and SMITH, 1976). Since the levels of these metabolites in the CSF depend on the state of functional activity of the transmitter systems concerned, their estimation can be of value for purposes of clinical investigation and research.

Changes in the composition of the CSF are also caused by membrane transport systems that effect the active clearance of anions and organic acids from the CSF. These transport systems are present in the choroid plexus and also in the brain capillaries including those near the subarachnoid surface; the pial capillaries may also play a part (KATZMAN, 1975). Thus, the concentrations of acids such as HVA and 5-HIAA in the CSF are found to be higher in the lateral ventricles than in the cisterna magna and higher in the cisterna magna than in the lumbar CSF. Their clearance from the CSF and the ventricular-lumbar gradient are reduced by probenecid, which blocks the transport mechanism. A different system, blocked by perchlorate, effects the clearance of Cl^+ and other halide ions from the CSF.

In newborn infants the protein concentration in the CSF (about 80 mg per 100 ml) is usually much higher than in later life, and the concentration falls to the adult level at about 4–6 months of age. The CSF protein level in premature infants is even higher than in those born at full term. The clinical observation that kernicterus occurs only in newborn infants suggests that the barrier system is less efficient in the neonatal period, since kernicterus implies the penetration of the barrier by the bilirubin-protein complex in the blood (ZETTERSTRÖM, 1959). The rate of uptake of labelled ions such as Cl^-, phosphate and thiocyanate into the brain is relatively high in young animals. Changes with age and regional differences in amino acid concentration in the CSF are due in part to the existence of several different transport systems that mature at different ages: transport systems for dibasic, neutral, imino and β-amino acids have been identified (KOROBKIN and CUTLER, 1977).

III. Metabolic Compartmentation

The neuronal plasma membrane is relatively impermeable to molecules that are neither of very small size nor lipid-soluble, but neurons can take in many substances including proteins by pinocytosis (invagination to form a vesicle). It has been shown by histochemical methods that certain sensory neurons and neurons of the visual cortex will take in foreign proteins such as a plant peroxidase at the nerve endings. These are then transported by cytoplasmic flow to the cell body and dendrites of the cell. Thus, horseradish peroxidase on a mouse's or a rabbit's tongue is taken in at the nerve endings and after travelling at some 3 mm/h it arrives in due course at the hypoglossal nucleus in the brain stem (KRISTENSSON, 1975). It is thought that this may be a physiological mechanism for assisting the recognition of toxic items of food. The uptake at a nerve ending and cytoplasmic transport of a modulator might also constitute a physiological mechanism for producing a type of delayed response (MCILWAIN, 1976).

Proteins and other metabolites are distributed by cytoplasmic flow in certain channels in the axons and dendrites of the neurons, but their entry into many parts of the cell is restricted by the membranes of the reticular endothelium, nucleus, mitochondria and other organelles. The structural heterogeneity of the cells results in the coexistence of separate metabolic pools or compartments in which a given compound may be taken up and metabolized at different rates or in different ways. Similar considerations apply to the glia as well as to the neurons. Studies with labelled compounds have shown that while some metabolites, such as glucose and pyruvate, penetrate relatively freely into most regions of all types of cells, other metabolites, such as amino acids, have only limited entry into certain structures or cells in the brain.

When [^{14}C]glutamate is injected intravenously in the rat, it enters the liver and other organs where it is aminated to form [^{14}C]glutamine, but owing to the blood-brain barrier very little enters the brain. If the blood-brain barrier is bypassed by injecting [^{14}C]glutamate intracisternally, it is quickly converted into [^{14}C]glutamine in the brain. Of considerable interest is the observation that the specific radioactivity of the glutamine formed is as much as five times greater than that of the glutamate in the brain as a whole. This indicates that the [^{14}C]glutamate entering the brain does not mix with the rest of the glutamate in the tissue but enters a small metabolic compartment in which glutamine is synthesized from the highly labelled precursor [^{14}C]glutamate (BERL, 1973). Further work has provided evidence of a similar compartmentation in the brain of the metabolism of many other metabolites including GABA and other amino acids, the monoamine transmitters, and the metabolites of the tricarboxylic acid cycle (BALÁZS and CREMER, 1973).

Attempts to identify the structures associated with the metabolic compartment (I) in which there is rapid labelling of glutamine showed that it is different from a second compartment (II), located mainly in the synapses, in which glutamate is decarboxylated to form GABA. It is different again from a third compartment (III) located mainly in the nerve cell bodies and dendrites, in which protein synthesis occurs and most of the tissue glutamate is found. The careful characterization of these three glutamate-containing compartments indicated that the one containing the active glutamate-glutamine system is apparently located mainly in the glial cells (BALÁZS et al., 1973). Studies of the metabolism of glutamate in young animals showed that the compartmentation pattern is different from that in the adult. In the kitten the adult pattern does not develop until about 4 weeks of age in the brain as a whole or 6 weeks in regions, such as the cerebellum, which are late to mature (BERL, 1973).

Metabolic compartmentation implies the incomplete mixing of metabolites in a heterogeneous system, so that one fraction of a marker compound has a different fate from the rest; it may result not only from permeability barriers but also from differences in the rate of metabolism at different sites, with delay in equilibration. Compartmentation depends on structural organization, and in some cases a compartment may be attributed to the metabolic characteristics of a specific structure such as the synaptic membranes or the mitochondria; however, a metabolic compartment may also relate to a situation existing at numerous different anatomical sites in different types of cells.

E. Metabolism and Function

I. Metabolism of Growth

During early foetal life, the brain is undergoing rapid growth, and its metabolism is characterized by the high activity of the enzymes concerned in synthesizing the proteins and lipoproteins that together account for some 90% of the dry weight. The initial increase in the DNA content of the brain is due to the proliferation of neuroblasts, which are the first cells to appear in considerable numbers. There is then a proliferation of separate sets of cells destined to become 1) long-axoned macroneurons, 2) short-axoned interneurons and finally 3) glial cells (ALTMAN, 1969). There is also an uneven invasion by cells of vascular tissue, which reach a higher density in cortical and other regions of high metabolic activity. In considering the metabolic changes during development, we are dealing, therefore, not with the growth and differentiation of a single set of cells, but with tissues changing markedly in cell population as well as in structure, metabolism, and size. At various stages of development, processes of cell degeneration take place, and as cells of one kind disappear, their place is taken by cells of newer types with different physical and metabolic characteristics. The distribution of the various types of cells is also changed by cell migration. Thus, cells migrate out from the walls of the ventricles and take up new positions in the organized layers of the cerebral cortex. The nature of the guiding mechanism that directs the migrating cells is not yet clear, but it is thought that glial processes serve as guidelines and the glycoproteins at the cell surface play a part in the recognition and contact functions of the migrating cells (BARONDES, 1975).

The basic processes of protein synthesis – replication of DNA, transcription of DNA to RNA, and translation of RNA to protein – occur in the brain as in other organs. The development of cell-specific enzymes and structural proteins then gives each type of cell its own unique metabolic and physical character. In neural tissues, enzymes associated with transmitter function appear at an early age; three isoenzymes of acetylcholinesterase were identified in the 6-day-old chick embryo brain (SHARMA et al., 1975). Glutamate decarboxylase (GAD) has been shown by immunocytochemical techniques to be present in growing axons and their growth cones, and monoamines have been demonstrated in growing axons by fluorescence microscopy (SIDMAN, 1975).

The maturation of each region of the developing brain is marked by a similar sequence of events. As the proliferation of neuroblasts comes to an end, the differentiation of the nerve cells coincides with a sharp increase in activity of a number of enzymes related to functional activity (BALÁZS et al., 1975). At this point the glial cells rapidly increase in number, and there is a large increase in lipid content and overall weight of the tissue as myelination proceeds. It was observed by FLEXNER (1952) that the onset of differentiation, which he named the 'critical period,' is associated with an enlargement of the cell nucleus and an increase in RNA as the rapid sprouting of dendrites occurs. This is followed by the onset of spontaneous electrical activity. Besides serving as a developmental marker, the critical period is important in that the effects of nutritional, hormonal, and other environmental factors depend on whether they act before or after the critical period. Thus, protein calorie deficiency before the critical period reduces DNA synthesis and causes a permanent deficit in cell number in the brain (BALÁZS et al., 1975). Thyroid deficiency and steroid hormones at the time of cell differentiation influence the wiring pattern of the brain and hence the ultimate behaviour of the adult.

In each species the cycle of changes associated with the critical period is repeated successively in the different regional structures of the brain as they mature. Myelination starts in the brain stem in man at the end of the 5th month of foetal life, while other areas are still at the proliferative stage. In the ontogenetically newer structures of the brain, such as the association areas of the cerebral cortex, myelination does not start until 4 months after birth (YAKOVLEV and LECOURS, 1967). In comparing the course of maturation in different species, the time of birth is unsatisfactory as a reference point, since in some species, such as the guinea pig, birth occurs at a much later stage of maturation than in others. The so-called growth spurt of the brain as a whole is also imprecise, since it lumps together increases in weight due to proliferation of glial cells and deposition of myelin in the various structures that mature in different species at different rates and times. The critical period in the development of the cerebral cortex gives a more reliable basis for comparison. Convenient markers for the biochemical maturation of the brain are the development of metabolic compartmentation or the appearance of the adult enzyme pattern, which effects the rapid conversion of glucose carbon into glutamate. This can be observed by recording the labelling of the amino acids by [^{14}C]glucose. It occurs in the rat at about the 15th day after birth and marks the change from the 'metabolism of growth' to the 'metabolism of function' (GAITONDE and RICHTER, 1966; PATEL and BALÁZS, 1975).

The growth of the foetal brain is influenced by the level of growth hormone secreted by the mother, and there is evidence that this is mediated by a specific brain trophin in the mother's blood that promotes cell proliferation in the foetal brain (SARA et al., 1976). Besides nutritional and endocrine factors, the development of the brain is influenced by environmental stimuli of various kinds including those associated with normal activity and those producing stress (BENNETT et al., 1964; BALÁZS et al., 1977).

II. Protein Metabolism

During the maturation of the brain, the protein content increases and there is a shift from the synthesis of water-soluble proteins to synthesis of proteins that are membrane-bound. The rate of protein synthesis in the foetal brain, as indicated by the incorporation of labelled amino acids, is very high and greater at first than in the liver and most other organs. After the critical period, the rate decreases with the falling off in the rate of growth of the brain, but it still remains at a relatively high level in the brain, and protein synthesis continues throughout life at a rate comparable to that of secreting glandular tissue. The first estimates of the rate of protein turnover using [^{35}S]methionine gave a mean value of about 14 days for the half-life of the proteins of the adult rat brain (GAITONDE and RICHTER, 1956; LAJTHA et al., 1957), but it is not easy to know the specific activity of the precursor amino acid in a heterogeneous tissue such as brain in which there is compartmentation of metabolites. More recent estimates of protein turnover in the mouse brain, made by measuring the incorporation after long-term labelling with [^{14}C]tyrosine, gave as the closest approximation one compartment of high turnover rate containing 5.7% of the brain proteins, with a half-life of 15 h, and a second compartment containing 94.3% of the proteins, with a half-life of 10 days (LAJTHA et al., 1976).

Studies of the localization of protein synthesis by radioautographic methods showed that it is greater in the grey matter of the brain than in the white and most active in the bodies of the nerve cells. It is particularly active in the supraoptic nucleus and other hypothalamic nuclei containing secretory neurons (COHN et al., 1954). In subcellular fractions of brain tissue separated after administration in vivo of a labelled amino acid, the labelling was found to be relatively slow in the proteins of the cell nuclei, mitochondria and myelin but rapid in the microsomal fraction, which contains a liponucleoprotein with a half-life of the order of 50–100 min (CLOUET and RICHTER, 1958). While protein synthesis is most active in the cell body, it also takes place in the mitochondria that are present in other parts of the cell including the synapses, which contain about 6% of the total RNA in the tissue (BALÁZS and COCKS, 1967). The proteins of the synaptic plasma membranes are estimated to have a half-life of the order of 5 days (SABRI et al., 1974), and protein synthesis has been shown to take place in isolated synaptosomes (GAMBETTI et al., 1972; HERNANDEZ, 1974).

In considering the fate of the proteins synthesized in the brain, it is relevant that nervous tissues contain an active proteolytic system. A neutral proteinase that liberates amino acids from the cell proteins at pH 7.0 is more active in white matter than in grey; it appears to be associated with axon material since it is also present in peripheral nerve (ANSELL and RICHTER, 1954). If protein is synthesized in the cell body and broken down or released in the axon and nerve endings, this would agree with a net outward flow of axoplasm towards the periphery. This was suggested by the earlier observation of a damming of the flow in nerve fibres that had been artificially constricted (WEISS and HISCOE, 1948). Some of the protein formed in the cell body is likely to be used for the renewal of the structural proteins of the cell membranes. A part of the protein is also required for the synthesis of the transmitters that are released at the nerve endings. In the secretory neurons of the hypothalamus, a part of the axoplasmic protein is used for the formation of peptide hormones; there is also some evidence for secretion of specific proteins at the nerve endings when the transmitter is released from catecholaminergic or cholinergic neurons (DE POTTER et al., 1969; MUSICK and HUBBARD, 1972). The breakdown by proteolytic enzymes of proteins in the axons or in the synaptic clefts yields amino acids that are available for resynthesis of protein or for the energy metabolism of the cell. Glutamic acid is among the substrates most readily utilized by nervous tissues as a source of energy. It may, therefore, be relevant that the rapidly turning-over protein fraction in the brain includes one with a high content of glutamic acid (MINARD and RICHTER, 1968). The observation that the release of labelled amino acids in long-term experiments is less than might be expected from incorporation rates, provides evidence for a considerable reutilization of the locally released amino acids in the brain (LAJTHA and SHERSHEN, 1976).

The effect of stimulation on the protein metabolism of the brain is of interest in connection with various memory hypotheses involving proteins that have been proposed. There have been conflicting reports of increased or decreased protein turnover resulting from electrical stimulation; however, such changes in amino acid incorporation are difficult to interpret, since stimulation of the brain may cause changes in membrane permeability, size of amino acid precursor pool and circulation, which could affect the results (BHARUCHA and ELLIOTT, 1974; RICHTER, 1966). There is evidence that amino acid incorporation is reduced in narcosis, in insulin hypoglycemia and in hypothermia. Protein synthesis is also inhibited by puromycin, cycloheximide and other drugs. Inhibition of protein synthesis in the brain by puromycin has no significant effect on normal behaviour or on learning, but the permanent memory of what has been learned is completely blocked. It is concluded that memory fixation involves protein synthesis at synapses that have been sensitized by the signals they have received (AGRANOFF, 1975). The hypothesis that glycoproteins may play a part in this process has been under discussion in recent years (ESSMAN and NAKAJIMA, 1973). Much of the work on memory mechanisms has been done on the goldfish, and it has been reported that in goldfish learning new swimming skills the 'information-gathering' state is associated with the synthesis of a specific RNA with an altered base composition; this then mediates the synthesis of specific proteins related to the acquisition of new behaviour in the cytoplasmic fraction of the brain (SHASHOUA, 1976).

III. Lipid Metabolism

In the developing rat brain, a phase of rapid synthesis of gangliosides that coincides with the outgrowth of neuronal processes at about day 10 is followed by a phase of rapid synthesis of myelin lipids (cerebrosides, sulphatides, sphingomyelins, triphosphoinositide, etc.), maximal at about day 20, as myelination proceeds. The synthetic pathways of the brain lipids are similar in general to those in other organs. During myelination cholesterol can enter the brain from the blood, but cholesterol is also synthesized in the brain, and desmosterol, which is the precursor of cholesterol, is found in the brain at the start of myelination. Once deposited in the myelin, the cholesterol is relatively inert, and there is little turnover of labelled cholesterol in the myelin fraction of the brain.

Glucose, glycerol and acetate can be utilized for the synthesis of lipids in the brain. It has been reported that in the developing mammalian brain ketone bodies (acetoacetate and 3-hydroxybutyrate) are utilized in preference to glucose as precursors of brain lipids (PATEL and OWEN, 1977). The influx of ketone bodies from the blood into the brain is high in the rat in the first 3 weeks of life but falls with increasing age, owing to reduced blood level and decreased activity of a carrier-mediated transport system (DANIEL et al., 1977).

In contrast to cholesterol, the phospholipids show a high degree of metabolic activity, and in the mouse brain they have a mean half-life of about 35 h. The rate of incorporation of ^{32}P into the phospholipids is decreased in nembutal narcosis, hypothermia, insulin hypoglycemia and electrically induced convulsions; it was also shown to be decreased by 25% under normal physiological conditions in animals subjected to the stress of exposure in a slowly rotating drum, while in control animals that had been accustomed to the treatment there was no change (DAWSON and RICHTER, 1950). The phospholipids are a heterogeneous group, and the individual components do not all behave in the same way. Studies of the incorporation of ^{32}P in the isolated superior cervical ganglion of the rat have indicated that electrical stimulation decreases the incorporation into phosphatidylethanolamine but increases the labelling of phosphatidylinositol (BURT and LARRABEE, 1976). The turnover of phosphatidylinositol in brain slices was also found to be increased by treatment with acetylcholine (LUNT et al., 1971). There is evidence that the prostaglandins play a part in the central nervous system in mediating the responses to stimuli.

IV. Energy Metabolism and Function

The energy requirement of the brain is indicated by the oxygen consumption in vivo, which is about 3.5 ml O_2 per 100 g per minute in the adult. That means that the brain takes about one-fifth of the total oxygen used by the body in the normal resting state. In childhood the oxygen consumption of the brain is higher still, and in the child of 5 or 6 it may account for more than half the total basal oxygen consumption of the body (KENNEDY and SOKOLOFF, 1957). Analysis of the blood entering and leaving the brain has established that glucose is the main source of energy. Under normal conditions, about 85% of the glucose is oxidized to CO_2, while 13% is returned to the blood as lactate and 2% as pyruvate. In the foetal brain, glucose is utilized mainly by glycolysis to form lactate and pyruvate, a process that is less efficient than oxidation to CO_2 as a means of obtaining energy; however, obtaining energy by glycolysis makes it possible for the foetus and the newborn infant to survive anoxia considerably longer than the adult. The energy requirement of the foetal brain is considerably smaller than that of the adult. FLEXNER (1952) observed a sharp increase in the activity of the cytochrome oxidase, succinate dehydrogenase and other enzymes concerned in energy metabolism at the 'critical period,' and other investigators noted that the rate of respiration increases first in those parts of the brain that first become functionally mature. Thus, the medulla reaches maximum activity early and the cerebellum late, corresponding to the pattern of ontogenetic development (HIMWICH, 1951; RICHTER, 1955).

Although glucose is the main source of energy for brain metabolism, ketone bodies (acetoacetate and 3-hydroxybutyrate) are also utilized to a considerable extent by the brain in the foetus and in young animals. The decreased utilization of ketone bodies in the adult is due partly to the fall in their concentration in the blood and partly to their exclusion from the brain by the blood-brain barrier. There is also some falling off with age in the activity of the enzymes that metabolize ketone bodies in the brain (PAGE et al., 1971). Brain slices in vitro will oxidase mannose, lactate, succinate, octanoate, and a large number of other substances, but they are not utilized appreciably in vivo since the blood-brain barrier restricts their access to the brain.

A part of the glucose entering the brain is converted into glycogen, which is also continually being utilized and which serves as a local reserve of utilizable carbohydrate. Another part of the glucose is quickly converted into amino acids and their derivatives. The brain differs from other organs in the high level of dicarboxylic amino acids in the free amino acid pool. When [^{14}C]glucose is metabolized in the adult brain, a large proportion of the ^{14}C appears in the glutamate, glutamine, GABA and aspartic acid, and the immediate source of the CO_2 that is liberated is not the labelled glucose that is being metabolized. This characteristic is due largely to the activity of the transaminases, which effect the exchange of amino groups between amino acids and the ketoacids (α-ketoglutarate and oxaloacetate) of the citric acid cycle. The main pathways of energy metabolism in the brain are similar to those in other organs. There is a rapid flux of metabolites through the citric acid cycle, but the amination of α-ketoglutarate to form glutamate provides an alternative route to succinate through what is known as the GABA shunt (Fig. 4). The oxidation of glucose in the pentose phosphate pathway, which is more active in the developing brain, serves to provide pentose for nucleotide synthesis and produces the NADPH (reduced nicotinamide adenine dinucleotide phosphate) required for the processes of lipid synthesis. Most of the energy derived from the oxidation of glucose is made available for the functional metabolism of the brain in the form of high-energy phosphate bonds ($\sim$P) in ATP. A reserve of high-energy phosphate is maintained in the form of phosphocreatine.

Energy is required by the brain for the synthesis of neurotransmitters, proteins, and other metabolites. It is needed for cytoplasmic transport in the neurons and especially for the active transport of ions in maintaining the state of polarization of membranes discharging many times a second. Measurements of the oxygen consumption of the brain in human subjects have shown little overall change with changes of functional activity during mental exertion or sleep, but there is an increase in the regional blood flow in cortical association areas during abstract thinking, and regional increases are also found during REM sleep (INGVAR and LASSEN, 1975). The oxygen consumption of the brain is reduced in states of coma and anaesthesia, and it is increased in epileptic seizures and convulsions induced by electroshock or convulsant drugs (SOKOLOFF, 1973).

In animal experiments significant changes have been observed in metabolites in the brain, not only in anaesthesia and convulsions but also in sleep and in arousal under normal physiological conditions. Thus, the lactic acid level found in the brains of young rats killed during sleep by immersion in liquid air was 12.2 mg%, which is close to the level in anaesthetized animals and significantly lower than that (18.8 mg%) in the normal waking state. Rats excited by withdrawing their support gave a mean lactic acid level of 37.5 mg%, and the level was 65 mg% in animals taken during electroshock convulsions (RICHTER and DAWSON, 1948). Similar changes associated with functional activity of the brain have been observed for a number of other metabolites including phosphocreatine, inorganic phosphate, ammonia, and acetylcholine (RICHTER, 1952).

V. Pathological Deviations

The belief that metabolic factors may be involved in certain forms of mental illness is consistent with the observation that mental symptoms occur in conditions such as myxoedema, pellagra and Wilson's disease, in which biochemical factors are known to operate. Biochemical abnormalities have also been shown to be present in many conditions characterized by mental disorder including galactosemia, acute porphyria, the lipidoses, phenylketonuria, and the aminoacidurias. Hallucinations and other symptoms found in the psychoses can be produced by relatively simple chemical compounds such as mescaline or LSD, and psychotic states can be produced by administering compounds such as the amphetamines, which are simple derivatives of phenylethylamine. The idea that mental illness might be caused by an abnormal metabolite has been current for many years.

In considering the ways in which a metabolic abnormality can arise, it is evident that the normal metabolism depends on the pattern of enzymes resulting from genetic data encoded in the DNA. Some enzymes have a feedback mechanism to keep their activity within normal limits, but others show a large biological variation in different genetic strains and in different members of the same species. The complete absence of an essential enzyme would be lethal, but often we find a partial deficiency or overactivity that brings the concentration of a metabolite close to, or into, the pathological range. Such 'inborn errors' of metabolism have been identified in more than 50 conditions associated with mental retardation, including disorders of amino acid, carbohydrate, and lipid metabolism (RICHTER, 1967). Generally, as in the heterozygous carriers of a defective gene, the resulting metabolic imbalance is insufficient to produce overt symptoms, but it may produce symptoms under conditions of stress and the enzymatic defect may be shown by applying loading tests. It is estimated that the average individual is heterozygous for at least eight seriously detrimental genes, which give each individual his own characteristic pattern of inherited vulnerability (MULLER, 1950).

Since genetic factors are known to operate only through biochemical mechanisms, in the synthesis of enzymes and other proteins, it is evident that biochemical factors must play a part in any type of neurological or mental disorder in which genetic factors are involved. The importance of environmental factors such as vitamin deficiencies and toxic substances of exogenous origin is also clear. Different aspects of the pathology of nervous and mental disorders are reviewed in other chapters in this Volume (JELLINGER, 1978; MATUSSEK, 1978; ZERBIN-RÜDIN, 1978).

Pathological conditions can arise through the formation of antibodies that react with tissue proteins as an allergic response. It has been shown in animal experiments that injection of tissue preparations from the central nervous system produces an allergic response, experimental allergic encephalomyelitis (EAE) due to sensitization to the myelin basic protein. Myasthenia gravis is now known to involve an autoimmune response to the patient's acetylcholine receptor protein at the neuromuscular junctions, and it is believed that similar mechanisms may operate in multiple sclerosis and other neurological and mental disorders.

The demonstration of a local deficiency of dopamine in the basal ganglia in Parkinson's disease has drawn attention to the possibility that local defects in the transmitter mechanisms in other brain areas may be responsible for other neurological and mental conditions. It has now been shown that a decreased concentration of GABA in the basal ganglia in Huntington's chorea is associated with an 80% decrease in the activity of glutamic acid decarboxylase (GAD) in the same areas (BIRD and IVERSEN, 1974). The hyperkinetic condition characteristic of this disease can thus be related to a biochemical deficiency involving the GABA-containing inhibitory interneurons of the basal ganglia. The discovery of the opiate receptor system and the encephalins in the brain has again opened up a promising new field for investigation. It appears not unreasonable to hope that further neurochemical research will be helpful in revealing the mechanisms that operate in other pathological conditions and in elucidating many further problems in the neuropsychiatric field.

References

Abdel-Latif, A.A., Abood, L.G.: Biochemical studies on mitochondria and other cytoplasmic fractions of developing rat brain. J. Neurochem. **11**, 9–16 (1964)

Abood, L.G.: Brain mitochondria. In: Handbook of Neurochemistry. Lajtha, A. (ed.). New York: Plenum 1969, Vol. 2, pp. 303–326

Agranoff, B.W.: Biochemical strategies in the study of memory formation. In The Nervous System. Tower, D.B. (ed.). Vol. 1: The Basic Neurosciences. Brady, R.O. (ed.). New York: Raven 1975, pp. 585–590

Allen, W.S., Otterbein, E.C., Varma, R., Varma, R.S., Wardi, A.H.: Non-dialyzable sulfated sialoglycopeptide fractions derived from bovine heifer brain glycoproteins. J. Neurochem. **26**, 879–885 (1976)

Allweis, C., Magnes, J.: The uptake and oxidation of glucose by the perfused cat brain. J. Neurochem. **2**, 326–336 (1958)

Altman, J.: DNA metabolism and cell proliferation. In: Handbook of Neurochemistry. Lajtha, A. (ed.). New York: Plenum 1969, Vol. 2, pp. 137–182

Andén, N.-E., Carlsson, A., Häggendal, J.: Adrenergic mechanisms. Annu. Rev. Pharmacol. **9**, 119–134 (1969)

Ansell, G.B., Hawthorne, J.N.: Phospholipids: Chemistry, Metabolism and Function. Amsterdam: Elsevier 1964

Ansell, G.B., Richter, D.: Evidence for a 'neutral proteinase' in brain tissue. Biochem. Biophys. Acta **13**, 92–97 (1954)

Appel, S.H., Day, E.D., Mickey, D.D.: Cellular and subcellular fractionation. In: Basic Neurochemistry. Albers, R.W., Siegel, G.J., Katzman, R., Agranoff, B.W. (eds.). Boston: Little and Brown 1972, pp. 425–448

Axelrod, J.: The pineal gland. A model to study the regulation of the β-adrenergic receptor. In: The Nervous System. Tower, D.B. (ed.). Vol. 1: The Basic Sciences. Brady, R.O. (ed.). New York: Raven 1975, pp. 395–400

Bakay, L.: Dynamic aspects of the blood-brain barrier. In: Metabolism of the Nervous System. Richter, D. (ed.). Oxford: Pergamon 1957, pp. 136–149

Balasubramanian, K.A., Bachhawat, B.K.: Partial purification, properties and glycoprotein nature of arylsulphatase B from sheep brain. J. Neurochem. **27**, 485–492 (1976)

Balázs, R., Cocks, W.A.: RNA metabolism in subcellular fractions of brain tissue. J. Neurochem. **14**, 1035–1055 (1967)

Balázs, R., Cremer, J.E. (eds.): Metabolic Compartmentation in the Brain. London: Macmillan 1973

Balázs, R., Machiyama, Y., Hammond, B.J., Julian, T., Richter, D.: The operation of the GABA bypath of the tricarboxylic acid cycle in brain tissue in vitro. Biochem. J. **116**, 445–467 (1970)

Balázs, R., Patel, A.J., Richter, D.: Metabolic compartments in the brain. Their properties and relation to morphological structures. In: Metabolic Compartmentation in the Brain. Balázs, R., Cremer, J.E. (eds.). London: Macmillan 1973, pp. 167–186

Balázs, R., Lewis, P.D., Patel, A.J.: Effects of metabolic factors on brain development. In: Growth and Development of the Brain. Brazier, M.A.B. (ed.). New York: Raven 1975, pp. 83–115

Balázs, R., Patel, A.J., Lewis, P.D.: Metabolic influences on cell proliferation in the brain. In: Biochemical Correlates of Brain Structure and Function. Davison, A.N. (ed.). New York: Academic Press 1977, pp. 43–83

Banks, P.: ATP hydrolase activity associated with microtubules reassembled from bovine splenic nerve – a cautionary tale. J. Neurochem. **27**, 1465–1471 (1976)

Barondes, S.H.: Neuronal recognition. New York: Plenum 1975

Barondes, S.H., Dutton, G.R.: Protein metabolism in the nervous system. In: Basic Neurochemistry. Albers, R.W., Siegel, G.J., Katzman, R., Agranoff, B.W. (eds.). Boston: Little and Brown 1972, pp. 229–244

Bartlett, S.F., Lagercrantz, H., Smith, A.D.: Gel electrophoresis of soluble and insoluble proteins of noradrenergic vesicles from ox splenic nerve. Neuroscience **1**, 339–344 (1976)

Bennett, E.L., Diamond, M.C., Krech, D., Rosenzweig, M.R.: Chemical and anatomical plasticity of brain. Science **146**, 610–619 (1964)

Berl, S.: Glutamate compartmentation in developing cat brain. In: Metabolic Compartmentation in the Brain. Baláźs, R., Cremer, J.E. (eds.). London: Macmillan 1973, pp. 73–79

Berl, S., Puszkin, S., Nicklas, W.: Actomyosin-like protein in brain. Science **179**, 441–446 (1973)

Besser, G.M.: Hypothalamus as an endocrine organ. Br. Med. J. **3**, 613–615 (1974)

Bharucha, A.D., Elliott, K.A.C.: Effects of electrically induced convulsions and transmitter substances on RNA turnover in brain slices. Exp. Brain Res. **19**, 119–123 (1974)

Bird, E.D., Iversen, L.L.: Huntington's chorea. Post-mortem measurements of glutamic acid decarboxylase, choline acetyltransferase and dopamine in basal ganglia. Brain **97**, 457–472 (1974)

Bloom, F.E.: Central noradrenergic synaptic mechanisms. In: The Nervous System. Tower, D.B. (ed.). Vol. 1: The Basic Neurosciences. Brady, R.O. (ed.). New York: Raven 1975, pp. 373–380

Bock, E., Hamberger, A.: Immunoelectrophoretic determination of brain-specific antigens in bulk-prepared neuronal and glial cells. Brain Res. **112**, 329–335 (1976)

Bonkowski, L., Dryden, W.F.: The effects of putative neurotransmitters on the resting membrane potential of dissociated brain neurones in culture. Brain Res. **107**, 69–84 (1976)

Bradley, P.B.: Synaptic transmission in the central nervous system and its relevance for drug action. Int. Rev. Neurobiol. **11**, 1–56 (1968)

Bray, D.: Surface movements during the growth of single explanted neurons. Proc. Natl. Acad. Sci. USA **65**, 905–910 (1970)

Brostoff, S.W., Karkhanis, Y.D., Carlo, D.J., Reuter, W., Eylar, E.H.: Isolation and partial characterization of the major proteins of rabbit sciatic nerve myelin. Brain Res. **86**, 449–458 (1975)

Brunngraber, E.G.: Glycoproteins. In: Handbook of Neurochemistry. Lajtha, A. (ed.). New York: Plenum 1969, Vol. 1, pp. 223–244

Bunge, R.P.: Changing uses of nerve tissue culture 1950–1975. In: The Nervous System. Tower, D.B. (ed.). Vol. 1: The Basic Neurosciences. Brady, R.O. (ed.). New York: Raven 1975, pp. 31–42

Burnstock, G.: Do some nerve cells release more than one transmitter? Neuroscience **1**, 239–248 (1976)

Burt, D.R., Larrabee, M.G.: Phosphatidylinositol and other lipids in a mammalian sympathetic ganglion: effects of neuronal activity on incorporation of labelled inositol, phosphate, glycerol and acetate. J. Neurochem. **27**, 753–763 (1976)

Carlsson, A.: The impact of pharmacology on the problem of schizophrenia. In: Schizophrenia Today. Kemali, D., Bartholini, G., Richter, D. (eds.). Oxford: Pergamon 1976, pp. 89–103

Chang, M.M., Leeman, S.E., Niall, H.D.: Amino acid sequence of substance P. Nature New Biol. **232**, 86–87 (1971)

Changeux, J.-P., Kasai, M., Lee, C.Y.: Use of a snake venom toxin to characterize the cholinergic receptor protein. Proc. Natl. Acad. Sci. USA **67**, 1241–1247 (1970)

Clouet, D.H., Richter, D.: Incorporation of [^{35}S]-labelled methionine into the proteins of the rat brain. J. Neurochem. **3**, 219–229 (1958)

Coceani, F.: Prostaglandin system in developing and mature central nervous tissue. In: Brain Dysfunction in Infantile Febrile Convulsions. IBRO Monograph Series 2. Brazier, M.A.B., Coceani, F. (eds.). New York: Raven 1976, pp. 55–67

Cohn, P., Gaitonde, M.K., Richter, D.: The localization of protein formation in the rat brain. J. Physiol. **126**, 7 (1954)

Cotman, C.W.: Isolation of synaptosomal and synaptic plasma membrane fractions. In: Methods in Enzymology. Fleischer, L., Packer, L. (eds.). New York: Academic Press 1974, Vol. 31A, pp. 445–452

Coyle, J.T., Snyder, S.H.: Catecholamine uptake by synaptosomes in homogenates of rat brain: stereospecificity in different areas. J. Pharmacol. Exp. Ther. **170**, 221–231 (1969)

Curtis, D.R., Johnston, G.A.R.: Amino acid transmitters in the mammalian central nervous system. Rev. Physiol. **69**, 97–188 (1974)

Curtis, D.R., Watkins, J.C.: The excitation and depression of spinal neurones by structurally related amino acids. J. Neurochem. **6**, 117–141 (1960)

Curtis, D.R., Game, C.J.A., Lodge, D.: The in vivo inactivation of GABA and other inhibitory amino acids in the cat nervous system. Exp. Brain Res. **25**, 413–428 (1976)

Dahlström, A., Fuxe, K.: Evidence for the existence of monoamine neurons in the CNS. Acta Physiol. Scand. **62** [Suppl. 232], 1–55 (1965)

Daniel, P.M., Love, E.R., Moorhouse, S.R., Pratt, O.E.: The influence of age on the influx of ketone bodies into the brain of the rat. J. Physiol. (Lond.) **268**, 15–16 (1977)

David, G.B.: Cytoplasmic networks in neurons. In: Comparative Neurochemistry. Richter, D. (ed.). Oxford: Pergamon 1964, pp. 59–100

Davis, J.N., Lefkowitz, R.J.: β-Adrenergic receptor binding: synaptic localization in rat brain. Brain Res. **113**, 214–218 (1976)

Davison, A.N.: Lipid metabolism of nervous tissue. In: Applied Neurochemistry. Davison, A.N., Dobbing, J. (eds.). Oxford: Blackwell 1968, pp. 263–269

Dawson, R.M.C.: The metabolism of animal phospholipids and their turnover in cell membranes. In: Essays in Biochemistry. Campbell, P.N., Greville, G.D. (eds.). New York: Academic Press 1966, Vol. 2, pp. 66–78

Dawson, R.M.C., Richter, D.: The phosphorus metabolism of the brain. Proc. R. Soc. Lond. [Biol.] **137**, 252–267 (1950)

De Potter, W.P., De Schaepdryver, H., Moerman, E., Smith, A.D.: Evidence for the release of vesicle proteins together with noradrenaline upon stimulation of the splanchnic nerves. J. Physiol. (Lond.) **204**, 102–104 (1969)

De Robertis, E., Fiszer De Plazas, S.: Isolation of hydrophobic proteins binding amino acids. J. Neurochem. **26**, 1237–1243 (1976)

Droz, B.: Synthetic machinery and axoplasmic transport. Tower, D.B. (ed.). In: The Nervous System. Vol. 1: The Basic Neurosciences. Brady, R.O. (ed.). New York: Raven 1975, pp. 111–127

Dubcovich, M.L., Langer, S.Z.: Evidence against a physiological role of prostaglandins in the regulation of noradrenaline release in the cat spleen. J. Physiol. (Lond.) **251**, 737–762 (1975)

Du Vignaud, V.: Hormones of the posterior pituitary gland: oxytocin and vasopressin. In: The Harvey Lectures 1954–55. New York: Academic Press 1956, pp. 1–26

Eberhardt, N.L., Valeana, T., Timiras, P.S.: Hormone receptor interactions in brain: uptake and binding of thyroid hormone. Psychoneuroendocrinology **1**, 399–409 (1976)

Edström, A., Mattsson, H.: Fast axonal transport in vitro in the sciatic system of the frog. J. Neurochem. **19**, 205–221 (1972)

Eichberg, J., Hauser, G., Karnovsky, M.L.: Lipids of nervous tissue. In: The Structure and Function of Nervous Tissue. Bourne, G.H. (ed.). New York: Academic Press 1969, Vol. 3, pp. 185–287

Elde, R., Hökfelt, T., Johansson, O., Terenius, L.: Immunohistochemical studies using antibodies to leucine-enkephalin: initial observations on the nervous system of the rat. Neuroscience **1**, 349–351 (1976)

Elliott, K.A.C., Heller, I.H.: Metabolism of neurons and glia. In: Metabolism of the Nervous System. Richter, D. (ed.). Oxford: Pergamon 1957, pp. 286–290

Elliott, K.A.C., Page, I.K., Quastel, J.H.: Neurochemistry. Springfield: C.C. Thomas 1955 and 1962

Essman, W.B., Nakajima, S.: Current Biochemical Approaches to Learning and Memory. New York: Spectrum-Wiley 1973

Eylar, E.H.: The structure and immunologic properties of basic proteins of myelin. Ann. N.Y. Acad. Sci. **195**, 481–491 (1972)

Feldberg, W., Gupta, K.P.: Pyrogen fever and prostaglandin-like activity in cerebrospinal fluid. J. Physiol. (Lond.) **228**, 41–53 (1973)

Feldberg, W., Vogt, M.: Acetylcholine synthesis in different regions of the central nervous system. J. Physiol. (Lond.) **107**, 372–381 (1948)

Fewtrell, C.M.S.: The labelling and isolation of neuroreceptors. Neuroscience **1**, 249–273 (1976)

Flexner, L.B.: The development of the cerebral cortex. Harvey Lectures, Series 47. New York: Academic Press 1952, pp. 156–179

Flower, R.J., Vane, J.R.: Inhibition of prostaglandin synthetase in brain explains the antipyretic activity of paracetamol (4-acetamidophenol). Nature **240**, 410–411 (1972)

Folch-Pi, J.: Chemical Pathology of the Nervous System. Oxford: Pergamon 1961

Folch-Pi, J.: The history of research on proteolipids. In: The Nervous System. Tower, D.B. (ed.). Vol. 1: The Basic Neurosciences. Brady, R.O. (ed.). New York: Raven 1975, pp. 515–521

Folch-Pi, J., Stoffyn, P.: Proteolipids from membrane systems. Ann. NY Acad. Sci. **195**, 86–107 (1972)

Folch-Pi, J., Lees, M., Sloane-Stanley, G.H.: A simple method for the isolation and purification of total lipides from animal tissues. J. Biol. Chem. **226**, 497–509 (1957)
Frantz, A.G., Zimmerman, E.A.: Clinical Neuroendocrinology. In: The Nervous System. Tower, D.B. (ed.). Vol. 2: The Clinical Neurosciences. Chase, T.N. (ed.). New York: Raven 1975, pp. 183–191
Fuxe, K., Everitt, B.J., Agnati, L., Fredholm, B., Jonsson, G.: On the biochemistry and pharmacology of hallucinogens. In: Schizophrenia Today. Kemali, D., Bartholini, G., Richter, D. (eds.). Oxford: Pergamon 1976, pp. 135–157
Gaitonde, M.K.: Lipoproteins of brain. J. Neurochem. **8**, 234–242 (1961)
Gaitonde, M.K., Richter, D.: The metabolic activity of the proteins of the brain. Proc. R. Soc. Lond. [Biol.] **145**, 83–99 (1956)
Gaitonde, M.K., Richter, D.: Changes with age in the utilization of glucose carbon in liver and brain. J. Neurochem. **13**, 1309–1316 (1966)
Gambetti, P., Autilio-Gambetti, L.A., Gonatas, N.K., Shafer, B.: Protein synthesis in synaptosomal fractions. Ultrastructural radioautographic study. J. Cell. Biol. **52**, 526–535 (1972)
Garrod, A.E.: Inborn Errors of Metabolism. 2nd ed. London: Hodder and Stoughton 1923
Geiger, A.: Correlation of brain metabolism and function by use of a brain perfusion method in situ. Physiol. Rev. **38**, 1–20 (1958)
Gjessing, R.: Biological investigations in endogenous psychoses. Acta Psychiatr. Neurol. Scand. [Suppl.] **47**, 93–104 (1947)
Goodall, McC.: Metabolic products of adrealine and noradrenaline in urine. Pharmacol. Rev. **11**, 416–425 (1959)
Gray, E.G.: Presynaptic microtubules and their association with synaptic vesicles. Proc. R. Soc. Lond. [Biol.] **190**, 369–372 (1975)
Greenfield, S.A., Smith, A.D.: Changes in acetylcholinesterase concentration in rabbit cerebrospinal fluid following central electrical stimulation. J. Physiol. (Lond.) **258**, 108P–109P (1976)
Greengard, P.: Cyclic nucleotides, protein phosphorylation and neuronal function. In: Advances in Cyclic Nucleotide Research. Drummond, G.I., Greengard, P., Robison, G.A. (eds.). New York: Raven 1975, Vol. 5, pp. 585–601
Gross, G.W.: The microstream concept of axoplasmic and dendritic transport. In: Advances in Neurology. Vol. 12: Physiology and Pathology of Dendrites. Kreutzberg, G.W. (ed.). New York: Raven 1975, pp. 283–296
Guidotti, A., Cheyney, D.L., Trabucci, M., Doteuchi, M., Wang, C., Hawkins, R.A.: Focussed microwave radiation: a technique to minimize post mortem changes of cyclic nucleotides, DOPA and choline and to preserve brain morphology. Neuropharmacology **13**, 1115–1122 (1974)
Guillemin, R.: Physiological and clinical significance of hypothalamic and extra hypothalamic brain peptides. Triangle **15**, 1–7 (1976)
Guroff, G.: Some aspects of aromatic amino acid metabolism in the brain. In: The Nervous System. Tower, D.B. (ed.). Vol. 1: The Basic Neurosciences. Brady, R.O. (ed.). New York: Raven 1975, pp. 553–564
Hansson, H.-A., Hydén, H., Rönnbäck, L.: Localization of S-100 protein in isolated nerve cells by immunoelectron microscopy. Brain Res. **93**, 349–352 (1975)
Harvey, C.A., Milton, A.S.: Endogenous pyrogen fever, prostaglandin release and prostaglandin synthetase inhibitors. J. Physiol. **250**, 18–20 (1975)
Henry, J.L.: Substance P excitation of spinal nociceptive neurones. Neuroscience Abs. **1**, 390–391 (1975)
Hernandez, A.G.: Protein synthesis by synaptosomes from rat brain. Contribution by the intraterminal mitochondria. Biochem. J. **142**, 7–17 (1974)
Hess, H.H., Bass, N.H., Thalheimer, C., Devarakonda, R.: Gangliosides and the architecture of human frontal and rat somatosensory isocortex. J. Neurochem. **26**, 1115–1121 (1976)
Himwich, H.E.: Brain Metabolism and Cerebral Disorders. Baltimore: Williams and Wilkins 1951
Hökfelt, T., Elde, R., Johansson, O., Luft, R., Nilsson, G., Arimura, A.: Immunohistochemical evidence for separate populations of somatostatin-containing and substance P-containing primary afferent neurons in the rat. Neuroscience **1**, 131–136 (1976)
Hughes, J., Smith, T.W., Kosterlitz, H.W., Fothergill, L.A., Morgan, B.A., Morris, H.R.: Identification of two related pentapeptides from the brain with potent opiate agonist activity. Nature **258**, 577–579 (1975)

Huxtable, R.J., Barbeau, A.: Taurine. New York: Raven 1976
Hydén, H., Lange, P.: Differences in the metabolism of oligodendroglia and nerve cells in the vestibular area. In: Regional Neurochemistry. Kety, S.S., Elkes, J. (eds.). Oxford: Pergamon 1961, pp. 190–199
Ingvar, D.H., Lassen, N.A.: Regional cerebral blood flow. Acta Neurol. Scand. **41** [Suppl. 14], 1–250 (1965)
Ingvar, D.H., Lassen, N.A.: The Working Brain. The Coupling of Function, Metabolism and Blood Flow in the Brain. Copenhagen: Munksgaard 1975
Iversen, L.L.: Monoamines in the central nervous system and the actions of antidepressant drugs. In: Biochemistry and Mental Illness. Iversen, L.L., Rose, S.P.R. (eds.). London: Biochemical Society 1973 pp. 81–96
Iversen, L.L., Bloom, F.E.: Studies of the uptake of [^{3}H] GABA and [^{3}H] glycine in slices and homogenates of rat brain and spinal cord by electron microscopic autoradiography. Brain Res. **41**, 131–143 (1972)
Iversen, L.L., Iversen, S.D., Snyder, S.H.: Synaptic Modulators. In: Handbook of Psychopharmacology. New York: Plenum 1975, Vol. 5, p. 58
Jacquet, Y.F., Lajtha, A.: The periaqueductal gray: site of morphine analgesia and tolerance as shown by 2-way cross tolerance between systemic and intracerebral injections. Brain Res. **103**, 501–513 (1976)
Jasper, H.H., Koyama, I.: Rate of release of amino acids from the cerebral cortex in the cat as affected by brain-stem and thalamic stimulation. Can. J. Physiol. **47**, 889–905 (1969)
Joseph, M.H., Owen, F., Baker, H.F., Bourne, R.C.: Platelet serotonin concentration and monoamine oxidase activity in unmedicated chronic schizophrenic and in schizoaffective patients. Psychol. Med. **7**, 159–1962 (1976)
Kanazawa, I., Jessell, T.: Post mortem changes and regional distribution of substance-P in the rat and mouse nervous system. Brain Res. **17**, 362–367 (1976)
Karlin, A., Cowburn, D.A.: Molecular properties of membrane-bound and of solubilized and purified acetylcholine receptor identified by affinity labelling. In: Neurochemistry of Cholinergic Receptors. De Robertis, E., Schacht, J. (eds.). New York: Raven 1974, pp. 37–48
Katzman, R.: Cerebrospinal fluid physiology. In: The Nervous System. Tower, D.B. (ed.). Vol. 1: The Basic Neurosciences. Brady, R.O. (ed.). New York: Raven 1975, pp. 291–297
Kawakita, H.: Immunochemical studies on the brain specific protein. J. Neurochem. **19**, 87–94 (1972)
Kebabian, J.W., Clement-Cormier, Y.C., Petzold, G.L., Greengard, P.: Chemistry of dopamine receptors. In: Dopaminergic Mechanisms Calne, D., Chase, T.N., Barbeau, A. (eds.). New York: Raven 1975, pp. 1–11
Kennedy, C., Sokoloff, L.: An adaptation of the nitrous oxide method to the study of the cerebral circulation in children; normal values for cerebral blood flow and cerebral metabolic rate in childhood. J. Clin. Invest. **36**, 1130–1137 (1957)
Kety, S.S.: The theory and applications of the exchange of inert gas at the lungs and tissues. Pharmacol. Rev. **3**, 1–41 (1951)
Kety, S.S.: The general metabolism of the brain in vivo. In: Metabolism of the Nervous System. Richter, D. (ed.). Oxford: Pergamon 1957, pp. 221–237
Kety, S.S., Elkes, J.: Regional Neurochemistry. Oxford: Pergamon 1961
Kety, S.S., Schmidt, C.F.: The nitrous oxide method for blood flow in man: theory, procedure and normal values. J. Clin. Invest. **27**, 476–483 (1949)
Kirkpatrick, J.B., Hyams, L., Thomas, V.L., Howley, P.H.: Purification of intact microtubules from brain. J. Cell. Biol. **47**, 384–394 (1970)
Koelle, G.B.: Evidence for differences in primary functions of acetylcholinesterase at different synapses and neuroeffector junctions. In: Regional Neurochemistry. Kety, S.S., Elkes, J. (eds.). Oxford: Pergamon 1961, pp. 312–323
Koelle, G.B.: Microanatomy and pharmacology of cholinergic synapses. In: The Nervous System. Tower, D.B. (ed.). Vol. 1: The Basic Neurosciences. Brady, R.O. (ed.). New York: Raven 1975, pp. 363–371
Korobkin, R.K., Cutler, R.W.P.: Maturational changes of amino acid concentration in cerebrospinal fluid of the rat. Brain Res. **119**, 181–187 (1977)
Kosterlitz, H.W., Hughes, J.: Peptides with morphine-like action in the brain. Br. J. Psychiatr. **130**, 289–304 (1977)

Kristensson, K.: Retrograde axonal transport of protein tracers. In: The Use of Axonal Transport for Studies of Neuronal Connectivity. Cowan, W.M., Cuénod, M. (eds.). Amsterdam: Elsevier 1975, pp. 69–82

Krnjević, K.: Chemical nature of synaptic transmission in vertebrates. Physiol. Rev. **54**, 418–540 (1974)

Krnjević, K.: Electrophysiology of dopamine receptors. In: Dopaminergic Mechanisms. Calne, D., Chase, T.N., Barbeau, A. (eds.). New York: Raven 1975, pp. 13–24

Lagercrantz, H.: On the composition and function of large dense-cored vesicles in sympathetic nerves. Neuroscience **1**, 81–92 (1976)

Lajtha, A. (ed.): Handbook of Neurochemistry. Vol. 2: Structural Neurochemistry. New York: Plenum 1969

Lajtha, A. (ed.): Handbook of Neurochemistry. Vol. 3: Metabolic Reactions in the Nervous System. New York: Plenum 1970

Lajtha, A., Shershen, H.: Changes in the rates of protein synthesis in the brain of goldfish at various temperatures. Life Sci. **17**, 1861–1868 (1976)

Lajtha, A., Furst, S., Gerstein, A., Waelsch, H.: Amino acid and protein metabolism of the brain – I. J. Neurochem. **1**, 289–300 (1957)

Lajtha, A., Latzkovits, L., Toth, J.: Comparison of turnover rates of proteins of the brain, liver and kidney in mouse in vivo following long term labelling. Biochim. Biophys. Acta **425**, 511–520 (1976)

Lasher, R.S.: The uptake of ^{3}H-GABA and differentiation of stellate neurons in cultures of dissociated postnatal rat cerebellum. Brain Res. **69**, 235–254 (1974)

Levi, G., Raiteri, M.: Detectability of high and low affinity uptake systems for GABA and glutamate in rat brain slices and synaptosomes. Life Sci. **12**, 81–88 (1973)

Levi-Montalcini, R., Angeletti, P.U.: Nerve growth factor. Physiol. Rev. **48**, 534–569 (1971)

Levine, L.: Immunochemical approaches to the study of the nervous system. In: The Neurosciences. Quarton, G.C., Meinechuk, T., Schmitt, F.O. (eds.). New York: Rockefeller University Press 1967, pp. 220–230

Linton, E.A. Perkins, M.N., Whitehead, S.A.: Catecholamines and prostaglandins in the central control of ovulation. J. Physiol. (Lond.) **266**, 61–62 (1977)

Løvtrup-Rein, H., McEwen, B.S.: Isolation and fractionation of rat brain nuclei. J. Cell. Biol. **30**, 405–415 (1966)

Lowry, O.H.: Quantitative histochemistry. In: The Nervous System. Tower, D.B. (ed.). Vol. 1: The Basic Neurosciences. Brady, R.O. (ed.). New York: Raven 1975, pp. 523–533

Lumsden, C.E., Pomerat, C.M.: Normal oligodendrocytes in tissue culture. Exp. Cell. Res. **2**, 103–114 (1951)

Lunt, G.G., Canessa, O.M., De Robertis, E.: Association of the acetylcholine-phosphatidyl inositol effect with a 'receptor' proteolipid from cerebral cortex. Nature New Biol. **230**, 187–190 (1971)

Mandel, P., Dravid, A.R., Pete, N.: Poly C synthetase activity in the particulate fraction of rat brain nuclei. J. Neurochem. **14**, 301–306 (1967)

Margolis, R.K., Preti, C., Lai, D., Margolis, R.U.: Developmental changes in rat glycoproteins. Brain Res. **112**, 363–370 (1976)

Marks, N., Stern, F.: Novel enzymes involved in the inactivation of hypothalamo-hypophyseal hormones. In: Psychoneuroendocrinology. Workshop Conference, Mieken 1973. Basel: Karger 1974a, pp. 276–284

Marks, N., Stern, F.: Enzymatic mechanisms for the inactivation of luteinizing hormone-releasing hormone (LH-RH). Biochem. Biophys. Res. Commun. **61**, 1458–1463 (1974b)

Marks, N., Grynbaum, A., Benuck, M.: On the sequential cleavage of myelin basic protein by cathepsins A and D. J. Neurochem. **27**, 765–768 (1976)

Matus, A., Mughal, S.M.: Against synaptosomal localization of S-100 protein. Nature **258**, 746–748 (1975)

McBride, W.J., Van Tassel, J.: Resolution of proteins from subfractions of nerve endings. Brain Res. **44**, 177–187 (1972)

McCarthy, P.S., Walker, R.J., Woodruff, G.N.: Depressant actions of encephalins on neurones in the nucleus accumbens. J. Physiol. **267**, 40–41 (1977)

McEwen, B.S., De Kloet, R., Wallach, G.: Interactions in vivo and in vitro of corticoids and progesterone with cell nuclei and soluble macromolecules from rat brain regions and pituitary. Brain Res. **105**, 129–136 (1976)

McIlwain, H.: Translocation of neural modulators. A second category of nerve signal. Neurochem. Res. **1**, 351–368 (1976)
McIlwain, H., Bachelard, H.S.: Biochemistry and the Central Nervous System. London: Churchill 1971
Miani, N., Caniglia, A., Panetta, V.: A Brain-specific protein with affinity for DNA. J. Neurochem. **27**, 145–150 (1976)
Milton, A.S., Wendlandt, S.: Effects on body temperature of prostaglandins of the A, E, and F series on injection into the third ventricle of unanaesthetized cats and rabbits. J. Physiol. (Lond.) **218**, 325–336 (1971)
Minard, F.N., Richter, D.: Electroshock-induced seizures and the turnover of brain protein in the rat. J. Neurochem. **15**, 1463–1468 (1968)
Moore, B.W.: Chemistry and biology of two proteins, S-100 and 14-3-2, specific to the nervous system. Int. Rev. Neurobiol. **15**, 215–225 (1972)
Moore, B.W.: Membrane proteins in the nervous system. In: The Nervous System. Tower, D.B. (ed.). Vol. 1: The Basic Neurosciences. Brady, R.O. (ed.). New York: Raven 1975, pp. 503–514
Moore, B.W., McGregor, D.: Chromatographic and electrophoretic fractionation of soluble proteins of brain and liver. J. Biol. Chem. **240**, 1647–1653 (1965)
Morgan, I.G.: Synaptosomes and cell separation. Neuroscience **1**, 159–165 (1976)
Morell, P.: Myelin. New York: Plenum 1976
Muller, H.J.: Our load of mutations. Am. J. Hum. Genet. **2**, 111–176 (1950)
Murray, M.R.: Nervous tissue in vitro. In: Cells and Tissues in Culture. Willmer, F.M. (ed.). New York: Academic Press 1965, Vol. 2, pp. 373–455
Musick, J., Hubbard, J.I.: Release of protein from mouse motor nerve terminals. Nature **237**, 279–281 (1972)
Nelson, J.F., Holinka, C.F., Latham, K.R., Allen, J.K., Finch, C.E.: Corticosterone binding in cytosols from brain regions of mature and senescent male C57 Bl I 6J mice. Brain Res. **115**, 345–351 (1976)
Nelson, P., Peacock, J.: Electrical activity in dissociated cell cultures from fetal mouse cerebellum. Brain Res. **61**, 163–174 (1973)
Norton, W.T.: Myelin: structure and biochemistry. In: The Nervous System. Tower, D.B. (ed.). Vol. 1: The Basic Neurosciences. Brady, R.O. (ed.). New York: Raven 1975, pp. 467–481
Norton, W.T., Poduslo, S.E.: Neuronal soma and whole neuroglia of rat brain: a new isolation technique. Science **167**, 1144–1146 (1970)
Norton, W.T., Poduslo, S.E.: Myelination in rat brain. Changes in myelin composition during brain maturation. J. Neurochem. **21**, 759–773 (1973)
Ochoa, E.L.M., Bangham, A.D.: N-Acetylneuraminic acid molecules as possible serotonin binding sites. J. Neurochem. **26**, 1193–1198 (1976)
Ochs, S.: Axoplasmic transport. In: The Nervous System. Tower, D.B. (ed.). Vol. 1: The Basic Neurosciences. Brady, R.O. (ed.). New York: Raven 1975, pp. 137–146
Oesch, F., Otten, U., Thoenen, H.: Relationship between the rate of axoplasmic transport and subcellular distribution of enzymes involved in the synthesis of norepinephrine. J. Neurochem. **20**, 1691–1706 (1973)
Okun, L.M.: Isolated dorsal root ganglion neurons in culture. J. Neurobiol. **3**, 111–151 (1972)
Oldendorf, W.H.: Permeability of the blood-brain barrier. In: The Nervous System. Tower, D.B. (ed.). Vol. 1: The Basic Neurosciences. Brady, R.O. (ed.). New York: Raven 1975, pp. 279–289
Page, I.H.: Chemistry of the Brain. Springfield: C.C. Thomas 1937
Page, M.A., Krebs, H.A., Williamson, D.H.: Activities of enzymes of ketone body utilization in brain and other tissues of suckling rats. Biochem. J. **121**, 49–53 (1971)
Palacios, J.M., Mengod, G., Picatoste, F., Grau, M., Blanco, I.: Properties of rat brain histidine decarboxylase. J. Neurochem. **27**, 1455–1460 (1976)
Pardee, J.D., Bamburg, J.R.: Quantitation of Actin in developing brain. J. Neurochem. **26**, 1093–1098 (1976)
Pardridge, W.M., Oldendorf, W.H.: Transport of metabolic substrates through the blood-brain barrier. J. Neurochem. **28**, 5–12 (1977)
Patel, A.J., Balázs, R.: Factors affecting the development of metabolic compartmentation in the brain. In: Metabolic Compartmentation and Neurotransmission. Relation to Brain Structure and Function. Berl, S., Clark, D.D., Schneider, S. (eds.). New York: Plenum 1975, pp. 363–383

Patel, M.S., Owen, O.E.: Development and regulation of lipid synthesis from ketone bodies by rat brain. J. Neurochem. **28**, 109–114 (1977)
Patel, A.J., Johnson, A.L., Balázs, R.: Metabolic compartmentation of glutamate in GABA formation. J. Neurochem. **23**, 1271–1279 (1974)
Pert, C.B., Kuhar, M.J., Snyder, S.H.: Autoradiographic localization of the opiate receptor in rat brain. Life Sci. **16**, 1849–1854 (1975)
Pickel, V.M., Reis, D.J., Marangos, P.J., Zomely-Neurath, C.: Immunocytochemical localization of nervous system specific protein (NSP-R) in rat brain. Brain Res. **105**, 184–187 (1976)
Preston, E., Schönbaum, E.: Monoaminergic mechanisms in thermo-regulation. In: Brain Dysfunction in Infantile Febrile Convulsions. Brazier, M.A.B., Coceani, F. (eds.). New York: Raven 1976, pp. 75–87
Quarles, R.H.: Glycoproteins in the nervous system. In: The Nervous System. Tower, D.B. (ed.). Vol. 1: The Basic Neurosciences. Brady, R.O. (ed.). New York: Raven 1975, pp. 493–501
Quastel, J.H.: Metabolic activities of tissue preparations. In: Metabolism of the Nervous System. Richter, D. (ed.). Oxford: Pergamon 1957, pp. 267–285
Raichle, M.E., Posner, J.B., Plum, F.: Cerebral blood flow during and after hyperventilation. In: Brain and Blood Flow. Russell, R.W.R. (ed.). London: Pitman 1971, pp. 223–228
Rapoport, S.I.: Blood-Brain Barrier in Physiology and Medicine. New York: Raven 1976
Rassin, D.K.: Amino acids as putative transmitters: failure to bind to synaptic vesicles of guinea pig cerebral cortex. J. Neurochem. **19**, 139–148 (1972)
Richter, D.: Brain metabolism and cerebral function. Biochem. Soc. Symp. **8**, 62–76 (1952)
Richter, D.: Metabolism of the developing brain. In: Biochemistry of the Developing Nervous System. Waelsch, H. (ed.). New York: Academic Press 1955, pp. 225–250
Richter, D.: Metabolism of the Nervous System. Oxford: Pergamon 1957
Richter, D.: Comparative Neurochemistry. Oxford: Pergamon 1964
Richter, D.: Aspects of Learning and Memory. London: Heineman Medical Books 1966
Richter, D.: Biochemical aspects of mental retardation. Proceedings of IV World Congress of Psychiatry, Madrid 1966
Richter, D., Dawson, R.M.C.: Brain metabolism in emotional excitement and in sleep. Am. J. Physiol. **154**, 73–79 (1948)
Richter, D., Gaitonde, M.K., Cohn, P.: The localization of protein metabolism in the brain. In: Structure and function of the Cerebral Cortex. Tower, D.B., Schadé, J.P. (eds.). Amsterdam: Elsevier 1960, pp. 340–348
Roberts, E., Hammerschlag, R.: Amino acid transmitters. In: Basic Neurochemistry. Albers, R.W., Siegel, G.J., Katzman, R., Agranoff, B.W. (eds.). Boston: Little and Brown 1972, pp. 131–165
Roberts, P.J.: Glutamate receptors in the rat CNS. Nature **252**, 399–401 (1974)
Robison, G.A., Butcher, R.W., Sutherland, E.W.: Cyclic AMP. New York: Academic Press 1971
Roitbak, A.I., Bobrov, A.V.: Spreading depression resulting from cortical punctures. Acta Neurobiol. Exp. **35**, 761–768 (1975)
Rose, S.P.R.: Neurons and glia: separation techniques and biochemical inter-relationships. In: Handbook of Neurochemistry. Lajtha, A. (ed.). New York: Plenum 1969, Vol. 2, pp. 183–193
Rossiter, R.J.: Chemical constituents of brain and nerve. In: Neurochemistry. Elliott, K.A.C., Page, I.H., Quastel, J.H. (eds.). Springfield: C.C. Thomas 1962, pp. 10–54
Ruf, K.B., Kitchen, J.H., Wilkinson, H.: Synergistic effects of oestrogen and brain stimulation on precocious sexual maturation in the female rat. Acta Endocrinol. **82**, 225–237 (1976)
Sabri, M.T., Bone, A.H., Davison, A.N.: Turnover of myelin and other structural proteins in the developing rat brain. Biochem. J. **142**, 499–507 (1974)
Sachs, H.: Neurosecretion. In: Handbook of Neurochemistry. Lajtha, A. (ed.). New York: Plenum 1970, Vol. 4, pp. 373–428
Samuelsson, B.: Identification of a smooth muscle-stimulating factor in bovine brain. Prostaglandins and related factors. Biochim. Biophys. Acta **84**, 218–219 (1964)
Sara, V.R., King, T.L., Stuart, M.C., Lazarus, L.: Hormonal regulation of fetal brain cell proliferation. Endocrinology **99**, 90–97 (1976)
Sattin, A., Rall, T.W., Zanella, J.: Regulation of cyclic adenosine $3':5'$-monophosphate levels in guinea pig cerebral cortex by interaction of alpha adrenergic and adenosine receptor activity. J. Pharmacol. Exp. Ther. **192**, 22–32 (1975)

Schmitt, F.O., Dev, P., Smith, B.H.: Electrotonic processing of information by brain cells. Science **193**, 114–120 (1976)

Schubert, P., Kreutzberg, G.W.: Parameters of dendritic transport. In: Physiology and Pathology of Dendrites. Kreutzberg, G.W. (ed.). Advances in Neurology **12**, New York: Raven 1974, pp. 255–268

Sharma, N.C., Talwar, G.P.: Isolation and characterization of an organ-specific ribonucleoprotein from goat brain. J. Neurochem. **20**, 1625–1634 (1973)

Sharma, N.C., Shastri, N., Iqbal, Z., Jaffery, N.F., Talwar, G.P.: Ontogenesis of some key cellular components in the developing brain in the course of functional maturation. In: Growth and Development of the Brain: Nutritional, Genetic and Environmental Factors. Brazier, N.A.B. (ed.). New York: Raven 1975, pp. 17–32

Shashoua, V.E.: Brain metabolism and the acquisition of new behaviour. I. Evidence for specific changes in the pattern of protein synthesis. Brain Res. **111**, 347–364 (1976)

Sidman, R.L.: Cell interaction in mammalian brain development. In: The Nervous System. Tower, D.B. (ed.). Vol. 1: The Basic Neurosciences. Brady, R.O. (ed.). New York: Raven 1975, pp. 601–610

Siegel, G.J., Eisenman, J.S.: Hypothalamic-pituitary regulation. In: Basic Neurochemistry. Albers, R.W., Siegel, G.J., Katzman, R., Agranoff, B.W. (eds.). Boston: Little and Brown 1972, pp. 341–363

Simantov, R., Goodman, R., Aposhian, D., Snyder, S.H.: Philogenetic distribution of a morphine-like peptide 'enkephalin'. Brain Res. **111**, 204–211 (1976)

Snyder, S.H.: Catecholamines and serotonin. In: Basic Neurochemistry. Albers, R.W., Siegel, G.J., Katzman, R., Agranoff, B.W. (eds.). Boston: Little and Brown 1972, pp. 89–104

Snyder, S.H.: Amino acid neurotransmitters. Biochemical pharmacology. In: The Nervous System. Tower, D.B. (ed.). Vol. 1: The Basic Neurosciences. Brady, R.O. (ed.). New York: Raven 1975, pp. 355–361

Snyder, S.H., Simantov, R.: The opiate receptor and opioid peptides. J. Neurochem. **28**, 13–20 (1977)

Sokoloff, L.: Circulation and energy metabolism of the brain. In: Basic Neurochemistry. Albers, R.W., Siegel, G.J., Katzman, R., Agranoff, B.W. (eds.). Boston: Little and Brown 1973, pp. 299–325

Spohn, M., Davison, A.N.: Separation of myelin fragments from the central nervous system. In: Research Methods in Neurochemistry. Marks, N., Rodnight, R. (eds.). New York: Plenum 1972. Vol. 1, pp. 33–43

Stadler, H., Lloyd, K.G., Gadea-Ciria, M., Bartholini, G.: Enhanced striatal acetylcholine release by chlorpromazine and its reversal by apomorphine. Brain Res. **55**, 476–480 (1973)

Stein, L., Wise, C.D.: Possible etiology of schizophrenia. Science **171**, 1032–1036 (1971)

Suzuki, K.: Chemistry and metabolism of brain lipids. In: Basic Neurochemistry. Albers, R.W., Siegel, G.J., Katzman, R., Agranoff, B.W. (eds.). Boston: Little and Brown 1972, pp. 207–227

Suzuki, K.: Sphingolipids of the nervous system. In: The Nervous System. Tower, D.B. (ed.). Vol. 1: The Basic Neurosciences. Brady, R.O. (ed.). New York: Raven 1975, pp. 483–491

Tamir, H., Klein, A., Rapport, M.M.: Serotonin binding protein: enhancement of binding by Fe^{2+} and inhibition of binding by drugs. J. Neurochem. **26**, 871–878 (1976)

Tangri, K.K., Misra, N., Bhargava, K.P.: Central cholinergic mechanisms of pyrexia. In: Brain Dysfunction in Infantile Febrile Convulsions. Brazier, M.A.B., Coceani, F. (eds.). IBRO Monograph Series 2. New York: Raven 1976, pp. 89–106

Thudichum, J.W.L.: A Treatise on the Chemical Constitution of the Brain. London: Ballière, Tindall and Cox 1884

Toews, A.D., Horrocks, L.A., King, J.S.: Simultaneous isolation of purified microsomal and myelin fractions from rat spinal cord. J. Neurochem. **27**, 25–31 (1976)

Tregear, G.W., Niall, H.D., Potts, J.T., Leeman, S.E., Chang, M.M.: Synthesis of substance P. Nature New Biol. **232**, 87–89 (1971)

Twomey, S.L., Raeburn, S., Baxter, C.F.: Biochemical and immunological characterization of alkaloid-binding proteins from immature rat brain. J. Neurochem. **27**, 161–164 (1976)

Ueda, T., Maeno, H., Greengard, P.: Regulation of endogenous phosphorylation of specific proteins in synaptic membrane fractions from rat brain by adenosine 3′:5′-monophosphate. J. Biol. Chem. **248**, 8295–8305 (1973)

Usdin, E., Snyder, S.H.: Frontiers in Catecholamine Research. Oxford: Pergamon 1973
Vale, W., Brazeau, W., Rivier, C., Brown, M., Boss, B., Rivier, J., Burgus, R., Ling, N., Guillemin, R.: Somatostatin. Rec. Prog. Horm. Res. **31**, 365–392 (1975)
Van Harreveld, A., Crowell, J., Malhotra, S.K.: A study of extracellular space in central nervous tissue by freeze-substitution. J. Cell. Biol. **25**, 117–137 (1965)
Varon, S.: Humoral and cellular influences on neuronal development. In: The Nervous System. Tower, D.B. (ed.). Vol. 1: The Basic Neurosciences. New York: Raven 1975, pp. 621–630
Veech, R.L., Hawkins, R.A.: Brain blowing: a technique for in vivo study of brain metabolism. In: Research Methods in Neurochemistry. Marks, N., Rodnight, R. (eds.). New York: Plenum 1974, Vol. 2, pp. 171–182
Vogt, M.: Sympathomimetic amines in the central nervous system. Br. Med. Bull. **13**, 166–171 (1957)
Waelsch, H.: Biochemistry of the Developing Nervous System. New York: Academic Press 1955
Warburg, O.: The Metabolism of Tumours. (Translated by F. Dickens.) London: Constable 1930
Weiss, P., Hiscoe, H.B.: Experiments on the mechanism of nerve growth. J. Exp. Zool. **107**, 315–395 (1948)
Wellington, B.S., Livett, B.G., Jeffrey, P.L., Austin, L.: Biochemical and immunochemical studies on chick brain neurostenin. Neuroscience **1**, 23–34 (1976)
Westley, B.R., Thomas, P.J., Salaman, D.F., Knight, A., Barley, J.: Properties and partial purification of an oestrogen receptor from neonatal rat brain. Brain Res. **113**, 411–447 (1976)
Whittaker, V.P., Dowdall, M.J.: Current state of research on cholinergic synapses. In: Cholinergic Mechanisms. Waser, P.G. (ed.). New York: Raven 1975, pp. 23–42
Whittaker, V.P., Michaelson, I.A., Kirkland, R.J.A.: The separation of synaptic vesicles from nerve-ending particles. Biochem. J. **90**, 293–303 (1964)
Winkler, H.: The composition of adrenal chromaffin granules: an assessment of controversial results. Neuroscience **1**, 65–80 (1976)
Wolfgram, F.: A new proteolipid fraction of the nervous system. J. Neurochem. **13**, 461–470 (1966)
Wood, J.G., Dawson, R.M.C.: A major myelin glycoprotein of sciatic nerve. J. Neurochem. **21**, 717–719 (1973)
Woodbury, J.W.: Biophysics of nerve membrane. In: Basic Mechanisms of the Epilepsies. Jasper, H.H., Ward, A.A., Pope, A. (eds.). London: Churchill 1970, pp. 41–82
Woods, H.F., Graham, C.W., Green, A.R., Youdin, M.B.H., Grahame-Smith, D.G., Hughes, J.T.: Some histological and metabolic properties of an isolated perfused rat brain preparation with special reference to monoamine metabolism. Neuroscience **1**, 313–323 (1976)
Yakovlev, P.I., Lecours, A.-R.: The myelogenetic cycles of regional maturation of the brain. In: Regional Development of the Brain in Early Life. Minkowski, A. (ed.). Oxford: Blackwell Scientific 1967, pp. 3–70
Yalow, R., Berson, S.: Immunoassay of endogenous plasma insulin in man. J. Clin. Invest. **39**, 1157–1175 (1960)
Young, A.B., Snyder, S.H.: Strychnine findings associated with glycine receptors of the CNS. Proc. Natl. Acad. Sci. USA **70**, 2832–2836 (1973); **71**, 4002–4005 (1974)
Zetterström, R.: The blood-brain barrier system. In: Die physiologische Entwicklung des Kindes. Linneweh, F. (ed.). Berlin-Heidelberg-New York: Springer Verlag 1959, pp. 73–79

Stoffwechselpathologie der Zyklothymie und Schizophrenie

Von

N. Matussek

Inhalt

A. Zyklothymie	66
I. Biochemische Ergebnisse	66
1. Noradrenalin- und Serotoninsystem	66
2. Weitere Transmittersysteme, die im Zusammenhang mit affektiven Störungen diskutiert werden	74
II. Neuroendokrinologische Ergebnisse	75
1. Hypothalamus-Hypophysen-Nebennierenrinden-System	76
2. Hypothalamus-Hypophysen-Wachstumshormon (=STH)-System	81
3. Rezeptor-Hypothese der endogenen Depression	86
B. Schizophrenie	90
I. Dopamin-Hypothese	91
II. Transmethylierungs-Hypothese	94
III. Weitere Schizophrenie-Hypothesen bzw. Faktoren, die im Zusammenhang mit der Schizophrenie diskutiert werden	95
C. Schlußbemerkungen	97
Literatur	98
Ergänzende Hinweise und Literatur	109

Abkürzungen

A	Adrenalin	5-HT	Serotonin
ACH	Acetylcholin	5-HTP	5-Hydroxytryptophan
ACTH	Adrenocorticotropes Hormon	HVS	Homovanillinsäure
ATP	Adenosintriphosphat	MAO	Monoaminoxydase
DA	Dopamin	MHPG	3-Methoxy-4-hydroxyphenylglykol
DMPEA	3′4′-Dimethoxy-phenyläthylamin	NA	Noradrenalin
DMT	Dimethyl-tryptamin	O.M.B.	5-Methoxy-N-N-dimethyl-tryptamin
ES	Elektroschock	VMS	Vanillinmandelsäure
GABA	γ-Aminobuttersäure	ZNS	Zentralnervensystem
5-HIES	5-Hydroxyindolessigsäure		

Unsere Kenntnisse über Aufbau, Stoffwechsel und Regulationsmechanismen des Nervensystems sind in den letzten Jahren wesentlich erweitert worden. Je tiefere Einblicke wir jedoch in die Vorgänge im ZNS erhalten, um so klarer sehen wir, daß unsere Hirnfunktionen wesentlich komplizierter gesteuert werden, als wir noch vor wenigen Jahren annahmen. Wir sehen immer deutlicher, wie lückenhaft und unvollständig unser Wissen selbst heute noch ist. Das Ziel der biologischen Psychiatrie, Psychosen auf spezifische Stoffwechseldefekte zurückzuführen, ist immer noch nicht erreicht. Dennoch wäre es verfehlt daraus zu schließen, den Psychosen lägen keine neurobiologischen Defekte zugrunde, obwohl man sich jetzt schon einige Jahrzehnte um ihre Aufdeckung bemüht. Eine Reihe interessanter Ergebnisse, die mit unterschiedlichen Methoden von verschiedenen Arbeitsgruppen erhoben wurden, weisen auf Störungen in bestimmten neuronalen Systemen hin. Diese Ansätze müssen intensiv verfolgt werden.

Ganz sicher wäre unser Wissen über Stoffwechselveränderungen bei Psychosen wesentlich umfangreicher, wenn es brauchbare Tiermodelle für Depression oder Schizophrenie gäbe. Zwar besitzen wir einige pharmakologische und verhaltensbiologische Tiermodelle, vor allem für die Depression, doch lassen sich die damit gewonnenen Erkenntnisse nur mit Vorsicht und in Teilaspekten auf die Psychosen beim Menschen übertragen. Die Modelle trugen jedoch wesentlich dazu bei, Psychose-Hypothesen aufzustellen, um am Menschen gezielte Untersuchungen durchzuführen. Später wird darauf noch genauer eingegangen. Im Vordergrund des folgenden Beitrags stehen klinisch-biochemische und neuroendokrinologische Ergebnisse, die in den letzten Jahren an psychotischen Patienten erhoben wurden. Einige neuroendokrinologische Untersuchungen, vor allem bei der Depression, werden in diesem Beitrag deswegen abgehandelt, da sie im Zusammenhang mit den bestehenden biochemischen Hypothesen neue Aspekte aufzeigen (ausführliche Darstellung der Endokrinologie s. Beitrag von M. BLEULER in diesem Band).

Bei der Fülle von Ergebnissen, die seit der letzten Auflage der „Psychiatrie der Gegenwart" (1964) erzielt wurden, ist es hier nicht möglich, auf alle in der Zwischenzeit durchgeführten Untersuchungen einzugehen. Ich werde deshalb nur mir bedeutsam erscheinende Schwerpunkte ausführlich erörtern, andere Ansätze kürzer besprechen und auf Zusammenfassungen zu den betreffenden Problemen mit weiterführender Literatur hinweisen. Dabei wird im ersten Teil die Zyklothymie, im zweiten die Schizophrenie behandelt.

A. Zyklothymie

I. Biochemische Ergebnisse

1. Noradrenalin- und Serotoninsystem

EVERETT und TOMAN (1959) wiesen aufgrund ihrer tierexperimentellen Untersuchungen bei der Umkehr der Reserpinwirkung als erste darauf hin, daß bei der Depression möglicherweise eine Störung im Katecholaminstoffwechsel eine entscheidende Rolle spielt. In der Mitte der sechziger Jahre formulierten dann weitere Autoren (BUNNEY u. DAVIS, 1965; SCHILDKRAUT, 1965; MATUSSEK, 1966) gleichzeitig und unabhängig voneinander die sog. Katecholamin-Hypothese der Depression. Von anderen Autoren wurde auf die Bedeutung des Serotonins bei der Depression hingewiesen (COPPEN, 1967; LAPIN u. OXENKRUG, 1969; VAN PRAAG, 1969). Beide Theorien beruhten anfänglich auf der Beobachtung, daß bei der Bluthochdruckbehandlung mit Reserpin bei einem Teil der Patienten depressive Zustände auftraten, die von einer echten endogenen Depression in ihrer Symptomatologie nicht zu unterscheiden waren. Besonders von den Arbeitsgruppen von B.B. BRODIE am National Institute of Health in Bethesda und von A. CARLSSON in Göteborg wurde tierexperimentell gezeigt, daß Reserpingaben zu einer Verarmung der biogenen Amine (Serotonin, Dopamin und Noradrenalin) in den Nervenendigungen führen. Diese Amine sind jedoch wichtige Übertragersubstanzen im ZNS, die für die Funktionsfähigkeit aminerger Neurone von entscheidender Bedeutung sind. Da das durch Reserpin und andere ähnlich wirkende Substanzen ausgelöste Verhalten wie Sedation, Temperaturabfall u.a.m. durch trizyklische Antidepressiva und MAO-Hemmer aufgehoben wird, nahm man bei der Depression einen Aminmangel an, der durch Antidepressiva auf verschiedenen Wegen – entweder durch Hemmung des Rücktransports in die Nervenzelle oder durch Inhibition des wichtigsten abbauenden Enzyms, der MAO – kompensiert wird (s. Beitrag von A. CARLSSON in diesem Band). Die klinisch-biochemische Forschung war also aufgerufen, diese Theorien zu beweisen. Im folgenden werden die verschiedenen Wege, die eingeschlagen wurden, dargestellt und kritisch diskutiert.

a) Autopsieuntersuchungen

Da Hirn-Biopsieuntersuchungen an depressiven Patienten nicht in Frage kommen, wurden von verschiedenen Arbeitsgruppen Hirn-Autopsieuntersuchungen an gestorbenen oder suizidierten depressiven Patienten und entsprechenden Kontrollen durchgeführt.

Die bisher erhaltenen Ergebnisse (Tabelle 1) sind nicht einheitlich. Abgesehen von BESKOW et al. (1976) und COCHRAN et al. (1976) finden die anderen Arbeitsgruppen in bestimmten Hirnregionen erniedrigte 5-HT- oder 5-HIES-Werte. Die 5-HIES soll post mortem jedoch labiler als die Amine sein, so daß für die 5-HIES die Zeitspanne zwischen Tod und Autopsie von besonderer Bedeutung ist. Bei Berücksichtigung des Zeitfaktors sind keine signifikanten Unterschiede zu beobachten (BESKOW et al., 1976). Im Gegensatz zu anderen Gruppen fanden BIRKMAYER und RIEDERER (1975) vor allem im Nucleus ruber erniedrigte NA-Konzentrationen. Aus der gleichen Wiener Arbeitsgruppe berichtete in einer Zusammenfassung RIEDERER (1977) auch von erniedrigten MHPG-Werten bei depressiven Patienten. In diesem Zusammenhang sollte ferner erwähnt werden, daß PERRY et al. (1977) in post mortem-Hirngeweben endogen depressiver Patienten eine signifikant geringere Glutaminsäuredecarboxylaseaktivität in manchen Hirnstrukturen fanden, d.h. daß auch GABA-erge Neurone möglicherweise betroffen sind.

Zweifellos wären eindeutige Autopsiebefunde bei depressiven Patienten eine wichtige Stütze der Amin-Hypothese der Depression. Da jedoch manche Patien-

Tabelle 1. Amine und 5-HIES-Bestimmungen in Gehirnen von Selbstmördern und verstorbenen Depressiven; in Anlehnung an GOODWIN und POST (1975), mit Hinzufügung weiterer Untersuchungen

Studien	Anzahl der Gehirne	Gehirnareale	Ergebnisse
SHAW et al. (1967)	28	unterer Hirnstamm	5-HT erniedrigt
BOURNE et al. (1968)	23	unterer Hirnstamm	5-HT normal 5-HIES erniedrigt NA normal
PARE et al. (1969)	26	unterer Hirnstamm	5-HT erniedrigt NA normal DA normal
LLOYD et al. (1974)	5	verschiedene Gehirnregionen einschließlich 6 Nuclei raphe	5-HT erniedrigt im Nucl. dorsalis, Cent. inferior d. Raphe
BIRKMAYER u. RIEDERER (1975)	3	verschiedene Gehirnregionen	5-HT erniedrigt 5-HIES erniedrigt NA erniedrigt
BESKOW et al. (1976)	23	verschiedene Gehirnregionen	5-HT normal 5-HIES normal
COCHRAN et al. (1976)	10	verschiedene Gehirnregionen	5-HT normal

ten, die in diese Untersuchungen einbezogen wurden, bis kurz vor ihrem Tod Medikamente, auch Antidepressiva, eingenommen hatten und außerdem die Todesursache bzw. die Art des Suizids unterschiedlich war, sind die bisher erhaltenen Ergebnisse mit aller Vorsicht zu interpretieren. Deshalb lassen sich daraus meiner Meinung nach keine endgültigen Schlüsse für oder gegen die Amin-Hypothese ableiten, worauf noch ausführlicher eingegangen wird.

b) Liquoruntersuchungen

Ein anderer Weg, Rückschlüsse auf den Stoffwechsel der Neurohormone im Hirn zu ziehen, sind Analysen der Aminmetaboliten im Liquor cerebrospinalis. Im Mittelpunkt des Interesses standen dabei 5-HIES, als Hauptmetabolit des 5-HT, und MHPG, als Hauptmetabolit des NA-Hirnstoffwechsels. In der Peripherie ist die VMS Hauptstoffwechselprodukt des NA.

Einerseits wurden Basiswerte der Aminmetaboliten im Liquor bestimmt. Andere Autoren, vor allem VAN PRAAG, glauben, daß sich Aminstoffwechselstörungen im Hirn bei der Liquoranalyse besser demonstrieren lassen, wenn der Abtransport der Metabolite vom Liquor ins Blut durch Probenecid gehemmt wird. Dazu müssen jedoch zwei Lumbalpunktionen in kurzem Zeitabstand durchgeführt werden, was zu einer starken Belastung der Patienten führt und Schwierigkeiten in der Durchführung der klinischen Versuche mit sich bringt.

Bei Basiswertuntersuchungen der 5-HIES im Liquor wurden bisher unterschiedliche Ergebnisse erzielt (Tabelle 2). Auch mit Probenecid sind die 5-HIES-

Tabelle 2. Basiswerte der 5-HIES-Konzentration im Liquor bei depressiven und manischen Patienten; in Anlehnung an GOODWIN und POST (1975)

Studien	Kontrollpersonen		Depressive		Maniker	
	N	Mittelwert ± Standardabweichung CSF 5-HIES (ng/ml)	N	Mittelwert ± Standardabweichung CSF 5-HIES (ng/ml)	N	Mittelwert ± Standardabweichung CSF 5-HIES (ng/ml)
ASHCROFT et al. (1966)	21	19,1 ± 4,4	24	11,1 ± 3,9	4	18,7 ± 5,4
DENCKER et al. (1966)	34	30 (gemittelt)	14	10 (gemittelt)	6	10 (gemittelt)
FOTHERBY et al. (1963)	11	11,5 ± 4,1	11	12,2 ± 8,2		
			6	16,6 ± 9,4		
COPPEN et al. (1972)	20	42,3 ± 14	31	19,8 ± 8,5	18	19,7 ± 6,8
ROOS u. SJÖSTRÖM (1969)	26	29 ± 7	17	31 ± 8	19	36 ± 9
BOWERS et al. (1969)	18	43,5 ± 16,8	8	34,0 ± 11,5	8	42,0 ± 10,3
VAN PRAAG u. KORF (1971)	11	40 ± 24	14	17 ± 17		
PAPESCHI u. MCCLURE (1971)	10	28 ± 3	12	22 ± 2		
MCLEOD u. MCLEOD (1972)	12	32,6 ± 11,4	25	20,5 ± 12,1		
GOODWIN u. POST (1972)	29	27,3 ± 1,6	85	25,5 ± 3	40	28,7 ± 2,5
ASBERG et al. (1976)			68	(bimodale Verteilung)		
BANKI (1977)	32	27,5 ± 1,2	55	16,4 ± 0,9	10	13,9 ± 2,9

Liquorbefunde nicht einheitlich (Zusammenfassung s. GOODWIN u. POST, 1975). Dies hängt möglicherweise damit zusammen, daß es verschiedenartige Patientengruppen gibt. Neuere Untersuchungen, sowohl mit Basiswerten (ÅSBERG et al., 1976; ÅSBERG, 1977), als auch mit der Probenecid-Technik (VAN PRAAG, 1977a, b), ergaben eine bimodale Verteilung der 5-HIES im Liquor depressiver Patienten (Abb. 1), d.h. es soll depressive Patienten mit normalem 5-HT-Stoffwechsel und andere mit einem signifikanter geringeren 5-HT-Umsatz im Hirn geben. Allerdings fanden sich bei einer erst kürzlich abgeschlossenen Untersuchung an 29 endogen depressiven Patienten erneut keine Hinweise auf eine bimodale Verteilung der 5-HIES im Liquor (VESTERGAARD et al., 1978). Auf die möglichen Ursachen der unterschiedlichen Ergebnisse werde ich später eingehen.

Nach VAN PRAAG (1977a, b) sprechen Patienten mit niedriger 5-HIES besser auf eine Behandlung mit 5-HTP, der Vorstufe des 5-HT, an (weitere Diskussionen zu diesem Thema s. VAN PRAAG, 1977b). Anderseits berichten ÅSBERG et al. (1973), daß Patienten mit höheren 5-HIES-Werten im Liquor therapeutisch besser auf eine Behandlung mit Nortriptylin reagieren als solche mit niedriger 5-HIES-Konzentration. Da Nortriptylin ein starker Hemmer der NA-Aufnahme in die Nervenendigungen ist, wird geschlossen, daß bei Patienten mit normal hohen 5-HIES-Konzentrationen im Liquor eher eine Störung im NA-Stoffwechsel vorliegt. Ich halte es jedoch für notwendig, daß diese Befunde weiter ge-

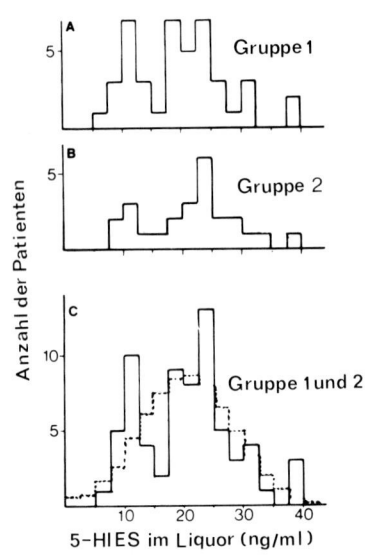

Abb. 1. Verteilung der 5-HIES-Konzentration im Liquor bei depressiven Patienten (nach ÅSBERG et al., 1976)

prüft und von anderen Autoren bestätigt werden, ehe man die 5-HIES-Bestimmung als Test für das Ansprechen auf eine bestimmte Therapie ansehen kann. Dies gilt sowohl für die van Praagschen als auch für die Ergebnisse von ÅSBERG.

Als es Anfang der siebziger Jahre möglich war, MHPG, den Hauptmetaboliten des NA im Hirn, im Liquor gaschromatographisch zu bestimmen, hoffte man, mit dieser Methode die NA-Hypothese der Depression eindeutig überprüfen zu können. Sollte nämlich bei der endogenen Depression ein NA-Mangel mit geringerem NA-Umsatz im Hirn vorliegen, müßten sich niedrigere MHPG-Konzentrationen im Liquor nachweisen lassen. Aber nur POST et al. (1973) fanden geringere MHPG-Mengen im Liquor bei depressiven Patienten, WILK et al. (1972) und SHAW et al. (1973) dagegen nicht.

Bei agitiert depressiven Patienten liegen die MHPG-Werte sogar eher höher (ASHCROFT et al., 1975). In der schon erwähnten 5-HIES-Untersuchung von VESTERGAARD et al. (1978) an endogen depressiven Patienten waren die MHPG-Liquorwerte bei uni- und bipolar Depressiven sogar signifikant höher als in der Kontrollgruppe und waren nicht von der Agitation der Patienten abhängig. Es wurde diskutiert, daß körperliche Aktivität in Beziehung zum MHPG-Liquorwert steht, doch läßt sich diese Frage noch nicht eindeutig beantworten (Übersicht s. GOODWIN u. POST, 1975). Die Frage, ob aufgrund der Liquor-MHPG-Untersuchungen die NA-Hypothese der Depression aufgegeben werden muß, wird später nochmals diskutiert.

c) Blutuntersuchungen

Sind Untersuchungen in der Körperperipherie, wie Blut- und Urinanalysen, überhaupt in der Lage, Hinweise auf Stoffwechselprozesse im ZNS zu geben?

Es ist nicht möglich, aus NA- oder 5-HT-Veränderungen im Blut auf Stoffwechselstörungen dieser Neurohormone im ZNS zu schließen. Vor allem ist ein großer Teil des in der Peripherie vorkommenden 5-HT nicht nervalen Ursprungs, sondern befindet sich in Thrombozyten. Da jedoch die NA- und 5-HT-Biosynthese im ZNS von der Zufuhr der jeweiligen Aminosäuren als Präkursoren (Tyrosin und Tryptophan) abhängig ist, wurden im Rahmen der Depressionsforschung derartige Analysen auch vorgenommen. Dies war besonders wichtig, weil die Biosynthese des Serotonins im ZNS vom peripheren Angebot an freiem Tryptophan abhängig ist (MOIR u. ECCLESTON, 1968; FERNSTROM u. WURTMAN, 1971). COPPEN et al. (1973 u. 1974), AYLWARD und MADDOCK (1973) und BAUMANN et al. (1975) fanden auch erniedrigte Plasmaspiegel von freiem Tryptophan, doch ließen sich diese Befunde von anderen Arbeitsgruppen nicht bestätigen (WIRZ-JUSTICE et al., 1975; PEET et al., 1976; NISKANEN et al., 1976; BLAZEK et al., 1977). Die Bestimmung des freien Tryptophans im Plasma bereitet methodisch gewisse Schwierigkeiten, so daß die Werte der einzelnen Laboratorien oft nicht übereinstimmen (BAUMANN et al., 1975).

Später zeigten WURTMAN et al. (1974), daß auch die Katecholaminsynthese im Hirn von der Hirn-Tyrosin-Konzentration abhängig ist. Nach diesen Untersuchungen kommt speziell der Nahrungszufuhr für die Biosynthese der Neurohormone im ZNS eine entscheidende Bedeutung zu (FERNSTROM, 1977; WURTMAN, 1977; WURTMAN et al., 1977).

Veränderungen der zirkadianen Tyrosin- bzw. Tryptophan-Plasmaspiegel wurden ebenfalls von verschiedenen Arbeitsgruppen gefunden (BIRKMAYER u. LINDAUER, 1970; BENKERT et al., 1971; KLEMPEL, 1972; CROMBACH et al., 1973). Es ist bis jetzt allerdings nicht sicher, inwieweit diese Ergebnisse klinische Relevanz besitzen und die postulierten Störungen im 5-HT- bzw. NA-Hirnstoffwechsel bei depressiven Patienten erklären. Für den Aminosäurentransport im ZNS ist das Verhältnis der verschiedenen Aminosäuren im Plasma von Bedeutung, da das Transportsystem der Blut-Hirn-Schranke nur eine begrenzte Kapazität besitzt. Auf die klinische Bedeutung dieser Befunde mit entsprechenden Tryptophan-Therapieversuchen machten erst kürzlich MØLLER et al. (1976) aufmerksam. Sie zeigten, daß depressive Patienten mit niedrigem Plasma-Tryptophanspiegel im Verhältnis zu anderen Plasmaaminosäuren, besonders Leucin, therapeutisch besser auf Tryptophangaben ansprachen als Depressive mit hohen Tryptophan-Plasmakonzentrationen. Auf diesem Gebiet müssen ebenfalls weitere Untersuchungen abgewartet werden, bevor sich endgültige Aussagen machen lassen. Besonders der periphere Tryptophanstoffwechsel unterliegt einer Reihe von wichtigen Steuerungsmechanismen, wie Aktivität der Tryptophanpyrrolase in der Leber, Verhältnis von freiem und gebundenem Tryptophan u.a.m., die heute von verschiedenen Arbeitsgruppen intensiv untersucht werden. Auch die verschiedenen Tryptophankompartimente werden einer eingehenden Analyse unterzogen (SHAW et al., 1975).

d) Urinuntersuchungen

Urinuntersuchungen an depressiven Patienten wurden vor allem im Hinblick auf Störungen im NA-Stoffwechsel durchgeführt, da 5-HT und DA mit ihren

Metaboliten 5-HIES und HVS im Urin zu einem großen Teil nicht nervalen Ursprungs sind. Da der NA-Metabolismus wegen verschiedener Enzymmuster im Hirn und in der Körperperipherie unterschiedlich gesteuert wird, lassen sich beim NA aus Urinanalysen mit aller Vorsicht Rückschlüsse auf das Stoffwechselgeschehen im ZNS ziehen. Im Hirn ist MHPG, in der Peripherie VMS Hauptmetabolit des NA. 25–60% des im Urin ausgeschiedenen MHPG sollen zentralen Ursprungs sein (MAAS u. LANDIS, 1968; SCHANBERG et al., 1968; MAAS et al., 1973; EBERT u. KOPIN, 1975). Da sich jedoch nicht immer Korrelationen zwischen MHPG-Werten im Liquor und Urin fanden (ACKENHEIL et al., 1974; SHOPSIN et al., 1974, dort auch ausführliche Diskussion dieser Fragestellung mit weiterer Literatur), läßt sich nicht sicher sagen, inwieweit Urin-MHPG-Werte auf Stoffwechselprozesse im Hirn schließen lassen oder nur ein Index für den Gesamtumsatz von NA und A sind (WALTER u. SHILCOCK, 1977). Unabhängig von dieser heute bestehenden Unsicherheit in der Interpretation der Ergebnisse brachten Urin-MHPG-Analysen in den letzten Jahren eine Reihe interessanter und viel beachteter Befunde.

Verschiedene Arbeitsgruppen stimmen darin überein, daß manische Patienten eine erhöhte Urin-MHPG-Ausscheidung gegenüber bipolaren Depressionen und Kontrollen haben (GREENSPAN et al., 1970; BOND et al., 1972; STODDARD et al., 1972; JONES et al., 1973). Dabei ist noch nicht eindeutig geklärt, inwieweit körperliche Aktivität die MHPG-Ausscheidung beeinflußt (HOWLETT u. JENNER, 1978). Darauf wird später nochmals eingegangen. In einer umfangreichen Studie fanden BECKMANN und GOODWIN (1975a) in der Urin-MHPG-Konzentration signifikante Unterschiede zwischen bipolaren und unipolaren Depressionen (Abb. 2). Werden alle depressiven Patienten zusammengenommen, unterscheiden sie sich nicht von der Kontrollgruppe. Eine kleine Gruppe von 5 schizophrenen Patienten zeigte ebenfalls niedrige MHPG-Ausscheidungen (s. neuere Arbeiten von SCHILDKRAUT et al., 1978a u. b und PICKAR et al., 1978 und kritische Stellungnahme HOLLISTER et al., 1978). Depressive mit Wahnideen zeigten eine signifikant geringere MHPG-Urinausscheidung als Patienten ohne Wahnideen (SWEENEY et al., 1978a). Von Interesse ist die MHPG-Ausscheidung auch im Hinblick auf eine antidepressive Behandlung mit trizyklischen Thymoleptika. Depressive Patienten, die wenig MHPG ausscheiden, sprechen besser auf Imipramin an, Patienten mit einer höheren MHPG-Ausscheidung reagieren therapeutisch besser auf Amitriptylin (MAAS et al., 1972; SCHILDKRAUT et al., 1973; BECKMANN u. GOODWIN, 1975a, b und 1979; BECKMANN, 1978). Da an den Nervenendigungen Imipramin stärker den NA-Stoffwechsel und Amitrptylin mehr den 5-HT-Stoffwechsel beeinflussen soll, wäre eine Beziehung zwischen MHPG-Ausscheidung und Ansprechbarkeit auf Antidepressiva denkbar. Aber auch diese Ergebnisse sind nicht unwidersprochen geblieben (COPPEN et al., 1979).

Daß sich aus Urinuntersuchungen auf NA und seine Metaboliten auch Hinweise bezüglich des Ansprechens einer Schlafentzugstherapie ziehen lassen, zeigte sich in unseren Untersuchungen an endogen depressiven Patienten. Patienten, die sich wesentlich unter einer Schlafentzugsbehandlung besserten, zeigten *in der Schlafentzugsnacht selbst* eine signifikant höhere NA- und VMS-Ausscheidung als die nicht gebesserten Patienten (MATUSSEK et al., 1974a; LOOSEN et al.,

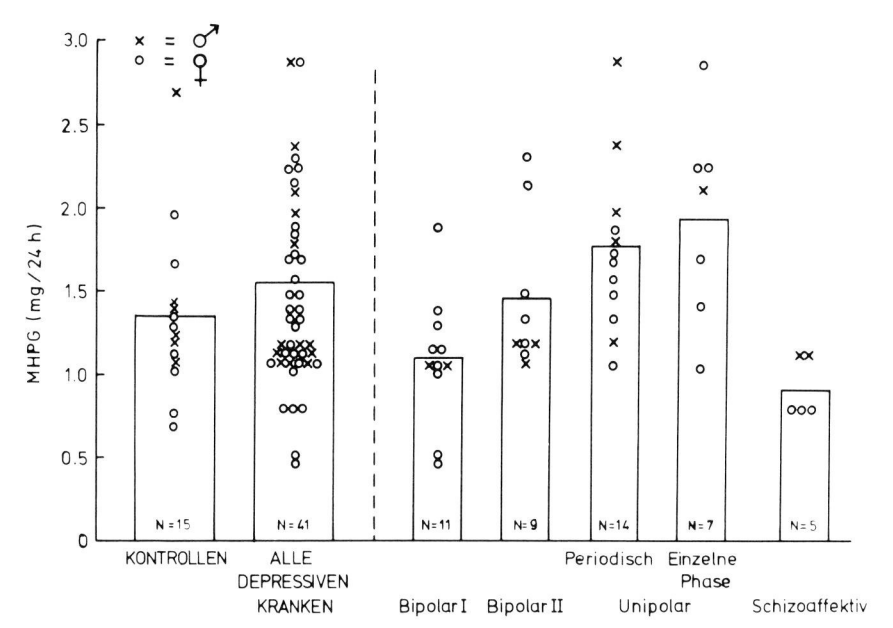

Abb. 2. MHPG-Mengen im 24 h-Urin von Kontrollen, depressiven und schizoaffektiven Patienten (nach BECKMANN u. GOODWIN, 1975a)

1974); *in der Nacht vor dem Schlafentzug* unterschied sich die gebesserte von der nicht gebesserten Gruppe durch eine signifikant höhere MHPG-Ausscheidung (MATUSSEK et al., 1977). In dieser Untersuchung nahm die MHPG-Ausscheidung in der Schlafentzugsnacht gegenüber der vorherigen im Bett verbrachten Nacht weder bei den Patienten noch bei den Kontrollen signifikant zu. Deshalb darf man annehmen, daß die MHPG-Urinausscheidung mit normaler motorischer Aktivität nicht in jedem Fall ansteigen muß (dazu s. SWEENEY et al., 1978b). In der Schlafentzugsnacht waren Probanden und Patienten körperlich aktiver, was auch aus den Bewegungsmesser-Werten hervorging. Aus diesem Grund ist es möglich, daß die oben beschriebene hohe MHPG-Ausscheidung bei Manikern nicht unbedingt auf eine größere motorische Aktivität zurückzuführen ist, sondern der spezifischen Stoffwechsellage der Manie entspricht. Ähnliche Ergebnisse wie wir bei der MHPG-Urinausscheidung unter Schlafentzug erhielten POST et al. (1976) in MHPG-Liquoranalysen. Sie fanden signifikant höhere MHPG-Liquorwerte in der durch Schlafentzug gebesserten Gruppe depressiver Patienten gegenüber der nicht gebesserten Gruppe. Wir schlossen aus unseren Ergebnissen, daß eine Schlafentzugsbehandlung nur dann erfolgreich ist, wenn die NA-Synthese im Organismus genügend gesteigert werden kann. Inwieweit dabei zentrale Mechanismen stärker als periphere betroffen sind, läßt sich anhand der bisher vorliegenden Befunde nicht sagen.

e) Therapieversuche mit Aminpräkursoren

Falls bei der Depression ein Amindefizit vorliegen sollte, wäre eine Substitutionstherapie mit den betreffenden Neurohormonen die Behandlung der Wahl.

Wegen der Undurchlässigkeit der Bluthirnschranke für die Amine müssen dazu die hirngängigen Vorstufen DOPA, 5-HTP oder Tryptophan herangezogen werden. Bei der Behandlung des Parkinsonismus, bei dem durch eine große Zahl voneinander unabhängiger Arbeiten die zuerst von EHRINGER und HORNYKIEWICZ (1960) erhobenen Befunde eines DA-Mangels in bestimmten Hirnstrukturen bestätigt werden konnten, fand dieses Behandlungsprinzip in der DOPA-Therapie eine glänzende Bestätigung (ausführliche Darstellung zu diesem Thema s. BIRKMAYER u. HORNYKIEWICZ, 1976). Trotz intensiver und zahlreicher Bemühungen gelang dies bisher bei der Depressionsbehandlung nicht. Auch nach der Entdeckung der peripheren Decarboxylasehemmstoffe, die dem Hirn mehr DOPA und 5-HTP zuführen, wurden bisher keine eindeutigen antidepressiven Effekte nach DOPA- bzw. 5-HTP-Gaben gefunden (INGVARSSON, 1965; MATUSSEK et al., 1966; MATUSSEK et al., 1970; POHLMEIER et al., 1970; GOODWIN et al., 1971; CARROLL, 1971; BUNNEY et al., 1972; SANO, 1972; MATUSSEK et al., 1974b; MENDELS et al., 1975; Übersicht s. WIRZ-JUSTICE, 1977). Es ist jedoch zu berücksichtigen, daß nach DOPA-Gaben mit oder ohne Decarboxylasehemmer der DA-Anstieg im Hirn beträchtlich ist, während die NA-Menge im Hirn nur geringfügig zu- und 5-HT sogar abnimmt (BENKERT et al., 1973a, b). Wenn für die NA-Synthese im Hirn, ebenso wie in der Peripherie, die Tyrosinhydroxylase der geschwindigkeitsbestimmende Schritt ist, sollte man nach DOPA auch einen eindeutigen NA-Anstieg erwarten. Das ist aber nicht der Fall, und daher ist im ZNS vielleicht die Dopamin-β-hydroxylase geschwindigkeitsbestimmend für die NA-Biosynthese (WISE et al., 1977).

Da, wie schon erwähnt, das Tryptophanangebot im Hirn die Biosynthese des Serotonins entscheidend beeinflußt, wurden auch Therapieversuche mit Tryptophan unternommen. Tryptophangaben bieten gegenüber der 5-HTP-Applikation den Vorteil einer selektiveren Anreicherung von 5-HT im Hirn, weil die Tryptophanhydroxylase, die Tryptophan in 5-HTP umsetzt, nur in serotonergen Neuronen vorkommt, während die Decarboxylase, die 5-HTP in 5-HT überführt, weniger spezifisch ist und auch in anderen Nervenzellen zu finden ist. Auf diese Weise beeinflussen 5-HTP und DOPA-Gaben auch andere aminerge Neurone, so daß spezifische, nur auf ein System gerichtete Effekte nicht zu erwarten sind. Behandlungsversuche mit Tryptophan allein waren bei depressiven Patienten widersprüchlich (COPPEN et al., 1967; CARROLL et al., 1970; MURPHY et al., 1974, dort weitere Literaturhinweise). Die antidepressive Wirkung von MAO-Hemmern soll durch zusätzliche Tryptophangaben gesteigert werden (COPPEN et al., 1963; PARE, 1963). Da MAO-Hemmer allein schon antidepressiv wirken und außer dem 5-HT-System auch katecholaminerge Neurone beeinflussen, lassen sich aus diesen Ergebnissen ebenfalls keine Schlüsse auf ein 5-HT-Defizit ziehen.

2. Weitere Transmittersysteme, die im Zusammenhang mit affektiven Störungen diskutiert werden

Im Vorangehenden wurden die heute immer noch im Mittelpunkt stehenden Störungen im NA- und 5-HT-Stoffwechsel diskutiert. Sicher ist es falsch, wegen der gegenseitigen Abhängigkeit und der vielfältigen Beziehungen zwischen verschiedenen Neuronensystemen bei der Depression nur an die Störung eines einzelnen Systems zu denken. Von manchen Seiten wird das Gleichgewicht zwischen NA- und 5-HT-System stärker in den Vordergrund gerückt (MAAS, 1975), obwohl es dafür bisher keine Beweise gibt. Von anderen Autoren werden weitere Transmittersysteme im Zusammenhang mit der Depression diskutiert.

Es gibt keinen Zweifel, daß das NA-System im Hirn auf das engste mit dem DA-System verbunden ist (ANDEN et al., 1973; STRÖMBOM, 1975, dort weitere Literaturhinweise). Vor allem scheint die Manie, die mit Neuroleptika, d.h. DA-Rezeptor-blockierenden Substanzen, therapeutisch beeinflußt wird, auf eine starke Beteiligung des Dopaminsystems hinzuweisen (SILVERSTONE, 1977). Ob dem DA-Stoffwechsel bei der Depression jedoch eine primäre Rolle zukommt, müssen weitere Untersuchungen zeigen (zusammenfassende Darstellung mit weiterer ausführlicher Literatur zur Dopaminhypothese s. RANDRUP et al., 1975; RANDRUP u. BAASTRUP, 1977; POST et al., 1978). Auf die Beziehungen vom DA zur Schizophrenie wird später ausführlich eingegangen.

Auch Phenyläthylamin (=PEA), eine den Katecholaminen sehr verwandte Substanz, wurde im ZNS gefunden und soll als Transmitter wirken. Nach Reserpin und Antidepressiva verhält es sich wie die anderen biogenen Amine. Der Vorstufe des Amins Phenylalanin werden auch antidepressive Eigenschaften zugeschrieben (s. BECKMANN et al., 1977a). E. FISCHER stellte aufgrund dieser und weiterer Daten die Phenylalanin-Hypothese der Depression auf (FISCHER, 1975, dort weitere Literatur). Bisher liegen zu wenige Untersuchungen vor, um zu dieser Hypothese sicher Stellung nehmen zu können (kritische Übersicht s. WYATT et al., 1977).

Von großem Interesse sind auch Untersuchungen, die die Bedeutung des cholinergen Systems bei Depression, Manie und Schizophrenie hervorheben (s. Zusammenfassung von DAVIS, 1975, mit weiterer Literatur). Gerade diese Arbeitsgruppe wies wiederholt darauf hin, daß eine Einzeltransmitter-Theorie den Gegebenheiten nicht gerecht wird. Sie demonstrierten die kurzdauernde antimanische Eigenschaft des Physostigmins, das durch Hemmung des Acetylcholin-Abbaus den Acetylcholin-Spiegel erhöht. Andererseits vertreten die Autoren die Ansicht, daß anticholinerge Eigenschaften sich günstig auf den antidepressiven Effekt verschiedener Antidepressiva auswirken. Einige neu entwickelte Antidepressiva zeigen jedoch nur geringe oder keine anticholinerge Wirkung (Übersicht dazu s. MATUSSEK u. GREIL, 1977). Es erscheint mir allerdings notwendig, diese Fragen weiterhin sorgfältig zu prüfen.

II. Neuroendokrinologische Ergebnisse

Die vorangehend dargestellten biochemischen Ergebnisse an depressiven Patienten führten bisher zu keinen eindeutigen Aussagen über eine Störung im Transmitterstoffwechsel. In den letzten Jahren entwickelte sich jedoch ein für die biologische Psychiatrie wichtiger neuer Forschungsansatz, der mit neuroendokrinologischen Methoden versucht, den Funktionsstörungen bei den Psychosen näherzukommen. Wir kennen heute eine Reihe von Neuronensystemen, die an der Steuerung der Hypophysenhormonsekretion beteiligt sind. Mit spezifischen Stimulationstests, die schon längere Zeit in der Endokrinologie angewendet werden, ist es möglich, bestimmte Hypophysenhormone freizusetzen und so die Funktionsfähigkeit der an der Hormonausschüttung beteiligten Neuronensysteme am Patienten direkt zu untersuchen. Methodisch ist dies dadurch möglich geworden, daß es gelang, die in kleinsten Konzentrationen im Blut vorkommenden Hormone radioimmunologisch zu bestimmen. Diese bahnbrechende Entwicklung, von der auch die Psychiatrie profitiert, wurde 1977 durch die Verleihung der Nobelpreise an ROSALYN YALOW, ROGER GUILLEMIN und ANDREW SCHALLY gewürdigt.

Von besonderem Interesse für die Depressionsforschung sind im Augenblick das Hypothalamus-Hypophysen-Nebennierenrinden-System und das Hypothalamus-Hypophysen-Wachstumshormon(=STH)-System. Da es bisher nicht möglich ist, alle Hypophysenhormone beim Menschen routinemäßig mit Hilfe geeigneter radioimmunologischer Tests zu untersuchen, auf diesem Gebiet jedoch weiterhin intensiv geforscht wird, kann man auch für die Zukunft mit einer Erweiterung dieser Forschungsrichtung rechnen.

1. Hypothalamus-Hypophysen-Nebennierenrinden-System

Bevor auf einige klinisch-neuroendokrinologische Befunde eingegangen wird, soll die zentralnervöse Regulation der Cortisolsekretion kurz besprochen werden (Abb. 3). Das Corticotropin-Releasing-Hormone (=CRH) gelangt über die Portalvene zur Hypophyse und setzt dort ACTH frei, das über die Blutzirkulation zur Nebennierenrinde gelangt und dort die Cortisolsekretion steuert. Aufgrund von in vitro- und in vivo-Studien stellen sich JONES et al. (1976) die CRH-Freisetzung heute folgendermaßen vor: Das Axon des CRH-enthaltenden Neurons endet an einer Kapillare der Portalvene. Eine Kollaterale des CRH-Neurons steht in Verbindung mit einem inhibitorischen GABA-Neuron, das als negativer

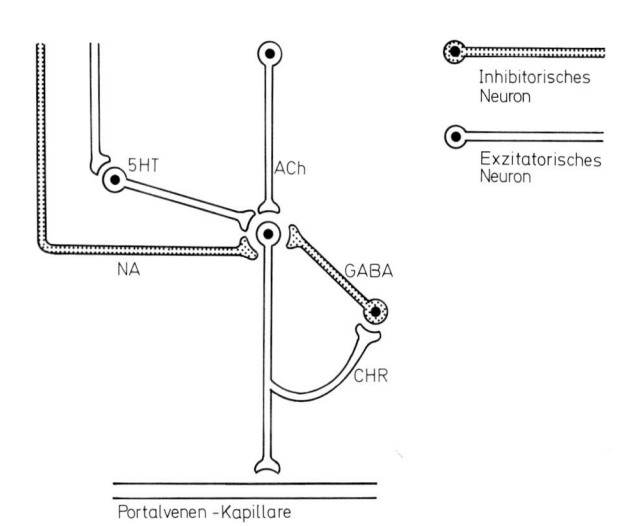

Abb. 3. Schematische Darstellung der CRH-Regulation (nach JONES et al., 1976). CRH=Corticotropin Releasing Hormone, ACH=Acetylcholin, 5-HT=5-Hydroxytryptamin=Serotonin, NA=Noradrenalin, GABA=γ-Aminobuttersäure

Rückkopplungsmechanismus die CRH-Aktivität hemmt. Andererseits hemmen auch bestimmte noradrenerge Neurone die CRH-Sekretion. Freigesetzt wird CRH dagegen einerseits über serotonerge Nervenbahnen und ein cholinerges Interneuron, andererseits von cholinergen Nervenfasern, die direkt am CRH-Neuron angreifen. Die an der CRH-Steuerung beteiligten Nervenzellen sind mit bestimmten limbischen Strukturen, die für das Affektleben von großer Bedeutung sind, eng verknüpft. Das komplizierte Zusammenspiel der einzelnen nervalen Strukturen ist jedoch noch nicht genau bekannt und wird in den nächsten Jahren weiter erforscht werden müssen.

Die Cortisolsekretion zeigt einen charakteristischen zirkadianen Rhythmus. Meist besteht ein inhibitorischer Einfluß auf die Cortisolsekretion, der vorwiegend in den Morgenstunden aufgehoben ist (CARROLL, 1972). Bei gesunden Probanden wird Cortisol nur über 6 Std im Tagesverlauf produziert. Am späten Abend oder nachts ist die Sekretion jedoch äußerst gering (HELLMANN et al., 1970). Schon 1964 zeigte GIBBONS, daß Patienten in der depressiven Phase mehr Cortisol produzieren als im freien Intervall. Bei depressiven Patienten treten häufiger Cortisolsekretionsepisoden auf als bei Gesunden oder im freien Intervall (Abb. 4 u. 5). Vor allem in den Nachmittags- und Nachtstunden ist die Differenz zwischen Depressiven und Gesunden besonders ausgeprägt. Von SACHAR et al. (1976) und von CARROLL und MENDELS (1976) wurden diese Befunde folgendermaßen interpretiert: Bei depressiven Patienten wird deswegen mehr Cortisol sezerniert, weil der zentrale hemmende Einfluß auf die Cortisolfreisetzung gestört ist.

Ein weiterer Hinweis auf eine Funktionsstörung in diesem System wurde im Dexamethason-Hemmtest gefunden. Dieser Test wird in der Endokrinologie

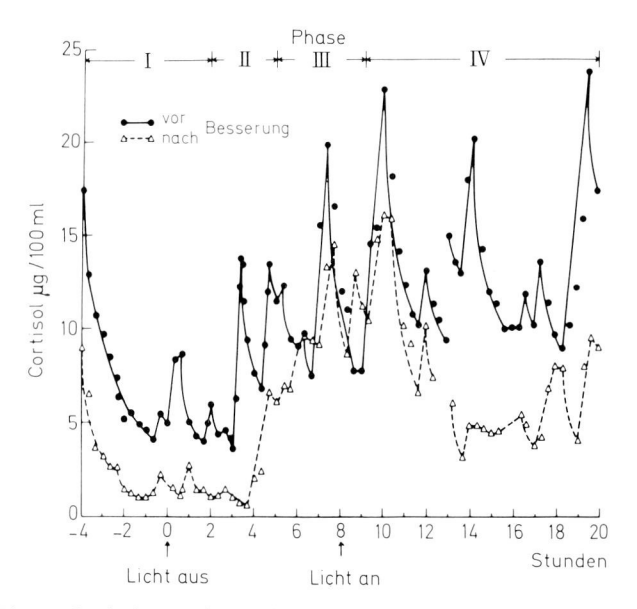

Abb. 4. 24 h-Plasma-Cortisolwerte einer unipolar depressiven 62jährigen Patientin vor und nach klinischer Besserung (nach SACHAR et al., 1976)

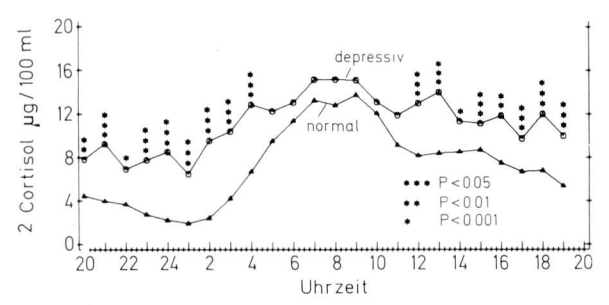

Abb. 5. Mittelwerte der Plasma-Cortisolkonzentration über 24 Std von 7 unipolar depressiven Patienten und 54 Kontrollen. Sterne geben die verschiedenen Signifikanzen zu den betreffenden Stunden zwischen den beiden Gruppen an (nach SACHAR et al., 1976)

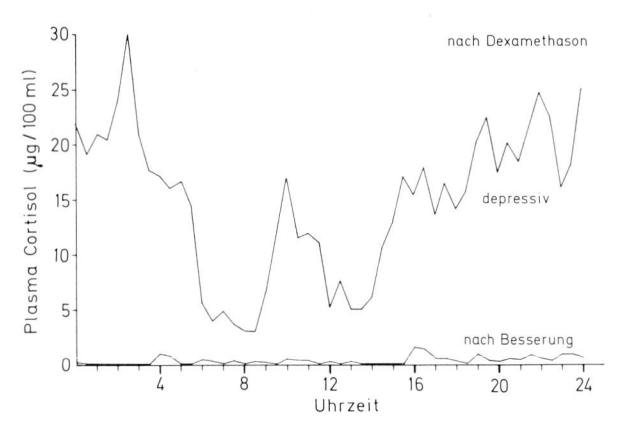

Abb. 6. Plasma-Cortisolkonzentration eines depressiven Patienten nach Dexamethason in der depressiven Phase und nach Besserung (nach CARROLL u. MENDELS, 1976)

schon seit längerer Zeit zur Prüfung der Steroidhormonproduktion der Nebennierenrinden herangezogen. Nach Gaben von Dexamethason, einem synthetischen Glucocorticoid, wird über einen Rückkopplungsmechanismus im ZNS die ACTH-Produktion gehemmt. Liegen Störungen in diesem Rückkopplungssystem vor, so hemmt Dexamethason die Cortisolsekretion nicht vollständig. Dies ist bei endogen depressiven Patienten in der depressiven Phase der Fall. Erst nach Besserung der Depression wird die Cortisolsekretion nach Dexamethasongabe wieder normal unterdrückt (Abb. 6). In diesem Dexamethason-Hemmtest unterscheiden sich auch neurotisch Depressive von gesunden Kontrollpersonen (KLEIN, 1974; CARROLL, 1977). Auch im Insulin- (PEREZ-REYES, 1972; CZERNIK, 1978) und im Methylamphetamin-Test (CHECKLEY u. CRAMMER, 1977) zeigen endogen depressive Patienten in der Phase signifikant niedrigere Cortisolstimulationswerte, die bei den meisten Patienten im freien Intervall wieder auf Werte von gesunden Probanden ansteigen (Abb. 7 u. 8). Sowohl mit Insulin als auch mit Methylamphetamin unterscheiden sich die endogenen von den neurotisch-reaktiven Depressionen (PEREZ-REYES, 1972; CZERNIK, 1978; CHECKLEY, 1979;

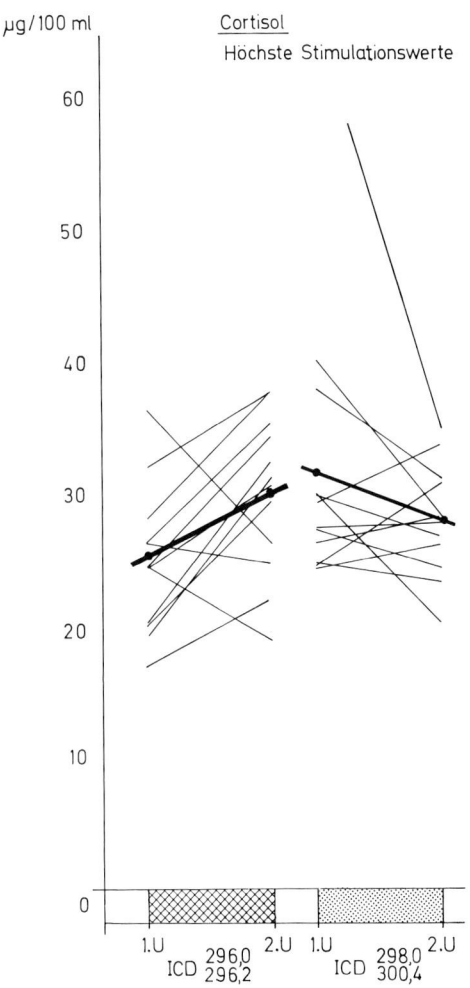

Abb. 7. Maxima der Plasmacortisolkonzentration nach Insulin (0,1 E/kg) bei endogenen (ICD 296,0 und 296,2) und reaktiv bzw. neurotisch depressiven Patienten (ICD 298,0 und 300,4) (nach CZERNIK, 1978)

Abb. 9). Die neurotisch-reaktive Gruppe zeigt nach Besserung häufiger eine Abnahme der Cortisolstimulationswerte (Abb. 7).

Im Zusammenhang mit der Cortisolsekretion soll folgendes festgehalten werden:
1. Die Cortisolsekretion verhält sich spontan und in verschiedenen Tests (Dexamethason, Insulin und Methylamphetamin) in der endogen depressiven Phase anders als im freien Intervall. Außerhalb der Phase normalisiert sich die Cortisolsekretion wieder. Sie ist also phasenabhängig.
2. Endogen depressive unterscheiden sich in ihrer Cortisolsekretion in den oben aufgeführten Tests signifikant von neurotisch-reaktiv depressiven Patienten

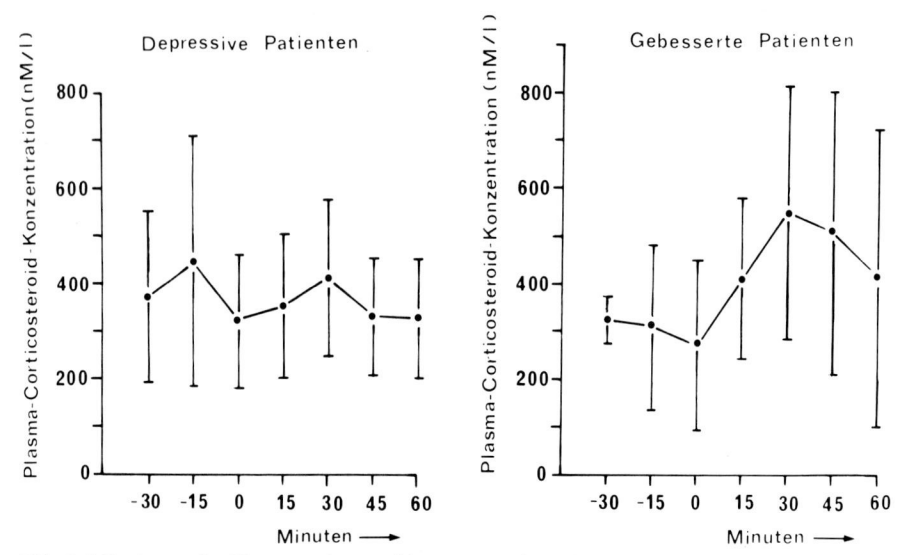

Abb. 8. Mittelwerte der Plasmacorticosteroid-Konzentration mit Standardabweichung nach Placebo (bei −30 min) und Methylamphetamin (15 mg/75 kg i.v.) zum Zeitpunkt 0 min bei 10 Patienten in der Depression und nach Besserung (nach CHECKLEY u. CRAMMER, 1978)

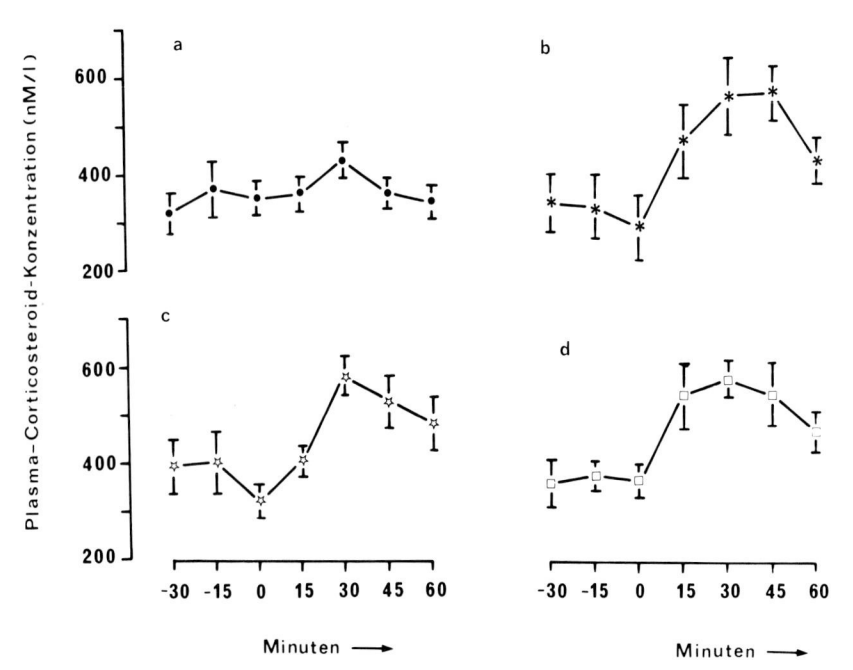

Abb. 9. Mittelwerte als Plasmacorticosteroid-Konzentration mit Standardabweichung nach i.v. Applikation von Placebo (−30 min) und Methylamphetamin (15 mg/75 kg) zum Zeitpunkt 0 bei Patienten mit (a) endogener Depression, (b) anderen funktionellen Psychosen, (c) reaktiver Depression, (d) anderen psychiatrischen Krankheiten (nach CHECKLEY, 1979)

und Kontrollen. Die neurotisch-reaktiven zeigen im Insulin-Test häufiger eine überschießende Reaktion, die sich mit Besserung normalisiert.

Also wäre eine Unterscheidung zwischen endogenen und neurotisch-reaktiven Depressionen durch diese Tests möglich.

2. Hypothalamus-Hypophysen-Wachstumshormon(=STH)-System

An der Steuerung der Wachstumshormonsekretion sind ebenfalls aminerge Neuronen beteiligt. Noradrenerge, dopaminerge und serotonerge Nervenzellen, die im Nucleus arcuatus im Hypothalamus enden, führen bei Aktivierung zu einer Freisetzung des STH-Releasing-Factors, der über den Blutweg im Vorderlappen der Hypophyse STH freisetzt (Abb. 10; Übersicht über STH-Regulation s. BROWN et al., 1978). Von besonderem Interesse für die Depressionsforschung sind die im Nucleus ventromedialis gelegenen Glukorezeptoren. Eine durch Insulin herbeigeführte Hypoglykämie setzt über den Releasing Factor STH frei. Diese Wirkung wird durch Phentolamin, einen α-adrenergen Rezeptorblocker, gehemmt (BLACKARD u. HEIDINGSFELDER, 1968). Man darf deshalb annehmen, daß noradrenerge Neurone die durch Insulin ausgelöste STH-Sekretion steuern. Gehemmt wird die STH-Sekretion ferner durch Somatostatin, einen Faktor, dessen Zusammenspiel mit dem Releasing Factor noch nicht genau geklärt ist. Von mehreren unabhängig voneinander arbeitenden Gruppen ist in den letzten Jahren gezeigt worden, daß bei unipolar depressiven Patienten die durch Insulin ausgelöste STH-Freisetzung signifikant verringert ist (MUELLER et al., 1969; ENDO, 1970; SACHAR et al., 1971; CARROLL, 1972; ENDO et al., 1974; CASPER et al., 1977; CZERNIK, 1978). Die in der endogenen Phase geringere STH-Sekretion steigt nach Besserung wieder an (MUELLER et al., 1969; ENDO

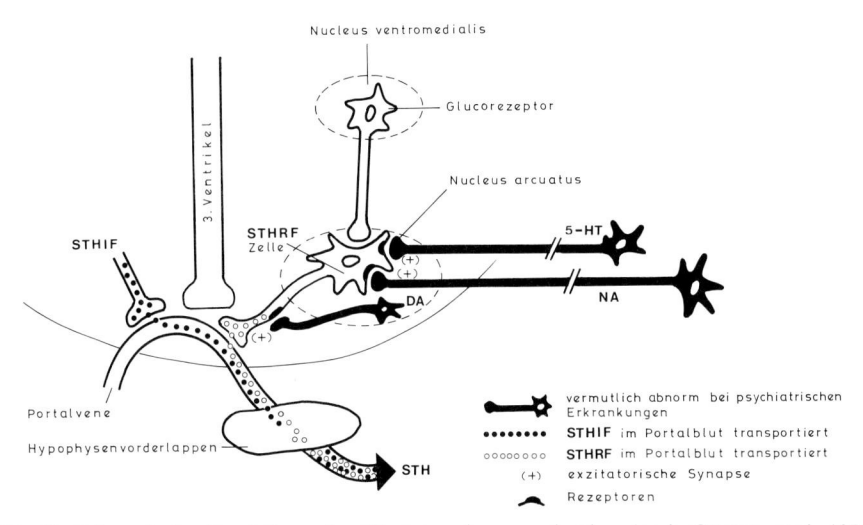

Abb. 10. Schematische Darstellung der Wachstumshormonsekretion (nach GARVER et al., 1975). STH = Wachstumshormon, STHRF = STH Releasing Factor, STHIF = STH Inhibiting Factor = Somatostatin, DA = Dopamin, NA = Noradrenalin, 5-HT = Serotonin

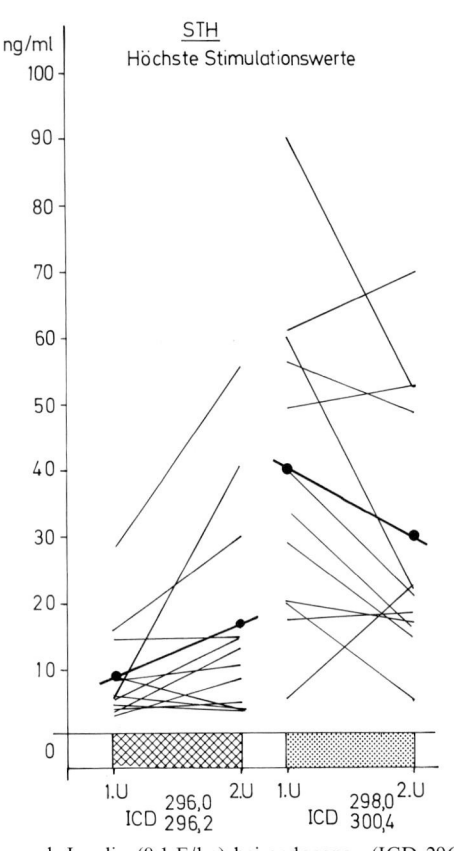

Abb. 11. STH-Maxima nach Insulin (0,1 E/kg) bei endogenen (ICD 296,0 und 296,2) und reaktiv bzw. neurotisch depressiven Patienten (ICD 298,0 und 300,4) (nach CZERNIK, 1978)

et al., 1974; CZERNIK, 1978), während die einer neurotisch-reaktiven Gruppe von einem signifikant höheren Ausgangsniveau später absinkt (Abb. 11). Im Zusammenhang mit biochemischen Befunden ist von Interesse, daß eine signifikante Korrelation zwischen MHPG-Ausscheidung im Urin und Höhe des STH-Maximums nach Insulin-Hypoglykämie gefunden wurde (GARVER et al., 1975). MHPG ist der Hauptmetabolit des NA im ZNS. Je niedriger das STH-Maximum, desto niedriger ist die MHPG-Ausscheidung im Urin (Abb. 12). Bipolare Patienten scheiden dabei, wie oben (Abb. 2) schon gezeigt, geringere MHPG-Mengen aus. Ob diese Befunde auf eine NA-Stoffwechselstörung im ZNS schließen lassen, ist heute noch fraglich, worauf schon hingewiesen wurde. Bei Untersuchungen an unserer Klinik über den Einfluß von Psychopharmaka auf die STH-Sekretion fanden LAAKMANN und BENKERT (1978) besonders nach Desmethylimipramin (=DMI) eine deutliche STH-Freisetzung, die bei neurotisch depressiven Patienten signifikant höher als bei endogenen ist, die praktisch kein STH ausschütten (LAAKMANN, 1979). Im Verlauf einer DMI-Behandlung geht die STH-Sekretion bei den neurotisch depressiven Patienten zurück, bei den endogenen bleibt sie dagegen unverändert gering. Auch im Schlaf (MAI et al., 1977) und nach Hitze-

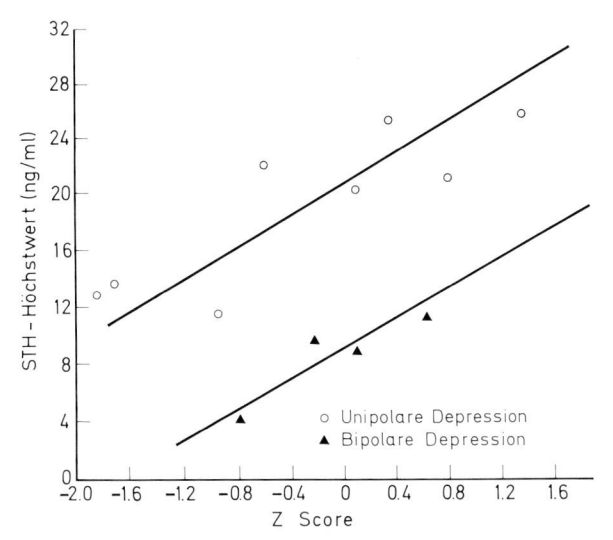

Abb. 12. Beziehungen zwischen Wachstumshormon-Maxima im Insulinhypoglykämie-Test und MHPG-Ausscheidung im Urin bei uni- und bipolar depressiven Patienten (nach GARVER et al., 1975). Z Score = Anzahl der Standardabweichungen über oder unter der erwarteten geschlechtsspezifischen 24 h-MHPG-Ausscheidung, MHPG = 3-Methoxy-4-hydroxyphenylglykol

stimulation (SCHILKRUT et al., 1975) zeigen endogen depressive Patienten eine gestörte STH-Sekretion.

Um die funktionellen Störungen der STH-Ausschüttung bei depressiven Patienten exakter zu erfassen, untersuchten wir ferner die Wirkung von Amphetamin auf die STH-Ausschüttung bei der Depression. Amphetamin ist eine Substanz, deren Angriffspunkt im ZNS weitgehend bekannt ist. Es wirkt vor allem durch Freisetzung von Noradrenalin und Dopamin und ist somit ein indirekt wirkender Stimulator. Gerade im Zusammenhang mit der Noradrenalin-Hypothese der Depression erschien uns Amphetamin als besonders geeignet. Es zeigte sich dabei, daß endogen depressive Patienten gegenüber gesunden Kontrollen signifikant weniger STH freisetzen, während reaktiv depressive im Mittelwert sogar mehr STH ausschütten (LANGER et al., 1975 u. 1976; Abb. 13). Eine kleine Gruppe von Schizophrenen und Alkoholikern verhielt sich im Amphetamintest ähnlich wie die Kontrollen. Endogen depressive Patienten zeigen im freien Intervall mit Amphetamin keine Zunahme der STH-Sekretion, was sich auch nach Methylamphetamin an 10 Patienten bestätigte (CHECKLEY u. CRAMMER, 1977). Darauf wird später nochmals eingegangen.

Wenn endogen depressive Patienten nach Amphetamin signifikant weniger STH freisetzen, liegt es bei dem bekannten Wirkungsmechanismus des Amphetamins nahe, die geringere Stimulation auf eine Funktionsstörung dopaminerger oder noradrenerger Neurone im ZNS zurückzuführen. Da Amphetamin, wie oben angedeutet, nur ein indirekter Stimulator ist und nicht direkt am Rezeptor angreift, stehen zwei Interpretationsmöglichkeiten offen:

1. Es besteht ein Amindefizit in den Nervenendigungen, wie es lange Zeit von der Noradrenalindefizit-Hypothese gefordert wurde.

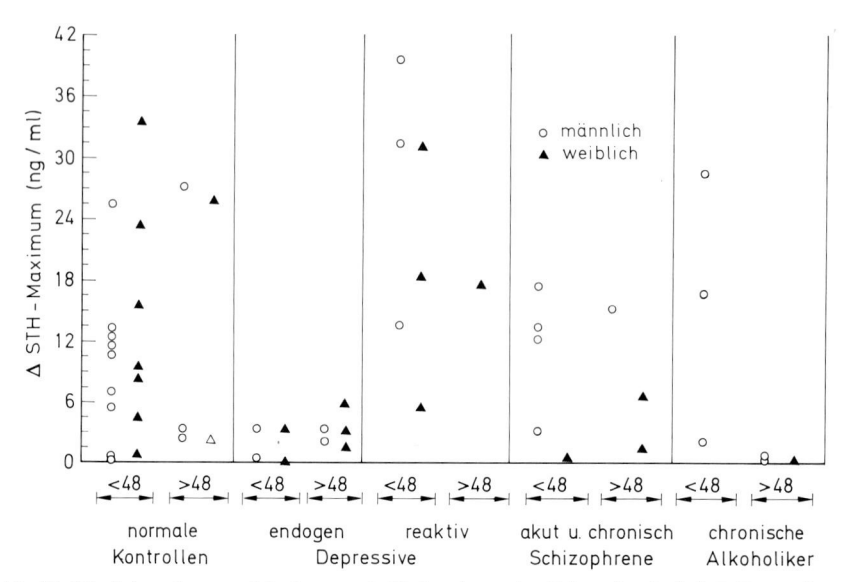

Abb. 13. Wachstumshormon-Maxima nach D-Amphetamin (0,1 mg/kg i.v.) bei Kontrollen und verschiedenen psychiatrischen Patientengruppen (nach LANGER et al., 1976). In den Gruppen wurde eine Unterteilung < bzw. > 48 Jahre alt vorgenommen

2. Der Aminrezeptor bestimmter Hirnareale ist bei endogen depressiven Patienten gegenüber Kontrollen oder neurotisch depressiven unempfindlicher.

Untersuchungen mit Apomorphin, einem Dopaminrezeptorstimulator, zeigten bei endogen Depressiven teils eine normale STH-Sekretion (MENDELS et al., 1974; CASPER et al., 1977; MAANY et al., 1979), bei einem Teil der Patienten auch eine geringere STH-Freisetzung (BALLDIN et al., 1978).

Wir prüften die Rezeptorempfindlichkeit mit Clonidin=Catapresan, einem α-adrenergen Rezeptorstimulator. Endogen depressive und Involutionsdepressionen zeigten im Vergleich zu reaktiv oder neurotisch depressiven Patienten nach Clonidin eine signifikant geringere STH-Freisetzung (MATUSSEK et al., 1979; Abb. 14). Da ein Teil der nicht-depressiven Kontrollen, überwiegend Frauen nach der Menopause, sich im Clonidin-Test ähnlich wie endogen depressive Patienten verhalten, nehmen wir an, daß die geringere α-Rezeptorempfindlichkeit in den für die STH-Sekretion verantwortlichen Hirnarealen bei der endogenen Depression nur einer von mehreren Faktoren ist, die bei der Depression zu berücksichtigen sind. Schizo-affektive Psychosen verhalten sich wie endogene Depressionen, während Schizophrene nach Clonidin meist eine deutliche STH-Freisetzung zeigen.

Hinsichtlich der Beziehungen zwischen Depression und dem Hypothalamus-Hypophysen-STH-System wollen wir zusammenfassend festhalten:

1. In den verschiedenen Stimulationstests (Insulin, Amphetamin, Clonidin) zeigen endogen depressive Patienten eine signifikant niedrigere STH-Sekretion als neurotisch-reaktive Patienten und Kontrollen.

2. Während die STH-Sekretion nach Insulin, ebenso wie die Cortisolsekretion, phasenabhängig verläuft, ist dies bei der Methylamphetamin- und Amphet-

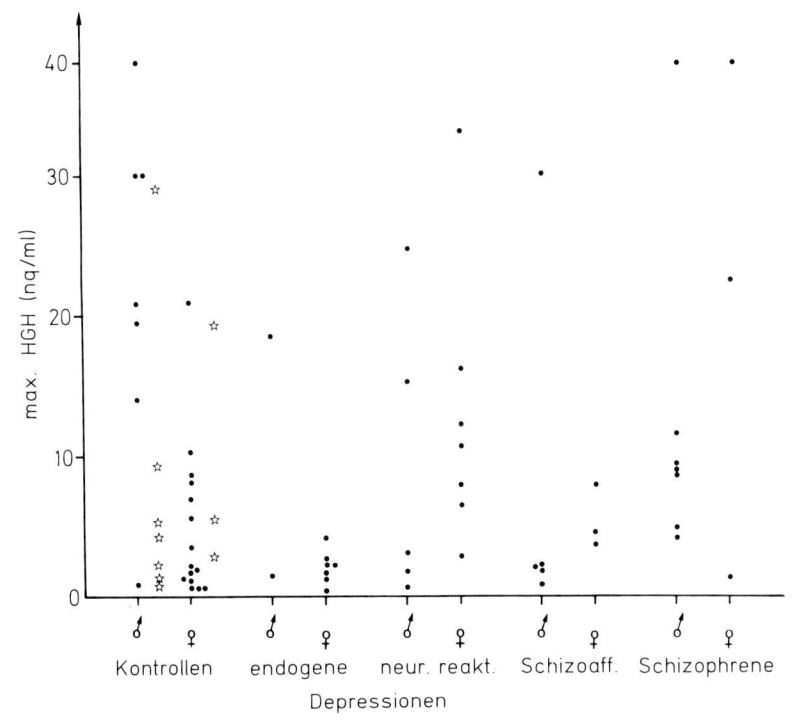

Abb. 14. Wachstumshormon-Maxima nach Clonidin (0,15 mg i.v.) bei männlichen ♂ bzw. weiblichen ♀ Kontrollen und verschiedenen psychiatrischen Patientengruppen (nach MATUSSEK et al., 1979). Sterne in der Kontrollgruppe sind Probanden, die angeben, regelmäßig 1 bis 2 l Bier zu trinken

aminwirkung auf die STH-Sekretion nicht der Fall; u.U. weist diese Reaktion auf einen Persönlichkeitsfaktor depressiver Patienten hin und könnte die Vulnerabilität für das Auftreten einer Depression anzeigen, zumal auch schizoaffektive Patienten mit paranoid-halluzinatorischer Symptomatik auf Clonidin vermindert STH sezernieren.

Von KENDLER und DAVIS (1977) wurde darauf hingewiesen, daß die erhöhte Corticosteroidkonzentration bei endogen depressiven Patienten Ursache für die geringere STH-Sekretion sein könnte. Dies ist bei manchen Krankheiten mit erhöhter Corticosteroidproduktion möglicherweise der Fall. Aber die phasenunabhängige niedrige STH-Sekretion nach Methylamphetamin (s.o.), wie auch die von uns nach Clonidingabe gefundenen Cortisolwerte bei Patienten und Probanden zeigen, daß die beiden Systeme auch unabhängig voneinander reagieren können. Wir fanden in unseren Clonidinuntersuchungen, ähnlich wie LAL et al. (1975), keine Beziehung zwischen Cortisol- und STH-Plasmawerten. Außerdem zeigten Probanden, bei denen auf Amphetamin- und Clonidingabe keine STH-Stimulation erfolgte, eine deutliche STH-Sekretion auf Insulin.

3. Rezeptor-Hypothese der endogenen Depression

In verschiedenen neuroendokrinologischen Untersuchungen unterscheiden sich, wie im Vorangehenden dargelegt, endogen depressive von neurotisch bzw. reaktiv depressiven Patienten, obwohl die verschiedenen depressiven Syndrome oft die gleiche Symptomatik zeigen. Die klinisch-neuroendokrinologischen Untersuchungen mit Clonidin, einem α-Rezeptor-Agonisten, ließen sich vielleicht so erklären, daß sich endogene von neurotisch-reaktiven Depressionen durch eine geringere Empfindlichkeit postsynaptischer α-Rezeptoren unterscheiden. Auch CHECKLEY und CRAMMER (1977) interpretieren ihre Methylamphetamin-Ergebnisse bei endogenen Depressionen mit einer reduzierten α-Rezeptorempfindlichkeit, da Thymoxamin, ein α-Rezeptorblocker, die Corticosteroidwirkung von Methylamphetamin hemmt (REES et al., 1970). Außerdem wurde von verschiedenen Arbeitsgruppen eine reduzierte STH-Sekretion bei endogenen Depressionen im Insulinhypoglykämietest gefunden (s.o.), und es wurde in diesem Zusammenhang darauf hingewiesen, daß Phentolamin, ein α-adrenerger Rezeptorblocker, die durch Insulin bedingte STH-Sekretion hemmt. Drei verschiedene Stimulationstests mit unterschiedlichen Angriffspunkten weisen also auf eine reduzierte α-adrenerge Rezeptorempfindlichkeit in bestimmten Hirnstrukturen bei endogen depressiven Patienten hin. Bei reaktiven und neurotischen Depressionen findet man im Gegensatz zu den endogenen in verschiedenen Stimulationstests normale oder sogar überhöhte Reaktionen, so daß die Annahme naheliegt, die Rezeptorempfindlichkeit bei diesen Patienten sei normal oder sogar gesteigert. Das verschiedenartige Verhalten der endogenen und der neurotisch-reaktiv depressiven Gruppe nach Besserung der Depression kommt in der Untersuchung von CZERNIK (1978) sehr eindrucksvoll zum Ausdruck (Abb. 11). Während die niedrigen STH-Werte bei den endogen depressiven Patienten nach Besserung zunehmen, fallen die bei der neurotisch-reaktiven Gruppe erhöhten Werte mit der Besserung ab. Wie läßt sich nun bei häufig gleicher Symptomatologie der Depressionsformen diese unterschiedliche Reaktion erklären?

Die Funktion einer Synapse läßt sich prä- oder postsynaptisch beeinflussen. An einer aminergen Synapse führt ein Aminmangel in den präsynaptisch gelegenen Speichern zum gleichen Verhalten, wie eine Abnahme der postsynaptischen Rezeptorempfindlichkeit. Bei endogen depressiven Patienten würden also eher Störungen auf der postsynaptischen Seite vorliegen, während neurotische und reaktive Depressionen eher mit einer Dysfunktion in präsynaptischen Prozessen in Verbindung zu bringen wären. Reserpin beispielsweise, greift an den präsynaptisch gelegenen Aminspeichern an und führt dort zu einer Entleerung. Die manchmal nach Reserpin auftretende Depression wäre damit als Modell einer neurotischen, reaktiven oder einer Erschöpfungsdepression nach KIELHOLZ anzusehen. Ein Aminmangel in den Nervenendigungen führt zu einer kompensatorischen Erhöhung der Rezeptorempfindlichkeit, was die oben angeführten Ergebnisse bei neurotisch-reaktiven Depressionen nach Insulin bzw. Amphetamin erklären könnte. Ein endogenes Depressionsmodell müßte nach diesen Überlegungen durch Blockade oder Herabsetzung der Empfindlichkeit postsynaptischer Rezeptoren herbeizuführen sein (Abb. 15).

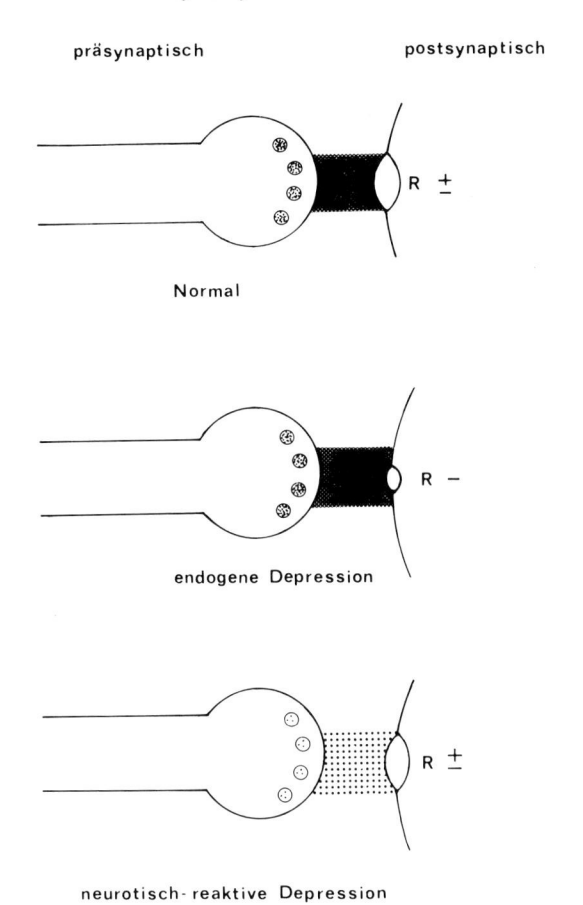

Abb. 15. Schematische Darstellung einer aminergen Nervenendigung. R = postsynaptischer Rezeptor, ± = normal funktionierender Rezeptor, − = Rezeptorempfindlichkeit reduziert, ⊛ = Speichergranula für Neurotransmitter, ▦ = Intensität der Transmitterfreisetzung zum postsynaptischen Rezeptor. In der untersten Darstellung ist durch den Mangel an Transmitter die Transmitterfreisetzung reduziert

Aufgrund schon länger vorliegender klinisch-biochemischer und tierexperimenteller Arbeiten kommen ASHCROFT et al. (1972) ebenfalls zu der Hypothese, daß es eine „lower-sensitivity"- und eine „low out-put"-Depression geben müßte, d.h. also, eine post- bzw. eine präsynaptische Depression. Die neuroendokrinologischen Ergebnisse stützen diese Annahme. Aufgrund theoretischer Überlegungen wiesen auch BUNNEY und MURPHY (1975) und BUNNEY und POST (1977) wiederholt auf die Bedeutung der Rezeptorempfindlichkeit bei affektiven Störungen hin.

Veränderungen der Empfindlichkeit postsynaptischer Rezeptoren spielten in den letzten Jahren auch bei der Erklärung der antidepressiven Wirkung eine zunehmend größere Rolle. Einerseits wurde tierexperimentell gezeigt, daß nur nach chronischer, nicht jedoch nach akuter ES-Behandlung postsynaptische Serotonin- und Dopaminrezeptoren empfindlicher werden (EVANS et al., 1976; GREEN u. GRAHAME-SMITH, 1976; GREEN u. KELLY, 1976). Andererseits kommen MODIGH (1975) und EDEN und MODIGH (1977) aufgrund ihrer Apomorphin- und Clonidinuntersuchungen an Ratten zu dem Ergebnis, daß wiederholte, nicht jedoch einzelne ES-Behandlung die Empfindlichkeit postsynaptischer Dopamin- und Noradrenalinrezeptoren oder neuronaler Strukturen, die mit diesen Rezeptoren verbunden sind, erhöht. Ähnliche Ergebnisse im Hinblick auf postsynaptische Rezeptorempfindlichkeit liegen mit trizyklischen Thymoleptika vor (MODIGH, 1976; SVENSSON, 1977). Allerdings wurde auch schon im Tierexperiment nach chronischer Behandlung mit Antidepressiva eine Abnahme der Rezeptorempfindlichkeit in corticalen (FRAZER u. MENDELS, 1977) und in limbischen Strukturen (VETULANI et al., 1976; SULSER et al., 1978) und bei β-adrenergen Rezeptoren (BANERJEE et al., 1977) gefunden. Während die vorangehenden tierexperimentellen Arbeiten alle Veränderungen der postsynaptischen Rezeptoren unter chronischer Pharmaka- oder ES-Behandlung beschrieben, werden in jüngster Zeit mehr und mehr auch die präsynaptischen Rezeptoren in die Untersuchungen über antidepressive Wirkungsmechanismen einbezogen. Es wird heute angenommen, daß Mianserin, ein neues von den trizyklischen Thymoleptika in Struktur und im pharmakologischen Wirkungsprofil abweichendes Antidepressivum, präsynaptische α-Rezeptoren hemmt und dadurch möglicherweise antidepressiv wirkt (BAUMANN u. MAITRE, 1977; LANGER, 1978). Es konnte ferner an Ratten demonstriert werden, daß durch chronische Behandlung mit Desmethylimipramin die präsynaptische α-Rezeptorempfindlichkeit abnimmt, wodurch mehr NA in der Nervenendigung freigesetzt wird (CREWS u. SMITH, 1978).

In den oben angeführten Tierexperimenten korreliert die Veränderung der Rezeptorempfindlichkeit wesentlich besser mit dem Zeitverlauf der antidepressiven Wirkung beim Patienten als mit der Wiederaufnahmehemmung der verschiedenen Neurohormone an den Nervenendigungen, die bisher als entscheidend für die antidepressive Wirkung angesehen wurde. Die Aufnahmehemmung der Amine an der Nervenendigung tritt momentan ein, während die antidepressive Wirkung beim Patienten erst nach einer Latenzzeit von 8–14 Tagen zu beobachten ist.

Im augenblicklichen Stadium der Untersuchungen über den Wirkungsmechanismus der antidepressiven Therapie läßt sich noch nicht genau sagen, welcher Effekt letztlich für die antidepressive Wirkung entscheidend ist. Die Einbeziehung der Rezeptorempfindlichkeit in die tierexperimentellen Untersuchungen, die nicht nur akut, sondern auch chronisch durchgeführt werden müssen, halte ich für einen wesentlichen Fortschritt auf diesem Gebiet.

Gibt es heute jedoch auch klinische Hinweise dafür, daß die postsynaptische Rezeptorempfindlichkeit unter antidepressiver Therapie erhöht wird? Die oben aufgeführten STH-Befunde, bei denen sich nach Abklingen der Depression unter der Behandlung die Stimulationswerte normalisieren, ließen sich mühelos mit einer erhöhten postsynaptischen Rezeptorempfindlichkeit bei endogenen Depressionen erklären. Ich möchte jedoch auch noch kurz auf einige neuere klinische Untersuchungen eingehen, die auf eine Steigerung der Rezeptorempfindlichkeit unter antidepressiver Therapie hinweisen bzw. demonstrieren, daß direkte Stimulation eines Rezeptors antidepressiv wirken kann.

1. CORSINI (1978) zeigten in einer sorgfältigen Doppelblindstudie, daß bei einer 7tägigen Zusatzmedikation von Haloperidol (3 mg) zu Chlorimipramin nach Absetzen von Haloperidol innerhalb von 2 Tagen eine schnelle Besserung der Depression eintritt, während die Chlorimipramin-Placebo-Gruppe sich wie üblich langsamer besserte. Wir wissen heute aus zahlreichen Untersuchungen, daß Haloperidol, wie auch andere Neuroleptika, vor allem Dopaminrezeptoren blockiert und dadurch nach Absetzen dieser Substanzen eine Rezeptorüberempfindlichkeit erzielt wird. Mit der Zunahme der DA-Rezeptorempfindlichkeit ließe sich also die schnellere Besserung der Depression erklären, doch stellt sich die Frage, ob ausschließlich DA-Rezeptoren für die Besserung verantwortlich zu machen sind. Die häufig in der Praxis mit gutem Erfolg angewandte Kombinationsbehandlung depressiver Patienten mit Neuroleptika und Thymoleptika würde über diese erhöhte Rezeptorempfindlichkeit eine theoretische Erklärung erfahren.

2. BALLDIN et al. (1978) untersuchten an endogen depressiven Patienten die postsynaptische DA-Rezeptorempfindlichkeit mit Apomorphin vor und nach elektrokonvulsiver Therapie. Ausgangspunkt dafür waren die oben erwähnten tierexperimentellen Untersuchungen von MODIGH (1975) und EDEN und MODIGH (1977). Bei den Patienten zeigte sich nach der elektrokonvulsiven Therapie eine starke Zunahme der STH-Sekretion, die von den Autoren zu Recht auf eine Zunahme der DA-Rezeptorempfindlichkeit zurückgeführt wird. Dieser Effekt ist jedoch nicht mit der Besserung signifikant korreliert. Es scheinen demnach außer DA-Rezeptoren noch andere Rezeptoren oder Mechanismen für den therapeutischen Erfolg verantwortlich zu sein.

3. KLEMPEL (1974) zeigte schon früher, daß depressive Patienten schneller auf trizyklische Thymoleptika ansprechen, wenn sie für wenige Tage zusätzlich mit α-Methyldopa behandelt werden. Es ist allerdings noch nicht sicher, ob durch α-Methyldopa die postsynaptische Rezeptorempfindlichkeit zunimmt.

4. Ein sensationelles Ergebnis für die Depressionsbehandlung ist erst jüngst aus Paris berichtet worden. Aufgrund pharmakologischer Überlegungen (FRANCES et al., 1977 u. 1978) wurde Salbutamol, ein β-adrenerger Rezeptoragonist, zur Therapie endogen depressiver Patienten herangezogen (JOUVENT et al., 1977). Schon nach 1–3 Tagen Infusionsbehandlung mit Salbutamol wurden bei den Patienten definitive Besserungen beobachtet. Bei veränderter postsynaptischer Rezeptorempfindlichkeit ließe sich dieser schnell eintretende antidepressive Effekt dadurch erklären, daß die Rezeptoren auch bei geringer Empfindlichkeit durch einen Agonisten stärker stimuliert werden. Es ist selbstverständlich, daß die vier zuletzt erwähnten klinischen Untersuchungen von anderen Arbeitsgruppen bestätigt werden müssen.

Die im Vorangehenden aufgeführten Ergebnisse zeigen, daß man bei der endogenen Depression sicherlich nicht nur von der reduzierten Empfindlichkeit des anfangs hervorgehobenen postsynaptischen α-adrenergen Rezeptors ausgehen darf, sondern auch andere Rezeptoren in die Überlegungen einbeziehen muß. Wir müssen uns bei der in der Rezeptorhypothese vorgelegten Darstellung darüber im klaren sein, daß es sich hier um einen ersten Versuch handelt, einige der bis heute erhaltenen Befunde zu interpretieren. Denn wir wissen bisher noch nicht genau, welche Systeme, welche Rezeptoren in welchen Hirnarealen bei dem komplexen psychischen Ablauf einer Depression betroffen sind. Wir stehen erst am Anfang, auch die Abhängigkeit verschiedener Transmittersysteme voneinander zu erforschen. Wir müssen uns auch darüber im klaren sein, daß die in den verschiedenen Studien verwendeten Pharmaka oft nicht nur an einem Rezeptor oder einem Transmittersystem angreifen, sondern auch andere Neurone beeinflussen. Die Überleitung eines Reizes von einer Nervenendigung auf ein anderes Neuron in der Synapse ist ständigen Regulationsprozessen unterworfen, in die auch präsynaptische oder Autorezeptoren mit Aktivierungen der verschiedenen Enzymsysteme u.a.m. einbezogen sind. Wir fangen erst an, einige Regelvorgänge zu verstehen. Auch Clonidin wirkt nicht nur an postsynaptischen, sondern in Abhängigkeit von der Konzentration auch an präsynaptischen Rezeptoren (STRÖMBOM, 1975). Es ist aber mit ziemlicher Sicherheit anzunehmen, daß die Clonidin-bedingte STH-Sekretion durch Stimulation postsynaptischer und nicht präsynaptischer Rezeptoren ausgelöst wird, da ein präsynaptischer Effekt die STH-Ausschüttung eher unterdrücken würde. Wichtig erscheint mir, zusammenfassend festzustellen, daß man heute bei Überlegungen über mögliche Stoffwechselstörungen bei einem depressiven Syndrom nicht mehr allein an ein Amindefizit zu denken hat, sondern daß auch eine veränderte Rezeptorempfindlichkeit in Betracht zu ziehen ist. Dies bedeutet, daß die ursprüngliche Aminhypothese zu erweitern ist.

Untersuchungen über die Rezeptorempfindlichkeit bei affektiven Erkrankungen und antidepressiven Mechanismen werden erst neuerdings in die neurobiologische Forschung einbezogen. Besonders bei klinisch-biochemischen Untersuchungen an depressiven Patienten ist es notwendig, diesen Überlegungen Rechnung zu tragen. Denn wir wissen heute, daß der Transmitterstoffwechsel bei postsynaptischen anders als bei präsynaptischen Störungen reguliert, ja teilweise sogar entgegengesetzt beeinflußt wird. So wird bei postsynaptischer Rezeptorblockade oder geringerer Rezeptorempfindlichkeit die Transmitterbiosynthese präsynaptisch gesteigert, bei Rezeptorüberempfindlichkeit dagegen ist sie verlangsamt. Dies könnte eine Ursache dafür sein, daß verschiedene Arbeitsgruppen bei depressiven Patienten unterschiedlicher Ätiologie keine einheitlichen biochemischen Ergebnisse erhielten, zumal sich auf der Syndromebene endogen depressive häufig nicht von neurotisch oder reaktiv depressiven Patienten unterscheiden lassen. Eine möglichst einwandfreie nosologische Zuordnung erscheint mir deshalb bei neurobiologischen Untersuchungen an depressiven Patienten unbedingt erforderlich, um den Funktionsstörungen bei den verschiedenen depressiven Syndromen besser als bisher auf die Spur zu kommen.

B. Schizophrenie

Während bis zum Beginn der sechziger Jahre das Hauptinteresse der biochemisch psychiatrischen Forschung der Schizophrenie galt und kaum über Depression und Manie gearbeitet wurde, hat sich dieses Verhältnis in den letzten 10 Jahren deutlich zugunsten der Depression verlagert.

Wie in der Depressionsforschung spielen heute Katecholamine und Indolamine auch in der biochemischen Schizophrenieforschung eine wichtige Rolle.

Bei den Katecholaminen handelt es sich vor allem um Dopamin. Bei den Indolaminen, zu denen das Serotonin gehört, werden bekannte Indolaminderivate im Zusammenhang mit der Schizophrenie diskutiert.

I. Dopamin-Hypothese

Von allen durch Pharmaka ausgelösten Psychosen weist das nach chronischem Mißbrauch von Amphetamin und ähnlich wirkenden Substanzen auftretende paranoid-halluzinatorische Syndrom die größte Ähnlichkeit mit der Schizophrenie auf (PANSE u. KLAGES, 1964, dort auch weitere Literaturhinweise; BELL, 1965). Aber auch akute hohe Amphetamingaben führen bei nicht-schizophrenen Probanden, die Amphetamin regelmäßig konsumieren, zu einem paranoid-halluzinatorischen Syndrom mit formalen Denkstörungen (ANGRIST u. GERSHON, 1970 u. 1971; ANGRIST et al., 1974, dort weitere Literatur zur Amphetaminpsychose). Wie schon im vorhergehenden Kapitel angeführt, wirkt Amphetamin im ZNS vorwiegend durch Freisetzung von Katecholaminen. Da L-DOPA gelegentlich bei Nichtschizophrenen (BIRKMAYER u. NEUMAYER, 1972; SATHANANTHAN u. ANGRIST, 1973) psychotische Zustände, aber auch bei schizophrenen Patienten eine Exazerbation der Symptomatik (DAVIS u. JANOWSKY, 1973; ANGRIST et al., 1973) hervorrufen kann, darf man annehmen, daß Störungen im Katecholaminstoffwechsel zumindest an den paranoid-halluzinatorischen Symptomen der Schizophrenie beteiligt sind. Diese Hypothese wird ferner dadurch gestützt und in Richtung des DA gelenkt, daß alle bisher bekannten antipsychotisch wirkenden Substanzen, wie Phenothiazine, Butyrophenone und Clozapin, vorwiegend DA-Rezeptoren blockieren (s. Beitrag von A. CARLSSON). Eine weitere Stütze für eine mögliche DA-Rezeptor-Überempfindlichkeit bei Schizophrenen erbrachten Untersuchungen mit Apomorphin und STH-Freisetzung. Wie Abb. 10 zeigt, sind DA-Neurone an der STH-Ausschüttung beteiligt. Nach Gaben von Apomorphin, einem DA-Rezeptor-Stimulator, kommt es bei akut Schizophrenen zu einer signifikant höheren (PANDEY et al., 1977; CASPER et al., 1977) und früheren (ROTROSEN et al., 1976) STH-Ausschüttung als bei Kontrollen. Dies wäre ein direkter Hinweis auf eine DA-Rezeptor-Überempfindlichkeit. Inwieweit diese Befunde bei den unbehandelten schizophrenen Patienten auf eine frühere neuroleptische Therapie zurückzuführen sind, müssen weitere Untersuchungen klären. Nach Absetzen von Neuroleptika kommt es zu einer länger anhaltenden Zunahme der DA-Rezeptorsensitivität, wodurch sich auch Spätdyskinesien und erhöhte STH-Freisetzung erklären lassen.

Diese neuroendokrinologischen Ergebnisse erhalten eine zusätzliche Stütze durch eine sorgfältig durchgeführte post mortem-Studie, in der die Spiroperidol-Bindung bei 19 Schizophrenen und 12 Kontrollen untersucht wurde (OWEN et al., 1978). Dabei zeigte sich in bestimmten Hirnstrukturen auch bei zwei Patienten, die noch nie mit Neuroleptika behandelt worden waren und bei 5 Patienten, die länger als ein Jahr von Neuroleptika frei waren, eine signifikant höhere Spiroperidol-Bindung. Spiroperidol ist, wie Haloperidol, ein Butyrophenonderivat und damit ein DA-Antagonist, der an DA-Rezeptoren gebunden wird. Eine erhöhte Bindung wird heute als ein Indikator für erhöhte Rezeptorempfindlichkeit angesehen. Ob damit aber nur postsynaptische Rezeptoren markiert werden, ist weiterhin zu prüfen, da nicht nur in der Präsynapse, sondern selbst in der Glia DA-Rezeptoren vorzukommen scheinen (Henn, 1978).

In einer erst kürzlich abgeschlossenen Studie unserer Klinik (Zander et al., 1978) zeigten jedoch schizophrene Patienten keine Zunahme ihrer psychotischen Symptomatik, wenn Neuroleptika für 30 Tage abgesetzt wurden, nachdem sie bis zu 15 Jahren chronisch damit behandelt worden waren. Wenn chronische Neuroleptikagabe, wie in Tierexperimenten demonstriert, zu einer Erhöhung der DA-Rezeptorempfindlichkeit und zu Spätdyskinesien führt und DA-Rezeptoren mit schizophrener Symptomatik in Beziehung stehen, sollten diese Patienten eigentlich wieder eine psychotische Symptomatik zeigen. Da dies jedoch nicht der Fall ist, müssen andere heute noch unbekannte Mechanismen an der Auslösung paranoid-halluzinatorischer Symptome beteiligt sein.

In diesem Zusammenhang sind auch erste Untersuchungen am Adenylat-Cyclase-System von Interesse. Dieses Enzym, das die Umwandlung von ATP in zyklisches 3'5'-AMP katalysiert, wird in enger Beziehung zum DA-Rezeptor diskutiert. Bei erhöhter DA-Rezeptorempfindlichkeit sollte man größere Mengen cAMP finden. Im Liquor schizophrener Patienten liegen die cAMP-Konzentrationen jedoch nicht höher als bei Kontrollen (Biederman et al., 1977). Fünf akute Schizophrene zeigen allerdings nach Prostaglandin-Stimulation eine signifikant höhere Adenylat-Cyclase-Aktivität in Thrombozyten (Pandey et al., 1977).

Andere Untersuchungen zeigten ebenfalls, daß nicht postsynaptische DA-Rezeptoren allein bei der Schizophrenie beteiligt sein können. Obwohl bei einem Parkinsonpatienten, allerdings unter DOPA-Medikation, durch Apomorphin eine exogene Psychose mit paranoiden Symptomen und Orientierungsstörungen auftrat (Strian et al., 1972), war es nicht möglich, mit Apomorphin bei Schizophrenen eine Symptomprovokation zu erreichen (Angrist et al., 1975; Smith et al., 1977). Allerdings gelang es Angrist et al. (1975) mit ET-495, einem anderen DA-Rezeptorstimulator, bei 4 von 7 schizophrenen Patienten ein paranoides Syndrom zu verstärken. Die Autoren weisen jedoch darauf hin, daß die Effekte nach ET-495 weniger ausgeprägt sind als nach Amphetamin, Methylphenidat oder L-DOPA, die ja nicht nur am DA-System angreifen. Die negativen Befunde mit Apomorphin bei Schizophrenen wurden zu Recht von Smith et al. (1977) damit erklärt, daß Apomorphin, abhängig von der Dosis, auch an den präsynaptischen DA-Rezeptoren angreift und daß evtl. dadurch keine Stimulation postsynaptischer Rezeptoren erzielt wird. Daß bei Schizophrenen auch eine NA-Rezeptorüberempfindlichkeit vorliegen könnte, ist aus unseren oben erwähnten Clonidinuntersuchungen erkennbar, in die wir auch schizophrene Patienten einbezogen haben. Bei ihnen fanden wir ein ähnliches Phänomen, wie in den zuvor erwähnten Arbeiten über Apomorphin. Einige Schizophrene setzen nach Clonidingaben signifikant größere Mengen STH frei (Abb. 14). Allerdings kam es nach Clonidinapplikation bei den schizophrenen Patienten in keinem Fall zu einer Zunahme der paranoid-halluzinatorischen Symptomatik, so daß die α-Rezeptoren damit nicht unmittelbar in Beziehung stehen können. Die Überempfindlichkeit noradrenerger Rezeptoren ließe sich auch mit den von Baker et al. (1976) im Urin schizophrener Patienten gefundenen MHPG-Sulfatmengen in Verbindung setzen, die, mit großer Vorsicht bei der Interpretation, auf einen niedrigeren NA-Umsatz im Hirn hinweisen könnten; denn erhöhte postsynaptische Rezeptorempfindlichkeit führt über Rückkopplungsmechanismen zu einer Abnahme der Transmittersynthese im präsynaptischen Neuron. Diese Befunde stehen jedoch wiederum nicht im Einklang mit den erhöhten NA-Werten im limbischen Vorderhirn, die in Autopsieuntersuchungen bei 4 chronisch paranoiden Schizophrenen gefunden wurden (FARLEY et al., 1978).

Das Auftreten bzw. eine Provokation schizophrener Symptome mit Substanzen, die die Verfügbarkeit von Katecholaminen am Rezeptor vergrößern, aber auch die Hemmung schizophrener Symptome durch Neuroleptika, die den Katecholaminstoffwechsel gegenteilig beeinflussen, sprechen für eine wichtige Rolle dieser Mechanismen bei der Schizophrenie. Eine gesteigerte Katecholaminsynthese liegt bei der Schizophrenie sicher nicht vor. Im Liquor finden sich keine erhöhten HVS- oder MHPG-Werte (PERSSON u. ROOS, 1969; RIMON et al., 1971; BOWERS, 1974; VAN PRAAG u. KORF, 1975) und eine Hemmung der Katecholaminsynthese mit α-Methyl-p-tyrosin führt zu keiner Besserung der psychotischen Symptomatik (GERSHON et al., 1967; CHARALAMPOUS u. BROWN, 1967).

Im Zusammenhang mit eventuellen Störungen im Katecholaminstoffwechsel wurde von WISE und STEIN (1973) aufgrund interessanter theoretischer Überlegungen die Dopamin-β-hydroxylase(=DBH)-Aktivität in verschiedenen Hirnarealen Schizophrener post mortem untersucht. Die Autoren fanden bei Schizophrenen in manchen Hirnarealen signifikant niedrigere DBH-Werte im Vergleich zu Kontrollhirnen (dazu s. WISE et al., 1977). Doch auch diese Ergebnisse ließen sich bisher nicht voll bestätigen (WYATT et al., 1975). Die Serum-DBH-Werte brachten bisher ebenfalls keine eindeutigen Ergebnisse bei Schizophrenen (SHOPSIN et al., 1972; DUNNER et al., 1973; MARKIANOS et al., 1976; OKADA et al., 1976; FUGITA et al., 1978). Doch wäre es wichtig, die DBH-Aktivität im Liquor bei Schizophrenen weiter zu untersuchen, wie von OKADA et al. (1976) begonnen.

Ausführlich setzt sich auch HARTMANN (1976) im Zusammenhang mit verschiedenen Auslösefaktoren für die Schizophrenie mit dem Katecholaminstoffwechsel und der Theorie von STEIN und WISE (1971) auseinander. Danach soll aufgrund der Ausschaltung oder Zerstörung noradrenerger Neurone das DA-System im ZNS dominieren. Eine Degeneration präsynaptischer noradrenerger Neurone oder Störungen in der NA-Biosynthese sollen zu einer Überempfindlichkeit postsynaptischer Rezeptoren führen. HARTMANN (1976) versuchte deshalb zunächst in einem eindrucksvollen Selbstversuch und später in einer Doppelblinduntersuchung an 12 freiwilligen Versuchspersonen (HARTMANN u. KELLER-TESCHKE, 1977) diese These zu überprüfen. Mit Fusarsäure wurde die DBH gehemmt und zusätzlich L-DOPA verabfolgt. Unsicherheit, begleitet von Denk- und Konzentrationsstörungen, stellte sich neben anderen psychischen Veränderungen ein. Diese Beobachtungen müssen natürlich in weiteren Studien abgeklärt werden, bevor sich endgültige Schlüsse ziehen lassen.

Sicher ist es zu früh, aufgrund der bisher vorliegenden Befunde die Schizophrenie als Katecholaminstoffwechselstörung zu beschreiben, an der vorwiegend das DA-System beteiligt ist. Allerdings weisen eine große Zahl unabhängig voneinander erhobener Befunde auf die Bedeutung dieses Systems für psychische Prozesse hin. Welche Hirnstrukturen, ob vorwiegend extrapyramidal-motorische, limbische oder cortikale Zentren betroffen sind, wissen wir heute nicht. Aber sehr wahrscheinlich spielen noch andere Faktoren, die für die Prädisposition entscheidend, aber heute noch weitgehend unbekannt sind, eine wichtige Rolle.

Im Zusammenhang mit der DA-Hypothese wurde auch daran gedacht, daß γ-Aminobuttersäure(=GABA)-Neurone bei der Schizophrenie beteiligt sind (ROBERTS, 1962 u. 1977; STEVENS et al., 1974; VAN KAMMEN, 1977; PLANTEY u. VAN KAMMEN, 1977). Die in dieser Richtung anfangs sehr interessanten klinisch-therapeutischen Untersuchungen mit Baclofen (FREDERIKSEN, 1975) ließen sich jedoch nicht voll bestätigen (BECKMANN et al., 1977b; BIGELOW et al., 1977). Es erscheint dennoch notwendig, weitere Untersuchungen in dieser Richtung zu unternehmen.

II. Transmethylierungs-Hypothese

OSMOND und SMYTHIES (1952) postulierten, daß der Schizophrenie eine Störung der Adrenalinbildung mit falscher N-Methylierung zugrunde liegt. Fast alle psychomimetisch wirkenden Drogen enthalten O- oder N-Methylgruppen wie Mescalin, Dimethyl-tryptamin (=DMT), 5-Methoxy-N-N-dimethyltryptamin (=O.M.B.), Bufotenin, Psylocybin, Psylocin oder LSD. Die durch diese Substanzen hervorgerufenen exogenen Psychosen sind vor allem wegen der vorherrschenden optischen Wahrnehmungsstörungen und der selten auftretenden akustischen Halluzinationen mit der Schizophrenie weniger vergleichbar als die Amphetaminpsychose. Auch eine Symptomprovokation bei schizophrenen Patienten gelingt mit diesen Substanzen nicht. Trotzdem wäre es denkbar, daß ein endogenes Stoffwechselprodukt durch falsche Methylierung in bestimmten Neuronensystemen schizophrene Symptome auslösen kann. Diese Vorstellungen wurden dadurch gestützt, daß durch Gaben allerdings recht hoher Dosen eines Methyldonators wie Methionin (20 g/Tag), teilweise in Gegenwart eines MAO-Hemmers, bei 40% chronisch schizophrener Patienten eine akute schizophrene Symptomatik ausgelöst werden kann. Dies ist von verschiedenen Arbeitsgruppen bestätigt worden (POLLIN et al., 1961; weitere Literatur und ausführlichere Diskussion der Ergebnisse s. SMYTHIES, 1976; NESTOROS et al., 1977).

Aufgrund der Hypothese einer möglicherweise falschen Methylierung wurden auch Therapieversuche mit Methylakzeptoren vorgenommen. Nikotinsäure und Nicotinamid wirken im Organismus als Methylakzeptoren. In Megadosen sahen manche Autoren gute therapeutische Effekte (HOFFER u. OSMOND, 1964; COTT, 1967; MASLOWSKI, 1967; ANANTH et al., 1970), während andere Arbeitsgruppen dies nicht bestätigen konnten (GALLANT et al., 1966; KLINE et al., 1967; MELTZER et al., 1969; BAN u. LEHMANN, 1970; WITTENBORN, 1974).

Wenn falsche Methylierungsprodukte im Organismus eines schizophrenen Patienten gebildet werden, sollte man sie im Liquor, Blut oder Urin dieser Patienten finden, nicht aber bei Kontrollen. Vor allem die Arbeitsgruppe von HIMWICH in den USA war intensiv bemüht, diesen Nachweis zu führen. Die Ergebnisse sind jedoch widersprüchlich (Übersicht mit weiterer Literatur dazu s. RIDGES, 1973). Auch im Liquor gelang es nicht, DMT oder O.M.B. spezifisch bei Schizophrenen mittels Gaschromatographie in Kombination mit Massenspektrometrie (= GC-MS) nachzuweisen. Man fand diese Substanzen sogar häufiger im Liquor nichtschizophrener Kontrollen (SMYTHIES, 1976; CORBETT et al., 1978). Auch im Blut konnten ANGRIST et al. (1976) mit der GC-MS-Methode keine signifikanten Unterschiede zwischen Schizophrenen und Kontrollen finden (weitere Literaturhinweise und kritische Diskussion dazu s. KOSLOW, 1977).

Ähnlich liegen die Ergebnisse von FRIEDHOFF und VAN WINKLE (1962) bei der O-methylierten Verbindung, dem 3′4′-Dimethoxy-phenyläthylamin (DMPEA). Auch hier halten sich positive und negative Ergebnisse die Waage (ausführliche Literatur dazu s. RIDGES, 1973 und FRIEDHOFF, 1977).

Im Zusammenhang mit den Methioninbefunden an schizophrenen Patienten werden auch andere Mechanismen als eine falsche Methylierung für die Symptomprovokation diskutiert. Einerseits entsteht aus Methionin durch Abspaltung des Methylrestes Homocystein, das sich mit Serin zum Cystathionin kondensiert. Da Serin im Tierexperiment bestimmte, durch Methionin ausgelöste Verhaltensänderungen hemmt, wird angenommen, daß möglicherweise größere Homocysteinmengen im Organismus psychotische Effekte auslösen (C_1-Cyclus-Hypothese, SMYTHIES, 1976). Andererseits hemmen hohe Methionindosen die Tryptophanaufnahme im Hirn und führen dadurch zu einer 5-HT-Erniedrigung im ZNS (Tryptophanaufnahme-Hypothese, SMYTHIES, 1976). Man sieht aus diesen verschiedenen Hypothesen, daß der Methionineffekt bei schizophrenen Patienten sich heute noch nicht eindeutig interpretieren läßt.

Wie am Anfang des Kapitels angedeutet, spielt bei den Theorien der Schizophrenie, ähnlich wie bei der Depression, auch ein gestörter 5-HT-Stoffwechsel eine wichtige Rolle. SMYTHIES (1976), aber auch GREEN und GRAHAME-SMITH (1976), vertreten die Auffassung, daß, zumindest bei manchen schizophrenen Patienten, das Gleichgewicht zwischen DA-System (überaktiv) und 5-HT-System (zu geringe Aktivität) gestört ist. Von SMYTHIES (1976) werden im Zusammenhang mit 5-HT-Bestimmungen im Blut Schizophrener zwei Typen der Schizophrenie diskutiert: ein Teil zeigt niedrige, der andere hohe 5-HT-Werte, also eine bimodale Verteilung, wie sie bei den Liquorstudien der Depression vorliegt (s. Kapitel Depression). Aber auch diese Befunde müssen noch überprüft werden. Auf die mögliche Überaktivität des DA-Systems wurde schon bei der Behandlung der DA-Hypothese ausführlich hingewiesen.

III. Weitere Schizophrenie-Hypothesen bzw. Faktoren, die im Zusammenhang mit der Schizophrenie diskutiert werden

Die Monoaminoxydase ist das Hauptabbauenzym sowohl für Katecholamine als auch für Serotonin. Niedrige Enzymaktivität hätte also theoretisch eine höhere Aminmenge zur Folge und könnte dadurch psychotische Symptome provozieren, wie es von HEINRICH (1966) unter MAO-Hemmern beschrieben wurde. Wir selbst fanden bisher jedoch im Blut keine Korrelation zwischen MAO-Aktivität und NA-Konzentration (unveröffentlichte Ergebnisse). Man kennt heute zwei Hauptformen des Enzyms (Typ A und Typ B). Typ B findet sich nicht nur im ZNS, sondern auch in Thrombozyten, so daß daher viele Untersuchungen an diesen Blutbestandteilen durchgeführt wurden. Die Enzymaktivität ist einerseits genetisch, andererseits von Umweltfaktoren, wie bestimmten Hormonen, Ernährung und Pharmaka abhängig. Besonders eine Gruppe am NIMH in Bethesda hat sich mit diesem Enzym in Beziehung zu psychiatrischen Erkrankungen umfassend und sorgfältig beschäftigt (s. Übersicht und kritische Diskussion mit weiteren Literaturangaben Murphy, 1976 und Murphy et al., 1977). Die bisher erhaltenen Ergebnisse zeigen, daß es keine einfache Korrelation zwischen MAO-Aktivität und irgendeiner psychiatrischen Erkrankung gibt, sondern eher eine Beziehung zwischen MAO-Aktivität und Vulnerabilität für verschiedene psychopathologische Auffälligkeiten, wie Suizidalität, Straffälligkeit und psychiatrische Hospitalisation (Buchsbaum et al., 1976). Die gemessene MAO-Aktivität hängt jedoch wesentlich vom Substrat ab, das bei den Untersuchungen verwendet wurde. Demisch et al. (1977), aber auch Potkin et al. (1978), zeigten erst kürzlich, daß paranoide schizophrene Patienten mit p-Tyramin bzw. Benzylamin signifikant niedrigere MAO-Aktivität aufweisen als Kontrollen, schizophrene Defektzustände und schizoaffektive Psychosen. Allerdings fand sich in diesem Zusammenhang auch bei affektiven Psychosen eine signifikant niedrigere MAO-Aktivität, was auch mit Benzylamin als Substrat bei Untersuchungen von Familien mit bipolaren affektiven Störungen durch Leckmann et al. (1977) festgestellt wurde.

Großes Interesse fanden schon Mitte der fünfziger Jahre die Aufsehen erregenden Befunde von Heath et al. (Leach et al., 1956) mit dem sog. Taraxein. Ausgehend von Coeruloplasmin-Untersuchungen sollte sich im Blut Schizophrener ein abnormes γ-Globulin befinden, das bei normalen Freiwilligen nach Injektion schizophrene Symptome auslösen würde. Verschiedene Arbeitsgruppen konnten die Heathschen Befunde nicht reproduzieren, und in den letzten Jahren ist es still um diesen Blutfaktor geworden (s. Ridges, 1973). Ein anderer spezifischer Plasmafaktor bei Schizophrenen soll das sog. S-Protein von Frohmann und Gottlieb sein. Dabei handelt es sich um ein α-2-Globulin, das bei Schizophrenen zu einem höheren Prozentsatz in einer α-Helixform gefunden wird als bei Kontrollen. Diese Konformationsänderung soll durch ein Tripeptid (Threonyl-valyl-leucin) verursacht werden (Frohmann, 1977). Auch diese Ergebnisse sind weiter abzuklären (s. Ridges, 1973).

In letzter Zeit wird dem Endorphin-Encephalin-System auch in der Psychoseforschung große Aufmerksamkeit zuteil. Es ist schon länger bekannt, daß Morphinagonisten abnorme psychische Reaktionen hervorrufen können. Nachdem man im ZNS Morphinrezeptoren nachwies und endogene Morphinagonisten – Encephaline und Endorphine – fand, wurden diese Substanzen auch für die Schizophrenieforschung aktuell. Chronisch Schizophrene sollen höhere Endorphinspiegel, die sich bei Besserung wieder normalisieren (Terenius et al., 1976) im Liquor aufweisen. Ferner soll Naloxon, ein Morphinantagonist, akustische Halluzinationen günstig beeinflussen (Gunne et al., 1977; Watson et al., 1978). Bisher ließ sich dieser Befund, auch mit höheren Dosen (4–24,8 mg/Tag) in Doppelblinduntersuchungen, nicht voll bestätigen (Volavka et al., 1977; Emrich et al., 1977 und 1979), doch wurden in einer offenen Studie an stuporösen und katatonen Schizophrenen, aber auch bei Alkoholintoxikationen mit Dosen bis zu 19,2 mg/Tag eindrucksvolle Effekte beobachtet (Schenk et al., 1978). Eine eindeutige Interpretation der Naloxonbefunde und damit auch eine Aussage über die Bedeutung der Endorphine für die Schizophrenie zu machen, ist augenblicklich noch nicht möglich. Während man anfangs annahm, daß ein Überschuß dieser Peptide bei der Schizophrenie eine Rolle spielen würde, wurde jüngst berichtet, daß β- (KLINE et al., 1978), aber auch γ-Endorphine (VERHOEVEN et al., 1978; VERHOEVEN et al., 1979; DE WIED u. VAN REE, 1978) bei Schizophrenen therapeutisch wirksam sind. Auf diesem aktuellen Gebiet wird augenblicklich von verschiedenen Gruppen intensiv gearbeitet, und man wird hoffentlich bald wissen, ob Endorphine für die Schizophrenie, ggf. auch für die Depression, von Bedeutung sind (weitere aktuelle Literaturhinweise dazu s. COSTA u. TRABUCCHI, 1978; VAN REE u. THERENIUS, 1978).

Wenn niedermolekulare Substanzen wie Encephalin, Endorphine, Taraxein oder das Frohmannsche Tripeptid eine wichtige Rolle in der Ätiologie oder Symptomatologie der Schizophrenie spielen, wäre es theoretisch denkbar, diese Stoffe durch Hämodialyse zu entfernen. Schon früher berichteten REITER (1938) und KIELHOLZ (1949) nach Austauschtransfusionen, später THÖLEN et al. (1960) nach Hämodialyse über eine wesentliche Besserung der psychotischen Symptomatik. Diesen Arbeiten wurde jedoch wenig Aufmerksamkeit gewidmet. Aber erst kürzlich erregte eine Untersuchung von WAGEMAKER und CADE (1977) nicht nur in den USA großes Aufsehen. Bei einer kleinen Gruppe von Schizophrenen, die in der Zwischenzeit erweitert wurde, ließen sich durch Hämodialyse dramatische Besserungen erzielen. Auf einer jüngst abgehaltenen Arbeitstagung über Hämodialyse, an der Nephrologen und Psychiater verschiedener europäischer Zentren teilnahmen, um ein gemeinsames Programm über den Gebrauch der künstlichen Niere zur Behandlung chronischer Schizophrenien zu erarbeiten, war man gegenüber den bisher in diesen Zentren mit diesem Verfahren erzielten therapeutischen Erfolgen wesentlich skeptischer als die oben genannten Autoren. Nur ein Drittel von insgesamt 22 schizophrenen Patienten hatte eine bemerkenswerte Besserung unter der Hämodialysebehandlung gezeigt (HIPPIUS et al., 1979). Bei einer Umfrage in verschiedenen amerikanischen Krankenhäusern zeigten von 50 Patienten, die an einer Schizophrenie litten und zusätzlich wegen Nierenversagens hämodialysiert werden mußten, nur 16% eine Besserung (PORT et al., 1978). Die Autoren weisen zu Recht darauf hin, daß diese Besserungsrate an die von KRAEPELIN schon früher beschriebene Spontanremission von 12,6% heranreicht (kritische Übersicht zur Hämodialyse bei schizophrenen Patienten s. PHILIPP, 1979). Von 10 Schizophrenen in unserer Klinik besserten sich bei einer Hämoperfusionsbehandlung auch nur zwei (NEDOPIL et al., 1979).

C. Schlußbemerkungen

Im Vorangehenden wurden die in meinen Augen wichtigsten biochemischen und neuroendokrinologischen Untersuchungen der letzten Jahre dargelegt und kurz kommentiert, mit denen man hofft, den Stoffwechselstörungen bei den Psychosen auf die Spur zu kommen.

Oft wurde bei den angeführten Untersuchungen an depressiven oder schizophrenen Patienten darauf hingewiesen, daß die vorliegenden Ergebnisse verschiedener Arbeitsgruppen nicht einheitlich waren. Zu einem großen Teil liegt dies an der unterschiedlichen Diagnostik der Krankheitsbilder, die oft schon von

Klinik zu Klinik, besonders jedoch zwischen Europa und den USA differiert. Solange kein besseres Diagnoseschema besteht, sollte man sich auf die ICD-Klassifikation der WHO einigen, damit die erhaltenen Ergebnisse international vergleichbar sind. Häufig wird nur aus der Querschnittssymptomatik eine Diagnose gestellt, ohne den Verlauf der Erkrankung zu berücksichtigen. Wie schwer es sein kann, eine Schizophrenie von einer schizo-affektiven Psychose oder eine neurotische von einer endogenen Depression allein anhand der Symptomatik abzugrenzen, wird jeder psychopathologisch erfahrene Psychiater einräumen. Ich habe eine Reihe von Untersuchungen angeführt, in denen sich die verschiedenen Krankheitsbilder biochemisch oder neuroendokrinologisch unterscheiden. Bei falscher diagnostischer Zuordnung würden sich derartige Unterschiede aufheben können. Im augenblicklichen Stadium biologisch-psychiatrischer Forschung ist eine eindeutige diagnostische Zuordnung besonders wichtig, und deshalb sollten nur diagnostisch klare Fälle in diese Untersuchungen einbezogen werden. Auf die dabei auftretenden Schwierigkeiten, vor allem auf dem Gebiet der Schizophrenieforschung, versuchten wir im gleichen Zusammenhang ausführlicher als hier hinzuweisen (ACKENHEIL et al., 1978). Vielleicht wird es eines Tages gelingen, aufgrund biochemischer oder neuroendokrinologischer Tests eindeutige Diagnosen und sichere Prognosen bei psychiatrischen Erkrankungen zu stellen und die adäquate Therapie einzuleiten.

Wir müssen uns jedoch darüber im klaren sein, daß das ZNS, besonders unser menschliches Hirn, wie schon eingangs erwähnt, uns in den meisten funktionellen, aber selbst auch in submikroskopisch-morphologischen Bereichen noch völlig unbekannt ist. Wir sind noch weit davon entfernt, selbst beim Tier primitive Reaktionen und Verhaltensweisen komplett neurobiologisch erklären zu können; um so weniger sind wir in der Lage, abnormes seelisch-menschliches Verhalten in seiner Vielfalt voll zu verstehen. Innerhalb der Biologie ist die Neurobiologie einer der jüngsten aber auch faszinierendsten Wissenszweige, der in den letzten Jahrzehnten einen ungeheuren Aufschwung und eine schnelle Entwicklung nahm. Manchmal könnte man verzweifeln, wenn immer neue Transmitter, Neuromodulatoren oder Regelmechanismen im Nervensystem entdeckt werden, wodurch unser begrenztes, einfältiges Verständnis über den Ablauf der Hirnprozesse wieder revidiert und so manche schon als bewiesen geltende Hypothese verlassen werden muß. Es ist sicher zu erwarten, daß bei der nächsten Auflage der „Psychiatrie der Gegenwart" in vielleicht wieder 15 Jahren unsere Kenntnisse über die neurobiologische Dysfunktion bei den Psychosen wesentlich erweitert sind. Die eine oder andere hier erwähnte Theorie wird man vielleicht schon vergessen haben. Die Untersuchungen zur Verifikation oder Falsifikation dieser Hypothesen wird in den kommenden Jahren unser Wissen über Hirnfunktionen bei Psychotikern in jedem Fall erweitern. Ob wir bis dahin allerdings den endogen oder exogen bedingten Stoffwechseldefekt bei Psychosen vollkommen erklären und verstehen werden, bleibt abzuwarten.

Literatur

Ackenheil, M., Hoffmann, G., Markianos, E., Nyström, I., Raese, J.: Einfluß von Clozapin auf die MHPG-, HVS- und 5-HIES-Ausscheidung im Urin und Liquor cerebrospinalis. Arzneim.-Forsch. **24**, 984–987 (1974)

Ackenheil, M., Hippius, H., Matussek, N.: Ergebnisse der biochemischen Forschung auf dem Schizophrenie-Gebiet. Nervenarzt **49**, 634–649 (1978)
Ananth, J., Ban, T.A., Lehmann, H.E., Bennett, J.: Nicotinic acid in the prevention in treatment of methionine-induced exacerbation of psychopathology in schizophrenics. Can. Psychiat. Ass. J. **15**, 15–20 (1970)
Anden, N.-E., Strömbom, U., Svensson, T.H.: Dopamine and noradrenaline receptor stimulation: reversal of reserpine-induced suppression of motor activity. Psychopharmacologia **29**, 289–298 (1973)
Angrist, B., Gershon, S.: The phenomenology of experimentally induced amphetamine psychosis – preliminary observations. Biol. Psychiatry **3**, 95–107 (1970)
Angrist, B., Gershon, S.: A pilot study of pathenogenic mechanisms in amphetamine psychosis utilizing differential effects of D and L amphetamine. Pharmakopsychiat. **2**, 64–75 (1971)
Angrist, B., Sathananthan, G., Gershon, S.: Behavioral effects of L-Dopa in schizophrenic patients. Psychopharmacologia **31**, 1–12 (1973)
Angrist, B., Sathananthan, G., Wilk, S., Gershon, S.: Amphetamine psychosis: behavioral and biochemical aspects. J. Psychiat. Res. **11**, 13–23 (1974)
Angrist, B., Thompson, H., Shopsin, B., Gershon, S.: Clinical studies with dopamine-receptor stimulants. Psychopharmacologia **44**, 273–280 (1975)
Angrist, B., Gershon, S., Sathananthan, G., Walker, R.W., Lopez-Ramos, B., Mandel, L.R., Vandenheuvel, W.J.A.: Dimethyltryptamine levels in blood of schizophrenic patients and control subjects. Psychopharmacology **47**, 29–32 (1976)
Åsberg, M.: Studies of monoamine metabolites in depressive illness. Symposia Medica Hoechst: Depressive Disorders. Rom, Mai 1977
Åsberg, M., Bertilsson, L., Tuck, D., Cronholm, B., Sjöqvist, F.: Indoleamine metabolites in the cerebrospinal fluid of depressed patients before and during treatment with nortriptyline. Clin. Pharmacol. Ther. **14**, 277–286 (1973)
Åsberg, M., Thorén, P., Träskman, L., Bertilsson, L., Ringberger, V.: "Serotonin depression" – a biochemical subgroup within the affective disorders. Science **191**, 478–480 (1976)
Ashcroft, G.W., Crawford, T.B.B., Eccleston, D., Sharman, D.F., MacDougall, E.J., Stanton, J.B., Binns, J.K.: 5-Hydroxyindole compounds in the cerebrospinal fluid of patients with psychiatric or neurological disease. Lancet **1966 II**, 1049–1052
Ashcroft, G.W., Eccleston, D., Murray, L.G., Glen, A.J., Crawford, T.B.B., Pullar, J.A., Shields, P.J., Walter, D.S., Blackburn, J.M., Chonnechan, J., Lonergan, M.: Modified amine hypothesis for the aethiology of affective illness. Lancet **1972 II,** 573–577
Ashcroft, G.W., Dow, R.C., Yates, C.M., Pullar, J.A.: Significance of lumbar CSF metabolite measurements in affective illness. Proceedings of the VI. International Congress of Pharmacology, Helsinki, 1975
Aylward, M., Maddock, J.: Plasma tryptophan levels in depression. Lancet **1973 I**, 936
Baker, J.M.H., Johnstone, E.C., Crow, T.J.: Determination of 3-methoxy-4-hydroxyphenylglycol conjugates in urine. Application to the study of central noradrenaline metabolism in unmedicated chronic schizophrenic patients. Psychopharmacology **51**, 47–51 (1976)
Balldin, J., Modigh, K., Wålinder, J., Wallin, L., Lindstedt, G.: Apomorphine induced growth hormone responses before and after ECT in endogenous depressed patients. IInd World Congress of Biological Psychiatry. Barcelona (1978)
Ban, T.A., Lehmann, H.E.: Nicotinic acid in the treatment of schizophrenia. Can. Psychiat. Ass. J. **15**, 499–500 (1970)
Banerjee, S.P., Kung, L.S., Riggi, S.J., Chanda, S.K.: Development of β-adrenergic receptor subsensitivity by antidepressants. Nature **268**, 455–456 (1977)
Banki, C.M.: Correlation between cerebrospinal fluid amine metabolites and psychomotor activity in affective disorders. J. Neurochem. **28**, 255–257 (1977)
Baumann, P., Maitre, L.: Blockade of presynaptic α-receptors and of amine uptake in the rat brain by the antidepressant mianserine. Arch. Pharmacol. **300**, 31–37 (1977)
Baumann, P., Schmocker, M., Reyero, F., Heimann, H.: Free and bound tryptophan in the blood of depressives. Acta Vitamin. Enzymol. **29**, 255–261 (1975)
Beckmann, H.: Biochemische Grundlagen der endogenen Depression. Nervenarzt **49**, 557–568 (1978)
Beckmann, H., Goodwin, F.K.: Renal MHPG excretion in depressed patients and normal controls. Exp. Brain Res. **23**, 17 (1975a)

Beckmann, H., Goodwin, F.K.: Antidepressant response to tricyclics and urinary MHPG in unipolar patients. Arch. Gen. Psychiatry **32**, 17–21 (1975b)
Beckmann, H., Goodwin, F.K.: Urinary MHPG in subgroups of depressed patients and normal controls. Neuropsychobiology (1979) (im Druck)
Beckmann, H., Strauss, M.A., Ludolph, E.: DL-phenylalanine in depressed patients: An open study. J. Neural. Transm. **41**, 123–134 (1977a)
Beckmann, H., Frische, M., Rüther, E., Zimmer, R.: Baclofen (para-chlorphenyl-GABA) in schizophrenia. Pharmakopsychiat. **10**, 26–31 (1977b)
Bell, D.S.: Comparison of amphetamine psychosis and schizophrenia. Brit. J. Psychiat. **111**, 701–707 (1965)
Benkert, O., Hippius, H.: Psychiatrische Pharmakotherapie. 2. Aufl. Berlin-Heidelberg-New York: Springer 1976
Benkert, O., Renz, A., Marano, C., Matussek, N.: Altered tyrosine daytime plasma level in endogenous depressive patients. Arch. Gen. Psychiatry **25**, 359–363 (1971)
Benkert, O., Gluba, H., Matussek, N.: Dopamine, noradrenaline and 5-hydroxytryptamine in relation to motor activity, fighting and mounting behaviour. I. L-Dopa and DL-threo-dihydroxyphenylserine in combination with Ro 4-4602, pargyline and reserpine. Neuropharmacology **12**, 177–186 (1973a)
Benkert, O., Renz, A., Matussek, N.: Dopamine, noradrenaline and 5-hydroxytryptamine in relation to motor activity, fighting and mounting behaviour. II. L-Dopa and DL-threo-dihydroxyphenylalanine. Neuropharmacology **12**, 187–193 (1973b)
Beskow, J., Gottfries, C.G., Roos, B.E., Winblad, B.: Determination of monoamines and monoamine metabolites in the human brain: post mortem studies in a group of suicides and in a control group. Acta Psychiat. Scand. **53**, 7–20 (1976)
Biedermann, J., Rimon, R., Ebstein, R., Belmaker, R.H., Davidson, J.T.: Cyclic AMP in the CSF of patients with schizophrenia. Brit. J. Psychiat. **130**, 64–67 (1971)
Bigelow, L.B., Nasrallah, H., Carman, J., Gillin, J.C., Wyatt, R.J.: Baclofen treatment in chronic schizophrenia: a clinical trial. Am. J. Psychiatry **134**, 318–320 (1977)
Birkmayer, W., Hornykiewicz, O.: Advances in Parkinsonism. Basel: Editiones Roche 1976
Birkmayer, W., Lindauer, W.: Störungen des Tyrosin- und Tryptophan-Metabolismus bei Depressionen. Arch. Psychiat. Nervenkr. **213**, 377 (1970)
Birkmayer, W., Neumayer, E.: Die Behandlung der DOPA-Psychosen mit L-Tryptophan. Nervenarzt **2**, 76–78 (1972)
Birkmayer, W., Riederer, R.: Biochemical post-mortem findings in depressed patients. J. Neural Transm. **37**, 95–109 (1975)
Blackard, W.G., Heidingsfelder, S.A.: Adrenergic receptor control mechanism for growth hormone secretion. J. Clin. Invest. **47**, 1407–1414 (1968)
Bond, P.A., Jenner, F.A., Sampson, G.A.: Daily variations of the urine content of 3-hydroxy-4-methoxyphenylglycol in two manic-depressive patients. Psychol. Med. **2**, 81–85 (1972)
Bourne, H.R., Bunney, W.E., Colburn, R.W., Davis, J.M., Davis, J.N., Shaw, D.M., Coppen, A.J.: Noradrenaline, 5-hydroxytryptamine, and 5-hydroxyindoleacetic acid in hindbrains of suicidal patients. Lancet **1968 II**, 805
Bowers, M.B.: Central dopamine turnover in schizophrenic syndromes. Arch. Gen. Psychiatry **31**, 50–54 (1974)
Bowers, M.B., Henninger, G.R., Gerbode, F.A.: Cerebrospinal fluid, 5-hydroxyindoleacetic acid, and homovanillic acid in psychiatric patients. Int. J. Neuropharmacol. **8**, 255–262 (1969)
Brown, G.M., Seggie, J.A., Chambers, H.W., Ettigi, R.G.: Psychoneuroendocrinology and growth hormone: A review. Psychoneuroendocrinology **3**, 131–153 (1978)
Buchsbaum, M., Coursey, R.D., Murphy, D.L.: The biochemical high-risk paradigm: behavioral and familial correlates of low platelet monoamine oxidase activity. Science **194**, 339–341 (1976)
Bunney, W.E., Davis, J.M.: Norepinephrine in depressive reactions. Arch. Gen. Psychiatry **13**, 483 (1965)
Bunney, W.E., Murphy, D.: Strategies for the systematic study of neurotransmitter receptor function in man. In: Pre- and Postsynaptic Receptors. New York: Marcel Dekker 1975
Bunney, W.E., Post, R.M.: Catecholamine agonist and receptor hypothesis of affective illness: Paradoxical drug effects. In: Neuroregulations and Psychiatric Disorders. New York: Oxford University Press 1977

Bunney, W.E., Goodwin, F.K., Murphy, D.: The 'switch process' in manic-depressive illness. III. Theoretical implications. Arch. Gen. Psychiatry **27**, 312–317 (1972)

Carroll, B.J.: Monoamine precursors in the treatment of depression. Clin. Pharmacol. Ther. **12**, 743–761 (1971)

Carroll, B.J.: The hypothalamic-pituitary-adrenal axis in depression. In: Depressive Illness: Some Research Studies. Springfield: Charles C. Thomas 1972

Carroll, B.J.: Neuroendocrine regulation in depression and mania. Symposia Medica Hoechst: Depressive Disorders. Rom, Mai 1977

Carroll, B.J., Curtis, G., Mendels, J., Sugerman, A.: Neuroendocrine regulation in depression. Arch. Gen. Psychiatry **33**, 1039–1058 (1976)

Carroll, B.J., Mendels, J.: Neuroendocrine regulation in affective disorders. In: Hormones, Behavior and Psychopathology. New York: Raven Press 1976

Carroll, B.J., Mowbray, R.M., Davies, B.M.: L-tryptophan in depression. Lancet **1970 II**, 776

Casper, R.C., Davis, J.M., Pandey, G.N., Garver, D.L., Dekirmenjian, H.: Neuroendocrine and amine studies in affective illness. Psychoneuroendocrinology **2**, 105–114 (1977)

Charalampous, K.D., Brown, S.: A clinical trial of α-methyl-para-tyrosine in mentally ill patients. Psychopharmacologia **11**, 422–429 (1967)

Checkley, S.A.: Corticosteroid and growth hormone responses to methylamphetamine in depressive illnes. Psychol. Med. **9**, 107–115 (1979)

Checkley, S.A., Crammer, J.L.: Hormone responses to methylamphetamine in depression: A new approach to the noradrenaline depletion hypothesis. Brit. J. Psychiat. **131**, 582–586 (1977)

Cochran, E., Robins, E., Grote, S.: Regional serotonin levels in brain: a comparison of depressive suicides and alcoholic suicides with controls. Biol. Psychiatry **11**, 283–295 (1976)

Coppen, A.: The biochemistry of affective disorders. Brit. J. Psychiat. **113**, 1237–1264 (1967)

Coppen, A., Rama Rao, V.A., Ruthven, C.R.J., Goodwin, B.L., Sandler, M.: Urinary 4-hydroxy-3-methoxyphenylglycol is not a predictor for clinical response to amitriptyline in depressive illness. Psychopharmacology **64**, 95–97 (1979)

Coppen, A., Eccleston, E.G., Peet, M.: Plasma tryptophan binding in depression. Adv. Biochem. Pharmacol. **11**, 325–333 (1974)

Coppen, A., Eccleston, E.G., Peet, M.: Total and free tryptophan concentration in the plasma of depressive patients. Lancet **1973 II**, 60–63

Coppen, A., Prange, A.J., Whybrow, P.C., Noguera, R.: Abnormalities of indoleamines in affective disorders. Arch. Gen. Psychiatry **26**, 474–478 (1972)

Coppen, A., Shaw, D.M., Farrell, J.P.: Potentiation of the antidepressive effect of a monoamine-oxidase inhibitor by tryptophan. Lancet **1963 I**, 79–81

Coppen, A., Shaw, D.M., Herzberg, B., Maggs, R.: Tryptophan in the treatment of depression. Lancet **1967 II**, 1178–1180

Corbett, L., Christian, S.T., Morin, R.D., Benington, F., Smythies, J.R.: Hallucinogenic N-methylated indoleamines in the cerebrospinal fluid of psychiatric and control populations. Brit. J. Psychiat. **132**, 139–144 (1978)

Corsini, G.U.: Antidepressant effect of haloperidol withdrawal during chlorimipramine therapy. IInd World Congress of Biological Psychiatry. Barcelona, 1978

Costa, E., Trabucchi, M.: The endorphins. Advances in Biochemical Psychopharmacology. New York: Raven Press 1978

Crews, F.T., Smith, C.B.: Presynaptic alpha-receptor subsentivity after long-term antidepressant treatment. Science **202**, 322–324 (1978)

Crombach, G., Berthold, A., Benkert, O., Matussek, N.: Further studies regarding altered tyrosine plasma levels in endogenous depressive patients. Proceedings of the V. Congress of Psychiatry, Mexiko 1971. Amsterdam: Excerpta Medica 1973

Czernik, A.: Veränderungen hypothalamisch-hypophysär gesteuerter Hormone bei Depressionen und durch Psychopharmaka. Südwestdeutsche Psychiater-Tagung, Baden-Baden 1978

Davis, J.M.: Critique of single amine theories: evidence of a cholinergic influence in the major mental illnesses. In: A Biology of the Major Psychoses: A Comparative Analysis. Vol. 54. New York: Raven Press 1975

Davis, J.M., Janowsky, D.S.: Amphetamine and methylphenidate in psychosis. In: Frontiers in Catecholamine Research. London: Pergamon Press 1973

Demisch, L., v.d. Mühlen, H., Bochnik, N., Seiler, N.: Substrate-typic changes of platelet monoamine oxidase activity in sub-types of schizophrenia. Arch. Psychiat. Nervenkr. **224**, 319–329 (1977)

Dencker, S.J., Malm, V., Roos, B.E., Werdenius, B.: Acid monoamine metabolites of cerebrospinal fluid in mental depression and mania. J. Neurochem. **13**, 1545–1548 (1966)

Dunner, D.L., Cohn, C.K., Weinsilboum, R.M., Wyatt, R.J.: The activity of dopamine-beta-hydroxylase and methionine-activating enzyme in blood of schizophrenic patients. Biol. Psychiatry **6**, 215–220 (1973)

Ebert, M., Kopin, J.J.: Differential labelling of origins of urinary catecholamine metabolites by dopamine-^{14}C. Trans. Assoc. Physicians **28**, 256–264 (1975)

Eden, S., Modigh, S.: Effects of apomorphine and clonidine on rat plasma growth hormone after pretreatment with reserpine and electroconvulsive shocks. Brain Res. **129**, 379–384 (1977)

Ehringer, H., Hornykiewicz, O.: Verteilung von Noradrenalin und Dopamin (3-Hydroxytyramin) im Gehirn des Menschen und ihr Verhalten bei Erkrankungen des extrapyramidalen Systems. Klin. Wschr. **28**, 1236–1239 (1960)

Emrich, H.M., Cording, C., Piree, S., Kölling, A., Zerssen, D. v., Herz, A.: Indication of an antipsychotic action of the opiate antagonist naloxone. Pharmakopsychiat. **10**, 265–270 (1977)

Emrich, H.M., Cording, C., Piree, S., Kölling, A., Möller, H.-J., Zerssen, D. v., Herz. A.: Actions of Naloxone in Different Types of Psychoses. In: Endorphins in Mental Health Research. London: MacMillan Press 1979

Endo, M.: Plasma growth hormone levels during insulin hypoglycemia in atypical psychosis. Folia Endocr. Jap. **45**, 1295–1296 (1970)

Endo, M., Endo, J., Nishikubo, M., Yamaguchi, T., Hatotani, N.: Endocrine studies in depression. In: Psychoneuroendocrinology. Basel: Karger 1974

Evans, J.P.M., Grahame-Smith, D.G., Green, A.R., Tordoff, A.F.C.: Electroconvulsive shock increases the behavioral responses of rats to brain 5-hydroxytryptamine accumulation and central nervous system stimulant drugs. Brit. J. Pharmacol. **56**, 193–199 (1976)

Everett, G.M., Toman, J.E.P.: Mode of action of Rauwolfia alkaloids and motor activity. In: Biological Psychiatry. Vol. I. New York-London: Grune & Stratton 1959

Farley, I.J., Price, K.S., MacCullough, E., Deck, J.H.N., Hordynski, W., Hornykiewicz, O.: Norepinephrine in chronic paranoid schizophrenia: above-normal levels in limbic forebrain. Science **200**, 456–458 (1978)

Fernstrom, J.: Dietary precursors, brain neurotransmitters and depressive illness. Symposia Medica Hoechst: Depressive Disorders. Rom, Mai 1977

Fernstrom, J., Wurtman, R.J.: Brain serotonin content: Increase following ingestion of carbohydrate diet. Science **174**, 1023–1025 (1971)

Fischer, E.: The phenylethylamine hypothesis of thymic homeostasis. Biol. Psychiatry **10**, 667–673 (1975)

Fotherby, K., Ashcroft, G.W., Affleck, J.W., Forrest, A.D.: Studies on sodium transfer and 5-hydroxyindoles in affective illness. J. Neurol. Neurosurg. Psychiatry **26**, 71–73 (1963)

Frances, H., Puech, A., Simon, P.: Stimulants β-adrénergiques: un profil psychopharmacologique voisin de celui des antidépresseurs. J. Pharmacol. **4**, 524 (1977)

Frances, H., Puech, A.J., Simon, P.: Profil psychopharmacologique de l'isoprenaline et du salbutamol. J. Pharmacol. **1**, 25–34 (1978)

Frazer, A., Mendels, J.: Do tricyclic antidepressants enhance adrenergic transmission. Am. J. Psychiat. **134**, 1040–1042 (1977)

Frederiksen, P.K.: Baclofen in the treatment of schizophrenia. Lancet **1975 I**, 702

Friedhoff, A.J.: Biosynthesis of endogenous hallucinations. In: Neuroregulators and Psychiatric Disorders. New York: Oxford University Press 1977

Friedhoff, A.J., Winkle, E. van: Isolation and characterization of a compound from the urine of schizophrenics. Nature **194**, 897–898 (1962)

Frohman, C.E.: Tripeptide plays a role in schizophrenia. Ref.-Chem. & Eng. News **55**, 35 (1977)

Fujita, K., Ito, T., Maruta, K., Teradaira, R., Beppu, H., Nakagami, Y., Kato, Y., Nagatsu, T., Kato, T.: Serum-dopamine-β-hydroxylase in schizophrenic patients. J. Neurochem. **30**, 1569–1572 (1978)

Gallant, D.M., Bishop, M.P., Steele, C.A.: DPN (NAD-oxidized form): a preliminary evaluation in chronic schizophrenic patients. Curr. Ther. Res. Clin. Exp. **8**, 542 (1966)

Garver, D.L., Pandey, G.N., Dekirmenjian, H., Deleon-Jones, F.: Growth hormone and catecholamines in affective disease. Am. J. Psychiatry **132**, 1149–1154 (1975)

Gershon, S., Hekimian, L.J., Floyd, A., Hollister, L.E.: α-Methyl-p-Tyrosine (AMT) in Schizophrenia. Psychopharmacologia **11**, 189–194 (1967)

Gibbons, J.L.: Cortisol secretion rate in depressive illness. Arch. Gen. Psychiatry **10**, 572–575 (1964)

Goodwin, F.K., Post, R.M.: Studies of amine metabolites in affective illness and in schizophrenia: a comparative analysis. In: Biology of the Major Psychoses: A Comparative Analysis. Vol. 54. New York: Raven Press 1975

Goodwin, F.K., Murphy, D.L., Brodie, H.K.H., Bunney, W.E.: Levodopa: alterations in behavior. Clin. Pharmacol. Ther. **12**, 383–396 (1971)

Green, A.R., Grahame-Smith, D.G.: Effects of drugs on the processes regulating the functional activity of brain 5-hydroxytryptamine. Nature **260**, 487–491 (1976)

Green, A.R., Kelly, P.H.: Evidence concerning the involvement of 5-hydroxytryptamine in the locomotor activity produced by amphetamine or tranylcypromine plus L-dopa. Brit. J. Pharmacol. **57**, 141–147 (1976)

Greenspan, K., Schildkraut, J.J., Gordon, E.K., Baer, L., Aronoff, M.D., Durell, J.: Catecholamine metabolism in affective disorders. III. J. Psychiat. Res. **7**, 171–183 (1970)

Gunne, L.M., Lindström, L., Terenius, J.: Naloxone-induced reversal of schizophrenic hallucinations. J. Neural Transm. **40**, 13–19 (1977)

Hartmann, E.: Schizophrenia: a theory. Psychopharmacology **49**, 1–15 (1976)

Hartmann, E., Keller-Teschke, M.: Biology of schizophrenia: mental effects of dopamine-β-hydroxylase inhibition in normal men. Lancet **1977 I**, 37–38

Heinrich, K.: Die gezielte Symptomprovokation mit monoaminoxydasehemmenden Substanzen in Diagnostik und Therapie schizophrener Psychosen. Nervenarzt **31**, 507 (1960)

Hellmann, L., Nakada, F., Curtis, J., Weitzman, E.D., Kream, J., Roffwarg, H., Ellman, S., Fushukima, D.K., Gallaher, T.F.: Cortisol is secreted episodically in normal man. J. Clin. Endocrinol. Metab. **30**, 411–422 (1970)

Henn, F.A.: Dopamine and schizophrenia. A theory revisited and revised. Lancet **1978 II**, 293–295

Hippius, H., Matussek, N., Nedopil, N., Strauss, A., Zerssen, G.D. von, Emrich, H., Kolff, W.J., Gurland, H.J.: Recommendations for the evaluation of possible therapeutic effects of blood purification methods in chronic schizophrenic patients. Artificial Organs: Thoughts and Progress. Vol. 3, No. 1 (1979).

Hoffer, A., Osmond, H.: Treatment of schizophrenia with nicotinic acid. Acta Psychiat. Scand. **40**, 171–189 (1964)

Hollister, L.E., Davis, K.L., Overall, J.E., Anderson, T.: Excretion of MHPG in normal subjects. Arch. Gen. Psychiatry **35**, 1410–1415 (1978)

Howlett, D.R., Jenner, F.A.: Studies relating to the clinical significance of urinary 3-methoxy-4-hydroxyphenylethylene glycol. Brit. J. Psychiat. **132**, 49–54 (1978)

Ingvarsson, C.G.: Orientierende klinische Versuche zur Wirkung des Dioxyphenylalanins (L-Dopa) bei endogener Depression. Arzneim.-Forsch. **15**, 849 (1965)

Jones, F.D., Maas, J.W., Dekirmenjian, H., Fawcett, J.A.: Urinary catecholamines during behavioural changes in a patient with manic-depressive cycles. Science **179**, 200–202 (1973)

Jones, M.T., Hillhause, E., Burden, J.: Secretion of corticotropin-releasing hormone in vitro. In: Frontiers in Neuroendocrinology. Vol. 4. New York: Raven Press 1976

Jouvent, R., Lecrubier, Y., Puech, A.-J., Frances, H., Simon, P., Wildlocher, D.: De l'étude expérimentale d'un stimulant beta-adrénergique à la mise en évidence de son activité antidépressive chez l'homme. Encephale **3**, 285–293 (1977)

Kammen, D. v.: γ-Aminobutyric acid (GABA) and the dopamine hypothesis of schizophrenia. Am. J. Psychiatry **134**, 138–143 (1977)

Kendler, K.S., Davis, K.L.: Elevated corticosteroids as a possible cause of abnormal neuroendocrine function in depressive illness. In: E. Usdin (Ed.), Communications in Psychopharmacology. Oxford-New York: Pergamon 1977

Kielholz, P.: Über Ergebnisse der Behandlung akuter Katatonien mit der Durchblutungsmethode. Ein Beitrag zum Versuch, die endotoxische Genese gewisser Formen der Schizophrenie abzuklären. Schweiz. Arch. Neurol. Psychiat. **63**, 230–245 (1945)

Klein, D.F.: Endogenomorphic depression. Arch. Gen. Psychiatry **31**, 447–454 (1974)

Klempel, K.: Orientierende Untersuchung des zirkadianen Plasma-Tyrosin-Rhythmus depressiver Syndrome unterschiedlicher Ätiologie. Arch. Psychiat. Nervenkr. **216**, 131–152 (1972)

Klempel, K.: Die partielle neuronale Denervation als Behandlungsprinzip affektiver Erkrankungen. Eine vorläufige Mitteilung. Nervenarzt **45**, 330–334 (1974)

Kline, N.S., Barclay, G.L., Cole, J.O., Esser, A.H., Lehmann, H., Wittenborn, J.R.: Controlled evaluation of nicotinamide adenine denucleotide in the treatment of chronic schizophrenic patients. Brit. J. Psychiat. **113**, 731–742 (1967)

Kline, N.S., Lehmann, H.E., Li, C.H., Cooper, T.B.: Pioneer work on endorphins in psychiatry. 11. CINP-Kongress, Wien, 1978

Koslow, S.H.: Biosignificance of N- and O-methylated indoles to psychiatric disorders. In: Neuroregulators and Psychiatric Disorders. New York: Oxford University Press 1977

Laakmann, G., Benkert, O.: Neuroendokrinologie und Psychopharmaka. Arzneim.-Forsch. (Drug Res.) **28**, 1277–1280 (1978)

Laakmann, G.: Neuroendocrine differences between endogenous and neurotic depression as seen in stimulation of growth hormon secretion. In: Neuroendocrine Correlates in Neurology and Psychiatry. Elsevier Holland 1979

Lal, S., Tolis, G., Martin, J.B., Brown, G.M., Guyda, H.: Effect of clonidine on growth hormone, prolactin, luteinizing hormone, follicle-stimulating hormone, and thyroid-stimulating hormone in the serum of normal men. J. Clin. Endocrinol. Metab. **41**, 827–832 (1975)

Langer, G., Heinze, G., Reim, B., Matussek, N.: Growth hormone response to d-amphetamine in normal controls and in depressive patients. Neurosci. Letters **1**, 185–189 (1975)

Langer, G., Heinze, G., Reim, B., Matussek, N.: Reduced growth hormone responses to amphetamine in endogenous depressive patients. Arch. Gen. Psychiatry **33**, 1471–1475 (1976)

Langer, S.Z.: Presynaptic receptors and the regulation of transmitter release in the peripheral and central nervous system: Physiological and pharmacological significance. In: Catecholamines: Basic and Clinical Frontiers. London-New York: Pergamon 1978

Lapin, I.P., Oxenkrug, G.F.: Intensification of the central serotonergic processes as a possible determinant of the thymoleptic effect. Lancet **1969 I**, 132

Leach, B.E., Cohen, M., Heath, R.G., Martens, S.: Studies of the role of ceruloplasmin and albumin in adrenalin metabolism. AMA Arch. Neurol. Psychiat. **76**, 635–642 (1956)

Leckmann, J.F., Gershon, S., Nichols, A.S., Murphy, D.L.: Reduced MAO activity in first-degreee relatives of individuals with bipolar affective disorders. A preliminary report. Arch. Gen. Psychiatry **34**, 601–606 (1977)

Lloyd, K.G., Farley, I.J., Deck, J.H.N., Hornykiewicz, O.: Serotonin and 5-hydroxy-indoleacetic acid in discrete areas of the brainstem of suicide victims and control patients. In: Advances in Biochemical Pharmacology. Vol. 2. New York: Raven Press 1974

Loosen, P., Ackenheil, M., Athen, D., Beckmann, H., Benkert, O., Dittmer, Th., Hippius, H., Matussek, N., Rüther, E., Scheller, M.: Schlafentzugsbehandlung endogener Depression. 2. Mitteilung: Vergleich psychopathologischer und biochemischer Parameter. Arzneim.-Forsch. **24**, 1075–1077 (1974)

Maany, I., Mendels, J., Frazer, A., Brunswick, D.: A study of growth hormone release in depression. Neuropsychobiology **5**, 282–289 (1979)

Maas, J.W.: Biogenic amines and depression. Arch. Gen. Psychiatry **32**, 1357–1361 (1975)

Maas, J.W., Dekirmenjian, H., Garver, D., Redmond, D.E., Landis, D.H.: Excretion of catecholamine metabolites following intraventricular injection of 6-hydroxydopamine in the macaca speciosa. Eur. J. Pharmacol. **23**, 121–130 (1973)

Maas, J.W., Fawcett, J.A., Dekirmenjian, H.: Catecholamine metabolism, depressive illness, and drug response. Arch. Gen. Psychiatry **26**, 252, 262 (1972)

Maas, J.W., Landis, D.H.: In vivo studies of metabolism of norepinephrine in the central nervous system. J. Pharmacol. Exp. Ther. **163**, 147–162 (1968)

Mai, F.M., Jenner, M.R., Shaw, B.F., Giles, D.E.: Nocturnal Growth Hormone (HGH) secretion in depressed and control subjects. IRCS Med. Sci. **5**, 568 (1977)

Markianos, E.S., Nyström, I., Reichel, H., Matussek, N.: Serum dopamine-β-hydroxylase in psychiatric patients and normals. Effect of d-amphetamine and haloperidol. Psychopharmacology **50**, 259–267 (1976)

Maslowski, J.: Zastosowanie keasu nikotynowego w leczeniu schizofrenii przewleklej. Psychiat. Pol. **1**, 307–311 (1967)

Matussek, N.: Neurobiologie und Depression. Med. Wschr. **20**, 109 (1966)

Matussek, N., Ackenheil, M., Athen, D., Beckmann, H., Benkert, O., Dittmer, Th., Hippius, H., Loosen, P., Rüther, E., Scheller, M.: Catecholamine metabolism under sleep deprivation

therapy of improved and not improved depressed patients. Pharmakopsychiat. **7**, 108–114 (1974a)
Matussek, N., Ackenheil, M., Hippius, H., Schröder, H.-Th., Schultes, H., Wasilewski, B.: Effect of clonidine on HGH release in psychiatric patients and controls. Psychiatry Research, 1979 im Druck
Matussek, N., Angst, J., Benkert, O., Gmür, M., Papousek, M., Rüther, E., Woggon, B.: The effect of L-5-hydroxytryptophan alone and in combination with a decarboxylase inhibitor (Ro 4-4602) in depressive patients. Adv. Biochem. Pharmacol. **11**, 399–404 (1974b)
Matussek, N., Benkert, O., Schneider, K., Otten, H., Pohlmeier, H.: Wirkung eines Decarboxylasehemmers (Ro 4-4602) in Kombination mit L-Dopa auf gehemmte Depressionen. Arzneim.-Forsch. **20**, 934–937 (1970)
Matussek, N., Greil, W.: New antidepressants. In: Psychotherapeutic Drugs. New York: Marcel Dekker 1977
Matussek, N., Römisch, P., Ackenheil, M.: MHPG excretion during sleep deprivation in endogenous depression. Neuropsychobiology **3**, 23–29 (1977)
Matussek, N., Pohlmeier, H., Rüther, E.: Wirkung von Dopa auf gehemmte Depressionen. Klin. Wschr. **12**, 727–728 (1966)
McLeod, W.R., McLeod, M.: Indoleamine and Cerebrospinal Fluid in Depressive Illness: Some Research Studies. Springfield: Thomas 1972
Meltzer, H., Shader, R., Grinspoon, L.: The Behavioral Effects of Nicotinamide Adenine Dinucleotide in Chronic Schizophrenia. Psychopharmacologia **15**, 144–152 (1969)
Mendels, J., Frazer, A., Carroll, B.J.: Growth hormone response in depression. Am. J. Psychiatry **131**, 1154–1155 (1974)
Mendels, J., Stinnett, J.L., Burns, D., Frazer, A.: Amine precursors and depression. Arch. Gen. Psychiatry **32**, 22–30 (1975)
Modigh, K.: Electroconvulsive shock and postsynaptic catecholamine effects: Increased psychomotor stimulant action of apomorphine and clonidine in reserpine pretreated mice by repeated ECS. J. Neural Transm. **36**, 19–32 (1975)
Modigh, K.: Correlation between clinical effects of various depressant treatments and their effects on monoaminergic receptors in the brain. 10th CINP Congress, Quebec, 1976
Moir, A.T.B., Eccleston, D.: The effects of precursor loading in the cerebral metabolism of 5-hydroxyindoles. J. Neurochem. **15**, 1093–1108 (1968)
Møller, S.E., Kirk, L., Fremming, K.H.: Plasma amino acids as an index for subgroups in manic depressive psychosis: correlation to effect of tryptophan. Psychopharmacology **49**, 205–213 (1976)
Mueller, P.S., Henninger, G.R., McDonald, R.K.: Insulin tolerance test in depression. Arch. Gen. Psychiatry **21**, 587–594 (1969)
Murphy, D.L.: Clinical, genetic, hormonal and drug influences on the activity of human platelet monoamine oxidase. In: Monoamine Oxidase and its Inhibition. Ciba Foundation Symposium 39. Amsterdam: Elsevier, Excerpta Medica 1976
Murphy, D.L., Baker, M., Goodwin, F.K., Miller, H., Kotin, J., Bunney, W.E.: L-tryptophan in affective disorders: indoleamine changes and differential clinical effects. Psychopharmacologia **34**, 11–20 (1974)
Murphy, D.L., Belmaker, R., Carpenter, W.T., Wyatt, R.T.: Monoamine oxidase in chronic schizophrenia. Studies of hormonal and other factors affecting enzyme activity. Brit. J. Psychiat. **130**, 151–158 (1977)
Nedopil, N., Dieterle, D., Hillebrand, G., Gurland, H.-J.: Hemoperfusion in chronic schizophrenia. A critical report. Kli.Wo. (im Druck)
Nestoros, I.N., Ban, T.A., Lehmann, H.E.: Transmethylation hypothesis of schizophrenia: Methionine and nicotinic acid. Int. Pharmacopsychiat. **12**, 215–246 (1977)
Niskanen, P., Huttunen, M., Tamminen, T., Jääskeläinen, J.: The daily rhythm of plasma tryptophan and tyrosine in depression. Brit. J. Psychiat. **128**, 67–73 (1976)
Okada, T., Shinoda, T., Kato, T., Ikuta, K., Nagatsu, T.: Dopamine-β-hydroxylase activity in serum and cerebrospinal fluid in neuropsychiatric diseases. Neuropsychobiology **2**, 139–144 (1976)
Osmond, H., Smythies, J.: Schizophrenia: A new approach. J. Ment. Sci. **98**, 309–315 (1952)
Owen, F., Cross, A.J., Crow, T.J., Longden, A., Poulter, M., Riley, G.J.: Increased dopamine receptor sensitivity in schizophrenia. Lancet **1978 II**, 224–226
Pandey, G.N., Garver, D.L., Tamminga, C., Ericksen, S., Ali, S.I., Davis, J.M.: Postsynaptic supersensitivity in schizophrenia. Am. J. Psychiatry **134**, 518–522 (1977)

Panse, F., Klages, W.: Klinisch-psychopathologische Beobachtungen bei chronischem Mißbrauch von Ephedrin und verwandten Substanzen. Archiv für Psychiatrie und Zeitschrift f. d. ges. Neurologie **206**, 69–95 (1964)

Papeschi, R., McClure, D.J.: Homovanillic acid and 5-hydroxyindole acetic acid in cerebrospinal fluid of depressed patients. Arch. Gen. Psychiatry **25**, 354–358 (1971)

Pare, C.M.B.: Potentiation of monoamine oxidase inhibitors by tryptophan. Lancet **1963 II**, 527–528

Pare, C.M.B., Yeung, D.P.H., Price, K., Stacey, R.S.: 5-Hydroxytryptamine, noradrenaline, and dopamine in brainstem, hypothalamus, and caudate nucleus of controls and of patients committing suicide by coal-gas poisoning. Lancet **1969 II**, 133

Peet, M., Moody, J.P., Worrall, E.P., Walker, P., Naylor, G.J.: Plasma tryptophan concentration in depressive illness and mania. Brit. J. Psychiat. **128**, 255–258 (1976)

Perez-Reyes, M.: Differences in the capacity of the sympathetic and endocrine systems of depressed patients to react to a physiological stress. In: Recent Advances in the Psychobiology of the Depressive Illnesses. Washington: Government Printing Office 1972

Perry, E.K., Gibson, P.H., Blessed, G., Perry, R.T., Tomlinson, B.E.: Neurotransmitter enzyme abnormalities in senile dementia. Choline acetyltransferase and glutamic acid decarboxylase activities in necropsy brain tissue. J. Neurol. Sci. **34**, 247–265 (1977)

Persson, T., Roos, B.E.: Acid metabolites from monoamines in cerebrospinal fluid of chronic schizophrenics. Brit. J. Psychiat. **115**, 95–98 (1969)

Philipp, M.: Hämodialyse und die Idee der Blutentgiftung in der Schizophreniebehandlung. Fortschr. Neurol. Psychiat. (1979)

Pickar, D., Sweeny, D.R., Maas, J.W., Heninger, G.R.: Primary affective disorder, clinical state change and MHPG excretion. A longitudinal study. Arch. Gen. Psychiatr. **35**, 1378–1383 (1978)

Plantey, F., Kammen, D.P. van: GBH and GABA. Am. J. Psychiatry **134**, 1045–1046 (1977)

Pohlmeier, H., Schön, I., Matussek, N.: Die Wirkung eines Decarboxylasehemmstoffs (Ro 4-4602) und L-Dopa auf gehemmte Depressionen. Arzneim.-Forsch. **20**, 932–933 (1970)

Pollin, W., Cardon, P.V., Kety, S.S.: Effects of amino acid feedings in schizophrenic patients treated with Iproniazid. Science **133**, 104–105 (1961)

Port, F.K., Kroll, P.D., Swartz, R.D.: The effect of hemodialysis on schizophrenia: A survey of patients with renal failure. Am. J. Psychiatry **135**, 743–744 (1978)

Post, R.M., Gerner, R.H., Carman, J.S., Gillin, J.C., Jimerson, D.C., Goodwin, F.K., Bunney, W.E., Jr.: Effects of a dopamine agonist piribedil in depressed patients. Arch. Gen. Psychiatry **35**, 609–615 (1978)

Post, R.M., Gordon, E.K., Goodwin, F.K., Bunney, W.E., Jr.: Central norepinephrine metabolism in depressed patients: 3-methoxy-4-hydroxy-phenyl-glycol in the cerebrospinal fluid. Science **179**, 1002–1003 (1973)

Post, R.M., Kotin, J., Goodwin, F.K.: Effects of sleep deprivation on mood and central amine metabolism in depressed patients. Arch. Gen. Psychiatry **33**, 627–632 (1976)

Potkin, S.G., Cannon, H.E., Murphy, D.L., Wyatt, R.J.: Are paranoid schizophrenics biologically different from other schizophrenics. New Engl. J. Med. **298**, 61–66 (1978)

Praag, H.M. van: Monoamines and depression. Pharmakopsychiat. **2**, 151–160 (1969)

Praag, H.M. van: Significance of biochemical parameters in the diagnosis, treatment and prevention of depressive disorders. Biol. Psychiatry **12**, 101–131 (1977a)

Praag, H.M. van: New evidence of serotonin deficient depression. Symposia Medica Hoechst: Depressive Disorders. Rom, Mai 1977b

Praag, H.M. van, Korf, J.: A pilot study of some kinetic aspects of the metabolism of 5-hydroxytryptamine in depression. Biol. Psychol. **3**, 105–112 (1971)

Praag, H.M. van, Korf, J.: Biochemical research into psychosis. Results of a new research strategy. Acta Psychiat. Scand. **51**, 268–284 (1975)

Randrup, A., Baastrup, C.: Uptake inhibition of biogenic amines by newer antidepressant drugs: Relevance to the dopamine hypothesis of depression. Psychopharmacology **53**, 309–314 (1977)

Randrup, A., Munkvad, I., Fog, R., Gerlach, J., Molander, L., Kjellberg, B., Scheel-Krüger, J.: Mania, depression and brain dopamine. In: Current Developments in Psychopharmacology. Vol. 2. New York: Spectrum Publications Inc. 1975

Ree, J.M. van, Terenius, L.: Characteristics and function of opioids. Developments in neuroscience. Amsterdam: Elsevier (1978)

Rees, L., Butler, P.W.P., Gosling, C., Besser, G.M.: Adrenergic blockade and corticosteroid and growth hormone responses to methylamphetamine. Nature **228**, 565–566 (1970)
Reiter, P.J.: Untersuchungen zur Beleuchtung der Intoxikationstheorie bei der Dementia praecox mit besonderer Berücksichtigung der Versuche mit Totaltransfusionen. Z. ges. Neurol. Psychiat. **160**, 598–614 (1938)
Ridges, A.P.: Abnormal metabolites in schizophrenia. Biochem. Soc. Spec. Publ. **1**, 175–188 (1973)
Riederer, P.: The distribution of free 4-hydroxy-3-methoxyphenylglycol in post mortem brains of parkinsonian and depressed patients. Ges. Biol. Chemie **358**, 292–293 (1977)
Rimon, R., Roos, B.E., Rakkolainen, V., Alanen, Y.: The content of 5-HIAA and HVA in the CSF of patients with acute schizophrenia. J. Psychosom. Res. **15**, 375–378 (1971)
Roberts, E.: A hypothesis suggesting that there is a defect in the GABA system in schizophrenia. Neurosci. Res. Program Bull. **10**, 468–482 (1972)
Roberts, E.: The γ-Aminobutyric Acid System and Schizophrenia. In: Neuroregulators and Psychiatric Disorders. New York: Oxford University Press 1977
Roos, B.E., Sjöström, R.: 5-Hydroxyindoleacetic acid (and homovanillic acid) levels in the CSF after probenecid application in patients with manic-depressive psychosis. Pharmacol. Clin. **1**, 153–155 (1969)
Rotrosen, J., Angrist, B.M., Gershon, S., Sachar, E.J., Malpern, F.S.: Dopamine receptor alteration in schizophrenia: neuroendocrine evidence. Psychopharmacology **51**, 1–7 (1976)
Sachar, E.J., Finkelstein, J., Hellmann, L.: Growth hormone responses in depressive illness. I. Response to insulin tolerance test. Arch. Gen. Psychiatry **25**, 263–269 (1971)
Sachar, E.J., Roffwarg, H.P., Gruen, P.H., Altmann, N., Sassin, J.: Pharmakopsychiat. **9**, 11–17 (1976)
Sano, I.: L-5-Hydroxytryptophan (L-5-HTP)-Therapie bei endogener Depression. Münch. Med. Wschr. **114**, 1713–1716 (1972)
Sathananthan, G., Angrist, B.: Response threshold to L-dopa in psychiatric patients. Biol. Psychiatry **7**, 139–146 (1973)
Schanberg, S.M., Schildkraut, J.J., Breese, G.R.: Metabolism of normetanephrine-H^3 in rat brain, identification of conjugated 3-methoxy-4-hydroxyphenylglycol as the major metabolite. Biochem. Pharmacol. **17**, 247–254 (1968)
Schenck, G.K., Enders, P., Engelmeier, H.-M., Ewert, T., Herdemerten, S., Köhler, K.-H., Lodemann, E., Matz, D., Pach, J.: Application of the morphine antagonist Naloxone in psychic disorders. A preliminary report about explorative pilot studies. Arzneim.-Forsch. **28**, 1274–1277 (1978)
Schildkraut, J.J.: The catecholamine hypothesis of affective disorders: a review of supporting evidence. Am. J. Psychiatry **122**, 509 (1965)
Schildkraut, J.J.: Norepinephrine metabolites as biochemical criteria for classifying depressive disorders and predicting responses to treatment: preliminary findings. Am. J. Psychiatry **130**, 695–698 (1973)
Schildkraut, J.J., Orsulak, P.J., Schatzberg, A.F., Gudeman, J.E., Cole, J.O., Rohde, W.A., LaBrie, R.A.: Toward a biochemical classification of depressive disorders. I. Differences in urinary excretion of MHPG and other catecholamine metabolites in clinically defined subtypes of depression. Arch. Gen. Psychiatry **35**, 1427–1433 (1978a)
Schildkraut, J.J., Orsulak, P.J., LaBrie, R.A., Schatzberg, A.F., Gudeman, J.E., Cole, J.O., Rohde, W.A.: Toward a biochemical classification of depressive disorders. II. Application of multivariate discriminant function analysis to data on urinary catecholamines and metabolites. Arch. Gen. Psychiatry **35**, 1436–1439 (1978b)
Schilkrut, R., Chandra, O., Osswald, M., Rüther, E., Baarfüsser, B., Matussek, N.: Growth hormone release during sleep and with thermal stimulation in depressed patients. Neuropsychobiology **1**, 70–79 (1975)
Shaw, D.M., Camps, F.E., Eccleston, E.G.: 5-Hydroxytryptamine in the hindbrain of depressive suicides. Brit. J. Psychiat. **113**, 1407 (1967)
Shaw, D.M., Johnson, A.J., Tidmarsh, S.F., MacSweeny, D.A., Hewland, H.R., Woolcock, N.E.: Multicompartimental analysis of amine acids. Psychol. Med. **5**, 206–213 (1975)
Shopsin, B., Freedman, L.S., Goldstein, M., Gershon, S.: Serum dopamine-β-hydroxylase activity and affective states. Psychopharmacologia **27**, 11–16 (1972)
Shopsin, B., Wilk, S., Sathananthan, G., Gershon, S., Davis, K.: Catecholamines and affective disorders revised: a critical assessment. J. Nerv. Ment. Dis. **158**, 369–383 (1974)

Silverstone, T.: Dopamine, mood and manic depressive psychosis. Symposia Medica Hoechst: Depressive Disorders. Rom, Mai 1977

Smith, R.C., Tamminga, C., Davis, J.M.: Effect of apomorphine on schizophrenic symptoms. J. Neural Transm. **40**, 171–176 (1977)

Smythies, R.J.: Recent progress in schizophrenia research. Lancet **1976 II**, 136–139

Stein, L., Wise, C.D.: Possible etiology of schizophrenia: progressive damage to the noradrenergic reward system by 6-hydroxydopamine. Science **171**, 1032–1036 (1971)

Stevens, J., Wilson, K., Foote, W.: GABA blockade, dopamine and schizophrenia: Experimental studies in the cat. Psychopharmacologia **39**, 105–119 (1974)

Stoddard, F.J., Post, R.M., Gillin, J.C., Buchsbaum, M.S., Carman, J.S., Bunney, W.E.: Phasic changes in manic-depressive illness. Annual Meeting. American Psychiatric Association, Detroit, Mai 1972

Strian, F., Micheler, E., Benkert, O.: Tremor inhibition in parkinson syndrome after apomorphine administration under L-dopa and decarboxylase inhibitor basic therapy. Pharmakopsychiat. **5**, 198–205 (1972)

Strömbom, U.: On the functional role of pre- and postsynaptic catecholamine receptors in brain. Acta Physiol. Scand., Suppl. 431. Göteborg, 1975

Sulser, F., Vetulani, J., Mobley, P.L.: Mode of action of antidepressant drugs. Biochem. Pharmacol. **27**, 257–261 (1978)

Svensson, T.H.: Central α-adrenoreceptors and affective symptoms and disorders. Symposia Medica Hoechst: Depressive Disorders. Rom, Mai 1977

Sweeney, D., Nelson, C., Bowers, M., Maas, J., Heninger, G.: Delusional versus non-delusional depression: neurochemical differences. Lancet **1978**a **II**, 100–101

Sweeney, D.R., Maas, J.W., Heninger, G.R.: State anxiety, physical activity, and urinary 3-methoxy-4-hydroxyphenethylene glycol excretion. Arch. Gen. Psychiatry **35**, 1418–1423 (1978b)

Terenius, L., Wahlström, A., Lindström, L., Widerlöv, E.: Increased CSF levels of endorphins in chronic psychosis. Neurosci. Letters **3**, 157–162 (1976)

Thölen, H., Stricker, E., Feer, H., Massini, M.-A., Staub, H.: Über die Anwendung der künstlichen Niere bei Schizophrenie und Myasthenia gravis. Dtsch. med. Wschr. **85**, 1012–1013 (1960)

Verhoeven, W.M.A., Praag, H.M. van, Botter, P.A., Sunier, A. Ree, J.M. van, Wied, D. de: Des-tyr[1]-endorphin in schizophrenia. Lancet **1978 I**, 1046–1047

Verhoeven, W.M.A., van Praag, H.M., van Ree, J.M., de Wied, D.: Improvement of schizophrenic patients treated with (des-tyr[1])-γ-endorphin (DTγE). Arch. Gen. Psychiatry **36**, 294–298 (1979)

Vestergaard, P., Sørensen, T., Hoppe, E., Rafaelsen, O.J., Yates, C.M., Nicolaou, N.: Biogenic amine metabolites in cerebrospinal fluid of patients with affective disorders. Acta Psychiat. Scand. **58**, 88–96 (1978)

Vetulani, J., Stawarz, R.J., Dingell, J.V., Sulser, F.: A possible common mechanism of action of antidepressant treatments: Reduction in the sensitivity of the noradrenergic cyclic AMP generating system. Naunyn-Schmiedeberg's Arch. Pharmacol. **293**, 109–114 (1976)

Volavka, J., Mallya, A., Baig, S., Perez-Cruet, J.: Naloxone in chronic schizophrenia. Science **196**, 1227–1228 (1977)

Wagemaker, H., Cade, R.: The use of hemodialysis in chronic schizophrenia. Am. J. Psychiatry **134**, 684–685 (1977)

Walter, D.S., Shilcock, G.M.: Urinary 3-methoxy-4-hydroxyphenylglycol, an index of peripheral rather than central adrenergic activity in the rat. J. Pharm. Pharmacol. **29**, 626–667 (1977)

Watson, S.J., Berger, P.A., Akil, H., Mills, M.J., Barchas, J.D.: Effects of naloxone on schizophrenia: Reduction in hallucinations in a subpopulation of subjects. Science **201**, 73–75 (1978)

Wied, D. de, Ree, J.M. van, Verhoeven, W.H., Praag, H.M. van: Endorphins and schizophrenia. II. World Congress of Biological Psychiatry. Barcelona, 1978

Wilk, S., Shopsin, B., Gershon, S., Suhl, M.: Cerebrospinal fluid levels of MHPG in affective disorders. Nature **235**, 440–441 (1972)

Wirz-Justice, A.: Theoretical and therapeutic potential of indoleamine precursors in affective disorders. Neuropsychobiology **3**, 199–233 (1977)

Wirz-Justice, A., Pühringer, W., Hole, G., Menzi, R.: Monoamine oxidase and free tryptophan in human plasma: normal variations and their implications for biochemical research in affective disorders. Pharmakopsychiat. **8**, 310–317 (1975)

Wise, C.D., Stein, L.: Dopamine-β-hydroxylase deficits in the brains of schizophrenic patients. Science **181**, 344–347 (1973)
Wise, C.D., Belluzzi, J.D., Stein, L.: Possible role of dopamine-β-hydroxylase in the regulation of norepinephrine biosynthesis in rat brain. Pharmacol. Biochem. Behav. **7**, 549–553 (1977)
Wittenborn, J.R.: A search for responders to niacin supplementation. Arch. Gen. Psychiatry **31**, 547–552 (1972)
Wurtman, R.J.: Relation between choline availability, acetylcholine synthesis and cholinergic function. Symposia Medica Hoechst: Depressive Disorders. Rom, Mai 1977
Wurtman, R.J., Larin, F., Mostafapour, S., Fernstrom, J.D.: Brain catechol synthesis: Control by brain tyrosine concentration. Science **185**, 183–184 (1974)
Wurtman, R.J., Cohen, E.L., Fernstrom, J.D.: Control of Brain Neurotransmitter Synthesis by Precursor Availability and Food Consumption. In: Neuroregulators and Psychiatric Disorders. New York: Oxford University Press 1977
Wyatt, R.J., Schwartz, T.Z., Schwartz, M.A., Erdelyi, E., Barchas, J.: Dopamine-β-hydroxylase activity in brains of chronic schizophrenics. Science **187**, 368–370 (1975)
Wyatt, R.J., Gillin, J.C., Stoff, D.M., Majo, E.A., Tinklenberg, J.R.: β-Phenylethylamine and the Neuropsychiatric Disturbances. In: Neuroregulators and Psychiatric Disorders. New York: Oxford University Press 1977
Zander, K.J., Ackenheil, M., Zimmer, R.: Biochemical Psychopathological Features in Chronic Schizophrenic Patients treated with Sulpiride. 7th International Congress of Pharmacology IUPHAR. Paris, Juli 1978

Ergänzende Hinweise und Literatur, die nach Manuskriptabgabe erschienen ist

Zur Zyklothymie

Noradrenalin- und Serotoninsystem: Im Kapitel „Zyklothymie" wurde unter Liquoruntersuchungen auf die Befunde von van Praag (1977a und b) hingewiesen, nach denen depressive Patienten mit niedriger 5-HIES-Konzentration im Liquor besser auf eine Behandlung mit 5-HTP ansprechen. Diese Untersuchungen sind in der Zwischenzeit von van Praag und Mitarbeitern erweitert worden. Es wurde gezeigt, daß bei depressiven Patienten mit niedriger 5-HIES-Liquorkonzentration nicht nur eine gute therapeutische, sondern sogar eine gute prophylaktische Wirkung mit 5-HTP in Kombination mit einem Decarboxylasehemmer zu erzielen ist (van Praag, 1979). Dieser Befund würde die 5-HT-Defizit-Hypothese stützen, doch bleiben bei den meisten Patienten auch nach Besserung die Liquor-5-HIES-Werte erniedrigt. Van Praag schließt daraus auf eine Prädisposition für Depressionen bei erniedrigter 5-HIES-Konzentration im Liquor. Nicht so eindeutig zugunsten der Bedeutung des 5-HT für die Depression läßt sich eine Untersuchung vom Karolinska-Institut mit Chlorimipramin interpretieren (Träskman et al., 1979). Dabei zeigte sich, daß Patienten mit „hohen" 5-HIES-Liquorwerten eine signifikante positive Korrelation zwischen Besserung der Depression und Plasmaspiegel von Desmethylchlorimipramin aufweisen. Desmethylchlorimipramin hemmt vorwiegend die NA-Aufnahme. In dieser Gruppe fand sich auch eine signifikante Beziehung zwischen Abnahme der MHPG-Konzentration und Besserung des psychopathologischen Zustands. Die

Autoren sehen darin eine weitere Stütze der Hypothese, daß Patienten mit „hohen" 5-HIES-Liquorwerten besser auf Antidepressiva ansprechen, die die NA-Aufnahme blockieren, also vorwiegend noradrenerge Neurone beeinflussen. Das würde bedeuten, daß bei diesen Patienten die Demethylierungsrate trizyklischer Thymoleptika für die antidepressive Therapie von Bedeutung ist, worauf auch die Liquorbefunde aus dem NIMH von MUSCETTOLA et al. (1978) mit Imipramin und unserer Klinik von JUNGKUNZ und KUSS (1978) mit Amitriptylin im Plasma bei unausgelesenen endogenen Depressionen hinweisen. In der Studie vom Karolinska-Institut mit Chlorimipramin ergab sich jedoch keine signifikante Beziehung in der Gruppe mit niedrigen 5-HIES-Liquorkonzentrationen zwischen Chlorimipraminplasmaspiegel und Besserung der Depression, was man fordern müßte, wenn die 5-HT-Aufnahmehemmung sich therapeutisch günstig bei depressiven Patienten mit einem niedrigen 5-HT-Umsatz auswirken würde.

Es fällt schwer, anhand der bisher vorliegenden Befunde die Bedeutung des Einflusses von Antidepressiva auf den 5-HT-Stoffwechsel für die Therapie einzuordnen. Erst kürzlich ist von MAJ et al. (1979), wie früher schon von FUXE et al. (1977) berichtet worden, daß Amitriptylin, ein anerkanntes und häufig verwendetes Antidepressivum, sogar postsynaptische Serotoninrezeptoren blockiert, was von Mianserin, Trazodone, Danitracen und Doxepin schon bekannt war (MAJ et al., 1977). Auch in der Studie von TRÄSKMAN et al. (1979) wird auf die 5-HT-blockierenden Eigenschaften des Chlorimipramins hingewiesen. Es wird deshalb auch überlegt, ob bei der Depression ein „überempfindlicher" postsynaptischer 5-HT-Rezeptor vorliegt (SHAW et al., 1977; APRISON et al., 1978). Wenn man auf der einen Seite bei endogen depressiven Patienten mit postsynaptischen 5-HT-Rezeptorblockern gute antidepressive Wirkung erzielt, auf der anderen Seite jedoch 5-HTP über ein zusätzliches 5-HT-Angebot am Rezeptor therapeutisch wirksam ist, muß es unterschiedliche Gruppen depressiver Patienten geben. Diese Frage gilt es in Zukunft zu klären.

Während MHPG bisher in klinisch-biochemischen Untersuchungen bei depressiven Patienten nur im Liquor bestimmt wurde (s. entsprechendes Kapitel bei der Zyklothymie), liegen jetzt auch erste interessante Plasma-MHPG-Befunde vor. Unter antidepressiver Therapie kommt es dabei in den ersten beiden Wochen zu einem signifikanten Anstieg der Plasma-MHPG-Spiegel, die in der 3. und 4. Woche wieder abfallen, jedoch noch über dem extrem niedrigen Ausgangswert vor Beginn der Therapie liegen (HALARIS und DEMET, 1979). Dies hängt mit den Stoffwechselveränderungen an den noradrenergen Nervenendigungen im Verlauf der Therapie zusammen, in die auch die Rezeptoren einbezogen sind. Das Plasma-MHPG verhält sich hierbei entgegengesetzt als das Liquor-MHPG in der oben erwähnten Studie von TRÄSKMAN et al. (1979). Hirn und Peripherie werden also nicht gleichsinnig reguliert. Wegen der sehr schwierigen Plasma-MHPG-Bestimmung müssen noch weitere Untersuchungen abgewartet werden, obwohl sich die erhaltenen Ergebnisse zwanglos mit den nachstehenden Befunden in Übereinstimmung bringen lassen.

Rezeptor-Hypothese: In einer sehr interessanten Studie untersuchten COPPEN und GHOSE (1978) die periphere α-Adrenorezeptor- und die zentrale DA-Rezeptorempfindlichkeit. Dabei zeigten mit Tyramin, NA und Phenylephrin endogen depressive Patienten im Blutdrucktest (pressor response test) mit allen 3 Substanzen ein signifikant stärkeres Ansprechen gegenüber Kontrollen, d.h. bei Depressiven vermag eine signifikant geringere Dosis der 3 blutdrucksteigernden Mittel den systolischen Blutdruck um 30 mm/Hg anzuheben. Da Phenylephrin ein peripherer direkter α-Adrenorezeptoragonist mit geringer β-Wirkung ist, interpretieren die Autoren ihre Befunde mit Recht in dem Sinne, daß bei endogen depressiven Patienten eine erhöhte periphere α-Adrenorezeptorempfindlichkeit vorliegt. Erhöhte Rezeptorempfindlichkeit verringert über einen Rückkopplungsmechanismus die NA-Biosynthese, und HALARIS und DEMET (1979) fanden bei ihren Patienten auch extrem niedrige MHPG-Ausgangswerte, die auf einen geringen NA-Umsatz hinweisen. Unter der Therapie steigen die MHPG-Werte wieder an, und mit Besserung der Depression nimmt die Rezeptorempfindlichkeit im Blutdrucktest wieder ab. Die Blutdruckeffekte mit Phenylephrin sind kein Hinweis auf die Empfindlichkeit zentraler α-Rezeptoren, was von den Autoren auch ausdrücklich betont wird. Sie können daher nicht als Widerspruch zur geringen α-Rezeptorempfindlichkeit angesehen werden, die aus den oben angeführten neuroendokrinologischen Daten geschlossen wurde. Wir wissen heute, daß der Effekt einer Droge nicht nur in einzelnen Hirnarealen unterschiedlich sein, sondern auch entgegengesetzte periphere und zentrale Wirkungen hervorrufen kann. – Im 2. Teil der Arbeit zeigen COPPEN und GHOSE (1978) im Bromocriptin-Test, daß die zentrale DA-Rezeptorempfindlichkeit bei depressiven Patienten nicht verändert ist, worauf im neuroendokrinologischen Kapitel anhand anderer Arbeiten schon hingewiesen wurde.

Hypothalamus-Hypophysen-Nebennierenrinden-System: Weitere Ergebnisse sind in der Zwischenzeit mit dem Dexamethason-Hemmtest erhalten worden. CARROLL (1979) modifizierte diesen Test, so daß er jetzt leichter bei stationären, aber auch ambulanten Patienten durchzuführen ist. Zwischen 23.00 und 24.00 Uhr wird 1 mg Dexamethason verabfolgt. Am nächsten Tag erfolgt nur eine Blutabnahme zur Cortisolbestimmung zwischen 16.00 und 17.00 Uhr. Damit wurden die früher erhobenen Befunde an weiteren uni- und bipolaren Patienten erweitert und die Differenzierung zu neurotisch Depressiven erhärtet. Auch die in Iowa untersuchten verschiedenen genetischen Formen unipolarer Depressionen unterschieden sich im Dexamethason-Hemmtest (SCHLESSER et al., 1979). Bei der sog. familiär bedingten reinen Depression („familial pure depressive disease") findet bei 82% keine Cortisolsuppression nach Dexamethason statt, während nur bei 37% sporadisch auftretender Depressionen („sporadic depressive disease") und 4% der sog. „depression spectrum disease" keine Suppression gefunden wurde. Die erste Gruppe ist mit unserer unipolaren endogenen Depression vergleichbar, die also in einem hohen Prozentsatz nicht supprimiert. Bei bipolaren Depressionen, deren nosologische Zuordnung am sichersten ist, liegt der Anteil, der keine Suppression im Dexamethason-Hemmtest zeigt, noch höher.

Zur Schizophrenie

Dopaminrezeptorempfindlichkeit: Im Zusammenhang mit der erhöhten DA-Rezeptorempfindlichkeit bei schizophrenen Patienten wären weitere Arbeiten von Cross et al. (1978) und Lee et al (1978) an post mortem Hirnen zu erwähnen. Dabei zeigte sich im Caudatus, Putamen und Nucleus accumbens eine signifikant höhere Spiroperidol- bzw. Haloperidolbindung bei Schizophrenen gegenüber Kontrollen. Da die Zahl nicht mit Neuroleptika behandelter Fälle bisher gering ist, muß man mit der Interpretation der Befunde vorsichtig sein. Aus diesem Grund erscheint es wichtig, die DA-Rezeptorempfindlichkeit bei akuten unbehandelten Schizophrenen mit Apomorphin weiterhin zu untersuchen, um diese wichtige Frage eindeutig beantworten zu können.

β-Endorphin: In einer sorgfältigen Studie von Emrich et al. (1979) zeigten sich mit einem empfindlichen und weitgehend spezifischen β-Endorphin-Radioimmunoassay weder im Plasma noch im Liquor schizophrener Patienten erhöhte β-Endorphinkonzentrationen, worüber vorher Terenius et al. (1976) und Lindström et al. (1978) berichtet hatten. Auch bei anderen psychiatrischen und neurologischen Krankheiten wurden in dieser Studie keine signifikanten Endorphinveränderungen gefunden. Diese Diskrepanz hängt sicherlich mit der bis vor kurzem noch sehr unspezifischen Bestimmungsmethode für die Endorphine zusammen, die in der Zwischenzeit verbessert wurde. Die möglichen Beziehungen zwischen Endorphinen, Dopamin und Schizophrenie wurden ausführlich von Volavka et al. (1979) beschrieben und von Watson und Atil (1979) und Usdin (1979) kritisch diskutiert (s. dazu auch Davis et al., 1979).

Literatur

Aprison, M.H., Takahashi, R., Tachiki, K.: Hypersensitive serotonergic receptors involved in clinical depression – a therory. In: Neuropharmacology and Behavior. Plenum Publishing Corporation 1978

Carroll, B.J.: Biogenic amines and neuroendocrine disturbance in depression. Symposium on "Biogenic Amines and Affective Disorders", London: 1979

Coppen, A., Ghose, K.: Peripheral α-adrenoreceptor and central dopamine receptor activity in depressive patients. Psychopharmacology **59**, 171–177 (1978)

Cross, A.J., Crow, T.J., Longden, A., Owen, F., Poulter, M., Riley, G.J.: Evidence for increased dopamine receptor sensitivity in post mortem brains from patients with schizophrenia. J. Physiol. **280**, 37 (1978)

Davis, G.C., Buchsbaum, M.S., Bunney, W.E. jr.: Research in endorphins and schizophrenia. Schizophrenia Bulletin **5**, 244–254 (1979)

Emrich, H.M., Höllt, V., Kissling, W., Fischler, M., Laspe, H., Heinemann, H., v. Zerssen, D., Herz, A.: β-endorphin-like immunoreactivity in cerebrospinal fluid and plasma of patients with schizophrenia and other neuropsychiatric disorders. Pharmakopsychiat. **12**, 269–276 (1979)

Fuxe, K., Ögren, S.-O., Aganati, L., Gustafsson, J.K., Jonsson, G.: On the mechanism of action of the antidepressant drugs amitriptyline and nortriptyline. Evidence for 5-hydroxytryptamine receptor blocking activity. Neurosci. Letters **6**, 339–344 (1977)

Halaris, A.E., DeMet, E.M.: Effects of the potential antidepressant AHR-1118 on amine uptake and on plasma 3-methoxy-4-hydroxyphenylglycol in manic-depressive illness. Psychopharmacology Bulletin **15**, 95–97 (1979)

Jungkunz, G., Kuss, H.J.: Amitriptyline and its demethylation rate. Lancet II, 1263–1264 (1978)

Van Kammen, D.P.: The dopamine hypothesis of schizophrenia revisited. Psychoneuroendocrinology **4**, 37–46 (1979)

Lee, T., Seeman, P., Toutellotte, W.W., Farley, I.J., Hornykiewicz, O.: Binding of ^{3}H-neuroleptics and ^{3}H-apomorphine in schizophrenic brains. Nature **274**, 897–900 (1978)

Lindström, L.H., Widerlöv, E., Gunne, L.-M., Wahlström, A., Terenius, L.: Endorphins in human cerebrospinal fluid: Clinical correlations to some psychotic states. Acta psychiat. scand. **57**, 153–164 (1978)

Maj, J., Gancarczyk, E., Gorszczyk, A., Rantow, A.: Doxepin as a blocker of central serotonin receptors. Pharmakopsychiat. **10**, 318–324 (1977)

Maj, J., Lewandowska, A., Rantow, A.: Central antiserotonin action of amitriptyline. Pharmakopsychiat. **12**, 281–285 (1979)

Muscettola, G., Goodwin, F.K., Potter, W.Z., Claeys, M.M., Markey, S.P.: Imipramine and desipramine in plasma and spinal fluid. Relationship to clinical response and serotonin metabolism. Arch. Gen. Psychiatry **35**, 621–625 (1978)

Praag, H.M. van: Central serotonin. Its relation to depression and depression prophylaxis. In: Biological Psychiatry Today. Amsterdam: Elsevier 1979

Schlesser, M.A., Winokur, G., Sherman, B.M.: Genetic subtypes of unipolar primary depressive illness distinguished by hypothalamic-pituitary-adrenal axis activity. Lancet I, 739–741 (1979)

Shaw, D.M., Riley, G.J., Michalakeas, A.C., Tidmarsh, S.F., Blazek, R., Johnson, A.L.: New direction to the amine hypothesis. Lancet I, 1259–1260 (1977)

Träskman, L., Åsberg, M., Bertilsson, L., Cronholm, B., Mellström, B., Neckers, L.M., Sjöqvist, F., Thorén, P., Tybring, G.: Plasma levels of chlorimipramine and its demethyl metabolite during treatment of depression. Differential biochemical and clinical effects of the two compounds. Clin. Pharmacol. Therapy (im Druck)

Usdin, E.: Endorphins, dopamine, and schizophrenia. Schizophrenia Bulletin **5**, 242–243 (1979)

Volavka, J., Davis, L.G., Ehrlich, Y.H.: Endorphins, dopamine and schizophrenia. Schizophrenia Bulletin **5**, 227–239 (1979)

Watson, S.J., Akil, H.: Endorphins, dopamine, and schizophrenia. Schizophrenia Bulletin **5**, 240–241 (1979)

Elektroenzephalographie und Psychiatrie

Von

H. Künkel

Inhalt

A. Einleitung 116
B. Die Grundphänomene des Elektroenzephalogramms 117
    I. Die elektroenzephalographische Grundaktivität 118
    II. Modifikationen der Grundaktivität 120
    III. Diskontinuierlich auftretende Aktivitätsformen 124
    IV. Zur Epidemiologie von EEG-Aktivitätsmustern 126
    V. Chronobiologische Aspekte 130
    VI. Zur diagnostischen „Spezifität" elektroenzephalographischer Befunde 132
A. Aspekte der EEG-Analyse und ihrer Auswertung 133
    I. Entwicklung der EEG-Analyse und einige ihrer Voraussetzungen 133
    II. Amplituden-Integration 134
    III. Period Analysis 138
    IV. Spektral-Analyse 140
    V. Daten- und Informationsreduktion 145
D. Grundphänomene evozierter und ereignisbezogener Potentiale 147
    I. Anmerkungen zur Methodik 147
    II. Visuell evozierte Reizantworten (VER) 148
    III. Akustisch evozierte Reizantworten (AER) 151
    IV. Somatosensorisch evozierte Reizantworten (SSER) 152
    V. Contingent Negative Variation (CNV) 152
    VI. Bereitschaftspotentiale, motorische Potentiale 153
    VII. Ergänzende Bemerkungen 154
E. EEG und Koma 155
    I. Grundsätzliche EEG-Veränderungen, Klassifikation von Koma-Stadien 155
    II. EEG-Befunde im Koma 157
    III. Modifikationen durch ätiologische Besonderheiten 157
    IV. Modifikationen durch topographische Besonderheiten 158
    V. Evozierte Potentiale im Koma 158
    VI. Ergänzende Bemerkungen 159
F. Symptomatische Psychosen und EEG 160
    I. Stoffwechselstörungen, endokrine Störungen 160
    II. Gefäßprozesse, Hypoxidosen 162
    III. Entzündungen des ZNS 162
    IV. Hirntraumen, EKT 163
    V. Intoxikationen und Entzugs-Syndrome 164
    VI. Syndromgenetische und verlaufsdynamische Aspekte 165

G. Epileptische Dämmerzustände, Psychosen und Verstimmungen 166
    I. Das EEG im Anfall und Intervall 166
    II. Dämmerzustände, Petit mal-Status, Status psychomotoricus 167
    III. Epileptische Psychosen und Verstimmungszustände. 170
    IV. Verlaufsdynamische Aspekte 170
H. EEG und endogene Psychosen 171
    I. Das EEG bei Schizophrenien 171
    II. EEG-Analyse bei schizophrenen Psychosen 172
    III. Evozierte und ereignisbezogene Potentiale bei schizophrenen Psychosen 175
    IV. Das EEG bei depressiven und manisch-depressiven Psychosen 176
    V. Verlaufsdynamische und syndromgenetische Aspekte 176
    VI. EEG und Hypothesenbildung 177
I. Quantitative Pharmako-Elektroenzephalographie 179
    I. EEG und Veränderungen des Verhaltens sowie der Befindlichkeit unter Medikationswirkungen 179
    II. Elektroenzephalographische Wirkungsprofile psychotroper Substanzen 180
J. Schluß. 181
Literatur 182

A. Einleitung

Die Bedeutung des Elektroenzephalogramms für die Psychiatrie ist lange Zeit mit großer Skepsis beurteilt worden. Noch 1967 kommt JUNG in der 1. Auflage dieses Werkes zu der Feststellung, daß das EEG nur im Zusammenhang mit normalen Bewußtseinsänderungen und pathologischen Bewußtseinsstörungen, insbesondere bei epileptischen Psychosen, ferner bei organischen Psychosen und bei Somato-Therapien von Psychosen für den Psychiater eine Rolle spiele. Diese Situation hat sich jedoch inzwischen gewandelt. Hierfür waren zum einen methodische Neuerungen maßgeblich, wie die Entwicklung der EEG-Analyse und die Technik der Registrierung evozierter und ereignisbezogener Potentiale, zum anderen auf der klinisch-psychiatrischen Seite die Blickwendung von einer mehr nosologisch orientierten Betrachtungsweise mit ihrem fragwürdigen Begriff von Krankheitseinheiten und einem monokausalen Denken hin zu Syndrom-Begriffen, die das Bedingungsgefüge psychopathologischer Phänomene wie auch eine Verlaufstypologie einzubeziehen suchen. Diese beiden Elemente der in den letzten Jahren erreichten Fortschritte auf dem Gebiet zwischen Elektroenzephalographie und Psychiatrie sind noch nicht auf allen Teilbereichen wirksam geworden, werden jedoch in der folgenden Darstellung wiederholt anklingen.

Auf der Seite der Elektroenzephalographie hat sich eine Reihe von methodischen Problemen gestellt, deren ungenügende Berücksichtigung die Ergebnisse der in der überwiegenden Mehrzahl querschnittsorientierten Vergleichsuntersuchungen früherer Jahre bestenfalls als vorläufig zu akzeptieren erlaubt. So ist etwa der Einfluß von Alter und Geschlecht auf die Häufigkeit normaler und pathologischer EEG-Befunde – wohl auch wegen nicht genügend differenzierter Kenntnis hierzu – oft unberücksichtigt geblieben. Die ihrem Grunde nach statistische Natur unseres Wissens über die hirnelektrische Aktivität und ihre Modifikationen ist erst anhand der Datenfülle bewußt geworden, die von den verschiedenen Verfahren zur quantitativen EEG-Analyse angeboten wird. Ihre Bewältigung forderte die Auseinandersetzung mit Verfahren der analytischen, vor allem der multivariaten Statistik, die nicht nur Möglichkeiten zur Erforschung komplexer Bedingungsgefüge boten, sondern die – kritisch eingesetzt – auch den Blick von eindimensionalen Zusammenhängen hin zu Strukturbeziehungen in mehrdimensionalen Begriffsräumen lenken werden. Wenn auch heute noch die sehr komplexe Methodik aus statistischer Versuchsplanung, Stichprobendefinitionen, Kontrolle von bekannten und Ausgleich von unbekannten Einflußgrößen über die Untersuchungstechniken bis hin zur Extraktion relevanter Information aus der Fülle elektroenzephalographischer und klinischer Daten ungewohnt ist, so darf man doch auf eine zunehmende Vertrautheit mit diesen Methoden Hoffnungen setzen. Experimentelle Psychologie und empirische Soziologie haben einige methodische Schritte vorgezeichnet. Soweit heute zu beurteilen, werden wesentliche Determinanten künftiger Erfolge in der psychiatrisch-elektrophysiologischen Forschung zunächst vorwiegend im klinischen Bereich liegen.

Von elektroenzephalographischer Seite stehen einige Werkzeuge bereit. Zumindest für den mehr biologisch interessierten Psychiater ist eine Kenntnis wenigstens der Grundphänomene des normalen und pathologischen EEG erforderlich, die in Abschn. B zusammen mit einigen weiterführenden Aspekten erörtert werden. Gleiches gilt für die EEG-Analyse, die Einblicke in die strukturellen Beziehungen der hirnelektrischen Aktivität eröffnet, die der visuellen EEG-Auswertung verschlossen bleiben (Abschn. C). Die in Abschn. D dargestellten evozierten und ereignisbezogenen Potentiale erlauben das Studium von Prozessen der Reiz- und Informationsverarbeitung unter normalen und pathologischen Bedingungen, deren Gewicht für psychiatrische Fragen nicht gering zu schätzen ist. Die Abschn. E–I geben, bedingt durch den zur Verfügung stehenden begrenzten Raum, Überblicke über eine Auswahl von Sachgebieten, zu denen das EEG mehr oder weniger beigetragen hat.

Die EEG-Literatur auch nur zu diesen Bereichen mit annähernder Vollständigkeit darzustellen, ist weder möglich noch sinnvoll. Den meisten Abschnitten wurden Hinweise auf zusammenfassende Monographien oder Übersichtsarbeiten vorangestellt, die eine detailliertere Orientierung erlauben. Einen Überblick über die Gesamtheit des heutigen elektroenzephalographischen Wissens bietet, wenn auch nicht immer mit gleichem Schwergewicht, das von Rémond herausgegebene Handbook of Electroencephalography and Clinical Neurophysiology (1971–1977), auf dessen Bände an geeigneter Stelle jeweils hingewiesen wird. Eine vollständige Bibliographie der älteren EEG-Literatur wurde von M.A.B. Brazier (1950) herausgegeben; eine laufende Bibliographie der EEG-Literatur erscheint, nach Sachgebieten geordnet, regelmäßig im Journal of Electroencephalography and Clinical Neurophysiology.[1] Nach Schlüsselworten gegliederte Bibliographien sind in den Supplementen 29 und 30 zum EEG-Journal sowie von Bickford et al. (1965) verfügbar.

B. Die Grundphänomene des Elektroenzephalogramms

Eine umfassende Darstellung des EEG, seiner normalen Variationen und pathologischen Veränderungen ist hier nicht beabsichtigt.

Zur Orientierung steht eine Reihe von deutschsprachigen Lehrbüchern zur Verfügung, von denen hier die von Christian (1975), Dumermuth (1976), Kugler (1966), Simon (1977) genannt

---

[1] Anm. bei der Korrektur: Dieser Literaturdienst des Brain Information Service der University of California, Los Angeles, ist inzwischen eingestellt worden.

seien, während COOPER et al. (1974) die mehr technischen Aspekte der EEG-Registrierung und -Auswertung darstellen. Als Atlas noch kaum übertroffen ist das dreibändige Werk von F.A. GIBBS und E.L. GIBBS (1950–1964).

Im folgenden werden die elektroenzephalographischen Grundphänomene besprochen, soweit sie für ein allgemeines Verständnis des EEG und für die im Zusammenhang mit psychiatrischen Fragestellungen referierten Befunde erforderlich scheinen. Überwiegend neurologisch interessierende Fragen werden nur gelegentlich gestreift werden. Mehr Gewicht wird dagegen auf epidemiologische und chronobiologische Aspekte gelegt, die in den einschlägigen Lehrbüchern meist unzureichend behandelt werden, deren Kenntnis jedoch für die Bewertung von im Zusammenhang mit Psychosen mitgeteilten Befunden und für die Beurteilung der Tragfähigkeit aus ihnen gezogener Schlüsse bedeutsam ist.

I. Die elektroenzephalographische Grundaktivität

Sofern nicht eine äußerst schwere allgemein-zerebrale und damit auch elektroenzephalographische Funktionsstörung vorliegt, zeigt sich bei dem üblicherweise in 8–16 Kanälen registrierten EEG eine sowohl zeitlich, als auch topographisch differenzierte kontinuierliche Wellenfolge, die einem Frequenzbereich von etwa 0,5/s bis über 30/s entstammt. Ober- und Untergrenze dieses Bereiches werden wesentlich durch die technischen Parameter der EEG-Verstärker beeinflußt, die Obergrenze maßgeblich auch durch die elektrischen Leitungseigenschaften der Strukturen zwischen Hirnoberfläche und Elektroden. Für die „klassische", visuelle EEG-Auswertung hat sich die Aufteilung in eine Reihe von Frequenzbändern als praktisch erwiesen, die in Tabelle 1 dargestellt ist. (Mit der Entwicklung der Spektralanalyse des EEG's hat sich allerdings bald herausgestellt, daß solche starren Grenzen der Realität nicht immer entsprechen und z.B. bei der Beurteilung von zerebralen Medikationswirkungen irreführen können.) Diese kontinuierliche Wellenfolge des EEG wird als *Grund- oder Hintergrundaktivität* bezeichnet. Je nachdem ob Wellen aus einzelnen der genannten Frequenzbänder in ihrer zeitlichen Häufigkeit, ihrer „Ausprägung", überwiegen, läßt sich eine *Alpha-, Beta-, Theta- oder Delta-Aktivität* unterscheiden. Dabei ist nicht zu übersehen, daß sich – auch im „normalen" EEG des Erwachsenen – stets Anteile aus allen Frequenzbändern nachweisen lassen. Typischerweise zeigen diese einzelnen Aktivitäten Schwerpunkte der topographischen Verteilung, so etwa – grosso modo – Alpha-Aktivität über den hinteren, Beta-Aktivität über den vorderen, Theta-Aktivität über den temporalen Hirnabschnitten. Überwiegt in einem EEG eine dieser Aktivitäten so, daß sie die Grundaktivität

Tabelle 1. Frequenzbereiche des EEG

	Frequenz (Hz)
Delta	0,5–3,5
Theta	>3,5–7,5
Alpha	>7,5–13
Beta	>13–32

charakterisiert, so läßt sich das EEG eingliedern (JUNG, 1953) etwa als *EEG vom Alpha-Typ* (Abb. 1) oder *Beta-Typ* (Abb. 2). Entsprechend bildet ein Gemisch beider Aktivitäten ein EEG vom *partiellen Beta-Typ*. Tritt u.a. ein größerer Anteil an Theta-Wellen hinzu, so liegt ein *unregelmäßiges EEG* vor. Überschreiten schließlich die Amplituden der Wellen, gemessen von Spitze zu Spitze, 20 µV nicht und liegt kein EEG vom β-Typ vor, so wird das EEG als *flaches EEG* bezeichnet. Die genannten EEG-Typen stellen zwar nicht alle, aber mit einer Gesamthäufigkeit von etwa 95% die häufigsten Normvarianten der EEG-Grundaktivität dar, die sich bei gesunden Probanden unter Standardbedingungen (Untersuchung bei hinreichender körperlicher und psychischer Entspannung, im Wachzustand, bei geschlossenen Augen) registrieren läßt.

Der individuelle Typ der Grundaktivität ist offenbar genetisch bedingt, wenn auch nicht alle Faktoren schon hinreichend überschaubar sind. Offensichtlich gilt die Erblichkeit weitgehend für das Beta-EEG, wie auch für das flache EEG, von denen autosomal dominante Erblichkeit angenommen wird (VOGEL, 1958, 1962, 1963; VOGEL u. GÖTZE, 1959; RICHTER, 1960).

Wegen der Besonderheiten des kindlichen EEG und seiner Entwicklung bis zur Adoleszenz vergleiche DUMERMUTH (1976).

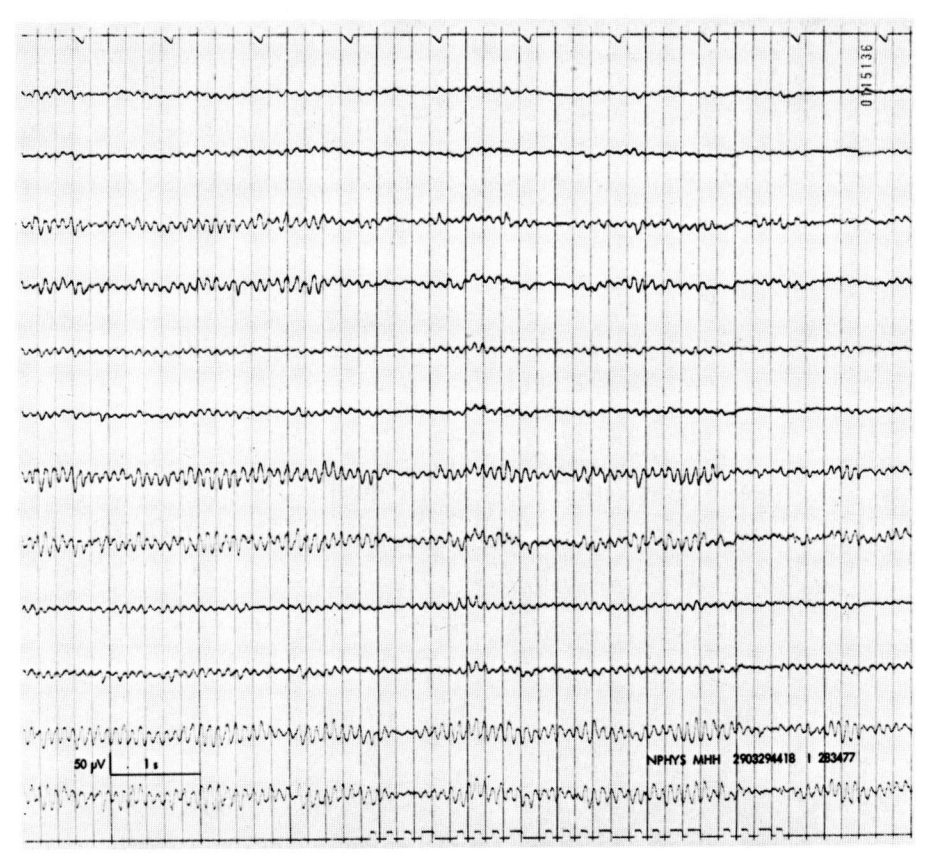

Abb. 1. EEG vom Alpha-Typ

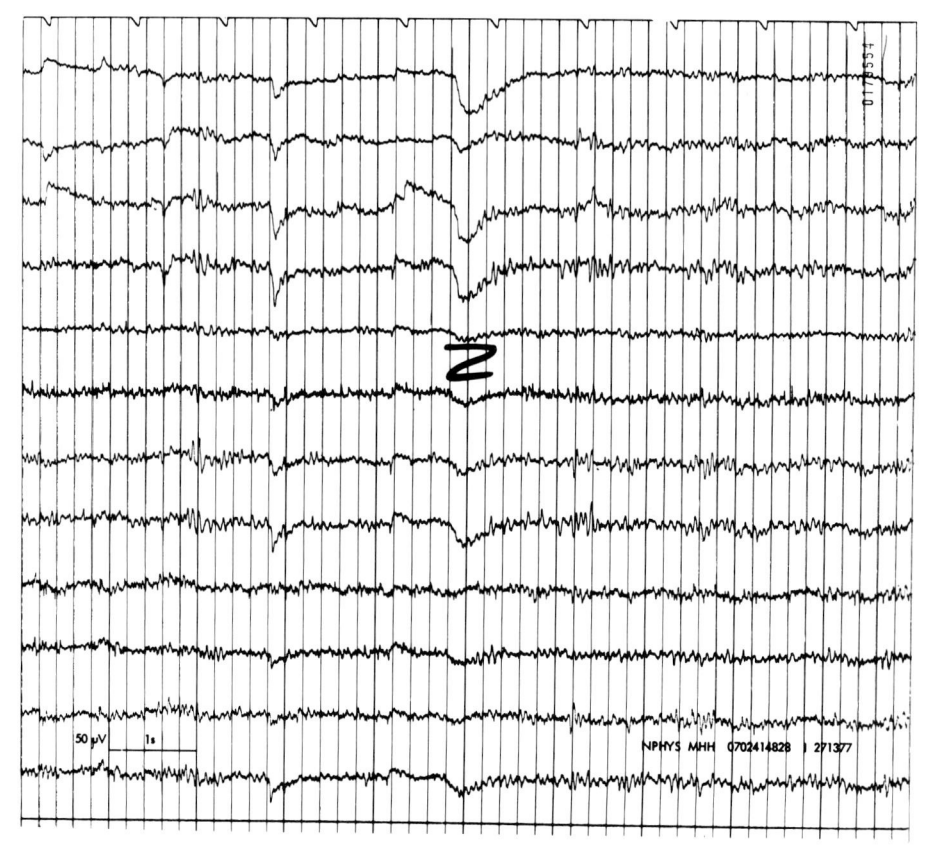

Abb. 2. EEG vom Beta-Typ

II. Modifikationen der Grundaktivität

Die Grundaktivität des EEG kann unter dem Einfluß sehr heterogener Faktoren in verschiedenen Richtungen modifiziert werden, von denen hier vornehmlich zwei, die Allgemeinveränderungen und die Herdbefunde, herausgegriffen seien.

Nimmt die Ausprägung von Theta-Wellen, schließlich auch von Delta-Wellen so zu, daß sie innerhalb der Grundaktivität zunehmend in den Vordergrund treten und endlich dominieren, so wird dies im deutschen Sprachgebrauch als *Allgemeinveränderung* bezeichnet. Dabei bleibt die annähernd seitengleiche Ausprägung zumindest bei visueller Auswertung weitgehend erhalten, während sich die topographischen Schwerpunkte von Theta- und Delta-Aktivität zunehmend verwischen und eine Ausbreitung über beide Hemisphären erfolgt. Im praktischen Gebrauch lassen sich mehrere Schweregrade von Allgemeinveränderungen gegeneinander abgrenzen, die gewissermaßen Abschnitte einer gleitenden Reihe darstellen. An ihrem Anfang steht die leichte Allgemeinveränderung, bei der zwar noch die „normale" Grundaktivität dominieren kann, indessen bereits eine deutliche Zunahme von Theta-Wellen über allen Hirnregionen ins Auge

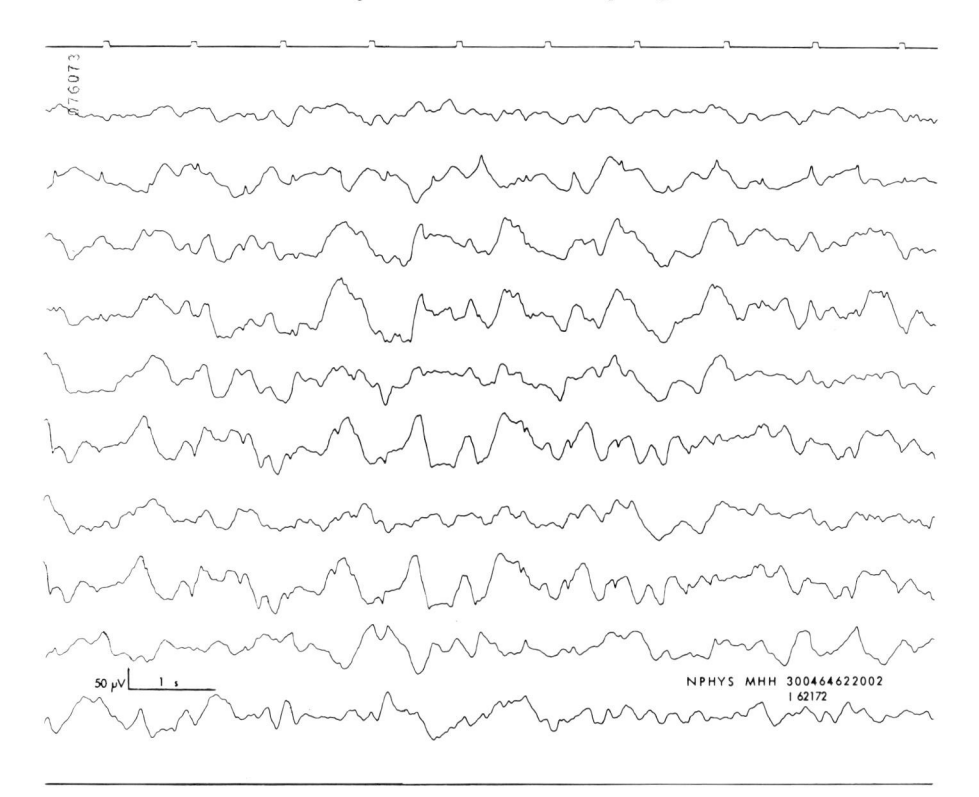

Abb. 3. Schwere Allgemeinveränderung

fällt, von ihrem temporalen Schwerpunkt ausgehend. Am anderen Ende steht die schwere Allgemeinveränderung (Abb. 3), bei der die Delta-Aktivität dominiert und Alpha- oder Beta-Wellen praktisch nicht mehr erkennbar sind. Qualitativ und quantitativ etwas andere Kriterien bietet die „burst-suppression"-Aktivität (Abb. 4), die gekennzeichnet ist durch Gruppen von Delta-Theta-Wellen, gelegentlich überlagert auch von rascheren Wellen. Diese Gruppen werden durch Strecken sehr niederamplitudiger EEG-Aktivität voneinander getrennt. Sie findet sich in tiefen Narkosestadien, aber auch bei schweren Intoxikationen; schließlich auch als Übergang zum sog. „Null-Linien-EEG", bei dem eine hirneigene elektrische Aktivität nicht mehr nachweisbar ist.

Einen gänzlich anderen Sachverhalt zeigt die *kontinuierliche Dysrhythmie*, die durch eine Vermehrung von Theta-Wellen, schließlich auch Delta-Wellen neben anderen Graphoelementen, wie steileren Abläufen, gekennzeichnet ist. Diese Aktivitätsform ist zwar grundsätzlich bilateral symmetrisch ausgeprägt, hebt sich aber durch ihren eindeutigen topographischen Schwerpunkt – beim Erwachsenen meist beiderseits temporo-frontal – von der fortbestehenden Grundaktivität des EEG ab (Abb. 5).

Der Gebrauch des Begriffes „Dysrhythmie" wird zwar von der Terminologie-Kommission der internationalen EEG-Föderation abgelehnt (CHATRIAN et al., 1974; BRAZIER et al., 1961), sie ver-

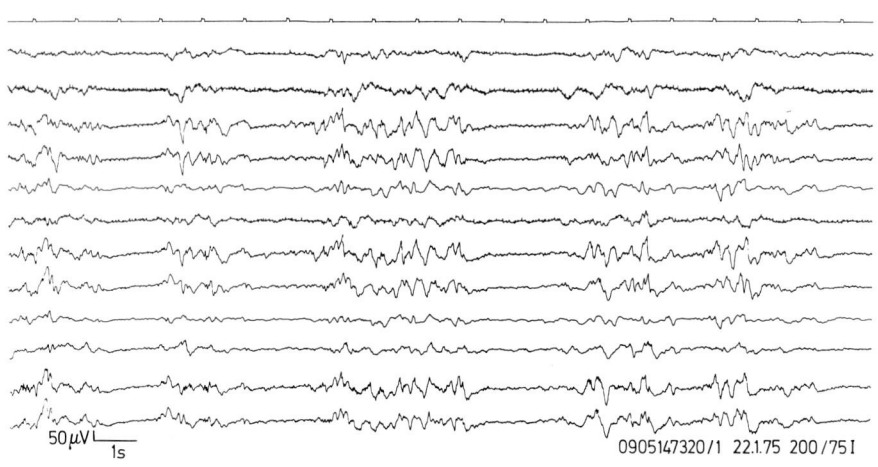

Abb. 4. „Burst-suppression"-Aktivität

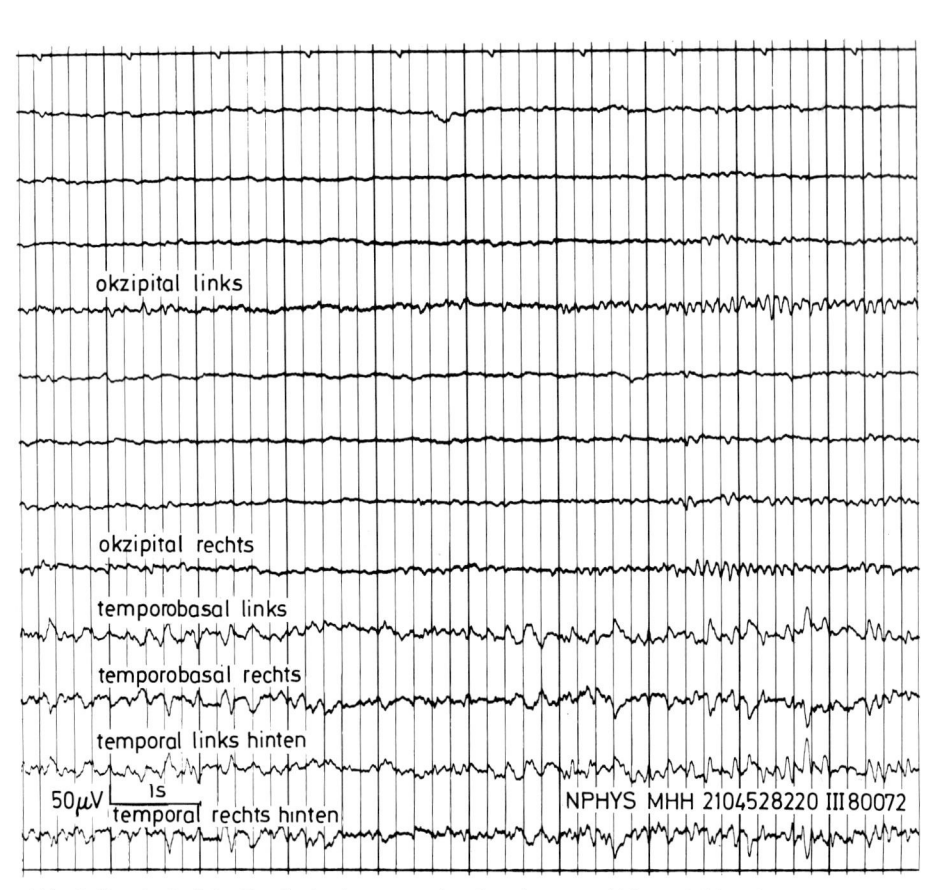

Abb. 5. Kontinuierliche Dysrhythmie temporobasal und temporal hinten beiderseits (vgl. den Kontrast zu den übrigen Kanälen, insbesondere auch okzipital beiderseits)

mochte sich indessen damit nicht durchzusetzen. Der so definierte Terminus beschreibt recht treffend die evidente Dys-Rhythmik dieser Form von EEG-Aktivität. Entsprechendes gilt für die gruppierte Dysrhythmie (s. unten).

Eine Abweichung vom Postulat der zwar topographisch differenzierten, aber bilateral symmetrisch ausgeprägten Grundaktivität wird als *Herdstörung* bezeichnet. Sie ist damit im Prinzip unilateral, zumindest eindeutig seitenbetont, innerhalb der betroffenen Hemisphäre wiederum mehr oder weniger umschrieben lokalisiert. Neben vielen anderen Formen von Graphoelementen spielt wiederum die Vermehrung von Theta- und Delta-Wellen eine wesentliche Rolle, die an der Stelle des Herdes die Grundaktivität des EEG unterlagern oder auch zunehmend verdrängen (Abb. 6). Ungeachtet ihres fokalen Schwerpunktes kann sich eine solche Herdaktivität auch auf benachbarte Regionen ausbreiten, mitunter auch eine ganze Hemisphäre mit annähernd gleicher Intensität erfassen. Auch bei Herdstörungen lassen sich, je nach dem Anteil von Theta- und Delta-Wellen, verschiedene Schweregrade für den praktischen Gebrauch unterscheiden.

Es kann nicht oft und deutlich genug betont werden, daß die genannten Modifikationen der Grundaktivität keineswegs notwendig als Ausdruck einer

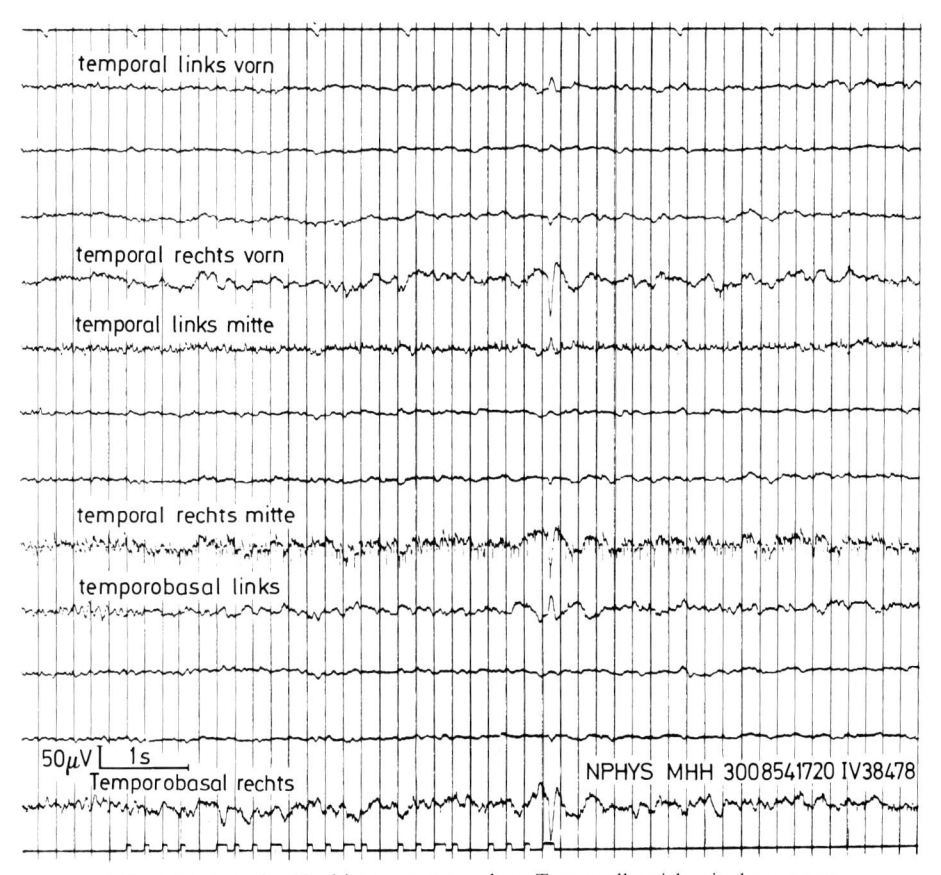

Abb. 6. Theta-Delta-Herd im gesamten rechten Temporalbereich mit sharp wave

morphologisch faßbaren Substanzschädigung des Gehirns zu interpretieren sind, wie es einem in der Geschichte der klinischen Anwendung der Elektroenzephalographie lange Zeit vorherrschenden und sich erst langsam zurückbildenden Mißverständnis entsprach. Zwar können Substanzschädigungen etwa durch Traumen, Entzündungsprozesse, vaskuläre Störungen, Tumoren, um nur einige zu nennen, im EEG zwar Allgemeinveränderungen wie auch Herdstörungen oder Kombinationen davon bewirken, indessen nur insoweit, als sie zu allgemeinen oder lokalen Änderungen oder Störungen der hirnelektrischen Funktionen führen. Störungen des zerebralen oder primär extrazerebralen Stoffwechsels können, ebenso wie zerebrale Medikationswirkung durch z.B. Psychopharmaka, vergleichbare Modifikationen der Grundaktivität bewirken. Davon unberührt bleibt die Tatsache, daß vor allem Bewußtseinsstörungen in besonderer Weise mit Allgemeinveränderungen korrelieren, so daß der Schweregrad einer Allgemeinveränderung vom Sopor bis hin zum tiefen Koma zunimmt. Auch hier bestätigen eher gewisse Ausnahmen diese Regel.

III. Diskontinuierlich auftretende Aktivitätsformen

Von der kontinuierlich ablaufenden Grundaktivität des EEG hebt sich eine Reihe von Potentialformen oder Graphoelementen ab, die einzeln oder gruppiert auftreten. Ihre Häufigkeit kann vom sporadischen Auftreten bis zu annähernd rhythmischer Wiederkehr im gleichen EEG wechseln. Sie überlagern meist, ersetzen aber auch nicht selten die dazwischen fortbestehende Grundaktivität. Im folgenden werden nur die für psychiatrische Fragestellungen bislang bedeutsamen Aktivitätsformen besprochen.

Die gruppierte Dysrhythmie ist charakterisiert durch abrupt auftretende Gruppen von polymorphen Graphoelementen (Theta-Delta-Wellen, steileren Abläufen) mit einer Dauer von meist weniger als 5 sec, die sich durch ihre Polymorphie und ihre deutlich höhere Amplitude von der Grundaktivität abheben (Abb. 7). Sie treten überwiegend beiderseits gleichzeitig, symmetrisch auf und haben im EEG des Erwachsenen, wie die kontinuierliche Dysrhythmie, ihren topographischen Schwerpunkt meist im temporo-frontalen Bereich. Nach ihrem Erscheinungsbild unterscheidet sich hiervon die *gruppierte abnorme Rhythmisierung*, die im Gegensatz zur gruppierten Dysrhythmie durch eine auffallende Monomorphie und Monofrequenz gekennzeichnet ist (Abb. 8). Sie wird nach dem treffenden Vorschlag von PENIN et al. (in ZEH, 1972) auch als „Parenrhythmie" bezeichnet und wurde, wie übrigens die meisten der klinisch bedeutsamen Aktivitätsformen, schon von BERGER (1931) gesehen. Gruppierte Dysrhythmie wie auch Parenrhythmie können lateralisiert, seltener auch einseitig fokal auftreten und erhalten dann die Bedeutung eines Herdbefundes.

Eine morphologisch, pathologisch und diagnostisch besondere Form diskontinuierlicher Aktivität ist die sog. *hypersynchrone Aktivität* (oft im deutschen Sprachgebrauch unter Vorwegnahme einer klinisch zu stellenden Diagnose auch als Krampfpotentiale bezeichnet). Sie umfaßt eine Reihe ihrer Gestalt nach heterogener Potentialformen, die als gemeinsames Charakteristikum die relativ enge diagnostische Beziehung zu cerebralen Anfallsleiden aufweisen. Hierzu gehören u.a. Graphoelemente wie spikes, spike-wave-Komplexe, sharp-waves und

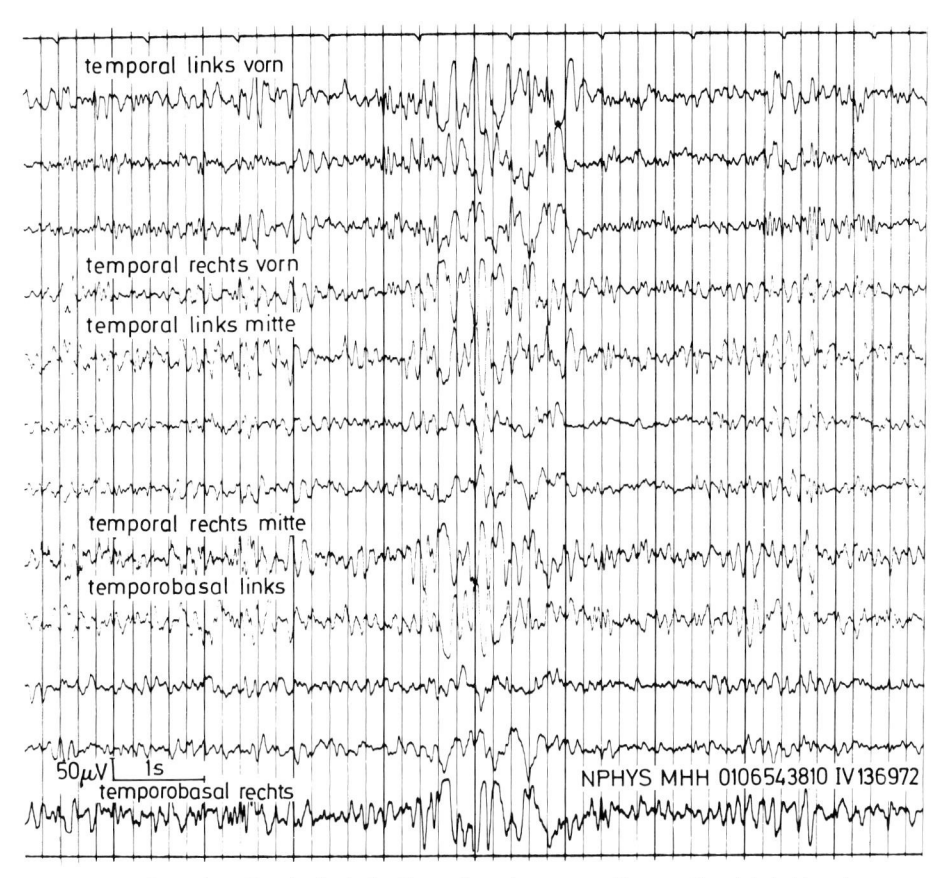

Abb. 7. Gruppierte Dysrhythmie im Frontal- und gesamten Temporalbereich beiderseits

steile Abläufe (Abb. 9, in Anlehnung an DUMERMUTH, 1976) sowie deren Kombinationen. Für ihr Auftreten im zeitlichen Ablauf gilt das für die gruppierte Dysrhythmie und Parenrhythmie Gesagte, allerdings mit der Einschränkung, daß für spikes und sharp waves das bilateral synchrone Auftreten eher die Ausnahme ist und diese Potentialformen häufig auch in umschriebener Lokalisierung auftreten und dann einen Herdbefund ausmachen, während bilateral synchrones Erscheinen für Züge von spike-wave-Komplexen eher die Regel ist.

Auch für die diskontinuierlich auftretenden Aktivitätsformen, am ehesten noch mit Ausnahme der hypersynchronen Aktivität, gilt das oben für die Modifikationen der Grundaktivität Gesagte: sie sind pathognostisch durchaus unspezifisch, finden sich bei einer großen Fülle verschiedenster klinischer Zustandsbilder (KÜNKEL, 1969) und sind nicht beweisende Zeichen einer morphologisch faßbaren Läsion, sondern eher Ausdruck eines besonderen Zustandes allgemeiner oder umschriebener zerebraler Reagibilität, der mit der Funktion von medialen Thalamuskernen (MORISON u. DEMPSEY, 1942; BUSER, 1964) sowie von Strukturen im unteren Hirnstammbereich (MAGNES et al., 1961) in Beziehung steht.

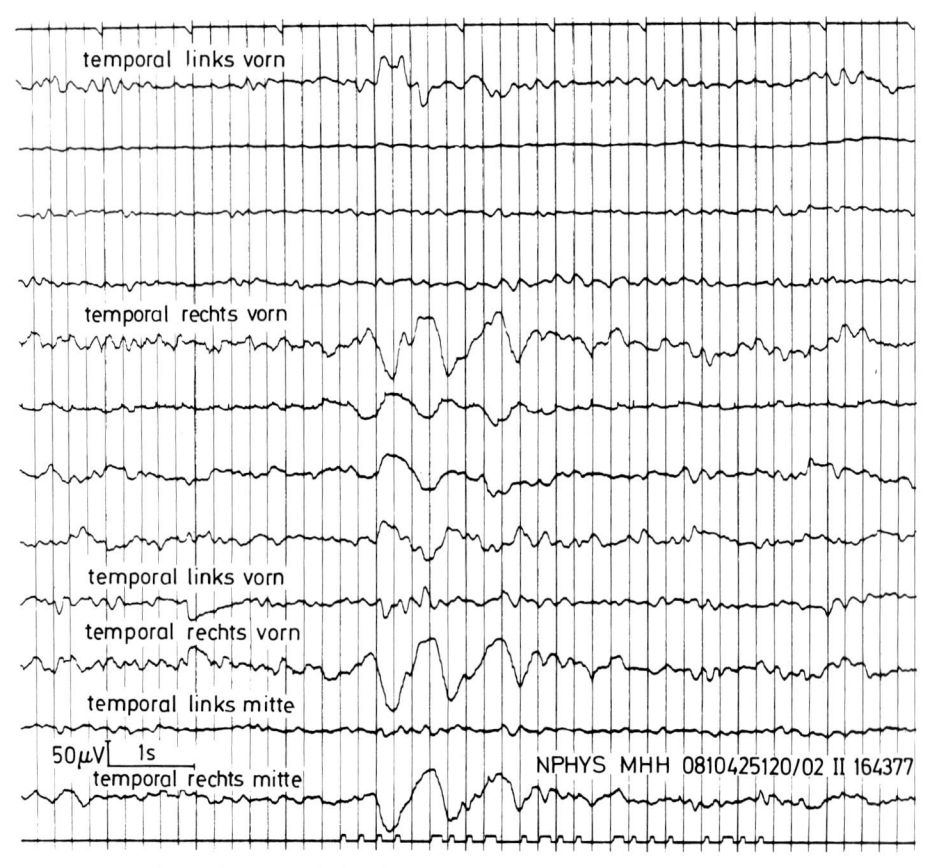

Abb. 8. Gruppierte abnorme Rhythmisierung (Delta-Parenrhythmie) temporal rechts vorn und Mitte mit Fortleitung nach temporal links vorn, bei mittlerer Allgemeinveränderung

Grundsätzlich das gleiche gilt für die hypersynchronen Potentialformen (zur Terminologie vgl. GASTAUT u. TASSINARI, 1975), denen abnorme Zustände der neuronalen Aktivität zugrunde liegen.

Zur Einführung in diese mehr experimentell-neurophysiologischen Problemkreise sei verwiesen auf BREMER (1958), FESSARD (1958), JUNG und TÖNNIES (1950), PENFIELD und JASPER (1954), WARD (1961), wo sich ausgezeichnete Literaturübersichten finden.

Die hypersynchrone Aktivität gehört zu den sehr wenigen Potentialformen, die eine relativ weitgehende diagnostische Spezifität aufweisen. Sie sind gemeinhin Ausdruck einer erhöhten zerebralen Krampfbereitschaft. Allerdings wurde früher ihre Beweiskraft für die Diagnose eines Anfallsleidens überschätzt; lediglich bei 65% erwachsener Merkmalsträger ist auch ein klinisch manifestes Anfallsleiden aktuell oder anamnestisch nachweisbar (GUTJAHR et al., 1979).

IV. Zur Epidemiologie von EEG-Aktivitätsmustern

Will man die Bedeutung von Befunden über die Häufigkeit verschiedener normaler oder pathologischer Merkmale bei psychischen Störungen beurteilen,

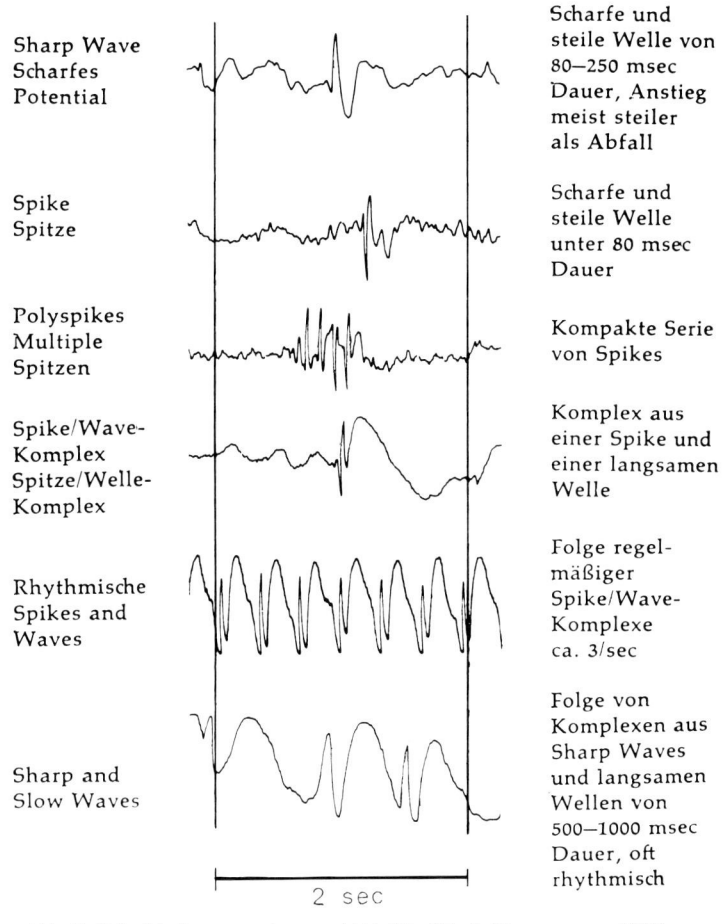

Sharp Wave Scharfes Potential		Scharfe und steile Welle von 80–250 msec Dauer, Anstieg meist steiler als Abfall
Spike Spitze		Scharfe und steile Welle unter 80 msec Dauer
Polyspikes Multiple Spitzen		Kompakte Serie von Spikes
Spike/Wave-Komplex Spitze/Welle-Komplex		Komplex aus einer Spike und einer langsamen Welle
Rhythmische Spikes and Waves		Folge regelmäßiger Spike/Wave-Komplexe ca. 3/sec
Sharp and Slow Waves		Folge von Komplexen aus Sharp Waves und langsamen Wellen von 500–1000 msec Dauer, oft rhythmisch

Abb. 9. Beispiele hypersynchroner Aktivität. (Nach DUMERMUTH, 1976)

so ist die Kenntnis ihrer Häufigkeit in Vergleichspopulationen unerläßlich, wobei insbesondere interferierende Faktoren wie Geschlecht und Alter zu berücksichtigen sind. Untersuchungen dieser Art, die sich auf ein umfangreiches Erfahrungsgut stützen können, sind eigenartigerweise selten. Ein Grund dafür ist zweifellos, daß Systeme einer standardisierten, in der klinisch-elektroenzephalographischen Routinediagnostik einsatzfähigen Befunddokumentation erst mit der Entwicklung moderner Verfahren der Datenerfassung und -verarbeitung möglich geworden sind (HELMCHEN et al., 1968; PENIN et al., 1972). Eine der wenigen Ausnahmen bildet die Untersuchung von F.A. GIBBS und E.L. GIBBS (1971), die sich auf ein Material von über 30000 EEG-Befunden stützt. Sie richtet sich allerdings mehr auf den Zusammenhang zwischen EEG-Merkmalen und diagnostischen Kategorien.

Bei allen solchen Studien erhebt sich allerdings die Frage, ob und inwieweit solche Befunde verallgemeinerungsfähig sind. Der Kliniker kann sich praktisch

Tabelle 2. Häufigkeit von EEG-Befunden in Abhängigkeit vom Geschlecht (p: Signifikanzstufe der Häufigkeitsdifferenz zwischen Männern (M) und Frauen (F); AV: Allgemeinveränderung; STP: hypersynchrone Aktivität). Untersucht an einer Population von 12500 Erst-EEG

	Häufigkeit (%)			
	Mittel	M	F	p
Alpha-Typ	49,0	52,6	44,6	+++
Part. Beta-Typ	12,3	10,5	14,5	+++
Beta-Typ	12,1	9,5	15,3	+++
Unregelm. EEG	10,8	10,0	11,7	+
7–8 s	1,3	1,6	0,9	+
AV	6,9			
Kontin. Dysrh.	10,6	9,6	11,7	++
Grupp. Dysrh.	9,7	7,4	12,5	+++
Parenrhythmie	6,1			
STP	3,5	2,8	4,2	++
Herd li.	14,7	14,2	15,4	
Herd re.	6,0			

$+ = P \leq 0{,}01$; $++ = P \leq 0{,}001$; $+++ = P \leq 0{,}0001$

nie die Situation eines demoskopischen Institutes schaffen, welches auf für die Gesamtpopulation repräsentative Stichproben zurückgreifen kann. Seine Stichproben, wie groß sie auch sein mögen, sind bestenfalls repräsentativ für den Teil der Gesamtpopulation, der irgendwann einmal klinisch untersucht wird. Entsprechendes gilt für die Untersuchungen über die Häufigkeit von EEG-Merkmalen, die nicht ohne weiteres über den Rahmen der Klientel extrapoliert werden können, die – aus welchen Gründen auch immer – zu einer EEG-Untersuchung überwiesen wird.

Tabelle 2 gibt einen Überblick über die Häufigkeit einiger Formen von EEG-Grundaktivitäten sowie anderer EEG-Merkmale, nach Geschlechtern getrennt. Dabei zeigen sich zunächst teilweise beträchtliche *geschlechtsabhängige Häufigkeitsunterschiede*. EEG vom Alpha-Typ, die den größen Anteil an EEG-Grundaktivität ausmachen, finden sich häufiger bei Männern, während partielle Beta-EEG und solche vom Beta-Typ bei Frauen wesentlich häufiger sind. Das gleiche gilt für die kontinuierlichen sowie für die gruppierten Dysrhythmien, während auffallenderweise bei Parenrhythmien ein solcher Unterschied nicht zu sichern ist. (Dieser Sachverhalt unterstreicht die Notwendigkeit, beide Formen diskontinuierlicher Aktivität voneinander zu unterscheiden, wie es ursprünglich aus Gründen der formalen Morphologie erfolgte.) Auch eine hypersynchrone Aktivität ist bei Frauen deutlich häufiger als bei Männern. Das beträchtliche Überwiegen von linksseitigen gegenüber rechtsseitigen Herdstörungen ist bereits mehrfach beschrieben wie auch gelegentlich bestritten worden (HELMCHEN et al., 1967). Als Deutung bietet sich der Hinweis auf den linksseitig anderen Abgang der A. carotis an, mit der Möglichkeit, daß es hier eher zu veränderten Strömungsverhältnissen aufgrund atherosklerotischer Plaques mit relativem Durchblutungsmangel kommen kann, wie die deutliche Zunahme von Linksherden mit dem Alter vermuten läßt. Eine plausible Deutung dieser geschlechtsabhängi-

Tabelle 3. Altersabhängigkeit der Häufigkeit von EEG-Merkmalen bei Männern (M) und Frauen (F) (p: Signifikanzstufe der Altersabhängigkeit; J: die Altersabhängigkeit ist für Männer und Frauen mit einer Signifikanzstufe von 0,01 verschieden; N: nicht verschieden; AV: Allgemeinveränderung; STP: hypersynchrone Aktivität)

	Altersabhängigkeit		Diff.
	M	F	M/F
Alpha-Typ	+++	+++	N
Part. Beta-Typ	+++	+++	J
Beta-Typ	+++	+++	J
Unregelm. EEG	+++	+++	N
7–8 s	+++	+++	J
AV	+++	+++	N
Kontin. Dysrh.	+++	+++	N
Grupp. Dysrh.	–	++	J
Parenrhythmie	+++	+++	J
STP	+++	+++	N
Herd li.	+++	+++	N
Herd re.	+++	+++	J

+ = $P \leq 0,01$; ++ = $P \leq 0,001$; +++ = $P \leq 0,0001$

gen Häufigkeitsunterschiede fehlt bislang, auch wenn der Einfluß genetisch bedingter Faktoren naheliegt.

Diese Zusammenhänge werden noch kompliziert durch die *Altersabhängigkeit* der relativen Häufigkeit von EEG-Merkmalen, die sich für fast alle von ihnen als hochsignifikant erweist (Tabelle 3). Wiederum ergeben sich eindeutige Geschlechtsdifferenzen auch für diese Altersabhängigkeit bei einer Reihe von Merkmalen. Als Beispiel sei diejenige für die relative Häufigkeit des EEG vom Beta-Typ herausgegriffen (Abb. 10, 11). Seine relative Häufigkeit nimmt bei beiden Geschlechtern bis zum Ende des 6. Lebensjahrzehnts linear zu, liegt allerdings bei Frauen stets höher als bei Männern, um dann wieder linear abzunehmen, bei Frauen indessen nur geringfügig. Derartige Zusammenhänge dürfen offensichtlich nicht unberücksichtigt bleiben, wenn Aussagen über die Häufigkeit verschiedener EEG-Merkmale, z.B. bei Kranken mit schizophrenen Psychosen, gemacht werden.

Die Mehrzahl der hiermit befaßten Untersuchungen läßt nicht erkennen, ob und wie solche Faktoren bei der Auswahl einer Kontrollgruppe berücksichtigt wurden. Auch die wenigen Studien, die „matched samples", nach Alter und Geschlecht angepaßte Vergleichsgruppen, heranziehen, lassen die Frage unbeantwortet, ob diese durch eine strikte Zufallsauswahl aus einer hinreichend großen Population unter Berücksichtigung dieser Einflußgrößen gebildet wurden. Ist dies nicht der Fall, so kann in der Kontrollgruppe ein systematischer Fehler („bias"), eingeführt werden, über dessen Richtung und Größe grundsätzlich kaum eine Aussage möglich ist, der aber sehr wohl Häufigkeitsdifferenzen vortäuschen, wie auch tatsächlich vorhandene Differenzen verwischen kann. Dieser Mangel kann auch durch einen oft beeindruckenden statistischen Aufwand, etwa durch den Einsatz von Diskriminanzanalysen oder multiplen Regressionen, nicht wettgemacht werden. Eine Voraussetzung für die Erfüllung dieser Bedingungen ist wiederum die Verfügbarkeit einer zugriffsfähigen, nach standardisierten EEG-Kriterien dokumentierten Population.

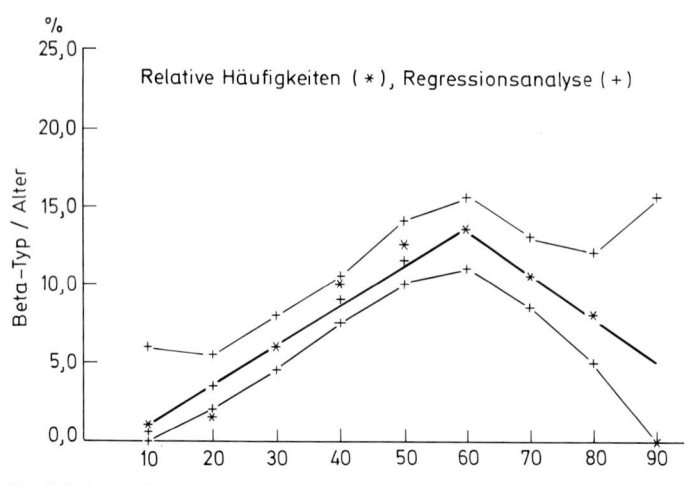

Abb. 10. Häufigkeit des EEG vom Beta-Typ bei Männern in Abhängigkeit vom Lebensalter

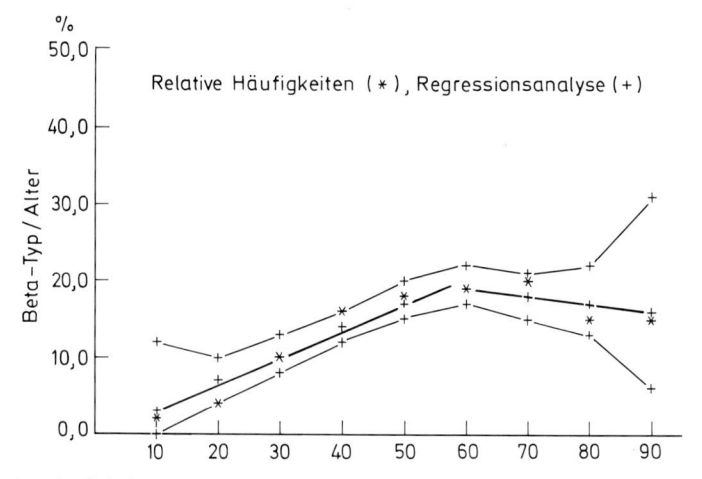

Abb. 11. Häufigkeit des EEG vom Beta-Typ bei Frauen in Abhängigkeit vom Lebensalter

V. Chronobiologische Aspekte

Es ist bereits gesichertes Wissen, daß fast jeder Parameter bei Mensch, Tier oder Pflanze zeitlichen Veränderungen unterliegt, indem er häufig offenkundigen, meist aber erst mit geeigneten statistischen Verfahren der Zeitreihenanalyse nachweisbaren Rhythmen folgt. Das Spektrum dieser Rhythmen läßt sich in einen ultradianen, zirkadianen und infradianen Bereich unterteilen, je nachdem ob ihre Periodenlängen kürzer als 24 Std, annähernd 24 Std oder aber wesentlich länger sind. Zu letzteren gehören auch die zirkannualen Rhythmen von etwa Jahreslänge.

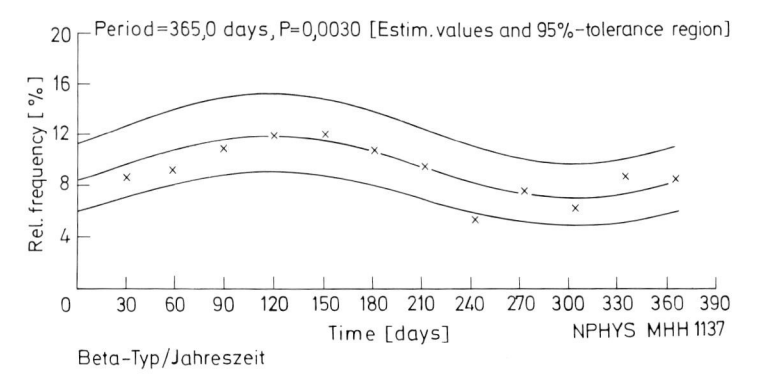

Abb. 12. Häufigkeit des EEG vom Beta-Typ bei Männern in Abhängigkeit von der Jahreszeit, gemittelt über 5 Jahre

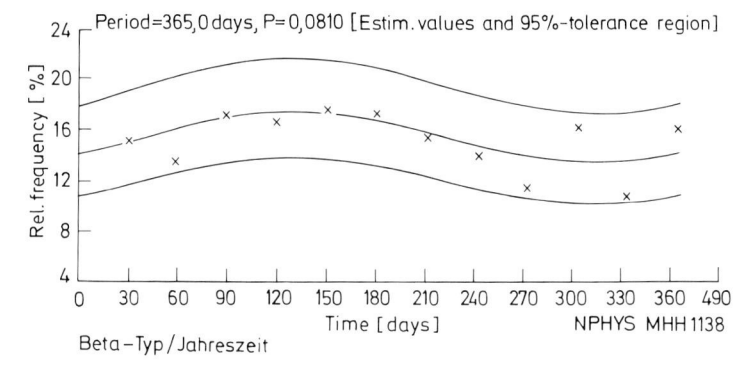

Abb. 13. Häufigkeit des EEG vom Beta-Typ bei Frauen in Abhängigkeit von der Jahreszeit, gemittelt über 5 Jahre (keine signifikante Periodik)

Einen Überblick über Begriffe und Methoden der Chronobiologie mit illustrativen Beispielen gibt HALBERG (1969, 1973, 1977). Dort finden sich auch Hinweise auf eine einführende Literatur. Die elektroenzephalographische Literatur hierzu ist noch spärlich. Es sei beispielsweise verwiesen auf ADEY et al. (1967), ENGEL et al. (1952), KRIPKE (1972), KÜNKEL et al. (1977).

Derartige Rhythmen lassen sich auch für die verschiedenen Phänomene des EEG nachweisen. So folgen die einzelnen Formen diskontinuierlicher Aktivität ultradianen Rhythmen, die der Atemrhythmik entsprechen, aber auch Periodenlängen von einigen Minuten und mehr aufweisen (KÜNKEL, 1969). Das gleiche gilt für die Ausprägung z.B. des Alpha- und Theta-Bandes (MACHLEIDT, 1975). Diese Rhythmen verschiedener Periodenlänge überlagern sich und ergeben damit das Bild einer differenzierten Zeitstruktur hirnelektrischer Aktivität. Dabei scheint es sich um ein tiefliegendes, vitales Phänomen zu handeln, zumal diese ultradianen Rhythmen auch durch eine massive medikamentöse Therapie, etwa eine Pharmakotherapie von Psychosen, nicht nennenswert beeinflußt werden, obgleich damit eine oft beträchtliche Veränderung der EEG-Grundaktivität einhergeht (SCHWEITZER, 1971; M. STERNBERG, 1971; P. STERNBERG, 1971). Die bislang nicht bewiesene Vermutung liegt nahe, daß auch die „suppression-burst"-Aktivität (s. oben) der schweren Intoxikationen Ausdruck dieser noch bis kurz vor dem Erlöschen der elektrischen Hirnaktivität persistierenden Rhythmik ist. Der physiologische Wechsel von Wach- und Schlafaktivität ist ein evidentes Beispiel zur zirkadianen EEG-Rhythmik. Aber auch im diurnalen (über die Wachphase sich erstreckenden) Ablauf läßt sich ein systematischer Rhythmus im EEG nachweisen, mit einem Maximum der Ausprägung aller Frequenzbänder etwa gegen 14 Uhr. Dabei stellt sich allerdings heraus, daß die topographische Differenzierung des EEG auch hierbei eine wesentliche Rolle spielt. Alpha- und Theta-Ausprägung zeigen das Maximum ihrer Ausprägung im fronto-präzentralen Bereich etwa 3 Std früher als im temporalen und okzipitalen Bereich (KÜNKEL et al., 1977). Die Frage, ob und inwiefern diese topographisch differenzierte Zeitstruktur der EEG-Aktivität bei psychotischen Erkrankungen verändert ist, muß vorderhand noch offen bleiben.

Chronobiologische Aspekte dürften auch für die Häufigkeit von EEG-Phänomenen im Jahresablauf von Bedeutung sein. Als Beispiel sei wiederum die Häufigkeit des EEG vom Beta-Typ im Jahresablauf herausgegriffen (GUTJAHR u. KÜNKEL, 1978). Sie zeigt bei Männern eine hochsignifikante Rhythmik mit einem Maximum etwa im April und einer geschätzten Häufigkeit von 12%, entsprechend ein Minimum im Oktober mit einer Häufigkeit von 7%. Bei Frauen läßt sich hingegen eine solche zirkannuale Rhythmik, obgleich angedeutet, nicht sichern (Abb. 12, 13). Offensichtlich müssen auch chronobiologische Faktoren künftig berücksichtigt werden, wenn abweichende Häufigkeiten von EEG-Befunden bei psychotisch Kranken diskutiert werden sollen.

VI. Zur diagnostischen „Spezifität" elektroenzephalographischer Befunde

Das auch heute noch eine Grundlage der klinischen Elektroenzephalographie bildende Werk von HANS BERGER schien in seinem Beginn einen faszinierenden neuen Weg zu eröffnen, die Natur veränderter Hirnfunktionen bei psychischen Erkrankungen zu studieren. BERGER selbst war zwar zu kritisch, für Schizophrenien oder depressive Störungen spezifische Wellenformen oder auch komplexere Phänomene zu erwarten, dennoch wäre eine solche Hoffnung wohl verständlich gewesen. Die Erfahrung lehrte indessen bald, daß es solche „spezifischen" EEG-Phänomene nicht gibt. Dies gilt, wie sich alsbald herausstellte, auch für rein neurologische Störungen, die mit morphologisch faßbaren Substanzschädigungen einhergehen. Es gibt keine Wellen- oder Aktivitätsformen, die für eine bestimmte neurologische oder psychische Störung oder gar für ein Krankheitsbild spezifisch wäre, vielleicht mit alleiniger Ausnahme der Panenzephalitiden (RADERMECKER, 1957), sowie – mit der oben gemachten Einschränkung – der zerebralen Anfallsleiden. Es gibt kaum einen EEG-Befund, der sich nicht gelegentlich bei jedem neurologischen oder psychiatrischen Krankheitsbild und bei manchen primär extrazerebralen Erkrankungen finden ließe, teilweise auch bei klinisch sonst anscheinend Gesunden (letzteres allenfalls mit Ausnahme schwererer Formen von Allgemeinveränderungen). Eine diagnostische „Spezifität" des EEG ist deshalb im wesentlichen zu verneinen. Dies besagt indessen keineswegs, daß das EEG sich nicht zunehmend als wichtiges Mittel zur Beschreibung, ja zur Definition von zerebralen Funktionszuständen und ihrer Veränderungen erweisen wird. Vor allem aus der psychiatrischen Forschung sind hierzu wesentliche Impulse gekommen und die Erwartung erscheint berechtigt, daß das klinisch-psychiatrische EEG, von modernen Verfahren, etwa der EEG-Analyse, profitierend, sich für diese Grundlagenforschung als nützlich erweisen wird.

C. Aspekte der EEG-Analyse und ihrer Auswertung

Die quantitative, computergestützte Analyse des EEG hat sich bei der Definition zerebraler Medikationswirkungen einen festen Platz geschaffen. Teile der Pharmako-Psychiatrie stützen sich in ihren methodischen Grundlagen darauf; auch in die Schizophrenie-Forschung haben die verschiedenen Analyseverfahren neue Anregungen eingebracht. Wenn das EEG heute und in Zukunft für die klinische Psychiatrie eine größere Bedeutung gewinnt, als noch vor einem oder zwei Jahrzehnten, so ist dies auch der differenzierteren Information zu verdanken, die von der EEG-Analyse für die Beurteilung zerebraler Funktionszustände bereitgestellt wird. Eine kritische Bewertung der bereits vorliegenden Befunde sowie der damit neu aufgeworfenen Fragen setzt allerdings ein grundsätzliches Verständnis der verschiedenen Analyseverfahren sowie ihrer Aussagemöglichkeiten voraus.

Nachfolgend wird eine kurze Übersicht über einige Verfahren der EEG-Analyse gegeben. Ihr tieferes Verständnis setzt eine enge Vertrautheit mit den Begriffen der statistischen Zeitreihenanalyse, der Signaltheorie und den Verfahren der multivariaten analytischen Statistik voraus. Eine Reihe von Symposiumsbänden und Monographien der letzten Jahre erlaubt eine Übersicht über die rasche Entwicklung von methodischen Grundlagen und experimentellen, teils auch klinischen Anwendungen (COBB u. VAN DUIJN, 1978; DOLCE u. KÜNKEL, 1975; ÉTEVENON, 1977; KELLAWAY u. PETERSEN, 1973, 1976; MATEJCEK u. SCHENK, 1975; RÉMOND, 1977; SCHENK, 1973).

I. Entwicklung der EEG-Analyse und einige ihrer Voraussetzungen

Hier soll anhand der Entwicklung der EEG-Analyse nur kurz dargestellt werden, wie die Versuche zur Lösung des Problems, den Informationsgehalt des EEG auszuschöpfen, über die Anwendung zunächst einfacherer, dann komplizierterer elektronischer Geräte, schließlich einerseits zum Einsatz von Computern, andererseits aber auch von Verfahren der statistischen Signalanalyse führen mußten, ohne die der heutige Stand und die künftigen Möglichkeiten undenkbar wären. Eine etwas ausführliche Erörterung findet sich an anderer Stelle (KÜNKEL, 1977).

Die ersten Ansätze zu einer quantitiativen EEG-Analyse reichen bereits in die Frühzeit der Elektroenzephalographie zurück. BERGER (1932) erkannte, daß eine visuelle EEG-Auswertung durch eine objektive Analyse-Methode unterstützt werden sollte und veranlaßte DIETSCH (1932), auf einige Kurvenstücke eine Fourier-Analyse anzuwenden. Für das klinische EEG blieben diese Arbeiten ohne Bedeutung, da ihre Fortsetzung wegen des damit verbundenen, kaum vorstellbaren Rechenaufwandes nicht möglich war. Ein erster Fortschritt ergab sich durch die Amplituden-Integration, die von DROHOCKI (1938, 1948) entwickelt wurde und die ein Maß für den mittleren Energiegehalt der EEG-Aktivität und seine zeitliche Variabilität lieferte. Diese Methode, die sich durch relativ geringen apparativen Aufwand und unmittelbare Anschaulichkeit ihrer Resultate auszeichnete, wird auch heute noch, z.B. in der elektroenzephalographischen Schizophrenieforschung, mit interessanten Resultaten angewendet. Ihr Nachteil ist, daß sie die Differenzierung der EEG-Aktivität im Frequenzbereich nicht berücksichtigt. Dies wurde erst mit den Frequenzanalysatoren möglich, die auf den Pionierarbeiten von BALDOCK und GREY WALTER (1946) beruhen und die von ULETT und LOEFFEL (1953) und SHIPTON (1956) fortgesetzt wurden. Die EEG-Analyse empfing damit neue Impulse, wenn auch der breitere Einsatz dieser Geräte durch ihre Instabilität sehr behindert wurde. Mit ihnen konnte der Bereich der EEG-Frequenzen in 24 Bänder aufgespalten werden, deren Energieinhalt und seine Veränderungen im Zeitablauf verfolgt werden konnten. Eine weitere Differenzierung der EEG-Frequenzen erlaubte die „period analysis", die von BURCH et al. (1964) entwickelt wurde. Sie ermittelt die Frequenz jeder einzelnen EEG-Welle und liefert somit weit mehr Informationen über die EEG-Aktivität, als etwa die Amplituden-Integration nach DROHOCKI. Dieses Verfahren findet bis heute breite und erfolgreiche Anwendung in der Psychopharmakologie. Es markiert gleichzeitig etwa den Zeitpunkt, von dem ab sich die EEG-Analyse der inzwischen auch für Laborzwecke verfügbar gewordenen Computer bediente. Die sich hierhin ausdrückende technische Entwicklung sowie die Entwicklung der Theorie von Zufallsprozessen stellten schließlich die Voraussetzungen dar für den Einsatz der Spektral-Analyse (D.O. WALTER, 1963). Weitere methodische Verbesserungen (DUMERMUTH u. FLÜHLER, 1967) erlauben heute die gleichzeitige Spektral-Analyse von 12 oder mehr Kanälen während der laufenden EEG-Registrierung, so daß die Resultate bereits bei ihrem Ende zur Verfügung stehen (KÜNKEL, 1972b). Bei diesem Entwicklungsstand der EEG-Analyse konnte endlich, nach vier Jahrzehnten, der Faden wieder aufgenommen werden, der nach den ersten Versuchen von BERGER und DIETSCH zunächst fallengelassen werden mußte.

Nachfolgend werden einige Analyse-Verfahren besprochen, auf deren Ergebnisse in späteren Abschnitten Bezug genommen wird. Dabei handelt es sich ausschließlich um Verfahren zur Analyse der Grundaktivität, während Methoden zur automatischen Erkennung diskontinuierlich auftretender EEG-Aktivität („Mustererkennung") unberücksichtigt bleiben. Sie haben in der klinisch-psychiatrischen Elektroenzephalographie bislang noch kaum Anwendung gefunden. Eine eingehendere Diskussion von Methoden und Problemen findet sich bei GOTMAN und GLOOR (1976), JACOB (1976), LOPES DA SILVA et al. (1977), MCGILLIVRAY (1977).

II. Amplituden-Integration

Eine ausführliche Darstellung der Methode, ihrer Entwicklung und ihrer Modifikationen sowie der mit ihr erlangten Resultate insbesondere bei psychiatrischen Fragestellungen findet sich bei GOLDSTEIN (1975). In ihrer heute gebräuchlichen Form werden nach geeigneter Verstärkung des Signals zunächst

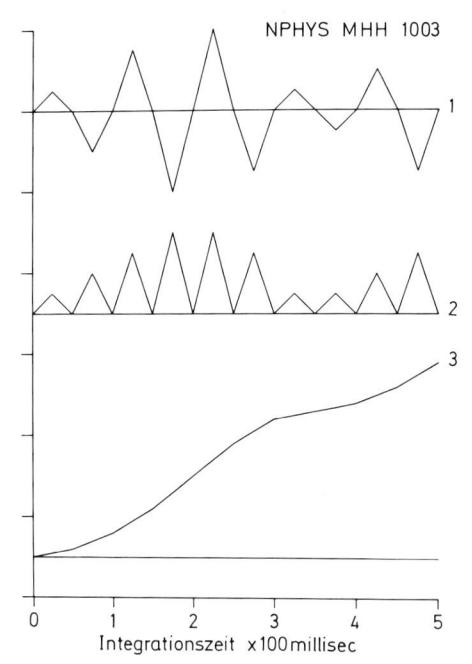

Abb. 14. Prinzip der Amplitudenintegration nach DROHOCKI (schematisch). 1: EEG-Kurve, 2: gleichgerichtete Kurve, 3: Zeitverlauf des Integrationswertes im Integrationsintervall

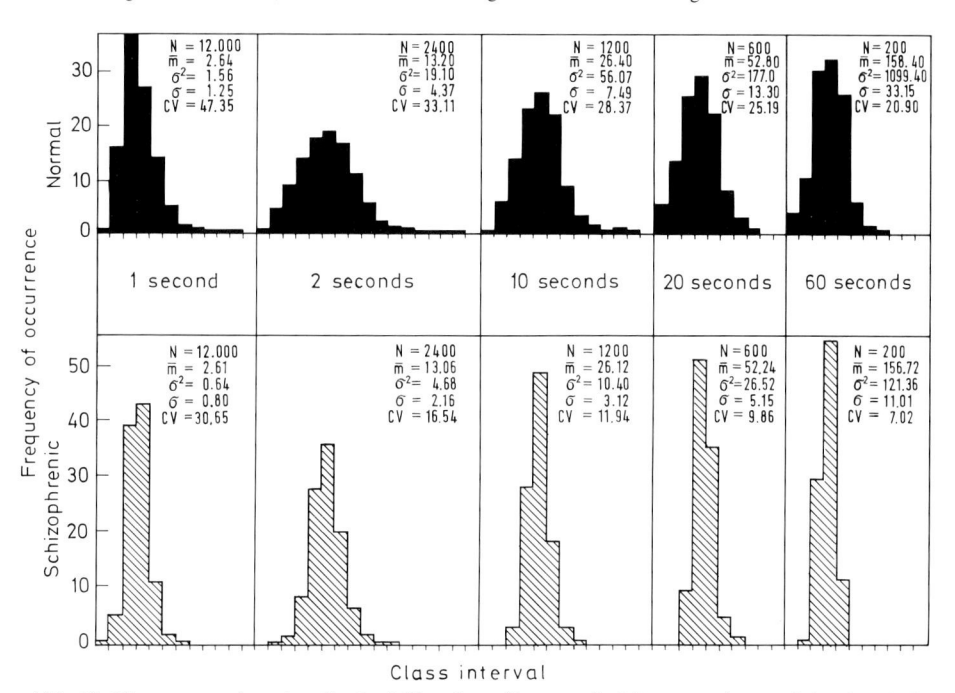

Abb. 15. Histogramm der „Amplituden"-Verteilung für gesunde Männer und männliche chronisch Schizophrene, für Integrationsintervalle von 1–60 s. (Aus GOLDSTEIN, 1975.) (CV = 100 $\sigma/\bar{m}$, Variationskoeffizient in %)

Frequenzen unter 0,75 Hz herausgefiltert, sodann erfolgt eine Zweiweg-Gleichrichtung mit anschließender Integration über frei wählbare Zeitspannen. Für jede dieser Integrations-Epochen liefert die Analyse demnach einen Zahlenwert, der der Fläche unter der gleichgerichteten EEG-Kurve proportional ist (Abb. 14). Die dem zeitlichen EEG-Ablauf entsprechende Folge von Integrationswerten („Amplituden", „Energiegehalt") kann dann durch einfache statistische Maße, wie Mittelwert, Streuung, Variationskoeffizient (Verhältnis von Streuung zum Mittelwert) und Verteilungshistogramme beschrieben werden.

Ein Beispiel für letztere stellt Abb. 15 dar (aus GOLDSTEIN, 1975). Hierbei fällt auf, daß die Patientengruppe eine geringere Streuung der Amplituden-Integrationswerte um einen Mittelwert aufweist, als die gesunde Kontrollgruppe. Die Folge der Integrationswerte läßt sich auch auf periodische Komponenten untersuchen (Abschn. B.V, ultradiane Rhythmen der EEG-Aktivität). Schließlich können Zusammenhänge zwischen z.B. Mittelwert der „Amplituden" und Variationskoeffizient bei Gruppen von Probanden studiert werden. Abb. 16 zeigt dies an zwei Gruppen von Männern verschiedenen Alters sowie einer Gruppe von Frauen. Bei jungen Männern ist der Variationskoeffizient offenbar von der mittleren Amplitude unabhängig, während er bei älteren Männern und bei Frauen zunimmt, allerdings verschieden stark. Dies kann als Hinweis darauf gewertet werden, daß die dynamische Struktur der EEG-Grundaktivität bei Männern und Frauen quantitativ verschieden ist. Allerdings bedarf diese Hypo-

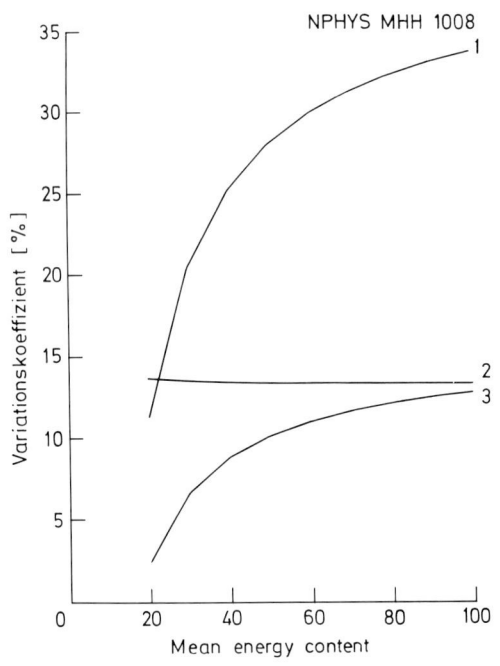

Abb. 16. Zusammenhang zwischen Variationskoeffizient und Mittel der „Amplituden". 1: Männer im Alter von 20–54 Jahren, 2: Männer im Alter von 17–21 Jahren, 3: Frauen im Alter von 19–46 Jahren. (Berechnet nach Daten von BURDICK et al., 1967)

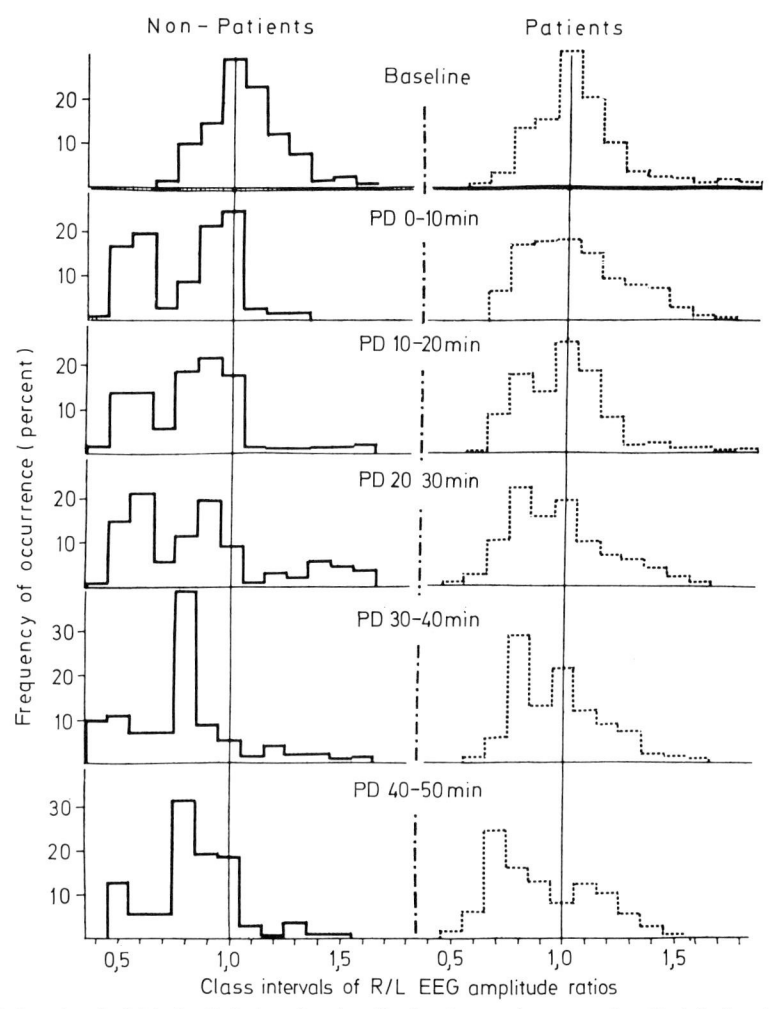

Abb. 17. Interhemisphärische Relation der Amplituden-Integrationswerte im Okzipitalbereich bei gesunden Probanden und bei Schizophrenen unter sensorischer Deprivation (PD). (Aus GOLDSTEIN, 1975)

these, die auf Befunde von BURDICK et al. (1967) zurückgeht, noch der genaueren Nachprüfung. Ferner scheint eine Altersabhängigkeit dieses Zusammenhanges vorzuliegen. Diese Befunde deuten erneut darauf hin, daß der Einfluß von Geschlecht und Alter beim Vergleich von gesunden Probanden und Kranken nicht außer acht gelassen werden darf (vgl. Abschn. B.IV). Schließlich kann auch das Seitenverhältnis der Amplitudenverteilung, etwa beim Vergleich des rechten und linken okzipitalen Kanals, unter verschiedenen Bedingungen untersucht werden. Ein Beispiel stellt in Abb. 17 die interhemisphärische Relation der „Amplituden" bei sensorischer Deprivation dar. Normale Probanden zeigen unter dieser Bedingung ein markantes Überwiegen der EEG-Aktivität über dem linken Okzipitalbereich, welches bei unbehandelten chronisch Schizophrenen wesentlich weniger ausgeprägt ist. Die Beispiele sollen einen Eindruck davon vermitteln, daß bereits diese einfach zu handhabende Methode, die auch an die statistische Auswertung keine besonderen Ansprüche stellt, trotz der nur geringen Nutzung der im EEG enthaltenen Information schon Einblicke in die strukturelle Organisation der EEG-Aktivität und ihre Veränderungen erlaubt, die einer nur visuellen EEG-Beurteilung nicht mehr möglich sind.

III. Period Analysis

Der englische Ausdruck wird hier verwendet, da der Terminus Perioden-Analyse bereits durch ältere Verfahren der Zeitreihen-Analyse besetzt ist, die einer statistischen Grundlage ermangeln und die heute nicht mehr im Gebrauch sind.

Eine zusammenfassende Erläuterung der Methoden sowie eine Reihe von Anwendungen auf psychiatrische und psychopharmakologische Fragen findet sich z.B. bei FINK (1977) und bei ITIL (1975). Die Abb. 18 und 19 geben eine vereinfachte, schematische Darstellung des Grundprinzips. Das EEG-Signal wird auf Null-Durchgänge in gleicher Richtung untersucht. Ihre zeitlichen Abstände definieren Periodenlängen von Wellen, die in verschiedene Frequenzklassen unterteilt werden können. Üblicherweise werden Frequenzklassen von 0,5–3,5 Hz, 3,5–7,5 Hz, 7,5–13 Hz, 13–20 Hz, 20–26,6 Hz, 26,6–40 Hz sowie über 40 Hz verwendet, in gewisser Analogie zu den Frequenzbändern der visuellen EEG-Auswertung. Da die Dauer jeder Welle bekannt ist, läßt sich berechnen, welcher Prozentsatz der gesamten Registrierzeit auf die einzelnen Frequenzbänder entfällt, was dann in einem Frequenzprofil (Abb. 19) dargestellt werden kann. Auch die Amplituden der Wellen lassen sich dabei unschwer berücksichtigen, etwa in der Art der Amplituden-Integration. Abb. 18 läßt erkennen, daß rasche, überlagerte Wellen, die die Null-Linie nicht schneiden, auf diese Weise nicht erfaßt werden. Zu diesem Zweck wird der Differentialquotient des Signals gebildet und diese Kurve dann in gleicher Weise analysiert (die Differentialquotientenbildung hebt gleichsam die raschen Wellen der Originalkurve hervor).

Die so gewonnenen Frequenzprofile lassen sich statistisch miteinander vergleichen oder auch mitteln. Auch hier gelangt man mit relativ einfachen statistischen Verfahren zu Aussagen. Dies soll am Beispiel der Abb. 20 aus ITIL (1975) veranschaulicht werden. Drei Versuchsgruppen erhielten Chlorpromazin, Imipramin und Diazepam. Die Frequenzprofile der Probanden jeder Gruppe wurden vor und drei Stunden nach Medikation gemittelt und diese mittleren Frequenzprofile vor und nach Medikation voneinander subtrahiert. Die so erhaltenen Differenzen sind in Abb. 20 dargestellt; sie werden anhand des t-Tests auf Signifikanz geprüft (gestrichelte Grenzen). Es zeigt sich, daß z.B. Imipramin zu einer Vermehrung von Wellen oberhalb von 20 Hz und zu einer Verminderung von Wellen des Alpha-Bandes führt. Auf diese Weise lassen sich für verschiedene Substanzklassen charakteristische Frequenzprofile gewinnen.

An dieser Stelle sind allerdings einige kritische Anmerkungen angebracht. Zunächst muß die Berechtigung zur Anwendung des einfachen t-Tests angezweifelt werden, da eine Anzahl von Variablen (die Anteile der Frequenzbänder) gleichzeitig auf Signifikanz geprüft werden. Eine multivariate Varianzanalyse wäre hier angemessener. Sodann wird ein Medikationseffekt gegen das Frequenzpro-

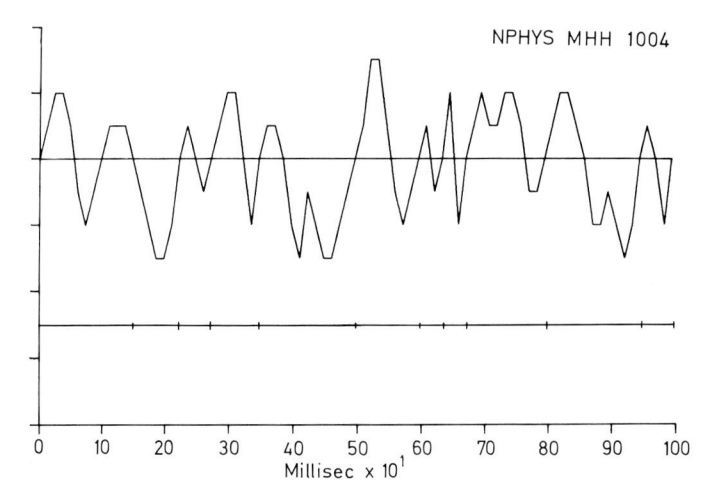

Abb. 18. Prinzip der period analysis (schematisch, Erläuterung s. Text)

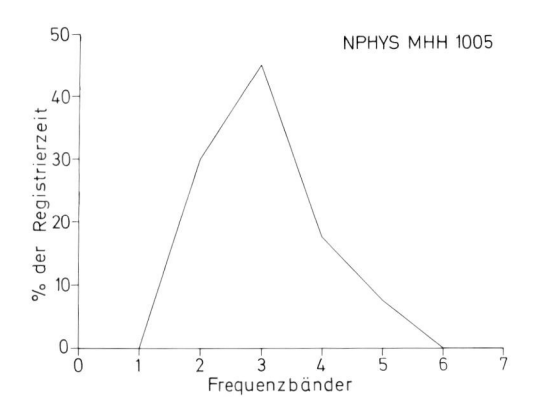

Abb. 19. Frequenzprofil der period analysis aus Abb. 18 (schematisch, Erläuterung s. Text).

fil vor Medikation geprüft. Dies ist im Hinblick auf seine Interpretation jedoch nur dann zulässig, wenn eine spontane zirkadiane Variation des EEG ausgeschlossen ist, was aber nicht zutrifft (s. Abschn. B.V), oder wenn nachgewiesen wird, daß dieses Analyseverfahren gegenüber der spontanen Variation unempfindlich ist. Anderenfalls könnte der als Medikationswirkung interpretierte Effekt ganz oder teilweise hierdurch bedingt oder verfälscht werden. Dieser Einwand würde entfallen, wenn nicht gegen einen Leerwert vor Medikation, sondern gegen einen Placebo-Effekt zu den gleichen Zeitpunkten geprüft würde (KÜNKEL et al., 1976). Ferner ist die Wahl eines festen Zeitintervalles für die Beurteilung der Medikationswirkung einigermaßen willkürlich und wird der Verlaufsdynamik einer Medikationswirkung nicht gerecht. Sie kann dabei über- oder unterschätzt und auch gänzlich übersehen werden (vgl. hierzu das Anwendungsbeispiel im folgenden Abschnitt). Diese Einwände betreffen allerdings eher die Versuchsplanung und ihre Auswertung, nicht die Analyse-Methode selbst.

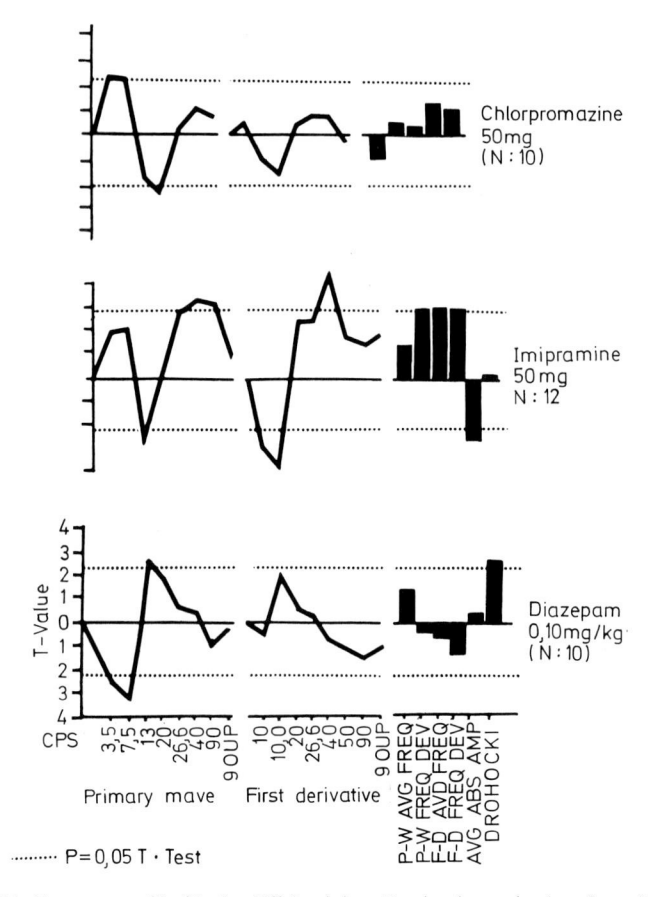

Abb. 20. Frequenzprofile für den Effekt einiger Psychopharmaka (aus ITIL, 1975)

IV. Spektral-Analyse

Die methodischen Grundlagen der EEG-Spektral-Analyse finden eine ohne besondere Voraussetzungen verständliche Beschreibung bei COOPER et al. (1974).

Jede Zeitreihe, also auch der Spannungsverlauf eines EEG-Kanals, läßt sich durch eine Summe von Funktionen mit bestimmten Eigenschaften darstellen. Die trigonometrischen Funktionen sind hierunter keineswegs die einzig möglichen (vgl. hierzu BÄUMLER et al., 1977), indessen ausgezeichnet durch Anschaulichkeit und dadurch, daß für sie eine solide statistisch fundierte Theorie vorliegt. Sie sind bislang fast ausschließlich für die Spektral-Analyse des EEG eingesetzt worden. Hier soll gleich auf einen Einwand gegen ihre Anwendung in der EEG-Analyse eingegangen werden, der auf einem Mißverständnis beruht: das Gehirn produziere keine Sinus-Wellen. Die Spektral-Analyse stellt lediglich eine unter gewissen Bedingungen erschöpfende, in ihren Eigenschaften genau bekannte, Beschreibung einer zufallsbedingten Funktion nach ihren Frequenzgehalten dar, ohne Aussagen über die Genese des EEG zu machen. So stützt sich die Spektral-

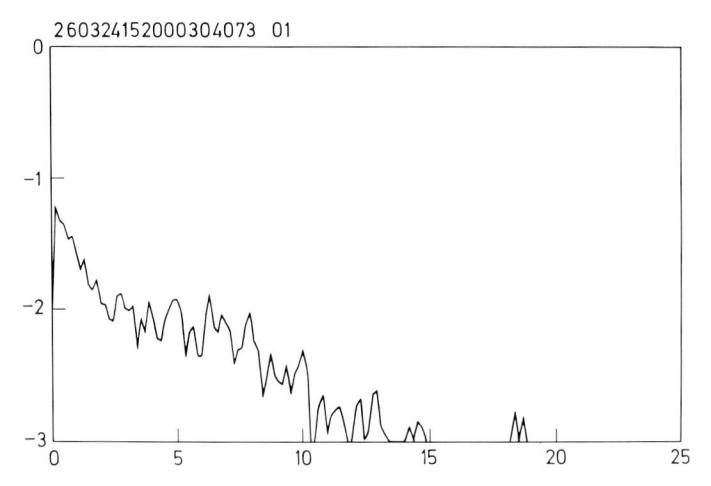

Abb. 21. Powerspektrum für einen EEG-Abschnitt von 3 min, präzentral links. (Abszisse: Frequenz in Hz, Ordinate: Leistung logarithmisch)

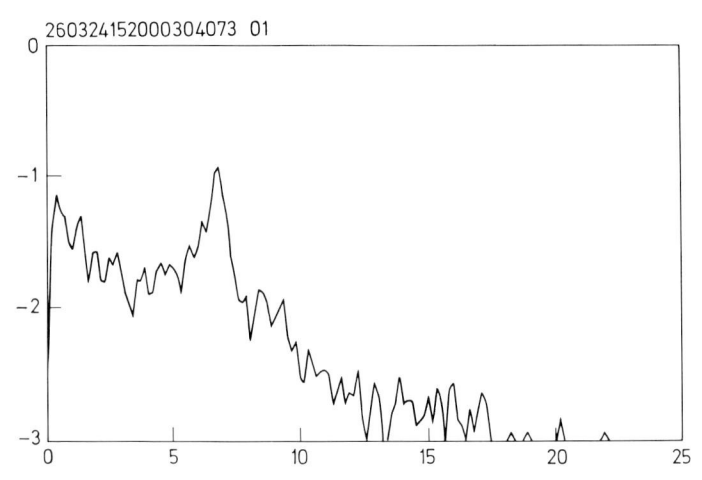

Abb. 22. Powerspektrum für einen EEG-Abschnitt von 3 min, präzentral rechts. (Abszisse: Frequenz in Hz, Ordinate: Leistung logarithmisch)

Analyse bezüglich des EEG im wesentlichen auf die Voraussetzung, daß es sich um eine in ihrem zeitlichen Verlauf zufallsbedingte, nicht vorhersagbare Funktion handelt, die sich z.B. durch ihren Mittelwert und ihre Varianz beschreiben läßt. Für diese Größen wird während des betrachteten Analyse-Intervalls zeitliche Konstanz angenommen (sog. Stationarität). (Diese Einschränkung läßt sich durch neuere Verfahren allerdings umgehen, worauf hier nicht eingegangen werden kann.) Die Varianz des EEG wird durch die Spektraldarstellung nach ihrem Frequenzgehalt aufgelöst. Hieraus erklärt sich die Bezeichnung Varianzspektrum. Da die Varianz physikalisch der Leistung oder Power eines Signales

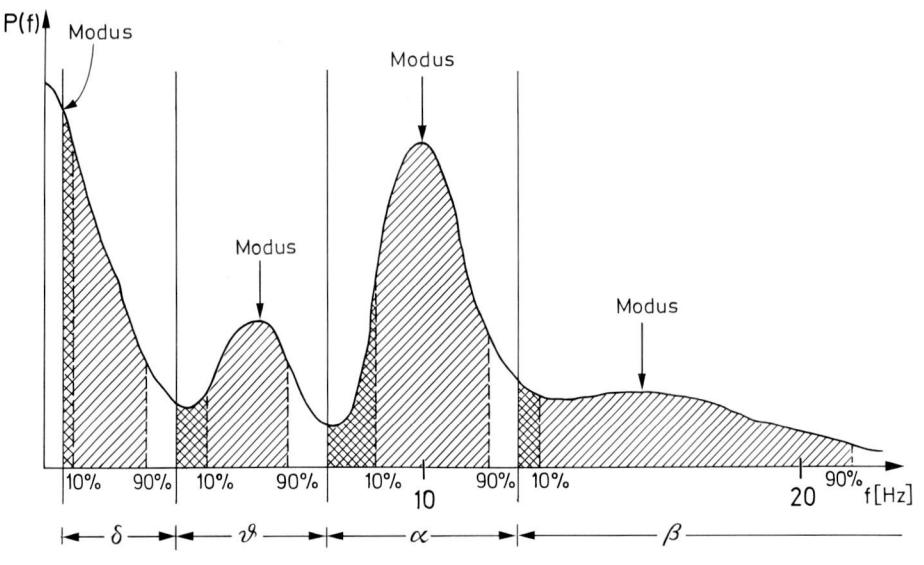

Abb. 23. Parameterextraktion aus EEG-Spektren. (Erläuterung s. Text)

äquivalent ist, wird auch die Bezeichnung Leistungs- oder Power-Spektrum verwendet.

Die Abb. 21 und 22 zeigen Spektren beider Präzentralregionen bei einem relativ flachen EEG mit Theta-Fokus präzentral rechts. (Der Ordinaten-Maßstab ist logarithmisch, um auch geringe Power-Anteile der höheren Frequenzen noch zu erkennen.) Der Abfall des Spektrums mit der Frequenz entspricht der Amplitudenabnahme mit zunehmenden Frequenzen. Überlagert ist auf der rechten Seite ein Gipfel bei etwa 6,75 Hz, der einen Herdbefund mit Theta-Wellen dieser Frequenz anzeigt.

Wie bei der period analysis ist auch hier erforderlich, die im allgemeinen recht komplexen Spektren durch eine Reihe von Meßgrößen, Parameter, objektiv zu beschreiben, da es nicht sinnvoll sein kann, die visuelle Auswertung von EEG lediglich durch die visuelle Beurteilung ihrer Spektren zu ersetzen. Dieses Problem ist bislang allerdings noch nicht in völlig zufriedenstellender Weise gelöst (KÜNKEL, 1972a; KÜNKEL, 1977). Eine Möglichkeit stellt Abb. 23 dar, die auf den „klassischen" Frequenzbändern des EEG (vgl. Tabelle 1) beruht. Für jedes Band wird die Fläche unter dem Spektrum als Band-Power berechnet. Ein Gipfel im Band definiert die dominante Frequenz; der Abschnitt, zwischen dem 10% und 90% der Bandleistung liegen, dient als Maß für die Frequenzvariabilität innerhalb des Bandes. Diese Parameter gehen dann in eine statistische Auswertung, z.B. durch eine Varianz-Analyse, ein. Abb. 24 zeigt aus einer vergleichenden Prüfung von Diazepam und Amitriptylin gegen Placebo die Veränderung der Theta-Power als einem der genannten Parameter im zeitlichen Verlauf der Medikationswirkung. Diazepam führt zu einer Abnahme, Amitriptylin zu einer Zunahme gegenüber dem Plazebo-Effekt, der mit als Ausdruck der spontanen zirkadianen EEG-Veränderungen interpretiert werden kann. Eine solche

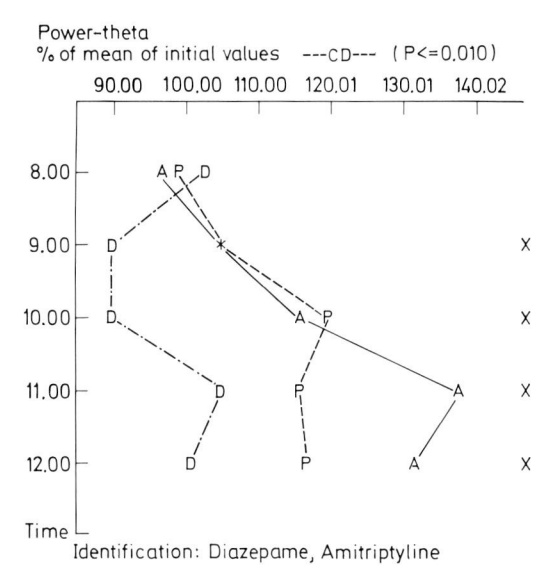

```
Power-theta
% of mean of initial values    ---CD---   ( P<=0.010 )
       90.00   100.00  110.00  120.01   130.01   140.02
```

Abb. 24. Zeitlicher Verlauf der Wirkung von Diazepam (D) und Amitriptylin (A) gegenüber Placebo (P) am Beispiel der Theta-Power. (CD: Kritische Differenz für $p \leq 0.01$)

Wirkungskurve läßt sich für jeden der genannten Parameter darstellen. Die vergleichende Analyse mehrerer EEG-Kanäle gibt Aufschluß über topographische Unterschiede der Medikationswirkung, wie Abb. 25 erkennen läßt. Bei dieser Untersuchung wurden auch mögliche Einflüsse von Aspekten der Persönlichkeitsstruktur auf die Medikationswirkungen untersucht, insbesondere der Neurotizismus-Score anhand des FPI-Tests. In dieser Form einer synoptischen Darstellung wurde auf die Einzelheiten des Zeitablaufs verzichtet, wie die Abb. 24 aufzeigt, und lediglich das Maximum der beobachteten Abweichung gegenüber Plazebo berücksichtigt, unabhängig vom Zeitpunkt seines Eintritts. Dennoch läßt sich auf diese Weise das EEG-Wirkungsprofil von Substanzen sehr differenziert gewinnen. Insbesondere läßt sich hier objektivieren, daß ein zerebraler Medikationseffekt qualitativ und quantitativ von psychosomatischen Faktoren abhängen kann (KÜNKEL et al., 1976; HEINZE u. KÜNKEL, 1979).

Die Mehrkanal-EEG-Spektral-Analyse erlaubt auch eine sychron-optische Darstellung der EEG-Verlaufsdynamik, die in solcher Differenzierung der visuellen Auswertung überhaupt nicht zugänglich ist (Abb. 26). Als hervorstechendes Merkmal zeigen die vier paarweise symmetrischen EEG-Kanäle einen Doppelgipfel im Alpha-Bereich. Die genauere Betrachtung über einen Zeitraum von 30 min zeigt, wie verwickelt die dynamischen Verhältnisse sich darstellen und daß sie in symmetrischen Kanälen durchaus unterschiedlich ablaufen. Diese Phänomene entziehen sich vorläufig noch einer zureichenden Beschreibung im konventionellen Begriffssystem der klinischen Elektroenzephalographie. Dieses Beispiel verdeutlicht, wie notwendig einerseits die Reduktion der in solcher Darstellung enthaltenen Datenmenge auf relevante Information ist. Andererseits

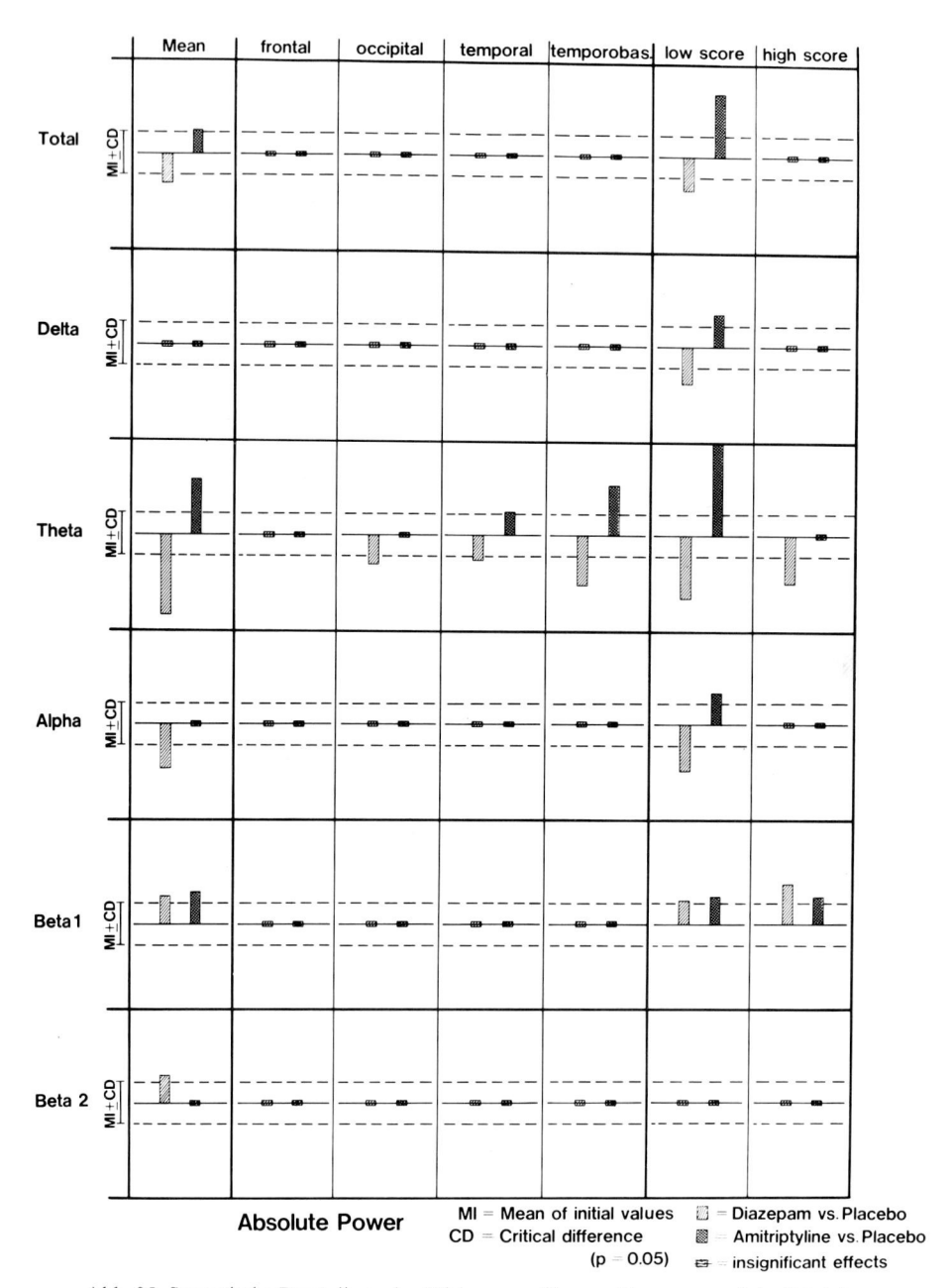

Abb. 25. Synoptische Darstellung des Wirkungsprofils von Diazepam und Amitriptylin

wird erkennbar, daß die Dimensionalität des elektroenzephalographischen Begriffssystems wesentlich erweitert werden muß, um die offensichtlich relevante Information auch fassen zu können.

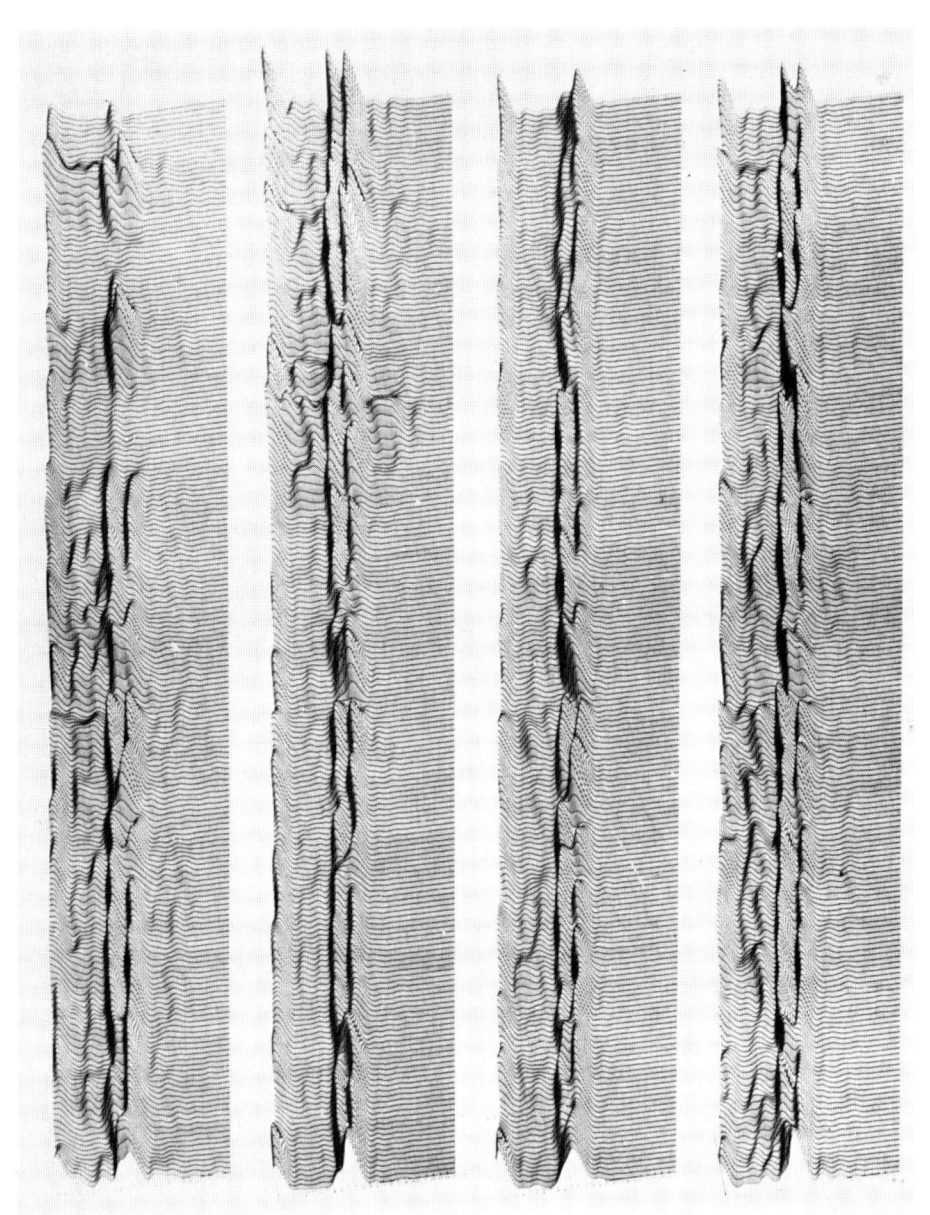

Aspekte der EEG-Analyse und ihrer Auswertung 145

Abb. 26. Verlaufsdynamik der EEG-Aktivität während 30 min. Von links nach rechts: temporobasal links, okzipital links, okzipital rechts, temporobasal rechts

V. Daten- und Informationsreduktion

Die in den Abschn. C.II–C.IV kurz dargestellten Beispiele von Verfahren der EEG-Analyse liefern eine in dieser Reihenfolge zunehmend differenzierte und umfangreiche quantitative Information über die dynamische Struktur der hirnelektrischen Aktivität und ihre topographische Differenzierung, die ohne Parameterextraktion und statistische Analyse rasch unübersehbar wird. Das Problem der EEG-Analyse liegt heute nicht mehr so sehr in der Methodik der einzelnen Verfahren, deren Zusammenhang untereinander mittlerweile theoretisch einigermaßen geklärt ist. Ein entscheidender Schritt auf dem Wege zu einer erfolgreichen Anwendung der EEG-Analyse auf klinisch-elektroenzephalographische Aufgaben bleibt die gezielte Reduktion der anfallenden Datenmengen auf die für die jeweilige Fragestellung relevante Information (KÜNKEL, 1978). Den wesentlichsten Anteil hieran hat die statistische Weiterverarbeitung der von der EEG-Analyse gelieferten Daten, sofern der Aspekt der Daten-Reduktion betrachtet wird. Damit nur z.T. parallel geht die gleichzeitige Informationsreduktion, die zum größeren Teil und überwiegend irreversibel durch das verwendete Analyse-Verfahren sowie die Parameter-Extraktion bewirkt wird. Der Vergleich der in den Abschn. C.II–C.IV erläuterten Verfahren läßt unschwer erkennen, daß die Amplituden-Integration nach DROHOCKI die stärkste, die Spektral-Analyse dagegen die am wenigsten eingreifende Informationsreduktion bewirkt, während die period analysis eine Mittelstellung einnimmt. Mit diesen Unterschieden der Informationsreduktion kann durchaus auch eine verschiedene Sensibilität von Analyse-Methoden gegenüber erwarteten EEG-Effekten verbunden sein. Beispielsweise vermochte die period analysis keine EEG-Effekte von einer dem Pyrithioxin chemisch verwandten Substanz aufzuzeigen, sehr wohl aber die Spektral-Analyse (FINK, 1977; KÜNKEL et al., 1976). Alle diese Aspekte müssen im Auge behalten werden, wenn EEG-analytische Befunde bei Psychosen oder bei der Klassifikation von Psychopharmaka beurteilt werden sollen.

Welches unerwartet große Maß von Datenreduktion etwa bei einer EEG-Spektral-Analyse von Medikationseffekten erforderlich wird, läßt sich am Beispiel des Vergleichs von Diazepam und Amitriptylin (Abb. 24, 25) veranschaulichen. Das Ausgangsmaterial waren 180 EEG, registriert in jeweils 8 Kanälen. Die in den Computer eingehende Datenmenge betrug dabei $3,6 \times 10^8$ bit (von „binary digit"; ein bit entspricht dem Informationsgehalt einer einfachen Ja-Nein-Entscheidung oder den Binär-Zahlen 0 oder 1). Mit dieser Datenmenge läßt sich der Druckinhalt von 15000 Seiten im Lexikonformat darstellen. Nach der Spektral-Analyse verbleiben 1440 Spektren mit einer Datenmenge von $2,4 \times 10^7$ bit, entsprechend einer Datenreduktion im Verhältnis von 15 zu 1. Die Extraktion der in Abschn. C.IV beschriebenen Parameter führt zu einer weiteren Datenreduktion im Verhältnis von etwa 28 zu 1. Die varianzanalytische Auswertung, etwa entsprechend dem Beispiel von Abb. 23, in der 6 von 18 Spektral-Parametern aufgeführt sind, führt zur Reduktion auf eine Datenmenge von 14 bit je Parameter (Anzahl von Ja-Nein-Entscheidungen bezüglich des Effektes von Diazepam bzw. Amitriptylin für die untersuchten Bedingungen), insgesamt also nur noch 252 bit. Vergleichsweise entspricht dies nur noch einem Druckgehalt von 42 Buchstaben.

Die Zusammenhänge zwischen EEG-Analyse- und Auswertungsverfahren einerseits sowie Daten- und Informationsreduktion andererseits sind noch wenig untersucht worden. Ihre nähere Kenntnis wäre jedoch von nicht zu unterschätzender Bedeutung, nicht nur für die Auswahl eines unter gegebener Fragestellung optimalen Verfahrens, sie würde auch unser Verständnis für die Funktionsstruktur des Gehirns und seine Informationsverarbeitung fördern, soweit sie sich im EEG ausdrücken. Heute gilt allerdings mehr denn je ein Zitat von D.O. WALTER aus dem Jahr 1963 (in freier Übersetzung): „Der Physiologe, der Computer und Statistik-Lehrbuch als ärgerlich empfindet, wird sich zugleich behindert sehen, wenn er die höchst organisierte Komplexität enträtseln will, die das Gehirn charakterisiert."

D. Grundphänomene evozierter und ereignisbezogener Potentiale

Eine Reihe von Monographien und Übersichtsarbeiten steht demjenigen zur Verfügung, der sich über evozierte und ereignisbezogene Potentiale informieren will. Hierzu sei verwiesen z.B. auf DESMEDT (1977), REGAN (1972, 1977), DAVIS (1977), VAN DER TWEEL (1977), LOW (1977), DONCHIN und LINDSLEY (1969), THOMPSON und PATTERSON (1974), STORM VAN LEEUWEN et al. (1975), McCALLUM und KNOTT (1973) (mit einer Bibliographie bis zum Jahre 1972).

Die Existenz von elektrischen kortikalen Antworten auf sensorische Reize hat bereits CATON (1875) in seinen Untersuchungen an der Hirnrinde von Versuchstieren nachgewiesen. Aber erst Jahrzehnte nach BERGERS ersten Arbeiten über das EEG des Menschen gelang es DAWSON (1954), Reizantworten auch im EEG des Menschen zu identifizieren. Seit der Entwicklung der Mittelungstechnik durch DAWSON steht der klinischen Neurophysiologie ein Verfahren zur Verfügung, welches der Untersuchung nicht nur von Vorgängen der Reizverarbeitung, sondern auch von anderen psychischen Vorgängen neue Wege eröffnet hat, die die Bedeutung des EEG für die Erforschung von Funktionsstrukturen des Gehirns und ihren Änderungen zunehmend unterstreichen. Dabei wird deutlich, daß eine Trennung von Grundaktivität und anderen Phänomenen des EEG einigermaßen willkürlich ist (WALTER, 1975), da sie oft eine Reaktion auf äußere Reize oder interne Prozesse darstellen.

Eine hervorstechende Eigenschaft evozierter Potentiale ist ihre beträchtliche inter- und intraindividuelle Variabilität, die ihre Interpretation stark beeinträchtigen kann. Dem Folgenden werden daher einige Anmerkungen zur Methodik vorangestellt, da sie in einem Umfang kritischen Einfluß auf die Ergebnisse der Registrierungen hat, der über den auf die Ableitung des EEG selbst weit hinausgeht. Antworten auf visuelle, akustische und sensorische Reize unterscheiden sich in wesentlichen Eigenschaften, so daß sie in gebotener Kürze dargestellt werden. Die „contingent negative variation" als Beispiel ereignisbezogener Potentiale spielt bei der Untersuchung von Psychosen eine zwar noch begrenzte, aber künftig sicher zunehmende Rolle, weshalb auch sie kurz besprochen wird, während das „Bereitschaftspotential" von motorischen Reaktionen nur gestreift werden kann.

I. Anmerkungen zur Methodik

Besonders bei *visueller Reizung* lassen sich verschiedene Reizformen einsetzen. In der Vergangenheit wurden am häufigsten Lichtblitze verwendet, entweder einzeln oder in Serien, mit einem Reizabstand von mindestens einer Sekunde, die sich einfach mit einer Gasentladungsröhre wie bei der Blinklichtbelastung im EEG erzeugen lassen. Meist wird dabei die gesamte Retina beleuchtet, während die Reizung lediglich von umschriebenen Retina-Arealen besondere technische Maßnahmen erfordert (ARMINGTON et al., 1961). Die Reizung mit sinusförmig moduliertem Licht bietet für die Analyse des optischen Systems Vorteile (van der Tweel et al., 1958), wurde bislang aber ebenso wie ein nach einer Zufallsfunktion intensitätsmoduliertes Licht wenig verwendet (van der Tweel, 1977). Schließlich gewinnt der Einsatz von strukturierten visuellen Reizen, insbesondere die Umkehr von Schachbrettmustern (Spehlmann, 1965), besonders in der Diagnostik der multiplen Sklerose (Halliday u. McDonald, 1977), zunehmende Bedeutung.

Akustische Reize werden üblicherweise über Kopfhörer oder Lautsprecher dargeboten, entweder als „clicks", wobei die Form der Flanken von Bedeutung ist, oder als Töne von kurzer Dauer. Hier wie bei *elektrischer Reizung* an peripheren Nerven zur Auslösung somatosensorischer Reizantworten sind bisher nur wenige Variationsmöglichkeiten untersucht worden.

Evozierte Potentiale besitzen in der Regel Amplituden von wenigen Mikrovolt, so daß sie in der spontanen Grundaktivität des EEG nicht ohne weiteres erkennbar sind. Zu ihrer Identifikation sind besondere Verfahren erforderlich, von denen die fortlaufende Summation und Mittelung gleichlanger EEG-Abschnitte nach gegebenem Reiz (Dawson, 1954) am häufigsten verwendet wird. Spezielle Rechner hierzu gehören heute zur Standardausrüstung vieler EEG-Labors. Mit zunehmender Anzahl summierter, reizsynchroner EEG-Abschnitte hebt sich das evozierte Potential gegenüber der fortlaufenden Grundaktivität immer deutlicher hervor. Die Zuverlässigkeit des Verfahrens hängt allerdings von Voraussetzungen ab, die offenbar nicht immer gültig sind (die Reizantwort sei deterministisch, die Grundaktivität stochastisch und reizunabhängig; Latenz, Form und Amplituden der Reizantwort bleiben in der Reizfolge konstant und zeigen keine Habituation; die Grundaktivität während der Reizfolge werde nicht durch Artefakte gestört).

Von noch stärkerem Einfluß auf evozierte Potentiale sind Faktoren, die durch die experimentellen Bedingungen häufig nur unvollkommen kontrolliert werden können, wie Vigilanz- und Aufmerksamkeitsänderungen der Probanden, Änderung des Muskeltonus, zunehmende Unbequemlichkeit der Versuchssituation, psychische Anspannung. Durch sie wird ein beträchtlicher Anteil der bekannten Variabilität evozierter Potentiale bedingt, so daß strikte Kontrolle und Einhaltung einer ganzen Reihe von Versuchsbedingungen unabdingbare Voraussetzungen darstellen.

Die Auswertung evozierter Potentiale beschränkt sich bislang, mit wenigen Ausnahmen, auf die Ausmessung von Latenz und Amplitude einzelner „peaks". Weitergehende Analyse-Methoden stützen sich auf statistische Verfahren, wie Faktoren-Analysen, Diskriminanz-Analysen oder Verfahren der Signal-Analyse. Für eine kurze Übersicht mit einschlägiger Literatur sei auf Lopes da Silva und van Rotterdam (1975) verwiesen.

II. Visuell evozierte Reizantworten (VER)

Eine typische evozierte Reizantwort auf Lichtblitz, registriert von der Okzipitalregion gegen das gleichseitige Ohr, zeigt Abb. 27. Hier wie in den folgenden Abbildungen weist die Negativität nach oben. Die Bezeichnung der einzelnen „peaks" mit römischen Ziffern folgt dem Vorschlag von Ciganek (1961). Die Komponenten I bis III werden häufig als „spezifische", die folgenden als „unspezifische Reizantwort" bezeichnet. Komponente III findet sich fast stets, während

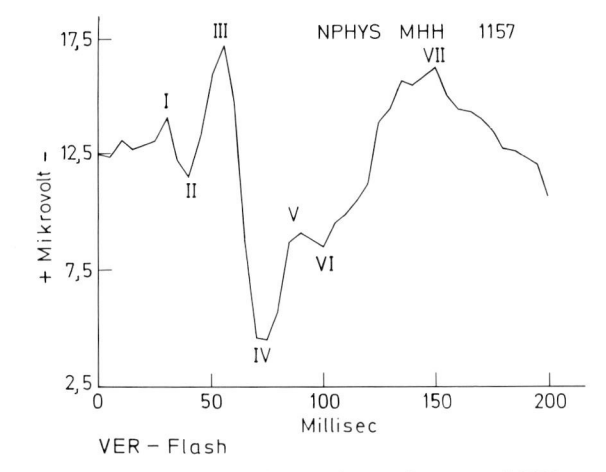

Abb. 27. Durch Lichtblitz evozierte Reizantwort (VER)

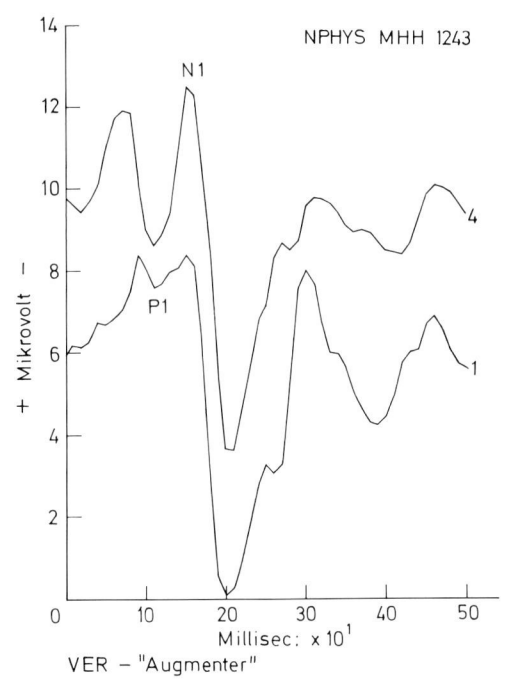

Abb. 28. Visuell (durch Lichtblitz) evozierte Reizantwort mit Zunahme der Amplitude P1-N1 bei Zunahme der Reizintensität im Verhältnis 1:4 („augmenter", s. Text)

I und II interindividuell labiler sind. Nach 800 bis 1000 msec beginnt häufig eine oszillierende Nachschwankung, die jedoch nur bei Alpha-Grundaktivität beobachtet wird und durch deren Summation zustande kommt (HELMCHEN et al., 1965).

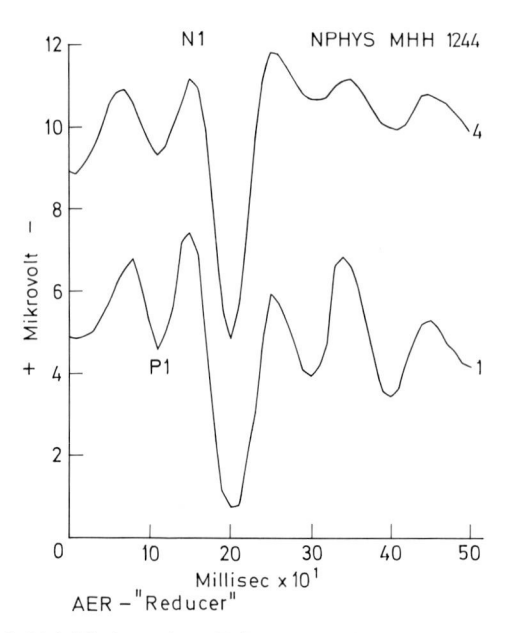

Abb. 29. Visuell (durch Lichtblitz) evozierte Reizantwort mit Abnahme der Amplitude P1-N1 bei Zunahme der Reizintensität im Verhältnis 1:4 („reducer", s. Text)

Reproduzierbare Versuchsbedingungen vorausgesetzt, bleibt der „spezifische" Anteil der Reizantwort intraindividuell einigermaßen konstant. Allerdings sind zirkadiane Schwankungen individuell verschieden deutlich ausgeprägt (HENINGER et al., 1969), auch ultradiane Variationen mit Perioden von 60 bis 120 min sind nachweisbar (KUGLER, 1965). Die „unspezifische" Reizantwort weist im allgemeinen eine große interindividuelle Variabilität auf. Die Altersabhängigkeit der VER ist u.a. von ELLINGSON (1966) und von WEINMANN et al. (1965) im Kindesalter untersucht worden. Danach entwickelt sich die für den Erwachsenen typische Form langsam vom 3. bis hin zum 16. Lebensjahr. Vom 50. Lebensjahr an nimmt die Variabilität der VER deutlich zu (JONKMAN, 1967). Geschlechtsdifferenzen sind offenbar nur geringfügig (SHAGASS et al., 1965), allerdings scheint die Entwicklung hin zur voll ausgebildeten Form bei Mädchen rascher zu verlaufen, als bei Knaben (ENGEL, 1967).

Ein Aspekt der individuellen Variabilität sei im Hinblick auf seine Bedeutung bei endogenen Psychosen erwähnt. Die Amplituden der Reizantwort auf Lichtblitz zeigen eine deutliche Abhängigkeit von der Intensität des Lichtreizes. BUCHSBAUM (1975) beobachtete, daß die Amplitudendifferenz zwischen P1 und N1 (nach seiner Nomenklatur, VI und VII nach CIGANEK) bei manchen Probanden mit zunehmender Reizintensität zunimmt, bei anderen dagegen abnimmt (Abb. 28, 29). Die erste Gruppe nennt er daher „augmenter", die zweite „reducer".

III. Akustisch evozierte Reizantworten (AER)

Abb. 30 zeigt die AER auf „click" bei einem Probanden mit besonders deutlicher Reizantwort. Die Bezeichnung der peaks folgt derjenigen von DAVIS und YOSHIE (1963), während SMITH et al. (1970) sie mit ihren Latenzen in Millisekunden bezeichnen. Die Form der AER sowie die Latenzen ihrer peaks zeigen eine noch größere inter- und intraindividuelle Variabilität als die VER, so daß bei ihrer Registrierung noch höhere Anforderungen gestellt werden müssen. Insbesondere Vigilanz- und Aufmerksamkeitsschwankungen sowie Ermüdung, die bei den notwendigen langen Versuchszeiten kaum zu vermeiden sind, wirken sich hier aus. Als relativ stabil erweisen sich die Potentialverläufe N1-P2 und P2-N2, die Werte zwischen 10 und 40 Mikrovolt erreichen können und die sich daher noch am ehesten zur Auswertung eignen.

Inwieweit die AER als spezifische Reaktion anzusehen sei, ist noch immer umstritten. STORM VAN LEEUWEN (1975) kommt zu der Auffassung, daß die AER weitgehend eine unspezifische Aktivität der Hirnrinde widerspiegelt. Sie würde sich dann wesentlich vom spezifischen Anteil der VER unterscheiden und darin der somatosensorischen Reizantwort ähneln. Bezüglich Einzelheiten der Diskussion muß hier u.a. auf DAVIS et al. (1966), VAUGHAN und RITTER (1970) und KOOI et al. (1971) verwiesen werden.

Die Abhängigkeit der AER-Amplitude von der Lautstärke des Reizes stellt die Grundlage für die objektive Audiometrie dar, während die Tonfrequenz nur einen geringfügigen Einfluß besitzt (DAVIS et al., 1966; KEIDEL u. SPRENG, 1965; SHARRARD, 1971). Wesentlich ist dagegen die Intervalldauer zwischen aufeinanderfolgenden Reizen, die nicht kürzer als 6 sec sein darf, da es sonst zu einer deutlichen Amplitudenabnahme im Sinne einer Habituation kommt

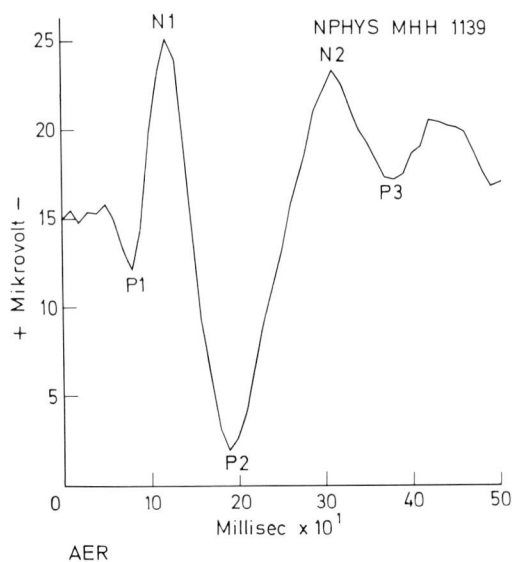

Abb. 30. Akustische evozierte Reizantwort (AER)

(DAVIS et al., 1966; FRUHSTORFER et al., 1970). Alters- und Geschlechtsabhängigkeit sind nicht so eingehend untersucht worden, wie bei der VER; jenseits der Kindheit scheint die AER einigermaßen entwickelt zu sein und konstant zu bleiben, während sie davor längere Latenzen und geringere Komplexität aufweist.

IV. Somatosensorisch evozierte Reizantworten (SSER)

Der erste Nachweis einer somatosensorisch ausgelösten Reizantwort nach elektrischem Reiz peripherer Nerven geht bereits auf die Pionierarbeit von DAWSON (1947) zurück. Die afferenten Impulse gehen offenbar über die Hinterstränge, den Lemniscus medialis und über Thalamuskerne (HALLIDAY u. WAKEFIELD, 1963; PAGNI, 1967). Trotz einer größeren Zahl systematischer Studien ist die Nomenklatur der einzelnen peaks durchaus noch kontrovers (HALLIDAY, 1975). Rein empirisch lassen sich in der SSER frühe und späte Komponenten abgrenzen. Erstere beginnen mit einer negativen Welle nach etwa 20 ms, gefolgt von ein oder zwei positiven Wellen mit Latenzen von 25–35 ms. Die letzteren beginnen mit einer Latenz von 50–65 ms und erstrecken sich etwa bis zu 250 ms. Am deutlichsten lassen sie sich kontralateral zur Reizseite nachweisen, finden sich aber auch ipsilateral. Generell läßt sich feststellen, daß beide Komponenten, besonders aber die späte, eine erhebliche Variabilität aufweisen, wie schon bei den AER erwähnt. Für eine ausführliche Übersicht über methodische, anatomische und physiologische Aspekte sei auf HALLIDAY (1975) verwiesen.

V. Contingent Negative Variation (CNV)

Von GREY WALTER et al. wurde 1964 ein Phänomen beschrieben, welches zunächst als „expectancy wave" oder mehr deskriptiv als „contingent negative variation" bezeichnet wurde. Diese Arbeit gab den Anstoß zur Entwicklung von Methoden, die ereignisbezogene zerebrale Potentiale in allgemeinerem Sinne zu untersuchen erlaubten und die damit neue Wege zur Erforschung höherer zentralnervöser Funktionen eröffneten. Abb. 31 zeigt die CNV in der ursprünglichen Versuchsanordnung. Im Zeitpunkt Null erfolgt ein Warnreiz (Lichtblitz), dem nach einer Sekunde ein Testreiz folgt (eine Serie von „clicks"). In dieser Versuchsanordnung wird der obere Potentialverlauf (I) registriert. Wird die Versuchsperson aufgefordert, den Testreiz („imperativer Reiz") durch Drücken eines Schalters möglichst rasch zu beenden, so resultiert typischerweise der Potentialverlauf der Kurve II mit einer negativen Auslenkung, die ein Ausmaß von 25–50 Mikrovolt erreicht, abhängig u.a. vom Ort der Registrierung. Die größte Amplitude findet sich dabei in Vertexnähe zwischen frontal bis präzentral.

Methodische Aspekte spielen bei der Registrierung der CNV eine entscheidende Rolle. Das Ausmaß der CNV hängt u.a. davon ab, ob im experimentellen Ablauf imperative Reize ausgelassen werden („equivocation", GREY WALTER et al., 1964), ob auf den imperativen Reiz andere Aufgaben gefordert werden oder ob verschiedene imperative Reize in nicht vorhersehbarer Reihenfolge gegeben werden, von denen nur ein bestimmter Reiz eine Reaktion erfordert. Auch die Registriereigenschaften der Verstärker sind wichtig: ihre Zeitkonstante sollte 8–10 s nicht unterschreiten. Dies bedeutet, daß die üblichen EEG-Verstärker normalerweise wenig geeignet sind. Eine ausführliche Darstellung dieser und weiterer kritischer Punkte gibt DONCHIN (1973).

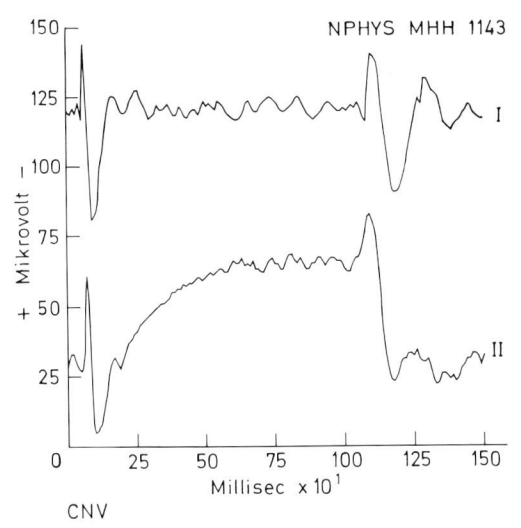

Abb. 31. Contingent Negative Variation (CNV, „Erwartungswelle")

Die CNV zeigt in Abhängigkeit von der speziellen Versuchssituation deutliche Geschlechtsunterschiede, die noch größer sind als die durch verschiedene Schwierigkeitsgrade der Reaktionsaufgabe bedingten Differenzen (DELSE et al., 1970). Die CNV in der in Abb. 31 gezeigten Form und unter den dort beschriebenen Bedingungen entwickelt sich offenbar im frühen Schulalter; ob später altersbedingte Variationen eine Rolle spielen, ist noch weitgehend unbekannt (COHEN, 1973). Die beträchtlichen methodischen Schwierigkeiten einer interindividuell reproduzierbaren Versuchssituation dürften solchen Untersuchungen auch große Hindernisse entgegenstellen.

Eine weitere Differenzierung ergibt sich bei Berücksichtigung der topographischen Verteilung der CNV, die anscheinend aus zwei negativ gehenden Potentialen besteht. Das eine erscheint unmittelbar nach dem Warnreiz mit größter Amplitude frontal, wie in Abb. 31, das andere unmittelbar vor dem imperativen Reiz mit größter Amplitude mehr fronto-präzentral (REGAN, 1977). Ersteres wird mit einem Aufmerksamkeitsanstieg in Zusammenhang gebracht, letzteres mit einer ansteigenden Reaktionsbereitschaft. Für eine Fülle von weiteren Befunden in Zusammenhang mit der CNV, die indessen für ihre Interpretation in Zusammenhang mit klinischen Fragestellungen von Bedeutung sind und hierbei beträchtliche Kontroversen bedingt haben, sei besonders auf die Übersichten bei DONCHIN und LINDSLEY (1969), LOW (1977), MCADAM (1974), MCCALLUM und KNOTT (1973, 1976), TECCE (1972) sowie THOMPSON und PATTERSON (1974) verwiesen.

VI. Bereitschaftspotentiale, motorische Potentiale

Jeder Willkürbewegung geht eine Folge von kortikalen Potentialen für eine Dauer bis zu einer Sekunde voraus, wie inzwischen hinreichend gesichert ist. Wohl als erste haben KORNHUBER und DEECKE (1965) sowie DEECKE et al. (1973)

das von ihnen so genannte Bereitschaftspotential beschrieben, welches als negative Potentialänderung mit größter Amplitude vertexnahe präzentro-parietal auftritt. Es findet sich bilateral, mit kontralateral zur innervierten Muskulatur etwas höherer Amplitude. Es ähnelt in der Form der CNV, ist mit ihr aber nicht identisch, wie Vaughan et al. (1968) annahmen. Etwa 80 ms vor dem elektromyographisch registrierten Bewegungsbeginn findet sich ein positiv gerichtetes, prämotorisches Potential, während das dem Einsetzen der Bewegung 50–60 ms vorausgehende motorische Potential wieder negativ gerichtet ist. Die Latenz des Bewegungsbeginns hängt von der innervierten Muskulatur ab und nimmt verständlicherweise in der Reihenfolge Gesichtsmuskulatur, Handmuskulatur, Fußmuskulatur zu. Dem motorischen Potential folgt wieder ein negatives, sog. Reafferenz-Potential. Auch das Bereitschaftspotential ist empfindlich gegenüber psychologischen Einflüssen der Versuchssituation. Die physiologische Bedeutung dieser bewegungsbezogenen Potentiale ist noch immer in der Diskussion.

Während die CNV und das Bereitschaftspotential negativ gerichtet sind, läßt sich nach Ablauf einer komplexen sensorischen Reizantwort auch oft ein positiv gerichtetes Potential registrieren, welches mit einer Latenz von 250–500 ms, häufig mit etwa 300 msec, nach dem Reiz auftritt und welches als „long latency potential" oder als „P 300" bezeichnet wird. Seine physiologischen Grundlagen und die Gründe für die große Variabilität seiner Latenz sind noch wenig geklärt (Low, 1977).

VII. Ergänzende Bemerkungen

Die Entdeckung der evozierten und ereignisbezogenen Potentiale hat gelehrt, daß jeder sensorische Reiz, jeder motorische Vorgang und offensichtlich jeder psychische Prozeß von kortikalen Potentialveränderungen begleitet, eingeleitet oder gefolgt wird. Sie sind oft von so kleiner Amplitude, daß sie in der spontanen Grundaktivität nicht ohne weiteres erkennbar sind oder nur mit besonderen Maßnahmen registriert werden können. Diese Potentiale kennzeichnet, mit gewisser Ausnahme vielleicht der VER, eine große Variabilität, die zu kritischen und subtilen Anforderungen an die Gesamtheit der Versuchssituation, nicht nur der speziellen Reizbedingungen führt. Der für ihr Studium erforderliche apparative Aufwand ist nicht gering und führt letztlich zum Einsatz von flexiblen Labor-Computern und recht komplexen Programmsystemen (Low, 1977; Regan, 1977). Diese Forschungsrichtung bleibt daher dem durchschnittlich ausgerüsteten EEG-Labor verschlossen. Dennoch eröffnet sie einen gänzlich neuen Blick in die Struktur höherer zentralnervöser Funktionen, der zugleich faszinierend und – vorläufig – verwirrend erscheint und dessen Möglichkeiten noch vor einem Jahrzehnt allenfalls geahnt werden konnten. Physiologische Grundlagen und Bedeutung dieser Phänomene sind noch immer teilweise unklar, ihre Labilität ist offenbar Ausdruck einer ebenfalls noch wenig verstandenen multifaktoriellen Bedingtheit. Andererseits ist sicher zu erwarten, daß die weitere methodische Entwicklung auf diesem Gebiet unser Verständnis psychischer Prozesse unter normalen und pathologischen Bedingungen fördern wird, auch wenn bislang trotz allen technischen und methodischen Aufwands noch immer nur erste Schritte in dieser Richtung möglich waren. Jedenfalls erscheint Bergers Hoffnung, das EEG als Abbild psychischer Vorgänge sehen zu können, nunmehr über jeden Zweifel hinaus begründet, wenn auch sein Code, mit dem es uns hierüber Aufschlüsse anbietet, von einer Entschlüsselung noch weit entfernt ist. Was uns als Variabilität, Labilität oder sogar Inkonsistenz dieser Erscheinungen beeindruckt, ist vielleicht eher Ausdruck unserer heutigen Unfähigkeit, die Vieldimensionalität ihrer Bedingungskonstellationen begrifflich zu erfassen. Dieser Aspekt wird im folgenden mehrfach wieder auftauchen, so bei der Diskussion von EEG-Befunden im Rahmen endogener Psychosen und bei EEG-Befunden im Verlauf psychiatrischer Pharmakotherapie.

E. EEG und Koma

Eine ausführliche Übersicht über die elektroenzephalographischen Aspekte der verschiedenen Komaformen wird von HARNER und NAQUET (1975) gegeben, wobei auch Probleme der Pathophysiologie erörtert werden. Ein älteres Standardwerk ist die Studie von FISCHGOLD und MATHIS (1959), die Koma-Probleme zwar vorwiegend von neurochirurgischer Sicht aus behandelt, indessen noch immer gültige Grundlagen vermittelt. Mehrere internationale Symposien haben das Bewußtsein und seine Störungen unter verschiedensten Gesichtswinkeln einigermaßen erschöpfend behandelt (ECCLES, 1966; GASTAUT, 1954; PENIN u. KÄUFER, 1965; PLUM u. POSNER, 1972). Eine Übersicht über die ältere Literatur gibt SILVERMAN (1963).

EEG-analytische Untersuchungen zum Thema sind vergleichsweise spärlich (BERGAMINI et al., 1966; FERILLO et al., 1969; FISCHGOLD u. MATHIS, 1959).

EEG-Veränderungen bei Bewußtseinsstörungen im Rahmen von symptomatischen Psychosen oder psychischen Störungen bei Epilepsie werden jeweils dort besprochen; hier stehen die EEG-Befunde bei Komaformen verschiedener Tiefe und Genese im Vordergrund. Bezüglich der Probleme des Hirntodes sei auf die von PENIN und KÄUFER (1969) herausgegebene Monographie verwiesen.

I. Grundsätzliche EEG-Veränderungen, Klassifikation von Koma-Stadien

Frühe Untersuchungen über den Zusammenhang zwischen Komatiefe und EEG gehen schon auf BERGER (1932, 1938), DAVIS und DAVIS (1939) zurück. Es schien damals einigermaßen gesichert, daß eine Zunahme von Theta- und Delta-Wellen im EEG einer zunehmenden Komatiefe parallel gehe. Das EEG wurde deshalb als zuverlässiger Indikator für die Beurteilung eines Komas angesehen (LINDSLEY, 1952; FISCHGOLD u. GASTAUT, 1957). Diese Regel bedarf allerdings der Präzisierung. Vermehrung von Theta-, Delta-Wellen kennzeichnet in unterschiedlicher Weise auch eine kontinuierliche Dysrhythmie, eine gruppierte Dysrhythmie oder Parenrhythmie, schließlich auch viele Herdbefunde (s. Abschn. B, S. 120ff.). Derartige Veränderungen finden sich indessen allein weniger bei deutlichen Bewußtseinsstörungen. Sie sollten besonders auch in diesem Zusammenhang von einer Allgemeinveränderung unterschieden werden, mit der sie in jeweils wechselnden Kombinationen auftreten können. Letztere, also die diffuse, kontinuierliche Vermehrung von Theta-, Delta-Wellen über beiden Hemisphären, ist für Bewußtseinsstörungen charakteristischer. Auch sie geht allerdings der Komatiefe nicht in einfacher Weise parallel, wie schon BERGER betont hat. Bei einem längerdauernden Koma können sich die EEG-Veränderungen durchaus – trotz klinischer Verschlechterung – teilweise zurückbilden (LUNDERVOLD et al., 1956). Jedenfalls lassen sich die diagnostischen Möglichkeiten des EEG besser nutzen, wenn die Befunde auf eine Klassifikation von Koma-Stadien bezogen werden, in deren Definitionen vorwiegend auch klinische Merkmale mit eingehen.

Als praktisch brauchbar erweist sich eine Klassifikation, die im wesentlichen auf die Studie von FISCHGOLD und MATHIS (1959) zurückgeht und die vier Stadien unterscheidet. (Eine Zweiteilung nur nach vorhandener oder fehlender Reaktion auf äußere Reize wird dem dynamischen Geschehen innerhalb des Komas nicht gerecht, eine Unterscheidung von bis zu 7 Stadien – z.B. BOZZA-MARRUBINI, 1964 – ist in der klinischen Praxis kaum praktikabel.) Im *Stadium I* ähnelt das klinische Bild äußerlich einer Hypersomnie mit Erweckbarkeit durch äußere Reize und der Reaktionsfähigkeit gegenüber äußeren Reizen. Spontaner Kontakt mit der Umgebung ist allerdings selten. Blink-, Korneal-, Pupillen- und Schluckreflexe sind noch ungestört, desgleichen die vegetativen Regulationen. Das EEG zeigt vorwiegend eine leichte bis mittlere Allgemeinveränderung mit deutlicher Reaktion auf Reize. Es unterscheidet sich meist von dem des physiologischen Schlafs, vor allem dadurch, daß nach Weckreizen rasch wieder Stadien deutlich vermehrter Theta- und Delta-Aktivität erreicht werden. Im *Stadium II* nimmt die Erweckbarkeit rasch ab, die Augen sind meist nicht mehr nach oben gerichtet, die Reaktion auf äußere Reize ist schwach oder erloschen. Die genannten Reflexe sind mehr oder weniger deutlich gestört, Veränderungen der Atmung treten auf. Das EEG zeigt in diesem Stadium nicht selten eine stärkere Labilität mit Fluktuation von mittlerer bis schwerer Allgemeinveränderung oder auch stärkere Amplituden-Reduktion, besonders in Atempausen. Äußere Reize provozieren, allerdings inkonstant, eine gruppierte Dysrhythmie oder auch Parenrhythmie. Wie im Stadium I können auch hier „Schlafspindeln" auftreten, spindelige Züge von langsamen Beta-Wellen im Frequenzbereich 13–15/s. Im *Stadium III* erlöschen Blink- und Schluckreflexe, Korneal- und Pupillenreflexe können noch erhalten sein. Die Spontanatmung kann bereits der Assistenz bedürfen. Die Reagibilität auf äußere Reize ist erloschen oder es kommt zu medullären Reflexen. Das EEG zeigt eine schwere Allgemeinveränderung ohne nennenswerte Fluktuation und ohne Reaktion auf äußere Reize. Im *Stadium IV* schließlich sind alle zerebralen Reflexe erloschen, die Spontanatmung sistiert und im EEG lassen sich keine Zeichen hirneigener elektrischer Aktivität mehr nachweisen (sog. „Null-Linien-EEG"). Der Übergang von Stadium III in Stadium IV wird nicht selten durch eine zunehmende Abflachung des EEG eingeleitet, wobei auch die dann prognostisch ungünstige „burst-suppression"-Aktivität (Abb. 4) für eine gewisse Zeit das EEG beherrschen kann.

Auch diese Klassifikation ist nicht voll befriedigend, weil sie in ein Kontinuum von Veränderungen aus praktischen Gründen Schnitte legt, die sich an klinischen und elektroenzephalographischen Kriterien orientieren. Insbesondere die Fluktuation der Komatiefe im Stadium II bringt Unsicherheiten für die Korrelation zwischen klinischen und elektroenzephalographischen Befunden.

II. EEG-Befunde im Koma

In der Praxis kann davon ausgegangen werden, daß eine schwere Allgemeinveränderung ohne Reagibilität auf äußere Reize und ohne erkennbare zeitliche Fluktuation die Annahme eines tiefen Komas des Stadium III rechtfertigt. Die Häufigkeit von Allgemeinveränderungen und ihr Schweregrad nehmen mit den Koma-Stadien im allgemeinen zu. LOEB (1964, 1975) fand bei 300 komatösen Kranken mit neoplastischen oder vaskulären zerebralen Prozessen im Stadium I in 25%, im Stadium II in 50% und im Stadium III in 60% mehr oder weniger schwere Allgemeinveränderungen. Herdstörungen dagegen fanden sich in etwa 70%, 50% und 25%. Ihr Auftreten hängt unmittelbar mit dem zerebralen Prozeß zusammen, der dem Koma zugrunde liegt. Diese Herde können durch eine zunehmende Allgemeinveränderung maskiert werden und dementsprechend im Stadium II in ihrer Ausprägung wechseln, entsprechend einer Fluktuation der Allgemeinveränderung.

Die *Reagibilität* des EEG auf äußere Reize kann im Stadium I noch der einer normalen Grundaktivität ähneln, wie der prompten Blockierung von noch in Resten vorhandener Alpha-Aktivität. Im Stadium II zeigt sich oft eine gruppierte Theta-, Delta-Aktivität nach einem Reiz, die meist schon zeitlich verzögert erscheint und besonders bei niedrigeren Amplituden der Grundaktivität deutlich wird. Im tiefen Koma kann, falls überhaupt eine Reaktion erfolgt, auch eine vorübergehende Abflachung provoziert werden. Die Bedeutung dieser interindividuell variablen Befunde liegt bei Verlaufsuntersuchungen darin, daß eine Reduktion und schließlich ein Erlöschen der EEG-Reagibilität – vom Koma bei Schlafmittel-Intoxikation abgesehen (KUBICKI, 1967; KUBICKI et al., 1970) – ein signum mali ominis darstellt.

Das Koma-EEG bietet mitunter Aspekte einer *Periodizität*, auf die in Abschn. B schon hingewiesen wurde. Sie zeigt sich in dem sog. „tracé alternant", in welchem mehrere Sekunden lange Phasen einer niedrigen, irregulären Aktivität mit Beta- oder auch Alpha-Wellen mit solchen hoher Theta-, Delta-Aktivität abwechselt. In ersteren Phasen finden sich bei polygraphischer Registrierung oft auch Störungen des Atem-Rhythmus bis hin zur Apnoe.

Die geschilderten Beziehungen zwischen EEG und Koma sind als Regeln zu werten, die durch klinisch-elektroenzephalographische Erfahrung zwar immer wieder bestätigt, im Einzelfall aber durchaus durchbrochen werden können. Grundsätzlich können komatöse Zustandsbilder sich mit den verschiedensten EEG-Befunden kombinieren, auch mit anscheinend „normalen" (LUNDERVOLD et al., 1956; SILVERMAN, 1963; RADERMECKER, 1967). Offensichtlich wird die Parellelität von Allgemeinveränderung und Koma-Stadium durch eine Reihe von Faktoren modifiziert, von denen Besonderheiten der Ätiologie und solche der Topographie eine wesentliche Rolle spielen.

III. Modifikationen durch ätiologische Besonderheiten

Eine Reihe von Störungen der Bewußtseinslage bei metabolischen Enzephalopathien zeigt Besonderheiten des EEG (HARNER u. KATZ, 1975). Hiervon seien nur einige herausgegriffen. Bei *urämischen Bewußtseinsstörungen* tritt neben der Allgemeinveränderung oft eine diskontinuierliche Aktivität mit gruppierter Dysrhythmie und auch hypersynchroner Aktivität, vor allem spikes und sharp waves, in den Vordergrund. Parallel dazu geht eine vermehrte Empfindlichkeit des EEG gegenüber Blinklichtbelastung, bis hin zu photokonvulsiven Reaktionen, ohne daß ein engerer Zusammenhang mit biochemischen Aspekten der Urämie immer erkennbar wird (KILEY, 1971, 1972; MERRILL u. HAMPERS, 1970; SPEHR et al., 1977). Das *hypoglykämische Koma* bietet im allgemeinen keine wesentlichen EEG-Besonderheiten. Eine besondere Form des hypoglykämischen Komas mit Hyperosmolarität ohne Ketose (MACCARIO, 1968; DANIELS et al., 1969) geht des öfteren auch mit fokalen Krampfanfällen und entsprechenden EEG-Befunden einher. Bei der hepatischen *Enzephalopathie* erweist sich das EEG für eine Früh-Diagnose und Prognose als bedeutsam, da EEG-Veränderungen noch vor anderen klinischen Zeichen auftreten können und sog. „triphasische Wellen", die langsamen hohen spikes ähneln, wichtige diagnostische Hinweise auf die Ätiologie liefern, obgleich sie auch bei anderen metabolischen Enzephalopathien auftreten können (SILVERMAN, 1962; PLUM und POSNER, 1972; PENIN, 1967).

IV. Modifikationen durch topographische Besonderheiten

Daß der einer Bewußtseinsstörung zugrunde liegende Prozeß durch seine Lokalisation das EEG im Sinne von Herdbefunden zumindest bei nicht allzu schwerer Allgemeinveränderung modifizieren kann, bedarf keiner näheren Erläuterung. Eine Besonderheit stellt indessen das EEG mit anscheinend „*normaler*" *Alpha-Aktivität* im Koma der Stufe III dar. Dieser zunächst befremdliche Befund wurde schon früh beschrieben (GASTAUT, 1954; LOEB u. MEYER, 1965). Er findet sich regelmäßig bei Läsionen im Hirnstamm, vorwiegend im Pons-Bereich, sofern das Mesenzephalon nicht betroffen ist. Diese „Pseudo-Alpha-Aktivität" ähnelt zwar nach Frequenz und topographischer Verteilung dem normalen Alpha-Rhythmus, zeigt indessen keine Reagibilität gegenüber äußeren Reizen. Sie zeigt jedenfalls fast ausnahmslos eine schlechte Prognose an, wie der Ort der Läsion erwarten läßt.

Schließlich sei noch auf das *apallische Syndrom* verwiesen, dessen klinische Aspekte von KRETSCHMER (1940) beschrieben wurden. Bezüglich der klinischen, neuropathologischen und elektroenzephalographischen Aspekte sei auf GERSTENBRAND (1967) sowie JELLINGER und SEITELBERGER (1970) und KLEE (1961) verwiesen. Die EEG-Befunde variieren hierbei von Fall zu Fall beträchtlich, von weitgehend normaler Grundaktivität über Herdveränderungen bis zu Allgemeinveränderungen. Der Übergang aus einem tiefen Koma in ein apallisches Syndrom wird häufig schon vor der klinischen Erkennbarkeit durch die zunehmende Ausprägung von Alpha-Aktivität signalisiert, zugleich mit wiederkehrender Reagibilität des EEG auf äußere Reize. Eine solche „Normalisierung" des EEG kann der klinischen Entwicklung indessen auch nachhinken oder auch gänzlich ausbleiben.

V. Evozierte Potentiale im Koma

Untersuchungen über die Bedeutung optisch evozierter Potentiale zur Bestimmung von Koma-Stadien und Prognose sind noch immer spärlich, die Deutung

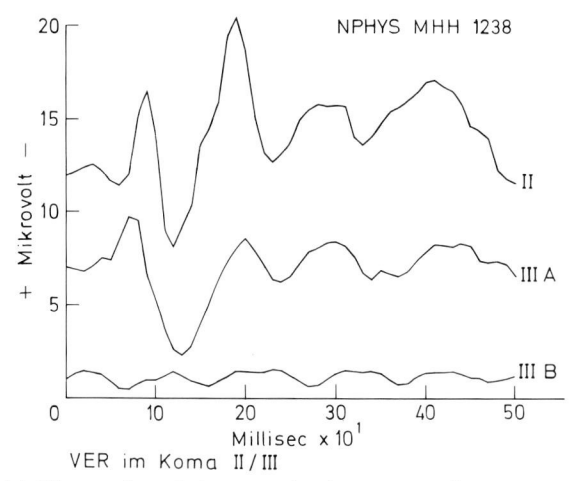

Abb. 32. Durch Lichtblitz evozierte Reizantwort in den Komastadien II und III (Erläuterung s. Text)

der vorliegenden Befunde widersprüchlich und unsicher (ARFEL, 1975; ARFEL u. WALTER, 1971; CORLETTO et al., 1966; LILLE et al., 1967). Als einigermaßen gesichert kann gelten, daß optisch wie auch akustisch evozierte Potentiale mit zunehmender Komatiefe in der Amplitude abnehmen und entdifferenziert werden. Abb. 32 zeigt eine eigene Beobachtung, bei der im Stadium III das optisch evozierte Potential zerfiel und schließlich eine Woche vor dem letalen Ausgang trotz unverändertem Schweregrades der Allgemeinveränderung bereits nicht mehr nachweisbar war. Umgekehrt zeigt das erneute Auftreten von evozierten Potentialen eine Besserung auch bei noch anscheinend unveränderter Koma-Tiefe an (ARFEL, 1967).

VI. Ergänzende Bemerkungen

Veränderungen des EEG sind nicht unmittelbarer Ausdruck von Veränderungen oder Störungen der Bewußtseinslage, auch wenn eine mehr statistische Parellelität zwischen Koma-Tiefe und Schweregrad von Allgemeinveränderungen des EEG recht gut durch die Erfahrung bestätigt wird. Im Einzelfall jedoch sind von dieser Regel auch Ausnahmen in verschiedener Richtung möglich, sei es, daß Herdstörungen das Bild modifizieren, sei es, daß im Verlauf der Schweregrad einer Allgemeinveränderung der Zunahme der klinisch bestimmten Koma-Tiefe zuwiderlaufen kann. Es darf dabei nicht übersehen werden, daß Bewußtseinsstörungen auf der einen, EEG-Veränderungen auf der anderen Seite verschiedene Aspekte der Manifestation des zugrunde liegenden zerebralen Prozesses sind, wie etwa eine Blutung, ein Trauma, eine Intoxikation oder eine Raumforderung. Durch eine solche im einzelnen unterschiedliche Ätiologie der Bewußtseinsstörung können deshalb verständlicherweise auch unterschiedliche elektroenzephalographische Manifestationen provoziert werden. Insoweit spielt auch eine Lokalisation nicht so sehr des zugrunde liegenden Prozesses, als der von ihm selbst oder von Fernwirkungen betroffenen Strukturen eine wesentliche Rolle. Unter diesem Aspekt läßt sich verstehen, daß ein „Pseudo-Alpha-EEG" auch bei Läsionen in anderen als Hirnstammregionen auftreten kann. Auch das andersartige EEG des apallischen Syndroms ist so zu sehen. Beim Problem der Beziehungen zwischen Bewußtseinsstörungen und EEG-Veränderungen ist im Auge zu behalten, daß nicht so sehr bestimmte zerebrale Prozesse, sondern die durch sie bewirkten zerebralen Funktionsänderungen zu bestimmten EEG-Veränderungen führen, unter denen Allgemeinveränderungen zwar eine wesentliche, aber nicht die alleinige Rolle spielen.

F. Symptomatische Psychosen und EEG

Der ätiologischen Vielfalt symptomatischer Psychosen steht eine relative Monotonie der möglichen Reaktionsformen im EEG gegenüber, die sich im wesentlichen lediglich in Modifikationen der Grundaktivität, wie Allgemeinveränderungen, kontinuierlichen Dysrhythmien oder Herdstörungen sowie in der Produktion der verschiedenen diskontinuierlich auftretenden Aktivitätsformen auszudrücken vermögen. Insoweit ist es wenig aufschlußreich, für das breite Spektrum symptomatischer Psychosen immer wieder gleiche oder ähnliche EEG-Veränderungen zu referieren, zumal im Einzelfall vom EEG her zu einer ätiologischen Diagnose meist nur wenig beigetragen werden kann. Ganz andere Zusammenhänge beginnen sich allerdings zu eröffnen, wenn Aspekte der Syndrom-Genese und der Verlaufsdynamik den begleitenden EEG-Veränderungen gegenübergestellt werden. Diese Betrachtungsweise wird auch bei den epileptischen Psychosen sowie bei den paranoid-halluzinatorischen Syndromen und Schizophrenien in verstärktem Maße zu berücksichtigen sein.

Ausführliche Darstellungen des Gegenstandes aus neuerer Zeit finden sich im Handbook of Electroencephalography and Clinical Neurophysiology, so in den Bänden 13b, 14 und 15, ferner bei FLÜGEL (1974), PENIN und ZEH (1964), PENIN (1971). Die ersten systematischen und umfassenden Studien dürften auf ENGEL und ROMANO (1944) zurückgehen.

I. Stoffwechselstörungen, endokrine Störungen

Übersichten über EEG-Veränderungen bei Stoffwechselstörungen und endokrinen Störungen finden sich zusammen mit ausführlichen Literaturübersichten bei CADILHAC et al. (1959), CADILHAC und RIBSTEIN (1961), FAURE (1961), FLÜGEL (1974), HESS (1954), ROHMER et al. (1969), THIÉBAUT et al. (1958); DUMERMUTH (1976) gibt diesbezüglich Kurvenbeispiele. Wie nicht anders zu erwarten, gibt es keine Befunde, die für bestimmte dieser Störungen pathognomonisch wären, selbst Korrelationen zwischen Blutspiegelwerten und EEG-Veränderungen sind im Einzelfall unsicher. Am deutlichsten finden sich Veränderungen bei Hypoglykämie und Alkalose, auch bei Hyperhydratation, während die gegensinnigen Zustände meist geringe oder keine EEG-Veränderungen bewirken. Die *Hypoglykämie* zeigt sich im EEG nach GIBBS et al. (1940) erst bei Glukosegehalten des Blutes von 40 mg-% und weniger als zunehmende Verlagsamung der Grundaktivität. Sie geht in eine zunehmend schwere Allgemeinveränderung beim hypoglykämischen Koma über, der anfangs auch eine gruppierte abnorme Delta-Rhythmisierung überlagert sein kann. Die Parallelität zum Blutzuckerspiegel ist allerdings keineswegs zwingend: ZIEGLER und PRESTHUS (1957) konnten zeigen, daß unter i.v. zugeführtem Insulin noch bei Glukosespiegeln von 15 mg-% wesentliche EEG-Veränderungen ausblieben. *Hyperglykämien* führen erst beim Coma diabeticum zu Allgemeinveränderungen (FLÜGEL u. DRUSCHKY, 1976). Bei der *Urämie* und ihren begleitenden psychotischen Störungen lassen sich keine einheitlichen Beziehungen zu EEG-Veränderungen herstellen, indessen kann das EEG bei der Dialyse auf ein drohendes „Dysäquilibrium-Syndrom" (KENNEDY et al., 1909; NADEL u. WILSON, 1976) mit Bewußtseinsstörungen,

Kloni und Krampfanfällen aufmerksam machen. Wesentlich ist hier offenbar der Gradient des Harnstoffspiegels, ebenso wie bei einer sich entwickelnden Urämie, bei deren schleichendem Verlauf das EEG relativ unauffällig bleibt (KILEY et al., 1976). Bei spektralanalytischen EEG-Untersuchungen fanden SPEHR et al. (1977) einen Zusammenhang zwischen der Erholung des psychischen Bildes und der Abnahme des Anteils langsamer Wellen, im Gegensatz zu KILEY und HINES (1965), KILEY et al. (1976). LEWIS et al. (1978) fanden bei 8 Kranken mit chronischer Hämodialyse eine Latenzverlängerung und höhere Amplituden visuell und somatosensorisch evozierter Potentiale. Nierentransplantation führte zu einer Normalisierung. Die *akute intermittierende Porphyrie* kann zu Allgemeinveränderungen führen (REYBELLET, 1964), desgleichen die *Vitamin-B_{12}-Mangelsyndrome*, ohne daß ein durchgehender Zusammenhang zwischen Blutbefunden und EEG erkennbar wird (WALLACE u. WESTMORELAND, 1976). Hier wie bei *Endokrinopathien* liegt die Bedeutung des EEG am ehesten mit in der Erfolgskontrolle einer Substitutionstherapie. Recht typische EEG-Veränderungen mit Frequenzverlangsamung, die meist noch nicht den Grad einer Allgemeinveränderung erreicht, begleiten ein endokrines Psychosyndrom, etwa bei *Hypothyreose* (LOGOTHETIS, 1963), während das Myxödemkoma als oft fatales Ereignis im EEG von einer rasch zunehmenden Allgemeinveränderung gekennzeichnet wird. Bei *Hyperthyreose* findet sich entsprechend eine Frequenzbeschleunigung (KOLLMANNSBERGER et al., 1967). Die thyreotoxische Enzephalopathie zeigt wiederum Allgemeinveränderungen wechselnden Ausmaßes; das gleiche gilt für die *hepatische Enzephalopathie* (PENIN, 1967; LANZINGER-ROSSNAGEL et al., 1977). Bei ihr sowie bei der urämischen Enzephalopathie können triphasische Wellen (vgl. Kap. E.III) diagnostische Hinweise geben. *Genetisch bedingte Stoffwechselstörungen* zeigen so gut wie immer stärkere EEG-Störungen mit Allgemeinveränderung, z.T. überlagert mit gruppierten Dysrhythmien und abnormen Rhythmisierungen (Einzelheiten der Literatur finden sich z.B. bei DUMERMUTH, 1976).

Mit den beschriebenen Modifikationen lassen sich für metabolische und endokrine Enzephalopathien vom EEG her einige allgemeingültige Feststellungen treffen (PENIN, 1971): Leichte Enzephalopathien lassen keine oder nur leichte EEG-Veränderungen in Form von Frequenzverlangsamungen der Grundaktivität oder kontinuierliche Dysrhythmien vorwiegend im temporobasalen Bereich erkennen. Bei mittleren Enzephalopathien pflegt sich eine gruppierte abnorme Rhythmisierung im Theta-Bereich oder eine gruppierte Dysrhythmie einzustellen, die bei zunehmendem Schweregrad der Enzephalopathie in eine Delta-Parenrhythmie oder ausgeprägte kontinuierliche Dysrhythmie mit topographischer Ausbreitung übergehen. Dabei ist zu betonen, daß eine solche Beziehung einlinig zu sehen ist: Diese EEG-Phänomene begleiten eine Enzephalopathie relativ häufig, sind dafür jedoch keineswegs beweisend. Anders bei den präkomatösen und komatösen Zuständen, bei denen Allgemeinveränderungen zunehmenden Schweregrades – mit den in Abschn. E dargestellten Modifikationen – so gut wie stets angetroffen werden. Hier ist der Zusammenhang auch umkehrbar: Allgemeinveränderungen in dem in Abschn. B definierten Sinn lassen Beeinträchtigungen oder Störungen in der Bewußtseinslage erwarten, die einer sorgfältigen Untersuchung nicht zu entgehen pflegen.

II. Gefäßprozesse, Hypoxidosen

Bei *chronischen zerebralen Gefäßprozessen* fand SPUNDA (1960) auffallend häufig Verlangsamungen des Alpha-Rhythmus bis hin zu leichten Allgemeinveränderungen. Dies galt besonders für Kranke mit psychischen Störungen, weniger für solche mit rein neurologischen Abweichungen, bei denen eher Herdstörungen zu beobachten waren. Hierbei blieb aber offen, inwieweit die Häufigkeit dieser Befunde sich von derjenigen einer altersentsprechenden Vergleichspopulation unterscheidet. Eine Untersuchung von MUNDY-CASTLE et al. (1954) ist hierzu auch heute noch aufschlußreicher, insofern zwei Gruppen von Probanden etwa gleichen Alters um 75 Jahre miteinander verglichen wurden, von denen die eine senile Psychosen aufwies. Frequenzlabile EEG, die für zerebrale Gefäßprozesse als bezeichnend gelten, sowie gruppierte Dysrhythmien, weniger auch Allgemeinveränderungen, fanden sich bei einem Viertel der Vergleichsgruppe ohne Psychosen, bei der anderen Gruppe dagegen zeigten sich in über der Hälfte vorwiegend Allgemeinveränderungen. Weitere Arbeiten hierzu (LUCE u. ROTHSCHILD, 1953), die bei Kranken mit psychotischen Störungen in 90% EEG-Abnormitäten fanden, müssen aus methodischen Gründen mit Zurückhaltung bewertet werden. Frequenzanalytische Untersuchungen von OBRIST und HENRY (1958) sowie OBRIST (1963) fanden einen Zusammenhang von verminderter zerebraler Sauerstoffaufnahme mit erniedrigter Grundfrequenz des EEG, was neuerdings von INGVAR et al. (1976) bestätigt wurde. Gewichtig sind die schon 1959 von ROTH erhobenen und später mehrfach bestätigten Befunde, wonach bei akuten Verwirrtheitszuständen Delta-Parenrhythmien auftraten, nicht aber bei chronischen dementiellen Verläufen. Die Rolle des EEG in der Verlaufs- und Therapiekontrolle zerebraler Gefäßprozesse gewinnt neben der rein neurologischen Diagnostik eine zunehmende Bedeutung (BRANDT et al., 1976). *Chronische zerebrale Hypoxidosen* bei respiratorischer Insuffizienz (PLANQUES et al., 1965), auch bei schweren generalisierten Myasthenien (PRÜLL et al., 1970), beim Pickwick-Syndrom, bei kongenitalen Vitien, gehen nur dann einigermaßen regelmäßig mit EEG-Befunden im Sinne von Allgemeinveränderungen einher, wenn gleichzeitig Störungen der Bewußtseinslage bestehen. *Akute Hypoxidosen*, etwa nach Strangulation (z.B. NIEDERMEYER, 1956; FÜNFGELD, 1967) oder Herzstillstand führen ausnahmslos zu den beim Koma typischen EEG-Veränderungen, insofern das Ereignis überhaupt überlebt wird. Dabei fällt auf, daß sich das EEG im Verlauf völlig normalisieren kann, während das psychopathologische Bild in einen chronischen Defektzustand übergeht.

III. Entzündungen des ZNS

Enzephalitiden und Meningitiden bieten im EEG unter psychiatrischen Aspekten keine Besonderheiten, die über die im Voranstehenden beschriebenen Zusammenhänge hinausgehen. Ausmaß von psychopathologischen und EEG-Veränderungen korrelieren nicht gesetzmäßig mit Ausnahme des auch hier wieder zu bestätigenden Zusammenhanges zwischen Bewußtseinsstörung und Allgemeinveränderung. Eine gelegentliche Ausnahme scheint, wie DUENSING schon 1949 betont hat, für die tuberkulöse Meningitis zu gelten, die durch vergleichsweise ausgeprägte Allgemeinveränderungen auffällt. Dies scheint besonders bei Kindern Gültigkeit zu haben (GARSCHE, 1954). Auch durch neuere Untersuchungen nicht überholt ist die sorgfältige Studie von HUBACH (1959) an 100 Kranken mit Enzephalitis, der bei einem Drittel der Kranken mit mittlerer Allgemeinveränderung keine Bewußtseinsstörungen fand, bei leichter Allgemeinveränderung sogar in über der Hälfte der Fälle. Bei der Verlaufsbetrachtung war nicht selten die Normalisierung des EEG gegenüber der klinischen Besserung verzögert, was auch durch MENSOKOVA (1958) gesehen wurde. Eine elektroenzephalographische Besonderheit bieten die Panenzephalitiden vom Typ Dawson, Pette-Döring, van Bogaert mit ihren fast pathognostischen EEG-Befunden (s. Abschn. B. VI), die wohl zuerst von BALTHASAR (1944) gesehen und später von RADERMECKER (1957) erschöpfend beschrieben wurden.

Eine gesonderte Besprechung erfordern Untersuchungen von PENIN und SCHAEFER (1964) sowie PENIN und MATIAR-VAHAR (1964) über das EEG der *Neurolues*. Die Querschnittsbetrachtung ergab bei den verschiedenen Formen der Neurolues keine sicheren Korrelationen etwa zwischen serologischen, psychischen und elektroenzephalographischen Befunden. Eine Ausnahme bildet das Syndrom des „akuten psychischen Leistungszerfalls" bei der progressiven Paralyse, bei dem sich ausnahmslos eine Delta-Parenrhythmie fand. (Eine gleichartige Beobachtung findet sich bereits bei BERGER, 1931.) Hier sind die in der Literatur nur zu oft vernachlässigten Verlaufsaspekte einer symptomatischen Psychose relevant: Eine Parenrhythmie, obwohl hierfür nicht spezifisch, entwickelt sich regelhaft, wenn sich die psychischen Störungen rasch zu einem besonderen Schweregrad entwickeln. Hierauf ist in Abschn. I.VI noch einzugehen.

IV. Hirntraumen, EKT

Die *EEG-Veränderungen bei Hirntraumen* und posttraumatischen Psychosen sind in noch heute gültiger Form von MEYER-MICKELEIT (1953) sowie SCHNEIDER und HUBACH (1962) dargestellt worden. Seit langem ist bekannt, daß nach einer Commotio nur minutenlange, allenfalls wenige Stunden anhaltende EEG-Veränderungen auftreten (DOW et al., 1944). Posttraumatische Allgemeinveränderungen finden sich stets beim Vorliegen einer traumatischen Psychose. Die EEG-Veränderungen, die durchaus mit Herdstörungen kombiniert sein können, bilden sich regelmäßig innerhalb von maximal 6 Monaten zurück, begleitet von einer Rückbildung auch der psychotischen Störung. In diesem Verlauf finden sich auch Phasen von abnormen Rhythmisierungen im Delta- und Theta-Bereich, die eine Allgemeinveränderung etwa bei leichter Bewußtseinsstörung überlagern können. Im Endverlauf kann die Normalisierung des EEG durchaus dem psychopathologischen Verlauf vorauseilen, ein leichtes amnestisches Korsakow-Syndrom kann noch monatelang trotz eines EEG mit allenfalls gering verlangsamter Grundfrequenz persistieren. Herdbefunde können unabhängig von einer neurologischen Symptomatik sehr viel länger überdauern, übrigens häufiger bei durch eine traumatische Psychose komplizierten Verläufen. Diskrepante Verläufe von EEG-Rückbildung und klinischer Besserung können gewisse Verlaufstendenzen zur Ausbildung eines Defektsyndroms signalisieren, in gewisser Ähnlichkeit mit den EEG-Verhältnissen bei der Entstehung eines apallischen Syndroms.

Von psychiatrischen Interesse sind auch die EEG-Veränderungen nach *EKT*, deren Darstellung sich u.a. bei CREMERIUS und JUNG (1947), JUNG (1950), LENNOX et al. (1951), MEYER-MICKELEIT (1949), SCANLON und MATHIAS (1967) finden. Dabei zeigen sich während des tonischen Stadiums hohe rasche Wellen und spikes, im klonischen Stadium hohe Delta-Wellen, danach für kurze Zeit eine starke Abflachung des EEG. In der postparoxysmalen Bewußtlosigkeit zeigt sich eine schwere Allgemeinveränderung mit Überwiegen hoher Delta-Wellen, dann eine Rückbildung zur leichten Allgemeinveränderung mit Ausgang in eine Normalisierung. Bemerkenswert ist, daß diese kontinuierliche Normalisierung mit zunehmender Anzahl von Krampfbehandlungen auch zunehmend protrahiert verläuft und Tage bis Wochen beanspruchen kann, parallel mit den sich zurückbildenden Störungen der Merkfähigkeit (FINK u. KAHN, 1957). Untersuchungen aus den letzten Jahren (MARJERRISON et al., 1975; STRÖMGREN u. JUUL-JENSEN, 1975) fügen diesem Bild zwar im Detail, nicht aber in den grundsätzlichen Zügen neue Aspekte hinzu.

V. Intoxikationen und Entzugs-Syndrome

Die psychischen Störungen bei chronischen Intoxikationen und bei Entzugs-Syndromen weisen bezüglich der sie begleitenden EEG-Veränderungen weitgehende Parallelen auf. Aus diesem Grunde soll hier vorwiegend auf alkoholtoxische und einige medikamentöse Syndrome eingegangen werden. Eine etwas weitergefaßte Übersicht gibt FLÜGEL (1974).

Die *akute Alkoholintoxikation* führt bei Blutspiegelwerten, die über 0,7–1,0$^0/_{00}$ liegen, zu einer leichten Allgemeinveränderung, die mit steigendem Blutalkoholspiegel kontinuierlich zunimmt, wobei allerdings erhebliche interindividuelle Differenzen zu finden sind (CASPERS u. ABELE, 1956; LORENZONI et al., 1968). Vermehrte Beta-Wellen, wie bei anderen Intoxikationen, finden sich dabei kaum. Die EEG-Veränderungen sind bei vergleichbaren Blutspiegeln im ansteigenden Teil der Alkoholkurve eher deutlicher als im abfallenden, verwertbare Korrelationen zu subjektiven und objektiven Ausfallserscheinungen finden sich jedenfalls bei Querschnittsuntersuchungen nicht. Evozierte Potentiale reagieren ebenfalls: bei Blutspiegeln von 1,5 $^0/_{00}$ zeigt sich bei akustisch evozierten Potentialen eine Verminderung der N1-P2-Amplitude ohne deutliche Veränderung der Latenzen (KROGH et al., 1978). Alkoholhalluzinosen zeigen im Querschnitt sehr variable EEG-Befunde (PRO u. WELLS, 1977; ALLAHYARI et al., 1976); im Prädelir und Delir herrschen flache EEG vor (FLÜGEL, 1974). Bei Alkoholentziehungen weniger häufig als bei *Medikamentenentzugssyndromen* kommt es zu wechselnd schweren EEG-Veränderungen und zum häufigen Auftreten von hypersynchronen Potentialen. Hierzu sind die systematischen Studien von WIKLER et al. (1955, 1956), ESSIG und FRASER (1958), WULFF (1959) aufschlußreich. Letzterer zeigte, daß bei Barbiturat-Entzug nicht nur der Serumspiegel, sondern auch sein negativer Gradient von Bedeutung ist. Bei rascher Ausscheidung fanden sich in 70% seiner Fälle Krampfpotentiale sowie schwere Entzugserscheinungen. Dies erklärt die bekannte Gefährlichkeit des Entzugs bei rasch ausgeschiedenen Barbituraten. Entsprechend finden sich auch im Barbiturat-Entziehungsdelir in drei von vier Fällen Krampfanfälle. HUBACH (1963) postuliert in einer interessanten Studie, daß die Trias von Dämmerzustand, Delir und Krampfanfall nach chronischer Einnahme und raschem Entzug bei allen Substanzen auftreten kann, denen eine krampfhemmende Wirkung zuzuschreiben ist.

VI. Syndromgenetische und verlaufsdynamische Aspekte

Ein Ergebnis der vorangegangenen Darstellung liegt darin, daß der Psychiater mit wenigen Ausnahmen enttäuscht sein wird, der vom EEG bei symptomatischen Psychosen eine ätiologische Klärung in seinen diagnostischen Bemühungen erwartet. Dies sollte indessen nicht verwundern, wenn die begrenzten hirnelektrischen Reaktionsmöglichkeiten auf unterschiedlichste Noxen bedacht werden, die weit weniger differenziert sind als das Spektrum der psychopathologischen Befunde. Auch sie allerdings sind in diesem Sinne nicht allzu spezifisch. Des weiteren konnten die in der Literatur überwiegenden Querschnittsuntersuchungen mit ihrer häufigen Vernachlässigung der verlaufsdynamischen und der oft unzureichenden Berücksichtigung epidemiologischer Aspekte von EEG-Befunden der psychiatrischen Forschung nur wenige Impulse vermitteln. Die verlaufsorientierten Studien weisen hingegen darauf hin, daß die Möglichkeiten des EEG zur Beurteilung von zerebralen Funktionszuständen und ihren Differenzierungen noch kaum ausgeschöpft wurden. PENIN (1971, 1974) hat zu Recht gefordert, daß die Bedingungskonstellationen der wohldefinierten EEG-Veränderungen im Rahmen symptomatischer Psychosen mit Blickrichtung auf psychopathologische Verlaufstypen untersucht werden müssen. Eine systematische Studie für symptomatische Psychosen, wie die von HELMCHEN (1968) für paranoid-halluzinatorische Syndrome, steht noch immer aus.

Einige Grundzüge lassen sich indessen bereits anvisieren. Die von PENIN herausgestellte gruppierte abnorme Rhythmisierung (Parenrhythmie) als umschriebenes EEG-Phänomen (vgl. Abschn. B) kann als Ausdruck einer besonderen Reaktion – und noch vorhandenen Reagibilität – mittelliniennaher Strukturen angesehen werden. Sie tritt u.a. dann auf, wenn sich eine Funktionsänderung in diesem Bereich – gleichgültig welcher Ursache – mit einem hinreichenden Gradienten entwickelt. Sie manifestiert sich allerdings nur in einem begrenzten Bereich einer Funktionsanomalie. Wird er zu schnell durchschritten oder kommt es dabei auch zu einer Funktionsstörung bewußtseinsregulierender Strukturen, so entwickelt sich eher, mitunter auch gewisse Zeit parallel dazu, eine Allgemeinveränderung. Die Parenrhythmie ist dabei nicht notwendig begleitendes Korrelat von psychopathologischen Veränderungen, wie es beim akuten Leistungszerfall der Paralyse der Fall ist, sondern kann durchaus auch etwa bei der Pharmakotherapie von Psychosen als prognostisch günstiges Phänomen auftreten (vgl. Abschn. H). Von dieser Blickrichtung aus kann verstanden werden, daß Parenrhythmie wie Allgemeinveränderung zwar ätiologisch unspezifisch, für bestimmte zerebrale Funktionszustände aber durchaus kennzeichnend sein können. Ihnen, insbesondere der Allgemeinveränderung, gehen unter Umständen psychopathologische Sachverhalte parallel. Die Bedingungen ihres gemeinsamen Auftretens bedürfen künftig noch der eingehenderen Erforschung in einer gemeinsamen elektroenzephalographischen und psychiatrischen Bemühung. Hierbei werden sich auch die noch offenen Fragen zur prognostischen Bedeutung des EEG bei symptomatischen Psychosen klären müssen. Bislang läßt sich hierzu nur die Differenzierung von reversibler symptomatischer Psychose und irreversiblem Defektsyndrom bei vorauseilender EEG-Normalisierung als annähernd gesichert betrachten.

G. Epileptische Dämmerzustände, Psychosen und Verstimmungen

Das EEG unter diesen Bedingungen bedarf einer gesonderten Beschreibung, da es, anders als bei symptomatischen Psychosen, nicht selten etwa bei Dämmerzuständen entscheidende differentialdiagnostische Hinweise zu geben vermag. Zu ihrem Verständnis ist indessen eine allgemeinere Kenntnis der EEG-Befunde bei einigen Anfallsformen sowie im Intervall zwischen Anfällen nützlich.

In der neueren Literatur ist das EEG der psychotischen Störungen im Rahmen von Anfallsleiden etwas vernachlässigt worden. So findet sich im Handbook of Electroencephalography weder in Band 13A (Epilepsien) noch in Band 13B (Psychische Erkrankungen) eine zusammenfassende Darstellung, allenfalls mehr verstreute Anmerkungen. Das EEG im Anfall und im Intervall wird dagegen ausführlicher dargestellt von LUGARESI und PAZZAGLIA (1975), GASTAUT und TASSINARI (1975a, b), sowie in der mit zahlreichen EEG-Beispielen illustrierten Monographie von JANZ (1969).

I. Das EEG im Anfall und Intervall

Im *generalisierten großen Anfall*, der im EEG-Labor eher zufällig zur Beobachtung kommt, ist aus technischen Gründen kaum eine Ableitung des EEG möglich. Seine Veränderungen sind jedoch aus den Untersuchungen bei der EKT gut bekannt; sie sind bereits in Abschn. F. IV erörtert worden. *Absencen* werden naturgemäß häufiger im EEG registriert, ihr gesetzmäßiges EEG-Korrelat sind Serien von typischen spike wave-Komplexen (s. Abschn. B.III) mit einer Frequenz von 3/sec, die generalisiert und symmetrisch mit frontal höchster Amplitude beginnen. Ihre Regularität sowie ihre Frequenzen nehmen gegen Ende der Absence meist ab; sie enden oft etwas weniger abrupt, als sie beginnen. Gelegentlich geht ihrem Beginn eine kurze Serie von spikes voraus. So beweisend dieses EEG-Phänomen für eine klinisch manifeste Absence ist, so wenig läßt sich hieraus rückschließen auf die jeweilige Ausgestaltung der Absence in Form von motorischen Automatismen oder vegetativen Phänomenen. Spike wave-Serien von weniger als 2–3 sec Dauer bleiben meist klinisch latent, jedoch lassen sich auch dabei meist Störungen der psychomotorischen Leistungsfähigkeit, z.B. eine Verlängerung der Reaktionszeit, nachweisen (JANZ, 1969; PENRY u. DREYFUSS, 1969). Dieses elektroenzephalographische Bild kann bei atypischen Absencen in verschiedener Weise variieren durch stärkere Irregularität der spike wave-Komplexe etwa mit wechselnden Frequenzen. Das Impulsiv-Petit mal geht einher mit poly-spike wave-Komplexen, bei denen der wave mehrere spikes vorausgehen. *Fokale klonische oder tonisch-klonische Anfälle* zeigen meist die EEG-Veränderungen des großen Anfalls, allerdings beschränkt auf die korrespondierenden Rindenareale, mit diffuser Ausbreitung bei sekundärer Generalisierung des Anfalls. So relativ eintönig das EEG-Bild der Absence ist, so differenziert ist dasjenige der *psychomotorischen Anfälle*. Am häufigsten, fast in der Hälfte der Fälle (GASTAUT et al., 1953) findet man regelmäßige, hohe Wellen aus dem Theta- oder raschen Delta-Bereich mit diffuser Verteilung, aber meist temporaler Prädilektion, auch mit Seitenbetonung. Im Anfall kann das EEG aber auch relativ unspezifisch nur eine kontinuierliche Dysrhythmie vorwiegend im temporalen Bereich aufweisen (CHRISTIAN, 1962) oder auch nur eine Abflachung aufweisen, wie GASTAUT (1953) sogar bei einem Fünftel seiner Fälle fand.

Im *Intervall* zwischen den Anfällen finden sich nur bei etwa 30% von Anfallskranken hypersynchrone Potentiale, die dann eine erhöhte Krampfbereitschaft beweisen. Bei einem weiteren Drittel von Anfallskranken finden sich unspezifische Veränderungen, Dysrhythmien oder auch Herdveränderungen, die bei Epileptikern bei Verlaufskontrollen nicht selten nach Intensität oder sogar Lokalisation wechseln können. Bei einem Drittel von Anfallskranken schließlich, besonders bei solchen mit seltenen und mit schlafgebundenen Anfällen, finden sich im Intervall-EEG normale oder allenfalls Grenzbefunde (JUNG, 1953). Im Intervall auftretende hypersynchrone Potentiale geben oft differentialdiagnostische Hinweise, wie sharp waves in temporalen Herden bei psychomotorischen Anfällen, spike wave-Komplexe bei Absencen, fokale spikes bei fokalen Anfällen, ohne daß die Typologie der hypersynchronen Potentiale, insbesondere im Erwachsenenalter, für bestimmte Anfallsformen beweisend wäre. Die in umgekehrter Richtung gestellte Frage, inwieweit hypersynchrone Potentiale ein Anfallsleiden beweisen, muß im Licht neuerer Untersuchungen zurückhaltender als früher beantwortet werden. In ihrer klassischen Studie fanden GIBBS, GIBBS und LENNOX (1943) bei 1000 gesunden Erwachsenen in weniger als 1% hypersynchrone Potentiale. Hieraus wurde oft der unzulässige Schluß gezogen, daß bei ihrem Auftreten mit einer Wahrscheinlichkeit von 99% Anfälle bestanden, noch bestehen oder demnächst auftreten werden. Tatsächlich sollen sich z.B. unter Blinklichtbelastung spikes oder spike wave-Komplexe bei 10–15% gesunder Mädchen zwischen 10 und 16 Jahren finden, bei Knaben nur 1–2%. Diese Häufigkeit nimmt mit zunehmendem Alter rasch ab (METRAKOS u. METRAKOS, 1961; RABENDING u. KLEPEL, 1970; WATSON u. MARCUS, 1962). GUTJAHR et al. (1978) fanden anhand einer klinischen Population, daß nur bei zwei Dritteln von Probanden mit hypersynchroner Aktivität Anfälle klinisch manifest oder anamnestisch eruierbar waren. Insoweit bleibt festzuhalten, daß solche Potentiale, sofern sie unter Standardbedingungen (s. Abschn. B) auftreten, zwar eine erhöhte Krampfbereitschaft beweisen, aber noch keinesfalls ein manifestes Anfallsleiden. Zur Diskussion dieses Sachverhaltes sei auch auf STEVENS (1977) verwiesen.

II. Dämmerzustände, Petit mal-Status, Status psychomotoricus

Postparoxysmale Dämmerzustände ergeben elektroenzephalographisch keine Probleme; sie zeigen die typische postparoxysmale Allgemeinveränderung mit rascherer oder langsamerer Rückbildung, annähernd parallel zur einsetzenden Orientierung. Häufiger, als früher angenommen, treten in solchen Dämmerzuständen, besonders bei protrahierter Rückbildung, auch generalisierte hypersynchrone Potentiale vom spike wave-Typ auf, vor allem bei Erwachsenen (JUNG, 1967), während dies bei Kindern seltener zu sein scheint. Ein ähnliches EEG-Bild bieten Dämmerzustände, die nicht in unmittelbarem zeitlichem Zusammenhang mit Anfällen auftreten, wobei hier Allgemeinveränderungen, oft kombiniert mit Dysrhythmien oder Herdbefunden, dominieren.

Andere Aspekte dagegen bietet der *Petit mal-Status*. Hier finden sich kontinuierliche, oft irreguläre, diffuse spike wave- oder poly-spike wave-Komplexe

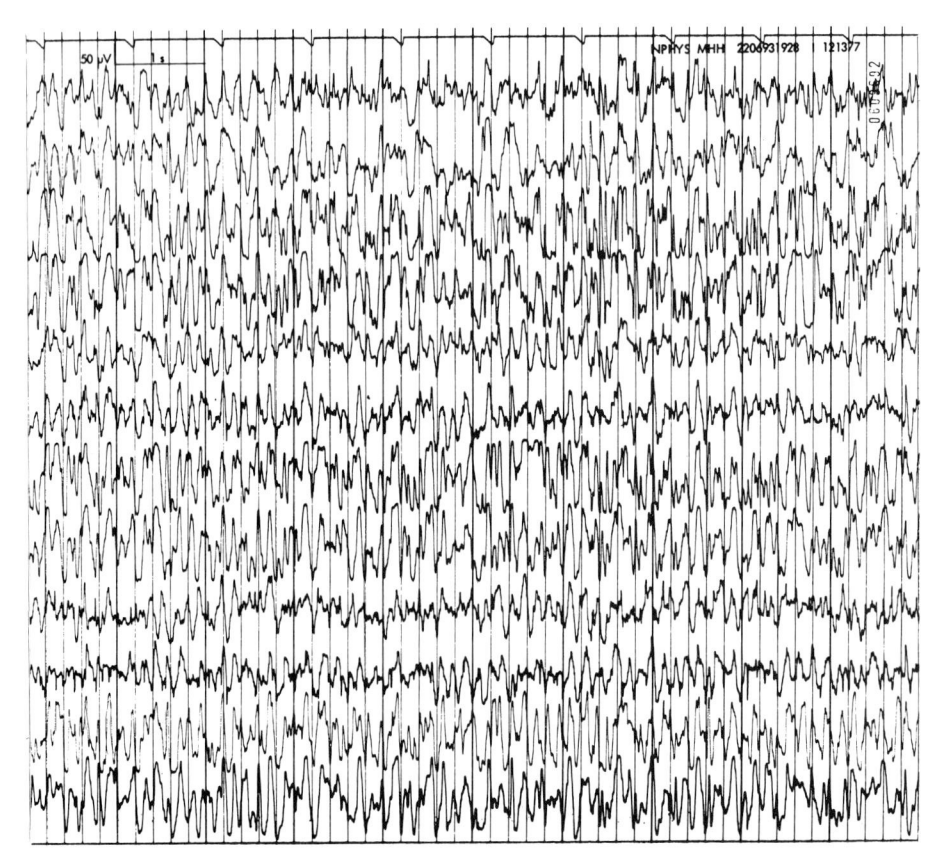

Abb. 33. Petit mal-Status bei einer 84jährigen Kranken. Kontinuierliche, irreguläre, meist polyphasische spike-wave-Komplexe. Ableitungen gegen das seitengleiche Ohr

mit frontaler Betonung, die auch in längeren Gruppen mit jeweils nur kurzer Unterbrechung auftreten können (GASTAUT et al., 1967; ROGER et al., 1973). Petit mal-Staten sind keineswegs an jugendliches Alter gebunden, finden sich aber häufiger bei männlichen Kranken unter 20 Jahren sowie bei weiblichen Kranken jenseits des 60. Lebensjahres (GASTAUT u. TASSINARI, 1975a). Abb. 33 zeigt ein solches typisches EEG-Bild. Fraglich bleibt allerdings, ob man GASTAUT und TASSINARI darin folgen soll, die auch solche Dämmerzustände zum Formenkreis des Petit mal-Status rechnen, die im EEG ganz dominierend eine Allgemeinveränderung mit überlagerter kontinuierlicher Dysrhythmie und vermehrter, gruppierter Beta-Aktivität zeigen und die nur gelegentlich Gruppen von spike wave-Komplexen aufweisen.

Differentialdiagnostisch größere Probleme bietet der seltene *Status psychomotorischer Anfälle*, dessen EEG-Dokumentation in der Literatur noch spärlich ist (DREYER, 1965; GASTAUT et al., 1956; JANZ, 1969; ROGER et al., 1973; LUGARESI et al., 1971; WOLF, 1970). Dies gilt besonders für die Formen, bei denen Orientierungs- und Bewußtseinsstörungen sowie Störungen der höheren Intelli-

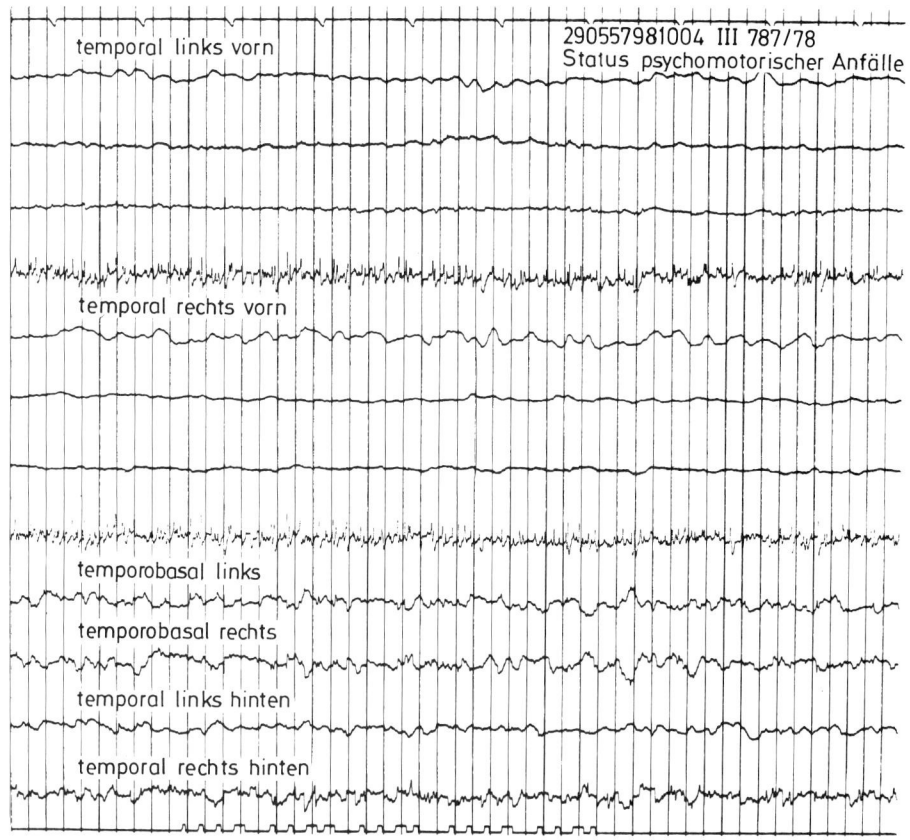

Abb. 34. EEG eines 21jährigen Patienten im Status psychomotorischer Anfälle. Flache Grundaktivität, kontinuierliche Dysrhythmie in beiden Temporalbereichen mit Schwerpunkt temporobasal

genzleistungen nicht dominieren und in deren Verlauf allenfalls Rudimente psychomotorischer Anfälle auftreten. Hierbei finden sich Allgemeinveränderungen leichter bis mittlerer Ausprägung, kontinuierliche Dysrhythmien oder gruppierte Dysrhythmien und Parenrhythmien, oft ohne daß hypersynchrone Potentiale etwa vom Typ der sharp waves registriert werden (Abb. 34). Schon klinisch leichter abgrenzbar sind die Staten psychomotorischer Anfälle, die im eigentlichen Sinne der Status-Definition durch eine stunden-, selten tagelange Folge von psychomotorischen Anfällen mit unvollständiger Aufhellung des Bewußtseins im Intervall gekennzeichnet sind. Im EEG finden sich die beschriebenen Korrelate der Anfälle, des öfteren auch im Temporalbereich fokal betonte sharp waves. WOLF (1970) hat hierfür die Bezeichnung „diskontinuierlicher Status psychomotorischer Anfälle" vorgeschlagen. Die des öfteren schwierige Differentialdiagnose zwischen Petit mal-Status und Status psychomotorischer Anfälle kann jedenfalls dann durch das EEG entscheidend erleichtert werden, wenn sich eine kontinuierliche spike wave-Aktivität registrieren läßt, wie sie für den Typ Petit mal-Status typisch ist.

III. Epileptische Psychosen und Verstimmungszustände

Es ist das Verdienst von LANDOLT (1955, 1958, 1963a, b), durch die etwas zugespitzte Interpretation seiner EEG-Beobachtungen bei epileptischen Psychosen der Forschung in diesem Bereich einen neuen Anstoß gegeben zu haben. Auf ihn geht der Begriff der „forcierten Normalisierung" zurück, der das weitgehend normale EEG innerhalb einer epileptischen Psychose oder eines Verstimmungszustandes bei zuvor pathologischer Aktivität bezeichnet. Dieser im Einzelfall immer wieder zu beobachtende und beeindruckende Sachverhalt ist jedoch unter Aspekten der relativen Häufigkeit für die Gesamtheit epileptischer Psychosen keineswegs repräsentativ, so daß LANDOLTs Auffassung hierzu manchen Widerspruch gefunden hat. DONGIER (1959/60) fand in seiner Untersuchung, die sich auf Befunde an 516 epileptischen Kranken mit psychotischen Störungen stützt, eine Rückbildung von hypersynchroner Aktivität nur in 24% der Fälle, ein normales EEG zeigten nur 16%. Zu vergleichbaren Befunden kamen SLATER et al. (1963). KÖHLER (1973) berichtet anhand eines Beobachtungsgutes von 66 Kranken mit schizoformen epileptischen Psychosen sowie 40 mit episodischen Verstimmungen und manisch-depressiv gefärbten Psychosen über lediglich 5% mit normalem EEG. Somit drängt sich der Schluß auf, daß normale Elektroenzephalogramme während epileptischer Psychosen nur ausnahmsweise zu beobachten sind. Von Interesse ist vielmehr die relative Häufigkeit bestimmter EEG-Befunde bei beiden Gruppen. Im Vordergrund steht eine paroxysmale Dysrhythmie mit einer Häufigkeit von rund 65%; sie ist somit hier eindeutig häufiger als bei Anfallskranken ohne Psychose. Das gleiche gilt für die hypersynchrone Aktivität mit einer Häufigkeit von 50%. Abnorme Rhythmisierungen schließlich zeigten sich bei den schizoformen Psychosen in rund 20%, bei der zweiten Gruppe nur in rund 8%.

IV. Verlaufsdynamische Aspekte

Die Feststellung von JUNG (1967), daß es gesetzmäßige Beziehungen zwischen EEG und epileptischen Psychosen nicht gebe, gilt sicher dann, wenn der Beurteilung Querschnittsbetrachtungen ohne Berücksichtigung des zeitlichen Verlaufes von psychotischen Bildern zugrunde gelegt werden. Die Verhältnisse stellen sich jedoch offenbar – wie bei den übrigen symptomatischen Psychosen und wie bei Schizophrenien – etwas anders dar, wenn EEG-Befunde in Längsschnitt-Untersuchungen zum jeweiligen Psychoseverlauf in Beziehung gesetzt werden. KÖHLER (1973) berücksichtigte bei seinen Untersuchungen die Prozeßaktivität zum Zeitpunkt der EEG-Ableitung, bestimmt nach den von HUBER und PENIN (1968) definierten Aktivitätskriterien von Psychosen. Dabei erwies sich die Häufigkeit einer gruppierten abnormen Rhythmisierung als eindeutig abhängig vom Aktivitätsgrad der Psychose. Sie war am häufigsten bei lebhafter Prozeßaktivität und nahm über subaktive bis hin zu inaktiven Prozeßkriterien signifikant ab. Dieser Zusammenhang war bei den schizoformen Psychosen am deutlichsten mit einer Irrtumswahrscheinlichkeit von 0,2% (ermittelt nach den Daten von KÖHLER). Die abnormen Rhythmisierungen bieten somit ein anderes Verhalten als die paroxysmalen Dysrhythmien, womit sich wiederum, wie schon bei den epidemiologischen Befunden (vgl. Abschn. B.4) erweist, daß beide Phänomene nicht nur von der EEG-Morphologie her zu unterscheiden sind, sondern trotz gewisser Gemeinsamkeiten – entgegen der Auffassung von HELMCHEN (1968) – verschiedene zerebrale Funktionszustände anzeigen.

Wenn auch die von KÖHLER mitgeteilten Befunde einige statistisch gesicherte Aussagen erlauben, so bleibt doch noch eine Reihe von Fragen offen. So ist zweifellos noch zu untersuchen, ob die Befunde über die abnormen Rhythmisierungen etwa durch eine antipsychotische Pharmakotherapie bedingt sind, ferner welchen Einfluß Alter und Geschlecht sowie Dauer der speziellen Anamnese haben und ob die Typologie des Anfallsleidens modifizierend wirkt. Die Bedeutung der hier ausführlicher referierten Befunde scheint vor allem darin zu liegen, daß sie die Notwendigkeit von Erhebungen an einem größeren Krankengut unter Einbeziehung differenzierter Kriterien der EEG-Befundung sowie der Prozeßaktivität belegen. Auch hier sind offenbar die begrenzten Möglichkeiten einer globalen elektroenzephalographisch-klinischen Querschnittsbetrachtung ausgeschöpft.

H. EEG und endogene Psychosen

Die Literatur über das EEG bei endogenen Psychosen, insbesondere bei Schizophrenien, hat in den letzten 10 Jahren einen Umfang angenommen, der hier eine Darstellung nur mit deutlicher Akzentsetzung erlaubt. Ausführliche Literaturübersichten aus neuerer Zeit finden sich bei BEEK et al. (1964), COLONY und WILLIS (1956), DONGIER (1973), ELLINGSON (1954), HELMCHEN (1968), KÜNKEL (1975), SHAGASS (1975, 1976, 1977) sowie SMALL und SMALL (1965). Ferner seien die bereits klassischen Studien von DAVIS und DAVIS (1939), DAVIS (1940, 1941, 1942), GREENBLATT et al. (1944), LEMERE (1941) und MACMAHON und WALTER (1938) erwähnt.

Der Einsatz des EEG in der psychiatrischen Forschung hat eine Reihe von Problemen evident gemacht, die bei der Mehrzahl älterer Untersuchungen kaum beachtet worden sind. Sie liegen zum einen auf der klinischen Seite. So wurden Patientengruppen mit verschiedenen Symptomkonstellationen häufig zusammengefaßt, obgleich sie durchaus in entgegengesetzter Richtung von Normalpopulationen abweichen können, wodurch fälschlich negative Resultate entstehen (GARMEZY, 1970). Auf elektroenzephalographischer Seite wurde ein unzulänglich definierter Begriff von Normalität und Nicht-Normalität verwendet (BENTE, 1965; LAIRY, 1956). Ferner wurde die Häufigkeit pathologischer EEG-Befunde bei Patientengruppen nicht nach den Einflüssen von Geschlecht und Alter korrigiert, was allerdings eine differenzierte statistische Methodik erfordert hätte. Schließlich wurden systematische Verlaufsuntersuchungen erst mit den Studien von HELMCHEN (1968) sowie HUBER und PENIN (1968) begonnen. Somit ist keineswegs verwunderlich, daß die Suche nach krankheitsspezifischen EEG-Mustern erfolglos bleiben mußte und das Urteil über die Rolle des EEG in der Psychiatrie negativ blieb (COLONY u. WILLIS, 1956; HILL, 1957; JUNG, 1967; SHAGASS, 1969).

I. Das EEG bei Schizophrenien

Querschnittsstudien des *Ruhe-EEG* berichten über äußerst diskrepante Häufigkeiten pathologischer Befunde mit einem Bereich von 5% bis zu 80% (BEEK et al., 1964; COLONY u. WILLIS, 1956; SHAGASS, 1977; SMALL u. SMALL, 1965). HESS (1963), HILL (1957) und JUNG (1967) kommen deshalb zu einer pessimistischen Auffassung bezüglich der elektroenzephalographischen Korrelate schizophrener Psychosen, die SHAGASS (1969) so formuliert: „Manche Aspekte hirnelektrischer Aktivität scheinen beim Schizophrenen von denjenigen des Normalen abzuweichen. Indessen sind die meisten positiven Befunde statistischer Natur und unspezifisch, manche sind unbestätigt und aus methodischen Gründen fragwürdig geblieben." Insbesondere gilt dies auch für die von DAVIS und DAVIS (1939) herausgestellte „choppy activity", eine niederamplitudige, diffuse, durch unregelmäßige höhere Frequenzen gekennzeichnete EEG-Aktivität geringer topographischer Organisation. IGERT und LAIRY (1962) haben darauf verwiesen, daß die Grundaktivität bei chronisch Schizophrenen durch eine „Hyperstabilität" mit geringer Amplitudenmodulation auffalle, was später von GOLDSTEIN et al. (1965) mit der Amplitudenintegration erneut beschrieben wurde. Diese Patienten lassen denn auch eine geringe Ansprechbarkeit auf eine Pharmakotherapie erwarten (ITIL, 1968; HELMCHEN u. KÜNKEL, 1964; IGERT u. LAIRY, 1962).

Aktivierungsmethoden des EEG sind schon frühzeitig zur Untersuchung der zerebralen Reagibilität bei Psychosen eingesetzt worden, so von LIBERSON (1944). Die bekannte Blockierung der Alpha-Grundaktivität bei visuellen Reizen (z.B. Augenöffnen) zeigt bei Schizophrenen keine Abweichung von normalen Kontrollen (HEIN et al., 1962). Eingreifendere Aktivierungsverfahren, wie die kombinierte Belastung mit Flickerlicht und Metrazolinjektionen (GASTAUT, 1950) ergeben bei Schizophrenen im Vergleich zu Normalen ebenfalls keine verwertbaren Unterschiede (LIEBERMANN et al., 1954), ebensowenig wie die EEG-Reaktionen auf intravenöse Pentothal-Injektionen (SILA et al., 1962). Diese Verfahren sind wegen ihrer schwer kontrollierbaren Risiken zu Recht bald wieder verlassen worden. SHAGASS (1954, 1956) definierte eine *„Sedierungs-Schwelle"* als die Menge intravenösen Amobarbitals, die eine maximale Steigerung der frontalen Beta-Produktion bewirkt. Sie soll bei chronisch Schizophrenen erhöht sein gegenüber akuten Schizophrenen und Normalen (SHAGASS, 1959). Im *Schlaf-EEG* auftretende sog. „Mitten"-Muster („Fäustling", langsamer spike mit nachfolgender, auf ihrer abfallenden Flanke „gekerbten" Welle) sollen sich bei Schizophrenen nach GIBBS und GIBBS (1963) in 37% der Fälle finden, bei Normalen dagegen weit seltener. Diese Befunde wurden von STRUVE et al. (1972) bestätigt, vor allem für akute Schizophrenien.

II. EEG-Analyse bei schizophrenen Psychosen

Mit der Anwendung der *Frequenzanalyse* nach GREY WALTER (s. Abschn. C.I) auf die EEG-Untersuchung von schizophrenen Psychosen ergaben sich zunächst sehr inkonsistente Befunde. KENNARD et al. (1955) fanden einen höheren Beta-Anteil, wie schon früher GIBBS (1939). Außerdem fanden sie bei Schizophrenen eine größere Frequenzvariabilität des Alpha-Rhythmus und eine geringere interhemisphärische Alpha-Synchronie (KENNARD u. SCHWARTZMAN, 1957). URYU und MORIYA (1969) fanden außer einem höheren Beta-Anteil auch eine erhöhte Alpha-Ausprägung. FINK et al. (1965) beobachteten dagegen keine Beta-Vermehrung, hingegen einen höheren Frequenzanteil im Delta-Bereich. VOLAVKA et al.

(1966) sahen dagegen bei Schizophrenen, ebenfalls mit der Frequenzanalyse, eine höhere Theta- sowie Alpha-Ausprägung.

Die *Amplituden-Integration* nach DROHOCKI (s. Abschn. C.II) ist vor allem von der Arbeitsgruppe um GOLDSTEIN für die Analyse von Schizophrenie-EEG verwendet worden. Es liegt in der Natur der Methode, daß damit besonders die dynamische Variabilität eines EEG in einfacher Weise untersucht werden kann. Ein damit erhaltener, grundsätzlich interessanter Befund zeigt für Schizophrene nicht nur einen durchschnittlich niedrigeren Variationskoeffizienten für die mittlere Energieproduktion im EEG (SUGERMAN et al., 1964; GOLDSTEIN et al., 1965; vgl. auch Abb. 15), sondern einen qualitativ verschiedenen funktionalen Zusammenhang: während der Variationskoeffizient für eine zunehmende mittlere Amplitude bei normalen männlichen Erwachsenen zunimmt und bei männlichen Jugendlichen konstant bleibt, nimmt er im Gegensatz hierzu bei männlichen Schizophrenen ab, wie Abb. 35 zeigt, deren Kurven nach Daten von BURDICK et al. (1967) berechnet wurden. (Zum Vergleich sei auch auf Abb. 16 verwiesen.) Zu gleichen Resultaten kamen MARJER-RISON et al. (1967). Diesen Sachverhalt, der die frühere Beobachtung einer „Hyperstabilität" des EEG Schizophrener bestätigt und präzisiert, haben GOLDSTEIN und SUGERMAN (1969) dahin interpretiert, daß bei den Kranken die Störung einer homöostatischen Hirnfunktion vorliege und die Schizophrenen ständig „hyperalert" seien mit mangelnder Fähigkeit zur Entspannung. Diese Hypothese soll später noch im Zusammenhang mit anderen diskutiert werden. Die Aspekte der EEG-Dynamik wurden von GOLDSTEIN (1975) auch unter sensorischer Deprivation untersucht (vgl. hierzu Abb. 17). Normale zeigten unter dieser Bedingung eine zunehmende Desorganisation der interhemisphärischen Amplitudenverteilung, die bei Schizophrenen deutlich geringer war.

Auch die „*period analysis*" ist von LESTER und EDWARDS (1966) auf EEG Schizophrener angewendet worden, wobei sich wiederum ein vermehrter Anteil rascher Beta-Aktivität im Vergleich zu Normalen ergab. ITIL et al. (1972) verglichen 100 unbehandelte Schizophrene mit 100 normalen Kontrollen bei differenzierter, psychopathologischer Definition ihrer Patientenstichprobe. Auch sie fanden mehr rasche Beta-Aktivität, aber auch mehr Theta-Delta-Aktivität als bei Normalen, dagegen weniger Alpha- und langsame Beta-Aktivität. Anhand einer Diskriminanzanalyse mit Variablen aus visueller Auswertung, „period analysis" und Frequenzanalyse untersuchten sie ferner, mit welcher Treffsicherheit zwischen den beiden Probandengruppen unterschieden werden konnte. Die Resultate der Frequenzanalyse waren mit einer Trefferrate von 55% enttäuschend, da sie über eine rein zufallsmäßige, blinde Zuordnung (50% Treffer) kaum hinausgingen. Die „period analysis" ergab 69% richtiger Zuordnungen, die visuelle Beurteilung der EEG sogar 86%. Der methodische Ansatz dieser Studie ist interessant, da er die Möglichkeiten der analytischen Statistik einsetzt, für die sich die quantitativen Daten der EEG-Analyse geradezu anbieten. Allerdings ergeben sich auch hier kritische Einwände bezüglich der Methodik (KÜNKEL, 1975), so daß die Validität der gemachten Aussagen vorläufig noch nicht gesichert erscheint.

Die *Spektralanalyse* des EEG hat, bedingt durch den methodischen Aufwand, erst relativ spät zu psychiatrischen Fragen beitragen können. LIFSHITZ und GRA-

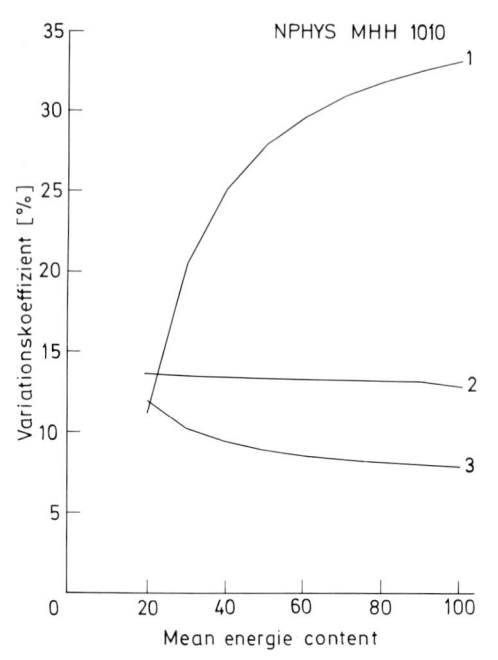

Abb. 35. Variationskoeffizient und „mean energy content" bei männlichen Erwachsenen (1), männlichen Jugendlichen (2) und erwachsenen chronisch Schizophrenen (S) (berechnet nach Daten von BURDICK et al., 1967)

DIJAN (1972, 1974) sahen hiermit bei Schizophrenen eine vermehrte Theta-Delta-Aktivität sowie eine vermehrte rasche Beta-Aktivität, ebenso wie GIANNITRAPANI und KAYTON (1974). SHAW (1976) hat die Arbeiten von GIANNITRAPANI und KAYTON, LIFSHITZ und GRADIJAN sowie ITIL et al. einer vergleichenden Analyse unterzogen. Nach GIANNITRAPANI und KAYTON, die ihre Untersuchung zwar in 16 EEG-Kanälen, indessen nur an 10 Kranken durchführten, diese aber wiederum unter psychopathologischen Aspekten sorgfältig homogen ausgewählt und einer nach Alter und Geschlecht angepaßten Kontrollgruppe gegenübergestellt haben, lag die mittlere Alpha-Frequenz bei Schizophrenen niedriger. Außerdem fand sich bei 5 der Kranken, jedoch bei keinem der Vergleichsgruppe ein Aktivitätsgipfel bei 29 Hz. GIANNITRAPANI glaubt, hier einen für schizophrene Psychosen charakteristischen Befund zu sehen. Von einer statistischen Sicherung kann bei dem genannten Stichprobenumfang allerdings noch nicht die Rede sein, so daß dieser Befund ebenfalls noch einer weiteren Überprüfung bedarf.

Als einigermaßen konsistente Befunde anhand der EEG-Analyse können somit die verminderte Amplitudenvariabilität, die veränderte interhemisphärische Amplitudenrelation, die vermehrte Ausprägung von Theta-, Delta- sowie rascher Beta-Aktivität und schließlich eine etwas verlangsamte dominante Frequenz der Grundaktivität angesehen werden (SHAGASS, 1977).

III. Evozierte und ereignisbezogene Potentiale bei schizophrenen Psychosen

Mit der sich entwickelnden Technik zur Registrierung evozierter und ereignisbezogener Potentiale und ihrem Einsatz zum Studium zerebraler Funktionsstrukturen ging bald auch die Anwendung auf psychiatrische Fragestellungen einher. Alle Formen dieser Potentiale wurden bei schizophrenen Kranken untersucht in der Hoffnung, Hinweise auf eine gestörte zerebrale Informationsverarbeitung zu finden. Hierzu existieren bereits mehrere monographische Übersichten (DONCHIN u. LINDSLEY, 1969; FESSARD u. LELORD, 1973; SHAGASS, 1972). *Visuell evozierte Potentiale* (VEP) können kürzere Latenzen und geringer ausgeprägte Nachschwankungen aufweisen (SHAGASS u. SCHWARTZ, 1965), ihr unspezifischer Anteil (vgl. Abschn. IV.2) zeigt eine größere Variabilität als bei normalen Kontrollen, was sich bei allen Typen evozierter Potentiale bestätigte (CALLAWAY et al., 1965; COHEN, 1973; LIFSHITZ, 1969; SHAGASS et al., 1974). Während der Vergleich von Amplituden inkonsistente Befunde ergab, scheint der individuell verschiedene Zusammenhang zwischen Reizintensität und Antwortamplitude eine Rolle zu spielen. BUCHSBAUM und PFEFFERBAUM (1971) sowie SOSKIS und SHAGASS (1974) und STARK und NORTON (1974) fanden bei zunehmender Reizintensität sowohl Zunahme, als auch Abnahme der Amplitude von N1-P2 (Abb. 28, 29) als individualtypisches Merkmal. Dementsprechend unterschieden sie zwischen „augmenter" und „reducer". Bei akuten Schizophrenen waren „reducer" eindeutig häufiger als bei normalen Kontrollen (BUCHSBAUM, 1975). *Akustisch evozierte Potentiale* (AER) zeigen bei Schizophrenen recht konsistent niedrigere Amplituden, oft auch kürzere Latenzen (COHEN, 1973; JONES u. CALLAWAY, 1970; SALETU et al., 1971). Auch für die „contingent negative variation" (CNV) werden bei Schizophrenen niedrigere Amplituden sowie eine verlängerte Negativität berichtet (DONGIER, 1973; MCCALLUM, 1973; SMALL u. SMALL, 1971; TIMSIT-BERTHIER, 1973), ferner ein weniger ausgeprägtes *Bereitschaftspotential* (DONGIER, 1974; TIMSIT-BERTHIER, 1973). DONGIER et al. (1974) sahen ein niedrigeres spätes positives Potential („P 300", s. Abschn. D.VI).

Die Menge der mit den neuen Techniken evozierter Potentiale erhobenen Befunde kann allerdings nicht darüber hinwegtäuschen, daß die Mehrzahl, wenn nicht alle, unspezifisch sind und daß bereits Aufmerksamkeitsänderungen der Versuchspersonen zu deutlichen Veränderungen meist der Amplitude führen (MCCALLUM u. WALTER, 1968). Die Deutung der Befunde muß deshalb vorläufig noch sehr vorsichtig erfolgen. SHAGASS (1977) zieht den Schluß, daß den Befunden bei Schizophrenie eine verminderte Aktivität von Strukturen der Formatio reticularis mesencephali zugrunde liegt, zumal er dabei vergleichbare Veränderungen wie bei Schizophrenen gefunden hat (SHAGASS u. ANDO, 1970). Der veränderte Funktionszustand dieser Strukturen wird dann als Korrelat für einen gestörten Mechanismus der Filterung afferenter Informationen verantwortlich gemacht (SHAGASS, 1976). Diese Hypothese ist zwar interessant, muß sich aber zweifellos erst noch an ausgedehnteren Untersuchungen bewähren.

IV. Das EEG bei depressiven und manisch-depressiven Psychosen

Es herrscht weitgehend Übereinstimmung darin, daß bei depressiven und manisch-depressiven Psychosen „abnorme" EEG-Befunde seltener sind, als bei schizophrenen Psychosen. Dies ergab sich schon aus den frühen Studien von DAVIS (1941, 1942). Sie fand in depressiven Phasen häufig einen langsameren Alpha-Rhythmus, als in manischen, in beiden war die Alpha-Ausprägung gemeinhin höher als bei Schizophrenen. GREENBLATT et al. (1944) kamen dagegen zu dem Schluß, daß bei affektiven Psychosen erhobene Befunde weitgehend durch ihre Altersabhängigkeit bedingt sind. Die Mehrzahl der Untersuchungen hierzu hat offensichtlich die Alters- und Geschlechtsabhängigkeit von EEG-Befunden (s. Abschn. B.IV) nicht berücksichtigt (MAGGS u. TURTON, 1956). Diesen schon jahrzehntealten Beobachtungen ist inzwischen kaum Neues hinzugefügt worden. *Aktivierungsmethoden* haben ebenfalls nur wenige Besonderheiten erkennen lassen, etwa eine verlängerte Alpha-Blockierung in der Depression (D'ELIA et al., 1974; WILSON u. WILSON, 1961), vermehrtes „photic driving" (Amplitudenzunahme von EEG-Wellen der Reizfrequenz; HURST et al., 1954). Im Schlaf zeigen Depressive häufiger „mitten"-Muster als Normale, indessen weniger als Schizophrene (GIBBS u. GIBBS, 1963). *Evozierte Potentiale* weisen auf gewisse Differenzen hin. So finden sich bei optischer Reizung mehr „reducer" (Abb. 29) bei rein depressiven Psychosen, mehr „augmenter" (Abb. 28) bei manisch-depressiven, wobei diese Differenz indessen nur bei männlichen Patienten nachweisbar war (BUCHSBAUM et al., 1971, 1973). SMALL und SMALL (1971) beschreiben eine verminderte CNV bei Manien wie bei Depressionen.

V. Verlaufsdynamische und syndromgenetische Aspekte

Die Entwicklungstendenz in der elektroenzephalographischen Psychoseforschung hat sich im angelsächsischen Bereich in den letzten Jahren einem zunehmenden Einsatz neuer methodischer Möglichkeiten der EEG-Analyse und der Registrierung evozierter und ereignisbezogener Potentiale zugewandt. Dabei haben sich auch differenzierte statistische Analyseverfahren als nützlich erwiesen, wie sie zur Bearbeitung der quantitativen Befunde der neueren Methoden unumgänglich sind. Es entsteht jedoch der Eindruck, als ob die Differenzierung der psychopathologischen Befunde bei psychiatrisch-elektroenzephalographischen Korrelationsuntersuchungen und teilweise auch die Berücksichtigung der individuellen Verlaufsdynamik von Psychosen nicht in gleichem Maße fortgeschritten sind – allenfalls wurde bei Schizophrenie zwischen akuten und chronischen Verläufen unterschieden, bei affektiven Psychosen zwischen depressiven und zyklothymen Verläufen.

HELMCHEN (1968) hat die Grenzen nosologischer Betrachtungsweise verlassen und den Blick auf die Bedingungskonstellationen und Verlaufsdynamik paranoid-halluzinatorischer Syndrome gerichtet. Dieser Ansatz erwies sich mit der Einbeziehung elektroenzephalographischer Befunde sogleich als fruchtbar, da er signifikante psychopathologisch-elektroenzephalographische Korrelationen im Verlauf einer Pharmakotherapie aufzeigen konnte. Schizophrene Defekte zeigten einen engen Zusammenhang mit Allgemeinveränderungen und rechtsseitigen EEG-Herden, hirnorganische Psychosyndrome als andere Facette eines psychischen Defizienz-Syndroms dagegen mit Frequenzlabilität und linksseitigen Herden. Paranoid-halluzinatorische Involutionspsychosen zeigen einen signifikanten Zusammenhang mit erhöhtem Beta-Anteil. Wesentlich erscheint weiter, daß sich Zusammenhänge von EEG-Merkmalen mit psychopathologischen Einzelmerkmalen nicht, sehr wohl aber mit dem psychopathologischen Verlaufsprofil nachweisen ließen. Während abklingender Wahnstimmung war das Auftreten einer gruppierten Dysrhythmie (oder Parenrhythmie?, zwischen beiden wurde in der Studie von HELMCHEN nicht unterschieden) charakteristisch, während eine unter Therapie überdauernde Wahnstimmung oder ein Wahn eher Zusammenhänge mit einer Allgemeinveränderung zeigte. Wesentlich erscheint, daß diese Korrelationen daraufhin geprüft wurden, ob sie durch den bekannten Alterszusammenhang dieser Merkmale vorgetäuscht sind, was indessen ausgeschlossen werden konnte, ebenso wie eine Abhängigkeit von der Dosis der Pharmakotherapie. Die Prüfung auf Einfluß des Geschlechts war allerdings nicht möglich, da ausschließlich Frauen untersucht wurden. Der von HELMCHEN gezogene Schluß, „daß auch im Bereich der sog. endogenen Psychosen differenzierbare zentral-nervöse, also somatische Funktionsänderungen mit bestimmten psychopathologischen Phänomenen korreliert sind", hätte in der Zwischenzeit Anlaß sein sollen, diese Blickrichtung mit Hilfe der EEG-Analyse und der Techniken evozierter Potentiale zu erweitern und zu differenzieren.

In die gleiche Richtung wie HELMCHEN zielen HUBER und PENIN (1968) und PENIN (1971). Auch sie betonen, daß es sinnlos sei, Schizophrenien schlechthin oder ihre herkömmlichen Unterformen mit elektroenzephalographischen Befunden zu korrelieren und stellen vielmehr die Rolle der Prozeßaktivität heraus. So fand PENIN (1971) bei 41 unbehandelten Schizophrenen, bei denen die Prozeßaktivität eindeutig bestimmbar war, eine klare Korrelation zwischen Prozeßaktivität und Auftreten von Parenrhythmie, während bei den prozeßinaktiven Kranken normale EEG registriert wurden. Hier ergeben sich somit bei schizophrenen Psychosen vergleichbare Zusammenhänge wie bei den symptomatischen und den epileptischen Psychosen. Die einigermaßen enttäuschenden Resultate der umfangreichen EEG-Literatur zur Schizophrenie dürften zu einem guten Teil darin begründet sein, daß die Dimensionen der Verlaufsdynamik und der Prozeßaktivität von Psychosen weitgehend unberücksichtigt geblieben sind.

VI. EEG und Hypothesenbildung

Die Literatur über die Beziehungen zwischen EEG und endogenen Psychosen fordert auch zu einigen kritischen Anmerkungen heraus, die die Hypothesenbildung anhand der erhobenen Befunde betreffen (KÜNKEL, 1975). Dies soll nur am Beispiel der vermehrten Beta-Aktivität bei Schizophrenen erörtert werden, einem der relativ konsistenten Befunde bei den verschiedenen Untersuchern. ITIL et al. (1972) interpretieren dies als Ausdruck eines „hyper-arousal", ohne sich darüber zu äußern, ob es sich dabei um einen erhöhten Aktivitätszustand des aktivierenden retikulären Systems handelt, was „ein genetisch orientiertes Konzept der Schizophrenie" aufweisen könnte, oder ob im Hinblick auf den hemmenden Einfluß des Hippokampus auf das aktivierende retikuläre System eher eine Unterfunktion des Hippokampus anzunehmen ist. LIFSHITZ und GRA-

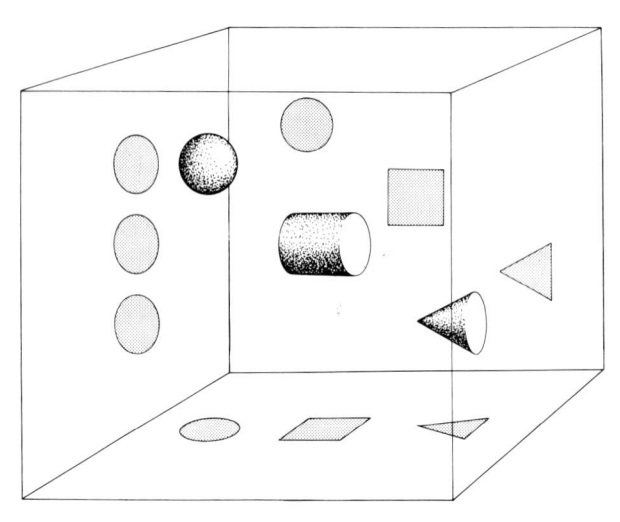

Abb. 36. Projektion eines dreidimensionalen Merkmalsraums auf verschiedene Ebenen

DIJAN (1972) nehmen im Gegensatz dazu eher ein „hypo-arousal" an. GIANNITRAPANI und KAYTON (1974) hingegen beziehen sich auf die von PITTS und MCCULLOCH (1947) entwickelte und auch von W.G. WALTER (1950) vertretene Hypothese, daß der Alpha-Rhythmus Ausdruck eines „scanning mechanism" sei, eines endogenen Rhythmus für die Suche nach Stimuli, der beim Vorhandensein eines weiten Bereichs von externen oder internen „Wahrnehmungen" sistiere. Die vermehrte Alpha-Frequenzlabilität, die GIANNITRAPANI und KAYTON im EEG Schizophrener beobachteten, deuten sie als Ausdruck einer gestörten „scanning activity" und damit als Hinweis auf eine Störung in der Verarbeitung interner oder externer Wahrnehmungen. In die gleiche Richtung zielt die Interpretation der Befunde über evozierte Potentiale durch SHAGASS (1976, s. Abschn. H.III). Dagegen ließe sich allerdings einwenden, daß sich frequenzlabile EEG auch bei nicht-psychotischen Probanden finden und gemeinhin als Ausdruck einer gestörten Hirndurchblutung gelten (JUNG, 1953; ROBERTS u. WALKER, 1954). Die spektralanalytisch nachweisbaren Gipfel im Beta-Band sind nach GIANNITRAPANI und KAYTON so schmalbandig wie bei Barbiturateffekten (SHAGASS, 1956) und nicht breitbandig wie beim „arousal" (GIANNITRAPANI, 1970). Ähnlich wie LIFSHITZ und GRADIJAN (1972) interpretieren GIANNITRAPANI und KAYTON daher die Beta-Vermehrung als Ausdruck einer gestörten Wachheit, eines „hypo-arousal".

Diese widersprüchlichen Deutungen der anhand von Schizophrenie-EEG erhobenen Befunde legen den Schluß nahe, daß die Dimensionalität des Begriffssystems, innerhalb dessen wir die Befunde zu erfassen suchen, zu gering und der Komplexität der Phänomene und ihrer Wechselbeziehungen nicht angemessen ist. Abb. 36 soll diesen Gedanken an einem einfachen Beispiel verdeutlichen, in dem sich ein im dreidimensionalen Raum eindeutiger Sachverhalt bei der Projektion auf verschiedenen Ebenen verschieden und teilweise widersprüchlich darstellt.

Die Fülle der quantitativen Daten aus der EEG-Analyse und der Registrierung evozierter und ereignisbezogener Potentiale zwingt dazu, durch statistische Analyseverfahren eine Datenreduktion auf relevante Informationen anzustreben (s. Abschn. C.V); offensichtlich muß aber auch die Dimensionalität unseres Begriffssystems erweitert werden, nicht zuletzt auch durch funktionsdynamische Kategorien, die sich aus den Kriterien psychopathologischer Verläufe herleiten.

I. Quantitative Pharmako-Elektroenzephalographie

Die elektroenzephalographische Untersuchung und Definition zerebraler Medikationseffekte hat im letzten Jahrzehnt eine rasche Entwicklung genommen, nachdem einerseits die computergestützte EEG-Analyse laborfähig geworden ist, andererseits geeignete statistische Analyseverfahren zur Auswertung der anfallenden quantitativen Daten eingesetzt wurden. Zwar reichen die Versuche zur Quantifizierung der Beziehungen zwischen EEG und Medikationswirkung schon weit zurück (ENGEL u. ROSENBAUM, 1945; HOAGLAND et al., 1946), indessen war die visuelle Beurteilung und die allenfalls von Hand betriebene Ausmessung von EEG-Kurven zu mühsam und ungenau, die Frequenzanalyse mit dem Grey Walter-Analysator (ULETT u. JOHNSON, 1957) durch Schwerfälligkeit und technische Instabilität belastet. Die Amplituden-Integration, die „period analysis" und die Spektral-Analyse, von denen die beiden letzteren erst mit der Verfügbarkeit von Laborcomputern praktische Bedeutung erlangten, haben eine neue Disziplin begründet, die ITIL (1972) als „quantitative Pharmakoelektroenzephalographie", FINK et al. (1967) als „EEG-Profil-Analyse" bezeichnen. Hiermit war die Klassifikation psychotroper Substanzen und die Vorhersage ihres klinischen Wirkungsprofils anhand von Ergebnissen der EEG-Analyse gemeint. FINK (1975) hat später diese Aufgabe erweitert auf die elektroenzephalographische Definition von Dosis-Wirkungskurven sowie der „zerebralen Bio-Verfügbarkeit" und die Gesamtheit der komplexen Methodik, die von der statistischen Versuchsplanung über die Bestimmung von Verhaltens- und subjektiven Befindlichkeitsänderungen bis zur multivariaten statistischen Analyse reicht, „zerebrale Elektrometrie" genannt.

Im folgenden können nur einige Aspekte dieser neuen Disziplin erörtert werden. Übersichten über den Stand von Methoden und Ergebnissen finden sich in der von ITIL (1974a) herausgegebenen Monographie, ferner bei FINK (1975, 1977) und ITIL (1974b), solche über die ältere Literatur gibt FINK (1963, 1964).

I. EEG und Veränderungen des Verhaltens sowie der Befindlichkeit unter Medikationswirkungen

Die Voraussage des klinischen Wirkungsprofils einer psychotropen Substanz anhand der von ihr provozierten EEG-Veränderungen scheint vorauszusetzen, daß ein regelhafter Zusammenhang besteht zwischen Befindlichkeits- und Verhaltensänderungen einerseits und definierbaren EEG-Veränderungen andererseits (FINK, 1975, 1977). Dies wurde längere Zeit allgemein abgelehnt, obgleich einzelne gezielte EEG-Studien gegen eine solche „Dissoziationshypothese" sprachen (BECKER, 1972; dort auch weitere Literatur) und mehrfach kritische Einwände gegen sie vorgebracht wurden (BRADLEY u. FINK, 1968; FINK, 1963). FINK (1975) beschreibt z.B. verminderte Wahrnehmungs-Diskrimination, verlangsamte Motorik, angehobene Stimmung und verlangsamten Gedankenablauf bei vermehrter Theta-Aktivität, eine Stimmungsanhebung und vermehrte Wahrnehmungsschärfe bei Zunahme niederamplitudiger Beta-Aktivität. Auch ITIL (1975) beschreibt Korrelationen zwischen EEG und Verhalten, vorwiegend unter Medikamentenwirkung. Aufgrund der Beurteilung des klinischen Wirkungsprofils einer Reihe von elektroenzephalographisch definierten Substanzklassen (FINK, 1967) ergab sich, daß Substanzen mit ähnlichem EEG-Profil auch ähnliche klinische Effekte besaßen. Daraus formulierte FINK (1977) die Hypothese, daß erstens die EEG-Veränderungen in direktem Zusammenhang mit den biochemischen Veränderungen stehen, die von Medikamenten im Gehirn bewirkt werden, und zweitens die Verhaltens- und Befindlichkeitsänderungen ebenfalls in direkter Beziehung zu diesen biochemischen Wirkungen stehen. Implizit wird der Schluß nahegelegt, daß EEG- und Verhaltensänderungen unter Medikationswirkung auf diese Weise miteinander zusammenhängen.

FINK betont selbst, daß diese Hypothese noch der kritischen Überprüfung bedarf. Vorläufig scheinen die Verhältnisse so einfach nicht zu liegen. So ließ sich bei vergleichender spektralanalytischer Prüfung verschiedener Substanzen zeigen (HEINZE u. KÜNKEL, 1979; KÜNKEL et al., 1976), daß Merkmale der Persönlichkeitsstruktur von Probanden die EEG-Effekte nicht nur quantitativ verändern (vgl. Abb. 25), sondern auch qualitativ umkehren können, daß ferner – wiederum in Abhängigkeit von Persönlichkeitsmerkmalen – Befindlichkeits- und Verhaltensänderungen mit gleichartigen EEG-Effekten korrelieren, die bei klinisch so unterschiedlich wirksamen Substanzen, wie etwa Diazepam und Amitriptylin, registriert werden. Dennoch ist unbestreitbar, daß die EEG-Effekte von Substanzen im Akut-Versuch eine Vorhersage der klinischen Langzeitwirkungen von Substanzen erlauben. Offensichtlich handelt es sich aber bei diesem Sachverhalt um keine eindimensionale Beziehung.

II. Elektroenzephalographische Wirkungsprofile psychotroper Substanzen

Anhand der „period analysis" des EEG im Akut-Versuch bei gesunden Probanden wurden zunächst 9 Substanzklassen definiert, je nach dem Verhalten der Frequenzen in den einzelnen Bändern sowie nach der Veränderung der mittleren Amplitude (vgl. hierzu die Frequenzprofile in Abb. 19, 20 sowie die Erläuterungen in Abschn. C.III). Tabelle 4 (in Anlehnung an FINK, 1977), gibt eine Übersicht über die beobachteten EEG-Effekte. Die aufgeführten Substanzen gelten als charakteristische Vertreter von ganzen Substanzklassen. Abb. 20 zeigt typische EEG-Frequenzprofile für Neuroleptika, Thymoleptika und Anxiolytika. Die sozusagen retrospektive EEG-Klassifikation von in ihrem klinischen Wirkungsprofil bekannten Substanzen erwies sich schließlich als erfolgreich in der Vorhersage des Effektes neuer Substanzen. FINK (1977) berichtet, daß von 53 geprüften und klinisch wirksamen Substanzen bei 19 auch ein klinisches Wir-

Tabelle 4. Elektroenzephalographische Wirkungsprofile. (In Anlehnung an FINK, 1977)

	Delta	Theta	Alpha	Beta 1	Beta 2	Ampl.
Chlorpromazin	+	+ +	+/−	0	−	+
Butaperazin	+	+ +	+ +	0	+/−	+
Reserpin	+	+	−	0	0	+
Amobarbital	0	+	0	+ +	+	+
Amphetamin	0	−	−	+	+ +	−
Ditran	+ +	+	−	+	+ +	−
Imipramin	+	+ +	−	+	+	−
Morphin	0	0	+ +	0	0	−
Iproniazid	0	+	−	0	0	+

+ = Zunahme; − = Abnahme; 0 = keine Veränderung; +/− = variable Effekte

kungsprofil untersucht wurde, welches ausnahmslos die Vorhersage durch die vorangegangenen EEG-Studien bestätigt habe. Ein Beispiel hierfür unter mehreren ist Mianserin (ITIL, 1972), welches im pharmakologischen Screening Antihistamin- und Antiserotonin-Eigenschaften zeigte. Seine durch das EEG-Profil postulierte antidepressive Wirkung war zuvor unbekannt, wurde aber in klinischen Studien bestätigt. Schließlich sei noch darauf hingewiesen, daß sich hierbei auch neue Möglichkeiten eröffnen, die Bio-Verfügbarkeit psychotroper Substanzen sowie die Pharmakodynamik ihrer zerebralen Wirkungen zu erfassen (FINK, 1975). Dies ist deswegen bedeutsam, weil die pharmakologischen Methoden hierzu wegen des Einflusses der Blut-Hirnschranke nur mit Einschränkung verwertbar sind, die EEG-Analyse dagegen eine empfindliche, objektive und nicht belastende Methode darstellt (ITIL, 1975).

J. Schluß

R. JUNG hat am Ende seines Beitrages „Neurophysiologie und Psychiatrie" in der 1. Auflage dieses Werkes u.a. die Frage gestellt, ob sich die zunehmend spezialisierte neurophysiologische Forschung nicht immer weiter von der klinischen Praxis entferne. Die Entwicklung des letzten Jahrzehnts hat gezeigt, daß sich zumindest die Elektroenzephalographie nicht nur methodisch differenziert hat, indem sie sich in zunehmendem Maße neuer Methoden der analytischen Statistik, der EEG-Analyse und der Untersuchung von Prozessen der Informationsverarbeitung bediente, sondern daß sie sich mit diesen Werkzeugen auch zunehmend wieder der klinischen Psychiatrie zugewandt hat. Wenn auch der Überblick über 4 Jahrzehnte elektroenzephalographischer Arbeit an psychiatrischen Fragen zunächst enttäuschend ausfallen mag, so ist hoffentlich erkennbar geworden, daß das EEG zu mehr taugt als nur zur Vermehrung der Zahl kurzlebiger Hypothesen mit unzureichender oder fragwürdiger Befundbasis. Eine nicht geringe Anzahl ermutigender Befunde war das Ergebnis eines noch immer anhaltenden technischen und methodischen Fortschritts, der sich schon bald unausweichlich des Computers bedienen mußte. Dabei bot sich erstmals die Möglichkeit, die Datenmengen der Elektroenzephalographie und die differenzierter gewordenen Befunde der klinischen Psychopathologie auf ihre gegenseitigen Strukturbeziehungen hin zu untersuchen. Die heutige klinische Elektroenzephalographie ist mit derjenigen noch vor einem Jahrzehnt nur noch bedingt vergleichbar, ihre Rolle als Mittel einer zerebralen Funktionsdiagnostik ist deutlicher geworden. Je besser unser Verständnis dieses Aspektes wird, desto tiefer wird auch unser Einblick nicht nur in die dynamische Struktur der hirnelektrischen Aktivität, sondern auch in die zerebrale Funktionsstruktur und ihre Modifikationen im Zusammenhang mit psychischen Störungen. Wir werden allerdings nicht erwarten dürfen, einfache Relationen zwischen psychopathologischen Phänomenen und elektroenzephalographischen Einzeltatsachen zu finden. Es wird bereits offenkundig, daß wir damit beginnen müssen, die Dimensionalität des neurophysiologischen und elektroenzephalographischen Begriffssystems neu zu überdenken und zu erweitern, in dem wir unsere Beobachtungen bislang zu deuten gewohnt sind. Die Fragen der Psychiatrie an die Elektroenzephalographie stellen noch immer eine Herausforderung dar; ihre Beantwortung wird die Hoffnungen rechtfertigen, in denen sich HANS BERGER einstmals enttäuscht sah.

Literatur

Adey, W.R., Kado, R.T., Walter, D.O.: Analysis of brain wave records from Gemini flight GT-7 by computation to be used in a thirty day primate flight. Life Sci. Space Res. **5**, 65–93 (1967).
Allahyari, H., Deisenhammer, E., Weiser, G.: EEG examination during delirium tremens. Psychiat. Clin. (Basel) **9**, 21–31 (1976).
Arfel, G.: Stimulations visuelles et silence cérébral. Electroenceph. clin. Neurophysiol. **23**, 172–175 (1967).
Arfel, G.: Introduction to clinical and EEG-studies. In: Altered states of consciousness, coma, cerebral death. Handbook of electroencephalography and clinical neurophysiology, Vol. 12. Harner, R.; Naquet, R. (eds.). Amsterdam: Elsevier 1975.
Arfel, G., Walter, S.: Potentiels évoqués et comas. Acta neurol. belg. **71**, 345–359 (1971).
Armington, J.C., Tepas, D.J., Kropfl, W.J., Hengst, D.W.H.: Summation of retinal potentials. J. opt. Soc. Amer. **51**, 877–886 (1961).
Bäumler, H., Wernecke, K.-D., Michel, J.: Die diskrete Walsh-Transformation zur Spektralanalyse des Elektroencephalogramms bei psychophysiologischen Untersuchungen. Elektron. Inform. Verarb. u. Kybernetik (EIK) **13**, 561–570 (1977).
Baldock, G.R., Walter, W.G.: A new electronic analyzer. Electronic Engn. **18**, 339–344 (1946).
Balthasar, K.: Zur Kenntnis der Panencephalitis nodosa (Pette). Arch. Psychiat. Nervenkr. **117**, 667–681 (1944).
Becker, D.: Hirnstromanalyse affektiver Verläufe. Ein experimenteller Beitrag zur neuropsychologischen Affektforschung. Göttingen: Hogrefe 1972.
Beek, H.H., von Bork, I.I., Herngreen, H., van der Most van Spijk, D.: Considerations of electroencephalography in schizophrenics with reference to a survey in 25 dutch mental hospitals. Psychiat. Neurol. Neurochir. **67**, 95 (1964).
Bente, D.: Das EEG bei Psychosen: Befunde und Probleme. Hippokrates **21**, 817–823 (1965).
Bergamini, L., Bergamasco, B., Mombelli, A.M., Mutani, R.: Autocorrelation analysis of EEG in coma. Schweiz. Arch. Neurol. Neurochir. Psychiat. **97**, 11–20 (1966).
Berger, H.: Über das Elektrenkephalogramm des Menschen. III. Mitteilung. Arch. Psychiat. Nervenkr. **94**, 16–60 (1931).
Berger, H.: Über das Elektrenkephalogramm des Menschen IV. Arch. Psychiat. Nervenkr. **97**, 6–26 (1932).
Berger, H.: Über das Elektrenkephalogramm des Menschen XIV. Arch. Psychiat. Nervenkr. **108**, 407–431 (1938).

Bergmann, L., Bergamasco, B.: Cortical evoked potentials in man. Springfield, Ill.: Thomas 1967.
Bickford, R.G., Jacobson, J.L., Langworthy, D.: A KWIC index of EEG-Literature. Amsterdam: Elsevier 1965.
Bozza-Marrubini, M.L.: Resuscitation treatment of the different degrees of unconsciousness. Acta neurochir. (Wien) **12**, 352–365 (1964).
Bradley, P., Fink, M. (eds.): Anticholinergic drugs and brain functions in animals and man. Progress in Brain Research, Vol. **28**. Amsterdam: Elsevier 1968.
Brandt, H.A., Metts, J.C., Kendrick, J.F., Fuster, B., Carney, A.: Cerebrovascular disease: electroencephalography in assessment and management. Clin. Electroencephalogr. (Chic.) **7**, 162–183 (1976).
Brazier, M.A.B.: Bibliography of Electroencephalography 1875–1948. Internat. Fed. Electroenceph. Clin. Neurophysiol. Montreal 1950
Brazier, M.A.B., Cobb, W.A., Fischgold, H., Gastaut, H., Gloor, P., Hess, R., Jasper, H., Loeb, C., Magnus, O., Pampiglione, G., Rémond, A., Storm van Leeuwen, W., Walter, W.G.: Preliminary proposal for an EEG terminology by the terminology commitee of the International Federation of Societies for electroencephalography and Clinical Neurophysiology. Electroenceph. clin. Neurophysiol. **13**, 646–650 (1961).
Bremer, F.: Les processus d'excitation et d'inhibition dans les phénomènes épileptiques. In: Bases physiologiques et aspects cliniques de l'épilepsie. Alajouanine, Th. (ed.). Paris: Masson 1958.
Buchsbaum, M.: Average evoked Response. Augmenting and reducing in schizophrenia and affective disorders. In: Biology of the major psychoses, Friedman, D.X. (ed.), pp. 129–142. Res. Publ. Assoc. Res. Nerv. Ment. Dis., Vol. 54. New York: Raven Press 1975.
Buchsbaum, M., Goodwin, F., Murphy, D., Borge, G.: AER in affective disorders. Amer. J. Psychiat. **128**, 51–57 (1971).
Buchsbaum, M., Goodwin, F., Murphy, D., Borge, G.: Average evoked response in bipolar and unipolar affective disorders: Relationship to sex, age of onset, and monoamine oxidase. Biol. Psychiat. **7**, 199–212 (1973).
Buchsbaum, M.A., Pfefferbaum, A.: Individual differences in stimulus intensity response. Psychophysiology **8**, 600–611 (1971).
Burch, N.R., Nettleton, W.I., Sweeney, J., Edwards, R.J.: Period analysis of the electroencephalogram on a general-purpose digital computer. Ann. N.Y. Acad. Sci. **115**, 827–843 (1964).
Burdick, J.A., Sugerman, A.A., Goldstein, L.: The application of regression analysis to quantitative EEG-analysis in man. Psychophysiology **3**, 249–254 (1967).
Buser, P.: Thalamic influences on the EEG. Electroenceph. clin. Neurophysiol. **16**, 18–26 (1964).
Cadilhac, J., Ribstein, M.: The EEG in metabolic disorders. World Neurol. **2**, 296–308 (1961).
Cadilhac, J., Ribstein, M., Jean, R.: EEG et troubles métaboliques. Rev. neurol. (Paris) **100**, 270–296 (1959).
Callaway, E., Jones, R.T., Layne, R.S.: Evoked responses and segmental sets of schizophrenia. Arch. Gen. Psychiat. **12**, 83–89 (1965).
Caspers, H., Abele, G.: Hirnelektrische Untersuchungen zur Frage der quantitativen Beziehungen zwischen Blutalkoholgehalt und Alkoholeffekt. Dtsch. Z. ges. gerichtl. Med. **45**, 492–509 (1956).
Caton, R.: The electric currents of the brain. Brit. med. J. **2**, 278 (1875).
Chatrian, G.E., Bergamini, L., Dondey, M., Klass, D.W., Lennox-Buchthal, M., Petersen, I.: A glossary of terms most commonly used by clinical electroencephalographers. Electroenceph. clin. Neurophysiol. **37**, 538–548 (1974).
Christian, W.: EEG-Veränderungen bei der psychomotorischen Epilepsie. Dtsch. Z. Nervenheilk. **183**, 218–244 (1962).
Christian, W.: Klinische Elektroencephalographie. 2. Aufl. Stuttgart: Thieme 1975.
Ciganek, L.: The EEG response (evoked response) to light stimulus in man. Electroenceph. clin. Neurophysiol. **13**, 165–172 (1961).
Cobb, W.A., van Duijn, H.: Contemporary Clinical Neurophysiology. Electroenceph. clin. Neurophysiol. Suppl. 34 (1978).
Cohen, J.: Developmental aspects of the CNV. In: Eventrelated slow potentials of the brain, McCallum, W., Knott, J.R. (eds.), pp. 133–137. Electroenceph. clin. Neurophysiol. Suppl. 33 (1973).
Cohen, R.: The influence of task-involvement stimulus variations on the reliability of auditory evoked responses in schizophrenia. In: Human neurophysiology, psychology, psychiatry. Average

evoked responses and their conditioning in normal subjects and psychiatric patients, Fessard, A., Lelord, G. (eds.), pp. 373–388. Paris: Inserm 1973.
Colony, H.S., Willis, S.E.: Electroencephalographic studies of 1000 schizophrenic patients. Am. J. Psychiat. **113**, 163–169 (1956).
Cooper, R., Osselton, J.W., Shaw, J.C.: Electroencephalographie. (Übersetzt von P. Rappelsberger.) Stuttgart: Fischer 1974.
Corletto, F., Gentilomo, A., Rosadini, G., Rossi, G., Zattoni, J.: Corrélations entre niveau de conscience, EEG et potentiels évoqués chez l'homme. Rev. Neurol. (Paris) **115**, 5–14 (1966).
Cremerius, J., Jung, R.: Über die Veränderungen des Elektroencephalogramms nach Elektroschockbehandlung. Nervenarzt **18**, 193–205 (1947).
Daniels, J.C., Shokroverty, S., Barron, K.: Anacidotic hyperglycemia and focal seizures. Arch. intern. Med. **124**, 701–705 (1969).
Davis, H.: Human auditory evoked potentials. In: Currents concepts in clinical neurophysiology, van Duijn, H., Donker, D.N.J., van Hoffelen, A.C. (eds.), pp. 49–62. Didactic lectures of the 9th Int. Congr. of Electroencephalography and Clinical Neurophysiology, Amsterdam 1977.
Davis, H., Yoshie, N.: Human evoked cortical responses to auditory stimuli. Physiologist **6**, 164 (1963).
Davis, H., Zerlin, S., Bowers, C., Spoor, A.: The slow responses of the human cortex to auditory stimuli: recovery process. Electroenceph. clin. Neurophysiol. **21**, 105–113 (1966).
Davis, P.A.: Evaluation of the electroencephalograms of schizophrenic patients. Amer. J. Psychiat. **96**, 851–860 (1940).
Davis, P.A.: Electroencephalograms of manic-depressive patients. Amer. J. Psychiat. **98**, 430–433 (1941).
Davis, P.A.: A comparative study of the EEGs of schizophrenic on manic-depressive patients. Am. J. Psychiat. **99**, 210–217 (1942)
Davis, P.A., Davis, H.: The electrical activity of the brain: its relation to physiological states and to states of impaired consciousness. Res. Publ. Ass. nerv. ment. Dis. **19**, 50–80 (1939).
Davis, P.A., Davis, H.: Electroencephalograms of psychiatric patients. Amer. J. Psychiat. **95**, 1007–1025 (1939).
Dawson, G.D.: Cerebral responses to electrical stimulation of the peripheral nerve in man. J. Neurol. Neurosurg. Psychiat. **10**, 134–140 (1947).
Dawson, G.D.: A summation technique for the detection of small evoked potentials. Electroenceph. clin. Neurophysiol. **6**, 65–84 (1954).
Deecke, L., Becker, W., Grözinger, B., Scheid, P., Kornhuber, H.: Human brain potentials preceding voluntary limb movements. In: Eventrelated slow potentials of the brain, McCallum, W., Knott, J.R. (eds.), pp. 87–94. Electroenceph. clin. Neurophysiol. Suppl. 33 (1973).
D'Elia, G., Laurell, B., Perris, C.: EEG photically elicited alpha-blocking responses in depressive patients before and after convulsive therapy. Acta psychiat. scand. (Suppl.) **255**, 159–172 (1974)
Delse, F., Marsh, G., Thompson, L.: The contingent negative variation as a pre-motor potential. Psychophysiology **6**, 619 (1970).
Desmedt, J. (ed.): Visual evoked potentials in man: new developments. Oxford: Clarendon Press 1977.
Dietsch, G.: Fourier-Analyse von Elektroencephalogrammen des Menschen. Pflügers Arch. ges. Physiol. **230**, 106–112 (1932).
Dolce, G., Künkel, H. (eds.): CEAN – Computerized EEG Analysis. Stuttgart: Fischer 1975
Donchin, E.: Methodological issues in CNN research, a review. In: Eventrelated slow potentials of the brain, McCallum, W., Knott, J.R. (eds.), pp. 3–17. Electroenceph. clin. Neurophysiol. Suppl. 33 (1973).
Donchin, E., Lindsley, D.B. (eds.): Average evoked potentials: methods, results and evaluations. NASA SP-91. Washington, D.C.: US Government Printing Office 1969.
Dongier, M.: Event related slow potential changes in psychiatry. In: Biological diagnosis of brain disorders, Bogoch, S. (ed.), pp. 47–59. New York: Spectrum 1973.
Dongier, M. (ed.): Mental diseases. Handbook of electroencephalography and clinical neurophysiology, Vol. XIII B. Amsterdam: Elsevier 1974
Dongier, M., Dubrowsky, B., Garcia-Rill, E.: Slow cerebral potentials in psychiatry. Amer. Psychiat. J. **19**, 177–183 (1974).
Dongier, S.: Statistical study of clinical and electroencephalographic manifestations of 536 psychotic

episodes occurring in 516 epileptics between clinical seizures. Epilepsia (Amst.) **1**, 117–142 (1959/60).
Dow, R.S., Ulett, G., Raaf, J.: EEG-studies immediately following head injury. Amer. J. Psychiat. **101**, 174–178 (1944).
Dreyer, R.: Zur Frage des Status epilepticus mit psychomotorischen Anfällen. Ein Beitrag zum temporalen Status epilepticus und zu typischen Dämmerzuständen und Verstimmungen. Nervenarzt **36**, 221–223 (1965).
Drohocki, Z.: L'électrospectrographie du cerveau. C.R. Soc. Biol. (Paris) **129**, 889–893 (1938).
Drohocki, Z.: L'intégrateur de l'électroproduction cérébrale pour l'électroencéphalographie quantitative. Rev. Neurol. (Paris) **80**, 619 (1948).
Duensing, F.: Das Elektroencephalogramm bei Störungen der Bewußtseinslage. Befunde bei Meningitiden und Hirntumoren mit Bemerkungen zur Pathophysiologie der Bewußtseinsstörungen. Arch. Psychiat. Nervenkr. **183**, 71–115 (1949).
Dumermuth, G.: Elektroencephalographie im Kindesalter. Einführung und Atlas. 3. Aufl. Stuttgart: Thieme 1976.
Dumermuth, G., Flühler, H.: Some modern aspects in numerical spectrum analysis of multi-channel electroencephalographic data. Med. biol. Eng. **5**, 319–331 (1967).
Eccles, J. (ed.): Brain and conscious experience. Berlin-Heidelberg-New York: Springer 1966.
Ellingson, R.J.: Development of visual evoked responses in human infants recorded by a response averager. Electroenceph. clin. Neurophysiol. **21**, 403–404 (1966).
Ellingson, R.J.: The incidence of EEG abnormality among patients with mental disorders of apparently non-organic origin: a critical review. Amer. J. Psychiat. **111**, 263–275 (1954).
Engel, G.L., Romano, J.: Delirium. II. Reversibility of the electroencephalogram with experimental procedures. Arch. Neurol. Psychiat. (Chic.) **51**, 378–421 (1944).
Engel, G.L., Rosenbaum, M.: Delirium. III. Electroencephalographic changes associated with acute alcoholic intoxication. Arch. Neurol. Psychiat. (Chic.) **53**, 44–50 (1945).
Engel, R.: Electroencephalographic responses to sound and to light in premature and fullterm neonates. Lancet **1967 87**, 181–186.
Engel, R., Halberg, F., Gurly, R.: The diurnal rhythm in EEG discharge and in circulating eosinophils in certain types of epilepsy. Electroenceph. clin. Neurophysiol. **4**, 115–116 (1952).
Essig, C.F., Fraser, H.F.: Electroencephalographic changes in man during use and withdrawal of barbiturates in moderate dosage. Electroenceph. clin. Neurophysiol. **10**, 649–656 (1958).
Étevenon, P.: Étude méthodologique d'électroencéphalographie quantitative. Application à quelques examples. Paris: Thèse 1977.
Faure, J.: L'activité électrique du cerveau. World Neurol. **2**, 879–894 (1961).
Ferillo, F., Rivano, C., Rosadini, G., Rossi, G.F., Turelka, C.: EEG spectral analysis in coma. Electroenceph. clin. Neurophysiol. **27**, 700 (1969).
Fessard, A.: Les mécanismes de synchronisation interneuronique et leur intervention dans la crise épileptique. In: Bases physiologiques et aspects cliniques de l'épilepsie. Alajouanine, Th. (ed.). Paris: Masson 1958.
Fessard, A., Lelord, G. (eds.): Human neurophysiology, psychology, psychiatry. Average evoked responses and their conditioning in normal subjects and psychiatric patients. Paris: Inserm 1973.
Fink, M.: Cerebral Electrometry–Quantitative EEG applied to human psychopharmacology. In: CEAN–Computerized EEG analysis, Dolce, G., Künkel, H. (eds.), pp. 271–288. Stuttgart: Fischer 1975.
Fink, M.: Quantitative EEG analysis and psychopharmacology. In: EEG informatics. A didactic review of methods and applications of EEG data processing, Rémond, A. (ed.), pp. 301–318. Amsterdam: Elsevier 1977.
Fink, M.: Quantitative electroencephalography in human psychopharmacology. II. Drug patterns. In: EEG and Behavior. Glaser, G. (ed.). New York: Basic Books 1963.
Fink, M.: A selected bibliography of electroencephalography in human psychopharmacology 1951–1962. Electroenceph. clin. Neurophysiol. Suppl. **23**, (1964).
Fink, M.: EEG Classification of psychoactive compounds in man: Review and theory of behavioral associations. In: Psychopharmacology – A review of progress 1957–1967. Efron, D., Cole, J.O., Levine, J., Wittenborn, J.R. (eds.). Washington, D.C.: Government printing office 1967.

Fink, M., Itil, T.M., Clyde, D.: A contribution to the classification of psychoses by quantitative EEG-measures. Proc. Soc. biol. Psychiat. **2**, 5–17 (1965).
Fink, M., Itil, T.M., Shapiro, D.: Digital computer analysis of the human EEG in psychiatric research. Compr. Psychiat. **8**, 521–538 (1967).
Fink, M., Kahn, R.L.: Relation of electroencephalographic delta activity to behavioral responses in electroshock. Arch. Neurol. Psychiat. (Chic.) **78**, 516–525 (1957).
Fischgold, H., Gastaut, H.: Conditionnement et réactivité en électroencéphalographie. Electroenceph. clin. Neurophysiol. Suppl. 6 (1957).
Fischgold, H., Mathis, P.: Comas, obnubilations et stupeurs. Études électroencéphaliques. Electroenceph. clin. Neurophysiol., Suppl. 11 (1959).
Flügel, K.A.: Die Elektroencephalographie der Funktionspsychosen. Stuttgart: Thieme 1974
Flügel, K.A., Druschky, K.F.: Elektroencephalographische und neurologische Befunde beim hyperosmolaren nicht-ketoazidotischen Coma diabeticum. Nervenarzt **47**, 723–736 (1976).
Fruhstorfer, H., Soveri, P., Järvilehto, T.: Short-time habituation of the auditory evoked response in man. Electroenceph. clin. Neurophysiol. **28**, 153–161 (1970).
Fünfgeld, E.W.: Étude à la récupération de l'EEG après hypoxie par strangulation avec rigidité de décérébration. Rev. neurol. **117**, 88–90 (1967).
Garmezy, N.: Process and reactive schizophrenia. Some conceptions and issues. Schizophrenia Bull. **2**, 30–74 (1970).
Garsche, R.: Das Elektroencephalogramm bei der Meningitis tuberculosa im Kindesalter. Untersuchungen bei 103 Erkrankungsfällen. Beitr. Klin. Tberk. **111**, 353–376 (1954).
Gastaut, H.: Combined photic and metrazol activation of the brain. Electroenceph. clin. Neurophysiol. **2**, 249–261 (1950).
Gastaut, H.: So-called „psychomotor" and „temporal" epilepsy. A critical study. Epilepsia (Boston) **2**, 57–78 (1953).
Gastaut, H.: The brain stem and cerebral electrogenesis in relation to consciousness. In: Brain mechanism and consciousness, Delafresnaye, J.F. (ed.), pp. 249–279. Springfield, Ill.: Thomas (1954).
Gastaut, H., Naquet, R., Vigourox, R., Roger, A., Badier, M.: Étude électrographique chez l'homme et chez l'animal des décharges épileptiques dits „psychomotrices". Rev. Neurol. **88**, 310–354 (1953).
Gastaut, H., Roger, J., Roger, A.: Sur la signification de certaines fugues épileptiques. À-propos d'une observation électro-clinique d',,état de mal temporal". Rev. Neurol. (Paris) **94**, 298–301 (1956).
Gastaut, H., Roger, J., Lob, H.: Les états de mal épileptiques. Paris: Masson 1967.
Gastaut, H., Tassinari, C.A.: The significance of ictal and interictal discharges with respect to epilepsy. In: Handbook of electroencephalography and clinical neurophysiology, Vol. III A. Gastaut, H., Tassinari, C.A. (eds.). Amsterdam: Elsevier 1975.
Gastaut, H., Tassinari, C.A.: Ictal discharges in different types of seizures. In: Handbook of electroencephalography and clinical neurophysiology, Vol. 13A, Gastaut, H., Tassinari, C.A. (eds.), pp. 20–45. Amsterdam: Elsevier 1975a.
Gastaut, H., Tassinari, C.A.: The ictal and interictal EEG in different types of epilepsy. In: Handbook of electroencephalography and clinical neurophysiology, Vol. 13 A, Gastaut, H., Tassinari, C.A. (eds.), pp. 46–64. Amsterdam: Elsevier 1975b.
Gerstenbrand, F.: Das traumatische apallische Syndrom. Wien: Springer 1967.
Giannitrapani, D.: EEG changes under differing auditory stimulus. Arch. gen. Psychiat. **23**, 445–453 (1970).
Giannitrapani, D., Kayton, L.: Schizophrenia and EEG spectrum analysis. Electroenceph. clin. Neurophysiol. **36**, 377–386 (1974).
Gibbs, F.A.: Cortical frequency spectra of schizophrenic, epileptic and normal individuals. Trans. Amer. neurol. Ass. **65**, 141–144 (1939).
Gibbs, F.A., Gibbs, E.L.: The mitten pattern: An electroencephalographic abnormality correlating with psychosis. J. Neuropsychiat. **5**, 6–13 (1963).
Gibbs, F.A., Gibbs, E.L.: Atlas of electroencephalography. Vol. I: Methodology and Controls. Cambridge: Addison-Wesley 1950 Vol. II: Epilepsy. Cambridge: Addison-Wesley 1952. Vol. III: Neurologiy and psychiatric disorders. Cambridge: Addison-Wesley 1964.
Gibbs, F.A., Gibbs, E.L.: Elektroencephalographie. Übersetzt von H. Künkel. Stuttgart: Fischer 1971.

Gibbs, F.A., Gibbs, E.L., Lennox, W.G.: Electroencephalographic classification of epileptic patients and control subjects. Arch. Neurol. Psychiat. (Chic.) **50**, 111–128 (1943).

Gibbs, F.A., Williams, D., Gibbs, E.L.: Modification of the cortical frequency spectrum by changes in CO_2, blood sugar and CO_2. J. Neurophysiol. **3**, 49–58 (1940).

Goldstein, L.: Time domain analysis of the EEG: The integrative method. In: CEAN-Computerized EEG analysis, Dolce, G., Künkel, H. (eds.), pp. 251–270. Stuttgart: Fischer 1975.

Goldstein, L.A., Sugerman, A.A.: EEG-correlates of psychopathology. In: Neurophysiological aspects of psychopathology, Zubin, J., Shagass, C. (eds.), pp. 1–19. Prov. Am. Psychopathol. Assoc., Vol. XXV. New York: Grune and Stratton 1969.

Goldstein, L., Sugerman, A.A., Stolberg, H., Murphre, H.B., Pfeiffer, C.C.: Electrocerebral activity in schizophrenics and non-psychotic subjects: Quantitative EEG amplitude-analysis. Electroenceph. clin. Neurophysiol. **19**, 350–361 (1965).

Gotman, J., Gloor, P.: Automatic recognition and quantification of interictal epileptic activity in the human scalp EEG. Electroenceph. clin. Neurophysiol. **41**, 513–529 (1976).

Greenblatt, M., Healy, M.M., Jones, G.A.: Age and electroencephalographic abnormality in neuropsychiatric patients: a study of 1593 cases. Amer. J. Psychiat. **101**, 82–90 (1944).

Gutjahr, L., Künkel, H.: Jahreszeitliche Einflüsse auf die Häufigkeit von EEG-Befunden. Arzneimittel-Forsch. (Drug Res.), **28**(II), 1857–1861 (1978).

Gutjahr, L., Machleidt, W., Ferber, C.: Die diagnostische Bedeutung von „steilen Potentialen" für die Erkennung von epileptischen Anfallsleiden. Methods Inf. Med. **18**, 25–30 (1979).

Halberg, F.: Chronobiology. Ann. Rev. Physiol. **31**, 675–725 (1969).

Halberg, F., Carendente, F., Cornelissen, G., Katinas, G.S.: Glossary of chronobiology. Chronobiologia **4**, Suppl. 1, 1977.

Halberg, F., Katinas, G.S., Chiba, Y., Garcia Sainz, M., Kováts, T.G., Künkel, H., Montalbetti, N., Reinberg, A., Scharf, R., Simpson, H.: Chronobiologic glossary. Int. J. Chronobiol. **1**, 31–63 (1973).

Halliday, A.M.: Somatosensory evoked responses. In: Evoked responses. Handbook of electroencephalography and clinical neurophysiology, Vol. 81. Storm van Leeuwen, W., Lopes da Silva, F.H., Kamp, A. (eds.). Amsterdam: Elsevier 1975.

Halliday, A.M., McDonald, W.I.: Pathophysiology of demyelinating disease. Brt. med. Bull. **33**, 21–27 (1977).

Halliday, A.M., Wakefield, G.S.: Cerebral evoked potentials in patients with dissociated sensory loss. J. Neurol. Neurosurg. Psychiat. **26**, 211–219 (1963).

Harner, R., Katz, R.I.: Electroencephalography in metabolic coma. In: Altered states of consciousness, coma, cerebral death. Handbook of electroencephalography and clinical neurophysiology, Vol. 12. Harner, R., Naquet, R. (eds.). Amsterdam: Elsevier 1975.

Harner, R., Naquet, R.: Altered states of consciousness, coma, cerebral death. Handbook of electroencephalography and clinical neurophysiology, Vol. 12. Amsterdam: Elsevier 1975.

Hein, P.L., Green, R.L., Wilson, W.P.: Latency and duration of the photically elicited arousal responses in the electroencephalograms of patients with chronic regressive schizophrenia. J. nerv. ment. Dis. **135**, 361–364 (1962).

Heinze, H.J., Künkel, H.: The significance of personality traits in EEG evaluation of drug effects. Pharmacopsychiatry **12**, 155–164 (1979).

Helmchen, H.: Bedingungskonstellationen paranoid-halluzinatorischer Syndrome. Monogr. Gesamtgeb. Psychiatr. (Berlin) 122. Berlin-Heidelberg-New York: Springer 1968.

Helmchen, H., Kanowski, S., Künkel, H.: Die Altersabhängigkeit der Lokalisation von EEG-Herden. Arch. Psychiat. Nervenkr. **209**, 474–483 (1967).

Helmchen, H., Künkel, H.: Der Einfluß von EEG-Verlaufsuntersuchungen unter psychiatrischer Pharmakotherapie von Psychosen. Arch. Psychiat. Nervenkr. **205**, 1–18 (1964).

Helmchen, H., Künkel, H., Oberhoffer, G., Penin, H.: EEG-Befund-Dokumentation mit optischem Markierungsleser. Nervenarzt **39**, 408–413 (1968).

Helmchen, H., Künkel, H., Selbach, H.: Zur Entstehung der „Rhythmischen Nachschwankung" (Rhythmic After-Activity) bei optisch ausgelösten Reizantworten (Evoked Responses) im EEG des Menschen. In: Clinical Neurophysiology: EEG, EMG. Proc. 6th Int. Congr. Electroenceph. Clin. Neurophysiol. pp. 517–522. Wien: Wiener medizin. Akademie 1965.

Heninger, G., McDonald, R.D., Goff, W.R., Sollberger, A.: Diurnal variations in the cerebral evoked response and EEG. Arch. Neurol. Psychiat. (Chic.) **21**, 330–337 (1969).

Hess, R.: Das Elektroencephalogramm bei endokrinen Störungen. In: Endokrinologische Psychiatrie. Bleuler, M. (ed.). Stuttgart: Thieme 1954.
Hess, R.: Elektrische Hirnaktivität und Psychopathologie. Schweiz. med. Wschr. **93**, 449–462 (1963).
Hill, D.: Das EEG bei Schizophrenie. In: Schizophrenie. Richter, D. (ed.). Stuttgart: Thieme 1957.
Hill, D.: The EEG in psychiatry. In: Electroencephalography: A symposium on its various aspects, Hill, D., Parr, G. (eds.), pp. 368–428. London: Macdonald 1963.
Hoagland, H., Malamud, W., Kaufman, I.C., Pincus, G.: Changes in the EEG and in the excretion of 17-ketosteroids accompanying electroshock therapy of agitated depression. Psychosom. Med. **8**, 246–251 (1946).
Hubach, H.: Über elektroencephalographische Befunde bei Encephalitis unter Berücksichtigung klinischer Gesichtspunkte. Dtsch. Z. Nervenheilk. **180**, 94–124 (1959).
Hubach, H.: Veränderungen der Krampferregbarkeit unter Einwirkung von Medikamenten und während der Entziehung. Fortschr. Neurol. Psychiat. **31**, 177–201 (1963).
Huber, G., Penin, H.: Klinisch-elektroencephalographische Korrelationsuntersuchungen bei Schizophrenen. Fortschr. Neurol. Psychiat. **36**, 641–659 (1968).
Hurst, L.A., Mundy-Castle, A.C., Beerstecher, D.M.: The electroencephalogram in manic-depressive psychosis. J. ment. Sci. **100**, 220–240 (1954).
Igert, C., Lairy, G.C.: Prognostic value of the EEG in course of the development of schizophrenics. Electroenceph. clin. Neurophysiol. **14**, 183–190 (1962).
Ingvar, D.H., Sjölund, B., Ardö, A.: Correlation between dominant EEG frequency, cerebral oxygen uptake and blood flow. Electroenceph. clin. Neurophysiol. **41**, 268–276 (1976).
Itil, T.M.: Digital computer period analyzed EEG in psychiatry and psychopharmacology. In: CEAN–Computerized EEG Analysis, Dolce, G., Künkel, H. (eds.), pp. 289–308. Stuttgart: Fischer 1975.
Itil, T.M.: Electroencephalography and pharmaco-psychiatry. In: Modern problems in pharmacopsychiatry, Vol. I, Freyhan, F.A., Petrilowitsch, N., Pichot, P. (eds.), pp. 163–194. Basel: Karger 1968.
Itil, T.M.: Quantitative pharmaco-electroencephalography in the discovery of a new group of psychotropic drugs. Dis. nerv. Syst. **33**, 557–559 (1972).
Itil, T.M. (ed.): Psychotropic drugs and the human EEG. Modern problems of pharmacopsychiatry, Vol. 8. Basel: Karger 1974a.
Itil, T.M.: Quantitative pharmaco-electroencephalography. Use of computerized cerebral biopotentials in psychotropic drug research. In: Psychotropic drugs and the human EEG, Itil, T.M. (ed.), pp. 43–75. Modern problems of pharmacopsychiatry, Vol. 8. Basel: Karger 1974b.
Itil, T.M., Saletu, B., Davis, S.: EEG-findings in chronic schizophrenics based on digital computer period analysis and analog power spectra. Biol. Psychiat. **5**, 1–13 (1972).
Jacob, H.: Ein Beitrag zur automatischen in Echtzeit ablaufenden Analyse von kontinuierlichen und intermittierenden Aktivitäten im Elektroencephalogramm. Dissert. TU Hannover 1976.
Janz, D.: Die Epilepsien. Spezielle Pathologie und Therapie. Stuttgart: Thieme 1969.
Jellinger, K., Seitelberger, F.: Protracted post-traumatic encephalopathy: pathology, pathogenesis and clinical implications. J. neurol. Sci. **10**, 51–94 (1970).
Jones, R.T., Callaway, E.: Auditory evoked responses in schizophrenia. A reassessment. Biol. Psychiat. **2**, 291–298 (1970).
Jonkman, E.J.: The average cortical response to photic stimulation. Amsterdam: Thesis 1967.
Jung, G.: Das Elektrencephalogramm (EEG). In: Handbuch der inneren Medizin, 4. Aufl., Bd. V/1, v. Bergmann, E., Frey, W., Schwiegk, H. (Hrsg.), S. 1216–1325. Berlin-Göttingen-Heidelberg: Springer 1953.
Jung, R.: Neurophysiologie und Psychiatrie. In: Psychiatrie der Gegenwart, Bd. I A, 1. Aufl. Gruhle, H.W., Jung, R., Mayer-Gross, W. (Hrsg.). Berlin-Heidelberg-New York: Springer 1967.
Jung, R.: Das EEG bei der psychiatrischen Schockbehandlung. Schweiz. Arch. Neurol. Psychiat. **66**, 421–423 (1950).
Jung, R.: Neurophysiologische Untersuchungsmethoden. In: Handbuch der inneren Medizin, Bd. V/1, v. Bergmann, G., Frey, W., Schwiegk, H. (Hrsg.), S. 1206–1420. Berlin-Göttingen-Heidelberg: Springer 1953.
Jung, R.: Neurophysiologie und Psychiatrie. In: Psychiatrie der Gegenwart, Bd. I A, 1. Aufl. Gruhle, H.W., Jung, R., Mayer-Gross, W. (Hrsg.). Berlin-Heidelberg-New York: Springer 1967.

Jung, R.: Neurophysiologische Untersuchungsmethoden. II: Das Elektroencephalogramm. In: Handbuch der Inneren Medizin, Bd. V. Berlin: Springer 1953.

Jung, R., Tönnies, F.: Hirnelektrische Untersuchungen über Entstehung und Erhaltung von Krampfentladungen. Arch. Psychiat. Nervenkr. **185**, 701–735 (1950).

Keidel, W.D., Spreng, M.: Computed audioencephalography in man (a technique of objective audiometry). Int. Audiol. **4**, 56–60 (1965).

Kellaway, P., Petersen, I. (eds.): Automation of clinical electroencephalography. New York: Raven Press 1973.

Kellaway, P., Petersen, I. (eds.): Quantitative analytic studies in epilepsy. New York: Raven Press 1976.

Kennard, M.A., Rabinovitch, M.S., Fister, W.P.: The use of frequency analysis in the interpretation of the EEG's of patients with psychological disorders. Electroenceph. clin. Neurophysiol. **7**, 29–38 (1955).

Kennard, M.A., Schwartzman, A.G.: A longitudinal study of electroencephalographic frequency patterns in mental hospital patients and normal controls. Electroenceph. clin. Neurophysiol. **9**, 263–274 (1957).

Kennedy, A.C., Linton, A.L., Luice, R.G., Renfrew, S.: Electroencephalographic changes during hemodialysis. Lancet **1909 I**, 408–411

Kety, S.S., Evarts, E.V., Williams, H.L. (eds.): Sleep and altered states of consciousness. Res. Publ. Ass. nerv. ment. Dis. **45** (1967).

Kiley, J., Hines, O.: Electroencephalographic evaluation of uremia. Arch. int. Med. **116**, 67–73 (1965).

Kiley, J.E.: Electronic EEG frequency analysis for evaluation of uremia. In: Proc. 4th Ann. Contractors Conf. of the Nat. Inst. of Arthritis and Metabolic Diseases. Krueger, K.K. (ed.), pp. 146–147. Washington: 1971.

Kiley, J.E.: Electronic EEG frequency analysis for evaluation of uremia. In: Proc. 5th Ann. Contractors Conf. of the Nat. Inst. of Arthritis and Metabolic Diseases, Krueger, K.K. (ed.), pp. 152–153. Washington: 1972.

Kiley, J.E., Woodruff, M.W., Pratt, K.L.: Evaluation of encephalopathy by EEG frequency analysis in chronic dialysis patients. Clin. Nephrol. **5**, 245–250 (1976).

Klee, A.: Akinetic mutism: review of the literature and report of a case. J. nerv. ment. Dis. **133**, 536–553 (1961).

Köhler, G.-H.: Hirnelektrische Untersuchungen bei epileptischen Psychosen unter besonderer Berücksichtigung der Prozeßaktivität. In: Psychische Störungen bei Epilepsie. Psychosen, Verstimmungen, Persönlichkeitsveränderungen, Penin, H. (Hrsg.), S. 41–50. Stuttgart, New York: Schattauer 1973.

Kollmannsberger, A., Kugler, J., Eymer, K.P.: Über Encephalopathien bei Lebererkrankungen (unter besonderer Berücksichtigung elektroencephalographischer Befunde). Verh. dtsch. Ges. inn. Med. **72**, 230–238 (1967).

Kooi, K.A., Tipton, A.C., Marshall, R.E.: Polarities and field configurations of the vertex components of the human auditory evoked response: a reinterpretation. Electroenceph. clin. Neurophysiol. **31**, 166–169 (1971).

Kornhuber, H.H., Deecke, L.: Hirnpotentialänderungen bei Willkürbewegungen und passiven Bewegungen des Menschen: Bereitschaftspotential und reafferente Potentiale. Pflügers Arch. ges. Physiol. **284**, 1–17 (1965).

Kretschmer, E.: Das apallische Syndrom. Z. ges. Neurol. Psychiat. **169**, 576–579 (1940).

Kripke, D.F.: An ultradian biologic rhythm associated with perceptual deprivation and REM sleep. Psychosom. Med. **34**, 221–234 (1972).

Krogh, H.J., Khan, M.A., Fosvig, L., Jensen, K., Kellerup, P.: N1-P2 component of the auditory evoked potential during alcohol intoxication and interaction of pyrithioxine in healthy adults. Electroenceph. clin. Neurophysiol. **44**, 1–7 (1978).

Kubicki, St.: Depth of coma and EEG changes in narcotic poisoning. Electroenceph. clin. Neurophysiol. **23**, 282 (1967).

Kubicki, St., Rieger, H., Busse, G.: EEG in fatal and near-fatal poisoning with soporific drugs. Clin. Electroenceph. **1**, 5–13 (1970).

Künkel, H.: Die Periodik der paroxysmalen Dysrhythmie im Elektroencephalogramm. Stuttgart: Thieme 1969.

Künkel, H.: Quantitative EEG-Analyse und schizophrene Psychosen. In: Entwicklungstendenzen biologischer Psychiatrie, Helmchen, H., Hippius, H. (Hrsg.), S. 41–50. Stuttgart: Thieme 1975.
Künkel, H.: Die Spektraldarstellung des EEG. EEG-EMG **3**, 15–24 (1972 a).
Künkel, H.: Simultane Vielkanal-on line-EEG-Analyse in Echtzeit. EEG-EMG **3**, 30–38 (1972 b).
Künkel, H.: Historical review of principal methods. In: EEG Informatics. A didactic review of methods and applications of EEG data processing, Rémond, A. (ed.), pp. 9–25. Amsterdam: Elsevier 1977.
Künkel, H.: Frequency analysis. Electroenceph. clin. Neurophysiol., Suppl. (1978) (im Druck).
Künkel, H., Luba, A., Niethardt, P.: Topographic and psychosomatic aspects of spectral EEG analysis of drug effects. In: Quantitative analytic studies in epilepsy. Kellaway, P., Petersen, I. (eds.), pp. 207–223. New York: Raven Press 1976 a.
Künkel, H., Machleidt, W., Niethardt, P.: Circadian variation of physiological and spectral EEG-parameters. Proc. XII. Int. Conf. Internat. Soc. Chronobiol. Washington, 1975, pp. 549–560. Milano: Il Ponte 1977.
Kugler, J.: Elektroencephalographie in Klinik und Praxis. 2. Aufl. Stuttgart: Thieme 1966.
Kugler, J.: Einflüsse von Medikamenten auf die okzipitale Reizantwort des EEG. In: Clinical Neurophysiology: EEG, EMG. Proc. 6th Int. Congr. Electroenceph. Clin. Neurophysiology, pp. 389–391. Wien: Wiener medizin. Akademie 1965.
Lairy, G.C.: Organisation de l'électroencephalogramme normal et pathologique. Aspect clinique. Rev. neurol. **94**, 749–801 (1956).
Landolt, H.: Über Verstimmungen, Dämmerzustände und schizophrene Zustandsbilder bei Epilepsie. Schweiz. Arch. Neurol. Psychiat. **76**, 313–371 (1955).
Landolt, H.: Serial electroencephalographic investigations during psychotic episodes in epileptic patients and schizophrenic attacks. In: Lectures on epilepsy, Lorentz de Haas (ed.), pp. 134–167. Amsterdam: Elsevier 1958.
Landolt, H.: Über einige Korrelationen zwischen Elektroencephalogramm und normalen und pathologischen psychischen Vorgängen. Schweiz. med. Wschr. **93**, 107–136 (1963 a).
Landolt, H.: Die Dämmer- und Verstimmungszustände bei Epilepsien und ihre Elektroencephalographie. Dtsch. Z. Nervenheilk. **185**, 411–430 (1963 b).
Lanzinger-Rossnagel, G., Christian, W., Kommerell, B.: Prä- und postoperative EEG-Verläufe bei shunt-operierten Leberzirrhotikern. Dtsch. med. Wschr. **102**, 725–731 (1977).
Lemere, F.: Cortical energy production in the psychoses. Psychosom. Med. **3**, 152–156 (1941).
Lennox, M.A., Ruch, T.C., Guterman, B.: The effect of benzedrine on the post-electroshock EEG. Electroenceph. clin. Neurophysiol. **3**, 63–69 (1951).
Lester, B.K., Edwards, R.J.: EEG fast activity in schizophrenic and control subjects. Int. J. Neuropsychiat. **2**, 143–156 (1966).
Lewis, E.G., Dustman, R.E., Beck, E.C.: Visual and somato-sensory evoked potential characteristics of patients undergoing hemodialysis and kidney transplantation. Electroenceph. clin. Neurophysiol. **44**, 223–231 (1978).
Liberson, W.T.: Functional electroencephalography in mental disorders. Dis. nerv. Syst. **5**, 357–364 (1944).
Lieberman, D.M., Hoenig, J., Hacker, M.: The metrazol-flicker threshold in neuropsychiatric patients. Electroenceph. clin. Neurophysiol. **6**, 9–18 (1954).
Lifshitz, K.: An examination of evoked potentials as indicators of information processing in normal and schizophrenic subjects. In: Average evoked potentials. Methods, results and evaluation, Donchin, E., Lindsley, D.B. (eds.), pp. 318–319, 357–362. Washington, D.C.: NASA 1969.
Lifshitz, K., Gradijan, J.: Relationship between measures of the coefficient of variation of the mean absolute EEG voltage and spectral intensities in schizophrenic and control subjects. Biol. Psychiat. **5**, 149–163 (1972).
Lifshitz, K., Gradijan, J.: Spectral evaluation of the electroencephalogram: Power and variability in chronic schizophrenics and control subjects. Psychophysiology **11**, 479–490 (1974).
Lille, F., Borlone, M., Lérique, A., Scherrer, J., Thieffry, S.: Evaluation de la profondeur du coma chez l'enfant par la technique des potentiels évoqués. Rev. neurol. **117**, 216–217 (1967).
Lindsley, D.B.: Psychological phenomena and the electroencephalogram. Electroenceph. clin. Neurophysiol. **4**, 443–456 (1952).
Loeb, C.: Electroencephalogram during coma. Acta neurochir. (Wien) **12**, 270–281 (1964).
Loeb, C.: Correlative EEG and clinico-pathological studies of patients in coma. In: Altered states

of consciousness, coma, cerebral death. Handbook of electroencephalography and clinical neurophysiology, Vol. 12, Harner, R., Naquet, R. (eds.). Amsterdam: Elsevier 1975.
Loeb, C., Meyer, J.C.: Strokes due to vertebro-basilar disease. Springfield, Ill.: Thomas 1965.
Logothetis, J.: Psychotic behavior as the initial indicator of adult myxoedema. J. nerv. ment. Dis. **136**, 561–568 (1963).
Lopes da Silva, F.H., van Rotterdam, A.: Analysis of evoked responses. In: Evoked responses. Handbook of electroencephalography and clinical neurophysiology, Vol. 8 A, Storm van Leeuwen, W., Lopes da Silva, F.H., Kamp, A. (eds.). Amsterdam: Elsevier 1975.
Lopes da Silva, F.H., van Hulten, K., Lommen, J.G., Storm van Leeuwen, W., van Vellen, C.W.M., Vliegenthart, W.: Automatic detection and localization of epileptic foci. Electroenceph. clin. Neurophysiol. **43**, 1–13 (1977).
Lorenzoni, E., Lechner, H., Geyer, N., Manowarda, K., Mauser, H.: Rheoencephalographische und EEG-Untersuchungen unter Hypoxie und Alkohol. Nervenarzt **39**, 25–31 (1968).
Low, M.D.: Event-related potentials and the CNV. In: EEG Informatics. A didactic review of methods and applications of EEG data processing, Rémond, A. (ed.), pp. 347–364. Amsterdam: Elsevier 1977.
Luce, R.A., Rothschild, D.: The correlation of electroencephalographic and clinical observations in psychiatric patients over 65. J. Geront. **8**, 167–172 (1953).
Lugaresi, E., Pazzaglia, P.: Interictal electroencephalogram. In: Handbook of electroencephalography and clinical neurophysiology, Vol. 13 A, Gastaut, H., Tassinari, C.A. (eds.), pp. 7–19. Amsterdam: Elsevier 1975.
Lugaresi, E., Pazzaglia, P., Tassinari, C.A.: Differentiation of „absence status" and „temporal lobe status". Epilepsia (Amsterdam) **12**, 77–87 (1971).
Lundervold, A.: Anoxia cerebri. An electroencephalographic investigation. Acta psychiat. scand. **31**, 160–161 (1956).
Lundervold, A., Hauge, T., Löken, A.C.: Unusual EEG in unconscious patient with brain stem atrophy. Electroenceph. clin. Neurophysiol. **8**, 665–670 (1956).
Maccario, M.: Neurologic dysfunction associated with nonketotic hyperglycemia. Arch. Neurol. Psychiat. (Chic.) **19**, 525–534 (1968).
Machleidt, W.: Tagesrhythmik und periodische Komponenten der Zeitstruktur des Alpha- und Theta-Bandes im Ruhe-EEG. Inaug. Dissert. FU Berlin 1975.
MacMahon, J.F., Walter, W.G.: The electro-encephalogram in schizophrenia. J. ment. Sci. **84**, 781–787 (1938).
Maggs, R., Turton, E.: Some EEG findings in old age and their selectionship to affective disorders. J. ment. Sci. **102**, 812–818 (1956).
Magnes, J., Moruzzi, G., Pompeiano, O.: EEG-synchronizing structure in the brain stem. Ciba Foundation Symposium on „the nature of sleep", pp. 57–78. London: Churchill 1961.
Marjerrison, G., Krause, A.E., Keogh, R.P.: Variation of the EEG in schizophrenia: Quantitative analysis with a modulus voltage integrator. Electroenceph. clin. Neurophysiol. **24**, 35–41 (1967).
Marjerrison, G., James, J., Reichert, H.: Unilateral and bilateral ECT: EEG-findings. Canad. psychiat. Ass. J. **20**, 257–266 (1975).
Matejcek, M., Schenk, G.K. (eds.): Quantitative analysis of the EEG. Konstanz: AEG-Telefunken, EDP Division 1975.
McAdam, D.W.: The contingent negative variation. In: Bioelectric recording techniques. Part B: Electroencephalography and human brain potentials, Thompson, R.F., Patterson, M.M. (eds.), pp. 245–257. New York: Academic Press 1974.
McCallum, W., Knott, J.R. (eds.): Event-related slow potentials of the brain: their relations to behavior. Electroenceph. clin. Neurophysiol. Suppl. 33 (1973).
McCallum, W.C.: Some psychological, psychiatric and neurologic aspects of the CNN. In: Human neurophysiology, psychology, psychiatry. Average evoked responses and their conditioning in normal subjects and psychiatric patients, Fessard, A., Lelord, G. (eds.), pp. 295–324. Paris: Inserm 1973.
McCallum, W.C., Knott, J.R. (eds.): The responsive brain. Bristol: Wright 1976.
McCallum, W.C., Walter, W.G.: The effects of attention and distraction on the contingent negative variation in normal and neurotic subjects. Electroenceph. clin. Neurophysiol. **25**, 319–323 (1968).
McGillivray, B.: The application of automated EEG analysis to the diagnosis of epilepsy. In:

EEG Informatics. A didactic review of methods and applications of EEG data processing. Rémond, A. (ed.). Amsterdam: Elsevier 1977.
Mensokova, Z.: The electroencephalogram in acute comatose meningoencephalitis. Čs. Neurol. **21**, 90–98 (1958).
Merrill, J.P., Hampers, C.L.: Uremia (part I). New Engl. J. Med. **282**, 953–961 (1970).
Metrakos, K.O., Metrakos, J.D.: Genetics of convulsive disorders. II. Genetic and electroencephalographic studies in centrencephalic epilepsy. Neurology (Minneap.) **11**, 474–483 (1961).
Meyer-Mickeleit, R.W.: Das Elektrencephalogramm beim Elektrokrampf des Menschen. Arch. Psychiat. Nervenkr. **183**, 12–33 (1949).
Meyer-Mickeleit, R.W.: Das Elektrencephalogramm nach gedeckten Kopfverletzungen. Dtsch. med. Wschr. **78**, 480–484 (1953).
Morison, R.S., Dempsey, E.W.: A study of thalamo-cortical relations. Amer. J. Physiol. **135**, 281–292 (1942).
Mundy-Castle, A.C., Hurst, L.A., Beerstecher, D.M., Prinsloo, T.: The electroencephalogram in the senile psychoses. Electroenceph. clin. Neurophysiol. **6**, 245–252 (1954).
Nadel, A.M., Wilson, W.P.: Dialysis encephalopathy: a possible seizure disorder. Neurology (Minneap.) **26**, 1130–1134 (1976).
Niedermeyer, E.: EEG-Untersuchungen bei suizidalem Erhängen. Wien. klin. Wschr. **68**, 555–556 (1956).
Obrist, W.D.: The EEG of healthy males. In: Human aging: a biological and behavioral study. Birren, J.E. et al. (eds.). Public Health Serv. Publication 986, pp. 77–93. Washington, D.C.: Government Print. Office 1963.
Obrist, W.D., Henry, C.E.: Electroencephalographic frequency analysis of aged psychiatric patients. Electroenceph. clin. Neurophysiol. **10**, 621–632 (1958).
Pagni, C.A.: Somato-sensory evoked potentials in thalamus and cortex of man. Electroenceph. clin. Neurophysiol. Suppl. **26**, 147–155 (1967).
Penfield, W., Jasper, H.H.: Epilepsy and the functional anatomy of the brain. Boston: Little, Brown 1954.
Penin, H.: Klinisch-elektroencephalographische Korrelationen bei endogenen Psychosen. In: (ohne Hrsg.): Ergebnisse biologischer Forschung bei endogenen Psychosen. Köln: Tropon-Werke (ohne Jahr)
Penin, H.: Die Bedeutung der Elektroencephalographie für die Schizophrenieforschung. In: Aetiologische Schizophrenien. Huber, G. (ed.). Stuttgart: Schattauer 1971.
Penin, H.: Über den diagnostischen Wert des Hirnstrombildes bei der hepato-portalen Encephalopathie. Zugleich ein klinisch-statistischer Beitrag zur Frage neurologischer und psychischer Veränderungen bei Leberzirrhosen und porto-cavalen Anastomose-Operationen. Fortschr. Neurol. Psychiat. **35**, 173–234 (1967).
Penin, H.: Über den diagnostischen Wert des Hirnstrombildes bei der hepato-portalen Enzephalopathie. Fortschr. Neurol. Psychiat. **35**, 173–234 (1967).
Penin, H.: Das EEG der symptomatischen Psychosen. Nervenarzt **42**, 242–252 (1971).
Penin, H.: Klinisch-elektroencephalographische Korrelationen bei endogenen Psychosen. Das ärztl. Gespräch **23**, 78–98 (1974).
Penin, H., Käufer, C. (eds.): Der Hirntod. Todeszeitbestimmung bei irreversiblem Funktionsverlust des Gehirns. Stuttgart: Thieme 1969.
Penin, H., Käufer, C. (eds.): Physiology of the states of consciousness. Acta neurochir. (Wien) **12**, 161–378 (1965).
Penin, H., Matiar-Vahar, H.: Das EEG der Neurolues. II. Mitteilung. Arch. Psychiat. Nervenkr. **205**, 449–464 (1964).
Penin, H., Schaefer, C.H.: Das EEG der Neurolues. I. Mitteilung. Arch. Psychiat. Nervenkr. **205**, 433–447 (1964).
Penin, H., Zeh, W.: Das Elektroencephalogramm der akuten symptomatischen Psychosen. Dtsch. med. Forsch. **2**, 17 (1964).
Penin, H., Helmchen, H., Jacobitz, K., Kanowski, S., Künkel, H., Zenker, K.: Anwendung einer EEG-Befunddokumentation auf wissenschaftliche Fragestellungen. EEG-EMG **3**, 6–15 (1972).
Penry, J.K., Dreyfuss, F.E.: A study of automatisms associated with the absence of petit mal. Epilepsia (Amst.) **10**, 417–418 (1969).

Pitts, W., McCulloch, W.S.: How we know universals: the perception of auditory and visual forms. Bull. math. Biophys. **9**, 127–147 (1947).
Planques, I., Grézes-Rueff, C., Bollinelli, R., Darrusio, J., Chabourne, M.: Tolérance cérébrale à l'anoxie chronique. Rev. neurol. **112**, 282–283 (1965).
Plum, F., Posner, J.B.: Diagnosis of stupor and coma. 2. Aufl. Philadelphia: Davis 1972.
Pro, J.D., Wells, C.E.: The use of the electroencephalogram in the diagnosis of delirium. Dis. nerv. Syst. **38**, 804–808 (1977).
Prüll, G., Krämer, W., Rompel, K.: EEG-Veränderungen bei Myasthenien. EEG-EMG **1**, 122 (1970).
Rabending, G., Klepel, H.: Photoconvulsive and photomyoclonic responses: age dependent variations of genetically determined photosensitivity. Neuropädiatrie **2**, 164–172 (1970).
Radermecker, J.: Das Elektroencephalogramm der subakuten sklerosierenden Leukoencephalitis. Wien. Z. Nervenheilk. **13**, 204–223 (1957).
Radermecker, J.: Das Elektroencephalogramm der subakuten sklerosierenden Leukoencephalitis und seine Variationsbreite. Wien. Z. Nervenheilk. **13**, 204–223 (1957).
Radermecker, J.: Severe acute necrosis of the pons with long survival. Electroclinical symptoms and absence of cerebral lesions. Electroenceph. clin. Neurophysiol. **23**, 281–282 (1967).
Regan, D.: Evoked potentials in psychology, sensory physiology and clinical medicine. London: Chapman and Hall 1972.
Regan, D.: Evoked potentials in brain and clinical research. In: EEG informatics. A didactic review of methods and applications of EEG data processing, Rémond, A. (ed.), pp. 319–346. Amsterdam: Elsevier 1977.
Rémond, A. (ed.): EEG Informatics. A didactic review of methods and applications of EEG data processing. Amsterdam: Elsevier 1977.
Rémond, A. (ed.): Handbook of Electroencephalography and Clinical Neurophysiology. Vol. 1–16. Amsterdam: Elsevier 1971–1977.
Rey-Bellet, J.: L'EEG dans la porphyrie aïgue intermittente. Schweiz. med. Wschr. **94**, 1134–1143 (1964).
Richter, K.: Über Anlagefaktoren im EEG. Fortschr. Neurol. Psychiat. **28**, 332–350 (1960).
Roberts, J.A., Walker, M.: The electroencephalogram in essential hypertension and chronic cerebrovascular disease. Electroenceph. clin. Neurophysiol. **6**, 461–468 (1954).
Roger, J., Lob, H., Tassinari, C.A.: Status epilepticus. In: Handbook of clinical neurology, Vol. 15, Vinken, P.J., Bruyn, G.W. (eds.), pp. 145–188. Amsterdam: North-Holland 1973.
Rohmer, F., Wackenheim, A., Kurtz, D.: L'EEG dans les syndromes endocriniens hypophysaires, thyroidiens, surrenaux et dans la tétanie de l'adulte. Rev. neurol. **100**, 297–314 (1969).
Romano, J., Engel, G.L.: Delirium I. Electroencephalographic data. Arch. Neurol. Psychiat. (Chic.) **51**, 336–377 (1944).
Roth, M.: Some diagnostic and aetiological aspects of confusional states in the elderly. Gerontologia (Basel) **1**, 83–95 (1959).
Saletu, B., Itil, T.M., Saletu, M.: Auditory evoked response, EEG, and thought processes in schizophrenics. Amer. J. Psychiat. **128**, 336–344 (1971).
Scanlon, W.G., Mathias, J.: Electroencephalographic and psychometric studies of Indoklon convulsive treatment and electroconvulsive treatment. Int. J. Neuropsychiat. **3**, 276–281 (1967).
Schenk, G.K. (ed.): Die Quantifizierung des Elektroencephalogramms. Konstanz: AEG-Telefunken, EDP Division 1973.
Schneider, E., Hubach, H.: Das EEG der traumatischen Psychosen. Dtsch. Z. Nervenheilk. **183**, 600–627 (1962).
Schweitzer, D.: Periodische Komponenten im Zeitablauf der Theta-Ausprägung. Inaug. Dissert. FU Berlin 1971.
Shagass, C.: The sedation threshold: A method for estimating tension in psychiatric patients. Electroenceph. clin. Neurophysiol. **6**, 221–233 (1954).
Shagass, C.: Sedation threshold: a neurophysiological tool for psychosomatic research. Psychosom. Med. **18**, 410–419 (1956).
Shagass, C.: A neurophysiological study of schizophrenia. Rep. 2nd Int. Congr. for Psychiatry Vol. **2**, 248–254 (1959).
Shagass, C.: Neurophysiological studies. In: The schizophrenic syndrome, Bellak, L., Loeb, L. (eds.), pp. 172–204. New York: Grune and Stratton 1969.

Shagass, C.: Evoked brain potentials in psychiatry. New York: Plenum Press 1972.
Shagass, C.: EEG and evoked responses in the psychoses. In: Biology of the major psychoses, Freedman, D.X. (ed.), pp. 101–127. Res. Publ. Assoc. Res. Nerv. Ment. Dis., Vol. 54. New York: Raven Press 1975.
Shagass, C.: An electrophysiological view of schizophrenia. Biol. Psychiat. 11, 3–30 (1976).
Shagass, C.: Twisted thoughts, twisted brain waves? In: Psychopathology and brain dysfunction, Shagass, C., Gershon, S., Friedhoff, A.J. (eds.), pp. 353–378. New York: Raven Press 1977.
Shagass, C., Ando, K.: Septal and reticular influences on cortical evoked responses recovery function. Biol. Psychiat. 2, 3–18 (1970).
Shagass, C., Schwartz, M.: Visual evoked response characteristics in a psychiatric population. Amer. J. Psychiat. 121, 979–987 (1965).
Shagass, C., Schwartz, M., Krishnamoorti, S.R.: Some physiologic correlations of cerebral responses evoked by light flash. J. psychosom. Res. 9, 223–231 (1965).
Shagass, C., Soskis, D.A., Straumanis, J.J., Overton, D.A.: Symptom patterns related to psychiatric illness. Biol. Psychiat. 9, 25–43 (1974).
Sharrard, G.A.W.: Evoked response audiometry in compared groups of normally hearing adults, normally hearing and deaf children and multiple-handicapped children. Electroenceph. clin. Neurophysiol. 30, 366–367 (1971).
Shaw, J.C.: Cerebral function and the EEG in psychiatric disorder: a hypothesis. Psychol. Med. 6, 307–311 (1976).
Shipton, H.W.: A transportable low frequency wave analyzer. Electroenceph. clin. Neurophysiol. 8, 705 (1956).
Sila, B., Mowrer, M., Ulett, G., Johnson, M.: The differentiation of psychiatric patients by EEG changes after sodium pentothal. In: Recent advances in biological psychiatry, Vol. IV, Wortis, J. (ed.), pp. 191–203. New York: Plenum Press 1962.
Silverman, D.: Some observations on the EEG in hepatic coma. Electroenceph. clin. Neurophysiol. 14, 53–59 (1962).
Silverman, D.: Retrospective study of the EEG in coma. Electroenceph. clin. Neurophysiol. 15, 486–503 (1963).
Simon, O.: Das Elektroencephalogramm. München: Urban & Schwarzenberg 1977.
Slater, E., Beard, W., Glithero, E.: The schizophrenia-like psychoses of epilepsy. Brit. J. Psychiat. 109, 95–150 (1963).
Small, J.G., Small, I.F.: Re-evaluation of clinical EEG-findings in schizophrenia. Dis. Nerv. Syst. 26, 345–349 (1965).
Small, J.G., Small, I.F.: Contingent negative variation correlations with psychiatric diagnosis. Arch. gen. Psychiat. 25, 550–554 (1971).
Smith, D.B.D., Donchin, E., Cohen, L., Star, A.: Auditory averaged evoked potentials in man during selective binaural listening. Electroenceph. clin. Neurophysiol. 28, 146–152 (1970).
Soskis, D.A., Shagass, C.: Evoked potential test of augmenting – reducing. Psychophysiology 11, 175–190 (1974).
Spehlmann, R.: The averaged electrical responses to diffuse and to patterned light in man. Electroenceph. clin. Neurophysiol. 19, 560–567 (1965).
Spehr, W., Sartorius, H., Berglund, K., Hjorth, B., Kablitz, C., Plog, U., Wiedemann, P.H., Zapf, K.: EEG and hemodialysis. A structural survey of EEG spectral analysis, Hjorth's EEG descriptors, blood variables and psychological date. Electroenceph. clin. Neurophysiol. 43, 787–797 (1977).
Spunda, Ch.: Das EEG bei akuten und chronischen zerebrovaskulären Erkrankungen. Wien. Z. Nervenheilk. 18, 79–94 (1960).
Stark, L.H., Norton, J.C.: The relative reliability of average evoked response parameters. Psychophysiology 11, 600–602 (1974).
Sternberg, M.: Periodische Komponenten im Zeitablauf der Beta-Ausprägung. Inaug. Dissert. FU Berlin 1971.
Sternberg, P.: Periodische Komponenten im Zeitablauf der Alpha-Ausprägung. Inaug. Dissert. FU Berlin 1971.
Stevens, J.R.: All that spikes is not fits. In: Psychopathology and brain dysfunction, Shagass, C., Gershon, S., Friedhoff, A.J. (eds.), pp. 183–198. New York: Raven Press 1977.
Storm van Leeuwen, W.: Auditory evoked responses. In: Evoked responses. Handbook of elec-

troencephalography and clinical neurophysiology, Vol. 8 A. Storm van Leeuwen, A., Lopes da Silva, F.H., Kamp, A. (eds.). Amsterdam: Elsevier 1975.

Storm van Leeuwen, W., Lopes da Silva, F.A., Kamp, A. (eds.): Evoked responses. In: Handbook of electroencephalography and clinical neurophysiology, Vol. 8 A, Rémond, A. (ed.). Amsterdam: Elsevier 1975.

Strömgren, L.S., Juul-Jensen, P.: EEG in unilateral and bilateral electroconvulsive therapy. Acta psychiat. scand. **51**, 340–360 (1975).

Struve, F.A., Becka, D.R., Klein, D.F.: β-mitten pattern and process and reactive schizophrenia. Arch. gen. Psychiat. **26**, 189–192 (1972).

Sugerman, A.A., Goldstein, L., Murphree, H.B., Pfeiffer, C.C., Jenney, E.H.: EEG and behavioral changes in schizophrenie. Arch. gen. Psychiat. **10**, 340–344 (1964).

Tecce, J.J.: Contingent negative variation (CNV) and psychological processes in man. Psychol. Bull. **77**, 73–108 (1972).

Thiébaut, F., Rohmer, F., Wackenheim, A.: Contribution à l'étude électroencéphalographique des syndromes endocriniens. Electroenceph. clin. Neurophysiol. **10**, 1–30 (1958).

Thompson, R.F., Patterson, M.M. (eds.): Bioelectric recording techniques. Part B: Electroencephalography and human brain potentials. New York: Academic Press 1974.

Timsit-Berthier, M.: CNV, slow potentials and motor potential studies in normal subjects and psychiatric patients. In: Human neurology, psychology, psychiatry. Average evoked responses and their conditioning in normal subjects and psychiatry patients, Fessard, A., Lelord, G. (eds.), pp. 327–366. Paris: Inserm 1973.

Ulett, G., Das, K., Hornung, F., Davis, D., Johnson, M.: Changes in the photically driven EEG following convulsive therapy. J. Neuropsychiat. **3**, 186–189 (1962).

Ulett, G.A., Johnson, M.W.: Effect of atropine and scopolamine upon electroencephalographic changes induced by electro-convulsive therapy. Electroenceph. clin. Neurophysiol. **9**, 217–224 (1957).

Ulett, G.A., Loeffel, R.G.: A new resonator-integrator unit for an automatic brain wave analyzer. Electroenceph. clin. Neurophysiol. **5**, 113–115 (1953).

Uryu, K., Moriya, A.: A frequency analyzing study of electroencephalogram in schizophrenic psychoses. Dynamic observation with the overlapping method. Proc. 6th An. Meeting Jap. EEG-Society **12**, 1957, zit. nach Goldstein, L., Sugerman, A.A., 1969.

Van der Tweel, L.H.: Visual evoked potentials, a methodological panorama. In: Current concepts in clinical neurophysiology, van Duijn, H., Donker, D.N.J., van Huffelen, A.C. (eds.), pp. 35–48. Didactic lectures of the 9th Int. Congr. of Electroencephalography and Clinical Neurophysiology Amsterdam 1977.

Van der Tweel, L.H., Sem-Jacobsen, C.W., Kamp, A., Storm van Leeuwen, W., Veringa, F.T.H.: Objective determination of response to modulated light. Acta physiol. pharmacol. neurol. **7**, 528 (1958).

Vaughan, H.G., Ritter, W.: The sources of auditory evoked responses recorded from the human head. Electroenceph. clin. Neurophysiol. **28**, 360–367 (1970).

Vaughan, H.G., Costa, L.D., Ritter, W.: Topography of the human motor potential. Electroenceph. clin. Neurophysiol. **25**, 1–10 (1968).

Vogel, F.: Über die Erblichkeit des normalen Elektroencephalogramms. Stuttgart: Thieme 1958.

Vogel, F.: Untersuchungen zur Genetik der Beta-Wellen im EEG des Menschen. Dtsch. Z. Nervenheilk. **184**, 137–173 (1962).

Vogel, F.: Genetische Aspekte des Elektroencephalogramms. Dtsch. med. Wschr. **88**, 1748–1759 (1963).

Vogel, F., Götze, W.: Familienuntersuchungen zur Genetik des normalen Elektroencephalogramms. Dtsch. Z. Nervenheilk. **178**, 668–700 (1959).

Volavka, J., Matousek, M., Roubicek, J.: EEG frequency analysis in schizophrenia. Acta psychiat. scand. **42**, 237–245 (1966).

Wallace, P.W., Westmoreland, B.F.: The electroencephalogram in pernicious anemia. Mayo Clin. Proc. **51**, 281–285 (1976).

Walter, D.O.: Spectral analysis for electroencephalograms: mathematical determination of neurophysiological relationships from records of limited duration. Exp. Neurol. **8**, 155–181 (1963).

Walter, P.L.: A KWIC index to EEG and allied literature 1966–1969. Electroenceph. clin. Neurophysiol. Suppl. 29 (1970).

Walter, W.G.: The twenty-fourth Maudsley lecture: The functions of the electrical rhythms in brain. J. ment. Sci. **96**, 1–31 (1950).
Walter, W.G.: Evoked response general. In: Evoked responses. Handbook of electroencephalography and clinical neurophysiology, Vol. 8A, Storm van Leeuwen, W., Lopes da Silva, F.H., Kamp, A. (eds.). Amsterdam: Elsevier 1975.
Walter, W.G., Cooper, R., Aldridge, V.J., McCallum, W.C., Winter, A.L.: Contingent negative variation: An electric sign of sensorimotor association and expectancy in the human brain. Nature (Lond.) **203**, 380–384 (1964).
Ward, A.A.: The epileptic neurone. Epilepsia **2**, 70–80 (1961).
Watson, C.S., Marcus, E.M.: The genetics and clinical significance of photogenic cerebral electrical abnormalities, myoclonus, and seizures. Trans. Amer. neurol. Ass. **87**, 251–253 (1962).
Weinmann, H., Creutzfeldt, O., Heyde, G.: Die Entwicklung der visuellen Reizantwort bei Kindern. Arch. Psychiat. Nervenkr. **207**, 323–341 (1965).
Wikler, A., Fraser, H.F., Isbell, H., Pescor, F.T.: Electroencephalograms during cycles of addiction to barbiturates in man. Electroenceph. clin. Neurophysiol. **7**, 1–13 (1955).
Wikler, A., Pescor, F.T., Fraser, H.F., Isbell, H.: Electroencephalographic changes associated with chronic alcoholic intoxication and the alcohol abstinence syndrome. Amer. J. Psychiat. **113**, 106–114 (1956).
Wilson, W.P. (ed.): Applications of electroencephalography to psychiatry. Durham, North Carolina: Duke Univ. Press 1965.
Wilson, W.P., Wilson, N.J.: Observations on the duration of the photically elicited arousal responses in depressive psychoses. J. nerv. ment. Dis. **133**, 438–440 (1961).
Wineburgh, M., Walter, P.L.: A KWIC to EEG and allied literature 1964–1966. Electroenceph. clin. Neurophysiol. Suppl. 30 (1971).
Wolf, P.: Zur Klinik und Psychopathologie des Status psychomotoricus. Nervenarzt **41**, 603–610 (1970).
Wulff, M.H.: The barbiturate withdrawal syndrome. Electroenceph. clin. Neurophysiol. Suppl. 14. Kopenhagen: Munksgaard 1959.
Zeh, W.: Progressive Paralyse. Verlaufs- und Korrelationsstudien. Stuttgart: Thieme 1964.
Ziegler, D.K., Presthus, J.: Normal electroencephalogram at deep levels of hypoglycaemia. Electroenceph. clin. Neurophysiol. **9**, 523–526 (1957).

Psychopharmacology: Basic Aspects

By

A. Carlsson

Contents

A. Introduction	198
B. Basic Aspects of Neurohumoral, Especially Monoaminergic, Transmission in the CNS	198
C. Monoaminergic Pathways in the CNS	200
D. Functional Aspects of the Monoaminergic Pathways	200
E. The Various Steps in Monoaminergic Transmission as Targets for Psychotropic Drugs	202
I. Monoamine-Synthesizing Enzymes	202
II. Monoamine-Degrading Enzymes	204
III. Storage in the Synaptic Vesicles	205
IV. Release by the Nerve Impulse	205
V. Re-Uptake	205
VI. Receptor Activation	206
VII. The Secondary Messengers	207
F. Some Aspects of the Regulation of Monoaminergic Neuronal Activities	207
G. Antipsychotic or Neuroleptic Agents	209
I. Introduction	209
II. Reserpine	210
III. Neuroleptics Not Depleting Monoamine Stores	210
1. Historical Note	210
2. Dopamine-Receptor Blockade: Functional Evidence	211
3. Dopamine-Receptor Blockade: Biochemical Evidence	212
4. The Possible Role of α-Adrenoceptor Blockade	212
5. Regional Aspects: Striatal vs Limbic Dopamine	212
6. The Possible Role of Dopaminergic Autoreceptors	215
7. Effect on Dopamine-Sensitive Adenylate Cyclase	216
8. In-Vitro Studies on Dopamine Binding and Release	216
9. Pharmacokinetic Aspects of Dopamine-Receptor Blockade	217
IV. Neuroleptic Properties of α-Methyltyrosine	218
V. Effects of Neuroleptics on Noncatecholaminergic Systems	219
1. 5-HT	219
2. Acetylcholine	219
3. GABA	219
VI. Endocrine Aspects of Neuroleptic Action	220
VII. Acutevs Long-Term-Effects of Neuroleptics	220
VIII. Effects of Neuroleptics on Developing Brain	221
IX. The Possible Role of Dopamine and Other Neurotransmitters in Psychosis	222

H. Antidepressant Agents. 223
      I. Introduction 223
      II. Monoamine Oxidase Inhibitors 224
      III. Inhibitors of Monoamine Re-Uptake 224
      IV. Interaction Between Monoamine Oxidase Inhibitors and Tricyclic Antidepressants 226
      V. Monoamine Precursors as Antidepressant Agents 226
      VI. Antidepressant Agents With Unknown Modes of Action 227
      VII. Effect of Electroconvulsive Treatment on Monoaminergic Mechanisms 228

I. Psychotomimetic Agents. 228
      I. Introduction 228
      II. LSD-25 and Other Psychotomimetic Indole Derivatives 229
      III. Amphetamines and Related Agents 229
      IV. Dopa 230
      V. Anticholinergic Agents With Psychotomimetic Activity 231

J. Sedatives, Hypnotics, and Anxiolytics 231

K. Ethyl Alcohol – Mechanisms Underlying Drug Dependence 232

L. Concluding Remarks 233

References 234

A. Introduction

The rational use of drugs requires knowledge about their mode of action. Besides, such knowledge will often initiate research toward unraveling physiologic and pathogenetic mechanisms. When KRAEPELIN (1892) coined the term pharmacopsychology, he emphasized this aspect: "From the particular effect of an already well-known drug on a particular mental process, the possibility exists to better recognize the true nature of the latter." It is interesting that SIGMUND FREUD (1914, 1930) has expressed similar lines of thought; in fact, he is not only the father of psychoanalysis but also one of the early prophets of modern psychopharmacology. However, it did not become possible to approach this problem in a fruitful manner until the 1950s, when the antipsychotic and antidepressant drugs were discovered. In addition, the discoveries that the clinical pictures of schizophrenia and depression can be faithfully mimicked by drugs also greatly helped to promote this research field.

B. Basic Aspects of Neurohumoral, Especially Monoaminergic, Transmission in the CNS

More than half a century has elapsed since neurohumoral transmission was demonstrated in the peripheral nervous system. It is only during the last two decades that this concept has gained entrance into CNS research. In this development the monoamines have played a decisive role. Noradrenaline, adrenaline, and 5-hydroxytryptamine (5-HT) were detected in the brain around 1950, and dopamine somewhat later (CARLSSON, 1972). The most important criteria for monoaminergic transmission in the CNS are the following (see CARLSSON, 1972):

1. The monoamines occur intraneuronally with the same intracellular distribution as that of noradrenaline in the peripheral nervous system, i.e., they are mainly stored in the synaptic vesicles (or granules), which occur abundantly in the so-called varicosities. Here synaptic contact is made between the nerve terminals and other neurons;
2. The monoamines are synthesized by means of intraneuronal enzymes, largely in the nerve terminals;
3. The monoamines are released through depolarization by the nerve impulses or excess K^+ ions, a process depending on Ca^{2+} ions;
4. Receptors, specific for the different monoamines, occur on the postsynaptic membranes and are activated by the release of monoamines. The postsynaptic neuron responds to the activation of monoaminergic receptors by inhibition or excitation. This will lead to changes in CNS functions, e.g., blood pressure regulation, spinal reflexes, motor behavior, or mental activity.
5. Efficient mechanisms for the inactivation of monoamines are capable of terminating the neurotransmission process.
6. The synthesis and turnover of monoamines are closely dependent on the nerve impulse.

For obvious reasons the different steps in neurotransmission are not as readily accessible for study in the central as in the peripheral nervous system. However, an abundance of data has accumulated during the last two decades demonstrating the role, of monoamines as transmitters in the CNS, and this role is hardly questioned today.

The monoamines are probably responsible for but a very small part of the neurohumoral transmission in the CNS. The great importance of acetylcholine as a central neurotransmitter can hardly be questioned, and in certain cases an intimate interaction between central cholinergic and monoaminergic neurons has been detected (SCHEEL-KRÜGER, 1969; BARTHOLINI and STADLER, 1975). A number of amino acids serve as putative transmitters, with inhibitory functions, e.g., γ-aminobutyric acid (GABA), glycine, and perhaps also taurine, or excitatory functions, e.g., glutamic or aspartic acid (ROBERTS et al., 1976; IVERSEN and OTSUKA, 1975; HUXTABLE and BARBEAU, 1976).

A vast and rapidly expanding research field is centered around peptides in the CNS. In neuroendocrinology several peptides with hormone-releasing functions are well established, e.g., TRH (thyrotropin-releasing hormone), a tripeptide that in addition to its well-established hormone-releasing function in the median eminence may serve as neurotransmitter in other parts of the CNS. TRH, like thyroxine and thyrotropin, has been reported to possess antidepressant properties, but the observations in this area are partly contradictory. TRH has been found to potentiate the central action of dopa in animal experiments. An intimate relationship appears to exist between several hormone-releasing or inhibitory factors in the median eminence and monoaminergic mechanisms. In fact, PIF (= prolactin inhibitory factor) is possibly not a peptide but may be identical with dopamine, which occurs abundantly in the median eminence (KAMBERI and THORN, 1975).

Another interesting peptide serving as a putative transmitter is substance P, an undecapeptide now available in synthetic form. Substance P occurs in especially high concentration in substantia nigra and in the basal ganglia (POWELL, 1973; HÖKFELT et al., 1975). It has recently been shown to stimulate the synthesis and metabolism of dopamine, noradrenaline, and 5-HT in the CNS (MAGNUSSON et al., 1976). Substance P may well serve as an excitatory transmitter with an input, inter alia, on monoaminergic neurons. However, it probably has other important transmitter functions, e.g., in primary sensibility afferents (OTSUKA et al., 1975).

Somatostatin is another putative peptide transmitter (KAMBERI and THORN, 1975), capable of stimulating the synthesis and turnover of monoamines in the CNS (GARCIA SEVILLA et al., 1978).

C. Monoaminergic Pathways in the CNS

The majority of the cell bodies of the central monoaminergic systems is localized in the lower brain stem, from which pathways ascend to various parts of the cerebrum and cerebellum or descend to the spinal cord. Some pathways are entirely confined to the lower brain stem (UNGERSTEDT, 1971).

The largest dopamine pathway, i.e., the nigrostriatal tract, has its cell bodies in the pars compacta of the substantia nigra, with the axons ascending in the lateral hypothalamus and the internal capsule to the caudate nucleus and putamen. The second largest dopamine pathway is called the mesolimbic pathway. Its cell bodies are located in the brain stem just medially to the substantia nigra. The terminals are located in various parts of the limbic system, e.g., the olfactory tubercle, the nucleus accumbens, the central nucleus of the amygdala, and certain parts of the paleocortex, e.g., the gyrus cinguli and the entorhinal cortex. In addition, many other parts of the CNS, e.g., neocortex, brain stem, and spinal cord, receive a sparse supply of dopaminergic nerve terminals. The tuberoinfundibular dopaminergic pathway is fairly large with cell bodies in the arcuate nucleus and terminals in the median eminence. Some of the so-called amacrine cells of the retina appear to be dopaminergic.

Noradrenergic pathways in the CNS originate in several nuclei in the lower brain stem, e.g., the locus ceruleus, and terminate in practically all parts of the CNS, including the spinal cord. The ascending pathways form a dorsal bundle, with terminals for example, in the cortex and hippocampus, and a ventral bundle innervating for example, the hypothalamus and other parts of the brain stem.

Adrenaline-carrying pathways are sparse and less well known, with apparently strongest representation in the brain stem.

The 5-HT pathways originate in the lower brain stem with the cell bodies in the so-called raphe nuclei close to the midline. Ascending and descending pathways innervate practically all parts of the CNS.

D. Functional Aspects of the Monoaminergic Pathways

The occurrence of monoaminergic nerve terminals in practically all parts of the CNS indicates involvement in a great variety of functions. The global importance of these pathways is illustrated by the reserpine syndrome, where the general loss of monoamine stores results in profound changes in sensory and motor functions, intake of food and fluid, endocrine functions, temperature regulation, central control of the autonomic nervous system, etc. (CARLSSON, 1965).

The detailed analysis of the functions of the various monoaminergic pathways has proved to be a complicated task. Some pathways are, however, more readily accessible for research than others. For example, the descending spinal pathways have proved useful models for investigating noradrenaline and 5-HT neurotransmission. Both monoamines have been found to influence, inter alia, spinal motor reflexes. For dopaminergic mechanisms the nigrostriatal pathway has been much employed, utilizing the turning resulting from unilaterally induced changes in dopaminergic activity. With such models it has, for example, been possible to demonstrate that dopaminergic, noradrenergic, and serotoninergic receptors have different structural requirements. The noradrenergic (and adrenergic) receptors appear to be largely of α-type, even though the existence also of central β-adrenergic receptors appears probable (ANDÉN et al., 1966, 1969).

The approach utilized for investigating the various transmitters and pathways from the functional point of view is the classic one, i.e., the consequences of their removal (by surgical lesions or drug treatment), replacement or excessive activation (e.g., by treatment with precursors or receptor agonists) are investigated. Psychotropic drugs serve as important tools in these studies. Another important aspect is the correlation between behavioral and other functional changes with variations in the turnover of transmitters in different brain regions.

Among the more conspicuous functions of the monoamines, especially the catecholamines, in the CNS are stimulating actions on motility, alertness, exploratory behavior, and conditioned reactions, and thus presumably the acquirement and maintenance of intellectual functions (CARLSSON, 1972). The role of dopamine appears to be fundamental in the sense that complete dopamine deficiency appears to bring these functions down to an extremely low level. To be able to demonstrate any purposeful function, e.g., of noradrenaline, a certain dopaminergic activity thus often seems a prerequisite. For example, severe dopamine deficiency leads to Parkinson-like motor disturbance with, inter alia, almost complete akinesia. In this condition, an α-adrenergic noradrenaline receptor agonist, such as clonidine, is practically devoid of motility-inducing activity. However, if motility is stimulated beforehand with apomorphine, a dopamine-receptor agonist, a further stimulating action of clonidine on motility can be readily demonstrated (ANDÉN et al., 1973). A similar relationship between dopamine and noradrenaline probably exists in other connections, e.g., in the control of exploratory and conditioned behavior (ENGEL and CARLSSON, 1976). Although the role of 5-HT for motility, alertness, etc., is less obvious, it is clear that excessive stimulation of 5-HT receptors leads to central excitation, hypermotility, changes in muscle tone, and tremors (MODIGH, 1974).

Aggressive behavior and sexual activity appear to be stimulated by the catecholamines but inhibited by 5-HT. The pain threshold appears to be elevated by a central action of 5-HT (COSTA et al., 1974c). In general the monoamines appear to cause elevation of seizure thresholds, although the role of the individual monoamines in this regard has not been fully elucidated (KILIAN and FREY, 1973).

Central α-adrenergic mechanisms appear to play an important role for the control of cardiovascular functions. Several blood pressure-lowering drugs appear to act by activating α-adrenergic receptors in the lower brain stem, e.g., α-methyldopa, dopa, and clonidine (HENNING, 1975).

The monoamines probably take part in the control of the sleep-wakefulness rhythm although the specific role of the different monoamines is a controversial issue (COSTA et al., 1974b). This also applies to some extent to their participation in temperature regulation (MODIGH and SVENSSON, 1972). Excessive 5-HT receptor activation leads to hyperthermia, whereas activation of dopamine receptors appears to have the opposite effect (FUXE and SJÖQUIST, 1972).

The functional role of the various monoaminergic pathways will be further discussed in subsequent sections dealing with the different classes of psychotropic drugs.

E. The Various Steps in Monoaminergic Transmission as Targets for Psychotropic Drugs

I. Monoamine-Synthesizing Enzymes
(USDIN and SNYDER, 1973; COSTA et al., 1974a)

The first step in the synthesis of catecholamines is the conversion of tyrosine to dopa by means of tyrosine hydroxylase (Fig. 1). α-Methyltyrosine is a fairly specific inhibitor of this enzyme. It has a neuroleptic-like action on behavior which can be reversed by rather small doses of L-dopa (for further discussion see below Sect. G.).

The first step in the synthesis of 5-HT is the conversion of tryptophan to 5-hydroxytryptophan by means of tryptophan hydroxylase (Fig. 2). p-Chlorophenylalanine is a relatively specific inhibitor of this enzyme. In animal experiments it has been shown to stimulate aggressiveness, irritability (with a lowering of pain threshold), and sexual behavior. Similar actions have been reported in man but are not equally well documented. The effects observed in animals are reversed by 5-hydroxytryptophan and are therefore presumably due to 5-HT deficiency.

The transport of tyrosine and tryptophan from blood to brain mainly occurs by a saturable carrier-mediated mechanism shared by large neutral L-aminoacids, which can thus compete with each other for this transport. A high concentration of tyrosine in plasma may thus lead to a reduced level of tryptophan in brain, and vice versa. Since tryptophan hydroxylase is not fully saturated with its substrate tryptophan, a high level of tyrosine, phenylalanine, isoleucine, etc., may thus lead to a retardation of 5-HT synthesis. Tyrosine hydroxylase is more fully, though probably not completely saturated with tyrosine. It is probable that catecholamine synthesis in the brain can be influenced to some extent by the concentrations of amino acids competing with tyrosine for carrier sites. This mechanism may be relevant for understanding, e.g., the retarded intellectual development in phenylketonuria.

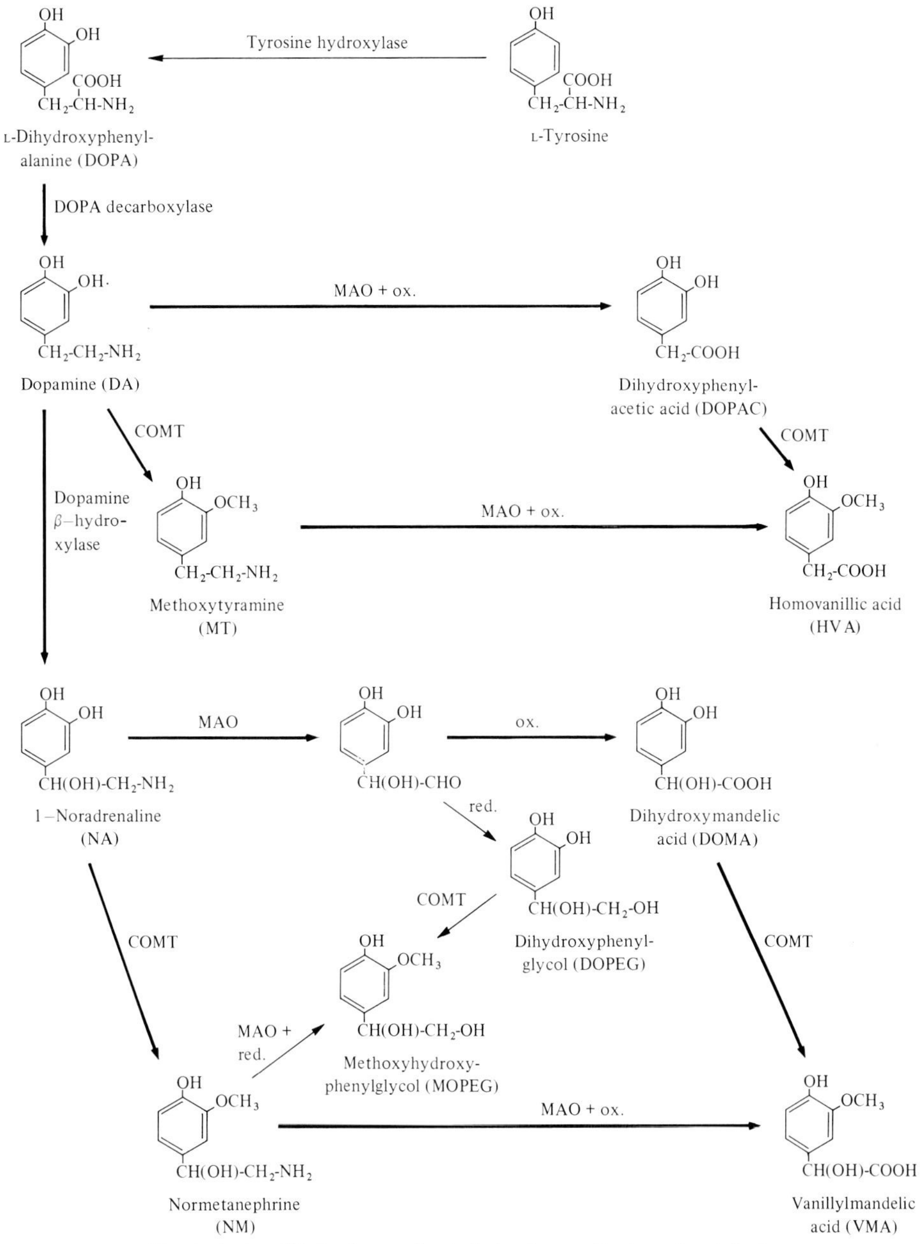

Fig. 1. A simplified scheme of catecholamine synthesis and metabolism

The second step in the synthesis of monoamines, i.e., the decarboxylation of dopa and 5-hydroxytryptophan to dopamine and 5-HT, respectively, by means of the aromatic L-amino acid decarboxylase, can be blocked by certain drugs. α-Methyldopa was once believed to act by inhibiting the decarboxylase, but its actions are probably mainly mediated by its decarboxylation products. Carbi-

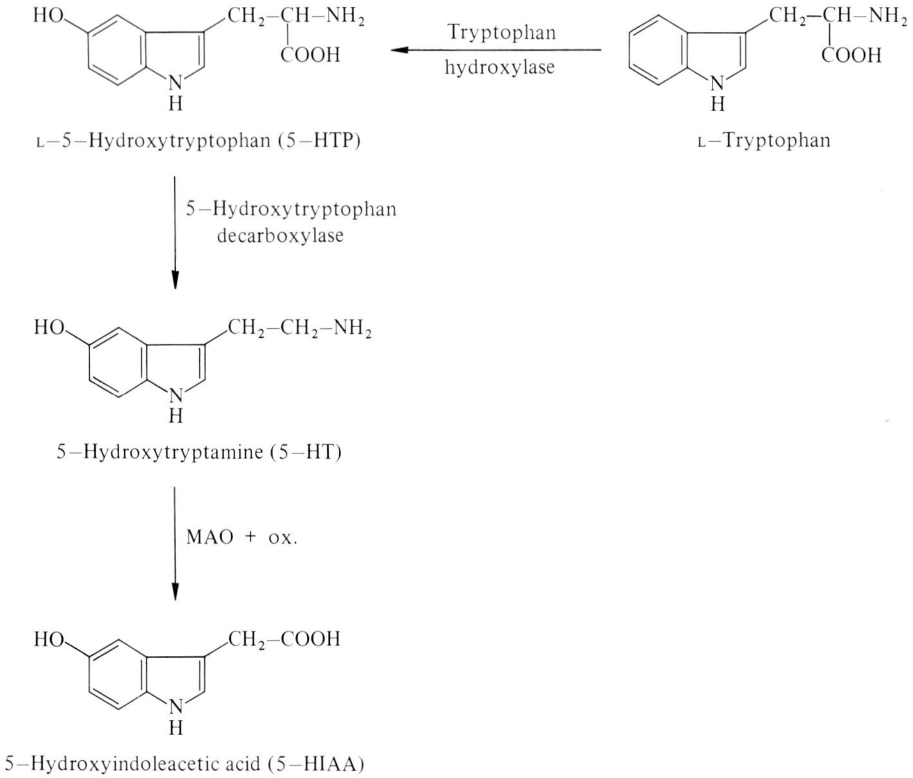

HO―[indole]―CH₂―CH(NH₂)―COOH ⟵ Tryptophan hydroxylase ⟵ [indole]―CH₂―CH(NH₂)―COOH

L-5-Hydroxytryptophan (5-HTP)   L-Tryptophan

↓ 5-Hydroxytryptophan decarboxylase

HO―[indole]―CH₂―CH₂―NH₂

5-Hydroxytryptamine (5-HT)

↓ MAO + ox.

HO―[indole]―CH₂―COOH

5-Hydroxyindoleacetic acid (5-HIAA)

Fig. 2. A simplified scheme of 5-hydroxytryptamine synthesis and metabolism

dopa (MK 486) and benserazid are decarboxylase inhibitors, which do not readily pass into the brain from the blood. They potentiate the central actions of L-dopa by blocking its decarboxylation in peripheral tissues and are used in combination with L-dopa for the treatment of Parkinsonism. In animal experiments centrally active decarboxylase inhibitors, particularly NSD 1015 (3-hydroxybenzylhydrazine), are used for measuring the first step in the synthesis of catecholamines and 5-HT. After inhibition of the enzyme dopa and 5-hydroxytryptophan accumulate in the brain, and the rate of accumulation can be taken as a measure of catecholamine and 5-HT synthesis, respectively (CARLSSON et al., 1972a).

Dopamine-β-hydroxylase catalyzes the conversion of dopamine to noradrenaline. This enzyme, in contrast to the other synthetic enzymes occurring in the cytoplasm, is located in the synaptic vesicles. Specific inhibitors are available but essentially for animal use. Disulfiram inhibits this enzyme, and this may play a role for some of its actions (GOODMAN and GILMAN, 1975).

II. Monoamine-Degrading Enzymes

Monoamine oxidase is the quantitatively most important degrading enzyme for the catecholamines (Fig. 1) and even more so for 5-HT (Fig. 2). Inhibitors of this enzyme cause accumulation of the monoamines, the consequences of which will be further discussed in a subsequent section.

Catechol-O-methyltransferase is the second enzyme involved in the degradation of catecholamines. In contrast to monoamine oxidase, which is mitochondrial and occurs, inter alia, within the monoamine-synthesizing neurons, catechol-O-methyltransferase appears to occur in the cytoplasm of the postsynaptic cells and perhaps also in glia cells, implying that the transmitter has to be released into the synaptic cleft and taken up by another cell in order to become available for degradation by this enzyme (JONASON, 1969). Inhibitors of this enzyme are used only in animal experiments.

III. Storage in the Synaptic Vesicles (CARLSSON, 1965)

To become available for release by the nerve impulse the newly synthesized transmitter must be taken up by the synaptic vesicles (Fig. 3), where it is incorporated together with adenosine triphosphate (ATP) and a protein called chromogranin. The uptake of transmitter by the vesicles is brought about by a specific ATP-dependent mechanism, which can be selectively blocked by low concentrations of reserpine and certain other drugs to be further discussed below.

IV. Release by the Nerve Impulse

The physiologic transmitter release by the nerve impulse is dependent on Ca^{2+} ions. The release is presumably preceded by a fusion between the vesicle and the plasma membranes and an increased permeability of the fused membrane, permitting release of the transmitter and the ATP with which it is stored. A varying proportion of stored material with higher molecular weight appears to be released along with the transmitter. In so far as all the intravesicular components are released in stoichiometric proportions, the release is said to occur by means of exocytosis (USDIN and SNYDER, 1973b). The amount of transmitter released per nerve impulse does not appear to be constant but is controlled, inter alia, by a feedback mechanism, involving a pre- or postsynaptic receptor. This problem will be further discussed below.

V. Re-Uptake

The final inactivation of transmitter occurs by enzymatic degradation, but this process is probably always preceded by uptake into one of the cells lining the synaptic gap. The most important or at least best-known uptake mechanism is the re-uptake by the presynaptic monoaminergic nerve terminal (Fig. 3). This uptake occurs by a specific ATP-dependent carrier mechanism with a high affinity to the transmitter. This mechanism is blocked, inter alia, by tricyclic antidepressant agents. Such blockade leads to an increased concentration or prolonged stay of transmitter in the synaptic cleft, which potentiates the action of the nerve impulse. This important mechanism will be further discussed under Sect. G.

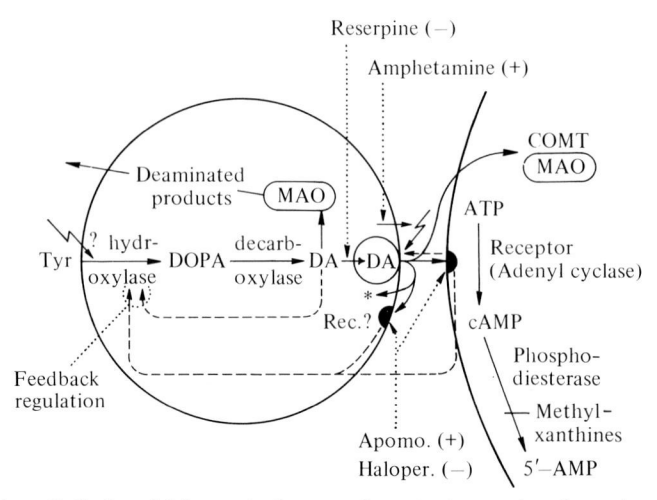

Fig. 3. A partly hypothetical model demonstrating some important events in a dopaminergic synapse. The *circle* to the *left* represents a dopaminergic nerve terminal which innervates the nerve cell to the *right*. In the nerve terminal tyrosine is enzymatically converted to dopamine (DA) via dopa. DA is taken up by synaptic vesicles (=granules) and will thus become available for release by the nerve impulse. After release DA activates postsynaptic dopaminergic receptors, intimately linked to adenyl cyclase, which is activated. The cyclic AMP thus formed induces a change in the postsynaptic cell membrane, presumably via activation of protein kinase. The cyclic AMP is degraded by phosphodiesterase, which can be inhibited, for example, by methylxanthines. The inactivation of DA, as of other monoamines, occurs partly by re-uptake, indicated by the *arrow close to the asterisk*. Degradation of DA can be performed by monoamine oxidase, part of which occurs within the monoaminergic neurons, or by catechol-O-methyltransferase (COMT), which is located in the postsynaptic neuron or an adjacent glia cell. The synthesis of DA is controlled by at least two different feedback mechanisms: end-product inhibition of tyrosine hydroxylase and a receptor-mediated mechanism. The dopaminergic receptors involved in this feedback regulation are probably located on the presynaptic cell membrane ("autoreceptors"). The sites of attack of four different types of psychotropic drugs are indicated: (1) *reserpine*, blocking the uptake of monoamines by synaptic vesicles; (2) *amphetamine*, causing release of catecholamine transmitters into the synaptic cleft; (3) *apomorphine*, causing activation; and (4) *haloperidol* causing blockade of dopaminergic receptors. Concerning blockade of re-uptake, the tricyclic antidepressants, e.g., imipramine, can inhibit this uptake in noradrenaline and 5-HT nerve terminals but is not active in dopaminergic nerve terminals

VI. Receptor Activation

In the synaptic gap the transmitter exerts its function by influencing specific postsynaptic receptors; their activation causes inhibition or excitation of the postsynaptic neuron. An increased activation of the receptors can be brought about in several different ways:

a. Release of transmitter by nerve impulse.
b. Administration of direct receptor agonists. The physiologic monoamines cannot penetrate readily through the blood-brain barrier but can be applied locally, e.g., by microiontophoresis. Certain synthetic substances can penetrate from the blood into the brain and activate monoaminergic receptors. For example, apomorphine is a directly acting dopamine-receptor agonist,

clonidine, an α-adrenergic agonist, and LSD-25, a serotoninergic receptor agonist.

c. Administration of a precursor, e.g., L-dopa, causing increased intraneuronal formation and overflow of dopamine into the synaptic cleft.
d. Reduced inactivation, e.g., through inhibition of monoamine oxidase or blockade of re-uptake.
e. Administration of drugs capable of releasing transmitter into the synaptic cleft. For example, amphetamine causes release of catecholamines, to be further discussed below.
f. For the sake of completeness, substances capable of stimulating the impulse generation in monoaminergic neurons should also be touched upon. As mentioned, substance P appears to have such an effect. Cholinergic drugs, e.g., the muscarinic receptor agonist oxotremorine, the cholinesterase inhibitor physostigmine, and thus probably also the endogenous agonist acetylcholine, appear to possess such activity. Apomorphine, and thus probably endogenous dopamine, appear to stimulate the impulse generation in noradrenaline and 5-HT neurons by activating dopamine receptors on these neurons or on interneurons. Diethyl ether, ethanol, and choral hydrate appear to stimulate impulse generation in catecholamine neurons through an indirect mechanism to be further discussed below.

The action of the transmitter on the receptor can be blocked by substances that bind to the receptor without activating it, so-called receptor antagonists. The clinically most important antipsychotic agents appear to act by blocking dopamine and to some extent also α-adrenergic noradrenaline receptors (see below). Selective 5-HT-receptor antagonists with strong influence on the central nervous system have not yet been discovered.

VII. The Secondary Messengers

The dopaminergic receptor, e.g., in the striatum, appears to be closely linked to the enzyme adenylate cyclase, which catalyzes the conversion of ATP to cyclic AMP. This process is activated by dopamine, and the action of dopamine can be blocked by dopamine-receptor antagonists (Fig. 3) (GREENGARD, 1975; ALMGREN et al., 1975; Section G). The cyclic AMP thus formed probably serves as a secondary messenger by activating a protein kinase in the cell membrane, leading to phosphorylation of a membrane protein. This in turn will lead to changes in ion permeability and membrane potential. In accordance with this hypothesis, inhibitors of the enzyme phosphodiesterase, e.g., caffeine, which catalyzes the degradation of cyclic AMP, have been shown to potentiate the behavioral actions of dopaminergic receptor agonists (WALDECK, 1975).

Cyclic AMP appears to serve as secondary messenger also in noradrenaline neurons.

F. Some Aspects of the Regulation of Monoaminergic Neuronal Activities

In classic physiology the nerve impulse flow is considered to be by far the most important variable in the physiologic activity of nerve cells. We now realize, however, that the amount of transmitter released per nerve impulse is variable and subject to regulation. The transmitter synthesis, too, is variable and is controlled not only by the impulse flow. Moreover, receptor sensitivity appears to be subject to regulation.

The physiologic activity of monoaminergic neurons is largely regulated by feedback mechanisms. The basic mechanism regulating the synthesis of catecholamines is probably a so-called end-product inhibition of tyrosine hydroxylase, leading to synthesis inhibition as the transmitter stores get filled. Through this mechanism the synthesis is increased when transmitter is released by nerve impulses. However, the nerve impulses can probably stimulate transmitter synthesis by some other, unknown influence on tyrosine hydroxylase. In 5-HT neurons a direct end-product inhibiton of transmitter synthesis does not seem to exist but, not withstanding, also here the transmitter synthesis is controlled to some extent by the nerve impulses (CARLSSON, 1976).

Another feedback mechanism, apparently operating independently of end-product inhibition, is mediated via the monoaminergic receptors (CARLSSON, 1975a). Thus, blockade of dopamine and noradrenaline (α-adrenergic) receptors by phenothiazines, clozapine, or other neuroleptics induce an increased impulse generation and an increased release, metabolism and synthesis of dopamine and noradrenaline. Conversely, dopamine-receptor agonists have an inhibitory influence on these mechanisms in dopaminergic neurons. This receptor-mediated feedback occurs in dopamine and noradrenaline as well as 5-HT neurons.

In part the receptor-mediated feedback is regulated via neuronal loops feeding the information back to the cell bodies or dendrites where the impulses are generated. However, feedback can also occur via local mechanisms confined to the nerve-terminal area and still operating after the nerve impulse flow is interrupted by cutting the axons. The receptors involved in the local feedback do not seem to be identical with the classic postsynaptic receptors, because the sensitivity of the two sets of receptors to agonists, for example, do not seem to be identical. Apomorphine is capable of inhibiting dopamine synthesis in doses 10–100 times lower than those required for classic postsynaptic receptor activation, as indicated by the typical signs of excitation with stereotypies, etc. In fact, these very low apomorphine doses cause inhibition of motility. The simplest explanation of these various observations is that the dopamine neurons possess receptors sensitive to their own transmitter, dopamine. Direct support for this view has been obtained by the demonstration of dopaminergic receptors on nigral dopaminergic cell bodies. Activation of these receptors by means of dopamine or apomorphine causes a prompt and pronounced inhibition of impulse generation. The dose of apomorphine required for this inhibition of firing is very low and comparable to that causing inhibition of dopamine synthesis and motility, as described above. The effect can be blocked by receptor antagonists such as chlorpromazine and haloperidol. Analogous observations on other neuronal systems indicate that similar conditions prevail in other monoaminergic systems (USDIN and SNYDER, 1973b). The receptors involved in this local feedback are often called presynaptic, but this may give rise to confusion if they are partly located on dopaminergic cell bodies, where they appear to be neither pre- nor postsynaptic: no dopaminergic innervation of nigral dopaminergic cells appears to exist. For this reason the term "autoreceptors" has been suggested to emphasize the basic feature, i.e., sensitivity to the neuron's own transmitter.

The autoreceptor theory should still be considered a working hypothesis, justified by permitting the explanation of some otherwise obscure, paradoxical phenomena, e.g., the increased dopamine synthesis in nerve terminals following axotomy or drug-induced inhibition of impulse generation by dopaminergic cell bodies (by treatment with, for example, γ-hydroxybutyric acid). The most interesting aspect of this theory is the possible preferential activation or blockade of these receptors, which would lead to actions opposite to those expected by a receptor agonist or antagonist. As mentioned previously, there is already some evidence supporting the view that low doses of apomorphine cause preferential activation of dopaminergic autoreceptors. Moreover, there are clinical reports on paradoxical actions of apomorphine, e.g., a sedative antipsychotic and antidelirious action, inhibition of choreatic phenomena, for example, in tardive dyskinesia and Gilles de la Tourette's disease, reduced craving for alcohol and other euphoriants. Extending this line of thought to other receptors, it cannot be excluded that the small doses required for inducing hallucinations by LSD-25 act by preferentially activating 5-HT autoreceptors and thus inhibiting 5-HT neurons. Also the α-adrenergic receptor agonist clonidine lowers blood pressure by preferential activation of α-adrenergic autoreceptors, leading to inhibition of noradrenaline and adrenaline neurons, for example, in the lower brain stem. It is obvious that the possible existence of autoreceptors and their preferential activation will complicate the analysis of drug actions, while at the same time opening up interesting new perspectives.

G. Antipsychotic or Neuroleptic Agents

I. Introduction

The term "neuroleptic" was coined by DELAY and DENIKER (1957) to emphasize the similar pharmacologic profile of two drugs with entirely different chemical structure, i.e., chlorpromazine and reserpine, and to distinguish these drugs from general depressants such as the classic sedative-hypnotics. Especially prominent features are: a state of affective indifference with depression of vigilance and initiative; a decrease in locomotor, especially exploratory activity and inhibition of conditioned behavior in animals; alleviation of excitation, agitation, and aggressiveness; a true antipsychotic action observed in patients with acute as well as chronic psychoses, e.g., schizophrenia and mania. These effects are obtained without any clouding of consciousness or impairment of intellectual functions, and larger doses do not cause ataxia or anesthesia as occurs after treatment with barbiturates. On the other hand, motor disturbances are produced by the neuroleptic agents, with Parkinsonian and other extrapyramidal symptoms, including the catalepsia observed in animals. Neurovegetative, e.g., antiemetic and endocrine, effects, especially galactorrhea due to increased secretion of prolactin, are also characteristic features.

II. Reserpine

Soon after the discovery of the first neuroleptic agents reserpine was shown to cause depletion of monoamine stores in brain as well as in other tissues. Interest was first focused on 5-HT and later on noradrenaline. However, the picture changed after the discovery of dopamine in the brain, with high levels in the basal ganglia, the depletion of dopamine by reserpine, and the antireserpine action of dopa, evidently related to the accumulation of dopamine in the brain (CARLSSON, 1965). More recently it has become possible to protect the stores of individual monoamines selectively against the action of reserpine (CARLSSON, 1975b). These observations indicate that the catecholamines, notably dopamine, are responsible for the most important features of the reserpine syndrome, even though 5-HT appears to play a contributory role.

The use of drugs as tools for elucidating biologic mechanisms is hampered by the limited specificity of drug actions in general. Admittedly the only primary action of reserpine established so far is that on the monoamine storage mechanism, but we cannot disregard the great variety of biochemical and functional changes induced by reserpine. There are different approaches to the specificity problem. One is to interfere with the effect on the monoamines in various ways and look for a correlation between biochemical and functional changes. This has been done in extensive studies, and the outcome has invariably been in favor of a causative role of monoamine depletion. Another approach is to investigate drugs having a pharmacologic profile similar to that of reserpine although differing in chemical structure. One example is tetrabenazine and a number of other benzoquinolizines, which have been found to deplete monoamines by blocking the storage mechanism reversibly, in contrast to the irreversible action of reserpine and its congeners on this mechanism.

On the basis of the data thus accumulated it is safe to conclude that the major pharmacologic actions of reserpine and its congeners are due to monoamine depletion. Moreover, the data indicate that catecholamines, notably dopamine, play a more important role than 5-HT for the gross behavioral syndrome induced by reserpine (CARLSSON, 1974).

III. Neuroleptics Not Depleting Monoamine Stores

1. Historical Note

Despite the similarity in pharmacologic profile, chlorpromazine, haloperidol, and their congeners differ from reserpine in causing little or no depletion of monoamines. Doubt was thus expressed as to the role of monoamines in neuroleptic action in general (JARVIK, 1965). During the last two decades numerous hypotheses have been advanced seeking to explain this action. During the last decade considerable evidence has accumulated, showing that the common denominator of those neuroleptics that do not deplete the monoamine stores is blockade of dopamine receptors. Many of the most frequently used neuroleptics are capable of blocking also α-adrenergic receptors, but this action does not appear to be a prerequisite for neuroleptic activity, even though it may play a contributory role. This concept of receptor blockade goes back to 1963 when CARLSSON and LINDQVIST described a specific action of chlorpromazine and haloperidol on catecholamine metabolism. These authors observed that low doses of chlorpromazine and haloperidol but not promethazine stimulated the accumulation of the O-methylated basic metabolites of dopamine and noradrenaline following monoamine oxidase inhibition. Since the catecholamine levels were uninfluenced by the neuroleptics, it was inferred that not only the metabolism but also the synthesis of the catecholamines was accelerated by the neuroleptic agents. It was known at this time that the awakening action of dopamine and noradrenaline (administered via their precursor dopa) was weakened by chlorpromazine and haloperidol, in contrast to reserpine, and thus the hypothesis was advanced that the former two neuroleptics act by blocking dopamine and noradrenaline receptors. The acceleration of the synthesis and metabolism of these agents was suggested to be due to feedback activation of the respective catecholamine-carrying neurons, ensuing upon the receptor blockade. This hypothesis has later been extensively investigated by means of a great variety of techniques and approaches and has received considerable support.

2. Dopamine-Receptor Blockade: Functional Evidence

As previously mentioned, the functional effects of dopamine (administered locally, systemically via the precursor dopa, or released into the synaptic cleft, e.g., by amphetamine) or other dopamine-receptor agonists, e.g., apomorphine, are antagonized by neuroleptic agents in a dose-dependent manner (ANDÉN, 1973; ANDÉN et al., 1970; JACKSON et al., 1975; PIJNENBURG et al., 1973). A rough correlation between the antagonistic effect and clinical antipsychotic potency is evident. The clinical significance of the experimental data is emphasized by studies in which inadequate behavior in a discrimination test has been produced in rats by excessive stimulation of dopamine receptors, by means of L-dopa, amphetamine, or apomorphine: the behavior could be normalized by neuroleptics, such as haloperidol or pimozide. Interestingly, the doses required for restoring essentially normal behavior caused severe inhibition of behavior when given alone, thus illustrating the competition between dopaminergic agonists and antagonists for receptor sites (AHLENIUS and ENGEL, 1975).

It may be recalled that psychotic patients, according to general clinical experience, tolerate higher doses of neuroleptic agents than nonpsychotic individuals, a fact suggesting that their dopaminergic receptor activity was elevated.

Microiontophoretic ejection of dopamine or apomorphine has a powerful inhibitory effect on the firing of identified dopaminergic cells in the lower brain stem, whereas α- and β-adrenergic receptor agonists are inactive. The inhibition is associated with an increase in the amplitude of action potentials recorded extracellularly, indicating a hyperpolarization of the neuronal membrane potential (AGHAJANIAN and BUNNEY, 1973; BUNNEY et al., 1973). The effect can be blocked by neuroleptic drugs applied microiontophoretically or systemically, but not by α- or β-adrenergic receptor antagonists (AGHAJANIAN and BUNNEY, 1974).

These observations indicate the presence of dopaminergic receptors on dopaminergic cells ("autoreceptors," see above). When given systemically most neuroleptics appear capable of stimulating the firing of dopaminergic cells.

3. Dopamine-Receptor Blockade: Biochemical Evidence

All neuroleptics investigated have been found to stimulate the synthesis and turnover of dopamine (ANDÉN et al., 1970; ANDÉN et al., 1972a; ANDÉN et al., 1964; CARLSSON and LINDQVIST, 1963, 1978a; DA PRADA and PLETSCHER, 1966; HYTTEL, 1974; NYBÄCK and SEDVALL, 1970; O'KEEFE et al., 1970; SEDVALL and NYBÄCK, 1972; STILLE and LAUENER, 1971). Also the release of dopamine is enhanced (BARTHOLINI et al., 1976b). The doses required for this effect are similar to those used in the functional studies referred to above. In fact, a close correlation ($r = 0.96$) has been found between the stimulating action of neuroleptics on dopamine synthesis in the striatum and their apomorphine-antagonistic action in the rat. Moreover, the ED 50s for the two actions were approximately the same, suggesting similar affinity of the receptors involved in the two actions. When stimulation of dopamine synthesis was compared with inhibition of food-reinforced lever pressing, the threshold doses of most neuroleptics were again similar. In the latter comparison, however, clozapine seemed to be an exception in having a clearly lower threshold dose for inhibition of lever pressing (for review and references, CARLSSON, 1977a). An effect so far unidentified may thus contribute to the neuroleptic action of clozapine (a strong α-adrenergic blockade (?), see below).

4. The Possible Role of α-Adrenoceptor Blockade

Chlorpromazine and several other neuroleptics are fairly potent α-adrenoceptor-blocking agents and appear to exert such an action also centrally (ANDÉN, 1976; ANDÉN et al., 1970). These neuroleptics stimulate noradrenaline synthesis and turnover in the brain, presumably via a receptor-mediated feedback mechanism (ANDÉN et al., 1970; CARLSSON and LINDQVIST, 1963, unpublished data; HYTTEL, 1974; NYBÄCK and SEDVALL, 1970). However, the correlation between neuroleptic activity and the effects on noradrenaline functions and turnover is poor. In fact, certain neuroleptics appear to lack α-adrenoceptor-blocking activity. Conversely, phenoxybenzamine, a centrally active α-adrenoceptor-blocking agent, appears to lack antipsychotic activity. It would thus appear that α-adrenergic blockade is not essential for the antipsychotic action. It has been suggested that the "unspecific" sedative component of neuroleptics is related to α-adrenergic blockade (NYBÄCK and SEDVALL, 1970). Such blockade may, however, play a contributory role for the antipsychotic action, too.

5. Regional Aspects: Striatal vs Limbic Dopamine

Schematically, we can distinguish three main dopamine-carrying neuronal pathways in the brain: the nigrostriatal, the mesolimbic, and the tuberoinfundibular pathway, the latter originating in the arcuate nucleus and terminating in the median eminence (UNGERSTEDT, 1971; see Sect. C). Similarly, we can distinguish three main components in the classic neuroleptic profile: the extrapyramidal, the antipsychotic, and the endocrine actions. These actions can be clearly separated from each other. It is a well-established clinical fact that anticholinergic agents efficiently antagonize the extrapyramidal actions while leaving the antipsychotic action more or less unchanged. Similarly, in experimental animals catalepsy is very efficiently antagonized by anticholinergics. Moreover, neuroleptics differ greatly in the ratio of extrapyramidal (and cataleptic) to antipsychotic activity. It is thus reasonable to assume that the two actions reside in different structures, i.e., the extrapyramidal effects in the striatum and the antipsychotic action in the limbic structures. In support of this, ANDÉN (1972) observed a differential action of anticholinergics in combination with neuroleptics on dopamine turnover in the two structures. Similarly, ANDÉN and STOCK (1973) found a stronger effect of clozapine on dopamine turnover in the limbic area than in the striatum when using haloperidol as a reference drug. Clozapine as compared to, for example, haloperidol is known to produce little or no extrapyramidal side effects (or catalepsy in animals) in doses which are equipotent with respect to antipsychotic activity. Several investigators have obtained results supporting a relationship between neuroleptics' liability to cause extrapyramidal side effects and their relative efficacy on striatal vs limbic dopamine turnover (BARTHOLINI et al., 1975; BARTHOLINI et al., 1976; STAWARZ et al., 1975; ZIVKOVIC et al., 1975).

Table 1 shows the effect of 11 neuroleptics and two other compounds (promethazine and phenoxybenzamine) on the formation of dopa in two dopamine-

Table 1. Effect of neuroleptics on catecholamine synthesis in rat brain regions[a]

	Maximal increase (%)			ED 50 (mg/kg)		
	Striatum	Limbic	Hemispheres	Striatum	Limbic	Hemispheres
Chlorpromazine	194	94	20	0.58	0.60	[c]
Thioridazine	146	90	45	2.46	2.53	3.00
Perphenazine	170	100	27	0.03	0.03	[c]
Promethazine	20[b]	< 10[b]	< 20[b]	[c]	[c]	[c]
Haloperidol	206	114	47	0.07	0.07	0.42
Spiroperidol	200	114	0	0.02	0.02	–
Pimozide	330	190	24	0.23	0.29	[c]
Clozapine	192	154	100	14.1	13.2	19.0
Chlorprothixene	140	80	19[b]	0.95	0.75	[c]
Clopenthixol	236	166	56	0.19	0.13	0.20
Sulpiride	130	95	85	21	20	[c]
Metoclopramide	190	120	21	2.8	2.8	[c]
Reserpine	200	125	150	0.2	0.2	0.1
Phenoxybenzamine	< 20[b,d]	30[d]	20	[c]	[c]	[c]

[a] Catecholamine synthesis was determined by measuring the rate of dopa accumulation induced within 30 min by an inhibitor of the aromatic L-amino acid decarboxylase (NSD 1015 = 3-hydroxybenzylhydrazine HCl, 100 mg/kg i.p.). The neuroleptics were injected 1 h before NSD 1015. Shown are the maximal percentage increases in dopa formation above control values obtained after vehicle plus NSD 1015, and the doses necessary for half-maximal increase (ED 50). The values obtained from striatum and limbic forebrain indicate effects on dopamine synthesis, and those from hemispheres on noradrenaline synthesis (unpublished data from Carlsson and Lindqvist)
[b] Not significant
[c] Data do not allow estimation of ED 50
[d] Maximal decrease

predominated brain areas, i.e., the striatum and the dopamine-rich limbic areas, and in the remaining part of the cerebral hemispheres, in which noradrenaline is the predominating catecholamine. The maximal increase in dopa formation and the ED 50s were derived from dose-response curves. It can be seen that all the neuroleptics, in contrast to the two non-neuroleptic agents, caused a marked increase in dopa formation in the dopamine-rich parts, indicating an increase in dopamine synthesis. However, the neuroleptics differed markedly with respect to ED 50 and maximal increase. The correlation of ED 50s for increase in dopa formation to ED 50s for apomorphine antagonism has already been mentioned (see above).

For most compounds the maximal increase in striatal dopa was approximately 200%. Pimozide showed a higher (333%) and thioridazine, chlorprothixene, and sulpiride, a lower (about 140%) increase. The low efficacy of thioridazine in increasing dopamine metabolite levels has been pointed out earlier (BÜRKI et al., 1975). For each agent the dopa formation was lower in the limbic areas than in the striatum. However, the ratio of striatal to limbic dopa varied among the neuroleptics and was lowest, i.e., 1.2, for clozapine as compared to about 1.8 for the majority of the other agents. Thus, the four neuroleptics known to have a low incidence of extrapyramidal side effects differed from the others in causing a low increase in striatal dopa formation, expressed in maximal percentage increase (thioridazine, chlorprothixene, and sulpiride) or as ratio of striatum to limbic system (clozapine). These results are thus in line with those quoted above. It should be pointed out, however, that ED 50s for the increase were approximately the same in the striatum as in the limbic areas for each compound, suggesting similar affinity to the dopaminergic receptors of the two areas. The regional differences in percentage increase are thus probably not due to different receptor affinities. Theoretically, the low maximal increases caused, e.g., by thioridazine and chlorprothixene, might be due to low intrinsic activity, i.e., mixed agonist-antagonist properties, of these agents. Alternatively and perhaps more likely, the feedback response to receptor blockade could be modified, owing to other actions of the neuroleptics, e.g., blockade of other receptors, such as muscarinic and α-adrenergic receptors.

Table 1 also shows the increase in dopa formation in the noradrenaline-predominated hemisphere portion. In general this increase was slight, if at all present, and generally did not exceed 50%. Clozapine was exceptional in causing a 100% increase. This is in line with other observations indicating a strong α-adrenergic blocking action of this compound (ANDÉN, 1976; HYTTEL, 1974). In cases where ED 50s could be estimated they tended to be higher than in the dopamine-rich regions. The difference was especially striking for haloperidol with ED 50s that were 0.42 and 0.07 mg/kg for the noradrenaline and dopamine regions, respectively. Reserpine differed from the other neuroleptics in causing a strong increase, 150%, in dopa formation in the noradrenaline-predominated region, and having a lower ED 50 (0.1 mg/kg) in this region than in the dopamine-rich areas (0.2 mg/kg). These reserpine data suggest that feedback activation can be quite strong also in noradrenaline neurons. The slight response to treatment with receptor-blocking neuroleptics observed in these neurons may therefore be due to poor α-adrenergic receptor blockade. However, also phenoxybenzamine, which is generally recognized as a potent α-adrenergic blocking agent capable of penetrating into the brain, caused only a moderate increase in dopa formation in the noradrenaline area. This agent may not be quite specific, since it caused a significant decrease in dopa formation in the limbic areas.

In conclusion, the available evidence suggests that the low liability to extrapyramidal side effects, which is characteristic for certain neuroleptics such as clozapine and thioridazine, is not due to differential affinities of striatal vs limbic dopamine receptors, but rather to some other factors that modify the consequences of dopamine-receptor blockade in the striatum and in the limbic forebrain. Factors possibly involved here are blockade of muscarinic or α-adrenergic receptors, differentially mixed dopaminergic agonist-antagonist properties, etc.

6. The Possible Role of Dopaminergic Autoreceptors

Receptor-mediated feedback activation of dopaminergic neurons might be brought about by a neuronal loop, feeding back the information from the postsynaptic neurons to the presynaptic (dopaminergic) cell bodies or dendrites. Lesion experiments supporting the existence of such a loop have been reported (BUNNEY and AGHAJANIAN, 1976). However, the problem is complicated by the existence of dopamine receptors on the dopaminergic neuron itself, so-called autoreceptors (see Sect. F). As mentioned, microiontophoretic application of dopamine or apomorphine on dopaminergic cell bodies inhibits their firing, and this effect can be blocked by a neuroleptic (AGHAJANIAN and BUNNEY, 1977). Moreover, the inhibitory effect of systemically administered apomorphine on dopamine synthesis in dopaminergic nerve terminals persists after cutting the dopaminergic axons, thus disconnecting the neuronal feedback loop. This inhibitory effect of a dopaminergic agonist on transmitter synthesis can be blocked by a neuroleptic agent (KEHR et al., 1972, 1977).

Apparently dopaminergic autoreceptors are located on various parts of the neuron. It seems possible to activate autoreceptors preferentially, e.g., by low doses of apomorphine, leading to a paradoxical inhibition of motility which can be blocked by a neuroleptic agent (STRÖMBOM, 1977). Low doses of certain neuroleptics are known to cause stimulatory phenomena, which can be recorded experimentally (AHLENIUS and ENGEL, 1971a). The possibility must be considered that neuroleptics may differ in their relative activities on pre- versus postsynaptic receptors, and that such differences may influence their pharmacologic profiles. Evidence in favor of such an assumption has been reported (WALTERS and ROTH, 1976).

Long dopaminergic dendrites projecting from the pars compacta to the pars reticulata of the substantia nigra have been described (BJÖRKLUND and LINDVALL, 1975). The possibility exists that these dendrites take synaptic contact with other dopaminergic or nondopaminergic dendrites. Such synapses might inter alia be involved in receptor-mediated feedback regulation and in the presynaptic actions of neuroleptic agents (GROVES et al., 1975). From a clinical viewpoint liability to extrapyramidal side effects, including tardive dyskinesia, may be related to relative receptor affinities in these various locations.

Inhibition of dopamine synthesis by dopamine-receptor agonists and reversal of this effect by neuroleptics have been demonstrated on synaptosomes in vitro. Presumably this action is mediated via autoreceptors (CHRISTIANSEN and SQUIRES, 1974; GOLDSTEIN et al., 1973; IVERSEN et al., 1976).

7. Effect on Dopamine-Sensitive Adenylate Cyclase

As previously mentioned, GREENGARD and his colleagues (GREENGARD, 1975; KEBABIAN and GREENGARD, 1971) have discovered a dopamine-sensitive adenylate cyclase in homogenates of caudate nucleus and limbic forebrain. The apparently specific stimulatory action of dopamine or apomorphine on this enzyme is specifically antagonized by neuroleptic agents, and a certain correlation seems to exist between the inhibitory activities on the enzyme and those on dopaminergic receptors as assessed in vivo (CLEMENT-CORMIER et al., 1974; MILLER et al., 1974). However, the butyrophenones showed lower enzyme inhibition than expected. These results are extremely interesting and may ultimately lead to the demonstration of the primary molecular changes underlying neuroleptic action.

8. In-Vitro Studies on Dopamine Binding and Release

SNYDER et al. (CREESE et al., 1976; SNYDER et al., 1976) have investigated the ability of various neuroleptics to displace [^{3}H]-dopamine and [^{3}H]-haloperidol from the binding sites of membranes from the corpus striatum and dopamine-rich structures in the limbic forebrain. The affinities of various neuroleptics to these binding sites were expressed as K_i and were found to correlate closely with ED 50s for antagonism of apomorphine stereotypies and with average daily clinical dosage. [^{3}H]-Haloperidol displacement showed a better correlation than [^{3}H]-dopamine displacement. Differences between the two sets of displacement data were suggested to be due to the occurrence of binding sites in two different states with preferential affinity for agonists and antagonists, respectively. Similar observations have been reported by SEEMAN et al. (1976).

SEEMAN and LEE (1975) also reported a close correlation between clinical potency and in-vitro data, though this time the latter referred to neuroleptic-induced inhibition of electrically stimulated release of [^{3}H]-dopamine from rat striatal slices. These observations are somewhat confusing, because (a) earlier experiments with the same technique had shown the opposite effect, i.e., enhancement of [^{3}H]-dopamine release by neuroleptics (FARNEBO and HAMBERGER, 1971), and (b) in-vivo data likewise show enhancement of [^{3}H]-dopamine release from brain, as revealed by push-pull cannula technique (BARTHOLINI et al., 1976a). The latter results are of course in line with an overwhelming amount of experimental evidence, briefly referred to above, indicating that neuroleptics stimulate the firing and the transmitter release, metabolism, and synthesis in dopaminergic neurons. Subsequent studies of SEEMAN and his colleagues (1976) showed that the concentrations of neuroleptics required for inhibition of dopamine release are higher than those required for displacement of [^{3}H]-dopamine from receptor sites.

9. Pharmacokinetic Aspects of Dopamine-Receptor Blockade

Against the background of the in-vitro data quoted above, the question may be raised whether it is possible to obtain an estimate of K_i on the basis of in-vivo data. This would have to involve certain assumptions, because the concentration of a neuroleptic in the water phase in contact with the receptor site cannot be measured. However, since we are dealing with lipid-soluble compounds that seem to permeate easily through biologic membranes, the assumption may be justified that this concentration is not far from that of the cerebrospinal fluid or the plasma ultrafiltrate, if time is allowed for equilibration. Many neuroleptics have a complex metabolism with several active metabolites, which of course complicates the matter considerably. Moreover, accurate pharmacokinetic data are sparse for many neuroleptics. Haloperidol does not seem to have any active metabolites. Recently a sufficiently sensitive method for determination of haloperidol in plasma has been developed, and some data on its pharmacokinetics are available (FORSMAN et al., 1974). In psychotic patients treated with 6 mg haloperidol daily a median total plasma level of 13 nM was recorded. With a protein binding of 8% (FORSMAN and ÖHMAN, 1977) the concentration of free haloperidol would thus be 1 nM. How far is this concentration from the K_i? We know that haloperidol in clinical dosage (6 mg daily) causes a considerable increase in the homovanillic acid level of the cerebrospinal fluid (240%) (SEDVALL et al., 1975). This increase is comparable to the maximal increase seen in haloperidol-treated rats (see above), suggesting that if anything the concentration at clinical dosage should be above IC 50. This assumption is supported by data from rats showing that at ED 50 plasma levels of similar magnitude are obtained (ÖHMAN et al., 1977). It therefore seems reasonable to conclude that K_i for haloperidol is probably not larger than 1 nM but possibly lower.

Table 2. Various in vitro activities of haloperidol and thioridazine as compared to steady-state total and free plasma levels in patients

	Haloperidol (nM)	Thioridazine (nM)
^{3}H dopamine binding, K_i	650[a]	1780[b]
^{3}H haloperidol binding, K_i	1.5[a]	14[b]
Adenylate cyclase activity, K_i	118[c]	36[c]
Inhibition of ^{3}H dopamine release, IC$_{50}$	90[d]	800[d]
Phrenic nerve block, IC$_{50}$	125[g]	152[g]
Plasma level, total	13[e]	2000[f]
Plasma level, free	1[e]	4[f]

[a] SNYDER et al. (1976)
[b] CREESE et al. (1976)
[c] CLEMENT-CORMIER et al. (1974)
[d] SEEMAN and LEE (1975)
[e] FORSMAN and ÖHMAN (1977); FORSMAN et al. (1974)
[f] NYBERG et al., (1979)
[g] SEEMAN et al. (1974)

Table 2 shows the K_is for haloperidol obtained in binding studies using [^{3}H]-dopamine and [^{3}H]-haloperidol and in measurements of adenylate cyclase activity, as compared to the plasma levels. It can be seen that all the K_is are higher than the level of free haloperidol in plasma. The closest K_i is that for [^{3}H]-haloperidol binding, which is only slightly higher than the plasma level. In the other cases the values differ by about two orders of magnitude. The corresponding data have been compiled for thioridazine, likewise shown in Table 2. In this case similar discrepancies are found. Thioridazine has active metabolites, but they do not seem to contribute greatly to the overall effect (AXELSSON, 1977). Several factors can account for the discrepancies:

1. The time allowed for equilibration is longer under in-vivo conditions, which may yield a lower K_i.
2. Active transport occurring in vivo but not, or less so, in vitro cannot be disregarded. The concentration of haloperidol in brain is much higher than in plasma and appears to be closely correlated to the pharmacologic actions (ÖHMAN et al., 1977). However, this high level may be due to high lipid solubility and binding and may thus not necessarily influence the level of haloperidol in the water phase of the brain.
3. The receptors occur in different states or have changed during the preparation of the homogenates, resulting in lower affinities.
4. The binding sites studied under the different experimental conditions are not identical and represent the true receptors only in part.

Further investigation is needed to settle these very interesting problems.

IV. Neuroleptic Properties of α-Methyltyrosine

In animals α-methyltyrosine, a rather potent and specific inhibitor of tyrosine hydroxylase, has many properties similar to those of a neuroleptic agent (CORRODI and HANSSON, 1966). However, its efficacy appears to be limited by the nephrotoxicity observed in larger doses. In schizophrenic patients no antipsychotic activity could be demonstrated (GERSHON et al., 1967).

During treatment with neuroleptics, the feedback activation of dopaminergic neurons, resulting from the dopamine receptor blockade, should serve to counteract the neuroleptic effects, at least if the dose of the neuroleptic agent is moderate and its action surmountable. If this asssumption is correct, it should be possible to demonstrate potentiation of neuroleptics by α-methyltyrosine. Such potentiation has indeed been shown in experimental animals (AHLENIUS and ENGEL, 1971b).

The failures of α-methyltyrosine to potentiate an α-adrenergic blocking agent and of a dopamine-β-hydroxylase inhibitor to potentiate neuroleptics support the view that dopamine is predominantly involved in this potentiation (AHLENIUS and ENGEL, 1977). In chronic schizophrenic patients α-methyltyrosine has been found to potentiate the antipsychotic action of subthreshold doses of neuroleptic agents (WÅLINDER et al., 1976a). Also the extrapyramidal actions are potentiated (WÅLINDER and CARLSSON, 1973).

The failure of α-methyltyrosine as an antipsychotic agent per se may be explained by its nephrotoxic action, which prevents the drug from being used in sufficiently high dosage. The ability of nontoxic doses of α-methyltyrosine to potentiate the antipsychotic action of neuroleptic agents provides additional support for a role of the catecholamines, especially dopamine, in the pathogenesis of, e.g., schizophrenic psychosis.

V. Effects of Neuroleptics on Noncatecholaminergic Systems

1. 5-HT

As mentioned above, the pharmacologic profile of reserpine is probably to a certain extent due to 5-HT depletion, even if the role of catecholamine depletion predominates. Receptor-blocking neuroleptics are generally not very effective in counteracting central effects of 5-HT induced, e.g., via 5-hydroxytryptophan administration (ANDÉN, 1971). Likewise, many of them fail to influence 5-HT turnover. In the study on the effect of neuroleptic agents on monoamine synthesis referred to above we found only a few compounds having a clear-cut effect – inhibition or stimulation – on 5-hydroxytryptophan formation. For example, chlorprothixene caused inhibition of synthesis. Such an effect is seen after antidepressant agents, e.g., chlorimipramine, presumably owing to feedback adjustment resulting from blockade of 5-HT re-uptake (CARLSSON, 1977). However, no such effect of chlorprothixene has been reported (FELGER, 1965). The action of chlorprothixene and other neuroleptics on 5-HT synthesis and turnover warrants further investigation.

2. Acetylcholine

Neuroleptic agents have been found to stimulate the turnover and release of acetylcholine in the caudate nucleus (LADINSKY et al., 1975; McGEER et al., 1974; SETHY and VAN WOERT, 1974; STADLER et al., 1973; TRABUCCHI et al., 1975). Presumably, the short cholinergic neurons in the striatum are under inhibitory dopaminergic control, which is released by dopamine-receptor blockade. In a dopamine-rich limbic area this effect was not seen, indicating a stronger dopaminergic control on cholinergic neurons in the striatum than in limbic areas (BARTHOLINI et al., 1975). These observations are interesting in view of the fact that extrapyramidal side effects of neuroleptics, in contrast to their antipsychotic action, are efficiently counteracted by anticholinergic agents. Similarly, feedback-induced stimulation of dopamine metabolism is counteracted by anticholinergics more efficiently in the striatum than in the limbic areas (see above).

It is still an open question to what extent the scarcity of extrapyramidal side effects of neuroleptic agents such as clozapine and thioridazine can be accounted for by anticholinergic activity (BARTHOLINI et al., 1975; MELTZER and STAHL, 1976).

It should be pointed out that cholinergic mechanisms may influence dopamine neurons at several levels (JAVOY et al., 1974).

3. GABA

A striatonigral GABA pathway has been described, which presumably constitutes an important part of a feedback loop (OKADA, 1976). Local application of GABA on nigral dopaminergic neurons causes inhibition of firing which in contrast to the action of dopamine persists after pretreatment with a neuroleptic agent (AGHAJANIAN and BUNNEY, 1977). The inhibition is accompanied by the appropriate biochemical changes (ANDÉN and STOCK, 1973). Similar changes are induced by intracerebroventricular injection of GABA (BISWAS and CARLSSON, 1977a) or systemic administration of GABA-ergic drugs (COTT et al., 1976). Even though GABA is unable to penetrate grossly through the blood-brain barrier, systemic administration of GABA causes biochemical changes in dopamine synthesis and metabolism similar to those observed after local administration, suggesting that blood-borne GABA can reach dopaminergic neurons in sufficient concentration to inhibit firing (BISWAS and CARLSSON, 1977b). The biochemical changes are accompanied by behavioral actions, which are potentiated by neuroleptic agents or by ethanol (BISWAS and CARLSSON, 1978a).

Since GABA and GABA-ergic drugs influence not only the nigrostriatal but also the mesolimbic dopamine system, they might possess antipsychotic activity. In a preliminary report, FREDERIKSEN (1975) described an antipsychotic action of baclofen in schizophrenic patients. Baclofen (p-chlorophenyl-GABA) is a GABA-derivative with somewhat GABA-like actions, although its mode of action has not been precisely defined. Unfortunately, other investigators have not been able to confirm FREDERIKSEN's observations (DAVIS et al., 1976; SIMPSON et al., 1976). However, in the experimental "psychosis model" of AHLENIUS and ENGEL (1975) baclofen was able to restore the abnormal behavior induced by excessive stimulation of dopaminergic receptors (AHLENIUS et al., 1975).

Further work is warranted to assess the action of GABA.

VI. Endocrine Aspects of Neuroleptic Action

Hypothalamic monoamines are involved in several neuroendocrine mechanisms. Of special interest is the inhibitory action of the tuberoinfundibular dopamine neurons on prolactin secretion either via release of prolactin inhibitory factor into the pituitary portal vessels or through a direct action on the pituitary by dopamine reaching the gland via the pituitary portal system (MACLEOD and LEHMEYER, 1974; MCCANN et al., 1972; MEITES et al., 1972; SCHAAR and CLEMENS, 1974). Consequently, dopaminergic receptor agonists decrease and antagonists increase prolactin levels in plasma and cerebrospinal fluid (SEDVALL et al., 1975). These changes in prolactin level are of special clinical interest because they offer the possibility to measure a "postsynaptic" dopamine action, which might be closely related to the antipsychotic effect. In rats a close correlation between haloperidol-induced increase in prolactin, on the one hand, and brain haloperidol levels and inhibition of a conditioned avoidance response, on the other, has been observed (ÖHMAN et al., 1977). More work is necessary to establish the clinical usefulness of this interesting approach (for review see MELTZER and STAHL, 1976).

VII. Acute vs Long-Term Effects of Neuroleptics

According to general clinical experience, the full therapeutic response to a neuroleptic agent may require several weeks and may last for a considerable time after cessation of therapy. There are thus reasons to believe that the primary actions of neuroleptics, as observed in short-term experiments, induce a series of important secondary effects, the nature of which has not yet been fully clarified.

Experimentally an increased sensitivity to dopamine-receptor agonists has been observed after cessation of treatment with neuroleptic agents. Supersensitivity has also been found after destruction of dopaminergic neurons, and may thus be related to the well-known denervation supersensitivity observed in peripheral tissues (MÖLLER-NIELSEN et al., 1974; SMITH and DAVIS, 1976; UNGERSTEDT et al., 1975). However, the problem is complicated to some extent by the existence of both pre- and postsynaptic receptors. Loss of the former receptors as a consequence of denervation should influence the dose-response curve of a receptor agonist apart from changes in postsynaptic receptor sensitivity. Nevertheless, increased sensitivity of both pre- and postsynaptic receptors appears to be a probable consequence of chronic treatment with neuroleptics.

A logical consequence of supersensitivity to receptor agonists would be reduced sensitivity to antagonists. In fact, extrapyramidal side effects tend to diminish in the course of therapy, suggesting that tolerance to this action develops more rapidly than the antipsychotic action (KLEIN and DAVIS, 1969). The increase in prolactin levels shows no clear-cut signs of tolerance, suggesting that this action is more like the antipsychotic effect (MELTZER and FANG, 1976). The feedback response of the dopaminergic neurons to neuroleptic treatment generally tends to diminish, and this reduction may be less marked in the limbic than in the striatal system (BOWERS and ROZITIS, 1974). However, adaptation has been observed also in the limbic system (ÖHMAN et al., 1977).

When adaptation or tolerance to a pharmacologic action occurs, it seems logical to expect the appearance of abstinence or rebound phenomena after cessation of long-term treatment. ENGEL et al. (1976) observed a hyperkinetic syndrome lasting for 2 weeks following cessation of chronic treatment of rats and mice with penfluridol. This syndrome could be prevented by α-methyltyrosine and appeared to be due partly to increased receptor sensitivity, partly to increased activity of the presynaptic striatal dopamine neurons.

This withdrawal syndrome may possibly serve as model for the clinically observed tardive dyskinesia. This extrapyramidal side effect differs from the classic ones in the following respects: it occurs only after chronic treatment and is not always fully reversible; it is counteracted by a new neuroleptic dose and is worsened by anticholinergics (MELTZER and STAHL, 1976). Further elucidation of tardive dyskinesia is urgently needed.

VIII. Effects of Neuroleptics on Developing Brain

The dopamine neurons appear to mature relatively late in ontogenesis. Neurons are generally assumed to be particularly vulnerable during the growth and maturation process. These considerations led LUNDBORG and ENGEL (1976) to investigate the effect of neuroleptics on monoaminergic mechanisms during development. Nursing rat mothers were given, for example, penfluridol in low dosage on days 1, 3, and 5 after delivery. Four weeks after birth, i.e., long after the neuroleptic had been eliminated, the young animals displayed an impaired acquisition of a conditioned avoidance response. The brains of these 4-week-old animals showed biochemical abnormalities, e.g., a reduced synthesis of dopamine and noradrenaline in the limbic areas and in the cerebral cortex.

These observations are of considerable theoretical and practical interest. Further studies are needed to clarify the mechanisms involved and the significance of the observations with respect to the use of centrally acting drugs pre- and postnatally.

IX. The Possible Role of Dopamine and Other Neurotransmitters in Psychosis

It is generally recognized that neuroleptics exert a true antipsychotic action, e.g., in schizophrenia and mania. In other words, we are not merely dealing with a suppression, but with an actual normalization of disturbed behavior. Experimental observations quoted above support this view. It is therefore probable that the neuroleptics have a site of action very strategically located with respect to those functions that are disturbed under certain psychotic conditions.

The neuroleptic agents can be divided into classes differing fundamentally in their actions at the molecular level as well as in chemical structure. Nevertheless, it would appear from the data referred to above that they have one characteristic in common: they all reduce the activity of dopaminergic receptors. In addition, most of them have a similar action on α-adrenergic receptors, but this action is less strikingly correlated to neuroleptic activity.

Reduction of dopaminergic receptor activity can be brought about either by pre- or postsynaptic effects. Reserpine and its congeners interfere with the intraneuronal storage and thus with the availability of transmitter for release by nerve impulse. α-Methyltyrosine, which has clear-cut antipsychotic activity in the presence of a subthreshold dose of a dopamine-receptor blocking agent, acts by inhibiting tyrosine hydroxylase. The most important groups of neuroleptic agents in all probability act by blocking dopamine receptors. It should be pointed out that this group is very heterogeneous with respect to chemical structure.

In view of this heterogeneity in chemical structure and site of action at the molecular level, it seems very unlikely that the neuroleptic agents should have in common an additional, thus far unidentified site of action unrelated to the effect on dopamine. It appears safe to conclude that the neuroleptic action is brought about by inhibition of dopaminergic functions. However, the pharmacologic profile of individual neuroleptics may be modified by additional effects, e.g., on α-adrenergic, cholinergic, or histaminergic receptors, or on 5-HT metabolism. Some of these actions may contribute to the antipsychotic activity. But this does not detract from the conclusion that inhibition of dopaminergic functions is the fundamental mode of action of the neuroleptics known so far.

To establish the exact site of the antipsychotic action within the dopaminergic system in the brain requires further investigation. The evidence available so far points to the mesolimbic dopamine system, including those parts of this system terminating in paleocortical areas, as the most likely site.

A pathogenetic role of dopamine in schizophrenia is suggested by the ability of amphetamine and its congeners to release dopamine and to aggravate or reproduce faithfully schizophrenia of the paranoid type (MELTZER and STAHL, 1976). A similar change in behavior may be induced by dopa (GOODWIN et al., 1971).

So far, no consistent change in catecholamine metabolism has been detected in schizophrenia (MELTZER and STAHL, 1976). This does not exclude the possibility that such a disturbance exists. For example, increased dopamine release in a small brain area, decreased transport into sites of metabolic breakdown, or receptor supersensitivity may have escaped detection. However, it seems almost equally probable that the primary disturbance does not reside in the dopaminergic synapse but in a system intimately related with dopamine neurons. Several transmitters may therefore be looked upon as candidates for primary involvement in schizophrenia: GABA, substance P, 5-HT, etc. Needless to say, we urgently need to deepen our knowledge of the interaction between dopamine and other transmitter systems. The only reasonably safe conclusion we can draw today is that dopamine offers an important clue to unraveling the psychopathology underlying schizophrenia.

H. Antidepressant Agents

I. Introduction

The first observations on the mood-elevating action of iproniazid were made in 1951 while testing the drug along with isoniazid for tuberculostatic activity (BOSWORTH, 1959). The following year iproniazid was discovered to be a potent inhibitor of monoamine oxidase (ZELLER et al., 1959), and about 5 years later the ability of iproniazid to antagonize the action of reserpine was described. This was shortly after the discovery that reserpine causes depletion of monoamine stores (for review, SHORE, 1962). Since reserpine had been found capable of faithfully mimicking so-called endogenous depression, it did not seem far-fetched to speculate that iproniazid might have antidepressant activity. A systematic clinical trial performed by KLINE and his colleagues revealed that this was indeed the case (LOOMER et al., 1957).

When KUHN (1958) discovered the antidepressant action of imipramine, the pharmacologists were first taken aback, because the primitive tests for psychopharmacologic activity available at that time had revealed only some chlorpromazine-like actions of imipramine, when given in large doses. However, already the following year SIGG (1959; also SIGG et al., 1963) discovered the ability of imipramine to potentiate the action of noradrenaline and of sympathetic nerve stimulation. Blockade of 5-HT uptake by imipramine was first observed in platelets (MARSHALL et al., 1960), and shortly afterward blockade of noradrenaline uptake was observed in adrenergic nerves (AXELROD et al., 1961; HERTTING et al., 1961) and in brain (DENGLER et al., 1961; GLOWINSKI and AXELROD, 1965).

Today we know of four classes of agents used in the treatment and prophylaxis of depression: (1) monoamine oxidase inhibitors, (2) inhibitors of monoamine re-uptake, (3) monoamine precursors, and (4) other agents, among which lithium is most important. The fact that at least three of these classes have their main actions on monoamine metabolism strongly favors an involvement of monoamines in the mechanism underlying the depression and has initiated intensive and partly successful research to find a disturbance in monoamine metabolism in this disorder.

II. Monoamine Oxidase Inhibitors

Monoamine oxidase inhibitors have now but limited clinical use, mainly due to their severe side effects. The most important side effect is hypertensive crisis, due to potentiation of the sympathomimetic agent tyramine, which occurs in certain foods and beverages, e.g., cheese, canned anchovies, wine. Tyramine is an excellent substrate for monoamine oxidase, and its bioavailability and half-life are considerably increased after inhibition of this enzyme. In addition, its activity as an indirectly acting sympathomimetic is markedly increased by the accumulation of noradrenaline in the adrenergic nerves induced by monoamine oxidase inhibition.

Monoamine oxidase is not a uniform enzyme but consists of at least two isoenzymes. Theoretically, it seems possible to develop inhibitors of the enzyme(s) responsible for the deamination of monoamines in brain while leaving the enzyme catalyzing the deamination of tyramine, e.g., in the digestive tract, unaffected. Work along these lines is in progress in several laboratories and may lead to a renaissance of this class of agents.

III. Inhibitors of Monoamine Re-Uptake

The different types of monoaminergic neurons possess a mechanism by means of which the transmitter released into the synaptic cleft can be partially recaptured and reprocessed within the neuron. This mechanism has different structural requirements in the dopaminergic, noradrenergic, and serotonergic neurons, the affinity being highest for the neuron's own transmitter. The activity of uptake-blocking agents is similarly differential, depending on the chemical structure. Imipramine and other tricyclic antidepressants in general use appear to lack uptake-blocking activity in dopaminergic neurons. In noradrenaline neurons the highest activity is exerted by secondary amines such as desipramine and protriptyline, whereas tertiary amines, e.g., imipramine, amitriptyline, and especially chlorimipramine, tend to have their highest activity in 5-HT neurons. This is particularly interesting in view of the difference in clinical activity tending to exist between secondary and tertiary amines among the tricyclic antidepressants. The former drugs tend to cause predominantly psychomotor activation, and the latter, mood elevation. This suggests that noradrenaline is primarily involved in the control of psychomotor activity, and 5-HT, in the control of mood (CARLSSON et al., 1969a, b). It should be realized, however, that the differences between tertiary and secondary amines tend to be blurred, owing to the fact that the latter amines occur as metabolites of the former and may thus build up rather high concentrations in the body fluids in the course of therapy. The ratio of secondary to tertiary amines during therapy with the latter amines is partly dependent on the route of administration. The highest ratios are obtained after oral administration, owing to first-pass deamination in the intestinal mucosa and liver.

Some tricyclic antidepressants, e.g., amitriptyline and trimipramine, have a sedative and anxiolytic action component, probably due to partial blockade of dopamine and/or noradrenaline receptors. There is thus no sharp demarcation line between the antidepressants and the neuroleptics. In fact, Parkinson-like side effects occasionally occur during treatment with certain antidepressants.

At present considerable efforts are made to develop antidepressant agents acting more selectively on either noradrenaline or 5-HT uptake. Such agents will probably be available for general use within a few years. In the search for new drugs blocking monoamine uptake the tricyclic structure has been found not to be essential for activity. Certain analgesics, e.g., pethidine and methadone, and antihistaminics, e.g., brompheniramine (with the activity residing in the dextrorotatory enantiomer), have been found to be active inhibitors of monoamine uptake. However, no correlation appears to exist between blockade of monamine uptake and analgesic or antihistaminic activity.

Among recently developed, rather selective inhibitors of monoamine uptake may be mentioned maprotiline and zimelidine, which inhibit noradrenaline and 5-HT uptake, respectively. Such agents will probably prove helpful in elucidating the roles of the different monoamines for antidepressant activity. In addition, the possibility exists that different types of depression may respond more favorably to either type of agent. A further advantage with the new generation of antidepressants is their relative lack of anticholinergic side effects and of cardiotoxicity.

Blocking re-uptake should cause an increased concentration of transmitter in the synaptic cleft. Unfortunately, it is not possible to measure this concentration directly, especially not in the intact animal. One indirect way of approaching this problem is to investigate the feedback response induced by the increased receptor activation in the synaptic cleft. Thus, compounds blocking preferentially noradrenaline and 5-HT re-uptake have been found to inhibit firing and transmitter synthesis and turnover preferentially in noradrenaline and 5-HT neurons, respectively (CORRODI and FUXE, 1969; MEEK and WERDINIUS, 1970; NYBÄCK, 1975; NYBÄCK et al., 1975; SAMANIN et al., 1975; SEDVALL et al., 1975). These observations support the view that inhibition of noradrenaline and 5-HT re-uptake does indeed lead to activation of noradrenaline and 5-HT receptors, respectively. This feedback response provides an opportunity for checking the activity of uptake inhibitors in patients undergoing treatment with these drugs: antidepressant agents have been found to cause a decrease in noradrenaline and 5-HT metabolites in the cerebrospinal fluid of patients treated with these drugs. Moreover, drugs preferentially blocking noradrenaline and 5-HT re-uptake induce the corresponding differential changes in metabolite levels (BERTILSSON et al., 1974; SEDVALL et al., 1975; SIWERS, 1976; WÅLINDER et al., 1976). An important bridge between animal experimental data and clinical observations has thus been established.

It should be emphasized that many of the antidepressant drugs in current use have actions in additon to blockade of uptake and that these additional actions probably contribute significantly to the individual profile of each drug. Examples of additional actions are blockade of muscarinic-cholinergic, dopaminergic, and α-adrenergic receptors. When the feedback response on the synthesis of the different monoamines is studied, such actions may influence the results. For example, large doses of amitriptyline cause an increased synthesis of dopamine in rat brain, presumably as a result of dopamine receptor blockade. Mianserin, a tetracyclic, and trimipramine, a tricyclic antidepressant with strong sedative properties, were found to stimulate both dopamine and noradrenaline synthesis. On the other hand, nomifensine, a drug with stimulant properties reported to block dopamine and noradrenaline re-uptake, caused a decrease in the synthesis of both these catecholamines (CARLSSON and LINDQVIST, 1978c). Remarkably enough, certain agents selectively blocking 5-HT re-uptake, e.g., zimelidine, norzimelidine, and chlorimipramine, caused, besides inhibition of 5-HT synthesis, an increase in dopamine synthesis in the absence of any detectable sedation. A possible explanation may be stimulation of dopamine neurons as a result of 5-HT receptor activation.

The picture thus emerging is that the antidepressant agents in current use, and those being introduced, represent a very heterogeneous group, where blockade of re-uptake of one or more monoamines is an important feature, but where additional actions contribute significantly to the individual profiles of activity. From the practical point of view this implies that in cases where an antidepressant agent has not yielded a satisfactory result, it may well prove worthwhile to try another agent. There are reasons to hope that in the future it will be possible to predict on the basis of clinical symptoms or laboratory findings which type of agent will be most suitable in the individual case.

IV. Interaction Between Monoamine Oxidase Inhibitors and Tricyclic Antidepressants

A dramatic interaction between monoamine oxidase inhibitors and tricyclic antidepressants has been observed in experimental animals as well as in patients, which show excitation and hyperthermia, sometimes ending fatally. This interaction is probably due to overflow of monoamines into the extraneuronal space when monoamine oxidase is inhibited and amine re-uptake is subsequently blocked (CARLSSON, 1976). A dominating role in the development of this syndrome seems to be played by 5-HT. A similar interaction has been described after treatment with monoamine oxidase inhibitors and pethidine, which also blocks 5-HT re-uptake.

Simultaneous treatment with monoamine oxidase inhibitors and tricyclic antidepressants appears to be possible and sometimes therapeutically active without serious side effects, provided that doses are kept low.

V. Monoamine Precursors as Antidepressant Agents

Tyrosine hydroxylase appears to be about 75% saturated with tyrosine under normal conditions, and thus tyrosine treatment will cause but a slight increase in catecholamine synthesis. However, tryptophan hydroxylase appears to be at most half saturated with tryptophan, and additional tryptophan administration may thus cause a doubling or more of 5-HT synthesis in the brain. In case precursor levels are below normal, even stronger effects on monoamine synthesis may be expected.

Dopa decarboxylase and 5-hydroxytryptophan (5-HTP) decarboxylase are closely related, if not identical, and are often referred to as aromatic L-amino acid decarboxylase. Pyridoxal phosphate (formed from vitamin B_6) serves as cofactor. This enzyme is greatly undersaturated with its substrates, and thus administration of dopa or 5-HTP may lead to a considerable increase in the synthesis of the respective monoamines.

An antidepressive action of dopa has been observed occasionally, but depression has also been reported in Parkinsonian patients undergoing dopa therapy. It appears that under certain conditions dopa treatment will interfere with the intestinal absorption of tryptophan (LEHMANN, 1973).

Treatment of depressed patients with tryptophan has yielded conflicting results. Paradoxically, the best results have been obtained in studies using relatively low doses of tryptophan (YOUNG and SOURKES, 1977). Higher doses have been suggested to cause induction of tryptophan pyrrolase and hence lower tryptophan levels in plasma and brain. Alternatively, high doses interfere with brain uptake of other amino acids, and this may weaken the therapeutic response, e.g., by reducing the concentration of tyrosine in the brain, which in turn will retard the synthesis of noradrenaline and dopamine (CARLSSON and LINDQVIST, 1978b). When given in combination with monoamine oxidase inhibitors, tryptophan appears to have a more consistent therapeutic effect in depression. Similarly tryptophan plus clomipramine, a relatively potent inhibitor of 5-HT uptake, proved more active than placebo plus clomipramine in elevating mood and in reducing anxiety in a controlled study on depressed patients. Retardation was equally reduced in the two treatment groups (WÅLINDER et al., 1976b). These observations provide some support for the speculation (see above) that 5-HT is more closely associated with mood and noradrenaline with drive.

Opinions differ about the antidepressant activity of 5-HTP. Most promising results appear to have been obtained in a study in which 5-HTP was combined with clomipramine and carbidopa to prevent decarboxylation of 5-HTP in extracerebral tissues (VAN PRAAG, 1974; VAN PRAAG et al., 1974).

p-Chlorophenylalanine, an inhibitor of tryptophan hydroxylase, has been reported to prevent the antidepressant response to imipramine, whereas α-methyltyrosine, an inhibitor of tyrosine hydroxylase, was unable to prevent the response (SHOPSIN et al., 1975).

VI. Antidepressant Agents With Unknown Modes of Action

The three groups of antidepressant agents briefly described above have the common property of promoting monoaminergic transmission by inhibiting the inactivation or enhancing the synthesis of monoamines. However, in view of the complex neuronal phenomena probably underlying the control of mood and related functions, it can hardly be expected that all antidepressant agents should necessarily act by influencing monoaminergic mechanisms. Iprindole and mianserin may be cited as possible examples, although they are not entirely devoid of actions on monoamines.

The lithium ion may also be mentioned in this context. Lithium differs from other antidepressants with the possible exception of tryptophan (YOUNG and SOURKES, 1977) in being able to alleviate mania. Besides, lithium is capable of preventing rather than alleviating depression. The question arises whether lithium could act by influencing some monoaminergic mechanisms. Certain observations may be quoted in support of this possibility. For example, lithium has been found to enhance the uptake of tryptophan by brain synaptosomes (KNAPP and MANDELL, 1975) and to act like α-methyltyrosine in certain behavioral experimental models (BERGGREN et al., 1978). However, more work is obviously needed to settle this point.

VII. Effect of Electroconvulsive Treatment on Monoaminergic Mechanisms

Electroconvulsive treatment (ECT) is still considered superior to other treatments for depression. It is capable of stimulating brain-monoamine turnover, but the effect is temporary. However, recently an increase in the sensitivity of monoaminergic receptors has been demonstrated after ECT treatment. This effect is long-lasting and cumulative and thus resembles the clinical response to ECT (MODIGH, 1975). This link between the experimental and clinical observations is strengthened by the finding that depressed Parkinsonian patients respond to ECT with an improvement also of the motor dysfunction (LEBENSOHN and JENKINS, 1975).

I. Psychotomimetic Agents

I. Introduction

The ability of certain drugs to mimic the symptomatology of psychosis has attracted a great deal of interest over a period of several centuries. Mescaline, an active component of the Mexican peyote, is one of the early prototypes of a so-called psychotomimetic agent. In the 1940s the highly active LSD-25 (lysergic acid diethylamide) was discovered, and we now know several other natural and synthetic compounds with similar properties. Most of them are indoles, e.g., LSD-25, psilocybin and dimethyltryptamine, whereas mescaline (3,4,5-trimethoxyphenethylamine) is more closely related to the catecholamines. All these compounds are potent hallucinogens and are capable of producing severe psychotic conditions somewhat similar to schizophrenia. However, it is generally not difficult to distinguish between these drug-induced conditions and schizophrenia. This is also true of certain anticholinergic agents with hallucinogenic properties, e.g., Ditran and other glycolate esters. Most interesting among the psychotomimetic agents are the amphetamines, because they are capable of faithfully mimicking paranoid schizophrenia and of aggravating pre-existing schizophrenic symptoms without distorting the symptomatology. Apart from the amphetamines, dopa appears to be the only agent capable of faithfully mimicking schizophrenic symptomatology, and indeed the paranoid form (GOODWIN et al., 1971; for general review, BERGER et al., 1978).

The mode of action of the various types of psychotomimetic agents will be briefly discussed below.

II. LSD-25 and Other Psychotomimetic Indole Derivatives

LSD-25, psilocybin, and dimethyltryptamine appear to influence monoaminergic mechanisms in about the same manner. In functional tests on, for example, spinal mechanisms in the rat these derivatives produce the picture of 5-HT-receptor activation. The effect on the receptors appears to be direct, since it persists after removal of endogenous 5-HT stores by treatment with reserpine plus inhibitors of 5-HT synthesis. Biochemically these hallucinogens inhibit the turnover of 5-HT in brain, presumably via a receptor-mediated feedback mechanism (ANDÉN et al., 1971). LSD-25 has been shown to inhibit the firing of serotonergic raphe neurons even in very low dosage (AGHAJANIAN et al., 1968).

These hallucinogens also stimulate noradrenaline turnover in brain; the effect is possibly secondary to the activation of 5-HT receptors. In addition, it appears that LSD-25 is a partial dopamine-receptor agonist (PERSSON and JOHANSSON, 1978; KEHR et al., 1978).

The mechanism underlying the psychotomimetic effect of these indoles is by no means clear. In case 5-HT-receptor activation is involved, the question arises as to whether presynaptic "autoreceptors" are primarily activated, leading to inhibiton of serotonergic transmission, or if activation of postsynaptic 5-HT receptors is required for psychotomimetic action. Moreover, the possible involvement of the catecholamines remains to be clarified.

III. Amphetamines and Related Agents

The central stimulation induced by the amphetamines and certain (though not all) related agents persists or is even enhanced after pretreatment with reserpine. This led to the assumption that amphetamines are capable of activating catecholamine receptors directly. However, it was subsequently shown that the action of amphetamines can be prevented by α-methyltyrosine and restored by additional treatment with small doses of dopa. These observations suggest that amphetamines are capable of releasing catecholamines from a small, reserpine-resistant pool occurring in the cytoplasm outside the synaptic vesicles and highly dependent on the rate of synthesis. Biochemical support for this view is available, but the exact mechanism by which release is induced by amphetamines is not known. Blockade of re-uptake by amphetamines occurs only after relatively large doses and can thus not explain the release (CARLSSON, 1970; CARLSSON, 1975c).

In contrast to α-methyltyrosine, an inhibitor of dopamine-β-hydroxylase proved ineffective in preventing the central stimulation by dexamphetamine in reserpine-pretreated animals, indicating that dopamine rather than noradrenaline is important for the stimulating action. However, in animals not pretreated with reserpine inhibition of dopamine-β-hydroxylase appears to attenuate the amphetamine-induced central stimulation somewhat, suggesting that also noradrenaline may be involved (SVENSSON, 1970).

The amphetamines referred to above are the racemic mixture of amphetamine as well as the dextro and levo enantiomers and their N-methylated derivatives (SVENSSON, 1971). The dextro-rotatory enantiomer of amphetamine is considerably more potent than the levo form in releasing dopamine and in inducing central stimulation, whereas the two forms appear to be equipotent as noradrenaline releasers. Phenmetrazine appears to act essentially as the amphetamines, whereas certain other amphetamine-like drugs seem to act by releasing vesicle-bound catecholamines; their action is blocked by reserpine, but not α-methyltyrosine pretreatment (SCHEEL-KRÜGER, 1971, 1972).

Amantadine, which is used in the treatment of Parkinsonism, can have amphetamine-like mental side effects and seems to act essentially like the amphetamines (STRÖMBERG et al., 1970; SVENSSON, 1973; SVENSSON and STRÖMBERG, 1970).

The central stimulating action of amphetamine can be considerably reduced by α-methyltyrosine pretreatment also in man (JÖNSSON et al., 1969). Whether this is also true of the psychotomimetic action has not been investigated, but this seems probable, since the two actions are presumably closely related to each other.

IV. Dopa

Irrespective of etiology, Parkinsonism appears to be due to insufficient activation of striatal dopaminergic receptors. The underlying cause may be degeneration of dopaminergic neurons, as in cryptogenic or postencephalitic Parkinsonism, depletion of vesicular dopamine stores, as after reserpine treatment, or blockade of dopaminergic postsynaptic receptors, as after treatment with neuroleptics of phenothiazine, thiaxanthene, or butyrophenone type (CARLSSON, 1972). Mental changes appear to accompany the motor disturbance not only in drug-induced Parkinsonism. L-Dopa often appears to influence also these changes favorably. As is well known the degeneration of monoaminergic neurons in Parkinsonism is not strictly limited to the striatal dopaminergic system. The mental changes are thus not necessarily located to the striatum but may also be due to disturbances, e.g., in the limbic system.

Dopa treatment of Parkinson patients may, on the other hand, cause mental side effects. Besides depression, which has already been mentioned, confusion, manic conditions and the picture of paranoid schizophrenia have been described (GOODWIN et al., 1971). The last-named phenomenon is especially interesting since it supports the view that paranoid psychosis can be induced by activating central catecholamine receptors. In animal experiments such activation, induced by dopa, amphetamine, or apomorphine, can lead to inadequate behavior with loss of discrimination between different conditioning stimuli, and this can be restored by neuroleptics. Since selective dopamine-receptor agonists and antagonists appear to be effective in this model, dopamine receptors appear to be especially important in this type of inadequate behavior (AHLENIUS and ENGEL, 1976).

V. Anticholinergic Agents With Psychotomimetic Activity

It is well known that most anticholinergics in clinical use can induce psychotic conditions with hallucinations. However, the psychotomimetic activity is especially prominent in certain anticholinergics. This is true of Ditran and related glycolate esters. These esters have no very marked effect on the turnover of monoamines (ANDÉN et al., 1972b). Perhaps these agents act by causing an imbalance between antagonistic cholinergic and monoaminergic systems. Such an antagonism is generally recognized in the striatum (BARTHOLINI and STADLER, 1975; SCHEEL-KRÜGER, 1969) but may occur also in other parts of the brain. However, the fact that the extrapyramidal side effects can be antagonized by anticholinergics, while leaving the antipsychotic action more or less unaffected, argues for a special organization of the cholinergic-dopaminergic balance in the striatum.

J. Sedatives, Hypnotics, and Anxiolytics

Ethyl alcohol is the oldest representative of this group but will be treated separately.

Classic pharmacology used to apply the term "indifferent narcotics" to emphasize some remarkable features of this group. Thus, they have certain physicochemical properties in common, with high lipophilia and low specificity as regards chemical structure. A number of theories on the mechanism underlying general anesthesia are based on different physicochemical properties. It has been proposed, for example, that indifferent narcotics exert a general unspecific action on the metabolism and activity of cells by accumulating in certain interphases in biologic membranes. This view probably grasps an important aspect of this type of drugs. However, the demarcation line between these drugs and agents with a high structural specificity and a selective affinity for receptors, enzymes, or transport mechanisms is not always sharp. For example, the barbiturates have many properties in common with the lower aliphatic alcohols and would thus appear to belong to the indifferent narcotics. However, small changes in chemical structure may lead to drastic changes in pharmacologic profile, suggesting a more specific mode of action. The benzodiazepines are even supposed to act by combining with specific receptors (SQUIRES and BRAESTRUP, 1977) and to facilitate GABA transmission by some as yet undefined mechanism (COSTA et al., 1976; GUIDOTTI, 1978), although the latter hypothesis is not supported by all the available data (BISWAS and CARLSSON, 1978b).

The profile of activity is by no means the same for all the sedative-anxiolytic drugs. Certain alcohols, e.g., ethanol and chloral hydrate, as well as diethyl ether and many other inhalation anesthetics, cause a pronounced excitation stage in subanesthetic concentrations, whereas barbiturates are generally, though not always, devoid of this property. The benzodiazepines are stronger anxiolytics than the barbiturates in relation to general sedative effects and have a more favorable therapeutic index.

Hopefully the current rapid progress in basic brain research will aid in clarifying the mode of action of this important group of drugs.

K. Ethyl Alcohol –
Mechanisms Underlying Drug Dependence

The actions of ethanol and other dependence-producing agents on the brain neurotransmitters represent a fascinating research area. The extent to which monoamines and other transmitters are involved in euphoria, drug dependence, and secondary changes like dementia induced by ethanol is not clear. However, certain observations suggest that important changes in these systems occur after acute as well as chronic ethanol administration.

Like many other anesthetics, ethanol in subanesthetic doses can give rise to excitation, its degree and character showing considerable individual variation. Whether this excitation is due to release of subcortical mechanisms from cortical inhibition or to a genuine excitatory action of low ethanol concentrations on nerve cells, has not been established.

An excitatory action of ethanol can be demonstrated also in experimental animals. For example, in mice an increased motility is evident, and in rats avoidance acquisition is facilitated (CHESHER, 1974). These actions can be prevented by α-methyltyrosine, in doses which have no obvious action on the motility per se (CARLSSON et al., 1972b). Endogenous catecholamines thus appear to be essential for the stimulating action of ethanol. Certain observations indicate that ethanol is capable of stimulating synthesis and turnover of catecholamines (CARLSSON and LINDQVIST, 1973). However, more recent findings suggest that the action of ethanol on catecholamine metabolism is more complex (unpublished data of this laboratory).

In man, it has been shown that the stimulant and euphoriant action of ethanol can be antagonized by pretreatment with α-methyltyrosine (AHLENIUS et al., 1973b). The "primary reinforcing properties" of ethanol may thus involve activation or at least require a certain activity of central catecholamine receptors. Similar mechanisms may operate for other dependence-producing organic solvents as well as for amphetamines and opiates (ENGEL and CARLSSON, 1976). It should be recalled that catecholaminergic neuronal pathways appear to be involved in self-stimulation, a phenomenon probably closely related to drug addiction (STEIN, 1964).

Apomorphine has for decades been ascribed a favorable influence in alcoholism and other forms of drug dependence, even though this point is controversial (SCHLATTER and LAL, 1972; WADSTEIN et al., 1978). In animal experiments apomorphine is capable of preventing the stimulating action of ethanol (CARLSSON et al., 1974), possibly due to preferential activation of dopaminergic autoreceptors (see Sect. F).

β-Adrenergic receptor antagonists appear to have a favorable influence on anxiety in alcoholics. It has not yet been decided whether this action is mediated via central or peripheral β-adrenergic receptors. Certain observations argue in favor of a central involvement (ENGEL and LILJEQUIST, 1976a).

In animals under chronic ethanol exposure and withdrawal various changes in catecholamine metabolism have been reported. Most striking is an increased apparent sensitivity of dopamine receptors in nucleus accumbens (ENGEL and LILJEQUIST, 1976b).

In the brains of chronic alcoholics examined post mortem a reduction of monoamine levels has been observed (unpublished data of an ongoing Swedish investigation).

The various observations quoted above suggest that the brain monoamines are fundamentally involved in the acute and chronic actions of alcohol and other dependence-producing drugs. However, the nature of this involvement requires further investigation.

L. Concluding Remarks

The mode of action of psychotropic drugs has been investigated with great intensity during the 25-year era of modern psychopharmacology. This research has been successful not only with regard to its immediate purpose, but has opened new important research fields, not least by initiating the entrance of the concept of chemical transmission into CNS research.

The rapid progress made thus far justifies some optimism as regards the development during the next decade. Extrapolation from current activities indicates that the various amine, amino acid, and peptide transmitters, will be studied intensely to clarify the synaptic mechanisms and interactions at a morphologic as well as functional level.

It is only natural that in the study of the mode of action of psychotropic drugs emphasis was initially placed on the acute and immediate effects. In recent years it has been increasingly realized, however, that important secondary changes follow upon the primary effects. Therapeutic responses to psychotropic drugs are often delayed by a couple of weeks or more and may, in fact, be more closely correlated to secondary than to primary neuronal changes. The secondary changes are not well understood, but probably involve increases or decreases in the number of relevant macromolecules, such as receptors, enzymes, and carrier molecules. Such changes might be loosely referred to as "trophic." It may be in this area that we have to look for explanations of various obscure phenomena, such as the delayed therapeutic response to antidepressants, neuroleptics and L-dopa, tardive dyskinesias, altered drug responses in abusers, and the cumulative, long-lasting therapeutic response to ECT. The coupling between the short- and long-term synaptic changes is no doubt an important aspect of neurobiology, and research in this area will probably increase our understanding not only of drug responses but also of the natural history of mental disorders.

Another new research area of considerable interest deals with the specific sensitivity of neurons under development, e.g., perinatally, to various chemical and noxious influences; even moderate exposure during a short critical period may lead to persistent neuronal changes and disturbances in brain function (AHLENIUS et al., 1973a; ENGEL and LUNDBORG, 1974).

Finally, we can anticipate considerable progress in research on age-related neuronal deficiencies, which may lead to senile dementia and other disturbances of old age. The possible substitution therapy in cases of transmission failure, in analogy to L-dopa therapy in Parkinson's disease, is a real challenge. The increasing sophistication of clinical neurochemistry may help to identify specific transmitter deficiencies and guide basic research in this area.

References

Aghajanian, G.K., Bunney, B.S.: Central dopaminergic neurons: neurophysiological identification and responses to drugs. In: Frontiers in catecholamine research. Snyder, S.H., Usdin, E. (eds.), pp. 643–648. New York: Pergamon Press 1973

Aghajanian, G.K., Bunney, G.S.: Pre- and postsynaptic feedback mechanisms in central dopaminergic neurons. In: Frontiers of neurology and neuroscience research. Seeman, P., Brown, G.M. (eds.), pp. 4–11. Toronto: University of Toronto Press 1974

Aghajanian, G.K., Bunney, B.S.: Dopamine autoreceptors: pharmacological characterization by microiontophoretic single cell recording studies. Naunyn Schmiedebergs Arch. Pharmacol. **297**, 1–8 (1977)

Aghajanian, G.K., Foote, W.E., Sheard, M.H.: Lysergic acid diethylamide: sensitive neuronal units in the mid brain raphe. Science **161**, 706–708 (1968)

Ahlenius, S., Engel, J.: Effects of small doses of haloperidol on timing behaviour (Letters to the Editor). J. Pharm. Pharmacol. **23**, 301–302 (1971a)

Ahlenius, S., Engel, J.: Behavioural effects of haloperidol after tyrosine hydroxylase inhibition. Eur. J. Pharmacol. **15**, 187–192 (1971b)

Ahlenius, S., Engel, J.: On the interaction between pimozide and α-methyl-tyrosine. J. Pharm. Pharmacol. **25**, 172–174 (1973)

Ahlenius, S., Engel, J.: Antagonism by haloperidol of the L-dopa-induced disruption of a successive discrimination in the rat. J. Neural Transm. **36**, 43–49 (1975)

Ahlenius, S., Engel, J.: Normalization by antipsychotic drugs of biochemically induced behaviour in rats. Psychopharmacology **49**, 119–123 (1976)

Ahlenius, S., Engel, J.: Potentiation by α-methyltyrosine of the suppression of food-reinforced leverpressing behaviour induced by antipsychotic drugs. Acta Pharmacol. Toxicol. (Kbh.) **40**, 115–125 (1977)

Ahlenius, S., Brown, R., Engel, J., Lundborg, P.: Learning deficits in 4 weeks old offspring of the nursing mothers treated with the neuroleptic drug penfluridol. Naunyn Schmiedebergs Arch. Pharmacol. **279**, 31–37 (1973a)

Ahlenius, S., Carlsson, A., Engel, J., Svensson, T., Södersten, P.: Antagonism by α-methyltyrosine of the ethanol-induced stimulation and euphoria in man. Clin. Pharmacol. Ther. **14**, 586–591 (1973b)

Ahlenius, S., Carlsson, A., Engel, J.: Antagonism by baclophen of the d-amphetamine-induced disruption of a successive discrimination in the rat. J. Neural Transm. **36**, 327–333 (1975)

Almgren, O., Carlsson, A., Engel, J. (eds.): Chemical tools in catecholamine research. II. p. 249–304. Amsterdam: North-Holland 1975

Andén, N.-E.: Monoamines and synaptic transmission. In: Monoamines, noyaux gris centraux et syndrome de Parkinson. de Ajuriaguerra, J., Gauthier, G. (eds.), pp. 61–72. Geneva: George 1971

Andén, N.-E.: Dopamine turnover in the corpus striatum and the limbic system after treatment with neuroleptic and anti-acetylcholine drugs. J. Pharm. Pharmacol. **24**, 905–906 (1972)

Andén, N.-E.: Catecholamine receptor mechanisms in vertebrates. In: Frontiers in catecholamine research. Snyder, S.H., Usdin, E. (eds.), pp. 661–665. New York: Pergamon Press 1973

Andén, N.-E.: The interaction of neuroleptic drugs with striatal and limbic dopaminergic mechanisms. In: Antipsychotic drugs, pharmacodynamics and pharmacokinetics. Sedvall, G., Uvnäs, B., Zotterman, Y. (eds.), pp. 217–225. New York: Pergamon Press 1976

Andén, N.-E., Stock, G.: Effect of clozapine on the turnover of dopamine in the corpus striatum and in the limbic system. J. Pharm. Pharmacol. **25**, 346–348 (1973)

Andén, N.-E., Roos, B.-E., Werdinius, B.: Effects of chlorpromazine, haloperidol and reserpine on the levels of phenolic acids in rabbit corpus striatum. Life Sci. **3**, 149–158 (1964)

Andén, N.-E., Dahlström, A., Fuxe, K., Larsson, K.: Functional role of the nigro-striatal dopamine neurons. Acta Pharmacol. Toxicol. (Kbh.) **24**, 263–274 (1966)

Andén, N.-E., Carlsson, A., Häggendal, J.: Adrenergic mechanisms. Annu. Rev. Pharmacol. **9**, 119–134 (1969)

Andén, N.-E., Butcher, S.G., Corrodi, H., Fuxe, K., Ungerstedt, U.: Receptor activity and turnover of dopamine and noradrenaline after neuroleptics. Eur. J. Pharmacol. **11**, 303–314 (1970)

Andén, N.-E., Corrodi, H., Fuxe, K.: Hallucinogenic drugs of the indolealkylamine type and central monoamine neurons. J. Pharmacol. Exp. Ther. **179**, 236–249 (1971)

Andén, N.-E., Corrodi, H., Fuxe, K.: Effect of neuroleptic drugs on central catecholamine turnover assessed using tyrosine- and dopamine-β-hydroxylase inhibitors. J. Pharm. Pharmacol. **24**, 177–182 (1972a)

Andén, N.-E., Corrodi, H., Fuxe, K.: The effect of psychotomimetic glycolate esters on central monoamine neurons. Eur. J. Pharmacol. **17**, 97–102 (1972b)

Andén, N.-E., Strömbom, U., Svensson, T.H.: Dopamine and noradrenaline receptor stimulation: Reversal of reserpine-induced suppression of motor activity. Psychopharmacologia **29**, 289–298 (1973)

Axelrod, J., Whitby, L.G., Hertting, G.: Effect of psychotropic drugs on the uptake of ^{3}H-norepinephrine by tissues. Science **133**, 383–384 (1961)

Axelsson, T.: On the serum concentrations and antipsychotic effects of thioridazine, thioridazine side-chain sulfoxide and thioridazine side-chain sulfone in chronic psychotic patients. Curr. Ther. Res. **21**, 587–605 (1977)

Bartholini, G.: Differential effect of neuroleptic drugs on dopamine turnover in the extrapyramidal and limbic system. J. Pharm. Pharmacol. **28**, 429–433 (1975)

Bartholini, G., Stadler, H.: Cholinergic and GABA-ergic influence on the dopamine release in extrapyramidal centers. In: Chemical tools in catecholamine research. II. Almgren, O., Carlsson, A., Engel, J. (eds.), pp. 235–239. Amsterdam: North-Holland 1975

Bartholini, G., Stadler, H., Lloyd, K.: Cholinergic-dopaminergic interregulations within the extrapyramidal system. In: Cholinergic mechanisms. Waser, P.G. (ed.), pp. 411–418. New York: Raven Press 1975

Bartholini, G., Stadler, H., Gadea-Ciria, M., Lloyd, K.G.: The use of the push-pull cannula to estimate the dynamics of acetylcholine and catecholamines within various brain areas. Neuropharmacology **15**, 515–519 (1976a)

Bartholini, G., Stadler, H., Gadea-Ciria, M., Lloyd, K.G.: The effect of antipsychotic drugs on the release of neurotransmitters in various brain areas. In: Antipsychotic drugs, pharmacodynamics and pharmacokinetics. Sedvall, G., Uvnäs, B., Zotterman, Y. (eds.), pp. 105–116. New York: Pergamon Press 1976b

Berger, P.A., Glen, R.E., Barchas, J.D.: Neuroregulators and schizophrenia. In: Psychopharmacology: A generation of progress. Lipton, M.A., DiMascio, A., Killam, K.F. (eds.), pp. 1071–1082. New York: Raven Press 1978

Berggren, U., Tallstedt, L., Ahlenius, S., Engel, J.: The effect of lithium on amphetamine-induced locomotor stimulation. Psychopharmacology **59**, 41–45 (1978)

Bertilsson, L., Åsberg, M., Thorén, P.: Differential effect of chlorimipramine and nortriptyline on metabolites of serotonin and noradrenaline in the cerebrospinal fluid of depressed patients. Eur. J. Clin. Pharmacol. **7**, 365–368 (1974)

Biswas, B., Carlsson, A.: The effect of intracerebroventricularly administered GABA on brain monoamine metabolism. Naunyn Schmiedebergs Arch. Pharmacol. **299**, 41–46 (1977a)

Biswas, B., Carlsson, A.: The effect of intraperitoneally administered GABA on brain monoamine metabolism. Naunyn Schmiedebergs Arch. Pharmacol. **299**, 47–51 (1977b)

Biswas, B., Carlsson, A.: Effect of intraperitoneally administered GABA in the locomotor activity of mice. Psychopharmacology **59**, 91–94 (1978a)

Biswas, B., Carlsson, A.: On the mode of action of diazepam on brain catecholamine metabolism. Naunyn Schmiedebergs Arch. Pharmacol. **303**, 73–78 (1978b)

Björklund, A., Lindvall, O.: Dopamine in dendrites of substantia nigra neurons: suggestions for a role in dendritic terminals. Brain Res. **83**, 531–537 (1975)

Bosworth, D.M.: Iproniazid: A brief review of its introduction and clinial use. Ann. N.Y. Acad. Sci. **80**, 809–820 (1959)

Bowers, M.B., Jr., Rozitis, A.: Regional differences in homovanillic acid concentration after acute and chronic administration of antipsychotic drugs. J. Pharm. Pharmacol. **26**, 743–745 (1974)

Bunney, B.S., Aghajanian, G.K.: d-Amphetamine-induced inhibition of central dopaminergic neurons: mediation by a striato-nigral feedback pathway. Science 192, 391–393 (1976)

Bunney, B.S., Walters, J.R., Roth, R.H., Aghajanian, G.K.: Dopaminergic neurons: effects of antipsychotic drugs and amphetamine on single cell activity. J. Pharmacol. Exp. Ther. 185, 560–571 (1973)

Bürki, H.R., Ruch, W., Asper, H.: Effects of clozapine, thioridazine, perlapine and haloperidol on the metabolism of the biogenic amines in the brain of the rat. Psychopharmacology 41, 27–33 (1975)

Carlsson, A.: Drugs which block the storage of 5-hydroxytryptamine and related amines. In: Handbuch der experimentellen Pharmakologie. Ergänzungswerk, Bd. XIX. Erspamer, V. (Hrsg.), S. 529–592. Berlin: Springer 1965

Carlsson, A.: Amphetamine and brain catecholamines. In: Proceedings of the Mario Negri Institute for Pharmacological Research. Costa, E., Garattini, S. (eds.), pp. 289–300. New York: Raven Press 1970

Carlsson, A.: Biochemical and pharmacological aspects of parkinsonism. Proceedings of the Twentieth Congress of Scandinavian Neurologists, Oslo, 1972. Acta Neurol. Scand. 48, Suppl. 51, 11–42 (1972)

Carlsson, A.: Antipsychotic drugs and catecholamine synapses. J. Psychiatr. Res. 11, 57–64 (1974)

Carlsson, A.: Dopaminergic autoreceptors. In: Chemical tools in catecholamine research. II. Almgren, O., Carlsson, A., Engel, J. (eds.), pp. 219–225. Amsterdam: North-Holland 1975a

Carlsson, A.: Monoamine-depleting drugs. Pharmacol. Ther. [B] 1 (3), 393–400 (1975b)

Carlsson, A.: Drugs acting through dopamine release. Pharmacol. Ther. [B] 1 (3), 401–405 (1975c)

Carlsson, A.: The contribution of drug research to investigating the nature of endogenous depression. Pharmakopsychiatrie 1, 2–10 (1976)

Carlsson, A.: Does dopamine play a role in schizophrenia? Psychol. Med. 7, 583–597 (1977a)

Carlsson, A.: The influence of antidepressants on central monoaminergic systems. In: Neurotransmission and disturbed behaviour. van Praag, H.M. (ed.), pp. 19–33. Amsterdam: Erven Gohn B.V. 1977b

Carlsson, A., Lindqvist, M.: Effect of chlorpromazine or haloperidol on formation of 3-methoxytyramine and normetanephrine in mouse brain. Acta Pharmacol. Toxicol. (Kbh.) 20, 140–144 (1963)

Carlsson, A., Lindqvist, M.: Effect of ethanol on the hydroxylation of tyrosine and tryptophan in rat brain in vivo. J. Pharm. Pharmacol. 25, 437–440 (1973)

Carlsson, A., Lindqvist, M.: Effect of reserpine on monoamine synthesis and on apparent dopaminergic receptor sensitivity in rat brain. In: Neuropharmacology and behaviour. Haber, B., Aprison, M.H. (eds.), pp. 89–102. New York: Plenum 1978a

Carlsson, A., Lindqvist, M.: Dependence of 5-HT and catecholamine synthesis on concentrations of precursor amino-acids in rat brain. Naunyn Schmiedebergs Arch. Pharmacol. 303, 157–164 (1978b)

Carlsson, A., Lindqvist, M.: Effects of antidepressant agents on the synthesis of brain monoamines. J. Neural Transm. 43, 73–91 (1978c)

Carlsson, A., Corrodi, H., Fuxe, K., Hökfelt, T.: Effect of antidepressant drugs on the depletion of intraneuronal brain 5-hydroxtryptamine stores caused by 4-methyl-α-ethyl-meta-tyramine. Eur. J. Pharmacol. 5, 357–366 (1969a)

Carlsson, A., Corrodi, H., Fuxe, K., Hökfelt, T.: Effects of some antidepressant drugs on the depletion of intraneuronal brain catecholamine stores caused by 4,α-dimethyl-meta-tyramine. Eur. J. Pharmacol. 5, 367–373 (1969b)

Carlsson, A., Davis, J.N., Kehr, W., Lindqvist, M., Atack, C.V.: Simultaneous measurement of tyrosine and tryptophan hydroxylase activities in brain in vivo using an inhibitor of the aromatic amino acid decarboxylase. Naunyn Schmiedebergs Arch. Pharmacol. 275, 153–168 (1972a)

Carlsson, A., Engel, J., Svensson, T.H.: Inhibition of ethanol-induced excitation in mice and rats by α-methyl-p-tyrosine. Psychopharmacology 26, 307–312 (1972b)

Carlsson, A., Engel, J., Strömbom, U., Svensson, T.H., Waldeck, B.: Suppression by dopamine-agonists of the ethanol-induced stimulation of locomotor activity and brain dopamine synthesis. Naunyn Schmiedebergs Arch. Pharmacol. 283, 117–128 (1974)

Chesher, G.B.: Facilitation of avoidance acquisition in the rat by ethanol and its abolition by α-methyl-p-tyrosine. Psychopharmacology 39, 87–95 (1974)

Christiansen, J., Squires, R.F.: Antagonistic effects of apomorphine and haloperidol on rat striatal synaptosomal tyrosine hydroxylase. J. Pharm. Pharmacol. **26**, 367–368 (1974)

Clement-Cormier, Y.C., Kebabian, J.W., Petzold, G.L., Greengard, P.: Dopamine-sensitive adenylate cyclase in mammalian brain: a possible site of action of antipsychotic drugs. Proc. Natl. Acad. Sci. U.S.A. **71**, 1113–1117 (1974)

Corrodi, H., Fuxe, K.: Decreased turnover in central 5-HT nerve terminals induced by antidepressant drugs of the imipramine type. Eur. J. Pharmacol. **7**, 56–59 (1969)

Corrodi, H., Hanson, L.C.F.: Central effects of an inhibitor of tyrosine hydroxylation. Psychopharmacology **10**, 116–125 (1966)

Costa, E., Gessa, G.L., Sandler, M. (eds.): Serotonin – New Vistas. Biochemistry and behavioral and clinical studies. In: Advances in biochemical psychopharmacology. Vol. XI, pp. 1–168. New York: Raven Press 1974a

Costa, E., Gessa, G.L., Sandler, M. (eds.): Serotonin – New Vistas. Biochemistry and behavioral and clinical studies. In: Advances in biochemical psychopharmacology. Vol. XI, pp. 169–216. New York: Raven Press 1974b

Costa, E., Gessa, G.L., Sandler, M. (eds.): Serotonin – New Vistas. Biochemistry and behavioral and clinical studies. In: Advances in biochemical psychopharmacology. Vol. XI, pp. 217–264. New York: Raven Press 1974c

Costa, E., Guidotti, A., Mao, C.C.: A GABA hypothesis for the action of benzodiazepines. In: GABA in nervous system function. Kroc Foundation Series, Vol. V. Roberts, E., Chase, T.N., Torver, D.B. (eds.), pp. 413–426. New York: Raven Press 1976

Cott, J., Carlsson, A., Engel, J., Lindqvist, M.: Suppression of ethanol-induced locomotor stimulation by GABA-like drugs. Naunyn Schmiedebergs Arch. Pharmacol. **295**, 203–209 (1976)

Creese, I., Burt, D.R., Snyder, S.H.: Dopamine receptor binding predicts clinical and pharmacological potencies of antischizophrenic drugs. Science **192**, 481–483 (1976)

Da Prada, M., Pletscher, A.: Acceleration of cerebral dopamine turn-over by chlorpromazine. Experientia **22**, 465–466 (1966)

Davis, K.L., Hollister, L.E., Berger, P.A.: Baclofen in schizophrenia. Lancet **1976I**, 1245

Delay, J., Deniker, O.: Charactéristiques psychophysiologiques des médicaments neuroleptiques. In: Psychotropic drugs. Garattini, S., Ghetti, V. (eds.), pp. 485–501. Amsterdam: Elsevier 1957

Dengler, H.J., Spiegel, H.E., Titus, E.O.: Uptake of tritium-labelled norepinephrine in brain and other tissues of cat *in vitro*. Science **133**, 1072–1073 (1961)

Engel, J., Carlsson, A.: Catecholamines and behaviour. Curr. Dev. Psychopharmacol. **4**, 1–32 (1976)

Engel, J., Liljequist, S.: Behavioural effects of β-receptor blocking agents in experimental animals. In: Neuro-psychiatric effects of adrenergic beta-receptor blocking agents. Clin. Pharmacol. **12**, 45–52 (1976a)

Engel, J., Liljequist, S.: The effect of long-term ethanol treatment on the sensitivity of the dopamine receptors in the nucleus accumbens. Psychopharmacology **49**, 253–257 (1976b)

Engel, J., Lundborg, P.: Regional changes in monoamine levels and in the rate of tyrosine and tryptophan hydroxylation in 4 week old offspring of nursing mothers treated with the neuroleptic drug penfluridol. Naunyn Schmiedebergs Arch. Pharmacol. **282**, 327–334 (1974)

Engel, J., Liljequist, S., Johannesen, K.: Behavioural effects of long-term treatments with antipsychotic drugs. In: Antipsychotic drugs, pharmacodynamics and pharmacokinetics. Sedvall, G., Uvnäs, B., Zotterman, Y. (eds.), pp. 63–71. Oxford: Pergamon Press 1976

Farnebo, L.-O., Hamberger, B.: Drug-induced changes in the release of [^{3}H]-monoamines from field stimulated rat brain slices. Acta Physiol. Scand. **84**, Suppl. 371, 35–44 (1971)

Felger, H.L.: Depressed hospitalized psychiatric patients treated with chlorprothixene concentrate. J. N. Drugs **5**, 240–248 (1965)

Forsman, A.: Individual differences in clinical response to an antipsychotic drug. Theses, pp.1–33. University of Göteborg 1977

Forsman, A., Öhman, R.: Studies on plasma protein binding of haloperidol. Curr. Ther. Res. **21**, 245–255 (1977)

Forsman, A., Mårtensson, E., Nyberg, G., Öhman, R.: A gas chromatographic method for determining haloperidol. Naunyn Schmiedebergs Arch. Pharmacol. **286**, 113–124 (1974)

Frederiksen, P.K.: Baclofen in the treatment of schizophrenia. Lancet **1975I**, no. 7908, 702–703

Freud, S.: On narcissism – An introduction. (Trans. 1962 J. Strachey), p. 73. London: Hogarth Press 1914

Freud, S.: Letter to Marie Bonaparte, 15 January 1930. Cited by Jones, E. (1957). In: The life and work of Sigmund Freud. Vol. III, p. 449. New York: Basic Books 1930
Fuxe, K., Sjöqvist, F.: Hypothermic effect of apomorphine in the mouse. J. Pharm. Pharmacol. **24**, 702–705 (1972)
Garcia-Sevilla, J.A., Magnusson, T., Carlsson, A.: Effect of intracerebroventricularly administered somatostatin on brain monoamine turnover. Brain Res. **155**, 159–164 (1978)
Gershon, S., Heikimian, L.J., Floyd, A., Jr., Hollister, L.E.: Methyl-p-tyrosine (AMT) in schizophrenia. Psychopharmacology **11**, 189–194 (1967)
Glowinski, J., Axelrod, J.: Effects of drugs on the uptake, release and metabolism of norepinephrine in the rat brain. J. Pharmacol. Exp. Ther. **149**, 43–49 (1965)
Goldstein, M., Anagnoste, B., Shirron, C.: The effect of trivastal, haloperidol and dibutyryl cyclic AMP on ^{14}C dopamine synthesis in rat striatum. J. Pharm. Pharmacol. **25**, 348–351 (1973)
Goodman, L.S., Gilman, A. (eds.): The pharmacological basis of therapeutics, 5th ed. pp. 148–149. New York: Macmillan 1975
Goodwin, F.K., Murphy, D.L., Brodie, H.K.H., Bunney, W.E.: Levodopa: alterations in behaviour. Clin. Pharmacol. Ther. **12**, 383–396 (1971)
Greengard, P.: Presynaptic and postsynaptic roles of cyclic AMP and protein phosphorylation at catecholaminergic synapses. In: Chemical tools in catecholamine research. Almgren, O., Carlsson, A., Engel, J. (eds.), Vol. II, pp. 249–256. Amsterdam: North-Holland 1975
Groves, P.M., Wilson, C.J., Young, S.J., Rebec, G.V.: Self-inhibition by dopaminergic neurons. Science **190**, 522–529 (1975)
Guidotti, A.: Synaptic mechanisms in the action of benzodiazepines. In: Psychopharmacology: A generation of progress. Lipton, M.A., DiMascio, A., Killam, K.F. (eds.), pp. 1349–1357. New York: Raven Press 1978
Henning, M.: Central sympathetic transmitters and hypertension. Clin. Sci. Mol. Med. **48**, 195–203 (1975)
Hertting, G., Axelrod, J., Kopin, I.J., Whitby, L.G.: Lack of uptake of catecholamines after chronic denervation of sympathetic nerves. Nature **189**, 66 (1961)
Hökfelt, T., Johansson, O., Fuxe, K., Löfström, A., Goldstein, M., Park, D., Ebstein, R., Fraser, H., Jeffcoate, S., Effendie, S., Luft, R., Arimura, A.: Mapping and relationship of hypothalamic neurotransmitters and hypothalamic hormones. In: Proceedings of the Sixth International Congress of Pharmacology. Tuomisto, J., Paasonen, M.K. (eds.), Vol. III, p. 93–110. Helsinki, Finland: 1975
Huxtable, R., Barbeau, A. (eds.): Taurine. New York: Raven Press 1976
Hyttel, J.: Effect of neuroleptics on the disappearance rate of ^{14}C labelled catecholamines formed from ^{14}C tyrosine in mouse brain. J. Pharm. Pharmacol. **26**, 588–596 (1974)
Iversen, L.L., Otsuka, M.: Symposium on novel transmitter substances. In: Proceedings of the Sixth International Congress of Pharmacology. Tuomisto, J., Paasonen, M.K. (eds.), Vol. III, pp. 35–102. Helsinki, Finland: 1975
Iversen, L.L., Rogawski, M.A., Miller, R.J.: Comparison of the effects of neuroleptic drugs on pre- and postsynaptic dopaminergic mechanisms in the rat striatum. Mol. Pharmacol. **12**, 251–262 (1976)
Jackson, D.M., Andén, N.-E., Dahlström, A.: A functional effect of dopamine in the nucleus accumbens and in some other dopamine-rich parts of the rat brain. Psychopharmacology **45**, 139–149 (1975)
Jarvik, M.E.: Drugs used in the treatment of psychiatric disorders. In: The pharmacological basis of therapeutics, 3rd ed. Goodman, L.S., Gilman, A. (eds.), pp. 159–214. New York: Macmillan 1965
Javoy, F., Agid, Y., Bouvet, D., Glowinski, J.: Changes in neostriatal dopamine metabolism after carbachol or atropine microinjections into the substantia nigra. Brain Res. **68**, 253–260 (1974)
Jonason, J.: Metabolism of dopamine and noradrenaline in normal atrophied and postganglionically sympathectomized rat salivary glands *in vitro*. Acta Physiol. Scand. **76**, 299–311 (1969)
Jönsson, L.-E., Gunne, L.-M., Änggård, E.: Effects of α-methyltyrosine in amphetamine-dependent subjects. Pharmacol. Clin. **2**, 27–29 (1969)
Kamberi, I.A., Thorn, N.A.: Symposium on interactions of neurotransmitters and the hypothalamic releasing hormones. In: Proceedings of the Sixth International Congress of Pharmacology. Tuomisto, J., Paasonen, M.K. (eds.), Vol. III, pp. 93–167. Helsinki, Finland: 1975

Kebabian, J.W., Greengard, P.: Dopamine-sensitive adenyl cyclase: possible role in synaptic transmission. Science **174**, 1346–1349 (1971)

Kehr, W., Speckenbach, W.: Effect of lisuride and LSD on monoamine synthesis after axotomy or reserpine treatment in rat brain. Naunyn Schmiedebergs Arch. Pharmacol. **301**, 163–169 (1978)

Kehr, W., Carlsson, A., Lindqvist, M., Magnusson, T., Atack, C.: Evidence for a receptor-mediated feedback control of striatal tyrosine hydroxylase activity. J. Pharm. Pharmacol. **24**, 744–747 (1972)

Kehr, W., Carlsson, A., Lindqvist, M.: Catecholamine synthesis in rat brain after axotomy: interaction between apomorphine and haloperidol. Naunyn Schmiedebergs Arch. Pharmacol. **297**, 111–117 (1977)

Kilian, M., Frey, H.H.: Central monoamines and convulsive thresholds in mice and rats. Neuropharmacology **12**, 681–692 (1973)

Klein, D.F., Davis, J.M.: Diagnosis and drug treatment of psychiatric disorders. Baltimore: Williams and Wilkins 1969

Knapp, S., Mandell, A.J.: Effects of lithium chloride on parameters of biosynthetic capacity for 5-hydroxytryptamine in rat brain. J. Pharmacol. Exp. Ther. **193**, 812–823 (1975)

Kraepelin, E.: Über die Beeinflussung einfacher psychischer Vorgänge durch einige Arzneimittel, S. 227. Jena: Gustav Fischer 1892

Kuhn, R.: The treatment of depressive states with G 22355 (imipramine hydrochloride). Am. J. Psychiatry **115**, 459 (1958)

Ladinsky, H., Consolo, S., Bianchi, S., Samanin, R., Ghezzi, D.: Cholinergic-dopaminergic interaction in the striatum: the effect of 6-hydroxydopamine or pimozide treatment on the increased striatal acetylcholine levels induced by apomorphine, piribedil and d-amphetamine. Brain Res. **84**, 221–226 (1975)

Lebensohn, Z.M., Jenkins, R.B.: Improvement of parkinsonism in depressed patients treated with ECT. Am. J. Psychiatry **132**, 283–285 (1975)

Lehmann, J.: Tryptophan malabsorption in levodopa-treated parkinsonian patients. Acta Med. Scand. **194**, 181–189 (1973)

Loomer, H.P., Saunders, J.C., Kline, N.S.: A clinical and pharmacodynamic evaluation of iproniazid as a psychic energizer. Am. Psychiatr. Assoc. Psychiatric Res. Rep. **8**, 129 (1957)

Lundborg, P., Engel, J.: Learning deficits and selective biochemical brain changes in 4-week-old offspring of nursing rat mothers treated with neuroleptics. In: Antipsychotic drugs, pharmacodynamics and pharmacokinetics. Sedvall, G., Uvnäs, B., Zotterman, Y. (eds.), pp. 261–269. Oxford: Pergamon Press 1976

MacLeod, R.M., Lehmeyer, J.E.: Studies on the mechanism of the dopamine-mediated inhibition of prolactin secretion. Endocrinology **94**, 1077–1085 (1974)

Magnusson, T., Carlsson, A., Fisher, G.H., Chang, D., Folkers, K.: Effect of synthetic substance P on monoaminergic mechanisms in brain. J. Neural Transm. **38**, 89–93 (1976)

Marshall, E., Stirling, G.S., Tait, A.C., Todrick, A.: The effect of iproniazid and imipramine on the blood platelet serotonin level in man. Br. J. Pharmacol. **15**, 35–41 (1960)

McCann, S.M., Kaira, P.S., Donoso, A.P., Bishop, W., Schneider, H.P.G., Fawcett, C.P., Krulich, L.: The role of monoamines in the control of gonadotropin and prolactin secretion. In: Median eminence: Structure and function. Knugge, K.M., Scott, D.F., Weendl, A. (eds.), pp. 224–235. Basel: Karger 1972

McGeer, P.L., Grewaal, D.S., McGeer, E.G.: Influence of non-cholinergic drugs on rat striatal acetylcholine levels. Brain Res. **80**, 211–217 (1974)

Meek, J., Werdinius, B.: Hydroxytryptamine turnover decreased by the antidepressant drug chlorimipramine. Letter to the Editor. J. Pharm. Pharmacol. **22**, 141–143 (1970)

Meites, J., Lu, K.-H., Wuttke, W., Welsch, C.W., Nagasawa, H., Quadri, S.K.: Recent studies on functions and control of prolactin secretion in rats. Recent Prog. Horm. Res. **28**, 471–526 (1972)

Meltzer, H.Y., Fang, V.S.: Serum prolactin levels in schizophrenia: effect of antipsychotic drugs. A preliminary report. In: Hormones, behaviour and psychopathology. Sachar, E.J. (ed.). New York: Raven Press 1976

Meltzer, H.Y., Stahl, M.: The dopamine hypothesis of schizophrenia: a review. Schizophrenia Bull. **2**, 19–76 (1976)

Miller, R.J., Horn, A.S., Iversen, L.L.: The action of neuroleptic drugs on dopaminestimulated adenosine cyclic 3′,5′monophosphate production in rat neostriatum and limbic forebrain. Mol. Pharmacol. **10**, 759–766 (1974)

Miller, R.J., Horn, A.S., Iversen, L.L.: Effect of butaclamol on dopamine-sensitive adenylate cyclase in rat striatum. J. Pharm. Pharmacol. **27**, 212–213 (1975)

Modigh, K.: Functional aspects of 5-hydroxytryptamine turnover in the central nervous system. Acta Physiol. Scand., Suppl. 403, 5–56 (1974)

Modigh, K.: Electro-convulsive shock and postsynaptic catecholamine effects: Increased psychomotor stimulant action of apomorphine and clonidine in reserpine-pretreated mice by repeated ECS. J. Neural Transm. **36**, 19–32 (1975)

Modigh, K., Svensson, T.H.: On the role of central nervous system catecholamines and 5-hydroxytryptamine in the nialamide-induced behavioural syndrome. Br. J. Pharmacol. **46**, 32–45 (1972)

Möller-Nielsen, I., Fjalland, B., Pedersen, V., Nymark, M.: Pharmacology of neuroleptics upon repeated administration. Psychopharmacology **34**, 95–104 (1974)

Nybäck, H.: On the relation between transmitter turnover and impulse flow in brain catecholamine neurons. In: Chemical tools in catecholamine research. II. Almgren, O., Carlsson, A., Engel, J. (eds.), pp. 127–134. Amsterdam: North Holland 1975

Nybäck, H., Sedvall, G.: Further studies on the accumulation and disappearance of catecholamines formed from tyrosine-^{14}C in mouse brain. Effect of some phenothiazine analogues. Eur. J. Pharmacol. **10**, 193–205 (1970)

Nybäck, H.V., Walters, J.R., Aghajanian, G.K., Roth, R.H.: Tricyclic antidepressants: effects on the firing rate of brain noradrenergic neurons. Eur. J. Pharmacol. **32**, 302–312 (1975)

Nyberg, G., Axelsson, R., Mårtensson, E.: On the binding of thioridazine and thioridazine metabolites to serum proteins in psychiatric patients. Eur. J. Clin. Pharmacol. (1979) (in press)

Öhman, R., Larsson, M., Nilsson, I.M., Engel, J., Carlsson, A.: Neurometabolic and behavioural effects of haloperidol in relation to drug levels in serum and brain. Naunyn Schmiedebergs Arch. Pharmacol. **299**, 105–114 (1977)

Okada, Y.: Role of GABA in the substantia nigra. In: GABA in nervous system function. Roberts, E., Chase, T.N., Tower, D.B. (eds.), pp. 235–243. New York: Raven Press 1976

O'Keefe, R., Sharman, D.F., Vogt, M.: Effect of drugs used in psychoses on cerebral dopamine metabolism. Br. J. Pharmacol. **38**, 287–304 (1970)

Otsuka, M., Konishi, S., Takahaski, T.: Hypothalamic substance P as a candidate for transmitter of primary afferent neurons. Fed. Proc. **34**, 1922–1928 (1975)

Persson, S.-Å., Johansson, H.: The effect of lysergic acid diethylamide (LSD) and 2-bromo-lysergic acid diethylamide (BOL) on the striatal DOPA accumulation: influence of central 5-hydroxytryptaminergic pathways. Brain Res. **142**, 505–513 (1978)

Pijnenburg, A.J.J., Woodruff, G.N., van Rossum, J.M.: Ergometrine induced locomotor activity following intracerebral injection into the nucleus accumbens. Brain Res. **59**, 289–302 (1973)

Powell, D., Leeman, S.E., Tregear, G.W., Niall, H.D., Potts, J.T.: Radioimmunoassay for substance P. Nature [New Biol.] **241**, 252–254 (1973)

van Praag, H.M.: Therapy-resistant depressions: biochemical and pharmacological considerations. Psychother. Psychosom. **23**, 169–178 (1974)

van Praag, H.M., van den Burg, W., Bos, E.R.H., Dols, L.C.W.: 5-Hydroxytryptophan in combination with clomipramine in "therapy-resistant" depressions. Psychopharmacology **38**, 625–648 (1974)

Roberts, E., Chase, T.N., Tower, D.B. (eds.): GABA in nervous system function. In: Kroc Foundation Series, vol. V. New York: Raven Press 1976

Samanin, R., Bernasconi, S., Garattini, S.: The effect of nomifensine on the depletion of brain serotonin and catecholamines induced respectively by fenfluramine and 6-hydroxydopamine in rats. Eur. J. Pharmacol. **34**, 377–380 (1975)

Schaar, C.J., Clemens, J.A.: The role of catecholamines in the release of anterior pituitary prolactin *in vitro*. Endocrinology **95**, 1202–1212 (1974)

Scheel-Krüger, J.: Pharmacological studies on a counterbalancing adrenergic-cholinergic system in the brain. Acta Physiol. Scand. 77, Suppl. 330, 66 (1969)

Scheel-Krüger, J.: Comparative studies of various amphetamine analogues demonstrating different interactions with the metabolism of the catecholamines in the brain. Eur. J. Pharmacol. **14**, 47–59 (1971)

Scheel-Krüger, J.: Some aspects of the mechanisms of action of various stimulant amphetamine analogues. Psychiatr. Neurol. Neurochir. **75**, 179–192 (1972)

Schlatter, E.K.E., Lal, S.: Treatment of alcoholism with Dent's oral apomorphine method. Q. J. Stud. Alcohol. **33**, 430–436 (1972)

Sedvall, G., Nybäck, G.: Neuroleptikabehandling vid schizofreni. Nord. Psyk. Tidskr. **26**, 323–340 (1972)

Sedvall, G., Alfredsson, G., Bjerkenstedt, L., Eneroth, P., Fyrö, B., Härnryd, C., Swahn, C.-G., Wiesel, F.-A., Wode-Helgodt, B.: Selective effects of psychoactive drugs on levels of monoamine metabolites and prolactin in cerebrospinal fluid of psychiatric patients. In: Proceedings of the Sixth International Congress of Pharmacology. Tuomisto, J., Paasonen, M.K. (eds.), Vol. III, pp. 255–267. Helsinki, Finland: 1975

Seeman, P., Lee, T.: Antipsychotic drugs: direct correlation between clinical potency and presynaptic action on dopamine neurons. Science **188**, 1217–1219 (1975)

Seeman, P., Staiman, A., Lee, T., Chang-Wang, M.: The membrane actions of tranquillizers in relation to neuroleptic-induced Parkinsonism and tardive dyskinesia. In: The phenothiazines and structurally related drugs. Forrest, S., Carr, C.J., Usdin, E. (eds.), pp. 137–148. New York: Raven Press 1974

Seeman, P., Lee, T., Chan-Wong, M., Wong, K.: Antipsychotic drug doses and neuroleptic dopamine receptors. Nature **261**, 717–719 (1976)

Sethy, V.H., van Woert, M.H.: Modification of striatal acetylcholine concentration by dopamine receptor agonists and antagonists. Res. Commun. Chem. Pathol. Pharmacol. **8**, 13–28 (1974)

Shopsin, B.S., Gershon, S., Goldstein, M., Friedman, E., Wilk, S.: Use of synthesis inhibitors in defining role for biogenic amines during imipramine treatment in depressed patients. Psychopharmacol. Commun. **1** (2), 239–249 (1975)

Shore, P.A.: Release of serotonin and catecholamines by drugs. Pharmacol. Rev. **14**, 531–550 (1962)

Sigg, E.B.: Pharmacological studies with tofranil. Can. Psychiatr. Assoc. J. **45**, 75–85 (1959)

Sigg, E.B., Soffer, L., Gyermek, L.: Influence of imipramine and related psychoactive agents on the effect of 5-hydroxytryptamine and catecholamines on the cat nictitating membrane. J. Pharmacol. Exp. Ther. **142**, 13–20 (1963)

Simpson, G.M., Branchey, M.H., Shiwastava, R.K.: Baclofen in schizophrenia. Lancet **1976 I**, 966–967

Siwers, B.: Clinical pharmacological assessment of some antidepressant drugs. Thesis Stockholm 1976

Smith, R.C., Davis, J.M.: Behavioural evidence for supersensitivity after chronic administration of haloperidol, clozapine, and thioridazine. Life Sci. **19**, 725–732 (1976)

Snyder, S.H., Burt, D.R., Creese, I.: The dopamine receptor of mammalian brain: direct demonstration of binding to agonist and antagonist states. Soc. Neurosci. Symp. **1**, 28–49 (1976)

Squires, R.F., Braestrup, C.: Benzodiazepine receptors in rat brain. Nature **266**, 732–734 (1977)

Stadler, H., Lloyd, K.B., Gadea-Ciria, M., Bartholoni, G.: Enhanced striatal acetylcholine release by chlorpromazine and its reversal by apomorphine. Brain Res. **55**, 476–480 (1973)

Stawarz, R.J., Hill, H., Robinson, S.E., Settler, P., Dingell, J.V., Sulser, F.: On the significance of the increase in homovanillic acid (HVA) caused by antipsychotic drugs in corpus striatum and limbic forebrain. Psychopharmacology **43**, 125–130 (1975)

Stein, L.: Self stimulation of the brain and central stimulant action of amphetamine. Fed. Proc. **23**, 836–850 (1964)

Stille, G., von, Lauener, H.: Zur Pharmakologie katatonigener Stoffe, I. Mitteilung: Korrelation zwischen neuroleptischer Katalepsie und Homovanillinsäuregehalt im C. striatum bei Ratten. Arzneim.-Forsch. **21**, 252–255 (1971)

Strömberg, U., Svensson, T.H., Waldeck, B.: On the mode of action of amantadine. J. Pharm. Pharmacol. **22**, 959–962 (1970)

Strömbom, U.: Antagonism by haloperidol of locomotor depression induced by small doses of apomorphine. J. Neural Transm. **40**, 191–194 (1977)

Svensson, T.: The effect of inhibition of catecholamine synthesis on dexamphetamine induced central stimulation. Eur. J. Pharmacol. **12**, 161–166 (1970)

Svensson, T.: Functional and biochemical effects of d- and l-amphetamine on central catecholamine neurons. Naunyn Schmiedebergs Arch. Pharmacol. **271**, 170–180 (1971)

Svensson, T.: Dopamine release and direct receptor activation in the central nervous system by D-145, an amantadine derivative. Eur. J. Pharmacol. **23**, 232–238 (1973)

Svensson, T., Strömberg, U.: Potentiation by amantadine hydrochloride of L-DOPA-induced effects in mice. J. Pharm. Pharmacol. **22**, 639–640 (1970)

Trabucchi, M., Cheney, D.L., Racagni, G., Costa, E.: In vivo inhibition of striatal acetylcholine turnover by L-dopa, apomorphine and (+)-amphetamine. Brain Res. **85**, 130–134 (1975)

Ungerstedt, U.: Stereotaxic mapping of the monoamine pathway in the rat brain. Acta Physiol. Scand. **82**, Suppl. 367, 1–48 (1971)

Ungerstedt, U., Ljungberg, T., Hoffer, B., Siggins, G.: Dopaminergic supersensitivity in the striatum. Adv. Neurol. **9**, 57–65 (1975)

Usdin, E., Snyder, S. (eds.): Frontiers in catecholamine research, pp.1–106. New York: Pergamon Press 1973a

Usdin, E., Snyder, S. (eds.): Frontiers in catecholamine research, pp. 399–626. New York: Pergamon Press 1973b

Wadstein, J., Öhlin, H., Stenberg, P.: Effects of apomorphine and apomorphine-L-dopa-carbidopa on alcohol post-intoxication symptoms. Drug Alcohol Dependence (1978) (in press)

Waldeck, B.: Effect of caffeine on locomotor activity and central catecholamine mechanisms: A study with special reference to drug interaction. Acta Pharmacol. Toxicol (Kbh.) **36**, Suppl. 4, 1–23 (1975)

Wålinder, J., Carlsson, A.: Potentiation of neuroleptics by catecholamine inhibitors. Br. Med. J. **1973 I**, 551–552

Wålinder, J., Skott, A., Carlsson, A., Roos, B.-E.: Potentiation by metyrosine of thioridazine effects in chronic schizophrenics. Arch. Gen. Psychiatr. **33**, 501–505 (1976a)

Wålinder, J., Skott, A., Nagy, A., Carlsson, A., Roos, B.-E.: Potentiation of the antidepressant action of chlomipramine by tryptophan. Arch. Gen. Psychiatr. **33**, 1384–1389 (1976b)

Walters, J.R., Roth, R.H.: Dopaminergic neurons: an in vivo system for measuring drug interactions with presynaptic receptors. Naunyn Schmiedebergs Arch. Pharmacol. **296**, 5–14 (1976)

Young, S.N., Sourkes, T.L.: Tryptophan in the central nervous system: regulation and significance. Adv. Neurochem. **2**, 133–191 (1977)

Zeller, E.A., Blanksma, L.A., Burkard, W.P., Pacha, W.L., Lazanas, J.C.: In vitro and in vivo inhibition of amine oxidases. Ann. N.Y. Acad. Sci. **80**, 583–590 (1959)

Zivkovic, B., Guidotti, A., Revuelta, A., Costa, E.: Effect of thioridazine, clozapine and other antipsychotics on the kinetic state of tyrosine hydroxylase and on the turnover rate of dopamine in striatum and nucleus accumbens. J. Pharmacol. Exp. Ther. **194**, 37–46 (1975)

Psychopharmakotherapie

Von

J. Angst und B. Woggon

Inhalt

A. Einleitung	244
B. Antipsychotika	248
I. Kurzwirksame Antipsychotika	248
II. Depotneuroleptika	255
C. Antidepressiva	258
I. Tri- und tetrazyklische Antidepressiva (Thymoleptika)	259
II. Monoaminooxydasehemmer	264
D. Psychostimulantien	268
E. Lithium	270
F. Anxiolytika	275
G. Betarezeptoren-Blocker	278
H. Hypnotika	280
I. Behandlung psychiatrischer Notfallsituationen	284
I. Allgemeines	284
II. Erregungszustände	285
III. Delirien	285
IV. Stupor	286
V. Dysleptische Krisen	286
J. Nebenwirkungen von Psychopharmaka	286
I. Kardiovaskuläre Nebenwirkungen	286
II. Vegetative Nebenwirkungen	288
III. Pigmentablagerungen in den Augen	289
IV. Gastrointestinale Nebenwirkungen	289
V. Unerwünschte Effekte auf Körpergewicht und Körpergröße	290
VI. Leberveränderungen	290
VII. Hämatologische Nebenwirkungen	291
VIII. Dermatologische Nebenwirkungen	292
IX. Endokrinologische Nebenwirkungen	292
X. Sexuelle Störungen	293
XI. Gravidität und Puerperium	293
XII. Stoffwechselveränderungen	295
XIII. Unerwartete Todesfälle	295
XIV. Neurologische Nebenwirkungen	295

XV. Epileptische Anfälle 298
XVI. Psychische Nebenwirkungen................ 298
XVII. Vergiftungen mit Psychopharmaka............. 299

Literatur 302

A. Einleitung

Die vorliegende zusammenfassende Darstellung der Psychopharmakotherapie kann auf 50 Seiten lediglich einen groben Überblick vermitteln. Eine größere Zahl wichtiger Themen muß unberücksichtigt bleiben, beispielsweise methodische Grundprobleme, Beziehung zur Pharmakopsychologie, Regeln für die Behandlung von Kindern und Alterspatienten, Vorgehen beim Umstellen von einem Psychopharmakon auf ein anderes, Pharmakogenetik, ethische und juristische Probleme (ANGST u. DINKELKAMP, 1974; CAMPBEL u. SHAPIRO, 1975; CORNU, 1963; MÖLLER, 1976).

1. Klassifikation

Von verschiedenen Einteilungsprinzipien der Psychopharmaka hat sich für den Kliniker am besten dasjenige nach der Wirkung bewährt (PÖLDINGER, 1967; PÖLDINGER u. SCHMIDLIN, 1972): 1. Psychopharmaka im engeren Sinne (Antipsychotika, Anxiolytika, Antidepressiva), 2. Psychopharmaka im weiteren Sinne (Hypnotika, Sedativa, Antiepileptika, Psychostimulantien) und 3. Psychopharmaka mit psychotomimetischer Wirkung (Psycholytika oder Psychodysleptika).

Wir haben uns auf die Darstellung folgender Gruppen beschränkt: Antipsychotika, Antidepressiva, Psychostimulantien, Lithium, Anxiolytika, Betarezeptorenblocker und Hypnotika. Besonderes Gewicht wird auf die Beschreibung der Nebenwirkungen gelegt (KLINE u. ANGST, 1979).

Innerhalb der einzelnen Gruppen werden die Psychopharmaka entsprechend bestimmten Wirkungskomponenten oder chemischer Ähnlichkeit unterteilt. Auf einzelne Substanzen konnte im Text nicht eingegangen werden; sie wurden auszugsweise in Tabellen zusammengestellt (generic name, Handelsname in der Bundesrepublik Deutschland, Österreich und der Schweiz, Dosierungsbereich). Die den generic names in Klammern beigefügte Zahl bezieht sich auf die von USDIN und EFRON (1972) zusammengestellte Übersicht der Psychopharmaka (mit Strukturformeln). Ausführliche und bezüglich der einzelnen Präparate detailliertere Darstellungen der Therapie mit Psychopharmaka finden sich bei ANGST (1969), BENKERT und HIPPIUS (1974), DEGKWITZ (1967), HEINRICH (1976), MEYERS und SOLOMON (1974).

2. Indikationsstellung

Aufgrund der weitgehend fehlenden Kenntnis über die Ursachen psychiatrischer Erkrankungen, insbesondere der endogenen Psychosen, ist eine kausale Behandlung bisher nicht möglich. Psychopharmaka haben keinen nachgewiesenen Einfluß auf den eigentlichen Krankheitsprozeß, sondern lindern oder unterdrücken die subjektiv empfundenen und objektiv beobachtbaren Symptome.

Entsprechend erfolgt die Indikationsstellung in der Regel nicht anhand der nosologischen Diagnose, sondern aufgrund der vorhandenen Symptome oder Syndrome. Eine spezifische Indikationsstellung, d.h. die Auswahl des für einen bestimmten Patienten richtigen Medikamentes, ist kaum möglich, weil Kriterien fehlen, die eine Voraussage des Therapieerfolges erlauben würden. In diesem Zusammenhang ist darauf hinzuweisen, daß es recht unterschiedliche Definitionen der Begriffe „Therapieerfolg" und „Therapieresistenz" gibt.

3. Prognostika

BIELSKI und FRIEDEL (1976) haben eine kritische Literaturübersicht zum Thema „Voraussage des Therapieerfolges von trizyklischen Antidepressiva" zusammengestellt und dabei nur recht grobe Prädikatoren gefunden: höhere Gesellschaftsschicht, plötzlicher Beginn, Appetitlosigkeit, Gewichtsverlust, Durchschlafstörungen und psychomotorische Störungen. Eine ausführliche Darstellung des heutigen Wissensstandes über Therapieprädikatoren findet sich bei ANGST (1976).

Vielleicht sind die bisherigen Bemühungen, Therapieprädikatoren zu finden, unter anderem daran gescheitert, daß vor allem der Ausgangsbefund vor Behandlungsbeginn berücksichtigt wurde. Künftige Forschungen sollten versuchen, von den in den ersten Stunden und Tagen der Psychopharmakabehandlung beobachteten Veränderungen von Symptomen, Gefühlen und Leistungen auszugehen.

4. Bedeutung der Psychopharmakotherapie

Im Gesamtbehandlungsplan nehmen die Psychopharmaka bei schweren psychischen Störungen einen zentralen Platz ein und werden in ihrer Wirkung durch andere Behandlungsverfahren, zum Beispiel Beschäftigungstherapie, unterstützt. Häufig ermöglicht erst eine medikamentös erzielte Symptomreduktion den Einsatz anderer Therapieformen, zum Beispiel Psychotherapie oder Rehabilitationsverfahren. Schematisch ausgedrückt besteht die Wirkung der Psychopharmaka vor allem in einem Abbau von Symptomen oder negativen Verhaltensweisen, wodurch nicht automatisch ein Aufbau oder ein neues Erlernen positiver („lebensbewältigender") Verhaltensweisen einsetzt, jedoch ermöglicht wird. Eine zu frühe, d.h. vor einer ausreichenden Symptomreduktion einsetzende Konfliktkonfrontation und Forderung nach „gesundem Verhalten" kann gerade bei endogenen Psychosen (Schizophrenie, Affektpsychosen) nicht nur erfolglos bleiben, sondern schwerste Rückfälle provozieren. Individuelles Wohlbefinden, soziale Integration, Bewältigung lebensgeschichtlich und situationsbedingter Konflikte und Probleme können oft nicht allein durch eine Symptomreduktion erreicht werden, setzen diese aber voraus.

5. Kombinationstherapien

Beim gleichzeitigen Vorhandensein unterschiedlicher Symptome werden häufig mehrere Psychopharmaka verordnet. Solche Kombinationstherapien können aufgrund möglicher Interaktionen nicht nur mehr oder auch weniger Nebenwirkungen verursachen als es aus der Addition der Substanzen abzuleiten ist, sondern können auch zu einer Verminderung oder unbeabsichtigten Verstärkung der Wirkung führen. Die früher nachgewiesenen, kasuistisch belegten oder denkbaren Interaktionen der verschiedenen Psychopharmaka sind kaum überschaubar (AYD, 1977; GRANT u. WALLER, 1972). Daher sollten Kombinationen nur bei dringendem Bedarf verordnet werden.

6. Dosierung, Applikation

Dosierung, Applikationsmodus und Applikationshäufigkeit von Psychopharmaka sollten theoretisch auf der Basis pharmakokinetischer Befunde bestimmt werden, die jedoch leider nur für einen kleinen Teil der Substanzen zur Verfügung stehen und deren Wert durch eine ausgeprägte interindividuelle Variabilität stark relativiert wird. Dosis-Wirkungs-Beziehungen können selten festgestellt und noch seltener reproduziert werden. Bezüglich der Relevanz des Plasmaspiegels von Psychopharmaka für deren therapeutische Wirksamkeit liegen sehr unterschiedliche und teilweise widersprüchliche Befunde vor (ÅSBERG et al., 1971; BRAITHWAITE et al., 1972; KANE et al., 1976; PEREL, 1976); die darauf gesetzten Hoffnungen haben sich nicht erfüllt. Noch immer gilt es, sich bei der Behandlung jedes einzelnen Patienten an die optimale Dosierung „heranzutasten", häufig auf dem viel zitierten Wege der „einschleichenden Dosierung". Neben der Ausprägung der eine Behandlung erfordernden Symptome sollte die Dosierung von Psychopharmaka durch den allgemeinen Grundsatz „so wenig wie möglich" bestimmt werden. Die notwendige Dauer der Behandlung richtet sich weitgehend nach vorliegenden klinischen Erfahrungen mit dem betreffenden Krankheits- bzw. Zustandsbild. Abgesehen von wenigen Ausnahmen, wie der Behandlung psychiatrischer Notfallsituationen und der Verordnung von Schlafmitteln, wird eine wirksame Psychopharmakotherapie meist längere Zeit nach Erreichen des Therapiezieles (Symptomfreiheit oder Symptomreduktion) fortgesetzt und nur langsam wieder abgebaut, falls es sich nicht um eine Langzeitbehandlung im weiteren Sinne des Prophylaxebegriffes handelt. Die starke Ausrichtung jeder einzelnen Psychopharmakabehandlung auf den individuellen Einzelfall ist demnach weniger durch einen Individualitätsdrang der Psychiater zu erklären als vielmehr dadurch begründet, daß beim weitgehenden Fehlen gültiger allgemeiner Behandlungsregeln jede Therapie Ähnlichkeit mit einem Experiment hat.

7. Methodik

Vor der Einführung in den Handel wird die Wirkungsweise neuer Substanzen zunächst im Rahmen klinischer Prüfungen an möglichst großen Patientengruppen bestimmt. Die Problematik klinischer Psychopharmakaprüfungen soll hier nur kurz angedeutet werden. Detaillierte Darstellungen finden sich u.a. bei HEIMANN (1975, 1977), PICHOT (1975) und WOGGON (1977). Die Ergebnisse von Psychopharmakaprüfungen sind in zweierlei Hinsicht unbefriedigend:
1. Der globale Wirkungsnachweis eines Psychopharmakons ist zwar möglich, es können aber keine spezifischen Indikationen für einzelne Präparate bestimmt werden. Bisher konnten keine zuverlässigen prognostischen Kriterien erarbeitet werden, so daß bei der Behandlung des einzelnen Patienten die Möglichkeit

fehlt, das für ihn richtige Antidepressivum oder Neuroleptikum auszuwählen. Die Beurteilung, ob ein verordnetes Präparat dem Patienten wirklich helfen kann, ist meist erst nach zwei bis drei Wochen möglich. 2. Wirkungsunterschiede zwischen ähnlichen Präparaten lassen sich in der Regel nicht nachweisen oder nicht zuverlässig reproduzieren.

Die unbefriedigende Aussagekraft klinischer Prüfungen läßt sich weitgehend auf folgende Problemkreise zurückführen: Fehlen differenzierter Hypothesen, ungenügende Kontrolle wirkungsmodifizierender Faktoren, Stichproben-Heterogenität, Beschränkung auf Fremdbeurteilung psychopathologischer Symptome, uneinheitliche Dosisveränderungen und Zusatzmedikation. Die Formulierung differenzierter Hypothesen über die mögliche Wirkung eines Psychopharmakons auf psychische Funktionen läßt sich auf der Basis tierexperimenteller Befunde kaum vornehmen. Detaillierte pharmakopsychologische Untersuchungen zur Veränderung definierter Verhaltens-, Leistungs- und Stimmungsvariablen liegen jedoch in der Regel nicht vor oder werden nicht berücksichtigt, da ihre Bedeutung leider bisher von der Mehrzahl der klinischen Prüfer nicht anerkannt wird (DEBUS, 1977; DITTRICH, 1974; JANKE, 1973; JANKE u. DEBUS, 1975; LEHMANN u. HOPES, 1977).

Bei der Durchführung klinischer Prüfungen werden wirkungsmodifizierende Faktoren meist nicht beachtet oder es wird bei Doppelblindstudien zu Unrecht angenommen, daß sie durch randomisierte Patientenzuordnung kontrolliert werden. Als Beispiele für wirkungsmodifizierende Faktoren sollen genannt werden: Placeboeffekte, Erwartungshaltung von Untersucher und Patient, Milieueinflüsse, interindividuelle Variabilität der Dosiswirkungsbeziehung, Persönlichkeit und individuelle Verarbeitung primärer Pharmakawirkungen.

Die in eine Psychopharmakaprüfung aufzunehmenden Patienten werden nach klinischen Gesichtspunkten ausgewählt wie Diagnose, Symptommuster und bisheriger Krankheitsverlauf. Psychophysiologische Reaktivität, Vorhandensein und Ausprägung umschriebener Veränderungen psychischer Funktionen wie z. B. Störungen der Wahrnehmung und der Filterung des Informationszuflusses werden bisher bei der Patientenauswahl nicht berücksichtigt. Bezüglich psychischer und physiologischer Störungen, die neben der psychopathologischen Symptomatik vorhanden sein können und vielleicht mit dieser in ursächlichem Zusammenhang stehen, sind die Stichproben der klinischen Prüfungen demnach ausgesprochen heterogen. Die Wirkung von Psychopharmaka wird meist ausschließlich aufgrund der Veränderung psychopathologischer Symptome beurteilt. Diese Symptome stellen jedoch zum Teil recht komplexe Phänomene dar, deren unmittelbare Beeinflussung durch ein Psychopharmakon kaum vorstellbar ist. Als Beispiel soll das Symptom „Gedankenentzug" dienen, dessen Entstehung man sich folgendermaßen vorstellen kann: Ausgehend von der Erfahrung, daß seine Gedankenfolgen häufig abreißen und der Beobachtung, daß er sich nicht dagegen wehren kann, kommt der Patient zur Feststellung, daß seine Gedanken ohne bzw. gegen seinen Willen abbrechen. Die Interpretation, daß seine Gedanken ihm von außen oder von einer Person entzogen werden, stellt demnach ein komplexes Verarbeitungsprodukt dar.

Psychopathologische Symptome werden meist durch Fremdbeurteilung erfaßt. Die Einbeziehung anderer Informationsebenen zusätzlich zur Fremdbeurteilungsebene (Selbstbeurteilung, objektive Testverfahren, psychophysiologische Untersuchungen) würde nicht nur eine umfassendere Beurteilung der Pharmakonwirkung ermöglichen, sondern auch die Beeinflußbarkeit der erhobenen Befunde vermindern (LEHMANN, 1975a, b).

Bei klinischen Prüfungen ist die Einhaltung fixer Dosierungsschemata meist nicht möglich, da eine klinisch notwendige Dosissteigerung bei ausbleibender Wirkung sinnvoll ist. Werden jedoch zwei zu vergleichende Präparate in Anpassung an Wirkung und Nebenwirkungen dosiert, so ist nicht gesichert, daß zwei äquivalent dosierte Substanzen miteinander verglichen werden.

Auch die zusätzliche Verordnung von psychoaktiven Substanzen (z. B. Hypnotika, Tranquilizer) kann Verfälschungen der eigentlichen Wirkung der Prüfsubstanz bedingen. Obwohl bei klinischen Prüfungen solche Zusatzmedikationen aus methodischen Gründen nicht erlaubt sind, lassen sie sich nicht immer ausschließen.

8. Ausblick

Die verschiedenen erwähnten Problemkreise klinischer Prüfungen können vielleicht zum Teil mit Hilfe einer strengen experimentellen Versuchsanordnung in Akutversuchen (Überprüfung der Wirkung einer Einzeldosis) kontrolliert werden. Zur Validierung der Aussagekraft solcher pharmakopsychiatrischer Akutversuche sollen Kriterien erarbeitet werden, die es erlauben, aus den Resultaten im Akutversuch eine Voraussage des therapeutischen Erfolges nach 20–30 Behandlungstagen (mittlere übliche Prüfungszeit in Phase I und II) abzuleiten. Die Einführung von Akutversuchen in den Bereich klinischer Psychopharmakaprüfungen soll einerseits eine rasche und aussagekräftige Bestimmung der Wirkungsprofile von Psychopharmaka ermöglichen, andererseits die Möglichkeit schaffen, bei der Behandlung eines einzelnen Patienten nach einem oder wenigen Tagen den wahrscheinlichen Therapieerfolg voraussagen zu können.

B. Antipsychotika

Kurzwirksame Antipsychotika und Depotneuroleptika werden getrennt dargestellt, obwohl sie zu den gleichen chemischen Gruppen gehören und bezüglich Wirkung und Nebenwirkungen mehr Ähnlichkeiten als Unterschiede aufweisen. Diese Aufteilung wurde wegen der verschiedenen Indikationen und teilweise recht abweichenden Behandlungstechnik gewählt.

I. Kurzwirksame Antipsychotika

1. Terminologie und Klassifikation

Neuroleptika werden heute zunehmend auch im deutschen Sprachgebrauch als Antipsychotika bezeichnet, wodurch ihre spezifische Wirkung auf Halluzinationen, Wahngedanken und andere psychotische Symptome betont wird. Chemisch handelt es sich um Phenothiazine, Thioxanthene, Butyrophenone, Diphenylbutylpiperidine, Dibenzodiazepine und Rauwolfiaalkaloide. Klinisch hat sich bisher am besten die Einteilung nach der Ausprägung der zusätzlich vorhandenen dämpfenden Wirkungskomponente bewährt. Levomepromazin, Clopenthixol und Clozapin sind Beispiele für initial stark dämpfende Antipsychotika. Phenothiazine mit Piperazinyl-Seitenkette und Butyrophenone wirken weniger dämpfend. Die früher geltende Auffassung, daß stark dämpfende Neuroleptika eine schwächere antipsychotische Wirkung haben als weniger dämpfende Substanzen, wird heute nicht mehr als richtig angesehen.

2. Klinische Wirkung

Antipsychotika bewirken eine Antriebs- und Affekthemmung und führen so zu einer relativen Indifferenz gegenüber Innen- und Außenwelt. Sie vermindern die psychomotorische Aktivität, wirken beruhigend, entspannend und besonders initial schlafanstoßend. Ihre antipsychotische Wirkung zeigt sich in einer Beeinflussung produktiver psychotischer Symptome (Halluzinationen, Wahn, Denk- und Affektstörungen), aber auch der sog. schizophrenen Minussymptome (Apathie, Interesselosigkeit und Autismus). In letzter Zeit wurde vermehrt über eine antidepressive Wirkungskomponente verschiedener Neuroleptika berichtet; eine gewisse antidepressive Wirkung wird Chlorprothixen, Levomepromazin und Thioridazin zugeschrieben. Antipsychotika erhöhen die Streßtoleranz, wirken antiemetisch, antiallergisch und rufen weder psychische noch körperliche Abhängigkeit hervor.

3. Wirkungseintritt

Bei der Betrachtung des Wirkungseintrittes von Antipsychotika muß man zwischen akuten und chronischen Zustandsbildern streng unterscheiden. Beobachtet man die Neuroleptikawirkung bei akuten Psychosen, so fällt auf, daß sich die einzelnen Wirkungskomponenten unterschiedlich rasch auswirken. Der dämpfende und entspannende Effekt wird sehr schnell deutlich, meist schon nach wenigen Stunden. Die antipsychotische Wirkung ist in der Regel erst nach einigen Tagen zu beobachten. Allerdings ist darauf hinzuweisen, daß sich mittels einer detaillierteren Erfassung psychopathologischer Symptome meist schon nach 3 bis 5 Tagen eine deutliche antipsychotische Wirkung nachweisen läßt.

4. Indikation

Die Indikationsstellung für die Behandlung mit Neuroleptika richtet sich in erster Linie nach dem vorhandenen Symptommuster und erst in zweiter Linie nach der nosologischen Diagnose. Die Zielsymptome und Zielsyndrome der neuroleptischen Behandlung lassen sich aus den Wirkungskomponenten der Antipsychotika ableiten. Die dämpfende Wirkungskomponente bedingt die Verwendung von Neuroleptika zur Behandlung von Angetriebenheit und Erregungszuständen. Ausgeprägte emotionale Spannungen und Angst werden durch die affektiv distanzierende oder abschirmende Wirkung der Neuroleptika günstig beeinflußt. Der sedierende und initial schlafanstoßende Effekt erweist sich als nützlich in der Behandlung schwerer Schlafstörungen. Die antipsychotische Wirkungskomponente ist vor allem wichtig für die Behandlung paranoider Denkinhalte, halluzinatorischer Erlebnisse und psychotischer Denkstörungen, wirkt sich jedoch auch günstig aus auf die sog. schizophrene Minussymptomatik, die gekennzeichnet ist durch Antriebsarmut, Interesselosigkeit und affektive Nivellierung.

Gültige Kriterien für eine spezifische Indikation einzelner Präparate konnten bisher nicht aufgestellt werden. Für die klinische Anwendung der Neuroleptika hat sich die Einteilung in stark dämpfende, mittelgradig dämpfende und wenig dämpfende Substanzen am besten bewährt. Stark dämpfende Antipsychotika sind vor allem bei Erregungszuständen, ausgeprägter psychischer und motorischer Angetriebenheit und Panik indiziert. Dementsprechend werden sie vor allem bei Manie und akuter Schizophrenie verwendet, häufig in Form einer Notfalltherapie.

Mittelstark dämpfende Neuroleptika werden am häufigsten zur Behandlung produktiver psychotischer Symptome bei Psychosen des schizophrenen Formenkreises verwendet.

Wenig dämpfende Antipsychotika sind vor allem zur Behandlung chronisch schizophrener Psychosen geeignet. Die bei diesen Krankheitsbildern zentrale Bemühung um Rehabilitation und dauerhafte soziale Integration wird häufig erst durch die stabilisierende Wirkung der Neuroleptika ermöglicht. Neben einer Reduktion der Hospitalisierungsdauer verhindert oder verzögert ihre langfristige Anwendung psychotische Rückfälle.

5. Kontraindikationen

Absolute Kontraindikationen sind kaum bekannt, ausgenommen die Gabe von Rauwolfiaalkaloiden bei Ulkusanamnese. Besondere Vorsicht ist notwendig bei Patienten mit Glaukom, Harnverhalten, Pylorusstenose, Prostatahypertrophie, kardiovaskulären Erkrankungen und organischen Hirnschäden. Bei Vorliegen dieser körperlichen Störungen ist eine langsam einschleichende Dosierung zu empfehlen. Während der Schwangerschaft ist die Einnahme von Neuroleptika möglichst zu vermeiden.

6. Nebenwirkungen

Eine detaillierte Darstellung der Nebenwirkungen findet sich in Kapitel J. Hier soll nur eine kurze Aufstellung der häufigeren Nebenwirkungen gegeben werden, die sich während der Behandlung mit einem Neuroleptikum entwickeln können.

Besonders wichtig und störend sind die extrapyramidalen Nebenwirkungen. Frühdyskinesien oder Dystonien können schon in der ersten Behandlungswoche auftreten. Etwas später kann sich ein neuroleptisch bedingtes Parkinsonsyndrom entwickeln. Die Akathisie stellt eine subjektiv besonders unangenehme Begleiterscheinung der neuroleptischen Behandlung dar. Spätdyskinesien werden erst nach längerer neuroleptischer Therapie beobachtet und können auch nach Absetzen der Antipsychotika persistieren.

Die anticholinerge und adrenerge Wirkungskomponente der Neuroleptika führen zu verschiedenen vegetativen Nebenwirkungen: Trockenheit der Schleimhäute (Mund, Nase, Vagina), Blutdrucksenkung, Tachykardie und Akkommodationsstörungen. Miktionsstörungen, Heißhunger, Exantheme und Galaktorrhoe werden nicht selten beobachtet. Nach langdauernder Gabe kann es zu einer Verminderung von Libido und Potenz kommen. Durch eine Senkung der Krampfschwelle können epileptische Anfälle provoziert werden. Überdosierungen können Delirien hervorrufen. Entzugserscheinungen, die auf eine mögliche Suchtkomponente hinweisen würden, sind nicht bekannt.

Bei 0,1 bis 1,0 $^0/_{00}$ der mit trizyklischen Neuroleptika behandelten Patienten werden Agranulozytosen beobachtet. Durch das im Südwesten von Finnland gehäufte Auftreten von Agranulozytose-Erkrankungen unter Clozapinbehandlung wurde diese Nebenwirkung trizyklischer Psychopharmaka in letzter Zeit sehr intensiv diskutiert. Aufgrund der Erfahrung, daß die frühzeitige Erkennung einer beginnenden Knochenmarkdepression durch die Diagnosestellung im klinisch asymptomatischen Stadium für die Prognose der Agranulozytose entscheidend ist, sind wöchentliche Leukozytenzählungen während der ersten 18 Behandlungswochen dringend zu empfehlen, am besten ergänzt durch tägliche Temperaturmessungen. Leider hat sich gezeigt, daß diese technisch einfachen Vorsichtsmaßnahmen nicht ausreichend befolgt werden, so daß Clozapin nach dem 1. November 1977 in der Schweiz nur noch an Klinikapotheken geliefert wird.

7. Applikation und Dosierung

Antipsychotika werden in der Regel per os verabreicht. Die parenterale Applikation (vor allem intramuskulär, selten intravenös) ist folgenden Situationen vorbehalten:

a) Parenterale Applikation kurzwirkender Neuroleptika

Bei Verweigerung oder Unmöglichkeit der oralen Einnahme, speziell zur notfallmäßig dringend erforderlichen Ruhigstellung bei Erregungszuständen und aggressivem Verhalten mit Selbst- und Fremdgefährdung. Die zur parenteralen Behandlung am häufigsten verwendeten Substanzen sind Perphenazin, Trifluoperazin, Fluphenazin, Haloperidol, Promazin und Thiothixen. Aufgrund der raschen Resorption tritt die beruhigende Wirkung verhältnismäßig schnell ein. Bezüglich der Dosierung gibt es zwei Möglichkeiten: a) niedrigere Dosierung, die im Abstand von $^1/_2$ bis 1 Stunde mehrmals wiederholt werden kann, b) einmalige Applikation einer hohen Dosierung. Es werden dabei teilweise recht große Tagesdosierungen verwendet, beispielsweise 60–100 mg Haloperidol. Sicher ist die intramuskuläre Anwendung für erregte Patienten geeigneter als die intravenöse Applikation, deren Überlegenheit bezüglich Wirkungseintritt und Wirkungsgrad bisher auch nicht nachgewiesen werden konnte. In diesem Zusammenhang ist eine multizentrische Prüfung von Fluphenazinhydrochlorid zur Akutbehandlung interessant, bei der kein wesentlicher Wirkungsunterschied zwischen intravenöser und intramuskulärer Applikationsweise gefunden wurde (PIESCHL et al., 1976). Bei der parenteralen Anwendung von Neuroleptika zur Akutbehandlung wird in der Regel recht hoch dosiert, was eine sorgfältige

Kreislaufüberwachung und Beachtung extrapyramidaler Nebenwirkungen notwendig macht. Neben den schon erwähnten Präparaten sind auch andere Neuroleptika, z. B. die stark dämpfenden Substanzen Levomepromazin und Clozapin, zur Akutbehandlung mit intramuskulären Injektionen geeignet.

b) Parenterale Applikation von Depotneuroleptika

Die Mehrzahl der zur Verfügung stehenden Depotneuroleptika (ausführliche Darstellung siehe Kapitel B.II.) liegt nicht in oral applizierbarer Form vor, sondern wird intramuskulär injiziert. Bei der Behandlung mit diesen Substanzen geht es um eine langfristige Therapie, die sich meist über viele Jahre erstreckt und bei der im Vergleich zur oralen Behandlungsform kleinere Dosierungen verwendet werden.

Bezüglich der Dosierung einzelner Präparate sei auf Tabelle 1 hingewiesen. Als Regel kann gelten, daß vor allem bei der langfristigen Behandlung mit Neuroleptika möglichst niedrige Dosierungen angestrebt werden sollen, d. h. die beste Einstellung auf ein Neuroleptikum ist diejenige mit der niedrigsten noch wirksamen Dosis. Zur Vermeidung extrapyramidaler und vegetativer Nebenwirkungen empfiehlt es sich, initial eher niedrig zu dosieren und im Verlauf einiger Tage die Dosis langsam bis zum Erreichen der Erhaltungsdosis zu steigern. Bei der Behandlung akut-psychotischer Patienten mit ausgeprägter Erregung muß von dieser Dosierungsregel abgewichen werden.

In letzter Zeit wurde in speziellen Indikationen versuchsweise eine *Behandlung mit sehr hohen Dosen von Neuroleptika* durchgeführt. Dabei handelt es sich vor allem um die Präparate Fluphenazin (100–1200 mg), Flupenthixol (60–300 mg), Haloperidol (60–300 mg), Perphenazin (120–600 mg) und Trifluoperazin (120–600 mg). Offenbar kommt es bei derart hohen Dosierungen weniger zur Entwicklung extrapyramidaler Nebenwirkungen als in einem mittleren Dosisbereich, wofür es bisher keine sichere pharmakologische oder biochemische Erklärung gibt. Eine mögliche Erklärung könnte darin zu finden sein, daß bei derart hohen Dosen die anticholinerge Wirkungskomponente der Neuroleptika so stark ausgeprägt ist, daß die Entwicklung extrapyramidaler Nebenwirkungen unterdrückt wird. Allerdings ist diese Behandlungsmethode noch nicht genug erprobt, um etwas über die Häufigkeit von Spätdyskinesien aussagen zu können. Daher empfiehlt GERLACH (1977) in einer Literaturzusammenstellung die zeitliche Begrenzung der Gabe hoher Neuroleptikadosen auf 2 bis 3 Monate. Er führt folgende Kontraindikationen auf: spezielle Neuroleptikaempfindlichkeit bei älteren Patienten, Patienten mit intrazerebralen Affektionen, endogenen Depressionen und Patienten mit schweren Herz-, Leber- und Nierenleiden. Wegen der bisher noch nicht sicher abgeklärten Verträglichkeit wird eine begrenzte Anwendung bei therapieresistenten Patienten empfohlen.

Nicht nur bei Therapiebeginn, sondern auch beim Umstellen auf ein anderes Neuroleptikum ergibt sich die Schwierigkeit, adäquate bzw. äquivalente Dosierungen verschiedener Neuroleptika anzugeben. Eine Doppelblindstudie zur Frage des Umstellungseffektes konnte eine vermehrte Rückfallhäufigkeit bei denjenigen schizophrenen Patienten nachweisen, die auf ein anderes Neuroleptikum umgestellt worden waren, im Vergleich zu den Patienten, die weiterhin ihre neuroleptische Dauermedikation eingenommen hatten (GARDOS, 1974).

Das Auftreten feinmotorischer Veränderungen (Handschrift) wird von HAASE et al. (1974) als Zeichen für eine wirksame neuroleptische Dosis gewertet und dient zur Bestimmung der von ihm beschriebenen „neuroleptischen Schwelle", deren Bedeutung jedoch umstritten ist, besonders seit der Einführung des Clozapin, dessen antipsychotische Wirksamkeit nicht von extrapyramidalen Nebenwirkungen begleitet ist.

8. Behandlungsdauer

Die Behandlungsdauer ist in erster Linie vom Verlauf des zu behandelnden Zustandsbildes und von der Definition des Therapiezieles abhängig. Will man z. B. einen Patienten, der wegen eines Erregungszustandes notfallmäßig psychiatrisch hospitalisiert werden muß, medikamentös ruhigstellen, so ist dieses Therapieziel innerhalb von Stunden oder wenigen Tagen zu erreichen. Auch in der Behandlung der Manie werden Neuroleptika für relativ kurze Zeiträume verwendet. Anders sieht es bei der Behandlung schizophrener Schübe aus. Hier sollte auch nach Erreichen einer ausgeprägten Besserung der Symptomatik oder gar Symptomfreiheit die Medikation noch einige Zeit weitergeführt werden. Von verschiedenen Autoren werden feste Zeiträume für diese Fortsetzung der Neuroleptikagabe empfohlen, was jedoch äußerst problematisch ist. Am besten ist es, wenn im Einzelfall nach Stabilisierung des symptomfreien Zustandes oder Habitualzustandes ganz langsam eine vorsichtige Dosisreduktion vorgenommen wird. Auf diese Weise ist es jederzeit möglich, eine eventuell beginnende Verschlechterung durch Dosiserhöhung aufzufangen.

Für die Langzeitbehandlung chronisch schizophrener Psychosen werden in erster Linie Depotneuroleptika verwendet, da so eine gewichtige Dosiseinsparung möglich ist.

Unklar ist die Behandlungsdauer, die man bei ausbleibendem therapeutischen Erfolg eines Neuroleptikums einhalten sollte. Auch dafür lassen sich keine festen Regeln aufstellen.

Aufgrund der Beobachtung, daß chronisch schizophrene Patienten unter Langzeitbehandlung mit Neuroleptika eine Affekt- und Antriebsverminderung aufweisen, wurden mehrfach sog. Absetzstudien durchgeführt, um die Notwendigkeit der weiteren Neuroleptikabehandlung und die Rückfallgefährdung zu überprüfen (ANDREWS et al., 1976; BLACKBURN u. ALLEN, 1961; BURNETT et al., 1975; DENBER u. BIRD, 1955; DIAMOND u. MARKS, 1960; GOOD et al., 1958; GROSS et al., 1960; LUTZ, 1965; MEADOW et al., 1975; MORGAN u. CHEADLE, 1974; OLSON u. PETERSON, 1960; PRIEN u. KLETT, 1972; PRIEN et al., 1971; RAVARIS et al., 1967; ROTHSTEIN, 1960; UHLÍŘ et al., 1973). Die Resultate der verschiedenen Absetzstudien ermöglichen keine einheitliche Aussage darüber, für welche Patienten eine Beendigung der Neuroleptikagabe oder aber eine intermittierende Behandlung am vorteilhaftesten sind. 40–70% chronisch schizophrener Patienten, bei denen die neuroleptische Dauermedikation abgesetzt wird, zeigen innerhalb von 6 Monaten einen Rückfall. Einige Autoren stellten eine erhöhte Rückfalltendenz bei Patienten fest, die vorher mit relativ großen Neuroleptikadosierungen behandelt worden waren.

Auch wenn sich bisher nicht mit Sicherheit sagen läßt, welche chronisch schizophrenen Patienten am ehesten von einer Unterbrechung der Neuroleptikatherapie profitieren, so sollte doch gerade bei nicht optimal gebesserten Patienten eine zumindest vorübergehende Unterbrechung dieser Behandlung in Erwägung gezogen werden.

9. Antipsychotisch wirksame Präparate

Die antipsychotisch wirksamen Substanzen sind mit generic name, Handelsnamen und üblicher Dosierung auszugsweise in Tabelle 1 zusammengestellt.

Tabelle 1. Antipsychotika

Internationale chemische Kurzbezeichnung (generic name)	Handelsnamen			Dosierung (per os, mg/Tag)	
	BRD	Österreich	Schweiz	klinisch	ambulant
1. Phenothiazine					
1.1. Aminoalkylphenothiazine					
Chlorpromazin (20)[a]	Largactil Megaphen	Largactil Chlorpromazin	Largactil Chlorazin	150–600	50–200
Levomepromazin (69)	Neurocil	Nozinan	Nozinan	100–600	50–200
Promazin (98)	Protactyl Verophen	–	Prazine	150–1000	50–200
Trifluopromazin (132)	Psyquil	Psyquil	Siquil	75–300	50–150
1.2. Piperazinylalkylphenothiazine (Phenothiazin-Derivate mit Piperazinylalkyl-Seitenkette)					
Fluphenazin (47)	Dapotum Lyogen Omca	Dapotum Lyogen Omca	Dapotum Permitil Lyogen Moditen	2–20	3–6
Perazin (84)	Taxilan	Taxilan	–	75–600	75–300
Perphenazin (86)	Decentan	Decentan	Trilafon	12–64	8–32
Prochlorperazin (95)	–	–	Stemetil	30–150	15–60
Thioproperazin (124)	Mayeptil	Majeptil	Majeptil	10–50	5–10
Thiopropazat (123)	Tonoquil Vesitan	–	Dartal Tonoquil Vesitan	20–60	10–30
Trifluoperazin (130)	Jatroneural	Jatroneural	Eskazinyl Terfluzine	6–30	2–10
1.3. Piperidylalkylphenothiazine (Phenothiazin-Derivate mit Piperidylalkyl-Seitenkette)					
Mepazin (64)	Pacatal	Pacatal	–	50–400	25–150
Mesoridazin (65) (=Sulforidazin)	Inofal	Lidanil	Lidanil	150–600	75–200
Propericiazin (100) (=Periciazin)	Aolept	Neuleptil	Neuleptil	50–150	20–60
Thioridazin (125)	Melleril	Melleril	Melleril	200–600	75–200

Tabelle 1 (Fortsetzung)

Internationale chemische Kurzbezeichnung (generic name)	Handelsnamen			Dosierung (per os, mg/Tag)	
	BRD	Österreich	Schweiz	klinisch	ambulant
2. Thioxanthene					
Chlorprothixen (168)	Taractan Truxal	Taractan Truxal	Taractan Truxal	150–600	50–150
Clopenthixol (173)	Ciatyl	Sordinol	Sordinol	100–300	20–150
Flupenthixol (191)	Fluanxol	Fluanxol	Fluanxol	2–10	1–3
Thiothixen (243)	Orbinamon	Orbinamon	–	20–80	10–30
3. Butyrophenone					
Benperidol (608)	Glianimon	–	–	1–6	0,25–1,5
Bromperidol (609)	noch in Entwicklung			6–10 mg	
Floropipamid (616)	Dipiperon	Dipiperon	Dipiperon	160–360	80–160
Haloperidol (621)	Haldol	Haldol	Haloperidol	2–20	1–6
Methylperidol (623)	Luvatrena	Luvatren	Luvatren	15–30	10–20
Trifluoperidol (633)	Triperidol	Triperidol	Triperidol	2–8	1–4
4. Diphenylbutylpiperidine					
Pimozid (925)	Orap	Orap	Orap	4–10	3–6
5. Dibenzodiazepine					
Clozapin (199)	Leponex	Leponex	Leponex	25–600	12,5–150
6. Dibenzothiazepine					
Clotiapin (174)	–	Entumin	Entumine	120–200	60–120
7. Rauwolfiaalkaloide					
Reserpin (318)	Sedaraupin Serpasil	Serpasil	Serpasil	2–8	1–3
8. Andere Strukturen					
Sulpirid (982)	Dogmatil	–	Dogmatil	300–600	100–300

[a] Die in Klammern den generic names beigefügte Zahl bezieht sich auf die von Usdin und Efron (1972) herausgegebene Zusammenstellung psychotroper Substanzen

II. Depotneuroleptika

1. Terminologie und Klassifikation

Depot- oder Langzeitneuroleptika sind Substanzen mit neuroleptischem Wirkungsprofil, deren Wirkung mindestens einige Tage anhält. Chemisch handelt es sich um Substanzen aus der Gruppe der Phenothiazine, Thioxanthene und Diphenylbutylpiperidine.

2. Klinische Wirkung

Die Depotneuroleptika weisen das gleiche Wirkungsprofil auf wie die kurzwirksamen Neuroleptika. Sie beeinflussen produktive psychotische Symptome wie Denkstörungen, Halluzinationen und Wahnbildung, aber auch Autismus, affektive Nivellierung und Interesselosigkeit, wirken beruhigend, spannungslösend und kontaktfördernd. Ihre insgesamt ausgleichende und stabilisierende Wirkung erleichtert die Rehabilitation, soziale Anpassung und Integration. In der Literatur beschriebene Wirkungsunterschiede zwischen den Präparaten konnten nur selten reproduziert werden und scheinen sich vor allem auf die Ausprägung extrapyramidaler Nebenwirkungen und die teilweise subjektiv als sehr unangenehm empfundene Dämpfung zu beziehen. Als wenig dämpfend werden Flupenthixoldecanoat und Penfluridol beschrieben (JOHNSON u. MALIK, 1975; TANGHE u. VEREECKEN, 1972; ZAPLETÁLEK et al., 1973).

3. Indikationen

Depotneuroleptika sind vor allem für die Langzeittherapie chronisch schizophrener Psychosen indiziert. Als chronisch bezeichnen wir eine Schizophrenie, die eine minimale Krankheitsdauer von 2 Jahren ohne symptomfreies Intervall aufweist. Sowohl produktive psychotische Symptome als auch sogenannte Minussymptome sprechen auf die Behandlung mit Depotneuroleptika gut an (WOGGON, 1975; WOGGON u. ANGST, 1977). Eine relative Indikation stellen subakute Schizophrenien dar, bei denen die Symptomatik länger als $^1/_2$ Jahr vorhanden ist. Außerdem werden Depotneuroleptika versuchsweise auch bei Alkoholismus, schweren Neurosen, Affektpsychosen, sexuellen Verhaltensstörungen oder Aggressionen angewendet (BARTHOLOMEW, 1966, 1968; HARRIOT u. RESCHE-RIGON, 1972; MAY, 1975).

4. Vorteile der Behandlung mit Depotneuroleptika

Die Behandlung mit Depotneuroleptika führt zu einer Verkürzung der Hospitalisierungsdauer, Senkung der Behandlungskosten, Verminderung der Rückfälle und Wiederaufnahmen ins psychiatrische Krankenhaus (DE MORAIS et al., 1972). Die Rehospitalisationsquote ist unter Depotneuroleptika überraschend niedrig und sogar kleiner als unter peroraler Behandlung mit Neuroleptika. Die Angaben schwanken zwischen 5 und 10% (CARNEY u. SHEFFIELD, 1975; HIRSCH et al., 1973; IMLAH u. MURPHY, 1973). Die größere Sicherheit bezüglich der Rückfallprophylaxe ist wahrscheinlich größtenteils darauf zurückzuführen, daß die Einnahme des Medikamentes nicht allein vom Patienten abhängt. Für Patienten, die mit Injektionen nicht einverstanden sind, steht das oral applizierbare Penfluridol zur Verfügung.

5. Beginn einer depotneuroleptischen Medikation

Die wichtigste Voraussetzung für den Erfolg einer depotneuroleptischen Langzeitbehandlung ist die Kooperation des Patienten. Diese kann nur durch eingehende Aufklärung des Patienten über Vor- und Nachteile der depotneuroleptischen Behandlung gewonnen werden. Auch nach der eigentlichen Einstellung auf das Depotneuroleptikum ist eine dauernde Motivationsarbeit zur Fortführung der Langzeittherapie notwendig. Es hat sich gezeigt, daß eine mindestens einmal monatliche Konsultation notwendig ist.

Anfänglich wurde die Einstellung auf Depotneuroleptika vor allem stationär begonnen, was heute jedoch nicht mehr so verbreitet ist. Bei einschleichender Dosierung kann man auch ambulant eine Einstellung vornehmen, sogar ohne orale Vormedikation. Immer wieder wird in der Literatur betont, daß sowohl die initiale Dosierung als auch das Injektionsintervall individuell bestimmt werden müssen und daß die Anpassung der Dosierung im Behandlungsverlauf wichtig ist. Meistens ist mit zunehmender Behandlungsdauer eine Dosisreduktion nicht nur möglich, sondern notwendig.

6. Nebenwirkungen

Unter der Behandlung mit Depotneuroleptika können die gleichen Nebenwirkungen beobachtet werden wie bei der Behandlung mit kurzwirksamen Neuroleptika. Die Nebenwirkungen zeigen große interindividuelle Schwankungen und sind abhängig von der Dosierung und dem Applikationsintervall, scheinen in manchen Familien gehäuft vorzukommen und nehmen mit der Dauer der Behandlung ab. Die extrapyramidalen Nebenwirkungen, insbesondere das Parkinsonsyndrom, sind durch Gabe von Antiparkinsonmitteln gut kontrollierbar. Gut bewährt hat sich die Selbstapplikation von Antiparkinsonmitteln durch den Patienten, der im Bedarfsfall die verordnete Dosierung einnimmt. Absetzversuche von Antiparkinsonmitteln haben veranschaulicht, daß eine Dauermedikation dieser Substanzen in der Regel nicht nötig ist (ANGST u. WOGGON, 1975; KLETT u. COLE, 1971; ORLOV et al., 1971).

Bei persistierenden Dyskinesien und Akathisie empfiehlt es sich, das Depotneuroleptikum abzusetzen. Die lokale Verträglichkeit der injizierbaren Depotneuroleptika ist gut. Bei subjektiv unangenehm stark empfundener Dämpfung sind Dosisreduktion und Intervalldehnung indiziert.

Im Verlauf von etwa 5–25% depotneuroleptischer Behandlungen werden depressive Verstimmungen beobachtet, die teilweise ein so starkes Ausmaß annehmen, daß die Verschreibung von Antidepressiva nötig wird. Es liegen auch Berichte über Suizide vor. Der Zeitpunkt, zu dem sich diese Depressionen entwickeln, ist offenbar sehr unterschiedlich (DE ALARCÓN u. CARNEY, 1969; CARNEY u. SHEFFIELD, 1975; DICK, 1972; GAMKRELIDZE u. PUTKORADZE-GAMKRELIDZE, 1973; SCHMIDT, 1975; WOGGON u. ANGST, 1976). Die Ursache depressiver Verstimmungen unter neuroleptischer Medikation ist nicht geklärt. Einige Autoren sprechen von einer „pharmakogenen Depression". Andererseits gibt es Studien, die eine Abnahme depressiver Symptome im Verlauf neuroleptischer Behandlungen aufzeigen (HUCKER et al., 1976; WOGGON et al., 1976). Die als Nebenwirkung der Neuroleptika auftretende Akinese kann mit Depressionen verwechselt werden (RIFKIN et al., 1975b). Reaktive Depressionen nach Abklingen schizophrener Schübe sind auch aus der präneuroleptischen Zeit bekannt. Krankheitseinsicht und wiedergewonnene Realitätskontrolle lassen es verständlich erscheinen, daß bei der häufig recht schwierigen sozialen Situation chronisch schizophrener Patienten reaktive Depressionen entstehen können.

7. Applikation und Dosierung

Mit Ausnahme von Penfluridol und des noch im Prüfungsstadium befindlichen Clopimozid werden Depotneuroleptika intramuskulär injiziert. Auf die Notwendigkeit einer individuellen Anpassung der Dosierung und des Applikationsintervalles wurde schon hingewiesen. Im Vergleich zu den üblichen Tagesdosierungen kurzwirksamer Neuroleptika werden Depotneuroleptika sehr niedrig dosiert.

8. Behandlungsdauer

Bisher konnte nicht nachgewiesen werden, daß eine mehr als dreijährige neuroleptische Behandlung den Verlauf der Schizophrenie entscheidend verändert (Pritchard, 1967). Im Einzelfall hat es sich jedoch bewährt, den Patienten mehrere Jahre lang mit Depotneuroleptika zu behandeln, weil nur so eine individuelle Verlaufsbeurteilung möglich ist.

Bei Absetzen von Depotneuroleptika können Rückfälle bis zu 6 Monaten nachher eintreten. Behandlungsabbrüche scheinen bei injizierbaren Depotneuroleptika seltener zu sein als bei oraler Applikation kurzwirksamer Neuroleptika (Crawford u. Forrest, 1974). Im Verlauf längerer Behandlungen spielen sie jedoch eine nicht zu unterschätzende Rolle. So beobachtete Dick (1972), daß die Hälfte der untersuchten Patienten nach einem Jahr die Depotneuroleptika-Medikation abgebrochen hatte.

Am häufigsten werden Behandlungen mit Depotneuroleptika auf Wunsch des Patienten beendet. Dabei ist es oft schwierig, die Gründe zu erfahren, die den Patienten zur Äußerung dieses Wunsches veranlassen. Verminderte Kooperation bei Verschlechterung des Zustandsbildes, Nebenwirkungen oder der Wunsch, frei von Medikamenten zu sein, können eine Rolle spielen. Manchmal ist es nicht möglich, diese Gründe mit dem Patienten näher zu diskutieren, da er sich ohne Kommentar aus der therapeutischen Beziehung zurückzieht. Ist dies nicht der Fall, so sollte dieser Wunsch Anlaß zu einer intensiven Besprechung mit dem Patienten sein.

9. Präparate

Die in Deutschland, Österreich und der Schweiz verfügbaren Präparate und die in Entwicklung befindlichen Depotneuroleptika sind mit Dosierung und Applikationsintervall in Tabelle 2 zusammengestellt.

C. Antidepressiva

Im Mittelpunkt der antidepressiven Behandlung steht die Anwendung trizyklischer und tetrazyklischer Antidepressiva, gelegentlich kombiniert mit Anxiolytika oder kleineren Dosen von Antipsychotika. Monoaminooxydasehemmer werden vor allem zur Behandlung gehemmter Depressionen verwendet. Zur Behandlung therapieresistenter Depressionen werden Psychostimulantien, Schlafentzug und Elektroschock herangezogen. Außerdem werden gelegentlich Behandlungs-

Tabelle 2. Depotneuroleptika

Internationale chemische Kurzbezeichnung (generic name)	Handelsname in BRD, Österreich, Schweiz	Mittlere Wirkungsdauer (Wochen)	Applikations- modus	Durchschnittliche Dosierung pro Applikation (mg)
1. Im Handel				
α-Clopenthixoldecanoat	–	2	i.m.	100–150
Flupenthixoldecanoat	Fluanxol Depot	2–3	i.m.	40
Fluphenazindecanoat (46)[a]	Dapotum D Lyogen Depot	3–4	i.m.	12,5–25
Fluspirilen (753)	Imap	1	i.m.	2–6
Penfluridol (909)	Semap	1	p.o.	20–40
Perphenazinoenanthat	Decentan-Depot	2	i.m.	100
2. In Entwicklung				
Clopimozid	–	1	p.o.	10–20
Fluphenazinoenanthat (48)	–	2	i.m.	25–50
Pipothiazinpalmitat	–	4–5	i.m.	25

[a] Die in Klammern den generic names beigefügte Zahl bezieht sich auf die von Usdin und Efron (1972) herausgegebene Zusammenstellung psychotroper Substanzen

versuche mit Vorstufen von biogenen Aminen, mit Hormonen oder mit „Releasing-Factors" von Hormonen unternommen.

Als Antidepressiva im engeren Sinne gelten tri- und tetrazyklische Antidepressiva (Thymoleptika) und Monoaminooxydasehemmer (Thymeretika). Antidepressiva wirken nicht euphorisierend, sondern bessern die Depression als Ganzes.

Bei der Darstellung der Antidepressiva werden wir uns auf die Antidepressiva im engeren Sinne beschränken und die Gruppe der tri- und tetrazyklischen Antidepressiva und die Gruppe der Monoaminooxydasehemmer getrennt beschreiben.

I. Tri- und tetrazyklische Antidepressiva (Thymoleptika)

1. Klassifikation

Fast allen tri- und tetrazyklischen Antidepressiva ist eine sedierende Wirkungskomponente zuzuschreiben, deren Ausprägung bei den verschiedenen Substanzen unterschiedlich ist. Diese sedierende Wirkungskomponente erweist sich als vorteilhaft bezüglich der schweren depressiven Schlafstörung, der inneren Unruhe oder der depressiven Agitiertheit.

Außerdem bewirkt eine leichte Sedierung häufig auch eine Anxiolyse. Die anxiolytische Wirkung von sedierenden Antidepressiva ist jedoch nicht mit derjenigen von eigentlichen Anxiolytika (z. B. Benzodiazepine) vergleichbar, welche auch ohne wesentliche Sedierung anxiolytisch wirken.

Eine Klassifikation der Antidepressiva aufgrund einer relativ spezifischen Wirkung auf den Antrieb ist jedoch problematisch. Es gibt keine aussagekräftigen empirischen Untersuchungen, welche gestützt auf getrennte Messungen von Antrieb, Stimmung und anderer Symptome die Möglichkeit einer spezifischen Differenzierung nachweisen. Wahrscheinlicher ist es, daß die sogenannten aktivierenden Antidepressiva wegen ihrer kaum oder wenig sedierenden Wirkung als antriebssteigernd beschrieben werden, um sie von den sedierenden Antidepressiva abzugrenzen. Zwischen den hypothetisch vorstellbaren Polen Trimipramin (sedierend) und MAO-Hemmer (nicht sedierend) lassen sich die Antidepressiva entsprechend der Ausprägung ihrer sedierenden Wirkungskomponente folgendermaßen anordnen (HEINRICH, 1976; KIELHOLZ, 1966): Trimipramin, Doxepin, Amitriptylin, Melitracen, Dibenzepin, Dimetracin, Noxiptilin, Imipramin, Clomipramin, Protriptylin, Nortriptylin, Desipramin, MAO-Hemmer.

Im allgemeinen sind die Gemeinsamkeiten zwischen den Präparaten bedeutend größer als ihre Unterschiede. Die individuelle Reagibilität des Patienten ist wahrscheinlich im Vergleich zu substanzeigenen Wirkungsqualitäten von ausschlaggebender Bedeutung dafür, ob der Patient sich eher sediert oder stimuliert fühlt. Dementsprechend ist die Behandlungsanamnese als außerordentlich wichtig anzusehen.

Aufgrund einer Vielzahl methodischer Schwierigkeiten ist die wissenschaftliche Differenzierung der Wirkung einzelner Antidepressiva in den üblichen klinischen Prüfungen kaum möglich. Eine zunehmend größere Zahl neuer Antidepressiva erweist sich als nicht differenzierbar von den Standardpräparaten Imipramin oder Amitriptylin. Daraus ist jedoch nicht abzuleiten, daß sie gleich wirksam sind wie die Standardpräparate.

2. Klinische Wirkung

Als Abkömmling der trizyklischen Antipsychotika wurde das erste Antidepressivum Imipramin als sedativ-hypnotische oder antipsychotische Substanz klinisch geprüft. Es ist KUHNs bleibendes Verdienst (KUHN, 1957), die antidepressive Wirkung von Imipramin erkannt zu haben.

Tri- und tetrazyklische Antidepressiva wirken nicht nur antidepressiv, sondern haben ein sehr breites pharmakologisches Wirkungsspektrum (siehe CARLSSON), wobei einzelne dieser zusätzlichen Wirkungskomponenten für die Therapie der depressiven Symptomatik nützlich sein können; dies gilt im besonderen für die sedierende Wirkungskomponente.

Die Vermutung, daß eine pharmakologisch bedingte vorübergehende Antriebssteigerung vor der Remission des depressiven Zustandsbildes zu einer Zunahme der Suizidgefahr am Beginn der antidepressiven Behandlung führt, muß als unbewiesen angesehen werden. Kasuistische Berichte über Suizide liegen für alle Phasen einer antidepressiven Behandlung vor. Kontrollierte Studien zeigen, daß unter der antidepressiven Behandlung eine lineare Rückbildung der Suizidalität erfolgt, wobei diese Rückbildung nicht nur mit dem Antrieb, sondern vor allem mit dem Schweregrad des ganzen depressiven Zustandsbildes korreliert ist.

Die Bedeutung genetischer Faktoren für die Wirksamkeit von Antidepressiva ist nicht sicher nachgewiesen, jedoch wahrscheinlich aufgrund der Beobachtung, daß Blutsverwandte eine ähnliche Ansprechbarkeit auf bestimmte Antidepressiva zeigen (ANGST, 1964).

3. Wirkungseintritt

Der Wirkungseintritt der einzelnen Wirkungskomponenten ist unterschiedlich. Am schnellsten macht sich die sedierende Wirkungskomponente der Antidepressiva bemerkbar, die häufig mit einem angstlösenden Effekt verknüpft ist. Daher fühlen sich die Patienten oft durch ein sedierendes Antidepressivum rascher gebessert als durch ein nicht sedierendes. Es ist jedoch nicht angemessen, den sedierenden Substanzen eine schnellere antidepressive Wirkung zuzuschreiben, da sie die depressive Kernsymptomatik (Antriebsverlust, Initiativelosigkeit, Gedächtnisstörungen, Konzentrationsstörungen und depressive Grundbefindlichkeit) nicht schneller beeinflussen als die nicht oder kaum sedierenden Präparate.

Bezüglich der eigentlichen antidepressiven Wirkung wird von vielen Autoren eine Wirkungslatenz von 2 bis 4 Wochen beschrieben. Diese auch in einigen Lehrbüchern enthaltene Behauptung beruht nicht auf den Ergebnissen seriöser klinischer Prüfungen und wird durch eine Reihe von Befunden entkräftet. Bei genauer Untersuchung der Patienten bestätigt die klinische Erfahrung den schon in der ersten Arbeit von KUHN (1957) beschriebenen Befund, daß unter Antidepressiva schon innerhalb von 1 bis 7 Tagen eindrückliche Besserungen beobachtet werden können. Kontrollierte Studien zeigen, daß bereits nach 5tägiger antidepressiver Behandlung eine signifikante Rückbildung depressiver Symptome nachweisbar ist. Die Ausprägung und Häufigkeit depressiver Symptome zeigt im Verlauf einer 20–30tägigen klinischen Prüfung eine lineare Rückbildung, was gegen die Annahme eines initialen Placeboeffektes spricht. In diesem Zusammenhang ist zu betonen, daß endogen depressive Patienten schlechte Placeboreaktoren sind.

Kontrollierte Prüfungen zeigen, daß diejenigen Patienten, die nach 20- bis 30tägiger Behandlung entscheidend gebessert sind, mehrheitlich bereits in den ersten 5 bis 10 Behandlungstagen eine beginnende Besserung erfahren. Diejenigen Patienten, die in den ersten 10 Behandlungstagen keine Besserung erleben, bleiben gehäuft auch nach längerer antidepressiver Behandlung therapieresistent.

Die Frage der Wirkungslatenz ist nicht nur von theoretischer Bedeutung, sondern von großer praktischer Wichtigkeit bezüglich der Frage, wie lange eine wirkungslose antidepressive Behandlung fortgesetzt werden muß und darf, bis sie als erfolglos bezeichnet werden kann. Zeichnet sich nach zweiwöchiger Antidepressivabehandlung keine Besserungstendenz ab, so darf auf ein anderes Präparat umgestellt werden.

Natürlich können bei einer mehr als zwei Wochen dauernden Behandlung noch Remissionen beobachtet werden. Diese Spätbesserungen können jedoch nicht sicher von Spontanremissionen abgegrenzt werden. Betrachtet man die Phasendauer endogener Depressionen (Median 6 Monate), so wird deutlich, daß mit zunehmender Behandlungsdauer die Wahrscheinlichkeit einer Spontanremission immer größer wird.

4. Indikationen

Unabhängig von der nosologischen Diagnose sind trizyklische und tetrazyklische Antidepressiva bei jedem depressiven Zustandsbild indiziert, das nicht durch eine andere kausale Therapie gebessert werden kann (ANGST u. THEOBALD, 1970). Antidepressiva sind indiziert bei organischen Depressionen, symptomatischen Depressionen, Depressionen bei Schizophrenien, schizo-affektiven Psychosen, endogenen Depressionen (monopolare und bipolare Affektpsychosen), neurotischen Depressionen, Erschöpfungsdepressionen und reaktiven Depressionen. Dieses vielfältige Indikationsspektrum kann auf zweierlei Weise interpretiert werden: Einerseits kann der antidepressive Effekt als unspezifisch gedeutet werden, andererseits liegt die Annahme einer allen depressiven Syndromen zugrunde liegenden biochemischen Störung nahe.

Für die differentielle Indikationsstellung der Antidepressiva gilt unabhängig von der Ätiologie die Syndromdiagnostik als wegweisend. Im einzelnen werden folgende Syndrome unterschieden: 1. gehemmt- bzw. apathisch-depressives Syndrom, 2. agitiert-depressives Syndrom, 3. hypochondrisches Syndrom, 4. phobisch-anankastisches Syndrom, 5. psychotisch-depressives Syndrom mit Wahnideen und/oder Halluzinationen, 6. larviert-depressives Syndrom, 7. organisch-depressives Syndrom.

Die Wahl eines bestimmten Antidepressivums hängt vor allem von der Ausprägung der depressiven Hemmung oder Agitiertheit ab. Bei ausgeprägter Angst ist eine Kombination mit Anxiolytika oder kleinen Dosierungen von Antipsychotika zu empfehlen. Bei therapieresistenten Depressionen kann in einzelnen Fällen die Kombination mit Trijodthyronin erfolgreich sein (nur für Frauen gesichert).

5. Kontraindikationen

Bei der Indikationsstellung sind Begleiterkrankungen, welche relative Kontraindikationen bilden, gebührend zu berücksichtigen. Als Kontraindikation wird am häufigsten das Glaukom, insbesondere das Schmalwinkelglaukom genannt; dieses stellt aber unter gleichzeitiger augenärztlicher Kontrolle nur noch eine relative Kontraindikation dar. In Zusammenarbeit mit einem Ophthalmologen können Antidepressiva (eher in kleineren Dosen) kombiniert mit Anxiolytika verabreicht werden.

Besonders zu beachten ist die Kardiotoxizität vieler Antidepressiva, so daß besonders Vorsicht bei Koronarsklerose, bei Arrhythmien und bei Herzinsuffizienz geboten ist; unmittelbar nach einem Herzinfarkt ist ein Antidepressivum kontraindiziert. Erhöhte Vorsicht ist schließlich geboten bei Epilepsien (Erniedrigung der Krampfschwelle durch Antidepressiva, ausgenommen das auf dem Kontinent noch nicht im Handel befindliche Viloxazin) sowie das Vorhandensein einer Arteriosklerose (vorsichtige Dosierung).

Absolut kontraindiziert ist die Kombination von trizyklischen und tetrazyklischen Antidepressiva mit Monoaminooxydasehemmern, wenn eine Vorbehandlung mit letzteren stattgefunden hat. Nach Abschluß einer Therapie mit einem MAO-Hemmer ist ein freies Intervall von mindestens 7–10 Tagen einzuschalten.

Eine gewisse Vorsicht mit höheren Dosen von Antidepressiva ist schließlich wegen der anticholinergen Begleiteffekte bei älteren Männern mit einer Prostatavergrößerung nötig, da hier die Gefahr der Harnverhaltung erhöht ist.

Wegen der erhöhten Bereitschaft zu pharmakogenen Delirien ist bei allen Formen von Hirnschädigungen eine besonders vorsichtige Antidepressivabehandlung indiziert.

6. Nebenwirkungen

Die Ausprägung vegetativer und insbesondere anticholinerger Nebenwirkungen ist bei den einzelnen Substanzen unterschiedlich. Mögliche Nebenwirkungen sind: Sedierung, Schwäche, Müdigkeit, Somnolenz; Störungen der visuellen Akkommodation; Trockenheit der Schleimhäute (Mund, Nase, Vagina); Mydriasis; Schwitzen; Tachykardie, Arrhythmie; EKG-Veränderungen (Abflachung der T-Welle); Hypotension (orthostatische); Konstipation, Diarrhoe; Hemmung der Miktion, Harnverhaltung; Nausea, Erbrechen; Körpergewichtszunahme; Eosinophilie; Leukopenie, Agranulozytose; Erhöhung der Blutsenkungsgeschwindigkeit; Thrombosen, Thrombophlebitiden; Ikterus, vorübergehender Anstieg von SGOT, SGPT oder alkalischer Phosphatase; allergische Hautreaktionen; Ödeme der Haut; Galaktorrhoe, Gynäkomastie, Amenorrhoe; Tremor; epileptische Krämpfe; Atonie des Darmes, im besonderen des Ileum, Ileus; Insomnie; Agitation, Angst; Delirien; Aktivierung schizophrener Symptome bei latenter oder manifester Schizophrenie.

7. Applikation und Dosierung

Antidepressiva werden in der Regel oral verabreicht und gut resorbiert. Innerhalb von 3 bis 5 Tagen sollte die Dosierung rasch auf die volle therapeutische Dosis gesteigert werden. Ausnahmen sind: 1. Patienten mit organischen Hirnschädigungen sollten niedrigere Dosen erhalten und die Dosissteigerung muß langsam durchgeführt werden. 2. Bei der Behandlung hypochondrischer Syndrome ist vor allem auf die Vermeidung von Nebenwirkungen zu achten, da diese die hypochondrischen Befürchtungen unterstützen können.

Aufgrund der langen Halbwertzeiten (PEREL, 1977) ist die 3mal tägliche Applikation von Antidepressiva nicht nötig und wird zunehmend durch eine 1- bis 2mal tägliche Applikation abgelöst (AYD, 1974a; SCHORER, 1973). Dabei haben sich besonders Retardformen bewährt, wie Imipramin-Pamoat (DOYLE, 1975; GOLDBERG u. NATHAN, 1972; HULL u. MARSHALL, 1975; MENDELS u. DIGIACOMO, 1973; MILLER et al., 1973) oder Saroten retard, deren Toxizität geringer ist, wodurch die Gefahr akzidenteller oder suizidaler Vergiftungen vermindert wird.

Bei der 1mal täglichen Applikation von Antidepressiva ist vor allem die abendliche Gabe direkt vor dem Schlafengehen zu empfehlen. Bei gleichbleibender Wirkung treten weniger Nebenwirkungen auf und die Schlafstörungen werden günstig beeinflußt (gilt auch für nicht sedierende Antidepressiva).

Vergleichsweise selten werden Antidepressiva parenteral verabreicht. Die *intravenöse Infusionsbehandlung* mit Antidepressiva (z.B. Maprotilin, Clomipramin, Dibenzepin Nomifensin) ist nicht nur bei therapieresistenten Depressionen indiziert, sondern sollte auch bei Vorliegen schwer gehemmter Depressionen durchgeführt werden.

8. Behandlungsdauer

Die meisten Patienten bessern sich unter einer antidepressiven Behandlung nicht bis zur Symptomfreiheit, sondern es bleiben in der Regel gewisse Restsymptome (Schlafstörung, Morgentief, Konzentrationsschwäche, verminderte Libido) hartnäckig über mehrere Monate bestehen, was als Ausdruck der durch die Medikation nur unvollständig beseitigten Symptomatik unter der noch im Gang befindlichen Phase interpretiert werden kann. Bei diesen Patienten ergibt es sich von selbst, daß die Antidepressivaeinnahme in Abhängigkeit von der Restsymptomatik auch nach der Klinikentlassung 3 oder mehr Monate lang fortgesetzt wird. Eine Dosisverminderung soll nur langsam vorgenommen werden.

Auch bei Vorliegen eines optimalen Behandlungserfolges (völlige Symptomfreiheit) sollte das Antidepressivum mehrere Wochen oder besser Monate weitergegeben werden, da wir auch bei diesen Patienten von der Vorstellung ausgehen müssen, daß das Medikament so lange weiterbenötigt wird, wie die Phase andauert und daß eigentliche Phasenverkürzungen nicht zu erzielen sind (ANGST u. FREY, 1978).

Die häufigsten Fehler bei der Behandlung mit Antidepressiva sind ein zu frühes Absetzen der Medikation oder eine zu niedrige Dosierung. Das Absetzen der Behandlung sollte ausschleichend erfolgen, ausgenommen im Falle eines Umschlages in Hypomanie oder Manie.

Erfahrungen mit mehrjähriger Gabe tri- und tetrazyklischer Antidepressiva zur Prophylaxe weiterer depressiver Phasen lassen vermuten, daß eine derartige Dauermedikation für monopolare Affektpsychosen eine gewisse Alternative zur Lithiumprophylaxe darstellt.

9. Präparate

Die im deutschsprachigen Teil Europas zur Verfügung stehenden Präparate sind in Tabelle 3 aufgeführt.

II. Monoaminooxydasehemmer

1. Klassifikation

Monoaminooxydasehemmer (Thymeretika) können eingeteilt werden in Hydrazin- und Nicht-Hydrazin-Derivate, sowie nach ihrer Spezifität der Blockierung der Monoaminooxydasen A und B. Doch ist aus klinischer Sicht nichts darüber bekannt, daß diese Differenzierung für die Praxis relevant wäre.

2. Klinische Wirkung

Um eine hinreichende klinische Wirkung bei depressiven Syndromen zu erreichen, muß die Aktivität der Monoaminooxydase in den Blutplättchen zu mindestens 80% gehemmt sein (NIES et al., 1975). Der Metabolismus der MAO-Hemmer läuft über eine Acetylierung, welche vererbt variiert, so daß langsame und rasche Acetylierer unterschieden werden können, welche auch unterschiedlich auf die Therapie ansprechen sollen (JOHNSTONE, 1975). Von großer klinischer Bedeutung ist die Tatsache, daß zwar MAO-Hemmer relativ rasch wieder eliminiert werden (innerhalb von 1-2 Tagen), daß die Enzymhemmung jedoch während 1-2 Wochen mittelüberdauernd persistiert, was zu einem anhaltenden Anstieg von biogenen Aminen im Gehirn und den Geweben führt.

Tabelle 3. Antidepressiva

Internationale chemische Kurzbezeichnung (generic name)	Handelsnamen			Dosierung (per os, mg/Tag)	
	BRD	Österreich	Schweiz	klinisch	ambulant
1.1. Trizyklische Antidepressiva					
Amitriptylin (156)[a]	Laroxyl Saroten Tryptizol	Saroten Tryptizol	Laroxyl Saroten Tryptizol	75–300	75–150
Clomipramin (165)	Anafranil	Anafranil	Anafranil	75–300	50–150
Desimipramin (182)	Pertofran	Pertofran	Pertofran	75–300	50–150
Dibenzepin (184)	Noveril	Noveril	Noveril	480–720	120–240
Dimetracin (186)	Istonil	Istonil	Istonil	75–600	75–200
Doxepin (187)	Aponal Sinquan	Sinquan	Sinquan	75–300	75–150
Imipramin (206)	Tofranil	Tofranil	Tofranil	75–200	75–150
Lofepramin (Clofepramin Lopramin) (171)	Gamonil	–	Gamonil	105–210	105–140
Melitracen (212)	Trausabun	Trausabun	Dixeran	75–250	75–150
Nortriptylin (223)	Nortrilen	Nortrilen	Nortrilen Sensival	30–100	30–75
Noxiptilin (224)	Agedal	Agedal	–	100–450	75–150
Opipramol (227)	Insidon	Insidon	Insidon	150–300	150–200
Protriptylin (236)	Maximed	Concordin	Concordin	20–60	15–30
Trimipramin (245)	Stangyl Surmontil	Stangyl	Surmontil	100–400	50–150
1.2. Tetrazyklische Antidepressiva					
Maprotilin (1252)	Ludiomil	Ludiomil	Ludiomil	75–200	75–150
Mianserin	Tolvin	Tolvon	Tolvon	30–120	10–40
1.3. Andere Strukturen					
Nomifensin	Alival	–	Alival	100–200	75–150
Trazodon (994)	–	–	Trittico	100–200	75–150
1.4. Monominooxydasehemmer					
Isocarboxazid (777)	–	Marplan	Marplan	30–90	10–30
Nialamid (867)	–	Niamid	–	100–300	75–150
Tranylcypromin (1192)	Parnate	–	–	20–100	10–20
– in Kombination mit Trifluoperazin (130)	Jatrosom	Jatrosom	Eskapar	3×1 Drg.	1–2 Drg.

[a] Die in Klammern den generic names beigefügte Zahl bezieht sich auf die von Usdin und Efron (1972) herausgegebene Zusammenstellung psychotroper Substanzen

Bei der Beschreibung der antidepressiven Wirkung der MAO-Hemmer wird von vielen Autoren weniger die stimmungsaufhellende als die antriebssteigernde Wirkungskomponente betont. Eine qualitative Wirkungsdifferenz gegenüber tri- und tetrazyklischen Antidepressiva ist aber nicht hinreichend überprüft. Als einziger MAO-Hemmer hat Tranylcypromin eine amphetaminähnliche Seitenkette, wodurch vielleicht seine stimulierende Wirkung zu erklären ist.

3. Wirkungseintritt

Klinisch ist der Wirkungseintritt erst innerhalb von 10–20 Behandlungstagen zu erwarten; eine Ausnahme bildet Tranylcypromin wegen seiner stimulierenden Wirkungskomponente.

4. Indikationen

MAO-Hemmer sind vor allem bei gehemmten Depressionen indiziert und werden zur Zeit in erster Linie bei Resistenz auf tri- und tetrazyklische Antidepressiva verschrieben, ausnahmsweise auch bei atypischen depressiven Syndromen, wie phobisch zwangshaften, ängstlichen Syndromen.

5. Kontraindikationen

Die Kontraindikationen für die Gabe von MAO-Hemmern ergeben sich vor allem bei der gleichzeitigen Verabreichung anderer Pharmaka und dem Genuß einiger Nahrungsmittel. MAO-Hemmer können zu einer Interaktion führen mit folgenden Substanzen: Aminopyrin, Acetanilid, Cocain, Meperidin, Reserpin, Tyramin. Nach HONIGFELD und HOWARD (1973) haben folgende Nahrungsmittel einen hohen Tyramingehalt: Camembert, Cheddar, Gruyère, Stilton, Boursalt, Chianti und Rollmöpse. Einen mittleren Gehalt an Tyramin haben: Emmentaler, Brie, Schmelzkäse, Roquefort und anderer Schimmelkäse (Blue), Romano, Sherry, Bier, Salz- und Trockenheringe sowie Hühnerleber. Wenig Tyramin enthalten: Amerikanischer Käse (American), Gouda, Parmesan, Riesling, Sauterne, Champagner und italienischer Rotwein (ausgenommen Chianti). Außerdem sollten folgende Produkte nicht genossen werden: konservierte Feigen, Rosinen, Saubohnen, Hefeprodukte und -extrakte, Sojasauce, Schokolade, saure Gurken, Gewürzgurken, Sauerkraut, Coffein in exzessiven Dosierungen und rezeptfreie Medikamente gegen Erkältungen und Heuschnupfen. Pharmakologisch ist eine Interaktion zu erwarten mit allen sympathomimetischen Substanzen wie Amphetamin, Fenfluramin, Ephedrin, Phenylpropanolamin, trizyklischen und tetrazyklischen Antidepressiva, Barbituraten, Hypnotika, Pethidin, Antihistaminica, Antihypertensiva, Hypoglykämika und Insulin. Diese Interaktionsmöglichkeiten erschweren die Verabreichung von MAO-Hemmern, insbesondere in der ambulanten Behandlung. Will man nach einem erfolglosen Therapieversuch mit MAO-Hemmern den Patienten mit einem tri- oder tetrazyklischen Antidepressivum behandeln, so sollte eine Medikamentenpause von 7–10 Tagen dazwischengeschaltet werden. Mit Ausnahme von Phenothiazinen können Neuroleptika gefahrlos im Anschluß an eine Behandlung mit MAO-Hemmern gegeben werden.

Eine Kombination von MAO-Hemmern mit trizyklischen Antidepressiva ist im Prinzip möglich, falls die Therapie mit beiden Substanzen gleichzeitig begonnen wird oder falls der MAO-Hemmer zeitlich verspätet hinzugegeben wird. Hingegen besteht eine absolute Kontraindikation gegen eine Vorbehandlung mit einem MAO-Hemmer und eine anschließende Kombination mit einem anderen Antidepressivum (trizyklisches oder tetrazyklisches). Eine Übersicht über die Kombinationstherapie mit trizyklischen Antidepressiva und MAO-Hemmern geben ANANTH und LUCHINS (1977). Die Inkompatibilität zwischen MAO-Hemmern und trizyklischen Antidepressiva wurde zuerst durch HARRER (1961, 1967) erwähnt, welcher toxische Effekte wie Schwindel, Nausea, Erbrechen, groben Tremor, Kopfschmerzen, profuses Schwitzen, Dyspnoe, Kollaps und in gewissen Fällen Delirien und Verwirrungen schilderte. Untersuchungen von MARKS (1965) zeigten die Wichtigkeit des Tyramin in der Pathogenese solcher Nebenwirkungen. Es kann dabei zu einem plötzlichen Abfall des Blutdruckes, gelegentlich aber auch zu einem Anstieg kommen. Da aber derartige Nebenwirkungen durch MAO-Hemmer allein auch erzeugt werden können, ist es bis heute unklar, inwieweit die Kombination mit trizyklischen Pharmaka ein besonderes Risiko darstellt.

In einer größeren Studie von SHOPSIN und KLINE (1974) an über 500 Patienten unter MAO-Hemmern, kombiniert mit trizyklischen Antidepressiva, wurde gezeigt, daß die Häufigkeit von Nebenwirkungen nicht größer ist als bei der Verabreichung der einen Substanzgruppe allein. Bei der Kombination sind im allgemeinen etwas niedrigere Dosen zu verwenden. Die Überlegenheit der Kombinationsbehandlung ist bis heute nicht genügend gesichert; obwohl sie wahrscheinlich ungefährlich ist, sollte sie nur von speziell mit diesem Behandlungsverfahren vertrauten Ärzten verordnet werden.

6. Nebenwirkungen

MAO-Hemmer können folgende Nebenwirkungen hervorrufen: Blutdrucksenkung, Kollaps, plötzlicher Blutdruckanstieg (hypertone Blutdruckkrisen), Kopfschmerzen, Schwindel, Insomnie, Impotenz, Libidoverlust, Orgasmusschwäche, Aktivation latenter oder manifester schizophrener Syndrome, toxische Verwirrungszustände, epileptische Anfälle (erniedrigte Krampfschwelle), Ikterus, Inkompatibilität mit gewissen Nahrungsmitteln und anderen Pharmaka (siehe Kontraindikationen).

7. Applikation und Behandlungsdauer

MAO-Hemmer werden oral appliziert. Die empfehlenswerte Behandlungsdauer entspricht den allgemeinen Grundsätzen der Verabreichung von Antidepressiva. Die minimale Behandlungsdauer dürfte im allgemeinen zwischen 2 und 4 Wochen liegen, um die therapeutische Ansprechbarkeit überhaupt beurteilen zu können.

8. Präparate

Die im deutschsprachigen Raum verfügbaren Präparate finden sich in Tabelle 3. Es fehlen darunter das weltweit intensiv verwendete Phenelzin sowie das Iproniazid, das wegen Ikterusgefahr aus dem Handel gezogen wurde, jedoch in Australien ohne nennenswerte Komplikationen verordnet wird. Die Entwicklung der Monoaminooxydasehemmer zur Behandlung der depressiven Erkrankungen ist in den letzten Jahren etwas zu Unrecht vernachlässigt worden, und entsprechend dürftig ist auch das Angebot von Präparaten.

D. Psychostimulantien

1. Terminologie und Klassifikation

Unter dem Begriff Psychostimulantien werden alle unspezifisch psychostimulierend und aktivierend wirkenden Substanzen zusammengefaßt. Andere Bezeichnungen sind Stimulantien, Psychotonika, Energetika und im angelsächsischen Sprachgebrauch „psychoenergizer". Als Prototyp der Psychostimulantien gelten die Amphetamine. Eine gebräuchliche Einteilung der Psychostimulantien besteht in der Abgrenzung von Amphetaminen (Weckamine) und Nicht-Amphetaminen, die jedoch durch die große Ähnlichkeit (Wirkung, Suchtgefahr) relativiert wird, die zwischen einigen Nicht-Amphetaminen (z.B. Methylphenidat, Phenmetracin) und den Weckaminen besteht.

2. Klinische Wirkung

Die aktivierende Wirkung der Psychostimulantien führt zu einer Unterdrückung von Müdigkeit und Schlafbedürfnis und einer vorübergehenden Steigerung der Konzentrations- und Leistungsfähigkeit. Das subjektive Gefühl der Leistungssteigerung ist häufig stärker ausgeprägt als der objektivierbare Leistungszuwachs. Einige Stimulantien können das Hungergefühl unterdrücken und werden daher als Appetitzügler verwendet.

3. Wirkungseintritt

Die subjektiv empfundene und objektiv beobachtbare Wirkung der Psychostimulantien setzt außerordentlich rasch (30–60 min) nach der Einnahme ein. Das Ausmaß der Wirkung ist offenbar abhängig von der Ausgangslage, d.h. um so größer, je stärker die vorhandenen Beschwerden, wie z.B. Müdigkeit oder Erschöpfung ausgeprägt sind.

4. Indikationen

Die Indikationen für Psychostimulantien leiten sich unmittelbar aus ihren Wirkungskomponenten ab: Erschöpfungssyndrome (beispielsweise postinfektiös) oder in außerordentlichen Belastungssituationen (Krieg, Bergtouren); Narkolepsie, Appetithemmung, Hyperkinese bei Kindern; gelegentlich organisch gefärbte depressive Erschöpfungssyndrome und therapieresistente Depressionen. Bei der Verwendung von Psychostimulantien zur Behandlung therapieresistenter Depressionen kann ein Kippen in Hypomanie oder Manie provoziert werden. Der Grund für die Anwendung von Stimulantien bei therapieresistenten Depressionen ist weniger in der euphorisierenden als vielmehr in der aktivierenden Wirkungskomponente dieser Substanzen zu sehen. Wegen der potentiellen Suchtgefahr empfiehlt sich eine möglichst enge Indikationsstellung. Die teilweise überspitzt formulierten Warnungen mancher Kollegen vor dem therapeutischen Einsatz von Psychostimulantien sind jedoch als übertrieben anzusehen, da Depressive wahrscheinlich ein biologisch erniedrigtes Suchtpotential aufweisen.

5. Kontraindikationen

Die Gabe von Stimulantien ist bei Vorliegen einer Sucht oder Abhängigkeit kontraindiziert. Versuche, ausgeprägt apathische chronisch Schizophrene durch Stimulantien zu aktivieren, müssen äußerst sorgfältig kontrolliert werden, da die Gefahr einer unerwünschten Aktivierung schizophrener Symptome besteht. Ebenfalls mit großer Vorsicht ist die Anwendung bei Epilepsie durchzuführen, da eine Provokation epileptischer Anfälle möglich ist.

6. Nebenwirkungen

Neben der schon erwähnten möglichen Provokation epileptischer Anfälle und Aktivierung schizophrener Symptome können Psychostimulantien vor allem folgende Nebenwirkungen verursachen: Tremor, Tachykardie, hypertensive Krisen, Mundtrockenheit, unerwünschte Gewichtsabnahme, Impotenz, Insomnie, Angst, Reizbarkeit, Unruhe, motorische Stereotypien und Zwangshandlungen. Besonders ist auf die nach chronischem Mißbrauch mögliche Entwicklung paranoider und paranoid-halluzinatorischer Psychosen hinzuweisen, deren Symptomatik von derjenigen einer paranoiden Schizophrenie nicht zu unterscheiden ist. Das Risiko für diese Komplikation besteht vor allem bei älteren Patienten und bei vorbestehender hirnorganischer Schädigung.

Eine besonders wichtige Nebenwirkung der Psychostimulantien stellt die potentielle Suchtgefahr dar, die vor allem auf die euphorisierende Wirkungskomponente zurückzuführen ist.

7. Applikation und Dosierung

Therapeutisch werden Stimulantien in der Regel oral appliziert. Der intravenöse Applikationsmodus ist vor allem bei Drogenabhängigen üblich (Fixer). Therapeutisch werden Dosierungen von 2mal 5–10 mg Amphetamin pro die verwendet. Beim Süchtigen führt die rasche Toleranzentwicklung schon nach kurzem Mißbrauch zu enormen Dosissteigerungen auf ein Vielfaches der initialen Tagesdosis.

8. Behandlungsdauer

Aufgrund der beschriebenen Nebenwirkungen, insbesondere der Suchtgefahr und der möglichen Entwicklung paranoider Psychosen, sollten Psychostimulantien möglichst nur kurzfristig verordnet werden. Als Ausnahme kann die Verwendung bei der Behandlung therapieresistenter Depressionen gelten, bei der auch nach mehrwöchiger bis monatelanger Gabe äußerst selten größere Dosissteigerungen oder gar die Entwicklung einer Abhängigkeit zu beobachten sind.

9. Präparate

Zur engeren Gruppe der Weckamine gehören Amphetamin (Elastonon), Dextroamphetamin (Maxiton, Dexedrine) und Methamphetamin (Pervitin, Gerobit). Propylhexedrin (Eventin), Fenetyllin (Captagon) und Amphetaminil (Aponeuron, AN_1) haben eine analoge Wirkung. Auch Methylphenidat (Ritalin) und Phenmetrazin (Preludin) sind in ihrer Wirkung und den Nebenwirkungen den Amphetaminen gleichzustellen. Auf schwächere Stimulantien, Kombinationspräparate und Appetitzügler kann hier nicht näher eingegangen werden.

E. Lithium

1. Terminologie und Klassifikation

Zusammenfassend wird die Therapie mit den 7 verschiedenen zur Verfügung stehenden Lithiumsalzen, mit kurzwirksamen und Retardpräparaten, als Lithiumbehandlung bezeichnet. Die mehr als 30 existierenden Präparate enthalten Lithium in Form verschiedener Salze, für die bisher kein Wirkungsunterschied nachgewiesen wurde. Leider enthalten die Tabletten der verschiedenen Präparate unterschiedliche Lithiummengen. Um falsche Dosierungen zu vermeiden, sollte die Dosierung in mäq Lithium angegeben werden. 1 mäq (= 1 mval = 1 mmol = 6,9 mg) Lithium sind enthalten in: 37 mg Lithium-Carbonat, 55 mg Lithium-Sulfat, 66 mg Lithium-Acetat, 94 mg Lithium-Citrat, 154 mg Lithium-Adipat, 154 mg Lithium-Glutamat und 200 mg Lithium-Gluconat (SCHOU, 1973). Die Einteilung der Lithiumpräparate kann nach den verschiedenen Salzen vorgenommen werden oder in kurzwirksame und Retard-Formen.

2. Klinische Wirkung

Lithium wirkt therapeutisch auf hypomanische und manische Symptome und prophylaktisch gegen Erkrankungen, die mit stärkeren Auslenkungen der Stimmungslage einhergehen, insbesondere auf Phasen der monopolaren und bipolaren Affektpsychosen sowie auf affektive Residualsymptome in den Intervallen (ANGST, 1970; BAASTRUP et al., 1970; COPPEN et al., 1971; JOHNSON, 1975).

3. Wirkungseintritt

Im Unterschied zur rasch einsetzenden therapeutischen Wirkung von Lithium bei der Behandlung der Manie ist eine sichere rezidiv-prophylaktische Wirkung erst nach 3–6monatiger Lithiumeinnahme zu erwarten.

4. Indikationen

Eine Lithiumprophylaxe ist bei periodischen endogenen Depressionen, Spätdepressionen, manisch-depressivem Kranksein und schizo-affektiven Psychosen indiziert, wenn innerhalb der letzten zwei Jahre 2–3 Phasen aufgetreten sind. Bei Erkrankungen mit weiter auseinanderliegenden Phasen oder bei einer Ersterkrankung sollte eine Lithiumprophylaxe nur eingeleitet werden, wenn eine ausgesprochen stark ausgeprägte Symptomatik (insbesondere gefährliche Suizidalität, Gefährdung der sozialen Stellung durch Manie) und/oder eine schwere familiäre Belastung (vor allem mit bipolaren Affektpsychosen) vorliegen. Es muß betont werden, daß aus nicht bekannten Gründen nicht bei allen Patienten eine 100%ige Rezidivprophylaxe (=Heilung) erreicht wird. Lithium bewirkt in diesen Fällen eine verminderte Symptomausprägung, Verkürzung der Phasen und Verlängerung der gesunden Intervalle. Die Wirkung ist bei schizoaffektiven Psychosen weniger gut als bei reinen Affektpsychosen.

Therapeutisch, im Sinne einer direkten Beeinflussung der Symptomatik, wirkt Lithium bei Manie. In der Regel ist wegen des etwas verzögert einsetzenden Effektes von Lithium und der Toxizität bei hoher Dosierung anfänglich eine Kombinationstherapie mit Neuroleptika nötig.

Eine verschiedentlich beschriebene antidepressive Wirkung von Lithium (BARON et al., 1975; WATANABE et al., 1975) konnte nicht sicher reproduziert werden (MORRIS u. BECK, 1974). Therapieversuche wurden bei folgenden Krankheitsbildern unternommen: chronischer Alkoholismus (insbesondere Dipsomanie), nicht-psychotische Aggressivität (beispielsweise bei Häftlingen), Neuroleptika-induzierte persistierende Dyskinesien (GERLACH et al., 1975; KLINE et al., 1974b; MARINI et al., 1976; MERRY et al., 1976; SHEARD, 1975; TUPIN et al., 1973; WORRALL et al., 1975; WREN et al., 1974). Die Ergebnisse können noch nicht als gesichert bezeichnet werden. Vereinzelte kasuistische Mitteilungen über eine Effektverminderung von Amphetamin bei gleichzeitiger Lithiumgabe deuten auf eine mögliche Anwendbarkeit von Lithium zur Behandlung der Amphetaminsucht hin (FLEMENBAUM, 1974; VAN KAMMEN u. MURPHY, 1975).

5. Kontraindikationen

Die Gabe von Lithium ist kontraindiziert bei ausgeprägter Niereninsuffizienz und kochsalzfreier Diät. Bei schweren Herz- und Kreislaufkrankheiten sowie bei Morbus Addison sollte kein Lithium gegeben werden. Eine besonders sorgfältige Überwachung ist notwendig bei Patienten mit zerebraler Krampfbereitschaft und bei geriatrischen Patienten.

Während der Schwangerschaft, insbesondere in den ersten 4 Monaten, ist Lithium kontraindiziert. Es gibt Hinweise auf ein erhöhtes Risiko kardiovaskulärer Mißbildungen (WEINSTEIN u. GOLDFIELD, 1975).

1968 wurde das Lithium-Baby-Register gegründet, um die Häufigkeit von Mißbildungen bei Kindern zu bestimmen, deren Mütter im ersten Schwangerschaftsdrittel Lithium eingenommen haben. Eine katamnestische Untersuchung (SCHOU, 1976) von 60 bei der Geburt unauffälligen Lithiumkindern ergab keine Häufung somatischer oder psychischer Störungen in den ersten Lebensjahren.

6. Nebenwirkungen

Unabhängig von den verschiedenen Salzformen machen die Retardpräparate wegen der längeren Absorptionsperiode (8–10 Std im Vergleich zu 3–6 Std) und dem daraus resultierenden weniger starken Konzentrationsanstieg deutlich weniger Nebenwirkungen als kurzwirksame Lithiumpräparate.

Zahl und Ausprägung der Nebenwirkungen sind interindividuell außerordentlich verschieden. Einige Nebenwirkungen treten vor allem kurz nach Beginn der Lithiumeinnahme auf und bilden sich später zurück (Übelkeit, leichte Diarrhoe, feinschlägiger Fingertremor, Polyurie und Polydipsie), andere werden erst nach längerer Lithiumbehandlung beobachtet (Gewichtszunahme, Kropf, Myxödem und Ödeme).

SHOPSIN und GERSHON (1973) haben eine 44 Nebenwirkungen umfassende Liste zusammengestellt, die mit der Abkürzung LTCL (Lithium Toxicity Checklist) bezeichnet wird. Eine genaue Kenntnis möglicher Nebenwirkungen ist nicht nur für den behandelnden Arzt, sondern vor allem auch für den Patienten wichtig, da er möglichst Nebenwirkungen und Vergiftungssymptome kennen und voneinander unterscheiden sollte.

Die unter Lithium beobachteten Nebenwirkungen sollten nur in Ausnahmefällen einen Abbruch der Prophylaxe zur Folge haben.

Subjektiv besonders unangenehm kann der feinschlägige Tremor der Hände sein. Die verschiedentlich empfohlene Behandlung dieses Tremors mit Betarezeptorenblockern (z. B. 40–80 mg Propranolol pro Tag; FLORU, 1971; KIRK et al., 1973; SCHOU et al., 1973b) ist nicht immer erfolgreich und war in einer interessanten experimentellen Untersuchung von KELLETT et al. (1975) deutlich weniger wirksam als Placebo.

Die bei einigen Patienten recht drastische Gewichtszunahme (VENDSBORG et al., 1976b) kann in der Regel durch Kalorienbeschränkung erfolgreich behandelt werden, bildet jedoch in seltenen Fällen einen berechtigten Grund zur Beendigung der Lithiumprophylaxe.

Bei etwa 10% der Lithiumpatienten werden Veränderungen der Schilddrüsenfunktion oder Schilddrüsengröße beobachtet (euthyreote und hypothyreote Struma, Myxödem). Bei genauer Untersuchung hat sich feststellen lassen, daß in der Regel vorbestehende Schilddrüsenveränderungen vorhanden waren. Da es sich um reversible Veränderungen handelt, die durch zusätzliche Thyroxingabe ausgeglichen werden können, stellen Schilddrüsenveränderungen keine Kontraindikation für den Beginn oder die Weiterführung einer Lithiumprophylaxe dar. Empfehlenswert ist eine Kontrolle der Schilddrüsenfunktion vor der Einstellung auf Lithium und eine regelmäßige Wiederholung derselben, besonders in der 12. bis 16. Woche (Palpation, Bestimmung von PBI und T_4). Vorübergehende Leukozytosen, Zunahme der Glucosetoleranz und EKG-Veränderungen stellen keine Abbruchgründe dar, sollten jedoch mit Hilfe einer jährlichen internistischen Untersuchung überwacht werden (VENDSBORG u. RAFAELSEN, 1973; WATANABE et al., 1974). Als psychische Nebenwirkungen können selten Konzentrationsschwäche und Müdigkeit auftreten (BAUER et al., 1973). Es liegen vereinzelte Berichte über die Entwicklung organischer Psychosyndrome (RIFKIN et al., 1973b; THORNTON u. PRAY, 1975; WALDMANN et al., 1974) oder akuter exogener Reaktionstypen (AGULNIK et al., 1972) vor.

Entzugserscheinungen wurden bei Absetzen von Lithium bisher nicht beobachtet (RIFKIN et al., 1975a).

Eine Lithiumvergiftung entwickelt sich in der Regel erst bei Blutspiegelwerten von 1,5–2,0 mäq/l. Dabei ist zu beachten, daß eine Zunahme der Lithiumkonzentration nicht nur durch eine Dosissteigerung bewirkt werden kann, sondern auch bei unveränderter Dosis durch eine Veränderung der Stoffwechselsituation und der Nierenfunktion entstehen kann. Die Symptomatik einer Lithiumvergiftung entwickelt sich meist langsam. Weil eine Lithiumvergiftung mit einer relativ komplexen internistischen Therapie behandelt werden muß (Überwachung der Plasmaelektrolyte, forcierte Diurese, Peritonealdialyse, Hämodialyse), sollte sofort eine Einweisung in eine medizinische Klinik erfolgen. Als tödlich gelten Blutspiegelwerte von 4–6 mäq/l.

Bei Patienten in höherem Lebensalter (nach dem 65. Lebensjahr) kann auch bei normalem Lithiumspiegel eine dosisabhängige Dysarthrie auftreten, die der Sprachveränderung bei Beginn der Alkoholintoxikation ähnelt (SOLOMON u. VIKKERS, 1975).

7. Applikation und Dosierung

Die Applikation von Lithium erfolgt oral und zwar 3mal täglich bei Verwendung kurzwirksamer Präparate oder 2mal täglich bei Verordnung von Retardpräparaten. Bei Patienten, die trotz sorgfältiger Kontrolle des Serumspiegels unangenehme Nebenwirkungen haben, kann der größere Teil der Tagesdosis abends gegeben werden. Die oft empfohlene einmalige Gabe der gesamten Tagesdosis am Abend ist nur in seltenen Fällen (individuell sehr variable Halbwertszeit) und dann auch nur bei Verwendung von Retardpräparaten zu empfehlen. Vor der einmaligen Einnahme der Tagesdosis kurzwirksamer Präparate muß gewarnt werden, da teilweise toxische postabsorptive Konzentrationsanstiege erfolgen, die nach längerer Zeit eventuell Nierenschäden hervorrufen können.

Bezüglich der Dosierung ist zwischen der Behandlung der Manie und der prophylaktischen Dauermedikation zu unterscheiden. Die therapeutisch wirksame Lithiumdosis bei Manie beträgt bei ausschließlicher Gabe von Lithium 30–60 mäq tgl. und bei Kombination mit Neuroleptika (Neuroleptikadosis kann nach einer Woche langsam reduziert werden) 20–30 mäq. Die Lithiumbehandlung der Manie sollte auch bei Patienten, die anschließend nicht dauerhaft auf Lithium eingestellt werden sollen, 1–2 Monate lang durchgeführt werden, um das Aufflackern manischer Symptome zu vermeiden.

Der Beginn der Lithiumprophylaxe erfolgt am besten vor Beendigung einer depressiven Phase. Für die erfolgreiche Durchführung der Langzeitmedikation stellt die Aufklärung des Patienten über Wirkung und Nebenwirkungen von Lithium und die dadurch vermehrte Kooperationsbereitschaft die wichtigste Voraussetzung dar. Zur Vermeidung von Nebenwirkungen sollte die Prophylaxe möglichst einschleichend begonnen werden. d.h. mit einer initialen Tagesdosis von 6–8 mäq Lithium. Folgendes Procedere hat sich gut bewährt: vom 1. bis 3. Tag werden abends 6–8 mäq gegeben, vom 4. bis 6. Tag morgens und abends je 6–8 mäq und vom 7. bis 9. Tag morgens 6–8 und abends 12–16 mäq. Die Dosissteigerung sollte nur bei guter Verträglichkeit in 3-Tagesschritten vorgenommen werden, andernfalls langsamer.

Am 10. Tag sollte eine erste Blutspiegelkontrolle vorgenommen werden und anschließend die Dosis in der beschriebenen Weise weiter gesteigert werden bis zum Erreichen des notwendigen Serumspiegels von 0,7 bis 1,0 mäq/l. Die Blutentnahme zur Kontrolle des Lithiumspiegels sollte 10 oder mehr Stunden nach Einnahme der letzten Lithiumdosis erfolgen (nicht unbedingt nüchtern). Praktisch hat sich ein Intervall von 12 oder 18 Std zwischen der letzten Lithiumeinnahme und der Blutentnahme bewährt. Der Spiegel nach 18 Std ist etwa 0,1 bis 0,2 mäq/l niedriger als der Wert nach 12 Std.

Die für den beschriebenen Lithiumspiegel erforderliche Dosierung ist von Patient zu Patient individuell herauszufinden und kann zwischen 8–10 mäq pro die und 67–70 mäq pro die liegen. Ältere Patienten benötigen in der Regel niedrigere Dosierungen.

COOPER und SIMPSON (1976) haben ein Verfahren vorgeschlagen, mit dem sie aufgrund der Serumkonzentration 24 Std nach Einnahme einer Testdosis die benötigte Tagesdosis voraussagen können.

Im ersten Behandlungsmonat sollte der Lithiumspiegel wöchentlich, später monatlich kontrolliert werden. Längere Abstände zwischen den Kontrollen sind möglich bei kooperativen Patienten mit langfristig konstantem Lithiumspiegel.

Nach der Einstellungsphase soll außer den Routinekontrollen in folgenden Situationen der Lithiumspiegel bestimmt werden: 1. Auftreten von Vergiftungssymptomen, 2. Rückfall (zu niedrige Dosis?), 3. 7 Tage nach Dosisänderung und Präparatwechsel, 4. interkurrente körperliche Erkrankungen, z.B. Infekte, 5. Änderung der Kochsalzaufnahme und des Wasserhaushaltes, 6. Behandlung mit Kortikoiden und Diuretika, 7. Schwangerschaft (falls nicht abgesetzt, eigentlich Kontraindikation), da die glomeruläre Filtrationsrate bei Beginn um 30–50% ansteigt und kurz vor oder bei der Geburt wieder absinkt.

Die Kombination von Lithium mit anderen Psychopharmaka ist durchaus möglich, kann jedoch zu einer Verstärkung des Tremors führen. Einige kasuistische Mitteilungen haben vor der Kombination von Lithium und Haloperidol gewarnt wegen ausgeprägter Neurotoxizität (COHEN u. COHEN, 1973) sowie schweren extrapyramidalen Nebenwirkungen (MARHOLD et al., 1974). Eine kritische Betrachtung dieser Berichte zeigt jedoch, daß im Vergleich zur verbreiteten

Tabelle 4. Lithium-Präparate

Lithiumsalz	Handelsnamen			Lithiumgehalt pro Tablette	
	BRD	Österreich	Schweiz	mg Lithiumsalz	mäq Lithium
1. Kurzwirksame Präparate					
Lithium-Acetat	Quilonum	Quilonorm	Quilonorm	536	8,1
Lithium-Carbonat	–	Neurolepsin	–	300	8,1
2. Retard-Präparate					
Lithium-Carbonat	Quilonum retard	Quilonorm retard	Quilonorm retard	450	12,2
	Hypnorex	–	Hypnorex	400	10,8
Lithium-Sulfat	–	–	Lithiofor	660	12
	Lithium duriles	–	–	330	6

Anwendung von Lithium derart schwere Nebenwirkungen äußerst selten sind und daß in den beschriebenen Fällen die Durchführung der medikamentösen Therapie nicht als ganz kunstgerecht angesehen werden kann (AYD, 1975a).

8. Behandlungsdauer

Die Prophylaxe mit Lithium sollte mindestens ein Jahr lang, in der Regel jedoch auf unbeschränkte Dauer durchgeführt werden. Während eventuell auftretenden Krankheitsphasen sollte die Einnahme von Lithium weitergeführt werden. Kurzdauernde Unterbrechungen von wenigen Wochen beeinträchtigen die prophylaktische Wirkung nicht und sind bei Fieberzuständen und mit Diarrhoe verknüpften Erkrankungen indiziert.

9. Präparate

Eine Auswahl der im Handel befindlichen Lithiumpräparate ist in Tabelle 4 zusammengestellt.

F. Anxiolytika

1. Terminologie und Klassifikation

Unter Anxiolytika (Tranquilizer) werden diejenigen Psychopharmaka verstanden, welche in erster Linie zur Behandlung von Angstzuständen verschiedenster Ätiologie indiziert sind. Chemisch handelt es sich vorwiegend um Benzodiazepine, welche diesbezüglich den Markt beherrschen. Zu den Anxiolytika werden aber auch Substanzen mit anderer chemischer Struktur gezählt wie Carbaminsäure-Derivate, Diphenylmethan-Derivate, tri- und tetrazyklische Tranquilizer. Sedativa und Antipsychotika können in kleinen Dosen bei Angstzuständen erfolgreich angewendet werden, ohne daß sie deshalb direkt den Anxiolytika zuzurechnen wären.

2. Klinische Wirkung

Die psychotrope anxiolytische Wirkung ist unspezifisch gegen Angstsyndrome verschiedenster Ätiologie gerichtet. Angstzustände sind Syndrome mit innerer subjektiv erlebter Angst, Furcht oder Panik, psychischer oder motorischer Unruhe und vegetativen Begleitsymptomen wie Mundtrockenheit, Obstipation, Diarrhoe, Tachykardie, Mydriasis und Schwitzen. Reine Angstsyndrome kommen vorwiegend bei funktionellen Störungen vor, so bei Neurosen, psychosomatischen Erkrankungen, Depressionen und Sucht.

Die verschiedenen Präparate unterscheiden sich weniger in der Anxiolyse als in ihren sedierenden und muskelrelaxierenden sowie antikonvulsiven Eigenschaften. Diese sind bei der Differentialindikation zu berücksichtigen. Anxiolytika sind dadurch charakterisiert, daß sie im Gegensatz zu den Neuroleptika keine antipsychotische Wirkung aufweisen, keine extrapyramidalen Nebenwirkungen erzeugen und auch nur sehr milde vegetative Nebenwirkungen hervorrufen. Sie sind also außerordentlich gut verträglich.

3. Wirkungseintritt

In Abhängigkeit von der Art und Dauer der bestehenden Symptomatik ist mit einer unterschiedlichen Dauer bis zum Wirkungseintritt zu rechnen. Bei der parenteralen Anwendung im Rahmen psychiatrischer Notfallsituationen (z. B. Erregungszustände, Delirien, Panikzustände) wird eine sehr rasche (wenige Minuten bis Stunden) Wirkung beobachtet. Bei der Behandlung länger bestehender Angstsymptome (z. B. bei Neurosen) ist erst etwa nach 5 Tagen mit einer leichten Besserung zu rechnen, die die Wirksamkeit des Präparates anzeigt. Bleibt diese Besserung aus, so sollte die Dosierung gesteigert oder nach 8 bis 10 Tagen das Präparat gewechselt werden.

4. Indikationen

Bei der Indikationsstellung muß man berücksichtigen, daß die Therapie mit Anxiolytika eine symptomatische Behandlung zur gezielten Bekämpfung von Angstsymptomen darstellt. Die verläßliche Wirkung, die Häufigkeit von Angstsyndromen verschiedenster Ätiologie und die gute Verträglichkeit verleiten leicht zu einer kurzschlüssigen, eine genaue Diagnose überspringenden Verschreibung. Grundsätzlich sollte ein Anxiolytikum erst nach genauer körperlicher und psychischer Untersuchung und Diagnosestellung verschrieben werden, falls keine spezifischere Therapie (Psychotherapie, Antidepressiva, Antipsychotika) angezeigt ist.

Die Indikationsstellung ist heute sehr breit und umfaßt nicht nur Angstsyndrome bei Neurosen, psychosomatischen Störungen, Suchten und Depressionen, sondern Anxiolytika werden auch vielfach im Rahmen der somatischen Medizin zur Dämpfung reaktiver Angst, Spannung und Unruhe verabreicht; so zum Beispiel vor somatischen Eingriffen, zur Geburtsvorbereitung, bei gastrointestinalen Störungen, Allergien, Kopfschmerzen, rheumatischen Schmerzen und Schlafstörungen. Innerhalb der Psychiatrie stellen seltenere Indikationen das Delirium tremens, die arteriosklerotische Erregung und epileptische Verstimmungen dar, schließlich auch sexuelle Hyperaktivität.

Benzodiazepine wirken nicht antidepressiv, vermögen aber Angst und Erregung als Teilsymptome der Depression zu lindern und werden daher gelegentlich kombiniert mit Antidepressiva verordnet, zumal auch keine Enzyminduktion der letzteren stattfindet. Bei Manien oder Schizophrenien sind Tranquilizer in der Regel nicht indiziert. Viel diskutiert wurde die Wirkung gegen die Hostilität; entgegen den ursprünglichen Erwartungen wurde nicht selten eine Steigerung der Hostilität und des Kampfverhaltens am Tier und gelegentlich auch beim Menschen beobachtet. Dieser Effekt dürfte nicht einer direkten Steigerung der Hostilität durch die Anxiolytika zuzuschreiben sein, sondern eher einer Angstminderung und Enthemmung.

Neuromuskuläre Erkrankungen, gekennzeichnet durch Spasmen, Tonuserhöhung und Schmerzen, bilden eine besondere Indikation für Anxiolytika, da die periphere muskelrelaxierende Wirkung und die zentrale Entspannung kombiniert nutzbringend sind.

Anxiolytika wurden immer wieder empfohlen zur Milderung von Entzugserscheinungen, zum Beispiel bei Alkoholismus. Die hier auftretenden psychischen und vegetativen Entzugserscheinungen sind meist so milde und kurzdauernd, daß angesichts des vorhandenen Suchtpotentials besser nicht zu einer Anxiolytikatherapie gegriffen wird. Bei anamnestisch bekannter Gefahr von schweren Entzugserscheinungen (Delirien, epileptische Anfälle) hingegen sind Benzodiazepine indiziert. Das gleiche gilt für Entzugserscheinungen bei Hypnotikasucht oder bei Heroinsucht (so auch bei Neugeborenen von heroinsüchtigen Müttern). Benzodiazepine sind schließlich indiziert, um unerwünschte Symptome nach Einnahme von halluzinogenen Stoffen zu unterdrücken (z.B. LSD).

Benzodiazepine sind zum Teil wirksame Hypnotika. Sie können wie andere Schlafmittel einen Kater (Hangover) und psychomotorische Störungen hervorrufen. Bei psychoreaktiven Schlafstörungen (in der Regel erkennbar an Einschlafstörungen und um Konflikte kreisendes Denken) muß nicht unbedingt zum Hypnotikum gegriffen werden, sondern es kann ein Anxiolytikum allein schon genügend entspannen, um den Schlaf in Gang zu bringen. Der Schlaf selbst wird durch Benzodiazepine wie durch andere Hypnotika unphysiologisch im Sinne einer Unterdrückung der REM-Phasen verändert, mit einem anhaltenden Rebound nach Absetzen der Therapie. Einzelne Präparate machen hier gewisse Ausnahmen, so wurde nach Flurazepam kein Rebound gefunden, und therapeutische Dosen von Flurazepam scheinen den REM-Schlaf nur gering zu reduzieren. Charakteristisch ist im übrigen eine Reduktion des Stadiums 4 des orthodoxen Schlafes, was therapeutisch wichtig sein mag bei der Behandlung der Enuresis nocturna, des Somnambulismus und des Pavor nocturnus, von denen angenommen wird, daß sie vorwiegend im Stadium 4 auftreten.

5. Kontraindikationen

Als eigentliche Kontraindikation ist nur die Myasthenia gravis zu nennen. Besondere Vorsicht ist aber auch geboten bei Gravidität, Herzinsuffizienz, Leber- oder Niereninsuffizienz, zerebralen Schädigungen und bei Kombination mit Alkohol.

6. Nebenwirkungen

Die wichtigsten Nebenwirkungen bestehen in: Übersedierung, Schläfrigkeit, Somnolenz, Hangover; Schwindel, Ataxie, Dysarthrie, Diplopie, Visusstörungen; Muskelrelaxation, Muskelschwäche, plötzliches Zusammensacken; Verlust von Libido, Impotenz, Ejakulationsstörungen; Enuresis; Verwirrung; Agitation, Hostilität; Hypotension; Gewichtszunahme, Appetitzunahme; allergische Hautreaktionen, Ödeme; Obstipation, Diarrhoe, Nausea, Vomitus, Dysphagie.

Im Verhältnis zur enormen Verbreitung von Anxiolytika muß deren Suchtpotential als sehr niedrig bezeichnet werden. Erhöht ist natürlich die Gefahr bei Drogenabhängigen und Alkoholikern. Das Entzugssyndrom entspricht dem der Barbituratsucht: Schlaflosigkeit, Agitation, Appetitverlust, epileptische Anfälle, Myoklonien, psychotische Verwirrungen und Depressionen. Angesichts der engen pharmakologischen Verwandtschaft zum Alkohol addieren sich in kleineren Dosen die Wirkungen beider Substanzen, in höheren Dosierungen erfolgt eventuell sogar eine Potenzierung mit entsprechender Gefährdung z.B. im Straßenverkehr. Der Diphenylhydantoinspiegel kann durch Benzodiazepine erhöht werden. Eine Erklärung dafür steht noch aus.

7. Applikation und Dosierung

Die häufigste Applikationsform der Anxiolytika ist die orale Einnahme. In der psychiatrischen Klinik werden Anxiolytika in akuten Notfallsituationen auch intramuskulär oder Diazepam sogar intravenös injiziert (sorgfältige Kreislaufüberwachung, langsame Injektion!).

Dosierungsrichtlinien lassen sich für Anxiolytika kaum aufstellen, da die therapeutische Dosisbreite dieser Substanzen außerordentlich groß ist. Abgesehen von der Behandlung in Akutsituationen hat es sich bewährt, die bei dem betreffenden Patienten kleinste wirksame Dosis zu geben. Bei der individuell sehr unterschiedlichen Wirkung ist besonders in der ambulanten Behandlung initial die Gabe einer ganz kleinen Dosierung (beispielsweise 2 oder 5 mg Diazepam) vorteilhaft.

Die sedierende Wirkungskomponente der Anxiolytika ist recht unterschiedlich ausgeprägt. Daher ist bei vielen ambulanten Patienten die einmalige abendliche Gabe am günstigsten, was bei der langen Halbwertzeit (7 bis 30 Std) der meisten Anxiolytika auch aus pharmakokinetischen Gründen gerechtfertigt erscheint.

8. Behandlungsdauer

Anders als bei der Behandlung mit Antipsychotika und Antidepressiva sollten Anxiolytika möglichst kurzfristig eingenommen werden. Bei erreichter Symptomfreiheit oder bei deutlicher Besserung ist eine längere Fortführung der Anxiolytikagabe unnötig und ein langsames Absetzen indiziert. Eine mehrmonatige Anxiolytikabehandlung ist selten notwendig, beispielsweise bei Angstneurosen. In vielen Fällen ist während einer länger dauernden Anxiolytikabehandlung ein Präparatwechsel günstig.

In der Regel wird die Anxiolytikatherapie mit einem einzigen Präparat durchgeführt. Die gleichzeitige Verordnung mehrerer Anxiolytika sollte therapeutisch ungünstig zu beeinflussenden Ausnahmefällen vorbehalten bleiben.

9. Präparate

Die in Deutschland, Österreich und der Schweiz zur Verfügung stehenden Anxiolytika sind in Tabelle 5 zusammengestellt.

G. Betarezeptoren-Blocker

1. Terminologie und Klassifikation

Betablocker sind Substanzen, die reversibel und kompetitiv Betarezeptoren im sympathischen System zu blockieren vermögen, also Antagonisten von Noradrenalin und Adrenalin, vielleicht auch Dopamin. Chemisch sind alle Betablocker durch eine katecholaminähnliche Struktur charakterisiert; sie schalten die Wirkung der Katecholamine auf das zyklische AMP in den Rezeptoren aus. Die Betablocker können in kardiostimulierende und gefäßerweiternde Substanzen eingeteilt werden. Betablocker passieren die Bluthirnschranke in unterschied-

Tabelle 5. Anxiolytika

Internationale chemische Kurzbezeichnung (generic name)	Handelsnamen			Dosierung (per os, mg/Tag) klinisch und ambulant
	BRD	Österreich	Schweiz	
1. Benzodiazepine				
Chlorazepat (522)[a] (Dikalium-Chlorazepat)	Tranxilium	Tranxilium	Tranxilium	10–60
Chlordiazepoxid (523)	Librium	Librium	Librium	20–100
Diazepam (528)	Valium	Valium Umbrium	Valium	10–60
Lorazepam (533)	Tavor	Temesta	Temesta	2–10
Medazepam (534)	Nobrium	Nobrium	Nobrium	15–30
Oxazepam (538)	Adumbran Praxiten	Adumbran Anxiolit Praxiten	–	10–60
Prazepam (539)	Demetin	Demetin	–	10–30
2. Carbaminsäure-Derivate				
Guajokolglycerinäther (1362)	Reorganin	–	–	50–1500
Meprobamat (1446)	Meprosa Miltaun Urbilat Aneural Cyrpon Dabromat Meprobamat Meprocompren	Cyrpon Meprobamat Microbamat Pertranquil Epikur Miltaun	Meprodil Miltown Oasil Pertranquil Quanamane	400–1200
Phenoprobamat (1374)	Gamaquil	Gamaquil	–	400–800
3. Diphenylmethan-Derivate				
Hydroxin (768)	Atarax Masmoran	Atarax	Atarax	50–100
4. Tri- und tetrazyklische Tranquilizer				
Benzoctamin (1104)	Tacitin	Tacitin	Tacitin	10–40
Opipramol (227)	Insidon	Insidon	Insidon	75–200

[a] Die in Klammern den generic names beigefügte Zahl bezieht sich auf die von USDIN und EFRON (1972) herausgegebene Zusammenstellung psychotroper Substanzen

lichem Maße und sind auch unterschiedlich lipophil, was zu einer sehr variablen Verteilung im Gehirn führt.

2. Indikationen

Betablocker bewirken eine Blockierung peripherer neurovegetativer Symptome der Angst und werden aus diesem Grunde zur Behandlung folgender

Störungen verwendet: funktionelle kardiale Syndrome, periphere vegetative Symptome bei Depressionen (PÖLDINGER, 1967) und Angstsymptome bei Kindern.

FLORU (1977) hat auf die Vorteile der Betablocker gegenüber den Tranquilizern hingewiesen: weniger Nebenwirkungen, sehr geringe Leistungsbeeinträchtigung und keine Anzeichen für Gewöhnung. Endogene Psychosen, z. B. Schizophrenien, werden durch Betablocker nicht sicher gebessert. Wiederholt wurden Erfolge bei Psychosen des akuten endogenen Reaktionstyps kasuistisch mitgeteilt. v. ZERSSEN (1976) berichtete über die erfolgreiche Behandlung einer organischen Psychose bei Porphyrie und beobachtete bei mehreren manischen Patienten eine leichte bis deutliche Besserung.

Entzugserscheinungen bei Alkoholsucht können durch Betablocker gemildert werden (Tremor, Blutdruck, Puls, Befindlichkeit des Patienten). Hinweise auf eine mögliche Verhütung von Amphetaminpsychosen durch Betablocker bedürfen einer gründlichen Überprüfung.

FLORU wies 1971 auf günstige Behandlungserfolge mit Betablockern bei lithiumbedingtem Tremor hin. Bei Parkinsontremor haben sich Betablocker nicht als wirksam erwiesen.

Vegetative Nebenwirkungen (Blutdruckschwankungen, Arrhythmien) von Antidepressiva und adrenerge Nebeneffekte von Neuroleptika können durch Betablocker gebessert werden. Auch bei Vergiftungen mit tri- und tetrazyklischen Antidepressiva sowie MAO-Hemmern können Betablocker verwendet werden.

3. Nebenwirkungen

Betablocker können Müdigkeit, Kopfschmerzen, Paraesthesien und allgemeine Schwäche bewirken und toxische Psychosen auslösen. Herzinsuffizienz, Arrhythmie, latentes Asthma und Diabetes mellitus können sich unter der Behandlung mit Betablockern verschlechtern.

4. Präparate

Am häufigsten werden Oxprenolol, Pindolol und Propranolol verwendet.

H. Hypnotika

1. Terminologie und Klassifikation

Hypnotika oder Schlafmittel stellen eine chemisch ausgesprochen heterogene Gruppe dar. Eigentlich kann jedes Pharmakon als Hypnotikum bezeichnet werden, das eine schlaffördernde Wirkung hat. Kennzeichnend für Hypnotika im engeren Sinne ist das dosisabhängige Spektrum sedativ – hypnotisch – narkotisch. Darunter ist zu verstehen, daß Hypnotika in niedriger Dosierung sedierend wirken, in einer mittleren Dosierung ihre eigentliche Schlafmittelwirkung entfalten und in hohen Dosen narkotisch wirken. Entsprechend ihrer Zugehörigkeit zu bestimmten chemischen Substanzgruppen können die Schlafmittel eingeteilt werden in Alkohole, Harnstoffderivate, Barbitursäurederivate, Piperidinderivate, Chinazolinonderivate, Benzodiazepinderivate und Thiazolderivate.

Eine andere Einteilungsmöglichkeit besteht darin, die Schlafmittel in zwei Gruppen einzuteilen, nämlich in Barbiturate und Nichtbarbiturate. Diese Einteilung ist wegen der Suchtgefahr der Barbiturate sinnvoll.

In Abhängigkeit von der Wirkungsdauer werden die Hypnotika klinisch in Einschlafmittel (kurzwirksam, schneller Wirkungseintritt) und Durchschlafmittel (länger wirksam, verzögerter Wirkungseintritt möglich) eingeteilt. Diese Einteilung ist für die Verordnung eines bestimmten Schlafmittels vorzuziehen, da die Präparatwahl vor allem nach der Art der vorliegenden Schlafstörung erfolgt.

Es liegt eine Fülle von Kombinationspräparaten vor (barbiturathaltige und barbituratfreie), deren Anwendung aus pharmakologischer Sicht wegen der Gefahr unübersichtlicher Interaktionen und Potenzierungseffekte als problematisch anzusehen ist.

2. Klinische Wirkung

Wie schon erwähnt, wirken Hypnotika je nach der verwendeten Dosierung sedierend, hypnotisch oder narkotisch. Vor allem Barbiturate und Chlormethiazol haben außerdem eine antikonvulsive Wirkungskomponente, die zur Behandlung epileptischer Anfälle, des Status epilepticus und bei einigen Barbituraten auch zur antiepileptischen Dauermedikation eingesetzt wird.

3. Wirkungseintritt

Die in Tabelle 6 als Einschlafmittel gekennzeichneten Hypnotika zeigen einen raschen Wirkungseintritt und sollen daher erst kurz vor dem Schlafengehen eingenommen werden. Die Wirkung der Durchschlafmittel setzt in der Regel weniger prompt ein.

4. Indikationen

Bei den vielen unterschiedlichen Ursachen von Schlafstörungen ist eine genaue Anamnese und eine exakte Beschreibung der Schlafstörung sehr wichtig. Schlafstörungen können infolge somatischer Erkrankungen oder Störungen (Schmerzzustände, internistische Erkrankungen wie Herzinsuffizienz, neurologische Prozesse), inadäquate Umgebung, ungünstiger Tagesablauf (ausgeprägter Konsum erregender Mittel, Bewegungsmangel, abendliche große Mahlzeiten), psychiatrische Erkrankungen oder durch verschiedenste Konflikte und Beanspruchungen hervorgerufen werden. Eine große Zahl von Schlafstörungen ist durch eine kausale Therapie des Grundleidens besser zu behandeln als durch Verordnung von Hypnotika. Schlafstörungen bei zerebralsklerotischen Patienten werden durch Schlafmittel eher ungünstig beeinflußt, sprechen dagegen gut auf anregende Medikamente an, z.B. Coffein. Außerdem ist bei diesen Patienten die Möglichkeit schlafmittel-induzierter Verwirrungszustände (insbesondere nach Barbituraten) gegeben.

Erst nach Abklärung einer möglichen Kausaltherapie ist die Verordnung von Hypnotika indiziert. Die differentielle Indikationsstellung erfolgt vor allem in Abhängigkeit von der qualitativen und quantitativen Ausgestaltung der Schlafstörung.

Tabelle 6. Hypnotika

Internationale chemische Kurzbezeichnung (generic name)	Chemische Gruppe	Handelsnamen BRD	Österreich	Schweiz	Dosierung (per os, mg)
1. Einschlafmittel					
Bromisoval (1493)[a]	H	Bromural	–	Bromural	600–1 200
Chloralhydrat (1413)	A	Chloraldurat (rot)	Chloraldurat (rot)	Chloraldurat (rot)	1 000–2 000
Clomethiazol (708) (Chlormethiazol)	T	Distraneurin	Distraneurin	–	500
Ethinamat (1442)	U	Valamin	Valamin	Valamin	500–2 000
Flunitrazepam	Be	–	–	Rohypnol	2–8
Gluthetimid (758)	P	Doriden	Doriden	Doriden	250–400
Hexobarbital (576)	B	Evipan	–	Evipan	260–520
Methaqualon (843)	Ch	Revonal	Revonal	Revonal	200–400
Nitrazepam (536)	Be	Mogadan	Mogadon	Mogadon	5–10
Pentobarbital (583)	B	Repocal	Nembutal	Repocal	100–200
Pyrithyldion	P	Persedon	Persedon	Persedon	200–400
2. Durchschlafmittel					
Chloralhydrat (1413)	A	Chloraldurat (blau)	Chloraldurat (blau)	Chloraldurat (blau)	1 000–2 000
Cyclobarbital (570)	B	Phanodorm	Phanodorm	Phanodorm	100–200
Flurazepam (530)	Be	Dalmadorm	–	Dalmadorm	15–30
Flunitrazepam	Be	–	–	Rohypnol	2–8
Heptabarbital (574)	B	Medomin	Medomin	Medomin	100–200
Methyprylon (849)	P	Noludar	Noludar	Noludar	200–400
Phenobarbital	B	Luminal	Austrominal	Luminal	60–100

[a] Die in Klammern den generic names beigefügte Zahl bezieht sich auf die von USDIN und EFRON (1972) herausgegebene Zusammenstellung psychotroper Substanzen
A = Alkohol; B = Barbiturat; Be = Benzodiazepin; Ch = Chinazolinon-Derivat; H = Harnstoff-Derivat; P = Piperidin-Derivat; U = Urethan-Derivat; T = Thiazol-Derivat

Besonders hinzuweisen ist auf Chlormethiazol, das nicht nur in der Delirbehandlung eine große Rolle spielt, sondern sich auch als Schlafmittel vor allem bei Vorhandensein organischer Hirnschäden bewährt hat.

Bei psychotischen Patienten, die ohnehin unter neuroleptischer Medikation stehen, kann durch abendliche Gabe einer höheren Neuroleptikadosis oft eine ausreichende Schlafwirkung erzielt werden, so daß die gleichzeitige Gabe von Schlafmitteln vermieden werden kann. Gleiches gilt für Patienten mit leichter ausgeprägten depressiven Schlafstörungen, die mit sedierenden Antidepressiva behandelt werden.

Bei suchtgefährdeten Patienten empfiehlt sich an Stelle einer Schlafmittelverordnung die Applikation von Neuroleptika. Bei diesen Patienten muß jedoch beachtet werden, daß eventuell extrapyramidale Nebenwirkungen auftreten können.

Die Kombination von Barbituraten und Neuroleptika kann bei ganz schweren Schlafstörungen empfohlen werden, da die schlafanstoßende Wirkung der Barbiturate durch Neuroleptika unterstützt wird. Sind Schlafstörungen gleichzeitig mit Suizidalität oder drohender Fremdgefährdung (z. B. bei Psychosen) vorhanden, so müssen sie als zwingende Indikation für die Verordnung hoher Hypnotikadosen angesehen werden.

5. Kontraindikationen

Barbiturate sind absolut kontraindiziert bei intermittierender Porphyrie, da sie eine Vermehrung der Porphyrinkörper bewirken. Bei Vorliegen von Leber- und Nierenkrankheiten sollen Barbiturate und Chloralhydrat nicht gegeben werden. Letzteres sollte auch bei Herzbeschwerden und Gastritis vermieden werden. Bei chronischem Emphysem sollten Barbiturate nur mit größter Vorsicht verordnet werden, da sie die Tätigkeit des Atemzentrums hemmen, was bei körperlich gesunden Patienten in hypnotischen Dosen keine Rolle spielt.

Selbstverständlich ist die Gabe von Hypnotika wegen der starken Tendenz zur Abhängigkeit oder Sucht bei süchtigen Patienten genau zu prüfen.

6. Nebenwirkungen

Nicht als Nebenwirkung, jedoch als oft unerwünschte Wirkung der Barbiturate muß die Enzyminduktion angesehen werden, wodurch gleichzeitig verordnete Psychopharmaka (z. B. Antidepressiva und manche Neuroleptika) beschleunigt abgebaut werden.

Die wichtigsten Nebenwirkungen oder besser Gefahren der Hypnotika bestehen in der Toleranzentwicklung, der Ausbildung psychischer und physischer Abhängigkeit und der teilweise lebensbedrohlichen Toxizität höherer Dosierungen. Letztere spielt nicht nur eine Rolle bei Suizidversuchen und Suiziden, sondern auch bei unbeabsichtigten Überdosierungen. Hypnotika können aufgrund ihrer teilweise recht ausgeprägten Kumulationsneigung chronische Vergiftungen hervorrufen, die durch Sprachstörungen, Nystagmus, Ataxie, Apathie, Interesseneinengung, emotionale Nivellierung und Verlangsamung des Denkens gekennzeichnet sind.

Nach langfristiger Anwendung von Metaqualon sind Polyneuropathien beschrieben worden, beginnend mit Paraesthesien und motorischer Schwäche in den unteren Extremitäten.

Die wichtigsten Symptome der Barbituratvergiftung sind Bewußtlosigkeit (oft nach einem deliranten Erregungsstadium), zentrale Atemhemmung mit Sauerstoffmangelsymptomatik, spät einsetzendes Kreislaufversagen, Verminderung der Nierenfunktion und Temperaturabfall (Anstieg infolge Bronchopneumonie). Entsprechend dieser Symptomatik besteht die von KUSCHINSKY und LÜLLMANN (1974) empfohlene Behandlung vor allem in einer Beseitigung der zentralen Atemlähmung, Überwachung und Normalisierung des Kreislaufes und in einer Magenspülung. Bei schweren Vergiftungen sind forcierte osmotische Diurese, Austauschtransfusion und Hämodialyse indiziert. Die Anwendung von Analeptika ist Ausnahmefällen vorbehalten.

Folgende Entziehungssymptome kennzeichnen die Barbituratsucht: Angst, Schwäche, Nausea, Tremor, Delirien und sehr häufig epileptische Anfälle.

Es ist besonders auf die Gefahr des Bromismus bei chronischer Zufuhr von bromhaltigen Harnstoffderivaten hinzuweisen, die vor allem durch die fehlende Rezeptpflicht verstärkt wird. Die wichtigsten Symptome des Bromismus sind Akne, Schnupfen, Konjunktivitis und zentralnervöse Symptome wie Apathie, Ataxie und Depressionen.

7. Applikation und Dosierung

Zur Behandlung von Schlafstörungen werden die Hypnotika meist oral appliziert. Einige Präparate liegen als Suppositorien vor. Die parenterale Applikation (besonders intramuskulär) kommt vor allem zur Beruhigung erregter Patienten zur Anwendung. Bei der Behandlung von Delirien kann Chlormethiazol intravenös injiziert oder als Tropfinfusion verabreicht werden.

Die wirksame hypnotische Dosierung der gebräuchlichsten Hypnotika ist in Tabelle 6 zusammengestellt.

8. Behandlungsdauer

Hypnotika sollten so kurz wie möglich angewendet werden, im günstigsten Fall nur wenige Tage bis zwei Wochen. Ist eine längere Gabe von Schlafmitteln indiziert, so sollte von Zeit zu Zeit das Präparat gewechselt werden und ein Schlafmittel aus einer anderen chemischen Gruppe verordnet werden.

Bei Vorliegen einer Barbituratsucht ist zur Vermeidung ängstlicher Unruhe, epileptischer Anfälle und Delirien der Entzug nicht plötzlich sondern sukzessiv im Verlauf von etwa 10–20 Tagen durchzuführen. Noch besser hat sich der sofortige Ersatz des Suchtmittels durch Chlormethiazol bewährt.

9. Präparate

Die Hypnotika sind geordnet nach Einschlaf- und Durchschlafmitteln mit der wirksamen schlafanstoßenden Dosierung in Tabelle 6 zusammengestellt. Die einzelnen Präparate sind entsprechend ihrer Zugehörigkeit zu bestimmten chemischen Gruppen gekennzeichnet.

I. Behandlung psychiatrischer Notfallsituationen

I. Allgemeines

Als Wichtigstes ist zunächst eine genaue Zustandsbeschreibung mit Syndromdiagnose vorzunehmen. Die oft schwierige nosologische Diagnose kann erleichtert werden durch fremdanamnestische Angaben. Neben allgemeinmedizinischen Maßnahmen wie z.B. Lagerung bewußtloser Patienten, Überprüfung von Atmung, Blasenfüllung, Temperatur, Herz- und Kreislauffunktionen, kann eine symptomatische medikamentöse Therapie notwendig sein. Wird der Patient als hospitalisierungsbedürftig angesehen, so sollte im Einweisungszeugnis nicht nur eine möglichst genaue Beschreibung des Zustandes vor Gabe einer Medikation, sondern auch diese selbst angegeben werden. Bei bewußtlosen Patienten ist vor allem darauf zu achten, daß auch während des Transportes ins Krankenhaus eine genaue Überwachung und richtige Lagerung eingehalten wird.

II. Erregungszustände

Als Symptome können neben Angst, psychomotorischer Unruhe, starker Erregung und Aggressivität auch Desorientierung, Umdämmerung und Verwirrung auftreten. Es ist besonders auf das Vorhandensein und die Ausprägung von Bewußtseinsstörungen zu achten. Psychomotorische Erregungszustände können vor allem bei folgenden Grundkrankheiten vorkommen: Schizophrenie, Manie, schwere körperliche Erkrankungen, akute und chronische Hirnerkrankungen, Intoxikationen mit Alkohol, Psychopharmaka, Halluzinogenen, psychogene Erregungszustände.

Die Medikation bei akuten Erregungszuständen sollte nicht nur symptomgerichtet, sondern unter Beachtung der Grundstörung erfolgen. Erregungszustände bei Schizophrenie und Manie sprechen gut auf intramuskuläre Injektionen von Clozapin (50–75 mg, bis 500 mg/24 Std), Levomepromazin (25–50 mg, bis 200 mg/24 Std) und Promazin (50–100 mg bis 200 mg/24 Std) an. Bei ausbleibender oder ungenügender Wirkung können die Injektionen schon nach 30 min wiederholt werden. Haloperidol (5 mg i. m., bis 20 mg/24 Std) hat sich vor allem bewährt bei symptomatischen Psychosen bei körperlichen Krankheiten, psychoorganischem Syndrom, Alkoholrausch, akuten Intoxikationen mit Psychopharmaka und Halluzinogenen. Bei ganz schwerer Erregung kann Haloperidol auch intravenös injiziert werden. Bei ängstlich gefärbten Erregungszuständen, besonders bei psychogener Erregung und bei bad trips nach Halluzinogenen wird Diazepam (10 mg, bis 40 mg/24 Std) intramuskulär oder auch ganz langsam intravenös injiziert.

Die früher oft verwendete Kombination von Morphin und Scopolamin sollte nur im äußersten Notfall eingesetzt werden, da bei organischen Vorschädigungen lebensgefährliche Nebenwirkungen, insbesondere eine Atemdepression zu befürchten sind.

Bei diagnostischer Unklarheit kann entweder Chlormethiazol oder Haloperidol verwendet werden. Bei Intoxikationen mit Alkohol oder Schlafmitteln soll Chlormethiazol nicht gegeben werden.

III. Delirien

Zusätzlich zur motorischen Unruhe und Erregung sind Delirien durch Orientierungsstörungen, Verwirrtheit, Sinnestäuschungen und auch Wahngedanken gekennzeichnet. Im Vordergrund steht die organische Färbung des Zustandsbildes. Delirien können verschiedenste Ursachen haben: chronischer Alkoholismus, Medikamentensucht, Halluzinogenabusus, schwere körperliche Erkrankungen mit primärer oder sekundärer Hirnbeteiligung wie z. B. Infektionskrankheiten. Neuroleptika, Antidepressiva und Antiparkinsonmittel können in hoher Dosierung oder aber bei Patienten mit organischen Hirnschäden, zerebraler Arteriosklerose und im Alter zu Delirien führen.

Ungeachtet der Ursache ist die wichtigste therapeutische Maßnahme das Absetzen aller Medikamente, Suchtmittel und ärztlich verordneter Psychopharmaka. Bei Delirien im Rahmen körperlicher Erkrankungen ist die Behandlung der Grundkrankheit sofort aufzunehmen. Als Medikation der Wahl ist bei Delirien Chlormethiazol anzusehen (Ausnahme: Delir bei Chlormethiazol-Sucht, Behandlung mit Haloperidol). In der Regel wird Chlormethiazol oral appliziert (–8 g/24 Std), seltener (nur in Kliniken) intravenös infundiert. Vor Beginn der Chlormethiazol-Behandlung sollte außer Haloperidol kein dämpfendes Präparat gegeben werden, da sonst die Gefahr besteht, daß sich die dämpfende Wirkung verstärkt.

IV. Stupor

Differentialdiagnostisch kommen ein psychogener, katatoner oder depressiver Stupor in Frage. Ohne Anamnese ist diese Unterscheidung selten möglich. Wichtig ist vor allem die somatische Untersuchung, da eine mögliche Verwechslung mit Sopor, Koma oder Kollaps zu vermeiden ist. In der Regel wird bei denjenigen Patienten, deren Zustand nicht offenkundig psychogen ausgelöst wurde, eine Krankenhauseinweisung nicht zu umgehen sein. Für den Notfallarzt sollte die Regel gelten, daß er möglichst keine Medikamente applizieren sollte.

V. Dysleptische Krisen

Unter der Therapie mit Neuroleptika können Dyskinesien in Form von Krämpfen im oropharyngealen, okulären Bereich und in der Muskulatur von Schulter und Hals auftreten, die mit intramuskulärer oder sogar intravenöser Applikation von Antiparkinsonmitteln, vor allem Biperiden (2,5–5 mg) gut zu beherrschen sind. Diese auch als akute Dystonien oder extrapyramidale Frühdyskinesien bezeichneten Nebenwirkungen sind vor allem bei Betroffensein der Zungen- und Schlundmuskulatur aufgrund der entstehenden Erstickungsangst äußerst quälend und bedürfen einer sofortigen medikamentösen Behandlung.

J. Nebenwirkungen von Psychopharmaka

I. Kardiovaskuläre Nebenwirkungen

Angesichts der Häufigkeit von Herz- und Kreislauferkrankungen in der Bevölkerung sind die kardiovaskulären Nebenwirkungen der Psychopharmaka besonders wichtig. Patienten im Alter von mehr als 50 Jahren können vor allem während einer Langzeitmedikation mit Psychopharmaka langsam kardial dekompensieren. Bei der Behandlung älterer Patienten ist daher besonders sorgfältig auf Frühsymptome zu achten und im Bedarfsfall eine Herzmedikation einzuleiten.

Die nach therapeutischen Dosen von Psychopharmaka beobachteten *EKG-Veränderungen* (HATASHITA, 1974) sind meistens auf reversible Repolarisationsstörungen zurückzuführen (HIPPIUS u. MALIN, 1968; MALIN u. ROSENBERG, 1974). Trizyklische Antidepressiva werden rasch vom Myokard aufgenommen und verursachen starke anticholinerge Effekte (VOHRA u. BURROWS, 1974). Katecholamin-Wirkungen können geblockt werden. Nebeneffekte sind Sinustachykardien, Verlängerungen der atrioventrikulären und intraventrikulären Überleitungszeit, supraventrikuläre Tachykardien, ventrikuläre Arrhythmien, ausgesprochene Bradykardie und Asystolien sowie gelegentlich atrioventrikulärer oder sinuatriärer Block. Im EKG können Verlängerungen des QT-Intervalles und eine ST-Hebung beobachtet werden, wodurch Verwechslungen mit Myokardinfarkten möglich sind (BALLIN, 1975; CAMPICHE, 1973; ELIASEN u. ANDERSEN, 1975; KANTOR et al., 1975). In diesem Zusammenhang ist es erstaunlich, daß Kinder während der Behandlung mit den verschiedensten Psychopharmaka offenbar keine Repolarisationsstörungen im EKG zeigen (MARTIN u. ZAUG, 1975; WINSBERG et al., 1975; WOLPERT u. FARR, 1975). Eine quantitative Beziehung zwischen einer Dosierung von Psychopharmaka und T-Wellen-Veränderungen im EKG konnte bisher nicht gesichert werden (WENDKOS, 1967).

Ursächlich auf Psychopharmaka zurückzuführende pathologisch-anatomische Schädigungen des Myokards sind nicht bekannt.

Im Rahmen der vegetativen Nebenwirkungen von Psychopharmaka werden *Tachykardien* (am häufigsten unter Antidepressivamedikation) und *Bradykardien* (z.B. unter Reserpin) beobachtet.

Übersichten zum Thema der Kreislaufwirkung von Psychopharmaka geben die Arbeiten von MOCCETTI et al. (1971), PIESCHL (1973) und TÖLLE (1969).

Ein *Blutdruckanstieg* wird unter Psychopharmakamedikation selten beobachtet, am ehesten bei geriatrischen Patienten (BARUK u. PÉCHENY, 1965; BUFFA et al., 1963; MASTROGIOVANNI, 1964). Ein plötzlicher Blutdruckanstieg wurde gelegentlich beobachtet, wenn nach einer Vorbehandlung mit MAO-Hemmern ohne die vorgeschriebene Pause ein trizyklisches Antidepressivum verabreicht wurde.

Eine *Blutdrucksenkung* ist besonders zu Beginn einer Psychopharmakabehandlung häufig. Subjektive Symptome zeigen erfahrungsgemäß nur eine geringe Korrelation mit dem Ausmaß des Blutdruckabfalles (BUSFIELD et al., 1962).

Im Prinzip können alle Psychopharmaka, vor allem aber Antipsychotika und trizyklische Antidepressiva, aber auch Benzodiazepine einen Blutdruckabfall hervorrufen (BINEIK u. BORNSCHEUER, 1972a, b; GREENBLATT u. KOCH-WESER, 1973; LAMBERT et al., 1973; MAN u. CHEN, 1973; WOJDYSLAWSKA et al., 1975). Besonders häufig werden Blutdrucksenkungen bei älteren Patienten und bei Patienten mit labilem Blutdruck bei Hypertension beobachtet. Es wird nicht nur der systolische, sondern auch der diastolische Blutdruck erniedrigt. Ophthalmodynamographisch läßt sich die Blutdrucksenkung auch zentral nachweisen (BOJANOVSKY u. TÖLLE, 1973; TÖLLE, 1973).

In der Gruppe der Antipsychotika wird ein hypotensiver Effekt besonders den Phenothiazinen mit aliphatischer Seitenkette oder mit einer Piperidin-Gruppe zugeschrieben. Etwas günstiger sind Phenothiazine mit Piperazinylalkyl-Seitenkette. Neue tri- und tetrazyklische Antidepressiva wie Maprotilin, Mianserin, Nomifensin und Lofepramin weisen eine bessere kardiovaskuläre Verträglichkeit auf als die klassischen trizyklischen Antidepressiva.

Die Behandlung der Kreislaufnebenwirkungen erfolgt mit Betablockern (MAY, 1975), die vor allem die Tachykardie günstig beeinflussen (BESSUGES u. OURGAUD, 1972; BROWN et al., 1972; ISAC et al., 1972; MODESTIN, 1976; VOHRA u. BURROWS, 1974). Gegen die Hypotension werden Dihydroergotamin (BOJANOVSKY u. TÖLLE, 1974; TÖLLE, 1973), Methylphenidat (FLEMENBAUM, 1972) oder Mineralokortikoide (HOLLSTEIN, 1975) angewandt.

II. Vegetative Nebenwirkungen

Die meisten trizyklischen Antidepressiva und Phenothiazine wirken adrenerg und anticholinerg, die MAO-Hemmer hingegen nur adrenerg. Die von diesen psychotropen Pharmaka hervorgerufenen vegetativen Nebenwirkungen sind bei den allermeisten Patienten nur mild ausgeprägt und bilden sich nach 1- bis 2wöchiger Behandlung bereits zurück. Bei langsamer Steigerung der Initialdosis in den ersten 3 Tagen ist die vegetative Verträglichkeit der Psychopharmaka besser als bei sofortiger Gabe der vollen therapeutisch wirksamen Dosis.

Bei einigen psychischen Erkrankungen, insbesondere bei Depressionen, ist als Krankheitssymptom *Mundtrockenheit* vorhanden, die leider durch die Behandlung mit Antidepressiva noch verstärkt wird (durch Messungen der Speichelsekretion bestätigt). Ausnahmsweise können dadurch folgende Komplikationen verursacht werden: Glossitis, Stomatitis und Ulzera der Mundschleimhaut. Die Trockenheit der *Schleimhäute* kann sich auch auf die Schleimhäute der Nase und der Vagina erstrecken.

Als Teilsymptom eines neuroleptisch indizierten Parkinsonsyndroms können viele Antipsychotika eine *Hypersalivation* hervorrufen. Auch während der Behandlung mit Clozapin, das keine anderen Parkinsonsymptome erzeugt, wird häufig eine Hypersalivation beobachtet.

Einige Antipsychotika führen zur *Miosis,* andere zu Mydriasis. Durch Erschlaffung der Ziliarmuskeln können *Visus-Störungen* verursacht werden.

Durch die anticholinerge Wirkung vieler Psychopharmaka können sich *Akkommodationsstörungen* entwickeln, die subjektiv als verschwommenes Sehen wahrgenommen werden und zu Schwierigkeiten beim Lesen und Handarbeiten führen. Diese besonders für intellektuelle Patienten gelegentlich sehr hinderliche Nebenwirkung ist reversibel und sollte dem Patienten vor Therapiebeginn erklärt werden. Der Visus auf größere Distanz bleibt unbehindert, so daß die Fahrtüchtigkeit nicht eingeschränkt wird.

Bei vorbebestendem Glaukom besteht eine relative Kontraindikation gegen die Behandlung mit anticholinerg wirksamen Substanzen; in der Regel kann jedoch unter gleichzeitiger Kontrolle durch einen Ophthalmologen eine solche Behandlung (z. B. mit Antidepressiva) gut durchgeführt werden. Bei Glaukompatienten ist die Applikation von Substanzen ohne anticholinerge Wirkung (z. B. Mianserin, Anxiolytika) vorzuziehen.

Nach *Miktionsstörungen* sollte gezielt gefragt werden, da viele Patienten nicht spontan über diese Nebenwirkung zu klagen wagen. Sie leiden unter Harndrang, ohne die Blase komplett leeren zu können, und haben eine Pollakisurie oder sogar eine komplette *Harnverhaltung*. Die Dosierung und vor allem die individuelle Empfindlichkeit sind für die Ausprägung dieser Nebenwirkung entscheidend (MERRILL u. MARKLAND, 1972). Bei einer Harnverhaltung sollte nur ausnahmsweise katheterisiert werden; besser ist die Gabe von Dihydroergotamin oder Ubretid (HERTRICH, 1975). Gehäuft treten ausgeprägte Miktionsstörungen bei älteren Patienten auf, vor allem bei Männern mit Prostatahypertrophie. Unter dämpfend wirkenden Psychopharmaka kann ausnahmsweise eine Urininkontinenz auftreten (KIMBROUGH, 1972).

Schwitzen ist eine häufige Nebenwirkung von trizyklischen Antidepressiva, Antipsychotika und Anxiolytika.

Während die unter Phenothiazinen häufig zu beobachtende *Hypothermie* klinisch ohne Relevanz ist, ist die *Hyperthermie* von größter Bedeutung (HARDER et al., 1971). Sie kann das erste Symptom einer zentralen Intoxikation mit eventuell letalem Ausgang sein (AUBERT, 1973; JONCHEV u. ARIANOVA, 1974; OPPENHEIM, 1973).

Für die Behandlung anticholinerger Nebenwirkungen hat sich vor allem Dihydergot bewährt (BOJANOVSKY u. TÖLLE, 1974; CRISCUOLI, 1971; HEIBERG u. LINGJAERDE, 1972; LUMINEAU et al., 1972; MAROCCHINO u. SAVIO, 1973; PAUGET, 1972; SCHNETZLER u. ALLEON, 1974; SCHOU et al., 1973b).

III. Pigmentablagerungen in den Augen

Nach hochdosierter Langzeitbehandlung mit Phenothiazinen werden Pigmentablagerungen in der Haut, den inneren Organen und den Augen beobachtet, häufig verknüpft mit einer allgemeinen Steigerung der Photosensibilität der Haut. Die teilweise reversiblen Pigmentablagerungen betreffen vor allem die vorderen Partien der Augenlinse, weniger häufig das Endothel der Cornea, die Konjunktiva und die Vorderfläche der Iris (FORREST et al., 1966). Diese Nebenwirkungen wurden vor allem in den Vereinigten Staaten beobachtet, wo exzessive Phenothiazin-Dosierungen verordnet werden. Sie sind abhängig von der kumulativ verabreichten Dosis und damit auch von der Dauer der Medikation. Aufgrund der Häufung der beschriebenen Pigmentablagerungen bei schwarzen Patienten (ELIE et al., 1972), wird eine genetische Disposition in Erwägung gezogen.

3-Jahres-Katamnesen haben gezeigt, daß die Pigmentablagerungen weniger gefährlich sind als ursprünglich angenommen wurde (FORREST u. SNOW, 1968). Die Wirkung der Behandlung mit d-Penicillamin ist nicht gesichert (GUNN, 1967).

Durch Pigmentverschiebungen kann es zu einer *Retinopathie* kommen, die offenbar dosisabhängig ist und vor allem bei Langzeitbehandlungen mit Antipsychotika entsteht.

Durch Abspeicherung der Psychopharmaka oder ihrer Metaboliten können *Linsentrübungen* hervorgerufen werden. Auch Melaninablagerungen können Linsentrübungen bewirken; schizophrene Patienten haben gehäuft eine Störung der Melanogenese (GREINER, 1968a, b).

IV. Gastrointestinale Nebenwirkungen

Obwohl die meisten trizyklischen Psychopharmaka, insbesondere die Phenothiazine, antiemetische Eigenschaften haben, können sie vor allem in den ersten

Behandlungstagen Übelkeit oder Erbrechen hervorrufen. Die Entstehung dieser Nebenwirkungen ist nicht genau bekannt; diskutiert werden die anticholinerge Wirkung, die Hypomotilität und Relaxation des Magens, verknüpft mit Sekretionshemmung (BIRNBAUM u. KARMELI, 1974; FISCHBACH, 1973).

Eine seltene, aber gefährliche Komplikation der Reserpinbehandlung stellt die Perforation eines Ulcus ventriculi dar. Daher ist Reserpin bei Patienten mit Ulkusanamnese kontraindiziert.

Ein beträchtlicher Anteil der Bevölkerung, insbesondere Frauen, weist eine *Obstipation* auf, die außerdem ein Symptom von Depressionen, Spannungs- und Angstzuständen ist. Bei der Behandlung mit Antidepressiva kann sich dieses vorbestehende Symptom verstärken, so daß schwerere Obstipationen entstehen. Vor der Verordnung von Laxativa sollte eine möglichst genaue Abklärung bezüglich einer Regelmäßigkeit des Stuhlganges erfolgen, um die unnötige Verabreichung von Laxantien zu vermeiden. Die Obstipation kann mit einer verminderten Magensekretion und einer Dilatation von Darmteilen verknüpft sein (selten Ileus).

Mit Ausnahme von Lithium bewirken Psychopharmaka selten eine Diarrhoe (MITCHELL, 1975).

V. Unerwünschte Effekte auf Körpergewicht und Körpergröße

Besonders bei langfristiger Behandlung mit Antipsychotika und Lithium wird häufig eine unerwünschte Gewichtszunahme beobachtet (ÅBERG, 1975; BÍLÝ et al., 1973; DEMPSEY et al., 1976; MUELLER u. DE LA VERGNE, 1973; VENDSBORG et al., 1976a, b). Bisher gibt es keine spezifische Behandlung gegen diese unangenehme Nebenwirkung, die keineswegs nur auf eine verminderte motorische Aktivität der Patienten zurückzuführen ist.

Eine Sonderstellung nimmt die Gewichtszunahme während der Behandlung mit Antidepressiva ein. Depressive Patienten zeigen als Krankheitssymptome Appetitverlust und Gewichtsabnahme, so daß der unter der Behandlung zu beobachtende Gewichtsanstieg als ein Zeichen der Besserung interpretiert werden kann. Tatsächlich wurde eine positive Korrelation zwischen Therapieeffekt und Gewichtszunahme festgestellt (HOLDEN u. HOLDEN, 1970; SIMPSON et al., 1969; SINGH et al., 1970).

Bei hyperaktiven Kindern, die mit Dextroamphetamin oder mit Methylphenidat behandelt worden waren, wurde eine Reduktion des Längenwachstums festgestellt (SAFER u. ALLEN, 1973).

VI. Leberveränderungen

Trotz einer ausgedehnten Literatur über die Hepatotoxizität von Psychopharmaka sind keine genauen Zahlen erhältlich, die es erlauben würden, die Häufigkeit des pharmakogenen Ikterus abzuschätzen. Ikteruserkrankungen werden vor allem während der ersten 3 Monate von Psychopharmakabehandlungen beobachtet. Die 14 Tage anhaltenden Prodromalsymptome sind Fieber, Nausea, Magenbeschwerden und Übelkeit. Der in der Regel 3 Wochen dauernde Ikterus ist verbunden mit Inappetenz, Schwäche, Müdigkeit, Pruritus, acholischem Stuhl, dunklem Urin und gelegentlicher Vergrößerung der Leber. Alkalische

Phosphatase und SGOT sind erhöht, letztere jedoch nicht so stark wie bei Virushepatitiden. Bei meist normalem Serumprotein sind die Eosinophilen gelegentlich etwas erhöht. Die Prognose ist in der Regel günstig. Eine Korrelation zwischen Psychopharmakadosierung und Ikterusrisiko scheint nicht zu bestehen.

Häufiger werden während einer Psychopharmakabehandlung Veränderungen der *Leberenzyme* beobachtet, deren Kausalzusammenhang mit der Einnahme von Psychopharmaka nicht gesichert ist.

VII. Hämatologische Nebenwirkungen

In den ersten Wochen einer Behandlung mit trizyklischen Antipsychotika kann sich eine klinisch bedeutungslose *Leukopenie, Leukozytose* mit Linksverschiebung oder *Eosinophilie* entwickeln. Nach längerer Behandlung werden manchmal relative Lymphozytosen beobachtet. Eine seltene, aber gefährliche Nebenwirkung (0,1–1,0$^0/_{00}$ der mit trizyklischen Neuroleptika behandelten Patienten) ist die *Agranulozytose* (metabolischer Typ) (ANANTH u. BESZTERCZEY, 1973; ANANTH et al., 1973; PISCIOTTA, 1971). Unter trizyklischen Antidepressiva ist sie wesentlich seltener und nach Butyrophenonen kommt sie praktisch nicht vor. Offenbar gibt es Patienten, die eine spezielle Disposition für diese Nebenwirkung haben (PISCIOTTA, 1968). Die Symptome der Agranulozytose sind lokale Infektionen, Fieber, Pharyngitis, Ulzerationen im Mund, Dysphagie, Dermatitis, Enterokolitis und gelegentlich Ikterus. Wird die Diagnose rechtzeitig gestellt, ist die Prognose in der Regel gut, verglichen mit der aplastischen Anämie nach Chloramphenicol. Die Mortalität beträgt 0% bei Diagnose der Granulozytopenie (<3200) vor der Infektion, 30% bei Diagnose am Tag der Infektion und 30% für die 10% der Patienten, die erst nach $1^1/_2$ Jahren eine Granulozytopenie entwickeln (90% in den ersten 18 Behandlungswochen). Bei Diagnosestellung muß das Neuroleptikum sofort abgesetzt werden, da sonst die Mortalität zunimmt (AMSLER, 1977).

Nachdem unter Clozapin gehäuft Agranulozytosen beobachtet worden waren (IDÄNPÄÄN-HEIKKILÄ et al., 1975), die teilweise einen tödlichen Ausgang hatten, wurde zur Vorbeugung die wöchentliche Leukozytenzählung (nur bei pathologischem Wert Differentialblutbild nötig) in den ersten 18 Wochen der Therapie vorgeschlagen, die jedoch leider nicht von allen Ärzten durchgeführt wird.

Kasuistische Mitteilungen berichten über *Anämie* und *Purpura*, deren Kausalzusammenhang mit einer Psychopharmakabehandlung nicht gesichert ist (HUSSAIN et al., 1973; KOZAKOVA, 1971; LITVAK u. KAELBING, 1972). In den ersten Wochen einer Psychopharmakabehandlung wird häufig ein klinisch bedeutungsloser *Anstieg der Blutsenkungsgeschwindigkeit* festgestellt.

Es liegen Anhaltspunkte dafür vor, daß Chlorpromazin und andere Psychopharmaka gelegentlich durch Steigerung der antikoagulativen Eigenschaften eine *Hemmung der Blutgerinnung* hervorrufen können (Hämolyse von Erythrocyten) und daß nach längerer Applikation eine *erhöhte Gerinnungsneigung* entstehen kann (eventuell Hemmung der Thrombozyten-Phosphodiesterase) (NOVAK, 1972; RYSANEK et al., 1973).

MEIER-EWERT et al. (1967) fanden bei 2,9% von 1172 mit Psychopharmaka behandelten Patienten eine *thromboembolische Komplikation*, in der Kontrollgruppe dagegen nur bei 0,6%. Diese Komplikationen scheinen bei Frauen häufiger zu sein, und es werden Varikosis, Herzinsuffizienz und Fieberzustände als prädisponierende Faktoren angenommen. Sehr selten kann es zu einer tödlichen *Lungenembolie* kommen (SINGER et al., 1975).

VIII. Dermatologische Nebenwirkungen

Wie andere Medikamente können Psychopharmaka *Arzneimittelexantheme* hervorrufen, manchmal auf dem Boden einer Photosensibilisierung der Haut (HALMY, 1975). Dabei scheint eine gekreuzte Sensibilität auf verschiedene Psychopharmaka vorzukommen (JUNG et al., 1963). Für schwer ausgeprägte Hautläsionen ähnlich eines Lupus erythematodes oder der Dermatitis exfoliativa ist der Kausalzusammenhang nicht gesichert.

Vor allem unter Langzeitmedikation und nach außerordentlich hohen Dosen von Phenothiazinen und ähnlichen Substanzen werden graue oder metallische *Hautpigmentationen* beobachtet, vor allem an den lichtexponierten Stellen und häufig verknüpft mit Pigmentationen der Augen. Histologisch handelt es sich um Pigmentationen der Basalschicht der Haut mit Ablagerungen in der Dermis. Durch einen Tyndalleffekt kann die Haut einen blauen Schimmer annehmen. Eine Beziehung zwischen Hautpigmentationen und neurologischen oder gastrointestinalen Nebenwirkungen besteht nicht (VULPE, 1967; WARNER, 1967).

Lithium kann eine vorbestehende Akne verschlimmern und eine Dermatitis hervorrufen (DUBOIS et al., 1972; KURTIN, 1973; MÜLLER u. KRÜGER, 1975; RIFKIN et al., 1973a).

IX. Endokrinologische Nebenwirkungen

Antidepressiva und Antipsychotika können vor allem nach Langzeitapplikation und hoher Dosierung bei männlichen und weiblichen Patienten eine *Galaktorrhoe* und *Gynäkomastie* hervorrufen (SHADER u. DIMASCIO, 1970). Die Galaktorrhoe ist selten spontan und in der Regel nur durch Drücken der Brustdrüsen festzustellen. Gleichzeitig mit einer Galaktorrhoe wird bei Frauen häufig eine *Amenorrhoe* (FENASSE et al., 1972) und gelegentlich eine Abnahme der Libido beobachtet (BEUMONT et al., 1972; MARGAT u. BROUSSOT, 1968). Eine genaue Untersuchung des Sekrets ergab Ähnlichkeiten zur Muttermilch (LAZOS et al., 1972). Als Erklärungsmöglichkeiten werden eine Hemmung der Prolactinsekretion der Hypophyse, eine direkte Wirkung auf den Hypothalamus oder eine Hemmung der Sekretion des PIF (Prolactin-inhibitory-factor) des Thalamus diskutiert. Einige Antipsychotika bewirken einen *erhöhten Prolactinspiegel* im Plasma (BEN-DAVID et al., 1971; KOLAKOWSKA et al., 1975; WILSON et al., 1975). Eine kausale Beziehung zwischen Reserpinmedikation und Mammakarzinom konnte nicht nachgewiesen werden (Anonym, 1974a, b, c, 1975; ARMSTRONG et al., 1974; FAIGLE u. DÖRHÖFER, 1975; HEINONEN et al., 1974a, b; IMMICH, 1974; LASKA et al., 1975; O'FALLON et al., 1975; SAXÉN u. PETO, 1974; VENEZIAN et al., 1974).

Auch bei medikamentös nicht behandelten schwer ausgeprägten psychischen Erkrankungen (Schizophrenie, Depression, Manie, Neurosen) kann eine Amenorrhoe auftreten. Ihre gehäufte Beobachtung bei mit Psychopharmaka behandelten Patienten läßt es jedoch gerechtfertigt erscheinen, die Amenorrhoe als Nebenwirkung anzusehen.

Eine zusammenfassende Darstellung der Beeinflussung von Hypophyse und Nebennierenrinde durch Psychopharmaka findet sich bei SHADER et al. (1970b).

Veränderungen der *Schilddrüsenfunktion* sind nur für Lithium gesichert. Es können euthyreote und hypothyreote Strumen und in einzelnen Fällen auch ein Myxödem beobachtet werden. Es handelt sich um reversible und durch Thyroxin gut zu behandelnde Veränderungen, die einen Abbruch der Lithiumprophylaxe nicht nötig machen.

Untersuchungen zum Plasmaspiegel des luteotropen Hormons, der Oestrogene und des Wuchshormons bei mit Neuroleptika behandelten Patienten ergaben keine signifikanten Veränderungen (BEUMONT et al., 1974a, b; SALDANHA et al., 1972).

Nach längerer Lithiumbehandlung kann sich vorübergehend ein renaler *Diabetes insipidus* entwickeln (SØRENSEN et al., 1973).

Psychiatrische Patienten haben durchschnittlich einen eher höheren *Blutzuckerspiegel* als Gesunde (SHADER et al., 1970a). Die Induktion eines *Diabetes mellitus* durch Psychopharmaka ist nicht gesichert. Bei disponierten Patienten können Phenothiazine gelegentlich Hyperglykämien auslösen und unter Antidepressiva wurden Blutzuckersenkungen beobachtet. Über den Zusammenhang zwischen Chlorpromazin und Diabetes-Risiko haben KORENYI und LOWENSTEIN (1968) die Literatur zusammengefaßt. Eine Erhöhung der *Glucosetoleranz* wurde während der Behandlung mit Lithium (VENDSBORG u. RAFAELSEN, 1973) gefunden.

X. Sexuelle Störungen

Verschiedenste sexuelle Störungen wie Verminderung der Spermatogenese, Priapismus und Ejakulationsstörungen sind als Nebenwirkungen von Psychopharmaka beobachtet worden (BAŠTECKÝ u. GREGOVÁ, 1974; BLAIR u. SIMPSON, 1966; BOURGEOIS, 1972; SHADER, 1972).

Vor allem nach längerer Behandlung können Psychopharmaka, auch Anxiolytika, eine *Verminderung von Libido und Potenz* bewirken. Diese von sexuellen Symptomen psychischer Krankheiten oft nicht sicher abzugrenzenden Nebenwirkungen sind für die Patienten und deren Partner äußerst unangenehm, rufen häufig schwere Ängste und Insuffizienzgefühle hervor und sollten unbedingt vor Behandlungsbeginn mit dem einzelnen Patienten gründlich besprochen werden. Vor allem ist darauf hinzuweisen, daß es sich um vorübergehende Störungen handelt und nicht um bleibende organische Veränderungen.

XI. Gravidität und Puerperium

Die Gefahr teratogener Wirkungen von Psychopharmaka ist methodisch schwer zu untersuchen. Die Ergebnisse von Tierversuchen können kaum auf den Menschen übertragen werden. Teilweise werden Mütter, die Kinder mit Mißbildungen geboren haben, nachträglich über den Gebrauch von Psychopharmaka während der Schwangerschaft befragt. Dieses Vorgehen ist bezüglich seiner Aussagekraft als fragwürdig anzusehen. Die sicherste Methode stellen prospektive Studien dar. KULLANDER und KÄLLÉN (1976) haben in einer prospektiven

Studie 6376 schwangere Frauen untersucht. Sie fanden eine Beziehung zwischen Psychopharmakagebrauch während der Schwangerschaft und der Häufigkeit späterer Fehlgeburten oder legaler Aborte. Sie führen diesen Befund auf den vermehrten Psychopharmakakonsum während unerwünschter Schwangerschaften zurück. Sie fanden keine Beziehung zwischen Psychopharmakagebrauch und der Häufigkeit von Totgeburten oder Mißbildungen der Kinder. HARTZ et al. (1975) untersuchten prospektiv 50 282 schwangere Frauen und fanden keine Häufung von Mißbildungen und auch keine spezifische Form von Mißbildungen bei den 1870 Kindern, die in utero dem Einfluß von Meprobamat oder Chlordiazepoxyd ausgesetzt waren. Interessanterweise fanden sie auch keinen Unterschied bezüglich Mißbildungen beim Vergleich verschiedener Zeitpunkte, zu denen während der Schwangerschaft die erwähnten Substanzen eingenommen worden waren. Es wurde keine erhöhte Häufigkeit von Totgeburten oder Todesfällen bis zum 4. Geburtstag der Kinder festgestellt. Nach 8 Monaten wurden die Kinder gründlich untersucht bezüglich geistiger und motorischer Entwicklung und mit 4 Jahren ihr Intelligenzquotient bestimmt. Die Resultate ergaben keinerlei Anhaltspunkte für kindliche Hirnschäden nach Einnahme von Meprobamat oder Chlordiazepoxyd während der Schwangerschaft.

Übersichtsarbeiten zur teratogenen Wirkung von Psychopharmaka: AYD (1964a, b, c); SHADER (1970); VAN WAES u. VAN DE VELDE (1969). Es ist in diesem Zusammenhang daran zu erinnern, daß die früher weit verbreitete Einnahme von Chlorpromazin oder auch Haloperidol als Antiemetika während der Frühschwangerschaft nicht zu einem Anstieg kindlicher Mißbildungen geführt hatte. ANANTH (1976) beschreibt Entziehungssymptome bei Neugeborenen nach Einnahme von Opiaten, Hypnotika, Analgetika und trizyklischen Antidepressiva während der Schwangerschaft. Außerdem berichtet er über Nebenwirkungen bei Neugeborenen nach Gebrauch von Neuroleptika, Lithium, Antidepressiva, Anxiolytika, Antikonvulsiva und Bromiden während der Schwangerschaft. Er weist darauf hin, daß diese Stoffe im allgemeinen ungefährlich sind, daß sie schwangeren Frauen jedoch nur nach strenger Indikationsstellung verordnet werden sollten.

SCHOU et al (1973a, c; SCHOU u. AMDISEN, 1973) haben auf die Risiken einer Lithiumverabreichung während der Schwangerschaft hingewiesen. Es wäre möglich, daß durch die Hemmung der Thyroxinsynthese das Risiko eines Hypothyreoidismus des Neugeborenen erhöht würde (Kausalzusammenhang nicht gesichert). Es bestehen auch Anhaltspunkte für eine Vermehrung von kardiovaskulären Mißbildungen. Im ersten Trimester der Schwangerschaft gilt Lithium heute als kontraindiziert.

Die Verabreichung dämpfender Psychopharmaka (Antipsychotika, Hypnotika, Anxiolytika) vor der Geburt kann eine verminderte Respiration des Neugeborenen bewirken und eine oft monatelang anhaltende Sedierung des Kindes hervorrufen (DESMOND et al., 1968). Bei Neugeborenen wurden bis zu 6 Monaten extrapyramidale Neuroleptikanebenwirkungen beobachtet (HILL et al., 1966).

Eine gute Zusammenfassung über die Folgen des Psychopharmakagebrauchs während der Stillzeit wurde von AYD veröffentlicht (1973a). Auch während dieser Zeit kann es durch Einnahme dämpfender Substanzen zu einer unerwünschten Sedierung des Kindes kommen.

XII. Stoffwechselveränderungen

Einzelne Autoren (LOVETT-DOUST u. HUSZKA, 1973) nehmen an, daß Phenothiazine und Butyrophenone das Plasma-Kalium und die Kortikosteroide steigern können. Es ist auch berichtet worden, daß Phenelzin das Plasma-Natrium erhöhen und das Magnesium senken könne.

In künftigen Studien, vor allem bei Verabreichung trizyklischer Substanzen, ist besonders auf Veränderungen des Phospholipidstoffwechsels zu achten (LÜLLMANN et al., 1973).

XIII. Unerwartete Todesfälle

Plötzliche und unerwartete Todesfälle von mit Psychopharmaka behandelten Patienten werfen immer wieder die Frage nach einem Kausalzusammenhang zur Medikamenteneinnahme auf, vor allem wenn sich bei der Autopsie keine einleuchtende Erklärung für den Exitus ergibt (MOORE u. BOOK, 1970). Als Ursache kommen kardiovaskuläre Effekte, Autoimmunreaktionen oder individualspezifische Überempfindlichkeitsreaktionen auf Phenothiazine in Frage. Eine Analyse von 17 Todesfällen schizophrener Patienten (DYNES, 1969) zeigte, daß nur 5 dieser Patienten Phenothiazine erhalten hatten. Eine Untersuchung kardial vorgeschädigter Patienten unter Amitriptylinbehandlung im Vergleich zu einer Kontrollgruppe ergab keine erhöhte Mortalität unter der Pharmakotherapie.

Zusammenfassend läßt sich sagen, daß keine sicheren Anhaltspunkte dafür vorliegen, daß die Verabreichung von Psychopharmaka die Mortalität der Patienten erhöhen würde.

XIV. Neurologische Nebenwirkungen

Antipsychotika, Antidepressiva und Lithium können einen leichten oder schweren *Tremor* hervorrufen, ohne daß gleichzeitig extrapyramidale Nebenwirkungen auftreten müssen. Der Lithiumtremor kann mit Betablockern (Propranolol, Pindolol, Practolol) günstig beeinflußt werden (BROWN, 1976; FLORU, 1971; FLORU et al., 1974a, b; KÖNIG, 1975). Neuroleptisch induzierte *Parkinsonsyndrome* sind charakterisiert durch Akinese und Rigor. Subjektiv sind die verminderte Motilität und die Bradyphrenie äußerst unangenehm. Trizyklische Antidepressiva rufen keine Parkinsonsyndrome hervor, sondern scheinen diesbezüglich eher einen antagonistischen Effekt zu haben.

Ein plötzliches Absetzen der Neuroleptika und der begleitenden Antiparkinsonmittel kann zu einem vorübergehenden Anstieg extrapyramidaler Symptome führen, da das Antiparkinsonmittel wegen seiner kürzeren Halbwertszeit rasch wirkungslos wird, während die Antipsychotikawirkung länger erhalten bleibt.

Während der ersten Tage einer neuroleptischen Therapie kann es zu *akuten Dystonien* kommen, die vor allem kranial zu beobachten sind in Form von Muskelspasmen der Augen, der Gesichtsmuskulatur, der Mund-, Zungen- und Schlundmuskulatur, auch der Nackenmuskulatur und etwas weniger häufig an den oberen und noch seltener an den unteren Extremitäten. Meistens sind diese Anfälle unilateral. Ein dabei auftretender Opisthotonus mag mit einer Hysterie verwechselt werden. Jüngere Patienten sind besonders disponiert und Männer mehr gefährdet als Frauen. Das Risiko dystoner Reaktionen auf die Verabreichung von Antipsychotika mit hoher diesbezüglicher Potenz ist so groß, daß es für die ersten Wochen der Neuroleptikabehandlung eine Kombination mit einem Antiparkinsonmittel rechtfertigt, vor allem bei ambulanten Patienten. Akute Dystonien sprechen auf intravenös applizierte Antiparkinsonmittel (z.B. 5 mg Biperiden) meist innerhalb weniger Sekunden an.

Besonders bei Frühdyskinesien und beim neuroleptisch bedingten Parkinsonsyndrom hat sich die Gabe von anticholinerg wirksamen *Antiparkinsonmitteln* bewährt. Dagegen helfen sie wenig bei Akathisie und sind bei persistierenden Dyskinesien kontraindiziert.

Die dopaminergen Antiparkinsonmittel L-Dopa und Adamantan-Derivate können bei neuroleptisch bedingter Parkinsonsymptomatik nicht empfohlen werden, da bisher nicht sicher auszuschließen ist, ob durch eine Aktivierung dopaminerger Rezeptoren eine Provokation der psychotischen Symptomatik hervorgerufen werden kann.

Antiparkinsonmittel (siehe Tabelle 7) sollten möglichst nicht prophylaktisch, sondern erst nach Auftreten von extrapyramidalen Nebenwirkungen gegeben werden. Eine dauerhafte Verordnung ist nicht notwendig, wie verschiedene Absetzversuche gezeigt haben. Ein Absetzversuch von FLEISCHHAUER (1975) an 49 neuroleptisch behandelten Patienten zeigte bei 8% der Patienten ein erneutes Auftreten von extrapyramidalen Nebenwirkungen. Diese entwickeln sich 1 bis 3 Wochen nach Absetzen der Antiparkinsonmittel.

Die Wirksamkeit von oral oder parenteral applizierten Antiparkinsonmitteln bleibt auch nach längerer Applikationsdauer bestehen (KLINE et al., 1974a).

Die *Nebenwirkungen der Antiparkinsonmittel* sind denjenigen anticholinerg wirksamer Antidepressiva vergleichbar: Mydriasis, Trockenheit der Schleimhäute, Schwitzen, Tachykardie, Hypotonie und Hemmung der Miktion. Bei hochdosierter Gabe kann es zu Delirien kommen. Die Anwendung von Antiparkinsonmitteln muß bei Glaukom, Prostatahypertrophie, Harnverhalten und schweren kardiovaskulären Komplikationen mit besonderer Vorsicht gehandhabt werden.

Tabelle 7. Antiparkinsonmittel

Internationale chemische Kurzbezeichnung (generic name)	Handelsnamen			Dosierung (per os, mg/Tag)
	BRD	Österreich	Schweiz	
Benztropin (689)[a]	Cogentin	Cogentin	Cogentin	1–4
Biperiden (690)	Akineton	Akineton	Akineton	6–10
Dexetimid (721)	–	–	Tremblex	0,5–1
Orphenadrin (1254)	Norflex	Norflex	Norflex	150–400
Procyclidin (935)	Osnervan	Kemadrin	Kemadrin	7,5–30
Trihexyphenidyl (995)	Artane	Artane	Artane	2–15

[a] Die in Klammern den generic names beigefügte Zahl bezieht sich auf die von USDIN und EFRON (1972) herausgegebene Zusammenstellung psychotroper Substanzen

Die *psychische Eigenwirkung der Antiparkinsonmittel* kann als leicht euphorisierend beschrieben werden. Dadurch scheint eine gewisse Tendenz zur Abhängigkeit hervorgerufen zu werden.

Die unter Antipsychotikabehandlung auftretende *Akathisie* besteht in einer inneren Unruhe und Unfähigkeit des Patienten still zu sitzen. Er leidet oft unter einer Unruhe in den Beinen und ist gezwungen ständig aufzustehen, umherzugehen oder im Stehen die Fersen vom Boden wechselnd abzuheben. Diese Nebenwirkung ist sehr charakteristisch und darf nicht mit einer psychotischen Unruhe verwechselt werden. Am besten hilft das Absetzen des Neuroleptikums. Methylphenidat ist wirkungslos (CARMAN, 1972; FANN et al., 1973).

Zu den wichtigsten und schwersten Nebenwirkungen antipsychotischer Substanzen gehören die *persistierenden Dyskinesien*. Die Symptomatik variiert außerordentlich stark und kann sich nach Monaten oder Jahren einer Dauermedikation entwickeln und auch nach Absetzen derselben noch unbestimmt lange fortdauern oder abklingen. Das erste Auftreten wird unter der Medikation oder auch unverzüglich nach Absetzen derselben beobachtet (AYD, 1974b; JACOBSON et al., 1974; SIMPSON et al., 1965). Die Häufigkeit ist unterschiedlich und hängt vor allem von der Höhe der Dosierung und der Wahl des Präparates ab. Die häufigste Symptomatik besteht in klonischen Kontraktionen einzelner Muskeln oder Muskelgruppen vor allem um den Mund, Bewegungen der Zunge, Leckbewegungen, Lippenschmatzen, Augenzwinkern, kauenden Bewegungen, unwillkürlichen Bewegungen der Finger, Hände oder Schultern. In schweren Fällen kann es zur Ausbildung eines Hemiballismus oder größerer Bewegungsabläufe des Rumpfes kommen. Die gefährlichste Form persistierender Dyskinesien besteht in einem Spasmus der Glottis.

Beziehungen zwischen dem Risiko einer persistierenden Dyskinesie und der kumulativ verabreichten Dosis von Antipsychotika sind nicht gesichert. Frauen sind stärker gefährdet als Männer und ältere Kranke stärker als junge (BELLABARBA et al., 1967; HEINRICH et al., 1968; HERSHON et al., 1972; HIPPIUS u. LANGE, 1970; JUS et al., 1976a, b). Bei hirngeschädigten Patienten treten persistierende Dyskinesien gehäuft auf. In diesem Zusammenhang muß darauf hingewiesen werden, daß zufolge zerebraler altersbedingter Prozesse auch spontan recht häufig vor allem orale Dyskinesien auftreten, die nicht auf eine psychotrope Medikation zurückzuführen sind.

Die Pathogenese der persistierenden Dyskinesien ist unbekannt. Diskutiert wird eine striale dopaminerge Überempfindlichkeit der Rezeptoren (KLAWANS u. RUBOVITS, 1972); für diese Hypothese spricht eine Studie, bei der L-Dopa in Kombination mit einem Decarboxylasehemmer Dyskinesien auslöste oder verschlimmerte, Alpha-Methyl-p-Tyrosin dagegen die Symptome reduzierte. Eine Verschlimmerung der Symptomatik wurde nicht nur unter L-Dopa (HIPPIUS u. LOGEMANN, 1970), sondern auch unter Methylphenidat beobachtet (FANN et al., 1973). Es ist relativ gesichert, daß über eine Dopaminrezeptorenblockade die Entzugsdyskinesien wieder behoben werden können (FRANGOS u. CHRISTODOULIDES, 1975).

Die Behandlung persistierender Hyperkinesien ist äußerst schwierig (HELMCHEN, 1969). Zunächst muß das Neuroleptikum abgesetzt werden. Manchmal ist die Applikation eines anderen Antipsychotikums wirksam, z.B. Clozapin

(Simpson u. Varga, 1974), oft sind sie jedoch therapieresistent. Behandlungsversuche liegen vor mit Reserpin (Ayd, 1973b; Sato et al., 1971), Tetrabenazin (Gilligan et al., 1972; Kazamatsuri et al., 1972a, 1973; McLellan, 1972), Haloperidol (Frangos u. Christodoulides, 1975; Kazamatsuri et al., 1972b), Perphenazin (Fahn, 1972), Thiopropazat (Anonym, 1972; Bullock, 1972; Curran, 1973; Jonchev u. Mitkov, 1971), Pimozid (Claveria et al., 1975), Lioresal (Korsgaard, 1976), Deanol (Ayd, 1975b; Casey u. Denney, 1975; Curran et al., 1975; Fann et al., 1975; de Silva u. Huang, 1975), Alpha-Methyl-p-Tyrosin (Gerlach et al., 1974; Gerlach u. Thorsen, 1976; Viukari u. Linnoila, 1975), Apomorphin (Gessa et al., 1972), Cyproheptadin (Goldman, 1976), Lithium (Gerlach et al., 1975; Klawans u. Rubovits, 1972) und Imipramin (Levy, 1973).

XV. Epileptische Anfälle

Die meisten antipsychotischen und antidepressiven Pharmaka erniedrigen die zerebrale Krampfschwelle und können bei disponierten Individuen zu einer Provokation epileptischer Anfälle führen. Bei epileptischen Psychosen werden trotzdem Antipsychotika verwendet in Kombination mit Antiepileptika.

XVI. Psychische Nebenwirkungen

Da die meisten psychotropen Pharmaka eine sedierende Wirkungskomponente haben, besteht besonders bei Langzeitbehandlungen die Gefahr der *Übersedierung*. Sie wird vor allem bei Dauermedikation mit Neuroleptika, auch mit Depotneuroleptika beobachtet.

Unter langfristiger Einnahme von Lithium wurden Ermüdung, Konzentrations- und Merkfähigkeitsstörungen beobachtet (Bauer et al., 1973; Hofmann et al., 1974; Waldmann et al., 1974).

Als Nebenwirkungen von Antipsychotika werden oft sogenannte *pharmakogene Depressionen* beschrieben, deren Existenz jedoch nicht gesichert ist. Die nach Abklingen akuter schizophrener Symptomatik zu beobachtenden depressiven Syndrome konnten bisher nicht vom Spontanverlauf schizophrener und schizoaffektiver Psychosen abgegrenzt werden und können durchaus auch reaktiv ausgelöste Depressionen darstellen.

Bei depressiven Patienten können während einer antidepressiven Behandlung mit tri- oder tetrazyklischen Substanzen, MAO-Hemmern, Amphetamin und Elektroschock *manische Syndrome* auftreten, die oft als Prädikator einer antidepressiven Effizienz der Behandlung interpretiert wurden. Es existieren jedoch keine aussagekräftigen kontrollierten Vergleiche mit Krankheitsverläufen unter Placebo, die eine solche Interpretation gerechtfertigt erscheinen lassen. Als gesichert kann gelten, daß Patienten mit bipolaren affektiven Psychosen häufiger zu einem Umkippen in Hypomanie oder Manie neigen als unipolar Depressive (Angst, 1965).

Stimulierend wirkende Substanzen wie Amphetamin, MAO-Hemmer, aber auch trizyklische Antidepressiva können eine *Provokation psychotischer Symptome* bewirken.

Organische Verwirrungszustände sind seltene Komplikationen der Psychopharmakabehandlung. Am häufigsten werden sie durch Antiparkinsonmittel oder andere anticholinerg wirkende Psychopharmaka verursacht und treten ausnahmsweise auch als Entzugserscheinungen nach Benzodiazepin-Medikation auf (NERENZ, 1974). *Delirien* kommen unter allen möglichen anticholinerg wirksamen Psychopharmaka vor (Therapie: Absetzen des Psychopharmakons, Gabe von Dihydroergotamin und Chlormethiazol). Interessant ist die Beobachtung, daß nach durch Antidepressiva ausgelösten Delirien eine durchgreifende Besserung der depressiven Symptomatik erfolgen kann.

XVII. Vergiftungen mit Psychopharmaka

MATTHEW und LAWSON haben 1975 die 3. Auflage ihres Buches „Treatment of common acute poisonings" herausgegeben, in dem sie die Resultate ihrer langjährigen Erfahrung in Diagnose und Behandlung von Vergiftungen dargestellt haben. Im folgenden Kapitel sollen auszugsweise ihre Ausführungen über Vergiftungen mit Psychopharmaka wiedergegeben werden.

1. Vergiftungen mit trizyklischen Antidepressiva

Die Vergiftungssymptome treten 1 bis 2 Std nach Einnahme der Substanzen auf und bleiben selten länger als 18 bis 24 Std bestehen. Vereinzelt kommt es bis zu 6 Tagen nach der Einnahme zu plötzlichen Todesfällen, die wahrscheinlich auf Herzrhythmusstörungen zurückzuführen sind. Ernsthafte Vergiftungen kommen bei Erwachsenen in der Regel erst nach Einnahme von mehr als 1 g vor. Überlebt der Patient 18 Std, so ist die Prognose gut.

Symptome: Mundtrockenheit, erweiterte Pupillen, Tachykardie, Blutdruckabfall, Herzrhythmusstörungen, Hyperreflexie, tonisch-klonische Krämpfe (Ausweitung zum Status epilepticus möglich), Torticollis und Ataxien (vor allem bei Kindern), Rededrang, verschiedene Grade von Bewußtlosigkeit (selten schwerste Ausprägung), Atemdepressionen, Urinretention und fehlende Darmgeräusche. Halluzinationen (meist optisch) treten in der Regel erst nach Abklingen der übrigen Symptome auf und bleiben einige Tage erhalten.

Mit Physostigminsalicylat können Antidepressiva-Intoxikationen und pharmakogene Delirien erfolgreich behandelt werden (BURKS et al., 1974; CHOW u. SOUNEY, 1974; GRANACHER u. BALDESSARINI, 1975; HEISER u. WILBERT, 1974; NEWTON, 1975; SØRENSEN et al., 1973). Intravenös werden langsam innerhalb von 2 min 2 mg Physostigmin injiziert bis zu einer Gesamtdosis von 12 mg innerhalb von 5 Std; Bereithaltung von Atropin-Sulfat als Antidot. Weitere Literatur bei HOLINGER und KLAWANS (1976), KANAREK et al. (1973), MUNOZ und KUPLIC (1975).

2. Vergiftungen mit MAO-Hemmern

MAO-Hemmer sind höchst selten Ursache von Vergiftungen. Der Beginn der akuten Symptomatik kann bis zu 12 Std nach Einnahme verzögert auftreten. Dabei ist schwer zu unterscheiden, ob es sich um eine Überdosierung von MAO-Hemmern handelt oder um Auswirkungen einer Inkompatibilitätsreaktion zwischen MAO-Hemmern und anderen eingenommenen Substanzen oder Nahrungsmitteln. MAO-Hemmer werden schnell aus dem Gastrointestinaltrakt absorbiert und schnell ausgeschieden, haben aber wegen der länger dauernden Hemmung der Monoaminooxydase lang anhaltende Vergiftungserscheinungen zur Folge.

Symptome: 1. Bei Interaktion mit anderen Substanzen und Nahrungsmitteln: Kopfschmerzen, Fieber, hypertensive Krisen mit möglicher intrakranialer Hämorrhagie, Blutdruckabfall, zerebrale Erregung und epileptische Anfälle, Bewußtseinsverlust, kardiale Arrhythmien. 2. Bei akuter Überdosierung von MAO-Hemmern: Agitiertheit, Halluzinationen, Tachykardie, Hyperreflexie, Schwitzen, Hyperthermie oder Hypothermie, epileptische Anfälle, Blutdruckanstieg oder -abfall, Urinretention, Spastizität.

3. Vergiftungen mit Lithium

Lithium wird schnell absorbiert und vom Gewebe aufgenommen; Ausscheidung größtenteils durch die Nieren. Vergiftungen treten erst bei einem Blutspiegel von mehr als 1,5 mäq/l auf.

Symptome (meist langsame Entwicklung): Übelkeit, Erbrechen, Diarrhoe, Schläfrigkeit, Ataxie, positiver Rhomberg, verwaschene Sprache, Nystagmus, Dysdiadochokinese, grobschlägiger Tremor, Muskelzucken, Verwirrung, Bewußtlosigkeit, Muskelhypertonie mit hyperaktiven Sehnenreflexen, epileptische Krämpfe, Koma. Als tödlich werden Blutwerte von 4–6 mäq/l angesehen.

4. Vergiftungen mit Phenothiazinen

Werden gut absorbiert; lange Halbwertszeit; auch bei schwerer Überdosierung niedriger Blutspiegel. Von diagnostischem Wert ist die Bestimmung im Urin.

Symptome: Bewußtseinsverlust, Parkinsonismus, Dyskinesien, Akathisie, Blutdruckabfall, Tachykardie, Arrhythmien, äußerst selten Atemdepressionen, meist Hypothermie, selten leichte Hyperthermie.

5. Vergiftungen mit Benzodiazepinen

Langsame Absorption; bisher kein Exitus nach reiner Vergiftung mit Benzodiazepinen bekannt.

Symptome: meist milde; Schläfrigkeit, selten Bewußtlosigkeit, Schwindel, Ataxie, verwaschene Sprache, selten leichte Blutdrucksenkung, selten leichte Atemdepression.

6. Vergiftungen mit Barbituraten

Auch kurzwirksame Barbiturate können schwere Vergiftungen bewirken.
Symptomatik: Bewußtseinstrübung, zentrale Atemdepression, Hypovolämie, Hypothermie (Fieber nur bei Infektion), Abnahme oder Fehlen der Darmgeräusche, verminderte Nierenfunktion, Blasen auf der Haut (6% der Barbituratvergiftungen).

Vergiftungen mit nichtbarbiturathaltigen Schlafmitteln sehen ähnlich aus.

7. Vergiftungen mit Amphetaminen

Rasche Absorption, Nachweis im Urin.

Symptomatik: Rededrang, Ruhelosigkeit, Tremor, Reizbarkeit, Schlaflosigkeit sind sehr häufig. Außerdem können auftreten: Verwirrung, Aggressivität, Angst, Delirien, Halluzinationen, Panikzustände, Suizidtendenzen, Hyperreflexie der Beine. Nach initialer Stimulation können Dämpfung und Lethargie auftreten. Epileptische Krämpfe und tiefe Bewußtlosigkeit bei schweren Vergiftungen. Kopfschmerzen, Tachykardie, Flush, Arrhythmien, Angina pectoris, Hypertension, Hypotension, Kollaps, Mundtrockenheit, Nausea, Erbrechen, Diarrhoe, abdominale Koliken, Schwitzen.

8. Therapie von Psychopharmaka-Vergiftungen

Als wichtigste allgemeine *Notfallmaßnahmen* gelten: 1. Atemwege säubern, Seitenlage auch beim Transport, bei schwerer Bewußtlosigkeit Verwendung eines oropharyngealen oder endotrachealen Tubus mit Manschette. 2. Zur Schockprophylaxe sollen die Beine hochgelagert werden. 3. Eine weitere Absorption oral eingenommener Substanzen wird am besten durch Provokation von Erbrechen oder Magenspülungen verhindert. Erbrechen soll nur bei Patienten provoziert werden, die bei Bewußtsein sind. Dafür ist die beste Methode die mit dem Finger oder Löffelstiel; Salzlösungen haben sich wegen Veränderungen des Elektrolythaushaltes nicht bewährt, emetische Drogen sollten nicht verwendet werden.

Magenspülungen sind in der Regel nur bis zu 4 Std nach Einnahme des Giftes nützlich (Ausnahme: Salicylate und trizyklische Antidepressiva).

In der Behandlung von Vergifteten ist eine *allgemeine intensive Pflege* von größter Bedeutung und bei 97% aller Fälle allein völlig ausreichend und erfolgreich. Nur bei 3% müssen spezielle Methoden (forcierte Diurese, Peritonealdialyse, Hämodialyse) angewendet werden, auf die wir nicht näher eingehen wollen.

Bewußtlose Patienten sollten zur Vermeidung von Druckstellen alle $1/2$ Std umgelagert werden. Bei der Umlagerung sollte routinemäßig folgendes durchgeführt werden: passive Bewegung der Glieder, Abklopfen des Brustkastens, Absaugen der oberen Luftwege oder eines Tubus; Kontrolle von Puls, Blutdruck und Temperatur; Einstufung des Grades der Bewußtseinstrübung (Verschlimmerung des Intoxikationszustandes?).

Bei Fehlen von Austrocknungszeichen sind Flüssigkeitsinfusionen auch bei bewußtlosen Patienten in den ersten 12 Std nicht nötig. Bei Hypothermie (rektal 36° C) muß der weitere Wärmeverlust durch Aufenthalt in Räumen mit Zimmertemperatur von 36° C und Einwickeln des Patienten in Folie vermieden werden. Sinkt die Temperatur unter rektal 29,5° C, soll eine aktive Erwärmung durch Warmwasserbäder der Unterarme vorgenommen werden. Dabei soll die Körpertemperatur stündlich um 4° C steigen. Erst wenn dies nicht der Fall ist, werden Spezialmaßnahmen eingesetzt.

Die Einführung eines Katheters ist in der Regel unnötig und soll nur bei Patienten durchgeführt werden, die eine stark gefüllte Blase haben, die sich auf einfachen Handdruck nicht entleert. Tritt Inkontinenz auf, so ist zu erwarten, daß der Patient bald das Bewußtsein wieder erlangt.

Die routinemäßige Antibiotikaprophylaxe ist unnötig.

Häufigste Fehler bei der Behandlung von Vergiftungen: die Suche nach einem Antidot muß meist erfolglos bleiben, da nur bei weniger als 2% aller Vergiftungsformen ein spezifischer pharmakologischer Antagonist existiert. Der häufigste Fehler besteht in einer raschen und unnötigen Durchführung der erwähnten Spezialmaßnahmen, oft aus dem Gefühl der ärztlichen Hilflosigkeit heraus. In diesem Zusammenhang ist es wichtig zu wissen, daß man heute nicht in der Lage ist, vorauszusagen, wie lange ein Patient bewußtlos bleiben wird.

Literatur

Åberg, A.: Weight change and psychotropic drug treatment. Opusc. med. (Stockh.) **20**, 13–19 (1975)

Agulnik, P.L., Dimascio, A., Moore, P.: Acute brain syndrome associated with lithium therapy. Amer. J. Psychiat. **129**, 621–623 (1972)

Alarcón, R. de, Carney, M.W.P.: Severe depressive mood changes following slow-release intramuscular fluphenazine injection. Brit. med. J. **3**, 564–567 (1969)

Amsler, H.A.: Metabolische Granulozytopenien unter trizyklischen Psychopharmaka. Vortrag an der Psychiatrischen Universitätsklinik Zürich, 9. 7. 1977

Ananth, J.: Side effects on fetus and infant of psychotropic drug use during pregnancy. Int. Pharmacopsychiat. **11**, 246–260 (1976)

Ananth, J., Luchins, D.: A review of combined tricyclic and MAOI therapy. Comprehens. Psychiat. **18**, 221–230 (1977)

Ananth, J.V., Beszterczey, A.: Treatment of psychosis subsequent to phenothiazine-induced agranulocytosis. Comprehens. Psychiat. **14**, 319–324 (1973)

Ananth, J.V., Valles, J.V., Whitelaw, J.P.: Usual and unusual agranulocytosis during neuroleptic therapy. Amer. J. Psychiat. **130**, 100–102 (1973)

Andrews, P., Hall, J.N., Snaith, R.P.: A controlled trial of phenothiazine withdrawal in chronic schizophrenic patients. Brit. J. Psychiat. **128**, 451–455 (1976)

Angst, J.: Antidepressiver Effekt und genetische Faktoren. Arzneimittel-Forsch. (Drug Res.) **14**, 496–500 (1964)

Angst, J.: Zur Prognose antidepressiver Behandlungen. Anglogerm. med. Rev. **2**, 733–751 (1965)

Angst, J.: Die somatische Therapie der Schizophrenie. Stuttgart: Georg Thieme 1969

Angst, J.: Die Lithiumprophylaxe affektiver Psychosen. Ars Med. (Liestal) **1**, 29–40 (1970)

Angst, J.: Drug evaluation. In: Neuro-Psychopharmacology Proceedings of the 10th Congress of the Collegium Internationale Neuro-Psychopharmacologicum, Quebec July 1976. ed. by Deniker, P., Radouco-Thomas, C., Villeneuve, A., Vol. 2, Pergamon Press Oxford-New York-Toronto-Sidney-Paris-Frankfurt. 1023–1031, 1978

Angst, J., Dinkelkamp, Th.: Die somatische Therapie der Schizophrenie. Stuttgart: Georg Thieme 1974

Angst, J., Frey, R.: The course of affective disorders. I. Change of diagnosis of monopolar, unipolar and bipolar illness. Arch. Psychiat. Nervenkr. **226**, 57–64 (1978)

Angst, J., Theobald, W.: Tofranil (Imipramin). Bern: Stämpfli & Cie AG. 1970

Angst, J., Woggon, B.: Klinische Prüfung von fünf Depotneuroleptika. Vergleich der Wirkungsprofile von Fluphenazindecanoat, Fluspirilen, Penfluridol, Perphenazinenanthat und Pipothiazinpalmitat. Arzneimittel-Forsch. (Drug Res.) **25**, 267–270 (1975)

Anonym: Efficacy of thiopropazate dihydrochloride (dartalan) in treating persisting phenothiazine-induced choreo-athetosis and akathisia. Med. J. Aust. **2**, 629 (1972)

Anonym (Report from the Boston Collaborative Drug Surveillance Program, Boston University Medical Center): Reserpine and breast cancer. Lancet **1974a/II**, 669–671

Anonym: Rauwolfia derivatives and cancer. Lancet **1974b/II**, 701–702

Anonym: Rauwolfia-Alkaloide (Reserpin) und Mammakarzinom. Schweiz. Ärzteztg **45**, 1738 (1974c)

Anonym: Rauwolfia and breast cancer. Lancet **1975/II**, 312–313
Armstrong, B., Stevens, N., Doll, R.: Retrospective study of the association between use of rauwolfia derivatives and breast cancer in english women. Lancet **1974/II**, 672–675
Åsberg, M., Cronholm, B., Sjöqvist, F., Tuck, D.: Relationship between plasma level and therapeutic effect of nortriptyline. Brit. med. J. **3**, 331–334 (1971)
Aubert, C.: Les hyperthermies dues aux neuroleptiques. Essai d'interprétation physiopathologique. Encéphale **57**, 126–159 (1973)
Ayd, F.J., jr.: Perphenazine: A reappraisal after eight years. Dis. nerv. Syst. **15**, 311–317 (1964a)
Ayd, F.J., jr.: Children born of mothers treated with chlorpromazine during pregnancy. Clin. Med. **71**, 1758–1763 (1964b)
Ayd, F.J., jr.: Chlorpromazine: Ten year's experience. In: Neuropsychopharmacology (Bradley, P.B., Flügel, F., Hoch, P.H., eds.), Vol. 3. New York: Elsevier 1964c, pp. 572–574
Ayd, F.J., jr. (ed.): Excretion of psychotropic drugs in human breast milk. Int. Drug Ther. Newsl. **8**, 33–40 (1973a)
Ayd, F.J., jr. (ed.): The effectiveness of reserpine therapy for persistent dyskinesia. Int. Drug Ther. Newsl. **8**, 15 (1973b)
Ayd, F.J., jr.: Once-a-day dosage tricyclic antidepressant drug therapy: a survey. Dis. nerv. Syst. **35**, 475–480 (1974a)
Ayd, F.J., jr. (ed.): Neurological effects of abrupt withdrawal of neuroleptic medications in schizophrenic children. Int. Drug Ther. Newsl. **9**, 25–28 (1974b)
Ayd, F.J., jr. (ed.): Lithium – haloperidol for mania: Is it safe or hazardous? Int. Drug. Ther. Newsl. **10**, 29–36 (1975a)
Ayd, F.J., jr. (ed.): Deanol therapy for tardive dyskinesia. Int. Drug Ther. Newsl. **10**, 38–40 (1975b)
Ayd, F.J., jr. (ed.): Psychotropic drug combinations: Good and bad. Int. Drug Ther. Newsl. **12**, 13–16 (1977)
Baastrup, P.C., Poulsen, J.C., Schou, M., Amdisen, A.: Prophylactic lithium double-blind discontinuation in manic-depressive and recurrent-depressive disorders. Lancet **1970/II**, 326–333
Ballin, J.C.: Toxicity of tricyclic antidepressants. J. Amer. med. Ass. **231**, 1369 (1975)
Baron, M., Gershon, E.S., Rudy, V., Jonas, W.Z., Buchsbaum, M.: Lithium carbonate response in depression. Prediction by unipolar/bipolar illness, average-evoked response, catechol-O-methyl transferase, and family history. Arch. gen. Psychiat. **32**, 1107–1111 (1975)
Bartholomew, A.A.: A long-acting phenothiazine in the treatment of alcoholics in an outpatient clinic. Quart. J. Stud. Alcohol **27**, 510–513 (1966)
Bartholomew, A.A.: A long acting phenothiazine as a possible agent to control deviant sexual behavior. Amer. J. Psychiat. **124**, 917–929 (1968)
Baruk, H., Pécheny, J.: Essai clinique de l'imipramine 10 mg en thérapeutique géronto-psychiatrique. Ann. Moreau Tours **2**, 218–221 (1965)
Baštecký, J., Gregová, L.: Priapism as a possible complication of the chlorpromazine treatment. Activ. nerv. sup. (Praha) **16**, 175 (1974)
Bauer, H., Girke, W., Kanowski, S., Krebs, F.A., Müller-Oerlinghausen, B.: Ergebnisse zum Problem der psychophysischen Ermüdung unter Lithium-Dauertherapie. Activ. nerv. sup. (Praha) **15**, 89–90 (1973)
Bellabarba, U., Hippius, H., Kanowski, S.: Zur Differentialdiagnose hyperkinetisch-dystoner Begleitwirkungen von Psychopharmaka. Med. Welt **18**, 559–563 (1967)
Ben-David, M., Danon, A., Sulman, F.G.: Evidence of antagonism between prolactin and gonadotrophin secretion: Effect of methallibure on perphenazine induced prolactin secretion in ovariectomized rats. J. Endocrinol. **51**, 719–725 (1971)
Benkert, O., Hippius, H.: Psychiatrische Pharmakotherapie. Berlin-Heidelberg-New York: Springer 1974
Bessuges, J.M., Qurgaud, J.J.: Correction par le ‹praxinor› des hypotensions dues aux thérapeutiques psychiatriques. J. méd. Montpellier **7**, 320–323 (1972)
Beumont, P.J.V., Corker, C.S., Friesen, H.G., Kolakowska, T., Mandelbrote, B.M., Marshall, J., Murray, M.A.F., Wiles, D.H.: The effects of phenothiazines on endocrine function: II. Effects in men and post-menopausal women. Brit. J. Psychiat. **124**, 420–430 (1974a)
Beumont, P.J.V., Harris, G.W., Carr, P.J., Friesen, H.G., Kolakowska, T., MacKinnon, P.C.B., Mandelbrote, B.M., Wiles, D.: Some endocrine effects of phenothiazines: a preliminary report. J. psychosom. Res. **16**, 297–304 (1972)

Beumont, P.J.V., Gelder, M.G., Friesen, H.G., Harris, G.W., MacKinnon, P.C.B., Mandelbrote, B.M., Wiles, D.H.: The effects of phenothiazines on endocrine function: I. Patients with inappropriate lactation and amenorrhoea. Brit. J. Psychiat. **124**, 413–419 (1974)

Bielski, R.J., Friedel, R.O.: Prediction of tricyclic antidepressant response. A critical review. Arch. gen. Psychiat. **33**, 1479–1489 (1976)

Bílý, J., Hametová, M., Hanuš, H., Poláčková, J.: Prognosis of lithium prophylaxis. Activ. nerv. sup. (Praha) **15**, 88–89 (1973)

Bineik, E., Bornscheuer, B.: Zur Kreislaufwirkung von Neuroleptika im Alter. Akt. Gerontol. **2**, 287–290 (1972 a)

Bineik, E., Bornscheuer, B.: Zur Wirkung von Neuroleptika auf den kephalen Kreislauf bei psychiatrischen Alterspatienten. Pharmakopsychiat. **5**, 70–81 (1972 b)

Birnbaum, D., Karmeli, F.: The effect of psychopharmaca on uropeptic activity. Psychother. Psychosom. **24**, 102–105 (1974)

Blackburn, H.L., Allen, J.L.: Behavioral effects of interrupting and resuming tranquilizing medication among schizophrenics. J. nerv. ment. Dis. **133**, 303–308 (1961)

Blair, J.H., Simpson, G.M.: Effect of antipsychotic drugs on reproductive functions. Dis. nerv. Syst. **27**, 645–647 (1966)

Bojanovsky, J., Tölle, R.: Ophthalmodynamographische Untersuchungen während thymoleptischer Behandlung. Pharmakopsychiat. **6**, 178–185 (1973)

Bojanovsky, J., Tölle, R.: Dihydroergotamin gegen die Kreislaufwirkungen der Thymoleptika. Dtsch. med. Wschr. **99**, 1064–1069 (1974)

Bourgeois, M.: Priapismes sous neuroleptiques (trois cas). Nouv. Presse méd. **1**, 1161 (1972)

Braithwaite, R.A., Gouling, R., Théanu, G., Bailey, J., Coppen, A.: Plasma concentration of amitriptyline and clinical response. Lancet **1972/I**, 1297–1300

Brown, K.G.E., McMichen, H.U.S., Briggs, D.S.: Tachyarrhythmia in severe imipramine overdose controlled by practolol. Arch. Dis. Childh. **47**, 104–106 (1972)

Brown, W.T.: Side effects of lithium therapy and their treatment. Canad. psychiat. Ass. J. **21**, 13–21 (1976)

Buffa, P., Lacal, C.F., LoGullo, O., Pedretti, A., Armocide, C.C.: Sindrome depresivo involutivo y arterioescleroso. Notas Terapeuticas **8**, 1–6 (1963)

Bullock, R.J.: Efficacy of thiopropazate dihydrochloride (dartalan) in treating persisting phenothiazine induced choreo athetosis and akathisia. Med. J. Aust. **2**, 314–316 (1972)

Burks, J.S., Walker, J.E., Rumack, B.H., Ott, J.E.: Tricyclic antidepressant poisoning. Reversal of coma, choreoathetosis, and myoclonus by physostigmine. J. Amer. med. Ass. **230**, 1405–1407 (1974)

Burnett, G.B., Little, S.R.C.J., Graham, N., Forrest, A.D.: The assessment of thiothixene in chronic schizophrenia. A double-blind controlled trial. Dis. nerv. Syst. **36**, 625–629 (1975)

Busfield, B.L., Schneller, P., Capra, D.: Depressive symptom or side effect? A comparative study of symptoms during pre-treatment and treatment periods of patients on three antidepressant medications. J. nerv. ment. Dis. **134**, 339–345 (1962)

Campbell, M., Shapiro, T.: Therapy of psychiatric disorders of childhood. In: Manual of psychiatric therapeutics (Shader, R.I., ed.). Boston: Little, Brown & Co. 1975, pp. 137–162

Campiche, J.: Antidépressifs et myocarde. Recherche de la toxicité myocardique lors de traitements par les antidépressifs tricycliques administrés par voie intraveineuse. Rev. méd. Suisse rom. **93**, 461–479 (1973)

Carman, J.S.: Methylphenidate in akathisia. Lancet **1972/II**, 1093

Carney, M.W.P., Sheffield, B.F.: Forty-two months experience of flupenthixol decanoate in the maintenance treatment of schizophrenia. Curr. med. Res. Opin. **3**, 447–452 (1975)

Casey, D.E., Denney, D.: Deanol in the treatment of tardive dyskinesia. Amer. J. Psychiat. **132**, 864–867 (1975)

Charriot, G., Resche-Rigon, P.: Travaux cliniques sur le moditen-retard et le modecate; indications nouvelles, dans un secteur à nombre de lits restraint, impliquant une «équilibration» extrahospitalière des thérapeutiques. C.R. Congr. Psychiat. Neurol. langue franç. **70**, 1903–1909 (1972)

Chow, M., Souney, P.: Use of physostigmine in treatment of acute tricyclic antidepressant overdose. Hartford Hosp. Bull. **29**, 393–399 (1974)

Claveria, L.E., Teychenne, P.F., Calne, D.B., Haskayne, L., Petrie, A., Lodge-Patch, I.C.: Tardive dyskinesia treated with pimozide. J. neurol. Sci. (Amst.) **24**, 393–401 (1975)

Cohen, W.J., Cohen, N.H.: Combined lithium and haloperidol therapy: A dangerous combination producing irreversible brain damage. Excerpta med. (Amst.); Int. Congr. Ser. **296**, 42 (1973)
Cooper, T.B., Simpson, G.M.: The 24-hour lithium level as a prognosticator of dosage requirements: A 2-year follow-up study. Amer. J. Psychiat. **133**, 440–443 (1976)
Coppen, A., Noguera, R., Bailey, J., Burns, B.H., Swani, M.S., Hare, E.H., Gardner, R., Maggs, R.: Prophylactic lithium in affective disorders. Controlled trial. Lancet **1971/II**, 275–279
Cornu, F.: Psychopharmakotherapie. In: Psychiatrie der Gegenwart. Forschung und Praxis (Gruhle, H.W., Jung, R., Mayer-Gross, W., Müller, M., Hrsg.), Band I/2, S. 495–659. Berlin-Göttingen-Heidelberg: Springer 1963
Crawford, R., Forrest, A.: Controlled trial of depot fluphenazine in out-patient schizophrenics. Brit. J. Psychiat. **124**, 385–391 (1974)
Criscuoli, P.M.: Osservazioni cliniche controllate sull' effetto terapeutico associato (tioridazina e diidroergotamina) in pedopsichiatria. Neuropsichiat. infant. **122/123**, 363–370 (1971)
Curran, D.J., Nagaswami, S., Mohan, K.J.: Treatment of phenothiazine induced bulbar persistent dyskinesia with deanol acetamidobenzoate. Dis. nerv. Syst. **36**, 71–73 (1975)
Curran, J.P.: Management of tardive dyskinesia with thiopropazate. Amer. J. Psychiat. **130**, 925–927 (1973)
Debus, G.: Theoretische und methodische Aspekte der Wirkungsprüfung psychiatrischer Psychopharmaka bei gesunden Probanden. Pharmakopsychiat. **10**, 109–118 (1977)
Degkwitz, R.: Leitfaden der Psychopharmakologie für Klinik und Praxis. Stuttgart: Wissenschaftliche Verlagsgesellschaft 1967
Dempsey, G.M., Dunner, D.L., Fieve, R.R., Farkas, T., Wong, J.: Treatment of excessive weight gain in patients taking lithium. Amer. J. Psychiat. **133**, 1082–1084 (1976)
Denber, H.C.B., Bird, E.G.: Chlorpromazine in the treatment of mental illness. II. Side effects and relapse rates. Amer. J. Psychiat. **112**, 465 (1955)
Desmond, M.M., Rudolph, A.J., Hill, R.M., Claghorn, J.L., Dreessen, P.R., Burgdorf, I.: Behavioral alterations in infants born to mothers on psychoactive medication during pregnancy. Tex. Inst. ment. Sci. (1968/November), 20–23
Diamond, L.S., Marks, J.D.: Discontinuation of tranquilizers among chronic schizophrenic patients receiving maintenance dosage. J. nerv. ment. Dis. **131**, 247–251 (1960)
Dick, P.: Bilan comparatif et critique de notre expérience de trois neuroleptiques-retard. In: Institutions psychiatriques et neuroleptiques retards (Burner, M., publ.). Paris/Zürich: Squibb 1972, pp. 63–71
Dittrich, A.: Probleme der pharmakopsychologischen Forschung. In: Klinische Psychologie (Schraml, W., Baumann, U., Hrsg.), Band II, S. 523–558. Bern: Huber 1974
Doyle, L.N.: Imipramine pamoate in depression. Psychosomatics **16**, 129–131 (1975)
Dubois, E.L., Tallman, E., Wonka, R.A.: Chlorpromazine induced systemic lupus erythematosus. Case report and review of the literature. J. Amer. med. Ass. **221**, 595–596 (1972)
Dynes, J.B.: Sudden death. Dis. nerv. Syst. **30**, 24–28 (1969)
Eliasen, P., Andersen, M.: Sinoatrial block during lithium treatment. Europ. J. Cardiol. **3**, 97–98 (1975)
Elie, R., Morin, L., Tetreault, L.: Effets de l'ethopropazine et du trihexyphénidyle sur quelques paramètres du syndrome neuroleptique. Encéphale **61**, 32–52 (1972)
Fahn, S.: Treatment of choreic movements with perphenazine. Dis. nerv. Syst. **33**, 653–658 (1972)
Faigle, J.W., Dörhöfer, G.: Reserpine and chemical carcinogenesis. Lancet **1975/I**, 643
Fann, W.E., Davis, J.M., Wilson, I.C.: Methylphenidate in tardive dyskinesia. Amer. J. Psychiat. **130**, 922–924 (1973)
Fann, W.E., Sullivan, J.L. III, Miller, R.D., McKenzie, G.M.: Deanol in tardive dyskinesia: A preliminary report. Psychopharmacologia (Berl.) **42**, 135–137 (1975)
Fenasse, R., Mazet, M., Serment, H.: A propos de l'étiologie des syndromes aménorrhée galactorrhée. Rev. franç. Gynéc. **67**, 625–631 (1972)
Fischbach, R.: Die vegetativen Effekte der Antidepressiva im Bereich des Gastro-Intestinaltraktes. Wien. med. Wschr. **123**, Suppl. Nr. 5, 1–26 (1973)
Fleischhauer, J.: Open withdrawal of antiparkinson drugs in the neuroleptic induced parkinson syndrome. Int. Pharmacopsychiat. **10**, 222–229 (1975)
Flemenbaum, A.: Hypertensive episodes after adding methylphenidate (ritalin) to tricyclic antide-

pressants. Report of three cases and review of clinical adventages. Psychosomatics **13**, 265–268 (1972)
Flemenbaum, A.: Does lithium block the effects of amphetamine? A report of three cases. Amer. J. Psychiat. **131**, 820–821 (1974)
Floru, L.: Klinische Behandlungsversuche des lithiumbedingten Tremors durch einen Beta-Rezeptorenantagonisten (Propanolol). Int. Pharmacopsychiat. **6**, 197–222 (1971)
Floru, L.: Die Anwendung Beta-blockierender Substanzen in der Psychiatrie und Neurologie. Fortschr. Neurol. Psychiat. **45**, 112–127 (1977)
Floru, L., Floru, L., Tegeler, J.: Wirkung von Beta-Rezeptorenblockern (Pindolol und Practolol) auf den lithiumbedingten Tremor. Klinischer Versuch und theoretische Erwägungen. Arzneimittel-Forsch. (Drug Res.) **24**, 1122–1125 (1974a)
Floru, L., Floru, L., Tegeler, J.: Therapeutic value of beta receptor blocking substances in lithium induced tremor. Trials of therapy with pindolol and practolol. Med. Welt **25**, 450–452 (1974b)
Forrest, F.M., Snow, H.L.: Prognosis of eye complications caused by phenothiazines. Dis. nerv. Syst. **29**, Suppl. Nr. 3, 26–28 (1968)
Forrest, F.M., Snow, H.L., Erickson, G., Geiter, C.W., Laxson, G.O.: Incidence of late "melanosis" side effects in chronic mental patients after long-term phenothiazine therapy. Proc. West. Pharmacol. Soc. **9**, 18–20 (1966)
Frangos, E., Christodoulides, H.: Clinical observations on the treatment of tardive dyskinesia with haloperidol. Acta psychiat. belg. **75**, 19–32 (1975)
Gamkrelidze, Sh.A., Putkoradze-Gamkrelidze, N.A.: Our experience with moditene-depot in chronic schizophrenia. Activ. nerv. sup. (Praha) **15**, 169 (1973)
Gardos, G.: Are antipsychotic drugs interchangeable? J. nerv. ment. Dis. **159**, 343–348 (1974)
Gáspar, M., Poeldinger, W.: Betablocker in der Behandlung von ängstlich gefärbten Depressionen. Vergleichende Untersuchungen mit Clomipramin in Kombination mit Oxprenolol und Placebo in einer klinischen cross-over-studie bei Depressionen. In: Betablocker und Zentralnervensystem (Kielholz, P. Ed), Internationales Symposium St. Moritz, 5.–6. Januar 1976, pp. 134–138. Bern-Stuttgart-Wien: Hans Huber 1978
Gerlach, J.: Antipsychotische Behandlung mit Neuroleptika in sehr hohen Dosen. Ugeskr. Laeg. **139**, 959–961 (1977)
Gerlach, J., Thorsen, K.: The movement pattern of oral tardive dyskinesia in relation to anticholinergic and antidopaminergic treatment. Int. Pharmacopsychiat. **11**, 1–7 (1976)
Gerlach, J., Reisby, N., Randrup, A.: Dopaminergic hypersensivity and cholinergic hypofunction in the pathophysiology of tardive dyskinesia. Psychopharmacologia (Berl.) **34**, 21–35 (1974)
Gerlach, J., Thorsen, K., Munkvad, I.: Effect of lithium on neuroleptic-induced tardive dyskinesia compared with placebo in a double-blind cross-over trial. Pharmakopsychiat. **8**, 51–56 (1975)
Gessa, R., Tagliamonte, A., Gessa, G.L.: Blockade by apomorphine of haloperidol induced dyskinesia in schizophrenic patients. Lancet **1972/II**, 981
Gilligan, B.S., Wodak, J., Veale, J.L., Munro, O.R.: Tetrabenazine in the treatment of extrapyramidal dyskinesias. Med. J. Aust. **2**, 1054–1055 (1972)
Goldberg, H.L., Nathan, L.: A double-blind study of tofranil pamoate vs. tofranil hydrochloride. Psychosomatics **13**, 131–134 (1972)
Goldman, D.: Treatment of phenothiazine-induced dyskinesia. Psychopharmacologia (Berl.) **47**, 271–272 (1976)
Good, W.W., Sterling, M., Holtzman, W.H.: Termination of chlorpromazine with schizophrenic patients. Amer. J. Psychiat. **115**, 443–448 (1958)
Granacher, R.P., Baldessarini, R.J.: Physostigmine. Its use in acute anticholinergic syndrome with antidepressant and antiparkinson drugs. Arch. gen. Psychiat. **32**, 375–380 (1975)
Grant, B.R., Waller, R.H. (eds.): Drug interaction index. Kelowna, Canada: Meditec Publ. Ltd. 1972
Greenblatt, D.J., Koch-Weser, J.: Adverse reactions to intravenous diazepam: A report from the Boston collaborative drug surveillance program. Amer. J. Med. Sci. **266**, 261–266 (1973)
Greiner, A.C.: Schizophrenia melanosis: Iatrogenic-congenital defect. Dis. nerv. Syst. **29**, Suppl. Nr. 3, 14–15 (1968a)
Greiner, A.C.: Phenothiazines and diffuse melanosis. Agressologie **9**, 219–224 (1968b)
Gross, M., Hitchman, I.L., Reeves, W.P., Lawrence, J., Newell, P.C.: Discontinuation of treatment with ataractic drugs. A preliminary report. Amer. J. Psychiat. **116**, 931–932 (1960)

Gunn, D.R.: Skin pigmentation and the phenothiazines: A psychiatrist's comments. In: Toxicity and adverse reaction studies with neuroleptics and antidepressants (Lehmann, H.E., Ban, T.A., eds.). Verdun: Quebec Psychopharmacological Research Association 1967, pp. 72–74

Haase, H.J.: Therapie mit Psychopharmaka und anderen psychotropen Medikamenten. Stuttgart: Schattauer 1972

Haase, H.J., Floru, L., Knaack, M.: The clinical importance of the neuroleptic threshold and its fine motor determination by the handwriting test. J. int. med. Res. **2**, 321–330 (1974)

Halmy, K.: Exanthem induced by diazepam and sunlight. The etiology of fix exanthem cleared up by patch test applied to the site of the exanthem. Börgyögy. vener. Szle **51**, 71–75 (1975)

Harder, A., Modestin, J., Steiner, H.: Verlauf der Körpertemperatur bei Neuroleptika-Injektionskuren. Schweiz. med. Wschr. **101**, 828–831 (1971)

Harrer, G.: Zur Inkompatibilität zwischen Monoaminooxydase-Hemmern und Imipramin. Wien. med. Wschr. **111**, 551–553 (1961)

Harrer, G.: Inkompatibilitätserscheinungen bei Psychopharmaka. In: Neuropsychopharmacology. Proc. 5th Meeting C.I.N.P., Washington 1966. Int. Congr. Ser. **Nr. 129**, 588–594. Amsterdam: Excerpta medica 1967

Hartz, S.C., Heinonen, O.P., Shapiro, S., Siskind, V., Slone, D.: Antenatal exposure to meprobamate and chlordiazepoxide in relation to malformations, mental development, and childhood mortality. New Engl. J. Med. **292**, 726–728 (1975)

Hatashita, Y.: Experimental study of effects of psychotropic drugs on cardiac function. J. Kansai med. Univ. **26**, 203–231 (1974)

Heiberg, A., Lingjaerde, O.: A controlled study on the possible effect of dihydroergotamine against dryness of the mouth in patients treated with tricyclic antidepressants. Acta psychiat. scand. **48**, 353–359 (1972)

Heimann, H.: Methodologische Probleme bei der Effizienzprüfung von Psychopharmaka. Arch. Psychiat. Nervenkr. **220**, 281–288 (1975)

Heimann, H.: Allgemeine methodologische Probleme der klinischen Prüfung von Psychopharmaka. Pharmakopsychiat. **10**, 119–129 (1977)

Heinonen, O.P., Shapiro, S., Laurain, A.R. and The Boston Collaborative Drug surveillance Program Research Group: Rauwolfia derivatives and breast cancer. Lancet **1974a/II**, 1315–1317

Heinonen, O.P., Shapiro, S., Tuominen, L., Turunen, M.I.: Reserpine use in relation to breast cancer. Lancet **1974b/II**, 675–677

Heinrich, K.: Psychopharmaka in Klinik und Praxis. Stuttgart: Georg Thieme 1976

Heinrich, K., Wegener, I., Bender, H.-J.: Späte extrapyramidale Hyperkinesen bei neuroleptischer Langzeittherapie. Pharmakopsychiat. **1**, 169–195 (1968)

Heiser, J.F., Wilbert, D.E.: Reversal of delirium induced by tricyclic antidepressant drugs with physostigmine. Amer. J. Psychiat. **131**, 1275–1277 (1974)

Helmchen, H.: Die Gefahren einer zu intensiven Therapie mit psychisch wirksamen Pharmaka. Therapiewoche **19**, 212–218 (1969)

Hershon, H.I., Kennedy, P.F., McGuire, R.J.: Persistence of extrapyramidal disorders and psychiatric relapse after withdrawal of long-term phenothiazine therapy. Brit. J. Psychiat. **120**, 41–50 (1972)

Hertrich, O.: Therapie psychopharmakabedingter Nebenwirkungen mit Distigminbromid (Ubretid, BC 51). Nervenarzt **46**, 264–267 (1975)

Hill, R.M., Desmond, M.M., Kay, J.L.: Extrapyramidal dysfunction in an infant of a schizophrenic mother. J. Pediat. **69**, 589–595 (1966)

Hippius, H., Lange, J.: Zur Problematik der späten extrapyramidalen Hyperkinesen nach langfristiger neuroleptischer Therapie. Arzneimittel-Forsch. (Drug Res.) **20**, 888–890 (1970)

Hippius, H., Logemann, G.: Zur Wirkung von Dioxyphenylalanin (L-Dopa) auf extrapyramidalmotorische Hyperkinesen nach langfristiger neuroleptischer Therapie. Arzneimittel-Forsch. (Drug Res.) **20**, 894–896 (1970)

Hippius, H., Malin, J.-P.: Veränderungen des Elektrokardiogramms während der Behandlung mit trizyklischen Psychopharmaka. Pharmakopsychiat. **1**, 140–144 (1968)

Hirsch, S.R., Gaind, R., Rohde, P.D., Stevens, B.C., Wing, J.K.: Outpatient maintenance of chronic schizophrenic patients with long-acting fluphenazine: Double-blind placebo trial. Brit. med. J. **1**, 633–636 (1973)

Hofmann, G., Grünberger, J., König, P., Presslich, O., Wolf, R.: Die mehrjährige Lithiumtherapie affektiver Störungen. Langzeiteffekte und Begleiterscheinungen. Psychiat. clin. **7**, 129–148 (1974)

Holden, J.M.C., Holden, U.P.: Weight changes with schizophrenic psychosis and psychotropic drug therapy. Psychosomatics **11**, 551–561 (1970)

Holinger, P.C., Klawans, H.L.: Reversal of tricyclic-overdosage-induced central anticholinergic syndrome by physostigmine. Amer. J. Psychiat. **133**, 1018–1023 (1976)

Hollstein, H.: Astonin H bei der Behandlung psychopharmakabedingter hypotoner Kreislauf-Regulationsstörungen. Med. Welt **26**, 231–233 (1975)

Honigfeld, G., Howard, A.: Psychiatric drugs. A desk reference. New York-San Francisco-London: Academic Press 1973

Hucker, H., Woggon, B., Angst, J.: Präparatspezifische Ergebnisse der Auswertung. In: Schweizerische Studie über die Behandlung mit Depotneuroleptika. Zürich: Squibb AG. 1976

Hull, R.C., Marshall, J.A.: Single-dose imipramine pamoate in the treatment of depressive neurosis. Psychosomatics **16**, 84–87 (1975)

Hussain, M.Z., Khan, A.G., Chaudhry, Z.A.: Aplastic anemia associated with lithium therapy. Canad. med. Ass. J. **108**, 724–728 (1973)

Idänpään-Heikkilä, J., Alhava, E., Olkinuora, M., Palva, I.: Clozapine and agranulocytosis. Lancet **1975/II**, 611

Imlah, N.W., Murphy, K.P.: The clinical use of long acting psychotropic drugs. Therapie **28**, 587–594 (1973)

Immich, H.: Rauwolfia derivatives and cancer. Lancet **1974/II**, 774–775

Isac, M., Stern, S., Edelstein, E.L.: The treatment of phenothiazine-induced tachycardia by propanolol. Israel Ann. Psychiat. **10**, 272–277 (1972)

Jacobson, G., Baldessarini, R.J., Manschreck, T.: Tardive and withdrawal dyskinesia associated with haloperidol. Amer. J. Psychiat. **131**, 910–913 (1974)

Janke, W.: Methodologische Aspekte zur Relevanz von Psychopharmaka-Untersuchungen an Gesunden für die Pharmakotherapie. In: Psychopharmacology, sexual disorders and drug abuse (Ban, T.A., Boissier, J.R., Gessa, G.J., Heimann, H., Hollister, L., Lehmann, H.E., Munkvad, I., Steinberg, H., Sulser, F., Sundwall, A., Vinar, O., eds.). Amsterdam: North Holland Publ. Co. 1973, pp. 257–263

Janke, W., Debus, G.: Pharmakopsychologische Untersuchungen an gesunden Probanden zur Prognose der therapeutischen Effizienz von Psychopharmaka. Arzneimittel-Forsch. (Drug Res.) **25**, 1185–1194 (1975)

Johnson, D.A.W., Malik, N.A.: A double-blind comparison of fluphenazine decanoate and flupenthixol decanoate in the treatment of acute schizophrenia. Acta psychiat. scand. **51**, 257–267 (1975)

Johnson, F.N.: Lithium research and therapy. London-New York-San Francisco: Academic Press 1975

Johnstone, E.C.: The relationship between acetylator status and response to the monoamine oxidase inhibitor drug phenelzine in depressed patients. In: Neuropsychopharmacology (Boissier, J.R., Hippius, H., Pichot, P., eds.). Amsterdam: Excerpta Medica 1975, pp. 771–777

Jonchev, V., Arianova, L.: Case report of acute central vegetative dysregulation due to neuroleptic therapy. Savr. Med. **25**, 21–23 (1974)

Jonchev, V., Mitkov, V.: Traitement des hyperkinésies choréiques à la thiopropérasine (majeptil). Folia med. (Plovdiv) **13**, 339–344 (1971)

Jung, E.G., Schwarz-Speck, M., Kormany, G.: Beitrag zur Photoallergie auf Chlorphenothiazine. Schweiz. med. Wschr. **93**, 249–250 (1963)

Jus, A., Pineau, R., Lachance, R., Pelchat, G., Jus, K., Pires, P., Villeneuve, R.: Epidemiology of tardive gyskinesia. Part I. Dis. nerv. Syst. **37**, 210–214 (1976a)

Jus, A., Pineau, R., Lachance, R., Pelchat, G., Jus, K., Pires, P., Villeneuve, R.: Epidemiology of tardive dyskinesia. Part II. Dis. nerv. Syst. **37**, 257–261 (1976b)

Kammen, D.P. van, Murphy, D.L.: Attenuation of the euphoriant and activating effects of d- and l-amphetamine by lithium carbonate treatment. Psychopharmacologia (Berl.) **44**, 215–224 (1975)

Kanarek, K.S., Thompson, P.D., Levin, S.E.: The management of imipramine (tofranil) intoxication in children. S. Afr. med. J. **47**, 835–838 (1973)

Kane, J., Rifkin, A., Quitkin, F., Klein, D.F.: Antidepressant drug blood levels, pharmacokinetics and clinical outcome. In: Progress in psychiatric drug treatment (Klein, D.F., Gittelman-Klein, R., eds.). New York: Brunner/Mazel Publ. 1976, pp. 136–158

Kantor, S.J., Bigger, J.T., jr., Glassman, A.H., Macken, D.L., Perel, J.M.: Imipramine-induced heart block. J. Amer. med. Ass. **231**, 1364–1366 (1975)

Kazamatsuri, H., Chien, Ch.-P., Cole, J.O.: Treatment of tardive dyskinesia. I. Clinical efficacy of a dopamine-depleting agent, tetrabenazine. Arch. gen. Psychiat. **27**, 95–99 (1972a)

Kazamatsuri, H., Chien, Ch.-P., Cole, J.O.: Treatment of tardive dyskinesia. II. Short-term efficacy of dopamine-blocking agents haloperidol and thiopropazate. Arch. gen. Psychiat. **27**, 100–103 (1972b)

Kazamatsuri, H., Chien, Ch.-P., Cole, J.O.: Long-term treatment of tardive dyskinesia with haloperidol and tetrabenazine. Amer. J. Psychiat. **130**, 479–483 (1973)

Kellett, J.M., Metcalfe, M., Bailey, J., Coppen, A.J.: Beta blockade in lithium tremor. J. Neurol. Neurosurg. Psychiat. **38**, 719–721 (1975)

Kielholz, P.: Diagnose und Therapie der Depressionen für den Praktiker, 2. Aufl., München: J.F. Lehmanns Verlag 1966

Kimbrough, J.C.: Incontinence with doxepine. J. Amer. med. Ass. **221**, 510 (1972)

Kirk, L., Baastrup, P.C., Schou, M.: Propanololbehandlung bei Lithiumtremor. Nervenarzt **44**, 657–658 (1973)

Klawans, H.L., jr., Rubovits, R.: An experimental model of tardive dyskinesia. J. Neural Transm. **33**, 235–246 (1972)

Klett, C.J., Cole, J.O.: Principles and problems in establishing the efficacy of psychotropic agents. Section 2, 53–57: Methodology. Introduction. Public Health Service Publication No. 2138. Washington: U.S. Government Printing Office 1971

Kline, N.S., Angst, J.: Psychiatric syndroms and drug treatment. (Im Druck, 1979)

Kline, N.S., Mason, B.T., Winick, L.: Biperiden (akineton): Effective prophylactic and therapeutic anti-parkinsonian agent. Curr. ther. Res. **16**, 838–843 (1974a)

Kline, N.S., Wren, J.C., Cooper, T.B., Varga, E., Canal, O.: Evaluation of lithium therapy in chronic and periodic alcoholism. Amer. J. med. Sci. **268**, 15–22 (1974b)

König, L.: Lithiumtremor – Kombinationsbehandlung mit Beta-Rezeptorenblockern? Psychiat. Neurol. med. Psychol. (Lpz.) **27**, 720–724 (1975)

Kolakowska, T., Wiles, D.H., McNeilly, A.S., Gelder, M.G.: Correlation between plasma levels of prolactin and chlorpromazine in psychiatric patients. Psychol. Med. **5**, 214–216 (1975)

Korenyi, C., Lowenstein, B.: Chlorpromazine induced diabetes. Dis. nerv. Syst. **29**, 827–828 (1968)

Korsgaard, S.: Baclofen (lioresal) in the treatment of neuroleptic-induced tardive dyskinesia. Acta psychiat. scand. **54**, 17–24 (1976)

Kozakova, M.: Drug purpura after antidepressive drugs. Čsl. Derm. **46**, 158–160 (1971)

Kuhn, R.: Über die Behandlung depressiver Zustände mit einem Iminodibenzylderivat (G 22355). Schweiz. med. Wschr. **87**, 1135–1140 (1957)

Kullander, S., Källén, B.: A prospective study of drugs and pregnancy. I. Psychopharmaca. Acta obstet. gynec. scand. **55**, 25–33 (1976)

Kurtin, S.B.: Lithium carbonate dermatitis. J. Amer. med. Ass. **223**, 802 (1973)

Kuschinsky, G., Lüllmann, H.: Kurzes Lehrbuch der Pharmakologie, 6. Aufl. Stuttgart: Georg Thieme 1974

Lambert, P.A., Chaulaic, J.L., Cabrol, G.: Les troubles cardiovasculaires observés au cours des traitements par les antidépresseurs tricycliques. J. Méd. Lyon **54**, 1145–1154 (1973)

Laska, E.M., Siegel, C., Meisner, M., Fischer, S., Wanderling, J.: Matched-pairs study of reserpine use and breast cancer. Lancet **1975/II**, 296–300

Lazos, G., Kapetanakis, S., Photiades, H.: Lactation in male mammary glands after treatment with psychotropic drugs. Immunoelectrophoretic study of the secretion. Acta neurol. psychiat. hellen. **11**, 154–163 (1972)

Lehmann, E., Hopes, H.: Experimentelle Untersuchung der psychologischen Wirkung eines neuen Antidepressivums (Lofepramin) im Vergleich zu Imipramin und Placebo. Unveröffentlichtes Manuskript

Lehmann, H.E.: Psychobiological measures in psychiatry – review of the present status. In: Neuropsychopharmacology (Boissier, J.R., Hippius, H., Pichot, P., eds.). Amsterdam: Excerpta Medica 1975a, pp. 146–158

Lehmann, H.E.: Types and characteristics of objective measures of psychopathology. In: Experimental approaches to psychopathology (Kietzman, M.L., Sutton, S., Zubin, J., eds.). London: Academic Press 1975b

Levy, H.B.: Imipramine for the hyperkinetic syndrome. J. Amer. med. Ass. **225**, 527 (1973)
Litvak, R., Kaelbing, R.: Dermatological side effects with psychotropics. Dis. nerv. Syst. **33**, 309–311 (1972)
Lovett-Doust, J.W., Huszka, L.: Influence of some psychoactive drugs on mineral metabolism in man. Int. Pharmacopsychiat. **8**, 159–172 (1973)
Lüllmann, H., Lüllmann-Rauch, R., Wassermann, O.: Arzneimittel-induzierte Phospholipidspeicherkrankheit. Dtsch. med. Wschr. **98**, 1616–1625 (1973)
Lumineau, J.P., Garraud, M.J., Gaillard, A.: Action de la dihydroergotamine sur les complications salivaires des traitements psychotropes. Ouest méd. **25**, 85–89 (1972)
Lutz, E.G.: Dissipation of phenothiazine effect and recurrence of schizophrenic psychosis. Dis. nerv. Syst. **26**, 355–357 (1965)
Malin, J.P., Rosenberg, L.: Multidimensionale pharmakopsychiatrische Untersuchungen mit dem Neuroleptikum Perazin. 5. Mitteilung: Beeinflussung der ventrikulären Erregungsrückbildung im Elektrokardiogramm. Pharmakopsychiat. **7**, 41–49 (1974)
Man, P.L., Chen, C.H.: Severe shock caused by chlorpromazine hypersensitivity. Brit. J. Psychiat. **122**, 185–187 (1973)
Margat, M.-P., Broussot, T.: Application du chlorhydrate de fluphénazine, relavé par l'œnanthate de fluphénazine chez 40 schizophrènes et délirants chroniques. C.R. Congr. Psychiat. Neurol. langue franç. **66**, 602–606 (1968)
Marhold, J., Zimanová, J., Lachman, M., Král, J., Vojtěchovský, B.: To the incompatibility of haloperidol with lithium salts. Activ. nerv. sup. (Praha) **16**, 199–200 (1974)
Marini, J.L., Sheard, M.H., Bridges, C.I., Wagner, E., jr.: An evaluation of the double-blind design in a study comparing lithium carbonate with placebo. Acta psychiat. scand. **53**, 343–354 (1976)
Marks, J.: Interactions involving drugs used in psychiatry: Scientific basis of drug therapy in psychiatry. Symposium London 1964. Oxford: Pergamon Press 1965, pp. 191–201
Marocchino, R., Savio, P.A.: Studio clinico della diidroergotamina somministrata per via parenterale in associazione à psicofarmaci. Ann. Freniat. Sci. affini **86**, 66–70 (1973)
Martin, G.I., Zaug, P.J.: Electrocardiographic monitoring of enuretic children receiving therapeutic doses of imipramine. Amer. J. Psychiat. **132**, 540–542 (1975)
Mastrogiovanni, P.D.: Tofranil in gerontopsichiatria. Rass. Neuropsichiat. **18**, 107–121 (1964)
Matthew, H., Lawson, A.A.H.: Treatment of common acute poisoning, 3rd ed. Edinburgh-London: E. & S. Livingstone 1975
May, V.: Therapeutische Kombination von Psychopharmaka und Beta-Sympathicolytica. Nervenarzt **46**, 268–271 (1975)
May, V.: Zur Therapie von Alkoholikern mit oralen Neuroleptika und dem Depotneuroleptikum Dapotum D. Therapiewoche **25**, 972–980 (1975)
McLellan, D.L.: The suppression of involuntary movements with tetrabenazine. Scot. med. J. **17**, 367–370 (1972)
Meadow, A., Dunlon, P.T., Blacker, K.H.: Effects of phenothiazines on anxiety and cognition in schizophrenia. Dis. nerv. Syst. **36**, 203–208 (1975)
Meier-Ewert, K., Baumgart, H.H., Friedenberg, P.: Thromboembolische Komplikationen bei neuro- und thymoleptischer Behandlung. Dtsch. med. Wschr. **92**, 2174–2178 (1967)
Mendels, J., Digiacomo, J.: The treatment of depression with a single daily dose of imipramine pamoate. Amer. J. Psychiat. **130**, 1022–1024 (1973)
Merrill, D.C., Markland, C.: Vesical dysfunction induced by the major tranquilizers. J. Urol. **107**, 769–776 (1972)
Merry, J., Reynolds, C.M., Bailey, J., Coppen, A.: Prophylactic treatment of alcoholism by lithium carbonate. A controlled study. Lancet **1976/II**, 481–482
Meyers, F.H., Solomon, P.: Psychopharmacology. In: Handbook of psychiatry (Solomon, P., Patch, V.D., eds.). Los Altos, Calif.: Lange Medical Publ. 1974, pp. 427–463
Miller, W.C., jr., Marcotte, D.B., McCurdy, L.: A controlled study of single-dose administration of imipramine pamoate in endogenous depression. Curr. ther. Res. **15**, 700–706 (1973)
Mitchell, A.B.S.: Thioridazine induced diarrhoea. Postgrad. med. J. **51**, 182–183 (1975)
Moccetti, T., Lichtlen, P., Albert, H., Meier, E., Imbach, P.: Kardiotoxizität der trizyklischen Antidepressive. Phenothiazine und Imipraminderivate. Schweiz. med. Wschr. **101**, 1–10 (1971)

Modestin, J.: Diskussionsbemerkung zur Arbeit „Therapeutische Kombination von Psychopharmaka und Beta-Sympathicolytica" von V. May. Nervenarzt **47**, 54 (1976)
Möller, H.-J.: Methodische Grundprobleme der Psychiatrie. Stuttgart-Berlin-Köln-Mainz: Kohlhammer 1976
Moore, M.T., Book, M.H.: Sudden death in phenothiazine therapy: A clinicopathologic study of 12 cases. Psychiat. Quart. **44**, 389–402 (1970)
Morais, T.M. de, Pereira-Reis, M.J., Simao-Bines, J. et al.: O efeito economico do tratamento com o enantato de flufenazina em pacientes ambulatoriais. Folha méd. **64**, 1359–1364 (1972)
Morgan, R., Cheadle, J.: Maintenance treatment of chronic schizophrenia with neuroleptic drugs. Acta psychiat. scand. **50**, 78–85 (1974)
Morris, J.B., Beck, A.T.: The efficacy of antidepressant drugs. A review of research 1958 to 1972. Arch. gen. Psychiat. **30**, 667–674 (1974)
Müller, D., Krüger, E.: Nebenwirkungen der Lithiumtherapie. Psychiat. Neurol. med. Psychol. (Lpz.) **27**, 172–180 (1975)
Mueller, P.S., de la Vergne, P.M.: Amitriptyline, weight gain and carbohydrate craving: A side effect. Brit. J. Psychiat. **123**, 501–507 (1973)
Munoz, R.A., Kuplic, J.B.: Large overdose of tricyclic antidepressants treated with physostigmine salicylate. Psychosomatics **16**, 77–78 (1975)
Nerenz, K.: Ein Fall von Valium-Entzugsdelir mit Grand-mal-Anfällen. Ein kasuistischer Beitrag zum Valium-Mißbrauch und zur Valiumsucht. Nervenarzt **45**, 385–386 (1974)
Newton, R.W.: Physostigmine salicylate in the treatment of tricyclic antidepressant overdosage. J. Amer. med. Ass. **231**, 941–943 (1975)
Nies, A., Robinson, D.S., Lamborn, K.R., Ravaris, C.L., Ives, J.O.: The efficacy of the monoamine oxidase inhibitor, phenelzine: dose effects and prediction of response. In: Neuropsychopharmacology (Boissier, J.R., Hippius, H., Pichot, P., eds.). Amsterdam: Excerpta Medica 1975, pp. 765–770
Novak, E.N.: The effect of chlorpromazine on the blood coagulation. Farmakol. Toksikol. **35**, 717–720 (1972)
O'Fallon, W.M., Labarthe, D.R., Kurland, L.T.: Rauwolfia derivatives and breast cancer. A case/control study in Olmsted County, Minnesota. Lancet **1975/II**, 292–296
Olson, G.W., Peterson, D.B.: Sudden removal of tranquilizing drugs from chronic psychiatric patients. J. nerv. ment. Dis. **131**, 252–255 (1960)
Oppenheim, G.: Mutism and hyperthermia in a patient treated with neuroleptics. Med. J. Aust. **2**, 228–229 (1973)
Orlov, P., Kasparian, G., Dimascio, A., Cole, J.O.: Withdrawal of antiparkinson drugs. Arch. gen. Psychiat. **25**, 410–412 (1971)
Pauget, J.D.: Correction par la dihydroergotamine Sandoz des effets secondaires provoqués par les psychotropes. Psychol. Méd. **4**, 821–829 (1972)
Perel, J.M.: Tricyclic antidepressants: Relationship among pharmacokinetics: Metabolism and clinical response. Vortrag auf dem Hoechst-Symposium „Depressive Disorders", Rom, 9.–11. 5. 1977
Perel, J.M., Shostak, M., Gann, E., Kantor, S.J., Glassmann, A.H.: Pharmacodynamics of imipramine and clinical outcome in depressed patients. In: Pharmacokinetics of psychoactive drugs: Blood levels and clinical response (Gottschalk, L.A., Merlis, S., eds.). New York: Spectrum Publ. Inc. 1976, pp. 229–241
Pichot, P.: Methodik der Effizienzprüfung in der Psychopharmakologie. Arch. Psychiat. Nervenkr. **220**, 281–288 (1975)
Pieschl, D.: Die kardiovasculären Wirkungen der Neuroleptika nach dem heutigen Erkenntnisstand. Nervenarzt **44**, 212–215 (1973)
Pieschl, D., Kulhanek, F., Piergies, A.: Verbundstudie Dapotumacutum: Erfahrungen bei 660 Schizophrenen. Referat am DGPN-Kongreß, Düsseldorf, 27.11.1976
Pisciotta, A.V.: Mechanisms of phenothiazine induced agranulocytosis. In: Psychopharmacological Review of Progress, 1957–1976 (Efron, D.H., ed.). Public Health Service Publication No. 1836. Washington: U.S. Government Printing Office 1968, pp. 597–605
Pisciotta, A.V.: Studies on agranulocytosis. – IX. A biochemical defect in chlorpromazine sensitive marrow cells. J. Lab. clin. Med. **78**, 435–448 (1971)
Pöldinger, W.: Kompendium der Psychopharmakotherapie. Basel: F. Hoffmann-La Roche & Co. AG. 1967

Pöldinger, W., Schmidlin, W.: Index Psychopharmacorum. Bern-Stuttgart-Wien: Verlag Hans Huber 1972
Prien, R.F., Klett, C.J.: An appraisal of the long-term use of tranquilizing medication with hospitalized chronic schizophrenics: a review of the drug discontinuation literature. Schiz. Bull. **5**, 64–73 (1972)
Prien, R.F., Levine, J., Switalski, R.W.: Discontinuation of chemotherapy for chronic schizophrenics. Hosp. Community Psychiat. **22**, 4–7 (1971)
Pritchard, M.: Prognosis of schizophrenia before and after pharmacotherapy. II. Three-year follow-up. Brit. J. Psychiat. **113**, 1353–1359 (1967)
Ravaris, C.L., Weaver, L.A., Brooks, G.W.: Further studies with fluphenazine enanthate: II. Relapse rate in patients deprived of medication. Amer. J. Psychiat. **124**, 248–249 (1967)
Rifkin, A., Kurtin, S.B., Quitkin, F., Klein, D.F.: Lithium induced folliculitis. Amer. J. Psychiat. **130**, 1018–1019 (1973a)
Rifkin, A., Quitkin, F., Klein, D.F.: Organic brain syndrome during lithium carbonate treatment. Comprehens. Psychiat. **14**, 251–254 (1973b)
Rifkin, A., Quitkin, F., Howard, A., Klein, D.F.: A study of abrupt lithium withdrawal. Psychopharmacologia (Berl.) **44**, 157–158 (1975a)
Rifkin, A., Quitkin, F., Klein, D.F.: Akinesia. A poorly recognized drug induced extrapyramidal behavioral disorder. Arch. gen. Psychiat. **32**, 672–674 (1975b)
Rothstein, Ch.: An evaluation of the effects of discontinuation of chlorpromazine. New Engl. J. Med. **262**, 67–69 (1960)
Rysanek, K., Spankova, H., Mlejnkova, M.: Effect of tricyclic antidepressants on phosphodiesterase: Correlation between aggregability and thrombocyte metabolism. Activ. nerv. sup. (Praha) **15**, 126–127 (1973)
Safer, D.J., Allen, R.P.: Factors influencing the suppressant effects of two stimulant drugs on the growth of hyperactive children. Pediatrics **51**, 660–667 (1973)
Saldanha, V.F., Havard, C.W.H., Bird, R., Gardner, R.: The effect of chlorpromazine on pituitary function. Clin. Endocr. (Oxford) **1**, 173–180 (1972)
Sato, S., Daly, R., Peters, H.: Reserpine therapy of phenothiazine induced dyskinesia. Dis. nerv. Syst. **32**, 680–685 (1971)
Saxén, E.A., Peto, R.: Rauwolfia derivatives and breast cancer. Lancet **1974/II**, 833
Scharfetter, C.: Allgemeine Psychopathologie. Eine Einführung. Stuttgart: Georg Thieme 1976
Schmidt, P.: Zur ambulanten Behandlung von Psychosen mit Depot-Fluphenazin. Psychiat. Neurol. med. Psychol. (Lpz.) **27**, 231–238 (1975)
Schnetzler, J.P., Alleon, A.M.: La correction des effets végétatifs des psychotropes par les fortes doses de dihydroergotamine chez les vieillards et les adultes. Inform. psychiat. **50**, 779–781 (1974)
Schorer, C.E.: Single dose vs. divided dose imipramine. Psychopharmacologia (Berl.) **28**, 115–119 (1973)
Schou, M.: Preparations, dosage, and control. In: Lithium. Its role in psychiatric research and treatment (Gershon, S., Shopsin, B., eds.). New York-London: Plenum Press 1973, pp. 189–199
Schou, M.: What happened later to the lithium babies? A follow-up study of children born without malformations. Acta psychiat. scand. **54**, 193–197 (1976)
Schou, M., Amdisen, A.: Lithium and pregnancy. III. Lithium ingestion by children breast-fed by women on lithium treatment. Brit. med. J. **2**, 138 (1973)
Schou, M., Amdisen, A., Steenstrup, O.R.: Lithium and pregnancy. II. Hazards to women given lithium during pregnancy and delivery. Brit. med. J. **2**, 137 (1973a)
Schou, M., Baastrup, P.C., Kirk, L.: Hand tremor, Acta psychiat. scand. Suppl. **243**, 39 (1973b)
Schou, M., Goldfield, M.D., Weinstein, M.R., Villeneuve, A.: Lithium and pregnancy. I. Report from the Register of Lithium Babies. Brit. med. J. **2**, 135–136 (1973c)
Schuster, P., Gabriel, E., Kuefferle, B., Karobath, M.: Reversal by physostigmine of clozapine-induced delirium. Lancet **1976/I**, 37–38
Shader, R.I.: Pregnancy and psychotropic drugs. In: Psychotropic drug side effects (Shader, R.I., Dimascio, A., eds.). Baltimore: The Williams & Wilkins Company 1970, pp. 206–213
Shader, R.I.: Sexual dysfunction associated with mesoridazine besylate (serentil). Psychopharmacologia (Berl.) **27**, 293–294 (1972)
Shader, R.I., Dimascio, A.: Galactorrhea and gynecomastia. In: Psychotropic drug side effects (Shader, R.I., Dimascio, A., eds.). Baltimore: The Williams & Wilkins Company 1970, pp. 4–9

Shader, R.I., Belfer, M.L., Dimascio, A.: Glucose metabolism. In: Psychotropic drug side effects (Shader, R.I., Dimascio, A., eds.). Baltimore: The Williams & Wilkins Company 1970a, pp. 46–62

Shader, R.I., Giller, D.R., Dimascio, A.: Hypothalamic-pituitary-adrenal axis. In: Psychotropic drug side effects (Shader, R.I., Dimascio, A., eds.). Baltimore: The Williams & Wilkins Company 1970b, pp. 16–24

Sheard, M.H.: Lithium in the treatment of aggression. J. nerv. ment. Dis. **160**, 108–118 (1975)

Shopsin, B., Gershon, S.: Pharmacology-toxicology of the lithium ion. In: Lithium. Its role in psychiatric research and treatment (Gershon, S., Shopsin, B., eds.). New York-London: Plenum Press 1973, pp. 107–146

Shopsin, B., Kline, N.S.: Combined tricyclic and monoamine oxidase inhibitor (MAOi) therapy in depressed outpatients. C.I.N.P., IX Congr., Paris 1974; symposia abstracts in: J. Pharmacol. **5**, Suppl. Nr. 1, 103 (1974)

Silva, L. de, Huang, C.Y.: Deanol in tardive dyskinesia. Brit. med. J. **3**, 466 (1975)

Simpson, G.M., Varga, E.: Clozapine – a new antipsychotic agent. Curr. ther. Res. **16**, 679–686 (1974)

Simpson, G.M., Amin, M., Kunz, E.: Withdrawal effects of phenothiazines Comprehens. Psychiat. **6**, 347–351 (1965)

Simpson, G.M., Amin, M., Kunz-Bartholini, E., Salim, T., Watts, T.P.S.: Problems in the evaluation of the optimal dose of butyrophenone (trifluperidol). Int. Pharmacopsychiat. **2**, 59–70 (1969)

Simpson, G.M., Branchey, M.H., Lee, J.H., Voitashevsky, A., Zoubok, B.: Lithium in tardive dyskinesia. Pharmakopsychiat. **9**, 76–80 (1976)

Singer, L., Finance, F., Ruh, D.: A propos d'embolies pulmonaires survenues en un mois chez trois femmes agées atteintes de psychose maniaco dépressive. Discussion. Rôle étiopathogénique du traitement psychiatrique. Ann. méd.-psychol. **2**, 256–263 (1975)

Singh, M.M., Vergel de Dios, L., Kline, N.S.: Weight as a correlate of clinical response to psychotropic drugs. Psychosomatics **11**, 562–570 (1970)

Solomon, K., Vickers, R.: Dysarthria resulting from lithium carbonate. A case report. J. Amer. med. Ass. **231**, 280 (1975)

Sørensen, R., Jensen, J., Mulder, J., Schou, M.: Polyuria/polydipsia. Acta psychiat. scand. Suppl. **243**, 39 (1973)

Tanghe, A., Vereecken, J.L.T.M.: Fluspirilene, an injectable, and penfluridol, an oral long acting, neuroleptic. A comparative double blind trial in residual schizophrenia. Acta psychiat. scand. **48**, 315–331 (1972)

Thornton, W.E., Pray, B.J.: Lithium intoxication. A report of two cases. Canad. psychiat. Ass. J. **20**, 281–282 (1975)

Tölle, R.: Kreislaufwirkungen der Thymoleptika im Behandlungsverlauf. Pharmakopsychiat. **2**, 75–86 (1969)

Tölle, R.: Kreislaufregulation bei Depressiven und bei antidepressiver Behandlung. Therapiewoche **23**, 4412–4414 (1973)

Tupin, J.P., Smith, D.B., Clanon, T.L., Kim, L.I., Nugent, A., Groupe, A.: The long-term use of lithium in aggressive prisoners. Comprehens. Psychiat. **14**, 311–317 (1973)

Uhlíř, F., Kancucká, V., Lukačiková, E.: Placebo periods in chlorpromazine maintenance treatment. Activ. nerv. sup. (Praha) **15**, 83 (1973)

Usdin, E., Efron, D.H.: Psychotropic drugs and related compounds. 2nd. ed. Rockville, Maryland, Dep. of health, educ., and welfare 1972. (DHEW publ. no. "HSM" 72–9074)

Vendsborg, P.B., Rafaelsen, O.J.: Lithium in man: effect on glucose tolerance and serum electrolytes. Acta psychiat. scand. **49**, 601–610 (1973)

Vendsborg, P.B., Bach-Mortensen, N., Rafaelsen, O.J.: Fat cell number and weight gain in lithium treated patients. Acta psychiat. scand. **53**, 355–359 (1976a)

Vendsborg, P.B., Bech, P., Rafaelsen, O.J.: Lithium treatment and weight gain. Acta psychiat. scand. **53**, 139–147 (1976b)

Venezian, E.C., Casirola, G., Marini, G., Ippoliti, G., Invernizzi, R.: Rauwolfia derivatives and breast cancer. Lancet **1974/II**, 1266

Viukari, M., Linnoila, M.: Effect of methyldopa on tardive dyskinesia in psychogeriatric patients. Curr. ther. Res. **18**, 417–424 (1975)

Vohra, J., Burrows, G.D.: Cardiovascular complications of tricyclic antidepressant overdosage. Drugs **8**, 432–437 (1974)

Vulpe, M.: Skin pigmentation and the phenothiazines. Neurological aspects. In: Toxicity and adverse reaction studies with neuroleptics and antidepressants (Lehmann, H.E., Ban, T.A., eds.), Verdun: Quebec Psychopharmacological Research Association 1967, pp. 56–59

Waes, A. van, van de Velde, E.: Safety evaluation of haloperidol in the treatment of hyperemesis gravidarum. J. clin. Pharmacol. **9**, 224–227 (1969)

Waldmann, K.-D., Greger, J., Kluge, H., Gröschel, W., Zahlten, W., Hartmann, W.: Beitrag zur Lithiumintoxikation bei therapeutischer Lithium-Serum-Konzentration. Psychiat. clin. **7**, 56–62 (1974)

Warner, H.: Skin pigmentation and the phenothiazines. Gastroenterological aspects. In: Toxicity and adverse reaction studies with neuroleptics and antidepressants (Lehmann, H.E., Ban, T.A., eds.). Verdun: Quebec Psychopharmacological Research Association 1967, pp. 70

Watanabe, S., Ishino, H., Otsuki, S.: Double-blind comparison of lithium carbonate and imipramine in treatment of depression. Arch. gen. Psychiat. **32**, 659–668 (1975)

Watanabe, S., Taguchi, K., Nakashima, Y., Ebara, T., Iguchi, K., Otsuki, S.: Leukocytosis during lithium treatment and its correlation to serum lithium level. Folia psychiat. neurol. jap. **28**, 161–165 (1974)

Weinstein, M.R., Goldfield, M.D.: Cardiovascular malformations with lithium use during pregnancy. Amer. J. Psychiat. **132**, 529–531 (1975)

Wendkos, M.H.: Electrocardiographic changes with psychoactive drugs. Experiments with thioridazine. In: Toxicity and adverse reaction studies with neuroleptics and antidepressants (Lehmann, H.E., Ban, T.A., eds.). Verdun: Quebec Psychopharmacological Research Association 1967, pp. 143–155

Wilson, R.G., Hamilton, J.R., Boyd, W.D., Forrest, A.P.M., Cole, E.N., Boyns, A.R., Griffiths, K.: The effect of long term phenothiazine therapy on plasma prolactin. Brit. J. Psychiat. **127**, 71–74 (1975)

Winsberg, B.G., Goldstein, S., Yepes, L.E., Perel, J.M.: Imipramine and electrocardiographic abnormalities in hyperactive children. Amer. J. Psychiat. **132**, 542–545 (1975)

Woggon, B.: Depotneuroleptika – praktische Durchführung der Langzeitbehandlung und methodische Schwierigkeiten bei der klinischen Prüfung. Ther. Umsch. **32**, 501–506 (1975)

Woggon, B.: Schwierigkeiten bei der Planung von Psychopharmakaprüfungen aus der Sicht des klinischen Prüfers. Pharmakopsychiat. **10**, 140–146 (1977)

Woggon, B., Angst, J.: Einzelne Aspekte der Behandlung mit Depotneuroleptika. In: Therapie, Rehabilitation und Prävention schizophrener Erkrankungen (Huber, G., Hrsg.), S. 191–205. Stuttgart-New York: Schattauer 1976

Woggon, B., Angst, J.: Die Bedeutung der Depotneuroleptika für die Langzeitbehandlung schizophrener Patienten. Praxis **66**, 421–427 (1977)

Woggon, B., Hucker, H., Angst, J.: Allgemeine, nicht präparatspezifische Ergebnisse. In: Schweizerische Studie über die Behandlung mit Depotneuroleptika. Zürich: Squibb AG, 1976

Wojdyslawska, I., Siuchninska, H., Goraj, A.: Results of clozapine treatment in schizophrenics. Psychiat. pol. **9**, 45–50 (1975)

Wolpert, A., Farr, D.: Psychotropics and their effect on the EKG in children. Dis. nerv. Syst. **36**, 435–436 (1975)

Worrall, E.P., Moody, J.P., Naylor, G.J.: Lithium in non-manic-depressives: Antiaggressive effect and red blood cell lithium values. Brit. J. Psychiat. **126**, 464–468 (1975)

Wren, J.C., Kline, N.S., Cooper, T.B. et al.: Evaluation of lithium therapy in chronic alcoholism. Clin. Med. **81**, 33–36 (1974)

Zapletálek, M., Preiningerová, O., Bílý, J.: A contribution to the maintenance treatment of psychoses with depot neuroleptics. Activ. nerv. sup. (Praha) **15**, 87 (1973)

Zerssen, D. von: Beta-adrenergic blocking agents in the treatment of psychoses. A report on 17 cases. In: Neuro-psychiatric effects of adrenergic beta-receptor blocking agents (Carlsson, C., Engel, J., Hansson, L., eds.). München-Berlin-Wien: Urban & Schwarzenberg 1976, pp. 105–114

Convulsive Therapy

By

J.O. Ottosson

Contents

A. Frequency	316
B. Principle	316
C. Technique	317
I. Anesthesiologic Principles	317
II. Pharmacologic Convulsive Therapy	317
III. Electroconvulsive Therapy	318
1. Properties of Electric Stimulation	318
2. Distribution of Current	319
3. Treatment Intervals	319
D. Systemic Effects	320
E. Effects on the Central Nervous System	321
I. Electroencephalography	321
1. Seizure Activity	321
2. Postseizure Activity	321
3. Relation Between Postseizure EEG and Antidepressive Effect	322
II. Cerebral Circulation and Metabolism	322
III. Blood-Brain Barrier	323
IV. Neuropathology	323
V. Neurochemistry	324
F. Memory Disturbance	325
I. Relation to Antidepressive Effect	325
II. Memory Gap for Treatment Course	326
III. Anterograde Amnesia	326
1. Pathophysiologic Mechanisms	326
2. Duration	327
IV. Retrograde Amnesia	327
V. Subjective Experience of Memory	328
G. Indications and Outcome	328
I. Depressive Disorders	328
1. Comparative Outcome Studies	328
2. Prediction of Antidepressive Effect	330
3. Combination of ECT and Drugs in Treatment of Depression	332
II. Manic Disorders	333
III. Schizophrenic Disorders	333
IV. Confusional States	334

H. Complications and Contraindications 335
    I. Complications 335
    II. Cardiovascular Effects. 336
    III. Contraindications. 336
    IV. Influence of Age 336
I. Mechanisms of Action. 337
    I. Antidepressive Effect 337
        1. Unrelatedness to Organic Syndrome 337
        2. Psychologic Theories 337
        3. Involvement of Hypothalamus 338
        4. Amine Hypothesis 338
        5. Permeability Hypothesis. 340
        6. Electrolyte Hypothesis 340
    II. Antipsychotic and Antimanic Effects 340
    III. Anticonfusional Effect. 341
    IV. Amnestic Mechanism of Action. 341
References 341

A. Frequency

The use of convulsive therapy (CT) has decreased in the last 10–20 years (FLÅTTEN, 1975; APERIA et al., 1976; CLARE, 1976; D'ELIA and FREDRIKSEN, 1979). This may be the result of several factors combined: increasing supply of psychotropic drugs, more rational use of such drugs due to increased knowledge of their dynamics and kinetics, increased use of prophylaxis with lithium salts, and possibly negative attitudes to CT in mass media and public opinion. The use of ECT (electroconvulsive therapy) has become ever more restricted to severe depression for which no equivalent alternative has been proposed (STRÖMGREN, 1977b; APA Task Force, 1978). In 1975, 4% of Swedish psychiatric inpatients received ECT (D'ELIA and FREDRIKSEN, 1978).

B. Principle

The principle of CT is to induce grand mal seizures under controlled conditions. The therapeutic action of the treatment, at least in cases of depression, is related to the seizure and not to the inducing agent, electric current or a chemical substance. The treatment is therefore convulsive (or more specifically related to the cerebral seizure) and not an electric or a pharmacologic therapy. The amnestic side effects and other manifestations of an organic syndrome, however, are partly a direct effect of the electric stimulation. These relations can be visualized in the following way as far as electroconvulsive therapy is concerned:

```
              Electric stimulation
                  /       \
            Seizure activity   \
              /       \         \
   Therapeutic action   Organic syndrome
```

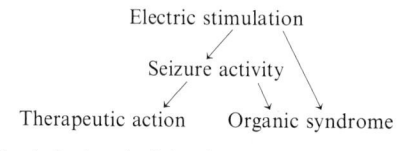

Fig. 1. Basic principle of electroconvulsive therapy

C. Technique

I. Anesthesiologic Principles

Modern treatment follows four anesthesiologic principles:
1. Premedication with atropine or methylscopolamine, given to diminish secretion of saliva, which may be aspirated, and to prevent abnormal cardiac activity in the vagal area.
2. Intravenous barbiturate narcosis to reduce anxiety and prevent discomfort from the subsequent muscular relaxation. The narcosis is kept superficial so as not to unnecessarily increase the seizure threshold and interfere with seizure activity. Since fewer electrocardiographic abnormalities have been recorded with methohexital than with thiopental, methohexital is the drug of choice (WOODRUFF et al., 1968).
3. Muscular relaxation with succinylcholine (HOLMBERG and THESLEFF, 1952). For routine use, a dose reducing but not abolishing muscular activity is usually chosen. Total abolition of muscular activity makes it difficult to ascertain if a grand mal seizure has been induced.
4. Artificial ventilation with 100% oxygen keeping the arterial oxygen saturation above 90% (HOLMBERG, 1953). If the patient is well ventilated before the induction of the seizure this oxygen saturation is maintained due to apneic diffusion oxygenation (HOLMDAHL, 1953) provided that the seizure activity does not last longer than 1 min. With durations above 1 min hypoxia and hypercapnia may develop. In some centers the patient is ventilated throughout the treatment, a procedure that should be routine at signs of cardiac disease. Extravagal arrhythmia such as premature ventricular contraction may be prevented if hypoxia and hypercapnia are avoided (McKENNA et al., 1970).

II. Pharmacologic Convulsive Therapy

MEDUNA's original treatment consisted of a pharmacologic convulsive therapy using camphor and later pentamethylenetetrazol as seizure-inducing agents. These agents are seldom used nowadays because they are less reliable in inducing one (and only one) seizure and cause the patient more discomfort in the form of preconvulsive anxiety and postconvulsive confusion than the electric method. Renewed interest in pharmacologic CT was aroused by the introduction of flurothyl (Indoklon), a volatile substance that can induce convulsive activity after administration via inhalation (ICT). Seizures induced by pharmacologic means usually last longer than electric seizures, obviously because the convulsive substance is left in the blood and forces the central nervous system to continued activity. Comparative studies of ECT and ICT show equal antidepressive efficacy (LAURELL, 1970). As expected with reference to Fig. 1 a reduced memory disturbance was recorded after a single treatment of ICT, whereas after a series of treatments the memory disturbance was of the same magnitude as after ECT. Probably the gain from the elimination of the electric current is outweighed by the longer seizures with more exhaustion of the central nervous system. Flurothyl treatment is technically more difficult than ECT and has never spread outside a few centers. The preparation itself is no longer on the market.

III. Electroconvulsive Therapy

1. Properties of Electric Stimulation

The use of electric stimulation as a seizure-inducing agent is now widespread. Stimulating the brain with a low dose of electricity effects only minor autonomic reactions. When the dose is increased unconsciousness and irregular muscular contractions of short duration (petit mal response) are evoked. Further increase effects a grand mal response of unconsciousness and tonic and clonic contractions. Atypical "dissociated" seizure patterns characterized by partially abolished consciousness and spontaneous breathing retained during the seizure, may be seen after an intermediate dose of electricity (LIBERSON, 1953). Increase of the electric current above the threshold for a grand mal seizure does not change the seizure activity further. According to Fig. 1, the aim of the therapy is to induce grand mal seizure activity with a minimal dose of electricity.

Three properties of electric stimulation can be modified so that the organic psychosyndrome can be minimized: the amount of energy, the type, and the mode of application. The organic psychosyndrome is increased as measured by retro- and anterograde amnesia by administering supraliminal energy (OTTOSSON, 1960; CRONHOLM and OTTOSSON, 1963a). Brief impulses of direct current (BST = brief stimulus technique) can induce seizure activity with a smaller amount of electric energy and hence a reduced organic syndrome compared with alternating current (LIBERSON, 1953; MAXWELL, 1968; VALENTINE et al., 1968; WEAVER et al., 1974, 1977). These observations have had astonishingly little influence on abandoning alternating current machines, which moreover give fewer possibilities to liminal stimulation (DAVIES et al., 1970). Several different BST machines on the market have variations in the duration, frequency, form, amplitude of the impulses as well as possibilities to modulate frequency and amplitude. The significance of all these parameters is insufficiently known. A lower limit seems to exist as far as duration of the pulses is concerned. A duration below 1 ms with correspondingly increased amplitude tends to give "dissociated" seizure patterns, which probably have a lower antidepressive efficiency (CRONHOLM and OTTOSSON, 1963b). The glissando technique, gradually increasing the current to give the seizure a subdued outset, makes the machines more expensive without fulfilling this purpose (BLACHLY and DENNEY, 1976). The use of muscular relaxation has made such modifications obsolete.

Unilateral application of the electric stimulation over one hemisphere is unanimously agreed to diminish both postconvulsive confusion and retro- and anterograde amnesia when compared with bilateral stimulation (see D'ELIA, 1970; STRÖMGREN, 1973). This is explained by a reduction of the amount of cerebral tissue in the direct path of current flow. The type of amnesia is dependent on the stimulated hemisphere. While stimulation of the nondominant hemisphere gives reduced verbal memory disturbance, stimulation of the dominant hemisphere reduces the disturbance for nonverbal material such as spatial relations, gestalts, and faces (DORNBUSH and WILLIAMS, 1974; D'ELIA et al., 1976). It should be emphasized that unilateral ECT does not imply unilateral seizure activity; only generalized bilateral seizure activity is induced with unilateral stimulation. If the seizure activity is not bilateral and maximal, the treatment does not have full theraputic effect. The reason for some psychiatrists' impression that unilateral treatment is less efficient is probably due to the induction of occasionally submaximal seizures. When the patient is totally paralyzed it is impossible to check the generalization of the seizure activity without EEG (STRÖMGREN and JUUL-JENSEN, 1975). A survey of well-controlled comparative studies with good treatment technique show comparable antidepressive efficacy (D'ELIA and RAOTMA, 1975).

2. Distribution of Current

The distribution of current in the brain is determined by the conductivity of the scalp and the resistance of the skull which interact to create a wide diffusion of the current. Using cadavers, SMITT and WEGENER (1944) estimated that only 5%–10% and HAYES (1950) in live spider monkeys that 20% of the voltage drop occurred in the brain. WEAVER et al. (1976) in a nonhomogeneous three-sphere computerized simulation model of the head estimated that 44% of the current never penetrates the brain in bilateral treatment and 64%, in unilateral treatment. All investigators thus agree that the output from the machine exceeds by far the input to the brain. Unilateral treatment on an average results in a one-third reduction in current density, the stimulated side having densities 1.5–3 times those of the opposite side. This measurement corresponds well to the reduced confusion and memory disturbance after unilateral stimulation.

The electric properties of the scalp and skull explain why variations in the unilateral placement of the electrodes do not result in variations in memory disturbance. The hope of reducing memory disturbance by avoiding the temporal region has consequently not been realized (INGLIS, 1970). On the whole it does not seem possible by further manipulation of the electric stimulation to reduce the direct effects of the current on the brain beyond those obtained by using BST, threshold-dose, and unilateral placement of the electrodes. However, it is important not to increase the seizure threshold by using anticonvulsive drugs before the treatment (e.g., diazepam) and by giving deeper narcosis than necessary.

3. Treatment Intervals

There are other ways of minimizing the organic psychosyndrome. Administration of abundant oxygen together with muscular relaxation prevents cerebral hypoxia. The establishment of a maximal number of seizures in a series (usually 10–12) and of intervals of at least 2–3 days between the treatments has the same motive. This endeavor to obtain the antidepressive effect in as pure a culture as possible is opposite to so-called regressive ECT, characterized by several and frequent treatments with the aim of inducing a confused, annihilated state from which a healthy condition will resurrect. The claim that such unphysiologic treatment is more advantageous than drug treatment in schizophrenia is not well founded (EXNER and MURILLO, 1973).

Quite another matter is the attempt to shorten the intervals between the treatments so as to obtain a more rapid remission of depression. STRÖMGREN

(1975) increased the frequency from two to four per week and reported higher antidepressant efficiency as measured by a shortening of the hospital stay by 11 days. However, since there is as yet no follow-up, the relapse rate is not known. Moreover the long-term retention of memory material should be compared.

BLACHLY and GOWING (1966) have gone even further by giving multiple (four–six–eight) treatments in one session only a few minutes apart. Remarkably the duration of the seizures did not decline; this was explained by an abundant oxygen supply. However, in most cases it was not possible to enhance the clinical efficacy. The antidepressive effect as well as the memory disturbance seem to depend on the evolution of processes that once established proceed relatively independently (ABRAMS, 1974). This may parallel observations that a prolonged seizure with total muscular relaxation, continued insufflation of oxygen, and administration of analeptic drugs has not been proven to be more efficient than a seizure that terminates spontaneously (HOLMBERG et al., 1956). Likewise, the effect of electrically and pharmacologically induced seizures is similar in spite of the fact that the latter last up to 70% longer (LAURELL, 1970). The duration of a self-sustained maximal seizure cannot be directly related to its antidepressive efficacy (OTTOSSON, 1962). A short (30 s) and a long seizure (120 s) may thus have equal antidepressive efficacy. However, submaximal seizures have decreased antidepressive efficiency (KALINOWSKY et al., 1942; HOLT and BORKOWSKI, 1951; CRONHOLM and OTTOSSON, 1960).

In summary, an optimal antidepressive effect is dependent on the induction of maximal cerebral seizure activity. The number of seizures required is usually six–ten. To obtain a cumulative effect intervals of at least 24–48 h seem optimal. Relief from depression by means of a one-session therapy does not seem possible.

D. Systemic Effects

ECT has a multitude of effects on the organism; indeed probably no single bodily function is not transiently influenced since the total involvement of the C.N.S. has repercussions everywhere in the periphery (review by HOLMBERG, 1963; OTTOSSON, 1974).

These systemic effects, the examination of which has depended on their putative relation to ECT's therapeutic action may be divided into three groups:
1. Direct effects of the seizure such as muscular convulsions, hypoxia, hypercapnia, increased blood pressure, increased pulse rate, and other expressions of a sympathetic and parasympathetic hyperactivity. Most of these effects are reduced or eliminated when ECT is given according to anesthesiologic principles and should be regarded as coincidental phenomena irrelevant as therapeutic factors.
2. Stress-related changes. Unspecific adaptational changes belong to the stress syndrome with increased pituitary-adrenocortical as well as adrenomedullary activity. These changes can also be considered coincidental since the stress syndrome initiated in other ways or by the administration of ACTH has no antidepressive effect.

3. Vegetative effects indicating diencephalic influence (body weight, appetite, sleep, digestion, libido, menstruation). Disturbances of these functions seem to reflect a basic disorder in affective disease, and ECT-induced changes in them may be cause or consequence of the antidepressive effect. Recent neuroendocrinologic evidence indicates that closely adjacent, related, or even the same diencephalic nuclei regulate mood, affect, and vegetative-hormonal functions. The mechanisms in the endocrinologic and autonomous nervous system regulating such functions thus deserve more attention if a closer understanding of the therapeutic action of ECT is desired.

E. Effects on the Central Nervous System

I. Electroencephalography

1. Seizure Activity

ECT makes feasible the study of the grand mal seizure pattern, which is seldom possible in epileptics. The pattern after bilateral stimulation reveals two components: a bilaterally synchronous rhythm throughout the seizure with a frequency declining from 5–7 to 2 cycles/s and an irregular fast activity at 18–22 cycles/s, which is superimposed on the slow activity and corresponds to the tonic phase. The seizure stops simultaneously in all leads (OTTOSSON, 1960).

The seizure pattern in unilateral ECT is similar, except for a somewhat higher voltage on the stimulated than on the nonstimulated side, especially when the dominant side is stimulated (D'ELIA, 1970).

Seizures induced with flurothyl last longer and have more fast activity and lower regularity and rhythmicity (i.e., less synchronization) compared with electrically induced seizures (LAURELL, 1970).

The duration of the maximal seizure und standard conditions varies among patients but is rather constant in the same patient except for the first treatment, which is the longest (HOLMBERG, 1954; FINNER, 1954). The duration is determined by circulatory and respiratory dimensions.

2. Postseizure Activity

In the comatose state immediately after the seizure periods of more-or-less complete electric silence last up to several minutes after the seizure. The silence is occasionally interrupted by bilaterally synchronous delta waves mostly frontally, single at first, then in short episodes, and finally continuous. The delta activity is gradually superimposed upon and later substituted by faster activity, and within 1 h the pattern has almost reverted to the preseizure appearance. The recovery of the EEG pattern is influenced only transiently by arousal stimuli (KIRSTEIN and OTTOSSON, 1960).

Unilateral ECT presents a similar pattern of restitution, except for a higher voltage amplitude on the stimulated side for the first postseizure minutes which agrees with higher involvement of that side during the seizure (D'ELIA, 1970).

In the further course of development asymmetric changes occur more frequently on the dominant side irrespective of right or left electric induction (SMALL, 1974).

After flurothyl-induced seizures the degree of disturbance is more pronounced and the restitution slower. These effects are probably secondary to the longer seizure, which results in a higher degree of metabolic exhaustion. The clinical correlate is a protracted confusion (LAURELL, 1970).

After series of 11–21 treatments visual ratings of EEG have returned to pretreatment status after 2–3 months (SMALL, 1974).

In summary, irrespective of the mode of induction a centrencephalic pacemaker corresponding to brain stem structures is evidenced by the bilateral synchrony of the seizure activity, the simultaneous discontinuation in all regions, and the likewise bilaterally synchronous, slow postseizure activity. This pacemaker is forced into action from the very beginning in bilateral ECT and at a somewhat later stage in unilateral treatment. Flurothyl therapy probably evokes cortical pacemakers in addition.

3. Relation Between Postseizure EEG and Antidepressive Effect

Since several symptoms in severe depression indicate a hypothalamic disturbance, the involvement of the brain stem in convulsive therapy is probably relevant (ROTH, 1951; OTTOSSON, 1962). A study by VOLAVKA et al. (1972) could ascertain no relation between the short-term antidepressive effect and the amount of postseizure delta activity. However, ROTH et al. (1957) showed that the thiopental-induced delta activity in the post-treatment EEG correlated with the stability of the long-term clinical outcome: the more delta activity, the smaller the probability of a relapse at 3 and 6 months after ECT. This need not imply that delta activity, or rather the cerebral change resulting in delta activity, is a component of the antidepressive process; rather a correlation is expected since both the antidepressive effect and the delta activity are related to the seizure activity. Interestingly delta activity may serve as a signal of sufficient treatment; however, this possibility of regulating the number of ECT is seldom utilized. Close attention to the clinical course is generally sufficient for deciding an appropriate, tailored series of treatments, but an additional method may be needed in cases with a high relapse rate. The practice in some quarters of additional "stabilizing" treatments following symptomatic relief was not substantiated in a controlled investigation (BARTON et al., 1973).

II. Cerebral Circulation and Metabolism

During convulsive activity in completely relaxed and oxygenated animals and man, the cerebral oxygen consumption is about doubled; however, the cerebral blood flow also increases. The fact that the arteriovenous oxygen content difference is reduced, i.e., a "luxury" perfusion occurs during seizure activity (PLUM et al., 1968, 1974; BERESFORD et al., 1969; POSNER et al., 1969), proves this compensatory mechanism sufficient. The central nervous system can adjust its vascular bed and the systemic blood pressure to meet its metabolic demands. Production of lactic acid (BRODERSEN et al., 1973) and increase of brain extracellular potassium (BOLWIG et al., 1977a) cause vasodilatation, which in additon to the blood pressure increase provides the necessary oxygen supply to the brain. The increase of cerebral blood flow has been observed to last for a week in depressed patients who were improved; schizophrenics who did not respond to the treatment showed a decrease of the cerebral blood flow (LOVETT DOUST and RASCHKA, 1975).

Whereas convulsive therapy following modern anesthesiologic principles does not create a general cerebral hypoxia, local hypoxia cannot be definitely excluded. Some part of the brain, for instance the hippocampus, may cause this due to its higher metabolic activity, so that even an increased cerebral blood flow may not meet the metabolic demands (LIBERSON and CADILHAC, 1953; BERLYNE and STRACHAN, 1968). A relative hypoxia may thus arise which may be a mechanism in memory disturbance. Spastic constriction of cerebral arteries during seizure activity has also been suspected (MATAKAS et al., 1977).

III. Blood-Brain Barrier

Studies of the blood-brain barrier with indicator-dilution technique do not give evidence for structural changes in the capillaries during ECT (BOLWIG et al., 1977c, d). The diffusion capacity of the capillaries increases as a consequence of the increased cerebral blood flow, but the transport of electrolytes and low molecular tracer substances changes only insignificantly. Similar changes and a corresponding increase of the cerebral blood flow can be recorded during hypercapnia. Therefore changes in the transport of substances from the blood to the brain probably depend on the increased perfusion of the brain and not on the seizure activity itself. Since carbon dioxide has no antidepressive effect the increased cerebral blood flow and consequent changes in the transport of substances are not likely to be significant therapeutic factors, at least not without some connection to seizure activity.

IV. Neuropathology

Whereas ECT is generally agreed to give rise to reversible changes in the neurons and glia, the question of permanent damage is a point of dissension. However, animal experiments have proven that electroconvulsive shocks if given in great number, at short intervals, without narcosis, relaxation, and oxygenation can cause permanent damage (HARTELIUS, 1952). This finding is hardly astonishing, but it does not apply to modern clinical administration of ECT following anesthesiologic principles, i.e., below 12 in number in a series and with at least 24–48 h intervals between. For obvious reasons no systematic neuropathologic studies have been conducted in man, but animal experiments striving to simulate clinical ECT as much as possible show no proof of permanent damage. Constriction of cerebral vessels has been observed in relaxed cats through a skull window to last up to 20 min (MATAKAS et al., 1977) after two–five probably suprathreshold electric stimulations given during a 5-min interval. Similar "vasospasm" may occur in ECT as a direct effect of the electric stimulation during the seizure period. Since significant changes in cerebral cells do not begin to appear in the monkey until 20 min after the middle cerebral artery has been totally occluded – the changes are reversible if the occlusion is removed during this timespan – a putative vasospasm during ECT is not likely to have any long-lasting effect on cerebral structures (GARCIA, 1978). This conclusion agrees with studies on unparalyzed baboons which required more than 1 h of practically continuous seizure activity to produce ischemic cell changes (MELDRUM et al., 1973a). After muscular paralysis the neuronal damage was less severe for comparable seizure durations (MELDRUM et al., 1973b).

Studies of the blood-brain barrier present similar findings. In relaxed, well-oxygenated cats a breakdown of the barrier function could be demonstrated only after seizure periods exceeding 5 min (LORENZO et al., 1975). Experiments simulating clinical ECT give evidence of extravasation of protein molecules, but this takes place by vesicular transport across intact vascular walls and is reversible within a few minutes after the seizure when the blood pressure is normalized. Vascular changes were not noted, nor was brain edema observed under electron microscope after ten consecutive electric stimuli (BOLWIG et al., 1977b). This may parallel the astonishingly small effect on sensorium and memory after multiple seizures in one session (BLACHLY and GOWING, 1966). The crucial protecting factors are probably an abundant supply of oxygen and the fact that the total cerebral blood flow is increased more than required for the increased cerebral metabolism.

Apart from effecting changes in the cerebral blood flow the electric current may have a damaging effect on the neurons. Using the same magnitude of electric stimulation in cats as in human ECT which implies a strong overdose, QUANDT and SOMMER (1966) found neuronal degeneration and gliosis along the current's presumed path. Such changes are neither expected nor recorded in human ECT which shows a more diffuse spread of current in the brain (WEAVER et al., 1976). Nevertheless, these findings underscore the importance of using threshold doses of electric energy.

These studies conclude that modern ECT induces only reversible changes in the cerebral circulation, consisting of a general increase of the blood flow and possibly local constrictions, which are not likely to result in permanent effects on neurons or glia. Threshold stimulation provides no evidence of direct adverse effects on the neurons from the electric current.

V. Neurochemistry

Two areas are in the center of current research because of their inherent possibilities of elucidating the action mechanism of ECT: influence on central monoaminergic activity and influence on neurohormonal activity of the hypothalamic-pituitary axis.

The pertinent question concerning the effect of ECT on monoamines and humoral transmission is whether or not its antidepressive action agrees with the catecholamine or indoleamine hypothesis. Acute effects of ECT are less interesting in this context since they may well be coincidental; effects that accumulate during a series of treatments and then remain are more likely to

be relevant. Recent animal research has established the following effects fulfilling these criteria:
1. Increase of the synthesis of noradrenaline (but not of dopamine or serotonin) (MODIGH, 1976).
2. Increase of the sensitivity of dopamine and possibly also noradrenaline receptors (MODIGH, 1975; EDÉN and MODIGH, 1977).
3. Increase of the sensitivity of serotonin receptors (EVANS et al., 1976; GREEN et al., 1977).

Whereas "low-output" depressions have been ascribed to noradrenaline, dopamine, and serotonin (POST and GOODWIN, 1975; ÅSBERG et al., 1976) the evidence for low-sensitivity depression is mainly indirect (Medical Research Council, 1972). However, if depression is associated with low functional activity in monoaminergic systems ECT seems to have the possibility of counteracting both low-output and low-sensitivity depression. ECT then has the property of a broad spectrum antidepressive treatment. This may explain the higher outcome rate in comparison with the more specifically acting antidepressant drugs.

No consistent biochemical data on ECT in depression has yet confirmed the animal findings. A fundamental problem is to decide whether increase of, e.g., the sensitivity of a neuron, is cause or consequence of the relief from depression.

Recent neuroendocrinologic research on severe depression has shown evidence of disturbance in several hypothalamic neuroendocrine cell systems regulating the secretion from the pituitary gland. This hypothalamic dysfunction is probably due to reduced noradrenergic activity (SACHAR et al., 1976) and implies that (1) the hypothalamic symptoms of severe depression (anorexia, decreased libido, menstrual disturbance, sleep disturbance, diurnal rhythm) have a neurochemical basis and (2) the endocrinologic and amine data fit into a consistent pattern. Several acute effects of ECT have been described on pituitary hormone outputs, some of which increase while some remain unchanged. So far only limited data on cumulative, sustained effects have been recorded, including an increased growth-hormone response to dopamine-noradrenaline agonists in rats (EDÉN and MODIGH, 1977).

In summary, the effect of ECT on monoaminergic systems agrees with the amine hypotheses for depressive disorders. The influence of ECT on depression with hypothalamic symptoms has been well established but its sustained effect on specific neuroendocrine systems is as yet not sufficiently known.

F. Memory Disturbance

I. Relation to Antidepressive Effect

Memory disturbance has been such a conspicuous feature of ECT that it has even been adduced a therapeutic factor. However, there is no relation between changes in memory and depression to support such a view; on the contrary, learning ability increases with amelioration of the depression (CRON-

HOLM and OTTOSSON, 1961; STRÖMGREN, 1977a). Moreover it is possible to dissociate the effects on memory from those on depression (OTTOSSON, 1968) and to obtain a maximal antidepressive effect with a minimal memory disturbance in unilateral, nondominant ECT.

II. Memory Gap for Treatment Course

Both a retrograde and anterograde amnesia result from each treatment and in the ordinary 48–72 h intervals they combine to form a continuous memory gap corresponding to the course of treatments. This is valid also for the least memory disturbing modifications. A reduced cognitive function due to the mental disturbance in itself may be an additional explanation of the memory gap, although it is rarely a source of complaints.

III. Anterograde Amnesia

In assessing *anterograde memory* function it is important to distinguish between learning (measured by immediate reproduction) and retention (measured by delayed reproduction). The typical disturbance after ECT is impairment of retention while learning is unchanged or improved (CRONHOLM and OTTOSSON, 1961). Tests aiming at estimating memory disturbance after ECT gain in validity with increasing intervals between immediate and delayed reproduction. SQUIRE and MILLER (1974), testing at intervals of 24 h, ascertained a cumulative increase of memory impairment during a series of four treatments which was not shown when an interval of only half an hour was used. Several studies have used the Wechsler memory scale, which only measures learning.

1. Pathophysiologic Mechanisms

There are important differences between learning and retention: learning is related to intelligence, retention is not; learning is influenced by depression, retention is not; learning is dependent on neocortical activity, retention, on activity in older parts of the brain, particularly the Papez' circuit or the limbic forebrain circuit comprising hippocampus, fornix, corpora mamillaria, thalamus, and cingulum, which is involved in the process of storing information (CRONHOLM et al., 1963; BARBIZET, 1963).

The anterograde amnesia following ECT has the characteristics of a Korsakoff syndrome, in which a lesion has been determined in the mamillary bodies. Therefore, it is probable that an involvement of Papez' circuit, also explains the impairment of retention in ECT. The following two mechanisms are conceivable:

1. The hippocampus has a lower epileptogenic threshold than the rest of the brain and during seizure activity is also characterized by a higher metabolic rate (LIBERSON and CADILHAC, 1953; BERLYNE and STRACHAN, 1968). A relative hypoxia possibly develops in the hippocampus due to the higher oxygen demand although the arteriovenous oxygen difference over the whole brain is not increased in ECT.
2. The hippocampus projects just at the site of the frontotemporal electrode, which is standard in practically all treatment modifications whether unilateral

or bilateral and may, therefore, receive a high density of current. However, attempts to avoid this site have not diminished the memory disturbance, since the current is diffusely spread due to the electric properties of skull and scalp (D'ELIA, 1976). Nor is a return to pharmacologic convulsive therapy a solution since the longer seizures impose a greater strain on the brain. The least disturbance is produced with unilateral stimulation and abundant oxygenation.

2. Duration

The duration of anterograde amnesia following a treatment series varies with number, frequency, technique of treatments, and with the test procedure. A test applied 1 week after a series of 2–7 bilateral treatments still showed a 30% reduction of the retention after 3 h, whereas a test at 1 month after 2–12 treatments showed that retention had returned to the pretreatment level (CRONHOLM and BLOMQUIST, 1959; CRONHOLM and MOLANDER, 1964). With the same tests full restitution had occurred 3–7 days after a series of 3–10 *unilateral* nondominant treatments (D'ELIA, 1970). Thus, whereas restitution occurs within a month with bilateral treatment it takes a week at the most with unilateral nondominant treatment. With intervals as long as 2 weeks between immediate and delayed reproduction no evidence of persisting memory impairment was determined 6–9 months after 5–17 bilateral or unilateral nondominant treatments given three times per week (SQUIRE and CHASE, 1975). Thus, normal use of ECT shows no evidence of permanent impairment, a conclusion agreeing with neuropathologic and neurophysiologic evidence. However, after series comprising 40–263 treatments (median number 58.5), a permanent impairment of cognitive functioning is possible (TEMPLER et al., 1973).

IV. Retrograde Amnesia

ECT can also cause *retrograde amnesia* both for events immediately before the treatment (CRONHOLM and MOLANDER, 1961; DORNBUSH and WILLIAMS, 1974) and for remote events (SQUIRE and SLATER, 1975). Programs broadcast on television 1–3 years previously were forgotten 1 h after the fifth bilateral ECT while programs broadcast 4–17 years in the past were remembered as well as before ECT. Full restitution occurred after 1–2 weeks. No such deficit occurred after unilateral nondominant ECT (SQUIRE et al., 1975). Even a brief, temporary loss of orientation in the past, however, may be troublesome. Some people lose their previous topographic schemata and get lost in long-familiar surroundings (A Practising Psychiatrist, 1965). Also autobiographic material relating to early schooling, job, and other life experiences has been reported lost for at least 14–18 weeks (JANIS, 1950). However, most of the lost memories belonged to the year preceding hospitalization, a fact agreeing with the pattern of greater influence on recent than on remote memories. It is impossible to give a precise statement for the duration of irreversible retrograde amnesia, but memories acquired during the few days before a course of ECT may be permanently lost.

V. Subjective Experience of Memory

The patient's experience of his memory may give information that is not revealed by traditional tests. (The experience of changes in connection with ECT refer, if not specified, both to anterograde and retrograde effects.) Patients who have recovered from a depressive disease seldom complain of bad memory, in spite of the fact that their retention is objectively impaired. This is explained by the fact that one experiences firsthand the learning ability, which has improved when depression is alleviated, and not the retention (Cronholm and Ottosson, 1963c). Patients belonging to the 6–9 month follow-up of Squire and Chase (1975) without objective memory disturbance could still evaluate their memory as impaired, both as regards current learning problems and difficulties in recalling familiar material (apart from the time of hospitalization). About two-thirds had complaints after bilateral ECT, one-third, after unilateral ECT, as opposed to one-sixth, in a no-ECT control group. More than half of those with subjective memory impairment ascribed it to ECT. The authors suggest that the impairment of recent and remote memory initially associated with bilateral ECT could cause some persons to become more alert to subsequent memory failures, which are erroneously attributed to ECT even if they occur at a normal frequency.

In summary, since even a temporary memory impairment may cause inconvenience, those ECT modifications minimizing this side effect should be used. These include brief stimuli at threshold intensity, unilateral application over the nondominant hemisphere, methohexital anesthesia, muscular relaxation with succinylcholine, oxygen ensuring arterial oxygen saturation of more than 90%, no treatments more than necessary for a remission, and at least 48-h intervals between the treatments. If these principles are followed memory disturbance no longer poses a major problem in convulsive therapy. The only remaining changes established are (1) a vague reminiscence of the time of treatment and preceding the disease (which partly may be explained by the disease itself) which occurs in nearly all patients although troubling only a few, and (2) a subjective memory impairment for up to 1 year which occurs in a few patients.

G. Indications and Outcome

I. Depressive Disorders

1. Comparative Outcome Studies

Soon after its introduction ECT seemed an effective antidepressive therapy showing the most conspicuous results in involutional melancholia with a previously chronic course (Huston and Locher, 1948a; Fishbein, 1949; Bond, 1954), but also in manic-depressive psychosis. In the latter, ECT shortened the duration of depression and reduced mortality (Huston and Locher, 1948b; Ziskind et al., 1945; Bond and Morris, 1954). With the advent of drug therapy the relative merits of the different therapies became the pertinent question. Two multicenter studies are outstanding due to the magnitude of the patient series.

GREENBLATT et al. (1964) compared ECT (a series of at least nine treatments) with imipramine (maximum daily dose 200–250 mg), two MAO=monoamine oxidase inhibitors, and placebo in 281 inpatients with severe depressions (irrespective of diagnosis). The rate of marked improvement, i.e., patients practically symptom-free and capable of functioning in the community after 8 weeks, was 76% in the ECT group, 49% with imipramine, 50% with phenelzine, and 46% with placebo. ECT was superior in all diagnostic groups except among psychoneurotic depressive reactions, which showed a very high percentage of marked improvement irrespective of treatment. A British study (Medical Research Council, 1965) of similar design had a similar outcome. In this study depression was described as primary, i.e., not secondary, arising from some other psychiatric illness. The condition for inclusion was a persistent alteration of mood exceeding customary sadness and accompanied by self-depreciation, retardation, agitation, sleep disturbance, or hypochondriasis. After random allocation 269 patients received either ECT (four–eight treatments), imipramine 200 mg, phenelzine, or placebo. The patients were hospitalized at least during the first 4 weeks of the study. After that time and eliminating patients who had received additional treatment which could be given at any time due to lack of progress or deterioration the rates of marked improvement were 71% for ECT, 52% for imipramine, 30% for phenelzine, and 39% for placebo. The British study thus agrees with the American, showing that ECT was superior and phenelzine of no value. In addition, the British study showed a significant antidepressive effect of imipramine, which moreover was most obvious in men. In the further course of the British study the difference between ECT and imipramine leveled out. Thus at 8 weeks the percentage discharged without any additional treatment and not readmitted were 48% in the ECT and 37% in the imipramine group, after 12 weeks, 52% and 54%, respectively, and after 24 weeks, 54% in both groups. Additional treatment (ECT in the imipramine group, ECT or antidepressants or some other treatment in the ECT group) had been given in in-patient or out-patient care, to 26% in the ECT group and 32% in the imipramine group at the final evaluation. Thus the marked superiority of ECT over all other treatments after 4 and 8 weeks was no longer apparent as far as imipramine was concerned after 12 and 24 weeks. It should be added that about one-third (36%) of the patients had a satisfactory outcome on placebo alone after 24 weeks.

Most studies comparing ECT and drugs reach similar conclusions although most concentrate on short-term effects where ECT has an obvious advantage. Consideration of the fairly high relapse rate after ECT (THOMAS, 1954) and the possibility of prolonging a drug treatment, tends to reduce the difference. In a study by KILOH et al. (1960a, b) 89% markedly improved after 3 weeks with ECT; however, at 6 months the improvement rate had fallen to 48%, a result approaching that obtained with iproniazid (40%), an outcome probably not significantly different from that of placebo.

These long-term effects after ECT must not promote an attitude of reserve and resignation concerning the efficacy of ECT. The main characteristic of the antidepressive effect of ECT is the rapidity of its action, which is literally of vital importance since severely depressed patients have a considerable mortality (suicidal and nonsuicidal). A 3-year follow-up of hospitalized depressed patients in Iowa (AVERY and WINOKUR, 1976) showed the ECT group to have a lower total mortality than groups treated with other methods. Myocardial infarctions in particular occurred more frequently in inadequately treated groups, showing the importance of rapidly eliminating the stress on the organism which a severely depressive disease causes.

On the other hand, the value of tricyclic antidepressants relative to ECT is probably underestimated for two reasons:

1. The conventional dose of imipramine, for example, has probably been too low, since 300 mg, unusual in comparative studies, gave a greater and more consistent improvement than 150 mg (SIMPSON et al., 1976).
2. Monitoring the dose from the plasma level has only rarely been utilized. At least with nortriptyline the outcome was increased to levels equal to ECT (KRAGH-SÖRENSEN et al., 1976). The question of whether or not high-dose monitored antidepressive drug therapy can approach the efficacy of ECT requires further evaluation.

The studies cited fulfil ordinary requirements of a scientific experiment except for the double-blind test of ECT treatment. Although this source of error can hardly explain more than a minor part of the superiority of ECT some attempts have been made with controls receiving "mock" ECT. The six studies in this category (reviewed by BARTON, 1977) were made in the year 1956–1966 and can hardly be replicated in view of ethical objections to withholding effective treatment. Taken together, these studies show the superiority of ECT over simulated ECT with or without antidepressant medication.

2. Prediction of Antidepressive Effect

Several studies show that ECT is more effective in cases of endogenous than reactive (neurotic) depression (ROSE, 1963; CARNEY et al., 1965; MENDELS, 1965; CARNEY and SHEFFIELD, 1974). The diagnoses refer here not only to absence or presence of adequate precipitants and psychogenesis for the depression but to certain features of the depressive syndrome. A good response was associated with the "endogenous features," adequate personality, history of previous episodes of depression or mania, terminal insomnia, morning aggravation, self-denigration, weight loss, retardation, and agitation. Conversely a bad response was associated with inadequately premorbid personality, reactivity, initial insomnia, evening deterioration, and prominent anxiety. NYSTRÖM (1965) showed typing of a depression as endogenous or reactive to be of limited predictive value. Instead he emphasized several prognostic factors, which should be considered irrespective of diagnosis. In addition to the above-mentioned positive indicators for ECT, NYSTRÖM mentions profound depression of mood, duration less than 6 months and previous ECT with good effect. The duration factor is seen from another point of view by KUKOPULOS et al. (1977) who claim that ECT is effective only when given within 6 months of the spontaneous end of the depression. FOLSTEIN et al. (1973) reported that one or more of the features of hopelessness, worthlessness, guilt, and family history of suicide or affective disorder was present more often in improved than in unimproved patients. Finally older patients tend to respond better to ECT than young patients (STRÖMGREN, 1973).

On the whole, the same variables are predictive of positive response to the tricyclic drugs imipramine and amitriptyline (review by BIELSKI and FRIEDEL, 1976). However, there are three important exceptions. Presence of delusions predicts a poor response to imipramine and amitriptyline (and likely to the rest of the antidepressant drugs), whereas the response to ECT is favorable (HORDERN et al., 1963, 1964; CARNEY et al., 1965; MENDELS, 1965; GLASSMAN et al., 1975; SIMPSON et al., 1976). Presence of suicidal ideation predicts a poor tricyclic response (ROBIN and LANGLEY, 1964). Older patients tolerate antidepressants poorly. Since this prevents increase of the doses to effective levels, electroconvulsive therapy may be considered the first choice in such patients.

The division of depressive cases into severe and moderate (Medical Research Council, 1965) elucidates the merits of ECT compared with drugs. The percentage of marked improvement after 4 weeks was as follows:

Table 1. A comparison of improvement rates effected by ECT and drugs (%)

	Severely ill	Moderately ill
ECT	66	77
Imipramine	42	59
Phenelzine	30	30
Placebo	44	37

In the severely ill, to which deluded and suicidal patients belong, imipramine is no better than placebo, whereas in the moderately ill ECT is still most effective and imipramine is superior to placebo.

The prognostic studies mentioned previously may be summarized in the following table:

Table 2. Positive indicators of biologic treatment

Etiology	Cryptogenic (endogenous)
Symptoms	Retardation
	Hypothalamic symptoms
	Loss of appetite
	Loss of weight
	Decreased libido
	Disturbance of menstruation
	Early awakening
Severity	Deep
Course	
macro	Periodic
micro	Diurnal rhythm
	Nonreactivity

The more these requisites are fulfilled the better the prospects for good results. In short, the indications may be summarized in endogenous (or cryptogenic) depression irrespective of type and depression of endogenous type irrespective of cause (endogenomorphic depression according to KLEIN, 1974). Some originally psychogenic depressions display a functional shift and gradually become characterized by features of retardation and hypothalamic disturbance (POLLITT, 1965). In some cases biologic treatment is alone sufficient, but generally it must be followed by other measures directed toward the causes and consequences of the disease.

The positive indicators of ECT can be summarized as severe depressive states, i.e., states with delusions, suicidal risk, stupor, and refusal of food. In such cases ECT should be the first coice, whereas in depression of moderate severity it can be chosen if the response to antidepressant drugs is poor. For older people ECT is usually more efficient and safe and can be offered as first choice also in moderately depressed patients.

3. Combination of ECT and Drugs in Treatment of Depression

Three combinations are possible: drugs given before, together with, or after ECT. Although tricyclics given before ECT would be expected to reduce the number of treatments required, NYSTRÖM (1965) found no significant difference between untreated and pretreated depressives. Neither do tricyclic drugs administered simultaneously with ECT reduce the number of treatments or improve the quality of the response (SEAGER and BIRD, 1962; WILSON et al., 1963; IMLAH et al., 1965). A comparison of ECT + amitriptyline with ECT + diazepam showed a difference in favor of the former combination (KAY et al., 1970), but this is probably explained by the anticonvulsive properties of diazepam which reduce the efficacy of ECT; diazepam possibly also has a depressant effect. ECT + chlorpromazine had, if anything, less effect on cognitive inhibition than ECT + placebo (ARFWIDSSON et al., 1973), other depressive symptoms being improved to a similar degree. Finally ECT + L-tryptophan had only a marginally better effect without practical importance on retardation symptoms when compared with ECT alone (D'ELIA et al., 1977).

Follow-up treatment with tricyclics after ECT has not been studied much, but available evidence indicates a stabilizing effect of imipramine (3×25 mg) up to 6 months (SEAGER and BIRD, 1962; IMLAH et al., 1965). The design of these studies does not permit a definite conclusion on whether or not the beneficial effects were due to the maintenance medication or to this in combination with simultaneous treatment of ECT and drug.

In summary, simultaneous administration of ECT and antidepressant drugs is at best superfluous and may be harmful by inducing a manic state (JOTKOWITZ, 1962; KAY et al., 1970). The antidepressive effect of ECT is so strong that it leaves little scope for further improvement. Maintenance follow-up treatment, however, may reduce the relapse rate. Such strategy felicitously combines the rapid effect of ECT with the long-term effect of drugs.

II. Manic Disorders

Retrospective studies indicate that ECT in manic patients improves discharge conditions and shortens the hospitalization when compared with an untreated, matched control group (McCabe, 1976). Manic conditions are reported to require more frequent and a greater number of treatments extending even to the stage of mental confusion than do depressive disorders (Schiele and Schneider, 1949). Such descriptions indicate that manic conditions were treated with the induction of an organic psychosyndrome, which is avoided in the treatment of depression. The early experience with ECT in mania has hardly any relevance today when the crucial issue is whether ECT has anything to offer in addition to lithium salts and haloperidol. Although no such comparative study has been conducted, it can safely be said that – except for cases not responding to antimanic drugs and threatened by manic exhaustion – manic disorders are rarely an indication for ECT.

III. Schizophrenic Disorders

Contrary to the proven use of ECT in severe depression, ECT is being used less and less in schizophrenic psychosis both in the United States (APA Task Force, 1978) and the Scandinavian countries (Strömgren, 1977b). Chronic schizophrenia has shown no positive effects to the treatment (Miller et al., 1953; Brill et al., 1959; Heath et al., 1964) or less effect than of neuroleptics (Gambill and Wilson, 1966). Acute schizophrenia may show some positive, short-term effects, but the study by Gottlieb and Huston (1951) found no difference from brief psychotherapy after 1–4 years. When compared with a neuroleptic drug and psychotherapy in acute schizophrenics, ECT had a lower release rate (79%) than trifluoperazine alone or with psychotherapy (95%–96%) but higher than with psychotherapy alone (65%) (May et al., 1976a). The follow-up results are difficult to interpret since all groups could have had access to drugs outside the hospital (May et al., 1976b). Other studies show equal effects from chlorpromazine and ECT (Langsley et al., 1959; King, 1960; Childers, 1964). The only argument in support of ECT was the poor compliance of medication (Baker et al., 1958), which should have no actuality when depot preparations are available. Moreover regressive ECT with as many as 26 treatments on an average given twice a day was reported to be somewhat better than unspecified drug therapy (Exner and Murillo, 1973) in a nonrandomized comparison. In agreement with this Kalinowsky and Hippius (1969) emphasized the necessity of long courses of ECT to obtain results in schizophrenic psychoses. A subsequent increase in psychopathology was reported after such intensive therapy (King, 1958), but this did not occur in the Exner and Murillo study.

Thus, little research supports the use of ECT as a primary treatment in schizophrenic psychoses; instead neuroleptic drugs with various sociopsychiatric measures are the treatment of choice (May, 1976). However, when such therapy failed a trial with ECT was sometimes reported successful (Wells, 1973). Patients with depressive or catatonic features in this study did best, but it is doubtful whether cases diagnosed as schizophrenics in Rochester would have been so labeled in Europe, e.g., only a minority of patients had thought disorder in the WELLS study. According to FOLSTEIN et al. (1973), patients with SCHNEIDER's (1959) "first-rank" symptoms are unlikely to improve with ECT in the absence of affective features.

Studies show that ECT in combination with neuroleptic drugs may have advantages over drugs alone (CHILDERS, 1964; SMITH et al., 1967). In the latter study the combined treatment (12 ECT + 400 mg chlorpromazine) resulted in a more rapid amelioration, especially with regard to hostility and ideas of persecution, and earlier release from the hospital. The benefits appeared to outweigh the transient confusion and memory deficit. No difference in global rating and social functioning was ascertained after 6 months or 1 year.

In summary, ECT is no longer an important treatment in schizophrenic psychosis. Cases not responding to an adequate neuroleptic medication but to subsequent ECT are not likely to be diagnosed as schizophrenia according to SCHNEIDER's definition, but rather as depressive or schizoaffective psychosis. Also syndromes with catatonic features and uncertain taxonomic position may improve. However, the value of combining ECT and neuroleptic drugs seems to be well established also in "core" schizophrenia.

This primarily negative evaluation of the use of ECT in schizophrenic psychosis should be qualified since its mechanism of action is unknown. In the absence of support for alternative opinions, it seems difficult to exclude the possibility that ECT in schizophrenic psychosis, as in manic states, has no specific effect as in depressive disorders but acts by inducing an organic psychosyndrome. However, this may form a basis for developing new adaptive patterns. A neurophysiologic-adaptive hypothesis has received experimental support in several studies by FINK and co-workers (FINK, 1974).

IV. Confusional States

Psychogenic (reactive) psychosis of confusional type often shows a dramatic acute phase with strong emotions, deep regression, psychomotor restlessness, delusions, and illusions or hallucinations. Attempts at suicide occur in at least 10% of cases. Due to this and vegetative overarousal ECT was considered necessary in about two-thirds of the cases in a Swedish series (BERGMAN, 1976). One or two treatments were sufficient for the patients' confused states to clear and make them communicable and subsequently responsive to psychotherapy.

Even more dramatic is the picture of delirium acutum (acute lethal catatonia, pernicious catatonia, catatonic excitement state, *akute tödliche Katatonie*). This rare state may occur in the course of psychogenic psychosis as well as in manic-depressive disease and schizophrenia. Such patients may bring themselves to a dangerous point of dehydration and exhaustion unless their symptoms are brought under control with ECT, which in this situation is life-saving. High fever and poor physical condition, common in these cases, should not be regarded as contraindications. Two to three treatments en bloc may be necessary. Although drug treatment usually prevents the development of serious delirium, it may, when such has developed, be less effective and even lead to collapse and death.

Also the periodic mixed confusional-affective states diagnosed as cycloid psychosis respond well to ECT administered in the same number and frequency as in depressions belonging to a unipolar or bipolar affective disease (PERRIS, 1974).

Finally ECT may occasionally be given in delirious states complicating organic illness, the prognosis of which may worsen with the persistence of the delirium (ROBERTS, 1963). Although alcoholic deliria are mainly treated with drugs having cross-tolerance to alcohol, successful treatment with ECT has been described from several quarters (e.g., DUDLEY and WILLIAMS, 1972). Illogical as it may seem, ECT has also been used in psychoses associated with epilepsy. ECT is a possible choice in two of the numerous psychotic manifestations in epilepsy. Mood changes and twilight states may appear as prodromal signs, which terminate in spontaneous convulsions. If a seizure is induced artificially, the prodromal phase may be shortened (KALINOWSKY and HIPPIUS, 1969). If, however, the same symptoms appear as paroxysmal or postparoxysmal manifestations, the administration of ECT does not seem rational. The second indication concerns the mood changes or paranoid and schizophrenialike psychotic states, which alternate with the fits and are associated with normalization of EEG (*Alternativ-Psychose* or *Normalisierungs-Psychose*, see LANDOLT, 1955; TELLENBACH, 1965; JANZ, 1969; cf. SLATER and BEARD, 1963). Since the normalization of EEG is often a consequence of antiepileptic medication the treatment in these cases should first consist of discontinued medication; reappearance of seizures may indicate the end of the psychotic episode. Residual symptoms may respond favorably to ECT if they have been of comparatively short duration and the personality is not too deteriorated.

However, ECT may accentuate the underlying organic disease by producing a cerebral edema, disturbing tenuous local metabolism by increasing the demands during the seizure, or causing neurophysiologic impairment. Therefore, ECT must be used with caution when organic brain disease is suspected (PAULSON, 1967; SMITH and MELLICK, 1975).

The mechanism of the anticonfusional ECT action is not known. Since the patients are often exhausted and intravenous narcosis may be effective in less severe cases, the induced sleep may possibly be the therapeutic factor.

Administration of ECT in bromide poisoning has the effect of removing the psychotic symptoms together with reducing the bromide level in the spinal fluid, perhaps due to increased membrane permeability (ARNESON and OURSO, 1965) that facilitates the elimination of bromide.

H. Complications and Contraindications

I. Complications

Modern ECT in accordance with anesthesiologic principles is a mild treatment, and complications are rare. Fractures and dislocations, common previously, practically never occur. Out of 25,000 treatments given in Sweden in 1975 there was one compression fracture of the spine, four circulatory insufficiencies, six laryngospasms, one status epilepticus, three loosenings of teeth, and one peroneal paresis. No death occurred. The incidence of fatal outcome based on nine large patient series from 1955–1978 in which treatments were given under anesthesia and muscular relaxation varied from 0–9 per 100,000 treatments, averaging 4. General anesthesia shows the same magnitude. Most of the deaths were in cardiac patients, and some occurred so late after treatment that the connection may be questioned (D'ELIA and FREDRIKSEN, 1978).

II. Cardiovascular Effects

A marked increase in blood pressure (systolic levels of 200–250 mm Hg) and pulse rate (up to 150/min) occurs in spite of total muscular relaxation which eliminates the Valsalva effect (PERRIN, 1961). These effects are explained by the intensive autonomic discharge. The venous pressure is practically unchanged. The blood-pressure increase can be eliminated with ganglionic blocking substances, which also obviate the increase of ocular pressure, conceivably important if convulsive treatment is given to patients with glaucoma (OTTOSSON and RENDAHL, 1963). On the whole, the cardiovascular effects in modern convulsive therapy are mild, and this is reflected in the small incidence of complications, even in bad risks.

III. Contraindications

There are few absolute contraindications. Even with anesthesia, total muscular relaxation, and oxygenation an increase of the blood pressure and intracranial pressure could be fatal in certain conditions, and these should not be treated (aneurysm of the aorta and aneurysm of cerebral arteries as manifested by subarachnoid hemorrhages, conditions of increased intracranial pressure). For the rest, the seriousness of the physical illness must be carefully weighed against the seriousness of the mental conditions. For example, a psychotic agitation may represent a strain on a diseased heart, e.g., due to a recent coronary infarct, and the elimination of this strain may be of vital importance. Similarly hypertension is partly caused by the mental condition, and in agitated depression increased blood pressure, instead of being a contraindication, may be seen as an indication for ECT (KALINOWSKY and HIPPIUS, 1969). To this may be added the risk of suicide which is much greater than the risk of fatal outcome with ECT. Pharmacotherapy may represent a choice, but the side effects of psychotropic drugs on the circulatory system are often more uncomfortable and more hazardous than ECT given under controlled conditions, especially in older people.

IV. Influence of Age

The period of the brain's greatest vulnerability for electric convulsive shocks in the rat seems to coincide with its peak of mitotic activity (WASTERLAIN and PLUM, 1973). The first year of life is the only period of active cell division in the postnatal human brain. However, there is evidence that epileptic fits have an adverse influence on cognitive functions also in the postmitotic phase in children. This together with the fact that the main indication for ECT, endogenous depression, is seldom present before the age of 18 has resulted in a very rare use of ECT in child psychiatry. It should be added that ECT in pregnant women has no adverse influence on the fetus (e.g., FORSSMAN, 1955).

However, in old age the opposite conditions prevail. Depression is common and responds particularly well to ECT (STRÖMGREN, 1973). Elderly people have an increased sensitivity to ECT concerning memory disturbance only because they have a lower initial memory function, but they do not suffer a greater impairment after treatment than young people (OTTOSSON, 1970; D'ELIA and RAOTMA, 1976). Since older people often suffer a longer-lasting posttreatment confusion, it is reasonable to prolong the interval between treatments. The confusion is reduced in unilateral treatment (LANCASTER et al., 1958; IMPASTATO and KARLINER, 1966; SUTHERLAND et al., 1968; D'ELIA, 1970).

I. Mechanisms of Action

I. Antidepressive Effect

1. Unrelatedness to Organic Syndrome

CT has been administered to various clinical conditions and has been shown to have a more-or-less positive effect on several of them. However, the antidepressive effect occupies an exceptional position for three reasons:

1) It is better than any other effect of CT (antipsychotic, antimanic, etc.).
2) It is better than any other antidepressive effect (e.g., drugs).
3) It is neither dependent on "organic" signs nor does it belong to an organic psycho-syndrome (confusion, deterioration, memory disturbance). The latter statement is based on experiments in which the antidepressive and organic effects have been dissociated from each other (unilateral ECT, supraliminal stimulation, drug modification of seizure activity (OTTOSSON, 1968)). These experiments have established that the antidepressive effect is related to generalized seizure activity and the organic effect to both seizure activity and direct influences of the current. The unrelatedness of antidepressive to the organic effects is of fundamental importance for the practical application of ECT which aims at optimizing the conditions for obtaining the antidepressive effect in as pure a culture as possible (few, not too frequent treatments, unilateral liminal stimulation, facilitation of seizure activity with oxygen, muscular relaxation, only superficial narcosis, and avoidance of drugs with anticonvulsive properties).

2. Psychologic Theories

An "organic," unspecific mechanism of the antidepressive action may thus be discarded. Similarly since seizure activity is a prerequisite for the antidepressive effect and simulated ECT is not effective, all psychologic theories can be refuted (fear, punishment, shock). Instead it is more fruitful to associate the antidepressive action of ECT with the action of antidepressive and depressiogenic drugs and formulate a hypothesis for all antidepressive treatments based in turn on a hypothesis for endogenous depression.

3. Involvement of Hypothalamus

Several studies converge to reveal the hypothalamus as an essential area in affective disorders and a focus of antidepressant therapies. Affective disorders have been observed in patients with hypothalamic lesions. Patients with endogenous depression develop anorexia, weight loss, decreased libido, menstrual disturbance, sleep disturbance, and diurnal variation, all symptoms indicating involvement of the hypothalamus. The basis of these hypothalamic symptoms has been elucidated by modern neuroendocrinologic research, which has shown disturbances in several hypothalamic neuroendocrine cell systems that regulate the secretion from the pituitary gland, e.g., of ACTH, growth hormone (HGH), and luteinizing hormone (LH) (SACHAR et al., 1976; CARROL et al., 1976a, b; ETTIGE and BROWN, 1977).

ECT administered to a patient under the influence of lidocaine results in seizure activity mainly in the brain stem; the duration of the seizure is directly related to the antidepressive effect (OTTOSSON, 1962). The post-treatment bilaterally synchronous delta activity in EEG which is presumably of diencephalic origin is related to the stability of the antidepressive effect (ROTH, 1951; ROTH et al., 1957). Thus, the antidepressive effect of ECT seems to depend on the seizure activity in the brain stem including the hypothalamus.

4. Amine Hypothesis

From delimiting the antidepressive effect in the hypothalamic area, we now proceed for several reasons to the level of neurons and humoral transmission.
1. The hypothalamus has a high concentration of the biogenic monoamines, noradrenaline and serotonin, serving as transmitters in the central nervous system (VOGT, 1962).
2. The hypothalamic dysfunction in endogenomorphic depression signals a disturbance in monoaminergic activity. For example, the continuous nonstress-related hypersecretion of cortisol, which is a most conspicuous finding in such depression, reflects ACTH hypersecretion, which in its turn reflects increased activity in hypothalamic neuroendocrine cells secreting corticotropin-releasing hormone. Evidence points to this resulting from disinhibition secondary to reduced noradrenergic activity. A noradrenergic deficit may also explain low levels of HGH and LH (SACHAR et al., 1976; GARVER et al., 1976).
3. The effects of antidepressive and depressiogenic drugs on monoaminergic systems have been well established.
4. The evidence for deviations in the levels of biogenic amines and their precursors and metabolites in affective disorders (critical review by BALDESSARINI, 1975) although it is at present rather equivocal. This evidence forms the basis

for the amine hypotheses of affective disorders (SCHILDKRAUT, 1965; COPPEN, 1967; LAPIN and OXENKRUG, 1969; CARLSSON, 1970; KETY, 1971).

Does the action of ECT agree with these hypotheses? Indirect evidence is obtained from a clinical observation: the hypothalamic symptoms represent a positive indicator of a good response to ECT and often improve early during treatment. Examination of the effect of ECT on amine metabolism and neuroendocrinologic function (OTTOSSON, 1978) is complicated by the difficulty of determining which effects are essential causal links in the antidepressive action, which are consequences of that action, and which are merely coincidental. Most of the short-term effects of ECT are likely to be coincidental consequences of the seizure. The long-term effects are more likely to be essential, but they may be consequences of the recovery from the depression. Animal experiments and clinical research should be combined to elucidate the cause-effect issue.

a) Animal Experiments. The biologic effects of electroconvulsive shocks can be isolated in animal experiments from the affective changes. Recent research has focused on cumulative and sustained effects, which are the obvious criteria if parallelling the antidepressive effect. The main results are both increase of the synthesis of noradrenaline and increase of the sensitivity of amine receptors (MODIGH, 1975, 1976; EVANS et al., 1976; GREEN et al., 1976).

b) Clinical Research. The results in animal experiments become relevant for the antidepressive action of ECT if the same functions are low in depressive disorders and normalize after recovery. A low synthesis rate of noradrenaline was shown by POST and GOODWIN (1975), but it remained low on recovery. Moreover evidence of a neuroendocrinologic dysfunction indicates indirectly a noradrenergic deficit, which partly normalizes on recovery. A failure to normalize may imply a relation to vulnerability to depressive illness rather than to manifest illness and need not contradict the relevance of these biologic changes. Low rates of the synthesis of dopamine and serotonin seem to characterize some depressive disorders (ASHCROFT et al., 1966; ÅSBERG et al., 1976; SJÖSTRÖM and ROOS, 1972; POST and GOODWIN, 1975), but they have no consistent counterpart in sustained ECT effects.

A low-sensitivity depression may be an alternative mechanism to low-output depression (Medical Research Council, 1972). The argument for this concept is at present mostly indirect since affective mood-swings have been difficult to derive from variations in the release of indole- or catecholamines as reflected by their metabolites in the urine or cerebrospinal fluid (BUNNEY et al., 1977). A clinical counterpart to the increase in receptor sensitivity in animals is the beneficial effect of ECT in Parkinson's disease, both on extrapyramidal and depressive symptoms (LEBENSOHN and JENKINS, 1975; ASNIS, 1977). As yet no increased, sustained neuroendocrinologic responses after ECT, which would signal increased receptor sensitivity, have been reported.

In summary, convincing evidence is lacking both for pre- and postsynaptic conditions in monoaminergic systems in depression and for the sustained effects of ECT. However, whereas current antidepressant drugs act by increasing the availability of transmitter to the receptor, ECT mainly acts by increasing receptor sensitivity (GRAHAME-SMITH et al., 1978). ECT seems to create conditions for counteracting both low-output and low-sensitivity depression. For instance, since it may relieve a depression due either to low output of serotonin or low sensitivity of serotonin receptors (if such depression exists) by increasing the sensitivity of these receptors, it represents a broad spectrum therapy for depression. This may explain the higher recovery rates in comparison with the more specifically acting antidepressive drugs.

5. Permeability Hypothesis

Although the amine hypothesis has received the most experimental support, two more hypotheses will be briefly considered. AIRD (1958) suggested on the basis of experiments with cocaine that increased permeability of the blood-brain barrier is a relevant mechanism in CT. The argument was strengthened by ANGEL and ROBERTS (1966), who showed increased permeability to cocaine after ECS as well as imipramine, amitriptyline, and nortriptyline, but not after chlorpromazine. Moreover ROSENBLATT et al. (1960) have shown that electroshock altered the permeability to noradrenaline, thereby making possible a combination of the permeability and monoamine hypotheses. However, in ECT combined with relaxation and oxygenation the permeability increased only minimally (BOLWIG et al., 1977c, d), as was the case during hypercapnia. The change of the cerebral blood flow, therefore, and not the epileptic activity appears responsible for the changes in permeability. Since hypercapnia has no definite antidepressive action these experiments seem to refute the belief that increased permeability of the blood-brain barrier is an antidepressive mechanism, at least without combination with seizure activity.

6. Electrolyte Hypothesis

There is some evidence of change in electrolyte and water distribution in depressive states. The research of GIBBONS (1960) and COPPEN (1960) shows increased intracellular sodium and water which normalize in the recovered, but not in the unrecovered patients. The improvement and increase of the extracellular fluid volume correlate with each other presumably due to a shift from intracellular spaces, both with ECT and imipramine treatment (BROWN et al., 1963). ECT has no definite acute effect (RUSSELL, 1960). At the present time it is not possible to decide whether the redistribution of fluid and electrolytes is a cause or a consequence of the antidepressive effect.

II. Antipsychotic and Antimanic Effects

Similar specific hypotheses for the antipsychotic and antimanic effects have not been formulated. In terms of receptor function all antipsychotic drugs block dopamine receptors, whereas ECT increases their sensitivity, therefore acting in the opposite way. Schizophrenic psychoses require a long series of treatments, which seldom cause remissions comparable to the ECT effect in depression but instead leave confusion and flattening of affect (provided that the disorder is not schizoaffective which responds to ECT as do depressive disorders). Also manic disorders often require frequent treatments and leave behind temporary organic signs. Both the antipsychotic and antimanic effects may, therefore, at least partly belong to an unspecific organic syndrome. However, this need not exclude a positive interaction with environmental factors, creating conditions for new adaptive patterns. Several studies by FINK and co-workers (FINK, 1974) have supported a "neurophysiologic-adaptive" hypothesis.

III. Anticonfusional Effect

The anticonfusional effect also has an unknown mechanism of action. Psychogenic confusion often needs only one or two treatments. Sleep may be the therapeutic factor since such confusions also clear up if sleep can be induced. In confusions due to bromide poisoning ECT probably acts by increasing membrane permeability, which accelerates the elimination of bromide (ARNESON and OURSO, 1965).

IV. Amnestic Mechanism of Action

Contrary to the antidepressive action in which the hypothalamus is involved the ECT effect on storage of memory material engages the mamillary bodies, fornix, hippocampus, and adjacent parts of the cingular cortex (the limbic forebrain circuit of Papez, BARBIZET, 1963). The relative importance of current and seizure has been discussed previously (see Sect. C III, p. 318–319). The neurochemical basis for the amnestic effects is probably involved with protein synthesis. Since the animal experiments in this area have been performed without oxygenation and relaxation, their significance for clinical ECT is uncertain. DUNN et al. (1974) have reported a decreased incorporation of leucine into protein as a direct result of the current. Good correlation is found between this effect and retrograde amnesia. ESSMAN (1968, 1974) has shown that serotonin in the brain is increased after a single electroshock, that serotonin injection into the brain produces amnesia, and that blocking the ECS-induced increase of serotonin with amitriptyline or nialamide antagonizes the amnestic effect. This parallels a recent observation by D'ELIA et al. (1978 b) that the combination of tryptophan and ECT produces more extensive amnesia than ECT alone and raises the possibility of also the amnestic effect being mediated by a biogenic amine.

References

A practising psychiatrist: The experience of electro-convulsive therapy. Br. J. Psychiatry **111**, 365–367 (1965)

Abrams, R.: Multiple ECT: What have we learned? In: Psychiobiology of convulsive therapy. Fink, M., Kety, S., McGaugh, J., Williams, T.A. (eds.), pp. 79–84. New York: John Wiley 1974

Aird, R.B.: Clinical correlates of electroshock therapy. Arch. Neurol. Psychiatry **79**, 633–639 (1958)

American Psychiatric Association (APA): Task force on ECT report. 1978

Angel, C., Roberts, A.J.: Effect of electroshock and antidepressant drugs on cerebrovascular permeability to cocaine in the rat. J. Nerv. Ment. Dis. **142**, 376–380 (1966)

Aperia, B., Rönnberg, E., Wetterberg, L.: Elektrokonvulsiv terapi. Utvecklingen under senaste decenniet i ABC-län (The frequency of ECT in three Swedish counties). Läkartidn. **73**, 4600–4602 (1976)

Arfwidsson, L., Arn, L., Beskow, J., D'Elia, G., Laurell, B., Ottosson, J.-O., Perris, C., Persson, G., Wistedt, B.: Chlorpromazine and the anti-depressive efficacy of electroconvulsive therapy. Acta Psychiatr. Scand. **49**, 580–587 (1973)

Arneson, G.A., Ourso, R.: Bromide intoxication and electroshock therapy. Am. J. Psychiatry **121**, 1115–1116 (1965)

Åsberg, M., Thorén, P., Träskman, L., Bertilsson, L., Ringberger, V.: "Serotonin depression" – a biochemical subgroup within the affective disorders? Science **191**, 478–480 (1976)

Ashcroft, G.W., Crawford, T.B.B., Eccleston, D., Sharman, D.F., MacDougall, E.J., Stanton, J.B., Binns, J.K.: Hydroxyindole compounds in cerebrospinal fluid of patients with psychiatric or neurological diseases. Lancet **1966/II**, 1049–1052

Asnis, G.: Parkinson's disease, depression, and ECT. A review and case study. Am. J. Psychiatry **134**, 191–195 (1977)

Avery, D., Winokur, G.: Mortality in depressed patients treated with electroconvulsive therapy and antidepressants. Arch. Gen. Psychiatry **33**, 1029–1037 (1976)

Baker, A.A., Game, J.A., Thorpe, J.G.: Physical treatment for schizophrenia. J. Ment. Sci. **104**, 860–864 (1958)

Baldessarini, R.J.: The basis for amine hypotheses in affective disorders. Arch. Gen. Psychiatry **32**, 1087–1093 (1975)

Barbizet, J.: Defect of memorizing of hippocampal-mammillary origin: a review. J. Neurol. Neurosurg. Psychiatry **26**, 127–135 (1963)

Barton, J.L.: ECT in depression: the evidence of controlled studies. Biol. Psychiatr. **12**, 687–695 (1977)

Barton, J.L., Mehta, S., Snaith, R.P.: The prophylactic value of extra ECT in depressive illness. Acta Psychiatr. Scand. **49**, 386–392 (1973)

Beresford, H.R., Posner, J.B., Plum, F.: Changes in brain lactate during induced cerebral seizures. Arch. Neurol. **20**, 243–248 (1969)

Bergman, W.: Om psykogena psykoser av konfusionstyp. En efterundersökning av 143 patienter (Psychogenic confusion of confusional type. A follow-up of 143 patients). M.D. Thesis, University of Stockholm 1976

Bielski, R.J., Friedel, R.O.: Prediction of tricyclic antidepressant response. A critical review. Arch. Gen. Psychiatry **33**, 1479–1489 (1976)

Berlyne, N., Strachan, M.: Neuropsychiatric sequelae of attempted hanging. Br. J. Psychiatry **114**, 411–422 (1968)

Blachly, P.H., Denney, D.D.: Sources of variability in electroconvulsive data. Convulsive Ther. Bull. **1**, 35–36 (1976)

Blachly, P.H., Gowing, D.: Multiple monitored electroconvulsive treatment. Compr. Psychiatry **7**, 100–109 (1966)

Bolwig, T.G., Astrup, J., Christoffersen, G.R.J.: EEG and extracellular K^+ in rat brain during pentylenetetrazol seizures and during respiratory arrest. Biomedicine **27**, 99–102 (1977a)

Bolwig, T.G., Hertz, M.M., Westergaard, E.: Acute hypertension causing blood-brain barrier breakdown during epileptic seizures. Acta Neurol. Scand. **56**, 335–342 (1977b)

Bolwig, T.G., Hertz, M.M., Paulson, O.B., Spotoft, H., Rafaelsen, O.J.: The permeability of the blood-brain barrier during electrically induced seizures in man. Eur. J. Clin. Invest. **7**, 87–93 (1977c)

Bolwig, T.G., Hertz, M.M., Holm-Jensen, J.: The permeability of the blood-brain barrier during electroshock seizures in the rat. Eur. J. Clin. Invest. **7**, 95–100 (1977d)

Bond, E.D.: Results of treatment in psychoses – with a control series. II. Involutional psychotic reaction. Am. J. Psychiatry **110**, 881–883 (1954)

Bond, E.D., Morris, H.H.: Results of treatment in psychoses – with a control series. III. Manic-depressive reactions. Am. J. Psychiatry **110**, 883–885 (1954)

Brill, N.D., Crumpton, E., Eiduson, S., Grayson, H.M., Hellman, I.I., Richards, R.A.: Relative effectiveness of various components of electro-convulsive therapy. Arch. Neurol. Psychiatry **81**, 627–635 (1959)

Brodersen, P., Paulson, O.B., Bolwig, T.G., Rogon, Z.E., Rafaelsen, O.J., Lassen, N.A.: Cerebral hyperemia in electrically induced epileptic seizures. Arch. Neurol. **28**, 334–338 (1973)

Brown, D.G., Hullin, R.P., Roberts, J.M.: Fluid distribution and the response of depression to E.C.T. and imipramine. Br. J. Psychiatry **109**, 395–398 (1963)

Bunney, W.E., jr., Post, R.M., Andersen, A.E., Kopanda, R.T.: A neuronal receptor sensitivity mechanism in affective illness (a review of evidence). Commun. Psychopharmacol. **1**, 393–405 (1977)
Carlsson, A.: Effects of drugs on amine uptake mechanisms in the brain. In: New aspects of storage and release mechanisms of catecholamines. Schümann, Hj., Kroneberg, S. (eds.), pp. 223–233. Heidelberg: Springer 1970
Carney, M.W.P., Sheffield, B.F.: The effects of pulse ECT in neurotic and endogenous depression. Br. J. Psychiatry **125**, 91–94 (1974)
Carney, M.W.P., Roth, M., Garside, R.F.: The diagnosis of depressive syndromes and the prediction of ECT response. Br. J. Psychiatry **111**, 659–674 (1965)
Carroll, B.J., Curtis, G.C., Mendels, J.: Neuroendocrine regulation in depression. I. Limbic system-adrenocortical dysfunction. Arch. Gen. Psychiatry **33**, 1039–1044 (1976)
Carroll, B.J., Curtis, G.C., Mendels, J.: Neuroendocrine regulation in depression. II. Discrimination of depressed from nondepressed patients. Arch. Gen. Psychiatry **33**, 1051–1058 (1976)
Childers, R.T.: Comparison of four regimens in newly admitted female schizophrenics. Am. J. Psychiatry **120**, 1010–1011 (1964)
Clare, A.: Psychiatry in dissent. London: Tavistock 1976
Coppen, A.: Abnormality of the blood-cerebrospinal-fluid barrier of patients suffering from a depressive illness. J. Neurol. Neurosurg. Psychiatry **23**, 156–161 (1960)
Coppen, A.: The biochemistry of affective disorders. Br. J. Psychiatry **113**, 1237–1264 (1967)
Cronholm, B., Blomquist, C.: Memory disturbances after electroconvulsive therapy. 2. Conditions one week after a series of treatments. Acta Psychiatr. Scand. **34**, 18–25 (1959)
Cronholm, B., Molander, L.: Memory disturbances after electroconvulsive therapy. 4. Influence of an interpolated electroconvulsive shock on retention of memory material. Acta Psychiatr. Scand. **36**, 83–90 (1961)
Cronholm, B., Molander, L.: Memory disturbances after electroconvulsive therapy. 5. Conditions one month after a series of treatments. Acta Psychiatr. Scand. **40**, 212–216 (1964)
Cronholm, B., Ottosson, J.O.: Experimental studies of the therapeutic action of electroconvulsive therapy in endogenous depression. Acta Psychiatr. Scand. **35** [Suppl. 145], 69–101 (1960)
Cronholm, B., Ottosson, J.O.: Memory functions in endogenous depression. Before and after electroconvulsive therapy. Arch. Gen. Psychiatry **5**, 193–199 (1961)
Cronholm, B., Ottosson, J.O.: The experience of memory function after electroconvulsive therapy. Br. J. Psychiatry **109**, 251–258 (1963a)
Cronholm, B., Ottosson, J.O.: Ultrabrief stimulus technique in electroconvulsive therapy. I. Influence on retrograde amnesia of treatments with the Elther ES electroshock apparatus, Siemens Konvulsator III and of lidocaine-modified treatment. J. Nerv. Ment. Dis. **137**, 117–123 (1963b)
Cronholm, B., Ottosson, J.O.: Ultrabrief stimulus technique in electroconvulsive therapy. II. Comparative studies of therapeutic effects and memory disturbance in treatment of endogenous depression with the Elther ES electroshock apparatus and Siemens Konvulsator III. J. Nerv. Ment. Dis. **137**, 268–276 (1963c)
Cronholm, B., Ottosson, J.O., Schalling, D.: The memory variables learning and retention in relation to intelligence and age in adults. Acta Psychiatr. Scand. **46** [Suppl. 219], 50–58 (1970)
Davies, R.K., Detre, T.P., Egger, M.D., Tucker, G.J., Wyman, R.J.: Electroconvulsive therapy instruments. Should they be reevaluated? Arch. Gen. Psychiatry **25**, 97–99 (1971)
D'Elia, G. (ed.): Unilateral electroconvulsive therapy. Acta Psychiatr. Scand. [Suppl. 215] (1970)
D'Elia, G.: Memory changes after unilateral electroconvulsive therapy with different electrode positions. Cortex **12**, 280–289 (1976)
D'Elia, G., Fredriksen, S.-O.: Elektrokonvulsiv terapi i Sverige. I. Behandlingsmetodik. (ECT in Sweden. I. Method of treatment.) Nord. Psykiat. Tidsskr. **32**, 534–542 (1978)
D'Elia, G., Fredriksen, S.-O.: Elektrokonvulsiv terapi i Sverige. III Utveckling 1966–1975 (ECT in Sweden. III. Development 1966–1975.) Nord. Psykiat. Tidsskr. **33**, 3–8 (1979)
D'Elia, G., Raotma, H.: Is unilateral ECT less effective than bilateral ECT? Br. J. Psychiatry **126**, 83–89 (1975)
D'Elia, G., Raotma, H.: Memory impairment after convulsive therapy. Influence of age and number of treatments. Arch. Psychiatr. Nervenkr. **223**, 219–226 (1977)

D'Elia, G., Lorentzson, S., Raotma, H., Widepalm, K.: Comparison of unilateral dominant and non-dominant ECT on verbal and non-verbal memory. Acta Psychiatr. Scand. **53**, 85–94 (1976)

D'Elia, G., Lehmann, J., Raotma, H.: Evaluation of the combination of tryptophan and ECT in the treatment of depression. Acta Psychiatr. Scand. **56**, 303–318 (1977)

D'Elia, G., Lehmann, J., Raotma, H.: Influence of tryptophan on memory functions in depressive patients treated with unilateral ECT. Acta Psychiatr. Scand. **57**, 259–268 (1978)

Dornbush, R., Williams, M.: Memory and ECT. In: Psychobiology of convulsive therapy. Fink, M., Kety, S., McGaugh, J., Williams, T.A. (eds.), pp. 199–207. New York: John Wiley 1974

Dudley, W.H.C., jr., Williams, J.G.: Electroconvulsive therapy in delirium tremens. Compr. Psychiatry **13**, 357–360 (1972)

Dunn, A., Giuditta, A., Wilson, J.E., Glassman, E.: The effect of electro-shock on brain RNA and protein synthesis and its possible relationship to behavioral effects. In: Psychobiology of convulsive therapy. Fink, M., Kety, S., McGaugh, J., Williams, T.A. (eds.), pp. 185–197. New York: John Wiley 1974

Edén, S., Modigh, K.: Effects of apomorphine and clonidine on rat plasma growth hormone after pretreatment with reserpine and electroconvulsive shocks. Brain Res. **129**, 379–384 (1977)

Essman, W.B.: Electroshock-induced retrograde amnesia and brain serotonin metabolism: Effects of several antidepressant compounds. Psychopharmacology **13**, 258–266 (1968)

Essman, W.B.: Effects of electroconvulsive shock on cerebral protein synthesis. In: Psychobiology of convulsive therapy. Fink, M., Kety, S., McGaugh, J., Williams, T.A. (eds.), pp. 237–249. New York: John Wiley 1974

Ettigi, P.G., Brown, G.M.: Psychoneuroendocrinology of affective disorder: An overview. Am. J. Psychiatry **134**, 493–501 (1977)

Evans, J.P.M., Grahame-Smith, D.G., Green, A.R., Tordoff, A.F.C.: Electroconvulsive shock increases the behavioural responses of rats to brain 5-hydroxytryptamine accumulation and central nervous system stimulant drugs. Br. J. Pharmacol. **56**, 193–199 (1976)

Exner, J.E., jr., Murillo, L.G.: Effectiveness of regressive ECT with process schizophrenia. Dis. Nerv. Syst. **34**, 44–48 (1973)

Fink, M.: Induced seizures and human behavior. In: Psychobiology of convulsive therapy. Fink, M., Kety, S., McGaugh, J., Williams, T.A. (eds.). New York: John Wiley 1974

Finner, R.W.: Duration of convulsion in electric shock therapy. J. Nerv. Ment. Dis. **119**, 530–537 (1954)

Fishbein, I.L.: Involutional melancholia and convulsive therapy. Am. J. Psychiatry **106**, 128–135 (1949)

Flåtten, Ö.: Bör elektrosjokkbehandlingen revalueres? (Should ECT be reevaluated?) Tidskr. norsk. lægefor. **95**, 1201–1206 (1975)

Folstein, M., Folstein, S., McHugh, P.R.: Clinical predictors of improvement after electroconvulsive therapy of patients with schizophrenia, neurotic reactions, and affective disorders. Biol. Psychiatr. **7**, 147–152 (1973)

Forssman, H.: Follow-up study of 16 children whose mothers were given electric convulsive therapy during gestation. Acta Psychiatr. Scand. **30**, 437–441 (1955)

Gambill, J.M., Wilson, I.C.: Activation of chronic withdrawn schizophrenics. Dis. Nerv. Syst. **27**, 615–617 (1966)

Garcia, J.: NIMH Conference on ECT: Efficacy and Impact. New Orleans, 1978

Garver, D.L., Pandey, G.N., Dekirmenjian, H., Davis, J.M.: Growth hormone responsiveness to hypoglycemia and urinary MHPG in affective disease patients: Preliminary observations. In: Hormones, behavior, and psychopathology. Sachar, E.J. (ed.), pp. 233–235. New York: Raven Press 1976

Gibbons, J.L.: Total body sodium and potassium in depressive illness. Clin. Sci. **19**, 133–138 (1960)

Glassman, A.H., Kantor, S.J., Shostak, M.: Depression, delusions, and drug response. Am. J. Psychiatry **132**, 716–719 (1975)

Gottlieb, J.S., Huston, P.E.: Treatment of schizophrenia. A comparison of three methods, brief psychotherapy, insulin coma, and electric shock. J. Nerv. Ment. Dis. **113**, 237–246 (1951)

Grahame-Smith, D.G., Green, A.R., Costain, D.W.: Mechanism of the antidepressant action of electroconvulsive therapy. Lancet **1978/I**, 254–257

Green, A.R., Heal, D.J., Grahame-Smith, D.G.: Further observations on the effect of repeated electroconvulsive shock on the behavioural responses of rats produced by increases in the functional activity of brain 5-HT and dopamine. Psychopharmacology **52**, 195–200 (1977)

Greenblatt, M., Grosser, G.H., Wechsler, H.: Differential response of hospitalized depressed patients to somatic therapy. Am. J. Psychiatry **120**, 935–943 (1964)

Hartelius, H.: Cerebral changes following electrically induced convulsions. An experimental study on cats. Acta Psychiatr. Scand. [Suppl. 77] (1952)

Hayes, K.J.: The current path in electric convulsion shock. Arch. Neurol. Psychiatr. **63**, 102–109 (1950)

Heath, E.S., Adams, A., Wakeling, P.L.G.: Short courses of ECT and simulated ECT in chronic schizophrenia. Br. J. Psychiatr. **110**, 800–807 (1964)

Holmberg, G.: The factor of hypoxemia in electroshock therapy. Am. J. Psychiatry **110**, 115–118 (1953)

Holmberg, G.: Effect on electrically induced convulsions of the number of previous treatments in a series. Arch. Neurol. Psychiatr. **71**, 619–623 (1954)

Holmberg, G.: Biological aspects of electroconvulsive therapy. Int. Rev. Neurobiol. **5**, 389–412 (1963)

Holmberg, G., Thesleff, S.: Succinyl-choline-iodide as a muscular relaxant in electroshock therapy. Am. J. Psychiatry **108**, 842–846 (1952)

Holmberg, G., Hård, G., Ramqvist, N.: Experiments in the prolongation of convulsions induced by electric shock treatment. Acta Psychiatr. Scand. **31**, 61–70 (1956)

Holmdahl, M., jr.: Apnoeic diffusion oxygenation in electroconvulsion therapy. Ups. J. Med. Sci. **58**, 269–280 (1953)

Holt, W.L., jr., Borkowski, W.: Drug-modified electric shock therapy. Clinical response to partial seizures facilitated by the anticonvulsant drugs diphenylhydantoin and mephenesin, alone and in combination. Psychiatr. Quart. **25**, 581–588 (1951)

Hordern, A., Holt, N.F., Burt, C.G., Gordon, W.F.: Amitriptyline in depressive states: phenomenology and prognostic considerations. Br. J. Psychiatry **109**, 815–825 (1963)

Hordern, A., Burt, C.G., Gordon, W.F., Holt, N.F.: Amitriptyline in depressive states: six month treatment results. Br. J. Psychiatry **110**, 641–647 (1964)

Huston, P.E., Locher, L.M.: Involutional psychosis. Course when untreated and when treated with electric shock. Arch. Neurol. Psychiatry **59**, 385–394 (1948a)

Huston, P.E., Locher, L.M.: Involutional psychosis. Course when untreated and when treated with electric shock. Arch. Neurol. Psychiatry **60**, 37–48 (1948b)

Imlah, N.W., Ryan, E., Harrington, J.A.: The influence of antidepressant drugs on the response to electroconvulsive therapy and on subsequent relapse rates. J. Neuropsychopharmacol. **4**, 438–442 (1965)

Impastato, D.J., Karliner, W.: Control of memory impairment in EST by unilateral stimulation of the non-dominant hemisphere. Dis. Nerv. Syst. **27**, 182–188 (1966)

Inglis, J.: Shock, surgery and cerebral asymmetry. Br. J. Psychiatry **117**, 143–148 (1970)

Janis, I.L.: Psychologic effects of electric convulsive treatments. J. Nerv. Ment. Dis. **111**, 359–382 (1950)

Janz, D.: Die Epilepsien. Spezielle Pathologie und Therapie. Stuttgart: Thieme 1969

Jotkowitz, M.W.: Manic reactions following combined "Tofranil" (imipramine) and electroconvulsive therapy. Med. J. Aust. **49**, 87–90 (1962)

Kalinowsky, L.B., Hippius, H.: Pharmacological, convulsive and other somatic treatments in psychiatry. New York, London: Grune & Stratton 1969

Kalinowsky, L.B., Barrera, S.E., Horwitz, W.A.: The "petit mal" response in electric shock therapy. Am. J. Psychiatry **98**, 708–711 (1942)

Kay, D.W.K., Fahy, T., Garside, R.F.: A seven-month double-blind trial of amitriptyline and diazepam in ECT-treated depressed patients. Br. J. Psychiatry **117**, 667–671 (1970)

Kety, S.S.: Brain amines and affective disorders: an overview. In: Brain chemistry and mental disease. Ho, B.T., McIsaac, W.M. (eds.). New York: Plenum Press 1971

Kiloh, L.G., Child, J.P., Latner, G.: A controlled trial of iproniazid in the treatment of endogenous depression. J. Ment. Sci. **106**, 1139–1144 (1960a)

Kiloh, L.G., Child, J.P., Latner, G.: Endogenous depression treated with iproniazid – a follow-up study. J. Ment. Sci. **106**, 1425–1428 (1960b)

King, P.D.: Regressive EST, chlorpromazine, and group therapy in treatment of hospitalized chronic schizophrenics. Am. J. Psychiatry **115**, 354–357 (1958)

King, P.D.: Chlorpromazine and electroconvulsive therapy in the treatment of newly hospitalized schizophrenics. J. Clin. Exp. Psychopathol. **21**, 101–105 (1960)

Kirstein, L., Ottosson, J.-O.: Experimental studies of electroencephalographic changes following electroconvulsive therapy. Acta Psychiatr. Scand. **35** [Suppl. 145], 49–67 (1960)

Klein, D.F.: Endogenomorphic depression. Arch. Gen. Psychiatry **31**, 447–454 (1974)

Kragh-Sörensen, P., Eggert-Hansen, C., Baastrup, P.C., Hvidberg, E.F.: Self-inhibiting action of nortriptyline's antidepressive effect at high plasma levels. Psychopharmacologia **45**, 305–312 (1976)

Kukopulos, A., Reginaldi, D., Tondo, L., Bernabei, A., Caliari, B.: Spontaneous length of depression and response to ECT. Psychol. Med. **7**, 625–629 (1977)

Lancaster, N., Steinert, R., Frost, I.: Unilateral electroconvulsive therapy. J. Ment. Sci. **104**, 221–227 (1958)

Landolt, H.: Über Verstimmungen, Dämmerzustände und schizophrene Zustandsbilder bei Epilepsie. Schweiz. Arch. Neurol. Psychiatr. **76**, 313–321 (1955)

Langsley, D.G., Enterline, J.D., Hickerson, G.: A comparison of chlorpromazine and EST in the treatment of acute schizophrenic and manic reactions. Arch. Neurol. Psychiatry **8**, 384–391 (1959)

Lapin, I.P., Oxenkrug, G.F.: Intensification of the central serotoninergic processes as a possible determinant of the thymoleptic effect. Lancet **1969/I**, 132–136

Laurell, B. (ed.): Flurothyl convulsive therapy. Acta Psychiatr. Scand. [Suppl. 213] (1970)

Lebensohn, Z.M., Jenkins, R.B.: Improvement of parkinsonism in depressed patients treated with ECT. Am. J. Psychiatry **132**, 283–285 (1975)

Liberson, W.T.: Current evaluation of electric convulsive therapy. Correlation of the parameters of electric current with physiologic and psychologic changes. Res. Publ. Assoc. Res. Nerv. Ment. Dis. **31**, 199–231 (1953)

Liberson, W.T., Cadilhac, J.G.: Electroshock and rhinencephalic seizure states. Confin. Neurol. **13**, 278–286 (1953)

Lorenzo, A.V., Hedley-Whyte, E.T., Eisenberg, H.M., Hsu, D.S.: Increased penetration of horseradish peroxidase across the blood brain barrier induced by Metrazol seizures. Brain Res. **88**, 136–140 (1975)

Lovett Doust, J.W., Raschka, L.B.: Enduring effects of modified ECT on the cerebral circulation in man. Psychiatr. Clin. **8**, 293–303 (1975)

Matakas, F., Cervós-Navarro, J., Roggendorf, W., Christmann, U., Sasaki, S.: Spastic constriction of cerebral vessels after electric convulsive treatment. Arch. Psychiatr. Nervenkr. **224**, 1–9 (1977)

Maxwell, R.D.H.: Electrical factors in electroconvulsive therapy. Acta Psychiatr. Scand. **44**, 436–448 (1968)

May, P.R.A.: When, what, and why? Psychopharmacotherapy and other treatments in schizophrenia. Compr. Psychiatry **17**, 683–693 (1976)

May, P.R.A., Tuma, A.H., Dixon, W.J.: Schizophenia – a follow-up study of results of treatment. I. Design and other problems. Arch. Gen. Psychiatry **33**, 474–478 (1976a)

May, P.R.A., Tuma, A.H., Yale, C., Potepan, P., Dixon, W.J.: Schizophrenia – a follow-up study of results of treatment. II. Hospital stay over two to five years. Arch. Gen. Psychiatry **33**, 481–486 (1976b)

McCabe, M.S.: ECT in the treatment of mania: a controlled study. Am. J. Psychiatry **133**, 688–691 (1976)

McKenna, G., Engle, R.P., jr., Brooks, H., Dalen, J.: Cardiac arrhythmias during electroshock therapy: significance, prevention, and treatment. Am. J. Psychiatry **127**, 530–533 (1970)

Medical Research Council: Clinical trial of the treatment of depressive illness. Br. Med. J. **1965/I**, 881–886

Medical Research Council Brain Metabolism Unit: Modified aminehypothesis for the aetiology of affective illness. Lancet **1972/II**, 573–577

Meldrum, B.S., Brierly, J.B.: Prolonged epileptic seizures in primates. Ischemic cell change and its relation to ictal physiological events. Arch. Neurol. **28**, 10–17 (1973a)

Meldrum, B.S., Vigouroux, R.A., Brierly, J.B.: Systemic factors and epileptic brain damage. Prolonged seizures in paralyzed, artificially ventilated baboons. Arch. Neurol. **29**, 82–87 (1973b)

Mendels, J.: Electroconvulsive therapy and depression. II. Significance of endogenous and reactive syndromes. Br. J. Psychiatry **111**, 682–686 (1965)

Miller, D.H., Clancy, J., Cumming, E.: A comparison between unidirectional current nonconvulsive electrical stimulation given with Reiter's machine, standard AC electroshock and pentothal in chronic schizophrenia. Am. J. Psychiatry **109**, 617–620 (1953)

Modigh, K.: Electroconvulsive shock and postsynaptic catecholamine effects: Increased psychomotor stimulant action of apomorphine and clonidine in reserpine pretreated mice by repeated ECS. J. Neural Transm. **36**, 19–32 (1975)

Modigh, K.: Long-term effects of electroconvulsive shock therapy on synthesis turnover and uptake of brain monoamines. Psychopharmacologia **49**, 179–185 (1976)

Nyström, S.: On relation between clinical factors and efficacy of ECT in depression. Acta Psychiatr. Scand. **40** [Suppl. 181] (1965)

Ottosson, J.O. (ed.): Experimental studies of the mode of action of electroconvulsive therapy. Acta Psychiatr. Scand. [Suppl. 145] (1960)

Ottosson, J.O.: Seizure characteristics and therapeutic efficiency in electroconvulsive therapy: An analysis of the antidepressive efficiency of grand mal and lidocaine-modified seizures. J. Nerv. Ment. Dis. **135**, 239–251 (1962)

Ottosson, J.O.: Memory disturbance after ECT; a major or minor side effect? Excerpta Med. Int. Congr. Ser. Psychosom. Med. **134**, 161–168 (1968)

Ottosson, J.O.: Influence of age on memory impairment after electroconvulsive therapy. Acta Psychiatr. Scand. [Suppl. 219], 154–165 (1970)

Ottosson, J.O.: Systemic biochemical effects of ECT. In: Psychobiology of convulsive therapy. Fink, M., Kety, S., McGaugh, J., Williams, T.A. (eds.), pp. 209–219. New York: Wiley 1974

Ottosson, J.O.: Mechanisms of action of convulsive therapy. Current status of concepts. NIMH Symposium on ECT: Efficacy and Impact. New Orleans 1978

Ottosson, J.O., Rendahl, I.: Effect of trimethaphan on intraocular pressure in electroconvulsive therapy. Arch. Ophthalmol. **70**, 466–470 (1963)

Paulson, G.W.: Exacerbation of organic brain disease by electroconvulsive treatment. NC Med. J. **28**, 328–331 (1967)

Perrin, G.M.: Cardiovascular aspects of electric shock therapy. Acta Psychiatr. Scand. **36** [Suppl. 152] (1961)

Perris, C.: A study of cycloid psychoses. Acta Psychiatr. Scand. [Suppl. 253] (1974)

Plum, F., Howse, D.C., Duffy, T.E.: Metabolic effects of seizures. In: Brain dysfunction in metabolic disorders. Plum, F. (ed.). Res. Publ. Assoc. Res. Nerv. Ment. Dis. **53**, 141–157 (1974)

Plum, F., Posner, J.P., Troy, B.: Cerebral metabolic and circulatory responses to induced convulsions in animals. Arch. Neurol. **18**, 1–13 (1968)

Pollitt, J.D.: Suggestions for a physiological classification of depression. Br. J. Psychiatry **111**, 489–495 (1965)

Posner, J.B., Plum, F., Van Poznak, A.: Cerebral metabolism during electrically induced seizures in man. Arch. Neurol. **20**, 388–395 (1969)

Post, R.M., Goodwin, F.K.: Studies on cerebrospinal fluid amine metabolites in depressed patients: conceptual problems and theoretical implications. In: The psychobiology of depression. Mendels, J. (ed.). New York: Spectrum 1975

Quandt, J., Sommer, H.: Zur Frage der Hirngewebsschädigungen nach elektrischer Krampfbehandlung. Eine tierexperimentelle Studie. Fortschr. Neurol. Psychiatr. **34**, 513–548 (1966)

Roberts, A.H.: The value of E.C.T. in delirium. Br. J. Psychiatry **109**, 653–655 (1963)

Robin, A.A., Langley, G.E.: A controlled trial of imipramine. Br. J. Psychiatry **110**, 419–422 (1964)

Rose, J.T.: Reactive and endogenous depressions – response to ECT. Br. J. Psychiatry **109**, 213–217 (1963)

Rosenblatt, S., Chanley, J.D., Sobotka, H., Kaufman, M.R.: Interrelationships between electroshock, the blood-brain barrier, and catecholamines. J. Neurochem. **5**, 172–176 (1960)

Roth, M.: Changes in the EEG under barbiturate anaesthesia produced by electro-convulsive treatment and their significance for the theory of ECT action. Electroencephalogr. Clin. Neurophysiol. **3**, 261–280 (1951)

Roth, M., Kay, D.W.K., Shaw, J., Green, J.: Prognosis and pentothal induced electroencephalographic changes in electro-convulsive treatment. Electroencephalogr. Clin. Neurophysiol. **9**, 225–237 (1957)

Russell, G.F.M.: Body weight and balance of water, sodium and potassium in depressed patients given electroconvulsive therapy. Clin. Sci. **19**, 327–336 (1960)

Sachar, E.J., Roffwarg, H.P., Gruen, P.H., Altman, N., Sassin, J.: Neuroendocrine studies of depressive illness. Pharmakopsychiatr. Neuropsychopharmacol. **9**, 11–17 (1976)

Schiele, B.C., Schneider, R.A.: The selective use of electroconvulsive therapy in manic patients. Dis. Nerv. Syst. **10**, 291–297 (1949)

Schildkraut, J.J.: The catecholamine hypothesis of affective disorders. A review of supporting evidence. Am. J. Psychiatry **122**, 509–522 (1965)

Schneider, K.: Clinical psychopathology. New York: Grune & Stratton 1959

Seager, C.P., Bird, R.L.: Imipramine with electrical treatment in depression. A controlled trial. J. Ment. Sci. **108**, 704–707 (1962)

Simpson, G.M., Lee, J.H., Cuculic, Z., Kellner, R.: Two dosages of imipramine in hospitalized endogenous and neurotic depressives. Arch. Gen. Psychiatry **33**, 1093–1102 (1976)

Sjöström, R., Roos, B.-E.: 5-Hydroxyindoleacetic acid and homovanillic acid in cerebrospinal fluid in manic-depressive psychosis. Eur. J. Clin. Pharmacol. **4**, 170–176 (1972)

Slater, E., Beard, A.W.: The schizophrenia-like psychoses of epilepsy. I. Psychiatric aspects. Br. J. Psychiatry **109**, 95–150 (1963)

Small, J.G.: EEG and neurophysiological studies of convulsive therapies. In: Psychobiology of convulsive therapy. Fink, M., Kety, S., McGaugh, J., Williams, T.A. (eds.), pp. 47–63. New York: Wiley 1974

Smith, J.S., Mellick, R.S.: Neuropsychiatric relapse following acute carbon monoxide poisoning – the contribution of electroconvulsive therapy. Med. J. Aust. **1**, 465–468 (1975)

Smitt, J.W., Wegener, C.F.: On electric convulsive therapy with particular regard to a parietal application of electrodes, controlled by intracerebral voltage measurements. Acta Psychiatr. Scand. **19**, 529–549 (1944)

Smith, K., Surphlis, W.R.P., Gynther, M.D., Shimkunas, A.M.: ECT-chlorpromazine and chlorpromazine compared in the treatment of schizophrenia. J. Nerv. Ment. Dis. **144**, 284–290 (1967)

Squire, L.R., Chase, P.M.: Memory functions six to nine months after electroconvulsive therapy. Arch. Gen. Psychiatry **32**, 1557–1564 (1975)

Squire, L.R., Miller, P.L.: Diminution of anterograde amnesia following electroconvulsive therapy. Br. J. Psychiatry **125**, 490–495 (1974)

Squire, L.R., Slater, P.C.: Forgetting in very long-term memory as assessed by an improved questionnaire technique. J. Exp. Psychol. [Hum. Learn.] **104**, 50–54 (1975)

Squire, L.R., Slater, P.C., Chase, P.M.: Retrograde amnesia: temporal gradient in very long-term memory following electroconvulsive therapy. Science **187**, 77–79 (1975)

Strömgren, L.S.: Unilateral versus bilateral electroconvulsive therapy. Investigations into the therapeutic effect in endogenous depression. Acta Psychiatr. Scand. [Suppl. 240] (1973)

Strömgren, L.S.: Therapeutic results in brief-interval unilateral ECT. Acta Psychiatr. Scand. **52**, 246–255 (1975)

Strömgren, L.S.: The influence of depression on memory. Acta Psychiatr. Scand. **56**, 109–128 (1977a)

Strömgren, L.S.: 4th World Congress of Psychiatry: Convulsive Therapy after 50 years. Honolulu 1977b

Strömgren, L.S., Juul-Jensen, P.: EEG in unilateral and bilateral electroconvulsive therapy. Acta Psychiatr. Scand. **51**, 340–360 (1975)

Sutherland, E.M., Oliver, J.E., Knight, D.R.: E.E.G., memory and confusion in dominant, non-dominant and bi-temporal E.C.T. Br. J. Psychiatry **115**, 1059–1064 (1969)

Tellenbach, H.: Epilepsie als Anfallsleiden und als Psychose. Über alternative Psychosen paranoider Prägung bei „forcierter Normalisierung" (Landolt) des Elektroencephalogramms Epileptischer. Nervenarzt **36**, 190–202 (1965)

Templer, D.J., Ruff, C.F., Armstrong, G.: Cognitive functioning and degree of psychosis in schizophrenics given many electroconvulsive treatments. Br. J. Psychiatry **123**, 441–443 (1973)

Thomas, D.L.L.: Prognosis of treatment with electrical treatment. Br. Med. J. **1954/II**, 950–1954

Valentine, M., Keddie, K.M.G., Dunne, D.: A comparison of techniques in electro-convulsive therapy. Br. J. Psychiatry **114**, 989–996 (1968)

Vogt, M.: The function of some pharmacologically active brain constituents. In: Aspects of psychiatric research. Richter, D., Tanner, J.M., Taylor, L., Zangwill, O.L. (eds.), pp. 343–364. London: Oxford University Press 1962

Volavka, J., Feldstein, S., Abrams, R., Dornbush, R., Fink, M.: EEG and clinical change after bilateral and unilateral electroconvulsive therapy. Electroencephalogr. Clin. Neurophysiol. **32**, 631–639 (1972)

Wasterlain, C.G., Plum, F.: Vulnerability of developing rat brain to electroconvulsive seizures. Arch. Neurol. **29**, 38–45 (1973)

Weaver, L.A., jr., Ives, J.O., Williams, R., Nies, A.: A comparison of standard alternating current and low-energy brief-pulse electrotherapy. Biol. Psychiatry **12**, 525–543 (1977)

Weaver, L., Ravaris, C., Rush, S., Paananen, R.: Stimulus parameters in electroconvulsive shock. J. Psychiatr. Res. **10**, 271–281 (1974)

Weaver, L., Williams, R., Rush, S.: Current density in bilateral and unilateral ECT. Biol. Psychiatry **11**, 303–312 (1976)

Wells, D.A.: Electroconvulsive treatment for schizophrenia. A ten-year survey in a university hospital psychiatric department. Compr. Psychiatry **14**, 291–298 (1973)

Wilson, I.C., Vernon, J.T., Guin, T., Sandifer, M.G.: A controlled study of treatments of depression. J. Neuropsychiatry **4**, 331–337 (1963)

Woodruff, R.A., jr., Pitts, F.N., jr., McClure, J.N., jr.: The drug modification of ECT. I. Methohexital, thiopental and preoxygenation. Arch. Gen. Psychiatry **18**, 605–611 (1968)

Ziskind, E., Somerfeld-Ziskind, E., Ziskind, L.: Metrazol and electroconvulsive therapy of the affective psychoses. Arch. Neurol. Psychiatry **53**, 212–217 (1945)

Psychosurgery

By

L. Laitinen

Contents

A. History 351
B. New Psychosurgery 357
   I. Surgical Approaches 359
      1. Cingulotomy 359
      2. Anterior Capsulotomy 363
      3. Kelly's and Richardson's Limbic Leukotomy 364
      4. Innominotomy 366
      5. Mesoloviotomy 367
      6. Posteromedial Hypothalamotomy 369
      7. Ventromedial Hypothalamotomy 370
      8. Thalamotomy 371
      9. Amygdalotomy 372
   II. Ethical Aspects of Psychosurgery 373
C. Recommendations for Selection of Psychosurgical Approach 374
References 374

A. History

The Swiss psychiatrist GOTTLIEB BURCKHARDT can be regarded as the father of psychosurgery. In 1891 he published in the *Allgemeine Zeitschrift für Psychiatrie* an essay entitled "Ueber Rindenexcisionen, als Beitrag zur operativen Therapie der Psychosen." He believed that specific psychotic symptoms could be eliminated by removal of the appropriate cortical area. For example, auditory hallucinations might be pacified by a lesion of the auditory temporoparietal cortex. He carried out such operations on six schizophrenics, all of whom were reported to have somewhat improved. The author defended his daring handling by declaring that he had never had as his guiding principle "primum est non nocere" but "melium anceps remedium quam nullam." His object was not to cure the patient but to change a dangerous personality into a harmless one. BURCKHARDT'S colleagues protested against his operations so much that he had to stop them, and his pioneer work was soon forgotten.

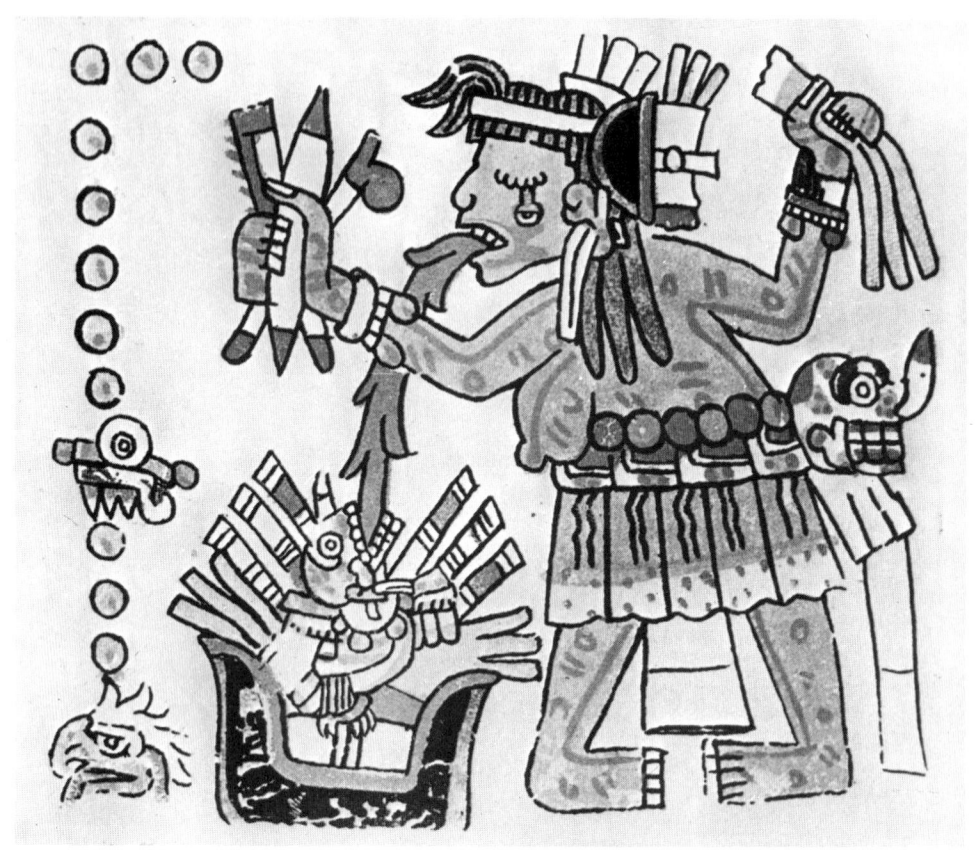

Fig. 1. Psychosurgery has long traditions. In pre-Columbian Mexico, the goddess Cihuateotl premedicates her young patient with a drug from her own mouth. The surgical instruments needed for trepanation are in her hand (Biblioteca Apostolica Vaticana)

In 1910 the great Estonian neurosurgeon Ludwig Puusepp, who at that time worked in St. Petersburg, carried out limited frontoparietal incisions on three psychiatric patients. The results were so poor that he did not publish them until 1937, 1 year after the Portuguese neurologist Egas Moniz had written his monograph on lobotomy.

It is difficult to assess the roles of Burckhardt and Puusepp in the later development of psychosurgery. Puusepp had worked for years with Bechterew and Pavlov and knew much about the anatomy and physiology of the frontolimbic brain. However, the true impetus that led to the creation of modern psychosurgery was to come from the United States.

In the early 1930s a broad interest in the localization of psychic functions and disorders in the brain began to develop. Psychiatrists, neurologists, and neuropathologists had become aware that tumors and vascular lesions of the frontal lobes often altered the patients' behavior. Neurophysiologists began to carry out animal experiments, mainly in primates, which more than other animals resemble man. The Yale University with JOHN FULTON as the leader of a research team became famous for their experiments. FULTON and JACOBSEN made bilateral ablations of the orbitofrontal cortex on trained chimpanzees. A normal chimpanzee when frustrated by a wrong choice in a discrimination task usually throws a temper tantrum; it kicks and screams like an angry child. Two chimpanzees, Becky and Lucy, lost this type of frustrational behavior completely after bilateral frontal ablations. If there still were moments of temper when the animal was repeatedly frustrated, they were short-lived, and after a few seconds the chimpanzee would forget most of what had happened. Overtrained normal chimpanzees easily develop an experimental neurosis, similar to that of PAVLOV's dogs, but Becky and Lucy showed neurotic behavior extremely seldom after the frontal ablations.

At the Second International Congress of Neurology in the summer of 1935 in London, FULTON and JACOBSEN (see FULTON 1952) presented a paper on these experiments. Another important paper on the topic of frontal lobes was read by BRICKNER (1936) who in great detail described the behavior of a patient whose frontal lobes had been removed and who, although less restrained, less inhibited, and less capable of complex synthesis, had little intellectual impairment. Among the participants at the congress was also EGAS MONIZ of Lisbon. He had already studied mental symptoms associated with the tumors of the frontal lobes and together with his neurosurgical colleague, Dr. ALMEIDA LIMA, he had considered the possibility of carrying out frontal ablations in agitated psychiatric patients. After listening to the paper of FULTON and JACOBSEN, MONIZ raised the question of whether a similar intervention that had been carried out on Becky and Lucy might relieve the anxiety and tension of certain psychiatric patients. FULTON became alarmed, he wrote later (1952), and stressed that the idea of bilateral frontal ablation was too hazardous a procedure in the human being. But MONIZ had evidently already made up his mind, and a few months later on 12 November 1935 the first frontal lobotomy was performed in Lisbon. In the first patients alcohol was injected into the frontal lobes. ALMEIDA LIMA soon designed a leukotome, a special instrument with a steel wire loop at the tip of a probe. By rotating the probe the protruding loop cut spherical pieces of frontal white matter (Fig. 2).

In 1936 MONIZ published his monograph *Tentatives opératoires dans le traitement de certaines psychoses* with the first results obtained in 20 agitated and depressed schizophrenic patients. Seven were reported to have recovered from their illness and another seven improved. In 1949 EGAS MONIZ shared with HESS the Nobel Prize in Physiology and Medicine. Dr. VIETS (1949) wrote in an editorial; "The 1949 Nobel Prize in Medicine":

The Nobel Prize for 1949 in medicine has been awarded... Dr. Egas Moniz, a former professor of neurology in the University of Lisbon (who)... devised the revolutionary brain operation of prefrontal leucotomy, later known as lobotomy, now widely used in the treatment of certain forms of mental disease. In the last thirteen years, since his report in 1936, thousands of such operations, now modified into various patterns, have been carried out in many parts of the world, greatly to the betterment of patients with the more serious and prolonged types of mental aberration. A new psychiatry may be said to have been born in 1935, when Moniz took his first bold step in the field of psychosurgery.

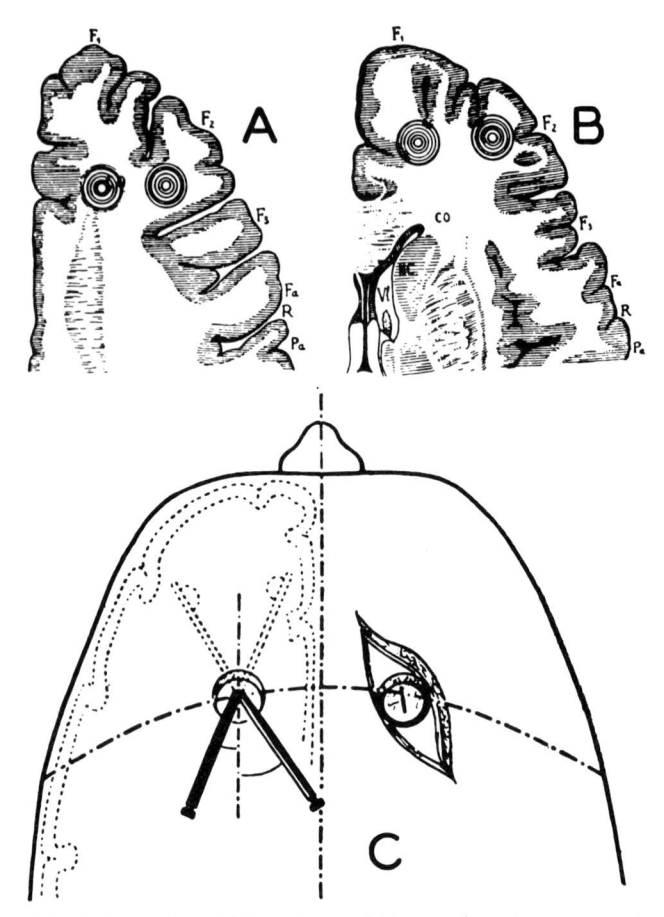

Fig. 2 A–C. Moniz technique of frontal leukotomy. *A* the location of the uppercuts; *B* location of the lower cuts; *C* the placement of the burr holes and leukotome

Frontal lobotomy soon became an important neurosurgical procedure, and VALENSTEIN (1973) has estimated that the number of lobotomized patients in the United States alone rose to a total of 40,000. An important factor leading to such a vast upsurge was the great number of American soldiers whose mental health had seriously suffered from World War II. According to VALENSTEIN, the Veterans Administration had directly encouraged American surgeons and psychiatrists to use lobotomy in these cases, because the new therapy was generally considered effective. Two neurosurgeons, WALTER FREEMAN and JAMES WATTS, developed the lobotomy technique further and operated on a large number of patients. By the end of 1950 the total number of their lobotomy patients had reached 1,000, and FREEMAN's total number of operations exceeded 3,500 patients.

Frontal lobotomy became one of the most common neurosurgical procedures. Apart from neurosurgeons, it was sometimes also practiced by general surgeons and psychiatrists. A notorious form of mass therapy could take place: many psychiatric hospitals had installed small, rather simple surgical theaters where a near-by or distant neurosurgeon operated, often during his weekend holiday, on many patients whom he had not met personally. A well-known English surgeon was said to fly to Malta, where during 1 hour in the afternoon he lobotomized four patients and then flew back to London. No wonder that lobotomy was often sharply criticized. *Medical Record* wrote in an editorial, "The Lobotomy Delusion" (1940):

> Of recent years, a type of meddlesome surgery, originally instituted in Spain, has been introduced into this country, frontal lobotomy by name. Lobotomy for frontal lobe malignant tumor we can understand, but by this extended lobotomy, one is supposed to be able to "pluck from the brain a hidden sorrow". It is claimed it can ameliorate or cure people suffering from obsessional and compulsion neuroses, and even bring restitution to the more cyclical and obstinate disorder – manic-depressive depression... The disorders mentioned for which there is claim of value are disorders of the entire personality, i.e., of the entire body, mental apparatus and all, and we recommend these aspirants for neurosurgical honors to read and digest Karl Menninger's remarks on polysurgical castration devices, not those of strictly phallic significance but those that maim and destroy the creative functions of a non-mutilated body.
>
> In the name of Madame Roland who cried aloud concerning the many crimes committed in the cause of "liberty" we would call the attention of these mutilating surgeons to the Hippocratic oath.

There is no reason to deny that many patients were operated on to pacify the ward. The neurosurgeon often had little chance to examine his patient preoperatively. Even the postoperative care was not seldom poor, which evidently led to an increased rate of surgical morbidity and mortality.

Surgical complications were not infrequent, not even in those series published from university departments. The mortality rate was about 2%. Postoperative epilepsy occurred in 10%, and emotional blunting was often recorded. These patients showed signs of tactlessness, emotional lability, euphoric traits, tendencies to outbursts, loss of memory, etc.

Lobotomy was, on the other hand, often a strikingly beneficial procedure. In a long-term follow-up study on 10,000 leukotomized patients, TOOTH and NEWTON (1961) showed that 47% of the patients with previously intractable mental disorders had been able to be discharged from the hospital. In 1948 The Connecticut Lobotomy Committee reported that in a series of 200 patients, 25% had been markedly improved and 90%, at least slightly. Anxiety and depression had been abolished in 75% of the patients.

In the late 1940s several neurosurgeons and psychiatrists began to seek specific surgical target areas in the frontal lobes, where lesions would result in beneficial effects without the above-mentioned side effects. Already in 1937 PAPEZ had asked himself: "Is emotion a magic product or is it a physiological process which depends on an anatomic mechanism?" He considered it such an important function that its mechanism, whatever it was, should be placed on a structural basis. He proposed that "the hypothalamus, the anterior thalamic nuclei, the gyrus cinguli, the hippocampus and their interconnections constitute a harmonious mechanism which may elaborate the functions of central emotion, as well as participate in emotional expression." In 1952 FULTON suggested that surgical interventions should be limited to the limbic brain, particularly to the cingulum and that, before the production of permanent lesions, physiologic functions of the target area should be studied by application of local anesthetics and electrical stimulation. A particular clinical report had possibly initiated this idea. In 1948 RYLANDER published a case report of a lobotomy patient who was obsessed with the idea that she had sinned against the Holy Ghost. RYLANDER and neurosurgeon OLOF SJÖQUIST noticed that the obsession persisted after a radical cut on one side, and it continued as cuts were gradually made on the opposite side until finally when the surgeon reached the fibers of the medial ventral quadrant, the patient's obsession suddenly disappeared. When she was asked about her sin against the Holy Ghost, she answered euphorically: "Oh, I don't believe in the Holy Ghost anymore." The patient's obsessions and psychotic behavior were reported to have disappeard completely and permanently.

There was also some indirect experimental evidence that some fibers in the cingulum might be associated with emotional and autonomic functions. SMITH (1945) had electrically stimulated the cingulum of monkeys and obtained vegetative reactions, such as dilatation of the pupils and changes in the heart rate. Surgical lesions in the area of stimulation made the animals tame and easy to handle. In 1948 WARD destroyed the anterior part of the cingulum in monkeys and observed that the animals, in addition to having become tame, also seemed to have become less neurotic than before surgery.

GRANTHAM (1951) was presumably the first neurosurgeon who aimed at placing small lesions in the cingulum. In 1951 he reported that his patients did not tend to suffer intellectual deficits afterward and that most of them exhibited marked therapeutic benefit. He had introduced thin probes into the area of the rostral cingulum and the knee of the corpus callosum and used electrocoagulation for lesion production.

Additional information about the beneficial lesion sites in the frontal brain was obtained from the comprehensive autopsy study of MEYER and BECK (1954). They made a clinico-pathologic association examination between the leukotomy lesion demonstrated at autopsy and the clinical state, pointing out that damage to the superior and lateral parts of the frontal lobes resulted in adverse effects of lobotomy. Success in the operation seemed to be related to the ventromedial quadrants of the thalamofrontal fibers.

Toward the end of the 1940s neurosurgeons were rather convinced that the psychosurgical lesions should be directed and restricted to certain strategic regions in the deep ventromedial frontal lobe. This led to the development of human stereotactic surgery (SPIEGEL et al., 1947; LEKSELL, 1949; TALAIRACH et al., 1949; RIECHERT and WOLFF, 1951; UCHIMURA and NARABAYASHI, 1951). Soon after the new stereotactic technique had become available for psychosurgeons, the rapid development in psychopharmacology seemed to relegate psychosurgery to the past. In the late 1950s it was practiced in only a very few places. LEKSELL (see HERNER, 1961) developed a stereotactic technique for making restricted lesions by thermocoagulation in the anterior branch of the internal capsule. KNIGHT (1964) placed radioactive yttrium-90 rods into the orbitofrontal white matter, which he called substantia innominata. His approach was a stereotactic modification of the orbitofrontal undercutting operation of SCOVILLE

(1949). Both LEKSELL and KNIGHT obtained good clinical results in many patients with intractable mental disorders. Side effects were shown to be clearly less frequent than after open lobotomies.

B. New Psychosurgery

In the mid 1960s it became clear that neither the new psychopharmaceutics nor the modern forms of psychotherapy had fulfilled the expectations. Although they gave relief to many patients and often prevented the disease from becoming chronic, the final result of treatment was sometimes poor. Some obsessive-compulsive states, certain forms of juvenile schizophrenia, anxiety states, recurrent depressions, and chronic pain states with addiction and/or depression often responded poorly to psychiatric treatment.

Some neurosurgeons, for example, SCOVILLE (1960) and DOWLING (see BAILEY et al., 1971), began to carry out open orbital undercutting operations and cingulate tractotomies, respectively. But the true impetus for development of the new psychosurgery came from stereotactic neurosurgery. The advantages of the stereotactic technique over open surgical approaches were numerous: the former could be performed easily under local anesthesia, enabling the psychosurgical team to administer physiologic and psychologic tests to the patient during the procedure. The stereotactic intervention was not particularly stressing, and the risk of hemorrhage was much lower than during open surgery. The stereotactic lesions could be placed and restricted to any subcortical area without much risk of cortical damage. These factors also contributed to a decreased surgical morbidity and mortality after stereotactic interventions.

For accurate determination of the surgical target areas, neuroradiologic assistance was necessary. Lumbar air encephalography or air ventriculography were often sufficient for good visualization of the cerebral ventricles and cortical sulci, but in some cases, for example, when the cingulum or the corpus callosum were the targets, carotid arteriography was used for accurate determination of the sulci of the cingulum and corpus callosum (Fig. 3). From stereotactic atlases (SCHALTENBRAND and BAILEY, 1959; TALAIRACH et al., 1957) it was possible to determine any desired brain area in relation to certain landmarks, as the anterior and posterior commissures and the midline of the third ventricle, which could be made visible in lateral and anteroposterior radiograms, respectively.

Electrophysiology affords valuable aid in accurately determining deep cerebral structures. With depth-EEG recording it is often possible to define the borderline of two neighboring regions. For example, the spontaneous electrical activity of the orbitofrontal cortex differs clearly from that of the adjacent white matter of the subcaudate region (substantia innominata). The regular callosal activity of low amplitude differs also from the irregular and often high-voltage activity of the neighboring cingulum. Recording the evoked responses to electrical stimulation of deep structures may also help the surgeon to determine the exact anatomic site of the stimulation target (Fig. 4).

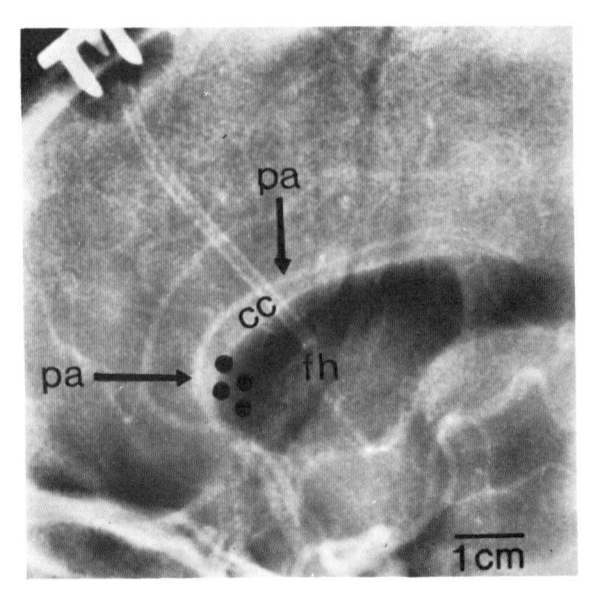

Fig. 3. Carotid arteriogram and air ventriculogram to show the site of the genu of the corpus callosum (*cc*). *pa*, pericallosal artery; *fh*, frontal horn. *Black dots* indicate the areas where 60-Hz stimulation caused a sensation of wellbeing and relaxation

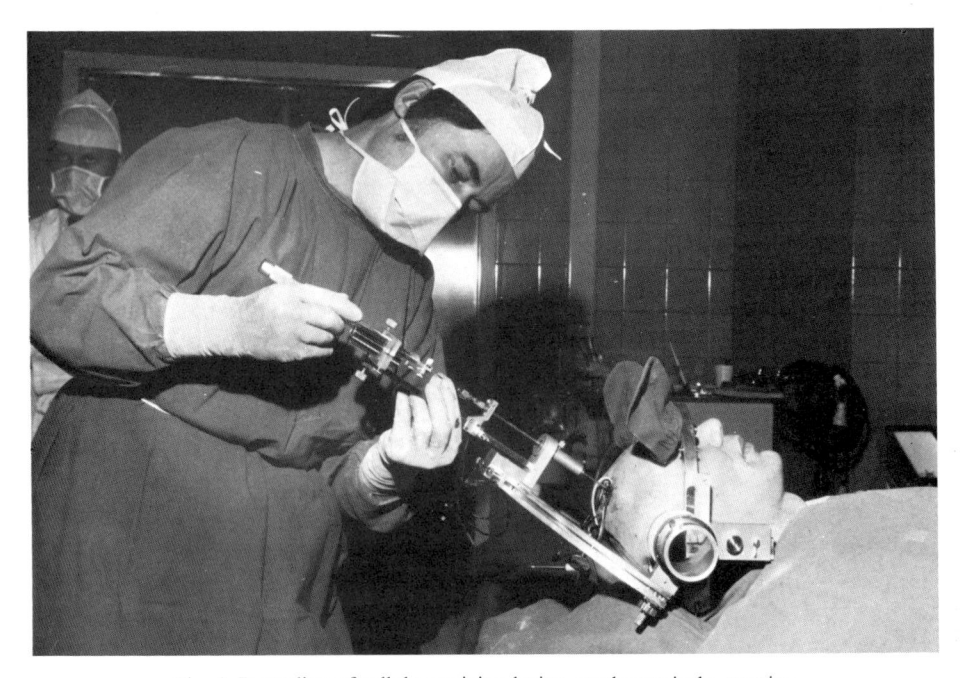

Fig. 4. Recording of cellular activity during psychosurgical operation

Brain lesions can be produced with electrocoagulation, cryothermia, ultrasound, mechanical leukotome, chemical agents, or irradiation.

Repeated electrical stimulation of some subcortical areas through chronically implanted probes, instead of destructive lesions, has been used recently by DELGADO et al. (1973). It is possible that this technique may eventually completely replace the destructive lesions.

One of the great advantages of the stereotactic technique over open surgery is that psychologic tests can be carried out during surgery (FEDIO and OMMAYA, 1970; KUKKA et al., 1976). The patients are only slightly sedated and cooperate with the examiner. Psychologic tasks are given the patient during ongoing electrical stimulation and during fake stimulation. It is important that neither the patient nor the examining psychologist know when true stimulation is being applied. The current intensity is just below the threshold for subjective sensation. The order of true and fake stimulations is randomized. The described technique affords valuable and reliable information about the functions of the limbic system.

I. Surgical Approaches

Today a large numer of specific stereotactic approaches are available for treating a patient with certain symptoms. The most commonly used methods are cingulotomy, anterior capsulotomy, innominotomy (subcaudate region), orbital undercutting, mesoloviotomy (knee of the corpus callosum), ventromedial tractotomy, intralaminar thalamotomy, amygdalotomy, and ventromedial and posteromedial hypothalamotomy (Fig. 5). Some investigators have combined at one session two approaches: ventromedial tractotomy and cingulotomy (KELLY and MITCHELL-HEGGS, 1973) or even three approaches: cingulotomy, innominotomy, and amygdalotomy (BROWN, 1973).

Selection of the surgical approach may be based on the symptomatology of the patient, but some psychosurgical teams operate on all patients in the same target. At present there is little objective evidence of the specificity of different approaches, although some recent clinical studies suggest that the surgical approach should be chosen according to the patient's symptoms (KULLBERG, 1977; TEUBER et al., 1977).

Since the open surgical approaches are becoming more and more unusual in the treatment of psychiatric illness I shall describe here only stereotactic methods and their results.

1. Cingulotomy

A large number of clinical studies have shown the importance of the cingulum for emotional disorders. In 1962 FOLTZ and WHITE reported on a series of 16 patients who had undergone cingulotomy for intractable pain. Five were classified as having "psychogenic" pain, and all of them showed at least "good" results. Five had organic diseases with paroxysmal pains precipitated by emotion, and two of them showed an exceedingly striking result. Six patients with malignancies and strong emotional factors showed at least

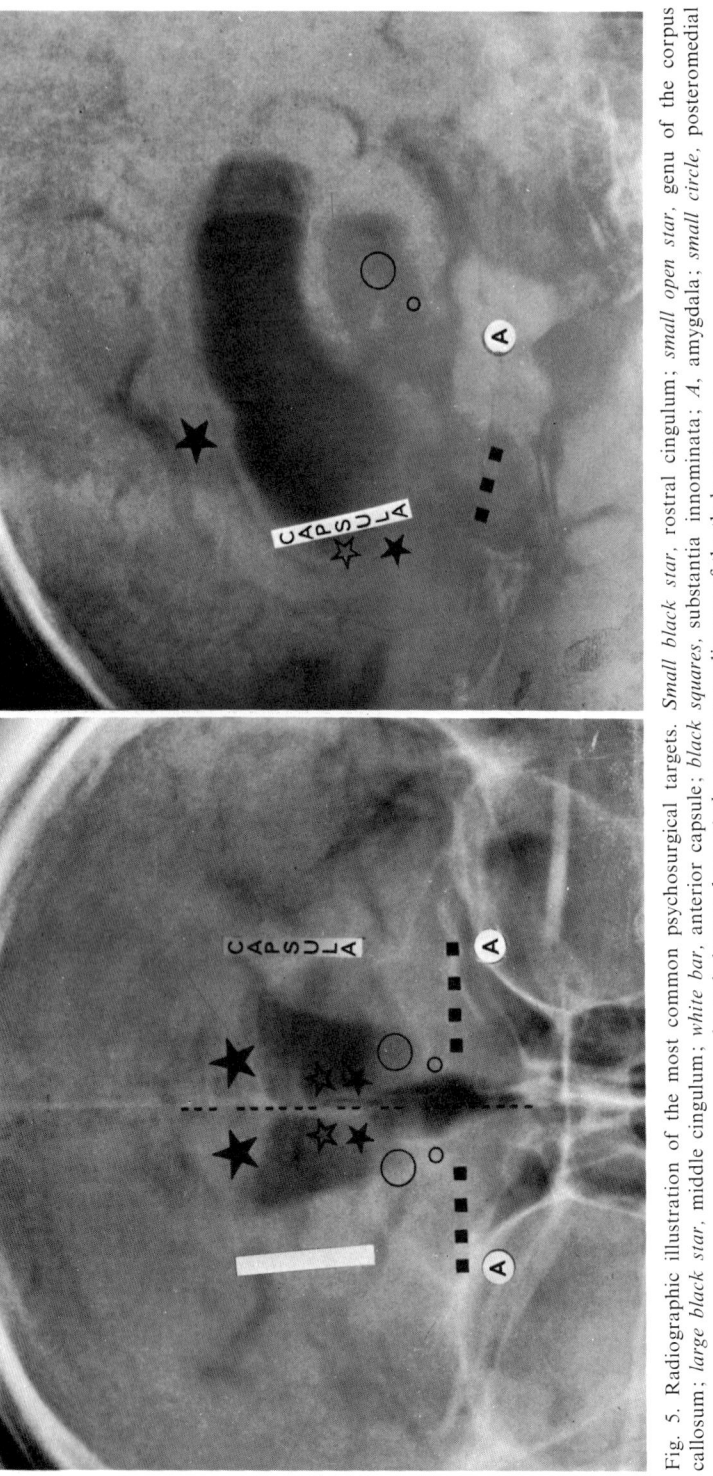

Fig. 5. Radiographic illustration of the most common psychosurgical targets. *Small black star*, rostral cingulum; *small open star*, genu of the corpus callosum; *large black star*, middle cingulum; *white bar*, anterior capsule; *black squares*, substantia innominata; *A*, amygdala; *small circle*, posteromedial hypothalamus; *large circle*, centrum medianum of the thalamus

"good" results. In 14 addicted patients an abrupt withdrawal of the drugs after operation resulted in slight withdrawal symptoms in five, but no symptoms were noticed in the remaining nine patients.

In 1972 BALASUBRAMANIAM et al. reported on 30 patients with drug addiction, who had undergone stereotactic cingulotomy. In 26 of them the operation resulted in the complete relief of addiction. In four the effect was transitory. No adverse effects were observed. The authors also studied the possible placebo effect of surgery in three patients, who only had burr holes, but had been told that cingulotomy had been carried out. None of them showed any improvement of addiction until a true cingulotomy had been performed.

In 1967 BALLANTINE et al. reported on a series of 69 patients who had undergone 95 operations in the cingulum. The stereotactic lesions were placed at a cingulate target 3–4 cm behind the tip of the frontal horn. In 75% of the patients, at least some improvement was observed after surgery. The best results were obtained in patients with manic-depressive illness (its phase was not stated): 77% of these patients (20 of 26 patients) showed a significant improvement. Equal results were obtained in their ten schizophrenic patients, seven of whom were clearly improved. In BALLANTINE's series neither the patients, their relatives, nor their psychiatrists had observed serious physical or psychologic complications of surgery. Two patients who had had a previous history of convulsions, had one postoperative seizure each, and one without previous history of epilepsy, had two convulsions in the postoperative follow-up period. Two patients with intractable pain were confused for 2–5 postoperative days, but both made a good recovery.

Five years later BALLANTINE et al. (1972) concluded that to be effective frontal cingulotomy must completely interrupt the cingulate bundle at a distance of 2–4 cm behind the tip of the frontal horns bilaterally. Even though minor parts of the corpus callosum or some supracingulate mediofrontal fibers had occasionally been damaged, in addition to the cingulotomy lesion, no detectable psychiatric worsening had been observed. The authors concluded that any patient who, despite intensive psychiatric treatment, has been totally incapacitated for a period of some months should be considered a possible candidate for cingulotomy.

BROWN and LIGHTHILL (1968) used a more anterior target than BALLANTINE et al. (1972) in the cingulum. They reported beneficial results in 92% of their 110 patients who had undergone 117 bilateral operations: 34% of the patients had obsessive-compulsive, 28% had affective disorders (manic-depressive psychosis), and 22% suffered from anxiety neurosis. Some radiograms in BROWN's paper may suggest that some lesions had at least partly destroyed the knee of the corpus callosum. Although the results of the operation were reported to have been good, BROWN (1973) later moved on to a three-target lesion, which included parts of the cingulum, substantia innominata, and amygdala. This approach was considered highly effective in schizophrenia and psychopathy.

In 1972 LAITINEN and VILKKI reported on 20 cingulotomy patients, who had suffered from various psychiatric disorders and in whom previous psychiatric treatments consisting of psycho-, pharmaco- and electrotherapy had proved ineffective. Half the patients were schizophrenic. LAITINEN's cingulate target was subrostral, i.e., lying in front of and below the knee of the corpus callosum. Analysis of the short-term clinical results showed that cingulotomy had had a very good anxiolytic effect in nine patients and a fair improvement in nine, while two patients obtained no benefit. The results were predominantly positive in the schizophrenic group. Seven of the ten patients became completely free from anxiety and fears, and four of them could be discharged from the mental hospital and return home without drugs within 2 months after surgery. There seemed to be consistent postoperative improvement in all performances on psychologic tests requiring manual and psychomotor speed. In some complicated visuomotor tasks (Digit Symbol, Block Design, and Purdue Pegboard Performance) the postoperative scores were significantly better than the preoperative scores. Although there might have been some training effect which improved the postoperative performances, the marked anxiolysis and the diminished need for drugs in the postoperative period were probably essential factors for the improved test performance.

MEYER et al. (1973) carried out 89 bilateral cingulotomies on 75 patients suffering from various forms of mental illness. Twelve patients were operated on twice and one patient with intractable pain, three times. There was no surgical mortality, but one patient had a subdural clot postoperatively; 70% of the patients showed a significant improvement. In the alcoholic patients the overall improvement was lower than in the remaining patients; 50% of the alcoholics benefited from surgery; 60% of the schizophrenic patients showed at least some improvement, which was still below the mean of the improved patients of the whole series (70%). The chronic pain states, depression (its type was not stated) and obsessive-compulsive disorders all did better than the mean for the series. Extensive pre- and postoperative psychologic testings were carried out in 30 patients. Fourteen of them showed excellent and seven moderate improvement, and three patients remained unchanged.

Since these and many other clinical studies on the effects of cingulotomy were solely conducted by neurosurgeons, the reliability of the reports was questioned. Therefore, it was widely welcomed when the United States National Commission for the Protection of Human Subjects of Biomedical and Behavioral Research in 1974 asked independent groups of highly qualified neuroscientists to conduct a retrospective study on clinical and psychologic effects of psychosurgery. One of these neuroscientists was HANS-LUKAS TEUBER (TEUBER et al., 1977), who carried out a clinical and psychologic study on 34 cases of cingulotomy drawn from a single hospital and a single neurosurgeon. The survey proceeded by means of extensive individual interviews with patients, their spouses, and their relatives; by observations of behavior in a research ward (which was completely independent of the referring psychiatrist and hospital); by repeated reviews of all available medical and surgical records; as well as by means of general physical and neurologic examinations and two dozen psychologic tests.

TEUBER et al. (1977) concluded that for the group of patients, who had a cingulotomy as a last resort and who had long-standing illness with many other therapeutic trials before surgery, no lasting additional deficits in behavioral capacities could be identified after the operation. Many patients with previous electroconvulsive treatments (ECT) had said spontaneously that they preferred the surgical procedure to ECT. Of the cingulotomized patients, those with chronic intractable pain did best: in nine of the eleven patients studied in depth, both the patients and their relatives claimed either complete or almost complete pain relief. Four of the patients who had been addicted to opiates or related drugs could be taken off the drugs without showing symptoms of drug withdrawal. The seven patients, who had suffered from depression, did not benefit as much from surgery, although five of them gave convincing reports of either full or partial relief. But two felt that they had not been helped at all.

Four patients with obsessive-compulsive disorders obtained no relief from cingulotomy. This is in contradiction to some cingulotomy reports referred to above, but in accordance with the recent findings of KULLBERG (1977), who carried out a comparative study on the effects of cingulotomy and anterior capsulotomy in obsessive and anxiety patients. She concluded that transient disturbances of cognitive and affective functioning were observed after both approaches, but they were much less marked after cingulotomy than after capsulotomy. On the other hand, more patients were improved in the capsulotomy group than in the cingulotomy group. Initial symptom relief following cingulotomy was temporary in several cases, whereas the effects of capsulotomy were better sustained. Cingulotomy had no positive effect on obsessive-compulsive states, but a moderate-to-excellent effect on anxiety states in 40% of the cases.

Specific adverse effects of cingulotomy seem to be rare. LAITINEN et al. (1973) found a slight reduction of imaginative productivity when their 46 cingulotomized patients were tested with the Holtzman Inkblot Technique (HOLTZMAN et al., 1961), but at the long-term follow-up examination (VILKKI, 1977) this deficit had disappeared almost completely. Neuroticism did not change after cingulotomy, whereas extraversion increased significantly ($p < 0.01$). A marked improvement was seen in the test for psychomotor performances (Purdue Pegboard Assembly Test, $p < 0.001$).

Additional evidence of the low risks of cingulotomy can be derived from a study of MITCHELL-HEGGS et al. (1977). This team, led by the psychiatrist DESMOND KELLY of London, England, combines cingulotomy with a tractotomy in the ventro-medial quadrant of the frontal lobes (see p. 364). Despite their large double bilateral lesions the mean scores on the Wechsler Adult Intelligence Scale show postoperative improvements of full scale ($p < 0.001$), performance ($p < 0.001$), and verbal IQ ($p < 0.01$).

2. Anterior Capsulotomy

In 1952 the Swedish neurosurgeon, LARS LEKSELL, developed a new surgical approach, which aimed at interruption of frontothalamic fibers at the level of the head of the caudate nucleus (HERNER, 1961). In his doctoral dissertation HERNER reported on 116 patients operated on by LEKSELL during the years 1952–57. The follow-up time ranged from 24 to 80 months. The lesions, made to interrupt the frontothalamic radiation, were placed ~20–25 mm lateral to the midline and 6–7 mm behind the tip of the frontal horn. The ventralmost part of the 20-mm long electrocoagulation lesion lay on the continued intercommissural line.

Half of the patients were schizophrenic, 19 suffered from various types of depression, 18 from obsessional, and 15 from anxiety neurosis. There was no surgical mortality. Postoperative epileptic fits occurred in four patients (3.4%).

The best results were obtained in obsessive states: 50% of the patients showing good and 28% fair improvement. Depressive patients had an outcome almost as positive: 53% had good and 21% fair relief of their symptoms. Also schizophrenic patients were found to be much improved after surgery: good improvement was observed in 27% and fair, in 58% of the cases. Only 16% had not benefited from capsulotomy.

Immediate side effects were relatively frequent, but they faded away during the follow-up period. Serious long-term side effects occurred in three patients, resulting in conflicts with the law (overt sexual behavior, alcohol addiction, and thefts, respectively). Urinary incontinence and mental confusion were often seen during the first postoperative days.

At the long-term follow-up examination it was found that the working capacity of the patients had improved in 69% of the cases of anxiety neurosis, in 61% of the obsessional, 56% of the depressive, and 56% of the schizophrenic group; 29% of all patients had regained full working capacity as compared to 3% before surgery.

BINGLEY et al. (1973, 1977) used a similar approach in obsessive-compulsive patients who had not benefited from conventional psychiatric treatment, including intensive supportive psychotherapy, group psychotherapy, behavioral therapy, and in some patients psychoanalysis. Their series of 1977 consisted of 35 patients. There was no surgical mortality and the morbidity was low: two patients had developed a transient hemiparesis. Postoperative epilepsy did not occur in any case. The follow-up time ranged from 4 to 55 months, with a mean of 35 months. Sixteen patients (46%) became free from symptoms, nine were much improved, and ten slightly improved. Before surgery three patients had full working capacity, but after surgery the number had increased to fourteen.

KULLBERG (1977) compared, as was mentioned in the cingulotomy part of this chapter, the effects of capsulotomy and cingulotomy on anxiety and obsessional neuroses. She concluded that the former was more effective than the latter, particularly in the obsessional group, but this improvement occurred at the cost of more serious side effects.

3. Kelly's and Richardson's Limbic Leukotomy

Limbic leukotomy consists of two bilateral lesions, one lying in the cingulum and the other in the medioventral quadrant of the frontal lobes. The coordinates of the cingulate target are as follows: 3 cm behind the tip of the frontal horn, 5 mm above the lateral ventricle, and 8 and 16 mm lateral to the midline (double lesions in the cingulum). The medioventral quadrant lesions lie in the frontal white matter 1 cm anterior to the base of the anterior clinoid, 1 cm above the floor of the anterior fossa, and 6 and 14 mm from the midline (even here double lesions in each hemisphere!). Therefore the total amount of brain tissue destroyed is rather large.

The rationale of this two-target approach is to interrupt the medial limbic circuit of PAPEZ (1937) in the cingulum bundle and additionally, by the medio-ventral quadrant lesions, to cut some frontolimbic circuits, which may deal with defense reactions (NAUTA, 1971). KELLY and his co-workers (KELLY et al., 1973) use electrical stimulation of the target area before producing permanent brain lesions in their anesthetized patients. The aim is to find out specific structures within the calculated target area where stimulation causes respiratory arrest or other vegetative reactions. Although it may be difficult to prove that the vegetative phenomena directly reflect the level of the emotional disorder, these authors have been able to demonstrate certain positive correlations between the occurrence of apnea during stimulation and the degree of clinical improvement (RICHARDSON et al., 1977).

The clinical results of KELLY's and RICHARDSON's limbic leukotomy have been good. In 1973 the London team (KELLY et al., 1973) reported on a series of 35 patients with mainly obsessional illnesses and stated that the operation had favorably influenced most symptoms of the patients (Table 1).

By 1977 the same team had operated on 66 patients (MITCHELL-HEGGS et al., 1977). The patients were examined 6 and 16 weeks after surgery. Their postoperative condition was grouped according to PIPPARD (1955): I, symptom-free; II, much improved; III, improved; IV, unchanged; V, worse. There was no difference found in the patients' clinical conditions between the postoperative examinations at 6 and 16 weeks, although the percentage of the improved patients with depression had declined from 100% to 78%. At the 16-week examination, the patients with obsessional neurosis showed the greatest improvement: 89% of them had benefited from surgery. Of the 27 patients in this group, seven were symptom-free, eleven much improved, and six improved, whereas two had become worse. The seven schizophrenic patients also seemed to have benefited from the operations: four were much improved, two improved,

Table 1. Psychometric mean values before and after limbic leukotomy, N=35 (KELLY et al., 1973)

		Pre	Post	p
MPI	Neuroticism	30.8	23.1	0.001
	Extraversion	12.9	14.2	NS
Depression,	Beck	26.4	18.7	0.001
	Hamilton	21.5	10.5	0.001
Anxiety,	Taylor	31.9	24.1	0.001
	Hamilton	22.2	12.3	0.001
MHQ	Anxiety	11.6	10.0	0.01
	Phobic	7.1	5.7	0.01
	Obsessional	11.3	10.2	0.05
	Somatic	8.2	5.5	0.001
	Depressive	10.6	7.9	0.001
	Hysteric	5.3	4.7	NS

while one had remained unchanged. Of the 15 patients with anxiety, 67% showed improvement at the 16-week examination: three were symptom-free, five much improved, two improved, and three unchanged. Two patients had become worse. The outcome of the nine depressive patients was also good: three symptom-free, two much improved, two improved, and two unchanged.

Despite the large bilateral lesions in the cingulum and the lower medial quadrant, serious side effects were rare. One of the 66 patients, who had previously had frontal lobotomy and whose lower quadrant lesion was therefore placed more posteriorly than usually, showed postoperatively "a transient neurological complication" and a memory deficit. Transitory confusion, anergia, urinary and bowel incontinence occurred sometimes, but they usually cleared up within a few weeks. Impairment of memory and mild lethargy occasionally might last for several months. Neither epilepsy nor weight gain were observed postoperatively.

4. Innominotomy

In 1960 KNIGHT (1964) had selected a subcortical supraorbital area, called substantia innominata by REICHERT, for a new stereotactic approach in the treatment of mental illness. Clinical observations and operative findings in a large series of restricted undercutting operations had drawn his attention to a concentration of important fibers in this area. He believed that the maximum benefit of orbital undercuttings was derived from the terminal few centimeters of the narrow incision which entered the substantia innominata beneath the head of the caudate nucleus and overlay the primitive cortex of areas 13 and 14 in the gyrus orbitalis and gyrus rectus.

KNIGHT began to insert yttrium-90 seeds stereotactically within this area. His aim was to produce a disk-shaped lesion having length and breadth, but little depth so as to avoid damage to the striatum. The bilateral lesions lay ~6 cm behind the frontal pole, just inside of the supraorbital cortex and were supposed to destroy an area ~20 mm long and 12 mm wide, lying 6–18 mm from the midline.

By 1969 KNIGHT had carried out bilateral innominotomies on 200 patients, most of whom had suffered from various types of depression. He concluded that the effects of surgery had been favorable. There had been no mortality, no postoperative epilepsy, and no serious personality changes.

In 1971 STRÖM-OLSEN and CARLISLE reported on 210 patients operated on by KNIGHT in the substantia innominata. The follow-up time of 150 patients ranged from 16 months to 8 years. Forty-six of them had suffered from anxiety states, 45 from recurrent depression, 24 from other types of depression, 20 from obsessional neurosis, 6 from involutional depression, 5 from schizophrenia, and 4 from other mental illnesses. Of the 150 patients, 49 (33%) recovered completely from their symptoms and an additional 24 (16%) had only minor residual symptoms and required no further psychiatric treatment. Thirty-five patients (23%) improved but still needed treatment, with persistent symptoms. Forty-one patients (27%) were unchanged, and one became worse.

The best results were obtained in depression, both recurrent and other forms; 56% became symptom-free or much improved. Favorable results were also obtained in obsessional neurosis (50% recovered and improved). In anxiety states the corresponding amount was 41%. None of the five schizophrenic patients benefited from this approach.

No patient showed a gross frontal lobe syndrome postoperatively. In 4 of the 150 patients (2.6%) there were some moderate and lasting sequelae. 17 (11.4%) displayed minor and trivial symptoms, which were not serious. In 129 patients (86%) there were no demonstrable personality changes whatsoever. Preoperatively only 1 patient had had full working capacity, whereas after surgery 72 had regained it. The capacity for enjoying leisure was in all patients impaired before surgery. A full capacity was regained by 74 of them after innominotomy. There was no surgical mortality. Postoperative epilepsy was observed in less than 1%.

In a later paper the same authors (STRÖM-OLSEN and CARLISLE, 1971) analyzed the effects of innominotomy on different symptoms. They found that loss of weight improved in 90%, aggressiveness in 89.5%, depression in 80.4%, phobias in 76.7%, obsessive ruminations in 76%, anxiety in 70%, tension in 68%, and obsessive compulsions in 62%. Hallucinations were improved in 75% of the patients.

VAERNET and MADSEN (1970) reported on two patients with frequent self-mutilations and reactive psychotic episodes who had not benefited from bilateral amygdalotomy. These symptoms disappeared after an additional innominotomy.

Basing his opinion on a personal series of over 600 innominotomies, KNIGHT (1973) stated that his subcaudate operation is particularly successful in chronic depression; those patients improving most are classified as anxiety states in whom a depressive element can be detected. Pure obsessional neurosis of early onset without depressive features always implies a worse prognosis. In eight patients, in whom innominotomy had failed, additional cingulotomy was carried out. One patient with phobic anxiety became symptom-free, and another patient with obsessional cleanliness who did not improve from cingulotomy after unsuccessful tractotomy, suddenly became symptom-free after a brain concussion! Two patients with depression and obsessional guilt feelings or obsessional violence were improved, whereas four remaining patients were not improved at all. These findings lend additional support to the impression that cingulotomy is not effective against obsessive-compulsive symptoms.

BRIDGES and GOKTEPE (1973) compared the surgical results in obsessional and depressive patients of STRÖM-OLSEN and CARLISLE (1971). They also analyzed the role of the patients' ages at onset of the illness and at operation. Their conclusion was that a relatively good prognosis can be expected after innominotomy in patients with primary obsessional symptoms if the age at onset of the illness is near 30 years or older, if there is depression present, if the onset of the obsessional symptoms was sudden, and particularly good prognosis is associated with illnesses occurring in relation to pregnancy.

5. Mesoloviotomy

In 1972 LAITINEN (1972) reported on 11 patients who had been operated on in the knee of the corpus callosum. Because the Greek name of the corpus callosum is *mesolovion*, he called his new operation anterior mesoloviotomy. Splitting of the corpus callosum had been used by neurosurgeons in the treatment of intractable epilepsy since 1939, and it was well known that incision of the anterior part of the corpus callosum did not cause serious side effects. The rationale for mesoloviotomy derived from the author's experience with rostral cingulotomies (LAITINEN and VILKKI, 1973b). Cingulotomies carried out under local anesthesia had permitted comprehensive electrophysiologic investigations during surgery. An interesting finding was that electrical stimulation of the rostral cingulum with 6 Hz below and in front of the genu of the corpus callosum gave rise to an evoked potential in the contralateral frontopolar scalp EEG. It seemed clear that the signal was mediated through the genu. During one such operation LAITINEN inserted an electrode into the rostral cingulum through the genu to investigate the transcallosal response. Electrical stimulation of the anterior layer of the genu with 60 Hz resulted in a sudden strong feeling of inner wellbeing and relaxation of the whole body of the patient, a 24-year-old woman with anxiety and obsessions of schizophrenic origin. The response was reproduced several times. A bilateral lesion, 6 by 6 mm in diameter, was produced in the anterior part of the genu; the center of the lesions lay 6 mm lateral to the midline. The postoperative course was good. All anxiety, fears, and obsessions were absent, and drug therapy could be terminated.

Seven of the 11 patients were schizophrenic, three suffered from anxiety neurosis, and one, from temporal lobe epilepsy with severe psychotic anxiety. Six patients were so improved that they could leave the mental hospital within 6–12 weeks, and some betterment was also seen in the remaining five.

By 1973 the number of mesoloviotomized patients had grown to 48 (LAITINEN and VILKKI, 1973a). The short-term clinical results were best in schizophrenia: of the 17 schizophrenics treated thus 4 were symptom-free, 10, much improved, 2, improved, and 1, unchanged. Of the 10 patients with anxiety neurosis, 2 were symptom-free, 3, much improved, 3, improved, and 2, unchanged. The authors stated that mesoloviotomy was effective against anxiety, tension, and fears of neurotic, schizophrenic, and epileptic origin. It was quite evident that the operation was ineffective against depression and obsessional symptoms.

A pleasant response of wellbeing and relaxation to high frequency stimulation was obtained in most patients who suffered from anxiety, tension, and fears of schizophrenic origin. Those patients suffering from depression or obsessional symptoms, even when accompanied by secondary anxiety, did not have any subjective sensation during stimulation, not even when the current intensity was increased to the maximum.

One patient had a postoperative subdural clot in the interhemispheric fissure. It caused a marked slowing of the immediate recovery, but subsequently the patient did well.

The comprehensive psychologic investigations indicated that mesoloviotomy immediately improved the emotional state and possibly also some memory functions of the patients. The psychomotor performance (Purdue Pegboard Assembly Test), short- and long-term memory (Recognition of Inkblots), and neuroticism (Eysenck Personality Inventory) were significantly improved.

Recently VILKKI (1977) reported on the long-term effects of mesoloviotomy in 31 patients whom he had been able to investigate psychologically before and after surgery. The patients had the following diagnoses: schizophrenia (ICD code 295.1, 3, 7, 8, 9), anxiety neurosis (300.0), depressive neurosis (300.4), obsessive-compulsive neurosis (300.3), involutional psychosis (296.0), and chronic pain with depression (304.3). The preoperative psychologic condition of the patients was usually miserable. The mean duration of illness was 10 years, and the age of the patients at operation, 37 years on the average. The operation was considered a last-resort therapy. The follow-up time ranged from 9 to 40 months, averaging 2 years. The test battery was comprehensive. The psychologic tests did not show average postoperative impairment in any performance, whereas improvements were noticed in the Culture Fair Intelligence Test, Memory Test for Recognition of Inkblots, and Neuroticism Test (Eysenck Personality Inventory). VILKKI also analyzed the clinical condition of the patients. Anxiety was improved in 72% of the patients, tension, in 71%, and fears, in 67%, whereas depression improved in only 37% of the patients. In the total series 10% of the patients were free from symptoms, 6%, much improved, 42%, slightly improved, and 35%, unchanged. Two patients (6%) had become worse, but worsening was, according to VILKKI, presumably caused by natural progression of the illness; there was no indication that surgery per se had caused the deterioration.

6. Posteromedial Hypothalamotomy

In 1962 SANO reported on six erethistic, idiotic, and epileptic patients who had had a bilateral stereotactic lesion in the posteromedial part of the hypothalamus. The surgical lesions lay 3–4 mm below the midpoint of the intercommissural line and 1–3 mm lateral to the wall of the third ventricle. During electrical stimulation of this target area the unanesthetized patients showed signs of increased wakefulness and a marked rise in blood pressure, tachycardia, mydriasis, and often flushing of the face. The estimated size of the lesions is 5 mm in diameter. The operation is first performed on one side and 7–20 days later on the other. Marked calming effects are observed after the second intervention. SANO et al. (1972) later reported on 53 patients operated on in the posteromedial hypothalamus. The procedure had produced marked calming effects in 95% of the patients. Postoperatively a tendency to a decreased sympathicotonia and an increased parasympathicotonia appeared. Of the intractable epileptic seizures 41% became controllable by medication after surgery.

These results were confirmed by SCHVARCZ et al. (1972), who had operated on 11 patients. Marked improvement with social readaptation and diminution of aggressiveness or violent behavior was achieved in 7 patients, improvement in 3, and no change in 1 patient. The best results were obtained in patients with normal intelligence and less satisfactory results in oligophrenic and hyperkinetic patients.

Postoperatively many patients were extremely sleepy for a few days. Other complications were reported to be infrequent. BALASUBRAMANIAM and KANAKA (1972) studied the effects of posteromedial hypothalamotomy and amygdalotomy in more than 200 restless patients. Both approaches were found to be effective against aggressiveness, assaultive behavior, and epileptic fits. Mere wandering or restlessness did not improve very much. The authors concluded that amygdalotomy is to be preferred as the first procedure for several reasons: bilateral amygdalotomy can be carried out in one session, whereas bilateral surgery in the hypothalamus requires two sessions. Another reason for the choice of amygdalotomy as the first operation is that there is often a primary pathologic tissue damage and physiologic disturbance (e. g., epileptic focus) in the amygdala, which should be eliminated if permanent cure is expected. The surgical mortality in the series of BALASUBRAMANIAM and KANAKA was 4.5% both in the amygdalotomy and hypothalamotomy groups. Transitory diabetes insipidus developed in 2 of the 42 hypothalamotomy patients and long-lasting hemiballism in 1 patient.

7. Ventromedial Hypothalamotomy

Neurosurgical treatment of sexual deviation has been practiced since 1962 in Germany (ROEDER, 1966; ROEDER and MUELLER, 1969; ROEDER et al., 1972; MUELLER et al., 1973; DIECKMANN and HASSLER, 1977), in the United States (HEATH, 1972), and in Czechoslovakia (NÁDVORNÍK et al., 1977). While there is a widespread criticism of psychosurgical treatment of criminal and sexually deviant patients, ROEDER and MUELLER (1969) defend their policy: „Es kann kein Zweifel bestehen, daß die experimentelle Verhaltensforschung grundsätzlich einen Weg gewiesen hat, wie sich mit Hilfe eines psychochirurgisch wirksamen Eingriffs im Bereich des ‚sex-behavior-center' die pädophile Homosexualität beseitigen oder eindämmen läßt. Forensische und juristische Schwierigkeiten bestehen hier grundsätzlich nicht, da es sich weder um eine operative noch chemische Kastration handelt."

By 1972 the Göttingen group (ROEDER et al., 1972) had performed ten ventromedial hypothalamotomies for sexual deviation. The coordinates of the lesions were as follows: 3–10 mm behind the anterior commissure, 6–15 mm below the intercommissural line, and 3–9 mm lateral to the midline of the third ventricle. The presumed size of the total lesion (comprising 3–4 electrocoagulations within the target area) was 70 mm^3, which was supposed to destroy three-quarters of the nucleus of Cajal.

Two of the ten patients were "cured" by the procedure, and a third patient, "homosexual by inclination" showed a complete loss of his abnormal drives, and an adjustment to normal life was achieved. Additionally, three patients were much improved and one slightly improved, while in three cases the result was not satisfactory. In general, the sexual potency was weakened but preserved after unilateral, and completely lost after bilateral hypothalamotomy. There was no deficiency of spermatozoa in the semen. The metabolites of the adrenocortical, gonadal, and corticoid hormones showed no changes. An 11th patient, who had been excluded from the series, was reported to have died from cerebral hemorrhage 7 days after surgery. Other side effects were not described.

By 1973 the total number of hypothalamotomized patients in Göttingen had reached 22. Of these patients 20 were sexually deviant, one suffered from neurotic "pseudo-homosexuality" and one, from intractable addiction to alcohol and drugs. The group of sexual deviants consisted of 14 cases of pedo- or ephebophile homosexuality and 6 cases with disturbances of heterosexual behavior (hypersexuality, exhibitionism, pedophilia). In 12 patients, the operation was unilateral in the nondominant hemisphere. Good or excellent relief from homosexuality was achieved in 15 patients with complete harmonization of their sexual and social behavior. Three more patients were slightly improved. Potency was preserved in all patients. No psycho-organic disturbances were detected after surgery.

The patient who suffered from neurotic "pseudo-homosexuality" did not improve. Nor did the patient with alcoholism and drug addiction benefit from hypothalamotomy.

DIECKMANN and HASSLER (1977) placed stereotactic lesions in the ventromedial nucleus of Cajal of the nondominant hypothalamus of four sexual offenders who had committed violent sexual crimes. In all of them the sexual drive was markedly reduced, and their sexual problems and activities were diminished; three were released from custody. Two patients felt constantly hungry postoperatively and gained weight. General psychic activity of two patients declined after surgery.

SCHNEIDER (1977) carried out psychologic investigations before and after surgery in six patients who underwent ventromedial hypothalamotomy for sexual delinquency. All of them complained of reduction of sexual potency after the operation. Correspondingly, psychologic concern with sexual problems and activity diminished. All patients had these complaints; there was no difference between patients demonstrating heterosexual hyperactivity or sexual deviation of the type homosexuality or pedophilia. Emotionally all six patients experienced an inner relaxation and calm after surgery. The concentration span improved. There was long-lasting reduction in visual retention, and dreaming activity was also definitely reduced. An important and long-lasting side effect was seen in the structure of thought, a change which appeared not earlier than 6–12 months after surgery. Thought had lost its flexibility; this was seen in projective tests, and there was a quantitative and qualitative change in the content of perception. Also an increased tendency to stereotypy, presumably linked to diminution of thought content, was found.

NÁDVORNÍK et al. (1977) reported on ten patients, three of whom had ventromedial hypothalamotomy for sexual hyperactivity, six, for alcoholism and nicotinism(!), and one, for hyperinsulinism. Surgery was always bilateral and was stated to have been successful. Increased appetite was noticed as side effects in two patients, and two showed abnormal excitement and euphoria, respectively. In the patient with hyperinsulinism the blood sugar level rose from 30 to 60 mg%.

8. Thalamotomy

Surgical lesions in the intralaminar and centromedian nuclei of the thalamus have been reported to exercise a favorable influence on the hyperresponsive syndrome (ANDY and JURKO, 1972), obsessive-compulsive disorders, phobias and tics (HASSLER and DIECKMANN, 1973), and erethistic idiocy and temporal lobe epilepsy (HASSLER and DIECKMANN, 1972).

ANDY and JURKO (1972) had carried out uni- and bilateral thalamotomies on 30 patients, who represented various types of abnormal behavior. These patients were operated on for hyperactivity (14 patients); aggression (2 patients); maladjustment (11 patients), and rhythmia "rocking" (3 patients). The surgical coordinates were as follows: 9 mm posterior to the midcommissural point, 1.3 mm above the intercommissural line, and 7 mm lateral to the midline of the third ventricle. Six patients were much improved, and 14, fairly improved, whereas ten patients did not benefit from surgery. Five patients died 3 weeks–6 months after the operation, suggesting a high surgical risk of intralaminar thalamotomy. The authors concluded that aggression benefited most from thalamotomy, bilateral operations were more effective than unilateral, and the optimum lesion site for good results appeared to be in the area of centromedian and intralaminar nuclei.

HASSLER and DIECKMANN (1972, 1973) carried out unilateral intralaminar, and medial thalamotomies on 27 patients and bilateral, on 13. They stated that thalamotomy always improved and often cured obsessive-compulsive neurosis, phobias, and motor compulsions like tics, cries, and coprolalia of Gilles de la Tourette's syndrome. Of the six patients who underwent bilateral thalamotomy for this syndrome, two developed a severe amnesia and akinesia, respectively, after surgery. Other side effects were not described. Of the 20 erethistic oligophrenic patients who had intralaminar or medial thalamotomy, ten obtained an almost complete relief from their aggression and violence, seven showed fair to good improvement, while in three the result was poor. The surgical target had been almost identical to that of ANDY and JURKO (1972).

Because of a high risk of side effects, NÁDVORNÍK et al. (1973) abandoned intralaminar thalamotomy.

9. Amygdalotomy

The Japanese physician NARABAYASHI (NARABAYASHI et al., 1963; NARABAYASHI, 1972; NARABAYASHI and SHIMA, 1973) introduced amygdalotomy in the treatment of restless behavior. By 1973 he had operated on 127 patients, the majority of whom suffered from epilepsy with various behavioral abnormalities, such as violence, uncontrollable explosive assaults, unsteadiness of mood, and poor concentration span. Almost all patients were younger than 20. The optimal target lay 17–19 mm from the midline, just above the tip of the temporal horn. About half of the patients had bilateral lesions, the size of which was presumed to be 8 by 8 mm in diameter.

Calming and marked reduction of aggressiveness, irritability, and unsteadiness occurred in 48% of the cases, and slight improvement was obtained in 37%. The follow-up ranged from 3 to 6.5 years. There was no mortality. Transient hemiparesis occurred once, and no case of detected memory deficit or Kluever-Bucy syndrome was determined.

MARK et al. (1972) carried out amygdalotomy on ten patients who suffered from episodic aggression or impulse dyscontrol. Three were completely free from their assaultiveness after unilateral amygdalotomy, and complete relief was also noticed in five of the seven patients who had bilateral operations. But 6–12 months later, four of these eight patients had a recurrence of their symptoms. Side effects were observed in five patients: transient visual field defect and dyslexia, impotence, hyperphagia, oculomotor palsy, and transient hemianopsia. The authors did not want to recommend amygdalotomy for widespread use in all patients with violent behavior, and they advocated a more extensive clinical trial under controlled conditions.

HITCHCOCK et al. (1972) also stressed the importance of pre- and postoperative assessment of patients undergoing amygdalotomy. ANDERSEN (1972), by examining selected aspects of psychologic testing, e. g., material specificity, learning and reproduction, and the course of the process, found selective differences in the ratio of the responses at the beginning of the task and the following responses. Thus, she found in her patients reduced ability to establish sets and also to protect the consolidation of learning process from registrations of irrelevant experience.

As was already reported in the part dealing with the posteromedial hypothalamotomy, BALASUBRAMANIAM and KANAKA (1972) found that amygdalotomy was more effective than hypothalamotomy in calming restless and violent patients.

II. Ethical Aspects of Psychosurgery

As was shown in this chapter, a relatively large number of clinical studies carried out by competent clinicians and psychologists all suggest that stereotactic operations may have a beneficial effect on some mental disorders without causing additional damage. In fact, this "last-resort" treatment has often proved superior to available conventional psychiatric therapy. Still there is a widespread criticism of psychosurgery, and many opponents consider it unethical. But the basic ethical problem of psychosurgery is only medical: whether psychosurgery can or cannot alleviate psychic illness without causing harmful side effects. Since pilot studies have not convinced the critics of psychosurgery, even when the patients' condition has been quantitatively assessed pre- and postoperatively, properly conducted controlled clinical studies are needed.

Such a controlled study was started in Helsinki in 1974 (LAITINEN, 1975). After definitive failure of psychiatric treatment, the patient was referred to the neurosurgical unit, where a multidisciplinary team tested him. The team consisted of a neurosurgeon, psychologist, psychiatrist, neurophysiologist, speech therapist, and social worker. The patient was first accepted for, or excluded from, the trial. At the time of admission, the patient was informed that the tests were given only to find out whether surgical treatment could be recommended. If he did not wish to be investigated for this purpose or if he did not understand the information, he was excluded from the trial. According to the dominant symptoms, one of the four stereotactic lesion targets – cingulum, genu of the corpus callosum, anterior capsule, or subcaudate region (substantia innominata) – was chosen. After the randomization, the surgical patients were informed of all the possible risks and benefits of surgery, and if they wished to have the operation it was carried out. Those patients who fell into the group of continued conservative therapy were told that surgery, at present at least, was not recommended because its effects were not sufficiently known. Follow-up examinations were undertaken at 3-, 6-, 12-, and 24-month intervals by the same multidisciplinary team, but the neurosurgeon was excluded from the assessment and the comparison of results. The psychiatrist of the team had had nothing to do with the pre-test treatment of the patients. After the randomization, he had to make every effort to guarantee that the two groups, surgical and conservative, received equally active psychiatric treatment.

A similarly controlled prospective trial was planned by the *Research Committee of the Royal College of Psychiatrists* (1977) in Great Britain.

There has been criticism of psychosurgery in the treatment of prisoners and children. Our practice has been, according to the Declaration of Helsinki of the World Medical Assembly, that prisoners, children, and severely psychotic patients must for now be excluded from psychosurgery. This issue is not one that will be easily resolved. Many have considered that to withhold psychosurgery totally from institutionalized patients, including prisoners, might in itself constitute an infringement of personal liberties. Nevertheless, psychosurgery is still an experimental therapy. Therefore its use in every single case requires an individual solution.

C. Recommendations for Selection of Psychosurgical Approach

It may have appeared from the figures presented in this chapter that different surgical approaches may lead to different results. An exact evaluation is difficult, however, because many neurosurgeons have used only one approach for all kinds of symptoms. Lack of control groups has made assessments more or less subjective. With all this in mind the final conclusions are drawn:
1. Chronic pain states with addiction and intractable manic-depressive illness can be effectively relieved by cingulotomy.
2. Obsessive-compulsive symptoms, neurotic anxiety, and phobias may be best influenced by anterior capsulotomy or by lower medial quadrant tractotomy combined with cingulotomy.
3. Recurrent depression is effectively alleviated by innominotomy.
4. Schizophrenic anxiety, tension, and catatonia can be abolished by mesoloviotomy.
5. Restless and violent behavior can be calmed by posteromedial hypothalamotomy or, when associated with temporal lobe epilepsy, by amygdalotomy.

Psychosurgery should be considered a "last-resort" treatment, but it should not be postponed to the extent that the patient has irreversibly lost his chance for social rehabilitation.

References

Andersen, R.: Differences in the course of learning as measured by various memory tasks after amygdalotomy in man. In: Psychosurgery. Hitchcock, E., Laitinen, L., Vaernet, K. (eds.), pp. 177–183. Springfield (Ill.): Charles C. Thomas 1972

References

Andy, O.J., Jurko, M.F.: Thalamotomy for hyperresponsive syndrome. Lesions in the centermedianum and intralaminar nuclei. In: Psychosurgery. Hitchcock, E., Laitinen, L., Vaernet, K. (eds.), pp. 127–135. Springfield (Ill.): Charles C. Thomas 1972

Bailey, H.R., Dowling, J.L., Swanton, C.H., Davies, E.: Studies in depression. I. Cingulo-tractotomy in the treatment of severe affective illness. Med. J. Aust. **1**, 8–12 (1971)

Balasubramaniam, V., Kanaka, T.S.: Amygdolatomy and hypothalamotomy – a comparative study. Proc. Inst. Neurol. Madras **3**, 67–74 (1972)

Balasubramaniam, V., Kanaka, T.S., Ramanujam, P.B.: Drug addiction and its management by surgery. J. Phys. Assoc. Madras **11**, 1–8 (1972)

Ballantine, H.T., Jr., Cassidy, W.L., Flanagan, N.B., Marino, R., Jr.: Stereotaxic anterior cingulotomy for neuropsychiatric illness and intractable pain. J. Neurosurg. **26**, 488–495 (1967)

Ballantine, H.T., Jr., Cassidy, W.L., Brodeur, J., Giriunas, I.: Frontal cingulotomy for mood disturbance. In: Psychosurgery. Hitchcock, E., Laitinen, L., Vaernet, K. (eds.), pp. 221–229. Springfield (Ill.): Charles C. Thomas 1972

Bingley, T., Leksell, L., Meyerson, B.A., Rylander, G.: Stereotactic anterior capsulotomy in anxiety and obsessive-compulsive states. In: Surgical approaches in psychiatry. Laitinen, L.V., Livingston, K.E. (eds.), pp. 159–164. Lancaster: Medical and Technical Publishing 1973

Bingley, T., Leksell, L., Meyerson, B.A., Rylander, G.: Long-term results of stereotactic anterior capsulotomy in chronic obsessive-compulsive neurosis. In: Neurosurgical treatment in psychiatry, pain, and epilepsy. Sweet, W.H., Obrador, S., Martín-Rodríguez, J.G. (eds.), pp. 287–299. Baltimore: University Park Press 1977

Brickner, R.M.: The intellectual functions of the frontal lobe. New York: Macmillan 1936

Bridges, P.K., Goktepe, E.O.: A review of patients with obsessional symptoms treated by psychosurgery. In: Surgical approaches in psychiatry. Laitinen, L.V., Livingston, K.E. (eds.), pp. 96–100. Lancaster: Medical and Technical Publishing 1973

Brown, M.H.: Further experience with multiple limbic targets for schizophrenia and aggression. In: Surgical approaches in psychiatry. Laitinen, L.V., Livingston, K.E. (eds.), pp. 189–195. Lancaster: Medical and Technical Publishing 1973

Brown, M.H., Lighthill, J.A.: Selective anterior cingulotomy: a psychosurgical evaluation. J. Neurosurg. **29**, 513–519 (1968)

Burckhardt, G.: Ueber Rindenexcisionen, als Beitrag zur operativen Therapie der Psychosen. Allg. Z. Psychiatr. **47**, 463–548 (1891)

Connecticut Lobotomy Committee: A co-operative clinical study of lobotomy. Res. Publ. Assoc. Res. Nerv. Ment. Dis. **27**, 769–794 (1948)

Delgado, J.M.R., Obrador, S., Martín-Rodríguez, J.G.: Two-way radio communication with the brain in psychosurgical patients. In: Surgical approaches in psychiatry. Laitinen, L.V., Livingston, K.E. (eds.), pp. 215–223. Lancaster: Medical and Technical Publishing 1973

Dieckmann, G., Hassler, R.: Treatment of sexual violence by stereotactic hypothalamotomy. In: Neurosurgical treatment in psychiatry, pain, and epilepsy. Sweet, W.H., Obrador, S., Martín-Rodríguez, J.G. (eds.), pp. 451–462. Baltimore: University Park Press 1977

Fedio, P., Ommaya, A.K.: Bilateral cingulum lesions and stimulation in man with lateralized impairment in short-term verbal memory. Exp. Neurol. **29**, 84–91 (1970)

Foltz, E.L., White, L.E.: Pain "relief" by frontal cingulumotomy. J. Neurosurg. **19**, 89–100 (1962)

Fulton, J.F.: The frontal lobes and human behaviour. pp. 1–23. Liverpool: University Press of Liverpool 1952

Grantham, E.G.: Prefrontal lobotomy for relief of pain. With a report of a new operative technique. J. Neurosurg. **8**, 405–410 (1951)

Hassler, R., Dieckmann, G.: Violence against oneself and against others as a target for stereotaxic psychosurgery. In: Present limits of neurosurgery. Fusek, I., Kunc, Z. (eds.), pp. 477–482. Prague: Avicenum 1972

Hassler, R., Dieckmann, G.: Relief of obsessive-compulsive disorders, phobias and tics by stereotactic coagulation of the rostral intralaminar and medial thalamic nuclei. In: Surgical approaches in psychiatry. Laitinen, L.V., Livingston, K.E. (eds.), pp. 206–212. Lancaster: Medical and Technical Publishing 1973

Heath, R.G.: Pleasure and brain activity in man. Deep and surface electroencephalograms during orgasm. J. Nerv. Ment. Dis. **154**, 3–18 (1972)

Herner, T.: Treatment of mental disorders with frontal stereotaxic thermo-lesions. Acta Psychiatr. Neurol. Scand. [Suppl. 158], **36**, 1–140 (1961)

Hitchcock, E., Ashcroft, G.W., Cairns, V.M., Murray, L.G.: Preoperative and postoperative assessment and management of psychosurgical patients. In: Psychosurgery. Hitchcock, E., Laitinen, L., Vaernet, K. (eds.), pp. 164–176. Springfield (Ill.): Charles C Thomas 1972

Holtzman, W.H., Thorpe, J.S., Swartz, J.D., Herron, E.W.: Inkblot perception and personality. Austin: University of Texas Press 1961

Kelly, D., Mitchell-Heggs, N.: Stereotactic limbic leucotomy – a follow-up study of thirty patients. Postgrad. Med. J. **49**, 865–882 (1973)

Kelly, D., Richardson, A., Mitchell-Heggs, N., Greenup, J., Chen, J., Hafner, R.J.: Stereotactic limbic leucotomy: a preliminary report on forty patients. Br. J. Psychiatry **123**, 141–151 (1973)

Knight, G.: The orbital cortex as an objective in the surgical treatment of mental illness. The results of 450 cases of open operation and the development of the stereotactic approach. Br. J. Surg. **51**, 114–124 (1964)

Knight, G.: Stereotactic surgery for the relief of suicidal and severe depression and intractable psychoneurosis. Postgrad. Med. J. **45**, 1–13 (1969)

Knight, G.: Additional stereotactic lesions in the cingulum following failed tractotomy in the subcaudate region. In: Surgical approaches in psychiatry. Laitinen, L.V., Livingston, K.E. (eds.), pp. 101–106. Lancaster: Medical and Technical Publishing 1973

Knight, G.C.: Bi-frontal stereotactic tractotomy: an atraumatic operation of value in the treatment of intractable psychoneurosis. I. Br. J. Psychiatry **115**, 257–266 (1969)

Kukka, E.-K., Vilkki, J., Laitinen, L.: Effects of subcortical stimulation and coagulation on subtraction performance. Neuropsychologia **14**, 137–140 (1976)

Kullberg, G.: Differences in effect of capsulotomy and cingulotomy. In: Neurosurgical treatment in psychiatry, pain, and epilepsy. Sweet, W.H., Obrador, S., Martín-Rodríguez, J.G. (eds.), pp. 301–308. Baltimore: University Park Press 1977

Laitinen, L., Toivakka, E., Vilkki, J.: Rostralnaya tsingulotomia pri psikhitseskih narusheniyah. Vopr. Neirokhir. **1**, 23–30 (1973)

Laitinen, L.V.: Stereotactic lesions in the knee of the corpus callosum in the treatment of emotional disorders. Lancet **1972 I**, 472–475

Laitinen, L.V.: Differential effects of various psychosurgical approaches. In: ICS No. 320. Recent progress in neurological surgery. Sano, K., Ischii, S. (eds.), pp. 256–260. Amsterdam: Excerpta Medica 1973

Laitinen, L.V.: Psychosurgery on trial. Lancet **1975 II**, 131–132

Laitinen, L.V., Vilkki, J.: Stereotaxic ventral anterior cingulotomy in some psychological disorders. In: Psychosurgery. Hitchcock, E., Laitinen, L., Vaernet, (eds.), pp. 242–252. Springfield (Ill.): Charles C. Thomas 1972

Laitinen, L.V., Vilkki, J.: Observations on the transcallosal emotional connections. In: Surgical approaches in psychiatry. Laitinen, L.V., Livingston, K.E. (eds.), pp. 74–80. Lancaster: Medical and Technical Publishing 1973a

Laitinen, L.V., Vilkki, J.: Electrophysiological and psychological studies on the function of the rostral cingulum and the knee of the corpus callosum in man. Psychiatr. Fenn. **3**, 249–259 (1973b)

Leksell, L.: A stereotaxic apparatus for intracerebral surgery. Acta Chir. Scand. **99**, 229–233 (1949)

Mark, V.H., Sweet, W.H., Ervin, F.R.: The effect of amygdalotomy on violent behaviour in patients with temporal lobe epilepsy. In: Psychosurgery. Hitchcock, E., Laitinen, L., Vaernet, K. (eds.), pp. 139–155. Springfield (Ill.): Charles C. Thomas 1972

Medical Record: Editorial **151**, 335 (1940)

Meyer, A., Beck, E.: Prefrontal leucotomy and related operations. Anatomical aspects of success or failure. Henderson Trust Lecture 17. Edinburgh, London: Oliver and Boyd 1954

Meyer, G., McElhaney, M., Martin, W., McGraw, C.P.: Stereotactic cingulotomy with results of acute stimulation and serial psychological testing. In: Surgical approaches in psychiatry. Laitinen, L.V., Livingston, K.E. (eds.), pp. 39–58. 1973 Lancaster: Medical and Technical Publishing

Mitchell-Heggs, N., Kelly, D., Richardson, A.E.: Stereotactic limbic leucotomy: clinical, psychological, and physiological assessment at 16 months. In: Neurosurgical treatment in psychiatry, pain, and epilepsy. Sweet, W.H., Obrador, S., Martín-Rodríguez, J.G. (eds.), pp. 367–379. Baltimore: University Park Press 1977

Moniz, E.: Tentatives opératoires dans le traitement de certaines psychoses. Paris: Masson 1936
Mueller, D., Roeder, F., Orthner, H.: Further results of stereotaxis in the human hypothalamus in sexual deviations. First use of this operation in addiction to drugs. Neurochirurgia (Stuttg.) 16, 113–126 (1973)
Nádvorník, P., Pogády, J., Šramka, M.: The results of stereotactic treatment of the aggressive syndrome. In: Surgical approaches in psychiatry. Laitinen, L.V., Livingston, K.E. (eds.), pp. 125–128. Lancaster: Medical and Technical Publishing 1973
Nádvorník, P., Šramka, M., Patoprstá, G.: Transventricular anterior hypothalamotomy in stereotactic treatment of hedonia. In: Neurosurgical treatment in psychiatry, pain, and epilepsy. Sweet, W.H., Obrador, S., Martín-Rodríguez, J.G. (eds.), pp. 445–449. Baltimore: University Park Press 1977
Narabayashi, H.: Stereotaxic amygdalotomy. In: Advances in behavioral biology. Elefteriou, B.E. (ed.), Vol. II, pp. 459–483. New York: Plenum 1972
Narabayashi, H., Shima, F.: Which is the better amygdala target, the medial or lateral nuclei? (For behaviour problems and paroxysm in epileptics.) In: Surgical approaches in psychiatry. Laitinen, L.V., Livingston, K.E. (eds.), pp. 129–134. Lancaster: Medical and Technical Publishing 1973
Narabayashi, H., Nagao, T., Saito, Y., Yoshida, M., Nagahato, M.: Stereotaxic amygdalotomy for behavior disorders. Arch. Neurol. 9, 1–16 (1963)
Nauta, W.J.H.: The problem of the frontal lobe: a reinterpretation. J. Psychiatr. Res. 8, 167–187 (1971)
Papez, J.W.: A proposed mechanism of emotion. Arch. Neurol. Psychiatr. 38, 725–743 (1937)
Pippard, J.: Rostral leucotomy: a report on 240 cases personally followed up after $1^{1}/_{2}$ to 5 years. Br. J. Psychiatry 118, 141–154 (1955)
Puusepp, L.: Alcune considerazioni sugli interventi chirurgici nelle malattie mentali. Gior. Accad. Med. Torino 100, 3–16 (1937)
Research Committee, The Royal College of Psychiatrists: Evaluation of the surgical treatment of functional mental illness: Proposal for a prospective controlled trial. In: Neurosurgical treatment in psychiatry, pain, and epilepsy. Sweet, W.H., Obrador, S., Martín-Rodríguez, J.G. (eds.), pp. 175–188. Baltimore: University Park Press 1977
Richardson, A.E., Kelly, D., Mitchell-Heggs, N.: Lesion site determination in stereotactic limbic leucotomy. In: Neurosurgical treatment in psychiatry, pain, and epilepsy. Sweet, W.H., Obrador, S., Martín-Rodríguez, J.G. (eds.), pp. 363–379. Baltimore: University Park Press 1977
Riechert, T., Wolff, M.: Zielgerät zur intrakraniellen elektrischen Ableitung und Ausschaltung mit besonderer Berücksichtigung der Eingriffe am Trigeminus. Nervenarzt 22, 437 (1951)
Roeder, F.: Stereotaxic lesions of the tuber cinereum in sexual deviation. Confin. Neurol. 27, 162–163 (1966)
Roeder, F., Mueller, D.: Zur stereotaktischen Heilung der pädophilen Homosexualität. Dtsch. Med. Wochenschr. 94, 409–415 (1969)
Roeder, F., Orthner, H., Mueller, D.: The stereotaxic treatment of pedophilic homosexuality and other sexual deviations. In: Psychosurgery. Hitchcock, E., Laitinen, L., Vaernet, K. (eds.), pp. 87–111. Sprinfield (Ill.): Charles C. Thomas 1972
Rylander, G.: Personality analysis before and after frontal lobotomy. Res. Publ. Assoc. Res. Nerv. Ment. Dis. 27, 691–705 (1948)
Sano, K.: Sedative neurosurgery. With special reference to postero-medial hypothalamotomy. Neurol. Med. Chir. (Tokyo) 4, 112–142 (1962)
Sano, K., Sekino, H., Mayanagi, Y.: Results of stimulation and destruction of the posterior hypothalamus in cases with violent, aggressive, or restless behaviours. In: Psychosurgery. Hitchcock, E., Laitinen, L., Vaernet, K. (eds.), pp. 57–75. Springfield (Ill.): Charles C. Thomas 1972
Schaltenbrand, G., Bailey, P.: Einführung in die stereotaktischen Operationen mit einem Atlas des menschlichen Gehirns. Stuttgart: Thieme 1959
Schneider, H.: Psychic changes in sexual delinquency after hypothalamotomy. In: Neurosurgical treatment in psychiatry, pain, and epilepsy. Sweet, W.H., Obrador, S., Martín-Rodríguez, J.G. (eds.), pp. 463–468. Baltimore: University Park Press 1977
Schvarcz, J.R., Driollet, R., Rios, E., Betti, O.: Stereotactic hypothalamotomy for behaviour disorders. Neurol. Neurosurg. Psychiatr. 35, 356–359 (1972)

Scoville, W.B.: Selective cortical undercutting as a means of modifying and studying frontal lobe function in man. J. Neurosurg. **6**, 65–73 (1949)

Scoville, W.B.: Late results of orbital undercutting: reports of 76 patients undergoing quantitative selective lobotomies. Am. J. Psychiatry **117**, 525–532 (1960)

Smith, W.K.: The functional significance of the rostral cingular cortex as revealed by its response to electrical stimulation. J. Neurophysiol. **8**, 241–255 (1945)

Spiegel, E.A., Wycis, H.T., Marks, M., Lee, A.J.: Stereotaxic apparatus for operations on the human brain. Science **106**, 349–350 (1947)

Ström-Olsen, R., Carlisle, S.: Bi-frontal stereotactic tractotomy. Br. J. Psychiatry **118**, 141–154 (1971)

Talairach, J., Hecaen, H., David, M., Monnier, M., de Ajuriaguerra, J.: Recherches sur la coagulation thérapeutique des estructures sous-corticales chez l'homme. Rev. Neurol. (Paris) **81**, 4–24 (1949)

Talairach, J., David, M., Tournoux, P., Corredor, H., Kvasina, T.: Atlas d'anatomie stéréotaxique. Paris: Masson 1957

Teuber, H.-L., Corkin, S.H., Twitchell, T.E.: Study of cingulotomy in man: a summary. In: Neurosurgical treatment in psychiatry, pain, and epilepsy. Sweet, W.H., Obrador, S., Martín-Rodríguez, J.G. (eds.), pp. 355–362. Baltimore: University Park Press 1977

Tooth, G.C., Newton, M.P.: Leucotomy in England and Wales 1942–1954. London: Her Majesty's Stationary Office (HMSO) 1961

Uchimura, Y., Narabayashi, H.: Stereotaxic instrument for operation on the basal ganglia. Psychiatr. Neurol. Jpn. **52**, 265–270 (1951)

Vaernet, K., Madsen, A.: Stereotaxic amygdalotomy and basofrontal tractotomy in psychotics with aggressive behaviour. Neurol. Neurosurg. Psychiatr. **33**, 858–863 (1970)

Valenstein, E.S.: Brain control. New York: Wiley & Sons 1973

Viets, H.R.: Editorial. N. Engl. J. Med. **1241**, 1025–1026 (1949)

Vilkki, J.: Late psychological and clinical effects of subrostral cingulotomy and anterior mesoloviotomy in psychiatric illness. In: Neurosurgical treatment in psychiatry, pain, and epilepsy. Sweet, W.H., Obrador, S., Martín-Rodríguez, J.G. (eds.), pp. 253–259. Baltimore: University Park Press 1977

Ward, A.A., Jr.: The anterior cingular gyrus and personality. Res. Publ. Assoc. Res. Nerv. Ment. Dis. **27**, 438–445 (1948)

Soziobiologie der Primaten

Von

D. Ploog

Inhalt

Einleitung	380
Perspektiven der Verhaltensbiologie	381
A. Kommunikationsprozesse	383
1. Soziale Signale der Primaten	383
2. Kommunikative Gesten	398
3. Vokale Signale bei Affen	425
4. Vokale Signale und Signalerkennung beim Menschen	434
B. Hirnstrukturen und -funktionen im Kommunikationsprozeß	444
1. Hirnevolution und Kommunikationsprozesse	444
2. Postulierte Determinanten für die zerebrale Erzeugung von Signalen	446
3. Einige Prinzipien der neuralen Organisation des Verhaltens	447
4. Zerebrale Korrelate emotionalen Verhaltens	452
C. Sozialisationsprozesse	487
1. Die Mutter-Kind-Dyade der Affen	488
2. Störungen der Sozialisation: Isolation und Deprivation bei Affen- und Menschenkindern	496
D. Von der Kommunikation zur Sprache	503
1. Das kommunikative Vermögen des Schimpansen	504
2. Gemeinsamkeiten bei Schimpanse und Kind im Erwerb von Zeichensprache und Sprache	515
3. Die phono-audio-visuelle Kommunikation des Säuglings	517
Literatur	523

„Der stammesgeschichtliche Aufbau der menschlichen Persönlichkeit hat sich in unendlich langsamer Entwicklung, in unzähligen feinen, kaum merklichen Fortschritten vollzogen; auch Rückschritte werden vorgekommen sein; Nebenwege wurden eingeschlagen und wieder verlassen. Das Endergebnis dieser unabsehbaren Entwicklung enthält naturgemäß Spuren und Überbleibsel aus den verschiedensten Abschnitten der Stammesgeschichte, mag auch die ungeheuere Mehrzahl einstmals herausgebildeter und dann überwundener Einrichtungen völlig verlorengegangen sein. Wenn wir daher heute versuchen, die Äußerungen des Irreseins mit den einzelnen Entwicklungsstufen der Persönlichkeit in Beziehung zu setzen, so fehlen uns dafür fast alle Voraussetzungen. Sollen diese Versuche über ein unsicheres Tasten hinausgelangen, so wird es notwendig sein, die Erscheinungen unseres Innenlebens überall auf ihre Wurzeln in der Seele des Kindes, des Naturmenschen, des Tieres zurückzuverfolgen, ferner zu prüfen, wieweit in Krankheitszuständen verschollene Regungen aus der Vorzeit der persönlichen und stammesgeschichtlichen Entwicklung neues Leben gewinnen. Die Ausblicke, die eine derartige Betrachtungsweise gewährt, scheinen mir trotz der Kümmerlichkeit unseres heutigen Wissens ermutigende zu sein; sie könnten mit dazu beitragen, uns unsere so unendlich schwierige Hauptaufgabe, das klinische Verständnis der Krankheitsformen, zu erleichtern."

EMIL KRAEPELIN, 1920

Einleitung

Die Psychiatrie ist in ihrer Theoriebildung über die Entstehung seelischer Störungen und Krankheiten auf sehr heterogene Wissensbestände angewiesen. Mehr als andere Disziplinen ist sie zudem Modeströmungen unterworfen, in denen zu Zeiten Akzente gesetzt werden, die von den theoriefördernden wissenschaftlichen Erkenntnissen ablenken. Trotz der raschen Zunahme unseres Wissens sind die Hauptgegenstände psychiatrischer Grundlagenforschung kontrovers: Die Bedeutung von Anlage und Umwelt – die Herkunft, Entstehung und Modifizierbarkeit der Triebe, Affekte und Gefühle – die Prozesse, die zur Wahrnehmung und zum Erkennen führen, die Gedächtnis und Lernen ermöglichen – die Determinanten des Sozialverhaltens und der Kommunikationsprozesse.

Zu diesen Themen kann die Verhaltensbiologie einen beträchtlichen Beitrag leisten und hat das Denken in der Psychopathologie während des vergangenen Jahrzehnts in neue Bewegung versetzt (WHITE, 1974; JANZARIK, 1974; KRANZ u. HEINRICH, 1975; McGUIRE u. FAIRBANKS, 1977). Im Kapitel „Verhaltensforschung und Psychiatrie" der 1. Auflage dieses Werkes (PLOOG, 1964c) habe ich eine Synthese aus Ethologie und vergleichender Psychologie (einschließlich dem Behaviorismus) versucht sowie Hirnstrukturen und neurophysiologische Prozesse beschrieben, die für angeborenes und erlerntes Verhalten in Betracht zu ziehen sind. Wenn auch das damals entwickelte Konzept nach wie vor höchst aktuell und dem heutigen Stand der Forschung angemessen geblieben ist, so sind doch die Ergebnisse der Forschung inzwischen so angewachsen, daß eine neue Darstellung dieser Art im gegebenen Rahmen zum Scheitern verurteilt wäre. Der Leser sei daher auf den früheren Beitrag und auf eine Reihe von inzwischen erschienenen Büchern mit ähnlicher Absicht (COUNT, 1970; HINDE, 1973; BATESON u. KLOPFER, 1975/76; v. CRANACH, 1976) verwiesen.

Wenn wir die Psychiatrie und Psychopathologie unter dem Gesichtspunkt der Verhaltensstörungen sehen, werden wir in der Forschung bestimmte Aspekte des Verhaltens besser an Tieren und speziell an nicht-menschlichen Primaten untersuchen, um unsere Fragestellung experimentell präziser fassen zu können. Damit verfahren wir hinsichtlich der Analyse des Verhaltens und seiner Störungen nicht anders als auch sonst in der experimentellen Medizin, in der das Tierexperiment zur Aufklärung von pathologischen Prozessen einen hervorragenden Platz hat. Doch anders als dort setzt man sich bei solchem Vorgehen in der psychiatrischen Forschung leicht dem Vorwurf des „Biologismus" aus. Damit ist gemeint, daß für die Erfassung menschlichen Verhaltens und Erlebens biologische Denk- und Erklärungsweisen unangemessen seien. Wenn auch der Mensch kein Affe, der Affe kein Hund und der Hund keine Ratte ist, so haben doch alle miteinander bestimmte seelische Eigenschaften gemeinsam, die für die menschliche Psychologie und Psychopathologie eine zentrale Rolle spielen: Ihre Verhaltensentwicklung ist stark umweltabhängig, sie zeigen den Ausdruck von Emotion und Affekten, ihr Verhalten ist durch ihre Lebensgeschichte mitbestimmt und durch Lernprozesse stark modifizierbar (SCOTT, 1964, 1967; HARLOW u. HARLOW, 1965a; MASON, 1965; MICHAEL u. CROOK, 1973). Beim Vergleich von Affe und Mensch ist die Liste der Gemeinsamkeiten am längsten. Wahrscheinlich gibt es überhaupt keine menschliche Fähigkeit, die nicht in einfacher Form und Gestalt auch beim Affen, speziell beim Schimpansen, aufgezeigt werden könnte, einschließlich Sprachelementen, Werkzeuggebrauch, Selbstwahrnehmung und Traditionen (GOODALL, 1965; KORTLANDT, 1965; GALLUP, 1970; EISENBERG u. DILLON, 1971; TELEKI, 1973; KURTH u. EIBL-EIBESFELDT, 1975; PREMACK, 1976a). Natürlich können wir Tiere nicht nach ihren Erlebnissen fragen. Introspektive oder verstehende Psychopathologie kann daher nicht die Domäne der Verhaltensforschung sein. Wohl aber kann man mit ihrer Hilfe die kausalen Zusammenhänge psychischer Störungen (i.S. Jaspers), soweit sie sich als Verhaltensstörungen fassen lassen, erstellen helfen.

Perspektiven der Verhaltensbiologie

Zunächst ist zu klären, was unter Verhaltensbiologie verstanden werden soll. In erster Linie ist die Betrachtungsweise der Ethologie zu nennen, die der Evolution des Verhaltens besondere Beachtung schenkt. Unter diesem Aspekt nimmt der Mensch seinen Platz als der am höchsten organisierte Primat ein. Seine einzigartigen artspezifischen Charakteristika können besser erklärt werden, wenn man sie in naturgeschichtlich vergleichendem Zusammenhang untersucht und als einen Jahrmillionen währenden Prozeß stammesgeschichtlicher Anpassung versteht (Abb. 1). So wie der vergleichende Morphologe und Physiologe sich für die Funktionen der Organe interessiert, fragt der vergleichende Verhaltensforscher nach der (arterhaltenden) Funktion von Verhaltensweisen im Hinblick auf die zu bewältigende Umwelt. Verhalten ist einerseits das Resultat aller inneren Vorgänge, die durch die Strukturen des Organismus hervorgebracht werden, andererseits eine geordnete Aktion in einer umweltbestimmten Situation. Jeder Schritt in der Entwicklung – phylogenetisch und ontogenetisch – kommt durch eine Modifikation der im Organismus vorgegebenen Strukturen als Folge der Interaktion mit der Umwelt zustande. Während in der Phylogenese Mutation und Selektion die Schöpfer und Schrittmacher der strukturellen Veränderungen sind, spielen in der Ontogenese außer den Reifungsvorgängen Lernprozesse die wichtigste – artspezifisch festgelegte – Rolle.

Neue Entwicklungen in der Evolution kommen nicht durch Addition neuer zu den alten Elementen zustande, sondern durch strukturelle Veränderungen des ganzen Organismus. Die sich daraus ergebenden Konsequenzen werden in dem anhaltenden Streitgespräch über „Tier und Mensch" nicht oder kaum je beachtet:

1. Neue Fähigkeiten des Menschen haben ihre spezielle Biologie, die für Homo sapiens charakteristisch ist, z.B. die Biologie der Sprache und des Sprechens mit ihren speziellen Hirnmechanismen und dem entsprechenden typisch menschlichen Stimmapparat.

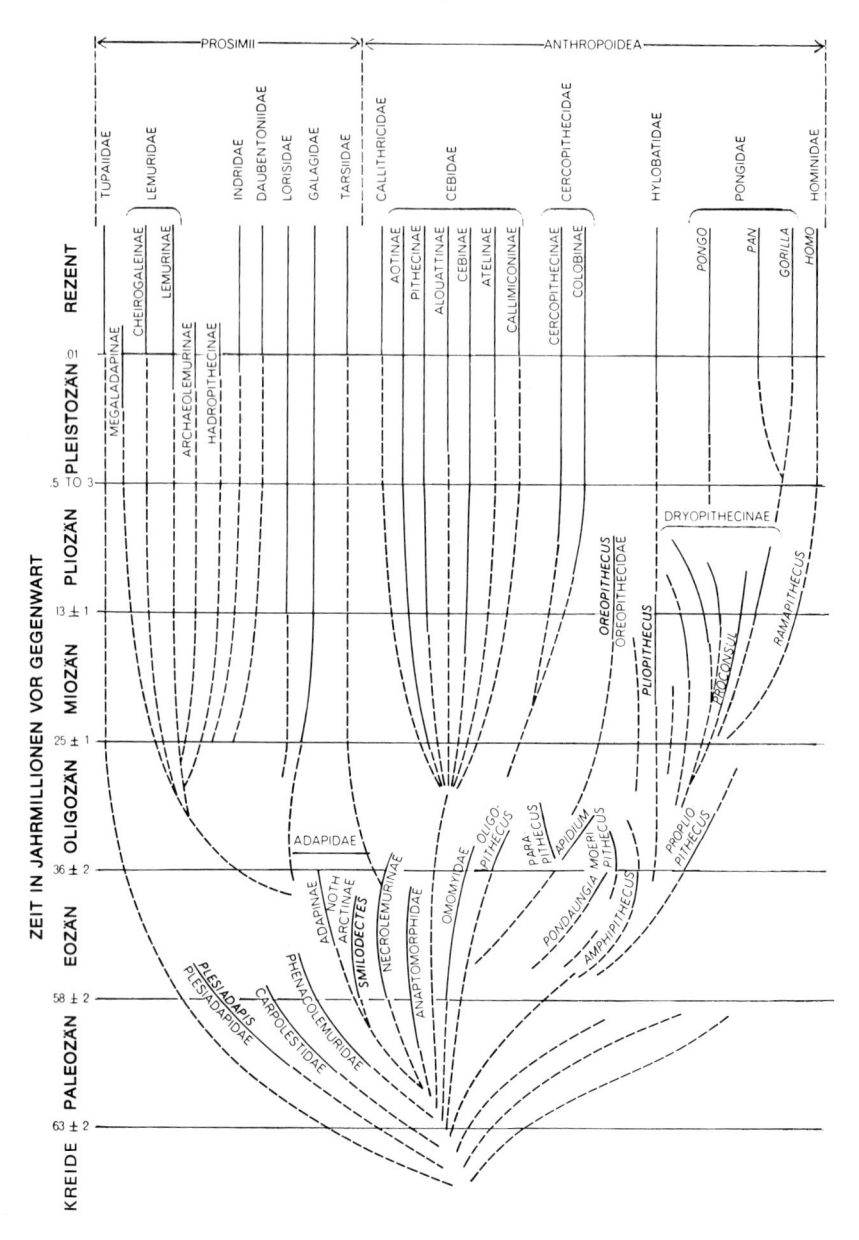

Abb. 1. Stammbaum der Primaten. Die Evolution begann in der Alttertiärzeit in der ersten Hälfte des Paleozäns mit den Subprimaten, die wahrscheinlich von Insektenfressern (Insectivora) abstammten. Die gestrichelten Linien zeigen hypothetische stammesgeschichtliche Verwandtschaften an, die im Zeitraum von Eozän bis zum Miozän besonders ungesichert sind. Einzelne Familien der Prosimii (Halbaffen) und der Anthropoidea kann man bis in das Miozän und das Ende des Oligozäns (25 Millionen Jahre) zurückverfolgen; noch nicht voll spezialisierte Vorformen der Menschenaffen haben vor etwa 15 Millionen Jahren gelebt (Dryopithecinae). Vorformen des Menschen sind wahrscheinlich im Beginn des Pliozäns vor rund 12 Millionen Jahren zuerst aufgetaucht (Ramapithecus). Gerade an der Evolution von Signalen lassen sich Entwicklungen, die zu Verhaltensänderungen führen, besonders gut erkennen. (Aus SIMONS, 1964)

2. Die neuen Fähigkeiten (z.B. Sprechen) nutzen den strukturellen Rahmen älterer Funktionen (z.B. Lautgebungen), deren Biologie dem neuen Entwicklungsschritt angepaßt worden ist.

3. Wo immer wir menschlichen Verhaltensweisen begegnen, die gemeinsame Züge mit nicht-menschlichen Primaten oder auch mit anderen höheren Säugern tragen, müssen wir bedenken, daß dieses Gemeinsamkeiten aufweisende Verhalten dennoch Teil der Gesamtstruktur menschlichen Verhaltens ist.

4. Als Resultat dieser Überlegungen kann man zugespitzt formulieren: Es gibt kein rein „animalisches" Verhalten des Menschen, das aus dem menschlichen Verhalten herausgelöst werden könnte, und umgekehrt gibt es kein rein menschliches Verhalten, das man vom tierischen Verhalten trennen kann.

Die Verhaltensbiologie kehrt die Fragen der Neurobiologie in gewisser Weise um. Während die Neurobiologie durch die Untersuchung von Membranen, Nervenzellen, neuronalen Verbänden und Hirnstrukturen das Verhalten eines Organismus erklären möchte, kommt die Verhaltensbiologie durch die Analyse des Verhaltens zur Erklärung organismischer Funktionen. In diesem Sinne ist auch die Evolution verlaufen, indem die Umwelt Anpassungen des Verhaltens forderte, was Änderungen des Organismus nach sich zog. Mit anderen Worten: man würde z.B. die Funktion eines Flugzeuges nicht durch die Analyse seiner Teile erklären können, wenn man nicht seine Flugeigenschaften untersuchte und wüßte, daß es zum Fliegen bestimmt ist.

Dementsprechend zählen wir alle Forschungsrichtungen zur Verhaltensbiologie, die zum Ziel haben, das Verhalten ganzer Lebewesen – in diesem Beitrag das Verhalten der Primaten – unter dem Gesichtspunkt der Interaktion von Organismus und Umwelt zu analysieren, vorherzusagen und gegebenenfalls zu verändern (WILSON, 1975). Dabei wollen wir uns wegen der engeren Beziehung zu psychopathologischen Fragestellungen auf die Kommunikation und Interaktion mit der sozialen Umwelt konzentrieren. Der Beitrag behandelt daher im wesentlichen die Soziobiologie der Primaten.

A. Kommunikationsprozesse

1. Soziale Signale der Primaten

Soziale Signale sind Mitteilungen von Artgenossen untereinander (LORENZ, 1935; TINBERGEN, 1948, 1952, 1955). Dazu können Bewegungen, Haltungen, Töne, Düfte und Berührungen, aber auch auffallende Farben und Muster dienen. Es ist sicher kein Zufall, daß die sozialen Signale zuerst an Vögeln und bald darauf auch an Fischen entdeckt und genauer untersucht worden sind. Abgesehen davon, daß deren Haltung und Beobachtung einfacher als bei Säugetieren und insbesondere bei Affen ist, nehmen fixierte, stereotype Verhaltensabläufe bei vielen Arten einen hervorragenden, für den Beobachter ins Auge springenden Anteil des Verhaltensrepertoires ein. Diese formstarren Bewegungen eignen sich besonders gut zur Unterscheidung von angeborenem und erworbenem Verhalten. Die Frage nach den angeborenen Formen des Verhaltens war für die sich in den 30er Jahren unter der Führung von LORENZ und TINBERGEN entwickelnde Ethologie von zentraler Bedeutung. Denn nur von dieser Fragestellung her war eine evolutionistisch orientierte Lehre vom Verhalten der Organismen möglich (MAYR, 1960; ANDREW, 1963; SIMONS, 1972) (s. Abb. 1). Das Verhalten der Säugetiere, besonders das der Affen, erschien zunächst schon wegen seines komplexen Aufbaus weniger zur Analyse geeignet. So erschienen die ersten systematischen Studien über das Ausdrucksverhalten von Säugetieren Ende der 40er Jahre, und erst Mitte der 50er Jahre fanden die „klassischen" Studien über das Sozialverhalten der Affen von ZUCKERMAN (1932) und von CARPENTER (1964) ihre Fortsetzung. Inzwischen sind zahlreiche Arbeiten und viele Bücher zu diesem Thema erschienen (BUETTNER-JANUSCH, 1963; SCHRIER et al., 1965, 1971; DE VORE, 1965; ALTMANN, 1967; MORRIS, 1967; CHANCE u. JOLLY, 1970; ROSENBLUM, 1970, 1971a, 1975; DAVIS, 1974; KONDO et al., 1975; JOLLY, 1975). Darin und in anderen Büchern über tierische Kommunikation (SEBEOK, 1977) ist ein großes Material über subhumane Primatenkommunikation zusammengetragen und unter verschiedensten, teils kontroversen Gesichtspunkten diskutiert worden. Unter den Kommunikationsformen hebt sich eine Gruppe heraus, die den Vorgang der Ritualisierung von sozialen Signalen (HUXLEY, 1923, 1966) besonders verdeutlicht.

a) Soziogenitale Signale der Affen

Das charakteristische gemeinsame Merkmal dieser Klasse von Signalen ist das Zurschaustellen der Genitalien und anderer Geschlechtsmerkmale in einer auf den Sozius bezogenen Situation. Diese Situation kann, muß aber nicht auf sexuelles Verhalten im engeren Sinne, d.h. auf die Kopulation, abgestellt sein. Oft besteht ein soziogenitales Signal nicht allein aus einer auffälligen Haltung und Bewegung; ein Farbmerkmal, ein Geruch, eine Berührung oder eine Vokalisation kann dazugehören, so daß auf seiten des Signalempfängers außer dem visuellen Sinn auch andere Sinnesmodalitäten wie Riechen, Fühlen und Hören angesprochen werden. Folgende Beispiele sollen diese Kommunikationsform veranschaulichen.

Der Totenkopfaffe (Saimiri sciureus), auch Totenköpfchen genannt, hat unter den Neuweltaffen wohl das auffälligste soziogenitale Signal entwickelt (PLOOG et al., 1963). Beide Geschlechter benutzen es in allen Altersstufen und in verschiedenen sozialen Situationen (Abb. 2). Das Grundmuster besteht in einer zur Pose erstarrten Bewegung. Beide Hände werden aufgestützt, ein Bein wird angewinkelt und weit abgespreizt. Die starke Auswärtsdrehung setzt sich von der Hüfte bis in den Fuß fort, so daß als eines der charakteristischen Zeichen die große Zehe weiter als sonst je beim Gebrauch des Greiffußes abgespreizt ist (s. Abb. 2a). Kurz vor oder während dieser Bewegung entwickelt sich bei voller Ausprägung des Signals eine maximale Erektion. In enger Stellung kann der Penis den Adressaten berühren (s. Abb. 2b). Bei Weibchen tritt die Klitoris hervor und schwillt sichtbar an. Der Körper ist gewöhnlich aufgerichtet und zeigt einen Buckel im Schulterblattbereich; in weiter Stellung (Abb. 2a) wird der Partner mit den Augen fixiert. Oft ist die Bewegung von je nach Situation

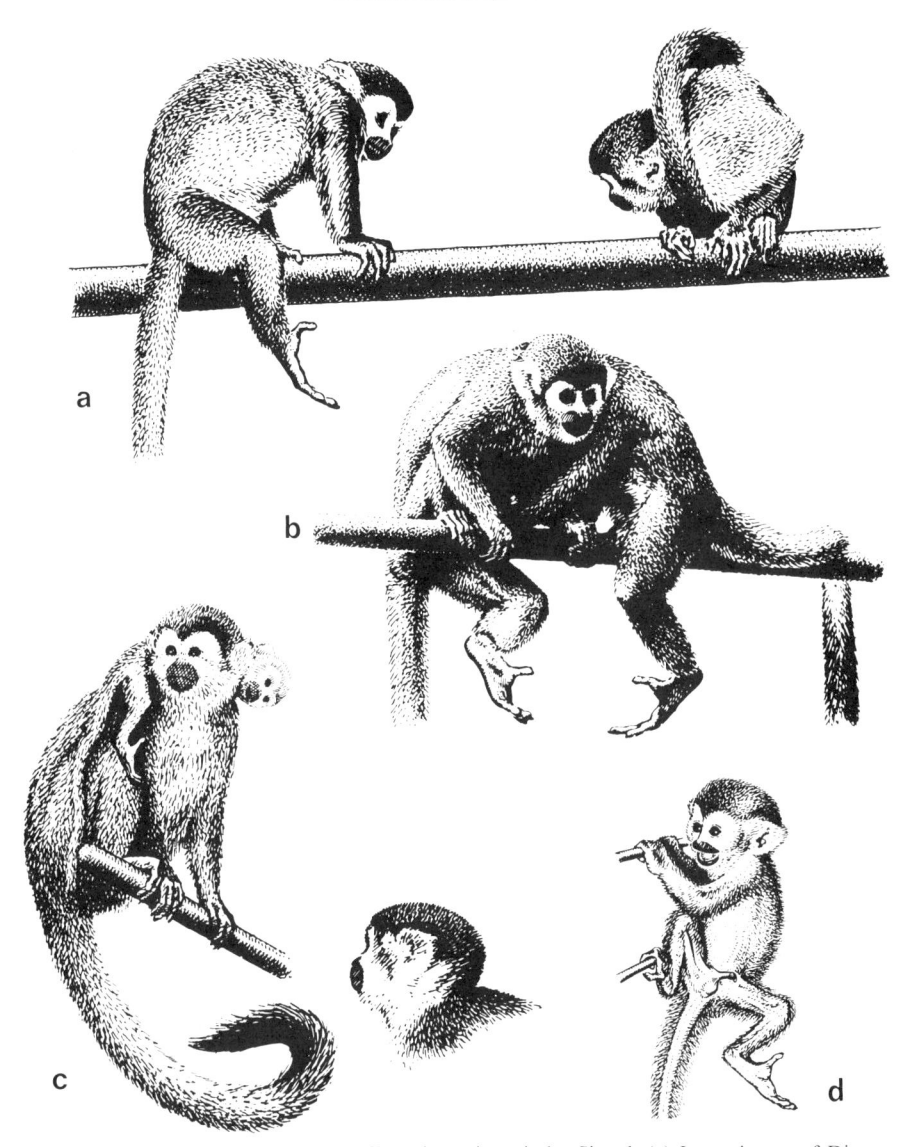

Abb. 2a–d. Imponieren des Totenkopfaffen, ein soziogenitales Signal. (a) Imponieren auf Distanz; imponierender Partner links auf den adressierten Partner rechts gerichtet. (b) Imponieren und Gegenimponieren in enger Stellung; die Tiere „messen sich". (c) Imponieren am zweiten Lebenstag, vom Rücken der Mutter auf einen Gruppengenossen gerichtet; Mund zur Vokalisation geöffnet. (d) 49 Tage altes Männchen imponiert sein Spiegelbild an und vokalisiert (a, b, d nach Photos, c nach Filmaufnahmen gezeichnet von HERMANN KACHER. (Aus PLOOG, 1972)

unterscheidbaren Vokalisationen begleitet. Manchmal, besonders bei Jungtieren, tritt ein Spritzer Urin aus. Das voll ausgeprägte Signal kann in besonderen Situationen minutenlang als Pose nahezu „stillstehen"; gewöhnlich hält es nur für einige Sekunden an, und manchmal tritt es nur andeutungsweise und flüchtig in Erscheinung. Der früheste Zeitpunkt in der Entwicklung, zu dem wir das

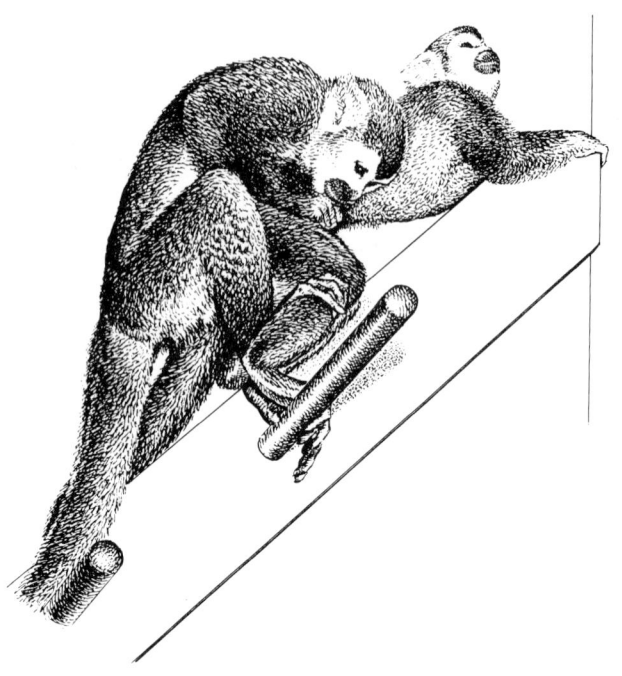

Abb. 3. Kopulationshaltung des Totenkopfaffen (nach Photo gezeichnet von HERMANN KACHER). (Aus LATTA et al., 1967)

Signal mit Sicherheit identifizieren konnten, war der 2. Lebenstag (s. Abb. 2c). Gewöhnlich wird es aber erst nach einigen Wochen beobachtet, wenn das Kind den Rücken der Mutter zeitweise verläßt (s. Abb. 2d). Dann kann es auch auf den Menschen oder auf das eigene Spiegelbild gerichtet sein (PLOOG u. MACLEAN, 1963b). Das weite Auswärtsrotieren des Beines kann man im ganzen Verhaltensrepertoire des Totenköpfchens sonst nur während einer vollen Kopulation sehen. Dabei macht es wie beim Imponieren einen leichten Buckel und gewinnt, wie die meisten Affen auch der alten Welt, durch Umgreifen der Unterschenkel des Weibchens Halt und spreizt beide Oberschenkel maximal (Abb. 3). Beim genitalen Imponieren ist das gesamte Spielbein maximal und das Standbein im Oberschenkel abgespreizt. Die Kopulationshaltung ist zu einem ins Auge springenden Signal abgewandelt. In der Beschreibung des Imponiergehabes beim Grauganter lesen wir bei LORENZ (1965a), daß auch der Unvoreingenommene den Eindruck von etwas Gespanntem, Geziertem empfängt. Das trifft ebenso auf das Totenköpfchen zu. Die sozialen Situationen, in denen das Signal benutzt wird, sind in der Tat immer gespannt.

Unterteilt man soziales Verhalten in zwei große Klassen, nämlich in Wettstreit und Zusammenhalt, in agonistisches und kohäsives Verhalten, so gehört das genitale Imponieren, wie alles Imponiergehabe bei Tier und Mensch, in die agonistische Kategorie. Innerhalb derer gibt es viele soziale Konstellationen, in denen genitales Imponieren angewandt wird, sei es unter Männchen und Weibchen oder Jugendlichen und Kindern. Alle denkbaren Kombinationen sind möglich; lediglich die Häufigkeitsverteilung, in der das Signal benutzt und empfangen wird, weist in einer gegebenen Sozietät signifikante Unterschiede auf. Der Empfänger des Signals, dessen Verhalten beeinflußt werden soll, hat, wie bei allen partnerbezogenen Signalen in Affengesellschaften, mehrere Möglichkeiten der Erwiderung. Das animponierte Totenköpfchen kann sich ducken und stillhalten (s. Abb. 2a), es kann das Imponieren mit Gegenimponieren erwidern (s. Abb. 2b), es kann den Imponierer attackieren, es hat verschiedene Möglichkeiten des Ausweichens, die wiederum von einer Anzahl von Faktoren abhängen. In bestimmten hormonabhängigen Phasen des Werbeverhaltens kann das Imponieren z.B. die sog. Kokettierflucht des Weibchens auslösen. Sicher ist, daß das Signal primär von der Sozietät „verstanden" wird, wenn auch die Antworten darauf verschieden ausfallen können. Das Signal enthält aggressive und defensive Elemente und reguliert die Distanz des Senders zum Empfänger des Signals. WICKLER (1967a) hat für den stammesgeschichtlich erklärbaren „Verständigungsprozeß", der sich zwischen Sender und Empfänger eines sozialen Signals abspielt, den Terminus Semantisierung vorgeschlagen.

Die für den Semantisierungsprozeß von ihm angegebenen charakteristischen Merkmale treffen fast alle auf das genitale Imponieren zu. Das vermutlich (phylogenetisch) ursprüngliche Verhalten als Teil der Kopulation hat einen Funktionswechsel erfahren und dient der Selbstbehauptung in der Gruppe. Die Bewegung bzw. Haltung hat sich von der sexuellen Motivation gelöst und eine eigene bekommen. Die Bewegung ist vereinfacht worden (keine oder nur wenige, eben angedeutete Hüftstöße, kein Umgreifen) und wirkt zugleich übertrieben. Das genitale Imponieren wird viel häufiger ausgelöst als das Kopulieren, so daß eine Schwellenerniedrigung anzunehmen ist. Das „Stillstehen" der Bewegung, wie es für ritualisierte Drohstellungen so typisch ist, fällt beim genitalen Imponieren des Totenköpfchens besonders auf. Sehr oft „erstarrt" auch der Signalempfänger in einer geduckten Haltung (s. Abb. 2a). Die ursprüngliche Orientierungsrichtung der Bewegung – Aufreiten von hinten – hat sich in ihr Gegenteil verkehrt. Der Sender richtet sich stets möglichst frontal auf den Empfänger, so daß er gut von ihm gesehen werden kann. Auch wenn das Signal gelegentlich über Distanzen von mehreren Metern gesendet wird, fühlt sich immer nur ein bestimmter Kumpan der Gruppe „angesprochen".

Eine andere Gruppe soziogenitaler Signale dient der Aggressionshemmung und Befriedigung. Auch hierfür gibt das Totenköpfchen ein anschauliches Beispiel. Bei Männchen und Weibchen dient das Rückenwälzen mit Rückenscheuern zum Felltrocknen und -reinigen. Es kann provoziert werden, indem man die Tiere naßspritzt. Man sieht Rückenwälzen außerdem nach der Geburt eines Babys, beim Spielen der Jungtiere und nach Erblicken des eigenen Spiegelbildes. Besonders häufig tritt es aber dann auf, wenn einander fremde Gruppen zusammengeführt werden und wenn ein fremdes Männchen in eine Gruppe eingesetzt wird (CASTELL et al., 1969). In diesem Zusammenhang entwickelt sich beim Wälzen häufig eine Erektion, während das fellreinigende Sichscheuern fehlt (Abb. 4). Das Präsentieren der Bauchseite hemmt die Flucht vor dem Eindringling und erleichtert ihm den Kontakt mit der neuen Gruppe.

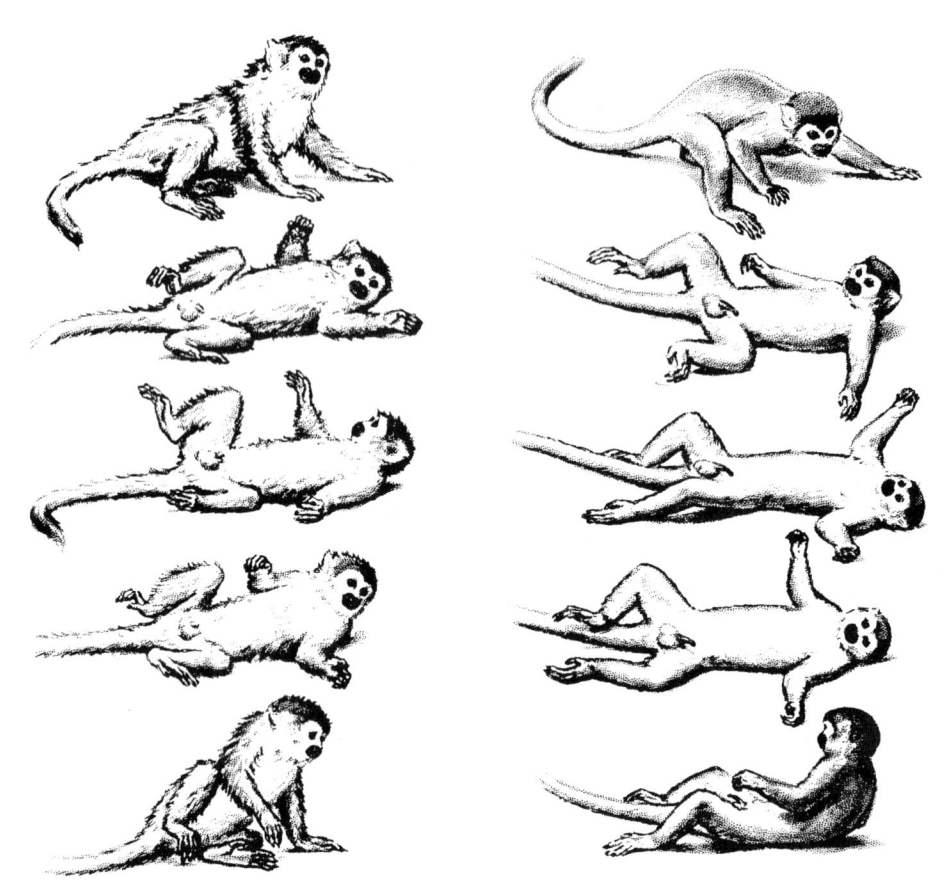

Abb. 4. Körperpflege und ritualisiertes Signal. Linke Bildfolge: Körperpflege: Rückenwälzen mit nassem Fell. Das Tier wälzt sich von einer Seite auf die andere und scheuert sich. Rechte Bildfolge: Soziales Signal: Präsentieren der Bauchseite in Rückenlage. Das Tier liegt, ohne sich zu scheuern, mit ausgebreiteten Armen auf dem Rücken und dreht sich etwas von einer Seite auf die andere. (Aus CASTELL et al., 1969). (Gezeichnet nach Filmaufnahmen von HERMANN KACHER)

Auch hier haben wir es wieder mit einem sozial wirksamen Signal zu tun, das, wie das genitale Imponieren, im Zustand einer Spannung zustande kommt. Die ambivalente Handlungsbereitschaft der Tiere schwankt zwischen Verteidigung und Aggression, zwischen Flucht und Annäherung. Das aus der Körperpflege stammende Signal wird in einer Bewegungsfolge vereinfacht, abgeschliffen und abgewandelt. Das Scheuern fehlt. Die Erektion kommt hinzu. Die Bewegung ist jetzt gerichtet, und zwar auf die fremden Artgenossen. Die auffällige, stereotype Wiederholung zeigt die Ritualisierung an. Es handelt sich um ein offenbar nur von dominierenden Männchen benutztes Fraternisierungssignal.

Dieser eminent soziale Vorgang der Hemmung von agonistischem und der Förderung von kohäsivem Verhalten findet seine besondere Ausprägung bei vielen Altweltaffen, denen allen das sog. Präsentieren gemeinsam ist. Der Schwanz wird erhoben und das Hinterteil dem Partner zugewendet. Mantelpaviane (Papio hamadryas) fallen jedem Zoobesucher durch ihr leuchtend rotes Hinterteil auf, das sich bei den Weibchen im Laufe des Menstruationszyklus in Größe, Form und Farbe ändert, bei den Männchen jedoch dauernd prominent und auffällig bleibt. Man fragt sich sofort, welchen Zweck dieses Phänomen hat. Die auch heute noch am weitesten verbreitete Meinung ist, daß die Schwellungen ein Nebenprodukt der hormonalen Vorgänge sind. Damit wären allenfalls die Veränderungen an der sog. Geschlechtshaut der Weibchen erklärt, nicht aber die Rötung und prominente Form bei den Männchen, die – äußerlich der den Weibchen sehr ähnlich, anatomisch aber eine reine Hauterscheinung – nicht in Zusammenhang mit den äußeren Geschlechtsorganen steht.

Einem unvoreingenommenen Beobachter kann es nicht entgehen, daß das auffallende Hinterteil dieser Affen eine Signalfunktion hat, über die sich übrigens schon DARWIN (1876) Gedanken machte. Weibchen in der follikulären (fertilen) Phase ihres Zyklus präsentieren den Männchen ihre Genitalregion am häufigsten. Mehrere Variationen dieses Präsentierens in verschiedenen Intensitätsstufen zeigt Abb. 5. Wie das Männchen auf dieses Signal reagiert, wird von seinem inneren Zustand (von Motivation, Stimmung oder Handlungsbereitschaft) und von verschiedenen sozialen Faktoren mitbestimmt, die in anderem Zusammenhang zur Sprache kommen. Das Signal kann unbeachtet bleiben, oder es kann sexuelle Handlungen verschiedener Dauer und Intensität auslösen. Es ist fraglich, ob es als solches überhaupt einen erkennbaren Einfluß auf die sexuelle Aktivität

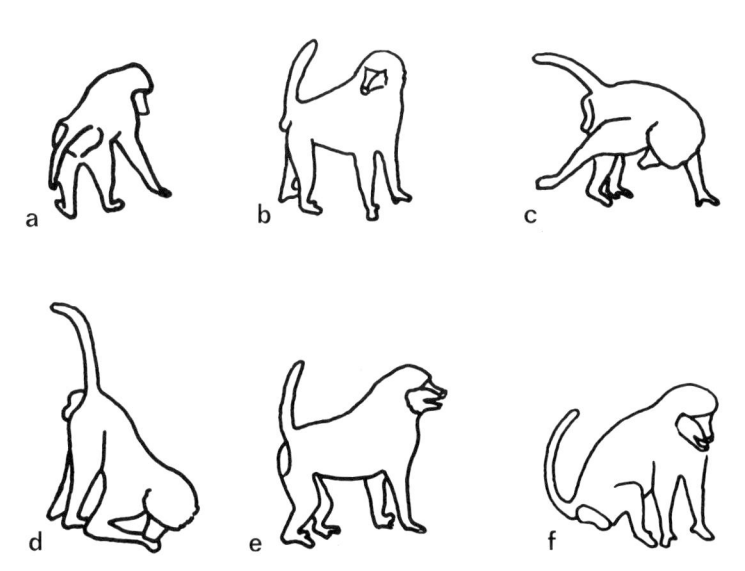

Abb. 5a–f. Verschiedene Variationen des Präsentierens. (a) Zuwendung des Genitalfeldes: Geste der Unterwerfungsbereitschaft und der Kopulationsaufforderung. Der Signalempfänger ist in allen Variationen stets links (hinter) dem präsentierenden Sender zu denken. (b) Steigerung der Intensität dieses Signals. (c) Präsentieren gegenüber vertrautem Partner, auch als Antwort auf dessen Zuwendung. (d) Intensive Kopulationsaufforderung. (e) Präsentieren mit Beinflexion als Ausdruck der Angst, meist vor dem Ranghöheren. (f) „Zweifrontenverhalten": Drohung nach vorn in Form des Brauenziehens, Unterwerfungsbereitschaft nach hinten durch Präsentieren in Sitzstellung. (Aus KUMMER, 1957)

des Männchens hat (ROWELL, 1967). Man sieht das Präsentieren nun aber keineswegs nur bei Weibchen im Östrus. Es kann von Männchen zu Männchen, von Weibchen zu Weibchen, ja auch bei Jungtieren beobachtet werden und wird nicht nur beim Mantelpavian, sondern auch bei anderen Pavianarten, bei verschiedenen Makakenarten, bei der grünen Meerkatze, ja auch bei Schimpansen als Geste der Unterwerfung angesehen. Diese submissive Geste zeigt also eine Rangordnung an und dient zur Beschwichtigung des möglicherweise aggressionsbereiten Ranghöheren. Auch wenn dieser keine Zeichen der Aggression zeigt, wird er mit dieser Geste gleichsam als Rückversicherung und Rangbestätigung „begrüßt". Das Präsentieren hat also eine aggressionshemmende Beschwichtigungsfunktion, die in zahlreichen sozialen Situationen angewendet wird.

WICKLER (1968) hat im Rahmen seiner Untersuchungen über die Mimikry eine neue Erklärung für das rote Hinterteil der Mantelpaviane und anderer Angehöriger dieser ganzen Unterfamilie der Cercopithecinae gegeben: das rote Hinterteil wird bei Männchen und Weibchen besonders beim Präsentieren sichtbar (Abb. 6). Es wirkt als Signalverstärkung. In einer streng hierarchisch gegliederten Gesellschaft, wie in der der Mantelpaviane (KUMMER, 1968), muß es von adaptivem Vorteil für die Männchen sein, möglichst effektive aggressionshemmende Signale aussenden zu können. Das Präsentieren der Weibchen, sei es als Kopulationsaufforderung oder als submissive Geste, besitzt diese Hemmungsfunktion. Die Männchen haben daher bei manchen Arten ein Hinterteil ausgebildet, das dem der Weibchen im Östrus stark ähnelt. Unter vielen Beispielen, die diese Erklärung von morphologischer und verhaltensphysiologischer Seite her untermauern, sind zwei besonders wichtig:

Die grau-grüne Meerkatze zeichnet sich durch besondere Farbenprächtigkeit aus. Das Perineum des Männchens ist bläulich und das Skrotum leuchtend blau. Von diesem Blau setzt sich der Penis in retrahiertem Zustand leuchtend rot ab. Diese blaurote „Kokarde" ist sowohl von vorne als auch beim Präsentieren von hinten sichtbar und ahmt zusammen mit dem Rot der Analgegend das anogenitale Muster des Weibchens im Österus auffällig nach (WICKLER, 1967b; EIBL-EIBESFELDT, 1978).

Eine Imitation des anogenitalen Musters, die noch unwahrscheinlicher ist, wurde schon in der Literatur des vorigen Jahrhunderts beschrieben. Das geschlechtsreife Weibchen des sog. Nacktbrustpavians oder Dschelada hat auf der Brust eine stundenglasförmige, nackte, rote Fläche, die von weißen, perlartigen Hautklunkern wie von einer Halskette umrandet ist (NAPIER u. NAPIER, 1967). Die Brustwarzen liegen rot gefärbt nahe der Mittellinie und imitieren in Farbe und relativer Lage die Vulva, während das ganze Brustmuster der weiblichen Anogenitalgegend gleicht. Hautklunker und Farbe beider Regionen treten im Östrus stärker hervor. Das Hinterteil des Männchens ähnelt in diesem Falle nicht dem des Weibchens, hingegen findet sich auch bei ihm der stundenglasförmige, nackte, rote Fleck auf der Brust, allerdings ohne die weißen Hautflekken (s. Abb. 6). Welche Signalfunktion diese Mimikry bei Weibchen und Männchen hat, ist noch unbekannt. Eine der Gesten, die beim Dschelada beobachtet worden ist, ist das Brustdarbieten gegenüber einem Opponenten (WICKLER, 1967b).

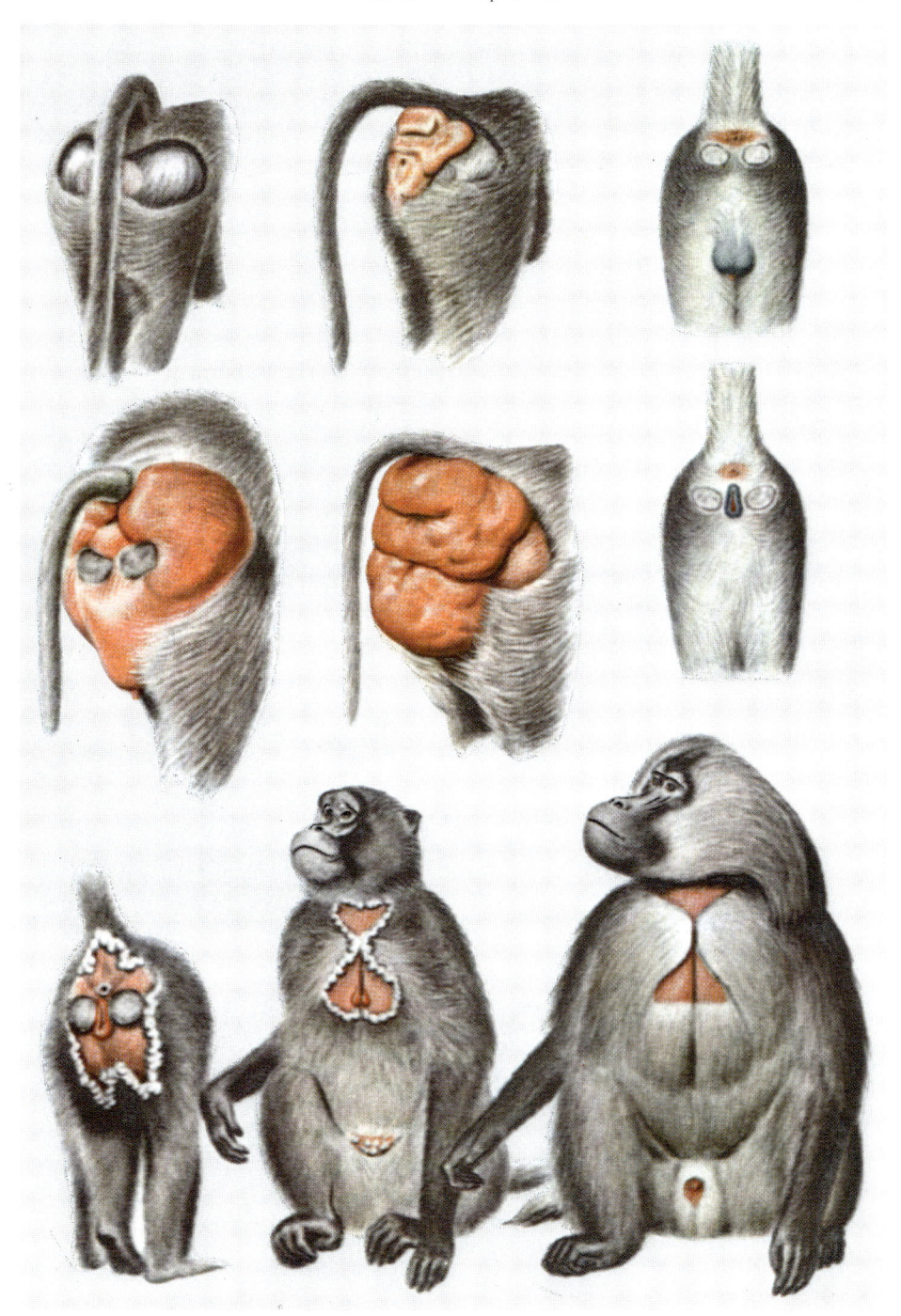

Abb. 6. Ano-genitale Muster und deren Imitation. Von links nach rechts: Oben: Anubis ♂; Anubis ♀ im Oestrus; Grüne Meerkatze ♂. Mitte: Mantelpavian ♀; Mantelpavian ♀ im Oestrus; Graugrüne Meerkatze ♀ im Oestrus. Unten: Nacktbrust-Pavian ♀ Hinterteil, ♀ und ♂ von vorne. (Aus WICKLER, 1967b)

Eine weitere wichtige Funktion des genitalen Imponierens ist bei „wachesitzenden" Pavianen, Meerkatzen, Husarenaffen und Nasenaffen beobachtet worden (HALL, 1960). Unter diesen Vertretern sehr verschiedener Gattungen der großen Altweltaffen-Familie der Schwanzaffen (Cercopithecidae) postiert sich ein männliches Gruppenmitglied an einem Ort mit guter Übersicht und blickt in der Umgebung herum, während der Rest der Gruppe der Nahrungssuche oder anderen Beschäftigungen nachgeht (Abb. 7). Da die Genitalien vieler Arten farbenprächtig hervorgehoben sind, werden sie in der Sitzstellung dieser „Wächter" weithin sichtbar. Bei einigen Arten scheint der Penis während des „Wachesitzens" über längere Zeit erigiert zu sein, bei anderen Arten treten mehrfache rasche Erektionen auf, wenn sich Artgenossen eines anderen Trupps nähern. Das Signal dient offensichtlich dazu, den fremden Trupps die Reviergrenzen anzuzeigen und sie vor dem Eindringen zu warnen (WICKLER, 1967b).

Unter den weit verbreiteten soziogenitalen Signalen haben wir einige ausgewählt, um das Prinzip der Ritualisierung und des Funktionswandels von Signalen im Dienste der Gruppenbildung und der Gruppenorganisation zu demonstrieren.

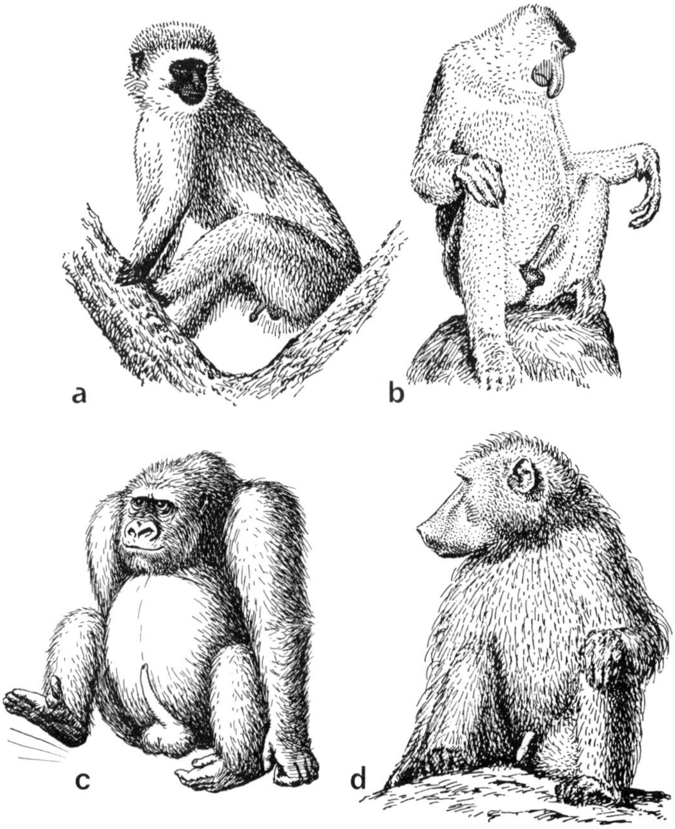

Abb. 7a–d. Genitales Imponieren der „Wächter". (a) Grüne Meerkatze (Cercopithecus aethiops), (b) Nasenaffe (Nasalis larvatus), (c) Anubis (Papio anubis), (d) Schimpanse in Werbe-Positur. (a, b, d aus WICKLER, 1967b; c nach VAN LAWICK-GOODALL, 1975)

Soziogenitale Signale werden auch von Halbaffen und anderen nicht zu den Primaten gehörenden Säugern benutzt, jedoch sind sie eng an das Verhaltensrepertoire gebunden, das zur Fortpflanzung der Art führt, während die soziogenitalen Signale der höheren Primaten (Anthropoidae) (s.Abb. 1) vor allem agonistischen und kohäsiven, damit gruppenformativen Zwecken dienen. Daher ist es oft außerordentlich schwer, den sexuellen Bereich im engeren Sinne abzugrenzen. Besonders bei Beachtung der Ontogenese der Signale gelangt man zu dem Schluß, daß die gruppenbildende Funktion das Primäre geworden ist, der die spätere sexuelle als eine mit der Pubertät einsetzende Spezialisierung und Differenzierung folgt.

b) Die Signalfunktion im Kontext des Verhaltens

Bereits an dieser Stelle sind Bemerkungen über die Kontext-Abhängigkeit einer Signalfunktion notwendig, weil es sich um ein grundsätzliches Prinzip handelt, das für alle Kommunikationsprozesse bis hin zur sprachlichen Mitteilung des Menschen gilt (PLOOG, 1970). Dieses Prinzip besagt, daß die Funktion eines sozialen Signals nur im Zusammenhang seines Auftretens und unter Berücksichtigung der Signalantwort verstanden werden kann. Dies bedeutet zugleich, daß Signal und Signalantwort nicht einem einfach determinierten Reiz-Reaktions-Muster folgen, sondern vielfach determiniert sind (MAURUS u. PRUSCHA, 1972; MAURUS et al., 1975; PRUSCHA u. MAURUS, 1976). Die Funktion eines Signals hängt davon ab, wie der Signalempfänger zu einem bestimmten Zeitpunkt im Laufe der fließenden Ereignisse den Informationsgehalt des Signals in einer bestimmten Situation beantwortet. Die Beantwortung ist von der Art der Wahrnehmung, vom jeweiligen Motivationszustand des Empfängers, von seinem sozialen Status, von seinem Reifegrad und von seiner Vorerfahrung (Lerngeschichte) abhängig. Dies läßt sich in den Grundzügen schon an den behandelten Beispielen soziogenitaler Signale zeigen (PLOOG, 1967, 1968; PLOOG u. MELNECHUK, 1969).

Daß das Signal wahrgenommen werden muß, um vom Empfänger beantwortet werden zu können, scheint selbstverständlich. Tatsächlich wird es aber nicht immer wahrgenommen, und oft mag es zwar wahrgenommen worden sein, wird aber nicht beantwortet. Der Sender muß es wiederholen, seine Position verändern oder eine weitere Sinnesmodalität des Empfängers ansprechen, z.B. dem visuellen Signal ein vokales hinzuzufügen. Die Distanz, aus der ein Signal wahrgenommen wird, spielt für seine Funktion eine wesentliche Rolle (MAURUS u. PLOOG, 1971).

Der Motivationszustand oder – was dasselbe bedeutet – die Stimmung oder Handlungsbereitschaft des Tieres hat einen wesentlichen Einfluß auf die Signalverarbeitung. Genitales Imponieren zwischen zwei Männchen kann z.B. kampfauslösend wirken, wenn die Männchen durch Weibchen im Östrus zur Kopulation motiviert sind; es kann aber unter den gleichen Bedingungen unbeachtet bleiben, wenn die Weibchen der Gruppe nicht im Östrus sind.

Der soziale Status von Sender und Empfänger ist für alle Kommunikationsprozesse von entscheidender Bedeutung. Das genitale Imponieren eines rangniedrigen Männchens gegenüber einem ranghöheren löst in den meisten Fällen aggressive Handlungen des ranghöheren Männchens aus. Ist aber das rangniedrigere Männchen der Adressat, bleibt es geduckt sitzen oder geht aus dem

Wege (PLOOG et al., 1963; MAURUS et al., 1975). Der Reifezustand bzw. das Alter eines Tieres bestimmt in hohem Grade die sozialen Interaktionen in der Gruppe. Das genitale Imponieren eines Neugeborenen (s.Abb. 2c) wird ohne Zweifel wahrgenommen, aber nicht darauf reagiert. Auch das Imponieren des älteren Kindes bleibt für längere Zeit unbeachtet. Spätestens mit dem Ende des ersten Lebensjahres reagiert aber das Alphatier – das ranghöchste Männchen – mit Drohen und auch Attacken gegen das jugendliche Männchen, wenn es

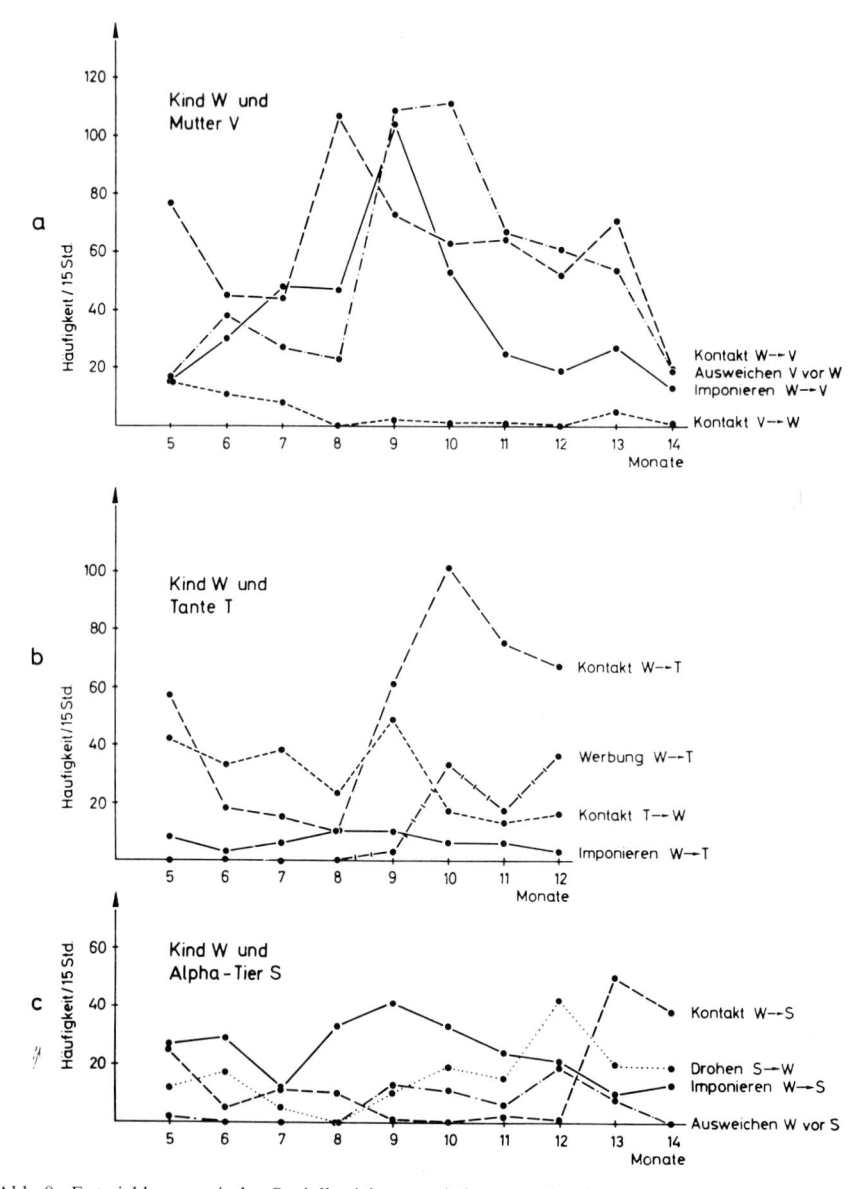

Abb. 8. Entwicklungstypische Sozialbeziehungen beim Totenköpfchen. (Aus PLOOG et al., 1967)

von ihm animponiert wird. Die rollenabhängigen Beziehungen, die das heranwachsende Junge seinen hauptsächlichen Partnern – Mutter, „Tante" und Alphatier – gegenüber zeigt, können wir dem Beispiel in Abb. 8 entnehmen (PLOOG et al., 1967; PLOOG, 1969b; HOPF, 1971, 1978).

c) Soziogenitale Signale des Menschen

Daß auch der Mensch – früher mehr als heute – soziogenitale Signale zur Kommunikation benutzt, lehren Beobachtung und zahlreiche kulturelle Dokumente (MACLEAN, 1962; PLOOG, 1966b; WICKLER, 1966; KOENIG, 1970; EIBL-EIBESFELDT, 1978). Dabei spielen männliche Signale, die den Penis direkt oder verborgen zur Schau stellen, die Hauptrolle, während für weibliche Signale nur sekundäre Geschlechtsmerkmale benutzt werden. Funktion und Bedeutung der männlichen Signale sind komplex und mehrfach determiniert. Eine Komponente besteht in der Demonstration von Herrschaft, Macht und Kraft. Herrscher und Gottheiten werden mit großem Phallus dargestellt, wie z.B. Amun-Re im Tempel von Karnak. Auf Abb. 9 empfängt der Herrscher den Segen der Gottheit. In anderem Zusammenhang hat das genitale Präsentieren eine defensive Komponente, wie z.B. bei den „Wächtern", die mit dem Rücken zum Feld oder Haus, das sie bewachen, gekehrt sind (WICKLER, 1966) (Abb. 10). HERODOT hält diese Hermen für sehr alt und aus Vorzeiten überbracht. In manchen Teilen der Erde, wie in Borneo und Nias, leben sie bis auf den heutigen Tag als Hauswächter fort; in Bali und auf den Nikobaren werden sie als Fetische gegen böse Geister benutzt (EIBL-EIBESFELDT u. WICKLER, 1968). In Neu-Guinea werden Penis-Futterale verschiedener Länge und Form getragen. Sie dienen zum „Imponieren" – als Schmuck und Rangabzeichen (WICKLER, 1970). Auch in Europa wurden Zeichen der Männlichkeit auf Rüstungen, Kriegerkleidung und Uniform bis in die jüngere Geschichte hinein ausgeschmückt und plastisch hervorgehoben (Abb. 11). Diese Tendenz setzte sich in den Husaren-Hosen vieler Nationen in Form von Stickereien und Fransenbesätzen fort und ist als Relikt z.B. im geschmückten Latz der bayerischen Lederhose zu erkennen. OTTO KOENIG (1970) schreibt in seiner Kulturethologie über die Regeln kultureller Abwandlungen

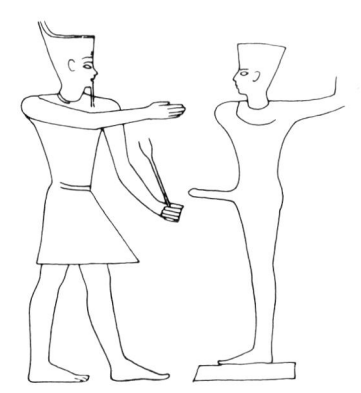

Abb. 9. Macht, Kraft und Segen. Ammun-Ré, XII. Dynastie. Karnak-Tempel Ägypten. (Aus WICKLER, 1967b)

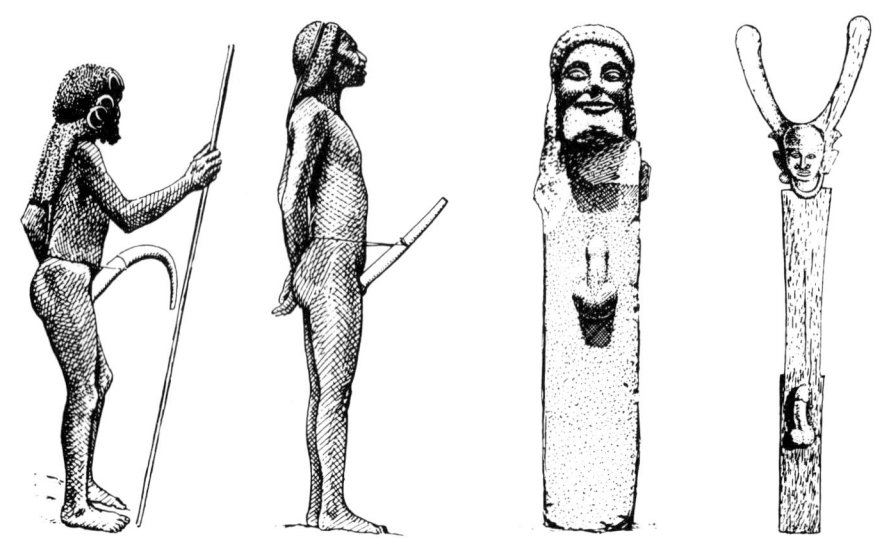

Abb. 10. Genitalpräsentieren beim Menschen. Links: zwei Papuas aus Kogume am Fluß Konca; daneben: Herme von Siphnos (490 v.Chr.), 66 cm hoch, Athen, Nationalmuseum. Rechts: Hauswächter („Siraha") der Eingeborenen der Insel Nias. Die mannshohen Figuren sind auch heute noch in Gebrauch. Bei der griechischen Statue wird der Bart als männliches Merkmal hervorgehoben, bei bartlosen Völkern betont man den männlichen Kopfputz. (Aus WICKLER, 1966)

von Uniformen und Landsknechtskleidung: „Auch hier waltet wiederum sichtbar das phylogenetisch-biologische Prinzip, funktionslos gewordenes Altes, sofern es sich nicht abträglich auswirkt, beizubehalten und, wo notwendig, in neuerlich Brauchbares umzuformen" (S. 78).

Bei der Diskussion über das genitale Imponieren taucht immer wieder die Frage auf, ob man daraus auch Erkenntnisse über den Exhibitionisten, seine Motivation und sein Verhalten gewinnen könne. Der Vergleich drängt sich geradezu auf, wenn man von Volksbräuchen liest, in denen Mädchen von Burschen durch das Präsentieren von Penisattrappen schockiert werden (UJVARY, 1966). Ohne auf die durchaus nicht so einheitliche Psychopathologie des Exhibitionismus einzugehen, sei doch so viel gesagt, daß beim Exhibitionieren ein soziogenitales Signal, das sonst nur noch ausnahmsweise im Dienste sexueller Funktionen steht, sekundär in einen sexuellen Akt zurückverwandelt wird. Das Gemeinsame von genitalem Präsentieren und Exhibitionieren liegt in der Ambivalenz zwischen Annäherung und Flucht, in der sich Imponierverhalten typischerweise abspielt. Penis-Präsentieren und Exhibitionieren geschehen in agonistischer Spannung und stehen im Zeichen der Selbstbehauptung. In beiden Fällen spielen Distanzen zum Partner eine große Rolle. Der Penis der „Wächter" erigiert, wenn der artgenössische fremde Trupp sich allzu sehr nähert. Das defensive genitale Imponieren der Totenköpfchen geschieht auf Distanz. Der Exhibitionist will die Distanz und scheut die Nähe, es sei denn, er befindet sich während des Aktes an sicherem Ort, z.B. am Flußufer, während Kanus mit Mädchen vorbeitreiben. JONES und FREI (1977) haben die Distanzempfind-

Kommunikationsprozesse 397

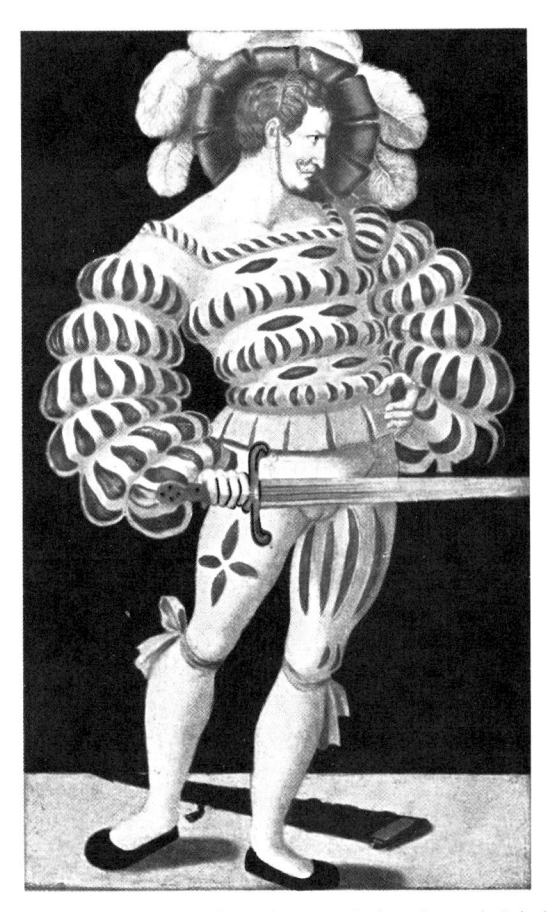

Abb. 11. Ein Landsknecht in imponierender Pose. Lukas Cranach-Schule, ca. 1545

lichkeit des Exhibitionisten zu einer einfachen und überraschend wirkungsvollen Verhaltenstherapie benutzt: Der Patient, der sich zuvor mit der ihm bevorstehenden Prozedur einverstanden erklärt hat, muß sich vor Ärzten und Schwestern ausziehen, während diese im Kreis um ihn herumsitzen und ihre Stühle näherrücken, bis der Patient, dann vollständig entkleidet, halt sagt. Nach einer bis mehreren Sitzungen sind viele Patienten auch nach vorangegangener jahrelanger Rückfälligkeit geheilt oder kommen selten zu prophylaktischen Wiederholungssitzungen freiwillig zur Behandlung zurück.

Ein wesentlicher Unterschied zwischen den hier besprochenen soziogenitalen Signalen und dem exhibitionistischen Verhalten liegt in der Wahl des Adressaten. WICKLER (1967b) betont mit Recht, daß die männlichen soziogenitalen Signale vorwiegend an männliche Artgenossen adressiert sind, während das Zur-Schau-Stellen der männlichen Genitalien weiblichen Artgenossen gegenüber keine erkennbare Wirkung hat oder jedenfalls nicht der Erhöhung der Paarungsbereitschaft dient. Neben den beschriebenen soziogenitalen Signalen gibt es noch andere Gesten, die sich auf die Genitalien beziehen, ohne eine sexuelle Funktion zu haben. So beschreibt JANE GOODALL (1965) z.B. von ihren Schimpansen am Gombe-Fluß, daß sie sich bei Begegnungen mit dem Finger oder der Hand wie zum Grüßen an den Lippen, dem Skrotum oder der Genitalgegend berühren. Es handelt sich um eine Berührungsgeste, mit der das begrüßte Tier gleichsam seines sozialen Status versichert wird. Auch in der menschlichen Gesellschaft wurden Versicherungen im Sinne von Schwüren durch Berührung der Genitalien des Ranghöheren abgegeben. MACLEAN (1962) weist in ähnlichem Zusammenhang auf das Alte Testament, Genesis 24 hin, wo Abraham alt geworden und wohlbetagt „zu seinem ältesten Knecht seines Hauses, der allen seinen Gütern vorstand", sprach: „Lege deine Hand unter meine Hüfte und schwöre mir bei dem Herrn, dem Gott des Himmels und der Erde, daß du meinem Sohn kein Weib nehmest von den Töchtern der Kananiter, unter welchen ich wohne". Daß die Hüfte stellvertretend für das Genitale steht, liest man auch bei THOMAS MANN in der Josefslegende. Vielleicht ist das Schwören bei dem Barte eine weitere Abwandlung dieser ursprünglichen Geste.

2. Kommunikative Gesten

Außer den soziogenitalen Signalen gibt es eine große Zahl von kommunikativen Gesten, deren stammesgeschichtlicher Ursprung zumindest wahrscheinlich gemacht werden kann (LORENZ, 1953). Diese Gesten betreffen samt und sonders die sozialen Beziehungen, die Individuen miteinander eingehen wollen oder miteinander haben und drücken gleichzeitig Wünsche oder Befürchtungen aus. Wie die sozialen Signale im allgemeinen, haben auch sie eine informative und eine emotionale Komponente. Die Funktionen der Gesten können in größere Klassen eingeteilt werden: Grüßen, Annäherung, Abwendung, Anerkennung, Ablehnung, Übereinstimmung, Dominanz und Submission, Werbung, Paarung und Aufzucht. Einige Beispiele sollen dies verdeutlichen.

Außer der Mimik und der Stimme, die in den nächsten Kapiteln behandelt werden, wird die Hand der Primaten (RENSCH, 1968) am häufigsten zur Kommunikation eingesetzt. Wenn das Kleinkind etwas haben möchte, streckt es die Hand mit nach oben geöffneter Fläche aus. Dasselbe tut das Schimpansenmädchen Washoe spontan; die Geste wurde dann von ihren Lehrern zum Erlernen der Zeichensprache als Zeichen für „gib mir mal" benutzt (s.S. 507). Die Hand wird auch in vielfachen Abwandlungen ihrer Stellung und Bewegung zum Grüßen verwendet (Abb. 12). Schimpansen strecken bei einer Begegnung die offene Hand aus. Man kommt jemandem mit offenen Händen entgegen oder kehrt beim Grüßen aus größerer Distanz die Handfläche des ausgestreckten Armes dem zu Grüßenden entgegen. Das Händeschütteln mag aus einer gemischten Motivation der Übereinstimmung und des ritualisierten Kraftmessens stammen. Außer den Händen werden auch Kopf und Körperhaltung für das Grüßen eingesetzt. KENDON und FERBER (1973) haben menschliche Begrüßungsszenen aus Filmen und Videoaufnahmen analysiert und zeigen können, daß die Kombination der Verhaltenselemente, die zum Grüßen eingesetzt werden, u.a. von der Distanz abhängt, in der die sich Grüßenden einander zuerst sehen, von der persönlichen Beziehung, in der sie miteinander stehen und von der Situation,

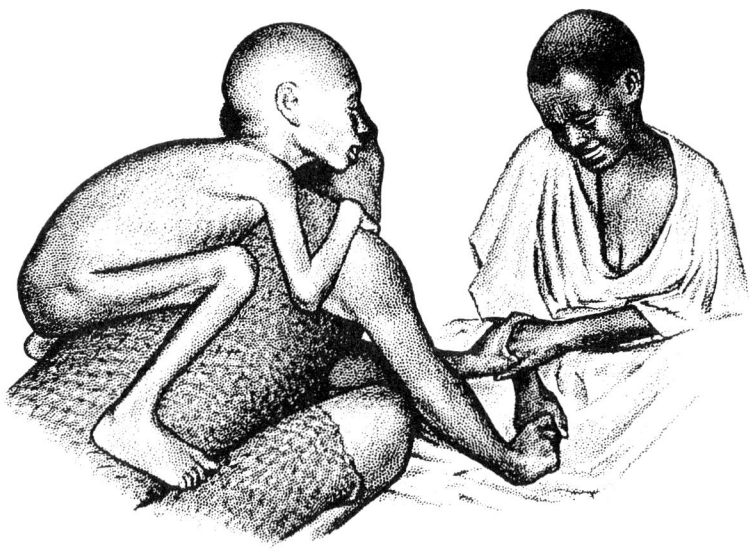

Abb. 12. Begrüßungsszene in Indien. Man beachte auch den Sitz des Kindes auf dem Rücken der Mutter. (Nach einem Zeitungsphoto „Hunger in Indien", gezeichnet von HERMANN KACHER)

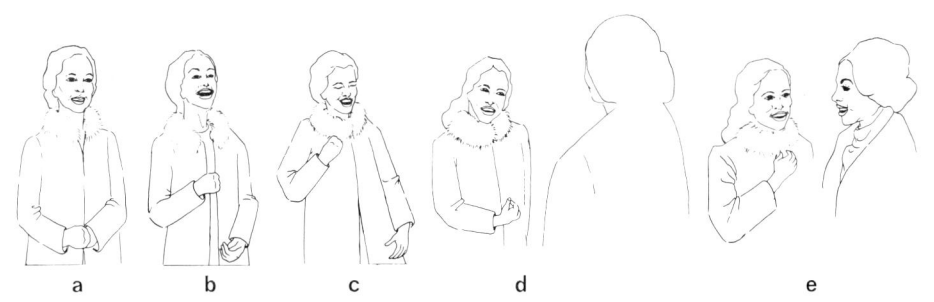

a b c d e

Abb. 13a–e. Begrüßungsszene (nach Filmaufnahmen gezeichnet): (a) Person P sichtet Person Q, (b) P wirft den Kopf zum Grüßen auf Distanz hoch, hebt die Augenbrauen und zeigt ein Offenes-Mund-Lächeln, (c) Kopfsenken und Augenschließen folgen, (d) Augenkontakt auf nahe Distanz mit Kopfneigung als Beispiel für die Endphase einer Grußzeremonie. (e) Nach der Begrüßung Wechsel von der vis-à-vis-Orientierung zur mehr rechtwinkligen Stellung. Ein Arm wird vor dem Körper gekreuzt (protektive Bewegung). (Aus KENDON u. FERBER, 1973)

in der die Begrüßung stattfindet. Diese drei Variablen bestimmen auch bei der Begegnung von nicht-menschlichen Primaten die Verhaltenselemente, die bei der Begegnung eingesetzt werden. Zum menschlichen Grüßen auf größere Distanz gehört das Kopfhochwerfen, das in anderem Zusammenhang und mit anderer Mimik bei Affen und Menschen Bestandteil einer Dominanzgebärde ist, zu der auch das Brauenheben und Mundoffen-Lächeln gehört (s.S. 402f.) (Abb. 13). Bei intimerer Begrüßung aus nächster Distanz kommt es zum Körperkontakt, man umschließt sich mit den Armen und küßt sich. Diese emotionsbetonte Geste kann beim Menschen zum reinen Ritual erstarren. Den Kuß zählt

BILZ (1971) zu den „Urszenen" des Menschen, in denen die Rollen des „Spielers" und „Gegenspielers" nach Art eines Textbuches festgelegt sind. Diese Rollen sind immer zugleich auch emotionale Rollen. In der Säuglingsaufzucht gibt es auch bei Affen das Vorkauen der Nahrung und die Mund-zu-Mund-Fütterung (Abb. 14), wie es beim Menschen wahrscheinlich über große Epochen üblich gewesen ist. Noch nach dem ersten Weltkrieg war in Holstein zu beobachten, wie Großmütter dem Säugling Buttermehlklöße vorkauten. Kommt die Mutter einem etwa dreimonatigen Säugling mit dem Mund zu nahe, so stülpt er schon bei Annäherung seine Lippen vor. Ist der Mund-zu-Mund-Kontakt vollzogen, schiebt das Kind seine Zunge vor und macht Leckbewegungen (PLOOG, 1964c, S. 337). Wie oft im Tierreich, sind Elemente des Mutter-Kind-Verhaltens und

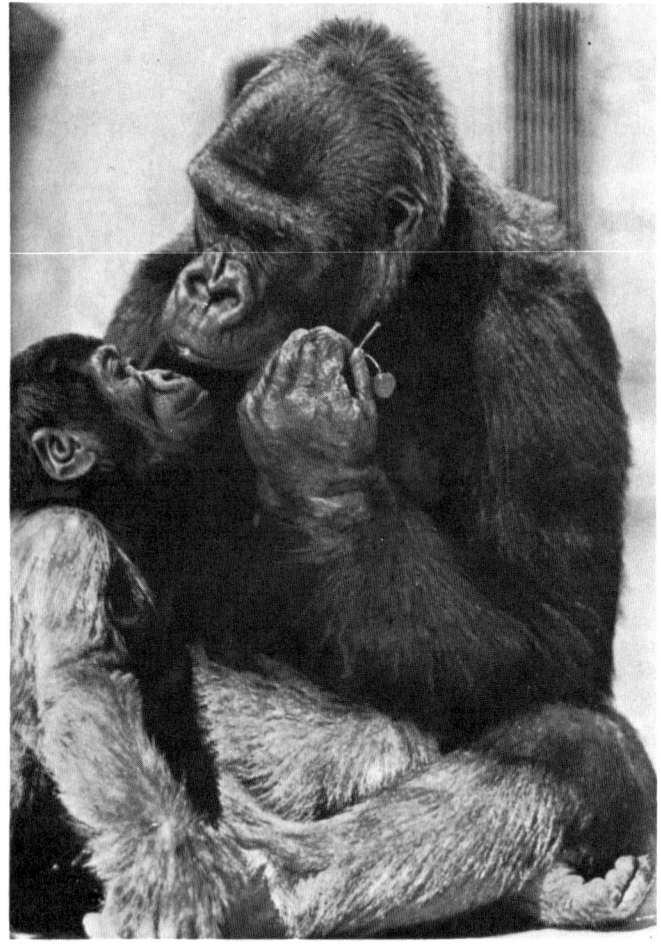

Abb. 14. Mund-zu-Mund-Fütterung. Eine Gorilla-Mutter füttert ihr Kind. (Aus LANG, 1964; Photo von PAUL STEINEMANN)

der Aufzucht mit in das menschliche Werbungsverhalten eingegangen. Nicht nur, daß Verliebte sich küssen und dabei die Zunge mitbenützen, sie stecken sich auch gerne gute Bissen in den Mund.

Ein Teil der Gesten stammt aus dem großen Repertoire der Verhaltensweisen, die zum Rangstreben und der Bereitschaft zur Unterordnung gehören. FREUD schrieb in einem Brief an EINSTEIN: „Es ist ein Stück der angeborenen und nicht zu beseitigenden Ungleichheit der Menschen, daß sie in Führer und Abhängige zerfallen. Die letzteren sind die übergroße Mehrheit, sie bedürfen einer Autorität, welche für sie Entscheidungen fällt, denen sie sich meist bedingungslos unterwerfen". Bei der Ausbildung von hierarchischen Strukturen, die in der einen oder anderen Form bei allen Primaten stattfindet, geht es nur ausnahmsweise um bedingungslose Unterwerfung. Jedes Individuum durchläuft in seiner Ontogenese einen Sozialisierungsprozeß, in dem es lernt, was „erlaubt" und was „verboten" ist. Die Signale, die in diesem „Erziehungsprozeß" eingesetzt werden, versteht der junge Affe in vielen Fällen von Geburt an. Welchen Platz er in der jeweiligen Gesellschaft einnimmt, hängt zu einem großen Teil von seiner Lebensgeschichte ab (s. weiteres dazu ab S. 487).

Ein zum Dominanzstreben benutztes Signal hatten wir schon im genitalen Imponieren kennengelernt. Der animponierte, rangniedrigere Affe duckt seinen Kopf (s. Abb. 2a). Ein ausschließlich zu den Dominanzsignalen gehöriges Verhalten ist das Kopfgreifen bei den Totenkopfaffen. Meist wird die flache Hand auf das Scheitelbein des Kontrahenten gelegt und der Kopf heruntergedrückt, seltener dabei in das Kopffell gegriffen. Ob diese Dominanzgeste auch bei den Menschenaffen eine wesentliche Rolle spielt, habe ich noch nicht herausfinden können. Der Kopf bzw. dessen Haltung ist jedenfalls beim Menschen ein äußerst wichtiges Ausdrucksmittel. Einige Redewendungen und ritualisierte Gesten weisen auf die Universalität ihrer Bedeutung hin. Dem Schüler wird der Kopf gewaschen. Man beugt sein Haupt in Demut, und man wird (oder wurde) an Haupt und Gliedern bestraft. Hocherhobenen Hauptes durchschreitet der Sieger die Menge, und der Zufluchtsuchende birgt sein Haupt an der Brust des Beschützenden. Dem Segen Erbittenden wird die Hand aufs Haupt gelegt. Der besiegte Gegner ist „aufs Haupt geschlagen".

EIBL-EIBESFELDT (1971b; 1973c) berichtet von den Waika-Indianern und JONES (1971) in gleicher Weise von den australischen Aborigines, daß sie sich mit meterlangen Holzkeulen in ritualisiertem Kampf in wohldosierter Stärke auf den Kopf schlagen, bis einer der Gegner bewußtlos zu Boden fällt. Todesfälle wurden nicht beobachtet. Zum Ausdruck der tiefsten Unterwerfung oder Verehrung wurde das Haupt an der Erde geborgen. In anderen Bezeugungen der Unterwerfung macht man sich klein. Odysseus umfaßt flehend die Knie der Arete, und Priamos fällt auf gleiche Weise vor Achilles nieder. „Alte Sozialgebärden" (BILZ, 1971) lösen zwingend eine von Emotion begleitete Antwort aus.

Die Liste der kommunikativen Gesten soll hier nicht vervollständigt werden. Einige dieser Bewegungen werden dauernd benutzt, z.B. die teils kulturabhängig bevorzugten Formen der Bejahung und Verneinung. DARWIN hielt das seitliche Abwenden des Kopfes, mit dem Säuglinge die Nahrung zurückweisen, für den ersten Akt der Verneinung. Auch das schon erwähnte blind-taube Mädchen schüttelte den Kopf, wenn es etwas nicht essen wollte oder etwas ablehnte

(s. Näheres bei EIBL-EIBESFELDT, 1973a, 1978 S. 557 ff.) Körperbewegungen und Körperhaltung mit abgestuften Zu- und Abwendungen des ganzen Körpers oder einiger seiner Teile müssen als ein integriertes Signalsystem betrachtet werden, dessen Mitteilungsfunktionen außerordentlich vielseitig und allen Primaten gemeinsam sind (v. CRANACH, 1971a; v. CRANACH u. VINE, 1972; HINDE, 1972a). Bei diesen kommunikativen Orientierungsbewegungen wirken Körper, Kopf und Auge gleichsinnig oder kontrastierend zusammen. Der Blickzuwendung kommt dabei eine besondere Bedeutung zu, auf die wir noch mehrfach zurückkommen werden. Unter den Orientierungsbewegungen hat die Blickzuwendung auf Grund ihrer Doppelfunktion eine Sonderstellung: Der Blick dient zum Empfang von visuellen Signalen, so auch zum Empfang des Blicks, und er ist selbst ein Signal (v. CRANACH, 1968, 1971b). In Affen- und Menschengruppen ist das Blickverhalten des einzelnen abhängig von Gruppenstruktur und Rangordnung; die Signalfunktion des Blickes ist damit in hohem Maße kontextabhängig (CHANCE, 1967, 1976). Der Blickkontakt kann bereits in den ersten Lebenstagen zwischen Mutter und Kind hergestellt werden (s.S. 415) und hat später im Erleben des Signalempfängers sowohl im kohäsiven wie im aggressiven Kontext einen hohen Bedeutungswert. Untersucht man aber, wie genau jemand einem ins Auge blickt, so wird das Urteil des Empfängers in der Distanz von 80–200 cm zunehmend ungenauer. Um sich in die Augen geblickt zu fühlen, genügt ein Blick auf das Gesicht (ELLGRING, 1970). Die wichtigste Funktion des Blickkontaktes in der sozialen Interaktion wird durch diese „egozentrische" Signalverarbeitung hervorgehoben. Der Mensch trägt damit die Bereitschaft, auf Blicke „sensitiv" zu reagieren, potentiell in sich (PLOOG, 1970).

a) Mimische Signale und Signalerkennung bei Affen

Ein aufmerksamer Zoobesucher, der sich zum Ziele setzt, nicht nur die Tiere, sondern auch die die Tiere beobachtenden Menschen mitzustudieren, wird vor den Affenkäfigen mehr fratzenschneidende Gesichter bemerken als irgendwo sonst. Das Verhalten der Menschen zeigt, daß sie spontan auf ein hervorstechendes Verhaltensmerkmal der Affen reagieren, nämlich deren mimische Beweglichkeit, die vom Menschen unmittelbar als Ausdrucksverhalten und damit als Mittel der Kommunikation aufgefaßt wird. Auch bei einigen niedrigeren Säugetieren gibt es eine einfachere Mimik, wie SCHENKEL (1947) am Wolf, LORENZ (1963) am Hund und LEYHAUSEN (1956/1973) an der Katze gezeigt haben. Darin kommen Flucht- und Angriffstendenzen oder, besonders beim Hund, auch differenziertere Handlungsbereitschaften zum Ausdruck. Doch erst bei den Affen tritt ein Formenreichtum der Gesichtsmotorik in Erscheinung, der die Ausdrucksbewegungen des Gesichts zur Mimik im engeren Sinne macht (Abb. 15). Um zunehmend differenzierte Gesichtsausdrücke hervorbringen zu können, ist eine entsprechend differenzierte Muskulatur mit der zugehörigen neuralen Versorgung notwendig. Ansätze dazu liegen bereits in der den Säugern eigenen Form der Nahrungsaufnahme, nämlich dem Saugen der Säuglinge und dem intensiven Kauen mit dem bezahnten Gebiß. Lippen und Wangen werden beweglicher. Schon bei primitiven Wirbeltieren können der Nahrungsaufnahme dienende Bewegungen kommunikative Funktionen bekommen, z.B. das Öffnen und

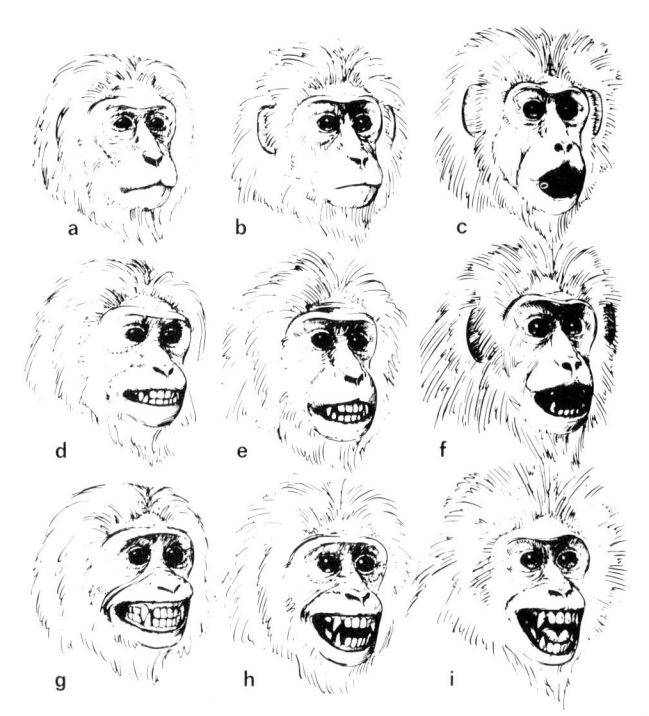

Abb. 15a–i. Mimische Signale des Bärenmakaken, gestuft nach Angriffsbereitschaft (von a nach c) und Fluchtbereitschaft (von a nach g) sowie deren Überlagerung in verschiedenen Intensitäten. Mit zunehmender Angriffsbereitschaft intensiviert sich das Starren, die Ohren steifen sich, die Haare sträuben sich, die Lippen werden schmaler und der Mund geöffnet; mit zunehmender Fluchtbereitschaft wendet sich der Blick ab, die Ohren legen sich an, die Lippen ziehen sich zurück und die Zähne werden gezeigt. (a) Neutraler Ausdruck, (b) Mildes Starren – selbstsichere Drohung, (c) Starren mit rundem Mund – intensiv-selbstsichere Drohung, (d) Leichtes Grimassieren – niedere Fluchtbereitschaft, (e) Angriff/Flucht-Überlagerung, (f) Starren mit offenem Mund – unsichere, intensive Drohung, (g) Starkes Grimassieren – intensive Fluchtbereitschaft, (h) Starren mit Zähnezeigen – starke Fluchtbereitschaft mit Angriffstendenz, (i) Starren und Zähne blecken – intensive Angriff/Flucht-Überlagerung. (Aus CHEVALIER-SKOLNIKOFF, 1973)

Schließen der Kiefer als Drohsignal. Mit dem Beweglicherwerden der Schnauze und der Lippen wird bereits das Entblößen der Zähne, insbesondere der Eckzähne, zur Drohung. Schließlich genügt ein leichtes Zurückziehen der Mundwinkel als Drohsignal niederer Intensität. Ursprünglich zusammengehörige Muskeln haben sich aufgesplittert und sind unabhängig voneinander beweglich geworden. Für die Augengegend hat das binokulare Sehen, die zunehmende Beweglichkeit der Augen und der Lider zur mimischen Differenzierung beigetragen. Für Tiere mit voll binokularem, scharfem Sehen bietet sich ein Vorteil für die Kommunikation, wenn die wesentlichen Ausdrucksbewegungen auf engem Raum mit einem Blick wahrgenommen werden können. Nach meinem Eindruck beachten Affenarten mit differenzierter Mimik auch das menschliche Gesicht mehr als solche mit ärmerem Ausdruck. Im ganzen gesehen und mit wichtigen Ausnahmen haben die Neuweltaffen eine weniger ausgeprägte Mimik als die Altweltaffen, und die Menschenaffen sind nicht zuletzt auch wegen ihres „sprechenden" Gesichts dem Menschen am ähnlichsten (Abb. 16).

Dennoch kann der Mensch die Mimik des Menschenaffen nicht in allen Variationen unmittelbar „lesen"; er braucht dazu einige Erfahrung. Um den Informationsgehalt eines mimischen Ausdrucks genauer bestimmen zu können, bedarf es einer eingehenden Analyse aller Situationen, in denen dieser Ausdruck vorkommt. Zu diesem Zwecke ist es sinnvoll, eine Klassifizierung der Mimik vorzunehmen, die auf möglichst viele Affenarten zutrifft. Dadurch kann die Funktion eines mimischen Signals besser beschrieben werden, und Vergleiche zwischen den Arten sind erleichtert.

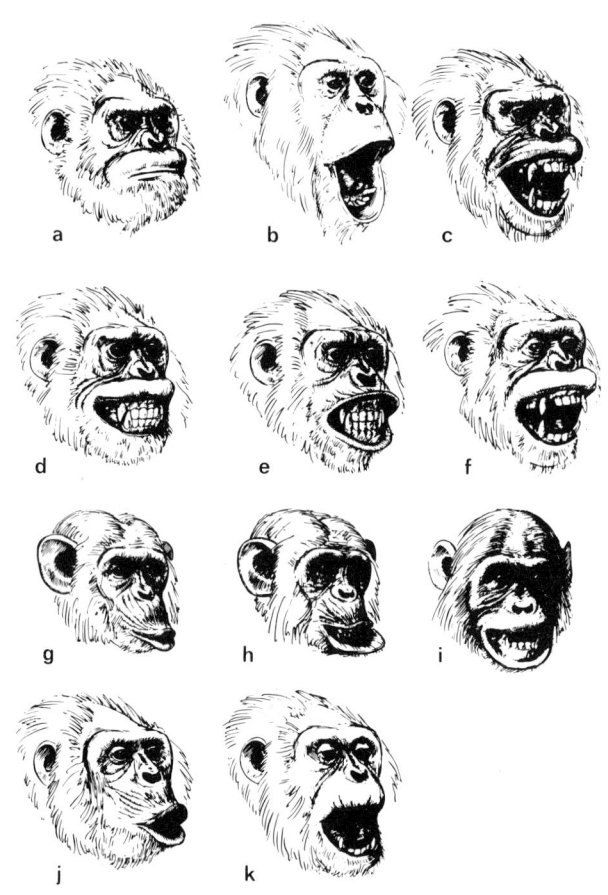

Abb. 16a–k. Einige Gesichtsausdrücke der Schimpansen. (a) Anstarren – „ärgerlich", (b) Waa-Gebell – „anschnauzen"/„schimpfen", (c) Kreischen – „ängstlich-ärgerlich", (d) Stummes Zähnezeigen mit zurückgezogenen Lippen – submissives Signal, (e) Stummes Zähnezeigen mit gewölbten Lippen – „ängstlich-zugeneigt(?)", (f) Stummes Zähnezeigen mit offenem Mund – „Zuneigung" (Lachen?), (g) Schnuteziehen – „Wunschenttäuschung", (h) Jammergesicht – „traurige Enttäuschung", (i) Heulgesicht – „Frustration" (bei Kindern), (j) Johlendes Gesicht – „aufgeregte Erwartung", (k) Spielgesicht – in Spiellaune. (Diagrammatische Zeichnungen von CHEVALIER-SKOLNIKOFF, 1973 nach VAN HOOFF, 1971 und VAN LAWICK-GOODALL, 1968a und b)

Klassifizierung mimischer Ausdrucksformen

Abb. 17 zeigt einen Klassifizierungsversuch für die Hundsaffen (Cercopithecinae) (VAN HOOFF, 1967): Die einzelnen mimischen Elemente, die zum Gesamtausdruck beitragen, sind Augen, Lider, Augenbrauen, Stirn- und Kopfhaut, Ohren, Kiefer, Mundwinkel und Lippen. Hinzu kommen nicht-mimische Elemente wie Kopf- und Körperbewegungen, -haltungen, Lautgebungen und vegetativ gesteuerte Zeichen, z.B. sich verändernde Pupillen oder sich sträubende Haare. Bei der Klassifizierung kann man von zwei Grundformen ausgehen, dem entspannten und dem aufmerksamen Gesicht. Beim entspannten Gesicht befinden sich alle mimischen Elemente in sozusagen neutraler Ausgangsposition. Alle Affen zeigen diesen Ausdruck, wenn sie herumsitzen oder liegen und nichts Besonderes tun. Das aufmerksame Gesicht drückt den Zustand der Aktionsbereitschaft aus und ist im Vergleich zum entspannten Gesicht an den weit geöffneten Augen mit voll sichtbarer Iris und erhöhtem Muskeltonus um die Mundgegend erkennbar.

Auf der Abbildung sind typische Gesichter schematisch dargestellt. Jedem Gesichtsausdruck kommt eine bestimmte Signalfunktion zu. Das Brauenziehen beim Mantelpavian ist z.B. ein Drohsignal mit niederer Intensität (KUMMER, 1957). Das Starren mit offenem Mund wird gewöhnlich vom dominanten Tier benutzt und hat die Flucht des Bedrohten zur Folge. Das Lippenspitzen kommt bei verschiedenen Genera vor, z.B. bei Makaken, Pavianen, beim Orang-Utan, auch beim Gorilla und besonders beim Schimpansen. In seiner typischen Ausprägung ist das Lippenspitzen ein Säuglingsausdruck, den man beobachtet, wenn das Baby nach seiner Mutter oder nach der Brust verlangt. Bei erwachsenen Tieren tritt es in Zusammenhang mit jeglichem Begehren auf, sei es Futter, seien es Artgenossen, Personen oder Objekte, häufig von ooch-artigen Lauten

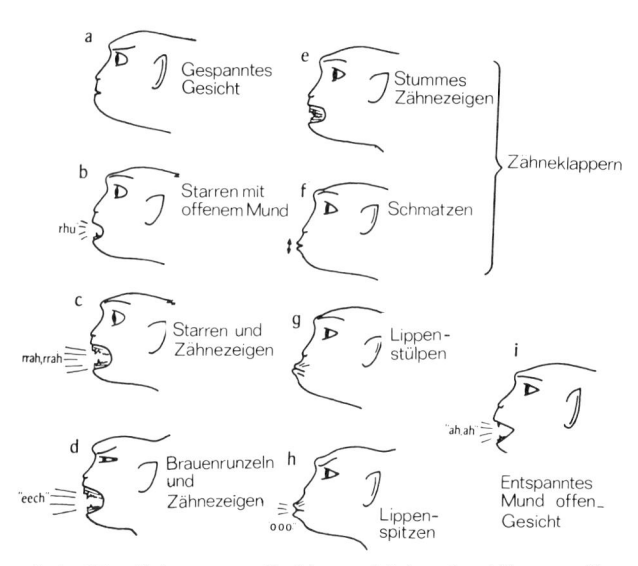

Abb. 17. Schematische Klassifizierung von Gesichtsausdrücken der Affen vom Typus Macaca. (Aus VAN HOOFF, 1967)

begleitet. Auf diese Weise kann es auch eine hinweisende Funktion erhalten, die die Kumpane in die Richtung des fixierten Objektes blicken läßt.

Beim Schimpansen, besonders bei Jungtieren, ist seit DARWIN (1872) immer wieder beschrieben worden, wie aus dem lippenspitzenden Begehren ein Wutanfall entstehen kann, wenn der Affe nicht erreicht, was er will (KÖHLER, 1921; YERKES u. YERKES, 1929; LADYGINA-KOHTS, 1935). Er reißt den Mund weit auf, zeigt alle Zähne und gerät in einen Bewegungssturm, stampft mit den Füßen auf, wirft sich auf den Boden und schlägt an Gegenstände.

Das Mund-offen-Gesicht wird bei vielen Arten während des Spielens beobachtet. Es ist deswegen auch als Spielgesicht bezeichnet worden. Das Spielen junger Affen, gleich ob es sich um Plattnasenaffen der Neuen Welt oder um Schmalnasenaffen der Alten Welt handelt, weist große Ähnlichkeiten zwischen den Arten auf. Es gibt das Balgen, das Jagen und das Fangen und das Kampfspiel, das mitunter in Ernst umschlagen kann und dann abbricht (LOIZOS, 1967; PLOOG et al., 1967). Das Mund-offen-Gesicht ist eine Intentionsbewegung zum Beißen. Dieses Scheinbeißen kommt im Spiel andauernd vor (Abb. 18). Dabei wird nur zart zugebissen und die Haut gezwickt. Viele Arten lassen während des Spielens auch typische Laute hören.

Beim Schimpansen ist dieser Gesichtsausdruck verschiedentlich mit dem menschlichen Lachen verglichen worden. DARWIN (1872) sah den Hauptunterschied darin, daß die obere Zahnreihe beim Schimpansen nicht entblößt ist. ANDREW (1963) beschrieb das Lachen des Schimpansen im Zusammenhang

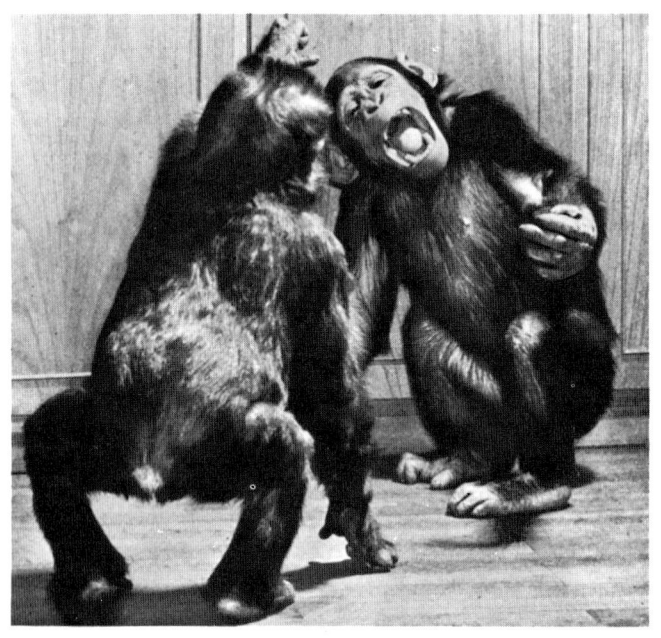

Abb. 18. Kampfspiel zwischen Gorilla- und Schimpansenjungen. Der Schimpanse zeigt das typische Spielgesicht in der Phase der Scheindrohung. (Photo von B. GRZIMEK, Zoologischer Garten, Frankfurt a.M.)

mit seinen kurzen, ziemlich tiefen Ä-ä-Lauten, wenn er gekitzelt wird. KOEHLER (1925) beobachtete leicht zurückgezogene Mundwinkel beim entspannten Betrachten von Objekten, die dem Schimpansen offensichtlich Freude bereiten, z.B. kleinen Menschenkindern. Spielende Berggorillas ziehen ihre Mundwinkel bei geöffnetem Mund weit zurück, ohne die Zähne zu zeigen (SCHALLER, 1963).

Im Rahmen der Biologie von Ausdruck und Eindruck (LEYHAUSEN, 1968) ist die Frage, welchen spezifischen Eindruck der mimische Ausdruck auf den Empfänger macht, in den letzten Jahren durch aufschlußreiche Experimente gefördert worden, die neues Licht auf die Psychobiologie des Sozialverhaltens werfen (PLOOG, 1969a). Drei Faktoren spielen eine entscheidende Rolle, nämlich das angeborene Schema (LORENZ, 1935, 1965), später von TINBERGEN (1952) angeborener Auslösemechanismus (AAM) genannt, die sozialen Bedingungen, unter denen der Affe aufwächst, und der Zeitpunkt, zu dem er seine ersten Erfahrungen mit Artgenossen sammelt.

HARLOW und seine Mitarbeiter, vor allem MASON (1965), veröffentlichten ab 1959 zahlreiche Experimente zur Veränderung des Sozialverhaltens durch frühe Isolierung von Artgenossen (HARLOW u. HARLOW, 1962a, 1965a). Ihnen folgten andere (HINDE et al., 1966; KAUFMAN u. ROSENBLUM, 1969). Nach den Ergebnissen besteht kein Zweifel, daß reger Sozialkontakt in den ersten Lebenswochen und -monaten unbedingt erforderlich ist, um später ein normales, voll ausgebildetes Sozial- und Sexualverhalten zu entwickeln. (Weiteres dazu s.S. 487ff.)

Um genauer zu untersuchen, welche Faktoren den Umgang mit anderen erschweren oder unmöglich machen, untersuchte SACKETT (1966) von Geburt an isoliert aufgezogene Rhesusaffen auf ihre Reaktionen gegenüber farbigen Diapositiven, auf denen Affen und andere Sehobjekte dargestellt waren (Abb. 19). Drückten die isolierten Affenkinder auf einen Hebel, konnten sie sich die Bilder selbst in ihren Käfig projizieren und durch die Zahl der Projektionen ihre Vorliebe für bestimmte Darstellungen anzeigen. Unter den 10 Kategorien von Bildern mit jeweils vier Variationen zur Auswahl waren die für das Experiment entscheidenden die Affenbabys, die mimisch drohenden erwachsenen Männchen, Affen in verschiedenen anderen Darstellungen und Kontrollbilder, z.B. eine Landschaft oder ein Mädchen. Von Tieren im ersten Lebensmonat wurden alle Bilder gleich häufig, im zweiten Monat alle Affenbilder häufiger und schließlich die Affenbabybilder am häufigsten gewählt. Die Wahlhäufigkeit der bis dahin bevorzugten Fotos mit mimisch drohenden Affen fiel plötzlich von zweieinhalb Monaten an stark ab und war nach insgesamt dreieinhalb Monaten unter die Wahlhäufigkeit der Kontrollbilder gesunken. Entsprechend der Versuchsanordnung sahen sich die Äffchen auch in dieser Zeit gelegentlich mit dem Drohbild konfrontiert. Dann schrien sie und zeigten ängstliches Verhalten. Erstaunlicherweise nahm die Aversion gegen das Drohbild im vierten Monat wieder ab und dessen Wahl stetig wieder zu, bis das Drohbild schließlich mit fünfeinhalb Monaten zusammen mit dem Babybild bei weitem bevorzugt wurde.

Nach Anlage des Experiments besteht kein Zweifel, daß die in einem bestimmten, begrenzten Zeitraum einsetzende heftige Reaktion auf das Drohgesicht angeboren ist. Das mimische Signal löst Furcht aus. Es bekommt zu einem

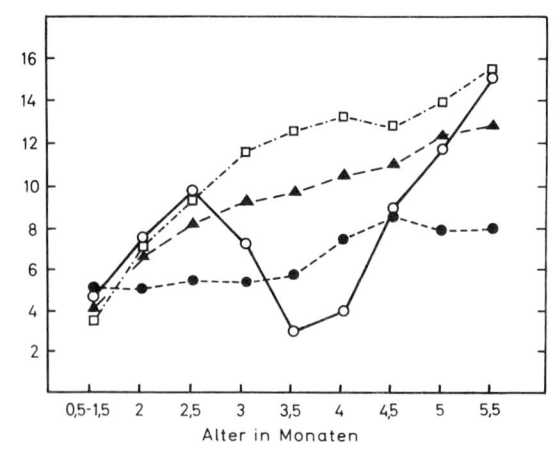

Abb. 19. Mimikerkennen bei isoliert aufgezogenen Rhesusaffen im Verlaufe des Reifungsprozesses. Auf der Ordinate ist die Häufigkeit (mittlere Anzahl aus fünfminütigen Testperioden) der Bilddarbietungen dargestellt, die durch Hebeldrücken selbst von den Affen ausgelöst werden. ○ Drohender erwachsener Artgenosse, □ Affenkind, ▲ andere Affen, ● Kontrollbilder. (Aus SACKETT, 1966)

prädeterminierten Zeitpunkt eine Bedeutung, die es vorher nicht gehabt hat, ohne daß für diesen Bedeutungswandel äußere Gründe vorhanden sind. Im Verhalten ändert sich etwas, das nicht gelernt worden ist. Eine derartige Veränderung der Reaktionsbereitschaft ist in anderen entwicklungsbiologischen Bereichen durchaus bekannt. Die Zeiten besonderer Empfindlichkeit für bestimmte Reize nennt man sensible Perioden.

LORENZ (1965) erkannte schon 1931/1935 die fundamentale Bedeutung solcher sensibler Perioden für das spätere Sozialverhalten und zeigte, daß bestimmte Erfahrungen innerhalb eines begrenzten Zeitraumes prägend auf bestimmte Verhaltensweisen wirken. Seine berühmt gewordene Dohle Tschok hatte ihn, der sie fütterte, als Elternkumpan angenommen. Als sie flügge wurde, brauchte sie Flugkumpane und fand die fliegenden Nebelkrähen; geschlechtsreif geworden, zeigte sich trotz der fortwährenden Gemeinschaft mit anderen, nichtfliegenden Dohlen, daß die vom Menschen bevorzugte Aufzucht Spuren hinterlassen hatte: Tschok balzte die Hausgehilfin an. Der erwachsene Pflegetrieb schließlich fand sein Objekt in der Fütterung eines Dohlenjungen. Seither sind viele Untersuchungen angestellt worden, um dem Vorgang der Prägung – diesem kurzfristigen Lernen auf einen Blick mit lang anhaltenden Folgen für das soziale Verhalten – auf den Grund zu kommen (Übersicht bei PLOOG, 1964c; HESS, 1975; EIBL-EIBESFELDT, 1978; SALZEN, 1979).

Die von der Drohmimik plötzlich beeindruckten Affen zeigten zwar eine sensible Periode für dieses Signal, doch anders als bei der Prägung erlosch die adäquate Reaktion auf diesen angeborenermaßen wirksamen Reiz nach einer gewissen Zeit. Dieser Befund ist für das Verständnis der sozialen Entwicklung der Primaten und damit für die Ontogenese der Kommunikationsprozesse von großer Bedeutung: Wenn einem sozialen Signal nicht die natürlicherweise eintretende, durch das Signal angekündigte Handlung folgt, ändert sich die Reaktion auf das Signal. Die isolierten Affen lernten niemals die sozialen Konsequenzen der Drohmimik kennen und erhielten keine Rückmeldung auf ihr ängstliches Verhalten. Anstelle der während der sensiblen Periode gezeigten Angstreaktion kam die vor dieser Zeit gezeigte positive Reaktion wieder hervor. Das ursprünglich unspezifische Signal mit dem allgemeinen Informationsgehalt „Affe" wurde während eines prädeterminierten Reifungsabschnittes spezifisch durch den Informationsgehalt „drohender Affe". Die angstauslösende Funktion des Signals wurde nicht durch entsprechende Partnerinteraktion genutzt. Nach ethologischer Vorstellung atrophiert auf diese Weise der neurosensorische Mechanismus (AAM), der eine spezielle angeborene Verhaltensweise auf ein passendes Signal hin freigibt, oder er verliert seine selektive Empfindlichkeit für eben dieses Signal.

Spätere Versuche mit den gleichen isolierten Affen, deren einzige visuelle Erfahrung in den projizierten Bildern bestand, zeigten nun in der Tat, daß diese nicht ausreichte, um ein normales Sozialverhalten herbeizuführen. Die Affen mit Bilderfahrung zeigten im Zusammenleben mit ihresgleichen ebenso schwere Störungen wie Affen, die total isoliert aufgewachsen waren. Sie unterschieden sich aber in einem überraschenden Punkt: Angstreaktionen gegenüber Artgenossen waren häufiger als bei allen Vergleichsgruppen, den total isolierten, den auf Sicht- und Hörkontakt beschränkten und den normal im Gruppenverband aufgewachsenen Affen (SACKETT, 1966). Daraus darf man schließen, daß die frühkindliche Erfahrung mit den Drohbildern nicht gänzlich ausgelöscht worden ist.

Daß die schweren Störungen des Sozialverhaltens nach isolierter Aufzucht mit Störungen des Mimikerkennens einhergehen, zeigen folgende Versuche:

Dressiert man Affen darauf, einen elektrischen Schlag durch Druck auf einen Hebel zu vermeiden (Konditionierte Reaktion, CR), nachdem in kurzem Zeitabstand ein Lichtzeichen (Konditionierender Stimulus, CS) gegeben worden ist, so lernen sowohl normal als auch isoliert aufgewachsene Tiere den schmerzhaften Schlag auch dann zu vermeiden, wenn der CS in unregelmäßigen Abständen gegeben wird. Diese CR ist bei beiden Gruppen von einer autonomen CR, nämlich der Erhöhung der Herzfrequenz, begleitet.

In dem folgenden Versuch werden jeweils zwei Affen in ein und dieselbe Konditionierungssituation eingespannt. Der eine führt den Versuch, wie beschrieben, in einem Versuchsraum durch, der zweite in einem anderen Raum, in dem er aber das Lichtzeichen nicht sehen kann. Statt dessen wird ihm auf einem Fersehschirm der erste Affe so gezeigt, daß er dessen Gesicht beobachten kann. Ein normal aufgewachsenes Tier erkennt schnell aus der Mimik seines Gegenübers, wann dieser das Lichtzeichen (CS) sieht, und kann den Schlag auf diese Weise vermeiden. Auch seine Herzschlagerhöhung entspricht der des mimischen Senders.

Ein isoliert aufgewachsenes Tier ist hingegen unfähig, in der Mimik seines Gegenübers zu lesen, und kann daher den Schmerzreiz nicht vermeiden; es zeigt dementsprechend keine konditionierte autonome Reaktion. Umgekehrt haben auch die normalen Tiere Schwierigkeiten, aus den Gesichtern der isolierten zu lesen; sie erhalten daher häufiger einen Schlag als während der Kommunikation mit ihresgleichen; der Herzschlag bleibt entsprechend unverändert. Daraus kann man schließen, daß die isoliert aufgewachsenen Affen nicht nur mimische Signale nicht erkennen können, sondern selbst auch in ihrem mimischen Ausdruck gestört sind (MILLER, 1967; MILLER et al., 1967).

b) Mimische Signale und Signalerkennung beim Menschen

DARWINS Erkenntnis, daß „der Ausdruck der Gemütsbewegungen bei Menschen und Tieren" (1872) eine gemeinsame Naturgeschichte hat und daher angeboren ist, hat sich in der psychologischen und anthropologisch orientierten Forschung lange Zeit nicht durchsetzen können. Allzusehr war man von der alleinigen Kulturbedingtheit des mimischen Verhaltens überzeugt (u.a. KLINEBERG, 1940; LABARRE, 1947) und ist es auch teilweise immer noch (BIRDWHISTELL, 1970). Von allen menschlichen Gesichtsausdrücken wurde das Lächeln der Säuglinge und Kinder am häufigsten studiert (WASHBURN, 1929; DENNIS u. DENNIS, 1937; SPITZ u. WOLF, 1946). Über die Frage, ob auch der Mensch über angeborene mimische Signale verfügt, ist viel gestritten worden. Heute besteht zunehmende Einigkeit darin, daß mimische Signale angeborene Ausdrucksbewegungen, also Instinktbewegungen i.S. von LORENZ (1937/1965, S. 283) und TINBERGEN (1948) sind, deren Anwendungsbereich und Ausgestaltung sich durch Erfahrung im soziokulturellen Milieu entwickelt und während des Heranwachsens unter voluntative Kontrolle kommt (PLOOG, 1964c; FREEDMAN, 1974; EIBL-EIBESFELDT, 1975, 1978).

Studien an Säuglingen und Kindern

Der erste, der am Beispiel des Lächelns auf den Instinktcharakter menschlicher Ausdrucksbewegungen hingewiesen hat, war OTTO KOEHLER (1954a). Seinen Beobachtungen folgten mehrere, teils umfangreiche Studien (AMBROSE, 1961; WOLFF, 1963; HERZKA, 1965). In den ersten Lebenstagen hat der Säugling meist beide Augen geschlossen. Dann bewegen sich bei seinem Lächeln nur Mund und Nasenpartie. Lächelt er bei offenen Augen, schließen sich die Lider ein wenig und am äußeren Augenwinkel können sich „Krähenfüße" bilden. Während der ersten ein oder zwei Wochen scheint Lächeln stärker an innere, zentralnervöse Vorgänge gebunden zu sein und tritt meist im irregulären Schlaf oder im Zustand der Schläfrigkeit, jedoch selten oder nie im regulären Schlaf oder im alerten Wachzustand auf (HERZKA, 1965; WOLFF, 1966). Da die Partnerbezogenheit meist noch fehlt und auslösende Reize nicht vorhanden sind, ist diese Form des Lächelns als Leerlaufaktivität einer Instinktbewegung anzusehen, wie sie von LORENZ für andere Erbkoordinationen beschrieben wurde.

Der Zeitpunkt des ersten Lächelns variiert stark und ist bereits bei Frühgeburten in der 42. Gestationswoche am 2. Lebenstag wiederholt beobachtet worden. Nicht selten tritt dieses Lächeln nur halbseitig auf. Bei voll ausgetragenen und genau auf das Lächeln beobachteten Kindern schwanken die Zeitangaben für halb- und beidseitiges Lächeln zwischen dem ersten und dem 17. Lebenstag (PLOOG, 1964c). Man hat viel darüber diskutiert, von welchem Zeitpunkt an das Lächeln zum sozialen Lächeln wird (RHEINGOLD, 1961, 1966, 1969). Das wichtigste Kriterium dafür ist wohl der Blickkontakt. DENNIS und DENNIS (1937) berichteten, daß in 20 von 40 Kindertagebüchern das Anlächeln zwischen der ersten und zehnten Woche vermerkt wurde.

Bei Erörterung der Ontogenese des Lächelns müssen die Auslösebedingungen sorgfältig mit in Betracht gezogen werden (SROUFE u. WATERS, 1976). AHRENS (1954) konnte in seinen Attrappenversuchen Lächeln während des ersten Lebensmonats mit zwei nebeneinanderstehenden Punkten oder nach Art eines übernormalen Schlüsselreizes mit drei untereinander angeordneten Punktpaaren auslösen. WOLFF (1963) fand, daß der früheste und verläßlichste Auslöser eine hohe menschliche Stimme ist. CHARLESWORTH und KREUTZER (1973) kamen in ihrer umfassenden Untersuchung wohl aller Arbeiten über die Gesichtsausdrücke von Säuglingen und Kindern zu dem Schluß, daß es keine feste Beziehung zwischen einer bestimmten Klasse von Auslösereizen und dem Lächeln gibt: Auditorische, taktile, visuelle und propriozeptiv-kinästhetische Reize können Lächeln hervorrufen.

Schließlich wäre auch nach der Funktion des Signals bzw. nach der Wirkung zu fragen, die das Lächeln auf die Artgenossen, zumeist die Mutter, ausübt. Nach Herodot entging Kypselos, der spätere Herrscher von Korinth, als Neugeborener der Tötung, indem er die Schergen anlächelte. Diese Sage zeigt sehr schön den wahren Sachverhalt, daß nämlich für dieses angeborene Ausdrucksverhalten keineswegs das Verhalten des Partners ausschlaggebend sein muß, daß diese Instinktbewegung aber eine mächtige Kraft auf ihn ausübt und stimmungsbeeinflussend wirkt. Wie entzückt selbst ganz unbeteiligte Menschen auf das Lächeln eines Babys reagieren, weiß jedermann aus Erfahrung. Für die Mutter bedeutet dieses Lächeln höchstes Glück. Wie bei allen sozialen Signalen wird beim Lächeln die enge Verschränkung zwischen Sender und Empfänger besonders deutlich. Die Instinktbewegung des Lächelns ist der angeborene Ausdruck der Freude, der seinerseits Freude auslöst. Gemeinsam mit anderen kohäsiven Signalen hat es eine Band-stiftende Funktion (EIBL-EIBESFELDT, 1978).

Den Vergleich des Lächelns mit den vermutlich homologen Instinktbewegungen junger Schimpansen wollen wir im Bilde demonstrieren (Abb. 20) und es dem Betrachter überlassen, ob er den Ausdruck im oberen Bild als Lächeln oder Lachen anerkennen will. Dem homologen Erwartungslächeln ist im unteren Teil des Bildes der homologe Ausdruck des Mißvergnügens gegenübergestellt.

Auch für das Lachen gibt es eine große Variation von auslösenden Reizen. Der am frühesten effektive Reiz ist Kitzeln. WOLFF (1969) löste Kichern und Lachen, wenn auch nicht bei allen Kindern, ziemlich regelmäßig durch Kitzeln unter den Armen, in der Leistenbeuge oder am Bauch gegen Ende des ersten Monats aus. Die meisten Studien über das Lachen stimmen darin überein, daß Lachen um Wochen bis Monate später als Lächeln zu beobachten und früher taktil als auf andere Weise auszulösen ist. KOEHLER (1957) faßte Lächeln, Lachen und Jauchzen als drei Intensitätsstufen der gleichen Instinktbewegung auf; eine der besten Auslösersituationen für die höhere Intensitätsstufe ist das Schaukeln. Sowohl Lachen als auch Jauchzen, das wir auch bei einem sich allein überlassenen Säugling von knapp 4 Monaten hörten (PLOOG, 1964c), treten zu einer Zeit auf, wo das Lachen Erwachsener das Baby nicht etwa ansteckt, sondern eher erschreckt und selbst dann noch zum Weinen bringen kann, wenn es selber gerade lacht.

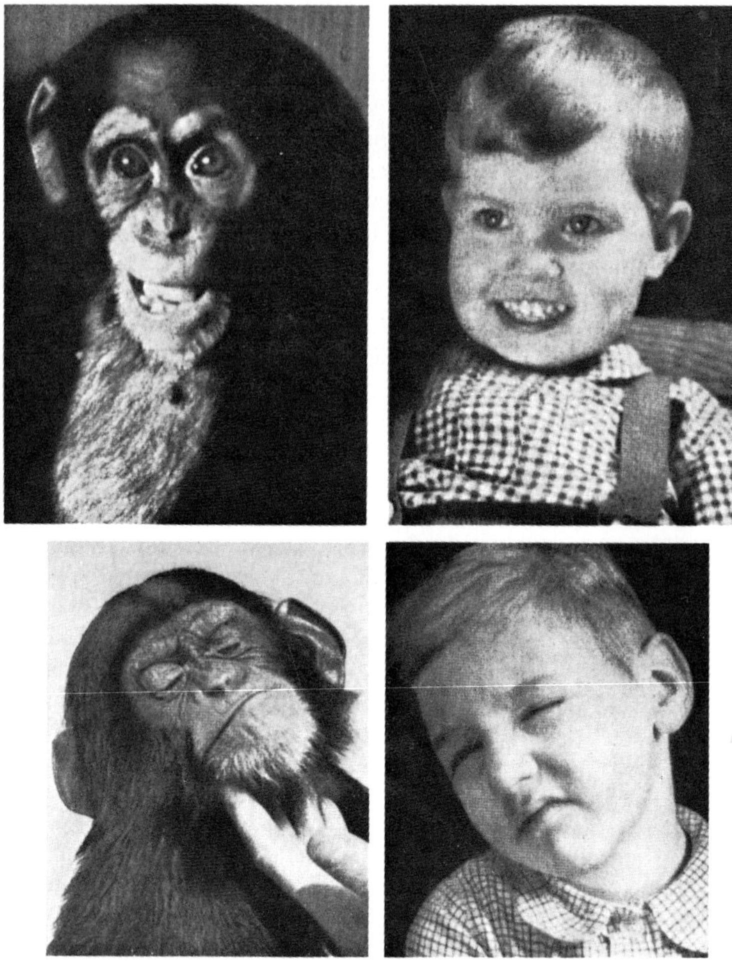

Abb. 20. Ausdrucksbewegungen: Homologe Instinktbewegungen bei Menschenaffe und Mensch. Oben: Erwartungslächeln einer jungen Schimpansin und eines kleinen Jungen. Unten: Mißvergnügen. (Photo von B. GRZIMEK)

Über die Ursprünge des menschlichen Lächelns und Lachens ist viel diskutiert worden, und manche Theorien sind entstanden (Übersicht bei ANDREW, 1963). Übereinstimmung besteht darin, daß es mindestens bei den Menschenaffen, vor allem beim Schimpansen, homologe Gesichtsausdrücke gibt, die dem Lächeln und Lachen entsprechen. Die Frage ist, ob Lächeln und Lachen lediglich verschiedene Intensitätsgrade ein und derselben Handlungsbereitschaft sind, wie z.B. LORENZ (1963) annimmt, oder ob beiden Ausdrucksweisen verschiedene Motivationen zugrunde liegen. Von manchen wird das Lächeln und Lachen als Dominanzgeste, von anderen als submissiver Ausdruck verstanden. VAN HOOFF (1967) beschreibt menschliche Situationen, in denen Lächeln adäquat, Lachen aber gänzlich fehl am Platze wäre, z.B. wenn man sich seinem künftigen Chef vorstellt oder eine Mutter ihr Kind tröstet. Umgekehrt mag in anderen Situationen, wo ein die kameradschaftlichen Bande stiftendes oder stärkendes Lachen erwartet wird, ein Lächeln befremdlich wirken. Beim Schimpansen jedenfalls glaubt van Hooff, zwei verschiedene Motivationen feststellen zu können. Die eine drückt sich im stummen Zähnezeigen aus und entspricht nach der Art der Mimik und den Situationen, in denen sie auftritt, dem menschlichen Lächeln. Die andere drückt sich im Mund-offen-Gesicht aus und entspricht besonders im Zusammenhang mit Stakkatolauten und lebhaften Körperbewegungen dem menschlichen Lachen. Während beim Menschen fraglos alle möglichen Übergänge vorhanden sind, bestehen diese beim Schimpansen nicht. Die Einbeziehung des Zähnezeigens in das Mund-offen-Gesicht, wie es der Mensch zeigt, mag mit der erweiterten, aber feiner abgestuften Signalfunktion zusammenhängen.

Schreien ist bekanntlich der am frühesten auftretende emotionale Ausdruck des Säuglings. Obwohl Gesichtsausdruck und Vokalisation recht variabel sind, kann man das Schreien doch klar von allen anderen Äußerungen des Säuglings unterscheiden. Wie Wolff (1969) gezeigt hat, ist die Zahl der Reizbedingungen, die Schreien hervorrufen, sehr groß. Gleich durch welche Ursache ausgelöst, hat es für die Pflegeperson einen starken Aufforderungscharakter und somit einen stark adaptiven Wert für den Säugling. Schon nach wenigen Wochen kann man verschiedene Formen des Schreiens unterscheiden, je nachdem, ob der Säugling Aufmerksamkeit erregen will („instrumentelles" Schreien), Hunger oder Schmerzen hat oder sonstiges Mißbehagen ausdrückt (Wolff, 1966). Die Differenzierungen des Schreiens sind lautspektrographisch objektivierbar; das Spektrogramm kann sogar zur Diagnostik, z.B. des Down-Syndroms eingesetzt werden (Wasz-Hoeckert et al., 1968; Lind et al., 1970).

Die weiteren emotionalen Äußerungen des Säuglings und die zugehörigen Gesichtsausdrücke sind fast alle auch schon von Darwin beschrieben worden. Jeder, der Säuglingsverhalten beobachtet, bemerkt die große Vielfalt von Gesichtsausdrücken im Vergleich zum verhältnismäßig limitierten Verhaltensrepertoire. Bisher hat nur Herzka (1965) den Versuch unternommen, diese Gesichtsausdrücke von der ersten Stunde bis zum Alter von 29 Wochen in 100 Fotografien zu dokumentieren. Jedes Foto ist kommentiert und die Reizbedingungen, die den Ausdruck hervorgerufen haben, sind – soweit möglich – angegeben. Die Vielfalt reicht vom „Engelslächeln" bis zum Gähnen, vom Ausdruck des Ergötzens bis zum Kummervollen und umfaßt Gesichtsausdrücke der Ablehnung und des Widerwillens – auslösbar übrigens durch salzige, saure und bittere Geschmacksstoffe, während Süßes einen behaglichen Ausdruck hervorruft (Steiner, 1974) – oder der Schläue und Weisheit des Erwachsenen. Dies weist auf die von Geburt an vorhandene große Gesichtsmuskelbeweglichkeit und den hohen Grad der neuromuskulären Organisation hin, die den der Menschenaffen noch übertrifft und für die spätere Sprachentwicklung entscheidend ist (s.S. 517ff.). Über diese Sammlung von Herzka hinaus gibt es bis jetzt keine befriedigende Taxonomie der Gesichtsausdrücke. Blurton Jones (1972) hat aus 500 Fotos 52 Komponenten der Gesichtsausdrücke abgeleitet und Ekman und Friesen (1976) haben einen Code entwickelt, der auf der Anatomie der Gesichtsmuskulatur aufbaut und dem früher von Leonhard (1968) und Heimann (1966) beschriebenen

Ansatz ähnelt, aber zum codierten Auswerten von mimischen Abläufen geeignet ist.

Durch bessere Methoden der Erfassung von Gesichtsausdrücken wird man in Zukunft auch mehr über deren Entwicklungsfolge aussagen können, an denen man emotionale Reifungsprozesse ablesen kann. CHARLESWORTH (1970) fand zum Beispiel, daß das Heben der Augenbrauen, wie es DARWIN beim Gesichtsausdruck der Überraschung beschrieben hat, bei Kindern im Alter von 4–12 Monaten in 132 Überraschungssituationen nicht beobachtet werden konnte, wohl aber manchmal der dazugehörige offene Mund. Der volle Gesichtsausdruck der Überraschung, schon sehr ähnlich dem des Erwachsenen, erscheint erst im Schulalter.

Außerordentlich aufschlußreiche Einblicke in die endogene Organisation des menschlichen Gemütslebens erhält man durch die Studien an blinden und blindtauben Kindern. DARWIN (1872) schrieb, daß viele Gesichtsausdrücke der kongenital Blinden angeboren sein müssen, da sie nicht durch Nachahmung erlernt werden können, und führte u.a. Lächeln und Lachen auf.

THOMPSEN (1941) studierte die Gesichtsausdrücke von 26 blinden Kindern, von denen 11 blind geboren wurden und 4 taub und blind waren; sie verglich diese Gruppe mit 29 sehenden Kindern gleicher Altersstufen von 7 Wochen bis zu 13 Jahren. Der einzige deutliche Gruppenunterschied bestand darin, daß die blind geborenen Kinder nach dem 6. Lebensjahr bedeutend weniger lächelten. Auch waren die individuellen Differenzen der Art zu lächeln größer. Beide Befunde sprechen dafür, daß die soziale Rückmeldung zur Aufrechterhaltung und Vereinheitlichung der Instinktbewegung beiträgt. Im übrigen fand THOMPSON, daß die Gesichtsausdrücke des Ärgers, des Schmollens und der Langeweile und Traurigkeit in beiden Gruppen ganz ähnlich sind und in angemessener Situation auftreten. Ein Kind wurde im Alter von 7 Wochen und dann wieder im 11. und 12. Monat gefilmt. Das zunächst gerade wahrnehmbare Zurückziehen der Mundwinkel beim Lächeln geschah im 11. Monat mit rundem Mund; im 12. Monat nahm der Mund eine eliptische Form an. Dieselbe Sequenz hatte auch WASHBURN (1929) bei sehenden Kindern gefunden. THOMPSON schloß daraus, daß das Lächeln bei blinden Kindern einen Reifungsprozeß durchmacht.

Experimentelle Untersuchungen zur Überraschungsreaktion an blindgeborenen und sehenden Kindern im Alter von 6–14 Jahren deckten keine Unterschiede im mimischen Ausdruck auf (CHARLESWORTH, 1970). Psychomotorisches und mimisches Verhalten konnte EIBL-EIBESFELDT (1973a, b) in Filmen von 2 taubblinden Kindern im Alter von 5 und 7 Jahren dokumentieren. Die Lachmotorik entsprach in allen Einzelheiten der gesunder Kinder. Sie warfen bei hoher Lachintensität in typischer Weise den Kopf zurück und öffneten dann auch den Mund. Das Lachen klang allerdings verhalten und mehr wie ein Kichern. Bei dem 7jährigen Mädchen konnten auch andere typische Ausdrucksbewegungen festgehalten werden. Bei Ärger stampfte es mit dem Fuß auf oder strampelte am Ort. Ablehnung geschah durch Kopfschütteln und Wegstoßen mit der Hand. Sie schmiegte sich gerne an und umarmte ihren Pfleger. Fremde unterschied sie von bekannten Personen durch Beriechen der Hand und wendete ihr Gesicht ab, ähnlich wie fremdelnde Kinder es tun.

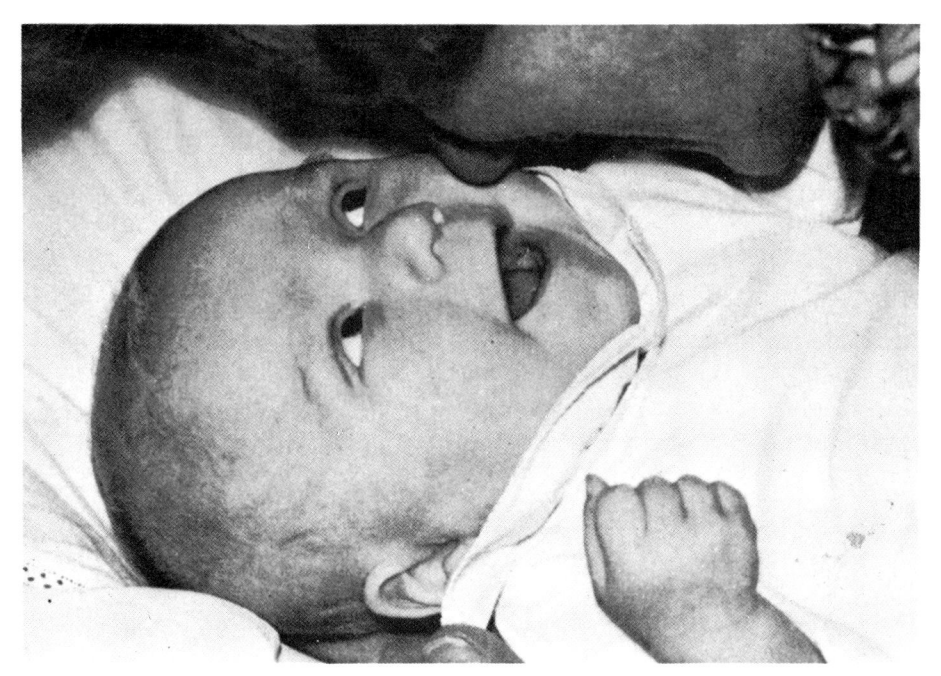

Abb. 21. Das Lächeln und Fixieren blinder Säuglinge. Von Geburt an blindes, 2 Monate und 20 Tage altes Mädchen, lächelnd; obgleich das Kind nichts sieht, blicken die Augen, die sich sonst nystagmisch bewegen, ruhig nach oben, als die über es gebeugte Mutter zu ihm spricht. (Aus FREEDMAN, 1964)

Unter den 4 kongenital blinden Kindern, die FREEDMAN (1964, 1965) studierte, war eines, das seinen Blick beim Lächeln auf die sich herabbeugende Mutter richtete, so daß der Ausdruck dieses 2 Monate und 20 Tage alten Mädchens kaum von dem eines sehenden Kindes zu unterscheiden war (Abb. 21). FREEDMAN (1965) scheint der einzige zu sein, der eine Zwillingsstudie über Verhaltensweisen während des ersten Lebensjahrs durchgeführt hat. 11 gleichgeschlechtliche ZZ und 9 EZ wurden in ihrem motorischen und expressiven Verhalten verglichen. EZ zeigten in bezug auf Lächeln und Furcht vor Fremden eine signifikant größere Ähnlichkeit als ZZ.

Mimikerkennen beim Menschen

Die Ontogenese des Mimikerkennes ist für die Säuglings- und frühe Kinderzeit aus methodischen Gründen schwierig zu erfassen. KAILA (1932) stellte im Laboratorium von CHARLOTTE BÜHLER die ersten Attrappen-Versuche am Säugling an. Ihm folgten RENÉ SPITZ und KÄTHE WOLF (1946). Sie stellten an 145 Kindern im Alter von 3–6 Monaten fest, daß rohe Gesichtsattrappen oder eine „sardonisch" verzerrte Fratze das Lächeln gerade so gut auszulösen vermögen wie das menschliche Gesicht. AHRENS (1954) stellte dann auf Grund seiner gründlicheren Attrappenversuche einen Entwicklungskalender auf, über den ich 1964 ausführlich berichtet habe:

Bis zum Beginn des 2. Monats kann Lächeln am besten durch zwei waagerecht oder senkrecht angeordente, augengroße Punkte auf einem grob ausgeschnittenen Kopfumriß ausgelöst werden. Mit dem 2. Monat ist die „Okula" (zwei waagerecht angeordnete Punkte) wirksamer. Mit drei Monaten bekommt die untere Gesichtshälfte eine mitwirkende Auslöserfunktion, ohne daß die Mundkonfiguration eine Rolle spielt. Die Okula muß differenzierter dargeboten werden. Im Alter von 4 Monaten können Mundbewegungen wirksam werden. Mit 5 Monaten läßt die Wirkung der Attrappen nach. Das auch von SPITZ hervorgehobene Breitziehen des Mundes entfaltet dieselbe auslösende Wirkung wie die volle bewegte Mundmimik des Erwachsenen. Beim 6 Monate alten Kind wirken Mundbewegungen, vor allem das Breitziehen, am stärksten. Im 8. Monat, wo nur das volle, lachende Erwachsenengesicht noch wirksam ist, beginnt sich das Ausdrucksverhältnis beim Säugling herauszubilden, das AHRENS bis zum Alter von 2 Jahren untersucht hat. Weitere Untersuchungen beziehen sich auf das Alter zwischen $2^1/_2$ und 6 Jahren (s. auch BÜHLER u. HETZER, 1928; HONKAVAARA, 1961; HÜCKSTEDT, 1965).

Die Stirnmimik, die ja zunächst keine Rolle spielt, kommt erst etwa mit 14 Monaten zur vollen Geltung. Dann nämlich dominiert die senkrechte Faltenbildung eindeutig über die waagrechte. Die Heimkinder reagierten darauf prompt mit Wegwenden des Kopfes, mit Fortlaufen, mit Weinen und Schreien; ja, es kam sogar vor, daß dem Untersucher ins Gesicht geschlagen wurde. Mit ziemlicher Sicherheit konnte Erfahrung ausgeschlossen werden, denn die Pflegepersonen waren spontan gar nicht imstande, eine „Drohmiene" zu machen. Sie mußte erst eingeübt werden. Die Erfahrung lehrt zudem, daß kaum je ein Erwachsener einem kleinen Kinde die Drohmiene zeigt. Fast durchwegs werden beim Schimpfen die Stimme und der Zeigefinger gehoben. Kinder in diesem Alter sind noch nicht in der Lage, eine Miene sinnvoll zu deuten. Selbst in einem Alter, in dem die Übertragung von Gegenständen auf eine Abbildung und ein korrektes Benennen einzelner Teile des Gesichtes sicher gelingen, kann der Gesichtsausdruck keineswegs sinnvoll gedeutet werden. Der zurechtweisende Blick wird nach unseren Erfahrungen frühestens mit 1,6 Jahren wirksam.

AHRENS' Untersuchungen sind in der Folgezeit aus methodischen Gründen angegriffen worden, doch ist es bisher niemandem gelungen, die Ontogenese des Mimikerkennens besser bzw. besser gesichert darzustellen. Bedenkt man alle Argumente gründlich, muß man zu dem Schluß kommen, daß es außerordentlich schwierig ist, bei Säuglingen mit solchen Experimenten zu schlüssigen Ergebnissen zu kommen. Mir scheint jedenfalls genügend klar zu sein, daß der Säugling mit zunehmender Organisation seiner visuellen Wahrnehmung auf zunehmend komplexere Reizkonstellationen des erwachsenen menschlichen Gesichts reagiert und daß in der Abfolge der am besten wirksamen Reizkonstellationen eine gewisse Regelhaftigkeit besteht. Die Frage, warum das Baby gerade mit Lächeln oder unter bestimmten Umständen auch mit Ablehnung und Weinen reagiert, läßt sich vermutlich mit Attrappen-Versuchen allein ebensowenig entscheiden, wie die Frage, ob es sich hier allein um die Reaktion auf ein angeborenes Schema handelt, wie LORENZ (1935) den angeborenen Auslösemechanismus (AAM) zunächst genannt hat, oder ob die Erfahrung eine entscheidende Rolle spielt. Wir werden uns diesem Problem noch auf andere Weise nähern.

Jedenfalls hat sich bereits DARWIN in diesem Zusammenhang über das Anlage-Umwelt-Problem – im Englischen als „nature-nurture-problem" bezeichnet – Gedanken gemacht. Während er vom Angeborensein des Gesichtsausdruckes überzeugt war, schien es ihm nicht so sicher, wie es mit der Entwicklung der Fähigkeit bestellt ist, die Gesichtsausdrücke anderer zu erkennen. BÜHLER und HETZER (1928) scheinen die ersten gewesen zu sein, die in systematischer Weise versucht haben, die Reaktionen von Kindern im ersten Lebensjahr auf zwei verschiedene Gesichtsausdrücke zu untersuchen. Sie boten drei Klassen von Reizen, erstens ein lächelndes und ein zorniges (lebendiges) Gesicht, zweitens eine liebevolle und eine schimpfende Stimme und drittens liebevolle und drohende Gebärden mit den Armen ohne stimmliche Äußerung und mit neutralem Gesicht. Die Reaktionen der Säuglinge wurden in zwei Klassen eingeteilt, nämlich positive (Lächeln, freudiges Strampeln) und negative (Bewegungslosigkeit, weinerliches Gesicht, Weinen). Die Ergebnisse zeigten, daß vom 3. bis zum Ende des 6. Monats keine neutralen Reaktionen auf das freundliche und auf das zornige Gesicht zu beobachten waren. Im 3. Monat waren 90% der Reaktionen auf das zornige Gesicht positiv! (vgl. S. 407f. und Abb. 19). Im 4. Monat waren 50% positiv und 50% negativ und vom 5. bis 7. Monat waren 100% negativ. Nach diesem Zeitpunkt nahmen die neutralen Reaktionen bis zu 40% zu, der Rest blieb in positive und negative Reizantworten geteilt. Die Ergebnisse in bezug auf die Stimmen waren nahezu identisch mit den Gesichtsausdrücken, während die Differenzierung der Gebärden erst später gelang.

Die Parallele zum Mimikerkennen isoliert aufgezogener Rhesusaffen ist hier unverkennbar. Das zornige Gesicht wird zunächst nicht von einem anderen Gesichtsausdruck getrennt – und dasselbe trifft auch für die Stimme zu –, von einem bestimmten Zeitpunkt an, nämlich am ausgeprägtesten vom 5. bis 7. Monat, wird scharf getrennt. Danach nimmt die Zahl der neutralen Reizantworten beträchtlich zu. Die auf S. 408 f. gegebene Interpretation dieser Ergebnisse trifft – mutatis mutandis – wohl auch auf den menschlichen Säugling zu.

Aus späteren, ähnlich angelegten, aber methodisch besser kontrollierten Studien (WILCOX u. CLAYTON, 1968; KREUTZER u. CHARLESWORTH, 1973) kann man nur schließen, daß das Baby in der Mitte seines 1. Lebensjahrs in der Lage ist, die Mimik Erwachsener in einigen Aspekten zu differenzieren. Auch die zahlreichen Arbeiten zur Differenzierung von Gesichtsausdrücken und den zugehörigen Emotionen, die an älteren Kindern vom 2. bis zum 14. Lebensjahr durchgeführt wurden, haben nicht viel mehr erbracht als die Erkenntnis, daß Kindern mit steigendem Alter zunehmend besser Emotionen von Erwachsenen dem entsprechenden Gesichtsausdruck zuordnen können (s. MCGREW, 1972; CHARLESWORTH u. KREUTZER, 1973).

Transkulturelle Studien an Erwachsenen

Bezüglich des Anlage-Umwelt-Problems, bzw. der Frage nach den angeborenen und erlernten Anteilen im Prozeß des Mimikerkennens, haben erst die Arbeiten von EIBL-EIBESFELDT (1970, 1976) und von EKMAN und seinen Mitarbeitern (1972) neue Wege geöffnet. EKMAN benutzte, wenn auch in elaborierter

Form, Techniken, die schon DARWIN und nach ihm andere angewandt hatten, nämlich Beobachtung von Kindern, Erwachsenen und psychisch Kranken, Kulturvergleiche, Wahl- und Zuordnungen von fotografierten Gesichtern und die Nachahmung von Gesichtsausdrücken.

Für transkulturelle Studien kann man zwei verschiedene Untersuchungsmethoden anwenden, von denen jede gewisse Vorteile und Nachteile hat. Im einen Fall sammelt man mit Hilfe von Film oder Videobändern mimisches Ausdrucksverhalten in bestimmten Situationen von Angehörigen verschiedener Kulturen und stellt auf irgendeine reproduzierbare Weise Ähnlichkeiten und Unterschiede der Gesichtsausdrücke in den zu vergleichenden Kulturen fest. Diese Methode hat vor allem EIBL-EIBESFELDT (1971a) für vergleichende Verhaltensstudien am Menschen verwendet und ist durch das Filmen mit einer Winkelkamera einem wesentlichen Einwand gegen diese Methode begegnet, daß nämlich das Verhalten der Gefilmten verfälscht würde, wenn sie sich beobachtet fühlten.

Die andere, in den Untersuchungen zum Mimikverständnis häufiger angewandte Methode benutzt das Urteilsvermögen von Versuchspersonen, die verbal oder auf andere Weise beschriebene Emotionen Fotografien von Gesichtsausdrücken zuzuordnen haben. Man kann dabei davon ausgehen, daß der Beurteilende auf seine eigene Erfahrung zurückgreift, sei es auf Selbst- oder Fremderfahrung, und die Zuordnung von mimischem Ausdruck und Emotion dementsprechend vornimmt. Wenn die eine bestimmte Emotion ausdrückende Mimik kulturbedingt wäre, dann müßten Angehörige verschiedener Kulturen auf verschiedene Erfahrungen zurückgreifen und dementsprechend zu verschiedenen Urteilen bei ihren Zuordnungen kommen. Wenn aber DARWIN recht hätte und die Gesichtsausdrücke der Gemütsbewegungen zu den Universalien der Menschheit gehörten, dann wäre auch transkulturell eine große Übereinstimmung der Urteile zu erwarten.

Bevor wir die wesentlichen Ergebnisse dieser Untersuchungen besprechen, müssen wir nochmals auf den Ausdrucksreichtum höherer Säuger zurückkommen (s.S. 402ff. und Abb. 15f.). Dieser hat, wie LORENZ zuerst erkannte, seine Wurzeln in der Überlagerung von Stimmungen verschiedener Intensität, die sich im Gesichtsausdruck widerspiegeln. In Abb. 22 hat EKMAN die Ausdrucksüberlagerungen beim Menschen auf ähnliche Weise dokumentiert. Er wählte die Überlagerungen von „Überraschung" und „Furcht". Seit DARWIN werden in den Mimikstudien am Menschen sog. primäre Gesichtsausdrücke verwendet, deren Mischungen dann den außerordentlichen Ausdrucksreichtum beim Menschen ergeben. Diese sind: Vergnügen, Mißvergnügen, Überraschung, Ärger (Wut), Angst (Furcht) und Trauer. TOMKINS Theorie der primären Affekte und Gesichtsausdrücke (1962, 1964) hat spätere Untersucher sichtbar beeinflußt. IZARD (1971) benutzte z.B. folgende Reihe in seinen transkulturellen Studien: Interesse – Erregung, Vergnügen – Freude, Überraschung – Erschrecken, Enttäuschung – Angst, Abscheu – Verachtung, Ärger – Wut, Scham – Demütigung, Furcht – Schrecken. Hier ist also jede Emotion in zwei Intensitätsstufen unterteilt. EKMAN (1973) teilt Emotionen in reine Emotionen („single emotions") und gemischte Emotionen („blended emotions") ein und glaubt, daß die reinen Emotionen für alle Menschen universal sind, während die gemischten in verschie-

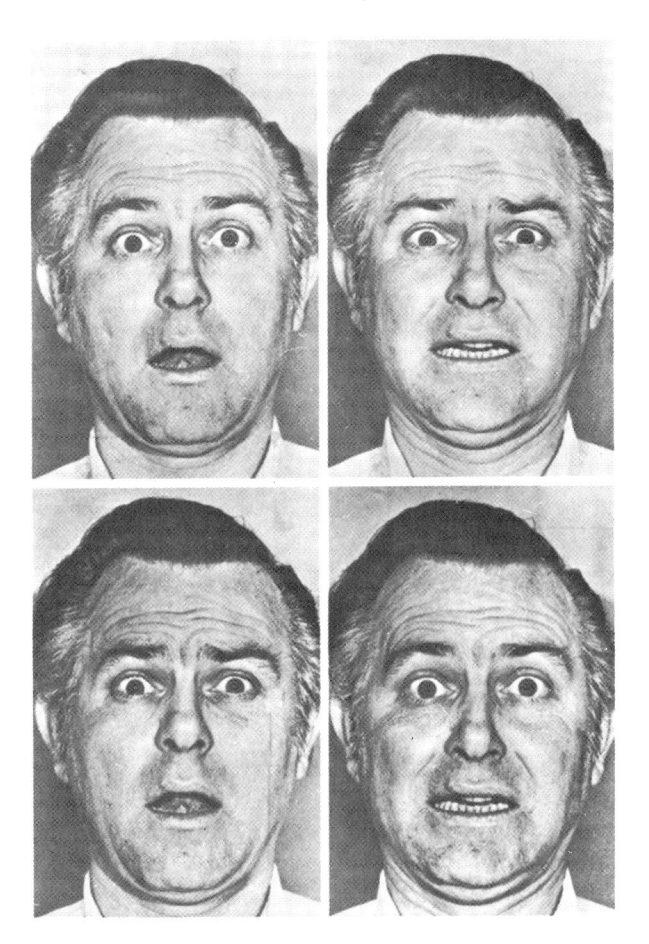

Abb. 22. Überlagerungen von Stimmungen im Gesichtsausdruck. Links oben: reiner Ausdruck der Überraschung; rechts oben: reiner Ausdruck der Furcht; links unten: im Ausdruck überlagert sich Überraschung (Mund) mit Furcht (Augen, Augenbrauen, Stirn); rechts unten: Überlagerung von Überraschung (Augenbrauen, Stirn) und Furcht (Mund). (Aus EKMAN, 1973)

denen Kulturen hinsichtlich der Häufigkeit ihres Auftretens variieren. Mit dieser Annahme versucht er, manche widersprüchlichen Ergebnisse in der Literatur zu erklären.

Studien in fünf Schriftkulturen

EKMAN und FRIESEN (1971) wählten aus 3000 Fotografien 30 Bilder von 14 verschiedenen Personen aus, deren Gesichter 6 verschiedene Emotionen ausdrückten. Tabelle 1 gibt das Ergebnis wieder. Wird das Gesamtmaterial einer statistischen Analyse unterzogen, findet sich weder ein signifikanter Unterschied zwischen den Urteilen aus allen 5 Ländern über alle Gesichtsausdrücke noch in bezug auf jeden einzelnen Ausdruck. IZARD (1971) testete auf ähnliche Weise 9 Schriftkulturen und kam zu nahezu gleichen Ergebnissen.

Tabelle 1. Übereinstimmung von Gesichtsausdruck und Emotion[a]

	Japan %	Brasilien %	Chile %	Argentinien %	USA %
Glücklich	87	97	90	94	97
Ängstlich	71	77	78	68	88
Überrascht	87	82	88	93	91
Ärgerlich	63	82	76	72	69
Widerlich/verächtlich	82	86	85	79	82
Traurig	74	82	90	85	73
Zahl der Beurteiler	29	40	119	168	99

[a] Den Beurteilern wurden 30 Photographien von 14 verschiedenen Personen vorgelegt, die sie entsprechend dem wahrgenommenen Gesichtsausdruck den sechs aufgeführten Emotionen zuzuordnen hatten. (Aus EKMAN u. FRIESEN, 1971)

Studien in analphabetischen Kulturen

Als ein Beispiel wählen wir einen Stamm im südöstlichen Bergland von Neuguinea, den EKMAN und FRIESEN (1971) untersuchten. Die Fore lebten 14 Jahre vor Beginn der Untersuchung in einer Steinzeitkultur. Seither hatten viele dieser Neuguineer intensiven Kontakt mit Missionaren und anderen Weißen. Es wurden daher solche ausgewählt, die möglichst keine Berührung mit westlichen Menschen hatten und weder englisch noch pidgin sprechen konnten. 189 Männern und Frauen wurden 3 Fotos für jeden Gesichtsausdruck vorgelegt, 130 Buben und Mädchen bekamen 2 Fotos. Zu den Fotos wurde eine kleine Geschichte erzählt, z.B. „seine Freunde sind gekommen und er ist glücklich", woraufhin die Versuchsperson das passende Foto zu wählen hatte. Tabelle 2 zeigt das Ergebnis. Es unterscheidet sich nicht von dem Vergleich der Schriftkulturen. Die Fore konnten nur Furcht nicht von Überraschung unterscheiden, vielleicht weil bei ihnen nur furchteinjagende Ereignisse auch diejenigen sind, die Überraschung erzeugen.

Andere Mitglieder aus dem Stamme der Fore, die an diesem Experiment nicht teilgenommen hatten, wurden gebeten, die Gesichter nachzuahmen, die sie machen würden, wenn sie die Personen in den Geschichten wären. (Auch diese Methode wurde schon von DARWIN benutzt.) Die Fotos dieser Gesichtsausdrücke wurden dann amerikanischen College-Studenten gezeigt. Obwohl diese nie Neuguineer gesehen hatten, bestand kaum eine Schwierigkeit, die nachgemachten Gesichtsausdrücke für Ärger, Abscheu, Traurigkeit und Vergnügen richtig einzuschätzen, während die Bilder für Furcht und Überraschung, ähnlich wie bei den Fore, häufiger verwechselt wurden.

Diese Studien zum Erkennen der emotionalen Bedeutung von Gesichtsausdrücken über sehr verschiedene Kulturen hinweg belegen ohne Zweifel – von anderen Denkansätzen bestimmt und unterschiedlich in den Methoden – die in der ethologisch orientierten Literatur immer wieder vertretene Auffassung von der Universalität menschlichen Ausdrucksverhaltens. Ein gut studiertes Beispiel ist der von EIBL-EIBESFELDT (1968, 1971b, 1978) beschriebene Augengruß.

Tabelle 2. Zuordnung eines Gesichtsausdrucks zu einer Emotion durch Steinzeitkulturmenschen[a]

In der Geschichte beschriebene Emotion	Bildwahlen in % Übereinstimmung mit gehörter Geschichte	
	Erwachsene	Kinder[b]
Glücklich	92	92
Traurig	79	81
Ärgerlich	84	90
Widerlich	81	85
Überrascht	68	98
Unterscheidung von ängstlich, widerlich und traurig	80	93
Unterscheidung von ängstlich und überrascht	43	—[c]
Zahl der Beurteiler	189	130

[a] Die Fore auf Neu-Guinea
[b] Die Erwachsenen hatten eine von drei vorgelegten Photographien zu wählen, die Kinder nur eine von zwei Photographien; daher die höheren % der richtigen Wahlen bei Kindern
[c] Diese Differenzierung wurde bei den Kindern nicht probiert. (Nach EKMAN u. FRIESEN, 1971)

Dieses Augengrüßen besteht in einem schnellen Anheben der Augenbrauen, das nur Bruchteile einer Sekunde dauert und dem stets ein Lächeln vorangeht. Verstärktes Lächeln und oft auch Kopfnicken schließen sich an. Es handelt sich um ein recht stereotypes, universelles Ausdrucksmuster, das EIBL-EIBESFELDT in vielen, ganz verschiedenen Kulturen fand, z.B. bei Balinesen, Papuas, Samoanern, Buschleuten, Waika-Indianern und Europäern. Beim Grüßen und Flirten, beim Schäkern mit Kindern und beim Danken tritt der Augengruß am häufigsten auf, kommt aber auch bei anderen Formen des Sozialkontaktes vor. Auf Samoa kann das Signal ein einfaches, zustimmendes Ja, in Griechenland ein ablehnendes Nein bedeuten.

Wie fast immer im Hin und Her der Argumente um das Anlage-Umwelt-Problem gibt es aber kein Entweder-Oder (PLOOG, 1979). Zweifellos wirken auch kulturelle Normen und Traditionen bis in die Mimik hinein. Die Muster der mimischen Signale sind dem Menschen angeboren wie die Gesichtsmuskeln, die sie ausführen und die neuronalen Programme, die sie erregen; der Kontext jedoch, in dem diese Signale gezeigt und beantwortet werden, die Regeln, unter denen ihre Benutzung erlaubt oder verboten ist, hängt vom Kanon der Kultur ab, in der das Individuum lebt, von seiner Stellung in der Gemeinschaft, von seinem Alter und seinem Geschlecht. Auch diese Abhängigkeit des Gebrauchs der Kommunikationsmittel von der Gemeinschaft, in der der Mensch lebt, teilt er, wenn auch in differenzierter Form, mit den übrigen Primaten (s.S. 393f.).

Ein Beispiel sei den Experimenten von EKMAN (1972) entnommen. Japanischen Studenten in Tokio und amerikanischen Studenten in Berkeley wurden Streßfilme gezeigt. Das Experiment wurde ihnen von ihrem Versuchsleiter als psychophysiologische Studie zur Messung von Streßreaktionen erklärt; entsprechende Vorkehrungen zur Ableitung des Elektrokardiogramms und des galvanischen Hautreflexes wurden getroffen. Nach der Instruktion verließ der japanische bzw. der amerikanische Versuchsleiter den Raum. Während jeweils ein Streßfilm und ein neutraler Filmstreifen liefen, wurden die Gesichter der Versuchspersonen unbemerkt gefilmt. Dann trat der Versuchsleiter wieder ein, befragte die Versuchsperson über ihre Gefühle, die sie während des Streßfilmes empfand, und setzte, während weiteres Streßmaterial gezeigt wurde, sein Interview fort. Mit Hilfe einer quantitativen Auswertetechnik für mimische Abläufe (EKMAN u. FRIESEN, 1976) wurden die beiden Gruppen in den verschiedenen Situationen verglichen. Die Übereinstimmung der mimischen Abläufe von Japanern und Amerikanern in der Streßsituation ohne Anwesenheit des Versuchsleiters war sehr groß. In der Interview-Situation fiel der Vergleich signifikant unterschiedlich aus. Die japanischen Studenten unterdrückten ihre negativen Gefühle weit mehr und lächelten dafür.

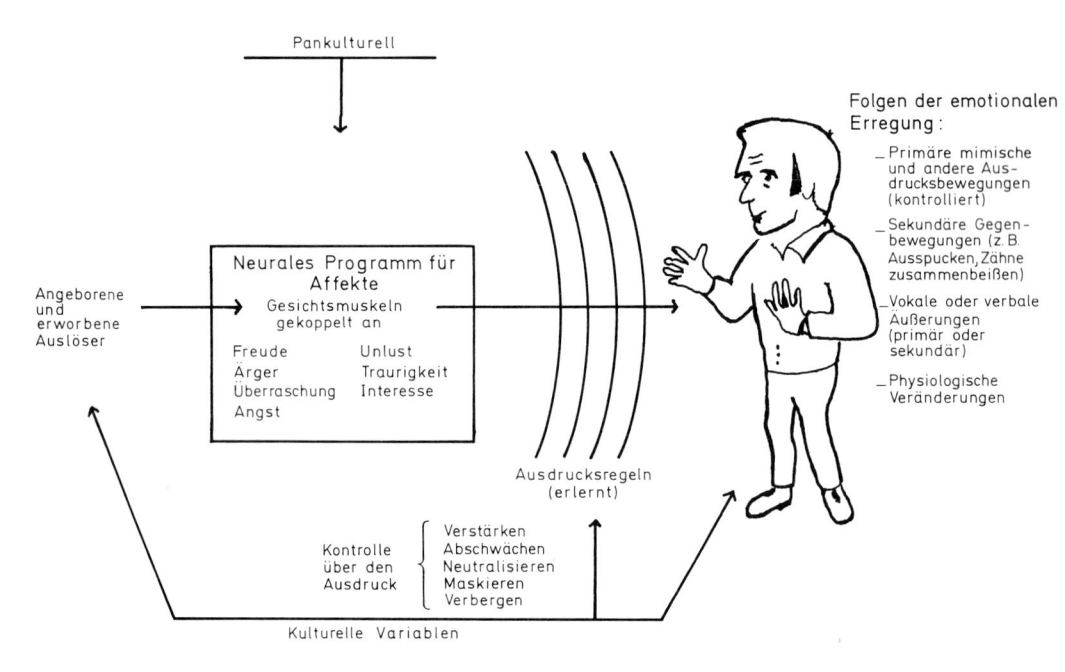

Abb. 23. Determinanten für den Gesichtsausdruck und andere Ausdrucksweisen des Menschen. (Aus EKMAN, 1971, modifiziert)

Abb. 23 faßt die Determinanten zusammen, die den menschlichen mimischen Ausdruck und mit ihm andere Antworten auf auslösende Ereignisse bestimmen, also psychomotorische, vokale, verbale und vegetative Reaktionen.

Die Beziehungen von angeborenen und erworbenen Auslösern zu den Emotionen

Mimische Abläufe sind, wie wir gezeigt haben, Erbkoordinationen im Sinne von LORENZ und damit Instinktbewegungen. Jedem mimischen Ausdruck entspricht – jedenfalls in den frühen Phasen der menschlichen Ontogenese – eine Stimmung, ein innerer Zustand, den man Emotion nennt (TOMKINS, 1962; TOMKINS u. MCCARTER, 1964; TOMKINS u. IZARD, 1965; HINDE, 1972a).

Sei es durch DARWINS Buch "The expression of the emotions in man and animals" oder aus anderen Gründen, werden im Schrifttum, besonders im englischsprachigen, die Worte Gesichtsausdruck (facial expression) synonym mit Gefühlsausdruck (facial expression of emotion) benutzt. Um aber über die Biologie von Ausdruck und Eindruck (LEYHAUSEN, 1968) sowie den inneren Zustand von Sender und Empfänger – die jeweiligen Emotionen – mehr Klarheit zu gewinnen, wollen wir die an sich untrennbaren Aspekte begrifflich trennen.

Nach dem ethologischen Grundmuster einer Instinkthandlung wird die Instinktbewegung durch einen passenden Reiz, den das Tier angeborenermaßen kennt, ausgelöst. Die Tatsache, daß ein bestimmtes, angeborenes Verhalten, z.B. das Lächeln, durch eine bestimmte, für jede Art typische Reizkombination ausgelöst werden kann, brachte LORENZ zu der fundamentalen Erkenntnis, daß jeder angeborenen Verhaltensweise ein „auslösendes angeborenes Schema" entspricht. Der heute eingebürgerte Ausdruck von TINBERGEN (1952) „angeborener Auslösemechanismus", kurz AAM genannt, besagt dasselbe. Man stellt sich darunter einen neurosensorischen Mechanismus nach Art eines Reizfilterapparates vor, der eine speziell angeborene Verhaltensweise auf passende Außenreize hin in Aktion setzt. Nun schleudert der Frosch, wenn er hungrig ist, seine Zunge zwar immer wieder auf eine Beuteattrappe und lernt nicht oder nur sehr schwer, daß die Attrappe keine wirkliche Fliege ist. Beim höheren Säuger und ganz besonders bei den Primaten kann man aber nachweisen, daß schon zu einem sehr frühen Zeitpunkt Lernen ins Spiel kommt. LORENZ (1935, 1965) hat dies von Anfang an betont und seine Vorstellungen vom Zusammenwirken angeborener und erworbener Bausteine des Verhaltens mit dem Terminus Instinkt-Dressurverschränkung gekennzeichnet (s. PLOOG u. GOTTWALD, 1974). Danach ist die Instinktbewegung das „movens" – der Verstärker – durch den Lernen ermöglicht wird. Das für unseren Zusammenhang Wesentliche ist aber die Abwandlung des AAM, in den sozusagen hineingelernt wird. Der AAM wird zum EAAM (dem durch Erfahrung veränderten AAM). Die Reizkonstellation, die ursprünglich die Instinktbewegung auslöste, hat sich durch Erfahrung spezifiziert (SCHLEIDT, 1962). Nicht mehr eine Attrappe mit Augenpunkten löst das Lächeln aus, sondern eine Attrappe mit Augenpunkten und Mund, später das ganze lebendige Gesicht, schließlich nur die Gesichtszüge bekannter Personen usw. Aber auch der rein erworbene Auslösemechanismus (EAM) kann eine Instinktbewegung auslösen. Dies ist für den Dressurvorgang bzw. für das Konditionieren von Verhaltensweisen typisch (PLOOG, 1964c, S. 331). Ein beliebiges Signal (CS), z.B. ein Geräusch, wird mit einem natürlichen (angeborenen) Signal (US), z.B. dem Anblick einer Maus, so gepaart, daß der US dem CS in kurzem Abstand folgt. Die Instinkthandlung, z.B. die Bewegungen des Beutefanges bei der Katze, wird zunächst vom US ausgelöst; nach einiger Erfahrung tritt der CS an die Stelle des US. (Die Katze setzt schon zum Beutefangen an, wenn sie das Geräusch hört.) Kann die Instinkthandlung erst durch dazwischengeschaltete Handlungen realisiert werden, spricht man von instrumentellem oder operantem Konditionieren. Es handelt sich um eine Dressur oder Selbstdressur durch Eigentätigkeit. Gelernt wird, was Erfolg bzw. Belohnung bringt. Das Belohnende ist die Ausführung der Instinkthandlung – im gewöhnlichen Laborversuch am häufigsten das Fressen von Nahrung.

Mit diesem Exkurs in die Lernpsychologie ist nicht die verkürzte Darstellung des recht komplizierten Lernens am Erfolg beabsichtigt, sondern die Beziehung zwischen Auslösern und Emotionen sollten analysiert werden. Das Lächeln des älteren Säuglings kann ebenso durch das lächelnde Angesicht der Mutter wie durch den Anblick eines vom Säugling selbst manipulierten Gegenstandes ausgelöst werden (s.S. 503). Die Instinktbewegung und die ihr zugehörige Emotion – das Gefühl der Freude – bleiben die gleichen, die Anzahl der Auslöser, die den EAAM in Gang setzen können, wächst und differenziert sich mit der Erfahrung. Schließlich kommen im Laufe der Ontogenese die Instinktbewegungen der Mimik unter voluntative Kontrolle, gegebenenfalls mit dem Effekt ihrer Unterdrückung, ohne daß die zugehörigen Emotionen mit unterdrückt werden müßten.

Beim erwachsenen Menschen läßt sich die direkte Beziehung zwischen dem zu einem bestimmten AAM gehörigen Auslöser und der vom AAM in Gang gesetzten Instinkthandlung nur noch selten herstellen. Am bekanntesten ist das von LORENZ (1943) beschriebene und analysierte Kindchenschema. Seine Hauptmerkmale sind ein im Verhältnis zum Rumpf zu großer Kopf, eine hohe, vorgewölbte Stirn über einem kleinen Gesicht, relativ große Augen, kleiner Mund, kurze Extremitäten, rundliche Körperformen und tolpatschige Bewegungen. Da die gleichen Merkmale nicht nur bei Menschenkindern, sondern auch bei vielen anderen Säugetierjungen vorkommen, lösen auch diese – insbesondere bei weiblichen Personen – die gleichen Brutpflegegefühle und -reaktionen wie menschliche Kinder aus (HÜCKSTEDT, 1965). Tierarten, die noch im ausgewachsenem Zustand solche Proportionsmerkmale zeigen, werden vom Menschen auch im adulten Stadium noch als besonders „niedlich" empfunden – was sich oft in der angehängten Verkleinerungssilbe -chen äußert (vgl. z.B. Spitzmaus und Eichhörnchen, Specht und Rotkehlchen).

Da nun aber Emotionen nicht allein an soziale Auslöser und Kommunikationsprozesse gebunden sind, sondern die Triebfeder des Handelns überhaupt darstellen, müssen wir weiter nach ihrer Herkunft fragen. Seit altersher werden die Gefühle, i.e.S. Emotionen, in die Nachbarschaft der Empfindungen gerückt. Die spezifischen Geschmacksempfindungen „süß" oder „salzig", die beim Neugeborenen mimische Reaktionen des Vergnügens oder Mißvergnügens auslösen, brauchen nicht gelernt zu werden (STEINER, 1977). Gelernt wird die Zuordnung vom Aussehen zuckriger Gegenstände zur spezifischen Geschmacksempfindung süß. Das gleiche gilt für alle übrigen Empfindungen wie Wärme, Kälte, Farben, sofern keine genetisch bedingten spezifischen Empfindungsausfälle vorliegen. Daß kochendes Wasser Schmerz verursacht, muß gelernt werden. Der Lernvorgang besteht hier – ähnlich wie bei der bedingten Reaktion – in einer direkten

Ankoppelung des zunächst neutralen Reizes (kochendes Wasser) an die angeborene Schmerzempfindung. Gerade beim Schmerz wird die neurobiologische Beziehung zwischen Empfindung und Gefühl am deutlichsten. Hier hat die Hirnchirurgie gezeigt, daß sich durch Ausschaltung von Hirngewebe die emotionale Komponente des Schmerzes, das Schmerzgefühl, beseitigen läßt, obwohl die Schmerzempfindung selbst weiter besteht. Der Patient sagt: „Es tut mir noch weh, aber es macht mir nichts mehr aus."

Da Sinnesempfindungen, abgesehen von der Tagesperiodik, normalerweise keine Schwankungen in der Reaktionsbereitschaft zeigen, sind sie den Reflexen gleichzusetzen. Ihnen gegenüber stehen die Emotionen oder Gefühle, die der Auslöser-Instinkthandlungs-Beziehung entsprechen. Vergnügen, Mißvergnügen, Überraschung, Ärger und Wut, Angst und Furcht, Trauer, Gefühle der Liebe und des Hasses und alle übrigen Emotionen sind allen Menschen eigen (EIBL-EIBESFELDT, 1970) und wie die Empfindungen angeborene subjektive Erscheinungen. Sie können in ihren spezifischen Qualitäten nicht erlernt werden, da weder Nachahmung noch sonst ein Modus des Lernens möglich ist. Unähnlich den Empfindungen sind die Emotionen jedoch für Instinkthandlungen charakteristischen Schwankungen in der Reaktionsbereitschaft unterworfen. Die Emotion erweist sich also als die subjektive Seite triebbedingten Verhaltens (JÜRGENS u. PLOOG, 1974). So außerordentlich variabel und zumeist erlernt die zum Triebziel führenden menschlichen Handlungen auch sind, die sich einstellenden Emotionen beim Verfolgen und Erreichen eines Zieles, beim Abgesperrtsein vom Ziel oder im Zielkonflikt sind erstaunlich universal und können als solche nicht an Vorbildern erlernt werden (PLOOG, 1977).

Wie wir im weiteren sehen werden, treffen wir im vokalen Bereich der Signalbildung und -übermittlung die gleichen Verhältnisse an: Der Informationsgehalt und der emotionale Gehalt sind im Kommunikationsprozeß nicht zu trennen. Wenn die Primaten auch vergleichsweise arm an formstarren Instinktbewegungen und reich an plastisch-adaptivem motorischen Verhalten sind, so trifft dies für mimische und vokale Bewegungsabläufe nicht in dem gleichen Maße zu. Hier bleibt die emotionale Komponente der Instinktbewegung an die motorischen Abläufe gekoppelt.

3. Vokale Signale bei Affen

Gerade im Hinblick auf die menschliche Sprache hat die Lautgebung der Tiere von jeher großes Interesse gefunden. Dabei spielte die Hoffnung, durch das Studium der Tierstimmen den Wurzeln der Sprache näherzukommen, ohne Zweifel eine Rolle. Der Artgesang der Vögel warf viele Probleme auf, die einer experimentellen Lösung zugänglich waren. Die einfache Möglichkeit zur isolierten Aufzucht, die oft hohe Artspezifität der Gesänge und ihre Abhängigkeit vom Hormonspiegel, die Möglichkeit, manche nahe verwandten Arten kreuzen zu können – um nur die wichtigsten Faktoren zu nennen –, schufen gute Voraussetzungen für die Untersuchung von Grundfragen der Ethologie (THORPE, 1961; MARLER, 1963; HINDE, 1969).

Alle diese Voraussetzungen bestehen bei Affen nicht. Das genauere Studium ihrer Vokalisationen hat eigentlich vor rund 20 Jahren begonnen, als sich durch eine verfeinerte Tonspektrographie die Möglichkeit ergab, auch weniger vokale, geräuschartige Laute in ihren Variationen und Übergängen genauer zu erfassen. Die Methode erlaubt, Laute von Tonbandaufnahmen so in fotografische Bilder umzusetzen, daß die Frequenzen nebst ihrer Intensitätsverteilung im Zeitverlauf sichtbar und damit leichter vergleichbar werden (ROWELL u. HINDE, 1962; ANDREW, 1963; MOYNIHAN, 1964, 1966; REYNOLDS u. REYNOLDS, 1965; WINTER et al., 1966; STRUHSAKER, 1967; MARLER, 1969).

Auch mit diesem wichtigen technischen Hilfsmittel stellen sich der Funktionsanalyse der Affenlaute große Schwierigkeiten in den Weg. Dies hängt vor allem mit der komplexen Struktur der Affengesellschaften zusammen, in der jedes Mitglied eine bestimmte Rolle einnimmt, die in der Kommunikation mit den Kumpanen ihren Ausdruck findet. Um den Informationsgehalt eines Lautes zu studieren, muß man erkennen können, in welchem Kontext er auftritt. Das gilt freilich genauso für Gesten, Haltungen und alle anderen Signale. Doch ist der flüchtige Laut, besonders wenn er in schnellem Austausch mit den anderen erfolgt, besonders schwer festzuhalten.

Ein einzelner Affe ist nur ein halber Affe. Lautäußerungen von ihm allein können zwar aus technischen Gründen bessere Tonspektrogramme liefern, doch ist die Aussage über die Bedeutung des Lautes sehr begrenzt, wenn man nicht denselben Laut schon unter möglichst natürlichen Bedingungen studiert hat. Da die weitaus meisten Laute auf spezielle Gruppensituationen oder auf individuelle Partner bezogen sind, kann man von einem einzelnen Affen wenig erfahren. Je größer seine sozialen Interaktionsmöglichkeiten sind, desto mehr wird der Beobachter über sein vokales Repertoire erfahren.

ROWELL und HINDE (1962) haben als erste eine spektrographische und funktionelle Beschreibung dieses Repertoires bei im Gruppenverband lebenden Rhesusaffen vorgenommen. Sie unterscheiden zwei große Gruppen von Lauten, nämlich geräuschartige mit rauhem, hartem Klang und klar klingende Rufe. Acht der rauhen Laute treten in verschiedenen Formen von Auseinandersetzungen (agonistisches Verhalten) und vier in „freundlichem Zusammenhang" auf.

Die klaren Rufe variieren bei gleichen Situationen stärker unter verschiedenen Individuen und sind daher vorläufig nicht genauer klassifiziert worden. Sie können mindestens fünf, vermutlich aber mehr Situationen zugeordnet werden, z.B. Ortsbewegungen von Gruppenmitgliedern, die neu in das Gesichtsfeld treten, Leuten, die kommen und gehen, oder gar der Sonne, die plötzlich durch die Wolken scheint. Die Richtung, in der die Veränderungen der Situation zu suchen ist, muß vom Hörer ermittelt werden; er blickt auf den Rufer und folgt seinem Blick. Andere Situationen, in denen klare Rufe vernommen wurden, sind dadurch gekennzeichnet, daß Tiere voneinander getrennt werden oder in Form von Ruf und Antwort Kontakt aufnehmen. Mehrere unterschiedliche Rufe sind mit verschiedenen Phasen der Fütterung und des Fressens verknüpft. Hier und auch unter anderen Umständen wird deutlich, daß die Laute nicht allein Ausdruck einer Stimmung sind, die sich auf andere Affen überträgt, sondern daß ein Laut auch zur individuellen Erkennung beitragen und bestimmten Rangordnungsstufen und Rollen zugeordnet sein kann. Jedenfalls sind manche Laute nur von rangniederen, andere von ranghohen Tieren zu hören. Eine besondere Kategorie wird durch die Babylaute gebildet.

Unter den rauhen Lauten gibt es verschiedene Bell- und Brüllaute, die unterschiedliche Intensitäten des Drohens ausdrücken und teils auch ranggebunden sind. Unter den Bellauten ist ein Warnlaut, der die Gruppe alarmiert und gegen den Feind hetzt. Es gibt das Angstgeschrei, das zu hören ist, wenn ein attackiertes Tier weder entwischen noch sich wehren kann. Unter den „freundlichen" Lauten sind solche, die Wohlbehagen ausdrücken oder im Zusammenhang mit sozialer Hautpflege auftreten. Eine genaue Zahl von abgrenzbaren Lauten – sie mag zwischen 20 und 30 liegen – ist schwierig anzugeben. Denn eine der hervorstechenden Eigenschaften der ganzen Rhesusaffenvokalisation ist die nahezu unbegrenzte Möglichkeit von Übergängen zwischen den Hauptlauten (Abb. 24a). Auf diese Weise können mit Hilfe eines relativ einfachen Grundsystems feine Abstufungen von Stimmungen ausgedrückt werden, die zusammen mit Mimik, Haltung und Bewegung zur weiteren Differenzierung der Mitteilung an die Gruppe oder an einzelne ihrer Mitglieder beitragen (ROWELL u. HINDE, 1962).

Abb. 24b soll dieses wichtige Prinzip der fließenden Übergänge von Vokalisation veranschaulichen (ROWELL, 1962). Die neun dargestellten Laute stellen ein System kontinuierlicher Übergänge dar, in dem einige Laute in mehrfacher Weise variieren. Die Keuchdrohung kann z.B. in Brüllen, Bellen und Knurren übergehen. Dieses Kontinuum von Variationen, das sich auf einen relativ schmalen, tieferen Frequenzbereich ähnlich dem der menschlichen Sprache erstreckt, ist für alle Makaken und Paviane, wahrscheinlich auch für andere Altweltaffen mit Ausnahme der Meerkatzen und Guerezas, vor allem aber für die Menschenaffen und insbesondere für den Schimpansen typisch (REYNOLDS u. REYNOLDS, 1965). Nirgendwo sonst im Tierreich gibt es derartige gleitende Abwandlungen. Vieles spricht dafür, daß dieses Vokalisationsprinzip eine der Voraussetzungen für die Evolution der menschlichen Sprache ist.

Im Gegensatz dazu steht ein Vokalisationsprinzip, in dem die verschiedenen Laute mit ihren entsprechenden Funktionen klarer gegeneinander abgegrenzt sind, wie man es aus der Vogelwelt kennt. Dies ist unter den Altweltaffen typisch für die Meerkatzen und Guerezas. STRUHSAKER (1967) konnte in freier Wildbahn bei der grünen Meerkatze mindestens 36 verschiedene Laute hören und die meisten davon spektrographisch dokumentieren. Diese Laute treten in 21 unterscheidbaren Situationen auf. Der Autor rechnet mit ungefähr 23 verschiedenen Nachrichten, die übertragen werden können und ungefähr ebenso vielen Antworten, die durch die Rufe hervorgerufen werden. Das Prinzip der disparaten Rufe ist auch für die meisten Neuweltaffen charakteristisch. Einige Arten, wie z.B. Callithrix und Saimiri, können wie die Vögel zwitschern. Der von ihnen benutzte Frequenzbereich liegt im ganzen höher als bei den Schmalnasenaffen und bestreicht den gesamten oberen Bereich unseres Hörvermögens. Die Disparität der einzelnen Laute und die Nutzung eines großen Frequenzbereiches haben vermutlich zur Artbildung und Artentrennung beigetragen.

Ein Beispiel dieses Prinzips gibt Abb. 25. Insgesamt sind 26 Laute aus dem Repertoire des Totenkopfaffen schematisch dargestellt und nach ihren klangphysikalischen Eigenschaften in fünf verschiedene Gruppen eingeteilt worden; eine sechste Gruppe besteht aus Kombinationen von Lauttypen aus diesen Gruppen. Bei der Funktionsanalyse der Laute stellte sich heraus, daß den fünf Gruppen jeweils eine allgemeine Funktion zugeordnet werden kann, die durch die einzel-

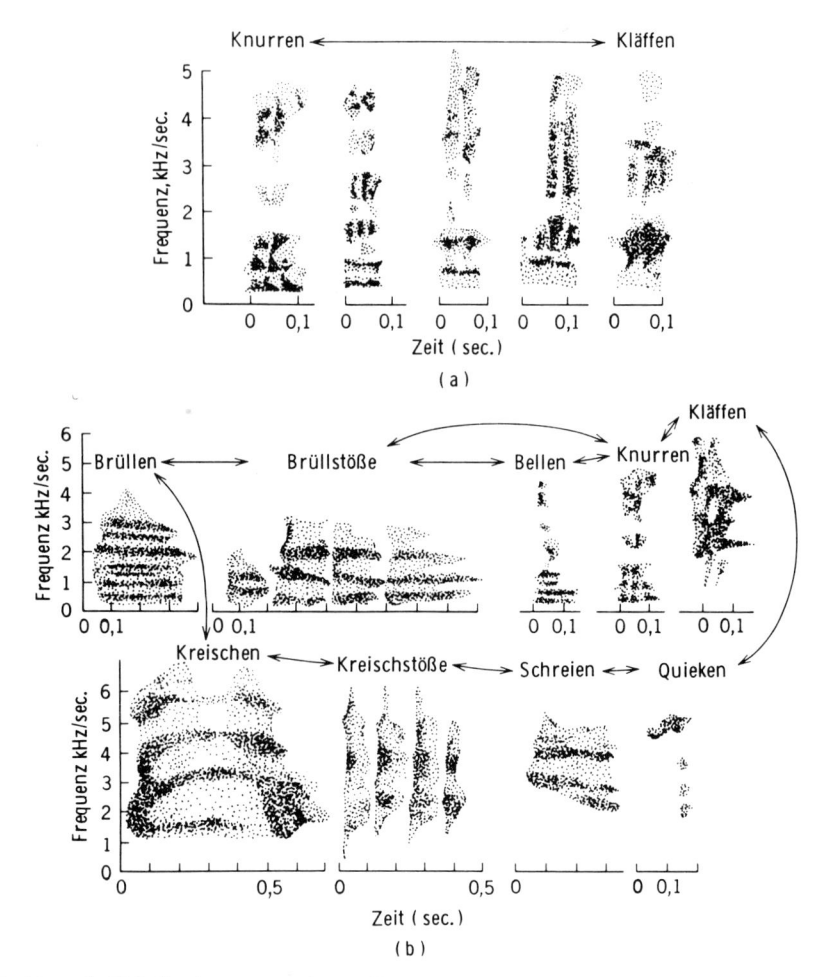

Abb. 24a u. b. Vokalisationen von Rhesusaffen (Macaca mulatta), gezeichnet nach Klangspektrogrammen. (a) Graduierte Übergänge vom Knurren über Bellen zum Kläffen (ROWELL u. HINDE, 1962). (b) Feingraduierte Übergänge innerhalb 9 verschiedener Rufe (ROWELL, 1962). Man beachte die vielfachen Beziehungen zwischen Brüllstoß, Brüllen, Bellen und Knurren (MARLER u. HAMILTON, 1966). Brüllen: Lautes, ziemlich langes Geräusch, das von sehr selbstsicheren Affen gemacht wird, wenn sie einen rangniedrigeren bedrohen. Brüllstöße: Abgehacktes Brüllen, das von einem weniger entschlossenen Affen gemacht wird, wenn er bei seiner beabsichtigten Attacke Gruppenunterstützung haben möchte. Bellen: Ähnlich dem kurzen Anschlag eines Hundes, ausgestoßen von einem drohenden Affen, der nicht genügend aggressiv motiviert ist, um auf den Bedrohten zuzulaufen. Knurren: Leiser und schriller als Bellen, von kurzen, rollenden R-Lauten unterbrochen; von Tieren abgegeben, die leicht alarmiert sind. Kläffen: Alarmruf des Rhesusaffen. Kreischen: Beim Bedrohen eines Ranghöheren; wenn erregt oder leicht alarmiert. Kreischstöße: Abgehacktes Kreischen; von Tieren erzeugt, wenn sie bedroht werden. Schreien: Tiere, die einen Kampf verlieren und gebissen werden. Quieken: Kurze, sehr hohe Stimmstöße, die von einem besiegten, erschöpften Tier am Ende eines Kampfes gemacht werden. (Aus MARLER u. HAMILTON, 1966)

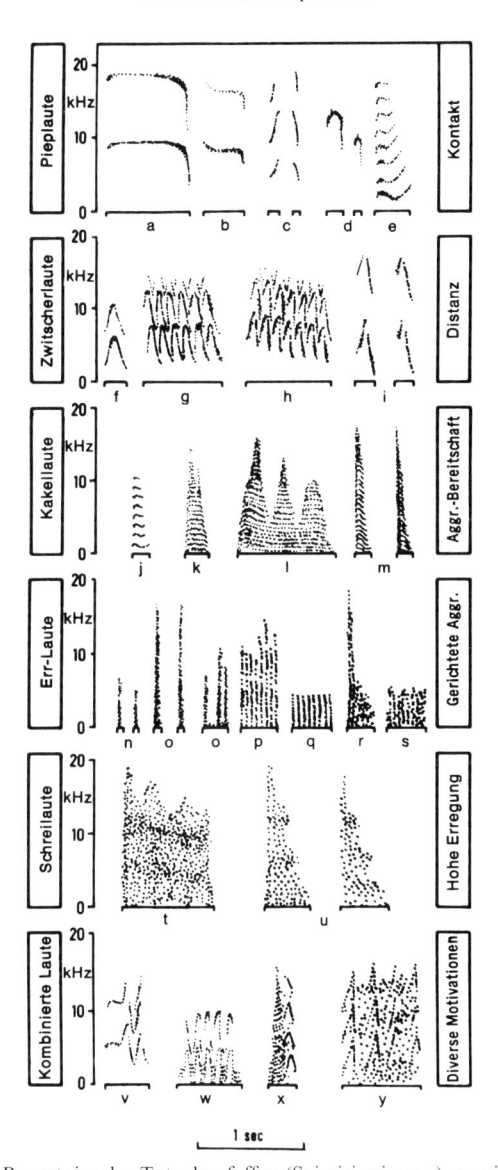

Abb. 25. Das vokale Repertoire des Totenkopfaffen (Saimiri sciureus), gezeichnet nach Klangspektrogrammen. (a) Fiepen, (b) Piepen, (c) Piepsen, (d) Alarmpieps, (e) Quieken, (f) Twit, (g) Trillern, (h) Zwitschern, (i) Tschacks, (j) Eh, (k) Kakeln, (l) Gackern, (m) Bellen, (n) Err, (o) Fauchen, (p) Tschörr, (q) Quarren, (r) Grunzen, (s) Ächzen, (t) Schreien, (u) Schrei, (v) Tschirpen, (w) Keckern, (x) Oink (Babylaut), (y) Kreischen. (Nach WINTER et al., 1966)

nen Lauttypen näher spezifiziert wird. So haben die Pieplaute eine Funktion, die dem Zusammenhalt der Gruppenmitglieder dient (Kontaktlaute). Darunter ist auch ein hoher, kurzer Warnlaut gegen Gefahr von oben (die Äffchen haben große Vögel als Luftfeinde). Ein anderer Laut kann regelmäßig bei Tieren ausgelöst werden, die man von der Sozietät trennt. Die zweite Gruppe umfaßt Laute, deren Funktion darin besteht, in bestimmten Situationen individuelle Distanz zwischen den Tieren zu schaffen. Eine dritte Gruppe drückt Erregung und eine allgemeine Aggressionsbereitschaft aus; darunter befindet sich ein bellender, sich wiederholender Warnlaut gegen Gefahr von unten (Bodenfeinde). Eine vierte Gruppe umfaßt Laute, die gezielte, auf ein Gruppenmitglied gerichtete Aggression ausdrücken. Eine fünfte enthält Laute hoher Erregung, wie sie z.b. Kämpfen vorausgehen oder sie begleiten können.

Fraglos sind in diesem Schema nicht alle Laute erfaßt. Auch bei diesen Affen gibt es zahllose Übergänge zwischen den Lauttypen (SCHOTT, 1975) und unterschiedliche Nuancen im Ausdruck, ja sogar unterschiedliche „Dialekte" bei zwei Rassen (WINTER, 1969; PLOOG et al., 1975). Es gibt Laute, die Dominanz ausdrücken und solche, die zu bestimmten Rollen im sozialen Gefüge gehören. Die Funktionsanalyse der Laute ist zwar noch lückenhaft, aber die relativ gute Unterscheidbarkeit der Lauttypen bildet eine günstige Voraussetzung zur experimentell kontrollierten Erforschung der Lautfunktionen. Der durch Lautgebung oder durch irgendein anderes Signal erzielte Effekt beim Empfänger ist durch mindestens drei Hauptfaktoren determiniert: 1. die Situation, in der das betreffende Signal abgegeben wird, vor allem die spezielle soziale Konstellation, andere äußere Faktoren wie Anwesenheit oder Abwesenheit von Futter, Feinden oder Menschen; 2. der Stimmungszustand (Motivation), in dem sich der Nachrichtenempfänger befindet; 3. die Rollen, die Sender und Empfänger in der sozialen Hierarchie einnehmen.

In Abb. 26a und b ist die äußere Situation konstant gehalten. Zwei miteinander bekannte Tiere bekommen zur üblichen Zeit Futter. Durch eine verlängerte Fastenzeit ist die Motivation der Tiere jedoch in b verändert. Das Resultat ist eine Verschiebung im Verteilungsmuster der Laute. Zwitschern, ein gewöhnlich mit Fütterung verbundener Distanzlaut, herrscht in a vor, während in

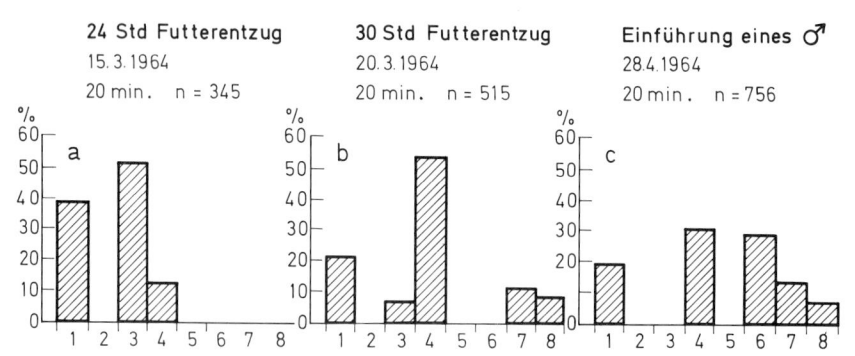

Abb. 26a–c. Vokalisation und Motivation. Häufigkeitsverteilung von Lauten (1–8) in drei verschiedenen Situationen (in Prozent der jeweiligen Stichprobe). a u. b: Fütterung von zwei eingesperrten Männchen nach 24 Std bzw. nach 30 Std Fastenzeit. Die Häufigkeit von Zwitschern (3) und Kakeln (4) kehrt sich um; Kakeln zeigt Aggressionsbereitschaft an; der Anteil der Kontaktlaute (1) geht zurück; Laute hoher Erregung kommen hinzu. c: Ein fremdes Männchen wird zu den nicht fastenden beiden Männchen gesetzt. Zwitschern fällt jetzt fort; zum Kakeln (4) kommt Tschörr (6) als Ausdruck gerichteter Aggression. Die Anzahl der registrierten Laute steigt von a nach c mit zunehmender Aggressionsbereitschaft von 345 auf 756 an. (Aus WINTER et al., 1966).

b Kakeln als ungerichteter Ausdruck der Aggressionsbereitschaft dominiert und von Lauten der Erregung, Keckern und Schreien, begleitet wird. In c wird die soziale Situation durch Einsetzen eines fremden Männchens entscheidend geändert. Jetzt sind erstmals Laute zu hören, die gerichtete Aggression signalisieren.

Die weitaus meisten Bedeutungen, die den Affenlauten bisher zugeschrieben wurden, stammen aus genauen Beobachtungen der natürlichen Situationen, in denen sie auftreten. Man kann bestimmte Bedeutungsklassen aufstellen, die die Primatenlaute mit anderen Tierlauten gemeinsam haben: feststellende, bewertende, vorschreibende und bestimmende Laute. Feststellende Laute veranlassen den Empfänger, seine Aufmerksamkeit in eine bestimmte Richtung zu lenken. Solche Laute aus naher Distanz können den Blick des Empfängers auf den Sender lenken, von dem er dann weitere Informationen durch gleichzeitig ausgesandte visuelle Signale erhält. Bewertende Laute scheinen häufig in Wiederholungssequenzen vorzukommen, wie z.B. das fortgesetzte Grunzen der Paviane, und zur Folge zu haben, daß der Empfänger eine von mehreren, gerade im Gang befindlichen Tätigkeiten bevorzugt. Die vorschreibenden Laute hingegen legen die Art der Antwort des Empfängers fest, z.B. in einer Rivalensituation oder im Alarm. Die bestimmenden Laute sind den vorschreibenden verwandt und zwingen den Empfänger zu bestimmten Handlungsfolgen, wie es etwa beim Schreien eines alleingelassenen Kindes beobachtet werden kann (MARLER, 1961, 1965).

Im ganzen gesehen ist die Information über die belebte und unbelebte Umgebung bei allen Affen sehr gering, wenn man sie mit dem erstaunlichen Aufwand vergleicht, der für die soziale Information benutzt wird. Jede feinste Stimmungsänderung findet ihren Ausdruck und zeigt spezifische Handlungsbereitschaften an, so daß die Partnerinteraktionen fortgesetzt abgestuft modifiziert werden können. Es gibt vokale Signale, auf die die ganze Gesellschaft reagiert, und andere, auf die nur der individuelle Empfänger antwortet. Die letzteren sind es vor allem, die auf nahe Distanz zum Partner im Zusammenspiel mit Mimik und Gestik einen Differenzierungsgrad der Kommunikation erreichen, der sonst in der Natur nicht vorkommt.

a) Ontogenese der Laute

Sowohl über die Ontogenese vokaler Signale als auch über deren Erkennung gibt es bisher nur spärliche Beobachtungen und kaum eine systematische Untersuchung. Die ersten Schreie gleich nach der Geburt sind bei mehreren Affenarten, u.a. auch beim Schimpansen, beschrieben worden. Rufe und Antworten von Neugeborenen und der Gruppe können schon während der ersten Lebensstunden und ausgeprägter während der ersten Lebenstage vernommen werden. Babyrufe, insbesondere „Hilfegeschrei", haben eine imperative Reaktion der Mutter zur Folge, selbst wenn diese zuvor noch nie ein Baby gesehen oder gehört hat. Auch bei anderen Mitgliedern einer Gruppe rufen Babyvokalisationen prompte Reaktionen hervor. Ein Schimpansenkind antwortet schon in den ersten Tagen auf verschiedene „Huut-Laute" mit unterscheidbaren „Huuts" (MARLER, 1969).

Bei einigen Affen sind spezielle Babylaute beschrieben worden, die man bei adulten Tieren nicht hört (ROWELL u. HINDE, 1962; ITANI, 1963; PLOOG et al., 1967; STRUHSAKER, 1967; WINTER, 1968b). Bei näherer Untersuchung wird sich vermutlich herausstellen, daß dies bei allen Affen der Fall ist. STRUHSAKER (1967) hat bei Meerkatzen in verschiedenen Altersklassen Unterschiede im Umfang des Repertoires gefunden; bei Kindern bis zu einem halben Jahr waren es 12 Laute, bei Jugendlichen bis zu anderthalb Jahren 18. Ob sich die Säuglingslaute differenzieren und auf diese Weise zu einem Erwachsenenrepertoire auswachsen oder ob einfach neue Laute hinzukommen und Säuglingslaute fortfallen, ob nach einer maximalen Repertoiregröße im Adoleszentenalter eine Reduzierung des Repertoires entsprechend der festgelegteren sozialen Rolle stattfindet – das sind alles ungeklärte Fragen, die in vergleichenden Untersuchungen auf Beantwortung warten. Der Totenkopfaffe kann schon vokalisieren, wenn er noch nicht einmal ganz den Mutterleib verlassen hat (BOWDEN et al., 1967). Bevor der erste Lebenstag vorüber ist, kann man Pieplaute, kurzes Zwitschern und ein spezifisch leises Quarren hören, das stets vor und im Zusammenhang mit dem Brusttrinken auftritt. Ein vier Wochen alter Säugling hat bereits ein Repertoire von mindestens 15 Lauten (PLOOG et al., 1967; WINTER, 1968a). Darunter sind einige typische Babylaute, die unter besonderen Bedingungen gelegentlich auch bei Erwachsenen gehört werden können. Ein Säugling, dessen Mutter starb, wurde vom 19. Lebenstag in Sicht- und Hörkontakt mit fremden Tieren, im übrigen aber allein mit einem ausgestopften Strumpf als Muttersurrogat aufgezogen (PLOOG, 1969b; HOPF, 1970). Er ließ, wenn er den Rücken erklommen und sich angeklammert hatte, den für Babys in diesem Alter typischen „Ortstriller" hören. In einer Bestandsaufnahme der Laute, die wiederholt in einer definierten Situation vor der Fütterung vorgenommen wurde, ließen sich keine Ausfälle im Repertoire feststellen (WINTER, 1968a).

Eine Beobachtung in bezug auf das Milchquarren legt die Vermutung nahe, daß manche Kinderlaute im wesentlichen ihre Form beibehalten, aber ihre Bedeutung ändern. Das Quarren kann später auf andere Partner als die Mutter gerichtet werden und insbesondere im Zusammenhang mit genitalem Imponieren (s.S. 394) eine aggressive Nebenbedeutung bekommen. Auch adulte Weibchen und insbesondere die „Tante" (PLOOG et al., 1967), die das Kind auf Mutters Rücken berühren und beriechen, lassen das Milchquarren hören. Vom „Tanten"-Verhalten der Rhesusaffen wird Vergleichbares berichtet (ROWELL et al., 1964).

Um herauszubekommen, welche Anteile eines bestimmten Verhaltens angeboren und welche erworben sind, haben die Ethologen seit langem die Aufzucht von Tieren unter Erfahrungsentzug, sog. Kaspar-Hauser-Versuche, vorgenommen (LORENZ, 1965). Dies ist hinsichtlich der Lautentwicklung bei Affen bisher nur beim Totenkopfäffchen gemacht worden (WINTER et al., 1973). Wenn man adulte Affen dieser Art vertaubt, kann man selbst nach Jahren keine Veränderungen der Lautgestalten feststellen (TALMAGE-RIGGS et al., 1972). Wenn man akustisch isoliert gehaltene, tragende Mütter während der Schwangerschaft operativ verstummt und das Neugeborene allein zusammen mit der Mutter aufzieht, mangelt es diesem an nichts außer der stimmlichen Erfahrung. Auch unter diesen Bedingungen wurden die meisten Laute bereits am ersten Lebenstag registriert und unterschieden sich nicht von denen normal aufgezogener Tiere. Der erste Ortstriller wurde am 3. Tage gehört. Eines der isolierten Tiere wurde am 5. Tage vertaubt und unterschied sich in seiner Lautgebung nicht von den normal aufwachsenden. Das erste Auftreten eines Lautes hängt bei diesen Tieren von den geeigneten Auslösebedingungen ab. Das Hören der eigenen Stimme zur Kontrolle der Lautproduktion scheint mindestens bei dieser Art zur Entwicklung der Lautgebung nicht nötig zu sein. Die Laute sind bei Geburt bereitliegende Aktionsmuster, die alle Charakteristiken von Instinktbewegungen (Erbkoordinationen) tragen. Bei Rhesusaffen, die im ersten Lebensmonat getrennt von ihren Müttern und später in Hör- und Sichtkontakt mit anderen Affen aufgezogen wurden, konnten allerdings im Alter zwischen 9 und 24 Monaten zusammen mit anderen Störungen des Sozialverhaltens auch deviante Vokalisationen registriert werden (NEWMAN u. SYMMES, 1974). Diese Abweichungen scheinen aber eher Folge emotionaler Störungen als Folge mangelnder akustischer Erfahrung zu sein. Immerhin muß man auch im Hinblick auf die Erfahrung mit der isolierten Aufzucht von Vögeln (WORDEN u. GALAMBOS, 1973; MARLER, 1977) in Rechnung stellen, daß es innerhalb der großen Primatenfamilie beträchtliche Artunterschiede gibt.

Zusammen mit der gut gesicherten Tatsache, daß kein Affe trotz seiner sonstigen Imitationsgaben auch nur den einfachsten Laut nachahmt und auch unter rigorosen experimentellen Bedingungen zu keinen nennenswerten Leistungen kommt, sprechen die bisherigen Beobachtungen an jungen Affen eher dafür, daß sowohl bei der Erzeugung als auch beim Verständnis der Laute Lernen eine untergeordnete Rolle spielt. Wie auch bei anderen sozialen Signalen wird hauptsächlich gelernt, wem gegenüber dieses oder jenes Signal besser benutzt oder nicht benutzt wird, weil es angenehme oder unangenehme Konsequenzen nach sich zieht (s.S. 393 ff.).

b) Erkennen der Laute

Wenn auch vieles für die Annahme spricht, daß der artspezifisch festgelegten Lautproduktion ein ebenfalls angeborener Erkennungsmechanismus zugrundeliegt, der die arteigenen Signale nach Art eines AAM erkennt, so sind damit die Probleme der Lauterkennung keineswegs gelöst. Wie schafft es dieser Erkennungsmechanismus, daß artfremde von arteigenen Lauten unterschieden werden? Wenn arteigene Laute angeborenermaßen verstanden werden, ohne daß sie gelernt werden müssen, wie wird dann andere akustische Information aus der Umgebung gelernt? Welche Feinheiten kann der Affe an einem Signal unterscheiden? Da die visuellen Signale in ihrer Funktion kontextabhängig, z.B. rang- oder rollenbezogen wirksam sind, und Sender und Empfänger eines Signals sich individuell kennen, sind für die vokalen Signale gleiche Feinheiten ihrer Wirkungsweise anzunehmen, die vom Empfänger der Mitteilung decodiert werden müssen. Eine gewisse Plastizität des Erkennungsapparates, der Erfahrung und Lernen ermöglicht, wird man voraussetzen können. Wir werden auf die Probleme der Lauterkennung noch mehrfach zurückkommen.

Hier sollen zwei Beispiele zeigen, wie man sich dem Problem der Lauterkennung nähern kann. Zunächst zur Rollen- und Rangabhängigkeit vokaler Signale: Sollten bestimmte Lauttypen einer Lautklasse bevorzugt von bestimmten Individuen einer Gruppe in bestimmten Situationen benutzt werden, wird man für diese Lauttypen bestimmte Funktionen (Signalbedeutungen) annehmen, die von den Empfängern erkannt werden. Solche Lauttypen werden typische spektrographisch erkennbare Eigenschaften (sog. features) haben, die Träger der dann mehrfach determinierten Lautbedeutung sind.

Die japanischen Makaken benutzen in ihrem vokalen Repertoire eine Klasse von Kuu-Lauten, die aus mindestens 7 Lauttypen besteht, die, distinkt in ihren spektrographischen Eigenschaften, hier ohne weitere Beschreibung Lauttypen A, B, C, D, E, F, G genannt werden. Der Laut A wurde fast ausschließlich von einem Männchen benutzt, das dem Haupttrupp ruhig in 50 m Abstand folgte und seinen Laut in Richtung des Trupps oder seiner Nachzügler sandte. Mehrere dominante Männchen benutzten fast ausschließlich den Laut C gegenüber subordinierten Tieren in nicht-aggressiver Kontaktsituation. Umgekehrt benutzten die subordinierten gegenüber den dominanten Tieren in ähnlicher Kontaktsituation überwiegend den Laut F, seltener E, selten D oder G. Paarungsbereite Weibchen benutzten überwiegend G, häufig auch F. Schließlich wurde der Laut D nur von Weibchen, meist von Mutter zu Kind geäußert (GREEN, 1975).

Ein weitaus schwierigeres Problem steckt in der Frage, ob der Affe dieselbe Klassifikation seiner arteigenen Laute vornimmt wie der hörende und beobachtende Mensch. Mit Hilfe der Zeichensprache der Schimpansen, die im Kapitel IV behandelt wird, hat man das akustische Unterscheidungsvermögen der Schimpansen näher untersuchen können.

Dem Schimpansen Bruno wurden die Handzeichen der amerikanischen Taubstummensprache (ASL) für „dasselbe" und für „verschieden" beigebracht. Durch zuerst simultane, dann sequentielle Vorlage von vielen gleichen und verschiedenen Objekten wurde sichergestellt, daß der Schimpanse die visuell richtigen Entscheidungen treffen und das entsprechende Zeichen signalisieren konnte. Dann wurde Bruno ein Tonband vorgespielt, auf dem Bell-Laute und Kreischlaute verschiedener Tiere – vom Menschen als deutlich verschiedene Laute klassifiziert – in Paaren geordnet zu hören waren.

Die Experimente zeigten, daß Bruno nicht wußte, ob er die beiden Laute eines Laut-Paares oder die lautgebenden Tiere unterscheiden sollte. Wenn das lautgebende Tier und das Laut-Paar identisch waren, antwortete er immer mit „dasselbe". Wenn das Tier und das Laut-Paar nicht identisch waren, hatte er ebenfalls keine Schwierigkeiten und signalisierte „verschieden". Wenn aber die Kombination: Gleiches Laut-Paar – verschiedenes Tier oder verschiedenes Laut-Paar und gleiches Tier verwendet wurde, gab Bruno beide Zeichen und gab damit zu erkennen, daß er die Sender-Tiere und die Signale unterscheiden konnte. Dieser auditorische Erkennungsprozeß ist für die kontextabhängige soziale Kommunikation eine notwendige Bedingung (BEATTY u. McDEVITT, 1975).

4. Vokale Signale und Signalerkennung beim Menschen

Auch beim Menschen gibt es nur wenige Studien über die ersten Lautproduktionen, während die Zahl der Arbeiten über Lauterkennung und die Anfänge des Sprechens und der Sprache außerordentlich groß ist (McNEILL, 1970; HINDE, 1974; BULLOCK, 1977). Der erste Laut, den der Mensch wenige Sekunden bis Minuten nach seiner Geburt produziert, ist noch am besten untersucht (PEIPER, 1964; WOLFF, 1969; WASZ-HOECKERT et al., 1968). Das Schreien ist wohl auch die Lautäußerung, die in den ersten Lebensmonaten bei weitem am häufigsten vorkommt und die Mitmenschen alarmiert. Wohl alle Säugetiere und Vögel verfügen über einen artspezifischen Notschrei, mit dem Zuwendung erzwungen wird. Er signalisiert einen Zustand, der dem Neugeborenen unzuträglich ist und zum Schaden werden kann, der beseitigt werden muß. Die Bedingungen, die Schreien hervorrufen können, sind recht verschieden. Dazu gehören Kälte oder Schmerzen aller Art, Hunger oder Unterbrechung des Fütterns. Schon im Alter von 5 Wochen kann der Säugling schreien, wenn eine Person, die er gerade angeschaut hat, verschwindet. Manche Mütter berichten, daß schon ihr 3 Wochen altes Kind schreit, um Zuwendung zu erhalten. Daß es verschiedene Formen des Schreiens und anderer Vokalisationen gibt, die verschiedene Stimmungen ausdrücken, wissen alle Mütter; man kann dies auch bis zu einem gewissen Grade durch Lautspektrogramme objektivieren (WOLFF, 1969; WASZ-HÖCKERT et al., 1968; MORATH, 1977).

Die zweite Lautform, die mit dem Beginn des Anlächelns auftritt, ist das aus verschiedenen Gaumen- und Lippengeräuschen bestehende Gurren (engl. cooing), das für die Person, an die es gerichtet ist, einen unwiderstehlichen Aufforderungscharakter hat, so daß mit Vergnügen hin- und hergegurrt wird. Das wechselseitige Abwarten und Gurren kann man bei Kindern im Alter zwischen 4–8 Wochen beobachten. Das Kind sucht die Gelegenheit zu diesem vokalen Dialog und zeigt Freude daran (WOLFF, 1963). Die Häufigkeit und Intensität des Gurrens hängt vom elterlichen Verhalten ab (RHEINGOLD et al., 1959). LENNEBERG (1967/1972) berichtet allerdings, daß das Gurren bei Kindern taubstummer Eltern genauso häufig ist wie bei Kindern normaler Eltern.

Wenn das soziale Lächeln voll ausgebildet ist, kommt eine variationsreichere, neue Vokalisationsform, das Lallen oder Babbeln, hinzu. Es besteht meist aus aneinandergereihten Konsonanten und Vokalen, ist weniger abhängig vom „Dialog" und kommt durchaus auch häufig vor, wenn das Kind alleine ist. Spricht ein Erwachsener zu ihm, hört es gewöhnlich auf und beginnt wieder, wenn der Erwachsene geendet hat. Auch so kommt eine „Konversation" zustande. Otto KOEHLER (1954b) hat in einer überhaupt nicht beachteten Arbeit „Vom Erbgut der Sprache" wohl als erster auf die Universalität der „Lallmonologe" hingewiesen. Spätere transkulturelle Vergleiche haben ihm darin rechtgegeben. Babys jeder Sprachgemeinschaft produzieren dieselben Laute oder Lautkombinationen in diesem Babbelalter (BROWN, 1965). In diesem Zusammenhang ist LENNEBERGS Befund, daß taube Kinder im Babbelalter mindestens während der ersten 6 Monate nicht von normalen zu unterscheiden sind, für die Theorie der Sprachentwicklung besonders wichtig. Offenbar ist in diesem Entwicklungsabschnitt die endogene Produktion von Lauten so vorprogrammiert, daß weder das Nachahmen eines Vorbildes noch die audiovokale Kontrolle eine Rolle spielt, obwohl die Lallmonologe so klingen als probiere der Säugling später für die Sprache benutzte Lautkombination aus. Die von LENNEBERG (1967/1972) mitgeteilte Beobachtung, daß Kinder, die im Babbelalter für mehrere Monate tracheotomiert wurden und daher keinerlei vokale „Übungen" machen konnten, später nach Wiederherstellung der Mundatmung keinerlei Sprachentwicklungsrückstände zeigten, haben PAPOUŠEK und ich (unveröffentlicht) an zwei Kindern bestätigen können. Da aber weder LENNEBERGS noch unsere Beobachtungen strengen experimentellen Kriterien standhalten, sollten solche Kinder unter besser kontrollierten Bedingungen untersucht werden. Sie könnten für die Frage beweisend sein, ob das Babbeln vorprogrammierten vokalen Bewegungen nach Art von Instinktbewegungen im Leerlauf entspricht oder ob es sich um „Fingerübungen" für das später einsetzende Sprechen handelt. Die eigentliche sprachliche Entwicklung beim Kleinkind ist weniger eine Phonations- als eine Artikulationsentwicklung. Höhere Anforderungen an den Phonationsmechanismus werden im Grunde erst im Singunterricht gestellt (JÜRGENS u. PLOOG, 1976). Das Kind lernt also zunächst bestimmte Wörter bzw. Silben willkürlich zu artikulieren. JAKOBSON (1944/1969) hat gezeigt, daß dabei bestimmte Phoneme leichter erlernt werden als andere; so wird von allen Vokalen zuerst /a/, erst später /e/ und /i/ und noch später /u/ und /o/ und erst zu allerletzt werden nasale Vokale gelernt. Für die Konsonanten gilt entsprechendes: die am frühesten gebildeten Konsonanten sind die Labiallaute /m/, /p/, /b/; ihnen folgen die Dentallaute /t/, /s/, /n/; die Nachhut bilden die Palatallaute /k/, /ch/, /j/. Innerhalb dieser Gruppe treten die Verschlußlaute vor den Reibelauten auf. JAKOBSON konnte wahrscheinlich machen, daß die Regeln, nach denen sich die Artikulation entwickelt, universalen Charakter haben: sie sind unabhängig von der zu erlernenden Sprache. Ferner gelten sie nicht nur für die ontogenetische Sprachentwicklung, sondern für die Sprachentwicklung allgemein. So hat in der Regel keine Sprache „spätere" Phonemformen (z.B. nasale Vokale) ohne die korrespondierenden „primitiveren" Phonemformen (nicht-nasale Vokale); auch läßt sich im aphatischen Sprachabbau beobachten, daß die späteren Phonemstufen stärker betroffen werden als die primitiveren (z.B. Umwandlung von palatalen Reibelauten /ch/ in palatale Verschlußlaute /k/). Die Entwicklung einer Sprache im eigentlichen Sinn, die unabhängig vom emotionalen Zustand des Sprechers und der Situation, in der sie hervorgebracht wird, auf erlernter Basis Informationen zu übermitteln vermag, schließt jedoch nicht aus, daß neben ihr auch noch beim Erwachsenen angeborenes Lautmaterial zur Kommunikation verwendet wird. Hierzu wären zum einen die nicht-verbalen, emotionalen Stimmungsäußerungen wie Lachen, Weinen, Schreien, Jauchzen, Stöhnen zu zählen, die funktionell den Tiervokalisationen entsprechen. Zum andern scheint auch die Intonation bei verbalen Äußerungen, soweit sie emotionalen Charakters ist, zumindest teilweise angeboren zu sein. So ließ KRAMER (1964) emotional gefärbte Schilderungen von Japanern in ihrer Sprache auf Tonband sprechen und anschließend von amerikanischen Studenten (ohne Japanisch-Kenntnisse) auf ihren Stimmungsausdruck beurteilen. Dabei waren jeweils 5 Kategorien zur Auswahl vorgegeben: Wut, Verachtung, Traurigkeit, Gleichgültigkeit, Verliebtheit. Bei der Auswertung zeigte sich eine statistisch gesicherte überzufällige Häufigkeit richtiger Beurteilungen. Emotionen drücken sich also nicht nur in den Worten aus, die der Sprecher wählt, sondern auch in der Art, wie er die Worte spricht. Dabei scheint die Art, wie sich Emotionen stimmlich manifestieren, transkulturell übereinzustimmen. Da jeder emotionale Ausdruck gleichzeitig eine kommunikative Funktion hat, heißt das, daß ein und demselben Wort, mit unterschiedlicher Emotion ausgesprochen, ein unterschiedlicher Informationsgehalt zukommt (Abb. 27).

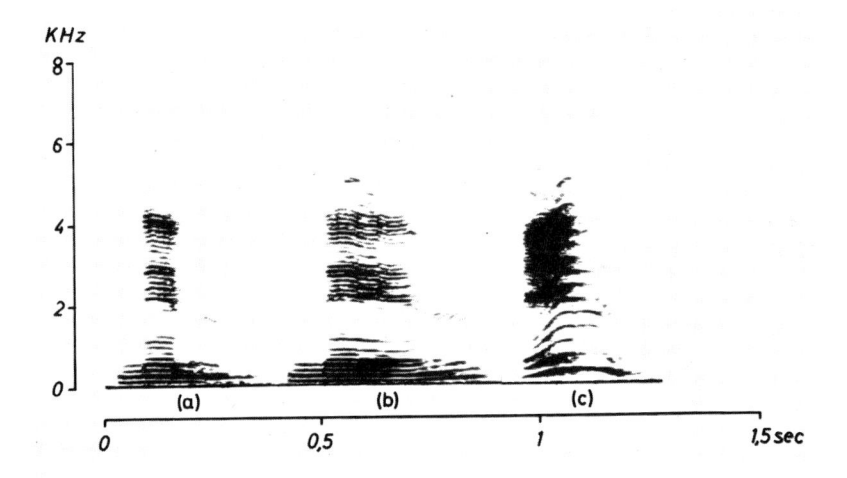

Abb. 27. Intonation der Stimme beim Sprechen. Frequenz-Zeit-Diagramme des Wortes „Nimm". (a) Ohne emotionalen Ausdruck, (b) zärtlich-lockend, (c) aggressiv-fordernd. (b) ist gegenüber (a) gekennzeichnet durch zeitliche Verlängerung des Vokals und leichten Anstieg der Grundfrequenz am Ende des Wortes; (c) unterscheidet sich von (a) durch ein starkes Ansteigen der Grundfrequenz im Mittelteil des Wortes und eine geräuschhafte (nicht-harmonische) Komponente am Vokalanfang zwischen 2 und 4 kHz. (Aus JÜRGENS, 1971)

TROJAN (1975) hat versucht, die Fülle nicht-verbaler, vokaler Stimmungsäußerungen durch drei Gegensatzpaare zu beschreiben: (1) gepreßte Stimme – nicht-gepreßte Stimme; diesem Gegensatzpaar entspricht auf der emotionalen Seite das Paar unangenehm – nicht unangenehm; lautspektrographisch äußert sich der Unterschied in einem erhöhten Anteil geräuschhafter (nicht-harmonischer) Komponenten beim gepreßten Sprechen, besonders in den Vokalen.

(2) Kraftstimme – Schonstimme: Dieses Paar gibt an, inwieweit das Geäußerte die Umwelt beeinflussen soll bzw. wie selbstbezogen es gemeint ist; klangspektrographisch entspricht der Kraftstimme eine hohe Schallintensität, der Schonstimme eine niedrige.

(3) Bruststimme – Kopfstimme: Dieses Paar gibt den Grad der Selbstsicherheit bzw. des Sich-Überwältigt-Fühlens an; ihm entspricht klangspektrographisch eine Verschiebung des Grundtons von höheren (Kopfstimme) zu tieferen Frequenzen (Bruststimme). Eine Zusammenstellung der Emotionen, mit jeweils einem Beispiel für die 8 Extrempositionen gibt Tabelle 3 (JÜRGENS u. PLOOG, 1976).

Die Erkennung von Sprachelementen während der ersten Lebenswochen des Säuglings konnte in den letzten Jahren mehrfach demonstriert werden (EIMAS et al., 1971; MOFFITT, 1971; MORSE, 1972; EIMAS, 1974). Diese Entdeckung ist für die Erforschung der biologischen Grundlagen der Sprache außerordentlich bedeutsam und gibt erste Hinweise auf spezies-spezifische angeborene zerebrale Mechanismen, die auf die im Fluß der Sprache verborgenen phonetischen Signale

Tabelle 3

	Kopfstimme	Bruststimme	
Gepreßte Stimme	Jammern	Verdruß	Schonstimme
Gepreßte Stimme	Angstschrei	Schimpfen	Kraftstimme
Nicht-gepreßte Stimme	Zärtlichkeit	Genießen	Schonstimme
Nicht-gepreßte Stimme	Jubeln	Imponieren	Kraftstimme

ansprechen und die Basis für das Sprachverständnis bilden, längst bevor das erste Wort gesprochen wird.

Welches sind nun aber diese Signale und wie kann man beweisen, daß das Baby darauf anspricht? Zur Beantwortung dieser Fragen ist ein wenn auch noch so rudimentärer Exkurs in die Phonetik notwendig, um die Natur dieser Signale beschreiben zu können.

Die artikulatorische Geste und die ihr zugrunde liegenden motorischen Prozesse sind die Bausteine für diese sozialen Signale (LIBERMAN et al., 1967). Es sind nicht die Worte der Syntax, sondern Sequenzen von sinnlosen Klangeinheiten, den sog. Phonemen, von denen es in jeder Sprache eine begrenzte Anzahl von einigen Dutzend gibt, die ausreichen, um zwischen den Worten einer Sprache zu unterscheiden. Die Phoneme sind durch eine gewisse Anzahl von Eigenschaften ausgezeichnet, z.B. /b/ und /p/, die durch Schließung der Lippen gebildet werden, haben die Eigenschaft „labial" gemeinsam, während die Phoneme /d/ und /t/ auf Grund ihrer Entstehung Alveolar-Laute genannt werden. Andererseits teilen die Phoneme /b/ und /d/ die Eigenschaften stimmhaft im Gegensatz zu den stimmlosen Lauten /p/ und /t/. Nimmt man die vier Laute zusammen, so bilden sie ein kleines System von Gemeinsamkeiten und Gegensätzen, so daß sich /b/:/d/=/p/:/t/ und /b/:/p/=/d/:/t/ verhält. Alle Sprachen haben eine phonologische Struktur, d.h. die Anordnung, in der Phoneme miteinander zu Worten verbunden werden können, ist begrenzt. Im Deutschen und Englischen ist z.B. ein Stoppkonsonant, der einem initialen /s/ folgt, immer stimmlos (z.B. Spur, stur bzw. spy, sky). Alle Sprachen haben eine Silbenstruktur, die sich aus Konsonanten und Vokalen zusammensetzt, was im allgemeinen Sinne auf zwei entgegengesetzten Bewegungsweisen, nämlich dem Schließen und Öffnen des Mundes bzw. des Vokaltraktes beruht. Hierdurch ist der größte Wahrnehmungskontrast gewährleistet. Die artikulatorische Funktion der Silbe kann man wahrscheinlich als eine neuronal gesteuerte Zeiteinheit zur Kontrolle der Sprechakte auffassen (FRY, 1964). Die Funktion, die die Silbe für die akustische Wahrnehmung hat, ist außerordentlich komplex und kann hier nicht beschrieben werden (s. STUDDERT-KENNEDY, 1976). Das Ergebnis sehr zahlreicher phonetischer Untersuchungen läuft jedenfalls darauf hinaus, daß die Silbenstruktur der Sprache eine außerordentliche Informationskompression gewährleistet, die dazu führt, daß mehrere phonetische Segmente – Konsonanten und Vokale – simultan von denselben akustischen Parametern getragen werden. Das phonetische Signal ist auf besondere Weise in der akusti-

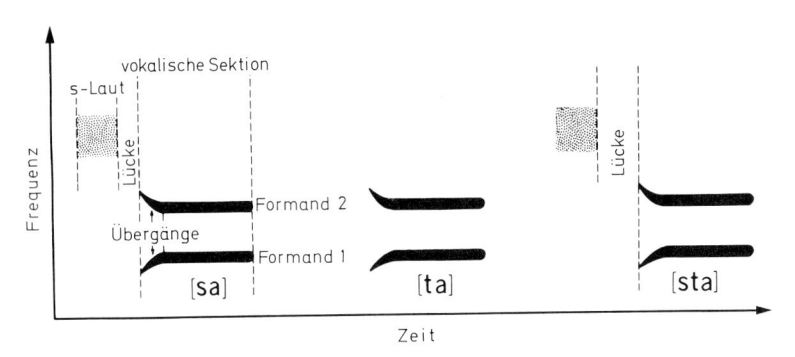

Abb. 28. Die Verschlüsselung des phonetischen Signals in der akustischen Engerie. Die Länge der dem scharfen /s/ folgenden Pause entscheidet über das wahrgenommene Phonem. (Aus LIBERMAN u. PISONI, 1977)

schen Energie verschlüsselt, die unser Ohr trifft. Es gibt keine direkte Korrespondenz zwischen phonetischen Segmenten und der Verteilung akustischer Energie im Zeitverlauf und somit auch keine akustischen Kriterien, nach denen man den Redefluß in Segmente einteilen könnte, die mit phonetisch relevanten Segmenten korrespondieren; mehr noch, die akustischen Kriterien können für jedes phonetische Segment variieren, je nach der Nachbarschaft zu anderen Segmenten, die gleichzeitig übertragen werden (LIBERMAN u. PISONI, 1977).

An zwei Beispielen können die recht komplizierten Sachverhalte vielleicht verständlich gemacht werden:

In Abb. 28 sind drei Lautspektrogramme von drei Silben schematisch aufgezeichnet, nämlich die Silben /sa/; /ta/; /sta/. Man sieht für das /s/ ein in seinem Frequenzband begrenztes Geräusch, das von einem stillen Intervall gefolgt ist. Dann beginnt der vokale Abschnitt mit einem kurzen Übergangsband des 1. und 2. Formanten, das durch die artikulatorische Bewegung der Sprechwerkzeuge von der Konsonantenstellung in die Vokalstellung zu erklären ist; es folgen die frequenzstabilen Bänder für ein langes /a/. Mit Hilfe eines Lautsynthese-Apparates kann man alle akustischen Parameter verändern. Läßt man das /s/ und damit auch das stille Intervall weg, hört der Mensch /ta/, obwohl nur der Übergang zu /a/, aber kein Konsonant geboten wurde. Setzt man zwischen das /s/ und den Vokal ein etwa doppelt so langes Intervall von ca. 60 ms, hört der Mensch nicht /sa/, sondern /sta/. In diesem Beispiel haben die akustischen Parameter einen differentiellen Effekt auf die Perzepte der drei Silben. Im folgenden Beispiel führen recht verschiedene akustische Ereignisse zur gleichen phonetischen Wahrnehmung (Abb. 29).

In den beiden Silben /did/ und /dud/, die je aus drei phonetischen Segmenten bestehen, wird ein Segment, der Vokal, geändert. Die unteren (ersten) Formanten in beiden Silben bleiben die gleichen. Die oberen Formanten in ihrer Stellung zu den unteren enthalten hinreichende Information darüber, daß es sich um die Vokale /i/ und /u/ handelt. Man sieht nun aber, daß die phonetische Differenz im mittleren Segment nicht auf Veränderungen im mittleren Anteil der Silbe

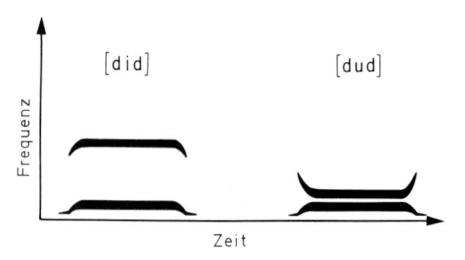

Abb. 29. Konsonantenbildung in Abhängigkeit vom Vokal (schematische Darstellung). Erklärung im Text. (Aus LIBERMAN u. PISONI, 1977)

beruht, sondern daß sich der ganze Formant ändert. Man sieht, daß sich die Übergangsbänder für /d/ an sehr verschiedenen Stellen des Spektrums befinden und in gegensinniger Richtung verlaufen, steigend und fallend in /did/, fallend und steigend in /dud/. Obwohl also die akustischen Merkmale für /d/ sehr verschieden sind, ist die artikulatorische Geste, nämlich die Berührung des Alveolarrandes mit der Zunge, die gleiche. Die unterschiedlichen akustischen Merkmale hängen also von der Koartikulation des Konsonanten mit dem jeweiligen Vokal ab. Die kontextbedingte Variation der akustischen Klangmerkmale wird sozusagen in Kauf genommen, um die gemeinsame artikulatorische Geste /d/ zu bewahren (LIBERMAN u. PISONI, 1977).

Auf diesem Hintergrund sind die oben (s.S. 435f.) erwähnten Entdeckungen an menschlichen Säuglingen zu verstehen. Welche Signale der Sprache sind es, die sie schon in den ersten Lebenswochen und Monaten zu unterscheiden verstehen?

Säuglinge im Alter von 1–6 Monaten sind in der Lage, synthetisch hergestellte Phoneme wie z.B. /b/ und /d/ voneinander zu unterscheiden (LASKY et al., 1975). Die Experimente zeigen, daß die Kinder genau die phonetische Eigenschaft erkennen, die den Ort der Lautbildung, also z.B. labial versus alveolar, anzeigt. Variationen der akustischen Parameter innerhalb eines Phonemes, z.B. /b/, werden auch dann nicht wahrgenommen, wenn die akustischen Unterschiede genauso groß sind wie bei der Unterscheidung zwischen labialen und alveolaren Konsonanten. Man nennt diese Unterscheidung daher kategorial, weil nicht die akustischen Unterschiede, sondern Kategorien von Phonemen (mit den zugrundeliegenden artikulatorischen Gesten) wahrgenommen werden.

Säuglinge können auch zwischen stimmhaften und stimmlosen Lauten wie /b/ und /p/ differenzieren (EIMAS et al., 1971; LASKY et al., 1975 u.a.). Das akustische Unterscheidungskriterium ist in diesem Falle die sog. Stimmanlautzeit (VOT); das ist die Zeit, die zwischen der Freisetzung des Lautes und dem Anschwingen der Stimmbänder vergeht (LISKER u. ABRAMSON, 1964). Je nach Konsonant kann sie zwischen 10 und 100 ms variieren. Die Zeit kann von der Verschiebung des 1. gegen den 2. Formanten gemessen werden (Abb. 30). Zur Prüfung der Differenzierungsfähigkeit von stimmhaften und stimmlosen Lauten wird den Säuglingen eine Reihe von Lauten präsentiert, bei der durch geeignete Lautsyntheseverfahren die Stimmanlautzeit kontinuierlich verändert

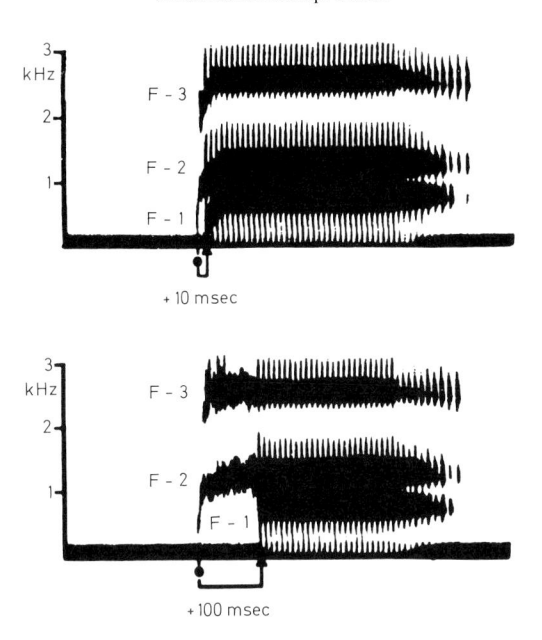

Abb. 30. Die Stimmanlaut-Zeit, ein Schlüssel für den Nachweis der Wahrnehmung von Sprachelementen beim Säugling. Spektrogramm eines synthetisch hergestellten Sprachlautes mit kurzer (oben) und langer (unten) Stimmanlaut-Zeit. F-1, F-2, F-3 die drei ersten informationtragenden Formanden (Frequenzbänder der akustischen Energie). Weitere Erklärung im Text. (Aus EIMAS et al., 1971; nach LISKER u. ABRAMSON, 1964)

wird. Im Laufe der Veränderung wird für den erwachsenen Hörer, gleich welcher Sprachgemeinschaft, an einer bestimmten Stelle des Kontinuums, sagen wir bis 60 ms, aus einem /b/ ein /p/, aus einem /d/ ein /t/, aus einem /g/ ein /k/.

Eine der Methoden, mit denen man Säuglinge nach ihrer Wahrnehmung befragt, beruht auf ihrer Saugfreudigkeit. Man gibt ihnen einen Lutscher und stellt die Grundfrequenz des Saugens fest; es sind gewöhnlich 20–30 Lutschbewegungen pro Minute. Dann wird der erste Sprachlaut über einen Lautsprecher gegeben und weitere Sprachlaute werden kontingent mit jeder Lutschbewegung präsentiert, wenn diese den zeitlichen Abstand von mindestens einer Sekunde von der vorangegangenen Bewegung hat. Der auditorische Reiz führt typischerweise zu einer Erhöhung der Lutschfrequenz und sinkt je nach Kind innerhalb von 4–15 min wieder ab. Wenn die Lutschfrequenz um mindestens 20% 2 min lang abgesunken ist, wird der zu diskriminierende Sprachlaut an Stelle des ersten 4 min lang gegeben, danach ist eine Testperiode beendet.

Abb. 31 stellt die Ergebnisse unter drei experimentellen Bedingungen dar. Gruppe D erhielt zwei verschiedene Testreize aus zwei verschiedenen phonemischen Kategorien /ba/ und /pa/. Die Differenz in der Stimmanlautzeit betrug 20 ms. Für die Gruppe S betrug die Differenz in der Stimmanlautzeit wiederum 20 ms, aber die Testreize stammten aus derselben phonemischen Kategorie /ba/ oder /pa/. In der dritten Kontrollgruppe 0 wurden zwar alle Reize des Experiments verwendet, doch wurde der Reiz während einer Sitzung nicht geändert.

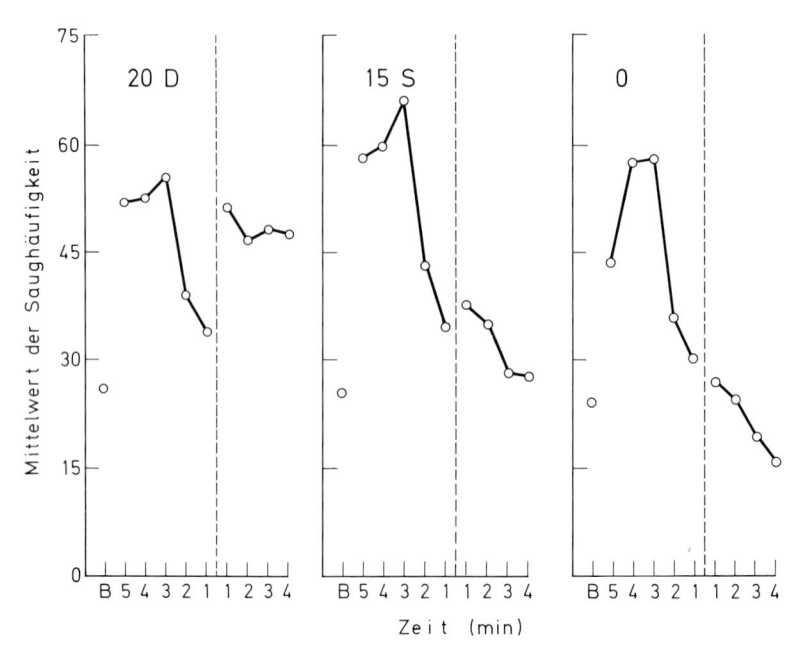

Abb. 31. Säuglinge zeigen ihre Unterscheidungsfähigkeit von harten und weichen Anlauten durch Veränderung ihrer Saugfrequenz an. 20 D, 20 S, O Verschiedene Versuchsbedingungen, s. Text. Gestrichelte Linie – Zeitpunkt des Lautwechsels. B 5–1 Habituation der Saugfrequenz vor Lautwechsel in Minuten; 1–4 Saugfrequenz nach Lautwechsel. (Aus EIMAS et al., 1971)

Die gestrichelte Linie gibt für die Bedingung D und S den Zeitpunkt des Reizwechsels an, und für die Kontrollgruppe 0 den Zeitpunkt, an dem ein Wechsel unter der Bedingung D und S stattgefunden hätte. Das Ergebnis zeigt klar, daß Säuglinge im Alter von 4 Monaten – die Ergebnisse für die 1 Monat alten sind fast identisch – die phonemische Kategorie stimmhaft von der Kategorie stimmlos trennen können. (Der kleine Anstieg nach Reizwechsel in Bedingung S ist nicht signifikant.) Die Ergebnisse wurden von anderen Untersuchern bestätigt (in BULLOCK, 1977), und weitere Diskriminationsfähigkeiten konnten aufgedeckt werden. EIMAS (1975a) fand sogar, daß Säuglinge im Alter von 2–3 Monaten /r/ und /l/ in nahezu kategorischer Weise unterscheiden konnten, eine Unterscheidung, die erwachsene Japaner nicht treffen können. Ob japanische Säuglinge zu dieser Differenzierung fähig sind, wird noch untersucht.

Durch diese Ergebnisse und eine ständig wachsende Anzahl von ähnlich ausgerichteten Arbeiten zur Sprachwahrnehmung auf phonetischer Ebene ist eine Diskussion über sog. Feature Detectors[1] in ähnlicher Art entstanden, wie man sie seit langem aus der visuellen Neurophysiologie kennt (s. BULLOCK, 1977; EIMAS et al., 1973; COOPER, 1974; EIMAS, 1975b; MILLER u. EIMAS, 1976). Man stellt sich darunter Nervenzellen oder Nervenzellverbände vor, die auf

---

[1] (=Merkmalentdecker, Merkmalerkenner – Übersetzung ins Deutsche ungebräuchlich)

spezifisch phonetische Eigenschaften ansprechen und aus dem Strom akustischer Information solche Ereignisse extrahieren, die linguistisch relevant sind.

Im Hinblick auf die Vielfalt der Meinungen und die zahlreichen ungelösten Probleme im gesamten Bereich akustischer Wahrnehmung kann man zum jetzigen Zeitpunkt über die Signalerkennung in einer vokalen Nachricht nur soviel sagen, daß Säuglinge in einem Alter, wo Erfahrung und Lernen im sprachlichen Bereich nicht in Betracht gezogen werden können, einige wesentliche phonetische Signale (artikulatorische Gesten) so wie erwachsene Hörer unterscheiden können. Aus ethologischer Sicht liegt es nahe, das Erkennen bzw. Unterscheiden dieser Signale auf angeborene Auslösemechanismen zurückzuführen. Daß die dem angeborenen Erkennen von Phonemen zugrundeliegenden Mechanismen neuronaler Natur sind, ist ein Postulat, das zunehmend an Konkretheit gewinnt. Am Beispiel der kategorialen Differenzierung von Phonemen läßt sich besonders gut zeigen, wie Lernen in einen angeborenen Mechanismus hineinwirkt. Die phonetischen Grenzen, z.B. zwischen /b/ und /p/, liegen nur in einem gewissen Bereich fest, können aber durch Erfahrung feiner differenziert oder verschoben werden. So gibt es im Vietnamesischen drei Härtegrade von /b/p/, die ein Erwachsener dieser Sprachgemeinschaft differenzieren kann. Die Grenzen von /b/ und /p/ liegen im Französischen anders als im Deutschen und sind z.B. im sächsischen Dialekt undifferenziert. Sollte sich herausstellen, daß japanische Kinder die Differenzierung von /r/ und /l/ vornehmen können, wäre dies ein weiterer Hinweis dafür, daß es außer einer feineren Einstimmung der Lauterkennung durch Erfahrung auch eine Entdifferenzierung durch Erfahrung gibt. In ethologischer Sicht sind dies Vorgänge, wie wir sie bei der Besprechung des AAM und EAAM kennengelernt haben (s.S. 423f.).

Man kann die kleinsten sprachlichen Segmente und deren einfache Kombination (dada, dudu, mama, papa) als eine Klasse von sozialen Signalen ansehen, die einen angeborenen Auslösemechanismus ansprechen und soziale Verhaltensweisen (Zuwendung, Blickkontakt, Lächeln) auslösen (PLOOG, 1971, 1972). Eine ähnliche Vermutung hat MATTINGLY (1972) geäußert: Sprechen habe während der Evolution der Sprache beim Frühmenschen zunächst als Schlüsselreiz zur Auslösung sozialer Verhaltensweisen funktioniert. Es könnte zur Erkennung zwischen Eltern und Kindern und zur Stiftung der Bindung zwischen Kind und Mutter beigetragen haben.

Kaum waren nun aber die Ergebnisse über das Phonem-Erkennen der Säuglinge bekannt geworden, tauchte die Frage auf, ob diese Fähigkeit nun wirklich eine spezifisch menschliche sei oder ob es nicht doch auch Tiere, zumal Affen gäbe, die in ähnlicher Weise in der Lage sind, menschliche Sprachelemente zu differenzieren. Tatsächlich erschienen kurz hintereinander mehrere Arbeiten zu diesem Thema mit teils widersprüchlichen Ergebnissen (MORSE u. SNOWDON, 1975; WATERS u. WILSON, 1976; SINNOTT et al., 1976). Die Ergebnisse stimmen darin überein, daß Affen die Fähigkeit besitzen, menschliche Sprachlaute zu unterscheiden, und zwar sowohl in der Dimension stimmhaft – stimmlos als auch in bezug auf den Ort der Artikulation, z.B. labial versus alveolar. Die Frage ist aber, ob diese Unterscheidungen auf Grund akustischer Merkmale oder phonetisch kategorial getroffen werden. Einerseits konnten die Affen zwar Unterschiede zwischen Kategorien treffen, doch waren ihre Diskriminationsleistungen bezüglich der akustischen Variationen innerhalb einer Kategorie gerade so gut (MORSE u. SNOWDON, 1975). Andererseits zeigten die Befunde eine bessere Diskriminationsfähigkeit zwischen Kategorien, aber die kategoriale Grenze änderte sich in Abhängigkeit von der Reizabstufung, was für die menschliche Diskriminationsleistung nicht zutrifft (WATERS u. WILSON, 1976). SINNOTT et al. (1976) wendeten eine Reiz-Diskriminationsmethode an, die Latenzzeitmessungen der Reizantworten erlaubte. Während sich die Latenzzeiten der Affen kontinuierlich mit zunehmender Verringerung der Reizunterschiede verlängerten, waren die Latenzzeiten der Menschen für alle interphonemischen Unterscheidungen gleich, stiegen aber bei intraphonemischen Unterscheidungen steil an. Aus diesen Ergebnissen muß man den Schluß ziehen, daß Affen und Menschen zwar ähnliche sensorische Kapazitäten im Hörbereich haben, daß der Mensch aber über eine darüber hinausgehende besondere Kapazität der Verarbeitung von Sprachlauten verfügt.

Eine phylogenetisch vergleichende Bemerkung ist hier angebracht. Die Natur macht bekanntlich keine Sprünge, sondern baut die Organismen und deren „Apparate" zur Umweltanpassung und erfolgreicheren Umweltbewältigung schrittweise um. Daß Affen, wie wir auf S. 478 ff. bei Besprechung der für den Kommunikationsprozeß verantwortlichen Hirnstrukturen näher beschreiben werden, ein außerordentliches Unterscheidungsvermögen für akustische Signale haben, ist bereits aus dem großen Variationsreichtum ihrer Vokalisationen zu schließen. Es ist daher durchaus denkbar, daß hier, wie in anderen Fällen, die Entwicklung des Signalempfangsapparates der Entwicklung des Signalproduktionsapparates vorausgeilt ist und der Affe über Hörbefähigungen verfügt, die als Vorstufen für die Wahrnehmung von phonetischen Signalen aufgefaßt werden können. Dies wiederholt sich in der menschlichen Ontogenese, wo, wie wir gesehen haben, das Erkennen von Sprachelementen dem Sprechen weit vorauseilt (s. weiteres auf S. 440ff.).

Dem wäre noch hinzuzufügen, daß die Natur nicht nur keine Sprünge macht, sondern manche Einrichtungen auch wiederholt entwickelt. Ein faszinierendes Kapitel dieser Art ist die Entwicklung des Vogelgesangs in ihren vielen Varianten. Für Dompfaffen (NICOLAI, 1959), Zebrafinken (IMMELMANN, 1969), Sperlinge (MARLER, 1970) und Buchfinken (NOTTEBOHM, 1972) gibt es z.B. eine Vorprogrammierung für das, was der Vogel bevorzugt wahrnimmt. Wenn man die jungen Männchen den Gesang ihrer eigenen Art und den Gesang anderer verwandter Arten hören läßt, wählen sie selektiv die Strophen der eigenen Art und speichern sie, ohne den Artgesang praktizieren zu können, bis zum nächsten Frühling in ihrem Gedächtnis, und singen sie dann als adulte Männchen. Wenn sie aber isoliert und ohne Gesangserfahrung aufwachsen, können sie ihre arteigenen Strophen nicht produzieren.

B. Hirnstrukturen und -funktionen im Kommunikationsprozeß

1. Hirnevolution und Kommunikationsprozesse

Der sich durch das vorangegangene Kapitel ziehende rote Faden wurde in den Perspektiven der Verhaltensbiologie beschrieben (S. 381ff.). Der in der

Evolution durch Mutation und Selektion erzielte Entfaltungsprozeß sozialer Kommunikationsformen ist durch zunehmend komplexer organisierte Nervensysteme realisiert worden. Das ZNS ist somit speziell auch in diesem Sinne ein Organ im Organismus, das dem Lebewesen zur Anpassung an die Umwelt dient, in der es lebt. So wie andere Organe und Organsysteme im Laufe der Jahrmillionen beträchtliche Veränderungen mit dem Ergebnis besserer Anpassung und effizienterer Leistung durchgemacht haben – man denke an die mehrfachen, umweltbezogenen Umwandlungen der Extremitäten von Wirbeltieren – so ist dies auch mit dem ZNS geschehen. Der dabei erreichte Zuwachs an Komplexität ist allerdings beispiellos größer als bei irgendeinem anderen Organsystem. Dies wird deutlich, wenn wir uns das erdgeschichtlich jüngste Produkt in der Entwicklungsreihe der Vertebraten, das Säugergehirn, anschauen (Abb. 32).

Die beschriebenen Kommunikationsformen sind also Leistungen eines höchstentwickelten ZNS, des Primatengehirns. Was wissen wir über die Hirnstrukturen, die kommunikatives Verhalten hervorbringen, und warum gebührt diesen Strukturen ein besonderes Interesse? Von dem wenigen, was wir wissen, soll einiges in diesem Kapitel berichtet werden. Besonderes Interesse müssen diese zerebralen Prozesse für die biologische Psychiatrie und für die nach kausalen Zusammenhängen forschende Psychopathologie haben. Denn weite Bereiche psychischer Störungen – von den endogenen Psychosen bis zu den Neurosen – lassen sich unter dem Gesichtspunkt der Störung kommunikativen Verhaltens begreifen. Die der Kommunikation dienenden Ausdrucksmittel – Mimik, Psychomotorik, Stimme und schließlich auch die sprachliche Mitteilung – sind in beobachtbarer und diagnostisch relevanter Weise gestört. Kommunikation und Affektivität stehen, wie wir gesehen haben, in einem unauflösbaren Zusammenhang, der in den Hirnprozessen seine Entsprechung haben muß. Nehmen

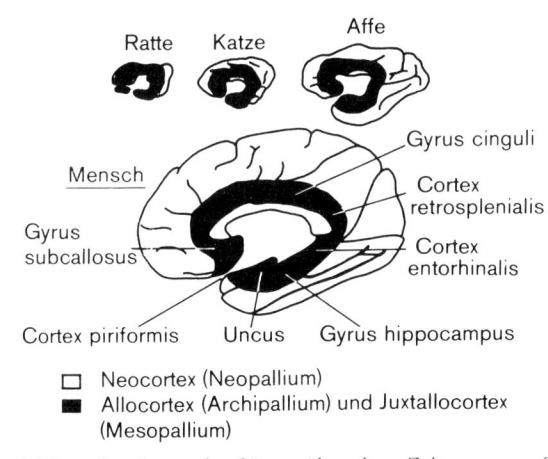

Abb. 32. Gehirnentwicklung der plazentalen Säuger über einen Zeitraum von 65 Millionen Jahren. Archipallium und Mesopallium umgeben den Hirnstamm und formen den allen Säugern gemeinsamen „großen limbischen Lobus" (schwarz), der seinerseits bei den höheren Säugern und schließlich den Primaten zunehmend vom Neocortex bedeckt und überlagert wird. Stark schematisierte mediale Seitenansichten in relativ proportionalen Größenverhältnissen. (Aus MacLean, 1954)

wir die Aphasien hinzu, die für die Theorien in der Psychopathologie eine so große Rolle gespielt haben, so bekommen die den Kommunikationsstörungen zugrundeliegenden Hirnstrukturen und -funktionen eine zentrale Bedeutung für die biologische Psychiatrie und erklärende Psychopathologie (SERBAN u. KLING, 1974; TOWER, 1975; STARTSEV, 1976; V. CRANACH, 1976; MOGENSON, 1977; SIEGMAN u. FELDSTEIN, 1978).

2. Postulierte Determinanten für die zerebrale Erzeugung von Signalen

Bei den Primaten beruht das Senden von sozialen Signalen im wesentlichen aus Bewegungen, die der Empfänger der Nachricht zu verstehen hat, insbesondere aus mimischen und vokalen Bewegungen. Visuelle Signale nach Art bleibender körperlicher Merkmale, z.B. eines roten Hinterteils, spielen eine vergleichsweise geringere Rolle.

Die Determinanten für ein aktuell gesendetes Signal, sei es ein mimisches oder vokales, stammen aus dem Zusammenwirken sehr verschiedener Einrichtungen des Organismus. Dies ist für das Verständnis der neuronalen Organisation von Signalen wichtig (s. Abb. 33).

Durch phylogenetisch-evolutionäre Anpassungsvorgänge hat jede Art das ihr eigene genetisch fixierte Potential zur artspezifischen Kommunikation. Sowohl für die Speicherung als auch für die Exekution der genetisch vorprogrammierten Bewegungsweisen muß es neuronale Strukturen geben.

Die angeborene Disposition zur artspezifischen Kommunikation kann durch Erfahrung verändert werden. Hierfür muß ein neuraler Mechanismus vorgesehen sein, der das vorhandene Bewegungsprogramm bzw. seine Anwendungsweise auf den jeweils neuesten Stand bringt. Hier greifen Wahrnehmungsprozesse, Lernprozesse und Maturationsprozesse eng ineinander und wirken sich auf die Kontrolle der Bewegungen aus. Der direkt wahrgenommene auslösende Reiz – das Signal – muß auf den AAM bzw. EAAM (s.S. 423f.) treffen, der die Ausdrucksbewegung – die Signalantwort – triggert. Dieser Mechanismus muß seine neuronale Vertretung haben.

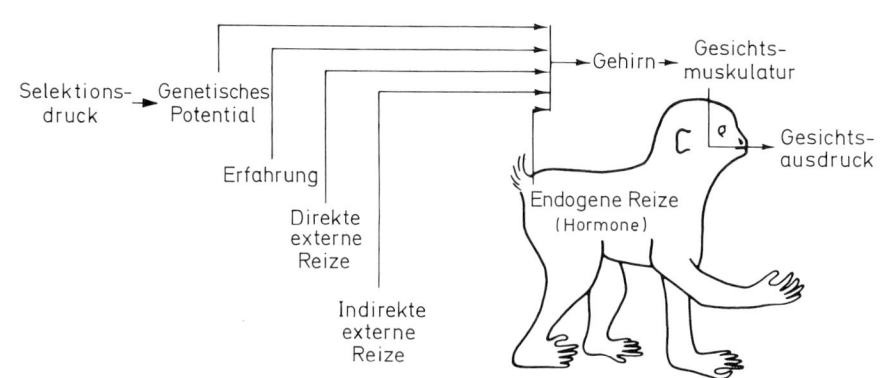

Abb. 33. Externe und interne Faktoren für die zerebrale Organisation der Ausdrucksbewegungen. (Diagramm von CHEVALIER-SKOLNIKOFF, 1973)

Andere, indirekte äußere Faktoren, wie z.B. Außentemperatur, Tageszeit, Nahrungsangebot, wirken auf die Handlungsbereitschaft ein. Auch diese externen Faktoren müssen neuronal ausgewertet werden. Schließlich spielt die Disposition des Senders aufgrund der Wirkung innerer Faktoren auf das ZNS eine wesentliche Rolle für die Generierung des Signals. Diese innere Faktoren, z.B. Hormone, biogene Amine und andere Überträgerstoffe, gehören daher zu den Determinanten für das gesendete Signal. Unter Disposition eines Lebewesens wollen wir die Gesamtheit aller Faktoren verstehen, aus denen sich der Organismus zu einem gegebenen Zeitpunkt konstituiert, seien es genetische, humorale, neuronale oder strukturell-morphologische Gegebenheiten. Zu diesen Faktoren gehören auch alle Folgen von Reizen, die je die Sinnesorgane oder das Nervensystem erregt haben, da nach neurophysiologischen und neurochemischen Detailergebnissen mindestens im Prinzip zu fordern ist, daß jeder Reiz die künftige Reaktionsbereitschaft des Organismus verändert.

Tatsächlich wissen wir wenig Spezielles über die neuralen Korrelate dieser den Kommunikationsprozeß determinierenden Faktoren. Klar wird aus diesen Überlegungen über die Determinanten, daß das Senden nicht vom Empfangen von Signalen und die Bewegungen nicht von den Wahrnehmungen zu trennen sind. Damit wird die Frage nach den zerebralen Grundlagen der Kommunikation aber zu einer Frage der neuralen Organisation des Verhaltens überhaupt (SZENTAGOTHAI u. ARBIB, 1974).

3. Einige Prinzipien der neuralen Organisation des Verhaltens

a) Das Prinzip der orientierten Handlung

Entsprechend der Tatsache, daß jegliches Verhalten und somit gerade auch das kommunikative einer Auseinandersetzung mit der Umwelt dient, muß eine Theorie der neuralen Organisation des Verhaltens handlungsorientiert sein. Um die Funktion eines Hirnsystems, z.B. des visuellen Systems, zu verstehen, müssen wir nach der Interaktion mit der Umwelt fragen, die dem Lebewesen durch das entsprechende System ermöglicht wird. Dementsprechend müssen wir annehmen, daß ein Lebewesen seine Umwelt in dem Maße wahrnimmt, wie es mit dieser Umwelt umgehen kann. Dieser Gedanke knüpft eng an die Lehren von J. v. UEXKÜLL (1956), UEXKÜLL und KRISZAT (1956) und H.S. JENNINGS (1906/1951) an, die als erste Interaktionen des Organismus und seines Lebensraumes als Systemganzes untersucht haben. Mit der Wahrnehmung eines Objektes, einer Bewegung, eines Signals, gewinnt der Organismus Zugang zu einem Aktionsprogramm, ohne daß dieses Programm jeweils ausgeführt werden müßte. Dieses potentielle Aktionsprogramm kann viele Unterprogramme haben, z.B. agonistische und kohäsive Verhaltensweisen, die jeweils in weitere Klassen aufgeteilt werden können (PRUSCHA u. MAURUS, 1976). Welches Programm die tatsächlich ablaufenden Aktionen dann kontrolliert, hängt von der Vorerfahrung mit dem Wahrgenommenen und der „Verrechnung" der anderen obengenannten Determinanten im Kontext des Verhaltens ab. ARBIB (1972) hat dieses theoretische Prinzip der aktionsorientierten Wahrnehmung auf kybernetischer Grundlage behandelt und experimentellen Befunden zugeordnet.

In der Tat gibt es eine große Zahl neurophysiologischer und entwicklungspsychologischer Befunde, die mit diesem Prinzip vereinbar oder besser erklärbar ist. Auf die Psychopathologie der Wahrnehmung angewandt, ergäben sich, wie mir scheint, neue Perspektiven, die bisherige Widersprüchlichkeiten beseitigen könnten.

b) Das Prinzip der Objekt- und der Ortswahrnehmung

Wie schon gesagt, dient die Objektwahrnehmung hauptsächlich der Interaktion mit den Objekten. Es kommt aber für diese Interaktion nicht nur darauf an, was wahrgenommen wird, sondern wo es wahrgenommen wird. Objekte werden also einerseits in ihrer Gestalt, andererseits in ihrer räumlichen Anordnung wahrgenommen. Für diese beiden grundlegend verschiedenen Weisen der visuellen Wahrnehmung (HELD, 1970) lassen sich zwei verschiedene neurale Systeme identifizieren, die u.a. beim Hamster (SCHNEIDER, 1969), beim Affen (HUMPHREY u. WEISKRANTZ, 1967) und beim Menschen (WEISKRANTZ et al., 1974; PÖPPEL et al., 1975) nachgewiesen wurden. Für die Kontur- und Gestaltwahrnehmung ist der visuelle Cortex erforderlich, während die oberen Vierhügel dafür entbehrlich sind; für die Ortswahrnehmung sind letztere erforderlich, während der Cortex entbehrlich ist. Wahrscheinlich gilt, mutatis mutandis, für das Was-Hören und Wo-Hören das gleiche. Das Prinzip soll verdeutlichen, daß integrierte Leistungen des Organismus, wie die Erkennung und räumliche Zuordnung von Objekten, auf zwei oder mehreren voneinander relativ unabhängigen neuralen Mechanismen beruhen können. Für die Kommunikation spielt das Was, oder besser das Wer, und das Wo eine außerordentliche Rolle, wie wir am Beispiel der Rangordnung und der Bedeutung räumlicher Distanz gezeigt haben.

c) Das Prinzip der räumlich-zeitlichen Abbildungsprozesse

Ein adaptives System muß in der Lage sein, Sinnesinformationen abzubilden und relevante Ereignisse in räumlich-zeitlicher Ordnung in das „Interne Modell der Welt" so einzubauen (MACKAY, 1956, 1965a; YOUNG, 1964), daß dieses laufend auf dem neuesten Stand gehalten wird. Diese fortgesetzte Synthese – von LASHLEY (s. BEACH et al., 1960) als neuropsychologische Aspekte schon vor mehr als 20 Jahren unübertrefflich gekennzeichnet – setzt Kurzzeit- und Langzeitgedächtnisprozesse voraus. Sie versetzt den Organismus in die Lage, vorauszuplanen und Entscheidungen zu treffen, ohne daß diese Prozesse notwendigerweise bewußt ablaufen müssen.

d) Das Prinzip der hierarchischen Organisation

Das Prinzip der hierarchischen Organisation des ZNS beschäftigt den Neurologen und Psychiater seit JACKSON wohl am meisten und wird auch im folgenden die wichtigste Rolle spielen. Gleichwohl muß es, wie jedes einzelne der Prinzipien, mit Reserve betrachtet werden. Es besagt, daß höhere Organisationsebenen des ZNS, wie der Cortex, niedere Ebenen, wie z.B. das Zwischenhirn kontrollieren, das wiederum das Mittelhirn unter Kontrolle hat (Abb. 34). JACKSON (1884)

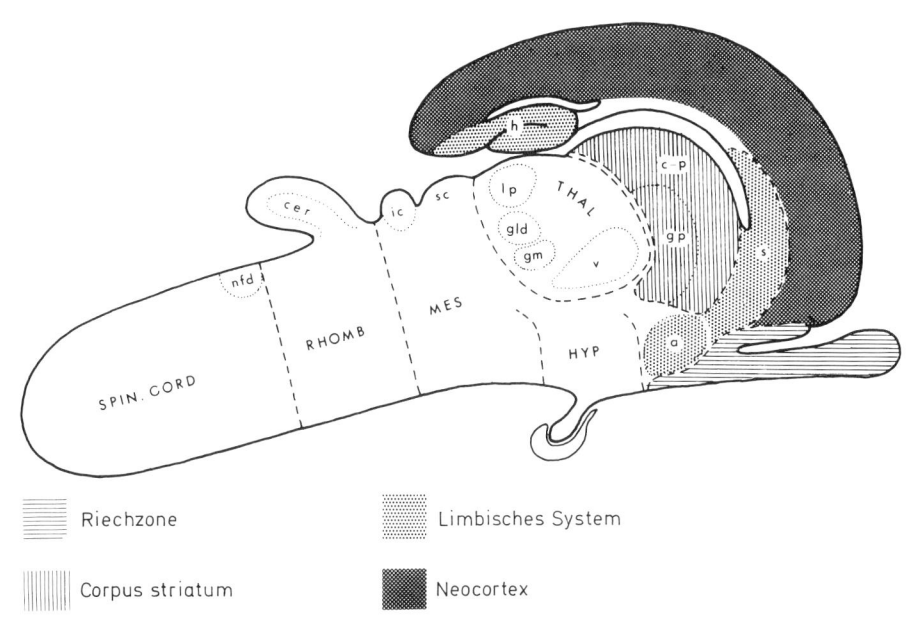

Abb. 34. Schematische Darstellung eines Säugerhirns. a = Amygdala; cer = Cerebellum; c-p = Caudo-putamen; gl = Corpus geniculatum lat.; gm = Corp. gen. med.; gp = Globus pallidus; h = Hippocampus (Ammonshorn); HYP = Hypothalamus; ic = Colliculus inferior; lp = Nucl. lat. post thalami; MES = Mesencephalon; nfd = Nuclei funiculi dors.; RHOMB = Rhombencephalon; S = Septum; sc = Colliculus superior; SPIN.CORD = Rückenmark; THAL = Thalamus. (Aus NAUTA u. KARTEN, 1971)

verwendete das von SPENCER (1862) stammende Konzept der hierarchischen Organisation des ZNS ganz im Sinne der Darwinschen Lehre und begründete es in drei Punkten:

– „Evolution is a passage from the most to the least organised – that is to say – from the lowest well organised centres to the highest least organised centres." (Dieses „am meisten" und „am wenigsten" Organisiert-Sein bedeutet die Festigkeit des funktionalen Verbandes der jeweiligen Zentren.)

– „Evolution is a passage from the most simple to the most complex; again from the lowest to the highest centres."

– „Evolution is a passage from the most automatic to the most voluntary."

Diese dreifache Definition bedeutet, so fährt JACKSON fort, daß die höchsten Zentren, welche den Gipfel der nervalen Entwicklung darstellen und das „organ of mind" oder die physische Basis des Bewußtseins bilden, am wenigsten organisiert sind, höchst komplex funktionieren und am meisten dem Willen unterworfen sind. Man beachte, daß es sich hier um eine rein funktionelle Definition handelt, in die keine anatomischen Zuordnungen eingeschlossen sind.

Die zentralen Fragen, die die Neurophysiologen seither beschäftigt haben, betreffen die Kontrollmechanismen im einzelnen und vor allem die Rückkoppelungssysteme von den niederen zu den höheren Organisationsebenen (HENATSCH, 1976). Denn es ist offensichtlich, daß ein hierarchisch aufgebautes Kommando-System nur funktionieren kann, wenn die höheren Ebenen eine Rückmeldung darüber erhalten, ob und wie die Kommandos ausgeführt worden sind. Einigkeit herrscht darüber, daß angeborene (vorprogrammierte) zentrale Bewegungsmuster die Basis für die motorische Organisation bilden. Es bedarf aber der laufenden und räumlich geordneten afferenten Rückmeldung, um Präzision der Bewegungen und adaptive Reaktionen auf sich ändernde Umweltbedingungen zu gewährleisten. Rückmeldungen sind ebenfalls für den Neuerwerb von (gelernten) Bewegungen erforderlich (JUNG, 1976). Wie aber die Rückmeldungen im Detail funktionieren, darüber gehen die Auffassungen auseinander. Weder das Reaffe-

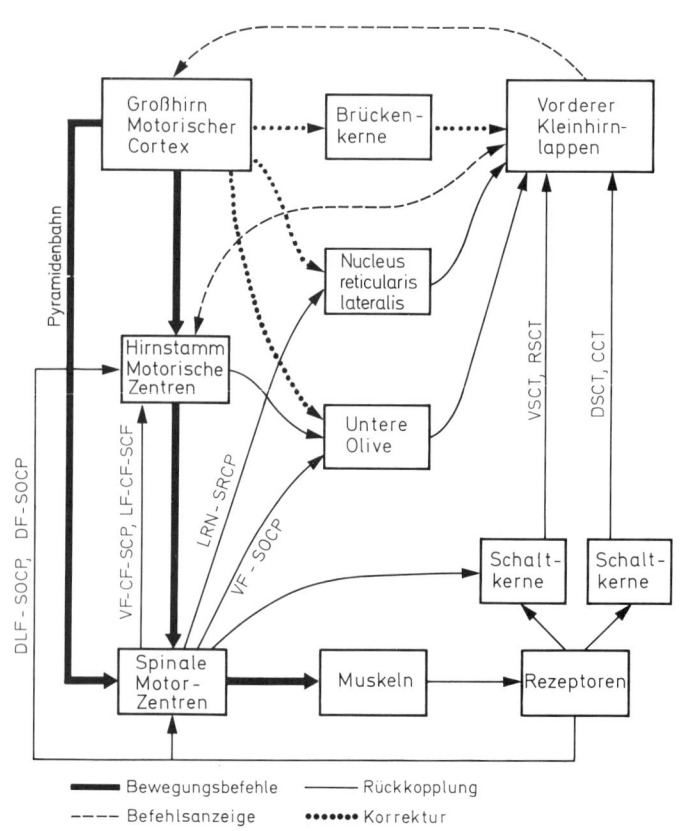

Abb. 35. Schema einiger Rückkoppelungskreise zwischen motorischem Cortex, Hirnstamm, Rückenmark und Kleinhirn. Vom Kleinhirnvorderlappen nimmt man Fehlerkorrekturen der vom Neocortex ausgelösten motorischen Aktivität an, die durch pyramidale und extrapyramidale Bahnen ausgeführt werden. Der Vorderlappen funktioniert als Monitor der Kommandosignale, die aus der unteren Olive und ponto-retikulären Kernen zu ihm gelangen. Die spino-cerebellären Bahnen dienen als Rückmeldeverbindungen, durch die die Aktivität niederer motorischer Zentren und der entstehenden Bewegungen überwacht werden. DSCT = propriozeptive und exterozeptive Fasern der dorsalen spinocerebellären Bahn; CCT = propriozeptive und exterozeptive Fasern des cuneo-cerebellären Trakts; VSCT = Tractus spinocerebellaris ventr.; RSCT = Tractus spinocerebellaris rostr.; LRN-SRCP = spinoreticulocerebelläre Bahn über Nucl. reticularis lat.; DF-SOCP = Tr. spino-olivocerebellaris dors.; DLF-SOCP = Tr. spino-olivocerebellaris dorsolat.; VF-SOCP = Tr. spino-olivocerebellaris ventr.; LF-CF-SCP = laterale spinocerebelläre Kletterfasern; VF-CF-SCP = ventrale spino-cerebelläre Kletterfasern. (Nach OSCARSSON, 1973)

renz-Prinzip (v. HOLST u. MITTELSTAEDT, 1950) noch der verwandte „Corollary Discharge" (TEUBER, 1967) reichen zur Erklärung der komplizierten Funktionszusammenhänge aus. Wahrscheinlich gibt es eine ganze Reihe verschiedener neuronaler Arrangements, die verschiedene Formen des Feedback gewährleisten. Schon ein stark simplifiziertes Schema (s. Abb. 35) weist auf die komplexen Zusammenhänge hin (SCHMITT u. WORDEN, 1974).

e) Das Prinzip der somatotopischen Repräsentation

Das Prinzip der somatotopischen Repräsentation von Motorik und somatischer Sensibilität ist auf allen Ebenen des ZNS realisiert und stellt sich am detailliertesten in den primären Rindenfeldern des sensomotorischen Cortex dar (Abb. 36). Dafür sind die Homunculi und Simisculi ein anschaulicher Ausdruck (KORNHUBER, 1972; HENATSCH, 1976). Zeichnungen dieser Art liegt die Tatsache zugrunde, daß die aus vertikal angeordneten Nervenzellsäulen bestehenden Funktionseinheiten des somatosensiblen Cortex über den Thalamus (HASSLER, 1967) Afferenzen von Hautrezeptoren bekommen. Jede Säule ist einem Rezeptor zugeordnet und stimmt in ihrer kortikalen Topographie mit der Topographie des rezeptiven Feldes an der Körperoberfläche überein. Umgekehrt gelingt es, durch feinste elektrische Reizungen des primären motorischen Cortex einzelne Muskeln zu erregen und so die topographischen Beziehungen zwischen Cortex und Bewegungsapparat herzustellen. Den größten Raum auf der Hirnoberfläche mit entsprechend zahlreichen Neuronen nehmen die Projektionen jener Muskeln ein, die zu besonders feinen und diskriminativen Bewegungen fähig sind, nämlich Lippen, Zunge, mimische Muskeln, dann der Daumen und die übrigen Finger der Hand. Der Cortex „denkt" in Bewegungen, hatte schon JACKSON argumentiert.

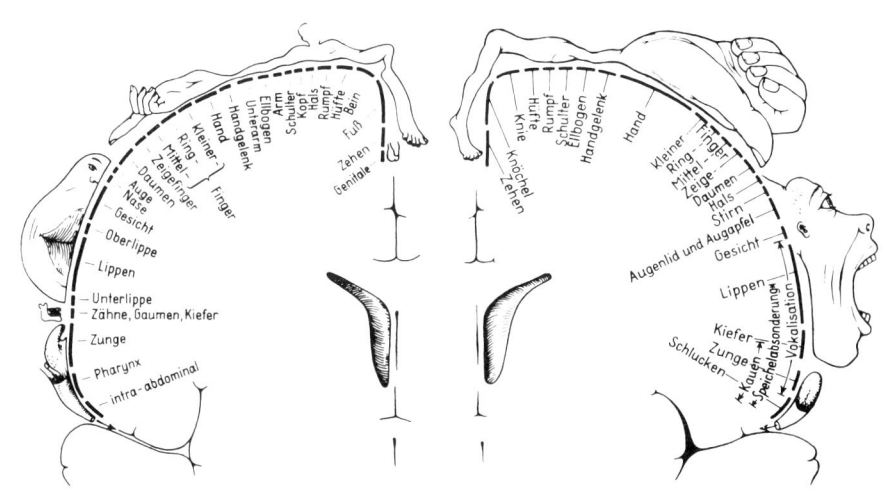

Abb. 36. Sensomotorischer „Homunculus": Die somatotope Repräsentation in der vorderen Zentralwindung (motorisch), rechts, und in der hinteren Zentralwindung (sensibel), links. (Aus PENFIELD u. RASMUSSEN, 1950)

Weitere, wesentlich kleinere somatotopisch undifferenzierter gegliederte Repräsentationsfelder finden sich in der motorischen Supplementärarea an der Medialfläche oberhalb des Gyrus cinguli, auf die wir im Zusammenhang mit der Vokalisation kommen (s.Abb. 50), und noch unschärfer in der Inselgegend (sog. II. sensomotorische Zone). Hier ist eine ipsilaterale Repräsentation der Gesichtsmuskulatur bekannt. In letzteren beiden Arealen sind beide Körperseiten repräsentiert, während vor allem die Extremitäten in den Zentralwindungen kontralateral vertreten sind. Muskeln jedoch, die nicht bisymmetrisch angelegt sind oder normalerweise beidseitig zusammenarbeiten, wie z.B. der weiche Gaumen, der Larynx und die Stimmbänder, werden bei Cortexreizungen bilateral beeinflußt (HENATSCH, s.oben; JÜRGENS, 1974).

Über die funktionale Zweckmäßigkeit und den Anpassungswert, den diese multiplen somatotopen Repräsentationen für das Verhalten haben, sind bisher nur Vermutungen angestellt worden. Bemerkenswert ist jedenfalls, daß die beiden Sinne, die die Abgrenzung des Organismus von seiner Umwelt bestimmen – das Tastgefühl als Nahsinn und das Sehen als Fernsinn – bei sonst großen Verschiedenheiten in ihrer Psychophysik – die quasi Punkt-für-Punkt-Abbildung vom Rezeptorfeld bis zum Cortex als Gemeinsames haben (PLOOG, 1973b). Von hier können Überlegungen zur sozio-biologischen Bedeutung dieses neuralen Organisationsprinzips ihren Ausgang nehmen.

4. Zerebrale Korrelate emotionalen Verhaltens

Soziale Kommunikation und Affektivität, so haben wir mehrfach betont, stehen in einem unauflösbaren Zusammenhang. Man muß daher annehmen, daß Hirnstrukturen, die emotionales Verhalten hervorbringen, auch die neurale Basis für Kommunikationsprozesse darstellen. Je besser dieser Nachweis gelänge, desto präziser könnte man die neuralen Prozesse beschreiben, die der Kommunikation zugrundeliegen. Damit würde auch ein hirnstrukturbezogener, neurobiologischer Zugang zu den Störungen der Kommunikation möglich. Zur Zeit können solche Störungen im Rahmen biologisch-psychiatrischer Behandlungsmethoden psychopharmakologisch beeinflußt werden, ohne daß eine präzise Vorstellung über die Wirkungszusammenhänge besteht. Neue Ansätze in der Psychopharmakologie zeigen allerdings, daß allgemein funktionale Konzepte über die Wirkungsmechanismen zunehmend mit Vorstellungen über Hirnstrukturen als „Targets" verbunden werden. Es geht also nicht nur um den allgemeinen Wirkungsmechanismus eines Transmitters, eines Peptides, eines Endorphins u.a.m., sondern um den Ort (die Orte) im neuronalen Systemverband, an dem diese Stoffe wirken. Hier eröffnen sich neue Wege zur Erforschung der Zusammenhänge zwischen Hirn und Verhalten.

Tatsächlich ist nun aber über die neurale Basis der Kommunikationsprozesse außerordentlich wenig bekannt. Dies hängt nicht zuletzt auch mit ihrer im vorigen Abschnitt beschriebenen Komplexität zusammen, aber auch mit mangelndem Wissen über die Funktion integrierter Systeme überhaupt. JUNG (1976) hat in seiner Einführung in die Bewegungsphysiologie nicht nur den Wissensstand, sondern auch die Wissenslücken festgestellt. Selbst das Wissen über die zerebralen Mechanismen „einfacher" Bewegungskoordinationen, z.B. des

Laufens, fehlt uns noch weitgehend, und um wieviel komplexere Koordinationen handelt es sich bei den sozialen Signalen, um die es bei der Beschreibung der Kommunikationsprozesse im wesentlichen geht. Vorläufig, so sagt JUNG, „ist für die Erfassung integrierter Bewegungsmuster die Verhaltensanalyse unentbehrlich" (S. 87).

Nehmen wir die eingehend beschriebenen mimischen Signale als Beispiel. Zwar wissen wir über die komplizierte Hirnanatomie der Gesichtsinnervation verhältnismäßig gut Bescheid. Es beteiligen sich 4 Hirnnerven (III, V, VII, XII) daran. Der Fazialiskern empfängt aber auch Impulse von den Basalganglien und vom Hypothalamus, die gerade für die unwillkürlichen mimischen Ausdrucksbewegungen entscheidend sind. Andere Einflüsse aus dem Hirnstamm sind wahrscheinlich. Von diesen anatomischen Verbindungen weiß man aber nichts, geschweige denn von der den mimischen Bewegungsmustern zugrundeliegenden Physiologie.

Es bleibt daher nichts anderes übrig, als die zerebralen Korrelate für emotionales Verhalten in allgemeiner Form zu beschreiben und dort, wo sich detailliertere Zusammenhänge zwischen kommunikativem Verhalten und Hirnstruktur aufzeigen lassen, exemplarisch ausführlicher zu werden. Dies soll am Beispiel soziogenitaler Signale und am Beispiel der Stimme geschehen.

a) Das limbische System

Wohl kein System des Gehirns hat während der letzten 25 Jahre mehr Beachtung gefunden als das limbische System. Die entstandene Literatur ist unübersehbar groß und voller Widersprüchlichkeiten (ADEY u. TOKIZANE, 1967; SMYTHIES, 1970; HOCKMAN, 1972; ELEFTHERIOU, 1972; DICARA, 1974). Dies ist, soweit es die Neurophysiologie des Verhaltens betrifft, kein Wunder, denn unter den Bedingungen der Verhaltensanalyse kann dieses System nicht unabhängig, sondern nur im Verband mit anderen Systemen funktionieren (PLOOG, 1964b). Zudem ist es nicht einheitlich organisiert, und seine Subsysteme dienen recht verschiedenen Funktionen. So mag bezweifelt werden, ob ein einheitlicher Nenner überhaupt existiert (ISAACSON, 1974).

Die Geschichte des limbischen Systems begann mit einem Konzept seiner Funktion; auch in diesem Abschnitt wird nur ein Konzept vorgetragen, das sich am Thema Kommunikation orientiert und das, wie Computeranalogien und andere Modelle des Nervensystems (ASHBY, 1960; YOUNG, 1964; MACKAY, 1965b) teilweise metaphorischen Charakter hat. Ein Modell soll möglichst viele Fakten in Rechnung stellen, darf aber selbst nicht mit den Fakten verwechselt werden. Die Bemühungen, die Funktionsleistung des limbischen Systems auf einen gemeinsamen Nenner zu bringen, sind seit den bahnbrechenden Untersuchungen von KLÜVER und BUCY (1937, 1938, 1939) sowie KLÜVER (1952) nicht abgerissen. Sie demonstrieren schwere Störungen emotionalen Verhaltens an Rhesusaffen, denen beide Schläfenlappen mit Uncus, Amygdala und größeren Hippocampusanteilen entfernt worden waren.

Das erste Funktionsmodell auf vergleichend neuroanatomischer Basis stammt von PAPEZ (1937): A proposed mechanism of emotion. PAPEZ machte den von ihm beschriebenen Neuronenkreis (Abb. 37; SMYTHIES, 1970) sowohl für Gefühlserlebnisse als auch für den Gefühlsausdruck verantwortlich und knüpfte damit schon an ältere Autoren an, die das Riechhirn als einen „inneren Apparat der allgemeinen körperlichen Einstellung, der Disposition und des affektiven Tonus" bezeichneten (HERRICK, 1933) oder wie KLEIST (1934) als Innenhirn, das „aufs engste mit den Innenempfindungen und den Gefühlen bei der Nahrungssuche, den Körperausscheidungen und den Geschlechtsvorgängen" verknüpft ist. MACLEAN (1969) griff die Idee von PAPEZ auf und brachte das „visceral brain" in einen Funktionszusammenhang mit psychosomatischen Erkrankungen. 1952 wurde in Anlehung an BROCAS (1878) „grand lobe limbique" der Ausdruck limbisches System von ihm geprägt (MACLEAN, 1952, 1954). Dieser Begriff ist anatomisch nicht unumstritten und wird mehr von Neurophysiologen, Psychologen und Neuropsychiatern gebraucht. Gemeint sind die Bereiche des Gehirns, die ringförmig wie ein Saum (Limbus) bilateral um den Hirnstamm angeordnet sind und eine Art Randzone zwischen Hirnstamm und Hypothalamus einerseits und Neocortex andererseits bilden (s. Abb. 32 und 34).

α) *Anatomie des limbischen Systems.* Auffällig ist, daß das limbische System bei den Säugern in Größe und Struktur relativ konstant geblieben ist; mit zunehmender Zerebralisation wird es durch den Neocortex umschlossen (s. Abb. 32). Seine Strukturen sind beidseitig ringförmig um den Hilus des Hirnstammes angeordnet und bilden einen inneren und einen äußeren Ring. Der innere Ring ist der phylogenetisch ältere Anteil des limbischen Systems (Archi-

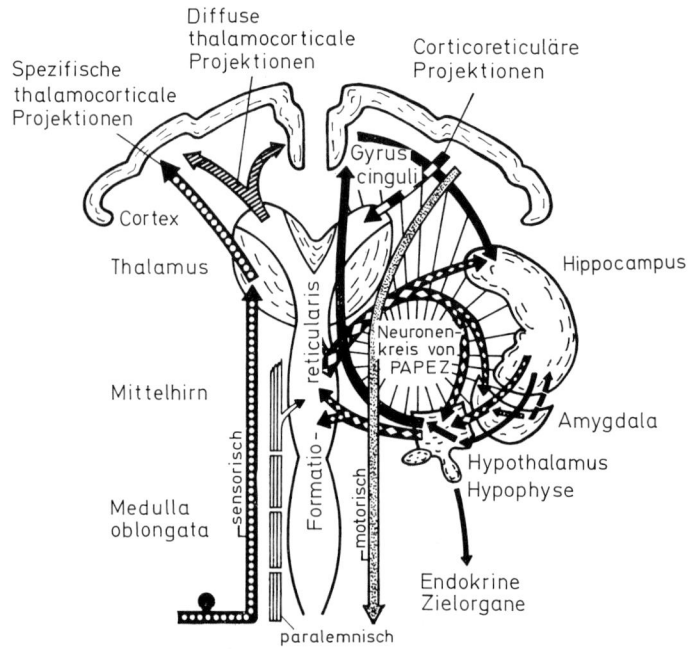

Abb. 37. Einige limbische Verbindungen nebst dem „Neuronen-Kreis für Emotionen" (PAPEZ): Hippocampus→Fornix→Septum→Corpora mamillaria→vorderer Thalamuskern→Gyrus cinguli →Hippocampus. (Aus SMITHIES, 1970)

pallium), er hat einen dreischichtigen Cortex (Allocortex). Zu ihm gehören die Strukturen mit olfaktorischen Verbindungen, der kortikomediale Anteil des Nucleus amygdalae und die gesamte Formatio hippocampi. Die Strukturen des äußeren Ringes liegen phylogenetisch zwischen Neo- und Archipallium, sie haben einen vierschichtigen Cortex (Mesocortex) und sind medial durch den Sulcus cinguli vom Neocortex getrennt. Zu ihnen gehören Gyrus cinguli, die Nuclei septi und der basolaterale Anteil der Amygdala. Manche Autoren rechnen auch den orbitoinsulotemporalen Cortex zum äußeren Ring des limbischen Systems (Abb. 38).

β) Afferente und efferente Verbindungen des limbischen Systems. Die afferenten und efferenten Verbindungen der Strukturen des limbischen Systems untereinander und mit Nachbarstrukturen sind sehr vielfältig und erst zum Teil bekannt (Abb. 38). Ihre funktionellen Bedeutungen können nur vage abgeschätzt werden. Es ist auffällig, daß dieses System über mächtige Faserstränge reziprok mit dem Hypothalamus verbunden ist. Die Formatio hippocampi und das Septum sind über den Fornix, der Mandelkern über die Stria terminalis und das ventrale amygdalofugale Bündel und die frontobasalen Anteile des limbischen Cortex über das mediale Vorderhirnbündel mit dem Hypothalamus verbunden. Diese und andere Verbindungen sind der anatomische Ausdruck dafür, daß der Hypothalamus der Kontrolle des limbischen Systems unterliegt (JAENIG, 1976). Generell sind die Strukturen des limbischen Systems, der Hypothalamus und das obere Mittelhirn (limbisches Mittelhirnareal), neuroanatomisch in multiplen Erregungskreisen organisiert (Abb. 39).

γ) Nucleus amygdalae und Hypothalamus. Der Mandelkern (Amygdala) ist ein subkortikales Kerngebiet des limbischen Systems, während der Hypothalamus nicht zum limbischen System gerechnet wird, aber doch anatomisch und funktional so enge reziproke Beziehungen zu ihm und insbesondere zu den Mandelkernen hat, daß eine Trennung verhaltensphysiologisch kaum möglich ist (Abb. 40).

Die Mandelkerne haben sich bei den Amphibien in enger Beziehung zum Riechhirn entwickelt und dienen bei ihnen zum Identifizieren der Nahrung, zur Feinderkennung und zum Aufspüren des Sexualpartners. Obwohl das Riechsystem bei höheren Säugern für die Steuerung des Verhaltens an Bedeutung verloren hat, ist der Mandelkern in seiner Funktion erhalten geblieben und übt auch bei Affe und Mensch eine unbezweifelbare Kontrolle auf das Verhalten, insbesondere auf aggressives Verhalten aus (MARK u. ERVIN, 1970; ELEFTHERIOU u. SCOTT, 1971; SWEET et al., 1977), spielt aber außerdem eine Rolle für die Regulation der Nahrungsaufnahme und der sexuellen Reifung. Über die Afferenzen zu den Amygdala ist wenig bekannt. Die beiden efferenten Fasersysteme mit offenbar antagonistischer Funktion sind denen der Amphibien homolog und konvergieren bei recht verschiedenem Verlauf auf den Nucleus ventromedialis des Hypothalamus, also jenem Kern, der sowohl für die sexuelle Maturation als auch für die Regulation der Nahrungsaufnahme – als sog. „Sättigungszentrum" – eine wichtige Rolle spielt. Zur Zeit wird über stereotaktische Eingriffe an diesem Ort, die zur Sozialisierung devianten sexuellen Verhaltens ausgeführt werden, heftig gestritten (MÜLLER et al., 1974; ROEDER et al., 1976; DIECKMANN

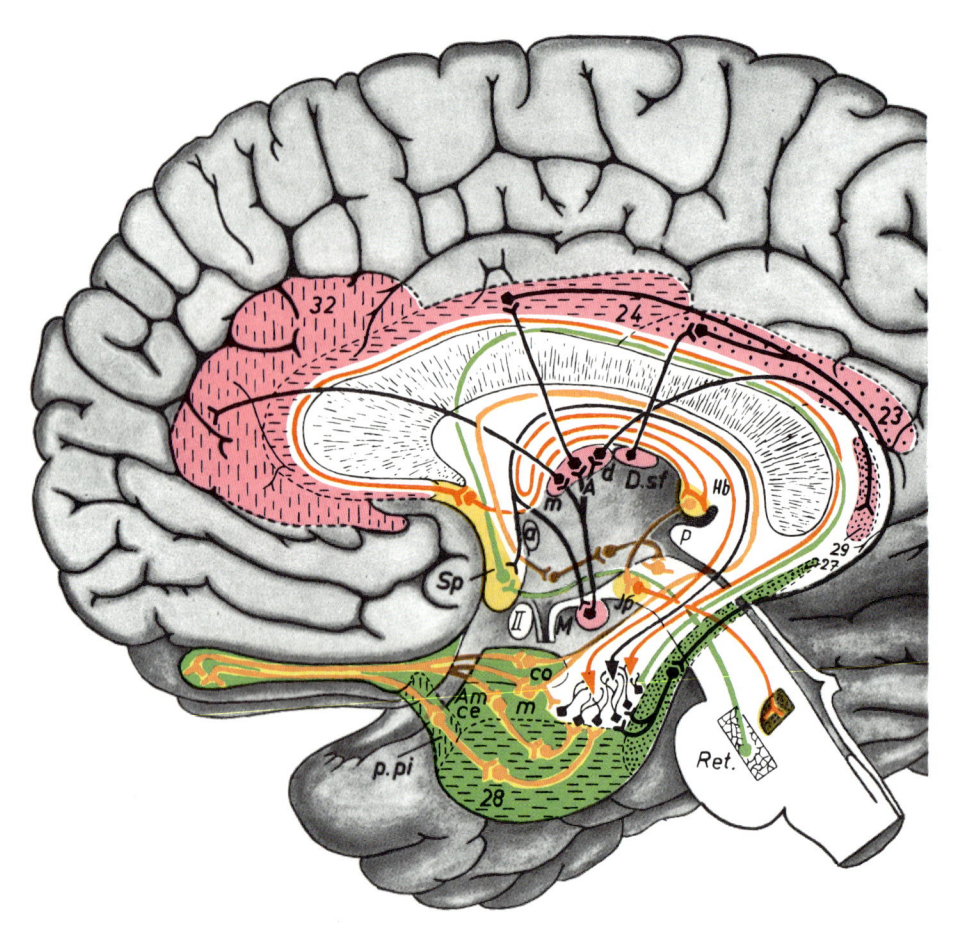

Abb. 38. Schema des limbischen Systems mit seinen olfaktorischen Zuflüssen. Alle seine Rindenfelder liegen an der Medialfläche des Gehirns und bilden einen „Saum" (limbus) um Balken und Stammganglien, der hier grün oder rot ist. Einige Kerne des Thalamus und des Mandelkernkomplexes sind durch Faserzüge (schwarz bzw. gelb) mit den limbischen Rindenfeldern verbunden. Dieses in sich geschlossene System hat ein Ausfallstor, nämlich zum Hirnstamm aus dem Nucleus interpeduncularis (Jp), und zwei Eingangspforten: eine von der Formatio reticularis (Ret in grün) und eine vom Riechorgan (Bulbus olfactorius in gelben Bahnen). Die olfaktorischen Afferenzen, die dem ganzen System den Namen Rhinenzephalon eingetragen hatten, verlaufen durch den Bulbus und Tractus olfactorius (links unten in gelb) nur zu zwei Endigungsstätten: der Area praepiriformis (p.pi) und drei Kernen der Amygdala (Am), nämlich dem kortikalen (co), dem zentralen (ce) und dem medialen (m) (in grün). Nur diese Strukturen sind sekundäre Riechfelder. – Aus dem kortikalen und medialen Kern der Amygdala entspringt das System der Stria terminalis (gelb; unter dem Balken). Die Stria terminalis erreicht über ihren „Bettkern" im Septumbereich (sp) das mediale Vorderhirnbündel, verschiedene Kerne des Hypothalamus und die dynamogene Zone in der Rückwand des III. Ventrikels. – Das sekundäre Riechfeld, Area praepiriformis (p.pi) ist, ebenso wie der zentrale Kern der Amygdala (ce), mit der Regio entorhinalis (28) verbunden. Von ihr gehen zwei efferente Verbindungen zum Ammonshorn bzw. Gyrus dentatus aus; der Tractus alvearis zum Feld h^1 und der Tractus perforans zu den Dendriten der Felder h^1 und h^2 und über den Gyrus dentatus (kleine schwarze Rhomben) zu den Feldern h^3 und h^4. – Unspezifische Afferenzen aus allen Sinnesgebieten erhält das Ammonshorn von der Formatio reticularis pontis (Ret) über eine Bahn zum Septum (Sp) bzw. Brocas Band. Von dort entspringen den Balken perforierende Fasern des Fornix longus (blasse grüne Bahn in der Abbildung), die im Gyrus dentatus

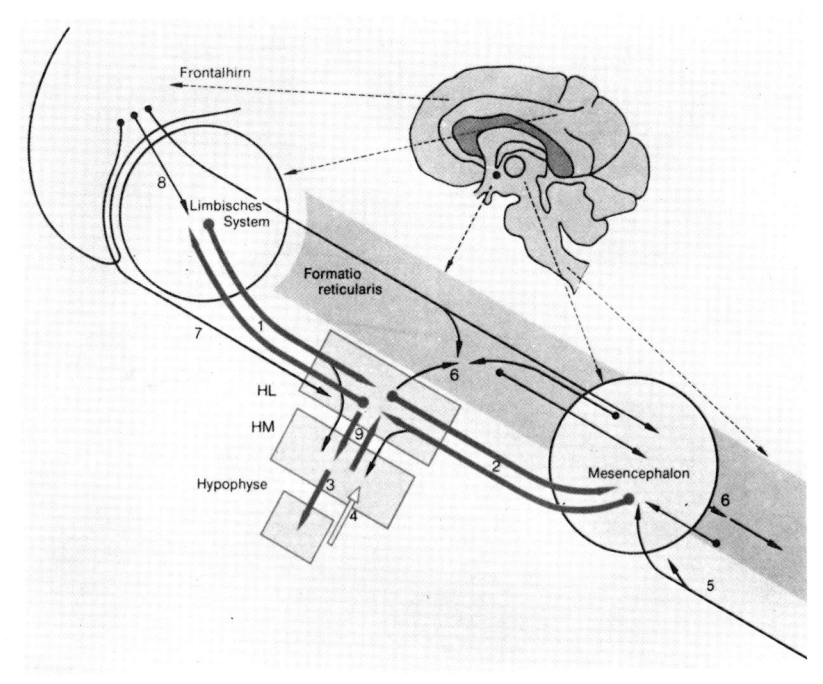

Abb. 39. Afferente und efferente Verbindungen des Hypothalamus. HM = Hypothalamus medialis, HL = Hypothalamus lateralis. (Aus JÄNIG, 1976)

u. HASSLER, 1976, 1977). Das eine Bündel entspringt im basolateralen Teil des Kernkomplexes der Amygdala und zieht als ventrales amygdalofugales, ziemlich breit gefächertes Faserbündel (VAF) medialwärts zur Basis des Septums (Brocas Diagonalband, s. Abb. 38), zur Area praeoptica und in den Hypothalamus zum Ventromedialkern. Das andere, dorsale Projektionssystem (ST) entspringt im kortikomedialen Anteil des Mandelkerns und zieht als Stria terminalis (s. Abb. 38) in großem Bogen zwischen Caudatum und Thalamus nach vorn

---

endigen und unspezifische Reaktionen des Ammonshorn ermöglichen. – Das Ammonshorn – durch 3 große Pyramidenzellen im weißen Feld dargestellt – ist der Ursprung von 3 Wirksystemen: 1. Fornixfasern (rote Pyramidenzelle mit roter Bahn) über Stria medullaris thalami zum Ganglion habenulae (Hb), welches auch Erregungen aus dem Septum empfängt. Vom Ganglion habenulae geht die Leitung über den Tractus retroflexus zum Nucleus interpedunculars (Jp) und zu medialen Kernen der Brückenhaube. 2. Die klassische Fornixbahn (in schwarz) zum Corpus mamillare (M) mit Nebenschluß zum Septum. Vom Corpus mamillare wird die Leitung direkt zu den 3 Kernen der vorderen Thalamusgruppe fortgesetzt (A, m, d). Diese Kerne projizieren unmittelbar zu limbischen Feldern auf dem Gyrus cinguli – roter Grund – und zwar Am zu Area 32, A zu Area 24 und Ad zu Area 29 (retrosplenialis). Das Cingulum-Feld 23 erhält seine spezifischen Projektionen von einem pallidär versorgten Thalamuskern D.sf. Von Area 24 und 23 gehen Fasern als Cingulum zurück über Area perirhinalis und praesubicularis (27) zum Ammonshorn und schließen den Erregungskreis. 3. Fasern des Fornix longus (rot) verlaufen über dem Balken zum Septum (gelb), um Anschluß an das 1. Fornix-System und – im Rückmeldekreis – an die septalen Afferenzen des Ammonshorns zu bekommen. (Aus HASSLER, 1967)

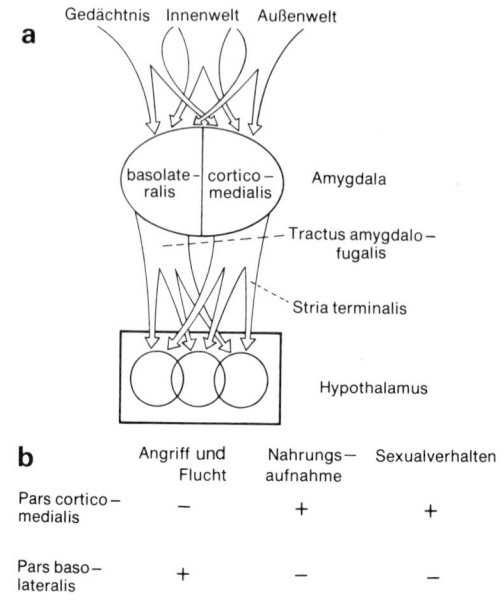

Abb. 40. Kontrolle hypothalamischer Verhaltensweisen durch den Nucl. amygdalae. + = Aktivierung, − = Hemmung. (Aus JÄNIG, 1976)

unter Abgabe von Fasern an Septum, Area praeoptica u.a. zum gleichen Hypothalamuskern. Das VAF übt einen exzitatorischen, die ST einen antagonistisch-hemmenden Einfluß aus. Ob diese dichotome Funktion nur für den Ventromedialkern oder auch für andere Terminalgebiete der beiden efferenten Amygdalabündel gilt, ist unbekannt. Jedenfalls besteht dieser Antagonismus auch in bezug auf die ACTH-Sekretion, wobei die kortikomediale Area inhibierend und die basolaterale Area fazilitierend auf die Ausschüttung des adreno-kortikotropen Hormons wirkt.

Was nun die Verhaltensstudien angeht, so wird durch elektrische Reizung des basolateralen Mandelkerns eine typische, umweltorientierte Defensivreaktion bei der Katze ausgelöst, während diese Reaktion ausbleibt, wenn man das VAF zerstört (HILTON u. ZBROZYNA, 1963). Diese Reaktion kann man zwar auch auslösen, wenn man die ST reizt (FERNANDEZ DE MOLINA u. HUNSPERGER, 1959, 1962), doch geschieht dies durch afferente Erregung der Amygdala. Auch Selbstreizungsverhalten bei Ratten konnte nur bei Implantation der Elektroden im kortikomedialen Bereich ausgelöst werden, während Reizung im basolateralen Teil Flucht hervorrief. Läsionen im basolateralen Teil hatten vermehrte Futteraufnahme, Läsionen im kortikomedialen Teil anorektisches Verhalten zur Folge. Durchtrennung der ST führt zu vorzeitiger sexueller Reife, tägliche Reizung der kortikomedialen Kerne verzögert sie. Schließlich gibt es Hinweise dafür, daß der kortikomediale Teil sexuelles Verhalten stimuliert. Ob der basolaterale Teil den gegenteiligen Effekt hat, ist unklar (GLOOR et al., 1972). Abb. 40 faßt die Amygdala-Hypothalamus-Beziehungen in vereinfachter Weise zusammen.

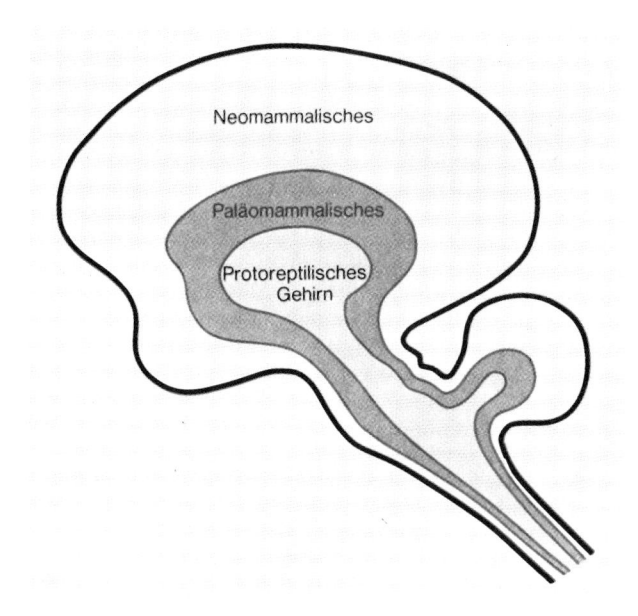

Abb. 41. Das „dreieinige Gehirn". Erklärung s. Text. (Aus MacLean, 1970)

b) Das „dreieinige Gehirn"

MacLean (1970, 1972a) geht in seinem Konzept wie Papez von vergleichend neuroanatomischen Vorstellungen aus und ordnet hypothetischen Evolutionsstadien des Gehirns entsprechende Verhaltensmuster zu. Das „Triune Brain" besteht aus drei Abschnitten, dem reptilischen Gehirn, dem paläomammalischen und dem neomammalischen Gehirn. Das „Reptil-Gehirn" ist aus der Matrix des oberen Hirnstammes geformt und schließt die ursprüngliche Substanz des retikulären Systems, des Mittelhirns und der Basalganglien ein. Das „Altsäuger-Gehirn" ist aus dem rudimentären Reptiliencortex gewachsen und entspricht dem limbischen System. Aus diesem heraus hat sich das „Neusäuger-Gehirn" entwickelt, das dem Neocortex entspricht, der in der Entwicklung der Primaten kulminiert (Abb. 41).

Natürlich handelt es sich hier um Prototypen von Gehirnen. Daß ein Reptil mit dem angenommenen protoreptilischen Gehirn existiert hat, kann empirisch nicht bewiesen werden. Die Einteilung bleibt daher spekulativ. Dennoch ist das „dreieinige Gehirn" als Modell wertvoll, weil sich daran mehrere der oben beschriebenen Prinzipien neuraler Organisation, vor allem das hierarchische, aufzeigen und zum Verhalten in Beziehung setzen lassen.

Das protoreptilische Gehirn produziert vorprogrammiertes Verhalten im Sinne von Instinkthandlungen (Lorenz, 1937; Tinbergen, 1952), die zum Überleben des Individuums wie auch zur Erhaltung der Art notwendig sind (MacLean, 1958; 1972b) und auf Artgedächtnis beruhen.

Das Altsäugergehirn stellt den ersten Versuch der Natur dar, das stereotype Verhalten plastischer zu gestalten, indem es dem Lebewesen sowohl ein besseres

Bild von seinen Innenvorgängen als auch von seiner Umgebung gibt, so daß es sich besser auf neue Situationen einstellen, ihre Bedeutung bewerten und aus ihnen lernen kann. Nach MACLEAN können sich Gedächtnisinhalte nur formieren, wenn sich innere und äußere Informationen verbinden. Diese Vorstellung paßt gut zu den Ergebnissen der Lern- und Motivationsforschung. Dem Hippocampus kommt für die Formierung von konditionierten Reaktionen und Gedächtnisinhalten bekanntlich eine wichtige Rolle zu (PLOOG, 1964a; ISAACSON, 1974). Zur Frage der Konditionierung von Hippocampuszellen hat MACLEAN (1972b) ein auf Einzelzellableitungen beruhendes Schema entworfen, das einen Mechanismus des Abgleichs von interozeptiven und exterozeptiven Reizen beschreibt (s. SCHMITT et al., 1970, S. 346).

Dem Neusäugergehirn erkennt MACLEAN die unemotionale Feinanalyse der physischen und sozialen Umwelt zu. Es arbeitet sozusagen unbehindert durch Signale aus der Innenwelt. Im Gegensatz zum Altsäugergehirn entwickelt es Handlungsstrategien und Konzepte. Es ist ein Gehirn, das in die Zukunft plant und, wie ISAACSON (1974) sagt, alteingeschliffenes Verhalten, sei es gelernt oder genetisch determiniert, modifiziert und unterdrückt.

Aufgrund von Tierexperimenten und klinischen Beobachtungen faßt MAC-LEAN (1972b; 1978) sein Konzept folgendermaßen zusammen: Das limbische System wird in drei Systemabschnitte mit unterschiedlichen Funktionen eingeteilt. Diese Systeme sind in Abb. 42 durch die feldförmig verteilten kleinen Zahlen gekennzeichnet und nach den drei „Knotenpunkten" Amygdala, Septum und vorderem Thalamuskern numeriert.

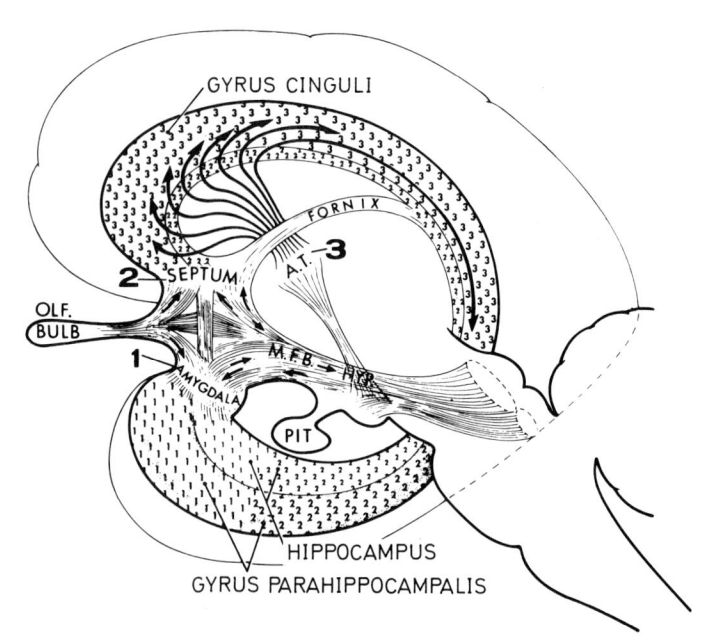

Abb. 42. Schema von drei Hauptabschnitten des limbischen Systems und deren Hauptverbindungen. Näheres im Text. Abkürzungen: AT = vordere Thalamuskerne, HYP = Hypothalamus, MFB = mediales Vorderhirnbündel, PIT = Hypophyse, OLF = Bulbus olfactorius. (Aus MACLEAN, 1978)

1. Das Amygdala-System ist für die oralen Aktivitäten – Fressen, Kämpfen und Selbstverteidigung – verantwortlich. 2. Das Septum-System besorgt das Fortpflanzungsverhalten (MacLean, 1958).

Bei Tieren führt die elektrische Reizung der Amygdala zum Fressen, zum Ausdruck der Wut, zum Angriff und zur Verteidigung (s.S. 455), während die Reizung des Septum-Systems sexuelles Verhalten und Bindungsverhalten bewirkt (s.S. 462). Wegen der engen reziproken Verbindungen dieser Systeme (vgl. Abb. 38) können die Erregungen von einem in das andere System überspringen – eine mögliche neurophysiologische Erklärung für das Übersprungverhalten (Tinbergen, 1940/1952) – und zu Kombinationen von oralen und sexuellen Verhaltensweisen führen. Die engen Beziehungen der beiden Systeme sind wahrscheinlich durch ihre Verbindungen mit dem Geruchssinn bedingt, der weit in die Stammesgeschichte zurückreicht und eine primäre Rolle bei der Nahrungssuche und beim Werbungs- und Kopulationsverhalten spielt, dem bei vielen Wirbeltieren der Kampf um das Weibchen vorausgeht. Hamstermännchen hören auf zu kopulieren und zu kämpfen, wenn ihnen der Bulbus olfactorius zerstört wird (Murphy u. Schneider, 1970). Ob dies auch auf den Rhesusaffen zutrifft, ist noch immer strittig (Michael et al., 1976a, b; Goldfoot, 1978).

Wie wir in vielfacher Hinsicht, so auch beim genitalen Imponieren des Totenkopfaffen (s. Abb. 2) gezeigt haben, spielen visuelle Signale für das sozio-sexuelle Verhalten der Affen eine dominierende Rolle. MacLean schreibt dem 3. System, das die Corpora mamillaria, den Tractus mamillothalamicus, die vorderen Thalamuskerne und den Gyrus cinguli einschließt, den Wandel im Sozialverhalten zu, der die Primaten und am ausgeprägtesten den Menschen kennzeichnet, nämlich die überragende Bedeutung visueller und die abnehmende Bedeutung olfaktorischer Reize. Dem entspricht die zunehmende Ausdehnung dieses Systems in der Primatenreihe mit der größten Entwicklung beim Menschen. Es hat keine Verbindung zum olfaktorischen System und existiert bei Reptilien noch nicht in dieser Form. Daß dieses System ebenfalls in sozio-sexuelles Verhalten (neben anderen sozialen Verhaltensweisen) involviert ist, wird im nächsten Kapitel beschrieben.

c) Die zerebrale Repräsentation sozio-sexuellen Verhaltens

Bei der Beschreibung soziogenitaler Signale hatten wir gezeigt, daß die Genitalfunktion in den Dienst der Kommunikation gestellt wird und nicht allein der Reproduktion der Art dient (s. Abb. 2 und Abb. 7). Dies muß man sich vor Augen halten, wenn man die nachstehend geschilderten elektrischen Hirnreizversuche richtig einschätzen will. Ziel der Hirnreizversuche war es, Orte im Gehirn aufzufinden, von denen beim Affen Erektionen des Penis auszulösen sind. Während dieser Experimente wurde gleichzeitig durch Beobachtungen einer Affenkolonie entdeckt, daß Erektionen als Komponenten eines kommunikativen Verhaltens auftreten können und als soziales Signal fungieren (Ploog et al., 1963). Während der Hirnreizversuche konnte der Affe sein natürliches Verhalten nicht zeigen. Er saß für die Dauer des Experiments wach und meist ruhig im Untersuchungsstuhl, an den er gewohnt war. Vor, während und nach der elektrischen Reizung wurden das Verhalten des Tieres und seine vegetativen

Reaktionen beobachtet. Durch systematische punktförmige Reizung des Gehirns wurde ein verzweigtes System gefunden, von dem Erektionen ausgelöst werden konnten (MACLEAN u. PLOOG, 1962).

Das System gruppiert sich wiederum in drei Hauptabschnitte, die große Teile des limbischen Systems und des Dienzephalons umfassen:

1. Die Lokalisationen für Auslösung von Erektionen (im folgenden positive Punkte genannt) folgen dem Projektionssystem des Hippocampus (VALENSTEIN u. NAUTA, 1959) zu Septum-, Thalamus- und Hypothalamus-Anteilen.

2. Sie liegen in solchen Strukturen, die die Corpora mamillaria, den Tractus mamillothalamicus, den Nucleus anterior thalami und den Gyrus cinguli umfassen.

3. Sie befinden sich im Gyrus rectus und im medialen Teil des Nucleus medialis dorsalis thalami wie auch in solchen Regionen, die als deren Verbindungen und Projektionen bekannt sind.

In den Hirndiagrammen (Abb. 43) folgt man den Symbolen für Erektionen vom Gyrus rectus (A 16) in den medialen Septumanteil (A 13.5) und dann in die mediale präoptische Region (A 12.5). Ungefähr auf halbem Wege durch die vordere Kommissur beginnen die positiven Punkte zu divergieren (A 11). Medial folgt man ihnen in den antero-medialen Teil des Hypothalamus; dort ist die Lokalisation inmitten des Nucleus paraventricularis besonders erwähnenswert (A 10.5; A 10). Lateralwärts ziehen die positiven Punkte über den Nucleus supraopticus hinweg und in den ventrolateralen Hypothalamus hinein. Auf der Ebene A 9.5 häufen sich die Loci oberhalb des Tractus opticus und lateral vom Fornix; aus den folgenden Diagrammen (A 9; A 8.5) ist zu ersehen, daß

▷

Abb. 43. Hirnkarten der cerebralen Repräsentation der männlichen Genitalfunktion von Saimiri sciureus. In 12 Diagrammen sind die Orte eingetragen, von denen an 29 erwachsenen Totenkopfaffen Erektionen durch elektrische Reizung ausgelöst werden konnten. Die schematischen Frontalabschnitte entsprechen Ebenen der stereotaktischen Koordinaten A 16 bis A 6. Diese Werte zeigen in Millimetern an, wie weit der jeweils repräsentative Schnitt oral von der Null-Linie (Zentrum der Ohrbolzen des stereotaktischen Gerätes) entfernt liegt. Buchstabe A (Anterior) und die zugehörige Zahl sitzen stets einer Linie auf, die 4 mm oberhalb der Null-Linie gelegen ist, womit neben der a-p-Ebene auch die Horizontalebene gekennzeichnet ist. Außerdem repräsentiert die Entfernung von aufeinanderfolgenden senkrechten Strichen jeweils 1 mm. Auf diese Weise können die stereotaktischen Koordinaten für die einzelnen Symbole geschätzt werden. – Senkrechte Striche entsprechen Orten, die bei der Hirnreizung negativ bezüglich der Erektionsauslösung waren. ◊ und □ entsprechen Orten, von denen Erektionen ausgelöst wurden (positive Punkte). ◊ Positive Punkte ohne Nachentladungen im Hippocampus. □ Positive Punkte mit begleitender oder folgender Hippocampus-Nachentladung. ◆ und ■ schwach ausgeprägte Erektion. ✦ und ▨ mittelstark ausgeprägte Erektion. ◆ und ■ starke bis maximale Erektion. ± Schwellung der Glans mit Vortreten des Penis aus dem Präputium. ● Erektionen nach Reizbeendigung in Verbindung mit Nachentladungen, die bioelektrische Aktivitätsveränderungen im Hippocampus nach sich ziehen. • Erektionen als Rebound-Phänomen nach Reizende ohne begleitende Hippocampus-Nachentladungen. – Abkürzungen: ad = Nucl. anterodorsalis thalami; al = Ansa lenticularis; av = Nucl. anteroventralis thalami; ca = Commissura anterior; cc = Corpus callosum; ci = Capsula interna; co = Chiasma opticum; db = Diagonalband von BROCA; f = Fornix; gc = Gyrus cinguli; gp = Globus pallidus; gr = Gyrus rectus; hc = Hypophysis cerebri; ld = Nucl. lateralis dors. thalami; m = Corpus mamillare; md = Nucl. medialis dors. thalami; mfb = Fasciculus medialis telencephali (medial forebrain bundle); mt = Fascicu-

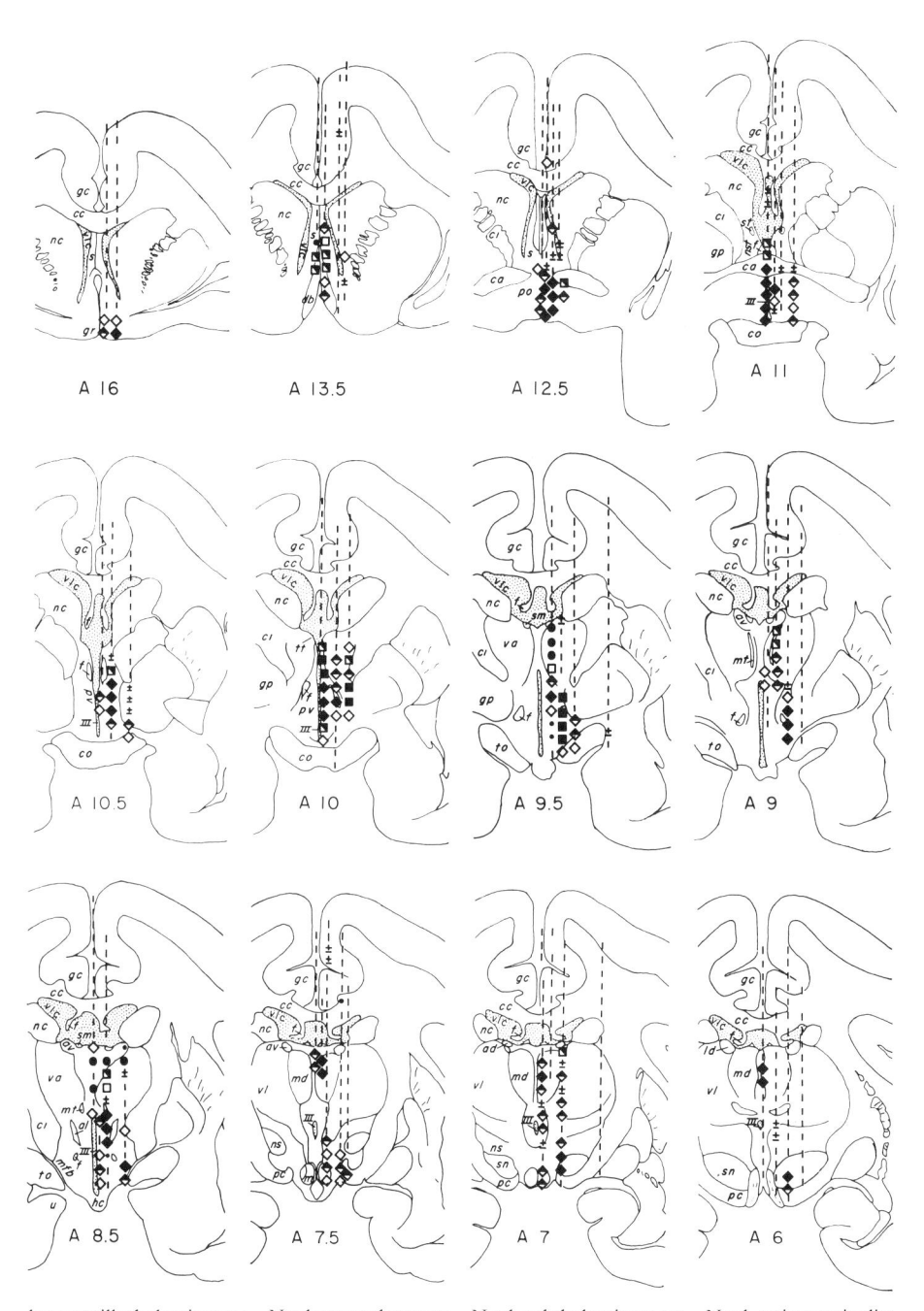

Hirnstrukturen und -funktionen im Kommunikationsprozeß   463

lus mamillothalamicus; nc = Nucleus caudatus; ns = Nucl. subthalamicus; nst = Nucl. stria terminalis; p = Putamen; pc = Pedunculus cerebri; po = Area praeoptica; pv = Nucl. paraventricularis hypothalami; s = Septum pellucidum; sm = Stria medullaris; sn = Substantia nigra; st = Stria terminalis; to = Tractus opticus; tt = Tuberculum thalami; u = Uncus gyri hippocampi; va = Nucl. ventralis anterior thalami; vl = Nucl. ventralis lateralis thalami; vlc = Ventriculus lateralis cerebri; III = Ventriculus tertius. (Aus MacLean u. Ploog, 1962) sie dem medialen Vorderhirnbündel (s. Abb. 38) folgen. Weiter kaudalwärts finden sich positive Punkte in den Corpora mamillaria und den medialen Anteilen des Nucleus subthalamicus und der Hirnschenkel (A 7.5; A 7). Für die Corpora mamillaria wurden positive Reizantworten in nicht weniger als 11 Tieren gefunden (MacLean u. Ploog, 1962; Ploog u. MacLean, 1963a). Während man am hinteren Pol der Corpora mamillaria noch positive Reaktionen erhält, sind unmittelbar kaudal davon gelegene Punkte der Mittellinie negativ. Die positiven Orte verschieben sich dann lateral und folgen tangential dem Verlauf der austretenden Okulomotoriusfasern durch den mittleren Teil der Substantia nigra ziehend (A 6) und weiter in die ventrolaterale Brücke (auf Abb. 43 nicht mehr dargestellt). Des weiteren findet man positive Punkte im Brückenarm. Von dieser Ebene ziehen die Punkte sich durch den ventrolateralen Teil der oberen Olive und wenden sich in Höhe des Austritts vom VI. Hirnnerven nach medial, wo man eben lateral von den Pyramiden Erektionen auslösen kann (MacLean et al., 1963a).

Die Befunde an den Corpora mamillaria lenken auf die positiven Loci entlang dem Tractus mamillo-thalamicus (A 9; A 8.5) und im vorderen Thalamus (A 10; A 7.5; A 7). Wie man auf A 10 sieht, können positive Reizantworten im Tuberculum thalami und im rostralen Thalamuspol ausgelöst werden. Andere Punkte finden sich an einer Stelle, wo die anteroventralen und anterodorsalen Kerne gerade kaudalwärts auslaufen (A 7). Besonders zu beachten sind die Lokalisationen im medialen Anteil des Nucleus medialis dorsalis thalami (A 7.5 bis A 6). Von hier scheint eine Bahn dem unteren Thalamusstiel in den lateralen Hypothalamus zu folgen und mit dem medialen Vorderhirnbündel in die Area ventralis tegmenti zu ziehen. Eine andere Verbindung erreicht den dorsomedialen Hypothalamus über das periventrikuläre Fasersystem (MacLean et al., 1963a). Im kaudalen Thalamus finden sich Punkte, die starkes Kratzen am Genitale und Ejakulation hervorrufen. Offenbar besteht hier eine somatotopische genitale Repräsentation. Die Ejakulation kann unabhängig von Kratzen und Erektion ausgelöst werden. Es werden dabei zweifellos sensorische Fasern erregt, die man entlang dem Tractus spinothalamicus verfolgen kann (MacLean et al., 1963b).

Wie auf Ebene A 8.5 und A 7 zu sehen, entstanden starke Erektionen bei Reizung nahe dem Dach des dritten Ventrikels; diese Area greift auf den Nucleus reuniens und die Gegend des dorsalen und posterioren Hypothalamus über. Auf A 10 sieht man positive Symbole auf der ganzen vertikalen Länge des Ventrikelwalles in der Ebene des Nucleus paraventricularis eingetragen. Eben kaudal davon erhält man hochgradig aversive Reizeffekte (ängstliches Gekreische usw.), sobald der Nucleus ventromedialis hypothalami einbezogen ist (s. dazu S. 455). Wiederum weiter kaudalwärts und rostral zu den Corpora mamillaria stößt man im Wall des 3. Ventrikels nochmals auf positive Punkte, die man bis in die Tubergegend[1] verfolgen kann. Nach den Befunden ist wahrscheinlich, daß Teile der periventrikulären Strukturen (mit deren Fortsetzung im Schützschen Bündel) in das Gesamtsystem einbezogen sind.

---

[1] s. hierzu Spatz, H.: Das Hypophysen-Hypothalamus-System in seiner Bedeutung für die Fortpflanzung [1953] sowie frühere Arbeiten dieses Autors zum gleichen Thema.

Schließlich sieht man auf A 12.5 und A 7.5, daß gelegentlich schwach positive Reizantworten im (oder gerade oberhalb vom) vorderen supracallosen Gyrus cinguli auszulösen waren. In späteren, hier noch nicht dokumentierten Versuchen fanden sich stark positive Punkte eben rostral vom Corpus callosum-Knie und in der Gegend des Gyrus subcallosus.

Der phylogenetisch jüngere Anteil des ganzen Systems, vor allem der Nucleus medialis dorsalis thalami mit seinen Projektionen zum orbitofrontalen und präfrontalen Cortex, spielt wahrscheinlich für die spezielle Entwicklung des Sexualverhaltens der Primaten eine entscheidende Rolle. Auch die anteriore Kerngruppe des Thalamus, die wiederum ein Teil des Hippocampus-Corpus mamillare-Cingulum-Systems ist, entwickelt sich bei den Primaten bis zum Menschen hinauf progressiv, während sich das Septum regressiv verändert.

Das die Erektionen begleitende Verhalten ist je nach Elektrodenlage verschieden. Strukturen, deren Reizung Angriffs-, Angst- oder Fluchtverhalten auslöst, können denen, die zur Erektion führen, ganz eng benachbart sein. Die entsprechenden Verhaltensweisen können sich durch Reizung überlagern. Die angewandte Technik erlaubte jedoch in den meisten Fällen, Elektrodenlage und Reizparameter so zu verändern, daß derartige Überlagerungen ausgeschaltet werden konnten. Aus den Ergebnissen darf man schließen, daß es außer dem Erektionen auslösenden System auch ein Erektionen hemmendes System gibt, das in Narkose früher ausfällt als das Erregungssystem. Nach Kastration bleiben die zerebralen Reiz-Effekte offenbar im wesentlichen unverändert erhalten. Umgebungseinflüsse, auf die das Tier ängstlich reagiert, können die Erektionen empfindlich hemmen, ja vollkommen unterdrücken.

Das genitale Imponieren, so hatten wir beschrieben (s.S. 384), kommt bei Männchen wie bei Weibchen vor. Bei Weibchen tritt an die Stelle der Erektion eine Schwellung der Klitoris. Stimuliert man das Gehirn von ovariektomierten Weibchen in der gleichen systematischen Weise wie gerade für Männchen beschrieben, erhält man eine vollkommene Übereinstimmung der Hirnorte, von denen eine Klitoris-Schwellung elektrisch auslösbar ist (MAURUS et al., 1966). Man kann daraus den Schluß ziehen, daß die Mechanismen für sozio-sexuelles Verhalten, soweit es die neuronale „Verschaltung" betrifft, bei beiden Geschlechtern die gleichen sind. Andererseits besteht nach den Ergebnissen der Verhaltensforschung an Primaten kein Zweifel darüber, daß sich männliches und weibliches Verhalten unterscheiden und daß diese Unterschiede schon sehr früh und lange vor der Pubertät deutlich sind (FRIEDMAN et al., 1974). Der Dimorphismus im Geschlechtsverhalten ist schon bei der Ratte und in weit differenzierteren Ausdrucksformen bei den Primaten kein absolut qualitativer, sondern ein quantitativer Unterschied: Verhaltensmuster, die typischerweise beim einen Geschlecht beobachtet werden, können gelegentlich auch beim anderen auftreten und umgekehrt. Dies gilt, soweit bekannt, für alle subhumanen Primaten und auf den gleichen psychobiologischen Grundlagen auch für den Menschen. Diese Unterschiede sind durch frühe, pränatale Differenzierung der involvierten Hirnstrukturen bedingt. Es kann hier nicht die Aufgabe sein, die umfangreichen neuroendokrinologischen, neurochemischen, neurophysiologischen und neuromorphologischen Ergebnisse der Geschlechtsdifferenzierung darzustellen (MICHAEL, 1968; FEDER u. WADE, 1974; GOY u. GOLDFOOT, 1974; HUTCHISON, 1974; MCEWEN et al., 1974; PFAFF et al., 1973, 1974). Es sollen aber die Zusammenhänge mit den diese Differenzierung tragenden Hirnstrukturen sichtbar werden.

In welchen Hirnstrukturen haben wir die hormonsensitiven Nervenzellen zu suchen, die männliches oder weibliches Sexualverhalten kontrollieren? Die genauesten Kenntnisse hierüber sind bislang an Ratten gewonnen worden. Soweit sie hier dargestellt werden, sind sie prinzipiell auf Primaten übertragbar.

Während einer kritischen Periode, die bei Ratten bis in die postnatale Zeit reicht, bei Primaten aber pränatal ist, nehmen die hormonsensitiven Hirnzellen die von den Gonaden des Embryos produzierten männlichen bzw. weiblichen Hormone auf und werden dadurch in ihrer Funktion „geprägt". Es gibt also einen Geschlechtsdimorphismus in der Feinstruktur gewisser Hirnregionen, vor allem der Area praeoptica, der durch frühe Androgenzufuhr bestimmt ist (RAISMAN u. FIELD, 1973). Ob es dieselben Zellindividuen sind, die entweder nur männliche oder nur weibliche Hormone aufnehmen oder verschiedene Zellindividuen in engster Nachbarschaft, von denen dann die nicht geprägten inaktiv bleiben, ist wohl noch ungewiß. Jedenfalls zeigen die Hirnregionen, die die höchste Aufnahme von radioaktivem Östradiol bei Weibchen zeigen, auch die höchste Aufnahme von radioaktivem Testosteron bei Männchen, wenn auch quantitativ weniger ausgeprägt.

Die Konzentrationen sind am besten für das Östradiol untersucht worden und finden sich im limbischen System, vor allem in den Septumkernen, in den kortikomedialen Amygdalakernen, in der medialen Area praeoptica, im medialen Hypothalamus und um die Außenränder des gesamten zentralen Höhlengraus. An Einzelzellableitungen in der Area praeoptica kann man zeigen, daß die Neurone männlicher Ratten auf Testosteron, die Neurone weiblicher Ratten auf Östrogene und Progesteron aktiviert werden (PFAFF et al., 1973).

Am Beispiel des Lordose-Reflexes der Ratte läßt sich das Zusammenspiel von Männchen und Weibchen bei der Kopulation mit den zugehörigen neuralen Mechanismen am besten demonstrieren. Diese Interdependenz von sensorischen Reizen und motorischen Antworten, abhängig von der Stärke des sensorischen Reizes und der Hormonkonzentration, kann als Modell für Interaktionssequenzen im allgemeinen dienen. Ähnlich dem in der Ethologie berühmt gewordenen Zickzack-Tanz der Stichlinge (TINBERGEN, 1952) ist hier das Kopulationsverhalten der Ratte, das in seinen Grundelementen allen Landsäugern gemeinsam ist, in schematischer Form dargestellt (Abb. 44).

Welches sind nun die notwendigen und hinreichenden Auslösereize für die Lordose? Experimente an Kaninchen, Ratten und Katzen haben gezeigt, daß die Fernsinne (Geruch, Sehen, Hören) nicht zur Auslösung der Kopulationshaltung nötig sind. Auch die vaginale Stimulierung ist nicht erforderlich. Notwendig und hinreichend sind alleine die Berührungen der Flanken, der Weichen und des Perineums. Anästhesiert man Perineum und Schwanzwurzel des Weibchens, sinkt bei Männchen-Weibchen-Begegnungen sowohl die Lordosehäufigkeit als auch die Intromissionshäufigkeit signifikant. Bei artifizieller Reizung der Flanken und des Perineums durch die Hand des Experimentators kann die Lordose ausgelöst werden. Die Stärke der Reizantwort hängt dabei von zwei Faktoren ab, nämlich erstens von der Reizstärke (Druck der Finger, Kratzen der Flanken) und zweitens von dem Östrogen-Progesteronspiegel. Zwischen sensorischem Reiz

♂ steigt von hinten auf, drückt Flanken des ♀ mit Vorderpfoten, berührt Schenkel mit Hinterpfoten, steigt hoch bis Becken den Steiß des ♀ berührt

♂ Beckenstöße gegen Leiste, Perineum und Vagina

♂ Intromission des Penis

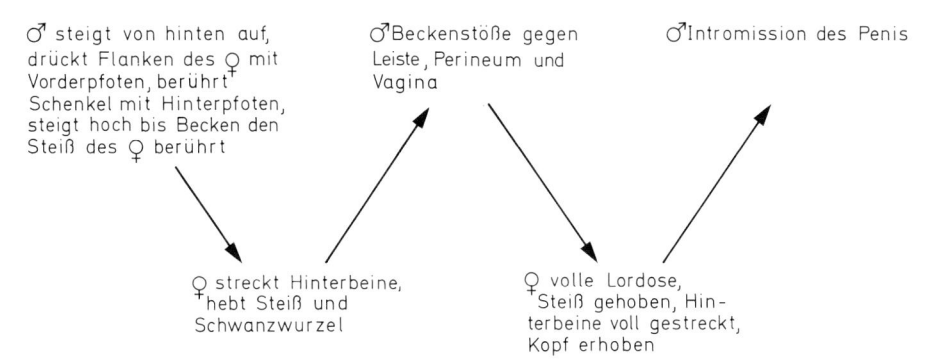

♀ streckt Hinterbeine, hebt Steiß und Schwanzwurzel

♀ volle Lordose, Steiß gehoben, Hinterbeine voll gestreckt, Kopf erhoben

Abb. 44. Simplifiziertes Modell der sensorischen (taktilen) Auslösung der weiblichen Kopulationshaltung (Lordose) der Ratte. Die minuziöse Reihenfolge der Bewegungen wurde mit Film und Röntgenkinematographie analysiert. (Nach Pfaff et al., 1973)

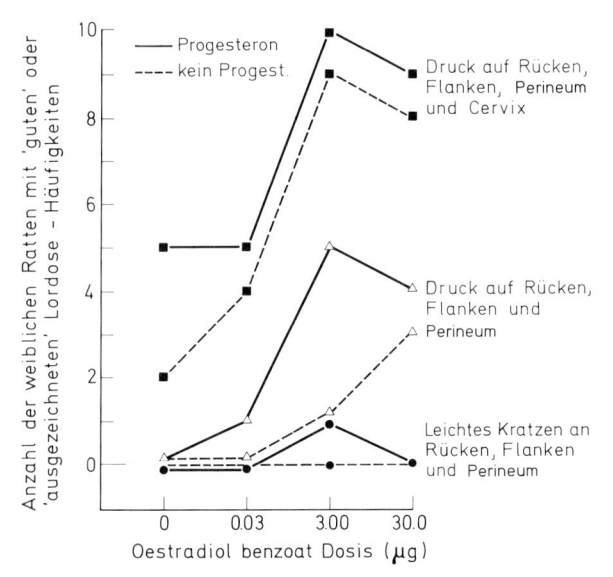

Abb. 45. Kopulationslordose der weiblichen Ratte in Abhängigkeit vom exterozeptiven Reiz und Östrogen-Progesteronspiegel. (Aus Pfaff et al., 1974)

und Disposition des Tieres besteht eine kompensatorische Beziehung (Abb. 45). Ein schwacher Reiz bei hohem Hormonspiegel kann die Lordose gleichermaßen auslösen wie ein starker Reiz bei niedrigem Hormonspiegel. Dieser, wenn auch nur in Grenzen mögliche Kompensationsmechanismus ist für die gesamte Verhaltensphysiologie – überall, wo es sich um Reiz-Antwort-Beziehungen handelt – von außerordentlicher Bedeutung. Auf die neuroendokrinneuronale Integration, die der Kopulationslordose zugrundeliegt, wollen wir kurz hinweisen:

Bereits auf peripherer Ebene bringen die neueren Ergebnisse eine Überraschung: Wird das Perineum mit Freyschen Haaren gereizt und von Fasern des zentralwärts durchtrennten N. pudendus abgeleitet, kann man bei einem sehr hohen Prozentsatz von ovariektomierten Ratten feststellen, daß sich das perineale rezeptive Feld erweitert und sich auf die dorsalen Schenkel ausdehnt, wenn die Ratten mit Östrogen behandelt werden. Aus Durchtrennungsversuchen auf verschiedenen spinalen Ebenen kann man schließen, daß die Lordosebewegung nicht allein auf spinaler Ebene organisiert wird. Hier scheint es allerdings Spezies-Differenzen zu geben. Läsionsversuche in verschiedenen Hypothalamusabschnitten zeigen, daß der mediale vordere Hypothalamus und die mediale präoptische Area, also Gegenden hoher Östrogenkonzentration, Kontrollinstanzen für die Kopulationslordose sind. Durch Hirnreizversuche konnten Steiß- und Schwanzbewegungen im ventrolateralen Hirnstamm und vor allem am lateralen und dorsolateralen Rand des mesenzephalen zentralen Höhlengraus ausgelöst werden. Im basalen Vorderhirn war die Auslösung dieser Bewegungen seltener; wenn sie aber mögkich war, dann lagen die Punkte im Bereich östradiolreicher Neuronenpopulationen.

Im Schema der Abb. 46 werden die der Kopulationslordose zugrundeliegenden Afferenzen und reizverarbeitenden Strukturen nochmals zusammengefaßt.

d) Die zerebrale Repräsentation audio-vokalen Verhaltens

Der vokale Ausdruck gehört bei Affe und Mensch zu den ersten Lebensäußerungen und hat von Anfang an eine kommunikative Funktion (s.S. 431 ff.). Was

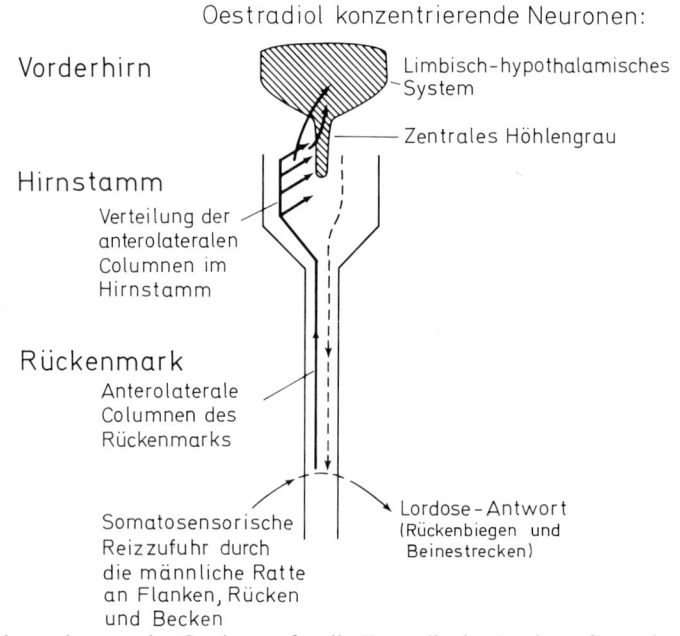

Abb. 46. Schema der neuralen Strukturen für die Kontrolle des Lordosereflexes der Ratte. (Aus PFAFF et al., 1974)

auch immer über die Einmaligkeit der Sprache, das souveränste Kommunikationsmittel des Menschen, zu sagen ist, es gibt keine natürliche Sprache ohne Vokalisation. In der Stimme drücken sich feinste Gemütsbewegungen aus, und das fließende Sprechen erfordert ein hohes Maß von motorischer Koordination. Soweit also Sprache lautgebender emotionaler Ausdruck ist, besteht kein grundsätzlicher Unterschied zum vokalen Ausdrucksvermögen der übrigen, nichtmenschlichen Primatenfamilie. Der erwachsene, gesunde Mensch macht von dieser Kommunikationsform nur in Ausnahmezuständen reinen Gebrauch, sonst kleidet er seinen vokalen Ausdruck in Worte. An den Lallmonologen der Kinder im vorsprachlichen Alter, am Singen ohne Worte bei den Erwachsenen sehen wir den Stimmungsausdruck und die kommunikative Funktion am reinsten.

α) Lautproduktion. Der periphere Apparat. Phylogenetisch betrachtet ist die Stimmgebung sehr alt und wurzelt in der Atmung. Entsprechend haben sich die stimmproduzierenden peripheren Strukturen und die generierenden, modulierenden und steuernden zerebralen Strukturen schrittweise zu immer komplexeren Systemen entwickelt. Was den peripheren Stimmapparat betrifft, so läßt sich auch innerhalb der Primatenfamilie noch eine bedeutsame Entwicklung nachweisen. Neben der fortschreitenden Differenzierung des Muskelapparates und der Umbildung des Knorpelskeletts ist für die Entwicklung der gesprochenen Sprache die Umformung des „Resonanzrohres" d.h. des supralaryngealen Trakts mit Glottis und Mund am wichtigsten. Die Bedeutung, die dem Kehlkopf einerseits und dem Resonanzrohr andererseits zukommt, steht bei nicht-verbalen und verbalen Äußerungen in umgekehrtem Verhältnis. Während die nicht-verbalen Lautäußerungen vorwiegend (und bei niedrigeren Vertebraten ausschließlich) auf unterschiedlicher Stimmlippenaktivität beruhen, ist die menschliche Sprache durch relativ gleichförmige Stimmlippenaktivität gekennzeichnet, in der Lautgestalten durch die Bewegungen von Lippen, Zunge und Gaumensegel geformt werden, wie das beim Flüstern deutlich wird. Das für die Artikulation entscheidende Resonanzrohr verlängert sich nun bei den Primaten und ganz besonders beim Menschen beträchtlich. Dadurch wächst die Vielfalt der Lautäußerungen enorm. Abb. 47 zeigt oben den morphologischen Hauptunterschied zwischen Schimpanse und Mensch: Der Winkel zwischen Pharynx und oberem Atmungstrakt ist beim Schimpansen bogenförmig flach, bei erwachsenen Menschen fast rechtwinklig, so daß Epiglottis und weicher Gaumen weit auseinanderliegen. Der untere Teil der Abbildung soll andeuten, daß es nur mit dem menschlichen Vokaltrakt möglich ist, die reinen Vokale /i/, /a/ und /u/ zu formen. Beim neugeborenen Menschen und beim erwachsenen Schimpansen liegt die Zunge gänzlich innerhalb der Mundhöhle; beim erwachsenen Menschen formt das hintere Zungendrittel in vertikaler Lage die Vorderwand des Pharynx. Diese nur dem Menschen eigene Konfiguration wird in der Ontogenese schon mit 6 Monaten deutlich und ist mit 2 Jahren, also während des Sprachentwicklungsalters, voll ausgebildet. Kinder mit ausgeprägtem Down-Syndrom behalten den Vokaltrakt des Neugeborenen und sind daher unfähig zum Sprechen (BENDA, 1969).

Die zerebralen Strukturen. Gleich ob es sich um den einfachen Paarungsruf des Frosches (CAPRANICA, 1965), das hunderte von Lautvarianten umfassende

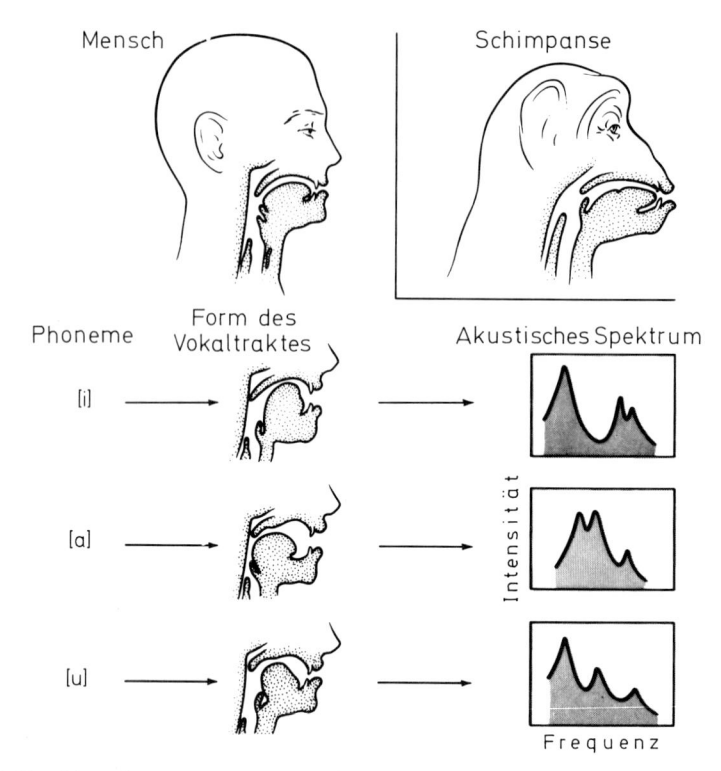

Abb. 47. Der Phonationsapparat von Mensch und Schimpanse. Erklärung im Text. (Aus WILSON, 1975)

Repertoire mancher Affenarten (GREEN, 1975; SCHOTT, 1975) oder die Stimmgebung des Menschen handelt, dieses Verhalten hat seine zerebrale Entsprechung. Tastet man beim Frosch das Gehirn mittels Elektroden nach Orten ab, deren elektrische Reizung Vokalisation hervorruft, so findet man zwei Gebiete, in denen artspezifische Laute auslösbar sind; das eine ist die mediale präoptische Region – von ihr lassen sich Paarungsrufe auslösen; das andere ist der Bereich zwischen Torus semicircularis und motorischem Trigeminuskern, also das dorsale Ponstegmentum – hier lassen sich Befreiungslaute produzieren (SCHMIDT, 1966). Zerstörung der präoptischen Region bringt die Paarungsrufe zum Verschwinden, läßt die Befreiungsrufe jedoch unbeeinflußt; nach Zerstörung des dorsalen Ponstegmentums geht sowohl die Fähigkeit zur Bildung von Paarungs- wie von Befreiungsrufen verloren. Da elektrische Reizung der präoptischen Region nicht nur Paarungsrufe, sondern auch andere Verhaltensweisen des Fortpflanzungsverhaltens zu aktivieren vermag, die betreffende Region außerdem zu den wenigen stark mit Androgenrezeptoren besetzten Gebieten im Froschhirn zählt (KELLY et al., 1975) und ihre Aktivierung bei der Auslösung des Paarungsrufes zu einer neuronalen Aktivitätsänderung im pontinen Vokalisationsgebiet führt, schloß SCHMIDT (1974) aus diesen Beobachtungen, daß der eigentliche neuronale Koordinationsmechanismus, sowohl für Paarungs- wie für Befreiungslaute, im Ponstegmentum sitzt. Der präoptischen Region würde in bezug auf die Auslösung des Paarungsrufes demnach nur eine bahnende Funktion zukommen.

Bei den Säugern wurden im wesentlichen drei Spezies mittels Hirnreizung genauer untersucht: Katze (MAGOUN et al., 1937; HUNSPERGER u. BUCHER, 1967), Totenkopfaffe (JÜRGENS u. PLOOG, 1970) und Rhesusaffe (ROBINSON, 1967). Im Unterschied zu den vorstehend genannten niederen Wirbeltierklassen bilden hier die vokalisationsauslösenden Hirnstrukturen ein weit ausgedehntes System. Beim Totenkopfaffen gelang es innerhalb dieses Systems außerdem, bestimmte Lauttypen bestimmten Strukturen zuzuordnen. So können gackerartige Laute (Abb. 48) (1) vom zentralen Höhlengrau und kaudolateral anschließenden Ponstegmentum ausgelöst werden; nach rostral lassen sich die „Gackerpunkte" dann entlang des 3. Ventrikels bis etwa auf Höhe der vorderen Kommissur verfolgen, wo ein Teil von ihnen dem unteren Thalamusstiel bis in den Mandelkern einerseits und zum medialen Nucleus ventralis anterior-Rand andererseits folgt, während der übrige Teil entlang des ventromedialen Capsula interna-Randes in den Gyrus rectus und Gyrus cinguli anterior zieht. Eine zweite Lautgruppe, die Schnurr- und Knurrlaute (2), zeigt eine zerebrale Repräsentation, die in einigen Abschnitten sich mit derjenigen der Gackerlaute überlappt; so z.B. im hinteren Höhlengrau und seitlich angrenzenden Tegmentum oder im Mandelkern. In anderen Abschnitten dagegen setzt sie sich von der der Gackerlaute klar ab, wie etwa im vorderen Gyrus cinguli und der darüberliegenden motorischen Supplementärarea, in der Stria terminalis und im ventrolateralen Mittelhirntegmentum. Ähnliches gilt auch für die beiden anderen in Abb. 48 dargestellten Lautgruppen (3) und (4) (JÜRGENS u. PLOOG, 1970).

Die beim Rhesusaffen gefundene, bisher allerdings noch nicht in natürliche Lautgruppen differenzierte Verteilung von Vokalisationspunkten ist im wesentlichen mit der des Totenkopfaffen identisch. Bei der Katze fehlen die mesokortikalen Vokalisationsgebiete (Supplementärarea, Gyrus cinguli anterior, Gyrus rectus).

Die große Anzahl der vokalisationsauslösenden Strukturen, deren enge Beziehung zum limbischen System, die Beobachtung, daß die ausgelösten Laute oft nicht isoliert, sondern in Begleitung anderer Reaktionen auftreten, wie auch die relativ lange Latenz der Laute machen wahrscheinlich, daß bei weitem nicht in allen vokalisationsauslösenden Strukturen die Lautäußerung direkt erzeugt wird. Vielmehr liegt die Annahme nahe, daß durch die Hirnreizung oft nur eine Stimmungsänderung bewirkt wird, auf die das Tier dann sekundär mit der Lautäußerung reagiert. Um diese Hypothese zu prüfen, wurden beim Totenkopfaffen sämtliche vokalisationsauslösenden Hirnstrukturen darauf getestet, ob ihre Reizung vom Tier als unangenehm, angenehm oder neutral empfunden wird (JÜRGENS, 1976). Die Untersuchung wurde in der Weise durchgeführt, daß die Tiere in einen Käfig gebracht wurden, der aus zwei Abteilen bestand: Aufenthalt im einen Abteil führte automatisch zu Reizung eines Vokalisationspunktes; Aufenthalt im anderen war reizfrei. Der mit dem Reiz beschickte und der reizfreie Teil des Käfigs wurde in vorprogrammierten, unregelmäßigen Zeitabständen ausgetauscht. Da das Tier frei beweglich war, bestimmte es durch seinen jeweiligen Aufenthaltsort selbst, ob es den Hirnreiz erhielt oder nicht.

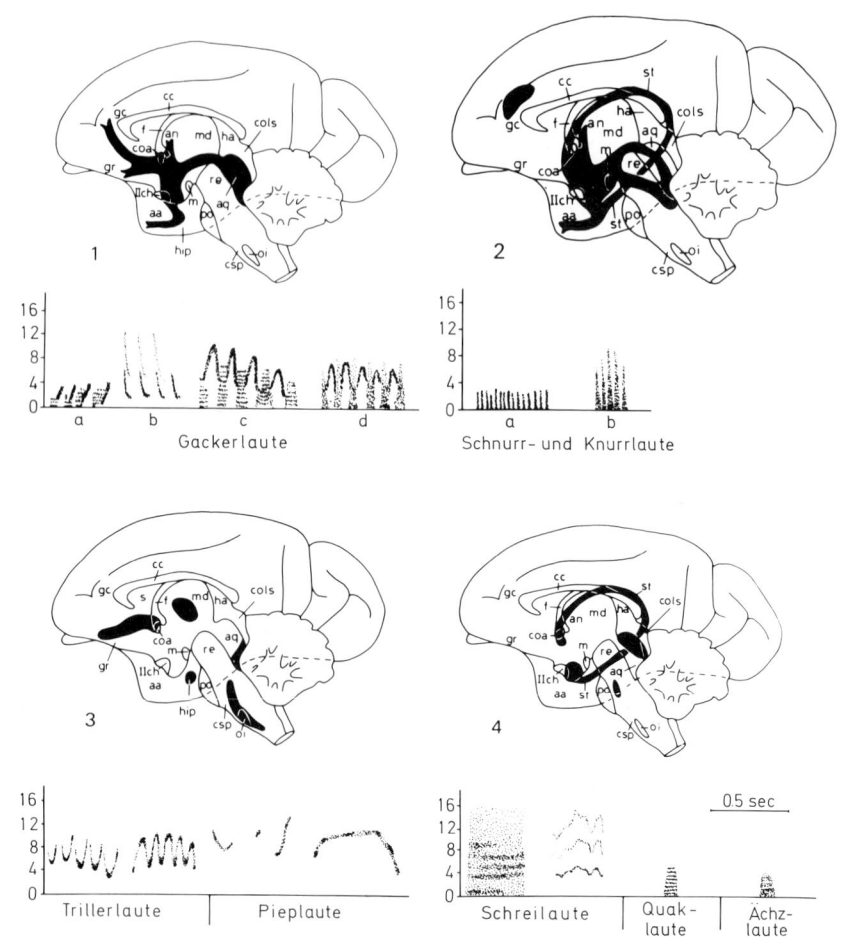

Abb. 48. Cerebrale Repräsentation der Lautgebung. Sagittaldarstellungen des Totenkopfaffengehirns mit Kennzeichnung (schwarz) der Strukturen, von denen Vokalisationen durch elektrische Hirnreize ausgelöst werden können. (1) Repräsentation der Gackerlaute, (2) der Schnurr- und Knurrlaute, (3) der Pieplaute, (4) der Schrei-Quak- und Ächzlaute mit den zugehörigen Sonagrammen dieser Lauttypen

Bei dieser Untersuchung zeigte sich, daß tatsächlich die Reizung der meisten vokalisationsauslösenden Strukturen vom Tier als unangenehm bzw. angenehm empfunden wird; neutrale Reizpunkte machen nur einen geringen Bruchteil aus. Lediglich in zwei Gebieten ist die ausgelöste Vokalisation nicht korreliert mit einer Stimmungsänderung – sei es, daß die Reizpunkte neutral sind oder daß eine gleichbleibende Vokalisation von variierenden Motivationseffekten begleitet wird: Das eine Gebiet erstreckt sich von der motorischen Supplementärarea durch den vorderen Gyrus cinguli bis in den Gyrus rectus, sowie ein Stück entlang des ventromedialen Capsula interna-Randes; das zweite Gebiet umfaßt das hintere Höhlengrau mit laterokaudal angrenzendem Ponstegmentum (Abb. 49). In diesen Gebieten läßt sich also die ausgelöste Lautäußerung mit

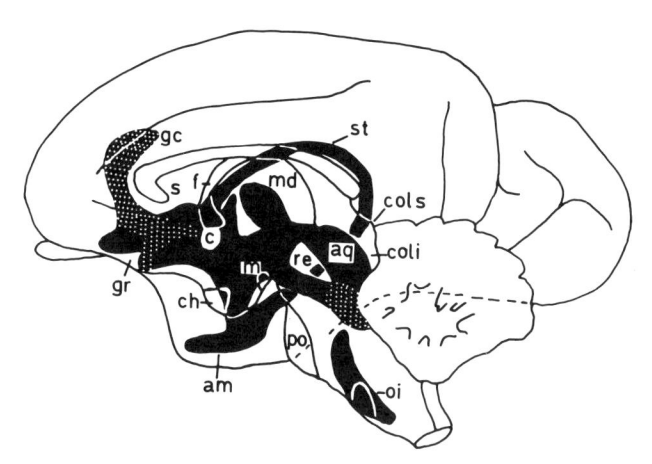

Abb. 49. Primäre und sekundäre Vokalisationsgebiete. Sagittaldarstellung sämtlicher vokalisationsauslösender Hirnstrukturen im Totenkopfaffengehirn (schwarz). Die gepunkteten Flächen geben Strukturen an, in denen der ausgelöste Laut unabhängig von etwaigen reizinduzierten angenehmen oder unangenehmen Empfindungsqualitäten ist. (Aus JÜRGENS u. PLOOG, 1976)

Sicherheit nicht auf etwaige unangenehme oder angenehme Reizqualitäten zurückführen. Die Interpretation, daß man es hier mit primären Vokalisationsgebieten zu tun hat, liegt nahe.

Noch von einer anderen Seite wurde das Problem des primären oder sekundären Charakters elektrisch ausgelöster Vokalisationen angegangen: Im präzentralen motorischen Cortex gibt es ein Areal nahe der Sylvischen Furche, dessen Reizung beim Affen Stimmlippenbewegungen, nicht aber Vokalisation hervorruft (JÜRGENS, 1974). In diesem Areal kann man sicher sein, daß die Stimmlippenbewegungen direkt und nicht motivationsbedingt ausgelöst werden. Es war deshalb von Interesse, die neuroanatomischen Verbindungen dieses Gebietes in bezug auf das vokalisationsauslösende „System" zu untersuchen – da eine direkte Verbindung zwischen kortikaler motorischer Stimmlippenarea einerseits und einem bestimmten Vokalisationsgebiet andererseits ebenfalls als ein Hinweis auf den primären Charakter des letzteren angesehen werden könnte. Bei der mit Hilfe der Autoradiographietechnik durchgeführten Studie (JÜRGENS, 1976) zeigte sich, daß die einzigen beiden Vokalisationsgebiete, zu denen die kortikale Stimmlippenarea direkt projiziert, nämlich der Cortex um den vorderen Sulcus cinguli und das Parabrachialgebiet im dorsalen Mittelhirn-Pons-Übergangsbereich, zu jenen Strukturen gehören, die auch im oben erwähnten Motivationstest als primäre Vokalisationsstrukturen wahrscheinlich gemacht werden konnten.

Das Vokalisationsgebiet in der dorsalen Mittelhirn-Pons-Übergangszone der Säuger, das sich weitgehend mit jenem der Amphibien und Reptilien homologisieren läßt, spielt demnach phylogenetisch bereits sehr früh bei der Lautproduktion eine Rolle. Diese Bedeutung behält es auch bei den Säugern bei, denn Läsionsversuche an Katzen haben gezeigt, daß Zerstörung dieser Zone, wie bei Fröschen, zur Stummheit führen kann (KELLY et al., 1946; ADAMETZ u. O'LEARY, 1959). Dieses stammesgeschichtlich alte Vokalisationsgebiet wird bei den Säugern jedoch offensichtlich durch jenes im Bereich des vorderen limbischen Cortex überlagert. Welche Rolle letzterem zukommt, läßt sich anhand von Ausschaltungsversuchen bei Rhesusaffen vermuten. SUTTON et al. (1974) trainierten Rhesusaffen, sich durch Vokalisieren Futterbelohnung zu verschaffen; dabei mußten die Laute eine bestimmte Mindestlänge und -lautstärke haben, wenn sie zur Belohnung (Apfelsaft) führen sollten. Als nach der Konsolidierung der Dressur eine bilaterale Abtragung des vorderen Gyrus cinguli vorgenommen wurde, zeigte sich, daß die Fähigkeit zum „willkürlichen" Vokalisieren weitgehend verloren war. Nicht verloren jedoch war die Fähigkeit, in stark emotionalen Situationen, z.B. auf angstauslösende Reize, normal mit entsprechenden Lautäußerungen zu reagieren. Auch waren die Tiere noch in der Lage, mit anderen als vokalen, andressierten Verhaltensweisen (z.B. Drücken eines Hebels), sich Futterbelohnung zu verschaffen.

Diese Ergebnisse legen die Annahme nahe, daß der vordere Gyrus cinguli-Bereich eine maßgebende Rolle bei der Regulierung der Bereitschaft spielt, sich stimmlich zu äußern; auf den Menschen übertragen würde dies einer Sprechantriebskontrolle entsprechen. Sieht man daraufhin die klinische Literatur durch, so scheint sich dieser Verdacht zu bestätigen. BOTEZ und BARBEAU (1971) haben in einer Übersichtsarbeit ein umfangreiches Patientenmaterial zusammengestellt, aus dem die enge Beziehung zwischen Läsionen im vorderen Gyrus cinguli und darüberliegenden motorischen Supplementärcortex einerseits und Sprechstörungen andererseits hervorgeht. Diese Sprechstörungen reichen von Fällen völliger Stummheit (meist in Form von akinetischem Mutismus) bis zu leichten Dysarthrien. RUBENS (1975), der zum gleichen Thema ebenfalls eine Reihe von Fällen gesammelt hat, fand, daß bei diesen Patienten ein deutlicher Unterschied zwischen der Fähigkeit des Spontansprechens und des Nachsprechens bestand. Während das Nachsprechen vorgesprochener Sätze oft nur geringfügig beeinträchtigt war, fehlten spontane Sprachäußerungen mitunter völlig. Das Nachsprechen klang intonationsmäßig ausdruckslos. Dieser letzte Aspekt wird auch von KONORSKI et al. (1961) betont, der den Verlust der Sprechdynamik in Richtung Monotonie und abgehacktem Sprechen als charakteristisches Symptom selbst unilateraler Läsionen des dorsomedialen Frontalcortex ansieht.

Diese Beobachtungen von sprachlichen Ausfallserscheinungen nach Läsionen im dorsomedialen Frontalcortex finden ihre sinngemäße Ergänzung in den Beobachtungen von BRICKNER (1940) und PENFIELD und WELCH (1951), die bei elektrischer Reizung des betreffenden Gebietes bei menschlichen Patienten impulsive Lautäußerungen und Wortrepetitionen hervorrufen konnten.

Die Untersuchung der Projektionen des homologen pericingulären Vokalisationsgebietes beim Totenkopfaffen ergab, daß direkte Verbindungen von hier zum dorsalen Mittelhirn-Pons-Vokalisationsgebiet existieren (MÜLLER-PREUSS u. JÜRGENS, 1976). Läsionen dieser Region können auch beim Menschen die Sprachantriebsstörung des akinetischen Mutismus auslösen. Ferner fanden sich Projektionen zu einer Reihe anderer vokalisationsauslösender Strukturen, wie dem vorderen zentralen Höhlengrau und dem rostral anschließenden periventrikulären Grau, dem Mittellinienthalamus, zentralen Mandelkern, Substantia innominata und entlang des unteren Thalamusstiels (JÜRGENS u. MÜLLER-PREUSS, 1977). Keine direkte Verbindung ließ sich zum Nucleus ambiguus, dem motori-

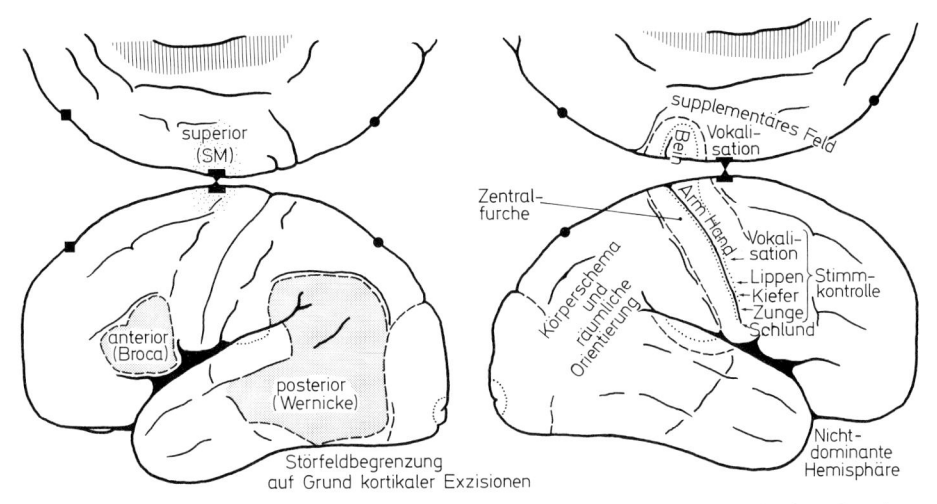

Abb. 50. Repräsentation von Vokalisation und Sprachfunktion in der Hirnrinde des Menschen. Rechts: Vokalisationen elektrisch ausgelöst unterhalb des Handbereiches der vorderen Zentralwindung *beider* Hemisphären (hier nur auf der nichtdominanten Hälfte dargestellt); supplementäre Vokalisationsfelder an den Innenkanten der Hirnhälften (hier nach oben umgeklappt). Links: Dominante Hemisphäre, vordere und hintere Sprachregion, von deren Funktion das Sprechen (BROCA) bzw. das Sprachverständnis (WERNICKE) abhängt; eine vorübergehende Störung des Sprechens entsteht auch bei Zerstörung des supplementären Feldes (S.M.) an der Innenkante der dominanten Hemisphäre. (Aus PENFIELD u. ROBERTS, 1959)

schen Hirnnervenkern für Stimmlippenbewegungen, nachweisen. Im Hinblick auf den Menschen ist von Interesse, daß sich eine massive Projektion zu dem der Broca-Area homologen Gebiet fand, sowie ein kräftiges Faserkontingent zum medialen Nucleus ventralis anterior thalami, von dem sich beim Menschen, ähnlich dem dorsomedialen Frontalcortex, ebenfalls Lautäußerungen durch elektrische Reizung auslösen lassen (HASSLER et al., 1960; SCHALTENBRAND, 1975). Wir erwähnten bereits, daß bei nicht-menschlichen Primaten im Fuß des präzentralen Cortex ein Gebiet liegt, dessen elektrische Reizung Stimmlippenbewegungen, nicht aber Lautäußerungen hervorruft. Reizt man das homologe Gebiet beim Menschen, lassen sich – im Gegensatz zum Affen – Lautäußerungen, wenn auch nicht-verbaler Art, auslösen (PENFIELD u. ROBERTS, 1959) (s. Abb. 50). Diese betreffenden Gebiete sind Teile des motorischen Gesichtscortex; sie sind umgeben von der motorischen Repräsentation anderer laryngealer, pharyngealer und oraler Muskeln. Zerstört man den motorischen Gesichtscortex beim Affen bilateral, so ist dies weder von Einfluß auf die Spontanvokalisation des Tieres, noch auf dessen „willkürliche" Vokalisation im Dressurversuch mit Futterbelohnung für jeden geäußerten Laut (SUTTON et al., 1974).

Wird der motorische Gesichtscortex jedoch beim Menschen geschädigt, so sind je nach Größe der Läsion mehr oder weniger schwerwiegende Sprechstörungen die Folge (CONRAD, 1948, 1954; BAY, 1957; BRAIN, 1961; KONORSKI et al., 1961; LURIA, 1964; HÉCAEN u. ANGELERGUES, 1964; BENSON, 1967; LECOURS u. LHERMITTE, 1976 u.a.). Diese Sprechstörungen äußern sich in Form von Artikulationsfehlern (Dysarthrie). Vermutlich sind diese als stimmliche Apraxie zu deuten. Noch ungeklärt ist, inwieweit der kaudal anschließende (postzentrale) sensorische Gesichtscortex bei der Dysarthrie beteiligt ist. Während LURIA eine postzentrale, sog. afferente motorische Aphasie (Dysarthrie durch Ausfall propriozeptiver Afferenzen) von einer präzentralen, sog. efferenten motorischen Aphasie (Schwierigkeit bei der seriellen Organisation von Phonemen) unterscheidet, differenziert HÉCAEN in bezug auf post- und präzentrale Läsionen nicht; andere Autoren (BAY; BENSON; BRAIN) scheinen dagegen mit der Dysarthrie ausschließlich präzentrale Läsionen zu verbinden. Klar zu unterscheiden ist jedoch die kortikale Gesichtsarea von der davorliegenden frontalen Broca-Area der dominanten Hemisphäre. Letztere scheint für die eigentliche Artikulation von untergeordneter oder vielleicht gar keiner Bedeutung zu sein; jedenfalls wurden schwerste Dysarthrien (Läsionen im unteren Gyrus praecentralis) bei völlig intakter Broca-Area beobachtet (LECOURS u. LHERMITTE, 1976). Dagegen sind Dysarthrien bei reinen Broca-Läsionen selten und nur zu beobachten, wenn die Herde tief ins Marklager und auf die Basalganglien übergreifen (HÉCAEN u. CONSOLI, 1973).

Aus den bisher geschilderten Befunden ergibt sich demnach für die zerebrale Organisation der Stimme folgendes Bild (Abb. 51): Die niedrigste Integrationsstufe für stimmliche Lautäußerungen scheint in der dorsalen Mittelhirn-Pons-Übergangszone (beim Säuger kaudales periaquäduktes Grau und parabrachiales Kerngebiet) zu liegen. Ihre Reizung führt bei allen daraufhin untersuchten, stimmfähigen Wirbeltieren zu artspezifischen Lautäußerungen, ihre Zerstörung zu Stummheit. Bei Transsektion des Hirnstammes unmittelbar oral von dieser Zone bleibt die Fähigkeit zu artspezifischen Lautäußerungen bei Säugern wie bei Amphibien erhalten (BAZETT u. PENFIELD, 1922; SCHMIDT, 1966). Eine direkte Verbindung sowohl vom periaquäduktalen Grau als auch den parabrachialen Kernen zum Nucleus ambiguus wurde beim Totenkopfaffen nachgewiesen (JÜRGENS, 1979). Die Aufgabe dieses ponto-mesenzephalen Gebietes besteht vermutlich in der Steuerung und Koordinierung von Stimmlippen-, Atem- und Oropharyngealbewegungen zu artspezifischen (angeborenen) Lautgestalten.

Dem Mittelhirn-Pons-Gebiet übergeordnet ist der Cortex um den vorderen Sulcus cinguli (Gyrus cinguli anterior und motorischer Supplementärcortex). Seine Reizung führt nur bei Primaten zu Vokalisation; seine Zerstörung bewirkt eine Reduktion des Sprachantriebes bzw., bei subhumanen Primaten, der willkürlich hervorgebrachten nicht streng reizgebundenen Vokalisation. Eine direkte Verbindung existiert zum ponto-mesenzephalen Vokalisationsgebiet, nicht jedoch zum Nucleus ambiguus.

Als höchste Integrationsstufe wäre dann der motorische und sensorische Gesichtscortex im Fuß der Zentralwindungen anzusetzen. Seine Reizung führt – abgesehen von wenigen zweifelhaften Fällen beim Schimpansen (LEYTON u. SHERRINGTON, 1917; HINES, 1940) – nur beim Menschen zur Vokalisation (PENFIELD u. ROBERTS, 1959). Seine Zerstörung ist beim Tier ohne Einfluß auf die Stimmgebung; beim Menschen zieht sie Sprechstörungen nach sich. Eine direkte Verbindung von der kortikalen Stimmlippenarea zum pericingulären und pontinen Vokalisationsgebiet, nicht jedoch zum Nucleus ambiguus, wurde am Totenkopfaffen nachgewiesen. Bei Schimpanse und Mensch scheint daneben eine direkte Verbindung Cortex – Nucleus ambiguus zu existieren (KUYPERS, 1958a,

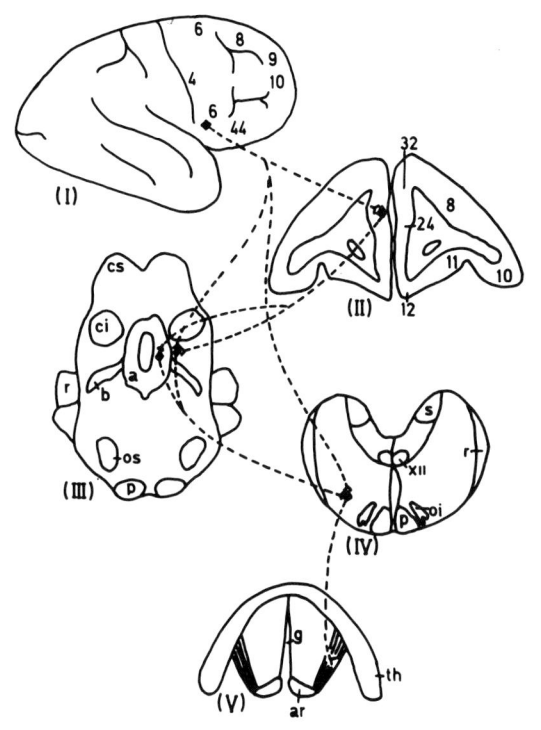

Abb. 51. Phonationsbahnen. Schema der neuronalen Verbindungen zwischen kortikaler Stimmlippenarea (I), peri-cingulärer Vokalisationsarea (II), dorsaler Mittelhirn-Pons-Übergangszone (III), Nucl. ambiguus (IV) und Kehlkopf (V) bei einem hochstehenden Primaten (Schimpanse, Mensch). Abkürzungen: a = periaquäduktes Grau; ar = Stellknorpel; b = Brachium conjunctivum; ci = Colliculus inferior; cs = Colliculus superior; g = Glottis; oi = untere Olive; os = obere Olive; p = Pyramidenbahn; r = Corpus restiforme; s = Nucl. tr. solitarii; th = Schildknorpel; XII = Nucl. n. hypoglossi; 4...44 = zytoarchitektonische Rindenfelder nach BRODMANN. (Aus JÜRGENS u. PLOOG, 1976)

b). Der perizentrale Gesichtscortex ist wahrscheinlich erst bei der willkürlichen Produktion erlernter Lautgestalten von Bedeutung.

Die drei hier beschriebenen Vokalisationsgebiete sind nicht die einzigen, die an der Stimmgebung beteiligt sind. So entwickelt sich parallel zur neokortikalen Stimmkontrolle die zerebelläre – über den Funktionskreis Cortex-Pons-Kleinhirn-Thalamus (Nucl. ventr. lat.) – Cortex (s. Abb. 35). Auch erwähnten wir bereits, daß dem medialen Nucleus ventralis anterior thalamis eine Funktion bei der Stimmgebung zuzukommen scheint. Doch glauben wir, daß es sich bei diesen Strukturen nicht um unabhängige, zusätzliche Funktionseinheiten handelt, sondern um solche, die in Abhängigkeit von den drei hier beschriebenen ihre stimmkontrollierende Bedeutung erhalten (JÜRGENS u. PLOOG, 1976).

Als neurologische Korrelate der menschlichen Sprache werden üblicherweise die Brocasche motorische und die Wernickesche sensorische Region der dominanten Hemisphäre verantwortlich gemacht. Alle Diagramme, die seit LICHTHEIM (1885) entworfen wurden, erklären die Aphasien letztlich durch Beeinträchtigung bzw. Zerstörung dieser „Zentren" selbst oder durch eine Unterbrechung zwischen ihnen. Wenn die „Diagram Makers" (HEAD, 1926) auch immer wieder wegen ihrer simplifizierenden Vorstellungen und der oft dem Schema widersprechenden klinischen Befunde kritisiert wurden, so besteht doch heute, vor allem unter dem Eindruck der Split-Brain-Experimente, allgemeine Übereinstimmung darin, daß anatomische Verknüpfungen eine wesentliche Voraussetzung für komplexe psychische Leistungen sind (PLOOG, 1973b).

Unser Diagramm (Abb. 51) kann zwar nichts zur Erklärung der hemisphärischen Spezialisierung beitragen – bezüglich der vokalisationsauslösenden Strukturen gibt es auch beim Menschen keine Dominanz einer Hirnhälfte –, doch tragen die im Diagramm zusammengefaßten Fakten zur Evolution der Stimme etwas zum Verständnis der subkortikalen Mechanismen bei, die zum ungestörten Sprechen notwendig sind. Im Gegensatz zum Lichtheimschen Horizontaldiagramm, das auf dem Konzept des Reflexbogens und der Assoziation von neuronalen Ereignissen beruht, stellt unser Diagramm eine vertikal-hierarchische Organisation dar, die im Sinne JACKSONS adäquat beschrieben werden kann, nämlich auf niederster Integrationsebene die automatische Steuerung von angeborenen Lautmustern, auf einer höheren Ebene der bedingte, d.h. nicht streng reizgebundene Einsatz der arteigenen Lautmuster und schließlich auf einer nächsthöheren Ebene die voluntative Produktion erlernter Lautfolgen. Dies gilt sowohl für die Phylogenese als auch für die Ontogenese der Lautproduktion. Elementare Charakteristika des Sprechens hängen von der Funktionsfähigkeit dieses Systems ab, z.B. der Antrieb zum Sprechen, Intonation, Timbre und Melodik der Sprache, ihre Flüssigkeit und Regelung der Lautstärke sowie wahrscheinlich auch eine Kontrolle über artikulatorische Sequenzen, die z.B. bei Müdigkeit einerseits und im Affekt andererseits Einbußen erleidet. Die Beteiligung des limbischen Systems am Sprachprozeß (RIKLAN u. LEVITA, 1969; ROBINSON, 1976) kommt auch bei schweren Formen der motorischen Aphasie heraus. Flüche und affektbesetzte Ausdrücke bleiben formelhaft als Sprachreste erhalten. Über die Beteiligung des limbischen Systems an sprachlicher Invention und Produktivität kann man im normalen und pathologischen Bereich, z.B. in bezug auf das Sprachverhalten in Psychosen, vorläufig nur Vermutungen anstellen. Insgesamt sind jedenfalls die subkortikalen Mechanismen, die zur Sprache bzw. deren Störungsmustern beitragen, bisher ungenügend erforscht (JÜRGENS u. PLOOG, 1976).

β) Lauterkennung. Seitdem WERNICKE (1874) die sensorische Aphasie beschrieb, gab es auf neuropsychologischer und neurophysiologischer Ebene Versuche, dem zerebralen Mechanismus der Lauterkennung auf die Spur zu kommen. Im Tierexperiment bediente man sich meistens einfacher akustischer Reize, um Aussagen über die auditorische Diskriminationsfähigkeit zu machen. Tiere mit einer totalen Abtragung des auditorischen Cortex können Töne verschiedener Höhe, Dauer und Intensität immer noch unterscheiden. Sie verlieren aber die Fähigkeit, kontinuierliches von unterbrochenem weißen Rauschen zu differenzieren. Je komplexer die Frequenz/Amplituden/Zeit-Charakteristiken der Testreize werden, desto schwerer ist die Diskriminationsstörung nach Läsionen des auditorischen Cortex (NEFF et al., 1975).

Erst in neuerer Zeit, unter dem Einfluß ethologischer Fragestellungen, trat die Bedeutung natürlicher Reizkonfigurationen für die Entschlüsselung auditorischer Information in den Vordergrund (PLOOG, 1971; WORDEN u. GALAMBOS, 1973). Wie bei den entsprechenden Untersuchungen im visuellen System (PÖPPEL et al., 1977) bieten sich zwei experimentelle Wege an, nämlich die Verarbeitung natürlicher Laute nach umschriebenen Hirnläsionen in kortikalen und subkortikalen Abschnitten des akustischen (auditorischen) Systems und die Antwort einzelner Nervenzellen auf arteigene artifizielle Laute. Für diese beiden Untersuchungsstrategien geben wir Beispiele. Dabei wollen wir im Auge behalten, daß es sich bei natürlichen Lauten um soziale Signale handelt. Könnte man die zentralnervöse Verarbeitung dieser Signale besser erklären, wäre man dem Verständnis der Kommunikationsprozesse (und den Störungen dieser Prozesse, mit denen wir es in der Psychopathologie zu tun haben) um ein gutes Stück näher gekommen.

Im ersten Beispiel müssen Affen lernen, arteigene von komplexen artifiziellen Lauten, die den arteigenen teils recht ähnlich sind, zu unterscheiden. Da die Affen ein und denselben Laut während einiger hundert Versuche nur 2mal zu hören bekommen, müssen sie über alle natürlichen gegenüber allen artifiziellen Lauten generalisieren. Die Aufgabe, mit der sie zeigen, ob sie die richtige Unterscheidung treffen, ist einfach: Wenn es sich um einen arteigenen Laut handelt, müssen sie von einer Stange nach unten springen und bekommen als Belohnung für eine kurze Zeit einen (stummen) Artgenossen durch eine Klappe zu sehen, während sie sonst für die Dauer der Versuche von anderen Affen isoliert sind. Wenn es sich um einen artifiziellen Laut handelt, müssen die Tiere auf der Stange sitzen bleiben.

Bei kleineren Läsionen der beiderseitigen ersten Schläfenlappenwindungen zeigt sich kein Defizit. Bei mittelgroßen bilateralen Läsionen, wo auch das temporale Operculum teilweise mitbetroffen ist, steigt die Fehlerzahl signifikant an; die Tiere treffen ihre Entscheidungen aber noch signifikant häufig richtig. Wenn die Läsionen ausgedehnt sind, so daß der auditorische Assoziationscortex vollständig fehlt und vom primären Hörcortex nur noch kleine Überbleibsel zu sehen sind (s. Abb. 52), geht das Diskriminationsvermögen für komplexe Lautmuster verloren, d.h. richtige und falsche Wahlen liegen im Zufallsbereich. Auch bei einem stark vereinfachten Test, wo die Tiere „Bellen" (s. Abb. 25) von weißem Rauschen zu unterscheiden hatten, versagten sie gänzlich, während die Tiere mit mittelgroßen Läsionen diese Aufgabe leicht meistern konnten. Demnach waren die Tiere mit den großen Läsionen keineswegs taub, denn sie sprangen beim Ertönen von Lauten herunter und blieben während der Reizintervalle auf ihrer Stange sitzen (HUPFER et al., 1977).

Wenn man hier das arteigene vokale Signal in Analogie zum Wort setzt, dann zeigen diese Ergebnisse, daß ein Analogon zur Worttaubheit durch Läsionsexperimente am Affen nicht produziert werden kann. Bei einem der sensorischen Aphasie vergleichbaren Defizit würde man erwarten, daß die Tiere bei sonst noch möglicher akustischer Diskriminationsfähigkeit speziell ihre arteigenen Laute nicht erkennen. Entweder konnten sie das aber noch, und sei es im vereinfachten Test, oder sie konnten überhaupt keine Geräusche mehr voneinander unterscheiden. Hierin gleichen die Tiere den beiden von LHERMITTE et al.

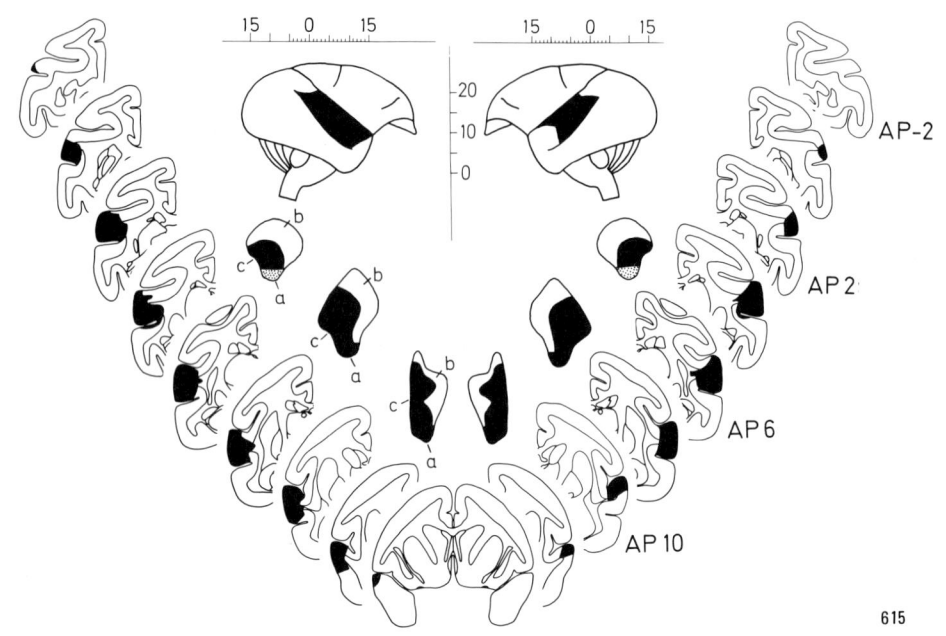

Abb. 52. Lauterkennung und Hörrinde beim Totenkopfaffen. Kortikale Läsion der Hörrinde (in schwarz) und retrograde Degeneration im Nucl. geniculatum mediale. (a) und (c) betreffen den parvozellulären, (b) betrifft den magnozellulären Anteil des Geniculatum mediale. Gepünktelte Areale bedeuten schwere, schwarze Areale totale Degeneration. (Aus HÜPFER et al., 1977)

(1971) beschriebenen Patienten mit einer sog. kortikalen Taubheit bei doppelseitiger, verifizierter ausgedehnter Läsion des Hörcortex. Diese Patienten konnten laut lesen und geschriebene Aufträge ausführen, aber sie konnten weder gesprochene Sprache verstehen noch Laute von Tieren, Musikinstrumente, Melodien oder Geräusche irgendwelcher Art identifizieren. Eine Patientin faßte ihre Störung in die Worte: „Je n'entends rien. C'est toujours le même bruit."

Beim Menschen bedarf es offenbar für das Sprachverständnis über die akustische Diskriminationsfähigkeit hinaus eines noch komplexeren Decodierungsmechanismus, der auf der Ebene der Phonem-Wahrnehmung liegt (s.S. 438f.). Während man akustische Ereignisse mit den Parametern Frequenz/Intensität/Zeitverlauf vollständig beschreiben kann, reichen diese Parameter für den phonetischen Code (LIBERMAN et al., 1967; LIBERMAN u. PISONI, 1977) nicht aus. Ob diese Ebene der Wahrnehmung akustischer Gestalten nur dem Menschen eigen ist, wissen wir nicht, weil wir so gut wie nichts über die spezifischen „Features" in einem Tierlaut wissen, die Träger des Informationsgehaltes eines Signals sind. Sicher ist nur, daß die Phoneme die arteigenen vokalen artikulatorischen Gesten des Homo sapiens sind. Um diese allen Sprachen gemeinsamen Gesten zu verstehen, bedarf es wahrscheinlich eines spezialisierten neuralen Mechanismus. Dieser kann dem von anderen Primaten ähnlich, aber nicht gleich sein.

Von der Vorstellung, daß es für arteigene Laute auch spezielle Detektoren im Hörcortex gibt, lassen sich auch die Versuche leiten, die Entladungsmuster

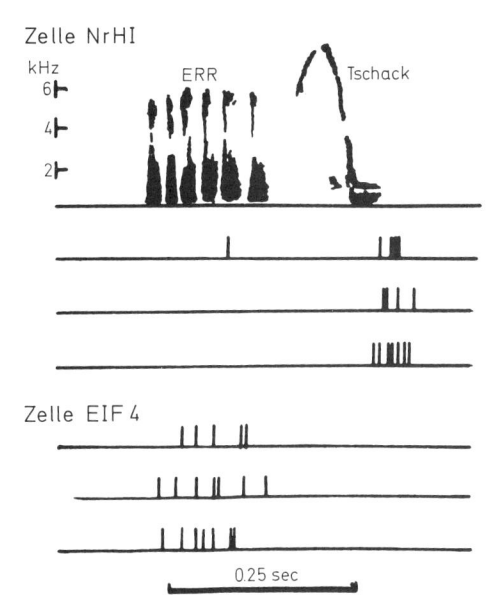

Abb. 53. Antworten einzelner Nervenzellen auf natürliche Laute. Ableitungen von Neuronen des primären Hörcortex. Oben: Das Lautspektrogramm eines zusammengesetzten natürlichen Lautes des Totenkopfaffen (Err-Tschack-Laut). Darunter: Die Antworten zweier Zellen zu jeweils einer Lautkomponente. (Aus WINTER u. FUNKENSTEIN, 1973)

einzelner Nervenzellen auf arteigene Laute zu untersuchen. Als WINTER und FUNKENSTEIN (1973) Neurone im primären Hörcortex des Affen fanden, die nur auf wenige oder gar nur auf einen arteigenen Laut, aber auf keine anderen akustischen Reize reagierten, schien die Hypothese vom „feature detector" nicht nur in der visuellen, sondern auch in der auditorischen Physiologie Bestätigung zu finden (s. Abb. 53). Inzwischen sind die Dinge sehr viel komplizierter geworden. Obwohl auch immer wieder Zellen mit sehr selektiver Ansprechbarkeit gefunden werden, wird man sicher nicht davon ausgehen können, daß die Erkennung einzelner artspezifischer Laute durch einzelne dafür spezialisierte Zellen herbeigeführt wird.

Ein hoher Prozentsatz von Zellen antwortet auf mehr als die Hälfte aller getesteten natürlichen Laute. Bestimmte Zellen zeigen auf sehr ähnliche Laute recht verschiedene Entladungsmuster. Die große Verschiedenheit der Zellantworten verschiedener Zellen auf dieselbe Vokalisation legt allein schon nahe, daß eine bestimmte Vokalisation nicht durch ein Zellentladungsmuster vercodet ist (WOLLBERG u. NEWMAN, 1972; WOLLBERG u. NEWMAN, 1973a, b; NEWMAN u. SYMMES, 1974b). Hinzu kommt, daß nicht wenige Zellen, die man für Stunden halten kann, über die Zeit hinweg variabel auf ein und dieselbe Vokalisation ansprechen, während andere Zellen in ihrer Antwort stabil bleiben (MANLEY u. MÜLLER-PREUSS, 1978). So sehr das „Feature-Konzept" auch die auditorische Physiologie stimuliert, bleibt es doch umstritten (NEWMAN, 1977). In der Aufklärung der Mechanismen für die Encodierung und Decodierung von Sinnesinformation befinden wir uns vor allem auf akustischem Gebiet ganz am Anfang.

e) Zerebral auslösbare Bewegungen mit Signalcharakter

Nicht nur Vokalisationen lassen sich durch intrazerebrale Reizung auslösen, sondern auch mimische Ausdrucksformen, Gesten, Haltungen und andere Bewegungen mit kommunikativer Funktion.

Um derartige Experimente in angemessener Weise durchführen zu können, benötigt man eine Methode, die erlaubt, Hirnreizungen an frei beweglichen Tieren im Gruppenverband durchzuführen. Die in das Hirn eingeheilten Drahtelektroden sind mit einem Transistorgerät verbunden, das so am Körper des Tieres (meist auf dem Kopf) angebracht ist, daß es nicht stört. Das Transistorgerät gibt auf einen Sendeimpuls von außerhalb des Gruppenkäfigs einen schwachen Strom frei, der genügt, um eine Verhaltensveränderung des Tieres herbeizuführen.

DELGADO (1963, 1965, 1967a, b, 1969) hat dieses technische Prinzip als erster angewandt, um vor allem aggressives Verhalten bei Rhesusaffen auszulösen und durch Kontrolle über dieses Verhalten Veränderungen in der sozialen Struktur der untersuchten Gruppe zu studieren. Ein Experiment soll erläutern, welche Möglichkeiten sich bieten, mit Hilfe der ferngesteuerten Hirnreizung die Beziehung zwischen Hirnfunktion und Hirnstruktur auf der einen Seite und das Sozialverhalten auf der anderen Seite zu untersuchen.

Die Äffin Lina wurde in drei verschieden zusammengesetzten Gruppen, wobei sie in der ersten Gruppe den niedrigsten Rang einnahm und in den beiden folgenden um jeweils eine Rangstufe aufstieg, an immer demselben Hirnort (Nucleus posterolateralis thalami) in jeder der drei Gruppen 120mal gereizt. Nach Reizende attackierte sie in der ersten Gruppe trotz Zeichen der Erregung andere Affen nur einmal und wurde selbst 15mal attackiert. In der zweiten Gruppe attackierte sie 6mal und wurde einmal angegriffen, in der dritten Gruppe attackierte sie 40mal und wurde kein einziges Mal angegriffen. Die Angriffe richteten sich überwiegend auf die Lina nachgeordneten Mitglieder der Gruppe. Außerhalb der Reizversuche waren die Beziehungen der Tiere friedlich oder mindestens frei von offenen Attacken (DELGADO, 1967b; DELGADO u. MIR, 1969).

Dieses Experiment und ähnliche Versuche zeigen, daß der Hirnreiz an geeigneter Stelle sich je nach sozialer Situation verschieden auswirkt (MAURUS et al., 1973; PRUSCHA u. MAURUS, 1976). Er bewirkt eine Veränderung der Handlungsbereitschaft. Die offenen Auseinandersetzungen werden aber durch die etablierte soziale Hierarchie bestimmt (ROBINSON et al., 1969).

Mit Hilfe der Fernauslösung von sozialen Signalen bietet sich also eine hervorragende Möglichkeit, Kommunikationsprozesse auf der Sender- und auf der Empfängerseite zu untersuchen. Auf der Senderseite sieht man nicht selten, daß Komponenten, die natürlicherweise zu einem sozial wirksamen Signal integriert sind, einzeln erscheinen und damit ihren Signalcharakter verlieren. Dies gilt z.B. für eine Komponente des genitalen Imponierens (s.S. 384): Von ausgedehnten subkortikalen Arealen kann man Erektionen auslösen (s.S. 461ff.), ohne daß diese körperliche Veränderung allein einen sichtbaren Einfluß auf das Verhalten des gereizten Tieres hat; das gleiche gilt für andere autonome Funktionen, die expressiv-emotionales Verhalten begleiten. Solche fraktionierten Anteile von natürlicherweise integriertem expressiven Verhalten rufen auf der Empfängerseite keine Verhaltensänderungen hervor. Die ferngesteuerte Hirnreizung gibt nun die Möglichkeit, die sozial wirksamen Komponenten expressiven Verhaltens zu studieren und deren Effekt auf den Empfänger in beliebig ausgewählten sozialen Situationen zu erfassen, so daß die Funktion sozialer Signale im Gruppenkontext präzise analysiert werden kann (MAURUS u. PRUSCHA, 1972, 1973; MAURUS et al., 1973, 1974, 1975).

In einer mit diesem Ziel geplanten Studie an Totenkopfaffen stellte sich z.B. heraus, daß Drohgesten niedriger Intensität nur von den Tieren beantwortet werden, die höher in der Rangordnung stehen als das drohende Tier, während sich bei den rangniedrigen Tieren keine sichtbare Reaktion auf die gleichen Drohgesten der Ranghöheren feststellen ließ. Drohgesten hoher Intensität, die offene Attacken einleiten, werden andererseits unabhängig von der Rangordnung von jedem Tier beantwortet (MAURUS u. PLOOG, 1971).

Die Modifikation des hirnphysiologischen Zustandes durch Reizung bestimmter Hirnorte bewirkt also eine Veränderung in den Hirnsystemen, die an der Signalerzeugung Anteil haben. Diese Veränderung wird gleichzeitig durch die gerade gegebene Gruppenkonstellation mitbestimmt, die das Tier wahrnimmt, während es gereizt wird. Wenn aus diesen beiden Komponenten ein Verhalten mit Informationsgehalt resultiert, wirkt dieses wieder auf die soziale Situation zurück. Auf diese Weise kann durch Manipulation des inneren Zustandes und Registrierung der resultierenden sozialen Interaktionen getestet werden, welche Hirnstrukturen an der Erzeugung der Kommunikation beteiligt sind und wie sich die zwischen Sendern und Empfängern ausgetauschten Informationen auf die einzelnen Gruppenmitglieder auswirken.

f) Zerebrale Selbstreizung

Die Entdeckung von OLDS und MILNER (1954), daß mit Hirnelektroden implantierte Ratten sich selbst reizen, wenn der Hebeldruck im Skinnerkäfig an Stelle des üblichen Futters einen elektrischen Stromimpuls auslöst, hat die Kenntnis von den neuronalen Substraten der Verstärkung („reinforcement") und der Verhaltensmotivation beträchtlich gefördert (OLDS, 1977; WAUQUIER u. ROLLS, 1976). Die Tiere (Ratten, Katzen, Hunde, Affen u.a.) streben so nach dem elektrischen Hirnreiz, als ob dieser das Triebziel, z.B. Futter oder Wasser ist oder als ob der Hirnreiz solche „Lust" erzeugt, daß das Verfolgen von Triebzielen irrelevant wird. Man hat daher das durch „intrakranielle Selbstreizung" erzeugte Verhalten mit süchtigem Verhalten verglichen (s. JUNG, 1958; PLOOG, 1964c, S. 416ff.; PLOOG, 1973b; JÜRGENS, 1978). Neben den neuronalen Substraten, die eine positive Verstärkung des Verhaltens bewirken, gibt es solche, deren Reizung eine negative Verstärkung herbeiführt. Das Tier vermeidet, den Hebel zu drücken, wenn es einmal die aversive Wirkung des Hirnreizes erfahren hat.

Den beiden antagonistisch wirkenden Systemen der positiven und negativen Verstärkung hat man verschiedene Namen gegeben, die jeweils gewisse verhaltensphysiologische Funktion kennzeichnen: Annäherungs- und Meidesystem (approach–avoidance), Belohnungs- und Bestrafungssystem (reward–punishment), System der Lust bzw. Unlust („pleasure centers") und der Verstärkung („reinforcement"). Das alte, oft kritisierte, in Philosophie und Psychologie häufig beanspruchte Lustprinzip hat durch die Selbstreizungsversuche eine hirnphysiologische Grundlage erhalten. Lust oder Befriedigung muß nicht stets sekundär durch Vermeidung von Unlust oder Entspannung eines Bedürfnisses (Triebreduktion) entstehen, sondern Lust und Unlust können auch primär durch entsprechende Hirnstrukturen aktiviert werden. Sie kommen zusammen ins Spiel und treten als Agonisten auf (PLOOG, 1964c, S. 416ff.). Die allgemeinste Formulierung, die man vom Verhalten her für diesen Antagonismus finden kann, ist auch am objektivsten feststellbar: Annäherung und Meidung – seien es Artgenossen, Sexualpartner, Futter, Wärme, Kälte oder Objekte der Erfahrung.

Die Hirnstrukturen mit positivem Reinforcement umfassen im niederen Säugergehirn das mediale Vorderhirnbündel, das olfaktorische und limbische Strukturen des Vorderhirns und Mittelhirnstrukturen verbindet, im höheren Säugergehirn das ganze limbische System mit seinen Zwischenhirn- und Mittelhirnverbindungen, Strukturen also, die emotionales Verhalten steuern (s.S. 452 und Abb. 38). Das Substrat mit negativem Verstärkungseffekt liegt mit seinen stärksten aversiven Effekten in einer schmalen Zone unterhalb und vor dem Tectum, wahrscheinlich der prätektalen Zone homolog, von der man schon bei der Kröte stärkste Fluchtreaktionen auslösen kann (EWERT, 1976). Das aversive System zieht sich periventrikulär in den medialen hinteren und vorderen Hypothalamus und in den unspezifischen Thalamus hinein. Ursprüngliche Vorstellungen, daß es sich durchwegs um topographisch-anatomisch getrennte Systeme handelt, haben sich nicht bestätigt. OLDS (1977) beschreibt eine breite intermediäre Zone im Hypothalamus, von der positive und negative Effekte auslösbar sind. Dies ist in Abb. 54 schematisch wiedergegeben. Es hatte sich nämlich herausgestellt, daß Annäherung oder Flucht u.U. von ein und derselben Elektrode mit gleichen Reizparametern auslösbar ist (VALENSTEIN, 1965), daß je nach vorausgegangener Nahrungsaufnahme vom gleichen Hirnort Fressen oder Trinken ausgelöst werden kann und daß das Angebot von Objekten im Käfig des Tieres darüber entscheidet, welches spezifische Verhalten durch den Hirnreiz induziert wird (VALENSTEIN, 1975). Seither ist die Diskussion über die Stabilität und Plastizität des „Motivationssystems" im Gange (VALENSTEIN, 1970; OLDS, 1977; WAUQUIER u. ROLLS, 1976). Für den in diesem Kapitel interessierenden Zusammenhang von Motivation und Kommunikation genügt es festzustellen, daß durch Selbstreizung bestimmter Hirnstrukturen triebhaftes Verhalten ausgelöst und spezifische Motivationen (Handlungsbereitschaften) induziert werden können. Die daran beteiligten Hirnstrukturen sind weitgehend mit denen identisch, von denen beim Affen Vokalisationen ausgelöst werden können (s. Abb. 49). Soziale Signale sind Mitteilungen und Ausdruck einer Stimmung (s.S. 383, 405, 423). Unter allen Signalen läßt sich die Entsprechung von Mitteilungen und Ausdruck der Stimmung bei den vokalen Signalen am besten erfassen. Dennoch kann das Tier dem menschlichen Beobachter nicht direkt mitteilen, wie ihm zu Mute ist. Hier bietet sich die Selbstreizung als eine Methode der Befragung an: Dem Tier wird die Gelegenheit gegeben, den vokalisationsproduzierenden elektrischen Hirnreiz durch Hebeldruck oder durch Wahl seines Aufenthaltsortes selbst an- oder auszuschalten. Auf diese Weise zeigt es an, ob es Hirnreize haben oder

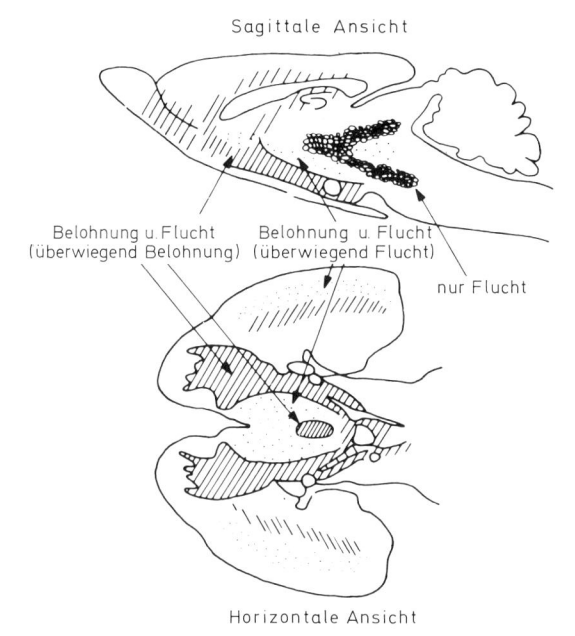

Abb. 54. Cerebrale Systeme für Verhaltensweisen der Annäherung und des Meidens. Sagittales und horizontales Schema eines Rattengehirns. In schraffierten Feldern bewirkt der elektrische Hirnreiz hauptsächlich einen Belohnungseffekt, in gepünktelten Feldern einen aversiven Effekt; in beiden Arealen kommen auch gemischte Wirkungen vor. Von der dunklen Zone konnte nur Flüchten ausgelöst werden. (Aus OLDS, 1977)

sie vermeiden will oder ob die Reize das Verhalten unbeeinflußt lassen (s.S. 473, Abb. 49). Besser als in sonstigen Selbstreizversuchen läßt sich darüber hinaus am Beispiel der Lautgebung zeigen, daß es sich bei dem Motivationssystem nicht um ein einheitliches System mit einer polaren Funktion (z.B. Annäherung/ Meidung) handelt, sondern um ein System mit Bereichen relativ selbständiger Funktionen, deren elektrische Reizung jeweils unterschiedliche Gestimmtheit hervorruft, ausgedrückt in Gackern, Schnurren, Piepen usw. (s. Abb. 48, S. 472).

Weiter ist zu bedenken, daß dieses System aufs engste mit den monaminergen Systemen verflochten oder identisch ist (WAUQUIER u. ROLLS, 1976; OLDS, 1977) und Steroid- und Peptidhormone hier vielfältig verhaltensmodifizierend einwirken (DE WIED, 1974). Dementsprechend haben sowohl die Psychopharmaka als auch süchtig machende Drogen, vor allem das Morphin (KUHAR et al., 1973; HERZ u. BLAESIG, 1974) ihre Angriffsorte innerhalb dieses Systems und wirken auf das Selbstreizungsverhalten und auf die Motivation der Tiere ein.

Daß sich diese Ergebnisse auch auf den Menschen übertragen lassen, ist durch entsprechende Untersuchungen im Rahmen neurochirurgischer Eingriffe am menschlichen Gehirn erwiesen. Die sich selbst reizenden Patienten beschreiben ganz eindeutig „positive" und „negative" lust- und unlustbetonte Gefühle, die sich mit Befriedigung, Behaglichkeit, Entspannung, Freude (mit Lächeln) auf der einen Seite und mit Angst, Ruhelosigkeit, Niedergeschlagenheit, Furcht und Schrecken auf der anderen Seite beschreiben lassen. Manche Patienten wünschten, sich selbst wiederholt reizen zu dürfen und gaben verschiedene Motive dafür an, z.B. aus Neugier, wegen des „ulkigen" Gefühls, wegen der erlebten Entspannung oder wegen des Vergnügens, das sie dabei empfanden (SEM-JACOBSEN u. TORKILDSEN, 1960; HASSLER, 1967; STEVENS et al., 1969; SEM-JACOBSEN u. STYRI, 1973). Auch wenn die Patienten nicht wissen, ob sie einen elektrischen Hirnreiz erhalten oder nicht, lassen sich differenziert beschriebene Emotionen auslösen und eindeutig dem Hirnreiz zuordnen (DELGADO, 1976). Eindrucksvoll und für den Zusammenhang von Kommunikation und Gestimmtheit von großer Bedeutung ist der oft plötzliche Stimmungsumschlag, der spontan und lebendig von den Patienten verbalisiert werden kann. Ein 11jähriger Patient DELGADOS (1976), der während der letzten 5 min vor dem unbemerkt gegebenen Hirnreiz geschwiegen hatte, rief sofort nach Reizbeginn aus: „Herr! Ihr könnt mich länger hier behalten, wenn Ihr mir das gebt, das mag ich gern!" Eine berühmt gewordene Beobachtung dieser Art stammt von FOERSTER und GAGEL (1934). Als FOERSTER anläßlich einer Tumorentfernung aus dem vorderen Hypothalamus einen leichten Druck auf benachbarte Strukturen ausübte, schlug die Stimmung des wie damals üblich nur lokal narkotisierten Patienten in Euphorie, Rededrang und witzelnde Ideenflucht um (s. HASSLER, 1967).

Diese Trias von Stimmungsänderung, Redeflußänderung und Veränderung des Gedankenablaufs ist seither unter elektrischem Hirnreiz bei wachen und voll orientierten Patienten so oft beschrieben worden, daß man den Zusammenhang als gesichert ansehen kann. HASSLER (1967) fand bei bipolaren Reizungen von medialen Anteilen der oralen Ventralkerne des Thalamus in 27,8% der Fälle ein herzhaftes, nicht unterdrückbares Lachen, während im medial benachbarten Kern häufiger ein unterdrückbares, zunächst kontralateral beginnendes Lächeln beobachtet wurde. Nach Gründen für ihre heitere Stimmung befragt, sagten Patienten z.B.: „Ich muß einfach lachen, ich habe ein lustiges Gefühl, von dem ich nicht sagen kann, wo es sitzt"; „es kommt mir immer wieder die gleiche verrückte Situation in den Sinn, deshalb muß ich lachen." Bei etwa 16% der Patienten mit stereotaktischen Operationen rief die Reizung der oralen Ventralkerne spontane Sprachäußerungen hervor: „Geh in den Keller und hole Kartoffeln." Nach längerer dauernder Reizung wurden die sprachlichen Äußerungen bis zur Unverständlichkeit beschleunigt. Dieser Rededrang war während der Reizung der oralen Ventralkerne dreimal häufiger als während der Pallidum-Reizungen. Ähnliche Lautproduktionen konnten bei Reizung des motorischen Supplementär-Cortex ausgelöst werden (s.S. 475). HASSLER (1967, S. 205) mißt diesen Befunden mit Recht erhebliche Allgemeinbedeutung zu. Es ist damit gesichert, schreibt er, daß auch komplizierte und hochintegrierte seelische Vorgänge, die sogar als rein menschliche Verhaltensweisen angesehen werden, von lokalisierten Hirnstrukturen aus in Gang gesetzt werden können. Dies wurde bis in die jüngste Zeit bestritten oder nur für den rein motorischen Mechanismus, nicht aber für die entsprechenden Gefühle zugegeben (VALENSTEIN, 1973).

Die Hirnreizversuche und ganz besonders die Selbstreiz-Versuche zeigen uns aber nicht nur die „endogen" (vom elektrischen Reiz in Gang gesetzten) entstehenden Emotionen, sondern auch die Verschränkung der Lernprozesse mit den Emotionen. Wie schon früher ausgeführt (s.S. 423ff.), sind es nicht die Emotionen, die gelernt werden können, sondern die Ereignisse, die bestimmte (der ganzen

Spezies gemeinsame) Emotionen auslösen. Genau dies belegen die Selbstreizversuche in den vielfältigsten Varianten: Unter der Bedingung des positiven Reinforcements (unter das eine große Vielfalt „positiver" Gefühle bzw. spezifischer Stimmungen zu subsumieren ist) kann nahezu jede beliebige Auslösersituation erlernt werden, die zum Erfolg, d.h. zur Belohnung durch Hirnreiz führt. Bringt zu einem bestimmten späteren Zeitpunkt die dann erworbene (erlernte) Auslösersituation nicht mehr den Erfolg – der Hirnreiz bleibt aus – wird diese Auslösersituation wieder irrelevant, d.h. sie wird verlernt oder, was das gleiche ist, sie wird ausgelöscht.

Heute, in einer Zeit, in der der Lustgewinn durch Drogen so weit verbreitet ist, bekommt die Erkenntnis, daß zwischen Säugetier und Mensch keine grundsätzlichen Unterschiede in den dem emotionalen Verhalten zugrunde liegenden Hirnprozessen bestehen, eine unmittelbare medizinische und psychologische Bedeutung. Annäherung und Meidung sind natürlicherweise mit äußeren Situationen verknüpft, an die sich das Verhalten anpaßt. Die Folgen (Konsequenzen) der Interaktionen mit der Umwelt, insbesondere der sozialen Umwelt, führen zu positiver und mit Lust verknüpfter oder zu negativer, mit Unlust verknüpfter Verstärkung derjenigen Aktionen, die die Konsequenzen herbeigeführt haben. Wird dieser natürliche Wirkungskreis durch Ausschaltung der äußeren Situation kurzgeschlossen und mit Hirnreiz oder neurotropen Drogen in das neuronale Substrat der Motivation eingegriffen, richtet sich das adaptive Verhalten nur noch auf die Quelle des Lustgewinns (auch als Quelle der Dämpfung von Unlust) und nicht mehr auf die Situationen, die natürlicherweise zu bewältigen sind, um positive Verstärkung zu bekommen oder negative in Kauf zu nehmen. Die Folge dieser Dissoziation von situationsorientierter Handlung und der damit verknüpften Emotion ist der Verlust der natürlichen (negativen) Rückkoppelung, die normalerweise ein triebbedingtes Verhalten beendet, z.B. durch Sättigungsgefühl im Verlauf der Nahrungsaufnahme, und die Bereitschaft für ein anderes Verhalten eröffnet. Süchtiges Verhalten ist durch die Außerkraftsetzung dieses höchst wichtigen homöostatischen Mechanismus gekennzeichnet (PLOOG, 1973a; PLOOG u. GOTTWALD, 1974, S. 147).

C. Sozialisationsprozesse

Alle sozial lebenden Säuger durchlaufen in ihrer Kindheit und Jugend eine Zeitspanne, in der sie sich an die Sozietät anpassen, in die sie hineingeboren werden. Dieser Prozeß besteht im wesentlichen aus Interaktionen zwischen dem Neuankömmling und den Mitgliedern der Sozietät, zuerst und insbesondere zwischen der Mutter und dem Kind. Der menschliche Säugling paßt sich durch „interaktive Rückkoppelung" innerhalb von 10 Tagen individuell an die für ihn sorgende Pflegeperson an (SANDER, 1969b, 1977a, b). Von ethologischer Seite bekam das Konzept der Sozialisation durch LORENZ (1935) einen lang anhaltenden Impuls, durch den unzählige Untersuchungen ausgelöst wurden (HESS, 1975). LORENZ beschrieb den erstmals von HEINROTH beobachteten Vorgang der Prägung von Graugänsen und mehreren Entenarten als eine Art Lernakt, bei dem die Jungen sich „auf den ersten Blick" gleich nach dem Schlüpfen ein „erworbenes Eltern-Kumpan-Schema" aneignen, wenn ihnen die rechten

Eltern fehlen. Sind solche geprägten Gänse erst einmal einem artfremden Adoptivelter – oder aber auch nur einem Objekt – gefolgt, kümmern sie sich nicht mehr um ihresgleichen und folgen ihren Artgenossen nicht nach. Ein derartiger Prägungsvorgang bezieht sich immer nur auf ein bestimmtes Verhalten, z.B. das Nachfolgen, dessen auslösende Reizsituation bestimmbar ist. Die Prägung eines bestimmten Verhaltens findet nur während einer sensiblen Periode in der Entwicklung statt; bei der Nachfolgereaktion der Entchen liegt sie z.B. in der 13. bis 16. Stunde nach dem Schlüpfen. Verstreicht diese kritische Zeit, kann das Tier nicht mehr geprägt werden. Die momenthaft erworbene Kenntnis des reaktionsauslösenden Objekts kann unter Umständen im Gegensatz zu den meisten Lernleistungen zeitlebens behalten werden.

Wenn auch die bei Vögeln gefundenen Regeln der Prägung nicht im gleichen Maße für Säuger gelten, so gibt es doch in bestimmten Abschnitten der Entwicklung sensible oder kritische Perioden, in denen prägungsähnliche, unter Umständen irreversible Lernvorgänge und prägungsartige Fixierungen stattfinden (s. EIBL-EIBESFELDT, 1978, S. 324). Besonders gut sind Hunde untersucht worden (SCOTT, 1962; SCOTT u. FULLER, 1965). Sie machen zwischen der 3. und 8. Lebenswoche eine kritische Periode der Entwicklung sozialer Beziehungen durch und knüpfen in diesem Zeitraum ein enges Band zu Artgenossen oder zum Menschen, gleichgültig, wie sie behandelt werden.

Unter den drei Hauptphänomenen, die sensible Perioden auszeichnen – optimale Lernfähigkeit, besondere Reizempfänglichkeit und Formierung der primären sozialen Bindung – kommt dem letzteren für den Sozialisationsprozeß der Primaten eine besondere Bedeutung zu. Sensible Perioden, soweit sie innerhalb der Kindheit und Jugend überhaupt für bestimmte Verhaltensbereiche abgrenzbar sind, nehmen entsprechend der langen Entwicklungs- und Reifungszeit der Primaten längere und weniger fixierte Zeiträume ein als bei allen übrigen Säugern.

Der Sozialisationsprozeß der Primaten ist durch eine Reihe biologischer Voraussetzungen mitbestimmt, die ihn, alle Faktoren zusammengenommen, von dem der übrigen gesellig lebenden Säuger abhebt. Die bei allen Primaten systematisch feststellbare Verlangsamung des postnatalen Entwicklungstempos ist vielleicht der wichtigste Faktor (H. SCHNEIDER, 1975). Mit dieser langen Wachstums- und Reifungsperiode, verbunden mit einer langen Abhängigkeit von der Mutter (oder einem Mutterersatz) steht eine verlängerte Periode des Lernens bereit, in der die Mitglieder der Gesellschaft Einfluß auf das Verhalten des Heranwachsenden nehmen. Nach Ablösung von der Mutter, einem bei allen näher studierten Primaten feststellbaren, hauptsächlich von der Mutter initiierten Prozeß, steht für erweiterte Interaktionen mit Artgenossen aller Altersklassen und Rangstufen ein mehrjähriger Zeitraum bis zum Erwachsenenalter zur Verfügung. Mit dem langsamen Reifungsprozeß hängt wahrscheinlich auch die große Flexibilität und Plastizität des Verhaltens zusammen, die eine große Anpassungsfähigkeit an ein weites Spektrum von sozialen Variablen erlauben (POIRIER, 1972; JOLLY, 1975).

1. Die Mutter-Kind-Dyade der Affen

Das Mutter-Kind-Verhalten für ungefähr 50 Genera mit mehreren Hundert lebenden Arten subhumaner Primaten gemeinsam auf wenigen Seiten abzuhandeln, bedarf einer kurzen Rechtfertigung. Tatsächlich sind die bereits viele Bände füllenden Beobachtungen „im Felde", d.h. in freier Wildbahn, nur an rund zwei Dutzend Arten gemacht worden, und für die kontrollierten Studien im Laboratorium schrumpft diese Zahl nochmals etwa um die Hälfte. Dabei nehmen die Studien an Makaken- und Pavianarten bei weitem den größten Raum ein. Uns soll es aber nicht auf die Vielfalt der Vergleiche oder eine umfassende Beschreibung des Mutter-Kind-Verhaltens, sondern auf das Gemeinsame in den Kommunikations- und Sozialisationsprozessen der Primaten ankommen. Soweit wie möglich ist dafür Sorge getragen, daß die Reduktion auf Gemeinsamkeiten sich nicht verfälschend auf den Inhalt auswirkt. Auch die Reduktion des Kommunikationsprozesses auf die Mutter-Kind-Dyade ist eine außerordentliche Vereinfachung der tatsächlichen Verhältnisse. Denn in den meisten der studierten Primatengesellschaften treten die männlichen Mitglieder recht früh in den Gesichtskreis der Kinder und tragen zu ihrer Protektion, aber auch zu ihrer Verhaltensentwicklung bei. Das gleiche gilt, wenn auch auf andere Weise, für die übrigen weiblichen Mitglieder und für die Kinder und Jugendlichen aller Altersklassen. Was für sozial lebende Säuger gilt, trifft in höchstem Maße für die Primaten zu: Es gibt kein unabhängiges Individuum, sondern nur das Mitglied als Teil von sozialen Beziehungen. Die kleinste Einheit eines solchen sozialen Systems ist die Mutter-Kind-Dyade. Das Studium dieser Beziehung zwischen zwei Individuen hat zum Ziel, Determinanten zu isolieren, die das Verhalten und die Entwicklung des Kindes bestimmen (HINDE u. WHITE, 1974; ROSENBLUM, 1971b) sowie Voraussagen über das dyadische Verhalten zu machen und damit Regeln aufzustellen zu können, die Teil eines multi-direktionalen Regelsystems sozialer Interaktionen sind (PLOOG, 1963; PLOOG et al., 1963; CARPENTER, 1973; SCOTT, 1977).

Die Ontogenese des Verhaltens von Tieren und Menschen wird üblicherweise in Stadien eingeteilt. Dabei ist man sich, besonders wenn es sich um Primaten handelt, darüber im klaren, daß sich diese Stadien teilweise überlappen können, daß sie für verschiedene Spezies sehr verschieden in ihrer zeitlichen Ausdehnung sind und größere interindividuelle Variationen aufweisen. Schließlich darf man bei der Aufteilung in Stadien nicht vergessen, daß die Entwicklung ein kontinuierlicher Prozeß ist. Einer Einteilung nach Stadien haftet aus diesen Gründen immer auch etwas Arbiträres an.

Von allen Primatenarten ist die Verhaltensentwicklung der Makaken, insbesondere der Rhesusaffen am ausgiebigsten untersucht worden (HARLOW u. HARLOW, 1965a, b; ROSENBLUM u. KAUFMAN, 1967; KAUFMAN u. ROSENBLUM, 1969; HINDE, 1971; JENSEN et al., 1973). HARLOW und HARLOW (1965a, b) haben die Mutter-Kind-Beziehungen in drei Stadien eingeteilt, das Stadium der mütterlichen Zuneigung und Beschützung (I), das der mütterlichen Ambivalenz (II) und das der Ablehnung (III).

Im I. Stadium verbringt die Mutter die meiste Zeit damit, das Baby nahe an Brust und Bauch zu halten oder es in ihren Armen oder zwischen ihren Beinen zu wiegen. Sie hält das Kind zurück, wenn es sich von ihr entfernen will. Das „Lausen" des Kindes – die soziale Hautpflege – nimmt sie über lange Strecken des Tages in Anspruch. Die meisten Affenarten wehren in dieser Zeit jeden sich annähernden Gruppengenossen oder auch den Menschen ab.

Der Versuch, am Kinde zu ziehen oder es gar wegzunehmen, führt mit ganz seltenen Ausnahmen zu heftiger Abwehr oder zum Angriff. Bei manchen Arten halten die Männchen sich in dieser ersten Zeit fern von den Babys, bei den meisten sind die erwachsenen Männchen uninteressiert. Die Weibchen, besonders die jungen, sind gleich nach der Geburt neugierig, versuchen das Kind zu beschnuppern, zu berühren und Hautpflege an ihm zu betreiben. Beim Rhesusaffen und bei anderen Arten, deren Neugeborene eine andere, meist schwarze Farbe im Unterschied zu den älteren Kindern und Erwachsenen haben, fällt auf, daß dieses erste Stadium so lange dauert, wie diese Kontrastfarbe erhalten bleibt. Während dieser Zeit findet zwischen Mutter und Kind keine mimische Kommunikation statt. Vokale Kommunikation scheint bei den meisten Arten wichtig zu sein, ist aber bisher nur selten systematisch untersucht worden (PLOOG, 1966b; PLOOG et al., 1967; WINTER et al., 1973). Obwohl Affenmütter verschiedener Arten, einschließlich Schimpansen (VAN LAWICK-GOODALL, 1967b) und Gorillas (SCHALLER, 1963) ihre toten Kinder in den ersten Tagen nach der Geburt stunden- und tagelang mit sich herumtragen können, spielt doch die Bewegung des Kindes zur Festigung des Bandes zwischen Mutter und Kind eine wichtige Rolle. Während unerfahrene Mütter ihre Kinder nicht selten während der ersten Tage wie fremde oder gar lästige Objekte behandeln, geben sie ihnen beim Krabbeln am Mutterkörper, vor allem wenn sie herabzufallen drohen, manuelle Hilfestellungen und taktile Orientierungshilfen.

Das Neugeborene bewegt sich im allgemeinen sofort oder doch innerhalb einer Minute. Es ist bei der Geburt motorisch weiter als das menschliche Baby, seine motorische Koordination und seine Reflexe sind besser entwickelt. Durch das Greifen in das Fell der Mutter hängt es fest an ihrem Bauch und beginnt nahezu unmittelbar durch seitliche und vertikale Kopfbewegungen nach den Brustwarzen zu suchen. Arten, die bald nach der Geburt auf den Rücken der Mutter krabbeln, finden ihren Weg, wenn auch zunächst mit gelegentlichen „Irrtümern", zur Brust zurück. Nach Sättigung zeigt der Affensäugling, von der Mutter unterstützt, ebenso wie der Menschensäugling eine entspannte, geöffnete Hand (Abb. 55). Beim Finden der Brust und bei der Orientierung am Körper der Mutter scheinen gewisse Merkmale wie die Lendenbeuge, die Achsel und der Hals als richtungsweisende Schlüsselreize zu fungieren. Dies wurde durch die Beobachtung von Orientierungsfehlern und deren Korrektur deutlich, vor allem aber auch durch das Verhalten eines auf einem ausgestopften Wollsokken handaufgezogenen Totenkopfäffchens (Abb. 56). Das Baby versuchte ungezählte Male die Brustwarzen auf der Unterseite des Sockens zu finden und stieß mit seiner Schnauze immer wieder in den Winkel zwischen Socken und Unterlage. Die Trennung der Nahrungsquelle (Milchflasche außerhalb des Sokkens) vom gesuchten Ort (Brustwarzen) bereitete dem Säugling die größten Schwierigkeiten und ließen ihn schwer zur Ruhe kommen (PLOOG, 1969b; HOPF, 1970; s. auch KING u. KING, 1970).

Diese Befunde passen sehr gut zu den früheren Ergebnissen von HARLOW und ZIMMERMANN (1959). Hatten die Rhesusäffchen die Wahl zwischen einer Mutterattrappe aus Draht, an der die Milchquelle angebracht war, und einer mit „haarigem" Tuch bedeckten Mutterattrappe, so verbrachten sie fast ihre ganze Zeit auf der Tuchmutter (Abb. 57). Unser Totenkopfäffchen ließ übrigens,

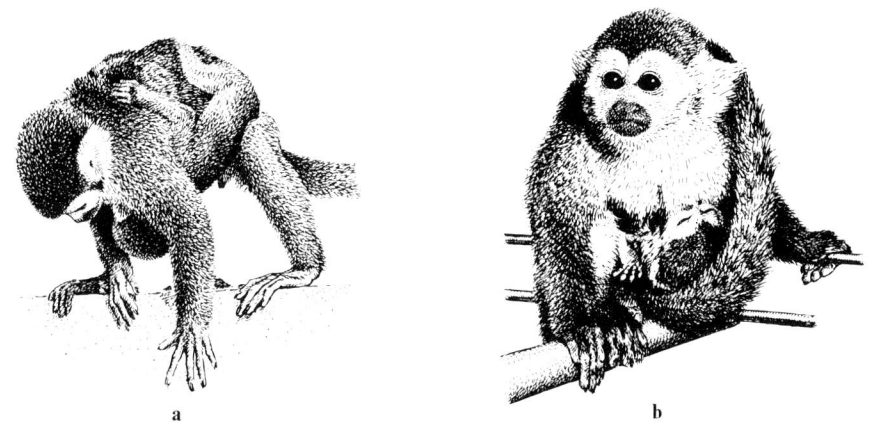

Abb. 55a u. b. Haltung des Kindes beim Trinken. Totenkopfaffe. (a) Kind 4 Wochen alt, (b) Kind 3 Wochen alt. Man beachte die nach Sättigung entspannte Hand des Säuglings. (Nach Photographien gezeichnet von HERMANN KACHER)

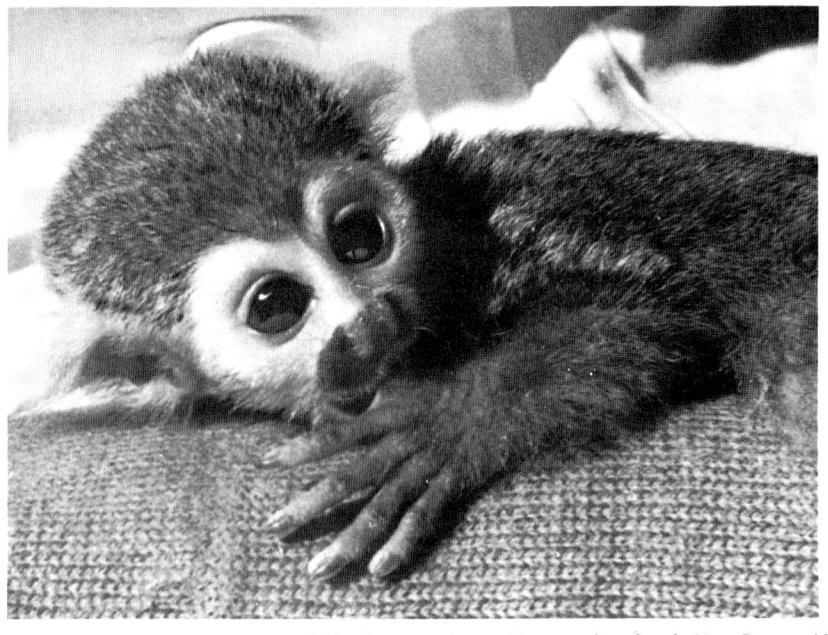

Abb. 56. Handaufgezogener Totenkopfaffe. 30 Tage alt, am Daumen lutschend. (Aus PLOOG, 1966)

wenn es den „Rücken" des Sockens erklommen hatte, gelegentlich den Ortstriller (s.S. 429) wie in der natürlichen Situation hören und steckte beim Defäzieren sein Hinterteil so heraus, daß der Socken nicht beschmutzt wurde. Auch wurde der Socken wie das Fell der Mutter in den ersten Tagen gekratzt. Nach wenigen Tagen kratzen die Babys nur noch sich selbst. Offenbar funktioniert die sensomotorische Rückmeldung noch nicht. Alle diese Befunde sprechen dafür, daß die Affenbabys eine Reihe von angeborenen Bewegungs- und kognitiven Fähigkeiten mit auf die Welt bringen, die für das Überleben wichtig sind. Denn die Affenmütter sind bald nach der nächtlichen Geburt wieder mobil und bewegen sich tagsüber mit dem Trupp ebenerdig oder in den Bäumen fort. HARLOW nennt dieses Entwicklungsstadium, das beim Rhesusaffen 10–20 Tage dauert, das Reflexstadium des Kindes, das mit der ersten Phase des Stadiums der mütterlichen Zuneigung und Protektion koinzidiert. Klammer- und Greifreflexe sind aber keine ausreichenden Kennzeichen für diese erste Entwicklungsphase. Sie sind vielmehr Teil eines höchst adaptiven Instinktverhaltens, in das innerhalb von wenigen Tagen, wie man aus den verbesserten Orientierungsleistungen und den effektiveren Bewegungen ableiten kann, Lernprozesse eingreifen. Bereits in den ersten Lebenstagen lernt der Säugling am Erfolg seiner eigenen Bewegun-

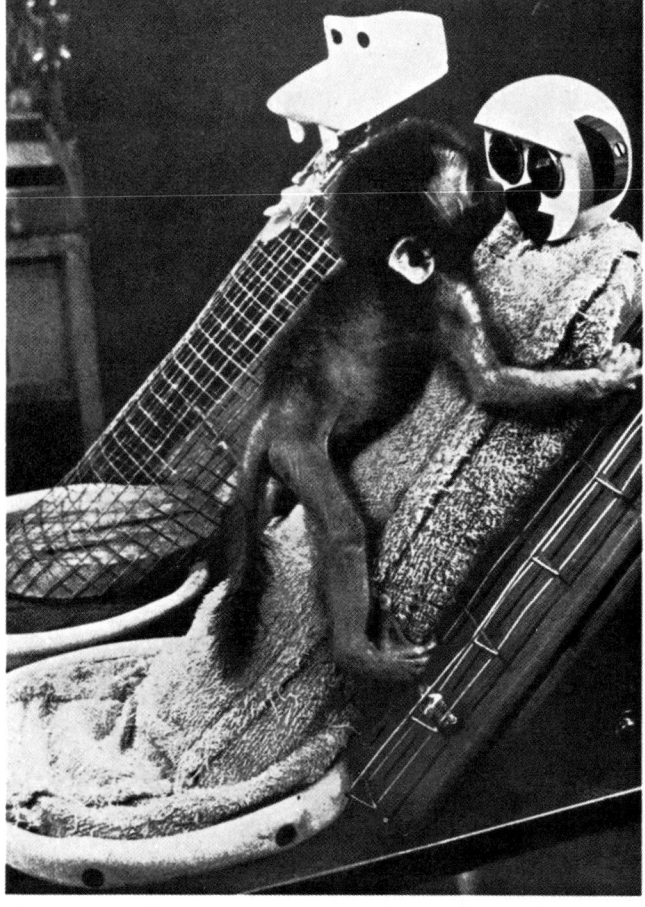

Abb. 57. Aufzucht mit Muttersurrogaten. Mit Stoff bezogene oder aus Draht gefertigte Mutterattrappen wurden verwendet um zu testen, welche dieser „Mütter" vom Rhesusäffchen bevorzugt wird. An der Drahtattrappe ist die Futterquelle (Milchflasche) angebracht. (Aus HARLOW, 1967)

gen und wird durch Nahrung belohnt. Natürlich muß man bei der rapiden Verhaltensentwicklung der ersten Wochen die Maturationsprozesse des ZNS in Rechnung stellen. Eine Abgrenzung von Lern- und Reifungsprozessen, die in ausgewählten Beispielen möglich wäre, wollen wir hier nicht vornehmen. Festzuhalten bleibt, daß der neugeborene Primat mit einem angeborenen Grundrepertoire von Verhaltensweisen und Fähigkeiten ausgestattet ist, das sich rasch und bereits in den ersten Lebenstagen erweitert.

Während des I. Stadiums der mütterlichen Zuneigung und Protektion entwickelt das Kind die starken Bande zur Mutter. Nach HARLOWs Laboratoriumsversuchen dauert diese Phase beim Rhesusaffen bis zum 60. oder 80. Lebenstag und ist für die späteren sozialen Beziehungen des Tieres entscheidend. Abgesehen vom Trinken und Schlafen verbringt das Kind die meiste Zeit auf dem Rücken oder Bauch der Mutter und krabbelt an ihrem Körper oder noch wackelig in ihrer unmittelbaren Reichweite herum. Die Mutter ist sehr besorgt um seine Sicherheit und verfolgt aufmerksam alle Aktivitäten des Kindes. In diesem Zeitraum spielt die visuelle (mimische) und vokale Kommunikation offenbar bei allen Primaten eine zunehmende Rolle. Nach MASON (1965) verhindert die dauernde mütterliche Präsenz in neuen und erschreckenden Situationen die Entwicklung von Stereotypien wie Fingerlutschen, Schaukeln und Selbstanklammern.

Im II. Stadium, der mütterlichen Ambivalenz, sind die Rollen zwischen Mutter und Kind vertauscht. Die Mutter paßt nicht mehr fortgesetzt auf das Kind auf, sondern das Kind bekommt Schutz und Hilfe, wenn es danach sucht, während die Mutter sich mehr und mehr anderen sozialen Aktivitäten zuwendet. Bei vielen Arten unterbricht die Mutter ihre Zuwendung erstmals vorübergehend, wenn sie wieder in den Östrus kommt und sexuell aktiv wird. Das Kind hat dann schon Kontakte und Unterstützung in der Gruppe, vor allem durch die sog. „Tanten" (HINDE, 1965; PLOOG et al., 1967; HOPF, 1971). Die Tante ist ein Weibchen der Gruppe, das sich von dem Neugeborenen besonders angezogen fühlt und über es wacht. Dieses Weibchen wird von der Mutter im Laufe der ersten Lebenswochen des Kindes geduldet. Nicht selten entsteht zwischen Kind, Mutter und Tante eine Bindung, die unabhängig vom Kind wird und sogar dessen Leben überdauern kann. Nach dem Östrus nimmt die Mutter ihr Kind wieder zur Brust und beschützt es, wenn es bedroht wird. Die Brustmilch ist zu diesem Zeitpunkt oft nicht mehr die Hauptnahrungsquelle für das Kind, aber das Brustnuckeln beruhigt das Kind, wenn es erregt ist – ähnlich der Wirkung des Schnullers beim menschlichen Säugling. Andererseits ist für dieses Stadium typisch, daß die Mutter aktiv mit der Entwöhnung beginnt. Sie entzieht sich dem Kinde zunehmend häufig, wenn es Brusttrinken will. Sowohl der Zeitpunkt des ersten Entwöhnungsverhaltens als auch die Mittel, die die Mutter wählt, sind arttypisch verschieden und innerhalb einer Art sehr variabel. Nicht selten drohen und schreien die Mütter ihre Kinder an und schlagen sie (SIMONDS, 1974; JOLLY, 1975).

Auf seiten des Kindes korrespondiert nach HARLOW und HARLOW (1965a) zur mütterlichen Ambivalenz das Stadium des Sicherheitsbedürfnisses. Das Kind sucht, wie gesagt, den Schutz der Mutter und benutzt sie als Zuflucht, wenn es bei seinen Explorationen der Umwelt in Bedrängnis gerät. Nach den Experimenten von HARLOW und seinen Mitarbeitern ist dieses Kind-Mutter-Verhalten nur dann gewährleistet, wenn die Mutter-Kind-Bindung während des I. Stadiums stattgefunden hat. Kinder, die mit plüschbedeckten Mutterattrappen aufgezogen waren, flüchteten bei Testuntersuchungen zur Begegnung mit neuen Objekten zur „Mutter" zurück und klammerten sich an sie, um sich nach einer Weile erneut der Exploration ihrer Umgebung zuzuwenden. Von Zeit zu Zeit kehrten sie zur „Mutter" zurück, als ob sie Rückversicherung und neuen Mut brauchten. Ganz anders die nur mit Drahtmüttern aufgezogenen Kinder. Wenn sie in neue Situationen mit unbekannten Objekten gebracht wurden, kauerten sie sich verschreckt zusammen, liefen nicht zu ihren Drahtattrappen (an denen sie ihre Nahrung erhielten) und machten keine weiteren Versuche, Objekte oder Umgebung zu explorieren. Die Kinder mit Plüschmüttern verhielten sich genauso, wenn ihre „Mütter" in der Testsituation nicht dabei waren.

Die inzwischen in größerer Zahl vorliegenden Feldstudien an verschiedenen Affen und Menschenaffen (DeVore, 1965; Kummer, 1968; van Lawick-Goodall, 1968a; Chance u. Jolly, 1970) haben diesen Grundsachverhalt bestätigt: Kinder kehren, während sie ihre Umgebung zu erkunden beginnen und mit neuen Situationen in Berührung kommen, häufig und regelmäßig zu ihren Müttern zurück. Die Nähe der Mutter wirkt angstreduzierend und bietet Sicherheit. Nur unter dieser Bedingung kann sich offenbar das Neugierverhalten entwickeln, das dem Kind die Exploration seiner physischen und sozialen Umgebung ermöglicht.

Das III. Stadium der mütterlichen Ablehnung und der Trennung von Kind und Mutter ist unter bestimmten Laboratoriumsbedingungen besonders kraß sichtbar und ereignet sich innerhalb eines kurzen Zeitraumes. In moderierter Form ist die Zurückweisung des Kindes durch die Mutter und Lockerung der engen Mutter-Kind-Beziehung aber in allen Primatensozietäten festzustellen. Die Trennung ist offenbar ein eingreifenderes Ereignis als die Entwöhnung und tritt bei einigen Arten bereits beim ersten Östrus der Mutter, meist aber erst mit der Geburt eines nachfolgenden Kindes auf. Besonders deutlich beim Rhesusaffen durchläuft die Mutter mit der neuen Geburt den vorher beschriebenen Zyklus und ist vollständig durch ihre mütterliche Zuwendung okkupiert. Das meist nur ein Jahr ältere Kind ist sozusagen über Nacht seines Schutzes, der Wärme und der Nähe der Mutter beraubt.

In der freien Wildbahn oder unter Laboratoriumsbedingungen, in denen größere Gruppen von Artgenossen zusammenleben, wird dieser Einschnitt durch die Sozietät, in der das Kind lebt, abgefangen oder tritt die besondere soziale Struktur, insbesondere beim Mantelpavian (Kummer, 1968) gar nicht in Erscheinung. Bei Schimpansen und Gorillas kann man ein Verhalten, das man mit mütterlicher Zurückweisung oder Ablehnung beschreiben könnte, nicht beobachten. Die Mutter wendet schon während der Entwöhnung keine Bestrafungsmethoden an. Auch wenn die Milch versiegt, darf das Kind weiter an der Brust nuckeln. Dennoch muß die Mutter das nachgeborene Geschwister vor den manchmal rauhen oder auch aggressiven Zugriffen des älteren Geschwisters schützen (van Lawick-Goodall, 1967a).

Auch bei weniger hoch entwickelten Affen, wie z.B. dem Totenkopfaffen, zieht sich die Zeit der schrittweisen Verselbständigung des Kindes über lange Zeit hin (Abb. 58). Nachdem das Kind zum ersten Mal vom Rücken der Mutter

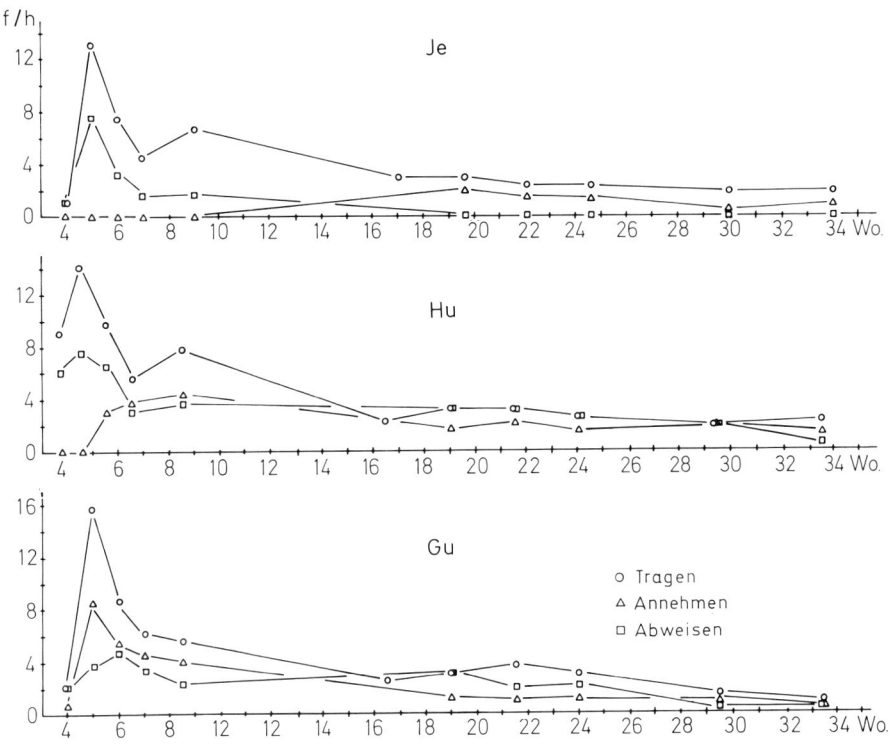

Abb. 58. Trennungsphase in der Kind-Mutter-Beziehung. Totenkopfaffe. Tragen, Annehmen und Abweisen im Verlauf von 34 Wochen bei drei Müttern mit ihren Kindern Je, Hu und Gu (drei gleichzeitige Aufzuchten in derselben Gruppe). Wo = Lebensalter des Kindes in Wochen; f/h = Häufigkeit pro Beobachtungsstunde. Typisch sind die hohen Traghäufigkeiten (= häufiger Wechsel zwischen Tragen und Alleinlaufen) um die 5. Woche und die allmähliche Abnahme aller drei Verhaltensweisen vom 3. bis 8. Lebensmonat. Beachte das individuell sehr unterschiedliche Einsetzen des Abweisens. (Aus HOPF, 1972)

gestiegen ist, läßt die Mutter es für einige Zeit kaum aus ihrer Reichweite. Später entsteht ein Wechselspiel, das den Eindruck einer ritualisierten Übung macht und oft von der Mutter begonnen wird. Mutter und Kind entfernen sich voneinander. Darauf läuft das Kind der Mutter zu. Diese weist es entweder auf verschiedene Art ab oder sie nimmt es an. Charakteristischerweise bietet sie dabei ihre niedergebeugte Schulter zum Aufsteigen an und läßt Tschack-Rufe hören. Wenn Gefahr droht, greift sie auch das schon größere Kind noch mit dem Arm auf.

Bei der Darstellung dieser frühen Sozialisationsprozesse haben wir uns auf die Mutter-Kind-Beziehung beschränkt, obwohl die Beziehungen des Kindes zu den Altersgenossen, zu den ranghöheren Männchen und später zu den Geschlechtspartnern eine wesentliche Rolle für die Sozialisation und die Organisation der jeweiligen Gesellschaft spielen. Dennoch scheint die Mutter-Kind-Beziehung in verschiedener Hinsicht die wichtigste zu sein. Obwohl nämlich bei jedem nachkommenden Geschwister eine sichtbare Ablösung des Kindes erfolgt, gibt es doch eine Reihe von Hinweisen, daß die Mutter-Kind-Beziehung Geburtenfolgen überdauert. Bei Schimpansen kann man den Zusammenhalt von Mutter und Kindern auf Lebenszeit beobachten. In einigen lang beobachteten Makaken-Gesellschaften scheinen sich Untergruppen nach der mütterlichen Abstammung zu formieren, so daß die Töchter und sogar deren Töchter und Kinder die Stamm-Mutter bis zu deren Tode als Zentrum haben (KAUFMAN, 1973; SIMONDS, 1974).

Entsprechend der sozialen Organisation von Primatengesellschaften bzw. als deren formende Kräfte unterscheiden HARLOW und seine Mitarbeiter (s. HARLOW u. HARLOW, 1965a) fünf verschiedene affektive Bindungssysteme, nämlich das System der Mutter-Kind-Bindung, der Mutter-Kind-Bindung, der Altersgenossen-Bindung, der heterosexuellen Bindung der Erwachsenen und der paternalen Bindung, womit die Bindung des dominanten Männchens an die Gruppe, seine Verteidigungsbereitschaft von Weibchen und Kindern und seine ordnenden Aufsichtsfunktionen gemeint sind. Die genannte Reihenfolge entspricht zugleich den Stadien im Reifungsprozeß des Individuums.

In den vorangegangenen Kapiteln ist von verschiedenen Seiten der Zusammenhang von Affektivität und Kommunikation beleuchtet worden. Im Mutter-Kind- bzw. Kind-Mutter-Verhältnis werden dafür und damit auch für den Sozialisationsprozeß die Grundlagen gelegt. Dies ist bisher am eindeutigsten durch die Isolations- und Deprivationsexperimente an Affenkindern bewiesen worden. Die Ergebnisse dieser Untersuchungen sind auch für den Aufbau menschlichen Sozialverhaltens und dessen Störungen von hoher Bedeutung.

2. Störungen der Sozialisation: Isolation und Deprivation bei Affen- und Menschenkindern

Seit RENÉ SPITZ 1946 über „anaclitic depression" bei Kleinkindern im Findelhaus und mit K.M. WOLF (1946) über "The smiling response; a contribution to the ontogenesis of social relations" berichtete, hat es lange gedauert, bis die Bedeutung dieser ersten empirischen, psychoanalytisch orientierten Studien an menschlichen Säuglingen und Kleinkindern in vollem Umfang erkannt wurde. 1957 und 1960 berichtete BOWLBY (1973b), teils auf den Untersuchungen seines Mitarbeiters ROBERTSON fußend, über Beobachtungen an einer großen Zahl von Kleinkindern, die von ihren Müttern getrennt worden waren. 1958 begann HARLOW, seine Versuche an von Geburt an isoliert aufgezogenen Rhesusaffenbabys zu veröffentlichen und 1962 erschien aus seinem Laboratorium der erste Bericht (SEAY et al., 1962) über Mutter-Kind-Trennungen nach einer Periode des Zusammenlebens, dem viele andere auch aus anderen Laboratorien folgten (HINDE et al., 1966; MASON, 1968; JONES u. CLARK, 1973; SUOMI et al., 1973; ERWIN et al., 1974).

Die von SPITZ beobachteten Kinder wurden in ihrem zweiten Lebenshalbjahr von ihren Müttern getrennt und reagierten mit Ängsten, Schreien und Abwendung, zeigten eine grobe Verhaltensretardierung, reagierten verzögert auf Reize, waren langsam in ihren Bewegungen, niedergeschlagen und stuporös. Sie litten an Anorexie, Gewichtsverlust und Schlaflosigkeit. Dieses Syndrom nannte SPITZ (in Anlehnung an FREUD, 1914) „anaklitische Depression". Wenn diese Reaktion auch nur bei 15% der Heimkinder in voller Ausprägung zur Beobachtung kam, so waren es gerade jene, die vor der Trennung ein besonders gutes Verhältnis zu ihren Müttern hatten. BOWLBY unterschied drei Phasen der Trennungsreaktion: 1. Die Protestphase, in der das Kind unruhig und oftmals weinend nach der Mutter sucht; 2. die Verzweiflungsphase, in der das Kind sich apathisch zurückzieht, und 3. schließlich die Phase des „Detachment", in der das Kind – wenigstens zunächst – die wieder mit ihm vereinigte Mutter ablehnt (BOWLBY, 1973a).

Die Kind-Mutter-Trennungen bei verschiedenen Makakenarten führten in ganz analoger Weise über eine Protestphase zur Verzweiflungsphase (KAUFMAN u. ROSENBLUM, 1967a). Nach lautem Schreien, Suchen, Umherrennen und allen Zeichen der Ruhelosigkeit setzt nach ein bis zwei Tagen bei den vier bis sieben Monate alten Tieren ein Zustand ein, der als „Depression" beschrieben wird. Sie sitzen in sich zusammengekrümmt, kaum Notiz von ihrer Umgebung nehmend. Dieser Zustand der Apathie entsteht auch dann, wenn die Trennung von Müttern und Kindern in einer Gruppe vorgenommen wird, so daß die miteinander aufgewachsenen Altersgenossen ohne ihre Mütter zusammenbleiben. Im Zustand der „Depression" kümmern sie sich nicht umeinander.

Ausprägung und Dauer der Verhaltensstörung hängen in voraussagbarer Weise von den näheren experimentellen Bedingungen ab. Bisher wurden folgende untersucht: die partielle Isolierung, in der das Affenbaby zwar von Geburt an andere Affen sehen und hören, sie aber nicht berühren kann; die totale Isolierung, entweder von Geburt an oder nach einer festgesetzten Periode sozialer Erfahrung; die Trennung von der Mutter bei fortbestehendem Zusammenleben mit den Altersgenossen; Trennung von den Altersgenossen; Variation des Alters, in dem die Isolierung oder Trennung vorgenommen wird; Variation der Zeitdauer der Isolierung oder Trennung und Variation der Häufigkeit der Trennung.

Die Ergebnisse mit den markantesten und theoretisch aufschlußreichsten Verhaltensstörungen sollen kurz beschrieben werden. Wenn man den Altersbeginn der Isolierung konstant hält, die Länge der Isolierung jedoch variiert, sind Art und Schwere der Störung mit der Isolationsdauer abstufbar. Affen, die von Geburt an 12 Monate isoliert waren, zeigen in der Gruppe die verschiedensten und ausgeprägtesten Abnormitäten, z.B. Selbstumklammern, Schaukeln und andere motorische Stereotypien, Kauen an den eigenen Extremitäten, Zurückgezogenheit und Kontaktunfähigkeit, aber auch schwere Störungen in der Interaktion, also beim Spiel, im sexuellen, aggressiven und submissiven Verhalten. Bei 6 Monate lang isolierten Tieren ist dieses Verhalten in qualitativ gleicher Form, aber weniger häufig zu beobachten. Während diese schwer „autistische" Störung des Sozialverhaltens bei den 6 bis 12 Monate isolierten Affen persistiert – falls keine therapeutischen Maßnahmen ergriffen werden –, gleicht sie sich bei einer nur 3monatigen Isolierung von selber aus.

Eine qualitativ andere Störung wird erzielt, wenn die Dauer der Isolierung konstant gehalten, aber das Entwicklungsalter, in dem die Isolierung einsetzt, variiert wird. Wird den Affen 6 Monate soziale Erfahrung gegeben, bevor sie für 6 Monate isoliert werden, zeigen sie später weniger die selbstbezogenen und stereotypen Verhaltensweisen, sondern sind passiv und bekunden kein Interesse an ihrer Umgebung. Die gestörte Affektlage drückt sich auch in heftigen und erregten Lautäußerungen der Tiere aus.

Die Form der sozialen Isolierung von Geburt an ist von GEWIRTZ (1961) mit dem Terminus „Privation" und die Isolierung nach einer Periode sozialer Erfahrung mit „Deprivation" gekennzeichnet worden. Aufgrund seiner Erfahrungen mit verhaltensgestörten Menschenkindern hat er auf den profunden Unterschied dieser beiden Isolationsformen hingewiesen (1969). Das einzige mir bekannte Deprivationsexperiment am Menschen stammt von PAPOUŠEK und PAPOUŠEK (1977) und zeigt, daß Störungen der Rückkoppelung des Verhaltens zwischen Mutter und Kind zu Störungen des emotionalen und kommunikativen Verhaltens des Kindes führen. Läßt die Mutter einen 4 Monate alten Säugling mehrfach für kurze Zeit allein, indem sie sich in üblicher Weise unter Blickkontakt und guten Worten in gewohntem Abschiedsritual von ihm zurückzieht, hat sie nach ihrer Rückkehr keine Schwierigkeiten, mit dem sich freundlich zuwendenden Kind den Kontakt zu erneuern. In dem Experiment entfernten sich die Mütter 6mal für nur 15 s in dieser Weise. Schalteten die Mütter, ohne das Kind vorzubereiten, für nur 3 s das Licht aus und kehrten unter sonst gleichen Bedingungen nach 15 s zum Kind zurück, reagierten die Säuglinge zunächst noch freudig bei der Rückkehr (Abb. 59a) und blieben während der Abwesenheit ruhig (Abb. 59b), lehnten dann aber zunehmend den Kontakt mit der Mutter ab (Abb. 59c, d). Bemühungen der Mütter, erneut Kontakt zu stiften, intensivierte die Abwendung der Säuglinge und führte bei einigen sogar zu verdrießlicher oder weinerlicher Ablehnung der Mütter. Die kurzen Perioden der Dunkelheit allein lösten solche Reaktionen der Kinder nicht aus, wie Kontrolluntersuchungen in weiteren Gruppen bewiesen. Es handelt sich hier um ein Separationsexperiment im kleinsten Zeitmaßstab, das Mütter und Beobachter überraschte und dessen Folgen zur Erleichterung beider rasch verschwanden. Die Untersuchungen zeigen aber, wie empfindlich der Säugling auf Unterbrechung der Rückkoppelung mit der Mutter reagiert. Die kommunikativen Verhaltensweisen in der Mutter-Kind-Dyade müssen auch für das Kind „voraussagbar" sein, wenn es die Mutter „verstehen" soll. Zerreißt dieser Zusammenhang, tritt eine affektive und damit kognitive Störung ein.

Die Isolationsexperimente mit Affenmüttern und ihren Kindern zeigten, daß die Störungen des Sozialverhaltens bis zu einem gewissen Grade – immer in Abhängigkeit von den experimentellen Bedingungen – durch eine zeitlich begrenzte Interaktion mit Gleichaltrigen kompensiert werden konnten: 20–30 min tägliches Spielen mit Altersgenossen verhinderte die unter den gegebenen Laborbedingungen meßbaren Schädigungen des Sozialverhaltens (HARLOW u. HARLOW, 1965a). Aus der Erfahrung, daß die Beziehung zu Alters- und Spielgenossen für die Entwicklung des Sozialverhaltens so wichtig sein kann wie die Mutter-Kind-Interaktion, wurde ein weiterer Typ der Trennungsexperimente entwickelt:

Trennt man „Freundschaftspaare" von 3 Monate alten Äffchen jeweils für 4 Tage, bringt sie dann für 3 Tage wieder zusammen und wiederholt diese Prozedur 20mal über eine Sechsmonatsperiode, so erhält man ein sehr überraschendes Ergebnis, nämlich einen nahezu vollständigen Stillstand der Verhaltensentwicklung (SUOMI et al., 1970; SUOMI u. HARLOW, 1972). Die Äffchen klammern sich aneinander, zeigen kein Neugierverhalten, haben kein Interesse an ihrer Umgebung und nutzen keine Gelegenheit zum Spielen. Bei jeder Trennung durchlaufen die Paare das Protest- und Verzweiflungsstadium, und jede Wieder-

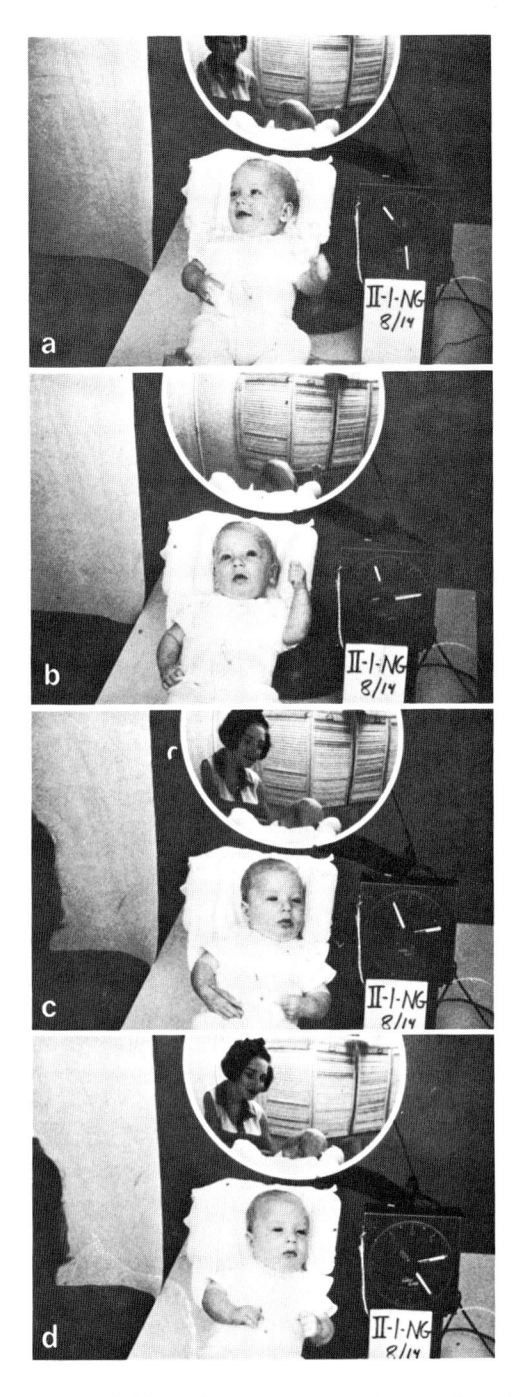

Abb. 59a–d. Störungen in der Rückkoppelung zwischen Mutter und Kind. Zuwendungs- und Abwendungsverhalten des Säuglings. (a) Nach der ersten Rückkehr der Mutter, (b) in Abwesenheit der Mutter, (c) und (d) Abwendung, nachdem sich die Mutter mehrmals entfernt hat. (Aus PAPOUŠEK u. PAPOUŠEK, 1977)

vereinigung führt zu neuer Bindung: Eine Entfremdung („Detachment"), wie sie von BOWLBY (1973a) bei Menschenkindern in den ersten 3 Lebensjahren beschrieben wird, kommt bei diesen (MCKINNEY et al., 1972) ebenso wie bei den von JENSEN und TOLMAN (1962) sowie von HINDE und Mitarbeitern (HINDE et al., 1966; HINDE u. SPENCER-BOOTH, 1971; HINDE u. MCGINNIS, 1977) angegebenen Mehrfach-Trennungsversuchen nicht vor.

Man kann aus diesen Versuchen schließen, daß der Verlust von Spielgefährten ebenso zum depressiven Syndrom führt wie der Verlust der Mutter. Die depressive Reaktion ist wahrscheinlich typisch für die Trennung früher enger sozialer Bindungen überhaupt. Neuere Versuche von EASTMAN und MASON (1975) und MASON (1979) zeigen allerdings, daß die das Sozialverhalten schädigenden Ursachen – jedenfalls in einem frühen Entwicklungsalter – letztlich basalerer Natur und nicht allein mit dem Mutter- oder Partnerverlust zu erklären sind. Allein mit beweglichen Mutterattrappen aufgezogene Rhesusäffchen, deren „Mütter" auf Aktionen des Babys mit Bewegungen reagierten und das Baby die Konsequenzen seines Handeln zu spüren bekam, zeigten kaum ein Verhaltensdefizit.

Nachdem nun von HARLOW und Mitarbeitern eine große Zahl von sozialen Variablen zur Auslösung eines depressiven Syndroms ausgetestet worden war, erfanden sie die sog. Senkrecht-Kammer und konnten damit relativ unabhängig von allen sozialen Variablen und sogar relativ unabhängig vom Lebensalter ein schweres, lang anhaltendes depressives Syndrom beim Rhesusaffen erzeugen (SUOMI u. HARLOW, 1972; HARLOW u. SUOMI, 1974). Die Senkrecht-Kammer ist ein vierkantiger Trichter aus Stahl, an dessen Boden der Affe hockt und sich kaum bewegen kann. Wird er nach 30 Tagen in durchaus noch gutem Ernährungszustand aus diesem furchtbaren Gefängnis befreit, bietet er dasselbe Bild wie nach den sozialen Trennungsexperimenten und dieser Zustand hält mindestens für 2 Monate an: der Affe bewegt sich kaum, zeigt keinerlei Interesse an seiner Umgebung, bleibt zusammengekauert und klammert sich an sich selbst an. Derartige Experimente sind nicht nur mit Affenkindern, sondern auch mit adoleszenten Affen im Alter von 3 Jahren nach vorangegangener normaler sozialer Erziehung gemacht worden – im wesentlichen immer mit dem gleichen Resultat.

Am Rande seien drei Prozeduren erwähnt, die zur Beseitigung des Syndroms ausprobiert wurden. Die erste ist eine sozio-therapeutische Methode. Die depressiven Affen wurden mit normal aufgewachsenen, möglichst jüngeren oder gleichaltrigen Tieren zusammengebracht. Unter ihrem Einfluß bildete sich das depressive Syndrom zurück (SUOMI et al., 1974, 1976). Die zweite Prozedur bestand in einer pharmakologischen Behandlung mit Chlorpromazin. Die Mehrzahl der verhaltensgestörten Tiere zeigte eine erhebliche Abnahme der pathologischen Verhaltensweisen. Die Zahl der behandelten Tiere ist allerdings klein (MCKINNEY et al., 1973). Drittens wurde über Effekte der Elektrokrampfbehandlung an Affen berichtet, die für zwei Monate in der Senkrecht-Kammer waren und ein schwer depressives Syndrom boten. Nach der Elektrokrampfbehandlung stiegen die umweltbezogenen Aktivitäten und verschiedene soziale Verhaltensweisen im Vergleich zur „Baseline" signifikant an, während die gleichen Verhaltensweisen bei den normalen, aber ebenfalls mit Elektrokrampf behandelten Kontrolltieren im Vergleich zu deren „Baseline" abnahmen (LEWIS u. MCKINNEY, 1976).

Den Schlußfolgerungen, die aus diesen Ergebnissen zu ziehen sind, muß die Bemerkung vorangeschickt werden, daß es nicht darum geht, das Affenmodell für affektive Störungen in eine kausal-genetische Parallele zum menschlichen depressiven Syndrom zu setzen, etwa in dem Sinne, wie man den Diabetes mellitus bei Affe und Mensch vergleichen kann. Es geht hier vielmehr darum, Parameter zur Auslösung affektiver Störungen experimentell zu isolieren und ihre Wirkungsweise zu erkennen (AKISAL u. MCKINNEY, 1973). Einer dieser Parameter ist offensichtlich die erzwungene Hilflosigkeit, die einen Kontrollverlust über alle wichtigen Verstärker nach sich zieht.

Nach den Experimenten von HARLOW, seinen Mitarbeitern und zahlreichen anderen Laboratorien besteht kein Zweifel, daß die Prozeduren der Isolation und der Trennung zu schweren Störungen der Affektivität führen, die sich vor allem im Sozialverhalten manifestieren. Störungen der Affektivität werden bei den Affen ganz ähnlich diagnostiziert und quantifiziert wie man das auch bei psychisch Kranken oder Abnormen tut, soweit es sich um sprachfreie Beurteilungsmethoden handelt.

Die Affenexperimente liefern zwei große Kategorien von Ergebnissen, nämlich einmal die Folgen von isolierter Aufzucht ohne vorangegangene soziale Erfahrung mit der Mutter oder mit anderen Artgenossen, zum anderen die Folgen der Trennung von Artgenossen nach mehr oder weniger langer Lebensperiode mit sozialer Erfahrung. Beide Kategorien unterscheiden sich beträchtlich voneinander (s.S. 498; DAVENPORT et al., 1973). Affen, die in die erste Kategorie gehören, zeigen eine Fülle von abnormen Verhaltensweisen, sei es im Spiel, im Sexualverhalten, im agonistischen Verhalten mit stark erhöhter Aggressions- und Angstbereitschaft, sei es in den Bewegungsweisen mit Schaukeln und vielen anderen Stereotypien. Die Affen in der zweiten Kategorie zeigen nach Ablauf der ersten Phase des Protests mit Schreien und allen Anzeichen der Erregung ein profundes Verhaltensdefizit, das sich vor allem in Passivität in allen Lebensbereichen äußert. Dies gilt auch für die Senkrecht-Kammer-Affen und auch für solche, die erstmals im 3. oder gar 5. Lebensjahr von ihren Genossen getrennt wurden, zu einer Zeit also, wo sie schon Adoleszente oder nahezu Erwachsene sind. Diese Differenzierung zwischen den beiden Kategorien ist aber keineswegs absolut. Es gibt Bereiche von Verhaltensstörungen, die beiden Kategorien gemeinsam sind, z.B. die Selbstanklammerung, die Mundmanipulationen am eigenen Körper und die mangelnde Umweltexploration. Vor allem aber gibt es auch große individuelle Unterschiede in der Ausprägung des Syndroms, speziell in der zweiten Kategorie, unter den gleichen experimentellen Bedingungen.

Dies bringt uns zurück zu einem Grundprinzip im Kommunikationsprozeß (s.S. 466f.): Disposition und Auslösesituation wirken kooperativ in der Aktualisierung eines bestimmten Verhaltens. Ein und dieselbe Auslösesituation kann je nach bestehender Disposition recht verschiedenes Verhalten in Gang setzen. Umgekehrt kann dies bei gleicher Disposition und verschiedener Auslösesituation geschehen. Schließlich können jeweilige Disposition und jeweilige Auslösesituation so zusammenwirken, daß das gleiche oder ein ähnliches Verhalten resultiert. Das Affenmodell gibt uns für alle drei Möglichkeiten zur Auslösung des depressiven Syndroms bei Affen Beispiele, wobei die Parameter, die zum aktuellen Verhalten führen, verhältnismäßig gut bestimmbar sind, ja sogar so dimensioniert werden können, daß Voraussagen über zukünftiges Verhalten möglich sind. Da die Affektivität und das Sozialverhalten des Menschen seinen nächsten Verwandten bei weitem am ähnlichsten ist, liegt die Annahme nahe, daß die Parameter, die bei der Auslösung der Affendepression entscheidend zusammenwirken, auch beim menschlichen depressiven Syndrom mit im Spiele sind. Dieses Modell schließt den unbezweifelbaren genetischen Aspekt, der für das menschliche (endogen) depressive Syndrom so wichtig ist, keineswegs aus. Ja, man kann sogar am Beispiel von zwei eng verwandten Makakenarten zeigen, daß verhältnismäßig geringe genetisch determinierte Differenzen in der Sozialstruktur und im Mutter-Kind-Verhalten zu deutlich verschiedenen Ergebnissen der Separationsversuche führen. Hutmakaken (M. radiata) hocken mehr hautnah zusammen, während Schweinsaffen (M. nemestrina) seltener Körperkontakte und eine größere individuelle Distanz zueinander haben. Während der Schwangerschaft und gleich nach der Geburt bleiben die Hutmakakenmütter eng mit der Gruppe zusammen, während Schweinsaffenmütter sich mit ihren Kindern absondern. Die Mütter beider Arten widmen den Kindern dieselbe intensive Pflege und Aufmerksamkeit, aber die Hutmakakenmutter tut dies im engen Kontakt mit anderen Gruppenmitgliedern, während die Schweinsaffenmutter sich dabei relativ isoliert hält. Dieser Artenunterschied machte sich bei Trennungsexperimenten, in denen den Kindern die Mütter fortgenommen wurden, dramatisch bemerkbar: Die Hutmakakenkinder wurden von allen Seiten bemuttert und von einer sog. Tante adoptiert, während die Schweinsaffenkinder sich selbst überlassen blieben und nicht selten davongejagt wurden. Die Schweinsaffenkinder entwickelten ein schweres depressives Syndrom wie bei den Rhesusaffen beschrieben, die Hutmakaken waren eine Weile erregt und jammerten, zeigten aber weiterhin Interesse an ihrer unbelebten und sozialen Umgebung. Ein depressives Syndrom entwickelte sich nicht (KAUFMAN u. ROSENBLUM, 1969; KAUFMAN, 1977). Kleine genetisch bedingte Unterschiede in der Verhaltensorganisation – so zeigt dieses Beispiel – können zu recht verschiedenen Reaktionen auf die gleiche Auslösesituation führen. Im Hinblick auf die außerordentliche Variabilität menschlichen bzw. menschenmütterlichen Verhaltens kann man auch im Hinblick auf neueste Ergebnisse in der Mutter-Kind-Interaktionsforschung schließen, daß die individuelle Disposition der Mutter und die individuelle Disposition des Säuglings recht verschiedene Interaktionsmuster hervorbringen und daher zu unterschiedlichen Reaktionsweisen auf Auslösesituationen, z.B. auf Trennung, führen (STERN, 1971; SCHAFFER, 1971; BLURTON JONES, 1972; FREEDMAN, 1974; HINDE, 1974; RICHARDS, 1974). BISCHOF (1975) hat – von BOWLBY (1969) ausgehend – ein Modell entwickelt, das die im ontogenetischen Prozeß der Bindung und Lösung hauptsächlich wirksamen Variablen miteinander in einem Wirkungsgefüge in Beziehung setzt.

Hier münden verhaltensbiologische Vorstellungen teilweise in psychoanalytische ein, und psychiatrisch-typologische Vorstellungen vom Primärcharakter oder von Persönlichkeitstypen schließen sich an. Die Beschreibung der Ontogenese des Verhaltens ist unter diesem Aspekt ein Weg zur Beschreibung der Persönlichkeit mit ihren individuellen Reaktionsmustern auf Auslösesituationen. Während die psychoanalytischen Theorien letztlich auf die innere Erfahrung, auf die Erlebnisse der Kinder und Erwachsenen zurückgreifen und die Lerntheoretiker den Organismus als zunächst unstrukturierten Reaktionsapparat auf Umweltreize auffassen, fußt die Verhaltensbiologie auf dem Konzept der Interaktion zwischen einem von Geburt an strukturierten, arttypischen Organismus und der Umwelt, für die er genetisch vorprogrammiert ist. Daß der menschliche Säugling mit einem kognitiven „Apparat" ausgestattet auf die Welt kommt und bereits in den ersten Lebenstagen differentiell auf Umweltreize antwortet, die er nicht gelernt haben kann, darf heute als erwiesen gelten (PIAGET, 1937/1954; BRUNER, 1968; OERTER, 1973; WOLFF, 1973). Ebenso erwiesen ist, daß der Säugling im Rahmen seiner angeborenen Ausstattung von Geburt an lernt und daß man den Lernerfolg bereits innerhalb der ersten Lebenswochen demonstrieren kann (PAPOUŠEK, 1961, 1977; SIQUELAND u. LIPSITT, 1966; PAPOUŠEK u. BERNSTEIN, 1969; MARTINIUS u. PAPOUŠEK, 1970; SAMAROFF, 1971). Das Erkennen von Regeln aus den Konsequenzen, die das eigene Handeln hervorruft, ist dabei ein entscheidender Faktor, der offenkundig Freude am eigenen Erfolg schon in den ersten Lebensmonaten hervorruft (WATSON, 1972; WATSON u. RAMEY, 1972; PAPOUŠEK u. PAPOUŠEK, 1975). Diese Voraussetzungen zur kognitiven Entwicklung sind unter Isolations- und Deprivationsbedingungen ausgeschlossen.

Weiteres zur Isolation, zur Deprivation, zu frühen Sozialisations- und Lernprozessen findet man in den Beiträgen von GROSS und KEMPE (s.S. 707) und ROBINS (s.S. 627) in Band I/1.

D. Von der Kommunikation zur Sprache

Die alte Frage nach der Herkunft der Sprache des Menschen* hat die Gemüter in jüngster Zeit erneut erregt. Von vielen Fähigkeiten, die allein dem Menschen zukommen sollten, war die Sprache die letzte Bastion, auf der die Einzigartigkeit des Menschen zu verteidigen war. Darüber sind jetzt Zweifel entstanden, nachdem bei Schimpansen Leistungen nachgewiesen worden sind, die mentalen Fähigkeiten bei Sprachprozessen gleichzukommen scheinen (s. PLOOG u. MELNECHUK, 1971).

Bei Theorien über die Wurzeln der Sprache (GEHLEN, 1940) hat von jeher einerseits die tierische Kommunikation in möglichst vielen Facetten (s. SEBEOK, 1977), andererseits die Ontogenese der menschlichen Sprache eine entscheidende Rolle gespielt (s. HARNAD et al., 1976). Erst in jüngster Zeit beginnt man zu sehen, daß die Ontogenese der Sprache längst vor dem ersten verstandenen oder gar gesprochenen Wort des Kindes beginnt und sich in einem vorsprachlichen Feld abspielt, das mit der Geburt beginnt (BRUNER, 1975; BULLOWA, 1979). In dieser „wortlosen", aber durchaus lautreichen Zeit des Lebens treffen wir auf die größten Gemeinsamkeiten, die der Mensch mit seinen nächsten Verwandten hat, aber auch schon auf die Unterschiede, die ihn vor allen anderen Primaten auszeichnen. Die Gemeinsamkeiten der soziobiologischen Ausstattung, die für

---

* Herodot, Buch 2, Kap. 2: Der Pharao Psammetich ließ 2 Kinder in völliger Abgeschiedenheit aufwachsen, um herauszufinden, welches die älteste Sprache der Welt sei. Als die Kinder das Wort „Bekos" sagten, was auf phrygisch Brot bedeutet, schloß der Pharao daraus, daß die Phryger älter als die Ägypter seien. – Eine Geschichte der biologischen Grundlagen der Sprache findet man bei OTTO MARX in LENNEBERG (1967/1972).

Kommunikationsprozesse erforderlich sind, sind für die Entwicklung der Sprache notwendige Bedingungen; die bisher erkannten Unterschiede, seien sie nur quantitativer oder auch qualitativer Art, sind allerdings keine hinreichenden Bedingungen, um das Phänomen der menschlichen Sprache erklären zu können. Die Erwartung, solches zu wollen, liefe letztlich auf die vollständige Erklärung menschlichen Verhaltens und Erkennens hinaus und ist daher Utopie. Im empirisch-pragmatischen Bereich der Wissenschaften hingegen – der menschlichen Entwicklung und ihrer Störungen –, in der Pädagogik und Sonderpädagogik, in der Psychiatrie, der Neuropsychologie und Psychotherapie, in den Konzepten der Sozialisation des Menschen und überall dort, wo es um menschliche Gesellung geht, geben empirisch gewonnene, detailliertere Einsichten in den Kommunikationsprozeß auch praktische Hilfen bei der Formulierung von realitätsbezogenen Zielen wie auch bei der Erklärung und Behandlung von Störungen der Kommunikation.

1. Das kommunikative Vermögen der Schimpansen

a) Verständigung

Alle Wissenschaftler, die sich mit Affengesellschaften befaßt haben, sind sich darüber einig, daß Affen sich untereinander verständigen. Der Gedanke, daß es sich bei dieser Verständigung um eine Sprache handelt, ist oft geäußert worden (GARNER, 1892/1900). Dennoch muß dieser Gedanke für alle bisher geschilderten Aspekte der Kommunikation verworfen werden, wenn man die einfachsten Formen der menschlichen Sprache als Definition für den Begriff Sprache benutzt. Die verschiedenen Gesichtspunkte, unter denen Kommunikationsprozesse bisher hier beschrieben worden sind, haben folgendes verdeutlicht: Die Verhaltensweisen, die auf das Verhalten Einfluß nehmen, sind allesamt Ausdrucksmittel, in denen sich ein bestimmter innerer Zustand, die Handlungsbereitschaft – auch Motivation genannt – widerspiegelt. Die Ausdrucksmittel des Senders machen Eindruck auf den Empfänger. Durch diese Wirkung haben die Ausdrucksmittel, die Signale, eine bestimmte Funktion, in der sich in Abhängigkeit vom Kontext ihres Auftretens und damit auch in Abhängigkeit der sozialen Rolle von Sender und Empfänger der spezifische Informationsgehalt des Signals ausdrückt (s.S. 393f.). Die Funktion eines Signals oder einer anderen definierbaren Verhaltenseinheit wird am besten aus der Reaktion des Informationsempfängers ersichtlich.

Die Hauptfunktion aller Verständigungsmittel besteht in der Regulierung der Beziehungen der Tiere untereinander. Die Interaktionen in der Gegenwart werden durch die Erfahrungen, die die Tiere in der Vergangenheit miteinander gehabt haben, beeinflußt. Insofern als jeder Partner einer Sozietät das Verhalten seiner Kumpane antizipieren und damit voraussagen kann, besteht eine Wirkung der Kommunikation in die unmittelbare Zukunft hinein. Kommunikation über Ereignisse in der Umgebung sind vergleichsweise selten. Sie beziehen sich auf Klassen von Objekten oder Ereignissen, die für die Gesellschaft relevant und unmittelbar gegenwärtig sind, z.B. Futter, fremde Artgenossen oder Feind in Sicht (z.B. Leopard, Schlange). Manche Informationen scheinen sich auch auf Veränderungen in der Natur, auf die Dämmerung, auf Sturm oder Regen zu beziehen.

Nach allen bisher gemachten Erfahrungen ist es aber nahezu sicher, daß bestimmte Gegenstände oder Klassen von Gegenständen nicht mit bestimmten Signalen, seien es Körperbewegungen oder Vokalisationen, bezeichnet werden, obwohl es nach zahlreichen Laboratoriumsuntersuchungen und Zirkus- und Zoodressuren klar ist, daß Affen ein außerordentlich feines Unterscheidungsvermögen für alle möglichen Formen, Farben und Konfigurationen und dazu ein vorzügliches Gedächtnis haben (KLÜVER, 1933, 1937; SCHRIER et al., 1965; STEBBINS, 1971; DAVIS, 1974). Mit anderen Worten: Affen analysieren ihre Umwelt nicht in der Form, daß sie den Dingen Zeichen zuordnen, d.h. den Dingen Namen geben.

Daß sich aber Schimpansen dennoch über gewisse, für sie anziehende oder abstoßende Objekte in ihrer Umgebung verständigen können, hat MENZEL mit 8 jungen, wildgefangenen, gut aneinander gewöhnten Tieren in einem größeren Gehege überzeugend gezeigt (MENZEL, 1975; MENZEL u. HALPERIN, 1975).

Einem der Affen wurden ein oder mehrere Plätze im Gelände gezeigt, wo Futter, Spielzeug, eine Schlange oder andere furchterregende Gegenstände versteckt wurden. Darauf wurde er in einen kleinen „Aufenthaltsraum" zu seinen Kumpanen zurückgebracht und die Tür zum Gehege einige Minuten nach der Rückkehr wieder geöffnet. Gewöhnlich ging das informierte Tier, der jeweilige „Anführer", ein paar Schritte in Richtung des Verstecks voraus und die anderen folgten ihm oder rannten auf dem Wege zum Ziel sogar einige Schritte voran. Bis zu 18 Verstecke konnten so von den Anführern mit ihrem Gefolge ausgemacht werden. Dabei wählten sie den kürzesten Weg zwischen den Zielen und nicht den, auf dem sie zu den Versteckplätzen geführt worden waren, so als hätten sie eine Lageplatzkarte im Kopf, nach der sie sich richteten.

Die Untersuchungen brachten eine Reihe von weiteren Überraschungen: Wenn dem Anführer niemand folgte, ging er zu keinem Versteckplatz, gleich, was versteckt war. Er versuchte, Kumpane mitzuzerren, lockte sie mit verschiedenen Mitteln oder gab schließlich auf, wenn er keine Gefolgschaft bekam. Aus dem Verhalten des Trupps während des Zielmarsches war klar zu erkennen, ob die Tiere Futter oder etwas anderes am Zielort erwarteten. Manchmal stoppte der Anführer, bellte und starrte auf den Ort, an dem eine Schlange versteckt war; einer aus dem Trupp ging dann mit einem Knüppel an den Versteckplatz und schlug darauf los. War die Schlange vorher unbemerkt entfernt worden, kletterten die Tiere auf einen Baum und verhielten sich so, als ob sie nach der außer Sicht geratenen Schlange suchten. Wenn Futter versteckt worden war, suchten sie aufgeregt und ohne Vorsicht mit den Händen danach. Wenn zwei Schimpansen als Anführer informiert wurden, hatte derjenige die größere Gefolgschaft, der das bessere Ziel hatte (mehr Futter, neueres Spielzeug)! Wenn man den Anführer nicht mitgehen ließ, jammerte er und seine Kumpane versuchten, seine Käfigtür zu öffnen, anstatt den Versteckplatz zu suchen. Nach MENZELS Beobachtungen sind die Zeichen des Anführers, nach denen sich der Trupp richtet, recht variabel und wirken zusammen: Marschrichtung, Hinzeigen, Hinsehen, Hinsehen von mehreren Standorten aus sind wohl die wichtigsten. Lautäußerungen werden außer dem Bellen, das durchaus den Bodenfeind anzeigen kann, nicht erwähnt und scheinen nicht besonders untersucht worden zu sein. Vorherrschend sind jedenfalls die visuell wahrnehmbaren Zeichen, soweit der

Beobachter sie überhaupt entdecken kann (s.S. 482f.). MENZEL spricht von der „Sprache der Augen". Die auf das Ziel hinweisenden Zeichen sind unabhängig vom emotionalen Zustand. Die dramatischsten und am menschenähnlichsten aussehenden Zeichen machten die kindlichsten und am wenigsten erfolgreichen Anführer. Wie JANE VAN LAWICK-GOODALL (1975) fand auch MENZEL, daß ältere Tiere Anzeichen ihrer Emotionen unterdrücken können und damit den anderen, besonders fremden oder ranghöheren Mitteilungen vorenthalten, ja, sie sogar irreleiten können, um dann auf Umwegen an das Futter zu gehen.

Die Versuche grenzen den Bereich und den Modus der Information ab, der über relevante Objekte in der Umwelt gegeben werden kann. Sie zeigen aber gleichzeitig die starke Gruppenbindung, von der die Handlungen mitbestimmt werden, so daß die Tiere in der freien Wildbahn vor Vereinzelung geschützt sind.

b) Werkzeuggebrauch und Selbsterkennung

Die Schimpansenversuche von KÖHLER (1921, 1925) sind in alle Lehrbücher eingegangen. Die Benützung von Objekten als Werkzeug ist dabei besonders herausgehoben worden. KLÜVER (1933, 1937) hat einem Cebusaffen über 200 Probleme aufgegeben, in denen das Tier die Objekte erst zurichten oder mehrere Objekte nacheinander benützen, Hindernisse beseitigen oder beide Hände gebrauchen mußte, um Futter zu erreichen. Die Arbeit am Problem, bei der der Affe sogar eine Ratte benutzte, um sein Ziel zu erreichen, dauerte von Sekunden bis fast zu einer Stunde. Dabei wechselte die Stimmung des Tieres von langer, besonnener Musterung der Situation bis zu wilden Affektausbrüchen. DÖHL (1966, 1968) hat in ausgeklügelten Versuchen mit Schimpansen deren Manipulierfähigkeit mit sequentiell zu Problemlösungen eingesetzten Werkzeugen bewiesen (Öffner verschiedener Art für Serien von geschlossenen Behältern u.ä.). Junge Orang-Utans setzen ebenfalls Werkzeuge für komplizierte Manipulationen ein, ohne übrigens für ihre Tätigkeit mit Futter, Spielzeug oder dergleichen unbedingt belohnt zu werden (RENSCH u. DÜCKER, 1966; DÖHL u. PODOLCZAK, 1973). JANE GOODALL (1965) hat vor einigen Jahren auch in freier Wildbahn beobachtet, daß Schimpansen Objekte zum Nahrungserwerb einsetzen und z.B. mit Stöcken nach Termiten angeln.

Ein anderes Vorrecht, das dem Menschen vorbehalten zu sein schien, war die Fähigkeit, sich selbst als Zeichen seiner Reflexionsfähigkeit im Spiegel zu erkennen. Inzwischen wurde der Beweis erbracht, daß Schimpansen ebenfalls dazu in der Lage sind (GALLUP, 1970, 1975). Auch die Schimpansin Washoe, von der sogleich die Rede sein wird, zeigt vor dem Spiegel auf sich selbst und meint sich selbst.

c) Namengeben

In den letzten Jahrzehnten ist immer wieder versucht worden, Schimpansen beizubringen, sich durch erlernte Laute ein geringes Vokabular zum Bezeichnen von Objekten anzueignen. Das ist niemandem geglückt. Von den im Hause aufgezogenen Menschenaffen hat es auch nach jahrelangem Training keiner so weit gebracht, daß man wirklich von solcher Fähigkeit sprechen kann (KEL-

LOGG u. KELLOGG, 1933/1967; LADYGINA-KOHTS, 1935; HAYES, 1951; KELLOGG, 1968). In letzter Zeit sind aber zwei ganz verschieden angelegte Versuche gelungen, die Anthropologen, Psychologen und Linguisten neue Fragen über die menschliche Sprache aufgegeben (BROWN, 1970) und die Welt in Erstaunen versetzt haben.

ALLEN und BEATRICE GARDNER (1969, 1971) wählten bei ihren Kommunikationsversuchen mit der Schimpansin Washoe bewußt eine Gestensprache, da frühere Erfahrungen gezeigt hatten, daß der Schimpanse, wie wohl alle Affen, unfähig ist, Laute nachzuahmen und seine Vokalisationen in erlernte Klangmuster umzuformen, die von seinen natürlichen nennenswert abweichen. Andererseits ist der Schimpanse reich an Gesten und neigt zur Imitation gesehener Bewegungen. Das Psychologenehepaar GARDNER wählte die Amerikanische Zeichensprache (ASL), die von vielen taubstummen Menschen mit allerlei Variationen benutzt wird. Man kann die verwendeten Zeichen als eine Art von Bildersprache ansehen, in der manches Zeichen eine „ikonische" Abbildung des Objekts ist – z.B. das Berühren beider Nasenlöcher mit den zusammengefügten Fingerspitzen einer Hand für den Gegenstand Blumen – und in der andere Zeichen nach willkürlicher Übereinkunft Gegenstände, Tätigkeiten oder Eigenschaften repräsentieren. Washoe war im Juni 1966, als die Experimente begannen, in einem auf 8–14 Monate geschätzten Alter. Ihr gewöhnlicher Tagesablauf wurde dem einem Menschenkind ensprechenden Alter weitgehend angepaßt. Nach 16monatigem Bemühen, längst nachdem ein hohes Maß an Anhänglichkeit gegenüber ihren Trainern offenkundig war, gelang es, eine gewisse Kontrolle über die Nachahmung von Zeichen zu erreichen. Nach 22 Trainingsmonaten wurden 34 Zeichen fest beherrscht (Tabelle 4). Im Mai 1970 wurde mir bei einem Besuch an Ort und Stelle berichtet, daß das Zeichenvokabular inzwischen auf weit über 100 angewachsen ist und schließlich 132 Zeichen betrug.

Washoe benutzt ihre Zeichen spontan im Umgang mit mehreren in der Zeichensprache unterrichteten Trainern und handelt sinngemäß auf deren Zeichen. Aus einer Serie von 64 Bildern benennt sie 56 korrekt, obwohl sie solche formalen „Sitzungen" nicht liebt. Sie kann auch einem Beobachter, der das vom Experimentator von einem anderen Raum aus projizierte Bild nicht sehen kann, durch entsprechende Zeichen mitteilen, was sie sieht. Man beachte in Tabelle 4, daß Washoe die Zeichen für „du", „ich-mich" auch als Antwort auf Fragen benutzt, daß sie das „Hundzeichen" auch macht, wenn sie den Hund nur bellen hört, und daß sie Zeichen in eigener Erfindung kombinieren kann (nicht in der Tabelle): „öffnen Essen-Trinken" (für Kühlschrank öffnen), „gehen süß" (Aufforderung, zu den Himbeeren getragen zu werden) oder „hören Essen" (auf das Hören des Klingelzeichens zum Essen). Sie hat auch eigene Zeichen, z.B. für ihr Lätzchen erfunden.

Washoe wurde 1970 in ein Primaten-Institut mit einer Schimpansenkolonie zu weiteren Studien gebracht. Dort wurde ihr u.a. das Zeichen für „Affe" beigebracht, das sie in einer Sitzung lernte und auf 2 Siamangs und einige Totenkopfaffen auf Befragen (in ASL) richtig anwendete. Vor Beginn der Sitzung hatte sie einen heftigen Drohkampf mit zwei Makaken in einem Käfig hinter sich. Auf Befragen, was diese Makaken seien, signalisierte sie das Zeichen für Dreck mit nachfolgendem Zeichen für Affe („Dirty" „Monkey"). „Dirty"

Tabelle 4. Ausgewählte Zeichen, die der weibliche Schimpanse Washoe nach 22 Monaten Training verläßlich benutzt. (Nach GARDNER u. GARDNER, 1969)

Zeichen	Beschreibung	Kontext
Süß (sweet)	Zeige- oder Zeige- und Mittelfinger berühren die wackelnde Zungenspitze	Für Nachtisch, spontan am Ende der Mahlzeit. Auch für Bonbons
Offen – öffnen (open)	Handflächen nebeneinander nach unten, dann Handflächen nach oben rotiert	Öffnen von Türen (Haus, Zimmer, Auto, Kühlschrank, Wandbord), Gefäßen, Wasserhähnen
Geh/Gehen (go)	Gegenbewegung zu „Komm – gib"	Während an der Hand oder auf der Schulter, gewöhnlich die gewünschte Richtung anzeigend
Essen (food – eat)	Mehrere Finger einer Hand werden in den Mund gesteckt	Während der Mahlzeit und bei deren Vorbereitung
Trinken (drink)	Der von der Faust abgespreizte Daumen berührt den Mund	Für Wasser, Medizin, Limonade usw. Bei Limonade oft mit „süß" kombiniert
Hund (dog)	Wiederholtes Schlagen auf den Schenkel	Für Hunde und für Bellen
Du (you)	Zeigefinger zeigt auf die Brust der Person	Wenn ein anderer beim Spielen drankommen soll. Auch als Antwort auf die Zeichen „Wer kitzeln?", „Wer bürsten?"
Ich/mich (I – me)	Zeigefinger deutet auf oder berührt die eigene Brust	Zeigt an, daß Washoe dran ist, wenn sie sich etwas (Essen, Trinken usw.) mit jemandem teilt

benutzte sie bis dahin für Exkremente und beschmutzte Sachen. Von da an benutzte sie das Dreck-Zeichen auch mitunter im Zusammenhang mit dem Namens-Zeichen ihres Trainers („Dirty" „Roger"), wenn er nicht tat, was sie wollte (FOUTS, 1973a).

Inzwischen haben weitere Schimpansen, ein Orang-Utan und ein Gorilla in anderen Laboratorien ein ASL-Repertoire erworben. Die individuellen Unterschiede im Zeichenerwerbstempo sind groß und betrugen bei 4 jungen Schimpansen für jedes der ersten 10 Zeichen zwischen 54 und 159 min (FOUTS, 1973b).

Ein wichtiger Punkt in der anhaltenden Auseinandersetzung über „Affensprache" und Menschensprache (PLOOG u. MELNECHUK, 1971; NOTTEBOHM, 1975; HARNAD et al., 1976; LIMBER, 1977) ist die Frage nach dem Spontangebrauch der ASL zur Kommunikation der Tiere untereinander. Washoe benutzt ihre ASL-Zeichen häufig gegenüber anderen Schimpansen, die aber entweder keine ASL können oder deren Zeichenschatz noch zu klein ist. Immerhin wurde intraspezifische ASL-Kommunikation beim gemeinsamen Fressen, z.B. beim Futterabgeben beobachtet, einem seltenen Akt, der aber auch unter natürlichen Bedingungen auf natürliche Gesten des Nahrungsverlangens beobachtet wurde (VAN LAWICK-GOODALL, 1975). Kitzeln-spielen ist in der Mensch-Schimpansen-Kommunikation sehr beliebt. Die beiden Schimpansen Booee und Bruno (zu der Zeit jeder mit 38 Zeichen) wurden bei einem Dialog beobachtet: Booee signalisierte zu Bruno „Kitzeln Booee". Bruno, der gerade Rosinen aus der Hand des Beobachters fraß, signalisierte zurück: „Booee, Booee mich Futter" und lehnte damit Booees Aufforderung ab (FOUTS, 1975).

Selbst das Verständnis für gesprochene Sprache scheint beim Schimpansen besser zu sein als bisher angenommen: Ally konnte auf das gesprochene Kommando, z.B. „bring mir den Löffel", aus verschiedenen Gegenständen den richtigen, z.B. den Löffel, auswählen. Dann wurde Ally das den gesprochenen Worten zugehörige ASL-Zeichen von einem Untersucher beigebracht, während ein anderer, der nicht wußte, was Ally gelehrt worden war, mit ASL „Was (ist) das" die Gegenstände, ohne deren Namen zu nennen, abfragte. Ally lernte, alle Zeichen zu übertragen. Er lernte mit anderen Worten eine gehörte Gegenstandsbezeichnung mit einem dafür stehenden sichtbaren Symbol, dem ASL-Zeichen, zu verbinden, wie der Mensch beim Erlernen einer Sprache die Vokabel Sombrero für das Wort Hut lernt und damit denselben Gegenstand meint (FOUTS et al., 1976).

Das Ehepaar GARDNER ist inzwischen dazu übergegangen, neugeborene Schimpansen von ihrem ersten oder zweiten Lebenstag an mit ASL aufzuziehen. Die Pflegepersonen sind perfekt in ASL, sind entweder selbst taub oder haben die Zeichensprache früh von ihren tauben Eltern gelernt. Die Schimpansenkinder Moja und Pili begannen ihre ersten Zeichen zu machen, als sie ungefähr 3 Monate alt waren; die ersten vier Zeichen wurden innerhalb weniger Tage erworben: Mit 6 Monaten waren es 15 bzw. 13 Zeichen. Während dieses Alter verglichen mit dem ersten Auftreten von gesprochenen Worten des Kindes früh zu sein scheint, wurde von Eltern tauber Kinder, die mit ASL aufwuchsen, berichtet, daß die ersten Zeichen mit 5 bis 6 Monaten zu beobachten sind.

d) Semantik, Syntax und Konzept

Es ist die Frage, ob die Grenzen zur menschlichen Sprache in weiteren Bereichen verschoben werden können. Dies ist PREMACK (1970, 1971) mit seinen Experimenten gelungen. Seine Schimpansin Sarah war vermutlich etwa 5 Jahre alt, als sie „lesen" und „schreiben" zu lernen begann. Auch sie hat wie Washoe und alle anderen erwähnten Schimpansen gezeigt, daß ein großer Grad von Vertrautheit und Anhänglichkeit vorhanden sein muß, wenn die „Schulaufgaben" mit ihren Lehrern – es waren im Laufe der Zeit 5 Trainer – überhaupt zustandekommen sollen. Sarah lebte seit längerer Zeit einzeln in einem Käfig und hatte täglich ihre Lernstunden. Sie erlernte das generelle Konzept, „X" ist der Name für „Y" beherrschen. Y ist eins von vielen Objekten, Tätigkeiten, Eigenschaften, Pronomen und X ist ein Stück Plastik von beliebiger Form und Farbe. Jedes bestimmte Stück X bedeutet ein bestimmtes Y. Die Plastikstücke, „Worte" genannt, sind auf der Unterfläche magnetisiert und können auf diese Weise an eine Metalltafel geheftet werden. Sarah „schreibt" und „liest" in senkrechten Kolumnen. Nach „Wort"-Kombinationen aus zwei Plastikstückchen hat sie zunehmend längere Kombinationen beherrschen gelernt, in denen die Reihenfolge der „Worte" die Bedeutung des „Satzes" bestimmt. Der erste komplizierte „Satz", den sie an die Tafel „schreiben" konnte, war von folgendem Typ: „Mary geben Apfel Sarah." Das heißt, Mary (oder ein anderer, ebenfalls anwesender Trainer), gib den Apfel (oder eine andere Frucht) Sarah. Es stellte sich bald heraus, daß des Trainers Zuwendung und Belobigung mit Gesten, Berührungen und Lauten wichtiger für den Erfolg war als die Belohnung mit

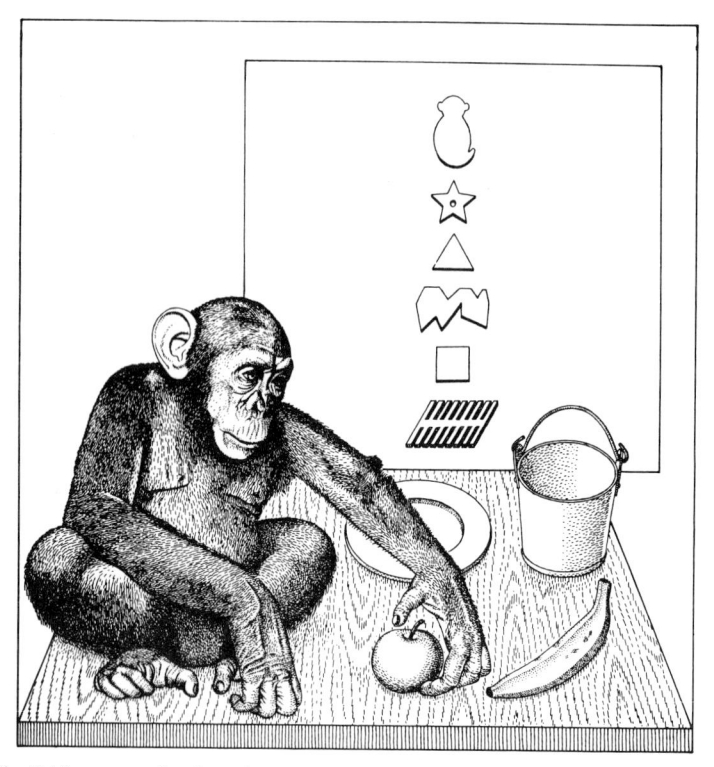

Abb. 60. Ein Schimpanse „liest" und „schreibt". Nachdem Sarah die Nachricht, „Sarah legen Apfel Eimer Banane Teller" aus den von oben nach unten geordneten, an der Wandtafel stehenden Symbolen für die oben angeführten Gegenstände entziffert hat, führt sie die Anweisung korrekt aus. (Aus PREMACK, 1972)

Futter. Der schwierige Aufforderungssatz, in dem sie etwas fortgeben muß, anstatt es zu bekommen, „Sarah geben Apfel Mary", konnte zunächst besser gemeistert werden, wenn sie anstelle des Apfels etwas Begehrteres zurückbekam.

Inzwischen beherrscht Sarah weitaus kompliziertere Zusammenhänge. Aufgaben vom Typ des Satzes „Sarah legen Apfel Eimer Banane Teller" (Sarah, lege den Apfel in den Eimer, die Banane auf den Teller) werden richtig gelöst (Abb. 60). Auch die Verneinung wird richtig verstanden: Sarah, lege Fruchtstückchen in den Eimer, nicht auf den Teller. Sowohl beim „Lesen" als auch beim „Schreiben" hält sie sich an die ihr in einzelnen Schritten beigebrachte Syntax und macht schließlich kaum noch Fehler bei der Wortfolge im Satzgefüge. Dabei hatte sie schließlich, ähnlich wie Washoe, ca. 130 „Worte" zur Verfügung Sie hat das Konzept von Einzahl und Mehrzahl begriffen und wendet die Symbole für „eins", „keins", „mehrere" und „alle" richtig an. Mit vier Farbkarten, denen sie bestimmte farblose Plastik-„Worte" zuordnen kann, lernt sie die Präpositionen Rot „auf" Grün, Rot „unter" Grün, Blau „neben" Gelb usw. Der Trainer legt Rot auf Grün, Rot neben Grün usw. Sarah „schreibt" das Gesehene mit entsprechenden „Worten" an die Tafel. Schließlich stört auch die Farbe des Plastikstückes die Farbbezeichnung nicht mehr, so daß selbst ein grünes Plastikstück, wenn es die richtige Form für „Rot" hat, zur Bezeichnung für Rot eingesetzt werden kann. Nachdem das Plastiksymbol für „Fragezeichen" beherrscht wird, kann sie Fragen nach dem Muster „A?A" mit „Ja" und „A?B" mit „Nein" beantworten. Dabei macht es keinen Unterschied, ob A und B Gegenstände oder Symbole (Plastikstücke) sind. Schließlich beherrscht sie das Konzept der Gleichheit und Verschiedenheit, so daß sie nach dem vorigen Muster („A gleich A"; „A nicht gleich B") mit den Worten „gleich" und „nein gleich" antwortet. Die außerordentlich schwierige Frage nach dem „Wort" als der mentalen Repräsentation des Gegenstandes hat PREMACK (1971) in ein Experiment gekleidet, das auf eine Eigenschaftsanalyse des Gegenstandes und seines Repräsentanten abzielt.

Abb. 61 zeigt in den beiden Spalten links unter A und B paarweise geordnete Eigenschaften, die auf den wahren Apfel oder das „Wort" für Apfel (blaues Dreieck) zutreffen oder nicht zutreffen. Die Paare von Eigenschaften sind ein roter (R) und ein grüner (G) Fleck; ein Kreis und ein Rechteck; ein Rechteck mit Stiel und ohne Stiel; ein Rechteck mit Stiel und ein Kreis. In der ersten Versuchsserie löst Sarah die Zuordnungsaufgaben richtig angesichts des wahren Objekts, in einer späteren Serie angesichts des Objektsrepräsentanten; das ist das „Wort" für Apfel.

Die hier ohne Schilderung der systematischen Methodik sehr gedrängt dargestellten Leistungen sind unerhört und mögen unglaublich klingen. Tatsächlich erhoben sich – ganz abgesehen von der Kritik der Linguisten und Psycholinguisten an PREMACKS Begriffen von Sprache – Zweifel an der Echtheit der von Sarah demonstrierten Intelligenzleistungen, die sämtlich von ungewollten und unbemerkbaren Fingerzeigen der Trainer abhängen könnten (s. PLOOG u. MELNECHUK, 1971). Diese Erklärung für scheinbar hohe Intelligenzleistungen von Tieren ist durch das rechnende Pferd, den „klugen Hans", berühmt geworden

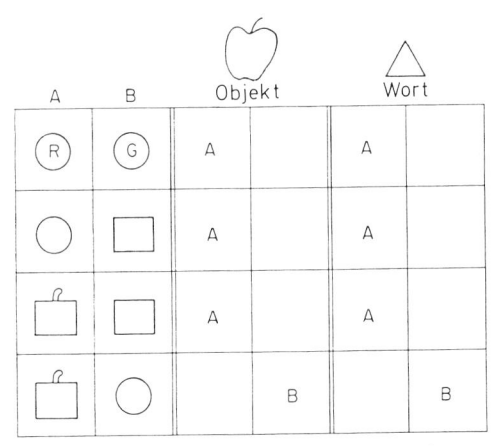

	A	B	Objekt	Wort
1	(R)	(G)	A	A
2	○	□	A	A
3	⌐□	□	A	A
4	⌐□	○	B	B

Abb. 61. Eigenschaftsanalyse eines Gegenstandes und eines diesen Gegenstand repräsentierenden Symbols durch einen weiblichen Schimpansen. Die Ergebnisse zur Gegenstandsanalyse und zur Symbolanalyse wurden in getrennten Versuchsreihen gewonnen. (R) und (G) sind ein roter und ein grüner Fleck; der Apfel ist rot, das Dreieck ist blau. (Aus PREMACK, 1976a)

(s. SOMMER, 1925), das fast unmerkliche Zeichen durch die sich bewegende Hutkrempe seines Dresseurs bekam. PREMACK konnte diesen Einwand, ähnlich wie bei Washoe geschehen, durch Blindversuche mit einem unerfahrenen Trainer und durch die statistische Analyse der Lernprozesse eindeutig widerlegen (A.J. PREMACK, 1976; PREMACK, 1976a). Das Kluge-Hans-Phänomen ist keine Erklärung für Sarahs „Sprache".

Während PREMACK drei weitere, wesentlich jüngere Schimpansen mit im Prinzip gleichem Erfolg trainierte, wurde auf seinen Methoden aufbauend am Yerkes-Primatenzentrum in Atlanta eine Maschinen-Sprache, genannt Yerkish, entworfen, der eine einfache Syntax zugrunde liegt, nach der die 75–125 möglichen Worte, genannt Lexigramme, geordnet werden müssen (GLASERSFELD u. PISANI, 1970). Lana, eine 3jährige Schimpansin, lernt auch hier „lesen" und „schreiben", indem sie über aufleuchtende Lexigramme, den Plastikstücken von Sarah vergleichbar, Instruktionen erhält und durch leichten Druck auf computergesteuerte Tasten ihre Antworten oder Wünsche „schreiben" kann. Auf den Tasten sind dieselben Symbole wie auf den Leuchtschirmen zu sehen. Sie wechseln jedoch ihren Ort, so daß Lana sich einen Satz, z.B. „Bitte Maschine gib Milch, Banane, Bonbon usw." oder „Bitte Maschine mache Musik, Dias, Kino, Fenster-auf usw." immer wieder neu zusammensuchen und in die syntaktisch richtige Reihenfolge bringen muß. Lana kann auf dieselbe Weise auch ihren Trainer aus dem Nebenzimmer rufen: „Bitte Tim kitzeln Lana" oder der Trainer kann sie über den Leuchtschirm auffordern: „Bitte Lana kitzeln Tim." Beide können auf eine Aufforderung „Ja" oder „Nein" signalisieren. Auf diese Weise kommt es zu kleinen Dialogen (RUMBAUGH et al., 1973, 1975). In ihren täglichen Sitzungen lernt Lana mehr und mehr Namen, kann vom Computer begonnene Sätze beenden und gelegentlich selbst neue Sätze erfinden. Sie überraschte eines Tages damit, daß sie auch nach dem Namen eines Gegenstandes fragt, dessen Namen sie nicht wußte. „Bitte Tim geben Lana Name von." Sie benutzte den ihr auf die Frage bekannt gemachten Namen (Lexigramm für eine Pappschachtel) sofort und fragte 15 min darauf nach dem ihr noch nicht bekannten Lexigramm für Tasse. Pappschachtel und Tasse enthielten ihre begehrten Bonbons (RUMBAUGH u. GILL, 1976). Wo und wie die Grenzen zwischen menschlicher Sprache und der Kommunikation dieser Schimpansen zu ziehen ist, wird für lange Zeit in der Debatte bleiben. Es besteht kein Zweifel, daß auch angesichts dieser Ergebnisse profunde Unterschiede vorhanden sind (BROWN, 1970, 1973; LENNEBERG, 1969, 1971; RUMBAUGH, 1975). Ungeachtet dessen wird es wieder um einen Schritt schwieriger, einfache Trennungslinien zu ziehen. Die alte Frage, was Sprache ist und wie sie entstanden ist (HERDER, 1772; W. v. HUMBOLDT, 1820/1915; GEHLEN, 1940; CHOMSKY, 1965; HOCKETT, 1963), wird neu überdacht werden müssen.

Offenbar verfügt der Schimpanse über mentale Konzepte, von denen er nach bisheriger Erfahrung in der Kommunikation mit seinesgleichen keinerlei Gebrauch macht. Unter phylogenetischen Gesichtspunkten kann man sich fragen, ob diese mentale Kapazität des Schimpansen eine Matrix, eine bestimmte Stufe vor der Entstehung der menschlichen Sprache widerspiegelt oder ob die Experimente einen verkümmerten Rest solcher Funktionen bloßlegen, die in der Stammesgeschichte des Menschen zum Zeitpunkt der Trennung von Hominiden und

Pongiden bereits vollkommener ausgebildet waren (s. Abb. 1). KORTLANDT und KOOIJ (1963) haben eine solche „Dehumanisierungs-Hypothese" aufgestellt. Für unsere Fragen nach den Ursprüngen der Kommunikation und ihrer Entwicklung ist dieser Unterschied nur von untergeordneter Bedeutung. Ob wir es beim Schimpansen mit Voraussetzungen oder mit Resten des Ursprungs der menschlichen Sprache zu tun haben, der Vergleich des tatsächlich Vorgefundenen hat der Suche nach den Gemeinsamkeiten und Unterschieden zwischen den Kommunikationssystemen der subhumanen Primaten und des Menschen einen neuen Elan verliehen.

e) Gestensprache oder Vokalsprache

Im Lichte der Zeichensprache der Menschenaffen scheint die alte, schon von PLATO im Kratylos und von AUGUSTIN in seinen Confessiones vertretene Hypothese wieder an Boden zu gewinnen, daß die Sprache der Frühmenschen eine Gestensprache gewesen und die Vokalsprache sich erst später, nachdem die anatomisch-physiologischen Voraussetzungen geschaffen waren (s.S. 469), zur menschlichen Sprech-Sprache entwickelt habe (HEWES, 1973a, 1976; STOKOE, 1976). HEWES, von dem diese Hypothese neuerlich am gründlichsten untersucht wurde, begründet sie unter anderem mit der Entstehung des aufrechten Gangs, dem Werkzeuggebrauch und der Werkzeugherstellung (1973a, b). Die Verfechter der Gestensprache stellen dabei durchaus in Rechnung, daß der Frühmensch auch verschiedene Laute zur Kommunikation eingesetzt hat, aber doch nur im Sinne des Ausdrucks von Gemütsbewegungen, um es mit DARWIN zu sagen. Die ersten Funktionen der Sprache hingegen, das Fordern, Hinweisen, Vorschlagen, Ablehnen, Annehmen und Fragen sei der Gestensprache entsprungen, die erst im Laufe der weiteren Evolution schrittweise, auch durch Umformung des supralaryngealen Apparates (s. Abb. 47), an Bedeutung gewonnen und schließlich wegen ihrer offensichtlichen Vorteile (u.a. Kommunikation auf Entfernung, unter Sichtbehinderung), nicht zuletzt auch wegen ihrer außerordentlichen Geschwindigkeit, die Gestensprache überflügelt habe und sie nunmehr unterdrücke, so daß diese jetzt als Relikt erscheine (STEKLIS u. HARNAD, 1976).

Ohne dieses vielschichtige, letztlich paläo-anthropologisch verankerte Argument hier vertiefen zu können, ist die gegenteilige Position ebenso vertretbar. Die letzten gemeinsamen Vorfahren von Affen und Menschen hatten ihre Gestensprache bereits entwickelt, vielleicht in ähnlicher Form wie die heutigen Menschenaffen unter natürlichen Bedingungen. Sie waren geschickt im Imitieren von Gesten, im Manipulieren von Gegenständen und ausdrucksreich mit ihren Händen (RENSCH, 1968). Sie hatten als primär visuell analysierende Tiere im wahrsten Sinne des Wortes Einsicht in komplexere Zusammenhänge (KÖHLER, 1921/1963; DÖHL, 1966), aber sie konnten ihre Stimme nicht von ihren Emotionen entkoppeln, sie konnten Laute nicht nachahmen und sie nicht zum Bezeichnen von Objekten, Kumpanen und Handlungen einsetzen. Gerade die (wahrscheinlich wiederum schrittweise) Emanzipation der Stimme von den Emotionen (PLOOG, 1970, 1972, 1975; JÜRGENS u. PLOOG, 1976), die Fähigkeit, Laute nachzuahmen und neuzubilden (wie die Schimpansen neue Handzeichen bilden können) und die Stimme unter voluntative Kontrolle zu bringen (s.S. 476), mag den entscheidenden Schritt zum Menschen gebracht und ihm damit einen außerordentlichen Selektionsvorteil verschafft haben (schnelle Verständigung ohne Sichtkontrolle, z.B. beim Jagen, in Gefahr, in Dunkelheit etc.). NOTTEBOHM (1975), ein Neuroornithologe, bringt in diesem Zusammenhang die Idee auf, daß diese menschlichen Vorfahren ihre Stimme zum individuellen Balzgesang eingesetzt haben könnten. Damit wäre bereits die Stimme des Frühmenschen bei der Attraktion des Sexualpartners und bei der Partnerwahl wirksam geworden; ein populationsgenetisch wirksames Mittel im Evolutionsprozeß, das bereits bei niederen Vertebraten seinen Ursprung hat (CAPRANICA, 1977).

Wie auch immer dieses Argument der Gesten- versus Vokalsprache weiter vorangetrieben werden kann, der entscheidende neurobiologische Unterschied zwischen der erlernbaren Gestensprache der Menschenaffen und der vokalen Menschensprache ist die Fähigkeit zu differenzierter Lautbildung und Lautnachahmung (s.S. 478). Damit wird der visuo-visuelle Kommunikationsprozeß, der allen Primaten eigen ist, um den audio-visuellen Kommunikationsprozeß in artspezifischer Weise bereichert. Diese bimodale audio-visuelle Rückkoppelung im Kommunikationsprozeß des Menschen ist wahrscheinlich die Wurzel für die Unterschiede in der Sprachkompetenz von Affe und Mensch und hat entsprechende zerebrale Grundlagen (s.S. 468ff.). Vorläufig können wir die Unterschiede der den beiden Kommunikationsformen zugrunde liegenden zerebralen Prozesse nicht genauer bestimmen. Zwar besteht kein Zweifel, daß die Hemisphärenspezialisierung beim Menschen wesentlich weiter fortgeschritten ist, ja, daß der überzeugende Nachweis einer Hemisphärendominanz beim Schimpansen noch fehlt. Aber wir wissen bisher nicht, ob der Schimpanse, wie dies beim taubstummen Menschen erwiesen ist, seine erlernte Zeichensprache bei Hirnläsionen in den dem Menschen homologen Sprachregionen einbüßt.

Wie wir früher beschrieben haben (s.S. 471), lassen sich Vokalisationen bei Affe und Mensch in beiden Hemisphären subkortikal durch elektrischen Hirnreiz auslösen, kortikal jedoch nur, und wiederum beiderseits, beim Menschen. Für die Emanzipation der Stimme von der Körpermotorik und von den Körpergesten muß ein kortikaler Hemmungsmechanismus entwickelt worden sein, der die Differenzierung der stimmlichen Feinstmotorik ermögliche und die Körpermotorik beim Gebrauch der Stimme hemmte. Diesen Entkoppelungsmechanismus – von GEHLEN (1940) klar bei der Beschreibung der „Lautgeste" erkannt – kann man nachweisen; er ist nicht vollständig.

Läßt man z.B. Versuchspersonen Stöckchen auf ihrem rechten oder linken Zeigefinger balancieren und sie dabei Sätze nachsprechen, gelingt Rechtshändern ohne linkshändige Verwandte das Balancieren des Stockes hochsignifikant kürzer mit der rechten als mit der linken Hand. Der Balanceakt verkürzt sich rechts (aber nicht links) noch erheblich, wenn phonetisch schwierige Sätze nachgesprochen werden müssen, und die Anzahl der versprochenen Worte nimmt zu. Bei Linkshändern verkürzte sich unter gleichen Bedingungen der Balanceakt in beiden Händen und bei Rechtshändern mit linkshändigen Verwandten variierten die Ergebnisse zwischen rechts und links. Auch Summen hatte bei Rechtshändern einen gewissen Einfluß auf den Balanceakt mit der rechten Hand (HICKS, 1975).

Wir können aus diesen Versuchen schließen, daß Stimmproduktion und Sprechen die Feinmotorik des Rechtshänders beeinträchtigt; die Entkoppelung ist nicht komplett. Daß dieser Mechanismus genetisch verankert ist, zeigen die Differenzen zwischen Links- und Rechtshändern mit Berücksichtigung von deren Verwandten. Es wäre interessant zu wissen, ob Schimpansen Stöckchen mit einer Hand balancieren können, während sie mit der anderen Zeichen machen.

2. Gemeinsamkeiten bei Schimpanse und Kind im Erwerb von Zeichensprache und Sprache

Mit Gemeinsamkeiten beim Vergleich von Schimpanse und Mensch sind hier nicht homologe Verhaltensweisen gemeint, sondern lediglich ein Vergleich von dem, was der Schimpanse und dem, was das Kind „kann", d.h. wofür beide kompetent sind. Die methodischen Schwierigkeiten eines solchen Vergleichs sind offensichtlich. Die hauptsächlichsten sind durch die unterschiedlichen Altersstufen bedingt, in denen Schimpanse und Kind mit der Zeichensprache bzw. Sprache ihre ersten Erfahrungen machen. Auch stehen die Menschenaffenuntersuchungen noch so am Anfang, daß sie untereinander methodisch schwer zu vergleichen sind. Schließlich gehen die wenigen Studien über den frühesten Spracherwerb beim Kind von verschiedenen methodischen und theoretischen Ansätzen aus.

Dennoch bringt der schlichte Vergleich der Phänomene eine gewisse Klärung der bisherigen Befunde. Die beschriebenen Affen beginnen mit ihren ersten Zeichen frühestens im 3. Monat und mit der Kombination von zwei Zeichen frühestens zwischen 4 und 6 Monaten. Kinder gebrauchen ihre ersten „Einwort-Sätze" ungefähr mit 20 Monaten und Zweiwort-Kombinationen mit ungefähr 2 Jahren (BROWN, 1973). Jedoch berichten verschiedene Autoren, daß taube Kinder und hörende Kinder von tauben Eltern ihre ersten Zeichen mit 5–6 Monaten und ihre ersten Zwei-Zeichen-Kombinationen mit etwa 14 Monaten machen (SCHLESINGER u. MEADOW, 1973; STOKOE, 1976). Sowohl taube Kinder (BELLUGI u. KLIMA, 1976) als auch Affen erfinden neue Zeichen (s. oben). Affen und Kinder lernen, ihre Zeichen bzw. Worte auf neue Objekte und Situationen anzuwenden (Generalisierung). Sehr interessant ist, daß Affen und taube Kinder Mittel haben, etwas in ihrer Aussage zu betonen oder eine Frage zu „intonieren". Will der Affe z.B. an einer bestimmten Stelle gekitzelt werden, macht er das Kitzelzeichen an der „grammatisch" falschen, aber auf den gewünschten Ort hinweisenden Stelle. Bei Fragen wird das Zeichen auch bei Kindern länger gehalten. Sprechende Kinder lernen erst die Frageintonation, bevor sie Frageformen benutzen.

BROWN (1973) hat den Spracherwerb bei Kindern in fünf Stufen gegliedert und als Einteilungsmaß die Wortzahl einer Äußerung benutzt. Auch hier fallen die Schimpansen in die Stufe 1 der 2–3jährigen Kinder mit der Länge einer Äußerung von knapp 2 bis höchstens 6 Zeichen.

Was nun das Befolgen von Satzregeln anbelangt, so haben wir darüber von Sarah und Lana berichtet. Auch Washoe, Ally und Booee zeigten eine deutliche Bevorzugung von Wortsequenzen (GARDNER u. GARDNER, 1975b; MILES, im Druck; RUMBAUGH u. GILL, 1976). Taube Kinder benutzen die Sequenz ihrer Zeichen ziemlich frei, während taube Kinder in englisch sprechender Umgebung ähnliche Sequenzpräferenzen zeigen wie die Affen. Welche Komplexität der Syntax aber schließlich doch beim Schimpansen demonstriert werden kann, zeigt Sarahs richtige Befolgung des nachstehenden Satzes: „Wenn rot auf grün (und nicht umgekehrt) dann Sarah nimm rot (und nicht grün)" (PREMACK, 1971). Derartige Wenn-dann-Beziehungen hat Sarah unter verschiedenen Bedingungen herstellen können. Daraus geht hervor, daß bei ihr (und anderen Schimpansen) Ursache-Wirkungs- bzw. Grund-Folge-Beziehungen nicht nur operational hergestellt (s.S. 509f.), sondern durch Symbole (Plastikstückchen) vermittelt werden können (PREMACK, 1976b). Dieses Stadium der Kompetenz reicht über die Stufe I in die Stufen II und III des Kindes hinein. Auch manche Leistungen Washoes auf „Wer"- und „Wo"-Fragen plazieren sie in die Stufe III (GARDNER u. GARDNER, 1974, 1975b). Hier paßt dann die Stufeneinteilung für das Kind nicht mehr für den Affe/Kind-Vergleich, um die Divergenzen und Limitierungen für den Affen einerseits und die rasch viel weiterreichende Kompetenz des Kindes adäquat beschreiben zu können.

Für Kinder der Spracherwerbsstufe I hat BROWN (1973) acht vorherrschende Bedeutungszusammenhänge beschrieben, die den Inhalt von über zwei Drittel ihrer Äußerungen ausmachen. Dazu gehören hinweisende, besitzanzeigende und ortsbezogene Ausdrücke mit Beziehungen zwischen dem, der die Handlung vollzieht (Agent), der Handlung selbst und dem Objekt. Für taube Kinder wird dasselbe berichtet (KLIMA u. BELLUGI, 1972). Die Affen benutzen ihre Zeichen in denselben Bedeutungszusammenhängen, die zwischen 68% und 75% der Dialoge ausmachten (MILES, 1979), so daß man sagen kann, daß die kommunikativen Akte auf dieser frühesten Stufe des Spracherwerbs die gleichen Funktionen (Bedeutungen) haben.

Damit kommen wir zur Äußerung von Absichten (Intentionalität), die in diesen kommunikativen Akten enthalten sind und deren Motivation erhellen. DORE (1975) fand, daß Handlungsaufforderung und Namengeben den größten Teil sprachlicher Äußerungen von Kindern unter 3 Jahren ausmachten. Dies trifft auch für die Affen zu. Ally z.B. verlangte nach Handlungen und Beachtung und fragte nach Zeichen (Namen) für neue Objekte. Die Absichtsäußerungen von Affen scheinen demnach ebenfalls den von Kindern der Stufe I zu entsprechen (MILES, 1976). Allerdings muß man bei der Bewertung der Intentionalität vorsichtig sein, weil sie in das von Menschen vorgegebene System der Zeichenakquisition eingebettet ist. Dies mag aber für Kinder der Akquisitionsstufe I genauso zutreffen. PREMACK (1976b) hat diesem Problem gesonderte Aufmerksamkeit gewidmet und untersucht, inwieweit der Schimpanse Information, die er hat, absichtlich nicht preisgibt oder den, der die Information haben möchte, absichtlich irreführt. In der experimentellen Situation kann Sarah ihre wahren Absichten nicht verbergen und verrät sich durch ihre unwillkürlichen Blicke, die sie nicht unterdrücken kann (PREMACK, 1976b; vgl. dazu S. 505). Ab wann können Kinder ihre Intentionen verbergen?

Im ganzen genommen fällt der Vergleich zwischen Schimpanse und Kind so aus, daß mit den künstlich geschaffenen Mitteln der Affenkommunikation kommunikative Akte produziert werden, die den frühesten Stufen des kindlichen Spracherwerbs außerordentlich ähnlich sind. Man kann daraus schließen, daß es eine gemeinsame Basis für die kognitiven Prozesse gibt, die die Kommunikation durch Symbole (Zeichen/Worte) ermöglicht.

3. Die phono-audio-visuelle Kommunikation des Säuglings

Der Vergleich von Schimpanse und Kind erlaubt den Schluß, daß den höheren Primaten eine kommunikative Kompetenz gemeinsam ist, deren Wurzeln in ihrer Soziobiologie zu suchen sind. Diese Wurzeln aufzuzeigen, war Gegenstand der vorangegangenen Kapitel. Neben den Gemeinsamkeiten in den Kommunikationsprozessen sollten die artspezifischen Unterschiede innerhalb der Primatenfamilie, insbesondere des Menschen zum Vorschein kommen, um die soziobiologischen Voraussetzungen zur Entwicklung der menschlichen Sprache beschreiben zu können.

Gehen wir von dem offenkundigsten Unterschied aus: Der Mensch benutzt den Vokaltrakt, um Lautgesten zu produzieren, die auf das Ohr des Rezipienten treffen und von dessen auditorischem System im Laufe einer frühen Entwicklungsperiode zu einer sprachlichen Mitteilung verarbeitet werden. Ist die auditive Eingangspforte durch Taubheit versperrt, kann der Mensch lernen, Körpergesten eines Senders mit Hilfe seines visuellen Systems zu einer sprachlichen Mitteilung zu verarbeiten. Er lernt dies auch, wenn er bei intaktem Hörsystem nur Körpergesten zu sehen bekommt (hörende Säuglinge taubstummer Eltern). Der Fall, daß der Mensch auch dann noch Sprache erwerben kann, wenn er nur über seinen Hautsinn Nachrichten empfängt, wie durch HELEN KELLER zuerst offenkundig wurde, soll hier außer Betracht bleiben, müßte aber bei jeder Theorie des Spracherwerbs gehörige Berücksichtigung finden.

Der Menschenaffe auf der anderen Seite benutzt zwar seinen Vokaltrakt zur Produktion arteigener (angeborener) Lautgesten, kann aber nicht lernen, diese Lautgesten in menschliche Phoneme (oder Morpheme) umzuformen. Hingegen kann er mit Hilfe seines visuellen Systems von Menschen gemachte Körpergesten oder Symbole erlernen und diese zu Mitteilungen formen, die einige essentielle Merkmale der menschlichen Sprache tragen.

Ist die Tatsache, daß der Mensch seine Stimme benutzt, um seine Sprache zu sprechen, eine unabdingbare Voraussetzung für die Evolution der Sprache? Gewinnt die Kommunikation durch den phono-auditorischen Modus eine neue Dimension oder handelt es sich beim visuo-visuellen Modus um einen äquivalenten Prozeß mit im Resultat gleicher Mitteilungsfunktion?

Aufschlüsse durch die Evolutionsforschung sind zu dieser Frage kaum möglich. Rückschlüsse von ontogenetischen auf stammesgeschichtliche Prozesse sind stets mit Unsicherheit behaftet. Dennoch fällt des Säuglings außerordentliche kommunikative Bereitschaft im phono-auditorischen Bereich stark ins Gewicht und muß bei einer soziobiologisch orientierten Abhandlung über die Voraussetzung zur Entwicklung der Sprache besondere Beachtung finden.

Wie kann die phono-auditorische Begabung des Säuglings präziser untersucht werden?

CONDON und SANDER (1974) haben mit Tonfilmaufnahmen eine Mikroanalyse des Säuglingsverhaltens durchgeführt, die den Zusammenhang zwischen Bewegungskonfigurationen des 12–48 Std alten Neugeborenen mit zu ihm gesprochener Sprache nachweist. Dabei handelt es sich um zweierlei Synchronisierungsvorgänge: Die während des aktiven Wachstadiums gesprochenen Worte des Erwachsenen bewirken eine Synchronisierung der kindlichen Bewegungen zu konfigurierten Bewegungsabläufen, und diese Abläufe sind mit den phonetischen Segmenten der gesprochenen Worte („come over and see who's over there") synchronisiert. Die Korrespondenz von Bewegungen und Sprache wurde bei allen 16 untersuchten Kindern festgestellt, gleich ob der Sprecher selbst zugegen war oder ob die Stimme vom Tonband kam. Chinesische Worte hatten bei den amerikanischen Kindern denselben Effekt wie englische Worte. Unterbrochene diskontinuierliche Vokale oder Klopflaute konnten nicht das gleiche Maß an Synchronisation hervorrufen wie die natürliche rhythmische Sprache. Bei einem Kind konnte der Synchronisationsprozeß über eine Sequenz von 89 Worten verfolgt werden.

Diese Synchronisierung bedeutet für die vorsprachliche Entwicklung des Kindes, daß der Organismus unzählige Male durch sprachliche Stimulierung Synchronisierungsprozesse durchläuft, bis er selbst das erste Wort produziert. Daß diese kommunikative Verhaltensbereitschaft des Neugeborenen mit der Fähigkeit des 4–12 Wochen alten Kindes zur kategorialen Perzeption von Phonemen ursächlich zusammenhängt (s.S. 440ff.), ist wahrscheinlich.

Aber nicht nur in perzeptiver Hinsicht zeigt sich der Säugling besonders empfänglich, sondern auch in seiner Anregbarkeit zur Lautproduktion. Schon früh hat man zu zeigen versucht, daß die Anzahl der vokalen Äußerungen des Kindes zunimmt, wenn das Vokalisieren von sozialer Stimulierung abhängig gemacht, d.h. durch soziale Stimulierung verstärkt wird (RHEINGOLD et al., 1959; WEISBERG, 1963). Die Experimente von KATHLEEN BLOOM (1975) zeigen, daß der Erwachsene als Auslöser für Lautäußerungen wirkt, unabhängig davon, ob der soziale Stimulus in (kontingente) zeitliche Abhängigkeit von der Vokalisation gebracht wird oder nicht.

Im ersten Experiment wurden 3 Monate alte Kinder in einer Gesicht-zu-Gesicht-Position alle 2 min für 2 s mit Lächeln, leichter Berührung auf den Bauch und „Hei Baby" angesprochen. Diese soziale Stimulierung verursachte einen starken Anstieg der Vokalisation während der ersten 30 s mit Gipfel während der ersten 15 s und einen rapiden Abfall in den folgenden 90 s vor dem Einsetzen des nächsten Reizes. Im zweiten Experiment wurde eine Auslösereigenschaft des Erwachsenen – nämlich der Blickkontakt – auf seine Funktion geprüft. Unter einer Versuchsbedingung trug der Stimulant Augengläser, unter der zweiten Versuchsbedingung hautfarbene Blenden mit einem kleinen zentralen Loch, das dem Experimentator gerade erlaubte, die Augen des Kindes zu sehen und die Gesicht-zu-Gesicht-Position einzuhalten. Die soziale Stimulierung wurde abhängig und unabhängig von einer vorangehenden Vokalisation durchgeführt. Unter dieser kontingenten und nicht-kontingenten Reizbedingung stieg die vokale Produktion des Babys hoch signifikant an, aber nur dann, wenn das Baby die Augen des Stimulanten sehen konnte.

Der Blickkontakt erweist sich hier als ein Katalysator der Lautproduktion. Der visuelle Reiz selbst löst das Vokalisieren nicht aus, aber er muß vorhanden sein, damit der soziale Reiz wirksam werden kann. Hier treffen wir auf einen entscheidenden Funktionszusammenhang in der vorsprachlichen Entwicklung: Die Verbindung der Lautäußerungen des Kindes mit dem wechselseitigen Blickkontakt in der sozialen Interaktion (PAPOUŠEK u. PAPOUŠEK, 1978) (s. Abb. 62). In einer Untersuchung zur Selbsterkennung bei 5 Monate alten Säuglingen

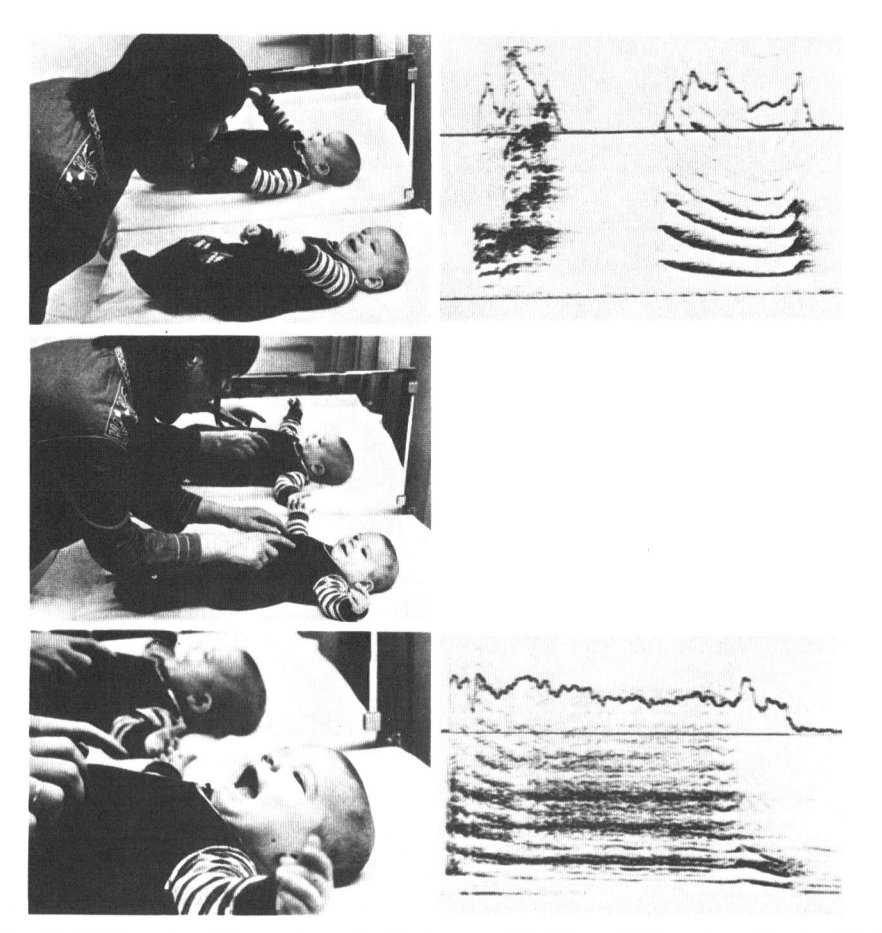

Abb. 62. Blickkontakt, Babysprache und Vokalisation. Die Mutter blickt und spricht das Kind an. Es antwortet mit Armestrecken, Lachen und einer fröhlichen Lautäußerung. Die Mutter macht ein „Spiel"; das Kind reagiert mit einer lustvollen Lautäußerung. (Filmsequenz und Sonagramme von PAPOUŠEK, unveröffentlicht)

gelang es sogar nachzuweisen, daß Babys, die sich selbst im Film betrachten, den Film vorziehen, in dem sie Blickkontakt mit sich selbst bekommen. Die Film-Analyse zeigt auch deutlich eine Veränderung im kindlichen Ausdrucksverhalten, wenn die Mutter im Beisein des Kindes plötzlich die Augen geschlossen hält (PAPOUŠEK u. PAPOUŠEK, 1974).

Erst in den letzten Jahren ist in den Interaktionsanalysen von Kind und Mutter oder Bezugsperson deutlich geworden, in welchem Maße die Mutter ihr Verhalten an das des Kindes anpaßt; das meiste tut sie, ohne es zu wissen oder lernen zu müssen, wenn auch Gewöhnungs- und Übungseffekte nachweisbar sind (STERN, 1971; KLAUS u. KENNELL, 1976; PAPOUŠEK u. PAPOUŠEK, 1977; SANDER, 1977a, b).

Für die Entwicklung von Interaktionsmustern im vorsprachlichen Bereich ist das Imitationsverhalten der Mutter besonders wichtig (s.S. 435), weil sich auf diese Weise schon in den ersten Lebenswochen phono-audio-visuelle Dialoge entwickeln und wie im Rollenspiel eingeübt werden. Die Mutter imitiert bevorzugt Gesichtsausdrücke, Nase-, Mund- und Zungenbewegungen sowie die Laute des Kindes. Sie verknüpft ihre Nachahmungen zeitlich eng mit dem bei ihrem Kind beobachteten Verhalten, das dadurch wiederum stimuliert wird. Eine für die Wirkung des Mutter-Verhaltens typische interaktive Sequenz beschrieben PAPOUŠEK u. PAPOUŠEK (1976) aufgrund von Filmaufnahmen: Zuerst macht die Mutter den Mund auf und streckt die Zunge heraus, und das Baby wiederholt die Bewegung. In einer zweiten Sequenz streckt das Baby die Zunge heraus und die Mutter imitiert es. Der Spaß, den das Kind dabei hat, ist evident. Besonders lebhaft wird neu auftretendes Verhalten imitiert und dadurch verstärkt.

Fast stets sind diese Blickkontakt-Bewegungsinteraktionen von „Reden" der Mutter begleitet. Dieser „Babysprache" kommt eine wichtige Funktion beim Spracherwerb zu. Gibt das Baby Laute von sich, imitiert und redet die Mutter mehr, und das Baby wird dadurch zu weiteren stimmlichen Äußerungen angeregt. Die Babysprache ist langsamer, die Zahl der immer wieder benutzten Worte ist gering, die Stimme ist hoch und sehr variabel in der Intonation. Eine wohldosierte Mischung von Wiederholung und Veränderung der Stimmlaute zieht offenbar die Aufmerksamkeit des Säuglings außerordentlich an. Nicht nur Mütter, sondern auch andere Erwachsene, ja auch 3–4 Jahre alte Kinder zeigen ein ähnliches Sprachverhalten gegenüber Babys (FERGUSON, 1964; SNOW, 1972; NEWPORT, 1977; PAPOUŠEK u. PAPOUŠEK, 1979; FERNALD, 1979).

Die Übertreibung der visuellen und vokalen Signale, die bei der sozialen Stimulierung des Säuglings benutzt werden, läßt sich besonders gut beim „Grüßen" der Mutter beobachten. Meist nach Blickkontakt beugt die Mutter den Kopf leicht zurück, hebt die Augenbrauen, macht große Augen, macht den Mund leicht auf, lächelt und sagt gern feststehende Worte in ähnlichem Tonfall (vgl. S. 518). Diese Szenen und andere ritualisierte audio-visuelle Kommunikationsformen machen es dem Kinde möglich, das Verhalten der Mutter oder anderer Bezugspersonen „vorauszusagen". Erst aus diesen herausgebildeten Formeln des Umgangs werden dann die vielfältigen Überraschungsspiele möglich, in denen das Kind bereits eine Erwartung über den Ablauf einer bestimmten Interaktion entwickelt hat.

Was nun die Entwicklung der Lautproduktion und der Artikulation des Kindes anbelangt, können wir an das Kapitel über die vokalen Signale des Menschen anknüpfen (s.S. 434 ff.): Die Lautäußerungen des Säuglings beginnen sich schon in den ersten Lebenswochen beim Schreien zu differenzieren und sind Ausdruck verschiedener Befindlichkeiten (Stimmungen, States). Bereits im 2. Monat werden Tonhöhe, Lautstärke, Frequenz- und Zeitverläufe moduliert; die Variationen der Lautäußerungen nehmen von Monat zu Monat zu. Nach dieser Phase des Gurrens kommt das Kind mit 6 Monaten ins Babbelalter; kürzere oder längere Frequenzen von Konsonanten und Vokalen (zuerst wie mama, bababa, maba, bamamama usw.) werden, auch wenn das Kind allein ist, geäußert, so als ob das Kind ohne kommunikative Absicht mit seinen Stimmwerkzeugen spielt. Die Zahl der konsonantischen und vokalen Elemente nimmt in regelhafter Abfolge zu. Das Sprechen des Erwachsenen zum Kinde oder auch nur seine Stimme regt die Lautproduktion an, beeinflußt sie aber nicht in ihrem in allen untersuchten Sprachgemeinschaften gleichen, regelhaften Entwicklungsablauf (LENNEBERG et al., 1965; LENNEBERG, 1967; TODD u. PALMER, 1968). Mit ungefähr 9 Monaten tritt ein Wendepunkt ein. Das Babbeln läßt deutlich nach oder hört für eine Weile sogar ganz auf. Das Kind beginnt bekannte Gesichter mit einfachen Lauten (/ae/, /ba/, u.ä.) zu adressieren. Es ist, als ob sich die Lautgebung reorganisiert und wieder mit scheinbar einfachen Lauten beginnt (NAKAZIMA, 1975). Erst mit ungefähr 10 Monaten beginnt das Kind, Sprachlaute der Erwachsenen wirklich zu imitieren, d.h. nachzuformen, und auch die ersten Worte zu verstehen. Mit 11 oder 12 Monaten beginnen die ersten Worte zu erscheinen. Damit setzt ein langer Prozeß der Artikulationsentwicklung ein, der sich wiederum durch eine Regelhaftigkeit im Auftreten bestimmter Phoneme auszeichnet, die zunächst noch unabhängig von der später gesprochenen Muttersprache ist. Vom ersten Wort zu den ersten Wortkombinationen – den Einwort- und Zweiwortsätzen – mit ungefähr 17 Monaten gibt es zahlreiche Übergänge und auch bezüglich der Anzahl von Worten sehr große individuelle Unterschiede. Damit setzt der Spracherwerb im engeren Sinne ein, der in diesem Beitrag nicht behandelt wird (MCNEILL, 1970; FERGUSON u. SLOBIN, 1973).

Die schrittweise Gewalt über das Wort beschreiben BULLOWA et al. (1964) bei dem Mädchen Dory anschaulich in 6 Stufen vom 9. bis 22. Lebensmonat:

1. (9–11 Monate): Die Mutter spricht das Wort „Schuh" während dieses Beobachtungsabschnitts immer wieder deutlich und klar im Zusammenhang mit Dorys Schuh aus.

2. (11 Monate und 14 Tage): Dory macht einen Versuch, das Wort Schuh zu imitieren, den die Mutter nicht akzeptiert. Nach Korrektur sagt das Kind „Tu". Wenig später, mit dem Rücken zum Kind gedreht, fordert die Mutter Dory auf, die Schuhe aus dem Mund zu nehmen; das Kind folgt der Aufforderung sofort.

3. (11 Monate und 21 Tage): Dory imitiert Mutters Wort „Schuh" erstmals zu deren Zufriedenheit, wenn es auch noch eine phonetisch schlechte Imitation war. Bald darauf kommt wieder „Tu Tu".

4. (11 Monate und 28 Tage sowie 12 Monate und 5 Tage): Dory benutzt das Wort Schuh in genügend klarer Aussprache spontan, ohne daß die Mutter das Wort vorspricht oder den Kontext dazu herstellt. Eine Woche später, während die Mutter mit ihr wegen nasser Hosen schimpft, versucht Dory, sie mit einem Schuh in der Hand abzulenken, hält die Schuhe hoch und sagt „Tschuh".

5. (16 Monate und 22 Tage): Dory benutzt das Wort Schuh spontan als Teil ihres sonstigen Einwort-Schatzes und in Kombination „Mama Tschuh" als Aufforderung an die Mutter, ihr die Schuhe zu geben. Etwas später wechselt sie mehrfach die Aussprache von Tsuh zu Tschuh bis zum schon gut ausgesprochenen „Schuh".

6. (22 Monate und 15 Tage): Dory beherrscht nun die adulte Aussprache fast immer und benutzt das „Sch" auch in anderem Zusammenhang jetzt richtig: „She go up". Sie hatte also zu diesem Zeitpunkt ihren Sprechapparat so unter Kontrolle, daß sie einen Vokallaut richtig formen und halten und einen Silben-

laut produzieren konnte, der mit einem Verschluß des Vokaltraktes beginnt und in offener Position endet.

Die Darstellung des Weges vom Vokalisieren zum Phonemisieren (vgl. S. 434 ff.) soll deutlich machen, daß die vokale Entwicklung des Menschen von Anbeginn grundsätzlich von der des Schimpansen oder eines anderen Menschenaffen verschieden ist, während die Wahrnehmungs- und Erkenntnisprozesse offenbar größere Ähnlichkeiten aufweisen. Würde Dory ein Schimpansenkind sein und ASL von ihrem Trainer lernen, könnte man die 6 Stufen des Zeichenerwerbs in ähnlicher Form, wenn auch in gerafftrem Zeitverlauf beschreiben. Die lange Zeit, die das Kind braucht, um das Kommando über seine Sprechwerkzeuge zu gewinnen, hängt selbstverständlich nicht von der Entwicklung seines Vokaltraktes ab (s.S. 469), die schon nach einem halben Jahr hinsichtlich der Form abgeschlossen ist.

Nur die frühkindliche zerebrale Entwicklung, die neuronalen Korrelate der Stimmbewegungen können für diesen Prozeß verantwortlich sein. LENNEBERGS fundamentale Beschreibung der spezies-spezifischen biologischen Grundlagen der Sprache (1967) treffen nicht allein auf die kognitiven, sondern auch auf die sensomotorischen Prozesse zu, die sich in den phono-artikulatorischen Bewegungen manifestieren. Der strenge Zeitplan der Entwicklung, der während des ersten Lebensjahres unabhängig von der jeweiligen Sprachkulturgemeinschaft abläuft, spricht allein schon für ein artspezifisches genetisch determiniertes Programm, das sich eingebettet in die übrige sensomotorische Entwicklung, aber doch in zunehmender Differenzierung als sich verselbständigender Teil der Motorik verwirklicht. Die Grundannahme von der Sprache als der Manifestation einer spezies-spezifischen kognitiven Disposition führt LENNEBERG (1967, S. 371 ff.) immer wieder zurück auf die Frage nach der Natur der zugrunde liegenden zerebralen Prozesse – Aktivitätszuständen, „die labil sind und von Bedingungen der Umgebung leicht affiziert oder moduliert werden" (LENNEBERG, 1975). Die ontogenetische Entwicklung hängt, wie letztlich jeder genetisch bedingte Prozeß, von einer großen Zahl interaktiver Faktoren ab. Nach einer anfänglichen Differenzierung einfacher Aktivitätszustände (z.B. Schreien), im wesentlichen als Folge der Hirnreifung, wird der wachsende Organismus zunehmend reagibel auf spezifische Umwelteinflüsse, die die weiteren Transformationen in zunehmend differenziertere Aktivitätszustände (z.B. die Gewalt über das erste Wort) mitbestimmen. Wenn die Umwelteinflüsse auch ohne Zweifel für die Entwicklung der kognitiven Sprachprozesse in hohem Grade wirksam sind – wie uns zudem in anderen Bereichen der Neurobiologie der Wahrnehmung, z.B. der Entwicklungsneurophysiologie des Sehens gezeigt wird – so können wir diesen neuronalen Differenzierungsprozeß an der Lautproduktion unmittelbar ablesen. Das spezifisch Menschliche der Sprache zeigt sich am klarsten zuerst auf seiten der Motorik eben im stimmlichen Verhalten, während das spezifisch Menschliche auf seiten des Wahrnehmens und Erkennens in diesem Stadium der Ontogenese nicht sicher abzugrenzen ist.

Daß für den motorischen wie für den kognitiven Sprachentwicklungsprozeß die ständige Interaktion des Kindes mit seiner sprachlichen Umwelt nötig ist, zeigen die Berichte über die sog. Wolfskinder oder „wilden Kinder" (ITARD, 1801; s. bei MALSON et al., 1972), von denen Kaspar Hauser im deutschen

Schrifttum am bekanntesten geworden ist (s. MERKENSCHLAGER u. SALLER, 1966). Sein Name wird in der ethologischen Literatur für Experimente verwendet, in denen Tiere unter Erfahrungsentzug, d.h. in teilweiser oder gänzlicher Isolation aufgezogen werden. Von allen diesen Kaspar-Hauser-Kindern wird berichtet, daß sie nie richtig sprechen lernten. Ein eingehend psycholinguistisch untersuchtes, mit $13^1/_2$ Jahren entdecktes, normal intelligentes Mädchen fast ohne Spracherfahrung wurde 1977 von SUSAN CURTISS beschrieben. Das Kind wuchs unter unvorstellbar grausamen Isolationsbedingungen auf und hatte auch 7 Jahre nach seiner Entdeckung und fortgesetzten pädagogischen Bemühungen mit fast 20 Jahren nur eine äußerst rudimentäre Sprache erworben.

Man kann in bezug auf den menschlichen Spracherwerb im Laufe der Evolution die Frage stellen, ob das Auftreten der phono-auditorischen Prozesse in der Tier-Mensch-Übergangszeit den damit begabten Vorfahren nicht nur durch ein differenzierteres Kommunikationssystem Selektionsvorteile entstanden sind, sondern ob diese spezifischen sensomotorischen Prozesse mit ihren sehr schnellen Zeitverläufen und hochkomplexen Zeitgestalten neue kognitive Fähigkeiten ermöglicht haben. Vielleicht führen hier Untersuchungen über die Abstraktionsfähigkeit der Taubstummen weiter.

Literatur

Adametz, J., O'Leary, J.L.: Experimental mutism resulting from periaqueductal lesions in cats. Neurology (Minneap.) **9**, 636–642 (1959)

Adey, W.R., Tokizane, T. (Hrsg.): Structure and function on the limbic system. Progress in brain research, Bd. 27. Amsterdam: Elsevier 1967

Ahrens, R.: Beitrag zur Entwicklung des Physiognomie- und Mimikerkennens. Z. Exp. Angew. Psychol. **2**, 412–454 (1954)

Akisal, H.S., McKinney, W.T.: Depressive disorders: Towards a unified hypothesis. Science **182**, 20–29 (1973)

Altmann, St.A. (Hrsg.): Social communication among primates. Chicago, London: The University of Chicago Press 1967

Ambrose, J.A.: The development of the smiling response in early infancy. In: Determinants of infant behavior. Foss, B. (Hrsg.), S. 179–196. London: Methuen 1961

Andrew, R.J.: The origin and evolution of the calls and facial expressions of the primates. Behaviour **20**, 1–109 (1963)

Arbib, M.A.: The metaphorical brain: An introduction to cybernetics as artificial intelligence and brain theory. New York: Wiley-Interscience 1972

Ashby, W.R.: Design for a brain: The origin of adaptive behavior, 2. Aufl. London: Science Paperbacks, Ass. Book Publ. 1960

Bateson, P.P.G., Klopfer, P.H. (Hrsg.): Perspectives in ethology. 2 Bde. New York, London: Plenum Press 1975/1976

Bay, E.: Die corticale Dysarthrie und ihre Beziehungen zur sogenannten motorischen Aphasie. Dtsch. Z. Nervenheilkd. **176**, 553–594 (1957)

Bazett, H.C., Penfield, W.G.: A study of the Sherrington decerebrate animal in the chronic as well as the acute condition. Brain **45**, 185–265 (1922)

Beach, F.A., Hebb, D.O., Morgan, C.T., Nissen, H.W. (Hrsg.): The neuropsychology of Lashley. (Selected papers of K.S. Lashley.) New York: McGraw-Hill 1960

Beatty, J., McDevitt, C.A.: Call discrimination in chimpanzees. Curr. Anthropol. **16**, 668–669 (1975)

Bellugi, K., Klima, E.S.: Two faces of sign: Iconic and abstract. Ann. N.Y. Acad. Sci. **280**, 514–538 (1976)

Benda, C.E.: Down's syndrome, mongolism and its management. New York: Grune and Stratton 1969

Benson, D.F.: Fluency in aphasia: Correlation with radioactive scan localization. Cortex **3**, 373–394 (1967)
Bilz, R.: Paläoanthropologie. Der neue Mensch in der Sicht einer Verhaltensforschung. 1. Bd., 1. Aufl. Frankfurt/Main: Suhrkamp 1971
Birdwhistell, R.L.: Kinesics and context. Philadelphia: University of Pennsylvania Press 1970
Bischof, N.: A systems approach toward the functional connections of attachment and fear. Child Dev. **46**, 801–817 (1975)
Bloom, K.: Social elicitation of infant vocal behavior. J. Exp. Child Psychol. **20**, 51–58 (1975)
Blurton Jones, N. (Hrsg.): Ethological studies of child behaviour. Cambridge: The University Press 1972
Botez, M.I., Barbeau, S.: Role of subcortical structures and particularly of the thalamus in mechanisms of speech and language. Int. J. Neurol. **8**, 300–320 (1971)
Bowden, D., Winter, P., Ploog, D.: Pregnancy and delivery behavior in the squirrel monkey (Saimiri sciureus) and other primates. Folia Primatol. (Basel) **5**, 1–42 (1967)
Bowlby, J.: An ethological approach to research in child development. Br. J. Med. Psychol. **30**, 230 (1957)
Bowlby, J.: Grief and mourning in infancy and early childhood. Psychoanal. Study Child **15**, 9 (1960)
Bowlby, J.: Attachment and loss. Bd. I, Attachment (The international psycho-analytical library). M. Masud, R. Khan (Hrsg.), Nr. 79. London: The Hogarth Press and the Institute of Psycho-Analysis 1969
Bowlby, J.: Attachment and loss, Bd. II, Separation and anger. (The international psycho-analytical library.) M. Masud, R. Khan (Hrsg.), Nr. 95. London: The Hogarth Press and the Institute of Psycho-Analysis 1973a
Bowlby, J.: Mütterliche Zuwendung und geistige Gesundheit. Kindler Taschenbücher „Geist und Psyche". München: Kindler 1973b
Brain, R.: Speech disorders: Aphasia, apraxia and agnosis. London, Washington, D.C.: Butterworth 1961
Brickner, R.M.: A human cortical area producing repetitive phenomena when stimulated. J. Neurophysiol. **3**, 128–130 (1940)
Broca, P.: Le grand-lobe limbique et la scissure limbique dans la serie des mammiferes. Rev. d'anthropol. Jg. 7, Bd. **1**, 385–498 (1878)
Brown, R.A.: Words and things. New York: Collier and MacMillan 1965
Brown, R.A.: Psycholinguistics, the first sentences of child and chimpanzee. In: Psycholinguistics, Brown, R. (Hrsg.). New York: MacMillan 1970
Brown, R.A.: A first language: The early stages. Cambridge, Mass.: Harvard University Press 1973
Bruner, J.S.: Processes of cognitive growth: Infancy Bd. III, Heinz Werner Lecture Series. Worcester: Clark University Press with Barre Publishers 1968
Bruner, J.S.: From communication to language – a psychological perspective. Cognition **3**, 255–287 (1974/75)
Bühler, C., Hetzer, H.: Das erste Verständnis für Ausdruck im ersten Lebensjahr. Z. Psychol. **107**, 50–61 (1928)
Buettner-Janusch, J.: Evolutionary and genetic biology of primates, Bd. I. New York: Academic Press 1963
Bullock, Th.H. (Hrsg.): Recognition of complex acoustic signals. Dahlem Konferenzen. Life sciences research report 5. Berlin: Abakon Verlagsgesellschaft 1977
Bullowa, M. (Hrsg.): Before speech. Cambridge: Cambridge University Press 1979
Bullowa, M., Jones, L.G., Duckert, A.R.: The acquisition of a word. Lang. Speech **7**, 107–111 (1964)
Capranica, R.R.: The evoked vocal response of the bullfrog. M.I.T. research monograph Nr. 33. Cambridge, Mass.: M.I.T. Press 1965
Capranica, R.R.: Auditory processing of vocal signals in anurans. In: The reproductive biology of amphibans, Taylor, D.H., Guttman, S.I. (Hrsg.), S. 337–355. New York: Plenum 1977
Carpenter, C.R.: Naturalistic behavior of nonhuman primates. University Park, Pa.: Pennsylvania State University Press 1964
Carpenter, C.R. (Hrsg.): Behavioral regulators of behavior in primates. Lewisburg: Bucknell University Press (Associated University Presses, Inc. Cranbury, New Jersey) 1973

Castell, R., Krohn, H., Ploog, D.: Rückenwälzen bei Totenkopfaffen (Saimiri sciureus): Körperpflege und soziale Funktion. Z. Tierpsychol. **26**, 488–497 (1969)
Chance, M.R.A.: Attention structure as the basis of primate rank orders. Man **2**, 503–518 (1967)
Chance, M.R.A.: Organization of attention in groups. In: Methods of inference from animal to human behaviour. Cranach, M.v. (Hrsg.), S. 213–235. Chicago, Mouton, Den Haag, Paris: Aldine 1976
Chance, M.R.A., Jolly, C.J.: Social groups of monkeys, apes and men. London: Jonathan Cape Thirty Bedford Square 1970
Charlesworth, W.R., Kreutzer, M.A.: Facial expressions of infants and children. In: Darwin and facial expression. Ekman, P. (Hrsg.), S. 91–168. New York: Academic Press 1973
Chevalier-Skolnikoff, S.: Facial expression of emotion in nonhuman primates. In: Darwin and facial expression, Ekman, P. (Hrsg.), S. 11–89. New York, London: Academic Press 1973
Chomsky, N.: Aspects of the theory of syntax. Cambridge, Mass.: MIT Press 1965. Deutsche Ausgabe: Aspekte der Syntax-Theorie. Frankfurt/Main: Suhrkamp Taschenbuch Wissenschaft 42, 1973
Condon, W.S., Sander, L.W.: Neonate movement is synchronized with adult speech: Interactional participation and language acquisition. Science **183**, 99–101 (1974)
Conrad, K.: Strukturanalysen hirnpathologischer Fälle. V. Mitteilung, Über die Brocasche motorische Aphasie. Dtsch. Z. Nervenheilkd. **158**, 132–187 (1948)
Conrad, K.: New problems of aphasia. Brain **77**, 491–501 (1954)
Cooper, W.E.: Contingent feature analysis in speech perception. Perception and Psychophysics **16**, 201–204 (1974)
Count, E.W.: Das Biogramm. Anthropologische Studien. Conditio humana. Ergebnisse aus den Wissenschaften vom Menschen. Frankfurt/Main: S. Fischer 1970
Cranach, M.v.: Über die Signalfunktion des Blickes in der Interaktion: In: Sozialtheorie und soziale Praxis. Albert, H., Irle, M., Lepsius, M.R., Matthias, E., Wildenmann, R. (Hrsg.) **3**, 201–224 (1968)
Cranach, M.v.: The role of orienting behavior in human interaction. In: Behavior and enviroment. Esser, A.H. (Hrsg.), S. 217–237. New York: Plenum Press 1971 a
Cranach, M.v.: Die nichtverbale Kommunikation im Kontext des kommunikativen Verhaltens. Jahrbuch der Max-Planck-Gesellschaft, S. 104–148. Göttingen: Hubert 1971 b
Cranach, M.v. (Hrsg.): Methods of inference from animal to human behaviour. (Proceedings of the conference on "The logic of inference from animal to human behaviour", held in Murten, Switzerland in March 1973). Paris: Mouton-Co., The Hague and Maison de l'Homme 1976
Cranach, M.v., Vine, J. (Hrsg.): Social communication and movement studies of interaction in man and chimpanzee. London: Academic Press 1972
Curtiss, S.: Genie. A psycholinguistic study of a modern-day "wild child". New York, London: Academic Press 1977
Darwin, Ch.: The expression of the emotions in man and animals. London: Murray 1872 (Der Ausdruck der Gemütsbewegungen bei Menschen und Tieren, Halle 1896)
Darwin, Ch.: Sexual selection in relation to monkeys. Nature **15**, 18–19 (1876)
Davenport, R.K., Rogers, M.R., Rumbaugh, D.M.: Long-term cognitive deficits in chimpanzees associated with early impoverished rearing. Dev. Psychol. **9**, 343 (1973)
Davis, R.T.: Monkeys as perceivers. In: Primate behavior. Developments in field and laboratory research, Rosenblum, L.A. (Hrsg.) Bd. 3. New York, London: Academic Press 1974
Delgado, J.M.R.: Cerebral heterostimulation in a monkey colony. Science **141**, 161–163 (1963)
Delgado, J.M.R.: Sequential behavior repeatedly induced by red nucleus stimulation in free monkey. Science **148**, 1361–1363 (1965)
Delgado, J.M.R.: Social rank and radio-stimulated aggressiveness in monkeys. J. Nerv. Ment. Dis. **144**, 383–390 (1967 a)
Delgado, J.M.R.: Aggression and defense under cerebral radio control. In: Aggression and defense. Neural mechanisms and social patterns. Clemente, C.D., Lindsley, D.B. (Hrsg.), S. 171–193. Berkeley: University California Press 1967 b
Delgado, J.M.R.: Physical control of the mind. Toward a psychocivilized society. New York: Harper and Row 1969
Delgado, J.M.R.: New orientations in brain stimulation in man. In: Brain stimulation reward.

Wauquier, A., Rolls, E.T. (Hrsg.), S. 481–503. Oxford: North-Holland Publ. Comp. Amsterdam 1976
Delgado, J.M.R., Mir, D.: Fragmental organization of emotional behavior in the monkey brain. Ann. N.Y. Acad. Sci. **159**, 731–751 (1969)
Dennis, W., Dennis, M.G.: Behavioral development in the first year as shown by forty biographies. Psychol. Rec. **1**, 349–361 (1937)
DeVore, I. (Hrsg.): Primate behavior. Field studies on monkeys and apes. New York: Holt, Rinehart and Winston 1965
DeWied, D.: Pituitary-adrenal system hormones and behavior. In: The neurosciences. Schmitt, F.O., Worden, F.G. (Hrsg.), Third Study Program, S. 653–666. Cambridge, Mass.: The MIT Press 1974
DiCara, L.V.: Limbic and autonomic nervous systems research. New York: Plenum Press 1974
Dieckmann, G., Hassler, R.: Psychochirurgie. Dtsch. Ärztebl. **18**, 1217–1223 (1976)
Dieckmann, G., Hassler, R.: Treatment of sexual violence by stereotactic hypothalamotomy. In: Neurosurgical treatment in psychiatry, pain and epilepsy. Sweet, W.H., Obrado, S., Martin-Rodriguez, J.G. (Hrsg.), S. 451–462. Baltimore: University Park Press 1977
Döhl, J.: Manipulierfähigkeit und „einsichtiges" Verhalten eines Schimpansen bei komplizierten Handlungsketten. Z. Tierpsychol. **23**, 77–113 (1966)
Döhl, J.: Über die Fähigkeit einer Schimpansin, Umwege mit selbstständigen Zwischenzielen zu überblicken. Z. Tierpsychol. **25**, 89–103 (1968)
Döhl, J., Podolczak, D.: Versuche zur Manipulierfreudigkeit von zwei jungen Orang-Utans (Pongo pygmaeus) im Frankfurter Zoo. Zool. Garten N.V. **43**, 81–94 (1973)
Dore, J.: Holophrases, speech acts and language universals. J. Child Lang. **2**, 21–40 (1975)
Eastman, R.F., Mason, W.A.: Looking behavior in monkeys raised with mobile stationary artificial mothers. Dev. Psychobiol. **8**, 213–221 (1975)
Eibl-Eibesfeldt, I.: Zur Ethologie des menschlichen Grußverhaltens. I. Beobachtungen an Balinesen, Papuas und Samoanern nebst vergleichenden Bemerkungen. Z. Tierpsychol. **25**, 727–744 (1968)
Eibl-Eibesfeldt, I.: Liebe und Haß. München: Piper 1970
Eibl-Eibesfeldt, I.: Das humanethologische Filmarchiv der Max-Planck-Gesellschaft. Homo **22**, 252–256 (1971a)
Eibl-Eibesfeldt, I.: Zur Ethologie menschlichen Grußverhaltens. II. Das Grußverhalten und einige andere Muster freundlicher Kontaktaufnahme der Waika (Yanoáma). Z. Tierpsychol. **29**, 1960–213 (1971b)
Eibl-Eibesfeldt, I.: The expressive behaviour of the deaf-and-blind-born. In: Social communication and movement. Cranach, M.v., Vine, I. (Hrsg.), European monographs in social psychology. Series Editor: Tajfel, H. London, New York Academic Press 1973
Eibl-Eibesfeldt, I.: Taubblind geborenes Mädchen (Deutschland) – Ausdrucksverhalten. Homo **24**, 39–47 (1973a)
Eibl-Eibesfeldt, I.: Taubblind geborenes Mädchen (Deutschland) – Explorierverhalten und Spiel. Homo **24**, 48–49 (1973b)
Eibl-Eibesfeldt, I.: Der vorprogrammierte Mensch. (Das Ererbte als bestimmender Faktor im menschlichen Verhalten.) Wien, München, Zürich: Molden 1973c
Eibl-Eibesfeldt, I.: Stammesgeschichtliche und kulturelle Anpassungen im menschlichen Verhalten In: Hominisation und Verhalten. Kurth, G., Eibl-Eibesfeldt, I. (Hrsg.). Stuttgart: Fischer 1975
Eibl-Eibesfeldt, I.: Menschenforschung auf neuen Wegen. Wien, München, Zürich: Molden 1976
Eibl-Eibesfeldt, I.: Grundriß der vergleichenden Verhaltensforschung. Ethologie. 1. Auflage 1967, 5. Auflage 1978. München: Piper 1978
Eibl-Eibesfeldt, I., Wickler, W.: Die ethologische Deutung einiger Wächterfiguren auf Bali. Z. Tierpsychol. **25**, 719–726 (1968)
Eimas, P.D.: Auditory and linguistic processing of cues for place of articulation by infants. Perception and Psychophysics **16**, 513–521 (1974)
Eimas, P.D.: Auditory and phonetic coding of the cues for speech: Discrimination of the (r-l) distinction by young infants. Perception and Psychophysics **18** (5), 341–347 (1975a)
Eimas, P.D.: Distinctive feature codes in the short-term memory of children. J. Exp. Child Psychol. **19**, 241–251 (1975b)
Eimas, P.D., Siqueland, E.R., Jusczyk, P., Vigorito, J.: Speech perception in infants. Science **171**, 303–306 (1971)

Eimas, P.D., Cooper, W.E., Corbit, J.D.: Some properties of linguistic detectors. Perception and Psychophysics **13**, 247–252 (1973)
Eisenberg, J.F., Dillon, W.S. (Hrsg.): Man and beast: Comparative social behavior. Smithsonian Annual III. Washington: Smithsonian Institution Press 1971
Ekman, P.: Universals and cultural differences in facial expressions of emotion. Nebraska symp. on motivation, S. 207–283. Lincoln, Nebraska: University of Nebraska Press 1972
Ekman, P. (Hrsg.): Darwin and facial expression. A century of research in review. New York, London: Academic Press 1973
Ekman, P., Friesen, W.V.: Constants across cultures in the face and emotion. J. Pers. Soc. Psychol. **17**, 124–129 (1971)
Ekman, P., Friesen, W.V.: Measuring facial movement. Environment. Psychol. Nonverb. Behav. **1**, 56–75 (1976)
Ekman, P., Friesen, W.V., Ellsworth, Ph.: Emotion in the human face: Guidelines for research and an integration of findings. New York, Toronto, Oxford, Sydney, Braunschweig: Pergamon Press 1972
Eleftheriou, B.E.: The neurobiology of the amygdala. (Proc. of a symposium on the neurobiology of the amygdala, Bar Harbor, Maine, June 6–17, 1971). New York, London: Plenum Press 1972
Eleftheriou, B.E., Scott, J.P. (Hrsg.): The physiology of aggression and defeat. London: Plenum Press 1971
Ellgring, J.H.: Die Beurteilung des Blicks auf Punkte innerhalb des Gesichtes. Z. Exp. Angew. Psychol. **17**, 600–607 (1970)
Erwin, T., Maple, T., Mitchel, G., Willott, T.: Follow-up study of isolation-reared and mother-reared rhesus monkeys paired with preadolescent conspecifics in late infancy: Cross-sex pairings. Dev. Psychol. **10**, 808–814 (1974)
Ewert, J.P.: Neuro-Ethologie. Einführung in die neurophysiologischen Grundlagen des Verhaltens. Berlin, Heidelberg, New York: Springer 1976
Feder, H.H., Wade, G.N.: Integrative actions of perinatal hormones of neural tissues mediating adult sexual behavior. In: The neurosciences. Third study program. Schmitt, F.O., Worden, F.G. (Hrsg.), S. 583–586. Cambridge, Mass.: The MIT Press 1974
Ferguson, C.A.: Baby talk in six languages. In: Ethnography of communication. Gumperts, J. Hymes, D. (Hrsg.). Suppl. Am. Anthropol. **66**, 103–114 (1964)
Ferguson, C.A., Slobin, D.I.: Studies of child language development. New York: Holt 1973
Fernald, A.: Rhythm and intonation in mothers' speech to newborns, in Vorbereitung
Fernandez de Molina, A., Hunsperger, R.W.: Central representation of affective reactions in forebrain and brain stem: Electrical stimulation of amygdala, stria terminalis, and adjacent structures. J. Physiol. **145**, 251–265 (1959)
Fernandez de Molina, A., Hunsperger, R.W.: Organization of the subcortical system governing defence and flight reactions in the cat. J. Physiol. **160**, 200–213 (1962)
Foerster, O., Gagel, O.: Ein Fall von Ependymcyste des 3. Ventrikels. Ein Beitrag zur Frage der Beziehungen psychischer Störungen zum Hirnstamm. Z. Neurol. **149**, 312–344 (1934)
Fouts, R.S.: Communication with chimpanzees. In: Hominisation und Verhalten. Eibl-Eibesfeldt, I., Kurth, G. (Hrsg.), S. 138–158. Stuttgart: Gustav Fischer 1973a
Fouts, R.S.: Acquisition and testing of gestural signs in four young chimpanzees. Science **180**, 978–980 (1973b)
Fouts, R.S.: Capacities for language in great apes. In: Socioecology and psychology of primates, Tuttle, R.H. (Hrsg.), S. 371–390. Den Haag, Paris: Mouton 1975
Fouts, R.S., Chown, B., Goodin, L.: Transfer of signed responses in American sign language from vocal English stimuli to physical object stimuli by a chimpanzee (Pan). Learning and Motivation **7**, 458–475 (1976)
Freedman, D.G.: Smiling in blind infants and the issue of innate vs. acquired. J. Psychol. Psychiatry **5**, 171–184 (1964)
Freedman, D.G.: Hereditary control of early social behavior. In: Determinants of infant behaviour III. Foss, B.M. (Hrsg.), S. 149–159. London: Methuen 1965
Freedman, D.G.: Human infancy: An evolutionary perspective. Hillsdale, New Jersey: Lawrence Erlbaum Associates 1974
Freud, S.: Drei Abhandlungen zur Sexualtheorie (1905). Gesammelte Werke, Bd. V. Frankfurt: Fischer 1963

Freud, S.: Zur Einführung des Narzißmus (1914). Gesammelte Werke, Bd. X. Frankfurt: Fischer 1963
Friedman, R.C., Richart, R.M., Vande Wiele, R.L. (Hrsg.): Sex differences in behavior. New York: Wiley 1974
Fry, D.B.: The function of the syllable. Z. Phonetik, Sprachwiss. und Kommunikationsforsch. **17**, 225–231 (1964)
Gallup, G.G., jr.: Chimpanzees: self-recognition. Science **167**, 86–87 (1970)
Gallup, G.G., jr.: Towards on operational definition of self-awareness. In: Socioecology and psychology of primates. Tuttle, R.H. (Hrsg.), S. 309–341. The Hague, Paris: Mouton 1975
Gardner, R.A., Gardner, B.T.: Teaching sign language to a chimpanzee. Science **165**, 664–672 (1969)
Gardner, B.T., Gardner, R.A.: Two-way communication with an infant chimpanzee. Behav. Non-Hum. Primates **4**, 117–184 (1971)
Gardner, B.T., Gardner, R.A.: Comparing the early utterances of child and chimpanzee. In: Minnesota symposium on child psychology **8**, 3–23. Pick, A. (Hrsg.). Minneapolis: University of Minnesota Press 1974
Gardner, R.A., Gardner, B.T.: Early signs of language in child and chimpanzee. Science **187**, 752–753 (1975a)
Gardner, B.T., Gardner, R.A.: Evidence for sentence constituents in the early utterance of child and chimpanzee. J. Exp. Psychol. Gen. **104**, 244–267 (1975b)
Garner, R.L.: The speech of monkeys. New York: Webster 1892. Die Sprache der Affen. Leipzig: Seemann 1900
Gehlen, A.: Der Mensch. Seine Natur und seine Stellung in der Welt. Berlin: Junker und Dünnhaupt 1940. (8. Aufl. Frankfurt: Athenäum 1966)
Gewirtz, J.L.: A learning analysis of the effect of normal stimulation, privation and deprivation on the acquisition of social motivation and attachment. In: Determinants of infant behaviour. Foss, B.M. (Hrsg.), S. 213. London: Methuen, New York: Wiley 1961
Gewirtz, J.L.: Mechanisms of social learning: Some roles of stimulation and behavior in early human development. In: Handbook of socialization, theory and research. Goslin, D.A. (Hrsg.), S. 57. Chicago: Rand Mc-Nally 1969
Glasersfeld, E.C. v., Pisani, P.P.: The multistore parser for hierarchical syntactic structures. Commun. Assoc. Computing Machinery **13**, 74–82 (1970)
Gloor, P., Murphy, J.T., Dreifuss, J.J.: Anatomical and physiological characteristics of the two amygdaloid projection system to the ventromedial hypothalamus. In: Limbic system mechanisms and autonomic function. Hockman, Ch.H. (Hrsg.), S. 60–77. Springfield, Ill.: Thomas 1972
Goldfoot, D.A.: Anosmia in male rhesus monkeys does not alter copulatory activity with cycling females. Science **199**, 1095–1096 (1978)
Goodall, J.: Chimpanzees of the gombe stream reserve: In: Primate behavior. DeVore, J. (Hrsg.) New York, Chicago, San Francisco, Toronto, London: Holt, Rinehart and Winston 1965
Goy, R.W., Goldfoot, D.A.: Experimental and hormonal factors influencing development of sexual behavior in the male rhesus monkey. In: The neurosciences. Third study program. Schmitt, F.O., Worden, F.G. (Hrsg.), S. 571–582. Cambridge, Mass.: The MIT Press 1974
Green, St.: Variation of vocal pattern with social situation in the Japanese monkey (Macaca fuscata): a field study. In: Primate behavior, developments in field and laboratory research. Rosenblum, L.A. (Hrsg.), Bd. 4, S. 2–99. New York: Academic Press 1975
Hall, K.R.L.: Social vigilance behaviour of the chacma baboon (Papio ursinus). Behaviour **16**, 261–284 (1960)
Harlow, H.F.: The nature of love. Am. Psychol. **12**, 673–685 (1958)
Harlow, H.F.: Love in infant monkeys. In: Psychobiology. The biological base of behavior. Readings from Scientific American, S. 100–106. San Francisco, London: W.H. Freeman 1967
Harlow, H.F., Harlow, K.: Social deprivation in monkeys. Sci. Am. **207**, 137–146 (1962)
Harlow, H.F., Harlow, M.K.: The affectional systems. In: Behavior of nonhuman primates. Schrier, A.M., Harlow, H.F., Stollnitz, F. (Hrsg.), Bd. II, S. 287–334. New York, London: Academic Press 1965a
Harlow, H.F., Harlow, M.K.: Effects of various mother-infant relationships in rhesus monkey behaviors. In: Determinants of infant behavior IV. Foss, B.M. (Hrsg.), S. 15–36, 283–293. London: Methuen 1965b

Harlow, H.F., Suomi, St.J.: Induced depression in monkeys. Behav. Biol. **12**, 273 (1974)
Harlow, H.F., Zimmermann, R.R.: Affectional responses in the infant monkey. Science **130**, 421–432 (1959)
Harnad, St.R., Steklis, H.D., Lancaster, J. (Hrsg.): Origins and evolution of language and speech. New York: New York Academy of Sciences 1976
Hassler, R.: Funktionelle Neuroanatomie und Psychiatrie. In: Psychiatrie der Gegenwart. Gruhle, H.W., Jung, R., Mayer-Gross, W., Müller, M. (Hrsg.), Bd. I/1 A, S. 153–285. Berlin, Heidelberg, New York: Springer 1967
Hassler, R., Riechert, T., Mundinger, F., Umbach, W., Ganglberger, J.A.: Physiological observations in stereotaxic operations in extrapyramidal motor disturbances. Brain **83**, 337–350 (1960)
Hayes, C.,: The ape in our house. New York: Harper and Row 1951
Head, H.: Aphasia and kindred disorders of speech. London: Cambridge University Press 1926
Hécaen, H., Angelergues, R.: Localization of symptoms in aphasia. In: Disorders of language. Reuck, A.V.S. de, O'Connor, M. (Hrsg.), S. 223–256. London: Churchill 1964
Hécaen, H., Consoli, S.: Analyse des troubles du langage au cours de lésions de l'aire de Broca. Neuropsychologia **11**, 377–388 (1973)
Heimann, H.: Die quantitative Analyse mimischer Bewegungen und ihre Anwendung in der Pharmako-Psychologie. Arzneim.-Forsch. **16**, 294–297 (1966)
Held, R.: Two modes of processing spatially distributed visual stimulation. In: The neurosciences, 2nd study program, Schmitt, F.O., Melnechuk, Th., Adelman, G. (Hrsg.), S. 317–324. New York: The Rockefeller University Press 1970
Henatsch, H.-D.: Bauplan der peripheren und zentralen sensomotorischen Kontrollen. In: Physiologie des Menschen. Bd. 14, Sensomotorik. Gauer, Kramer, Jung (Hrsg.), S. 193–420. München, Berlin, Wien: Urban und Schwarzenberg 1976
Herder, J.G.: Abhandlung über den Ursprung der Sprache. Berlin: Voss 1772
Herrick, C.J.: The functions of the olfactory parts of the cerebral cortex. Proc. Natl. Acad. Sci. USA **19**, 7 (1933)
Herz, A., Bläsig, J.: Neurobiologische Aspekte der Morphin-Abhängigkeit. Naturwissenschaften **61**, 232–238 (1974)
Herzka, H.S.: Das Gesicht des Säuglings: Ausdruck und Reifung. Basel, Stuttgart: Schwabe 1965
Hess, E.H.: Prägung. Die frühkindliche Entwicklung von Verhaltensmustern bei Tier und Mensch. München: Kindler 1975. Originalausgabe: Imprinting. Early experience and the developmental psychobiology of attachment. New York: Van Nostrand, Reinhold Comp. 1973
Hewes, G.W.: Primate communication and the gestural origin of language. Curr. Anthropol. **14**, 5–32 (1973a)
Hewes, G.W.: An explicit formulation of the relationship between tool-using, tool-making and the emergence of language. Visible Lang. **7**, 101–127 (1973b)
Hewes, H.: The current status of the gestural theory of language origin. Ann. N.Y. Acad. Sci. **280**, 482–504 (1976)
Hicks, R.E.: Intrahemispheric response competition between vocal and unimanual performance in normal adult human males. J. Comp. Physiol. Psychol. **89**, 50–60 (1975)
Hilton, S.M., Zbrozyna, A.W.: Amygdaloid region for defense reactions and its efferent pathways to the brainstem. J. Physiol. (Lond.) **165**, 160–173 (1963)
Hinde, R.A.: Rhesus monkey aunts. In: Determinants of infant behavior, Bd. III, Foss, B.M. (Hrsg.), S. 67–71. London: Methuen, New York: Wiley 1965
Hinde, R.A.: Bird vocalizations. London: Cambridge University Press 1969
Hinde, R.A.: Development of social behavior. In: Behavior of nonhuman primates. Modern research trends. Schrier, A.M., Stollnitz, F. (Hrsg.), S. 1–60. New York, London: Academic Press 1971
Hinde, R.A. (Hrsg.): Non-verbal communication. Cambridge: The University Press 1972a
Hinde, R.A.: Concepts of emotion. In: Physiology, emotion and psychosomatic illness. Ciba Foundation Symposium **8** (new series), S. 3–13. Amsterdam: Elsevier Excerpta Medica 1972b
Hinde, R.A.: Das Verhalten der Tiere I und II. Frankfurt: Suhrkamp 1973
Hinde, R.A.: Biological bases of human social behaviour. New York: McGraw-Hill 1974
Hinde, R.A., McGinnis, L.: Some factors influencing the effects of temporary mother-infant separation: some experiments with rhesus monkeys. Psychol. Med. **7**, 197–212 (1977)
Hinde, R.A., Spencer-Booth, Yv.: Effects of brief separation from mother on rhesus monkeys. Science **173**, 111–118 (1971)

Hinde, R.A., White, L.E.: Dynamics of a relationship: rhesus mother-infant ventro-ventral contact. J. Comp. Physiol. Psychol. **86**, 8–23 (1974)

Hinde, R.A., Spencer-Booth, Y., Bruce, M.: Effects of 6-day maternal deprivation on rhesus monkey infants. Nature **210**, 1021–1023 (1966)

Hines, M.: Movements elicited from precentral gyrus of adult chimpanzees by stimulation with sine wave currents. J. Neurophysiol. **3**, 442–466 (1940)

Hockett, C.F.: The problems of universals in language. In: Universals of language. Greenberg, J.H. (Hrsg.), S. 1–22. Cambridge, Mass.: MIT Press 1963

Hockman, Ch.H.: The limbic system mechanisms and autonomic function. Springfield, Ill.: Thomas 1972

Holst, E.v., Mittelstaedt, H.: Das Reafferenzprinzip. Naturwissenschaften **37**, 464–476 (1950)

Honkavaara, S.: The psychology of expression. Br. J. Physiol. Monogr. Suppl. **32**, 1–96 (1961)

Hooff, J.A.R.A.M., van: The facial display of the catarrhine monkeys and apes. In: Primate ethology. Morris, D. (Hrsg.), S. 7–68. London: Weidenfeld and Nicolson 1967

Hooff, J.A.R.A.M., van: Aspecten van Het Sociale Gedrag En De Communicatie Bij Humane En Hogere Niet-Humane Primaten. (Aspects of the social behaviour and communication in human and higher non-human primates.) Rotterdam: Bronder-Offset 1971

Hopf, S.: Report on a hand-reared squirrel monkey (Saimiri sciureus). Z. Tierpsychol. **27**, 610–621 (1970)

Hopf, S.: New findings on the the ontogeny of social behaviour in the squirrel monkey. Psychiat. Neurol. Neurochir. **74**, 21–34 (1971)

Hopf, S.: Sozialpsychologische Untersuchungen zur Verhaltensentwicklung des Totenkopfaffen. Inaugural-Diss. Marburg 1972

Hopf, S.: Huddling subgroups in captive squirrel monkeys and their changes in relation to ontogeny. Biol. of Behaviour **3**, 147–162 (1978)

Hückstedt, B.: Experimentelle Untersuchungen zum „Kindchenschema". Z. Exp. Angew. Psychol. **12**, 421–450 (1965)

Humboldt, W. v.: In: Werke Bd. IV (S. 14, 242); Bd. XVI (S. 177), Bd. VI (S. 21–27, 145). Hrsg. Königlich Preußische Akademie der Wissenschaften. Berlin: B. Behr 1915. Nachdruck: Berlin: de Gruyter 1968.

Humphrey, N.R., Weiskrantz, L.: Vision in monkeys after removal of the striate cortex. Nature **215**, 595–597 (1967)

Hunsperger, R.A., Bucher, V.M.: Affective behaviour produced by electrical stimulation in the forebrain and brain stem of the cat. Progr. Brain Res. **27**, 103–127 (1967)

Hupfer, K., Jürgens, U., Ploog, D.: The effects of superior temporal lesions of the recognition of species-specific calls in the squirrel monkey. Exp. Brain Res. **30**, 75–87 (1977)

Hutchison, J.B.: Differential hypothalamic sensitivity to androgen in the activation of reproductive behavior. In: The neurosciences. Third study program. Schmitt, F.O., Worden, F.G. (Hrsg.), S. 593–598. Cambridge, Mass.: The MIT Press 1974

Huxley, J.S.: Courtship activities in the red-throated diver (Colymbus stellatus Pontopp) together with a discussion of the evolution of courtship in birds. J. Linnean Society London. J. Zool. **35**, 253–292 (1923)

Huxley, J.S.: A discussion on ritualization of behavior in animals and man. Philos. Trans. R. Soc. Lond. **251**, 247–349 (1966)

Immelmann, K.: Song development in the zebra finch and other estrildid finches. In: Bird vocalizations. Hinde, R.A. (Hrsg.), S. 61–74. London, New York: Cambridge University Press 1969

Isaacson, R.L.: The limbic system. New York, London: Plenum Press 1974

Itani, J.: Vocal communication of the wild Japanese monkey. Primates **4**, 11–66 (1963)

Itard, C.E.: The face of emotion. New York: Appleton 1971

Jackson, J.H.: Croonian lectures on the evolution and dissolution of the nervous system. Lancet **8**, 555–558, 739–744, 649–652 (1884)

Jänig, W.: Das vegetative Nervensystem. In: Einführung in die Physiologie des Menschen. Schmidt, R.F., Thews, G. (Hrsg.), S. 114 ff. Berlin, Heidelberg, New York: Springer 1976

Jakobson, R.: Kindersprache, Aphasie und allgemeine Lautgesetze. Frankfurt: Suhrkamp 1969 (Nachdruck), Erstdruck in Uppsala 1944

Janzarik, W.: Themen und Tendenzen der deutschsprachigen Psychiatrie. Berlin, Heidelberg, New York: Springer 1974

Jennings, H.S.: The behavior of the lower organisms. New York: Wiley 1951 (1. Aufl. 1906)
Jensen, G.D., Tolman, C.W.: Mother-infant relationship in the monkey, Macaca nemestrina: The effect of brief separation and mother-infant specificity. J. Comp. Physiol. Psychol. **55**, 131 (1962)
Jensen, G.D., Bobitt, R., Gordon, B.N.: Mother and infant roles in the development of independence of Macaca nemestrina. In: Behavioral regulators in behavior in primates. Carpenter, C.R. (Hrsg.), S. 218–228. Lewisburg: Bucknell University Press 1973
Jolly, A.: Die Entwicklung des Primatenverhaltens. Stuttgart: G. Fischer 1975
Jones, I.H.: Stereotyped aggression in a group of Australian western desert aborigines. Br. J. Med. Psychol. **44**, 259–265 (1971)
Jones, B.C., Clark, D.L.: Mother-infant separation in squirrel monkeys living in a group. Dev. Psychobiol. **6**, 259–269 (1973)
Jones, I.H., Frei, D.: Provoked anxiety as a treatment of exhibitionism. Br. J. Psychiatry **131**, 295–300 (1977)
Jürgens, U.: Soziales Verhalten, Kommunikation und Hirnmechanismen. Umschau **71**, 799–802 (1971)
Jürgens, U.: The elicitability of vocalization from the cortical larynx area. Brain Res. **81**, 564–566 (1974)
Jürgens, U.: Reinforcing concomitants of electrically elicited vocalizations. Exp. Brain Res. **26**, 203–214 (1976)
Jürgens, U.: Intracranielle Selbstreizung – ein Modell zum Suchtverhalten. In: Sucht als Symptom. Keup, W. (Hrsg.), S. 19–23. Stuttgart: Thieme 1978
Jürgens, U.: Vocalization as an emotional indicator. A neuroethological study in the squirrel monkey. Behaviour **69**, 88–117 (1979)
Jürgens, U., Müller-Preuss, P.: Convergent projections of different limbic vocalization areas in the squirrel monkey. Exp. Brain Res. **29**, 75–83 (1977)
Jürgens, U., Ploog, D.: Cerebral representation of vocalization in the squirrel monkey. Exp. Brain Res. **10**, 532–554 (1970)
Jürgens, U., Ploog, D.: Von der Ethologie zur Psychologie. München: Kindler 1974
Jürgens, U., Ploog, D.: Zur Evolution der Stimme. Arch. Psychiatr. Nervenkr. **222**, 117–137 (1976)
Jung, R.: Selbstreizung des Gehirns im Tierversuch. Dtsch. Med. Wochenschr. **1958**, 1716–1721
Jung, R.: Einführung in die Bewegungsphysiologie. In: Physiologie des Menschen, Bd. 14, Sensomotorik. Gauer, O., Kramer, K., Jung, R. (Hrsg.), S. 1–98. München, Berlin, Wien: Urban und Schwarzenberg 1976
Kaila, E.: Die Reaktionen des Säuglings auf das menschliche Gesicht. Ann. Univ. Aboensis, Ser. B **17**, 114 (1932)
Kaufman, I.Ch.: The role of ontogeny in the establishment of species-specific patterns. In: Early development. Res. Publ. Assoc. Res. Nerv. Ment. Dis. **51**, 381–397 (1973)
Kaufman, I.Ch.: Developmental considerations of anxiety and depression. Psychobiological studies in monkeys. In: Psychoanalysis and contemporary science. Shapiro, T. (Hrsg.), S. 317–363. New York: Intern. University Press 1977
Kaufman, I.Ch., Rosenblum, L.A.: The reaction to separation in infant monkeys: anaclitic depression and conservation-withdrawal. Psychosom. Med. **29**, 648–675 (1967a)
Kaufman, I.Ch., Rosenblum, L.A.: Depression in infant monkeys separated from their mothers. Science **155**, 1030–1031 (1967b)
Kaufman, I.Ch., Rosenblum, L.A.: Effects of separation from mother on the emotional behavior of infant monkeys. Ann. N.Y. Acad. Sci. **159**, 681–695 (1969)
Kellogg, W.N.: Communication and language in the home-raised chimpanzee. Science **162**, 423–427 (1968)
Kellogg, W.N., Kellogg, L.A.: The ape and the child: A study of environmental influence upon early behavior. New York: McGraw-Hill 1933, Nachdruck 1967
Kelly, A.H., Beaton, L.E., Magoun, H.W.: A midbrain mechanism for facio-vocal activity. J. Neurophysiol. **9**, 181–189 (1946)
Kelly, D.B., Morell, J.I., Pfaff, D.W.: Autoradiographic localization of hormone concentrating cells in the brain of an amphibian, Xenopus laevis. I. Testosterone. J. Comp. Neurol. **164**, 47–62 (1975)
Kendon, A., Ferber, A.: A description of some human greetings. In: Comparative ecology and

behaviour of primates. Michael, R.P., Crook, J.H. (Hrsg.), S. 591–668. London, New York: Academic Press 1973

King, J.E., King, P.A.: Early behavior in hand-reared squirrel monkeys (Saimiri sciureus). Dev. Psychobiol. **2**, 251–256 (1970)

Klaus, M.H., Kennell, J.H.: Maternal-infant-bonding. Saint Louis: Mosby 1976

Kleist, K.: Gehirnpathologie. Leipzig: Barth 1934

Klima, E.S. Bellugi, U.: The signs of language in child and chimpanzee. In: Communication and affect: A comparative approach. Alloway, T., Krames, L., Pliner, P. (Hrsg.). New York: Academic Press 1972

Klineberg, O.: Social psychology. New York: Holt 1940

Klüver, H.: Behavior mechanisms in monkeys, S. 259–292. Chicago: University of Chicago Press 1933. Neuaufl. New York: Phoenix Science Series 1957

Klüver, H.: Re-examination of implement-using behavior in a cebus monkey after an interval of three years. Acta Psychol. **II**, 347–397 (1937)

Klüver, H.: Brain mechanisms and behavior with special reference to the rhinencephalon. Lancet **72**, 567–577 (1952)

Klüver, H., Bucy P.C.: "Psychic blindness" and other symptoms following bilateral temporal lobectomy in rhesus monkeys. Am. J. Physiol. **119**, 352 (1937)

Klüver, H., Bucy, P.C.: An analysis of certain effects of bilateral temporal lobectomy in the rhesus monkey with special reference to "psychic blindness". J. Psychol. **5**, 33–54 (1938)

Klüver, H., Bucy, P.C.: Preliminary analysis of functions of the temporal lobes in monkeys. A.M.A. Arch. Neurol. Psychiatry **42**, 979–1000 (1939)

Koehler, O.: Das Lächeln als angeborene Ausdrucksbewegung. Z. Menschl. Vererb. u. Konstit.-Lehre **32**, 390–398 (1954a)

Koehler, O.: Vom Erbgut der Sprache. Homo **5**, 97–104 (1954b)

Köhler, W.: Intelligenzprüfungen an Menschenaffen. Berlin, Göttingen, Heidelberg: Springer 1921, 2. Auflage 1963

Köhler, W.: The mentality of apes. New York: Brace and World 1925. Nachdruck London: Penguin 1957

Koenig, O.: Kultur und Verhaltensforschung. Einführung in die Kulturethologie. München: dtv 1970

Kondo, S., Kawai, M., Ehara, A.: Contemporary primatology. Proc. fifth internat. congr. primatol. Nagoya, August 1974. Basel: Karger 1975

Konorski, J., Kozniewska, H., Stepien, L., Subczynski, J.: Pathophysiological mechanism of disorder of higher nervous activity after brain lesions in man. Warschau: Poln. Akad. Wiss. 1961

Kornhuber, H.: Tastsinn und Lagesinn. In: Physiologie des Menschen, Bd. 11, Gauer, O., Kramer, K., Jung, R., (Hrsg.), S. 51–112. München, Berlin, Wien: Urban und Schwarzenberg 1972

Kortlandt, A.: How do chimpanzees use weapons when fighting leopards? Year book of the Am. Philosoph. Soc. **1965**, 327–332

Kortlandt, A., Kooij, M.: Protohominid behaviour in primates (preliminary communication). Symp. Zool. Soc., Lond. **10**, 61–88 (1963)

Kraepelin, E.: Die Erscheinungsformen des Irreseins. Z. gesamte Neurol. Psychiatr. **62**, 1–29 (1920)

Kramer, E.: Elimination of verbal cues in judgement of emotion from voice. J. Abnorm. Soc. Psychol. **68**, 390–396 (1964)

Kranz, H., Heinrich, K. (Hrsg.): Psychiatrische und ethologische Aspekte abnormen Verhaltens. 1. Düsseldorfer Symposium 1974. Stuttgart: Thieme 1975

Kreutzer, M.A., Charlesworth, W.R.: Infants' reaction to different expressions of emotions. Paper presented at the Society of Research in Child Development. Philadelphia, March 1973

Kuhar, M.J., Pert, C.B., Snyder, S.H.: Regional distribution of opiate receptor binding in monkey and human brain. Nature **245**, 447–450 (1973)

Kummer, H.: Soziales Verhalten einer Mantelpavian-Gruppe. Bern, Stuttgart: Huber 1957. Schweiz. Z. Psychol. Suppl. 33

Kummer, H.: Social organization of Hamadryas-baboons. A field study. Basel, New York: Karger 1968

Kurth, G., Eibl-Eibesfeldt, I. (Hrsg.): Hominisation und Verhalten. Stuttgart: Fischer 1975

Kuypers, H.G.J.M.: Some projections from the peri-central cortex to the pons and lower brain stem in monkey and chimpanzee. J. Comp. Neurol. **110**, 221–255 (1958a)

Kuypers, H.G.J.M.: Corticobulbar connexions to the pons and lower brain stem in man. Brain **81**, 364–388 (1958b)

LaBarre, W.: The cultural basis of emotions and gestures. J. Personal. **16**, 49–68 (1947)

Ladygina-Kohts, N.N.: Affenkind und Menschenkind, ihre Instinkte, Emotionen, Spiele, Gewohnheiten und Ausdrucksbewegungen. Moskau: Staatsverlag Museum Darwinianum, 1935

Lang, E.M.: Jambo – First gorilla raised by its mother in captivity. Natl. Geographic **125**, 446–453 (1964)

Lasky, R.E., Syrdal-Lasky, A., Klein, R.E.: VOT discrimination by four- and six-and-a-half monthold infants from Spanish environments. J. Exp. Child. Psychol. **20**, 215–225 (1975)

Latta, J., Hopf, S., Ploog, D.: Observation on mating behavior and sexual play in the squirrel monkey (Saimiri sciureus). Primates **8**, 229–246 (1967)

Lawick-Goodall, J., van: My friends, the wild chimpanzees. Washington: National Geographic Society 1967a

Lawick-Goodall, J., van: Mother-offspring relationships in free-ranging chimpanzees. In: Primate ethology. Morris, D. (Hrsg.), S. 365–436. London: Weidenfeld und Nicolson 1967b

Lawick-Goodall, J., van: A preliminary report on expressive movements and communication in the gombe stream chimpanzee. In: Primates: Studies in adaption and variability. Jay, P.C. (Hrsg.). New York: Holt 1968a

Lawick-Goodall, J., van: The behavior of free-living chimpanzees in the gombe stream reserve. Anim. Behav. Monogr. **1**, 161–311 (1968b)

Lawick-Goodall, J., van: The behaviour of the chimpanzee. In: Hominisation und Verhalten. Kurth, G., Eibl-Eibesfeldt, I. (Hrsg.), S. 74–136. Stuttgart: Fischer 1975

Lecours, H.R., Lhermitte, F.: The "pure form" of the phonetic disintegration syndrome (pure anarthria); anatomoclinical report of a historical case. Brain Lang. **3**, 88–113 (1976)

Lenneberg, E.H.: On explaining language. Science **164**, 635–643 (1969)

Lenneberg, E.H.: Of language knowledge, apes and brains. J. Psycholing. Res. **1**, 1–29 (1971)

Lenneberg, E.H.: Biological foundations of language. New York, London, Sidney: Wiley 1967. Deutsche Ausgabe: Biologische Grundlagen der Sprache. Frankfurt: Suhrkamp 1972

Lenneberg, E.H.: The concept of language differentiation. In: Foundations of language development. A multidisciplinary approach. Lenneberg, E.H., Lenneberg E. (Hrsg.), Bd. 1, S. 17–33. New York: Academic Press Inc. and Paris: The Unesco Press 1975

Lenneberg, E.H., Rebelsky, F.G., Nichols, I.A.: The vocalization of infants born to deaf and to hearing parents. Hum. Dev. **8**, 23–37 (1965)

Leonhard, K.: Der menschliche Ausdruck. Leipzig: Barth 1968

Lewis, J.K., McKinney, W.T., jr.: The effect of electrically induced convulsions on the behavior of normal and abnormal rhesus monkey. Dis. Nerv. Syst. **37**, 687–693 (1976)

Leyhausen, P.: Biologie von Ausdruck und Eindruck. In: Antriebe tierischen und menschlichen Verhaltens. Gesammelte Abhandlungen. Lorenz, K., Leyhausen, P. (Hrsg.), S. 297–436. München: Piper Paperback 1968

Leyhausen, P.: Verhaltensstudien an Katzen. 3. Aufl. Berlin, Hamburg: Parey 1973

Leyton, A.S.F., Sherrington, C.S.: Observations on the excitable cortex of the chimpanzee, orangutan, and gorilla. Q. J. Exp. Physiol. **11**, 135–222 (1917)

Lhermitte, F., Chain, F., Escourolle, R., Ducame, B., Pillon, B., Chedru, F.: Etude des troubles perceptifs auditifs dans les lésions temporales bilatérales. Rev. Neurol. **124**, 329–351 (1971)

Liberman, A.M., Pisoni, D.B.: Evidence for a special speech-perceiving subsystem in the human. In: Recognition of complex acoustic signals. Bullock, T.H. (Hrsg.), S. 56–76. Dahlem Konferenzen, Life Sciences Research Report 5, Berlin: Abakon Verlagsgesellschaft 1977

Liberman, A.M., Cooper, F.S., Shankweiler, D.P., Studdert-Kennedy, M.: Perception of the speech code. Psychol. Rev. **74**, 431–461 (1967)

Lichtheim, L.: Über Aphasie. Dt. Archiv Klin. Med. Leipzig S. 204–268 (1885)

Limber, J.: Language in child and chimpanzee? Am. Psychol. **32**, 280–295 (1977)

Lind, J., Vuorenkoski, V., Rosberg, G., Partanan, T.J., Wasz-Höckert, O.: Spectrographic analysis of vocal response to pain in infants with Down's syndrome. Dev. Med. Children Neurol. **12**, 478–486 (1970)

Lisker, L., Abramson, A.S.: A cross-language study of voicing in initial stops: acoustical measurements. Word **20**, 384–422 (1964)

Loizos, C.: Play behavior in higher primates: a review. In: Primate ethology. Morris, D. (Hrsg.), S. 176–218. London: Weidenfeld und Nicolson 1967
Lorenz, K.: Der Kumpan in der Umwelt des Vogels. J. Ornithol. **83**, 137–213, 289–413 (1935)
Lorenz, K.: Über die Bildung des Instinktbegriffes. Naturwissenschaften **25**, 289–300, 307–318, 324–331 (1937)
Lorenz, K.: Die angeborenen Formen möglicher Erfahrung. Z. Tierpsychol. **5**, 235–409 (1943)
Lorenz, K.: Über angeborene Instinktformen beim Menschen. Dtsch. Med. Wochenschr. **78**, 1566–1569, 1600–1604 (1953)
Lorenz, K.: Das sogenannte Böse. Wien: Borotha-Schoeler 1963
Lorenz, K.: Über tierisches und menschliches Verhalten. Aus dem Werdegang der Verhaltenslehre. Gesammelte Abhandlungen, 2 Bde. München: Piper 1965
Luria, A.R.: Factors and forms of aphasia. In: Disorders of language. Reuck, A.V.S. de, O'Connors, A. (Hrsg.), S. 143–167. London: Churchill 1964
MacKay, D.M.: The epistemological problem for automata. In: Automata studies. Shannon, C.E., McCarty, J. (Hrsg.), S. 235–251. Princeton, N.J.: Princeton University Press 1956
MacKay, D.M.: A mind's eye view of the brain. In: Cybernetics of the nervous system. Progress in brain research 17, Wiener, N., Schadé, J.P. (Hrsg.), S. 321–332. Amsterdam: Elsevier 1965a
MacKay, D.M.: Cerebral organization and the conscious control of action. In: Brain and conscious experience. Eccles, J.C. (Hrsg.), S. 422–445. New York: Springer 1965b
MacLean, P.D.: Psychosomatic disease and the "visceral brain". Psychosom. Med. **11**, 338–353 (1949)
MacLean, P.D.: Some psychiatric implications of physiological studies on fronto-temporal portion of limbic system (visceral brain). Electroencephalogr. Clin. Neurophysiol. **4**, 407–418 (1952)
MacLean, P.D.: The limbic system and its hippocampal formation: studies in animals and their possible application to man. J. Neurosurg. **11**, 29–44 (1954)
MacLean, P.D.: The limbic system with respect to self-preservation and the preservation of the species. J. Nerv. Ment. Dis. **127**, 1–11 (1958)
MacLean, P.D.: New findings relevant to the evolution of psychosexual functions of the brain. J. Nerv. Ment. Dis. **135**, 289–301 (1962)
MacLean, P.D.: The triune brain, emotion and scientific bias. In: The neurosciences. 2nd study program. Schmitt, F.O., Quarton, G.C., Melnechuk, Th., Adelman, G. (Hrsg.), S. 336–349. New York: The Rockefeller University Press 1970
MacLean, P.D.: Cerebral evolution and emotional processes: new findings on the striatal complex. Ann. N.Y. Acad. Sci. **193**, 137–149 (1972a)
MacLean, P.D.: Implications of microelectrode findings on exteroceptive inputs to the limbic cortex. In: Limbic system mechanisms and autonomic function. Hockmann, Ch.H. (Hrsg.). Springfield: Thomas 1972b
MacLean, P.D.: A mind of three minds: educating the triune brain. In: Education and the brain, 77th Yearbook of the National Society for the Study of Education, S. 308–342. Chicago, Ill.: The University of Chicago Press 1978
MacLean, P.D., Ploog, D.: Cerebral representation of penile erection. J. Neurophysiol. **25**, 29–55 (1962)
MacLean, P.D., Denniston, R.H., Dua, S.: Further studies on cerebral representation of penile erection: caudal thalamus midbrain and pons. J. Neurophysiol. **26**, 273–293 (1963a)
MacLean, P.D., Dua, S., Denniston, R.H.: Cerebral localization for scratching and seminal discharge. Arch. Neurol. **9**, 485–497 (1963b)
Magoun, H.W., Atlas, D., Ingersoll, E.H., Ranson, S.W.: Associated facial, vocal and respiratory components of emotional expression: An experimental study. J. Neurol. Psychopathol. **17**, 241–255 (1937)
Malson, L., Itard, J., Mannoni, O.: Die wilden Kinder. Frankfurt: Suhrkamp 1972. Originaltitel: Les enfants sauvages, Mythe et Réalité. Union Générale d'Editions 1964
Manley, J.A., Müller-Preuss, P.: Response variability of auditory cortex cells in the squirrel monkey to constant acoustic stimuli. Exp. Brain Res. **32**, 171–180 (1978)
Mark, H., Ervin, F.R.: Violence and the brain. New York: Harper and Row 1970
Marler, P.: The logical analysis of animal communication. J. Theor. Biol. **1**, 295–317 (1961)
Marler, P.: Inheritance and learning in the development of animal vocalizations. In: Acoustic behaviour of animals. Busnel, R.G. (Hrsg.), S. 228–243, 794–797. Amsterdam: Elsevier 1963

Marler, P.: Communication in monkeys and apes. In: Primate behavior. DeVore, I. (Hrsg.), S. 544–584. New York: Rinehart und Winston 1965
Marler, P.: Vocalization of wild chimpanzees. In: Proc. 2nd Internat. Congr. of Primatol. I: Behaviour. Carpenter, C.R. (Hrsg.), S. 94–100. Basel: Karger 1969
Marler, P.: A comparative approach to vocal learning: Song development in white-crowned sparrows. J. Comp. Physiol. Psychol. **71**, 1–25 (1970)
Marler, P.: Development and learning of recognition systems. In: Recognition of complex acoustic signals. Bullock, Th.H. (Hrsg.), S. 77–96. Dahlem Konferenzen. Life Sciences Research Report **5**, 1977
Marler, P., Hamilton, W.J.: Mechanisms of animal behavior. New York: Wiley 1966
Martinius, J.W., Papoušek, H.: Response to optic and exteroceptive stimuli in relation to state in the human newborn: habituation of the blink reflex. Neuropädiatrie **1**, 452–460 (1970)
Mason, W.A.: The social development of monkeys and apes. In: Primate behavior. DeVore, I. (Hrsg.), S. 514–543. New York: Holt, Rinehart und Winston 1965
Mason, W.A.: Early social deprivation in the nonhuman primates: Implication for human behavior. In: Biology and behavior. Environmental influences. Glass, D.C. (Hrsg.), S. 70–101. New York: The Rockefeller University Press and Russel Sage Foundation 1968
Mason, W.A.: Maternal attributes and primate cognitive development. In: Human ethology. Claims and limits of a new discipline. Cranach, M.v., Foppa, K., Lepenies, W., Ploog, D. (Hrsg.). Cambridge: Cambridge University Press 1979
Mattingly, I.G.: Speech cues and sign stimuli. Am. Sci. **60**, 327 (1972)
Maurus, M., Ploog, D.: Social signals in squirrel monkeys: analysis by cerebral radio stimulation. Exp. Brain Res. **12**, 171–183 (1971)
Maurus, M., Pruscha, H.: Quantitative analyses of behavioral sequences elicited by automated telestimulation in squirrel monkeys. Exp. Brain Res. **14**, 372–394 (1972)
Maurus, M., Pruscha, H.: Classification of social signals in squirrel monkeys by means of cluster analysis. Behaviour **47**, 106–128 (1973)
Maurus, M., Mitra, J., Ploog, D.: Cerebral representation of the clitoris in ovariectomized squirrel monkeys. Exp. Neurol. **13**, 283–288 (1966)
Maurus, M., Kühlmorgen, B., Hartmann, E.: Concerning the influence of experimental conditions on social interactions initiated by telestimulation in squirrel monkey groups. Brain Res. **64**, 271–280 (1973)
Maurus, M., Hartmann, E., Kühlmorgen, B.: Invariant quantities in communication processes of squirrel monkeys. Primates **15**, 179–192 (1974)
Maurus, M., Kühlmorgen, B., Hartmann-Wiesner, E., Pruscha, H.: An approach to the interpretation of the communicative meaning of visual signals in agonistic behavior of squirrel monkeys. Folia Primatol. (Basel) **23**, 206–226 (1975)
Mayr, E.: The emergence of evolutionary novelties. In: Evolution after Darwin. Tax, S. (Hrsg.), S. 349–380. Chicago: University of Chicago Press 1960
McEwen, B.S., Denef, C.J., Gerlach, J.L., Plapinger, L.: Chemical studies of the brain as a steroid hormone target tissue. In: The neurosciences. Third study program. Schmitt, F.O., Worden, F.G. (Hrsg.), S. 599–620. Cambridge, Mass.: The MIT Press 1974
McGrew, W.C.: An ethological study of children's behavior. New York, London: Academic Press 1972
McGuire, M.T., Fairbanks, L.A. (Hrsg.): Ethological psychiatry. Psychopathology in the context of evolutionary biology. Seminars in psychiatry. Milton Greenblatt, Series Editor. New York: Grune and Stratton 1977
McKinney, W.T., Suomi, St.J., Harlow, H.F.: Repetitive peer separations of juvenile-age rhesus monkeys. Arch. Gen. Psychiatry **27**, 200–203 (1972)
McKinney, W.T., Young, L.D., Suomi, St.J., Davis, J.M.: Chlorpromazine treatment of disturbed monkeys. Arch. Gen. Psychiatry **29**, 490–494 (1973)
McNeill, D.: The acquisition of language. New York: Harper and Row 1970
Menzel, E.W.: Natural language of young chimpanzees. New Scientist **65**, 127–130 (1975)
Menzel, E.W., Halperin, S.: Purposive behavior as a basis for objective communication between chimpanzees. Science **189**, 652–654 (1975)
Merkenschlager, F., Saller, K.: Kaspar Hauser. Ein zeitloses Problem. Nürnberg: Lorenz Spindler 1966

Michael, R.P. (Hrsg.): Endocrinology and human behaviour. Proc. of a conference held at the Institute of Psychiatry. London, 9 to 11 May 1967. London, New York, Toronto: Oxford University Press 1968

Michael, R.P., Crook, J.H. (Hrsg.): Comparative ecology and behaviour of primates. Proc. of a conference held at the Zool. Soc. London, November 1971. London, New York: Academic Press 1973

Michael, R.P., Bonsall, R.W., Zumpe, D.: Evidence for chemical communication in primates. Vitam. Horm. **34**, 137–185 (1976a)

Michael, R.P., Bonsall, R.W., Zumpe, D.: Letters to the Editor: "Lack of effects of vaginal fatty acids, etc." A reply to Goldfoot et al. Horm. Behav. **7**, 365–367 (1976b)

Miles, L.W.: The communicative competence of child and chimpanzee. Ann. N.Y. Acad. Sci. **280**, 592–597 (1976)

Miles, L.W.: Language acquisition in apes and children. In: An account of the visual mode: Man versus ape. Peng, F.C.C. (Hrsg.). Am. Assoc. Adv. Sci. (in press)

Miller, J.L., Eimas, P.D.: Studies on the selective tuning of feature detectors for speech. J. Phonetics **4**, 119–127 (1976)

Miller, R.E.: Experimental approaches to the physiological and behavioral concomitants of affective communication in rhesus monkeys. In: Social communications among primates. Altmann, S.A. (Hrsg.), S. 125–134. Chicago: University of Chicago Press 1967

Miller, R.E., Caul, W.F., Mirsky, I.A.: Communication of affects between feral and socially isolated monkeys. J. Pers. Soc. Psychol. **7**, 231–239 (1967)

Minde, K.: Persönliche Mitteilung 1978

Moffitt, A.R.: Consonant cue perception by twenty to twenty-four-week-old infants. Child Dev. **42**, 717–731 (1971)

Mogenson, G.J.: The neurobiology of behavior. An introduction. New Jersey: Hillsdale 1977

Morath, M.: Differences in the non-crying vocalizations of infants in the first four months of life. Neuropädiatrie (Suppl.) **8**, 543–545 (1977)

Morris, D.: Primate ethology. London: Weidenfeld and Nicolson 1967

Morse, P.A.: The discrimination of speech and non-speech stimuli in early infancy. J. Exp. Child Psychol. **14**, 477–492 (1972)

Morse, P.A., Snowden, C.T.: An investigation of categorical speech discrimination by rhesus monkeys. Perception and Psychophysics **17**, 9–16 (1975)

Moynihan, M.: Some behavior patterns of platyrrhine monkeys. I. The night monkey (Aotus trivirgatus). Smithson. Misc. Coll. **146**, 1–84 (1964)

Moynihan, M.: Communication in callicebus. J. Zool. Lond. **150**, 77–127 (1966)

Müller, D., Orthner, H., Roeder, F., König, A., Bosse, K., Kloos, G.: Einfluß von Hypothalamusläsionen auf Sexualverhalten und gonadotrope Funktion beim Menschen. Bericht über 23 Fälle. In: Endocrinology of sex. Dörner, G. (Hrsg.), S. 80–105. Leipzig: Barth 1974

Müller-Preuss, P., Jürgens, U.: Projection from the cingular vocalization area in the squirrel monkey. Brain Res. **103**, 29–43 (1976)

Murphy, M.R., Schneider, G.E.: Olfactory bulb removal eliminating mating behavior in the male golden hamster. Science **167**, 302–304 (1970)

Nakazima, S.: Phonemicization and symbolization in language development. In: Foundations of language development. A multidisciplinary approach, Bd. I, Lenneberg, E.H., Lenneberg, E. (Hrsg.), S. 181–187. London, New York: Academic Press 1975

Napier, J.R., Napier, P.N.: A handbook of living primates. New York: Academic Press 1967

Nauta, W.J.H., Karten, H.J.: A general profile of the vertebrate brain, with side lights on the ancestry of cerebral cortex. In: The neurosciences, 2nd study program. Schmitt, F.O. (Hrsg.), S. 11. New York: The Rockefeller University 1971

Neff, W.D., Diamond, I.T., Casseday, J.H.: Behavioral studies of auditory discrimination central nervous system. In: Handbook of sensory physiology Bd. V/2, Keidel, W.D., Neff, W.D. (Hrsg.), S. 307–400. Berlin, Heidelberg, New York: Springer 1975

Newman, J.D.: Biological filtering and neural mechanisms (Group report). In: Recognition of complex acoustic signals. Bullock, Th.H. (Hrsg.), S. 279–306. Dahlem Konferenzen, Life Sciences Research, Report 5. Berlin: Abakon Verlagsgesellschaft 1977

Newman, J.D., Symmes, D.: Vocal pathology in socially deprived monkeys. Dev. Psychobiol. **7**, 351–358 (1974a)

Newman, J.D., Symmes, D.: Arousal effects on unit responsiveness to vocalization in squirrel monkey auditory cortex. Brain Res. **78**, 125–138 (1974b)

Newman, J.D., Wollberg, Z.: Multiple coding of species-specific vocalizations in the auditory cortex of squirrel monkeys. Brain Res. **54**, 287–304 (1973a)

Newman, J.D., Wollberg, Z.: Responses of single neurons in the auditory cortex of squirrel monkeys of variants of a single cell type. Exp. Neurol. **40**, 821–824 (1973b)

Newport, E.L.: Motherese: The speech of mothers to young children. In: Cognitive theory, Bd. 2. Castellan, N.J., Jr., Pisoni, D.B., Potts, G.R. (Hrsg.), S. 177–217. New York: Wiley 1977

Nicolai, J.: Familientradition in der Gesangstradition des Gimpels (Pyrrhula pyrrhula L.). J. Ornithol. **100**, 39–46 (1959)

Nottebohm, F.: Neural lateralization of vocal control in a passerine bird. II. Subsong, calls and a theory of vocal learning. J. Exp. Zool. **179**, 35–50 (1972)

Nottebohm, F.: A zoologist's view of some language phenomena with particular emphasis on vocal learning. In: Foundations of language development. A multidisciplinary approach, Lenneberg, E.H., Lenneberg, E. (Hrsg.), S. 61–103. New York, London: Academic Press 1975

Oerter, R.: Moderne Entwicklungspsychologie. 13. Aufl. Donauwörth: Auer 1973

Olds, J.: Drives and reinforcements. Behavioral studies of hypothalamic functions. New York: Raven Press 1977

Olds, J., Milner, P.: Positive reinforcement produced by electrical stimulation of septal area and other regions of rat brain. J. Comp. Physiol. Psychol. **47**, 419–427 (1954)

Oscarsson, O.: Functional organization of spinocerebellar paths. In: Handbook of sensory physiology, Bd. II. Somatosensory system. Iggo, A. (Hrsg.), S. 339–380. Berlin, Heidelberg, New York: Springer 1973

Papez, J.W.: A proposed mechanism of emotion. Arch. Neurol. Psychiatry (Chicago) **38**, 725–743 (1937)

Papoušek, H.: Conditioned head rotating reflexes in infants in the first months of life. Acta Paediatr. (Uppsala) **50**, 565–576 (1961)

Papoušek, H.: Unveröffentlichte Befunde 1975

Papoušek, H.: Individual differences in adaptive processes of infants. In: Genetics, environment and intelligence. Oliverio, A. (Hrsg.), S. 269–283. Amsterdam: Elsevier/North-Holland Biomedical Press 1977

Papoušek, H., Bernstein, P.: The functions of conditioning stimulation in human neonates and infants. In: Stimulation in early infancy. Ambrose, A. (Hrsg.). London: Academic Press 1969

Papoušek, H., Papoušek, M.: Mirror image and self-recognition in young human infants: I. A new method of experimental analysis. Dev. Psychobiol. **7**, 149–157 (1974)

Papoušek, H., Papoušek, M.: Cognitive aspects of preverbal social interaction between human infant and adults. In: Parent-infant interaction. O'Connor, M. (Hrsg.), S. 241–260. Amsterdam: Elsevier 1975

Papoušek, H., Papoušek, M.: Mothering and the cognitive head-start: psychobiological considerations. In: Studies in mother infant interaction, The Loch Lomond Symp. Schaffer, H.R. (Hrsg.), S. 63–85. London: Academic Press 1976

Papoušek, H., Papoušek, M.: Die Entwicklung kognitiver Funktionen im Säuglingsalter. Der Kinderarzt **8**, 1071–1189 (1977)

Papoušek, H., Papoušek, M.: Early ontogeny of human social interaction: Its biological roots and social dimensions. In: Human ethology. Claims and limits of a new discipline. Cranach, M.v., Foppa, K., Lepenies, W., Ploog, D. (Hrsg.). Cambridge: Cambridge University Press 1979

Papoušek, H., Papoušek, M.: Die Frühentwicklung des Sozialverhaltens und der Kommunikation. In: Kinder- und Jugendpsychiatrie in Klinik und Praxis, Bd. 2. Remschmidt, H., Schmidt, M.H. (Hrsg.). Stuttgart: Thieme (im Druck)

Peiper, A.: Die Eigenart der kindlichen Hirntätigkeit. 3. Aufl. Leipzig: Edition Leipzig 1964

Penfield, W., Rasmussen, Th.: The cerebral cortex of man. New York: MacMillan 1950

Penfield, W., Roberts, L.: Speech and brain mechanisms. Princeton, N.J.: Princeton University Press 1959

Penfield, W., Welch, K.: The supplementary motor area of the cerebral cortex. Arch. Neurol. Psychiatr. (Chicago) **66**, 289–317 (1951)

Pfaff, D., Lewis, C., Diakow, C., Keiner, M.: Neurophysiological analysis of mating behavior responses as hormone-sensitive reflexes. Progr. Physiol. Psychol. **5**, 253–297 (1973)

Pfaff, D.W., Diakow, C., Zigmond, R.E., Kow, L.-M.: Neural and hormonal determinants of female mating behavior in rats. In: The neurosciences. Third study program. Schmitt, F.O., Worden, F.G. (Hrsg.), S. 621–646. Cambridge, Mass.: The MIT Press 1974
Piaget, J.: The construction of reality in the child. New York: Basic Books 1937/1954
Ploog, D.: Vergleichend quantitative Verhaltensstudien an zwei Totenkopffaffen-Kolonien. Z. Morph. Anthropol. **53**, 92–108 (1963)
Ploog, D.: Über experimentelle Grundlagen der Gedächtnisforschung. Nervenarzt **35**, 377–386 (1964a)
Ploog, D.: Vom limbischen System gesteuertes Verhalten. Nervenarzt **35**, 166–174 (1964b)
Ploog, D.: Verhaltensforschung und Psychiatrie. In: Psychiatrie der Gegenwart, Bd. I/1B. Gruhle, H.W., Jung, R., Mayer-Gross, W., Müller, M. (Hrsg.), S. 291–443. Berlin, Göttingen, Heidelberg: Springer 1964c
Ploog, D.: Experimentelle Verhaltensforschung. Nervenarzt **37**, 443–447 (1966a)
Ploog, D.: Biological bases for instinct and behavior: Studies on the development of social behavior in squirrel monkeys. In: Recent advances in biological psychiatry, Bd. VIII. Wortis, J. (Hrsg.), S. 199–223. New York: Plenum Press 1966b
Ploog, D.: The behavior of squirrel monkeys (Saimiri sciureus) as revealed by sociometry, bioacoustics, and brain stimulation. In: Social communication among primates. Altmann, S.A. (Hrsg.), S. 149–184. Chicago, Ill.: The University of Chicago Press 1967
Ploog, D.: Kommunikationsprozesse bei Affen. Homo **19**, 151–165 (1968)
Ploog, D.: Psychobiologie des Partnerschaftverhaltens. Nervenarzt **40**, 245–255 (1969a)
Ploog, D.: Early communication processes in squirrel monkeys. In: Brain and early behaviour. Development in the fetus and infant. Robinson, R.J. (Hrsg.), S. 269–298. London: Academic Press 1969b
Ploog, D.: Social communication among animals. In: The neurosciences. Second Study Program. Schmitt, F.O. (Hrsg.), S. 349–361. New York: The Rockefeller Press 1970
Ploog, D.: The relevance of natural stimulus patterns for sensory information processes. Brain Res. **31**, 353–359 (1971)
Ploog, D.: Kommunikation in Affengesellschaften und deren Bedeutung für die Verständigungsweisen des Menschen. In: Neue Anthropologie. Gadamer, H.G., Vogler, P. (Hrsg.), Bd. 2, S. 98–178. Stuttgart: Thieme 1972 u. dtv – Wissenschaftliche Reihe.
Ploog, D.: Comments on instinctive behavior, neural systems and reinforcement mechanisms. In: Psychic dependence – Bayer Symposium IV. Goldberg, L., Hoffmeister, F. (Hrsg.). S. 51–55. Berlin, Heidelberg, New York: Springer 1973a
Ploog, D.: Die cerebrale Repräsentation von Funktions- und Verhaltensweisen. S. 202–219. Verh. Dtsch. Zool. Ges. Stuttgart: Fischer 1973b
Ploog, D.: Vocal behavior and its "localization" as a prerequisite for speech. In: Cerebral localization. Zülch, K.J., Creutzfeldt, O., Galbraith, G.C. (Hrsg.), S. 230–237. Berlin, New York, Heidelberg: Springer 1975
Ploog, D.: Sozialverhalten und Hirnfunktion beim Menschen und seinen Verwandten. Klin. Wochenschr. **55**, 857–867 (1977)
Ploog, D.: Anlage und Umwelt. Dtsch. Ärztebl. **76**, 725–730; 815–819 (1979)
Ploog, D., Gottwald, P.: Verhaltensforschung. Instinkt – Lernen – Hirnfunktion. München: Urban und Schwarzenberg 1974
Ploog, D., MacLean, P.D.: On functions of the mamillary bodies in the squirrel monkey. Exp. Neurol. **7**, 76–85 (1963a)
Ploog, D., MacLean, P.D.: Display of penile erection in squirrel monkey (Saimiri sciureus). Anim. Behav. **11**, 32–39 (1963b)
Ploog, D., Melnechuk, T.: Primate communication. A report based on an NRP work session. Neurosci. Res. Program Bull. **7**, 419–510 (1969)
Ploog, D., Melnechuk, T.: Are apes capable of language? A report based on an NRP conference. Neurosci. Res. Program Bull. **9**, 599–700 (1971)
Ploog, D., Blitz, J., Ploog, F.: Studies on social and sexual behavior of the squirrel monkey (Saimiri sciureus). Folia Primatol. (Basel) **1**, 29–66 (1963)
Ploog, D., Hopf, S., Winter, P.: Ontogenese des Verhaltens von Totenkopf-Affen (Saimiri sciureus). Psychol. Forsch. **31**, 1–41 (1967)
Ploog, D., Hupfer, K., Jürgens, U., Newman, J.D.: Neuroethologic studies of vocalization in

squirrel monkeys, with special reference to genetic differences of calling in two subspecies. In: Growth and development of the brain. Brazier, M.A.B. (Hrsg.), S. 231–254. New York: Raven Press 1975

Pöppel, E., Cramon, D.v., Backmund, H.: Eccentricity-specific dissociation of visual functions in patients with lesions of the central visual pathways. Nature **256**, 489–490 (1975)

Pöppel, E., Held, R., Dowling, J.E. (Hrsg.): Neuronal mechanisms in visual perception. Neurosci. Res. Program Bull. **15**, 315–553 (1977)

Pöppel, E., Brinkmann, R., Cramon, D. v., Singer, W.: Association and dissociation of visual functions in a case of bilateral occipital lobe infarction. Arch. Psychiatr. Nervenkr. **225**, 1–21 (1978)

Poirier, F.E. (Hrsg.): Primate socialization. New York: Random House 1972

Premack, A.J.: Why chimps can read. New York: Harper and Row 1976

Premack, A.J., Premack, D.: Teaching language to an ape. Sci. Am. **227**, 92–99 (1972)

Premack, D.: A functional analysis of language. J. Exp. Anal. Behav. **14**, 107–125 (1970)

Premack, D.: Language in chimpanzee? Science **172**, 808–822 (1971)

Premack, D.: Intelligence in ape and man. Hillsdale: Lawrence Erlbaum Associates 1976a

Premack, D.: Language and intelligence in ape and man. Am. Sci. **64**, 674–683 (1976b)

Pruscha, H., Maurus, M.: The communicative function of some agonistic behavior patterns in squirrel monkeys. The relevance of social context. Behav. Ecol. Sociobiol. **1**, 185–214 (1976)

Raisman, G., Field, P.M.: Sexual dimorphism in the neuropil of the preoptic area of the rat and its dependence on neonatal androgen. Brain Res. **54**, 1–29 (1973)

Rensch, B. (Hrsg.): Handgebrauch und Verständigung bei Affen und Frühmenschen. Bern, Stuttgart: Huber 1968

Rensch, B., Dücker, G.: Manipulierfähigkeit eines jungen Orang-Utans und eines jungen Gorillas. Mit Anmerkungen über das Spielverhalten. Z. Tierpsychol. **23**, 874–892 (1966)

Reynolds, V., Reynolds, F.: Chimpanzees of the Budongo Forest. In: Primate behavior. DeVore, I. (Hrsg.), S. 368–424. New York: Rinehart and Winston 1965

Rheingold, H.L.: The effect of environmental stimulation upon social and exploratory behaviour in the human infant. In: Determinants of infant behaviour. Foss, B.M. (Hrsg.), S. 143–171. London: Methuen 1961

Rheingold, H.L.: Development of social behavior in the human infant. Monogr. Soc. Res. Child Dev. **31**, 1–17 (1966)

Rheingold, H.L.: The social and socializing infant. In: Handbook of socialization theory and research. Goslin, D. (Hrsg.), S. 779–790. Chicago: Rand McNally 1969

Rheingold, H.L., Gewirtz, J., Ross, H.: Social conditioning of vocalizations in the infant. J. Comp. Physiol. Psychol. **52**, 68–73 (1959)

Richards, M.P.M. (Hrsg.): The integration of a child into a social world. London, New York: Cambridge University Press 1974

Rieber, I., Meyer, A.-E., Schmidt, G., Schorsch, E., Sigusch, V.: Stellungnahme zu stereotaktischen Hirnoperationen an Menschen mit abweichendem Sexualverhalten. Sexualmed. **5**, 442–450 (1976)

Riklan, M., Levita, E.: Subcortical correlates of human behavior. Baltimore: Williams and Wilkins 1969

Robinson, B.W.: Vocalization evoked from forebrain in Macaca mulatta. Physiol. Behav. **2**, 345–354 (1967)

Robinson, B.W.: Limbic influences on human speech. In: Origins and evolution of language and speech. Harnad, St.R., Steklis, H.D., Lancaster, J. (Hrsg.), S. 761–771. Ann. N.Y. Acad. Sci. Bd. 280, New York: Acad. of Science 1976

Robinson, B.W., Alexander, M., Bowne, G.: Dominance reversal resulting from aggressive responses evoked by brain telestimulation. Physiol. Behav. **4**, 179–183 (1969)

Robinson, R.J. (Hrsg.): Brain and early behavior. London: Academic Press 1969

Rosenblum, L.A. (Hrsg.): Primate behavior. Developments in field and laboratory research. Bd. I. New York, London: Academic Press 1970

Rosenblum, L.A. (Hrsg.): Primate behavior. Developments in field and laboratory research. Bd. II. New York, London: Academic Press 1971a

Rosenblum, L.A.: Infant attachment in monkeys. In: The origins of human social relations. Schaffer, H.R. (Hrsg.), S. 85–108. New York: Academic Press 1971b

Rosenblum, L.A. (Hrsg.): Primate behavior. Developments in field and laboratory research. Bd. IV. New York, London: Academic Press 1975

Rosenblum, L.A., Kaufman, I.Ch.: Laboratory observations of early mother-infant relations in pigtail and bonnet macaques. In: Social communication among primates. Altmann, St.A. (Hrsg.), S. 33–42. Chicago, London: The University of Chicago Press 1967
Rowell, T.E.: Agonistic noises of the rhesus monkey (Macaca mulatta). Symp. Zool. Soc. Lond. **8**, 91–96 (1962)
Rowell, T.E.: Female reproductive cycles and the behavior of baboons and rhesus macaques. In: Social communication among primates. Altmann, S.A. (Hrsg.), S. 15–32. Chicago: University of Chicago Press 1967
Rowell, T.E., Hinde, R.A.: Vocal communication by the rhesus monkey. Proc. Zool. Soc. Lond. **2**, 279–294 (1962)
Rowell, T.E., Hinde, R., Spencer-Booth, Y.: Aunt-infant interaction in captive rhesus monkeys. Anim. Behav. **12**, 219–226 (1964)
Rubens, A.B.: Aphasia with infarction in the territory of the anterior cerebral artery. Cortex **11**, 239–250 (1975)
Rumbaugh, D.M.: The learning and symbolizing capacities of apes and monkeys. In: Socioecology and psychology of primates. Tuttle, R.H. (Hrsg.), S. 353–365. Den Haag, Paris: Mouton 1975
Rumbaugh, D.M., Gill, T.V.: Language and the acquisition of language skills by a chimpanzee (PAN). Ann. N.Y. Acad. Sci. **270**, 90–123 (1976), **280**, 562–578 (1976)
Rumbaugh, D.M., Gill, T.V., Glasersfeld, B.C.v.: Reading and sentence completion by a chimpanzee (PAN). Science **182**, 731–733 (1973)
Rumbaugh, D.M., Gill, T.V., Glasersfeld, E.v., Warner, H., Pisani, P.: Conversations with a chimpanzee in a computer-controlled environment. Biol. Psychiatry **10**, 627–641 (1975)
Sackett, G.P.: Monkeys reared in isolation with pictures as visual input. Evidence for an innate releasing mechanism. Science **154**, 1468–1473 (1966)
Salzen, E.A.: Social attachment and a sense of security. In: Human ethology. Claims and limits of a new discipline. Cranach, M.v., Foppa, K., Lepenies, W., Ploog, D. (Hrsg.). Cambridge: Cambridge University Press 1979
Samaroff, A.J.: Can conditioned responses be established in the newborn infant. Dev. Psychol. **5**, 1–12 (1971)
Sander, L.: Regulation of exchange in the infant caretaker system: A viewpoint on the ontogeny of "structures" In: Communicative structures and psychic structures. Freedman, N., Grand, S. (Hrsg.). New York: New York Plenum Press 1977a
Sander, L.W.: Regulation and organization in the early infant-caretaker system. In: Brain and early behavior. Robinson, R.J. (Hrsg.), S. 311–332. London: Academic Press 1969a
Sander, L.W.: The longitudinal course of early mother-child interaction – cross case comparisons in a sample of mother-child pairs. In: Determinants of infant behavior IV. Foss, B.M. (Hrsg.), S. 189–227. London: Methuen 1969b
Sander, L.W.: The regulation of exchange in the infant-caretaker system and some aspects of the context-content relationship. In: Interaction, conversation and development of language. Lewis, M., Rosenblum, L.A. (Hrsg.), S. 133–156. New York: Wiley 1977b
Scott, J.P.: Critical periods in behavioral development. Science **138**, 949–958 (1962)
Scott, J.P.: Genetics and the development of social behavior in dogs. Am. Zool. **4**, 161–168 (1964)
Scott, J.P.: Comparative psychology and ethology. Ann. Rev. Psychol. **18**, 65–86 (1967)
Scott, J.P.: The emotional basis of social behavior. Ann. N.Y. Acad. Sci. **159**, 777–790 (1969)
Scott, J.P.: Social genetics. Behav. Gen. **7**, 327–346 (1977)
Scott, J.P., Fuller, J.L.: Genetics and the social behavior of the dog. Chicago: University of Chicago Press 1965
Schaffer, H.R. (Hrsg.): The origins of human social relations. London, New York: Academic Press 1971
Schaller, G.B.: The mountain gorilla. Chicago: University of Chicago Press 1963
Schaltenbrand, G.: The effects on speech and language of stereotactical stimulation in thalamus and corpus callosum. Brain Lang. **2**, 70–77 (1975)
Schenkel, R.: Ausdrucksstudien an Wölfen. Behaviour **1**, 81–129 (1947)
Schleidt, W.: Die historische Entwicklung der Begriffe „angeborenes auslösendes Schema" und „angeborener Auslösemechanismus" in der Ethologie. Z. Tierpsychol. **19**, 697–722 (1962)
Schlesinger, H.S., Meadow, K.P.: Sound and sign. Berkeley, Cal.: University California Press 1973

Schmidt, R.S.: Central mechanisms of frog calling. Behaviour **26**, 251–285 (1966)
Schmidt, R.S.: Neural correlates of frog calling. J. Comp. Physiol. Psychol. **92**, 229–254 (1974)
Schmitt, F.O., Worden, F.G. (Hrsg.): The neurosciences. Third study program. Section on: Central processing of sensory input leading to motor output, S. 265–337. Cambridge, Mass., London: The MIT Press 1974
Schmitt, F.O., Quarton, G.C., Melnechuk, Th., Adelman, G. (Hrsg.): The neurosciences. 2nd study program. New York: The Rockefeller University Press 1970
Schneider, G.E.: Two visual systems. Science **163**, 895–902 (1969)
Schneider, H.: Entwicklung und Sozialisation der Primaten. Zur Psychologie der Entwicklung des Menschen aus dem interspezifischen Vergleich des Gebär- und Sterbealters. tuduv Studie, Reihe Kultur Wissenschaften Bd. 3. München: tuduv Verlagsgesellschaften 1975
Schott, D.: Quantititive analysis of the vocal repertoire of squirrel monkey (Saimiri sciureus). Z. Tierpsychol. **38**, 235–250 (1975)
Schrier, A.M., Harlow, H.F., Stollnitz, F. (Hrsg.): Behavior of nonhuman primates. Modern research trends. Bd. I u. II. New York, London: Academic Press 1965
Schrier, A.M., Harlow, H.F., Stollnitz, F. (Hrsg.): Behavior of nonhuman primates. Modern research trends. Bd. III. New York, London: Academic Press 1971
Seay, B., Hansen, E., Harlow, H.F.: Mother-infant separation in monkeys. J. Child Psychol. **3**, 123 (1962)
Sebeok, Th.A. (Hrsg.): How animals communicate. Bloomington, London: Indiana University Press 1977
Sem-Jacobsen, C.W., Torkildsen, A.: Depth recording and electrical stimulation in the human brain. In: Electrical studies on the unanesthetized brain. Ramay, E.R., O'Doherty, D.S. (Hrsg.). New York: Hoeber 1960
Sem-Jacobsen, C.W., Styri, O.B.: Manipulation of emotion. Electrophysiological and surgical methods. In: Symposium on parameters of emotion. Levi, I. (Hrsg.), S. 645–676. New York: Raven Press 1973
Serban, G., Kling, A. (Hrsg.): Animal models in human psychobiology. New York, London: Plenum Press 1974
Siegman, A.W., Feldstein, St. (Hrsg.): Nonverbal behavior and communication. Hillsdale, N.J.: Erlbaum 1978 (distributed by the Halsted Press Division of Wiley, New York, Toronto, London, Sydney)
Simonds, P.E.: The social primates. New York: Harper and Row 1974
Simons, E.L.: The early relatives of man. Sci. Am. **211**, 51–62 (1964)
Simons, E.L. (Hrsg.): Primate evolution. New York: MacMillan 1972
Sinnott, J.M., Beecher, M.D., Moody, D.B., Stebbins, W.C.: Speech sound discrimination by monkeys and humans. J. Acoust. Soc. Am. **60**, 687–695 (1976)
Siqueland, E.R., Lipsitt, L.P.: Conditioned head-turning behavior in newborn. J. Exp. Child Psychol. **3**, 356–376 (1966)
Smythies, J.R.: Brain mechanisms and behaviour, 2nd Ed. Oxford: Blackwell 1970
Snow, C.E.: Mother's speech to children learning language. Child Dev. **43**, 549–565 (1972)
Sommer, R.: Tierpsychologie. Leipzig: Quelle und Meyer 1925
Spatz, H.: Das Hypophysen-Hypothalamus-System in seiner Bedeutung für die Fortpflanzung. Verh. Anatom. Ges. 51. Versammlung, Mainz 1953
Spencer, H.: First principles. London: Williams and Norgate 1862
Spitz, R.A.: Anaclitic depression: an inquiry into the genesis of psychiatric conditions in early childhood. Psychoanal. Study Child **2**, 313 (1946)
Spitz, R.A., Wolf, K.M.: The smiling response: A contribution to the ontogenesis of social relations. Genet. Psychol. Monogr. **34**, 57–125 (1946)
Sroufe, L.A., Waters, E.: The ontogenesis of smiling and laughter: A perspective on the organization of development in infancy. Psychol. Rev. **83**, 173–189 (1976)
Startsev, V.G.: Primate models of human neurogenic disorders. New York: Wiley 1976
Stebbins, W.C.: Hearing. In: Behavior of nonhuman primates. Bd. 3. Schrier, A.M., Stollnitz, F. (Hrsg.), S. 159–192. New York, London: Academic Press 1971
Steiner, J.E.: Innate, discriminative human facial expressions to taste and smell stimulation. Ann. N.Y. Acad. Sci. **237**, 229–233 (1974)
Steiner, J.E.: Facial expressions of the neonate infant indicating the hedonics of food-related chemical

stimuli. In: Taste and development: The genesis of sweet preference. Weiffenbach, J.M. (Hrsg.), No. 77–1068, Chapt. 13, S. 173–189. Maryland: National Institutes of Health 1977

Steklis, H.D., Harnad, S.R.: From hand to mouth: Some critical stages in the evolution of language. Ann. N.Y. Acad. Sci. **280**, 505–513 (1976)

Stern, D.N.: A micro-analysis of mother-infant interaction behavior regulating social contact between a mother and her $3^1/_2$ month old twins. J. Am. Acad. Child Psychiatry **10**, 501–517 (1971)

Stevens, J.R., Mark, V.H., Ervin, F., Pacheco, P., Suematsu, K.: Deep temporal stimulation in man. Long latency, long lasting psychological changes induced by deep temporal stimulation in man. Arch. Neurol. (Chicago) **21**, 157–169 (1969)

Stokoe, W.C.: Sign language anatomy. Ann. N.Y. Acad. Sci. **280**, 505–513 (1976)

Struhsaker, T.T.: Auditory communication among vervet monkeys (Cercopithecus aethiops). In: Social communication among primates. Altmann, S.A. (Hrsg.), S. 281–324. Chicago: University of Chicago Press 1967

Studdert-Kennedy, M.: Speech perception. In: Contemporary issues in experimental phonetics. Lass, N.J. (Hrsg.), S. 243–293. New York: Academic Press 1976

Suomi, St.J., Harlow, H.F.: Depressive behavior in young monkeys subjected to vertical chamber confinement. J. Comp. Physiol. Psychol. **180**, 11 (1972)

Suomi, St.J., Harlow, H.F., Domek, C.J.: Effect of repetitive infant-infant separation of young monkeys. J. Abnorm. Soc. Psychol. **76**, 161 (1970)

Suomi, St.J., Collins, M.L., Harlow, H.F.: Effects of permanent separation from mother on infant monkeys. Dev. Psychol. **9**, 376–384 (1973)

Suomi, St.J., Harlow, H.F., Novak, M.A.: Reversal of social deficits produced by isolation rearing in monkeys. J. Hum. Evol. **3**, 527–534 (1974)

Suomi, St.J., Delizio, R., Harlow, H.F.: Social rehabilitation of separation-induced depressive disorders in monkeys. Am. J. Psychiatry **133**, 1279 (1976)

Sutton, D., Larson, C., Lindeman, R.C.: Neocortical and limbic lesion effects on primate phonation. Brain Res. **71**, 61–75 (1974)

Sweet, W.H., Obrador, S., Martin-Rodriguez, J.G.: Neurosurgical treatment in psychiatry, pain and epilepsy, Proc. of the 4th world congress of psychiatry surgery, Madrid 1975. Baltimore: University Park Press 1977

Szentágothai, J., Arbib, M.A.: Conceptual models of neural organization. Neurosci. Res. Program Bull. **12**, 307–510 (1974)

Talmage-Riggs, G., Winter, P., Ploog, D., Mayer, W.: Effects of deafening on the vocal behavior of the squirrel monkey (Saimiri sciureus). Folia Primat. (Basel) **17**, 404–420 (1972)

Teleki, G.: The predatory behavior of wild chimpanzees. Lewisburg: Bucknell University Press 1973. (Associated University Presses, Inc., Cranbury, New Jersey 1973)

Teuber, H.L.: Lacunae and research. Approaches to them. I. In: Brain mechanisms underlying speech and language. Darley, F.L. (Hrsg.), S. 204–216. New York: Grune and Stratton 1967

Thompson, J.: Development of facial expression of emotion in blind and seeing children. Arch. Psychol. **264**, 1–47 (1941)

Thorpe, W.H.: The biology of vocal communication and expression in birds. London: Cambridge University Press 1961

Tinbergen, N.: Social releasers and the experimental method required for their study. Wils. Bull. **60**, 6–52 (1948)

Tinbergen, N.: Instinktlehre. Berlin, Hamburg: Paul Parey 1952

Tinbergen, N.: Tiere untereinander. Berlin, Hamburg: Paul Parey 1955

Todd, G.A., Palmer, B.: Social reinforcement of infant babbling. Child Dev. **39**, 591–596 (1968)

Tomkins, S.S.: Consciousness, imagery and affect. Bd. I. New York: Springer 1962

Tomkins, S.S., Izard, C.E.: Affect, cognition and personality. Tavistock Publications. New York: Springer 1965

Tomkins, S.S., McCarter, R.: What and where are the primary affects? Some evidence for a theory. Percept. Mot. Skills **18**, 119–158 (1964)

Tower, D.B. (Hrsg.): The nervous system. Bd. 3. Human communication and its disorders. New York: Raven Press 1975

Trojan, F.: Biophonetik. Mannheim: Bibliograph. Inst. – Wissenschaftsverlag 1975

Uexküll, J. v.: Bedeutungslehre. 1. Auflage 1921. Hamburg: Rowohlts Deutsche Enzyklopädie 1956

Uexküll, J. v., Kriszat, G.: Streifzüge durch die Umwelten von Tieren und Menschen, Nr. 13. Hamburg: Rowohlts Deutsche Enzyklopädie 1956
Ujváry, Z.: Das Begräbnis parodierende Spiele in der ungarischen Volksüberlieferung. Österr. Z. Volkskd. **69**, 267–275 (1966)
Valenstein, E.S.: Independence of approach and escape reactions to electrical stimulation of the brain. J. Comp. Physiol. Psychol. **60**, 20–31 (1965)
Valenstein, E.S.: Stability and plasticity of motivation systems. In: The neurosciences. 2nd study program. Schmitt, F.O., Quarton, G.C., Melnechuk, Th., Adelman, G. (Hrsg.), S. 207–217. New York: The Rockefeller University Press 1970
Valenstein, E.S.: Brain control. A critical examination of brain stimulation and psychosurgery. New York, London, Sydney, Toronto: Wiley 1973
Valenstein, E.S.: Brain stimulation and behavior control. Nebraska symposium on motivation. S. 251–292, 1974. Lincoln, Nebraska: University of Nebraska Press 1975
Valenstein, E.S., Nauta, W.J.H.: A comparison of the distribution of the fornix system in the rat, guinea pig, cat and monkey. J. Comp. Neurol. **113**, 337–363 (1959)
Washburn, R.W.: A study of the smiling and laughing of infants in the first year of life. Genet. Psychol. Monogr. **6**, 398–537 (1929)
Wasz-Höckert, O., Lind, J., Vuorenkoski, V., Partanan, T., Vallane, E.: The infant cry: a spectrographic and auditory analysis. London: Heinemann 1968
Waters, R.S., Wilson, W.A.: Speech perception by rhesus monkeys: the voicing distinction in synthesized labial and velar stop consonants. Perception and Psychophysics **19**, 285–289 (1976)
Watson, J.S.: Smiling, cooing and "the game". Merrill-Palmer Quart. **18**, 323–339 (1972)
Watson, J.S., Ramey, C.T.: Reactions to response-contingent stimulation in early infancy. Merrill-Palmer Quart. **18**, 219–221 (1972)
Wauquier, A., Rolls, E.T. (Hrsg.): Brain stimulation reward. A collection of papers prepared for the first international conference on brain-stimulation reward at Janssen pharmaceutica, Beerse, Belgium on April 21–24, 1975. Amsterdam, Oxford: North-Holland Publ. Comp., New York: American Elsevier Publ. Comp. 1976
Weisberg, P.: Social and nonsocial conditioning of infant vocalization. Child Dev. **34**, 377–388 (1963)
Weiskrantz, L., Warrington, E.K., Sanders, M.D., Marshall, J.: Visual capacitiy in the hemianoptic field following a restricted occipital ablation. Brain **97**, 709–728 (1974)
Wernicke, C.: Der Aphasische Symptomenkomplex. Breslau: Cohn und Weigert 1874
White, N.F. (Hrsg.): Ethology and psychiatry. From the Clarence M. Hincks Memorial Lectures, held at McMaster University 1970. Toronto, Buffalo: University of Toronto Press 1974
Wickler, W.: Ursprung und biologische Bedeutung des Genitalpräsentierens männlicher Primaten. Z. Tierpsychol. **23**, 422–437 (1966)
Wickler, W.: Vergleichende Verhaltensforschung und Phylogenetik. In: Die Evolution der Organismen. 3. Aufl. Heberer, G. (Hrsg.), S. 420–508. Stuttgart: Fischer 1967a
Wickler, W.: Socio-sexual signals and their intra-specific imitation among primates. In: Primate ethology. Morris, D. (Hrsg.), S. 69–147. London: Weidenfeld and Nicolson 1967b, Chicago: Aldine 1967b
Wickler, W.: Mimikry. Nachahmung und Täuschung in der Natur. München: Kindler 1968
Wickler, W.: Stammesgeschichte und Ritualisierung. Zur Entstehung tierischer und menschlicher Verhaltensmuster. München: Piper 1970
Wilcox, B., Clayton, F.: Infant visual fixation on motion pictures of the human face. J. Exp. Child Psychol. **6** (1), 22–32 (1968)
Wilson, E.O.: Sociobiology. The new synthesis. Cambridge, Mass.: The Belknap Press of Harvard University Press 1975
Winter, P.: Verständigung durch Laute bei Totenkopfaffen. Umschau Wiss. Techn. **62**, 653–658 (1966)
Winter, P.: Lautäußerungen im Kommunikationssystem von Totenkopfaffen. Naturwiss. Rundschau **21**, 185–190 (1968a)
Winter, P.: Social communication in the squirrel monkey. In: The squirrel monkey. Rosenblum, L.A., Cooper, R.W. (Hrsg.), S. 235–253. New York: Academic Press 1968b
Winter, P.: Dialects in squirrel monkeys: vocalization of the Roman arch type. Folia Primatol. (Basel) **10**, 216–229 (1969)

Winter, P., Funkenstein, H.H.: The effect of species-specific vocalization on the discharge of auditory cortical cells in the awake squirrel monkey. Exp. Brain Res. **18**, 489–504 (1973)

Winter, P., Ploog, D., Latta, J.: Vocal repertoire of the squirrel monkey (Saimiri sciureus), its analysis and significance. Exp. Brain Res. **1**, 359–384 (1966)

Winter, P., Handley, P., Ploog, D., Schott, D.: Ontogeny of squirrel monkey calls under normal conditions and under acoustic isolation. Behaviour **47**, 230–239 (1973)

Wolff, P.H.: Observations on the early development of smiling. In: Determinants of infant behavior. II. Foss, B.M. (Hrsg.), S. 113–133. London: Methuen 1963

Wolff, P.H.: The causes, controls, and organization of behavior in the neonate. Psychol. Issues **5**, 1–99 (1966)

Wolff, P.H.: The natural history of crying and other vocalizations in early infancy. In: Determinants of infant behavior. IV. Foss, B.M. (Hrsg.), S. 81–109. London: Methuen 1969

Wolff, P.H.: Organization of behavior in the first three months of life. In: Biological and enviromental determinants of early development. Nurnberger, J.I. (Hrsg.), S. 132. Baltimore: Williams and Wilkins 1973

Wollberg, Z., Newman, J.D.: Auditory cortex of squirrel monkey: response patterns of single cells to species-specific vocalization. Science **175**, 212–214 (1972)

Worden, F.G., Galambos, R.: Auditory processing of biologically significant sounds. In: Neurosciences res. symposium summaries, Vol. 7. Schmitt, F.O., Adelmann, G., Worden, F.G. (Hrsg.), S. 1–119. Cambridge: MIT Press 1973

Yerkes, R.M., Yerkes, A.: The great apes. New Haven: Yale University Press 1929

Young, J.Z.: A model of the brain. Oxford: Clarendon Press 1964

Zuckerman, S.: The social life of monkeys and apes. New York: Harcout, Brace and Comp. 1932

Psychiatrische Genetik

Von

E. ZERBIN-RÜDIN

Inhalt

A. Allgemeiner Teil	545
B. Spezieller Teil	550
I. Exogene Psychosen	550
II. Die Schizophrenien	552
1. Familienbefunde	553
2. Kinder zweier schizophrener Eltern	554
3. Zwillingsbefunde	554
4. Adoptionsstudien	557
5. Erbgangshypothesen	561
6. Was gehört zur Schizophrenie?	563
7. Sind Einzelsyndrome erblich?	566
8. Was steckt dahinter? Zwischenglieder?	566
9. Anlage und Umwelt	571
10. Populationsgenetische Betrachtungen	576
III. Affektive Psychosen	577
IV. Atypische Psychosen und Beziehungen der Psychosen zueinander	584
V. Kindliche Psychosen	587
VI. Nicht-psychotische Persönlichkeits- und Verhaltensabweichungen	590
1. Neurosen und Psychopathien	591
2. Suizid	594
3. Hysterie	595
4. Kindliche Verhaltensstörungen	595
5. Kriminalität	596
6. Suchten	599
VII. Genetische Beratung	601
Literatur	602

A. Allgemeiner Teil

Dieses Kapitel schließt an STRÖMGRENs umfassende Übersicht über psychiatrische Genetik 1939–1964 in der 1. Auflage dieses Buches an. Wie STRÖMGREN schon damals betonte, kann es sich in Anbetracht der begrenzten Seitenzahl nicht um einen erschöpfenden Handbuchbeitrag handeln. Es wird vielmehr versucht, neue Befunde und neue Forschungsrichtungen in großen Zügen herauszuarbeiten. Dabei sind Kürze und Subjektivität der Darstellung unvermeidbar. Ältere Befunde und neue Details müssen bei STRÖMGREN (1967a), in BECKERS Handbuch der Humangenetik, Bd. V/1 (Krankheiten des Nervensystems) und Bd. V/2 (Psychiatrische Krankheiten), in einer der zusammenfassenden Darstellungen aus dem angelsächsischen Sprachraum (FIEVE et al., 1975; MEDNICK et al., 1974; ROSENTHAL, 1970; SLATER u. COWIE, 1971; SPERBER u. JARVIK, 1976), oder in den Originalarbeiten nachgelesen werden. Ausgeklammert bleiben genetische Befunde, die bereits andernorts in diesem Werk besprochen wurden, so die Genetik der Epilepsien (Bd. II/2, S. 691), der Oligophrenien und Genopathien (Bd. II/2, S. 799), und der psychiatrischen Erkrankungen des höheren Lebensalters (Bd. II/2, S. 1037).

In der Psychiatrie wie in der gesamten Medizin können wir Erbfaktoren auf 3 Ebenen erforschen: auf der molekularen, der chromosomalen und der phänotypischen (erscheinungsbildlichen) Ebene.

Auf die *molekulare Ebene* sind wir bei jenen Störungen vorgedrungen, die auf erblichen Stoffwechseldefekten beruhen. Ein Enzym ist durch eine, meist rezessive, Genmutation so verändert, daß es seine Funktionsfähigkeit ganz oder teilweise eingebüßt hat, oder es wird überhaupt nicht mehr gebildet. Eine Ansammlung toxischer Metaboliten vor dem Enzymblock, Vorkommen abnormer Metaboliten infolge ersatzweisen Abbaus über Stoffwechsel-Nebenwege oder das Fehlen notwendiger Stoffe hinter dem Block sind die Folge. Die beiden ersten Mechanismen scheinen häufiger zu sein. Nach der ein-Enzym-ein-Gen-Hypothese befinden wir uns hier bereits in recht gennahen Bereichen. Beispiele sind die Phenylketonurie (rezessiv erblicher Mangel des Enzyms Phenylalaninhydroxylase), die metachromatische Leukodystrophie (Mangel an Cerebrosidsulfatase) und die Sphingolipidosen, z.B. Morbus Tay-Sachs (Mangel an Acetylhexosaminidasen). Die Zahl der biochemisch aufgeklärten Erbleiden wächst ständig. Jedoch handelt es sich dabei meist um seltene Leiden.

Auf der zweiten Ebene liegen die *Chromosomenaberrationen*. Bei ihnen kennen wir die maßgeblichen biochemischen Veränderungen zwar nicht, sehen aber wenigstens im Lichtmikroskop handfeste Veränderungen des genetischen Materials in Gestalt von Umstrukturierungen der Chromosomen (Ringformen, Translokationen usw.) oder Mengenveränderungen (Verlust oder Überzahl von ganzen Chromosomen oder Chromosomenstücken). Die numerischen Chromosomenaberrationen sind von besonderer praktischer Bedeutung. Die autosomalen Aberrationen, sofern sie überhaupt mit dem Leben vereinbar sind, führen zu den verschiedensten Mißbildungen, reduzierter Lebenserwartung und Schwachsinn. Am bekanntesten und praktisch wichtigsten in dieser Gruppe ist der Mongolismus, bei dem das Chromosom 21 dreifach anstatt zweifach vorhanden ist (Trisomie 21). Bei Aberrationen der Geschlechtschromosomen (Klinefelter-Syndrom [XXY], Turner-Syndrom [XO], XYY-Syndrom, XXX-Syndrom, und manche Zwitterbildungen) finden sich teilweise funktionsunfähige Gonaden, Mißbildungen und Intelligenzminderung verschiedenen Grades. Leichtere psychische Störungen, besonders depressive Verstimmungen, paranoide Symptome, psychopathische und neurotische Bilder werden nicht allzu selten beobachtet.

Auf der dritten, der *phänotypischen Ebene* bewegen wir uns leider immer noch bei den meisten psychiatrischen Störungen und gerade bei den häufigsten.

Wir kennen keine gennahe metabolische Störung, keine Chromosomenanomalie, ja meist überhaupt keine somatische Grundlage und sind nach wie vor auf sorgfältige psychopathologische Untersuchungen angewiesen. Auch liegt in der Regel kein Mendelscher Erbgang vor.

Es gibt allerdings zwei Ausnahmen. Die Chorea Huntington zeigt eine allgemeine Atrophie des Gehirnes, insbesondere eine Schrumpfung der Basalganglien und folgt dem einfach dominanten Erbgang. Bei der Wilsonschen Krankheit (hepatolentikulären Degeneration) liegt ein Defekt des Caeruloplasmins und rezessiver Erbgang vor. In der Oligophrenieforschung liegen die Verhältnisse ein wenig günstiger. Wir kennen hier eine größere Zahl metabolischer und chromosomaler Schwachsinnsformen, ferner eine Gruppe syndromatischer Sonderformen, in der die geistige Behinderung u.a. mit Fehlbildungen des Gehirnes, Hautaffektionen oder Augenleiden einhergeht und gelegentlich einen klassischen Erbgang aufweist.

Da sich psychische Störungen im Verhalten zu äußern pflegen, rechnet man die psychiatrische Genetik heute häufig zur Verhaltensgenetik. Die klassische Verhaltensgenetik befaßt sich zwar traditionsgemäß mit experimentellen und beobachtenden Untersuchungen am Tier, doch finden sich in praktisch allen neueren verhaltensgenetischen Büchern als Beispiele aus dem Humanbereich psychische Erkrankungen, besonders die endogenen Psychosen (z. B. v. ABELEEN, 1974; EHRMAN et al., 1972; MCCLEARN u. DE FRIES, 1973; VANDENBERG, 1965). Das Buch von ROSENTHAL (1970) handelt ausschließlich von menschlichen Verhaltensstörungen.

Die Subsumierung der psychiatrischen Genetik unter die Verhaltensgenetik hat ihre Vor- und Nachteile (ZERBIN-RÜDIN, 1976). Einer der Vorteile liegt darin, daß Verhaltensweisen leichter zu beobachten sind als intrapsychische Vorgänge. Deshalb, aber nicht nur aus diesem Grund, hat die Auffassung der Psychiatrie als Verhaltenswissenschaft fruchtbare neue Denkanstöße und therapeutische Ansatzmöglichkeiten gegeben (PLOOG, 1964, 1969, 1973, 1975). Zu den Nachteilen gehört es, daß gleiches Verhalten höchst verschiedene Ursachen haben kann. Menschliche Verhaltensweisen können spontan und reaktiv, bewußt oder unbewußt, gezielt oder ungezielt ablaufen. Ferner kann gleiches Verhalten in verschiedenem Kontext verschiedene Wertigkeit besitzen. Die phänomenologische Verhaltensgenetik liegt also auf einer recht oberflächlichen Ebene und darf sich nicht selbst genügen. Die Frage stellt sich: Was steckt dahinter? Welche genetische Mechanismen sind es, die normale und pathologische Verhaltensweisen und Abläufe in Gang setzen, unterhalten und stoppen?

Die psychiatrische Genetik zeigt nicht nur zur Verhaltensforschung Beziehungen, sondern zu den verschiedensten Disziplinen: Neuroanatomie, -histologie, -chemie, -physiologie, Neurologie und klinischer Psychologie, Experimentalpsychologie, Epidemiologie und transkultureller Psychiatrie.

Mit den sattsam bekannten grundsätzlichen Schwierigkeiten bei der Objektivierung psychischer Phänomene hat auch die psychiatrische Genetik zu kämpfen. Bei Verhaltensweisen und intrapsychischen Vorgängen handelt es sich um äußerst komplexe, vielgestaltige und noch dazu zeitlich variable Merkmale. Sie lassen sich nicht eindeutig objektivieren und nicht präzise messen, obgleich die psychologischen Meßinstrumente – Tests aller Art, Fremd- und Selbstbeurteilungsskalen (v. ZERSSEN u. KOELLER, 1976) – laufend verbessert und durch experimentalpsychologische, neuropsychologische und neurochemische Untersuchungen ergänzt werden. Wir können Verhaltensweisen und psychische Phänomene nicht in einzelne Erbradikale auflösen und wir wissen nicht, sind sie das Endprodukt eines einzigen Genes oder ganzer Genkomplexe. Wir wissen auch nicht, ob und inwieweit die von der Psychologie erarbeiteten Kategorien und Grundphänomene und die in der Klinik beschriebenen Symptome und Syndrome genetischen Einheiten entsprechen.

Natürlich wird Verhalten nicht *nur* durch Gene bestimmt. Es wird durch Umwelteinflüsse aller Art mitgestaltet, unmittelbar durch die jeweilige Umwelt und den jeweiligen Partner, mittelbar durch früher gemachte Erfahrungen, Lernvorgänge und Prägungen. Überhaupt werden ja nicht fertige Merkmale vererbt, sondern kodierte Informationen. Die Erbanlage steckt den Kreis des Möglichen ab, die Umwelt bestimmt mit darüber, was davon realisiert wird und wie. Dabei gestattet die Erbanlage den Umwelteinflüssen jeweils einen größeren oder kleineren Spielraum: es gibt umweltlabile Eigenschaften (z. B. Körpergewicht) und umweltstabile (z. B. Körpergröße).

Anlage und Umwelt stehen nicht im Gegensatz zueinander, sie sind Partner, deren reibungsloses Zusammenspiel von grundlegender Wichtigkeit ist. Die wenigsten äußerlich wahrnehmbaren Eigenschaften sind rein anlagebedingt oder rein umweltbedingt, die meisten liegen zwischen diesen beiden Endpunkten, jeweils näher dem einen oder anderen Pol. Da psychische Eigenschaften und Verhaltensweisen ja gerade der Kommunikation und der Auseinandersetzung des Individuums mit der Außenwelt dienen, ist die Interaktion von Anlage und Umwelt hier besonders eng. Daher ist das Problem der Anlage – Umwelt – Interaktion in den Vordergrund gerückt, besonders in der psychiatrisch-genetischen Forschung, aber auch ganz allgemein (PLOOG, 1979; ZERBIN-RÜDIN, 1974).

Experimente am Menschen sind nur begrenzt durchführbar. Einen gewissen Ersatz für das geplante Experiment bieten Zwillinge und Adoptivkinder als sozusagen zufällige Experimente.

Die Zwillingsforschung geht bekanntlich von der Voraussetzung aus, daß eineiige ebenso wie zweieiige Zwillingspartner in gleicher oder sehr ähnlicher Umwelt aufwachsen. Die eineiigen Zwillinge (EZ) haben außerdem noch gleiches Erbgut, die zweieiigen (ZZ) nicht. Sind EZ für ein bestimmtes Merkmal häufiger konkordant als ZZ, so spricht dies für Erblichkeit. Andererseits sind Unterschiede zwischen EZ-Partnern Ausdruck der Spielbreite der Erbanlage und von nicht-erblichen Einflüssen.

Gegen dieses Konzept und die Beweiskraft der Zwillingsforschung werden zwei Einwände erhoben: 1. Die absolute Erbgleichheit der EZ sei fraglich. Dazu ist zu sagen: Erbungleiche Teilung einer befruchteten Eizelle kommt bei niedrigen Lebewesen vor. Menschliche EZ jedoch stimmen in allen untersuchten Erbmerkmalen (Blutgruppen, Serumfaktoren usw.) überein; daher heilen auch Haut- und Organtransplantate bei ihnen, und nur bei ihnen, komplikationslos ein. 2. EZ hätten nicht nur gleiches Erbgut, sondern wegen ihrer großen Gleichheit auch eine ähnlichere Umwelt als ZZ. Schon die intrauterine Umwelt kann aber gerade für EZ sehr verschieden sein. Die gemeinsame Plazenta führt gelegentlich zu einer derart ungleichen Blutverteilung, daß ein Zwilling hyperämisch und der andere anämisch geboren wird. Auch für die spätere und psychologische Umwelt findet der Einwand in neueren Untersuchungen keine Stütze (SHIELDS, 1978b). Fast ebenso viele ZZ (40%) wie EZ (50%) werden gleich gekleidet (COHEN et al., 1975). Hatten die Eltern eine falsche Meinung über die Eiigkeit ihrer Zwillingskinder, so stimmte die psychische Ähnlichkeit mit der tatsächlichen Eiigkeit überein und nicht mit der Meinung der Eltern (FREEDMAN, 1968; SCARR, 1968; SHIELDS, 1978b). Beim Vergleich von EZ- und ZZ-Partnern bezüglich Ähnlichkeit des Aussehens und Ähnlichkeit der Ergebnisse von Intelligenz- und Verhaltenstests fand sich keine systematische Beziehung. Die Vermutung, daß Zwillinge sich um so ähnlicher verhalten, je ähnlicher sie aussehen, bestätigt sich also nicht (MATHENY et al., 1976). Sogar ein „Kontrasteffekt" ließ sich feststellen (PLOMIN et al., 1976): Die Persönlichkeit von häufig verwechselten, also körperlich sehr ähnlichen EZ wurde von den Müttern weniger ähnlich beurteilt als die von selten verwechselten. EZ mögen sich eine ähnlichere Umwelt suchen, häufiger die gleichen Freunde wählen, inniger zusammenhalten als ZZ. Als man jedoch die Auswirkung der Unterschiede dieser „Mikroumwelt" systematisch untersuchte, fand man sie gering oder gar nicht vorhanden. Zwillinge, die sehr aneinander hingen, stimmten in Persönlichkeit, Intelligenz und neurotischen Erkrankungen nicht häufiger und stärker überein als Zwillinge mit geringerem Zusammenhalt (LOEHLIN u. NICHOLS, 1976; PARKER, 1964; SHIELDS, 1954; SHIELDS, 1978b).

Auch BECKER (1979) setzt sich mit dem Einwand auseinander, die ähnlichere Umwelt der EZ lasse die Erbkomponente psychischer Eigenschaften überschätzen und argumentiert u.a. wie folgt: Bei SHIELDS (1962) z.B. korrelieren die getrennt aufgewachsenen EZ höher für Neurotizismus und Extraversion als die zusammen aufgewachsenen. Das läßt sich am besten damit erklären, daß Polarisierung und Rollenteilung bei den zusammen aufgewachsenen EZ die Wirkung der unterschiedlichen Umwelt der getrennten EZ aufwiegt, oder sogar übertrifft. Identifikation hat nicht generell die Bedeutung, die ihr von psychoanalytischer Seite an Hand von Einzelkasuistiken beigemessen wird. Selbst Siamesische Zwillinge zeigen keine geringeren Charakterunterschiede als getrennt aufgewachsene EZ (LE GRAS, 1933). Auch hier liegt offenbar Polarisation vor. Aus dem Polarisierungseffekt folgt, daß die Diskordanz von EZ eher überschätzt und das Ausmaß der Erblichkeit im Zwillingsvergleich unterschätzt wird.

Die entscheidende Wirkung der drei oder sogar sechs ersten Lebensjahre auf die Persönlichkeitsentwicklung stellt BECKER ebenfalls in Frage. Statistisch gesehen sind sich EZ, die nach dem 3. Lebensjahr getrennt wurden, nicht ähnlicher als kurz nach Geburt getrennte.

Nach all dem scheint die Umwelt keinen so beherrschenden Einfluß auf die Persönlichkeitsbildung auszuüben, wie oft behauptet wird. Sicher sind nichterbliche Faktoren beteiligt, aber es sieht so aus, als ob es andere wären, als allgemein angenommen wurde.

Adoptionsstudien bilden eine wichtige Ergänzung der Zwillingsforschung. Sie nützen die Tatsache aus, daß bei Adoptivkindern biologische und soziale Familie verschieden sind und nicht identisch wie im Normalfall. Schienen die Adoptionsstudien zunächst als die ideale Methode, als das Ei des Kolumbus sozusagen, so haben doch auch sie ihre Grenzen und Fehlerquellen. Die Erfassung auslesefreier Serien ist mühsam und schwierig, die gewonnenen Fallzahlen bleiben trotzdem relativ klein. Die Adoptiveltern sind oft schwer zur Mitarbeit zu gewinnen, die biologischen Verwandten schwer ausfindig zu machen. Die Verhältnisse, die zu einer Adoption führen, sind außerordentlich komplex und die Siebungsvorgänge, denen Adoptiveltern, biologische Eltern und Kinder anläßlich einer Adoption unterzogen werden, können das Bild verfälschen.

Eine weitere Strategie bilden die prospektiven Längsschnittuntersuchungen. Sie gehen von der Annahme aus, daß Erkrankungen mit spätem Manifestationsalter (z.B. Schizophrenie) sich zumindest bei einem Teil der Kranken schon in der Kindheit irgendwie bemerkbar machen. Solche Symptome können diskret und retrospektiv nicht mehr faßbar sein. Man kann weiter vermuten, daß sie der genetischen Anlage näher stehen als die spätere, voll entwickelte Psychose und man hofft, durch frühe und wiederholte Untersuchungen Einsichten zu gewinnen, die durch eine spätere und einmalige Untersuchung nicht zu erlangen sind. Um den Aufwand möglichst gering zu halten, geht man von sog. „High-Risk-Kindern" aus, d.h. von Kindern, die auf Grund ihrer Verwandtschaft zu einem psychisch Kranken oder auf Grund irgendwelcher Auffälligkeiten erfahrungsgemäß ein erhöhtes Risiko haben, später zu erkranken.

Eine weitere Strategie: Man konstruiert auf Grund einiger empirischer Risikoziffern mathematisch-theoretische Erbgangsmodelle und testet sie an familiären Risikoziffern, die an verschiedenen Untergruppen gewonnen wurden. Diese bereits früher praktizierte Methode hat durch die Möglichkeiten der elektronischen Datenverarbeitung neuen Aufschwung bekommen, besonders in den angelsächsischen Ländern, die der Biomathematik seit je zugetan waren (FALCONER, 1965; FULKER, 1973; KIDD u. CAVALLI-SFORZA, 1973; REICH et al., 1975a, b).

Eine ziemlich neue Forschungsstrategie ist die Suche nach genetischen Markern, d.h. nach bekannten Genen, die mit einem unbekannten Gen gemeinsam vorkommen, es sozusagen markieren, und dadurch seine Identifikation erlauben. Dieser Weg wird besonders bei den Depressionen eingeschlagen.

In der Neurochemie ist kaum eine Untersuchung ausdrücklich genetisch orientiert, aber sehr viele schließen genetische Probleme mit ein. Fruchtbare Forschungsimpulse gehen z.B. von Substanzen aus, die beim Menschen psychoaktive Wirkungen besitzen und deren Stoffwechsel man aus dem Tierversuch kennt oder kennen zu lernen hoffen kann. Es handelt sich dabei hauptsächlich um 2 Gruppen: 1. Rauschdrogen, die in gewissem Sinn ein Analog zur Psychosenursache darstellen, und 2. Psychopharmaka, die als Antagonisten wirken. Beide Stoffgruppen beeinflussen die Neurotransmitter, bei denen hinwiederum erbliche Unterschiede in Menge und Aktivität gefunden wurden (BARCHAS et al., 1974).

B. Spezieller Teil

I. Exogene Psychosen

Traditionell unterscheidet man exogene und endogene Psychosen. Die exogenen Psychosen sind umweltbedingt und unterteilen sich in körperlich begründbare (symptomatische und organische) und psychoreaktive. Die endogenen Psychosen sind erblich.

Leider ist die Sache aber nicht so einfach und wird mit zunehmendem Wissen immer komplizierter. Rein psychopathologisch lassen sich exogene und endogene Psychosen nicht immer sicher unterscheiden. Exogene Psychosen verlaufen zwar häufig mit organischen Syndromen oder mit psychoreaktiver Symptomatik, aber sie zeigen sehr oft auch endogen gefärbte oder sogar klassisch endogene Bilder. Auch ursächlich gibt es keine klare Abgrenzung. Nicht alle Personen bekommen eine Psychose, wenn sie einem der als Psychoseursache angeschuldigten, oft weit verbreiteten, körperlichen oder seelischen Traumen ausgesetzt waren. Bedarf es vielleicht doch einer bestimmten Disposition, um auf solche „Anlässe" psychotisch zu reagieren? Andererseits sind eineiige Zwillinge für endogene Psychosen nicht immer konkordant, trotz ihres gleichen Erbgutes. Offenbar sind außer der erblichen Anlage noch Zusatzfaktoren notwendig.

Hier interessieren uns nur jene „exogenen" Psychosen, die unter dem Bild von „endogenen" verlaufen. Es fragt sich: Wirkt das Trauma tatsächlich ursächlich, indem es an derselben Stelle in die normalen Abläufe eingreift wie ein pathologisches Gen? Oder löst es eine latente Anlage aus? Oder sind gar ein Trauma und eine endogene Psychose rein zufällig zusammengetroffen?

Induzierte Psychosen s. S. 573, reaktive Depressionen S. 581, Suchtpsychosen S. 601, Anlage – Umweltprobleme bei Schizophrenie S. 571. Bei Wochenbettpsychosen werden hormonelle und psychoreaktive Faktoren als Ursache und als Auslöser diskutiert; grundsätzlich Neues ist seit den Ausführungen von ZERBIN-RÜDIN (1967) nicht hinzugekommen. Bei den Schizophrenie-ähnlichen Emotionspsychosen von LABHARDT (1963) treffen vermutlich alle 3 Faktoren zusammen: anlagebedingte, somatische und psychoreaktive. DAVISON und BAGLEY (1969) verdanken wir eine umfassende Übersicht über Schizophrenie-artige Psychosen bei Erkrankungen des Nervensystems, DIEBOLD (1974) eine Diskussion der genetischen Aspekte der organischen Psychosen und „organischen Pseudopsychopathien".

Symptomatische Psychosen, definiert als nicht-typische, fakultative Teilerscheinung oder Folge einer allgemeinen Erkrankung, treten besonders nach Infektionskrankheiten, Intoxikationen (z.B. ROEDER-KUTSCH u. SCHOLZ-WÖLFING, 1941) und endokrinen Störungen auf (z.B. BLEULER, 1948). Eine interessante und gründliche Untersuchung über psychotische Bilder nach Herzoperationen von MEYENDORF (1976) demonstriert die bei symptomatischen Psychosen auftretenden Probleme geradezu exemplarisch.

Bereits frühere Autoren (z.B. GERHARDT, 1865; TOWBIN, 1955) hatten Fälle von Psychosen nach Herzleiden und Hirnembolien berichtet und auf die Möglichkeit einer erblichen Prädisposition hingewiesen. MEYENDORF jedoch untersuchte erstmals eine systematisch gewonnene Serie von 150 herzoperierten Patienten. Postoperativ ließen sich 2 Gruppen schwerer psychischer Störungen beobachten: Gruppe 1: Unmittelbar postoperativ traten apathisch-stuporös-parkinsonartige Syndrome auf, die entweder nach 3 bis 5 Tagen wieder abklangen oder in Störungen der Gruppe 2 übergingen. Gelegentlich kamen bereits hier paranoide Vorstellungen vor, die aber erst nachträglich berichtet wurden. Gruppe 2: Am 3. bis 5. postoperativen Tag erschienen depressive, dysphorische oder produktiv psychotische (d.h. Schizophrenie-ähnliche) Bilder, die gewöhnlich nach 3 bis 7 Tagen ebenso abrupt wieder verschwanden, wie sie gekommen waren. Die Psychosen der Gruppe 2 sind es, die uns hier interessieren. Sie traten bei 87 der 150 Patienten auf, d.h. bei 58%. Die depressiven Syndrome waren mit 21,3% relativ häufig und schlossen sich meist, aber nicht immer, an eine Störung der Gruppe 1 an. 9,3% der Patienten zeigten dysphorische, 2,7% inkohärent zerfahrene Bilder. 15,3% legten ein delirant paranoides Syndrom und 9,3% ein paranoides Syndrom ohne Bewußtseins- und Orientierungsstörungen an den Tag. Diese beiden letzten delirant und nicht-delirant produktiv psychotischen Gruppen werden von MEYENDORF als die eigentlichen „kardiogenen" Psychosen angesehen. Die hierher gehörenden 37 Patienten hatten im Vergleich zu den übrigen 113 Patienten häufiger eine endogen psychotische Symptomatik in der Familienanamnese (1% Signifikanzniveau) und in der Eigenanamnese (1‰ Signifikanz).

Eine Reihe von Schlußfolgerungen und Problemen ergibt sich: 1. Hirnembolien müssen nicht mit neurologischen Symptomen einhergehen, sie können auch primär zu akuten Psychosen führen, die von depressiven und schizophrenen Psychosen nicht zu unterscheiden sind und in Unkenntnis der Embolie als solche diagnostiziert werden. Dies zeigen Mikroembolien, die erst autoptisch entdeckt werden. Allerdings weiß man nicht, wie viele Mikroembolien keine psychotischen Störungen verursachen und wie viele psychotische Störungen ohne Mikroembolie auftreten. 2. Als Ursache für die unmittelbar postoperativ und besonders für die nach 3-5 Tagen aufgetretenen psychotischen Störungen nimmt MEYENDORF Embolien im Bereich der Basalganglien „Basalganglien-Apoplexien" an. Diese Annahme wird gestützt durch die Tatsache, daß nicht nur Embolien und Mikroembolien nach Herzoperationen mit extrakorporalem Kreislauf häufiger auftreten als nach Herzoperationen ohne solchen, sondern auch kardiogene Psychosen (26% bzw. 18%). 3. Obwohl die durch die Herzoperation verursachten Noxen (Anämie, Embolie) relevant und als Erklärung für psychotische Störungen ausreichend sind, ist doch die Familien- und die Eigen-Anamnese bei den psychotisch reagierenden Herzpatienten häufiger auffällig als bei den nichtpsychotischen. „Man sieht diese Zustandsbilder in Zusammenhang mit den normalen psychologischen und körperlichen Reaktionen und Verhaltensweisen auf den operativen Stress... Daß eine Herzoperation jedoch nicht automatisch gleichzusetzen ist mit postoperativen psychischen Auffälligkeiten, sieht man schon daran, daß von 150 Herzoperierten 60 (40%) einen psychopathologisch unauffälligen Verlauf zeigten" (MEYENDORF). 4. Die postoperativen Störungen sind individuell verschieden. Warum? Ist die Verschiedenheit ausschließlich hirnlokalisatorisch zu erklären? Manches spricht dafür, daß dem nicht so ist. 5. Handelt es sich um Auslösung einer latenten Anlage, um somatische Phänokopien oder psychoreaktive Störungen? Dies ist für die depressiven Störungen besonders schwer zu entscheiden.

In Hamburg wird dem Problem psychischer Störungen nach Herzoperationen zur Zeit in einem Sonderforschungsprogramm mit erweiterter Fragestellung intensiv nachgegangen (DAHME et al., 1977; HUSE-KLEINSTOLL et al., 1976).

II. Die Schizophrenien

Zunächst seien einige der wichtigsten neueren Übersichten genannt, die sich mit den genetischen Aspekten der Schizophrenien befassen: ERLENMEYER-KIM-

LING (1972), FORREST und AFFLECK (1975), GOTTESMAN und SHIELDS (1972, 1976), KAPLAN (1972), MEDNICK et al. (1974), MITSUDA und FUKUDA (1974), ROSENTHAL (1970), ROSENTHAL und KETY (1968), Schizophrenia Bull. (1976, Heft 3), SHIELDS (1976b, 1978b), SLATER und COWIE (1971), ZERBIN-RÜDIN (1967, 1971a, b, 1978).

Nachdem seit den Befunden von RÜDIN (1916) und LUXENBURGER (1928) die Familien- und Zwillingsbefunde als Beweis für eine erbliche Grundlage der Schizophrenien gegolten hatten, nahmen um die Mitte des 20. Jahrhunderts rein umweltorientierte und lerntheoretische psychodynamische Theorien einen lebhaften Aufschwung. Man begann die erhöhten familiären Risikoziffern ausschließlich als Folge des gemeinsamen Milieus zu erklären. Die Erbtheorie hat jedoch alle Versuche der Widerlegung überlebt, und bisher ist kein Umweltfaktor bekannt geworden, der voraussagbar ein Erkrankungsrisiko von 10–15% produziert, so wie es der Faktor „Verwandtschaft 1. Grades zu einem Schizophrenen" tut (SHIELDS, 1976a). Die Behauptung der „Antipsychiatrie", eine Krankheit Schizophrenie gäbe es nicht, sie sei ein Märchen, kommentieren KETY et al. (1976) mit den Worten: "If schizophrenia is a myth, it is a myth with a substantial genetic component".

Die genetische Forschung ist heute von der traditionellen Feststellung globaler Risikoziffern zu differenzierteren Fragestellungen übergegangen. Frischen Aufwind verdankt sie dabei vor allem den Adoptions- und Prospektivstudien und der Zwillingsforschung. Da die unvollständige Zwillingskonkordanz zeigt, daß die Erbanlage allein für eine schizophrene Psychose nicht ausreicht, ist die Anlage-Umwelt-Interaktion in den Vordergrund des Interesses gerückt. Daneben steht das Problem der Heterogenität, der genetischen Verschiedenheit der Schizophrenien. Schließlich sucht man nach Symptomen, die möglicherweise dem Genotyp näher stehen als die voll entwickelte Psychose und klarere Erbverhältnisse zeigen. Dabei hat sich die psychiatrische Genetik genau wie die Psychiatrie mit diagnostischen und klassifikatorischen Problemen auseinanderzusetzen, hofft aber, mit ihren Mitteln zu deren Klärung beitragen zu können.

1. Familienbefunde

Das gleichartige Erkrankungsrisiko für Kinder und Geschwister eines Schizophrenen beträgt bekanntlich etwa 10%–15% (wobei es für die Kinder etwas höher ist als für die Geschwister), für die Eltern 5% oder etwas darüber, für die Verwandten 2. Grades (Vettern, Basen, Enkel usw.) 3%–4% und für die Durchschnittsbevölkerung 0,85%–1%. Neue Familienuntersuchungen aus verschiedenen Ländern haben diese empirischen Risikoziffern im wesentlichen bestätigt (Übersichten bei GOTTESMAN u. SHIELDS, 1976; HANSON et al., 1976; SHIELDS, 1976a, 1978b; Einzelarbeiten: z.B. BLEULER, 1972; KAY et al., 1975; LINDELIUS, 1970; REISBY, 1967; STEPHENS et al., 1975).

Die genannten Ziffern gelten für Untersuchungen, die sich einer klassischen Diagnostik im europäischen Sinne bedienen. Einige amerikanische Untersuchungen fanden wesentlich niedrigere Erkrankungsrisiken für die Verwandten 1. Grades (z.B. WINOKUR et al., 1974: 0,8%–2%), oder auch höhere (REED et al., 1973: 19%–25%). REED et al. mußten die Diagnosen der meist verstorbenen Probanden und Sekundärfälle nach dem Krankenblatt stellen und fanden so viele unklare Psychosen, daß sie meist von funktionellen Psychosen statt von Schizophrenien sprechen.

2. Kinder zweier schizophrener Eltern

Ihre Zahl dürfte in Zukunft steigen, denn die Erfolge der modernen Therapie und die Behandlung in offenen Abteilungen und ambulanter Gruppentherapie erleichtern die Eheschließung von und zwischen schizophrenen Patienten. Wie die 5 älteren Untersuchungen zeigen, erkranken die Kinder zweier Schizophrener zu etwa 50% an einer Psychose, vorwiegend an Schizophrenie (Zusammenfassung bei ERLENMEYER-KIMLING, 1968). Dazu kommt ein weites Spektrum psychischer und sozialer Auffälligkeiten. Immerhin bleiben 30%–40% der Kinder ganz normal, trotz Vernachlässigung, „broken home" und ausgiebigem „teaching of irrationality". Das ist ein sehr wichtiger Befund und ein Argument gegen die ausschließliche Umwelttheorie der Schizophrenie. Von den neueren „dual mating studies" (Übersicht bei GOTTESMAN u. SHIELDS, 1976) seien die zwei größten gegenwärtig laufenden genannt. Die prospektiv angelegte amerikanische Untersuchung von ERLENMEYER-KIMLING (1975), verfolgt 201 Kinder von 80 schizophrenen Elternpaaren. 32% der Kinder sind bereits mit Psychosen hospitalisiert worden und 19% zeigen andere psychische Auffälligkeiten. Die amerikanisch-dänische Untersuchung von GOTTESMAN und FISCHER (GOTTESMAN u. SHIELDS, 1976) umfaßt 400 erwachsene Nachkommen verschiedener psychiatrischer Patienten-Ehepaare. Bis jetzt wurden 25% der Nachkommen hospitalisiert. Doch die Untersuchung bezweckt nicht die Berechnung von Risikoziffern, sondern sie fragt: „Was kommt mit was vor?" „Gibt es antischizophrene Gene?" Mit anderen Worten, sie möchte herausfinden: Welche Störungen der Eltern können zu Schizophrenie bei den Kindern führen? Welche Störungen können bei den Kindern schizophrener Eltern auftreten? Kann ein schizophrenes Spektrum abgegrenzt werden? Gibt es Faktoren, die eine Schizophrenie ausschließen? Man glaubte z.B. früher, daß ein Epileptiker nicht an Schizophrenie erkranken könne. Die Theorie erwies sich zwar als falsch, führte aber zu der erfolgreichen Schocktherapie.

3. Zwillingsbefunde

Tabelle 1 zeigt die wichtigsten Zwillingsuntersuchungen. Die Konkordanzrate der EZ ist im großen und ganzen rund 4mal höher als die der ZZ, und diese Tatsache stellt einen Pfeiler der Erbtheorie dar. Die Einwände gegen die Beweiskraft der Zwillingsbefunde wurden bereits auf S. 548f. diskutiert. Für die genetische Theorie spricht es auch, daß Schizophrene nicht öfter aus Zwillingsgeburten stammen als dem Zufall nach zu erwarten ist (LUXENBURGER, 1928), und daß getrennt aufgewachsene EZ ungefähr ebenso oft konkordant erkranken wie zusammen aufgewachsene. Ferner haben die diskordanten, nicht-schizophrenen EZ-Partner mindestens ebenso viele schizophrene Nachkommen (12%) wie die schizophrenen Zwillingsprobanden selbst (9%) (FISCHER, 1971). Die Erklärung muß wohl in der elterlichen Erbanlage liegen, denn elterliches Erscheinungsbild und häusliches Milieu war für die Kinder verschieden: die einen hatten einen schizophrenen Elternteil, die anderen nicht.

Tabelle 1. Konkordanz für Schizophrenie bei eineiigen (EZ) und zweieiigen (ZZ) Zwillingspaaren. Die eingeklammerten Zahlen enthalten unsichere Fälle, bzw. Schizophrenien im weiteren Sinne

Autor		Herkunfts-land	Zahl der Paare		Konkordanz in %		Ver-hältnis EZ:ZZ
			ZZ	EZ	ZZ	EZ	
Luxenburger	1928	Deutschland	48	17	2,1	76,5	36,4
Rosanoff et al.	1934	U.S.A.	101	41	10,0	61,0	6,1
Essen-Möller	1941	Schweden	24	7	8,3 (16,7)	14,3 (71,4)	1,7 (4,3)
Essen-Möller	1970	Schweden	–	8	–	25,0 (75,0)	–
Kallmann	1946	U.S.A.	517	174	14,7	85,8	5,8
Kallmann (nach Shields et al.)	1967	U.S.A.	517	174	9,1 (10,3)	59,2 (69,0)	6,5 (6,7)
Slater	1953	England	115	41	11,3	68,3	6,0
Inouye	1961	Japan	17	55	11,8	60,0	5,1
Tienari	1963	Finnland	21	16	4,8	0	–
Tienari	1968	Finnland	–	17	–	6,0 (36,0)	–
Kringlen	1968	Norwegen	90	55	4,0 (10,0)	25,0 (38,0)	6,3 (3,8)
Fischer et al.	1969	Dänemark	41	21	9,8 (19,5)	23,8 (47,6)	2,4 (2,4)
Pollin et al.	1969	U.S.A.	146	80	4,1	13,8	3,4
Gottesman u. Shields	1972	England	33	22	9,1	50,0	5,5
Shields[a]	1976	–	–	28	–	63,3	–

[a] Sammelkasuistik getrennt aufgewachsener Paare

Die Spannweite der Konkordanzraten verschiedener Untersucher ist ziemlich groß. Nachdem Kallmann (1946) seine erfaßten amerikanischen Zwillinge zu 85% konkordant gefunden hatte, erregte der Finne Tienari (1963) beträchtliches Aufsehen, als er bei 16 EZ-Paaren eine Konkordanz von 0 berichtete. Bei näherem Zusehen ist die Diskrepanz allerdings nicht ganz so gewaltig. Kallmann hatte seine 85% mit stärkeren Alterskorrekturen errechnet und eine Neuberechnung nach der üblichen Methode ergab die wesentlich niedrigere Konkordanzziffer von 59%, bzw. 69% unter Einschluß wahrscheinlicher Schizophrenien (Shields et al., 1967). Andererseits mußte Tienari (1968) bei der Nachuntersuchung feststellen, daß 1 bzw. 6 Zwillingspartner auffällig geworden waren, was einer Konkordanz von 6% sichere Schizophrenie bzw. 36% einschließlich wahrscheinlicher Schizophrenie entspricht.

Trotz Korrektur der beiden Extremwerte bleiben Unterschiede zwischen den einzelnen Serien bestehen. Im allgemeinen liefern die neuen Serien niedrigere Werte als die älteren und die skandinavischen niedrigere als die übrigen. Man hat das damit zu erklären versucht, daß die älteren Serien Anstaltspatienten betrafen, also eine Auslese nach schweren Fällen mit hoher Konkordanz darstellen, während die neueren, besonders die skandinavischen Serien von ganzen Geburtsjahrgängen oder Populationen ausgehen, somit umfassender sind und der Wahrheit näher kommen. Allerdings bedarf der Wunderglaube an die überlegene Vollständigkeit und Genauigkeit solcher epidemiologischer Zwillingsstudien einiger Einschränkungen. Da es praktisch unmöglich ist, die mit viel Aufwand ermittelten Zwillinge dann mit noch mehr Aufwand auch wirklich alle individuell und intensiv zu verfolgen, wird entweder doch wieder nur eine Stichprobe untersucht, oder die Probanden werden durch Vergleich der Geburtenregister mit psychiatrischen Zentralregistern ermittelt, also doch wieder aus Krankenhauspatienten. Die Zwillingsserie von POLLIN et al. (1969) stellt, obgleich epidemiologisch angelegt, eine Auslese nach Gesundheit und spät erkrankten Fällen dar, und das erklärt wohl die niedrige Konkordanz. Die Arbeitsgruppe zog aus sämtlichen 15 909 Zwillingspaaren, die in der amerikanischen Wehrmacht gedient hatten, die schizophren Erkrankten heraus. Da beide Partner gedient haben mußten, fielen alle Paare weg, in denen ein oder beide Partner vor dem Musterungstermin erkrankt waren.

Weitere Erklärungsmöglichkeiten betreffen die Diagnostik. Erstens einmal wird die Schizophreniediagnose unterschiedlich aufgefaßt und gehandhabt. Sehen wir davon ab, so ist es aber überhaupt falsch zu meinen, es gäbe für eine bestimmte Serie nur eine einzige richtige und sinnvolle Konkordanzrate. GOTTESMAN und SHIELDS (1966) fanden die EZ-Partner 24 schizophrener Probanden zu 42% konkordant für stationär behandelte Schizophrenie, zu 54% für irgend eine stationär behandelte psychische Störung und zu 79% für irgend eine psychische Anomalie. Für die 33 ZZ lauteten die entsprechenden Zahlen 9%, 18% und 45%. Analog dazu betrug bei ESSEN-MÖLLER (1970) die EZ-Konkordanz für Schizophrenie 25%, für Hospitalaufenthalt 50% und für psychische Störungen insgesamt 75% (Gesamtzahl 8 Paare). Man geht also immer mehr dazu über, die Konkordanz feiner aufzugliedern, um so die Variationsbreite der schizophrenen Anlage besser zu fassen und vielleicht auch die Serien besser vergleichbar zu machen.

Die Psychosen eineiiger Zwillinge sind zwar in der Regel ähnlich und gehören der gleichen diagnostischen Kategorie an, individuelle Unterschiede sind aber praktisch immer vorhanden. Ein anschauliches Beispiel bilden eineiige Vierlingsschwestern, die konkordant an „Schizophrenie katatoner Färbung" erkrankten, aber deutliche Unterschiede im klinischen Bild boten (ROSENTHAL, 1963). Nur eine Schwester erlebte wiederholte Remissionen, während derer sie arbeitsfähig war und heiratete. Eine weitere Schwester war bereits als Kind auffällig gewesen, aber nicht als krank, sondern als böse und schlecht angesehen worden. Bei ihr nahm die Schizophrenie einen chronischen Verlauf, wie bei den beiden anderen später erkrankten Schwestern auch. Die fotografische Gleichheit von Zwillingsschicksalen, wie sie in der Laienpresse ausgiebig beschrieben und diskutiert wird, findet bei systematischer Betrachtung nur wenig Stütze. Ein unheimlicher Ausnahmefall: Zwillingsschwestern erkrankten gleichzeitig an Schizophrenie, wurden gemeinsam in eine psychiatrische Klinik aufgenommen, aber nach einiger Zeit aus therapeutischen Gründen getrennt und auf verschiedene Stationen verlegt. Die Schwestern stimmten der Trennung zu, litten jedoch sehr darunter. Ihr Gesundheitszustand war gut. Aber plötzlich starben sie zur gleichen Stunde, ohne Kontakt miteinander gehabt zu haben und ohne daß eine spezifische oder gar gewaltsame Todesursache zu finden gewesen wäre (WILSON u. REECE, 1964).

Eine dritte Erklärungsmöglichkeit liegt in zu kurzer Beobachtungsdauer, die zu niedrige Konkordanzen ergibt. Die Partner zweier Paare aus der dänischen Serie von FISCHER (1973) erkrankten mit einem Zeitabstand von 17 bzw. 29 Jahren. In der kleinen Serie von ESSEN-MÖLLER (1941) wurden 2 von 8 Partnern 11 und 23 Jahre nach dem ersterkrankten Zwilling eindeutig schizophren, was sich erst bei der Katamnese 1973 herausstellte. 2 weitere Partner hatten wegen Schizophrenie-ähnlicher Störungen kurze Krankenhausaufenthalte durchgemacht. Im Zuge der oben beschriebenen Untersuchung an amerikanischen Veteranenzwillingen hatte man Anfang der 60er Jahre sehr sorgfältig Schizophreniediskordante Zwillingspaare für bestimmte Fragestellungen ausgelesen. 10 Jahre später betrug die Konkordanz bereits 25% (BELMAKER et al., 1974). (Katamnestische Revision von TIENARI s. oben.)

Als vierte Erklärungsmöglichkeit schließlich gibt es vermutlich echte Unterschiede zwischen den einzelnen Serien und den Populationen, aus denen sie stammen. Umweltbedingungen und Genbestand könnten nach Ort und Zeit variieren.

Weitere Zwillingsbefunde s. S. 574–576.

4. Adoptionsstudien

Pionierarbeit leistete HESTON (1966). Er ging aus von 47 Kindern schwer schizophrener Mütter, die in einer psychiatrischen Klinik geboren, innerhalb von 3 Tagen von der Mutter getrennt wurden und in verschiedener Umgebung, in Heimen, Pflegestellen oder Adoptivfamilien aufwuchsen, aber niemals bei Verwandten mütterlicherseits. Dazu wurde eine Kontrollgruppe zusammengestellt. Im Alter von durchschnittlich 36 Jahren waren keine Kinder der Kontrollgruppe, aber 5 der Index-Kinder schizophren geworden. Das entspricht mit 16% genau dem Risiko, welches KALLMANN (1938, 1946) generell für die Kinder Schizophrener festgestellt hatte. Gleichsinnig fand HIGGINS (1976) für die Kinder Schizophrener ein etwa gleichhohes Erkrankungsrisiko, ob sie nun zu Hause oder in Pflegestellen aufgewachsen waren. In HESTONS Serie zeigten weiterhin 13 Kinder eine soziopathische Persönlichkeit und 9 neurotische Persönlichkeitsstörungen, was HESTON als Manifestation der schizophrenen Anlage ansieht. Andererseits gab es aber auch einige besonders „farbige" und positive Persönlichkeiten, wie sie in der Kontrollgruppe nicht zu verzeichnen waren.

In einer isländischen Untersuchung (KARLSSON, 1966) erkrankten die weggegebenen Kinder Schizophrener gar zu 29% (5 von 17). Die Serie ist sehr klein, einige Kinder waren von Verwandten aufgenommen worden und selektive Einflüsse mögen hereinspielen.

Außerordentlich einfallsreich und breit angelegt ist die amerikanisch-dänische Adoptionsstudie der Arbeitsgruppe um KETY, ROSENTHAL, SCHULSINGER und WENDER. 1962 begann man, 5483 Adoptionsfälle aus den Adoptionsregistern von Groß-Kopenhagen mit dem psychiatrischen Zentralregister zu vergleichen und diejenigen Fälle herauszuziehen, in denen leibliche Eltern, Adoptiveltern oder Adoptivkinder an Schizophrenie erkrankt waren. Die Autoren verfolgten 3 Hauptstrategien: Sie gingen aus 1. von schizophrenen Eltern, die ein Kind zur Adoption freigegeben hatten und verfolgten das Schicksal der Kinder, 2. von Kindern nicht-schizophrener Eltern, die von Schizophrenen adoptiert worden waren, 3. von Adoptivkindern, die schizophren geworden waren, und verglichen die biologischen Verwandten mit den Adoptivverwandten.

Erste Befunde erschienen 1968 (ROSENTHAL u. KETY, 1968). Weitere Veröffentlichungen folgten. Man bildete „gereinigte" und „erweiterte" Gruppen, ergänzte die ursprüngliche Beurteilung nach Aktenlage durch persönliche Interviews, berücksichtigte den psychischen Zustand des zweiten biologischen, nichtschizophrenen Elternteiles (ROSENTHAL, 1975) und sammelte Informationen über Familien, die Auskünfte verweigerten (PAIKIN et al., 1974). Die Untersuchungen sind noch im Gang, und das Material wird durch Ausdehnung auf ganz Dänemark vergrößert. All das brachte keine umwälzenden Änderungen, jedoch eine Fülle verschiedenartig berechneter Prozentzahlen. Einzelheiten müssen in den Originalen nachgelesen werden.

Unsicherheiten entstehen besonders für den europäischen Psychiater durch die weitherzige Handhabung der Schizophreniediagnose nach amerikanischem Muster und die Einführung des noch weitherzigeren Konzeptes der „Spektrumstörungen", welches reiche Gelegenheit für Spekulationen, aber auch für Kritik bietet. In dem vierstufigen Diagnoseschema bedeutet A nicht-schizophren. Sichere Schizophrenie umfaßt nicht nur chronische und Prozeßschizophrenien (B_1), sondern auch akute schizophrene Reaktionen (B_2), und „borderline"-Fälle, einschließlich pseudoneurotischer Schizophrenie, psychotischem Charakter und schwerem Schizoid (B_3). Zu den Spektrumstörungen (C) gehören „inadäquate", schizoide und paranoide Persönlichkeiten, sowie Störungen der Gruppe B_3 in leichterer Ausprägung. Sie werden nochmals unterteilt in „hard" und „soft". Die Kategorien $D_{1,2,3}$ umfassen unsichere und fragliche Fälle, entsprechend den drei B-Kategorien. Nicht immer wird ganz klar, welche Fälle noch zur Schizophrenie und welche zum Spektrum gehören, zumal die Autoren gelegentlich diagnostische Revisionen vornahmen. Im allgemeinen aber sind die Grunddaten so ausreichend dokumentiert, daß sie es ermöglichen, andere Prozentzahlen zu errechnen und andere Schlußfolgerungen zu ziehen als die Autoren selbst; eine Möglichkeit, von der GOTTESMAN und SHIELDS (1976) kritisch Gebrauch gemacht haben.

Ein so weites Schizophreniekonzept rechtfertigt sich insofern, als wir nicht wissen, was alles zur Schizophrenie gehört. Um einschlägige Fälle nicht zu übersehen, ist es sinnvoll, alle möglichen „verdächtigen" Störungen einzubeziehen, sofern dies ausdrücklich erläutert wird. Trotzdem hat die Einbeziehung der „Spektrumfälle" ihre Nachteile. Es handelt sich teilweise um recht unspezifische und häufige Störungen, die zwar gelegentlich Ausdruck einer Schizophrenie sein können, sehr oft aber wohl nichts damit zu tun haben, wie das häufige Vorkommen in den Kontrollgruppen zeigt. Man muß damit rechnen, daß sie durch den zweiten Ehepartner, also durch Heirat, in die Familien hereingekommen sind (GOTTESMAN u. SHIELDS, 1976) und die Situation eher komplizieren als klären. Im Gegensatz zu den früheren Befunden – nach Aktenlage – stützte die genauere Interview-Studie die Zugehörigkeit der akuten Schizophrenie (entfernt den schizoaffektiven Psychosen vergleichbar) zur Schizophrenie und die Zugehörigkeit des Schizoids zum schizophrenen Spektrum nicht mehr. Auch FOWLER et al. (1975) und STEPHENS et al. (1975) konnten die enge Zugehörigkeit der Spektrumstörungen zur Schizophrenie nicht bestätigen. Die Einführung der

Spektrumdiagnosen erschwert auch die Vergleichbarkeit mit anderen Untersuchungen. Das ist bedauerlich, auch wenn KETY et al. (1976) meinen, die Studie hätte eben ihre eigene Diagnostik; Vergleiche müßten zwischen den verschiedenen Probanden- und Kontrollgruppen innerhalb dieses einen großen Projektes gezogen werden und nicht mit den Ergebnissen anderer Autoren.

Nun zu den Ergebnissen: In der „Adoptees Study" (ROSENTHAL, 1972) erkrankten die wegadoptierten Nachkommen schizophrener Eltern zwar nur zu 4% an einer klassischen Schizophrenie, doch ist das immerhin das 5fache der Durchschnittserwartung von 0,85%. Weitere 28% litten an einer „Schizophrenie-Spektrumstörung". In der Kontrollgruppe (Adoptivkinder mit nicht-schizophrenen leiblichen Eltern) war kein einziges Kind an Schizophrenie erkrankt, aber 18% an Spektrumstörungen, was sehr hoch erscheint. In einer späteren Veröffentlichung (WENDER et al., 1974) wird angegeben, daß 18,8% der Indexfälle und 10,8% der Kontrollgruppe an Schizophrenie im weiteren Sinn („borderline" oder schwerer) litten.

Was bedeuten diese zunächst etwas verblüffenden Zahlen? Klassische Schizophrenien sind unter den wegadoptierten Nachkommen der Schizophrenen relativ selten, doch gehörten auch die „schizophrenen" Eltern zu einem guten Drittel der „borderline"- oder Spektrumgruppe an, hatten also möglicherweise keine „echte" Schizophrenie. Die Spektrumfälle dagegen sind in allen Gruppen zahlreich und das läßt mehrere Deutungen zu: a) Es handelt sich um allgemein häufige und relativ unspezifische Störungen. Im Bestreben, nur ja nichts zu übersehen, haben die Autoren alle möglichen Auffälligkeiten registriert und vielleicht überbewertet. b) Die Häufigkeit der Spektrumstörungen bei den Kontrollkindern könnte daraus resultieren, daß auch nicht-schizophrene Eltern, die ein Kind zur Adoption geben, ein erhöhtes Risiko für psychische Störungen (Spektrumstörungen?) besitzen. c) Die Spektrumstörungen in der Indexgruppe sind so zahlreich, weil bereits einige der „schizophrenen" Eltern an einer Spektrumstörung litten (s. oben), oder aber deren Ehegatten. Die Partner von Schizophrenen, die ein Kind zur Adoption geben, stellen insofern eine Auslese dar, als auch sie nicht willens oder fähig sind, ihr Kind aufzuziehen. Tatsächlich fand ROSENTHAL (1975) bei der Hälfte der Ehefrauen der schizophrenen Väter Spektrumstörungen, und die Kinder aus diesen Ehen litten häufiger wiederum an Spektrumstörungen als die übrigen Adoptivkinder.

Wie es auch sei, Schizophrenie und Schizophrenie-ähnliche Störungen traten bei den wegadoptierten Nachkommen schizophrener Eltern wesentlich häufiger auf als unter Adoptivkindern mit nicht-schizophrenen leiblichen Eltern. Mit intrauterinen mütterlichen Einflüssen läßt sich das nicht erklären. Denn nicht immer war die Mutter schizophren, wie bei HESTON, sondern in etwa einem Drittel der Fälle war es der Vater. Außerdem weisen die Halbgeschwister väterlicherseits eine beträchtliche Schizophrenierate auf, ja die höchste der ganzen Untersuchung (KETY et al., 1975). Auch eine Erwartungshaltung der Adoptiveltern im Sinne einer „self-fulfilling prophecy" kann keine Rolle gespielt haben; ein Großteil der leiblichen Eltern war erst nach der Adoption erkrankt, so daß die Adoptiveltern gar nichts davon wußten.

Die „Crossfostering Study" (WENDER et al., 1974) verfolgte das Schicksal von Kindern nicht-schizophrener Eltern, die von Schizophrenen adoptiert wor-

Tabelle 2. Häufigkeit (unkorrigierte Prozentziffern) von Schizophrenie und Schizophreniespektrumstörungen in den biologischen Familien und Adoptivfamilien von schizophren gewordenen Adoptivkindern und einer Kontrollgruppe. (Nach KETY et al., 1976)

	Biologische Eltern und Geschwister			Adoptiv-Eltern und Geschwister		
	Gesamt-zahl	Sichere Schizo-phrenie %	Schizo-phrenie +Spektrum %	Gesamt-zahl	Sichere Schizo-phrenie %	Schizo-phrenie +Spektrum %
Schizophrene Adoptierte	173	6,4	21,4	74	1,4	5,4
Nicht-schizophrene Adoptierte	174	1,7	10,9	91	2,2	7,7

den waren. Kein einziges Kind erkrankte an einer schweren Prozeßschizophrenie, aber 10,7% (3 von 28) an Schizophrenie im weitesten Sinn. In der Kontrollgruppe war die Erkrankungsziffer genau so hoch, nämlich 10,1%, unter den Adoptivkindern mit leiblichen schizophrenen Eltern dagegen höher, 18,8%.

Die „Adoptees Family Study" ging nicht von schizophrenen Eltern aus, sondern von Adoptivkindern, die später schizophren wurden, und untersuchte deren Verwandte (KETY et al., 1976). Tabelle 2 zeigt, daß wiederum Schizophrenie in den biologischen Familien weit häufiger vorkam als in den Adoptivfamilien. Auch hier waren klassische Schizophrenien bei den Verwandten relativ selten und die „schizophrenen" Adoptivkinder selbst litten ebenfalls nur zur Hälfte an einer klassischen Schizophrenie.

WENDER et al. (1968) verglichen in einer rein amerikanischen Studie die Psychopathologie von 10 Adoptiveltern schizophren gewordener Kinder mit der von 10 Adoptiveltern nicht-schizophrener Kinder und 10 leiblichen Eltern Schizophrener und fanden sie ungefähr in der Mitte zwischen den beiden Vergleichsgruppen. Sichere Aussagen über Ursache und Wirkung können nicht gemacht werden, doch liegt der Verdacht nahe, daß der Befund zumindest teilweise mit der Wirkung zu erklären ist, die vom Schizophrenen auf seine Umgebung, also auch auf die Adoptiveltern ausstrahlt (vgl. auch SCHULTE, 1968 u. WILLI, 1962).

Die Adoptionsstudien haben gezeigt, daß Schizophrenie in den biologischen Familien von Schizophrenen weit häufiger vorkommt als in den Adoptivfamilien und in Kontrollgruppen. Das steht mit der Erbtheorie im Einklang und nicht mit der Umwelttheorie. Die den Adoptionsstudien immanenten Fehlerquellen führen eher zu einer Unterschätzung des Erbeinflusses als zu einer Überschätzung (HORN et al., 1975). Ferner haben sie das Interesse an Schizophrenieverwandten Störungen neu belebt und sich nebenbei mit einer Reihe von Problemen befaßt, die schon früher in weniger spektakulären Serien behandelt worden waren. Zum Beispiel zeigte sich, daß Heimerziehung an sich das Schizophrenierisiko nicht vergrößert (HESTON u. DENNEY, 1968), daß niedrige soziale Schicht die Schizophrenieentstehung nicht begünstigt (WENDER et al., 1973) und daß zwischen gestörten Eltern-Kind-Beziehungen und Auftreten psychischer Störungen beim Kind nur eine schwache Korrelation besteht (ROSENTHAL et al., 1975).

5. Erbgangshypothesen

Modelle mit einem Hauptgen: Da die Mehrzahl der Schizophrenen von zwei nicht-schizophrenen Eltern abstammt, hatte man früher rezessive Vererbung angenommen (RÜDIN, 1916; KALLMANN, 1938). Die Nachkommen Schizophrener besitzen aber ein ebenso hohes Erkrankungsrisiko wie die Geschwister, und das paßt nicht zu Rezessivität. Daher werden heute dominante Theorien bevorzugt (HESTON, 1970; KARLSSON, 1972; SHIELDS et al., 1975; SLATER, 1958, 1972). Für sie spricht vor allem die Tatsache, daß die familiäre Belastung häufiger nur einseitig nachweisbar ist, d. h. entweder väterlicher- *oder* mütterlicherseits (SLATER u. TSUANG, 1968; TSUANG, 1971). Andere empirische Daten passen aber wiederum nicht dazu; vor allem sind die empirischen Risikoziffern für einfache Dominanz viel zu niedrig. Man muß also Hilfshypothesen, wie Manifestationsschwankungen, Umwelteinflüsse und Nebengene heranziehen.

Polygene bzw. multifaktorielle Modelle: Denkt man an Nebengene, so ist man nicht mehr weit entfernt von Polygenie, Vererbung durch mehrere Genpaare. Polygenie in ihren verschiedenen Varianten besitzt viele Anhänger (BLEULER, 1972; EDWARDS, 1972; FARLEY, 1976; KETY et al., 1968; KRINGLEN, 1967, 1968, 1976; ØDEGAARD, 1972). Die Gene werden mehr oder weniger spezifisch, die Erbkomponenten mehr oder weniger einflußreich gedacht. Praktisch alle polygenen Modelle beziehen Umweltfaktoren mit ein, sie sind multifaktoriell. Anlage- und Umweltfaktoren kombinieren sich von Fall zu Fall verschieden; die Gene sind zahlenmäßig begrenzt und besitzen verschiedenes Gewicht. Polygene Modelle kann man unterteilen in solche mit kontinuierlicher Verteilung und solche mit Schwellenwerten. Bei Vorliegen einer Schwelle bedarf es einer bestimmten Anzahl von Faktoren, bis die Schwelle überschritten wird und eine Wirkung auftritt. Neuerdings sind Modelle mit mehreren Schwellen aufgestellt worden (REICH et al., 1972, 1975a). Besonders GOTTESMAN und SHIELDS (1967, 1973, 1976) stellten triftige Überlegungen zugunsten spezifischer multifaktorieller Vererbung an und erzielten in der sorgfältig durchdachten Anwendung eines Zwei-Schwellen-Modells gute Übereinstimmung der Erwartungswerte mit den empirischen Daten.

Mit multifaktorieller Vererbung stehen viele Befunde in Einklang: die große Variationsbreite in Symptomatik und Schwere der schizophrenen Psychosen; das Ansteigen des Erkrankungsrisikos mit Zunahme der Zahl und der Erkrankungsschwere kranker Verwandter; das Vorkommen zahlreicher anderer psychischer Auffälligkeiten, wie Schizoid, Neurosen, soziale Anpassungsstörungen, in den Familien Schizophrener. Schließlich sind die Schizophrenien häufiger, als monogene Krankheiten zu sein pflegen und ihr Fortbestehen, trotz reduzierter Fruchtbarkeit der Kranken, ist leichter mit Polygenie als mit Monogenie vereinbar.

Doch auch Polygenie ist nicht ganz schlüssig. Insbesondere müssen auch hier teilweise extrem niedrige Manifestationsraten angenommen werden und die Erklärung der Diskordanz der EZ-Paare bereitet Schwierigkeiten. Daher hat

Essen-Möller (1977) einige Zweifel angemeldet, und Dalén (1972) hält die Theorie für so „weich", daß sie weder bewiesen, noch gegenbewiesen werden kann und daher auch von den Environmentalisten anerkannt wird, die jeder „harten" Erbtheorie feindlich gegenüberstehen. Monogene Theorien *sind* gegenbeweisbar; man sollte sie beibehalten und abwarten, was die Versuche, sie zu widerlegen, ergeben. Curnow und Smith (1975) hinwiederum halten zwar polygene Modelle ebenfalls für unwahrscheinlich, aber vorläufig als Arbeitshypothese für sehr nützlich!

Alle sind sich einig, wie schwierig es ist, den einen oder anderen Erbgang wahrscheinlicher zu machen. Trotzdem hat man versucht, durch Analyse der empirischen Risikoziffern mit verschiedenen mathematischen Methoden, wie Segregationsanalyse oder Schwellen-Modellen, Hinweise zu gewinnen (kurze Übersicht bei Smith u. Forrest, 1975). Aber schon die empirischen Daten variieren; die Ergebnisse der mathematischen Analysen und die Schlußfolgerungen der Autoren tun das erst recht, ja sie sind gelegentlich einander diametral entgegengesetzt. Elston und Campbell (1970) z.B. fanden gute Übereinstimmung der empirischen Daten mit einem monogenen Modell, Smith (1971) dagegen mit einem polygenen. Die von Gottesman und Shields (1976) errechneten Erwartungswerte aus einem polygenen Schwellen-Modell unterscheiden sich kaum von denen aus einem monogenen Modell mit unvollständiger Penetranz. Beide stehen einigermaßen mit den empirischen Daten in Einklang, die polygenen Werte jedoch etwas besser. Auch Kidd und Cavalli-Sforza (1973) fanden sowohl monogene als auch polygene Modelle mit den empirischen Daten vereinbar, jedoch die monogenen etwas beser. Matthysse und Kidd (1976) sowie Kessler (1976) dagegen stellen fest, daß sich die Voraussagen aus einem polygenen und einem monogenen Modell sehr deutlich voneinander unterscheiden, daß aber beide gleich schlecht zu den empirischen Befunden passen und diese nicht erklären können. Karlsson vertrat 1970 eine Zwei-Gen-Theorie, revidierte sie jedoch 1972 zugunsten von Monogenie, allerdings weniger auf Grund neuer mathematischer Modelle, als auf Grund neuer empirischer Familienbefunde.

Wenn ein Modell gut zu den empirischen Daten paßt, so läßt sich das zwar leicht feststellen, aber es ist ungewiß, inwieweit man damit eine reale biologische Tatsache erfaßt und inwieweit man lediglich die Gültigkeit der Statistik geprüft hat (Smith u. Forrest, 1975). Eine Entscheidung für oder wider Monogenie oder Polygenie ist also derzeit nicht möglich. Die Lösung wird wohl auch nicht von der Mathematik herkommen, sondern von der Verfügbarkeit besserer klinischer und genetischer Daten und von Fortschritten auf anderen Wissenschaftsgebieten, z.B. der Biochemie.

Alle Autoren ziehen mehr oder weniger Heterogenie, Uneinheitlichkeit, in Betracht. Sie ist um so wahrscheinlicher, als sich auch klinisch viel einheitlichere und besser definierte Krankheitsbilder wie Blindheit, Taubheit oder Muskeldystrophien, als genetisch uneinheitlich herausgestellt haben. Die Heterogenie bezieht sich in erster Linie auf die Schizophrenien insgesamt. Die klinischen Untergruppen hebephrener, paranoider und katatoner Färbung sind genetisch nicht scharf zu trennen, trotz der neu aufgeflammten Bemühungen (s. unten). Mitsuda (1967) hält die Schizophrenien für so uneinheitlich, daß statistische Erbgangsberechnungen an Serien überhaupt sinnlos und von vorneherein zum Scheitern verurteilt sind.

Auch LEONHARD betont die Heterogenität der Schizophrenien seit langem und sucht sie genetisch zu untermauern. Während er jedoch bei den Patienten die subtilsten klinischen Unterschiede herausarbeitete, machte er über die familiäre Belastung höchst summarische Angaben und verglich einfach die Anzahl „belasteter" Patienten in den einzelnen Gruppen. Generell fand er die „systematischen" (typischen) Schizophrenien niedriger belastet als die „unsystematischen" (atypischen) (LEONHARD, 1968). In neueren Untersuchungen gibt er die Zahl der Sekundärfälle an und seine Schülerin v. TROSTORFF (1975) berechnet korrigierte Prozentziffern. Die klinische Beschreibung der psychotischen Sekundärfälle ist jedoch weiterhin mangelhaft und Belastungsunterschiede werden mehr nach Höhe als nach Art gewertet. Wiederum sind die drei unsystematischen Schizophrenieformen höher belastet als die systematischen und innerhalb der unsystematischen sollen die affektvollen Paraphrenien rezessiven Erbgang zeigen, die periodischen Katatonien (die LEONHARD im Unterschied zu anderen europäischen Psychiatern immer noch häufig sieht) dominanten (LEONHARD, 1975a). „Um den mit meiner Diagnostik nicht vertrauten Autoren entgegenzukommen", nimmt LEONHARD (1975b) eine Zweiteilung in sporadische und familiäre Fälle vor, wobei sich die ersteren vorwiegend als systematische Schizophrenien, die letzteren als unsystematische erwiesen. Auch unterschiedliche Geschlechtsverteilungen ergaben sich.

Es gibt noch weitere Vererbungshypothesen, z. B. plasmatische, in den Mitochondrien lokalisierte Vererbung, wodurch die Diskordanz eineiiger Zwillingspaare erklärt würde (KANIG, 1973). Weitere Überlegungen finden sich in dem von KAPLAN (1972) herausgegebenen Buch. Hypothesen sind schnell aufgestellt, und sie bleiben straffrei, auch wenn sie noch so falsch sind! (GOTTESMAN u. SHIELDS, 1976).

In Anbetracht der unklaren Erbverhältnisse lassen sich verschiedene Überlegungen anstellen: 1. Was gehört überhaupt zu den Schizophrenien und was nicht? Lassen sich durch Aufspaltung der Schizophrenien in Untergruppen oder durch Ein- oder Ausschluß von fraglichen Schizophrenien, Randstörungen usw. Mendelziffern herausarbeiten? 2. Folgen Einzelsymptome oder -syndrome einem klaren Erbgang? 3. Was steckt hinter der Symptomatik der voll entwickelten Psychose und ist es möglich, Zwischenglieder zwischen der unbekannten, erblichen Grundlage (dem Genotyp) und dem Erscheinungsbild (dem Phänotyp) zu fassen? 4. Was muß zur erblichen Anlage noch hinzukommen, damit eine schizophrene Psychose entsteht?

6. Was gehört zur Schizophrenie?

Wir wissen nicht, ob von dem, was wir dazurechnen, nicht einiges abzutrennen wäre und andererseits Zustände, die als eigenständig gelten, im Grunde nicht doch dazugehören. Der Genetiker versucht also, ob er durch „splitting or lumping", durch Abspalten oder Zusammenwerfen, klare Verhältnisse zu finden vermag.

Schon früher war man bestrebt, eine reine Kerngruppe und damit den genetisch harten Kern herauszuschälen. Tatsächlich zeigten in manchen, aber nicht in allen Serien die atypischen und spät aufgetretenen Schizophrenien eine niedrigere familiäre Belastung als die typischen und frühen. KALLMANN (1938) fand die paranoiden Schizophrenien etwas niedriger belastet als die hebephrenen und die Simplexfälle. Neuerdings griff man dies wieder auf und versuchte genetische Unterschiede zwischen paranoiden und nicht-paranoiden, gut und schlecht remittierenden Schizophrenien herauszuarbeiten (MCCABE et al., 1971; WINOKUR et al., 1974). Die Unterschiede sind mehr quantitativer als qualitativer Art und man braucht sie nicht unbedingt mit einer Zwei-Krankheiten-Theorie zu erklären (TSUANG et al., 1974). SCHACHMATOWA (1977) unterscheidet in kontinuierlichen, schubförmig progredienten und rekurrenten Verläufen drei Untertypen, deren Verschiedenheiten sie betont. Zum Beispiel besitzen die schubförmigen Schizophrenien die höchste familiäre Belastung und die kontinuierlichen die niedrigste; die familiären Sekundärpsychosen sind meist gleichsinnig. Dennoch gibt es auch Gemeinsamkeiten. So finden sich die gleichen Persönlichkeitscharakteristika in allen drei Untergruppen gehäuft bei den Probanden und ihren Verwandten und es besteht ein Kontinuum von den kontinuierlichen zu den rekurrenten Verläufen und noch dazu keine scharfe Grenze gegen die manisch-depressiven Psychosen.

Alles in allem besitzen die schizophrenen Unterformen offenbar eine Neigung zu intrafamiliärer Ähnlichkeit und sie weisen Unterschiede in der Höhe der familiären Belastung auf. Trotzdem kommen sie auch gemeinsam in den Familien vor, und eine deutlich genetische Trennung besteht nicht.

Ein kleiner Teil der Schizophrenien könnte Phänokopien darstellen, nicht-erbliche Krankheitsbilder, die den erblichen völlig gleichen. Man kann sich vorstellen, daß ein nicht-erbliches Agens an der gleichen Stelle in die normalen Abläufe eingreift wie ein pathologisches Gen. Als Ursache kommen u. a. endokrine Störungen, Intoxikationen und Hirntraumen in Frage (DAVISON u. BAGLEY, 1969) aber sicher nur ausnahmsweise, denn unter Patienten mit derartigen Störungen findet sich nur eine geringe Erhöhung der Schizophreniehäufigkeit, wenn überhaupt eine. BLEULER schätzt den Anteil somatischer Phänokopien auf 1% (vgl. auch Abschn. B.I., S. 551).

Andererseits war seit jeher die beträchtliche Zahl nicht-psychotischer, aber psychisch auffälliger oder besonderer Persönlichkeiten in den Familien der Schizophrenen aufgefallen. Der Zustand der eineiigen Zwillingspartner von Schizophrenen reicht von ebenfalls schizophren über atypisch psychotisch, schizoid, neurotisch oder sonderlich bis zu zeitlebens ganz normal. Die Schizophrenieanlage kann sich offenbar verschieden manifestieren oder überhaupt stumm bleiben.

Um die Bedeutung des Schizoids führte die ältere Erbpsychiatrie hitzige Debatten. Man sah in ihm eine abortive Schizophrenie oder den Ausdruck von Teilanlagen (Übersicht bei PLANANSKY, 1966, 1972). Dann wurde es still darum, nicht zuletzt deshalb, weil Definition und Diagnose hier noch größerer Subjektivität unterliegen als bei den Schizophrenien. Neuerdings ist das Schizoid im Rahmen der Spektrumdiagnosen, besonders aber durch die Überlegungen von HESTON (1970) (modifiziert von SHIELDS et al., 1975) wieder aktuell geworden. HESTON sieht in der „schizophrenen und schizoiden Krankheit" eine Einheit, die sich dominant vererbt. Ob sie sich als Schizophrenie oder als Schizoid manifestiert, hängt von modifizierenden Faktoren ab. STEPHENS et al. (1975)

und KAY et al. (1975) konnten zwar das Vorkommen schizoider Verwandter in den Familien Schizophrener bestätigen, nicht aber das Hestonsche Dominanz-Modell. In ihrer Serie erreichten die empirischen Risikoziffern die für Dominanz erforderliche Höhe nur dann, wenn sie alle Spektrumdiagnosen mit einbezogen. Dann aber wurden die Risikoziffern in der Kontrollgruppe fast ebenso hoch, waren also nicht mehr spezifisch für die schizophrene Familie. Hier stellt sich die Frage: Wie oft beruhen Schizoid und Spektrumstörungen auf dem Schizophreniegen, wenn sie in Familien ohne einen schizophrenen Probanden vorkommen? Nicht alle Schizoiden werden schizophren und nicht alle Schizophrenen waren präpsychotisch schizoid. Vermutlich ist auch das Schizoid heterogen und es könnte sein, daß schizoide Persönlichkeit beim Verwandten eines Schizophrenen das Erkrankungsrisiko erhöht, also einen Prädiktor darstellt, nicht aber bei Personen ohne familiäre Schizophreniebelastung.

Mit erstaunlicher Sicherheit fand ESSEN-MÖLLER in einer internationalen Blindstudie (GOTTESMAN u. SHIELDS, 1972) als einziger alle EZ-Partner von schizophrenen Zwillingsprobanden heraus und zwar, wenn sie nicht selbst schizophren waren, nach Persönlichkeitsmerkmalen in Richtung des Schizoid. Damit ist sein Maßstab für so etwas wie Schizotyp oder Spektrumdiagnose der beste, und er besitzt ein sicheres „Schizophrenie-Gen-Gefühl", so wie RÜMKE sein berühmtes „Schizophreniegefühl".

Ferner bestehen symptomatologische Beziehungen zu den Neurosen. In einigen Serien zeigten sich neurotische Störungen besonders bei den weiblichen Verwandten Schizophrener vermehrt (CADORET, 1973; STEPHENS et al., 1975). In der Schweiz hatte man versucht, bei 70 stationär behandelten Neurotikerinnen eine eventuelle Weiterentwicklung zu Schizophrenie vorauszusagen. 20 Jahre später stellten sich 9 von 10 Verdachtsdiagnosen als falsch heraus, während 6 Patientinnen, von denen es niemand vermutet hatte, an Schizophrenie erkrankt waren (ERNST u. ERNST, 1965). MITSUDA et al. (1967) fanden unter den EZ-Partnern Schizophrener nicht selten Panneurosen, Zwangsneurosen und hypersensitive Neurosen. In den skandinavischen Serien fielen mehrere diskordante EZ-Partner als neurotisch auf. Freilich darf man nicht jede Neurose als verkappte Schizophrenie ansehen, denn geht man umgekehrt von neurotischen Probanden aus, so ist ihre Belastung mit Schizophrenie minimal. PLOOG (1969a) kommt durch verhaltensbiologische Überlegungen zu dem Schluß, daß Schizophrenie und Neurose wesensmäßig und ursächlich verschieden sind, daß aber die eine gelegentlich unter dem Bild der anderen verlaufen kann.

SHIELDS und GOTTESMAN (1972) packten das Problem einer genetisch relevanten Schizophreniediagnose sehr elegant in einer internationalen Studie an und ließen ihre eigene Zwillingsserie von 6 Psychiatern und Psychologen aus England, USA und Japan diagnostizieren. Die Teilnehmer an diesem höchst aufschlußreichen Experiment wurden „blind" gehalten hinsichtlich Eiigkeit und Diagnose der Zwillingspartner. Sie gehörten recht gegensätzlichen Schulen an und stellten die Schizophreniediagnose verschieden eng bzw. weit. Durch Diskussion wurden „Übereinstimmungsdiagnosen" erzielt, die etwa dem Kraepelinschen Konzept zuzüglich einiger Bleulerscher Kriterien entsprachen. Dieser mittelstrenge Schizophreniebegriff ließ die Konkordanzrate der eineiigen Zwillinge am stärksten über die der zweieiigen überwiegen und kommt somit der genetischen Grundlage am nächsten. Bekanntlich dient der Konkordanzunterschied als Maßstab für Erblichkeit; je größer er ist, um so wahrscheinlicher ist das betreffende Merkmal erblich. Die EZ nun waren zu 50% konkordant, die ZZ zu 9%, das gibt ein Verhältnis von 5,5:1. Die strengste diagnostische Fassung ergab mit 20% und 14% nicht nur die niedrigste Konkordanz der EZ, sondern mit einem Verhältnis von 1,4:1 auch die geringste Trennschärfe zwischen EZ und ZZ. Die Beschränkung auf Kernschizophrenie trifft das genetisch Wesentliche also offensichtlich nicht. Dazu paßt der Befund von BLEULER (1972), daß „Katastrophenverläufe", d.h. sehr rasch zu schwerem Enddefekt führende Prozesse kaum je zweimal in derselben Familie vorkommen, also nicht erbbedingt sind. Die weiteste Fassung der Diagnose ergab erwartungsgemäß die höchsten Konkordanzwerte, nämlich 58% und 24%, aber ebenfalls ein relativ niedriges Verhältnis, nämlich 2,4:1. Die Einbeziehung von Grenzfällen, Schizotypen und schizoiden Persönlichkeiten war also nicht sehr hilfreich bei dem Bemühen, einen deutlichen genetischen Faktor herauszuarbeiten.

In gewissem Widerspruch dazu scheinen die Adoptionsbefunde von KETY, ROSENTHAL et al. zu stehen. Sie ergaben die deutlichsten Unterschiede zwischen Bluts- und Adoptivverwandten gerade bei weitherziger Diagnose unter Einbeziehung des Spektrums. Jedoch wurden die beiden Probandenserien – Zwillinge und Adoptivkinder – mit verschiedener Methodik und Diagnostik gewonnen und allein das vermag manchen Widerspruch zu erklären.

7. Sind Einzelsyndrome erblich?

Denkt man an Polygenie, so scheint der Versuch sinnvoll, den Erbverhältnissen von einzelnen Syndromen und Teilleistungsschwächen nachzugehen. Eineiige Zwillinge erwiesen sich in Syndromen ähnlicher als im Gesamtbild der Psychose (ESSEN-MÖLLER, 1941). Psychisch kranke, stationär behandelte Geschwisterpaare verhielten sich jedoch gerade umgekehrt und stimmten im Gesamtbild der Erkrankung und in der diagnostischen Kategorie eher überein als in Einzelheiten (TSUANG, 1967). Wieder andere Untersuchungen ergaben eine familiäre Ähnlichkeit sowohl in einzelnen Symptomen und Syndromen als auch im Gesamtbild der Psychose (BARON u. STERN, 1976; DIEBOLD et al., 1977; ØDEGAARD, 1963).

Die noch spärlichen Untersuchungen über Teilleistungsschwächen, die auch „gesunde" d.h. klinisch unbehandelte und sozial angepaßte Verwandte der Schizophrenen mit einbeziehen, ergaben widersprüchliche Resultate. Mehrere Autoren fanden bei den Verwandten Störungen der kognitiven Funktionen vermehrt (ALANEN et al., 1963; MCCONAGHY, 1959; PHILLIPS et al., 1965), andere nicht (ROMNEY, 1969). An High-Risk-Kindern wurden die Bereitschaft zu Angstreaktionen (MEDNICK u. WILD, 1962) und Störungen der Aufmerksamkeit (ERLENMEYER-KIMLING et al., 1978; HECHT-ORZAK u. KORNETSKY, 1971; RUTSCHMANN et al., 1977) untersucht.

Alles in allem ergibt sich vorläufig für einzelne Syndrome kein klareres Erbbild als unter Beibehaltung der konventionellen Diagnose.

8. Was steckt dahinter? Zwischenglieder?

Vielleicht gelingt es, aus der Kette von Ereignissen, die vom Genotyp zum Phänotyp führen, psychodynamische, psychophysiologische, biochemische usw.

Zwischenglieder zu fassen, die einen deutlichen Erbgang erkennen lassen und somit genetisch relevant sind.

Bereits BLEULER und KRAEPELIN hatten vermutet, daß sich die ersten Anzeichen der schizophrenen Krankheit oft viele Jahre vor der eigentlichen Psychose bemerkbar machen und daß die dramatische, produktive Symptomatik „sekundär, in gewissem Sinne zufällig" sei und einen reaktiven Überbau der Persönlichkeit auf andere, grundlegende aber weniger in die Augen springende Störungen darstelle.

In retrospektiven Untersuchungen zeigt etwa die Hälfte der Schizophrenen prämorbid psychische Auffälligkeiten und soziale Anpassungsschwierigkeiten (Übersichten bei GARMEZY, 1974; KLORMAN et al., 1977a, b; KOKES et al., 1977; OFFORD u. CROSS, 1969; STRAUSS et al., 1977a, b). Den retrospektiven Erhebungen haften jedoch manche Fehlerquellen und Unsicherheiten an. Um sie zu vermeiden, plante man prospektive Projekte, die von (noch?) nicht-schizophrenen Personen mit erhöhtem Schizophrenierisiko ausgehen (PEARSON u. KLEY, 1957). Man fand sie bei Kindern mit sog. präschizophrenen Symptomen und bei Kindern schizophrener Patienten, für die sich die Bezeichnung „High-Risk-Kinder" eingebürgert hat.

Kinder mit präschizophrenen Symptomen wie Kontaktarmut, Schüchternheit, Introvertiertheit, Schulversagen, aber auch Aggressivität, Erregungszustände und Schulschwänzen, die über psychiatrische Kliniken oder Erziehungsberatungsstellen erfaßt worden waren und nicht auf Grund von Verwandtschaft zu einem Schizophrenen, erkrankten später weit seltener an Schizophrenie, als man erwartet hatte (MICHAEL et al., 1957; MORRIS et al., 1954).

Die Kinder schizophrener Eltern als die zweite und wichtigere Gruppe erkranken erfahrungsgemäß etwa 15mal häufiger an Schizophrenie als die Kinder nicht-schizophrener Eltern. Sie werden in größeren Abständen psychiatrischen, neurologischen, psychologischen und psychophysiologischen Untersuchungen unterzogen und man hofft, auf diese Weise wenigstens bei einigen der späteren Schizophrenen frühe Anzeichen der Schizophrenie zu finden, die Weiterentwicklung verfolgen zu können, auslösende und schützende Faktoren zu entdecken und schließlich Schlüsse auf die Ursache der Schizophrenien, aber auch Hinweise für Prognose, Prävention und Therapie zu gewinnen. Derzeit laufen in Skandinavien, USA und Israel etwa 20 prospektive Studien (ERLENMEYER-KIMLING, 1968, 1978; GARMEZY, 1974). Sie legen den Schwerpunkt teils mehr auf Vorläufersymptome bei den Kindern, teils mehr auf Auslösefaktoren aus der Umwelt.

Besonders populär geworden ist das engagierte und umfassende dänische Projekt von MEDNICK, SCHULSINGER u.Mitarb. Bereits 1958 hatte MEDNICK eine Lerntheorie der Schizophrenie veröffentlicht, nach der sich das autonome Nervensystem potentieller Schizophrener durch schnelle und überschießende Reaktionen auf Umweltreize auszeichnet. Konditionierbarkeit und Generalisierung von Reizen sind erhöht, die Erholungszeit der galvanischen Hautreaktion ist verkürzt. Diese Disposition ist vermutlich erblich, die Betroffenen neigen dazu, ein „avoidance thinking", d.h. eine schizophrene Denkstörung zu entwickeln.

1962 wurden 207 Nachkommen schwer schizophrener Mütter (High-Risk-Kinder) und eine Kontrollgruppe von 104 Low-Risk-Kindern mit einem Durchschnittsalter von 15 Jahren zusammengestellt. Die High-Risk-Kinder unterschieden sich von den Low-Risk-Kindern durch erhöhte autonome Responsivität, erhöhte Reizgeneralisierung, kürzere Latenz und raschere autonome Erholung; 5 Jahre später hatten 20 High-Risk-Kinder, die inzwischen 17–30 Jahre alt geworden waren, „einen schweren psychiatrischen Zusammenbruch" erlitten, darunter einige „sehr Schizophrenie-ähnliche Zustände". Sie hatten sich bei der Erstuntersuchung durch häufigeres Vorkommen von 5 Faktoren von den Kontrollen und den nicht erkrankten High-Risk-Kindern unterschieden: 1. Frühe Trennung von der Mutter durch deren Hospitalisierung, 2. abnorme Antworten im Assoziationstest, 3. störendes und aggressives Verhalten in der Schule, 4. schlechte Habituierung und langsame Extinktion konditionierter Reaktionen, 5. Schwangerschafts- und Geburtskomplikationen. Die wichtigsten Veröffentlichungen über diese Befunde und den ganzen Projektentwurf sind als Nachdrucke in dem Buch von MEDNICK et al. (1974) zusammengefaßt und außerdem bei SCHULSINGER und JACOBSEN (1975) kurz umrissen.

Nach weiteren 5 Jahren erfolgte die zweite Nachuntersuchung (SCHULSINGER, 1976). Die Diagnosen wurden durch klinisches Interview, durch zwei Computerprogramme (CAPPS u. CATEGO) und schließlich als Consensus-Diagnose gestellt. Alle vier Methoden ergaben eine außerordentlich hohe Zahl psychischer Auffälligkeiten, und zwar auch in der Kontrollgruppe. Die Untersucher betonen ihre „low threshold for diagnostic labeling". Als logische Folge des prospektiven Entwurfes wollten sie auch nicht die geringste psychopathologische Manifestation übersehen, da sie ja für die spätere Schizophrenie-Entwicklung von Bedeutung sein könnte. Die klinische Diagnose ergab in der High-Risk-Gruppe nur 13% psychisch völlig unauffällige Personen (23 von 173), in der Kontrollgruppe auch nur 30% (27/91). Immerhin fällt die Schizophreniehäufigkeit mit 7,5% (13/173) nicht aus dem Rahmen; in der Kontrollgruppe fand sich nur 1 Fall (1,1%). Die „borderline states" einschließlich schizoider und paranoider Persönlichkeiten dagegen erscheinen mit 41% (71/173) sehr hoch (Kontrollgruppe 5,5% = 5/91). Die CAPPS-Diagnose ergab mehr als doppelt soviele Schizophrenien (n=30), CATEGO um ein Drittel weniger (n=10), die Consensusdiagnose ungefähr gleich viel (n=15). Näher können wir auf die unterschiedlichen Ergebnisse der verschiedenen Systeme hier leider nicht eingehen.

Ein ausführlicher Bericht, der die Befunde dieser zweiten Nachuntersuchung mit den Anfangsbefunden vergleicht und frühere Auffälligkeiten mit späteren in Beziehung setzt, steht noch aus. Offenbar hatten sich nicht alle schizophren oder sonst auffällig gewordenen Nachkommen schon anfangs im auffälligen Teil der High-Risk-Gruppe befunden.

So interessant die psychophysiologischen Befunde von MEDNICK und SCHULSINGER sind, so konnten sie doch nicht allgemein bestätigt werden (ZAHN, 1977). VAN DYKE et al. (1974) konnten es nicht an adoptierten Kindern Schizophrener, und ERLENMEYER-KIMLING (1975) an den Kindern zweier schizophrener Eltern, „Super-High-Risk-Kindern" sozusagen, auch nicht.

In der Untersuchung an High-Risk- und Kontrollkindern von HANSON et al. (1976, 1977) zeigten fünf Kinder eine Symptomkombination von herabgesetzter motorischer Geschicklichkeit, großen Leistungsschwankungen bei Denkaufgaben und „präschizophrenen" Persönlichkeitsmerkmalen wie Autismus, flache und labile Emotionalität, Negativismus und Reizbarkeit. Auch waren lockere und bizarre Gedankenverbindungen und Angstbereitschaft zu eruieren, aber keine Halluzinationen und keine Ähnlichkeit zur Schizophrenie der Erwachsenen. Alle fünf Kinder stammten von schizophrenen Eltern und müssen als ernsthafte Anwärter auf eine schizophrene Psychose angesehen werden. Die Verifizierung kann erst die Katamnese bringen, wie überhaupt der Wert prospektiver Projekte mit der Katamnese steht und fällt.

Kindliche Schizophrenien (s. S. 588) wurden unter High-Risk-Kindern kaum beobachtet. ANTHONY (1968) sah relativ häufig passagere „mikroparanoide Psychosen" mit einer Dauer von 3 Tagen bis 3 Monaten. Sie waren aber offenbar nicht so schwer, daß sie ohne das intensive Forschungsprogramm registriert worden wären, geschweige denn, daß man die Kinder einem Arzt vorgestellt hätte.

HANSON et al. (1977), sowie SHIELDS (1977) verdanken wir eine hervorragende Diskussion der Möglichkeiten, Probleme und Grenzen von High-Risk-Studien. Eine Beschränkung der Methode liegt z. B. darin, daß die über High-Risk-Kinder erfaßten Schizophrenen nur einen Bruchteil der Kranken und somit eine Auslese darstellen; die meisten Schizophrenen stammen bekanntlich von zwei nichtschizophrenen Eltern ab. Insbesondere stellt sich die Frage: Was bedeuten die bei den Kindern Schizophrener gefundenen Auffälligkeiten überhaupt und inwieweit haben sich die Hoffnungen, Hinweise auf die Ursache der Schizophrenie und für die Prognose gefährdeter Personen zu erhalten, bis jetzt erfüllt? Die Befunde sind relativ unspezifisch, wie ja die bekannten retrospektiv gewonnenen Präkursoren der Schizophrenie auch. Trotzdem können auch unspezifische Auffälligkeiten Ausdruck eines spezifischen neurobiologischen Defizites und somit tatsächlich Indikatoren der Schizophrenieanlage sein. In diesem Fall müßten sie auch bei gesund bleibenden Trägern der Anlage, z. B. nicht erkrankenden High-Risk-Kindern und diskordanten EZ-Partnern nachweisbar sein. Sie können aber auch Auslöser oder Verstärker der Schizophrenieanlage darstellen. Sie wären dann bei Anlageträgern und Nichtanlageträgern zu finden. Weiterhin kann es sich um erste Symptome der bereits in Gang gesetzten Schizophrenie handeln. Sie dürften dann nur bei zukünftigen Schizophrenen vorkommen. Schließlich brauchen sie mit der Schizophrenie gar nichts zu tun zu haben, sondern können als Reaktion auf das gestörte häusliche Milieu entstanden sein. Selbst wenn einmal ein perfekter Indikator des Genotyps gefunden sein sollte, so kann auch er eine tatsächliche Erkrankung nicht gültig voraussagen, solange die relevanten Umweltauslöser unbekannt sind. Wie die eineiigen Zwillinge zeigen, erkranken viele Anlageträger überhaupt nicht. Daher ist ein allzu großer Enthusiasmus bezüglich prognostischer und präventiver Aufschlüsse verfrüht, und man sollte die Erwartungen nicht zu hoch spannen.

Ein weiteres Zwischenglied könnte in elektrophysiologischen Veränderungen faßbar sein. Die Ergebnisse von EEG-Untersuchungen sind jedoch vorläufig widersprüchlich. EEG-Anomalien, falls vorhanden, werden von vereinzelten Autoren, IVANITSKY und NATALEVICH (1969), z. B. als Ausdruck der Erbanlage gewertet, im allgemeinen aber eher als Symptom des schizophrenen Prozesses angesehen.

Auch immunbiologische Theorien haben Eingang in die Schizophrenieforschung gefunden. Russische Autoren sehen die Schizophrenie als eine Art Autoaggressionskrankheit, denn sie fanden Hirnantikörper und sensibilisierte Lymphozyten im Serum von Schizophrenen und einem Teil ihrer nächsten Blutsverwandten (VARTANIAN u. GINDILIS, 1972). Die Bestätigung steht aus. Immerhin hatte BURCH bereits in den 60er Jahren auf Grund mathematischer Überlegungen die Schizophrenie als Autoimmunkrankheit angesehen und komplizierte Vererbungsmodelle aufgestellt.

Große Hoffnungen gründen sich auf Fortschritte in der Neurochemie. Die Forschung befindet sich in Fluß und vorläufig gibt es zwar vielversprechende Ansätze, aber keine endgültigen Befunde. Die Neurotransmitter spielen offenbar nicht nur bei der normalen Impulsübertragung im Zentralnervensystem eine Rolle, sondern auch beim psychotischen Geschehen. Am intensivsten gearbeitet wird derzeit wohl über die zu den biogenen Aminen gehörenden Katecholamine und Indolamine.

Ein abweichender neurochemischer Befund bei einem Schizophrenen kann sowohl Ursache, als auch Folge der Psychose sein. Findet er sich jedoch auch beim diskordanten eineiigen Zwillingspartner, so liegt der Verdacht auf einen dispositionellen, der Erbanlage nicht zu fern stehenden Faktor nahe. Aufgrund dieser Überlegung befaßt sich die Arbeitsgruppe um POLLIN und STABENAU seit über 20 Jahren mit biochemischen Variablen bei konkordanten und diskordanten EZ-Paaren. Die meisten Untersuchungen erbrachten keine erbverdächtigen Abweichungen. Nur in einer Studie war die Urinausscheidung von 6 Katecholaminen und Katecholamin-Metaboliten bei den schizophrenen Zwillingen und ihren diskordanten Partnern ungefähr gleich erhöht (POLLIN, 1972). Die Erhöhung scheint also Ausdruck des Genotyps zu sein. Wie die Autoren selbst betonen, können jedoch mehrere Einwände gemacht werden. Die erhöhten Werte sind Gruppen-Mittelwerte und treffen nicht für jedes einzelne Paar zu; die Zahl der Paare ist noch dazu klein. Gerade der Metabolit, der den Katecholamin-Stoffwechsel des Gehirns am deutlichsten widerspiegeln soll, MHPG, verhielt sich anders. Schließlich ist ungewiß, inwieweit peripher nachweisbare Stoffwechselprodukte, wie Substanzen im Urin, den Metabolismus des Gehirns widerspiegeln; man denke an die Blut-Hirnschranke.

ARNOLD (1968) fand nach Succinylbelastung Veränderungen der energiereichen Phosphate in den Erythrozyten bei Schizophrenen und ihren Verwandten. Auch dies bedarf der Bestätigung.

Ein ernsthafter Anwärter auf Beteiligung am schizophrenen Geschehen ist die Monoaminooxydase (MAO), die eine wichtige Rolle im Stoffwechsel mehrerer Neurotransmitter spielt. Ihre Aktivität zeigte sich bei Schizophrenen erniedrigt (u.a. MURPHY u. WEISS, 1972; BERRETTINI et al., 1977), ebenso bei beiden Partnern Schizophrenie-diskordanter EZ-Paare (WYATT et al., 1973). Andere Autoren bestätigten dies jedoch nicht (BROCKINGTON et al., 1976) oder fanden eine reduzierte MAO-Aktivität bei manisch-depressiven Patienten (MURPHY u. WEISS, 1972; BELMAKER et al., 1976), so daß es sich wieder nicht um etwas Spezifisches zu handeln scheint.

Man beginnt das biochemische Problem noch von einer anderen Seite anzugehen, indem man bei gesunden Menschen, insbesondere Zwillingen und im Tierexperiment nach erblichen Unterschieden im Metabolismus der Neurotransmitter und Psychopharmaka sucht (z. B. BARCHAS et al., 1974). Ferner teilte man normale Individuen in solche mit niedriger und mit hoher MAO-Aktivität ein. Die Versuchspersonen mit MAO-Aktivitäten im unteren Bereich der Norm und ihre Familienangehörigen zeigten häufiger Aufenthalte in psychiatrischen Krankenhäusern, Suizide, Suizidversuche und Konflikte mit dem Gesetz als die Personen mit höherer MAO-Aktivität (BUCHSBAUM et al., 1976).

Bedenkt man die große Variabilität der schizophrenen Krankheitsbilder, die schubweisen Verläufe und wiederholten Remissionen, so wird man den genetischen Defekt in Regulationsmechanismen vermuten. Die Neurotransmitter sind offenbar nicht qualitativ verändert, vielleicht nicht einmal quantitativ. Manches spricht dafür, daß es sich um Veränderungen der Kompartmentierung (Verteilungsmuster) insgesamt gleichbleibender Transmittermengen handelt. Die Störungen sind eher funktionell als statisch, d.h. sie treten erst bei normaler oder vermehrter Beanspruchung auf. In dieser Sicht würde an bestimmten Orten ein Mangel oder Überschuß von Neurotransmittern entstehen und zwar nicht durch Defekte der auf- und abbauenden Enzyme, sondern durch Transport- und Verteilungsprobleme. Das genetische Problem läge in der prä- oder postsynaptischen Membran (JATZKEWITZ, 1968) oder bei den Zielorganen, den Rezeptoren (SEEMAN et al., 1975).

9. Anlage und Umwelt

Die Umwelttheorie sieht die Ursache der Schizophrenie ausschließlich in Umwelteinflüssen, in seelischen Traumen, psychodynamischen Mechanismen und Lernvorgängen. Um allgemeine Katastrophen, wie Krieg oder Wirtschaftsdepressionen, handelt es sich dabei nicht, denn die Schizophreniehäufigkeit nimmt in solchen Zeiten nicht zu. Wirksam sind individuelle Erlebnisse, insbesondere Familiendynamik, soziale Benachteiligung, seelische Isolierung, Liebesenttäuschungen und Verlust von Bezugspersonen. Alle diese Erfahrungen werden aber millionenmal gemacht, ohne daß der Betroffene an Schizophrenie erkrankt. Und wenn wirklich jemand schizophren wird, warum wird er dann gerade schizophren und nicht depressiv oder neurotisch? Die angeschuldigten Ursachen sind häufig die gleichen (BLOCK, 1969). Man muß auch damit rechnen, daß mißliche Erlebnisse im Vorfeld einer Psychose, wie gescheiterte Verlobung oder berufliche Schwierigkeiten schon Folge der beginnenden Psychose und nicht deren Ursache sind. Da Erb- und Umwelteinflüsse beteiligt sind und vielfach interagieren, haben auch die umweltorientierten Forschungsrichtungen wichtige Ergebnisse gebracht. Man muß sich nur davor hüten, Ursache und Wirkung zu verwechseln oder Kausalzusammenhänge zu konstruieren, wo keine vorhanden sind. Der Schizophrene *ist* krank und die Gesellschaft *ist* verlogen und keineswegs optimal; muß aber unbedingt ein Kausalzusammenhang bestehen (LINDINGER, 1975)?

Alle Befunde, die als Beweis für eine rein psychogene Ätiologie der Schizophrenie ins Feld geführt worden sind, lassen sich auch anders interpretieren. So wurde die Tatsache, daß Schizophrene ungefähr doppelt so oft eine schizophrene Mutter wie einen schizophrenen Vater haben, rein psychogenetisch im Sinne gestörter Mutter-Kind-Beziehungen als Schizophrenieursache gedeutet.

Sie erklärt sich jedoch großenteils als biostatistische Ausleseerscheinung. Heirat und Geburt von Kindern erfolgt meist vor Ausbruch einer manifesten Psychose. Die Frauen mit ihrem niedrigeren Heiratsalter und höheren Erkrankungsalter besitzen eine größere Chance als die Männer (rechnerisch eine doppelt so große), noch vor Ausbruch ihrer Schizophrenie zur Heirat und Fortpflanzung zu kommen (ESSEN-MÖLLER, 1963). Auch die „schizophrenogene" Mutter hat sich Abstriche an ihrer Bedeutung gefallen lassen müssen. ARIETI, einer ihrer eifrigsten Verfechter, revidierte 1971 seine Ansicht dahin, daß wohl nur 25% der Schizophrenen eine solche Mutter hätten. Die familiäre Transmission bestehe offenbar nicht nur in einer erlernten Denk- und Verhaltensstörung, sondern sei viel komplizierter. REISNER (1971) meint sogar, „die Ansicht, daß ein bestimmter Muttertyp, welcher sich charakterisieren ließe, schizophrenogen wäre, wird heute wohl allgemein abgelehnt" und knüpft an diese recht optimistische Feststellung sehr vernünftige gruppendynamische Betrachtungen der Reaktionen zwischen Kind, Mutter und Familie. Das Kind, und schon das Neugeborene, ist ja keineswegs nur ein Spielball des Verhaltens seiner Mutter. Es trägt seine eigenen Verhaltensmöglichkeiten in sich und beeinflußt seinerseits von Anfang an die Reaktionen seiner Umgebung (PAPOUŠEK u. PAPOUŠEK, 1974; SAMEROFF, 1978).

Manche Untersuchungen fanden unter Schizophrenen bevorzugt Erstgeborene, andere wieder Letztgeborene oder auch Einzelkinder. Die meist an geringen Fallzahlen gewonnenen Ergebnisse widersprechen sich und mögen selektiv zustande gekommen sein, beeinflußt durch lokale Verhältnisse. Nimmt man alle Untersuchungen zusammen, so entspricht die Stellung der Kranken in der Geschwisterreihe der zufälligen Erwartung (HARE u. PRICE, 1970; PRICE u. HARE, 1969).

Dagegen scheint erwiesen zu sein, daß die Geburtsmonate der Schizophrenen eine vom Durchschnitt abweichende Verteilung zeigen (DALÉN, 1968, 1975 für Schweden und Südafrika; HARE et al., 1974 für England und Wales; ØDEGAARD, 1974 für Norwegen; PARKER u. NEILSON, 1976 für Neu-Südwales/Australien). In der nördlichen Hemisphäre findet sich eine Häufung der Geburten Schizophrener in den Monaten Januar bis April, in der südlichen Hemisphäre von Mai bis Oktober (Südafrika), bzw. Juni bis August (Australien), also in beiden Fällen während der Wintermonate, eventuell noch im Frühjahr. Die Verschiebung läßt sich noch weiter aufgliedern. Generell zeigen die Schizophrenen der nördlichen Hemisphäre eine deutliche Häufung der Wintergeburten, die bei Männern und Frauen etwa gleich ist. In der südlichen Hemisphäre ist der winterliche Geburtengipfel nicht so deutlich und wird vorwiegend, in Australien fast ausschließlich, durch die weiblichen Patienten bewirkt. In Schweden weisen die im Norden geborenen Schizophrenen Geburtengipfel nicht nur im Januar und Februar, sondern auch im Juni auf. Bei Kranken mit günstigerem Verlauf ist die jahreszeitliche Verschiebung stärker als bei denen mit ungünstigem.

DALÉN hält die Möglichkeit von Artefakten durch Erfassungs- und Auswertungsfehler für unwahrscheinlich, und er diskutiert verschiedene Erklärungen, wie besonderes Zeugungsverhalten der Eltern, Alter der Mütter, jahreszeitlich bedingte Vermehrung von Infektionen, Frühgeburten, Geburtsschäden (Hämorrhagien). PARKER und NEILSON (1976) weisen darauf hin, daß sich auch die Geburten in der Allgemeinbevölkerung nicht ganz gleichmäßig über die Jahreszeiten verteilen. Die Schizophrenen zeigen offenbar prinzipiell gleichgerichtete, jedoch verstärkte jahreszeitliche Abweichungen wie der Durchschnitt. Man könnte die Hypothese aufstellen, die ganze Erscheinung sei ein Problem von Schwankungen der Konzeptionsbereitschaft. Zum Beispiel könnte die Konzeptionsfähigkeit der Frau durch die Außentemperatur über endokrine Vorgänge beeinflußt werden und die späteren Schizophrenen könnten gegenüber solchen physiologischen Faktoren besonders sensibel sein. Ähnliches gilt für das Geschlechtsverhältnis bei Geburt, welches ebenfalls jahreszeitliche Schwankungen aufweist. Letzten Endes sind aber alle diese Faktoren unbekannt und die Bedeutung der Befunde bleibt unklar.

Übrigens zeigen auch die manisch Depressiven bei HARE (1975a) einen deutlichen Geburtengipfel im Winter. In Schweden (DALÉN, 1975) ist diese Abweichung nur schwach und vorwiegend bei den bipolaren Psychosen zu beobachten, in Australien ist sie ebenfalls nicht signifikant und vorwiegend durch die Frauen bedingt.

Für neurotische Patienten hatte man eine normale Geburtenverteilung angenommen. PARKER und NEILSON (1976) jedoch fanden einen deutlichen Frühjahrsgipfel, besonders für Angstneurosen und am geringsten für depressive Neurosen, und sie wiesen eine gleichsinnige, allerdings schwache und nicht-signifikante Verschiebung auch in der Serie von HARE (1975b) nach.

Eine sorgfältige Untersuchung Schizophrenie-artiger Psychosen, die unter dem Einfluß schizophrener Patienten zustandekamen, zeigte, daß auch Folie à deux und induzierte Psychosen im allgemeinen einer genetischen Disposition bedürfen (SCHARFETTER, 1970). Induzent und Induzierter waren häufig blutsverwandt. Nichtblutsverwandte Induzierte, meist Ehegatten oder in Ehe-ähnlichen Bindungen lebende Personen, wiesen eine erhöhte familiäre Belastung mit Schizophrenie auf. Typische induzierte Psychosen sind unter Eheleuten nicht häufiger als dem zufälligen Zusammentreffen zweier Psychotiker entspricht. Das unterstreicht die Bedeutung der Erbanlage. Sie sind überhaupt selten, auch bei Blutsverwandten und trotz der relativen Häufigkeit der Schizophrenien. Damit sich solche seltene Fälle ereignen, muß also noch etwas hinzukommen, müssen besondere Verhältnisse vorliegen.

Der Mensch lebt nicht nur in der Familie und so hat man den Rahmen weiter gespannt und die Suche nach psychosozialen Ursachen auf Sozialschicht, Gesellschaft und Kultur ausgedehnt. Seit HOLLINGSHEAD und REDLICH (1958) in der untersten sozialen Klasse mehr Schizophrene fanden als in den oberen, waren viele von einer echten Kausalwirkung schlechter sozialer Verhältnisse überzeugt. Die Überrepräsentation der Schizophrenen in der untersten sozialen Klasse ist jedoch in USA nur in Großstädten über 50000 Einwohner zu beobachten, in mittleren Städten weniger deutlich und in Kleinstädten überhaupt nicht (KOHN, 1968). In Deutschland zeigt sie sich zwar in Mannheim (HÄFNER, 1971), nicht aber in älteren Untersuchungen im ländlichen Bayern. Außerdem scheinen manche Autoren den sozialen Stand *nach* Erkrankung und nicht den *vor* Erkrankung, bzw. den Stand des Vaters berücksichtigt zu haben. Offensichtlich gehören die Schizophrenen nach der Erkrankung vermehrt der sozialen Unterschicht an, nicht aber, wenn man den prämorbiden sozialen Stand und die Herkunft der Patienten analysiert (GOLDBERG u. MORRISON, 1963; HARE et al., 1972; HUBER et al., 1976). Es ist also doch wohl an ein soziales Absinken der Kranken zu denken.

DUNHAM, dessen frühere Untersuchung über die Kausalwirkung schlechter sozialer Verhältnisse zu den klassischen sozialpsychiatrischen Arbeiten gehört (FARIS u. DUNHAM, 1939), widerruft heute seine damalige Überzeugung (DUNHAM, 1976). Er fand in seiner ersten Studie methodische Fehler, die er in neuen Untersuchungsanordnungen vermied. Die Ergebnisse stützen die Hypothese der sozialen Kausalwirkung dann nicht mehr. Nr. 5 und Nr. 7 von DUNHAMS Schlußfolgerungen lauten: 5. Soziale Klasse ist kein ätiologischer Faktor in der Entwicklung der Schizophrenie. 7. Von keinem sozialpsychologischen Faktor konnte schlüssig gezeigt werden, daß er eine Rolle in der Entwicklung der Schizophrenie spielt (übersetzt v. Verf.).

In Bristol waren Schizophrene in bestimmten Stadtvierteln überrepräsentiert, und zwar nicht nur in Elendsvierteln, sondern auch in besseren Wohngegenden, die sich durch eine große Zahl von Einpersonenhaushalten und Wohnheimen auszeichneten. Daraus schloß man, daß Isolierung aus menschlichem und sozialem Kontakt Schizophrenie verursache (HARE, 1956). Es läßt sich aber nicht ausschließen, daß Schizophrene und zukünftige Schizophrene bevorzugt in diese Stadtviertel eingeströmt sind. Nicht die Einsamkeit hat Schizophrenie verursacht, sondern die (zukünftigen) Kranken haben Einsamkeit und Bindungslosigkeit gesucht. Wenn ferner Schizophrene überdurchschnittlich oft ledig oder geschieden sind, so mag dieser Familienstand zur Manifestation der Erkrankung beigetragen haben, er kann aber genausogut bereits Folge der Psychose oder der präpsychotischen Persönlichkeit sein. Die Schizophrenie hat offenbar schon vor ihrem klinischen Ausbruch weitreichende soziale Konsequenzen (KENNEDY, 1975).

Einwanderer in USA und Australien wiesen eine erhöhte Schizophrenierate auf (CADE, 1956; MALZBERG, 1962, 1964), und dafür soll der Streß der neuen, schwierigen Lebensbedingungen verantwortlich sein. Nach ØDEGAARD (1932, 1972) jedoch disponiert die präschizophrene Persönlichkeit vermehrt zur Auswanderung. Diese Meinung wird bestätigt durch die Tatsache, daß auch die bereits in der neuen Heimat geborenen Kinder vermehrt erkrankten, sowie durch eine dänische Zwillingsuntersuchung. Dänemark besitzt ein vorzügliches, für wissenschaftliche Forschungen angelegtes Zwillingsregister, aus dem mehrere aufschlußreiche Zwillingsuntersuchungen über verschiedene Krankheiten und Merkmale hervorgegangen sind (HAUGE et al., 1968). Von 25 Zwillingspaaren mit mindestens einem schizophrenen Partner waren 8 Zwillinge ausgewandert, die 6 Paaren angehörten. Der Prozentsatz der Ausgewanderten ist mit 16% höher als die sowieso recht hohe dänische Auswanderungsquote von etwa 5%. Bezüglich Auswanderung und Erkrankung ergaben sich nun die verschiedensten Kombinationen. Bei zwei Paaren waren beide Zwillinge ausgewandert, aber nur einer erkrankt. Bei zwei weiteren Paaren war nur ein Partner ausgewandert, aber beide, auch der zu Hause gebliebene, erkrankten; bei den beiden letzten Paaren schließlich blieb der ausgewanderte Partner gesund, aber der zu Hause gebliebene erkrankte (FISCHER, 1973). Man kann also nicht sagen, daß vorwiegend die ausgewanderten Zwillinge erkrankten.

Körperliche Schäden wurden weit seltener als seelische Belastungen zur Erklärung einer Schizophrenie herangezogen. Doch erhob sich immer wieder die

Behauptung, daß Schizophrene ein niedrigeres Geburtsgewicht hätten (POLLIN u. STABENAU, 1968; TORREY, 1977) und häufiger Komplikationen vor und während der Geburt durchmachten als ihre gesund gebliebenen Geschwister und Zwillingspartner. Schizophrenie sei das Resultat von vorgeburtlichen Entwicklungsstörungen und Geburtstraumen. Über den Umweg einer größeren Verwöhnung des leichteren, schwächlicheren Kindes wurde sogar eine psychogenetische Interpretation versucht. Einzelbeispiele lassen sich natürlich in beliebiger Zahl finden. In größeren, auslesefreien Zwillingsserien jedoch waren die Schizophrenen bei Geburt nicht viel öfter leichter als ihre gesunden Zwillingspartner. Und wenn sie leichter waren, so betrug der Unterschied oft nur wenige Gramm (FISCHER, 1972; GOTTESMAN u. SHIELDS, 1976; SHIELDS u. GOTTESMAN, 1977). Dazu kommt die Überlegung, daß bei konkordanten Paaren der leichtere und der schwere Partner erkrankt, während bei den rund 99% Zwillingspaaren, die frei von Schizophrenie bleiben, auch der leichtere Partner gesund bleibt. Schließlich neigen Zwillinge ganz allgemein zu Untergewicht, erkranken aber nicht häufiger als Einzelgeborene.

Nach perinatalen Komplikationen fahndete man retrospektiv besonders bei kindlichen Schizophrenien und was man so nannte (FISH, 1975; PASAMANICK et al., 1956; POLLACK u. WOERNER, 1966; TAFT u. GOLDFARB, 1964). Der Fragenkomplex hat große Aktualität gewonnen seit MEDNICK et al. an Hand ihrer Befunde an High-Risk-Kindern Schlußfolgerungen auf eine kausale Beziehung zwischen Schwangerschafts- und Geburtskomplikationen der (schizophrenen) Mütter und Auffälligkeiten, sowie späterer Schizophrenie der Kinder zogen (MEDNICK, 1970; MEDNICK et al., 1971, 1973). Es scheint aber, als ob perinatale Komplikationen erst bei Vorhandensein einer schizophrenen Anlage wirksam werden. Sie fanden sich nämlich gleich häufig bei den Kindern von schizophrenen, andersartig psychotischen und normalen Müttern. Nur in der schizophrenen Gruppe bestand eine Korrelation zu neurologischen Abweichungen und motorischen Rückständen der Kinder im ersten Lebensjahr (MCNEIL u. KAIJ, 1973; MIRDAL et al., 1977). Im allgemeinen pflegen Geburtstraumen unmittelbar postnatal zu organischen Symptomen und später zu Intelligenzausfällen zu führen.

Retrospektive Informationen über perinatale Komplikationen von Schizophrenen sind notgedrungen unvollständig, die prospektiven Befunde an High-Risk-Kindern können in ihrer Bedeutung erst katamnestisch nach 30 bis 40 Jahren beurteilt werden (SHIELDS, 1977; HANSON et al., 1976). Wie steht es überhaupt, wenn nicht die Mutter, sondern der Vater schizophren ist? Das Erkrankungsrisiko für Kinder schizophrener Väter und schizophrener Mütter ist gleichhoch. Die Deutung, der schizophrene Vater übe seine Wirkung durch Beunruhigung der Mutter während der Schwangerschaft aus, scheint an den Haaren herbeigezogen, man würde in diesem Fall eher eine depressive Verstimmung bei der Mutter, als eine Schizophrenie beim Kind erwarten.

Eher erscheint es plausibel, daß perinatale Faktoren eine schizophrene Anlage aktivieren und einen schwereren Verlauf der späteren Schizophrenie vorprogrammieren können. Die Erbanlage kann nicht allein verantwortlich sein für eine schizophrene Psychose, denn die eineiigen Zwillinge sind bekanntlich trotz ihres identischen Erbgutes nicht zu 100% konkordant, sondern zu rund 50%, oder höchstens 70%. Welche Auslöser kommen noch in Betracht? Man wird an die gleichen Ereignisse denken, wie sie in der psychoanalytischen Literatur als Alleinursache angeschuldigt worden sind. Letzten Endes sind sie aber genauso unbekannt wie die Erbfaktoren.

Im Einzelfall stehen ganz verschiedene Ereignisse und Belastungen in Beziehung zur Erkrankung gerade dieses oder jenes Patienten. Kein Faktor kommt einigermaßen konstant vor, jeder fehlt bei den meisten anderen Patienten und jeder wird millionenmal erlebt, ohne daß eine schizophrene Erkrankung folgt. Manche Ereignisse gehen etwas überdurchschnittlich oft einer Schizophrenie voraus, z.B. hormonelle Umstellungen, wie im Wochenbett und Klimakterium, und ein völlig zufälliges Zusammentreffen ist zu bezweifeln. Aber auch sie sind weder ausreichend, noch notwendig für eine schizophrene Erkrankung, und ein strikter Kausalzusammenhang ist ganz ausgeschlossen. Als Beispiel mögen 4 dänische eineiige Zwillingspaare dienen. Bei allen 4 Paaren erkrankte eine Zwillingsschwester nach einer Entbindung an Schizophrenie. Zwei Partnerinnen blieben gesund, obgleich auch sie Kinder hatten; die beiden anderen Partnerinnen erkrankten konkordant, aber ohne jemals schwanger gewesen zu sein (FISCHER, 1973).

Überhaupt haben sich die Hoffnungen, die man in das Studium von diskordanten und getrennt aufgewachsenen EZ-Paaren gesetzt hatte, nicht erfüllt. Die Befunde brachten eher eine Bestätigung der Erbtheorie, als Aufschluß über die beteiligten Umweltfaktoren. Getrennt aufgewachsene EZ erkrankten mit 60% ungefähr ebenso oft konkordant wie zusammen aufgewachsene. In diskordanten Paaren ließen sich dramatische Unterschiede in Lebensgeschichte und Gesundheitszustand praktisch niemals eruieren. Eine einzige sichere Aussage ergab sich: Der schizophrene Zwilling war als Kind ganz allgemein schwächlicher, er war introvertierter, submissiver und in der Schule weniger erfolgreich als sein gesund gebliebener Partner (FISCHER, 1972).

Die Auslösefaktoren sind offenbar weitgehend unspezifisch. Bei 100 normalen Männern ließ sich eine Fülle von Kindheitsereignissen erfragen, die gewöhnlich als Ursache einer Schizophrenie angesehen werden (RENAUD u. ESTESS, 1961). Die Manifestation der Anlage scheint durch mehr oder weniger zufällige Konstellationen von Alltagsbelastungen bewirkt zu werden. Jede normale und erst recht eine schwere Belastung kann die Schwelle zur Krankheit überschreiten lassen. Nach BLEULER (1948) muß der Auslöser zum Patienten passen „wie der Schlüssel ins Schloß". DIEBOLD (1969) vermutete, daß Ereignisse, die reales oder imaginäres Näherrücken bedeuten, Auslöser für Schizophrenien darstellen, Trennungs- und Verlustsituationen dagegen für Depressionen.

10. Populationsgenetische Betrachtungen

Bis vor kurzem war die Sterblichkeit der Schizophrenen auf das Dreifache erhöht und die Kinderzahl um ein Viertel bis zwei Drittel herabgesetzt. Wenn die Schizophrenie einerseits erbbedingt und andererseits einer so starken Gegenauslese unterworfen ist, warum ist sie dann nicht schon längst verschwunden? Nimmt man einfachen Erbgang und Ausgleich der Ausmerzrate durch Neumutationen an, so müßte die Mutationsrate so hoch sein, daß sie allen Erfahrungen der Humangenetik widerspricht. Wenn die Schizophrenien heterogen sind und durch verschiedene, jeweils seltene Gene zustande kommen, so könnte allerdings jedes einzelne dieser Gene eine realistische Mutationsrate besitzen (ERLENMEYER-KIMLING u. PARADOWSKI, 1966). Bei Annahme von polygenem Erbgang ist der Widerspruch zwischen Gegenauslese und Fortbestehen nicht ganz so kraß, besteht aber ebenfalls.

Daher wird immer wieder ein selektiver Vorteil der Schizophrenen oder der nicht manifest kranken Anlageträger, z.B. der Geschwister von Schizophrenen, diskutiert (HUXLEY et al., 1964). An Schizophrenen beobachtete man höhere Schmerztoleranz, herabgesetzte Infektionsanfälligkeit und verringerte Reaktion auf Histamin und vermutete, dies könnte ihnen in früheren Zeiten einen Überlebensvorteil gewährt haben. JARVIK und DECKARD (1977) glauben an bessere Überlebenschancen infolge einer paranoid-mißtrauischen Vorsichtshaltung, welche sie die „Odysseeische Persönlichkeit" nennen. Gegenwärtig kommt ein selektiver Vorteil eher für nicht-kranke Anlageträger in Betracht. Er wird aber durch die empirischen Befunde nicht gestützt: Die Geschwister Schizophrener haben keine erhöhte Fruchtbarkeit (BUCK et al., 1975; RIMMER u. JACOBSEN, 1976; LINDELIUS, 1970; LARSON u. NYMAN, 1973) und stehen mit ihrer Reproduktionsrate zwischen den Schizophrenen und dem Durchschnitt.

Selektive Vor- und Nachteile, Mortalitäts- und Reproduktionsraten können im Laufe der Zeit und unter verschiedenen Bedingungen wechseln. Die Nachkommenzahl der Schizophrenen ist nicht durch organische Behinderungen, durch den schizophrenen Genotyp an sich herabgesetzt, sondern infolge der Anpassungsstörungen und Interaktionsschwierigkeiten mit der Umwelt.

In New York und London nahmen während der letzten 20 Jahre Heiratshäufigkeit und Kinderzahl der Schizophrenen zu und die Differenz zur durchschnittlichen Geburtenrate verringerte sich. Die gleiche Tendenz zeigte sich auch bei den Geschwistern (ERLENMEYER-KIMLING et al., 1966, 1969; STEVENS, 1969). Als Gründe kommen in Betracht: verbesserte Therapieerfolge, kürzere Krankenhausaufenthalte und bessere Resozialisierung der Kranken; größere Toleranz der Bevölkerung; seltenere Anwendung der Geburtenkontrolle durch die Schizophrenen und ihre Familien bei gleichzeitigem Geburtenrückgang in der Allgemeinbevölkerung. Besonders die Londoner Untersuchung zeigte deutlich den Einfluß sozialer Faktoren. Die Fruchtbarkeit schizophrener Frauen lag höher, wenn sie katholisch waren und die Ehemänner körperlich arbeiteten, als wenn sie protestantisch waren und die Ehemänner Schreibtischberufe ausübten. Die Heiratshäufigkeit dagegen wurde am stärksten durch die präschizophrene Persönlichkeit beeinflußt: schizoide Personen heirateten seltener als nicht-schizoide.

III. Affektive Psychosen

Neuere Übersichtsarbeiten über die Genetik der affektiven Psychosen: ANGST (1972), CADORET (1976), GERSHON et al. (1971, 1976).

Nach den älteren Familienuntersuchungen besitzen die Verwandten 1. Grades manisch-depressiver und endogen depressiver Patienten ein Risiko von 10–15% ebenfalls an einer endogenen Affektpsychose zu erkranken (ZERBIN-RÜDIN, 1967). In den Untersuchungen seit 1967 liegen die familiären Risikoziffern eher darüber. Die wichtigste Entdeckung der neueren genetischen Depressionsforschung war jedoch die Feststellung von Unterschieden in Persönlichkeit und Familienbild von unipolaren (rein depressiven) und bipolaren (manisch-depressi-

Tabelle 3. Differenziertes Erkrankungsrisiko der Eltern und Geschwister von Probanden mit zyklischen (manisch-depressiven) und phasisch-depressiven Psychosen. (Nach ANGST u. PERRIS, 1968, aus ZERBIN-RÜDIN, 1971 a)

Probanden	Autor	Eltern und Geschwister		
		Zyklische und manische Psychosen	Phasisch-depressive Psychosen	Andere depressive Erkrankungen, Suizid
Zyklisch erkrankt	ANGST	3,70 ± 1,50	11,20 ± 2,50	3,1 ± 1,4
	PERRIS	10,80 ± 1,40	0,58 ± 0,03	8,6 ± 1,2
Phasisch-depressiv erkrankt	ANGST	0,29 ± 0,03	9,10 ± 1,60	2,3 ± 0,8
	PERRIS	0,35 ± 0,02	7,40 ± 1,10	6,8 ± 1,0

ven) Patienten (ANGST, 1966; PERRIS, 1966). Diese Entdeckung brachte die bis dahin stagnierende und weit hinter der Schizophrenieforschung zurückstehende Depressionsforschung in lebhaften Fluß. Eine Reihe von Serien wurde nach verschiedenen Gesichtspunkten gesammelt und je nach Fragestellung verschiedenartig aufgeschlüsselt, bearbeitet und ausgewertet.

Nach ANGST und PERRIS war die familiäre Belastung vorwiegend gleichsinnig, d.h. unipolare Patienten hatten unipolare Sekundärfälle in der Familie und bipolare Patienten wiederum bipolare. Die bipolaren Patienten waren höher mit affektiven Psychosen belastet als die unipolaren (Tabelle 3). Das weibliche Geschlecht überwog unter den unipolaren Patienten und ihren kranken Verwandten, nicht aber unter den bipolaren und ihren Sekundärfällen. Die prämorbide Persönlichkeit der Manisch-Depressiven war überwiegend synton, die der rein Depressiven ging in Richtung des asthenischen, „ordentlichen" Typus (ANGST, 1966; FREY, 1977; v. ZERSSEN, 1977). Die genetischen Unterschiede zwischen uni- und bipolaren Psychosen wurden in der Folge von mehreren Untersuchern bestätigt, neue Varianten und Untergruppen herausgearbeitet (GERSHON et al., 1975; MENDLEWICZ u. RAINER, 1974; SHIELDS, 1975; WINOKUR, 1973). Hereinnahme von Randgruppen und stärkere mathematische Alterskorrektur ergab für die Verwandten der Bipolaren Erkrankungsrisiken bis zu 50% (SHOPSIN et al., 1976; SUSLAK et al., 1976).

Die durchschnittliche Konkordanzrate affektpsychotischer Zwillingspaare beträgt rund 70% für die EZ und 19% für die ZZ. In konkordanten EZ-Paaren sind meistens, aber nicht immer, beide Partner entweder unipolar oder bipolar, vgl. Tabelle 4). In der Serie von BERTELSEN et al. (1977) sind übrigens alle 11 unipolar konkordanten Zwillingspaare weiblich; bei 9 Paaren wiesen die depressiven Phasen eine Beziehung zu Schwangerschaft, Entbindung oder Klimakterium auf.

Nun zeigt sich aber immer mehr, daß die Sache nicht so einfach ist. Das gemeinsame Vorkommen von uni- und bipolaren Psychosen in der gleichen Familie wird immer sicherer belegt, eine scharfe genetische Trennung besteht also nicht. ANGST hatte das schon 1966 gefunden. Es bestätigt sich auch in der ersten Adoptionsstudie über manisch-depressive Psychosen. MENDLEWICZ

Tabelle 4. Diagnostische Differenzierung ein- und zweieiiger Zwillingspaare nach uni- und bipolarer Psychose

	BERTELSEN et al. 1977		ZERBIN-RÜDIN 1969, 3 Serien	
	EZ %	ZZ %	EZ %	ZZ %
Beide unipolar depressiv	20,0	3,8	24,3	14,1
Beide bipolar oder manisch	25,4	3,8	10,8	2,8
1 unipolar, 1 bipolar oder manisch	12,7	9,6	5,4	7,0
Bedingt konkordant	25,4	17,3	18,9	11,3
Diskordant	16,3	65,4	40,5	64,8
Summe %	99,8	99,9	99,9	100
Gesamtzahl N	55	52	37	71

u. RAINER (1977) hatten in Brüssel und Umgebung 29 bipolare Patienten gesammelt, die im Alter von durchschnittlich 5,2 Monaten adoptiert worden waren. Endogen affektive Psychosen fanden sich unter den leiblichen Eltern 2,5mal häufiger als unter den Adoptiveltern, wobei die unipolaren Psychosen (12, bzw. 21%), die bipolaren (4, bzw. 7%) ums Dreifache überwogen. Insgesamt waren von den biologischen Eltern 29% erkrankt (16 von 58), von den Adoptiveltern aber auch nicht weniger als 12% (7/58) und zwar ohne Berücksichtigung von Spektrumstörungen! Eine Ergänzung mit sehr ähnlichen Resultaten bringt die kleine amerikanische Serie von CADORET (1978). Von den 8 adoptierten Kindern affektiv kranker Mütter (3 unipolar, 5 bipolar) erkrankten 3 an einer unipolaren Depression (37%). Die Erkrankungsrate der Adoptivkinder mit normalen biologischen Müttern (Vergleichsgruppe) ist mit 9% (4/43) erstaunlich hoch.

Für die Beziehungen zwischen uni- und bipolaren Psychosen gibt es drei Denkmöglichkeiten:

1. Die traditionelle, heute in Frage gestellte Auffassung sah die beiden Formen als genetische Einheit. Die Manie kann im Einzelfall latent bleiben; warum sollte sie das auch nicht können, wenn schon die ganze Psychose latent bleiben kann, wie die Zwillingsbefunde lehren. POST ist noch 1972 der Ansicht, daß seine Analyse das bimodale Modell nicht stützt.

2. Die zweite Möglichkeit ist die, daß uni- und bipolare Psychosen Teile ihrer Grundlage gemeinsam haben. GERSHON et al. (1975) stellten ein multifaktorielles Zwei- bzw. Drei-Schwellen-Modell auf. Die „Liability" (etwa zu übersetzen mit Krankheitsneigung oder Krankheitsdisposition) setzt sich aus Erb- und Umweltfaktoren zusammen und hat eine kontinuierliche Verteilung mit zwei Schwellen. Nach Überschreiten der ersten Schwelle tritt eine reine Depression auf, beim Überschreiten der zweiten Schwelle eine manisch-depressive Psychose. Die empirischen Daten der Autoren selbst, sowie die von ANGST, stimmen mit diesem Zwei-Schwellen-Modell überein, nicht aber die von PERRIS.

3. Die dritte Denkmöglichkeit sieht in uni- und bipolaren Psychosen zwei grundsätzlich verschiedene genetische Einheiten. Dies ist die in den letzten Jahren aufgestellte und von vielen Befunden gestützte Hypothese. Die Differenzierung

ist aber nur statistisch möglich und nicht im individuellen Fall. Wegen des gemeinsamen familiären Vorkommens muß ein Teil der unipolaren Depressionen wesensmäßig zu den bipolaren gehören, also „pseudo-unipolar" oder „kryptobipolar" sein. Wie kann man ihn erkennen?

PERRIS (1966) glaubte bei mehr als drei depressiven Phasen mit größter Wahrscheinlichkeit eine reine Depression annehmen zu können, ANGST et al. (1978) wiesen jedoch nach, daß die Sicherheit eines rein depressiven Verlaufes mit zunehmender Phasenzahl nur wenig zunimmt. KUPFER et al. (1975) versuchten es auf pharmakologischem Weg: Diejenigen reinen Depressionen, die auf Lithium ansprechen, sind pseudo-unipolar und gehören zu den bipolaren Psychosen; diejenigen, die auf Trizyklika ansprechen, stellen die echten unipolaren Depressionen dar. Aber selbst eindeutig bipolare Psychosen sprechen gelegentlich nicht auf Lithium an. Wir können also vorläufig echte und unechte unipolare Depressionen nicht unterscheiden (WEIL-MALHERBE, 1976). WINOKUR et al. suchen sich zu helfen, indem sie unipolare Depressionen kurzerhand dann als bipolar bezeichnen, wenn sie in Familien mit einem bipolaren Kranken vorkommen. Das mag stimmen, nimmt aber etwas vorweg, was erst bewiesen werden muß.

Wenn Heterogenität für die unipolaren Psychosen wahrscheinlich ist, so ist sie für die bipolaren Psychosen zumindest in Betracht zu ziehen. MENDLEWICZ et al. (1973) fanden, daß bipolare Patienten, die auf Lithium ansprachen, häufiger bipolare Sekundärfälle in der Familie hatten (15/24 = 63%) als die Lithiumversager (2/12 = 17%). Diese statistische Beziehung gilt im Einzelfall nicht: Es gibt belastete Fälle, die nicht auf Lithium ansprechen und unbelastete, die doch ansprechen. In ähnlicher Weise reagierten bipolar konkordante EZ-Paare am besten auf Lithium und Paare mit einem bipolaren und einem klinisch gesunden Partner am schlechtesten.

DUNNER und FIEVE (1975) unterteilten die bipolaren Psychosen nach Stärke und Sicherheit der manischen Komponente in zwei Gruppen, Bipolar I (mindestens einmal wegen Manie hospitalisiert) und Bipolar II (wegen Depression hospitalisiert mit manischen und hypomanischen Phasen in der Vorgeschichte). Wesentliche Belastungsunterschiede ergaben sich nicht. Der Manie wird überhaupt verstärkte Aufmerksamkeit gewidmet. HELZER und WINOKUR (1974), HELZER (1975) erfaßten die Probanden möglichst während einer manischen Phase, die teilweise die erste psychotische Phase überhaupt darstellte. Es bleibe dahingestellt, ob dieses Auswahlverfahren sehr glücklich ist. Die Autoren sehen auffallend viele Manien und zwei Fragen erheben sich: 1. Gehören wirklich alle Manien zu den manisch-depressiven Psychosen? 2. Inwieweit stellen die Probanden eine Auslese dar? Die Erfassung erfolgte über ehemalige Soldaten; es handelt sich also ausschließlich um Männer, z.T. um Neger. TAYLOR und ABRAMS (1973a) jedenfalls halten Manie für kein besonders stichhaltiges Auslesekriterium, um so weniger, als sie sicher heterogen ist. TAYLOR und ABRAMS arbeiteten eine früherkrankte Gruppe heraus mit Erkrankungsalter unter 30 Jahren, bipolarem Verlauf und hoher familiärer Belastung mit affektiven Psychosen und Spektrumstörungen und eine späterkrankte Gruppe mit Erkrankungsalter über 30 Jahren, unipolar manischem Verlauf und geringer Belastung.

Zur Bestätigung der Untergruppen suchte man die Hilfe von genetischen Markern, d.h. bekannten Genen, die mit dem unbekannten Gen gekoppelt vorkommen, es sozusagen markieren. Da das weibliche Geschlecht unter den Depressiven überwiegt, hatte man schon längst geschlechtsgebundenen Erbgang in Betracht gezogen. Es lag also nahe, jetzt X-chromosomal lokalisierte Markierungsgene zu wählen, nämlich Xg-Blutgruppe und Farbenblindheit. Tatsächlich war in einigen Familien mit bi- und unipolaren Psychosen die Psychose mit Farbenblindheit oder Xg gekoppelt, nicht aber in Familien mit ausschließlich unipolaren Erkrankungen. Man schloß daraus auf X-chromosomale Vererbung der bipolaren Psychosen (MENDLEWICZ u. FLEISS, 1974; WINOKUR u. TANNA, 1969). Andere Autoren konnten einen X-chromosomalen Erbgang jedoch nicht bestätigen. Vor allem dürfte sich ein X-chromosomales Leiden niemals vom Vater auf den Sohn vererben, denn nur die Töchter können das krankheitstragende X-Chromosom erhalten. Bei den bipolaren Psychosen kommt die Kombination kranker Vater – kranker Sohn aber oft genug vor (ANGST, 1966; DUNNER u. FIEVE, 1975; GOETZL et al., 1974; JAMES u. CHAPMAN, 1975; LORANGER, 1975; SMERALDI et al., 1977; TAYLOR u. ABRAMS, 1973a). Daher hatte man schon vor 40 Jahren die Hypothese geschlechtsgebundener Vererbung wieder fallen lassen. Vater-Sohn-Übertragungen stellen keine Rarität dar, sondern entsprechen in vielen Serien etwa der Erwartung und erscheinen vereinzelt sogar in den Serien der eifrigsten Verfechter X-chromosomalen Erbganges. Die Erklärungen, die väterliche Psychose sei reaktiv, oder neben dem Vater sei auch noch die Mutter bipolar psychotisch, wenn auch nur latent, scheinen an den Haaren herbeigezogen. In vielen Fällen ist nicht nur die Mutter gesund, sondern auch keine affektive Belastung in ihrer Familie nachweisbar, trotz sorgfältiger Untersuchung.

Ferner ist es merkwürdig, daß X-chromosomale Vererbung bei den bipolaren Psychosen vorliegen soll, während der Frauenüberschuß gerade bei den unipolaren besteht. Aus den Daten von ANGST geht X-chromosomale Vererbung – wenn überhaupt – eher für die unipolaren Psychosen hervor. X-chromosomale Vererbung scheint also zwar in einigen Familien vorzuliegen, aber sicher nicht generell.

Den bis jetzt beschriebenen Versuchen, klare Erbverhältnisse durch *Aus*gliederung von Untergruppen zu schaffen, stehen Bestrebungen gegenüber, der Wahrheit durch *Ein*gliederung „verwandter" Störungen näher zu kommen. Hier wird man in erster Linie an reaktive Depressionen und nicht-psychotische, insbesondere neurotische depressive Verstimmungen denken. STENSTEDT (1952) fand reaktive Depressionen in den Familien von endogen psychotischen Probanden vermehrt. Als er aber 1966 umgekehrt von reaktiv depressiven Probanden ausging, fand er in ihren Familien keine Vermehrung endogener Depressionen. Ferner gibt es Zwillingspaare, in denen ein Partner eine uni- oder bipolare Psychose aufweist, der andere aber nur leichtere depressive Verstimmungen oder Stimmungsschwankungen. Die psychotische Anlage kann sich offenbar auch in dieser Form manifestieren. Im übrigen sind die Zwillingsbefunde uneinheitlich. In einer englischen Serie (SHIELDS u. SLATER, 1966) ist die Konkordanz für neurotische Depressionen gleich Null, in einer skandinavischen immerhin vorhanden (JUEL-NIELSEN, 1964). Eine dänische Zwillingsserie von hospitalisierten, also sehr schweren psychoreaktiven Depressionen ergab eine niedrige Konkordanz für reaktive Depression, aber eine hohe für gestörte Persönlichkeitsentwicklung, d.h. für Neurosen überhaupt (SHAPIRO, 1970). Die deutsche Untersuchung von SCHEPANK (1974) erbrachte eine deutlich erkennbare Konkordanz für neurotisch-depressive Syndrome im weitesten Sinne.

Es verwundert nicht, wenn GUZE et al. (1975) feststellten, daß eine scharfe Trennung von psychotischen und nicht-psychotischen Depressionen nicht den Tatsachen entspricht und durch ihre Befunde an den Familien von „primär und sekundär depressiven Probanden" (wobei mit primär endogen psychotische und mit sekundär reaktive, nicht-psychotische Depressionen gemeint sind) nicht gestützt wird. Die reaktiven, neurotischen usw. Depressionen sind heterogen (SPICER et al., 1973). Ein Teil gehört zu den endogenen Depressionen, ein Teil hat andere Wurzeln. Die Überschneidung von Ätiologie und Symptomatologie kommt nicht nur bei psychischen Störungen vor, sondern ist in der Medizin ein allgemeines Phänomen.

In den USA spricht man neuerdings von „related disorders" und „spectrum disorders" und versteht darunter Alkoholismus, Soziopathie und Persönlichkeitsanomalien. AKISKAL et al. (1977) sahen bei 46 zyklothymen Patienten mit Diagnosen wie Hysterie und Soziopathie das gleiche Familienbild wie bei einer bipolaren Vergleichsgruppe und bei 35% Entwicklung regelrechter manischer und depressiver Phasen; sie schließen daraus, daß es ein bipolar-zyklothymes Spektrum gibt.

WINOKUR et al. (1971) glauben, daß die monopolaren Depressionen in „pure depression" und „spectrum depression" zerfallen. Völlig neu an dieser Einteilung ist, daß die Diagnose nicht für Einzelpersonen, sondern aus der Familienkonstellation gestellt wird. Bei „reiner Depression" müssen zwei Familienmitglieder depressiv sein, Spektrumstörungen dürfen nicht vermehrt vorkommen. Die Probanden wurden teilweise aus ehemaligen Soldaten erfaßt, sind also vorwiegend männlich; das Erkrankungsalter ist relativ hoch, die familiäre Belastung mit affektiven Störungen niedrig, Männer und Frauen sind gleich häufig erkrankt. Für die Diagnose einer Spektrum-Depression muß mindestens ein Familienmitglied depressiv und ein weiteres soziopathisch oder Alkoholiker sein. Die Gruppe zeichnet sich aus durch frühes Erkrankungsalter, hohe Belastung mit Depression und Soziopathien, Überwiegen des weiblichen Geschlechtes; die pathologische Anlage manifestiert sich nur bei den Frauen als Depression, bei den Männern als Alkoholismus. Koppelung einer der beiden Formen mit 20 verschiedenen genetischen Markern (Serumproteinen und sonstigen Serumfaktoren) ließ sich nicht sicher feststellen – man möchte sagen, wie zu erwarten! – höchstens ein gewisser Trend (TANNA et al., 1976a, b). Die Auslesemethode ist hoch selektiv und äußerst problematisch; der Auswertung und den Schlußfolgerungen drohen viele Fallgruben. Sie dürften eher familiäre Assoziationen als echte Koppelungen aufzeigen. Es muß zumindest offen bleiben, ob die Spektrumstörungen wirklich unmittelbarer Ausdruck der gleichen genetischen Grundlage sind und nicht vielmehr Ausdruck sekundärer Reaktionen und Resultat der Auswahlmethode oder selektiver Gattenwahl.

Die neurochemischen Befunde sind bis jetzt nicht eindeutig. Untersuchungen unter Einbeziehung der Verwandten sind wegen der praktischen Schwierigkeiten spärlich und ebenfalls alles andere als widerspruchsfrei. So fanden DUNNER et al. (1971) COMT (Catechol-O-Methyltransferase) bei unipolaren Frauen erniedrigt,

GERSHON u. JONAS (1975), die der gleichen Arbeitsgruppe angehören, bei affektpsychotischen Patienten und ihren Verwandten erhöht. Auch eine Erhöhung der MAO (Monoaminooxydase)-Aktivität bei Bipolaren ist nicht zweifelsfrei festgestellt (BELMAKER et al., 1976). Interessant und weiterführend scheinen Untersuchungen über erbliche Unterschiede der Lithiumresorption. Die Konzentration der Lithiumionen in Erythrozyten und Plasma ist bei eineiigen Zwillingen ähnlicher als bei zweieiigen. Man untersuchte dies zunächst an normalen Zwillingen (DORUS et al., 1974, 1975) und neuerdings an manisch-depressiven Zwillingen (MENDLEWICZ, persönliche Mitteilung).

Massive Traumen lösen depressive Phasen offenbar nur selten aus; häufiger sind leichte Operationen und fieberhafte Infekte und noch häufiger psychische Auslöser, besonders Veränderungs- und Verlustsituationen (WALCHER, 1971). Die Häufigkeit von Auslösern wird sehr verschieden angegeben, nämlich mit 3%–70%! Auch ihre Bedeutung wird unterschiedlich beurteilt. Besitzen die angeschuldigten Ereignisse im Vorfeld einer Depression wirklich auslösende oder gar pathogenetische Wirkung, oder ist die erhöhte Empfindlichkeit gegenüber Belastungen erstes Symptom der beginnenden Psychose? Die Auslöser sind offenbar unspezifisch. Manche kommen zwar etwas überdurchschnittlich häufig vor, z.B. hormonelle Umstellungen (Wochenbett und Klimakterium) sowie Verlustsituationen; aber auch sie sind für die Psychose weder notwendig, noch allein verantwortlich.

Im Erbgang scheint Dominanz eine Rolle zu spielen, ob man nun Monogenie oder Polygenie annimmt. Mehr noch als bei der Schizophrenie und auf Grund verschiedener Analysemethoden wird zur Zeit Polygenie für wahrscheinlicher gehalten (GOETZL et al., 1974; JAMES u. CHAPMAN, 1975; SLATER et al., 1971). PERRIS, der 1966 noch einem Hauptgen zugeneigt war, entschied sich 1971 ebenfalls für Polygenie. In der Serie von MENDLEWICZ et al. (1973) spricht die Verteilung der Sekundärfälle unter den Verwandten 1. Grades für einfache Dominanz, bei Einbeziehung der Verwandten 2. Grades aber wird Polygenie wahrscheinlicher.

Wie bei den Schizophrenien liegt der Erbfaktor vermutlich in Balance- und Verteilungsstörungen von Neurotransmittern oder Neurohormonen. Er könnte über Störungen von Reglermechanismen bei Transport- und Speicherungsvorgängen gehen und in der prä- oder postsynaptischen Membran lokalisiert sein.

Was für die gesamte psychiatrische Genetik gilt, demonstriert die Depressionsforschung in klassischer Weise. Auf der einen Seite bemüht man sich, die verschiedenen Konzepte – psychodynamische, klinische, neurobiologische – in das genetische Konzept zu integrieren (AKISKAL u. McKINNEY, 1975) und genetische Beziehungen zwischen verschiedenartigen Phänotypen aufzudecken. Auf der anderen Seite stellt sich zunehmend heraus, daß klinisch mehr oder weniger einheitliche Krankheitsgruppen, in diesem Fall die Depressionen, genetisch heterogen sind. Verschiedene Störungen münden über kurz oder lang in einen „common pathway", die Depression, ein, möge die gemeinsame Endstrecke im Bereich der psychischen Depression liegen oder schon früher bei neurochemischen Mechanismen beginnen. Daher werden die Forschungsergebnisse um so uneinheitlicher, je näher man an die Ursprünge der Ursachenketten gelangt (BEKKER, 1974).

IV. Atypische Psychosen und Beziehungen der Psychosen zueinander

Dieses wichtige Gebiet erfuhr lange eine ziemlich stiefmütterliche Behandlung. Als die Psychiatrie zur Wissenschaft wurde, ging sie zunächst einmal daran, ihr Gebiet zu ordnen, nach Typischem zu suchen, Zusammenhänge und Unterschiede herauszuarbeiten. Die Erbpsychiatrie konzentrierte sich auf Serien möglichst typisch erkrankter Probanden und hoffte, damit den Erbverhältnissen am schnellsten auf die Spur zu kommen. Dieser Weg war erfolgreich, ist aber bis zu einem gewissen Grad ausgeschöpft. Atypische Psychosen sind keineswegs seltene Randerscheinungen, sondern im Gegenteil recht häufig, und ihre Vernachlässigung führt zu einem unvollkommenen Bild der Wirklichkeit.

Als atypisch werden in erster Linie jene Psychosen bezeichnet, die schizophrene und affektive Elemente in sich vereinen, sei es im Querschnitt, sei es im Längsschnitt. Dazu kommen gelegentlich organische Komponenten. Der Kombinationen gibt es natürlich viele, und der individuellen Auffassung bei Gewichtung der Einzelsymptome und Stellung der Gesamtdiagnose sind kaum Grenzen gesetzt. Die atypischen Psychosen umfassen sehr heterogene Zustände und tragen viele Namen. In den USA ist für sie die Diagnose einer schizoaffektiven Psychose oder akuten schizophrenen Reaktion beliebt. In Skandinavien stecken sie teilweise in den „reaktiven" Psychosen, für die eine konstitutionelle Grundlage nicht auszuschließen ist, wie eigens betont wird. Außerdem gehören zu ihnen die Mischpsychosen, die schizophreniformen Psychosen, die benignen, remittierenden und geheilten Schizophrenien sowie die Schizophrenie-ähnlichen Emotionspsychosen.

Für alle gilt, was STRÖMGREN (1972) in seinen kurzen, prägnanten Ausführungen über die atypischen Psychosen bezüglich der schizoaffektiven Psychosen feststellt: Sie sind „eine Puffergruppe unbestimmten Inhaltes" und für schwer einzuordnende Fälle „sehr bequem". Alles in allem ist „die Verwirrung total". Zweifellos geht ein Teil der internationalen diagnostischen Diskrepanzen auf ihr Konto. Je enger die internationale Zusammenarbeit wird, um so notwendiger wird eine Klärung, damit die Vergleichbarkeit von Studien aus verschiedenen Ländern und Erdteilen gegeben ist.

So heterogen wie der ganze bequem/unbequeme Sektor der atypischen Psychosen sind die Serien, welche die Grundlage genetischer Untersuchungen bilden: Sie sind heterogen im Vergleich zueinander und heterogen in sich selbst. In einem Punkt aber stimmen sie mit wenigen Ausnahmen überein: Die familiäre Gesamtbelastung mit psychischen Störungen ist in diesen Familien sehr hoch, höher als bei schizophrenen und affektiven Psychosen, und sie ist äußerst bunt zusammengesetzt.

Man kann die atypischen Psychosen betrachten: 1. als Mischung klassisch-schizophrener und manisch-depressiver Psychosen, also als Mischpsychosen im wahrsten Sinn des Wortes; 2. als eigene Krankheitseinheiten; 3. als klassische Psychosen, die durch Persönlichkeitszüge, Erkrankungsalter oder sonstige Faktoren atypisch gefärbt sind. Offenbar kommt jede dieser drei Möglichkeiten vor.

Ad 1): SCHULZ (1940) fand unter den Kindern aus Ehen zwischen einem schizophrenen und einem affektpsychotischen Partner 3% Mischpsychosen, und das entspricht genau der theoretischen Erwartung einer Kombination der beiden Anlagen. Im übrigen aber sind Mischpsychosen mit gesicherter verschiedenartiger Belastung von väterlicher und mütterlicher Seite selten. FELDER (1977), der die mischpsychotische Gruppe von ANGST (1966) in etwas veränderter Zusammensetzung nachuntersuchte, teilte die 85 Probanden nach der Symptomatik in 4 Untergruppen auf: 1. Schizodominant, 2. Mitteltyp, 3. Schizophren plus manisch-depressiv, 4. Schizophren plus depressiv. Nach der familiären Belastung zu schließen, könnte Gruppe 2 echte Mischpsychosen enthalten. Die 3 übrigen Gruppen zeigen zwar gemischte Belastung mit schizophrenen, affektiven und atypischen Psychosen; diese ist aber nicht nach Elternseite aufgeschlüsselt und der Autor teilt lediglich mit, die Gruppen seien heterogen und gehörten weder zu den Schizophrenien, noch zu den affektiven Psychosen. ANGST (1966) hatte eine Tendenz gefunden, daß Probanden mit depressivem Beginn und schizophrener Weiterentwicklung, sowie Probanden mit gleichzeitiger depressiver und schizophrener Symptomatik ein eher schizophrenes Familienbild aufwiesen. Die Probanden mit schizophrenem Beginn und depressiver Weiterentwicklung standen mit ihrem Familienbild zwischen dem von schizophrenen und manisch-depressiven Probanden.

Ad 2): In manchen Familien kehren atypische Psychosen in gleicher oder ähnlicher Form immer wieder, und hier wird man an eigene Krankheitseinheiten denken (KAY, 1967). PERRIS (1974) nennt diese Gruppe „zykloide Psychosen" und kommt an Hand einer ausführlichen Literatur-Diskussion und eigener Familienuntersuchungen an 60 Probanden zu dem Schluß, daß es sich um Krankheiten sui generis handelt. Er betont die Notwendigkeit einer multifaktoriellen Betrachtungsweise. MITSUDA (1967) und seine Schüler in Japan sehen in den atypischen Psychosen selbständige Einheiten mit starker intrafamiliärer Homotypie. Bewußtseinsstörungen sind häufig, eine Minderwertigkeit des Zwischenhirn-Hypophysen-Systems wird erwogen. In den Familien kommen Zyklothymien vor, gelegentlich Epilepsien, aber Schizophrenien nur im Ausnahmefall. Die Japaner sahen auch kein einziges eineiiges Zwillingspaar mit einer typischen und einer atypischen Schizophrenie, während man in europäischen Serien solche Paare durchaus finden kann. Möglicherweise handelte es sich bei den japanischen und den europäischen atypischen Psychosen um verschiedene Dinge, obgleich FUKUDA dies verneint (persönliche Mitteilung).

Auch MCCABE (1975) betrachtet die reaktiven Psychosen als eigene „dritte funktionelle Psychose". Unter den Geschwistern von 40 reaktiv psychotischen Probanden fanden sich 6,7% ebenfalls reaktive Psychosen, 2,4% manisch-depressive Psychosen und 0,8% Schizophrenien. Erstaunlich hoch erwies sich bei den Eltern das Risiko für manisch-depressive Psychosen mit 7,4% (reaktive Psychosen 4,0%), allerdings bei kleiner Bezugsziffer. Zur Schizophrenie ist also keine genetische Beziehung erkennbar, die Beziehung zur manisch-depressiven Psychose hält MCCABE für unklar.

Immer wieder wird von manisch-depressiven Patienten berichtet, die schizophrene Nachkommen haben. Diese Kombination kann darauf beruhen, daß es sich bei Eltern wie Kindern im Grunde um atypische Psychosen handelt; es kann aber auch ein Fall auf Grund atypischer Phänomenologie fehldiagnostiziert worden sein (s. unten, Punkt 3). Zufälliges Zusammentreffen oder Übertragung durch den anderen Elternteil sind weitere Erklärungsmöglichkeiten. Gegen die Annahme einer Einheitspsychose spricht die ganz überwiegend gleichartige Belastung in den Familien Schizophrener und Affektpsychotischer.

TASCHEV und ROGLEV (1976) fanden unter 441 Patienten aus 210 Familien 11 Fälle, in denen die Eltern an Melancholie litten und die Kinder an Schizophrenie; das Umgekehrte kam nicht vor. In allen Fällen handelte es sich um atypische Psychosen und die psychopathologischen Bilder von Eltern und Kindern waren jeweils sehr ähnlich – trotz der verschiedenen Diagnose. Bei CAMMER (1970) litten 27% der 553 Kinder von 273 affektpsychotischen Eltern an Schizophrenie, 5,5% waren zwangsneurotisch und 14,3% emotional oder im Verhalten gestört; manisch-depressive Psychosen kamen anscheinend überhaupt nicht vor. Die Höhe der Belastung läßt an atypische Psychosen denken. Auch Geschwisterpaare zeigen gelegentlich die Kombination schizophrener und affektiver Psychosen (ØDEGAARD, 1972; SLATER, 1953; TASCHEV u. ROGLEV, 1976). Nach ELSÄSSER (1952) wäre ein Teil der als diskordant registrierten EZ-Paare konkordant, wenn man die Atypien der Krankheitsbilder als diagnostisches Hauptkriterium nehmen würde. Beim Probanden sind die Atypien schwächer ausgeprägt, so daß er gerade noch die Diagnose einer Schizophrenie oder manisch-depressiven Psychose erhalten hat. Beim Partner treten die Atypien derart in den Vordergrund, daß dies nicht mehr vertretbar ist.

Ad 3): Atypische Psychosen als Varianten schizophrener oder manisch-depressiver Psychosen. Das klinische Bild der Psychosen, wie praktisch aller Krankheiten, wird durch die verschiedensten Faktoren abgewandelt, z.B. Erkrankungsalter und Alter zum Zeitpunkt der Beobachtung, Geschlecht, organische Komponenten, Intelligenzgrad und Gesamtpersönlichkeit. Lehrbuchmäßige klassische Psychosen sind nicht so häufig wie sie sich der Diagnostiker wünscht, größere und kleinere Atypien sind die Regel. Bei genügender Sorgfalt und Beobachtungsdauer läßt sich aber ein Großteil der atypischen Psychosen auf den schizophrenen und manisch-depressiven Kreis aufteilen.

POST (1971) konnte ein Drittel seiner Patienten über 60 Jahre, die ein schizoaffektives Bild zeigten, im weiteren Verlauf einer der beiden großen Psychosen zuordnen. 29 Patienten blieben übrig; sie boten neben der schizophrenen und affektiven Symptomatik auch Zeichen zerebraler Schädigung, eine prämorbid auffällige Persönlichkeit und hohe familiäre Belastung. MORRISON et al. (1972) mußten nach 25–35 Jahren bei 63% ursprünglichen „Schizophrenen" die Diagnose revidieren. ABRAMS et al. (1974) fanden bei der Nachprüfung von 41 „paranoiden Schizophrenen" in der Hälfte der Fälle alle Kriterien einer Manie und auch eine familiäre Belastung wie bei manisch-depressiven Probanden.

BLEULERS (1941) „wellenförmig zur Heilung" verlaufende Schizophrenien und LANGFELDTS (1956) schizophrenieforme Psychosen hatten eine ebenso hohe Belastung mit Schizophrenie wie typische Schizophrenien, LEONHARDS atypische Psychosen sogar eine höhere. Bei den atypischen Schizophrenien von HALLGREN und SJÖGREN (1959), sowie den Schizophrenie-ähnlichen benignen Psychosen von WELNER und STRÖMGREN (1958), den „geheilten Schizophrenien" von WITTERMANS und SCHULZ (1950) und den Schizophrenie-ähnlichen Emotionspsychosen von LABHARDT (1963) dagegen war sie wesentlich niedriger. Wir sehen auch hier wieder Heterogenität.

Zum Schluß ein kurzer Hinweis auf Felduntersuchungen, die sämtliche psychische Störungen eines bestimmten Gebietes erfassen. Sie gehören zwar in das Reich der Epidemiologie, aber manche berücksichtigen auch genetische Gesichtspunkte, besonders die skandinavischen Untersuchungen und jene, die ihr Gebiet im Längsschnitt beobachten. Sie sind ganz besonders geeignet, unsere Kenntnis von den atypischen Psychosen, von der Entwicklung psychischer Störungen im Laufe der Zeit und von der Manifestation der Erbgrundlagen unter wechselnden Umweltbedingungen zu erweitern. Sie erfordern aber die Arbeit eines ganzen Lebens, ja zweier Generationen von Wissenschaftlern; daher sind die genetischen Ergebnisse vorerst noch nicht umfangreich.

Skandinavien ist durch seine geographischen Verhältnisse und ausgezeichneten Register besonders für solche Untersuchungen geeignet, und allein dort laufen an die 10 Projekte. Einen Überblick gab das Tromsø-Seminar (ANDERSEN et al., 1975), hier seien 3 exemplarische Studien herausgegriffen. ESSEN-MÖLLER und seine Mitarbeiter explorierten persönlich jeden der 2550 Einwohner zweier südschwedischer Pfarreien und stuften ihn zwischen den Endpolen „psychisch schwer verändert" und „psychisch unauffällig" ein. Die verschiedensten Aufschlüsselungen – nach Alter, Art der Störung, Schweregrad – wurden vorgenommen und können auf Grund der ausführlichen Dokumentation vom Leser nachvollzogen oder anders gemacht werden. Dieses „Lundby-Projekt" läuft bereits in dritter Wissenschaftler-Generation (ESSEN-MÖLLER, 1956; HAGNELL, 1966; HAGNELL u. ÖJESJÖ, 1975).

Das von STRÖMGREN et al. (1957) begonnene Samsø-Projekt ist verstärkt sozialpsychiatrisch orientiert und greift aus der Gesamtheit eine Fülle von Spezialthemen heraus, die gesondert bearbeitet werden (NIELSEN, 1976).

Das jüngste Projekt in dieser Reihe ist das von ASTRUP et al. Anfang der 70er Jahre ins Leben gerufene Berlevåg-Projekt (BJARNAR et al., 1975), welches eine unter extremen Bedingungen lebende kleine Fischer-Gemeinde nördlich des Polarkreises zum Gegenstand seiner Bemühungen gemacht hat.

V. Kindliche Psychosen

Das Studium kindlicher Psychosen dient in erster Linie dem Kind selbst (BOSCH, 1972). Außerdem hofft man, über die kindlichen Psychosen zu besserem Verständnis der Psychosen der Erwachsenen zu gelangen. Das Kind zeigt eine einförmigere Symptomatik und einen geringeren reaktiven Überbau als der Erwachsene, und es ist noch erkennbar eingebettet in das Familienmilieu, so daß Erb- und Umweltfaktoren vielleicht leichter zu identifizieren sind. Bis jetzt sieht es allerdings nicht so aus, als ob sich diese Hoffnung erfüllen würde. Es handelt sich doch um Sonderfälle, denn die meisten Erkrankungen erfolgen eben nicht im Kindesalter. Auch ist die Symptomatik zwar von jener der Erwachsenen verschieden und altersspezifisch, aber sehr wenig krankheitsspezifisch. Die kindlichen Symptome erlauben keine sichere Prognose für die spätere psychische Störung, und die endgültige Diagnose kann meist erst nach langer Verlaufsbeobachtung gestellt werden (DAHL, 1976). Zum Beispiel entwickeln sich Depressionen nicht allzu selten zu Schizophrenien und selbst schwere Störungen normalisieren sich mitunter.

Endogene Psychosen im Kindesalter sind selten, 1:2600 Kinder (HANSON u. GOTTESMAN, 1976) oder 1:100 Schizophrenien. Allerdings ist wohl mit einer gewissen Dunkelziffer zu rechnen. Das männliche Geschlecht ist überrepräsentiert. In der Mehrzahl handelt es sich um Schizophrenien und frühkindlichen Autismus, depressive Psychosen sind viel seltener. Um nichts zu präjudizieren, sprechen besonders amerikanische Autoren mit Vorliebe von kindlichen Psychosen, selbst wenn sie eigentlich Schizophrenien meinen. Zwei Gruppen lassen sich unterscheiden, nämlich frühkindliche (infantile) und spätkindliche (pubertäre und adoleszente) Fälle (HANSON u. GOTTESMAN, 1976). Die Altersverteilung bildet eine U-förmige Kurve mit Gipfeln im 1./2. und 13./14. Lebensjahr, die Grenze wird willkürlich beim 5. oder 7. Jahr gesetzt.

Eine gewisse Einigkeit besteht, daß die spätkindliche Gruppe enge Beziehungen zur Schizophrenie der Erwachsenen besitzt. Dafür sprechen die Katamnesen und die Familienbefunde. Die Serie von KALLMANN und ROTH (1956) umfaßt 50 einzelgeborene und 52 zwillingsgeborene Schizophrene im Alter von 7–11 Jahren. Die EZ sind zu 71%, die ZZ zu 17% für eine jugendliche Schizophrenie (unter 15 Jahren) konkordant. Unter Einbeziehung erwachsener Schizophrenieerkrankungen erhöhen sich die Konkordanzwerte auf 88% und 23%. Die Eltern sind zu 8,9±2,0% und die Geschwister zu 7,7±1,7% an Schizophrenie erkrankt. In der Serie von KOLVIN et al. (1971) (64 kindliche Schizophreniefälle über 5 Jahre) sind die Eltern zu 9,4±3,6%, die Geschwister jedoch nur zu 1,8±1,8% erkrankt. Aus den Daten von SPIEL (1961) und EGGERS (1973) läßt sich für die Eltern eine Schizophrenierate von 6% bzw. 4% errechnen.

Weit weniger Übereinstimmung herrscht bei den frühkindlichen Formen, die sich großenteils als frühkindlicher Autismus darstellen. Man hat das Wesen des frühkindlichen Autismus in extremer Abkapselung, sprachlicher Kommunikationsstörung, zwangshafter Veränderungsangst gesehen (KANNER, 1954), in einer Störung der Ego-Entwicklung (MAHLER, 1952), in einer Integrationsstörung zentralnervöser Funktionen auf verschiedenen Ebenen (FISH, 1975), in einer kognitiv-perzeptiv-sprachlichen Störung (RUTTER, 1971) und als Schizophrenievariante (FISH, 1975; BENDER, 1963, 1975).

Ebenso verschieden wie die theoretisch-klinischen Konzepte sind die genetischen Befunde und Schlußfolgerungen. KANNER selbst (1954) rechnete die Gruppe, trotz fehlender Schizophreniebelastung und mit Vorbehalt, zum schizophrenen Formenkreis. 3 von 131 Geschwistern von 100 frühautistischen Kindern waren ebenfalls autistisch, die sozial und intellektuell überdurchschnittlichen Eltern waren zu 85% kühle, schizoide Psychopathen, „emotionale Eisschränke". FISCHER (1965) stellt den frühkindlichen Autismus weit entschiedener zu den Schizophrenien. BENDER (1963, 1975), DAHL (1976), FISH (1975), MEYERS und GOLDFARB (1962) sehen in ihm Manifestationen einer echten Schizophrenie und belegen dies mit Katamnesen und Familienuntersuchungen.

In BENDERS Serie entwickelten sich die kindlichen Schizophrenien mit 63% etwa doppelt so oft wie die adoleszenten zu einer erwachsenen Schizophrenie. Die von BENDER auf Grund von pathologischen Reflexen und Tonusregulierungen, neurologischen Abweichungen usw. schon vor dem 2. Lebensjahr als Schizophrene diagnostizierten Kinder litten als Erwachsene sogar zu 72% an Schizophrenie. Die Eltern waren zu 11% (in anderen Serien sogar 30% und 43%!) schizophren, die Geschwister zu 13% (BENDER, 1963, 1975).

Auch FISH (1975) fand bei Kindern unter 2 Jahren Störungen von Sprechen, Denken und Motorik, sowie allgemeine Entwicklungsrückstände. Es handelte sich teils um Kinder, die später an kindlicher oder juveniler Schizophrenie erkrankten, teils um Kinder schizophrener Mütter. Wegen der teilweisen Erfassung über schizophrene Mütter können keine Risikoziffern der Eltern berechnet werden. FISH gründet ihre Theorie teils auf ihre eigenen Untersuchungen, teils auf die Befunde anderer Autoren. Sie sieht die Grundlage der Schizophrenie in einer Gehirnstörung, deren Symptomatik typisch für eine angeborene genetische Störung und völlig anders als bei traumatischen Hirnschäden ist. Sie besteht in einer zeitweisen Desintegration verschiedener Funktionsabläufe des Zentralnervensystems, Störungen von Entwicklungsmustern und Regulationen mit allgemeinem Entwicklungsrückstand und nicht in umschriebenen Störungen einzelner Merkmale und Funktionen. Die meisten Fälle von frühkindlichem Autismus gehören zur Schizophrenie und zeigen eine entsprechende familiäre Belastung. Von der frühkindlichen über die kindliche und juvenile Manifestation der Schizophrenieanlage bis zur Erwachsenenpsychose besteht ein Kontinuum. Der Verlauf ist um so maligner und die Prognose um so schlechter, je früher und schwerer die ersten Krankheitszeichen auftreten. Die familiären Sekundärfälle erkranken bevorzugt, aber nicht ausschließlich wiederum früh. Die grundlegende biologische Hirnstörung der Schizophrenie kann sich also bereits in frühester Kindheit, ja bei Geburt manifestieren, muß aber nicht. Man erinnere sich, daß nur etwa die Hälfte aller Schizophrenen Auffälligkeiten in der Kindheit zeigte und zwar meist unspezifische. Von erwachsenen Schizophrenen, die als Kinder wegen Verhaltensstörungen in eine Child Guidance Clinic gebracht worden waren, hatten nur 15% die Diagnose einer kindlichen Schizophrenie erhalten.

Die kindlichen Schizophrenien sind auch sicher kein Dosis- und Schwereproblem, denn sie kommen unter den Kindern schizophrener Elternpaare kaum vor (SCHULZ, 1940; ERLENMEYER-KIMLING, 1975). Bei dem einen Ausnahmefall von ELSÄSSER (1952) waren auch die beiden Eltern schon sehr jung erkrankt.

Andere Autoren fanden die Schizophreniebelastung bei frühkindlichem Autismus kaum oder gar nicht erhöht (KANNER, 1954; KOLVIN et al., 1971; RUTTER u. LOCKYER, 1967). Dies führt notgedrungen zu dem Schluß, der frühkindliche Autismus gehöre nicht zur Schizophrenie, wenn er auch organischen Ursprungs und möglicherweise genetisch beeinflußt ist (HANSON u. GOTTESMAN, 1976; RUTTER, 1974; SANKAR, 1976; STABENAU, 1975).

Die Zwillingsbefunde sind nicht sehr aussagekräftig. Es handelt sich um Einzelkasuistiken, die bekanntlich konkordante Paare überrepräsentieren. Zudem ist die symptomatologische Beschreibung oft ungenügend. In der Zusammenstellung von HANSON und GOTTESMAN (1976) sind 82% EZ (9 von 11 Paaren) und 25% ZZ (1 von 4 Paaren) konkordant; in der Übersicht von STABENAU (1975) beträgt die Konkordanz der EZ 93% (14 von 15 Paaren) und der ZZ 0% (5 Paare). Die einzige auslesefreie Serie von FOLSTEIN und RUTTER (nach HANSON u. GOTTESMAN, 1976) ergab die vorläufigen Konkordanzen EZ 36% (4 von 11 Paaren) und ZZ 0% (10 Paare).

Der frühkindliche Autismus ist also heterogen, und unter frühkindlicher Schizophrenie werden verschiedene Zustände verstanden. Verschiedene Autoren haben verschiedene Störungen bearbeitet und das ergibt verschiedene Befunde.

Jugendliche und kindliche Depressionen (Sammelband ANNELL, 1972) sind noch seltener als Schizophrenien und entwickeln sich zudem im weiteren Verlauf häufig zu Schizophrenien (DAHL, 1972; EGGERS, 1972; NISSEN, 1971). PÉNOT (1972) sah bei seinen symptomatologisch gemischten Fällen weitere Entwicklung zu Psychopathie; das häusliche Milieu war schlecht, die Mutter häufig depressiv. Im allgemeinen dominieren bei den kindlichen Depressionen somatische, besonders vegetative Beschwerden. Doch sollen auch in diesem frühen Stadium Schuldgefühle vorkommen, soll plötzlicher Phasenwechsel zwischen normalen und gestörtem Verhalten, zwischen Apathie und Erregung charakteristisch sein.

Die wenigen Serien, die Familienbefunde mitteilen, sind ebenso heterogen wie die kindlichen Depressionen überhaupt. Zudem wurden sie häufig selektiv nach bestimmten Gesichtspunkten erfaßt. Wenn z.B. familiäre Belastung zu den Auswahlkriterien gehört (REMSCHMIDT u. DAUNER, 1971; SCHMITZ, 1972), so besitzen familiäre Risikoziffern nur bedingten Aussagewert.

In der Serie von CEBIROGLU et al. (1972) hatten 27% von 85 depressiven Kindern ebenfalls depressive Eltern, doch waren nur knapp 10% der Kinder endogen depressiv. Bei MENDELSON et al. (1972) hatten „rein depressive" Kinder 66% depressive Mütter, „gemischt depressive" Kinder (Depression plus Angstzustände oder Aggression) 44%, und Kinder mit Angstzuständen 23% depressive Mütter.

Von 28 manisch-depressiv Erkrankten unter 19 Jahren (OLSEN, 1961) hatten 8 Patienten gleichartige Sekundärfälle unter Eltern und Geschwistern, weitere 6 Patienten andere Psychosen oder Schwachsinn. Manische Phasen waren viermal häufiger als depressive und nur einmal erfolgte Entwicklung zu Schizophrenie.

Die beiden aufschlußreichsten und aussagekräftigsten Serien sind wohl die von SPIEL (1961) und NISSEN (1971). Bei SPIEL waren 21,1% der Eltern endogen depressiver Kinder affektiv gestört, bei NISSEN 15,3% (einschließlich depressiver Verstimmungen, Suizidversuche und zykloider Psychopathie). Wenn NISSEN bei seinen 105 Probanden im Alter von 11–18 Jahren nach einer Beobachtungszeit von 9,1 Jahren 9 Schizophrenien, und 47 psychogene Depressionen, aber keine einzige endogene Depression sah, so mag das an dem jugendlichen Alter von 20–27 Jahren bei Beobachtungsabschluß liegen. Etliche „psychogene" Depressionen dürften sichere Anwärter auf eine „endogene" sein.

VI. Nicht-psychotische Persönlichkeits- und Verhaltensabweichungen

Diese Störungen zeigen fließende Übergänge zu normaler Persönlichkeit und normalem Verhalten – was immer man unter normal verstehen mag – und sind außerordentlich heterogen.

Früher pflegte man sie in Deutschland allgemein in Psychopathien und Neurosen zu unterteilen (umfassende Übersicht bei STRÖMGREN, 1967b). Heute orientiert man sich häufig am Verhalten (ROSENTHAL, 1970), insbesondere am sozialen Verhalten, und man spricht von Soziopathie, von asozialem, aggressivem, süchtigem, sexualabnormen usw. Verhalten. Dabei hat man es mit besonders uneinheitlichen Gruppen und komplexen Verhaltensmustern zu tun und was auf S. 547f. über die Problematik einer verhaltensorientierten Genetik und über die Schwierigkeit der Messung psychischer Phänomene gesagt wurde, gilt hier in verstärktem Maße.

Die derzeitige begriffliche und terminologische Verwirrung um die Psychopathie erklärt PICHOT (1978) aus nationalen Unterschieden und historischer Entwicklung. Das deutsche Konzept der psychopathischen Persönlichkeit von KURT SCHNEIDER (1923) ist psychologisch-strukturell orientiert. Im Gegensatz dazu ist der eingewurzelte angelsächsische Begriff der moral insanity operational. Es gab große Verwirrung, besonders in England, als man, im Bestreben eine moralische Verurteilung zu vermeiden, die Bezeichnung „moral insanity" durch „psychopathic disorders" ersetzte, das Kriterium des asozialen Verhaltens aber beibehielt. Um die Verwirrung vollständig zu machen, nannte man die psychologisch definierten Formen, also die psychopathischen Persönlichkeiten nach SCHNEIDER, nunmehr „personality disorders". Psychopathie und Soziopathie (moral insanity) überschneiden sich zwar, aber sie decken sich nicht (STRÖMGREN, 1977).

Die Unterteilung dieses Kapitels ist inkonsequent, da sie sich nach den verfügbaren Untersuchungen richten muß. Während der Abschnitt Neurosen und Psychopathien dem psychologischen Konzept folgt, beziehen sich die übrigen Abschnitte auf operational definierte Verhaltens- und Anpassungsstörungen.

Die immer wieder festgestellte familiäre Häufung gleicher oder ähnlicher derartiger Störungen läßt sich nicht ohne weiteres Anlagefaktoren zur Last legen, denn das familiäre und soziale Milieu ist häufig höchst ungünstig. Zwillings- und Adoptionsstudien haben jedoch gezeigt, daß abnorme Persönlichkeiten und Verhaltensweisen ebenso wie die normalen von Anlage- *und* Umweltfaktoren beeinflußt werden, wobei die beiden Größen bei verschiedenen Merkmalen und im individuellen Fall verschiedenes Gewicht besitzen (GOTTESMAN, 1963; SHIELDS, 1978a). Zum Beispiel sind Angst- und Zwangsneurosen deutlich erbabhängig, depressive und hysterische Zustände weniger oder gar nicht.

1. Neurosen und Psychopathien

Unter Psychoneurose versteht man gewöhnlich eine zeitlich begrenzte abnorme Persönlichkeitsreaktion, das Resultat fehlerhafter Verarbeitung eines Geschehnisses oder Tatbestandes, unter Psychopathie eine dauernde abnorme Persönlichkeitsstruktur oder -entwicklung. Bekanntlich können aber Neurosen chronifizieren und Psychopathien psychotherapeutisch gebessert werden. Auch ist eine abnorme Reaktion bevorzugt von einer abnormen Persönlichkeit zu erwarten, und so überschneiden sich die beiden Begriffe. K. SCHNEIDER kam zeitlebens weitgehend ohne die Diagnose „Neurose" aus, bei BECKER (1978) findet sich das Wort „Psychopathie" nur selten.

Neurotische und Psychopathie-artige Bilder kommen nicht nur eigenständig vor, sondern auch bei organischen Leiden, z.B. im Anfangsstadium von Hirntumoren, nach Hirnverletzungen und Enzephalitiden, bei Aberrationen der Geschlechtschromosomen, bei Chorea Huntington und schließlich zu Beginn von

Schizophrenien. Sind sie in solchen Fällen Symptom und direkte Folge des organischen Prozesses, also rein exogenen Ursprunges, oder kommen sie mittelbar, über eine Reaktion der Persönlichkeit auf das Krankheitsgeschehen zustande?

Die älteren Zwillingskonkordanzen für „Neurose" zeigen eine riesige Schwankungsbreite: EZ 0%–90%, ZZ 0%–50% (BECKER et al., 1970; SCHEPANK, 1973). Dies ist in erster Linie auf die Heterogenität der Neurosen und der Serien, sowie auf verschieden strenge Fassung des Konkordanzbegriffes zurückzuführen. Aufschlußreicher ist die gesonderte Betrachtung der verschiedenen Serien und Neuroseformen.

SHIELDS (1954) untersuchte neurotische Züge und Störungen bei „normalen" Zwillingen im Schulalter (36 EZ- und 26 ZZ-Paare). 63% der Knaben und 47% der Mädchen zeigten irgendwann neurotische Störungen, die meist noch im Bereich des Normalen lagen und die soziale Anpassung nicht wesentlich beeinträchtigten. Bei 23 EZ-Paaren (64%) und 18 ZZ-Paaren (68%) war mindestens 1 Partner auffällig. Bei den EZ-Paaren zeigten die Partner zu 26% sehr ähnliche, 35% im wesentlichen ähnliche und 13% verschiedene Symptome; 26% waren diskordant, d.h. 1 Partner war symptomfrei. Für die ZZ lauten die entsprechenden Werte 0%, 6%, 44%, 50%. Die Art der Störungen war stärker erblich beeinflußt als die Schwere, polygene Erbfaktoren sind anzunehmen.

SCHEPANK (1974) verband in seiner Zwillingsuntersuchung erstmals genetische Methoden mit psychoanalytischen Techniken. Er verglich nicht nur globale Diagnosen, sondern auch Einzelsymptome und Schweregrade. Nach dem „Leitsymptom" waren 52% EZ und 14% ZZ konkordant, für verschiedene Einzelsymptome betrug die Konkordanz bei der EZ 33% und den ZZ 17%. Bei Skalierung der neurotischen Störungen nach dem Schweregrad zeigten die EZ eine Differenz von 3,8 Punkten, die ZZ von 5,0 Punkten.

Die Zwillingsbefunde von SHIELDS und SLATER basieren auf dem von den Autoren 1948 angelegten Zwillingsregister des Maudsley Hospitals in London, welches laufend ergänzt wurde und gegenwärtig etwa 800 erwachsene und kindliche Zwillinge umfaßt. Die stärkste Erbkomponente zeigen Angst- und Zwangsneurosen (s. Tabelle 5). BECKER (1979) weist allerdings darauf hin, daß sich die Bezeichnungen „anxiety state" oder „reaction", „phobic reaction" einerseits und Angst- und Zwangsneurose andererseits nur teilweise entsprechen, ebenso wie Neurotizismus bei EYSENCK und CATELL zwar ähnliches meint, aber nicht dasselbe. Einige der Zwangsprobanden von SHIELDS (1978a) hatten zusätzlich Angstzustände und waren unter dieser Diagnose in der Serie von 1966 enthalten. Die Zwillinge mit Zwangssymptomen repräsentieren die erste auslesefreie Serie, die wir besitzen. Bis jetzt waren lediglich 17 konkordante und 7 diskordante EZ-Paare aus Einzelkasuistiken bekannt. Die daraus errechnete Konkordanz von 70% stimmt erstaunlich gut mit der Konkordanz von SHIELDS (74%) überein. Für Angstneurosen sind die EZ zu 41% konkordant, die ZZ nur zu 4%.

Depressive Neurosen machen einen Großteil der „anderen Neurosen" von SHIELDS und SLATER aus; ein Erbeinfluß ist nicht zu erkennen (Tabelle 5). Anders bei SHAPIRO (1970), wo die gleichartige Konkordanz der EZ nicht weniger als 60% beträgt. Das könnte allerdings auch bedeuten, daß einige seiner Fälle

Tabelle 5. Neuere Zwillingsbefunde bei neurotischen und phobischen Störungen

	Konkordanz								Diskordanz	
	Streng				Erweitert				EZ %	ZZ %
	EZ		ZZ		EZ		ZZ			
	Zahl	%	Zahl	%	Zahl	%	Zahl	%		
SHIELDS u. SLATER (1966)										
Angstneurosen[a]	7/17	41	1/28	4	1/17	6	5/28	14	53	82
Andere Neurosen[a]	0/12	0	0/21	0	3/12	25	5/21	24	75	76
SHIELDS (1978)										
Zwangsneurosen und Phobien[b]	14/19	74	4/22	18	2/19	10	9/22	41	16	41
SHAPIRO (1970)[a]										
Depressive Neurosen	6/10	60	1/9	11	1/10	10	0/9	0	30	89
Psychogene Depressionen	2/6	33	1/5	20	1/6	17	1/5	20	50	60
Zusammen	8/16	50	2/14	14	2/16	13	1/14	7	37	79

[a] Strenge Konkordanz: Gleichartige Störungen verschiedener Stärke. Erweiterte Konkordanz: Andersartige psychiatrische Diagnosen
[b] Strenge Konkordanz: Gleichartige Störungen von krankhaftem Ausmaß. Erweiterte Konkordanz: Gleichartige Symptome ohne wesentliche Beeinträchtigung

doch endogen sind (vgl. S. 581). Beide Autoren schließen, daß primär eine Persönlichkeitsstörung vorliegt, die sekundär zur nicht-endogenen Depression als einer von mehreren Manifestationsmöglichkeiten führt.

Diskordanzanalysen von EZ sind aufwendig, nur in besonders günstigen Fällen ergiebig (SCHEPANK, 1975) und erbrachten weniger relevante Umweltfaktoren, als erhofft (SHIELDS, 1978a).

SLATER (1964) betrachtet die Disposition zu Neurosen als kontinuierlich verteilte multifaktoriell bedingte Variable. Bei starker Disposition genügt ein geringer Streß zur Erkrankung, bei schwacher Disposition bedarf es einer starken Belastung. Vererbt wird eine neurotische Persönlichkeitsdisposition oder Reaktionsbereitschaft; Krankheitswert erlangt sie erst durch Umwelteinflüsse. Man hat versucht, diese Disposition und nicht die manifeste Neurose im sog. „neuroticism score" mittels Fragebogen und Test zu erfassen. Die Ergebnisse sind aber bis jetzt nicht eindeutig, jedenfalls nicht, was die Erbverhältnisse anbetrifft (EAVES u. EYSENCK, 1976).

Ein ähnliches Konzept entwickelt BECKER (1979) in seiner Übersicht über Wege und Probleme der Zwillingsforschung zu Persönlichkeit, Charakter und Neurosen. Er wägt Erb- und Umweltfaktoren, Struktur und Funktion, genetische und psychoanalytische Deutungen bei der Entstehung der Neurosen ab und unterscheidet neurotische Strukturen, die zumindest teilweise erbabhängigen „Persönlichkeitsqualitäten mit Zustandscharakter" entsprechen, und neurotische Reaktionen und Symptome, die eher „Haltungsperspektiven" verkörpern.

Die Verwirrung um Wort und Begriff der *Psychopathie* (vgl. S. 591) zeigte sich auch noch bei einer Arbeitstagung, die 1975 eben zu deren Klärung veranstaltet wurde (HARE u. SCHALLING, 1978). Drei Beiträge waren genetischen Aspekten gewidmet: Nach EYSENCK und EYSENCK (1978) bestimmen die drei Dimensionen Psychotizismus, Neurotizismus und Extraversion die Persönlichkeit. Sie sind voneinander unabhängig, weitgehend erbbestimmt und führen in pathologischen Varianten zu psychopathischem, antisozialem und psychotischem Verhalten. CLONINGER et al. (1978) orientieren sich in ihren Ausführungen weitgehend am Verhalten; MEDNICK und HUTCHINGS (1978) beschreiben psychophysiologische Befunde an Delinquenten.

Ältere, vorwiegend deutsche Untersuchungen zum psychologischen Psychopathiebegriff s. bei STRÖMGREN (1967b). Ganz allgemein kommen Psychopathie und Kriminalität in den Familien von Psychopathen vermehrt vor. Neuere Übersicht bei STRÖMGREN (1977). Schizoid s.S. 564, Soziopathie (Kriminalität) s.S. 596.

SLATER und SHIELDS (1969), die in etwa das Schneidersche Psychopathiekonzept verwenden, fanden EZ zu 33% komplett und zu 55% bedingt konkordant, die ZZ zu 6%, bzw. 29%.

SCHULSINGER (1972) erfaßte 57 Adoptivkinder mit späterer schwerer Psychopathie aus den gleichen dänischen Registern, die auch die Grundlage für die Schizophreniestudie bildeten. Psychopathie wurde definiert als unangemessenes, nicht-psychotisches, impulsives, an anderen abreagierendes („acting out") Verhalten. Psychopathie in diesem engeren Sinn fand sich unter den biologischen Verwandten fünfmal häufiger als in den Adoptivfamilien und Kontrollen, nämlich 3,9% gegenüber 0,8%. Bei Einbeziehung „psychopathischer Spektrumstörungen" (fragliche Psychopathie, Alkoholismus, Kriminalität, hysterische Züge) betrug der Unterschied nur das Doppelte, nämlich 14,4% zu 7,6%. Andere psychische Störungen waren nicht vermehrt.

2. Suizid

Suizid ist nach RINGEL (1965) zu etwa einem Viertel auf Neurosen und Psychopathien zurückzuführen, zu einem weiteren Viertel auf depressive Psychosen. Die Selbstmordhäufung in manchen Familien (z.B. BEICHL, 1965; HANHART, 1968/69) kann ebenso gut auf tradiertes Verhalten wie auf genetische Verankerung hinweisen, ob diese nun über eine Neurose oder Psychose geht oder nicht. Vorläufige Adoptionsbefunde von SCHULSINGER (1978) sind erstaunlich: „Reiner Suizid" (d.h. Suizid ohne erkennbare Psychose) fand sich in den biologischen Familien von Adoptivkindern, die später Suizid oder Suizidversuche begingen, weit häufiger als in den Adoptivfamilien. Das würde auf einen Erbfaktor hinweisen.

EZ sind nicht allzu oft für Suizid konkordant, ZZ niemals. In der Zusammenstellung von HABERLANDT (1967) betrugt die Konkordanz der EZ 9/51, der ZZ 0/98, in der auslesefreien Serie von JUEL-NIELSEN und VIDEBECH (1970) EZ 4/15, ZZ 0/15. Bei den konkordanten Fällen handelte es sich meist um psychotische Paare (JUEL-NIELSEN u. VIDEBECH, 1970; BERGER, 1964).

Geht man aber umgekehrt von psychotischen Zwillingen aus, so sind sie nur selten für Suizid konkordant. D'ELIA und PERRIS (1968/69) fanden das Selbstmordrisiko unter den Verwandten von manisch-depressiven Patienten, die

Suizid oder Suizidversuche begingen, nur minimal höher als unter den Verwandten von Selbstmord-freien Manisch-Depressiven. Eine Erbkomponente ist also unter psychotischen Bedingungen nur schwach zu erkennen, wenn überhaupt: Suizid kommt offenbar durch höchst individuelle Motivationen und einmalige Konstellationen endogener und exogener Faktoren zustande.

3. Hysterie

Die Diagnose Hysterie ist weder klinisch noch genetisch sehr nützlich, und die genetischen Befunde hängen weitgehend davon ab, was man unter Hysterie versteht und wie man sie definiert (SHIELDS, 1975). SLATER (1961) und SHIELDS (1978c) verneinen den Einfluß von Erbfaktoren zumindest von spezifischen, denn ihre EZ waren praktisch nie konkordant, jedoch war der Partner des öfteren neurotisch. LJUNGBERG (1957) fand abnorme Persönlichkeiten unter „Hysterischen" und ihren Verwandten vermehrt und schloß auf polygene Erbfaktoren. CLONINGER et al. (1975) benützen eine von ihrer Arbeitsgruppe aufgestellte Sonderform der Hysterie (Briquet-Syndrom) als Test- und Demonstrationsobjekt für ihr multifaktorielles Mehr-Schwellen-Modell der familiären Übertragung. Hysterie ist hier mit Soziopathie (Alkoholismus und Kriminalität) kombiniert; bei Überschreiten der ersten Schwelle äußert sich die multifaktorielle Faktorenkonstellation als Soziopathie beim Mann, bei Überschreiten der zweiten Schwelle als Hysterie bei der Frau und bei Überschreiten der dritten Schwelle als Soziopathie bei der Frau.

Eine ausführliche Diskussion genetischer Aspekte bei Hysterie gibt SHIELDS (in Druck).

4. Kindliche Verhaltensstörungen

Tabelle 6 gibt einen Überblick über Zwillingsbefunde bei einigen kindlichen Verhaltensstörungen. Die Konkordanz ist schon für die ZZ hoch: Zeichen für Umwelteinfluß; sie ist für die EZ wesentlich höher: Zeichen für Anlagewirkung. Dieser Trend dürfte allgemeine Gültigkeit besitzen, wenn auch die Höhe der

Tabelle 6. Neurotische Störungen bei kindlichen Zwillingen. Befunde von BAKWIN, nach SHIELDS (1975). (Aus ZERBIN-RÜDIN, 1978)

	Häufigkeit unter allen Zwillingen		Konkordanz in %		Häufigkeitsverhältnis Zwillingspartner: Zwillingspopulation	
	EZ	ZZ	EZ	ZZ	EZ	ZZ
Lesestörungen	14,0	14,9	91,2	45,0	6,5	3,1
Enuresis	21,7	21,4	80,9	52,6	3,7	2,5
Konstipation	9,5	7,4	82,3	30,0	8,7	4,1
Schlafwandeln	7,1	6,0	64,3	13,3	9,1	2,2
Reisekrankheit	20,2	19,2	85,0	44,4	4,2	2,3
Nägelbeißen	31,4	28,0	79,7	50,7	2,2	1,8
Fingerlutschen	30,9	23,6	74,6	60,3	2,4	2,6

Konkordanzziffern von örtlichen und zeitlichen Gegebenheiten, Familiengröße und Sozialschicht beeinflußt wird und daher schwankt.

Für Enuresis z.B. fand SHIELDS (1976b) 4 von 6 EZ-Paaren (66%) und 0 von 10 ZZ-Paaren konkordant. In der Familienuntersuchung von HALLGREN (1957) hatten 30% der Väter und Brüder (Erwartung 12%) und 18% der Mütter und Schwestern (Erwartung 8%) ebenfalls daran gelitten. 60% der nicht-stationär behandelten Kinder von KOLVIN et al. (1972) wiesen gleichartige familiäre Belastung auf. Weitere, in die gleiche Richtung gehende Daten s. bei LENZ (1974).

Stottern wurde von KAY (1964) untersucht. Die Familienbefunde demonstrieren außer Erbabhängigkeit eine allgemeine genetische Regel: Liegt bei einem Leiden Bevorzugung eines Geschlechtes und polygene Vererbung vor, besitzen die Verwandten des häufiger betroffenen Geschlechtes ein niedrigeres Erkrankungsrisiko als die Verwandten des seltener betroffenen Geschlechtes. Knaben stottern doppelt so oft wie Mädchen; ihre Eltern und Geschwister haben mit 6% (weibliche Personen) und 18% (männliche Personen) ein weit geringeres Erkrankungsrisiko als die Verwandten der stotternden Mädchen mit 13% (weibliche Personen) und 27% (männliche Personen). Vermutlich besitzen die Mädchen eine höhere Manifestationsschwelle und es bedarf einer größeren Anzahl von Genen zur Erkrankung; in der Verwandtschaft muß folglich eine größere Zahl von Genen und auch von Kranken vorhanden sein.

Nachdem man erkannt hat, daß „Ungezogenheit" von Kindern mitunter auf psychischen und neurologischen Störungen beruht, hat u.a. auch das hyperaktive Kind an Interesse gewonnen. Man fragt nicht nur nach der prognostischen Bedeutung dieses Syndroms, sondern auch nach seinen genetischen Beziehungen. CANTWELL (1975) fand die biologischen Familien hyperaktiver Kinder vermehrt mit dem gleichen Symptom, Alkoholismus und Soziopathie belastet, nicht aber die Adoptivfamilien. Biologische Familien und Adoptivfamilien wurden an zwei verschiedenen kindlichen Patientengruppen untersucht, dazu eine Kontrollgruppe. Affektive Psychosen waren mit 5% in allen drei Gruppen auffallend häufig. Umgekehrt fanden CADORET et al. (1975) bei den wegadoptierten Nachkommen antisozialer biologischer Eltern vermehrt behandlungsbedürftige Hyperaktivität im Kindesalter. STEWART und MORRISON (1973) stellten familiäre Belastung mit affektiven Störungen fest.

Über Dyslexie ist seit der großen Monographie von HALLGREN (1950) nichts grundsätzlich Neues erschienen (Übersichten WEINSCHENK, 1975; ZERBIN-RÜDIN, 1967). 45% der Geschwister litten ebenfalls an Dyslexie, 80% der dyslektischen Kinder hatten ebensolche Eltern, doch war die Anomalie bei den Eltern oft kompensiert und nur durch Spezialtests zu ermitteln. Dominante Vererbung ist wahrscheinlich.

5. Kriminalität

Wie Tabelle 7 zeigt, sind die EZ im allgemeinen mindestens doppelt so oft konkordant wie die ZZ, wenn auch die Zwillingsuntersuchungen jüngeren Datums niedrigere Konkordanzziffern zeigen als die früheren und die Serien von KRANZ (1936) sowie DALGARD und KRINGLEN (1976) Ausnahmen bilden. Pär-

Tabelle 7. Zwillingsbefunde bei Erwachsenen-Kriminalität. Nur gleichgeschlechtige Paare vorwiegend (bei DALGARD u. KRINGLEN ausschließlich) männlichen Geschlechts

Autor	Konkordanz der			
	EZ		ZZ	
	N	%	N	%
LANGE (1929)	10/13	77	2/17	12
KRANZ (1936)	21/32	66	23/43	53
STUMPFL (1936)	11/18	61	7/19	37
ROSANOFF (1941)	35/45	78	6/27	22
YOSHIMASU (1961)	17/28	61	2/18	11
CHRISTIANSEN (1974)				
Männliche Paare	25/71	35	15/120	12
Weibliche Paare	3/14	21	2/27	7
DALGARD u. KRINGLEN (1976)				
Nur schwere Delikte	8/31	26	8/54	15
Alle Delikte	11/49	22	16/49	18

chenzwillinge besitzen eine noch niedrigere Konkordanz als gleichgeschlechtige ZZ. Weibliche Paare sind unterrepräsentiert (Beispiel in Tabelle 7: Serie von CHRISTIANSEN, 1974), wie die Frauen unter Straftätern überhaupt.

Jedoch betonen alle Autoren, wie schwierig und unbefriedigend die rein statistische Erfassung und Deutung von Kriminalitätskonkordanzen ist, zumal sie sich ganz vorwiegend auf Strafakten und Verurteilung stützt. Man sucht also den wahren Verhältnissen durch die verschiedensten Überlegungen und Unterteilungen auf den Grund zu kommen.

LANGE (1929) und YOSHIMASU (1961) beschrieben drei getrennt aufgewachsene „diskordante" EZ-Paare, in denen der nicht straffällige Zwilling genau so asozial war wie sein abgeurteilter Bruder. Er hatte aber das Glück, Angehörige zu besitzen, die ihn in jeder Beziehung stützten und deckten. Wenn KRANZ alle individuellen Umstände würdigte, so schienen ihm einige seiner konkordanten Paare eher in die diskordante Gruppe zu gehören; da aber auch das Umgekehrte zutraf und manche Paare ihre Diskordanz nur einem Zufall verdankten, glichen sich die Verschiebungen weitgehend aus. Die Konkordanz der EZ blieb mit 66% gleich (21 ± 3 Paare), die der ZZ sank von 53% auf 44%. Die Konkordanz ist bei schweren Delikten ganz allgemein höher als bei leichten (Beispiel in Tabelle 7: Serie von DALGARD u. KRINGLEN, 1976). Ferner ist sie bei rückfälligen Straftätern höher als bei einmaligen und bei Frühkriminellen höher als bei Spätkriminellen (STUMPFL, 1936).

Die EZ erwiesen sich unter den verschiedensten Gesichtspunkten ähnlicher als die ZZ, z.B. nach Zahl der Verurteilungen, Strafmaß und Art des Deliktes (KRANZ, 1936). In solche Konkordanzunterschiede mögen auch nicht-erbliche Einflüsse eingehen; z.B. könnte der EZ-Partner eines aktenkundigen Straftäters ein höheres Risiko besitzen als ein ZZ-Partner, ebenfalls angeklagt und verurteilt zu werden. Alles in allem sind aber Anlagefaktoren offenbar doch beteiligt und DALGARD und KRINGLEN schließen sicher zu Unrecht, daß Heredität erwiesenermaßen gar keine Rolle spiele.

Tabelle 8. Zwillingsbefunde bei jugendlicher Kriminalität (nur Knaben). (Nach SHIELDS, 1976)

Autor	Konkordanz der			
	EZ		ZZ	
	N	%	N	%
ROSANOFF (1941)	29/29	100	12/17	71
HAYASHI (1967)	11/15	73	3/4	75
SHIELDS (1976b)	4/5	80	7/9	78

Dabei ist die Bedeutung der Umwelteinflüsse natürlich unbestritten, besonders bei der Jugendkriminalität (Tabelle 8). Die Zwillingskonkordanzen sind hier zwar hoch, aber für EZ und ZZ praktisch gleich. Erbeinflüsse lassen sich nicht erkennen. Dennoch muß wohl ein Teil genetisch beeinflußt sein, denn erwachsene Anlage-Straftäter pflegen ihre Karriere früh zu beginnen. Weiteres über Zwillingsbefunde s. bei CHRISTIANSEN (1974) und SHIELDS (1976b).

Deutlicher als in den Zwillingsuntersuchungen kommt der Anlagefaktor in den Adoptionsstudien heraus. In der dänischen Adoptionsstudie (HUTCHINGS u. MEDNICK, 1974) wurden Adoptivsöhne zu 10% straffällig, wenn weder der biologische, noch der Adoptivvater mit dem Gesetz in Konflikt gekommen war, Adoptivsöhne mit einem kriminellen Adoptivvater zu 11%, also nicht deutlich öfter. War aber der biologische Vater kriminell, stieg die Kriminalität auf das Doppelte, nämlich 21%, und waren gar beide Väter, biologischer *und* Adoptivvater kriminell, so wurden 36% der Adoptivsöhne straffällig. Anlage und Umwelt! Immerhin wurden trotz Anlage und Umwelt 64% nicht straffällig, jedenfalls nicht aktenkundig. Eine amerikanische Untersuchung verfolgte die zur Adoption gegebenen Babies weiblicher Strafgefangener, die meist zusätzlich noch einen kriminellen Vater hatten (CROWE, 1972, 1974). Sie wurden weit häufiger straffällig als Adoptivkinder von nicht-kriminellen biologischen Eltern. Die kleine Gruppe demonstriert wieder einmal, wie verwickelt und verschleiert die Anlage-Umwelt-Interaktion ist. Die straffälligen Adoptierten hatten vor Adoption deutlich länger in Heimen und Pflegestellen gelebt als die nicht-straffälligen, und man könnte den längeren Heimaufenthalt als Ursache der späteren Kriminalität ansehen. Doch in der Vergleichsgruppe von Kindern nicht-krimineller biologischer Eltern hatte eine vergleichbare Zahl vor Adoption ebenfalls eine vergleichbare Zeit in Heimen verbracht, aber ohne kriminell zu werden. Die ungünstigen Umweltverhältnisse entfalteten ihren Einfluß offensichtlich erst bei entsprechender Disposition.

Bei antisozialem Verhalten spielen offenbar polygen beeinflußte Persönlichkeitszüge wie Impulsivität oder Minderbegabung eine Rolle, wenn auch nur indirekt.

Immer wieder hat man versucht, für Kriminalität und Psychopathie physiologische oder somatische Korrelate zu finden. Zum Beispiel zeigen Kriminelle und Psychopathen vermehrt Auffälligkeiten im EEG (STRÖMGREN, 1967b; SYNDULKO, 1978) und EEG-Muster sind weitgehend erblich. Die Ergebnisse sind aber uneinheitlich und schwer zu interpretieren. In einer originellen Versuchsanordnung suchten MEDNICK und HUTCHINGS (1978) die Hypothese eines Lerndefektes für soziales Verhalten über einen psychophysiologischen Faktor (galvanische Hautreaktion) zu stützen. In den 4 Kombinationen Sohn kriminell – Vater nicht, Vater kriminell – Sohn nicht, beide kriminell, beide nicht kriminell zeigten die nicht-kriminellen Söhne krimineller Väter den höchsten IQ und die rascheste elektrodermale Erholung nach Stimulierung, die kriminellen Söhne nicht-krimineller Väter die langsamste. Die Probanden waren z.Z. der Untersuchung nicht inhaftiert.

Eine deutliche Beziehung zu Psychosen oder Geburtskomplikationen besteht nicht (SHIELDS, 1977). Auch die Chromosomenanomalie XYY wirkt nicht direkt kausal. Bekanntlich findet sich unter großwüchsigen, wegen Gewalttaten inhaftierten Männern eine überdurchschnittliche Anzahl der Chromosomenaberration XYY. Aber andererseits wird nur ein Bruchteil der XYY-Träger kriminell. Gleich bei dem ersten, 1961 veröffentlichten Fall handelte es sich um einen ganz unauffälligen Mann, den man wegen Chromosomenstörungen bei seinen Kindern untersucht hatte.

6. Suchten

Bei der Entstehung von Suchten spielen Umweltbedingungen, wie Kontakt mit einem Suchtmittel, Verführung, Modeströmungen usw. eine wesentliche Rolle, besonders bei Jugendlichen. Davon zeugt die epidemieartige Ausbreitung von Alkoholismus und Drogensuchten. Genetisch zur Sucht disponierte Personen können sich unmöglich in einem so kurzen Zeitraum so rapide vermehrt haben. Andererseits wird zum Glück nicht jeder süchtig, der einen Trip probiert oder einen Rausch gehabt hat und mit Opium behandelte depressive Patienten verfielen praktisch nie der Sucht. Es gibt offensichtlich Faktoren, die im Individuum selbst liegen und es zum Süchtigwerden disponieren oder davor schützen. Beim Alkoholismus (Übersichten bei SHIELDS, 1977; ZERBIN-RÜDIN, 1976) besteht eine deutliche familiäre Häufung. Da Definition und Häufigkeit des Alkoholismus nach Sozialstruktur und Trinksitten variieren, schwankt auch die Höhe der familiären Risikoziffern. Sie beträgt aber immer ein Vielfaches der Häufigkeit in der Gesamtbevölkerung (z.B. ÅMARK, 1951). Der Einwand, daß familiäre Häufung nicht grundsätzlich erbbedingt zu sein braucht, sondern auch milieubedingt sein kann, besteht zu Recht. Gegen die ausschließliche Milieutheorie sprechen jedoch die Befunde an Zwillingen und Adoptivkindern. Eineiige Zwillinge sind häufiger für Alkoholmißbrauch konkordant als zweieiige, nach KAIJ (1960) sind es 70% und 32% (nur männliche Paare). Die Zwillingsbefunde zeigen weiterhin, daß genetische Faktoren unterschiedlich an den einzelnen Komponenten des Alkoholgebrauchs und -mißbrauchs (z.B. Abstinenz, mittlerer Alkoholkonsum, hoher Alkoholkonsum mit und ohne Sucht, Trinkmenge, Trinkhäufigkeit) beteiligt sind, und daß für Umwelteinflüsse ein weiter Spielraum bleibt (PARTANEN et al., 1966; JONSSON u. NILSSON, 1968). Daher lassen sich aus den Zwillingsserien recht verschiedene Konkordanzen berechnen.

Die Adoptionsstudie von GOODWIN u.Mitarb. (1973, 1974) ergab Erstaunliches. Die in frühester Kindheit wegadoptierten Söhne von Alkoholikern verfielen später dem Alkohol ebenso oft wie Söhne, die bei ihrem trinkenden Vater aufgewachsen waren (um 20%) und viermal häufiger als Adoptivkinder, die von nichttrinkenden biologischen Eltern abstammten. Auch die Adoptionsstudie von CADORET und GATH (1978) weist deutlich auf die Beteiligung genetischer Faktoren hin. Allerdings sind die Zahlen sehr klein und die Methodik ist etwas ungewöhnlich. In Alkoholikerfamilien mit Stiefkindern erkrankten die leiblichen Kinder der Alkoholiker häufiger an Alkoholismus als die angeheirateten (SCHUKKIT et al., 1972).

Worin bestehen nun die Erbfaktoren? In Besonderheiten des Stoffwechsels? In Eigenarten der Persönlichkeit? Oder in beidem?

Schon der Appetit auf Alkohol weist erbliche Unterschiede auf. Es ist gelungen, Ratten- und Mäusestämme zu züchten, die bei freier Wahl alkoholische Getränke bevorzugen bzw. ablehnen. Die Alkoholpräferenz und -ablehnung zeigt Beziehungen zu Unterschieden der Enzymsteuerungen in Leber und Blut, und zu verschieden hohem Alkoholgehalt des Gehirnes bei Gabe gleicher Alkoholdosen (ERIKSSON, 1970, 1975); Kreuzungsversuche lassen auf polygene Vererbung schließen.

Auch beim Menschen dürften Stoffwechselfaktoren beteiligt sein. Asiaten z.B. vertragen Alkohol schlechter als Europäer. Auf Grund erblicher Besonderheiten ihres Enzymsystems besitzen sie eine niedrigere Toleranzgrenze und reagieren mit stärkeren vegetativen Beschwerden. Sie haben z.B. zu 85% eine erbliche Variante der Alkoholdehydrogenase, die nur 6% der Europiden besitzen. Ein erster Versuch wurde unternommen, genetische Marker für Alkoholismus in Gestalt von Serumfaktoren zu entdecken (HILL et al., 1975).

Interessant sind die Ergebnisse von Alkoholbelastungstests an normalen, also nicht alkoholsüchtigen Zwillingspaaren. PROPPING (1977) errechnete für die Alkohol-Absorptionsrate eine Heritabilität von 0,57, für die Abbaurate 0,41 und für die Eliminationsrate 0,46. VOGEL (1970) hatte bereits gezeigt, daß bestimmte EEG-Muster erblich sind. Dementsprechend fand PROPPING das EEG seiner normalen eineiigen Zwillingspaare ähnlich, und es blieb auch ähnlich in seiner Reaktion auf die Alkoholzufuhr, während das EEG der ZZ nach Alkoholzufuhr immer unähnlicher wurde. Die EEG-Reaktion zeigt keinen ersichtlichen Zusammenhang mit der Alkoholabsorptionsrate, sondern geht vermutlich über die Formatio reticularis des Hirnstammes.

In psychischer Hinsicht finden sich unter Süchtigen viele Personen mit Anpassungsschwierigkeiten. Freilich läßt sich retrospektiv oft nur schwer entscheiden, inwieweit die Persönlichkeitsanomalien bereits vor Suchtbeginn bestanden haben. Man weiß auch schon lange, daß Depressive gelegentlich Linderung beim Alkohol suchen. WINOKUR et al. (1970, 1971) glauben neuerdings, daß ein Teil des Alkoholismus auf einer Erbanlage beruht, die sich bei Frauen als Depression und bei Männern als Alkoholismus äußert (vgl. S. 582). Die Hypothese ist nicht sehr wahrscheinlich. REICH et al. (1975) wenden ihr multifaktorielles Schwellenmodell auch auf den Alkoholismus an.

Soweit Persönlichkeitsvariable als Anlagefaktoren im Spiel sind, dürften sie polygen bedingt sein. Für Stoffwechselvarianten kommt eher ein Hauptgen in Frage. Alkoholiker in abstinenten Populationen besitzen eine relativ starke genetische Veranlagung, solche in sehr trinkfreudigen Gesellschaften eine schwächere.

Erbschäden durch exzessiven Alkoholgenuß sind nicht sicher nachgewiesen. Wenn einige Untersuchungen unter den Nachkommen von Alkoholikern eine erhöhte Zahl von Hilfsschülern, Schulrepetenten und Kriminellen fanden, so besaß entweder der Alkoholiker selbst schon die Anlage zu diesen Merkmalen, oder sein Ehepartner brachte sie in die Familie oder es handelt sich um Milieuschäden. Alkoholismus der schwangeren Frau bedeutet eine hohe toxische Gefährdung der Leibesfrucht. Neben Tot- und Fehlgeburten kann es zur Alkohol-Embryopathie mit charakteristischen körperlichen und geistigen Schäden kommen (MAJEWSKI et al., 1976).

Für die Entstehung anderer Drogensuchten gilt ähnliches wie für den Alkoholismus. Zum Beispiel gibt es Rattenstämme, deren erblich verschiedene Neigung zu Morphiumaufnahme Beziehung zu Unterschieden in der Sensibilität gegenüber dem Morphin und in Resorption, Abbau und Ausscheidung des Morphins zeigt. Solche pharmakokinetischen und pharmakogenetischen Unterschiede bestehen zweifellos auch beim Menschen. Im psychischen Bereich weisen Drogensüchtige typische Charaktereigenschaften auf, die allerdings nur beschränkte Schlußfolgerungen auf die Persönlichkeit vor Suchtbeginn erlauben.

Der akute Drogengenuß führt ziemlich regelmäßig zu akuten Rauschzuständen. Darüber hinaus entwickeln sich mitunter psychotische Bilder anderer Färbung, die die direkte Drogenwirkung überdauern und eine gewisse Eigengesetzlichkeit entwickeln. Möglicherweise sind Träger einer psychotischen Anlage besonders anfällig für Drogenmißbrauch, der dann hinwiederum die manifeste Psychose auslöst und färbt. TATETSU (1960) fand japanische Patienten mit Schizophrenie-artigen Pervitinpsychosen erhöht, aber nicht ganz so hoch wie „echte" Schizophrene mit Schizophrenie belastet. DAVISON (1976) dagegen glaubt nicht an eine auslösende Drogenwirkung, sondern führt solche Psychosen ausschließlich auf die direkte toxische Wirkung zurück.

Drogensüchtige weisen nicht selten Chromosomenstörungen auf, Zeichen einer Schädigung der Erbsubstanz. Sie verschwinden wieder nach Aufhören der Drogenzufuhr. Die Befunde wurden an Lymphozyten gewonnen und es ist ungewiß, ob und inwieweit sie auch für die Geschlechtszellen gelten und somit das Risiko einer Erbschädigung der Kinder anzeigen.

VII. Genetische Beratung

Die genetische Beratung gewinnt zunehmend an Bedeutung und zwar auch gerade für die psychischen Störungen. Die Schizophrenien stehen in zwei ganz verschiedenen Beratungsstatistiken der Häufigkeit nach an 6. Stelle, nämlich in der Zusammenstellung von REED (1951) in Minneapolis und bei THEILE (1977) in der Beratungsstelle Marburg.

Während der letzten Jahre sind in englischer Sprache zahlreiche Veröffentlichungen über methodenkritische, ethische und juristische Aspekte der genetischen Beratung erschienen (z.B. LUBS und DE LA CRUZ, 1977; SKOGSTAD, 1978). Ausschließlich auf die Psychiatrie zugeschnitten ist das Buch von SPERBER und JARVIK (1976). Einige Probleme seien hier kurz angesprochen. Die ärztliche Schweigepflicht muß im Interesse des Patienten auf jeden Fall gewahrt bleiben; ihr steht ein moralischer Anspruch der Nachkommen auf Wissen um eine etwaige Gefährdung gegenüber. Dieses Problem entfällt bei der Beratung der Eltern von unmündigen, erblich kranken Kindern und tritt hauptsächlich bei den endogenen Psychosen mit ihrem hohen Erkrankungsalter auf. Es läßt sich aber auch hier fast immer befriedigend lösen. Weiter: Vorenthalten wichtiger Information kann strafbare Unterlassung sein; andererseits könnten gefährdete Personen durch das Wissen um ihr Risiko zu stark beunruhigt werden. Ja sogar die Möglichkeit einer „self-fulfilling prophecy" wird erwogen. Einer Aufklärungspflicht steht also die Möglichkeit einer iatrogenen Schädigung gegenüber. Inwieweit hat das Individuum ein Recht auf Wissen bzw. auf Nichtwissen? Inwieweit darf und soll der Berater Stellung beziehen und Entscheidungshilfen anbieten? Druck oder gar Zwang darf er nicht ausüben. Dagegen muß er alle möglichen Gesichtspunkte berücksichtigen und sich nicht ausschließlich auf die Risikoziffern konzentrieren. Man ging auch bereits daran, die Erfolge der genetischen Beratung katamnestisch nachzuprüfen (z.B. CARTER et al., 1971; LEONARD et al., 1972). Erfolgreich bedeutet dabei nicht unbedingt, daß die Beratenen das getan haben, was der Berater für vernünftig hielt. Es bedeutet vielmehr, daß die Beratung verstanden worden ist und den Beratenen geholfen hat, zu einer befriedigenden Entscheidung zu gelangen.

Weit schlechter ist es um Veröffentlichungen bestellt, die praktische Hilfen für die Beratungssituation an die Hand geben. Man muß die Grundlagen für den individuellen Beratungsfall meist mühsam aus weit verstreuten Veröffentlichungen in Fachzeitschriften zusammensuchen oder aus den umfangreichen genetischen Standardwerken beziehen, z.B. dem von P.E. BECKER herausgegebenen umfangreichen Handbuch der Humangenetik, in dem Band V/1 und V/II für Neurologie und Psychiatrie zuständig sind. In den handlicheren Kompendien, wie dem von FUHRMANN und VOGEL (1975), kommt die Psychiatrie zu kurz. Einige Anhaltspunkte geben KOCH (1977, 1978) und ZERBIN-RÜDIN (1979). DODINVAL (1974) ist neurologisch orientiert, schließt aber u.a. auch Chorea Huntington und Epilepsie mit ein. WITKOWSKI und PROKOP (1976) vermitteln im Telegrammstil gute Information für alle genetisch beeinflußten Leiden, nicht nur die psychiatrischen.

Auch der Psychiater sollte mit den Grundlagen der Vererbung und den Grundregeln der genetischen Beratung für sein Gebiet vertraut sein. MORACZEWSKI (1976) meint sogar, der Psychiater sei für jede genetische Beratung prädestiniert, da er auf Grund seiner Kenntnis der menschlichen Seele die Beratung am wirkungsvollsten und schonendsten vornehmen könne und außerdem die seelischen Schäden, die durch anderweitige, wenig taktvolle Aufklärung entstanden seien, wieder zu beheben vermöge!

Literatur

Abeleen, v. J.H.F. (ed.): The genetics of behaviour. Amsterdam-Oxford-New York: North Holland, Amer. Elsevier 1974
Abrams, R., Taylor, M.A., Gaztanaga, P.: Manic-depressive illness and paranoid schizophrenia. Arch. Gen. Psychiatry **31**, 640 (1974)
Akiskal, H.S., Djenderedjian, A.H., Rosenthal, R.H., Khani, M.K.: Cyclothymic disorder: Validating criteria for inclusion in the bipolar affective group. Am. J. Psychiatry **134**, 1227 (1977)
Akiskal, H.S., McKinney, T.M.: Overview of recent research in depression. Integration of ten models into a comprehensive clinical frame. Arch. Gen. Psychiatry **32**, 285 (1975)

Alanen, Y.O., Rekola, J., Stewen, A., Tuovinen, M., Takala, K., Rutanen, E.: Mental disorders in the siblings of schizophrenic patients. Acta Psychiatr. Scand. [Suppl.] **169**, 167 (1963)

Åmark, C.: A study in alcoholism. Acta Psychiatr. Scand. [Suppl.] **70** (1951)

Andersen, T., Astrup, C., Forsdal, A. (eds.): Social, somatic and psychiatric studies of geographically defined populations. The Tromsø Seminar in Medicine 1975. Acta Psychiatr. Scand. [Suppl.] **263** (1975)

Angst, J.: Zur Ätiologie und Nosologie endogener depressiver Psychosen. Monogr. Gesamtgeb. Neurol. Psychiatr. (Berlin) **112** (1966)

Angst, J.: Genetische Aspekte der Depression. In: Depressive Zustände. Kielholz, P. (Hrsg.). Int. Symp. St. Moritz. Bern: Huber 1972

Angst, J., Perris, C.: Zur Nosologie endogener Depressionen. Vergleich der Ergebnisse zweier Untersuchungen. Arch. Psychiatr. Nervenkr. **110**, 373 (1968)

Angst, J., Felder, W., Frey, R., Stassen, H.H.: The course of affective disorders. I. Change of diagnosis of monopolar, unipolar and bipolar illness. Arch. Psychiatr. Nervenkr. **226**, 57 (1978)

Annell, A.L. (ed.): Depressive states in childhood and adolescence. Stockholm: Almquist & Wiksell 1972

Anthony, E.J.: The developmental precursors of adult schizophrenia. In: The transmission of schizophrenia. Rosenthal, D., Kety, S. (eds.). Oxford-London-New York: Pergamon Press 1968

Arieti, S.: The origins of development of the pathology of schizophrenia. In: Die Entstehung der Schizophrenie. Bleuler, M., Angst, J. (Hrsg.). Bern: Huber 1971

Arnold, O.H.: Untersuchungen zum Erbgang des Morbus Schizophrenia. Wien. Klin. Wochenschr. **80**, 827 (1968)

Bakwin, H.: Zit. nach Shields, J., 1975

Barchas, J.D., Ciaranello, R.D., Dominic, J.A., Deguchi, T., Orenberg, E.K., Renson, J., Kessler, S.: Genetic differences in mechanisms involving neuroregulators. Z. Psychiatr. Res. **11**, 347 (1974)

Baron, M., Stern, M.: Familial concordance in schizophrenia: A comparative study of pairs of sibs. Compr. Psychiatry **17**, 461 (1976)

Becker, J.: Depression: Theory and research. Washington, D.C.: Winston 1974

Becker, P.E. (Hrsg.): Humangenetik. Ein kurzes Handbuch in 5 Bd. Stuttgart: Thieme 1966-1976

Becker, P.E.: Wege und Probleme der Zwillingsforschung. Persönlichkeit, Charakter und Neurosen. Ein historischer Überblick. Göttingen: Vandenhoeck u. Ruprecht 1979 (im Druck)

Becker, P.E., Schepank, H., Heigl-Evers, A.: 100 Zwillingspaare. Ein psychoanalytischer Beitrag zur Ätiologie neurotischer Erkrankungen. Fortschr. Psychoanalyse. Bd. IV. Göttingen: Hogrefe 1970

Beichl, L.: Über Selbstmordhäufung in einer Familie. Wien. Klin. Wochenschr. **77**, 727 (1965)

Belmaker, R.H., Ebstein, R., Rimon, R., Wyatt, R.J., Murphy, D.L.: Electrophoresis of platelet monoamine oxidase in schizophrenia and manic-depressive illness. Acta Psychiatr. Scand. **54**, 67 (1976)

Belmaker, R., Pollin, W., Wyatt, R.J., Cohen, St.: A follow-up of monozygotic twins discordant for schizophrenia. Arch. Gen. Psychiatry **30**, 219 (1974)

Bender, L.: Mental illness in childhood and heredity. Eugen. Quart. **10**, 1 (1963)

Bender, L.: Schizophrenic spectrum disorders in the families of schizophrenic children. In: Genetic research in psychiatry. Fieve, R., Rosenthal, D., Brill, H. (eds.). Baltimore: Johns Hopkins University Press 1975

Berger, H.: Manisch-depressive Psychosen bei eineiigen Zwillingen. Inaugural Dissertation, München 1964

Berrettini, W.H., Vogel, W.H., Clouse, R.: Platelet monoamine oxidase in chronic schizophrenia. Am. J. Psychiatry **134**, 805 (1977)

Bertelsen, A., Harvald, B., Hauge, M.: A Danish twin study of manic-depressive disorders. Br. J. Psychiatry **130**, 330 (1977)

Bjarnar, E., Reppesgaard, H., Astrup, C.: Psychiatric morbidity in Berlevåg. Acta Psychiatr. Scand. [Suppl.] **263**, 60 (1975)

Bleuler, M.: Krankheitsverlauf, Persönlichkeit und Verwandtschaft Schizophrener und ihre gegenseitigen Beziehungen. Sammlung psychiatrischer und neurologischer Einzeldarstellungen. Bd. XVI. Leipzig: Thieme 1941

Bleuler, M.: Untersuchungen aus dem Grengebiet zwischen Psychopathologie und Endokrinologie. Arch. Psychiatr. Nervenkr. **180**, 271 (1948)
Bleuler, M.: Die schizophrenen Geistesstörungen im Lichte langjähriger Kranken- und Familiengeschichten. Stuttgart: Thieme 1972
Block, J.: Parents of schizophrenic, neurotic, asthmatic, and congenitally ill children. A comparative study. Arch. Gen. Psychiatry **20**, 659 (1969)
Bosch, G.: Psychosen im Kindesalter. In: Psychiatrie der Gegenwart. Kisker, K.P., Meyer, J.E., Müller, M., Strömgren, E. (Hrsg.). Bd. II/1. Berlin-Heidelberg-New York: Springer 1972
Brockington, I., Crow, T.J., Johnstone, E.C., Owen, F.: An investigation of platelet monoamine oxidase activity in schizophrenia and schizo-affective psychosis. In: Monoamine oxidase and its inhibition. Wolstenholme, G.E., Knight, J. (eds.). CIBA Foundation Symposium No. 39. Amsterdam: Elsevier, Excerpta Medica, North-Holland 1962
Buchsbaum, M.S., Coursey, R.D., Murphy, D.L.: The biochemical high-risk paradigm: Behavioral and familial correlates of low platelet monoamine oxidase activity. Science **194**, 339 (1976)
Buck, C., Hobbs, G.E., Simpson, H., Wanklin, J.M.: Fertility of the sibs of schizophrenic patients. Br. J. Psychiatry **127**, 235 (1975)
Cade, J.F.: The aetiology of schizophrenia. Med. J. Aust. **2**, 135 (1956)
Cadoret, R.J.: Towards a definition of the schizoid state: Evidence from studies of twins and their families. Br. J. Psychiatry **122**, 679 (1973)
Cadoret, R.J.: Genetics of affective disorder. In: Biological foundations of psychiatry. Grenell, R.G., Gabay, S. (eds.). Vol. II. New York: Raven Press 1976
Cadoret, R.J.: Evidence for genetic inheritance of primary affective disorder in adoptees. Am. J. Psychiatry **135**, 463 (1978)
Cadoret, R.J., Gath, A.: Inheritance of alcoholism in adoptees. Br. J. Psychiatry **132**, 252 (1978)
Cadoret, R.J., Cunningham, L., Loftus, R., Edwards, J.: Studies of adoptees from psychiatrically disturbed biologic parents. J. Pediatr. **87**, 301 (1975)
Cammer, L.: Schizophrenic children of manic-depressive parents. Dis. Nerv. Syst. **31**, 177 (1970)
Cantwell, D.P.: Genetic studies of hyperactive children: Psychiatric illness in biological and adopting parents. In: Genetic research in psychiatry. Fieve, R.R., Rosenthal, D., Brill, H. (eds.). Baltimore-London: Johns Hopkins University Press 1975
Carter, C.O., Roberts, F.J.A., Evans, K.A., Buck, A.R.: Genetic clinic. A follow-up. Lancet **1971 I**, 281
Cebiroglu, R., Sümer, E., Polvan, Ö.: Etiology and pathogenesis of depression in Turkish children. In: Depressive states in childhood and adolescence. Annell, A.L. (ed.). Stockholm: Almquist & Wiksell 1972
Christiansen, K.O.: The genesis of aggressive criminality: Implications of a study of crime in a Danish twin study. In: Determinants and origins of aggressive behavior. De Wit, J., Hartup, W.W. (eds.). The Hague: Mouton 1974
Cloninger, C.R., Reich, T., Guze, S.B.: The multifactorial model of disease transmission: III. Familial relationship between sociopathy and hysteria (Briquet's Syndrome). Br. J. Psychiatry **127**, 23 (1975)
Cloninger, C.R., Reich, Th., Guze, S.B.: Genetic – environmental interactions and antisocial behaviour. In: Psychopathic behaviour. Hare, R.D., Schalling, D. (eds.). Chichester-New York-Brisbane-Toronto: Wiley 1978
Cohen, D.J., Dibble, E., Grawe, J.M., Pollin, W.: Reliable separating identical from fraternal twins. Arch. Gen. Psychiatry **32**, 1371 (1975)
Crowe, R.R.: An adoption study of antisocial personality. Arch. Gen. Psychiatry **31**, 785 (1974)
Curnow, R.N., Smith, C.: Multifactorial models for familial diseases in man. J. Roy. Statist. Soc. A, **138**, 131 (1975)
Dahl, V.: A follow-up study of a childpsychiatric clientele with special regard to manic-depressive psychosis. In: Depressive states in childhood and adolescence. Annell, A. (ed.). Stockholm: Almquist & Wiksell 1972
Dahl, V.: A follow-up study of a child psychiatric clientele with special regard to the diagnosis of psychosis. Acta Psychiatr. Scand. **54**, 106 (1976)
Dahme, B., Achilles, I., Flemming, B., Götze, P., Haag, A., Huse-Kleinstoll, G., Meffert, J., Polonius, J., Rosewald, G., Speidel, H.: Die psychische Bewältigung von Herzoperationen und Intensivpflege. Med. Psychologie **3**, 129 (1977)

Dalén, P.: Month of birth in schizophrenia. Acta Psychiatr. Scand. [Suppl.] **203**, 55 (1968)
Dalén, P.: One, two, or many? In: Genetic factors in schizophrenia. Kaplan, A.R. (ed.). Springfield, Ill.: Thomas 1972
Dalén, P.: Season of birth. A study of schizophrenia and other mental disorders. Amsterdam-Oxford: North Holland Publ. Comp. 1975
Dalgard, O.S., Kringlen, E.: A Norwegian twin study of criminality. Br. J. Criminology **16**, 213 (1976)
Davison, K.: Drug induced psychoses and their relationship to schizophrenia. In: Schizophrenia today. Kemali, D., Bartolini, G., Richter, D. (eds.). Oxford-New York: Pergamon Press 1976
Davison, K., Bagley, C.R.: Schizophrenia-like psychoses associated with organic disorders of the central nervous system: A review of the literature. In: Current problems in neuropsychiatry. Herrington, R.N. (ed.). Ashford-Kent: Brothers 1969
Diebold, K.: Zum Problem der Zusammenhänge von Anlage und Umwelt in der Psychiatrie. Nervenarzt **40**, 401 (1969)
Diebold, K.: Genetische Aspekte der organischen und endoformen Psychosen, der organischen Pseudopsychopathien und Pseudoneurosen. In: Das ärztliche Gespräch. Köln: Tropon-Werke 1974
Diebold, K., Arnold, E., Pfaff, W.: Statistische Untersuchungen zur Symptomatik und Syndromatik von 120 endogen psychotischen Elter-Kind- und Geschwisterpaaren. Fortschr. Neurol. Psychiatr. **45**, 349 (1977)
Dodinval, P.: La consultation génétique en neurologie. Acta Genet. Med. Gemellol. (Roma) **23**, 59 (1974)
Dorus, E., Pandey, G.N., Frazer, A., Mendels, J.: Genetic determinant of lithium ion distribution. An in vitro and in vivo monozygotic twin study. Arch. Gen. Psychiatry **31**, 463 (1974)
Dorus, E., Pandey, G.N., Davis, J.M.: Genetic determinant of lithium ion distribution. An in vitro and in vivo monozygotic-dizygotic twin study. Arch. Gen. Psychiatry **32**, 1097 (1975)
Dunham, H.W.: Society, culture, and mental disorder. Arch. Gen. Psychiatry **33**, 147 (1976)
Dunner, D.L., Fieve, R.R.: Psychiatric illness in fathers of men with bipolar primary affective disorder. Arch. Gen. Psychiatry **32**, 1134 (1975)
Dunner, D.L., Cohn, C.K., Gershon, E.S., Goodwin, F.K.: Differential catechol-O-methyltransferase activity in unipolar and bipolar affective illness. Arch. Gen. Psychiatry **25**, 348 (1971)
Dyke, van J., Rosenthal, D., Rasmussen, P.V.: Electrodermal functioning in adopted-away offspring of schizophrenics. J. Psychiatr. Res. **10**, 199 (1974)
Eaves, L., Eysenck, H.: Genetic and environmental components of inconsistency and unrepèatability in twins' responses to a neuroticism questionnaire. Behav. Genet. **6**, 145 (1976a)
Eaves, L., Eysenck, H.: Genotype × age interaction for neuroticism. Behav. Genet. **6**, 359 (1976b)
Edwards, J.H.: The genetical basis of schizophrenia. In: Genetic factors in schizophrenia. Kaplan, A. (ed.). Springfield, Ill.: Thomas 1972
Eggers, Ch.: Cyclothyme Phasen im Beginn und im Verlauf schizophrener Psychosen des Kindesalters. In: Depressionszustände bei Kindern und Jugendlichen. Annell, A.L. (ed.). Stockholm: Almquist & Wiksell 1972
Eggers, Ch.: Verlaufsweisen kindlicher und präpuberaler Schizophrenien. Monogr. Gesamtgeb. Psychiatr. (Berlin), Bd. 9. Berlin-Heidelberg-New York: Springer 1973
Ehrman, L., Omenn, G.S., Caspari, E. (eds.): Genetics, environment, and behavior. New York-London: Academic Press 1972
D'Elia, G., Perris, C.: Selbstmordversuche im Laufe unipolarer und bipolarer Depressionen. Arch. Psychiatr. Nervenkr. **212**, 339 (1969)
Elston, R.C., Campbell, M.A.: Schizophrenia: Evidence for the major gene hypothesis. Behav. Genet. **1**, 3 (1970)
Elsässer, G.: Die Nachkommen geisteskranker Elternpaare. Stuttgart: Thieme 1952
Eriksson, K.: Genetical analysis of the voluntary alcohol consumption in mice under quinine-saccharine motivation. Scand. L. Clin. Lab. Invest. **25**, 61 (1970)
Eriksson, K.: Alcohol imbibition and behavior: A comparative genetic approach. In: Psychopharmacogenetics. Eleftheriou, B.E. (ed.). New York: Plenum Publ. Co 1975
Erlenmeyer-Kimling, L.: Studies on the offspring of two schizophrenic parents. In: The transmission of schizophrenia. Rosenthal, D., Kety, S. (eds.). Oxford: Pergamon Press 1968
Erlenmeyer-Kimling, L. (ed.): Genetics and mental disorders. Int. J. Ment. Health **1**, 1 (1972)

Erlenmeyer-Kimling, L.: A prospective study of children at risk for schizophrenia: Methodological considerations and some preliminary findings. In: Life history research in psychopathology. Wirt, R., Winokur, G., Roff, M. (eds.), Vol. 4. Minneapolis: University of Minnesota Press 1975

Erlenmeyer-Kimling, L., Paradowski, W.: Selection and schizophrenia. Am. Nat. **100**, 651 (1966)

Erlenmeyer-Kimling, L., Rainer, J.D., Kallmann, F.J.: Current reproductive trends in schizophrenia. In: Psychopathology of schizophrenia. Hoch, P.D., Zubin, J. (eds.). New York: Grune & Stratton 1966

Erlenmeyer-Kimling, L., Nicol, S., Rainer, J., Deming, W.: Changes in fertility rates of schizophrenic patients in New York State. Am. J. Psychiatry **125**, 916 (1969)

Erlenmeyer-Kimling, L., Cornblatt, B., Fleiss, J.: High-risk research in schizophrenia. Psychiatr. Ann. **9**, 79 (1979)

Ernst, K., Ernst, C.: 70 zwanzigjährige Katamnesen hospitalisierter neurotischer Patientinnen. Schweiz. Arch. Neurol. Neurochir. Psychiatr. **95**, 359 (1965)

Essen-Möller, E.: Psychiatrische Untersuchungen an einer Serie von Zwillingen. Acta Psychiatr. Scand. [Suppl.] **23**, 1 (1941)

Essen-Möller, E.: Individual traits and morbidity in a Swedish rural population. Acta Psychiatr. Scand. [Suppl.] **100** (1956)

Essen-Möller, E.: Über die Schizophreniehäufigkeit bei Müttern von Schizophrenen. Schweiz. Arch. Neurol. Psychiatr. **91**, 260 (1963)

Essen-Möller, E.: Twenty-one psychiatric cases and their MZ cotwins. Acta Genet. Med. Gemellol. (Roma) **19**, 315 (1970)

Essen-Möller, E.: Evidence for polygenic inheritance in schizophrenia? Acta Psychiatr. Scand. **55**, 202 (1977)

Eysenck, H.J., Eysenck, S.B.G.: Psychopathic personality, and genetics. In: Psychopathic behaviour. Hare, R.D., Schalling, D. (eds.). Chichester-New York-Brisbane-Toronto: Wiley 1978

Falconer, D.S.: The inheritance of liability to certain diseases, estimated from the incidence among relatives. Ann. Hum. Genet. **29**, 51 (1965)

Faris, R.E.L., Dunham, H.W.: Mental disorders in urban areas. Chicago: University Chicago Press 1939

Farley, J.D.: Phylogenetic adaptations and the genetics of psychosis. Acta Psychiatr. Scand. **53**, 173 (1976)

Felder, W.: Katamnestische und genetische Untersuchung über 85 Patienten mit schizoaffektiver Mischpsychose. Zürich: Dissertation 1977

Fieve, R.R., Rosenthal, D., Brill, H. (eds.): Genetic research in psychiatry. Baltimore: Johns Hopkins University Press 1975

Fischer, E.: Der frühkindliche Autismus (Kanner). In: Jahrbuch f. Jugendpsychiatrie u. ihre Grenzgebiete. Stutte, H. (Hrsg.), Bd. IV. Bern: Huber 1965

Fischer, M.: Psychoses in the offspring of schizophrenic monozygotic twins and their normal co-twins. Br. J. Psychiatry **118**, 43 (1971)

Fischer, M.: Umweltfaktoren bei der Schizophrenie. Intrapaarvergleiche bei eineiigen Zwillingen. Nervenarzt **43**, 230 (1972)

Fischer, M.: Genetic and environmental factors in schizophrenia. Acta Psychiatr. Scand. [Suppl.] **228** (1973)

Fischer, M., Harvald, M., Hauge, M.: A Danish twin study of schizophrenia. Br. J. Psychiatry **115**, 981 (1969)

Fish, B.: Biologic antecedents of psychosis in children. In: Biology of the major psychoses. Freedman, D.X. (ed.). Res. Publ. Assoc. Res. Nerv. Ment. Dis. Vol. 54. New York: Raven Press 1975

Folstein, S., Rutter, M.: Infantile autism. A genetic study of 21 twin pairs. J. Child. Psychol. Psychiatry **18**, 297 (1977)

Forrest, A., Affleck, J. (eds.): New perspectives in schizophrenia. Edinburgh-London-New York: Churchill Livingstone 1975

Fowler, R.C., Tsuang, M.T., Cadoret, R.J., Monelly, E.: Non-psychotic disorders in the families of process schizophrenics. Acta Psychiatr. Scand. **51**, 153 (1975)

Freedman, D.G.: The ethological study of man. In: Genetic and environmental influences of behaviour. Thoday, J.M., Parkes, A.S. (eds.). Edinburgh: Oliver & Boyd 1968

Frey, R.: Die prämorbide Persönlichkeit von monopolar und bipolar Depressiven. Arch. Psychiatr. Nervenkr. **224**, 161 (1977)

Fuhrmann, W., Vogel, F.: Genetische Familienberatung. Heidelberger Taschenbücher Nr. 42. Berlin-Heidelberg-New York: Springer 1975

Fulker, D.W.: A biometrical genetic approach to intelligence and schizophrenia. Soc. Biol. **20**, 266 (1973)

Garmezy, N.: Children at risk: The search for the antecedents of schizophrenia. Part. I. Conceptual models and research methods. Part. II. Ongoing research programs, issues and intervention. Schiz. Bull. **1**, Experimental issue No. 8, 14 (1974), No. 9, 55 (1974)

Gerhardt, D.: Herzkrankheit und Geisteskrankheit. Wien. Med. Presse **7**, 155 (1865)

Gershon, E.S., Baron, M., Leckman, J.F.: Genetic models of the transmission of affective disorders. J. Psychiatr. Res. **12**, 301 (1975)

Gershon, E.S., Bunney, W.E., Leckman, J.F., van Eerdewegh, M., DeBauche, B.A.: The inheritance of affective disorders: A review of data and of hypotheses. Behav. Genet. **6**, 227 (1976)

Gershon, E.S., Dunner, D.L., Goodwin, F.K.: Toward a biology of affective disorders. Arch. Gen. Psychiatry **25**, 1 (1971)

Gershon, E.S., Jonas, W.Z.: Erythrocyte soluble catechol-O-methyltransferase activity in primary affective disorder. Arch. Gen. Psychiatry **32**, 1351 (1975)

Gershon, E.S., Mark, A., Cohen, M., Belizon, N., Baron, M., Knobe, K.E.: Transmitted factors in the morbid risk of affective disorders: A controlled study. J. Psychiatr. Res. **12**, 283 (1975)

Goetzl, U., Green, R., Whybrow, P., Jackson, R.: X linkage revisited. A further family study of manic-depressive illness. Arch. Gen. Psychiatry **31**, 665 (1974)

Goldberg, E.M., Morrison, S.L.: Schizophrenia and social class. Br. J. Psychiatry **109**, 785 (1963)

Goodwin, D.W., Schulsinger, F., Hermansen, L., Guze, S.B., Winokur, G.: Alcohol problems in adoptees raised apart from alcoholic biological parents. Arch. Gen. Psychiatry **28**, 238 (1973)

Goodwin, D.W., Schulsinger, F., Møller, N., Hermansen, L., Winokur, G., Guze, S.B.: Drinking problems in adopted and nonadopted sons of alcoholics. Arch. Gen. Psychiatry **31**, 164 (1974)

Gottesman, I.I.: Heritability of personality: A demonstration. Psychol. Monogr. **9** (whole No. 572), 77 (1963)

Gottesman, I.I., Shields, J.: Schizophrenia in twins: 16 years' consecutive admissions to a psychiatric clinic. Br. J. Psychiatry **112**, 809 (1966)

Gottesman, I.I., Shields, J.: A polygenic theory of schizophrenia. Proc. Natl. Acad. Sci. U.S.A. **58**, 199 (1967)

Gottesman, I.I., Shields, J.: Schizophrenia and genetics: A twin study vantage point. New York: Academic Press 1972

Gottesman, I.I., Shields, J.: Genetic theorizing and schizophrenia. Br. J. Psychiatry **122**, 15 (1973)

Gottesman, I.I., Shields, J.: A critical review of recent adoption, twin, and family studies of schizophrenia: Behavioral genetics perspectives. Schizophrenia Bull. **2**, 360 (1976)

Guze, S.B., Woodruff, R.A., Clayton, P.L.: The significance of psychotic affective disorders. Arch. Gen. Psychiatry **32**, 1147 (1975)

Haberlandt, W.: Der Selbstmord aus genetischer Sicht. In: Bericht 9. Tagung Dtsch. Ges. Anthrop. Freiburg 1965. Baitsch, H., Ritter, H. (Hrsg.). Berlin-Frankfurt-Zürich: Musterschmidt 1967

Häfner, H.: Der Einfluß von Umweltfaktoren auf das Erkrankungsrisiko für Schizophrenie. Nervenarzt **42**, 557 (1971)

Hagnell, O.: A prospective study of the incidence of mental disorder. Lund: Bonniers 1966

Hagnell, O., Öjesjö, L.: A prospective study concerning mental disorders of a total population investigated in 1947, 1957 and 1972. Acta Psychiatr. Scand. [Suppl.] 263 (1975)

Hallgren, B.: Specific dyslexia ("congenital word-blindness"): A clinical and genetic study. Acta Psychiatr. Neurol. Scand. [Suppl.] **65** (1950)

Hallgren, B.: Enuresis, a clinical and genetic study. Acta Psychiatr. Neurol. Scand. [Suppl.] **114** (1957)

Hallgren, B., Sjögren, T.: A clinical and genetico-statistical study of schizophrenia and low-grade mental deficiency in a large Swedish rural population. Acta Psychiatr. Scand. [Suppl.] **140** (1959)

Hanhart, E.: Zur Frage der Beteiligung genetischer Faktoren bei Selbstmorden anhand von temporären Häufungen familiärer Suizide in Schweizer Isolaten. Arch. Julius Klaus Stiftg. **43/44**, 1 (1968/1969)

Hanson, D.R., Gottesman, I.I.: The genetics, if any, of infantile autism and childhood schizophrenia. J. Autism Child. Schizo. **6**, 209 (1976)
Hanson, D.R., Gottesman, I.I., Heston, L.L.: Some possible childhood indicators of adult schizophrenia inferred from children of schizophrenics. Br. J. Psychiatry **129**, 142 (1976)
Hanson, D.R., Gottesman, I.I., Meehl, P.E.: Genetic theories and the validation of psychiatric diagnoses: Implications for the study of children of schizophrenics. J. Abnorm. Psychol. **86**, 575 (1977)
Hare, E.H.: Mental illness and social conditions in Bristol. J. Ment. Sci. **102**, 349 (1956)
Hare, E.H.: Manic-depressive psychosis and season of birth. Acta Psychiatr. Scand. **52**, 69 (1975a)
Hare, E.H.: Season of birth in schizophrenia and neurosis. Am. J. Psychiatry **132**, 1168 (1975b)
Hare, E.H., Price, J.S.: Birth rank in schizophrenia: With a consideration of the bias due to chances in birth-rate. Br. J. Psychiatry **116**, 409 (1970)
Hare, E.H., Price, J.S., Slater, E.: Parental social class in psychiatric patients. Br. J. Psychiatry **121**, 515 (1972)
Hare, E.H., Price, J.S., Slater, E.: Mental disorder and season of birth: A national sample compared with the general population. Br. J. Psychiatry **124**, 81 (1974)
Hare, R.D., Schalling, D. (eds.): Psychopathic behaviour. Chichester-New York-Brisbane-Toronto: Wiley 1978
Hauge, M., Harvald, B., Fischer, M., Gotlieb-Jensen, K., Juel-Nielsen, N., Raebild, I., Shapiro, R., Videbech, T.: The danish twin register. Acta Genet. Med. Gemellol. (Roma) **17**, 315 (1968)
Hayashi, S.: A study of juvenile delinquency in twins. In: Clinical genetics in psychiatry. Mitsuda, H. (ed.). Tokyo: Igaku Shoin 1967
Hecht Orzack, M., Kornetsky, C.: Environmental and familial predictors of attention behavior in chronic schizophrenics. J. Psychiatr. Res. **9**, 21 (1971)
Helzer, J.E.: Bipolar affective disorder in black and white men. Arch. Gen. Psychiatry **32**, 1140 (1975)
Helzer, J.E., Winokur, G.: A family interview study of male manic depressives. Arch. Gen. Psychiatry **31**, 73 (1974)
Heston, L.L.: Psychiatric disorders in foster home reared children of schizophrenic mothers. Br. J. Psychiatry **112**, 819 (1966)
Heston, L.L.: The genetics of schizophrenic and schizoid disease. Science **167**, 249 (1970)
Heston, L.L., Denney, D.: Interactions between early life experience and biological factors in schizophrenia. In: The transmission of schizophrenia. Rosenthal, D., Kety, S.S. (eds.). Oxford: Pergamon Press 1968
Higgins, J.: Effects of child rearing by schizophrenic mothers: a follow-up. J. Psychiatr. Res. **13**, 1 (1976)
Hill, S., Goodwin, D., Cadoret, R., Osterland, K., Doner, S.M.: Association and linkage between alcoholism and eleven serological markers. J. Stud. Alcohol **36**, 981 (1975)
Hollingshead, A.B., Redlich, F.C.: Social class and mental illness. New York: Wiley 1958
Horn, J.M., Green, M., Carney, R., Erickson, M.T.: Bias against genetic hypotheses in adoption studies. Arch. Gen. Psychiatry **32**, 1265 (1975)
Huber, G., Gross, G., Schüttler, R.: Konsequenzen der Verlaufsuntersuchungen für Therapie und Rehabilitation der Schizophrenien. In: Therapie, Rehabilitation und Prävention schizophrener Erkrankungen. Huber, G. (Hrsg.). Stuttgart-New York: Schattauer 1976
Huse-Kleinstoll, G., Dahme, B., Flemming, B., Haag, A., Meffert, J., Polonius, M.L., Rosewald, G., Speidel, H.: Einige somatische und psychologische Prädiktoren für psychopathologische Auffälligkeiten nach Herzoperationen. Thoraxchirurgie **24**, 386 (1976)
Hutchings, B., Mednick, S.A.: Registered criminality in the adoptive and biological parents of registered male adoptees. In: Genetics, environment and psychopathology. Mednick, S.A., Schulsinger, F., Higgins, J., Bell, B. (eds.). Amsterdam: North Holland, Amer. Elsevier 1974
Huxley, J., Mayr, E., Osmond, H., Hoffer, A.: Schizophrenia as a genetic morphism. Nature **204**, 220 (1964)
Inouye, E.: Similarity and dissimilarity of schizophrenia in twins. Proc. III. World Congr. Psychiatry Montreal **1**, 524 (1961)
Ivanitsky, A.M., Natalevich, E.S.: Comparative clinico-electroencephalographic investigation of schizophrenic patients with and without hereditary loading. Zit. nach Exc. Med. Amsterdam: Hum. Genet. **7**, 281 (1969)

James, N., Chapman, C.J.: A genetic study of bipolar affective disorder. Br. J. Psychiatry **126**, 449 (1975)

Jarvik, L.F., Deckard, B.S.: The odyssean personality. A survival advantage for carriers of genes predisposing to schizophrenia? Neuropsychobiology **3**, 179 (1977)

Jatzkewitz, H.: Biochemische Aspekte in der Psychiatrie. In: Jahrbuch d. Max-Planck-Ges. **138** (1968)

Jonsson, E., Nilsson, T.: Alkoholkonsumtion hos monozygota och dizygota tvillingpar. Nord. Hyg. T. **49**, 21 (1968). Zit. nach Exc. Med. Hum. Genet. **6**, 387 (1968)

Juel-Nielsen, N.: Individual and environment. A psychiatric psychological investigation of monozygotic twins reared apart. Acta Psychiatr. Scand. [Suppl.] **183** (1964)

Juel-Nielsen, N., Videbech, T.: A twin study of suicide. Acta Genet. Med. Gemellol. (Roma) **19**, 307 (1970)

Kaij, L.: Alcoholism in twins. Stockholm: Almquist & Wiksell 1960

Kallmann, F.J.: The genetics of schizophrenia. New York: Augustin 1938

Kallmann, F.J.: The genetic theory of schizophrenia. An analysis of 691 schizophrenic twin index families. Am. J. Psychiatry **103**, 309 (1946)

Kallmann, F.J., Roth, B.: Genetic aspects of pre-adolescent schizophrenia. Am. J. Psychiatry **112**, 599 (1956)

Kanig, K.: Einführung in die allgemeine und klinische Neurochemie. Stuttgart: Fischer 1973

Kanner, L.: To what extent is early infantile autism determined by constitutional inadequacies? Proc. Ass. Res. Nerv. Ment. Dis. **33**, 378 (1954)

Kaplan, A.R. (ed.): Genetic factors in "Schizophrenia". Springfield, Ill.: Thomas 1972

Karlsson, J.L.: The biologic basis of schizophrenia. Springfield, Ill.: Thomas 1966

Karlsson, J.L.: A double dominant genetic mechanism for schizophrenia. Hereditas **65**, 261 (1970)

Karlsson, J.L.: Type of dominance modification in schizophrenia. Hereditas **72**, 153 (1972)

Kay, D.W.K.: The genetics of stuttering. In: The syndrome of stuttering. Clinics in developmental medicine. No. 17, London: Heinemann 1964. Zit. nach Shields 1975

Kay, D.W.K., Roth, M., Atkinson, M.W., Stephens, D.A., Garside, R.F.: Genetic hypothesis and environmental factors in the light of psychiatric morbidity in the families of schizophrenics. Br. J. Psychiatry **127**, 109 (1975)

Kay, L.: Atypical endogenous psychosis. Br. J. Psychiatry **113**, 415 (1967)

Kennedy, P.F.: The ecology of schizophrenia. In: New perspectives in schizophrenia. Forrest, A., Affleck, J. (eds.). Edinburgh-London-New York: Churchill Livingstone 1975

Kessler, S.: Progress and regress in the research on the genetics of schizophrenia. Schizophrenia Bull. **2**, 434 (1976)

Kety, S.S., Rosenthal, D., Wender, P.H., Schulsinger, F.: The types and prevalence of mental illness in the biological and adoptive families of adopted schizophrenics. In: The transmission of schizophrenia. Rosenthal, D., Kety, S.S. (eds.). Oxford-London: Pergamon Press 1968

Kety, S.S., Rosenthal, D., Wender, P.H., Schulsinger, F.: Studies based on a total sample of adopted individuals and their relatives: Why they were necessary, what they demonstrated and failed to demonstrate. Schizophrenia Bull. **2**, 413 (1976)

Kety, S.S., Rosenthal, D., Wender, P.H., Schulsinger, F., Jacobsen, B.: Mental illness in the biological and adoptive families of adopted individuals who have become schizophrenic: A preliminary report based on psychiatric interviews. In: Genetic research in psychiatry. Fieve, R.R., Rosenthal, D., Brill, H. (eds.). Baltimore: Johns Hopkins University Press 1975

Kidd, K.K., Cavalli-Sforza, L.L.: An analysis of the genetics of schizophrenia. Soc. Biol. **20**, 254 (1973)

Klorman, R., Strauss, J., Kokes, R.: The relationship of demographic and diagnostic factors to measures of premorbid adjustment in schizophrenia. Schizophrenia Bull. **3**, 214 (1977a)

Klorman, R., Strauss, J., Kokes, R.: Some biological approaches in research on premorbid functioning in schizophrenia. Schizophrenia Bull. **3**, 226 (1977b)

Koch, G.: Genetische Beratung. In: Diagnostische und therapeutische Methoden in der Psychiatrie. Vogel, T., Vliegen, J. (Hrsg.). Stuttgart: Thieme 1977

Koch, G.: Genetische Beratungen bei neurologischen und psychiatrischen Erkrankungen. Allgemeine Richtlinien. In: Neurologische und psychiatrische Therapie. Flügel, K.A. (Hrsg.). Erlangen: Perimed 1978

Kohn, M.: Social class and schizophrenia: A critical review. In: The transmission of schizophrenia. Rosenthal, D., Kety, S.S. (eds.). Oxford: Pergamon Press 1968

Kokes, R., Strauss, J., Klorman, R.: Measuring premorbid adjustment: The instruments and their development. Schizophrenia Bull. **3**, 186 (1977)

Kolvin, I., Ounsted, C., Richardson, L., Garside, R.F. III: The family and social background in childhood psychoses. Br. J. Psychiatry **118**, 396 (1971)

Kolvin, I., Taunch, T., Currah, J., Garside, R.F., Nolan, J., Shaw, W.B.: Enuresis: A descriptive analysis and a controlled trial. Dev. Med. Child Neurol. **14**, 715 (1972)

Kopun, M., Propping, P.: The kinetics of ethanol absorption and elimination in twins supplemented by repetitive experiments in single subjects. Eur. J. Clin. Pharmacol. **11**, 63 (1977)

Kranz, H.: Lebensschicksale krimineller Zwillinge. Berlin: Springer 1936

Kringlen, E.: Schizophrenia in twins. Psychiatry **29**, 172 (1966)

Kringlen, E.: Heredity and environment in the functional psychoses. London: Heinemann Medical 1967

Kringlen, E.: An epidemiological-clinical twin study on schizophrenia. In: The transmission of schizophrenia. Rosenthal, D.S., Kety, S.S. (eds.). Oxford: Pergamon Press 1968

Kringlen, E.: Twins – still our best method. Schizophrenia Bull. **2**, 429 (1976)

Kupfer, D.J., Pickar, D., Himmelhoch, J.M., Detre, T.P.: Are there two types of unipolar depression? Arch. Gen. Psychiatry **32**, 866 (1975)

Labhardt, F.: Die schizophrenieähnlichen Emotionspsychosen. Monogr. Gesamtgeb. Psychiatr. (Berlin) **102**. Berlin: Springer 1963

Lange, J.: Verbrechen als Schicksal an kriminellen Zwillingen. Leipzig: Thieme 1929

Langfeldt, G.: The prognosis in schizophrenia. Acta Psychiatr. Scand. [Suppl.] **110** (1956)

Larson, C.A., Nyman, G.E.: Differential fertility in schizophrenia. Acta Psychiatr. Scand. **49**, 272 (1973)

Le Gras, A.M.: Psychose und Kriminalität bei Zwillingen. Z. Neurol. **144**, 198 (1933)

Lenz, W.: Enuresis. Antwort auf Umfrage. Pädiat. Praxis **14**, 60 (1974)

Leonard, C.O., Chase, G.A., Child, B.: Genetic counseling: A consumers view. N. Engl. J. Med. **287**, 433 (1972)

Leonhard, K.: Die Aufteilung der endogenen Psychosen. Berlin: Akademie-Verlag 1968

Leonhard, K.: Ein dominanter und ein rezessiver Erbgang bei zwei verschiedenen Formen von Schizophrenie. Nervenarzt **46**, 242 (1975a)

Leonhard, K.: Gegen die Auffassung einer Einheit Schizophrenie. Psychiatr. Neurol. Med. Psychol. (Leipz.) **27**, 65 (1975b)

Lindelius, R. (ed.): A study of schizophrenia: A clinical, prognostic, and family investigation. Acta Psychiatr. Scand. [Suppl.] **216** (1970)

Lindinger, H.: Kasuistische Mitteilungen zum Problem der Unrichtigkeiten in der psychiatrischen Außenanamnese. Nervenarzt **46**, 85 (1975)

Ljungberg, L.: Hysteria: A clinical, prognostic and genetic study. Acta Psychiatr. Scand. [Suppl.] **112** (1957)

Loehlin, J.C., Nichols, R.C.: Heredity, environment, and personality (a study of 850 sets of twins). Austin-London: University of Texas Press 1976

Loranger, A.W.: X-linkage and manic-depressive illness. Br. J. Psychiatry **127**, 482 (1975)

Lubs, H.A., de la Cruz, F. (eds.): Genetic counseling. New York: Raven Press 1977

Luxenburger, H.: Vorläufiger Bericht über psychiatrische Serienuntersuchungen an Zwillingen. Z. Gesamte Neurol. Psychiatr. **116**, 295 (1928)

Mahler, M.: On child psychosis in schizophrenia: Autistic and symbiotic infantile psychosis. In: Psychoanalytic study of the child. Vol. 7. New York: Internat. University Press 1952

Majewski, F., Bierich, J.R., Löser, H., Michaelis, R., Leiber, B., Bettecken, F.: Zur Klinik und Pathogenese der Alkohol-Embryopathie. Münch. Med. Wochenschr. **118**, 1635 (1976)

Malzberg, B.: Mental disease among Swedish-born and native-born of Swedish parentage in New York State 1949–1951. Acta Psychiatr. Scand. **38**, 79 (1962)

Malzberg, B.: Mental disease among native whites in New York State 1949–1951, classified according parentage. Ment. Hyg. (N.Y.) **48**, 517 (1964)

Matheny, A.P., Wilson, R.S., Dolan, A.B.: Relations between twins' similarity of appearance and behavioral similarity: testing an assumption. Behav. Genet. **6**, 343 (1976)

Matthysse, S.W., Kidd, K.K.: Estimating the genetic contribution to schizophrenia. Am. J. Psychiatry **133**, 185 (1976)
McCabe, M.: Reactive psychoses. Acta Psychiatr. Scand. [Suppl.] **259** (1975)
McCabe, M., Fowler, R.C., Cadoret, R.J., Winokur, G.: Familial differences in schizophrenia with good and poor prognosis. Psychol. Med. **1**, 326 (1971)
McClearn, G.E., DeFries, J.C.: Introduction to behavioral genetics. San Francisco: Freeman 1973
McConaghy, N.: The use of an object sorting test in elucidating the hereditary factor in schizophrenia. J. Neurol. Neurosurg. Psychiatry **22**, 243 (1959)
McNeil, T.F., Kaij, L.: Obstetric complications and physical size of offspring of schizophrenic, schizophrenic-like, and control mothers. Br. J. Psychiatry **123**, 341 (1973)
Mednick, S.A.: A learning theory approach to research in schizophrenia. Psychol. Bull. **55**, 316 (1958)
Mednick, S.A.: Breakdown in individuals at high risk of schizophrenia: Possible predispositional perinatal factors. Ment. Hyg. **54**, 50 (1970)
Mednick, S.A., Hutchings, B.: Genetic and psychophysiological factors in asocial behavior. In: Psychopathic behaviour. Hare, R.D., Schalling, D. (eds.). Chichester-New York-Brisbane-Toronto: Wiley 1978
Mednick, S.A., Mura, E., Schulsinger, F., Mednick, B.: Perinatal conditions and infant development in children with schizophrenic parents. Soc. Biol. [Suppl.] **18**, **1**, 103 (1971)
Mednick, S.A., Mura, E., Schulsinger, F., Mednick, B.: Erratum and further analysis: Perinatal conditions and infant development in children with schizophrenic parents. Soc. Biol. **20**, 111 (1973)
Mednick, S.A., Schulsinger, F., Higgins, J., Bell, B. (eds.): Genetics, environment and psychopathology. Amsterdam: North Holland 1974
Mednick, S.A., Wild, C.: Reciprocal augmentation of generalization and anxiety. J. Exp. Psychol. **63**, 621 (1962)
Mendelson, W.B., Reid, M.A., Frommer, E.A.: Some characteristic features accompanying depression, anxiety and aggressive behaviour in disturbed children under five. In: Depressive states in childhood and adolescence. Annell, A.L. (ed.). Stockholm: Almquist & Wiksell 1972
Mendlewicz, J., Fieve, R.R., Rainer, J.D., Cadaldo, M.: Affective disorder on paternal and maternal sides. Observations in bipolar (manic-depressive) patients with and without a family history. Br. J. Psychiatry **122** (1973a)
Mendlewicz, J., Fieve, R.R., Stallone, F.: Relationship between effectiveness of lithium therapy and family history. Am. J. Psychiatry **130**, 1011 (1973b)
Mendlewicz, J., Fleiss, J.L.: Linkage studies with X-chromosome markers in bipolar (manic-depressive) and unipolar (depressive) illnesses. Biol. Psychiatry **9**, 261 (1974)
Mendlewicz, J., Rainer, J.D.: Morbidity risk and genetic transmission in manic-depressive illness. Am. J. Hum. Genet. **26**, 692 (1974)
Mendlewicz, J., Rainer, J.D.: Adoption study supporting genetic transmission in manic-depressive illness. Nature **268**, 327 (1977)
Meyendorf, R.: Hirnembolie und Psychose. J. Neurol. **213**, 163 (1976)
Meyers, D., Goldfarb, W.: Psychiatric appraisals of parents and siblings of schizophrenic children. Am. J. Psychiatry **118**, 902 (1962)
Michael, C.M., Morris, D.P., Soroker, E.: Follow-up studies of shy, withdrawn children: II. Relativ incidence of schizophrenia. Am. J. Orthopsychiatry **27**, 331 (1957)
Mirdal, G.M., Rosenthal, D., Wender, P.H., Schulsinger, F.: Perinatal complications in offspring of psychotic parents. Br. J. Psychiatry **130**, 495 (1977)
Mitsuda, H. (ed.): Clinical genetics in psychiatry. Tokyo: Igaku Shoin 1967
Mitsuda, H., Fukuda, T. (eds.): Biological mechanisms of schizophrenia and schizophrenia-like psychoses. Tokyo: Igaku Shoin 1974. Stuttgart: Thieme 1974
Mitsuda, H., Sakai, T., Kobayashi, J.: A clinico-genetic study on the relationship between neurosis and psychosis. Bull. Osaka Med. Sch., Suppl. XII, 27 (1967)
Moraczewski, A.S.: Ethical aspects of genetic counseling. In: Psychiatry and Genetics. Sperber, M.A., Jarvik, L.F. (eds.) New York: Basic Books 1976
Morris, D.P., Soroker, E., Burrus, G.: Follow-up studies of shy, withdrawn children. Evaluation of later adjustment. Am. J. Orthopsychiatry **24**, 143 (1954)
Morrison, J., Clancy, J., Crowe, R.: The Iowa 500: I. Diagnostic validity in mania, depression, and schizophrenia. Arch. Gen. Psychiatry **27**, 457 (1972)

Murphy, D.L., Weiss, R.: Reduced monoamine oxidase in blood platelets from bipolar depressed patients. Am. J. Psychiatry **128**, 1351 (1972)

Nielsen, J.: The Samsø project from 1957 to 1974. Acta Psychiatr. Scand. **54**, 198 (1976)

Nissen, G.: Depressive Syndrome im Kindes- und Jugendalter. Monogr. Gesamtgeb. Psychiatr. (Berlin), Bd. 4. Berlin-Heidelberg-New York: Springer 1971

Ødegaard, Ø.: Emigration and insanity. Acta Psychiatr. Scand. [Suppl.] **4** (1932)

Ødegaard, Ø.: The psychiatric disease entities in the light of a genetic investigation. Acta Psychiatr. Scand. [Suppl.] **169**, 94 (1963)

Ødegaard, Ø.: The multifactorial theory of inheritance in predisposition to schizophrenia. In: Genetic factors in "Schizophrenia". Kaplan, A.R. (ed.). Springfield, Ill.: Thomas 1972

Ødegaard, Ø.: Season of birth in the general population and in patients with mental disorder in Norway. Br. J. Psychiatry **125**, 397 (1974)

Offord, D.R., Cross, L.A.: Behavioral antecedents of adult schizophrenia. Arch. Gen. Psychiatry **21**, 267 (1969)

Olsen, T.: Follow-up study of manic-depressive patients whose first attack occurred before the age of 19. In: Depression. Kristiansen, E. (ed.). Proc. Scand. Symp. Depression. Acta Psychiatr. Scand. [Suppl.] **162**, 45 (1961)

Paikin, H., Jacobsen, B., Schulsinger, F., Godtfredsen, K., Rosenthal, D., Wender, P., Kety, S.: Characteristics of people who refused to participate in a social and psychopathological study. In: Genetics, environment and psychopathology. Mednick, S.A., Schulsinger, F., Higgins, J., Bell, B. (eds.). Amsterdam: North Holland 1974

Papoušek, H., Papoušek, M.: Die Mutter-Kind-Beziehung und die kognitive Entwicklung des Kindes. In: Seelische Fehlentwicklung im Kindesalter und Gesellschaftsstruktur. Nissen, G., Strunk, P. (Hrsg.). Neuwied-Berlin: Luchterhand 1974

Parker, G., Neilson, M.: Mental disorder and season of birth – a southern hemisphere study. Br. J. Psychiatry **129**, 355 (1976)

Parker, N.: Close identification in twins discordant for obsessional neurosis. Br. J. Psychiatry **110**, 496 (1964)

Partanen, J.K., Bruun, T., Markanen, M.: Inheritance of drinking behavior; a study on intelligence, personality and use of alcohol in adult twins. Helsinki: The Finnish Foundation for Alcohol Studies 1966

Pasamanick, B., Rogers, M., Lilienfeld, A.M.: Pregnancy experience and the development of behavior disorder in children. Am. J. Psychiatry **112**, 613 (1956)

Pearson, J.S., Kley, I.B.: On the application of genetic expectancies as age-specific base rates in the study of human behavior disorders. Psychol. Bull. **54**, 406 (1957)

Pénot, B.: Charactéristiques et devenir des dépressions de la deuxième enfance. In: États dépressifs chez l'enfant et l'adolescent. Annell, A.L. (ed.). Stockholm: Almquist & Wiksell 1972

Perris, C.: A study of bipolar (manic-depressive) and unipolar recurrent depressive psychoses. Acta Psychiatr. Neurol. Scand. [Suppl.] **194** (1966)

Perris, C.: Abnormality on paternal and maternal sides: Observations in bipolar (manic-depressive) and unipolar depressive psychoses. Br. J. Psychiatry **118**, 207 (1971)

Perris, C.: A study of cycloid psychoses. Acta Psychiatr. Scand. [Suppl.] **253** (1974)

Phillips, J.E., Jacobsen, N., Turner, W.J.: Conceptual thinking in schizophrenics and their relatives. Br. J. Psychiatry **111**, 823 (1965)

Pichot, P.: Psychopathic behaviour. A historical overview. In: Psychopathic behaviour. Hare, R.D., Schalling, D. (eds.). Chichester-New York-Brisbane-Toronto: Wiley 1978

Planansky, K.: Conceptual boundaries of schizoidness. J. Nerv. Ment. Dis. **142**, 318 (1966)

Planansky, K.: Phenotypic boundaries and genetic specificity in schizophrenia. In: Genetic factors in "Schizophrenia". Kaplan, A.R. (ed.). Springfield, Ill.: Thomas 1972

Plomin, R., Willerman, L., Loehlin, J.C.: Resemblance in appearance and the equal environments assumption in twin studies of personality traits. Behav. Genet. **6**, 43 (1976)

Ploog, D.: Verhaltensforschung und Psychiatrie. In: Psychiatrie der Gegenwart. Gruhle, H.W., Jung, R., Mayer-Gross, W., Müller, M. (Hrsg.), Bd. I/1. Berlin-Göttingen-Heidelberg: Springer 1964

Ploog, D.: Verhaltensbiologische Hypothesen zur Entstehung endogener Psychosen. In: Schizophrenie und Zyklothymie. Huber, G. (Hrsg.). Stuttgart: Thieme 1969a

Ploog, D.: Psychobiologie des Partnerschaftsverhaltens. Nervenarzt **40**, 245 (1969b)

Ploog, D.: Die cerebrale Repräsentation von Funktions- und Verhaltensweisen. Verhandl. d. Deutsch. Zoolog. Ges. 66. Jahresvers. Stuttgart: Fischer 1973
Ploog, D.: Verhaltensbiologische Aspekte in der psychiatrischen Forschung. Dtsch. Med. Wochenschr. **100**, 2108 (1975)
Ploog, D.: Anlage und Umwelt. Dtsch. Ärztebl. **76**, 725 u. 815 (1979)
Pollack, M., Woerner, M.G.: Pre- and perinatal complications and "childhood schizophrenia": A comparison of five controlled studies. J. Child Psychol. Psychiatry **7**, 235 (1966)
Pollin, W.: The pathogenesis of schizophrenia. Arch. Gen. Psychiatry **27**, 29 (1972)
Pollin, W., Allen, M.G., Hoffer, A., Stabenau, J.R., Hrubec, Z.: Psychopathology in 15909 pairs of veteran twins: Evidence for a genetic factor in schizophrenia and its relative absence in psychoneurosis. Am. J. Psychiatry **126**, 597 (1969)
Pollin, W., Stabenau, J.R.: Biological, psychological and historical differences in a series of monozygotic twins discordant for schizophrenia. In: The transmission of schizophrenia. Rosenthal, D., Kety, S. (eds.). Oxford-London-New York: Pergamon Press 1968
Post, F.: Schizo-affective symptomatology in late life. Br. J. Psychiatry **118**, 437 (1971)
Post, F.: The management and nature of depressive illness in late life: A follow-through study. Br. J. Psychiatry **121**, 393 (1972)
Price, J.S., Hare, E.H.: Birth order studies: Some sources of bias. Br. J. Psychiatry **115**, 633 (1969)
Propping, P.: Genetic control of ethanol action on the central nervous system. An EEG study in twins. Hum. Genet. **35**, 309 (1977)
Reed, S.C.: Counseling in Human Genetics. Part. II; Bull. No. 7 of the Dight Institute. Minneapolis: University of Minnesota Press 1951. Zit. nach Koch 1977
Reed, S.C., Hartley, C., Anderson, V.E., Phillips, V.P., Johnson, N.A.: The psychoses: Family studies. Philadelphia: Saunders 1973
Reich, T., Cloninger, C.R., Guze, S.B.: The multifactorial model of disease transmission: I. Description of the model and its use in psychiatry. Br. J. Psychiatry **127**, 1 (1975a)
Reich, T., James, J.H., Morris, C.A.: The use of multiple thresholds in determining the mode of transmission in semi-continuous traits. Annals Hum. Genet. **36**, 163 (1972)
Reich, T., Winokur, G., Mullaney, J.: The transmission of alcoholism. In: Genetic research in psychiatry. Fieve, R.R., Rosenthal, D., Brill, H. (eds.). Baltimore-London: Johns Hopkins University Press 1975b
Reisby, N.: Psychoses in children of schizophrenic mothers. Acta Psychiatr. Scand. **43**, 8 (1967)
Reisner, H.: Die Mutter des Schizophrenen. In: Schizophrenie und Umwelt. Kranz, H., Heinrich, K. (Hrsg.). Stuttgart: Thieme 1971
Remschmidt, H., Dauner, I.: Zur Ätiologie und Differentialdiagnose depressiver Zustandsbilder bei Kindern und Jugendlichen. In: Jahrb. Jugendpsychiatrie u. ihre Grenzgebiete. Stutte, H. (Hrsg.). Bern-Stuttgart-Wien: Huber 1971
Renaud, H., Estess, F.: Life history interview with one hundred normal American males: "Pathogenicity" of childhood. Am. J. Orthopsychiatry **31**, 786 (1961)
Rimmer, J., Jacobsen, B.: Differential fertility of adopted schizophrenics and their half-siblings. Acta Psychiatr. Scand. **54**, 161 (1976)
Ringel, E.: Die psychologischen und psychiatrischen Hintergründe des Selbstmordes. Z. Alternsforsch. **18**, 76 (1965)
Roeder-Kutsch, T., Scholz-Wölfing, J.: Schizophrenes Siechtum auf der Grundlage ausgedehnter Hirnveränderungen nach Kohlenoxyd-Vergiftung. Z. Gesamte Neurol. Psychiatr. **173**, 702 (1941)
Romney, D.: Psychometrically assessed thought disorder in schizophrenic and control patients and in their parents and siblings. Br. J. Psychiatry **115**, 999 (1969)
Rosanoff, A.J., Handy, L.M., Plesset, J., Brush, R.: The etiology of so-called schizophrenic psychosis with special reference of their occurrence in twins. Am. J. Psychiatry **91**, 247 (1934)
Rosanoff, A.J., Handy, L.M., Plesset, I.R.: The etiology of child behavior difficulties, juvenile delinquency and adult criminality with special reference to their occurrence in twins. Psychiatric Monogr. (Calif.) No. 1, 1941. Sacramento, Dept. of Institutions. Zit. nach Shields 1976
Rosenthal, D.: The Genain quadruplets. New York: Basic Books 1963
Rosenthal, D.: Genetic theory and abnormal behavior. New York: McGraw-Hill 1970
Rosenthal, D.: Three adoption studies of heredity in the schizophrenic disorders. Int. J. Ment. Health **1**, 63 (1972)

Rosenthal, D.: Discussion: The concept of subschizophrenic disorders. In: Genetic research in psychiatry. Fieve, R.R., Rosenthal, D., Brill, H. (eds.). Baltimore: Johns Hopkins University Press 1975
Rosenthal, D., Kety, S.S. (eds.): The transmission of schizophrenia. Oxford: Pergamon Press 1968
Rosenthal, D., Wender, P.H., Kety, S., Schulsinger, F., Welner, J., Rieder, R.P.: Parent-child relationships and psychopathological disorders in the child. Arch. Gen. Psychiatry **32**, 466 (1975)
Rüdin, E.: Studien über Vererbung und Entstehung geistiger Störungen. I. Zur Vererbung und Neuentstehung der Dementia praecox. Monogr. Neurol. Psychiat. Berlin: Springer 1916
Rutschmann, J., Cornblatt, B., Erlenmeyer-Kimling, L.: Sustained attention in children at risk for schizophrenia. Arch. Gen. Psychiatry **34**, 571 (1977)
Rutter, M.: The description and classification of infantile autism. In: Infantile autism. Churchill, D.W., Alpern, G.D., DeMeyer, M.K. (eds.). Springfield, Ill.: Thomas 1971
Rutter, M.: The development of infantile autism. Psychol. Med. **4**, 147 (1974)
Rutter, M., Lockyer, L.A.: A five to fifteen year follow-up study of infantile psychosis. I. Description of the sample. Br. J. Psychiatry **113**, 1169 (1967)
Sameroff, A.J.: Caretaking or reproductive casualty? Determinants in developmental deviancy. In: Early developmental hazards: Predictors and precautions. Horowitz, F.D. (ed.). Washington, D.C.: AAAS 1978
Sankar, S.: Early infantile autism (EIA) is not primarily a psychiatric disorder. In: Mental health in children. Sankar, S. (ed.), Vol. II. Westbury, N.Y.: PJD Publ. 1976
Scarr, S.: Environmental bias in twin studies. Eugen. Quart. **15**, 34 (1968)
Schachmatowa, E.: Genealogische Untersuchungen. In: Schizophrenie. Sneshnewski, A.W. (ed.). Leipzig: Thieme 1977
Scharfetter, Ch.: Symbiontische Psychosen. Bern: Huber 1970
Schepank, H.: Erb- und Umweltfaktoren bei Neurosen. Nervenarzt **44**, 449 (1973)
Schepank, H.: Erb- und Umweltfaktoren bei Neurosen. Tiefenpsychologische Untersuchungen an 50 Zwillingspaaren. Monogr. Gesamtgeb. Psychiatr. (Berlin), Bd. 11. Berlin: Springer 1974
Schepank, H.: Diskordanzanalyse eineiiger Zwillingspaare. Z. Psychosom. Med. Psychoanal. **21**, 215 (1975)
Schizophrenia Bulletin (Dept. Health, Education and Welfare) **2**, issue 3 (1976)
Schmitz, W.: Nachlassen der Schulleistungen als Primärsymptom einer endogenen Depression. In: Depressive states in childhood and adolescence. Annell, A.L. (ed.). Stockholm: Almquist & Wiksell 1972
Schneider, K.: Die psychopathischen Persönlichkeiten. In: Handbuch der Psychiatrie. Aschaffenburg, G. (Hrsg.). Spez. Teil, 7. Abtl., 1. Teil. Wien: Deuticke 1923
Schneider, K.: „Der Psychopath" in heutiger Sicht. Fortschr. Neurol. Psychiatr. **26**, 1 (1958)
Schuckit, M., Goodwin, D., Winokur, G.: A study of alcoholism in halfsiblings. Am. J. Psychiatry **128**, 1132 (1972)
Schulsinger, F.: Psychopathy: Heredity and environment. Int. J. Ment. Health **1**, 190 (1972)
Schulsinger, F.: Suicide problems in the light of studies on adoptees. In: Origin, prevention and treatment of affective disorders. Schon, M., Strömgren, E. (eds.). London-New York-San Francisco: Academic Press 1979
Schulsinger, F., Jacobsen, B.: The heredity-environment issue in psychiatry. Perspectives from research at the Psykologisk Institut, Dept. of Psychiatry, Komunehospitalet. Acta Psychiatr. Scand. [Suppl.] **261**, 44 (1975)
Schulsinger, H.: A ten-year follow-up of children of schizophrenic mothers. Clinical assessment. Acta Psychiatr. Scand. **53**, 371 (1976)
Schulte, W.: Die Auswirkungen der Schizophrenie auf ihre Umwelt. Nervenarzt **39**, 98 (1968)
Schulz, B.: Kinder schizophrener Elternpaare. Z. Gesamte Neurol. Psychiatr. **168**, 332 (1940)
Schulz, B.: Kinder von Elternpaaren mit einem schizophrenen und einem affektpsychotischen Partner. Z. Gesamte Neurol. Psychiatr. **170**, 441 (1940)
Seeman, P., Chau Wong, M., Tedesco, J., Wong, K.: Brain receptors for antipsychotic drugs and dopamine direct binding assays. Proc. Natl. Acad. Sci. **72**, 4376 (1975)
Shapiro, R.W.: A twin study of non-endogenous depression. Aarhus: Universitetsforlaget, & Copenhagen: Munksgaard 1970
Shields, J.: Personality differences and neurotic traits in normal twin schoolchildren. Eugen. Rev. **45**, 213 (1954)

Shields, J.: Monozygotic twins brought up apart and brought up together. London: Oxford University Press 1962
Shields, J.: Some recent developments in psychiatric genetics. Arch. Psychiatr. Nervenkr. **220**, 347 (1975)
Shields, J.: Genetics in schizophrenia. In: Schizophrenia today. Kemali, D., Bartholini, G., Richter, D. (eds.). Oxford: Pergamon Press 1976a
Shields, J.: Polygenic influences. In: Child psychiatry. Rutter, M., Hersov, L.A. (eds.). Oxford-London-Edinburgh: Blackwell Scientific Publ. 1976b
Shields, J.: Genetics and alcoholism. In: Alcoholism: New knowledge and new responses. Edwards, G., Grant, M. (eds.). London: Croom Helm 1977
Shields, J.: High risk for schizophrenia: Genetic considerations. Psychol. Med. **7**, 7 (1977)
Shields, J.: The genetics of neurosis: Facts or fiction. Symposium in Stockholm "Facts about Neuroses", 1978a (in press)
Shields, J.: Genetics. In: Schizophrenia: Towards a new synthesis. Wing, J.K. (ed.). London: Academic Press 1978b
Shields, J.: Genetical studies of hysterical disorders. Submitted for publication
Shields, J., Gottesman, I.I.: Cross-national diagnosis of schizophrenia in twins. Arch. Gen. Psychiatry **27**, 725 (1972)
Shields, J., Gottesman, I.I.: Obstetric complications and twin studies of schizophrenia: Clarifications and affirmations. Schizophrenia Bull. **3**, 351 (1977)
Shields, J., Slater, E.: La similarité du diagnostic chez les jumeaux et le problème de la spécificité biologique dans les névroses et les troubles de la personnalité. Evolut. Psychiatr. **2**, 441 (1966)
Shields, J., Gottesman, I.I., Slater, E.: Kallmann's 1946 schizophrenic twin study in the light of new information. Acta Psychiatr. Scand. **43**, 385 (1967)
Shields, J., Heston, L.L., Gottesman, I.I.: Schizophrenia and the schizoid. The problem for genetic analysis. In: Genetic research in psychiatry. Fieve, R.R., Rosenthal, D., Brill, H. (eds.). Baltimore: Johns Hopkins University Press 1975
Shopsin, B., Mendlewicz, J., Suslak, L., Silbey, E., Gershon, S.: Genetics of affective disorders. II. Morbidity risks and genetic transmission. Neuropsychobiology **2**, 28 (1976)
Skogstad, W.: Genetische Beratung. Stuttgart: Ferdinand Enke 1978
Slater, E.: Psychotic and neurotic illnesses in twins. Med. Res. Council, Special Rep. Series No. 278. London: Her Majesty's Stat. Office 1953
Slater, E.: The monogenic theory of schizophrenia. Acta Genet. (Basel) **8**, 60 (1958)
Slater, E.: The thirty-fifth Maudsley lecture: "Hysteria 311". J. Ment. Sci. **107**, 359 (1961)
Slater, E.: Genetical factors in neurosis. Br. J. Psychol. **55**, 265 (1964)
Slater, E.: The case for a major partially dominant gene. In: Genetic factors in schizophrenia. Kaplan, A.R. (ed.). Springfield, Ill.: Thomas 1972
Slater, E., Cowie, V.A.: The genetics of mental disorders. London-New York: Oxford University Press 1971
Slater, E., Shields, J.: Genetical aspects of anxiety. In: Studies of anxiety. Lader, M.H. (ed.). Brit. J. Psychiatry Special Publ. No. 3. Ashford, Kent: Headley 1969
Slater, E., Tsuang, M.T.: Abnormality on paternal and maternal sides: Observations in schizophrenia and manic-depression. J. Med. Genet. **5**, 197 (1968)
Slater, E., Maxwell, J., Price, J.S.: Distribution of ancestral secondary cases in bipolar affective disorders. Br. J. Psychiatry **118**, 215 (1971)
Smeraldi, E., Negri, F., Melica, A.M.: A genetic study of affective disorders. Acta Psychiatr. Scand. **56**, 382 (1977)
Smith, C.: Recurrence risks for multifactorial inheritance. Am. J. Hum. Genet. **23**, 578 (1971)
Smith, C., Forrest, A.D.: The genetics of schizophrenia. In: New perspectives in schizophrenia. Forrest, A., Affleck, J. (eds.). Edinburgh-London-New York: Churchill Livingstone 1975
Sperber, M.A., Jarvik, L.F. (eds.): Psychiatry and genetics. New York: Basic Books Inc. 1976
Spicer, C.C., Hare, E.H., Slater, E.: Neurotic and psychotic forms of depressive illness: Evidence from age-incidence in a national sample. Br. J. Psychiatry **123**, 535 (1973)
Spiel, W.: Die endogenen Psychosen des Kindes- und Jugendalters. Bibl. Psychiat. Neurol. **113**. Basel-New York: Karger 1961
Stabenau, J.R.: Some genetic and family studies in autism and childhood schizophrenia. In: Mental health in children. Vol. I. Sankar, S. (ed.). Westbury, N.Y.: PJD Publ. 1975

Stenstedt, A.: A study in manic-depressive psychosis. Clinical, social and genetic investigation. Acta Psychiatr. Scand. [Suppl.] **79**, (1952)

Stenstedt, A.: Genetics of neurotic depression. Acta Psychiatr. Scand. **42**, 392 (1966)

Stephens, D.A., Atkinson, M.W., Kay, D.W.K., Roth, M., Garside, R.F.: Psychiatric morbidity in parents and sibs of schizophrenics and non-schizophrenics. Br. J. Psychiatry **127**, 97 (1975)

Stevens, B.: Marriage and fertility of women suffering from schizophrenia or affective disorders. Maudsley Monogr. **19**. London: Oxford University Press 1969

Stewart, M., Morrison, J.: Affective disorder among the relatives of hyperactive children. J. Child Psychol. Psychiatry **14**, 209 (1973)

Strauss, J., Klorman, R., Kokes, R., Sacksteder, J.: Premorbid adjustment in schizophrenia: Directions for research and application. Schizophrenia Bull. **3**, 240 (1977b)

Strauss, J., Kokes, R., Klorman, R., Sacksteder, J.: The concept of premorbid adjustment. Schizophrenia Bull. **3**, 182 (1977a)

Strömgren, E.: Psychiatrische Genetik. In: Psychiatrie der Gegenwart. Bd. I/1A. Gruhle, H.W., Jung, R., Mayer-Gross, W., Müller, M. (Hrsg.). Berlin-Heidelberg: Springer 1967a

Strömgren, E.: Neurosen und Psychopathien. In: Humangenetik. Bd. V/2. Becker, P.E. (Hrsg.). Stuttgart: Thieme 1967b

Strömgren, E.: Atypische Psychosen. Reaktive (psychogene) Psychosen. In: Psychiatrie der Gegenwart. Kisker, K.P., Meyer, J.-E., Müller, M., Strömgren, E. (Hrsg.). 2. Aufl., Bd. II/1. Berlin-Heidelberg-New York: Springer 1972

Strömgren, E.: Genetics of psychopathy. 6. World Congress of Psychiatry, Hawai 1977. (Im Druck)

Stumpfl, F.: Die Ursprünge des Verbrechens, dargestellt am Lebenslauf von Zwillingen. Leipzig: Thieme 1936

Suslak, L., Shopsin, B., Silbey, E., Mendlewicz, J., Gershon, S.: Genetics of affective disorders. I. Familial incidence study of bipolar, unipolar and schizo-affective illnesses. Neuropsychobiology **2**, 18 (1976)

Syndulko, K.: Electrocortical investigations of sociopathy. In: Psychopathic behaviour. Hare, E.D., Schalling, D. (eds.). Chichester-New York-Brisbane-Toronto: Wiley 1978

Taft, L., Goldfarb, W.: Prenatal and perinatal factors in childhood schizophrenia. Dev. Med. Child Neurol. **6**, 32 (1964)

Tanna, V.L., Winokur, G., Elston, R.C., Go, R.C.P.: A linkage study of depression spectrum disease: The use of the sib-pair method. Neuropsychobiology **2**, 52 (1976a)

Tanna, V.L., Winokur, G., Elston, R.C., Go, R.C.P.: A linkage study of pure depressive disease: The use of the sib-pair method. Biol. Psychiatry **11**, 767 (1976b)

Taschev, T., Roglev, M.: Vergleichende Untersuchungen an Psychosen von Eltern, Kindern und Geschwistern. Arch. Psychiatr. Nervenkr. **222**, 377 (1976)

Tatetsu, S.: Pervitin-Psychosen. Folia Psychiatr. Neurol. Jpn. [Suppl.] **6**, 25 (1960)

Taylor, M., Abrams, R.: Manic states. A genetic study of early and late onset affective disorders. Arch. Gen. Psychiatry **28**, 656 (1973a)

Taylor, M.A., Abrams, R.: The phenomenology of mania: A new look at some old patients. Arch. Gen. Psychiatry **29**, 520 (1973b)

Theile, U.: Genetische Beratung. Motivationsanalyse. München-Wien-Baltimore: Urban & Schwarzenberg 1977

Tienari, P.: Psychiatric illness in identical twins. Acta Psychiatr. Scand. [Suppl.] **171**, 39 (1963)

Tienari, P.: Schizophrenia in monozygotic male twins. In: The transmission of schizophrenia. Rosenthal, D., Kety, S.S. (eds.). Oxford: Pergamon Press 1968

Torrey, E.F.: Birth weights, perinatal insults, and HLA types: Return to "original din". Schizophrenia Bull. **3**, 347 (1977)

Towbin, A.: Recurrent cerebral embolism. Arch. Neurol. Psychiatr. **73**, 173 (1955)

Trostorff, S. v.: Verlauf und Psychose in der Verwandtschaft bei den systematischen und unsystematischen Schizophrenien und den zykloiden Psychosen. Psychiat. Neurol. Med. Psychol. (Leipz.) **27**, 80 (1975)

Tsuang, M.: A study of pairs of sibs both hospitalised for mental disorder. Br. J. Psychiatry **113**, 283 (1967)

Tsuang, M.: Abnormality on paternal and maternal sides in Chinese schizophrenics. Br. J. Psychiatry **118**, 211 (1971)

Tsuang, M., Fowler, R.C., Cadoret, R.J., Monelly, E.: Schizophrenia among first-degree relatives of paranoid and non paranoid schizophrenics. Compr. Psychiatry **15**, 295 (1974)

Vandenberg, S.G. (ed.): Methods and goals in human behavior genetics. New York-London: Academic Press 1965

Vartanian, M.A., Gindilis, V.M.: Genetic models and biological research in schizophrenia. In: Genetic factors in "schizophrenia". Kaplan A.R. (ed.). Springfield, Ill.: Thomas 1972

Vogel, F.: The genetic basis of the normal human electroencephalogram (EEG). Humangenetik **10**, 91 (1970)

Walcher, W. (Hrsg.): Probleme der Provokation depressiver Psychosen. Int. Sympos. Graz 1971. Wien: Hollinek 1971

Weil-Malherbe, H.: The biochemistry of affective disorders. In: Biological foundations of psychiatry. Grenell, R.G., Gabay, S. (eds.). New York: Raven Press 1976

Weinschenk, C.: Zum gegenwärtigen Stand der Legasthenie-Forschung. Fortschr. Med. **93**, 458 u. 550 (1975)

Welner, J., Strömgren, E.: Clinical and genetic studies on benign schizophreniform psychoses based on a follow-up. Acta Psychiatr. Scand. **33**, 377 (1958)

Wender, P.H., Rosenthal, D., Kety, S.S.: A psychiatric assessment of the adoptive parents of schizophrenics. In: The transmission of schizophrenia. Rosenthal, D., Kety, S.S. (eds.). Oxford: Pergamon Press 1968

Wender, P.H., Rosenthal, D., Kety, S.S., Schulsinger, F., Welner, J.: Social class and psychopathology in adoptees: A natural experimental method for separating the roles of genetic and experiential factors. Arch. Gen. Psychiatry **28**, 318 (1973)

Wender, P.H., Rosenthal, D., Kety, S.S., Schulsinger, F., Welner, J.: Cross-fostering: A research strategy for clarifying the role of genetic and experiential factors in the etiology of schizophrenia. Arch. Gen. Psychiatry **30**, 121 (1974)

Willi, J.: Die Schizophrenie in ihrer Auswirkung auf die Eltern. Schweiz. Arch. Neurol. Neurochir. Psychiatr. **89**, 426 (1962)

Wilson, J.C., Reece, J.C.: Simultaneous death in schizophrenic twins. Arch. Gen. Psychiatry **11**, 377 (1964)

Winokur, G.: The types of affective disorder. J. Nerv. Ment. Dis. **156**, 82 (1973)

Winokur, G., Tanna, V.L.: Possible role of X-linked dominant factor in manic-depressive disease. Dis. Nerv. Syst. **30**, 89 (1969)

Winokur, G., Reich, T., Rimmer, J., Pitts, F.N.: Alcoholism. III. Diagnosis and familial psychiatric illness in 259 alcoholic probands. Arch. Gen. Psychiatry **23**, 104 (1970)

Winokur, G., Rimmer J., Reich, T.: Alcoholism. IV. Is there more than one type of alcoholism? Br. J. Psychiatry **118**, 525 (1971a)

Winokur, G., Cadoret, R.J., Dorzab, J., Baker, M.: Depressive disease: A genetic study. Arch. Gen. Psychiatry **24**, 135 (1971b)

Winokur, G., Morrison, J., Clancy, J., Crowe, R.: Iowa 500: The clinical and genetic distinction of hebephrenic and paranoid schizophrenia. J. Nerv. Ment. Dis. **159**, 12 (1974)

Witkowski, R., Prokop, O.: Genetik erblicher Syndrome und Mißbildungen. Wörterbuch f.d. Familienberatung. Stuttgart: Fischer 1976

Wittermans, W., Schulz, B.: Genealogischer Beitrag zur Frage der geheilten Schizophrenien. Arch. Psychiatr. Nervenkr. **185**, 211 (1950)

Wyatt, R.J., Murphy, D.L., Belmaker, R., Cohen, S., Donnelly, C.H., Pollin, W.: Reduced monoamine oxidase activity in platelets: A possible genetic marker for vulnerability to schizophrenia. Science **179**, 916 (1973)

Yoshimasu, S.: The criminological significance of the family in the light of the studies of criminal twins. Acta Criminol. Leg. Jpn. **27**, 117 (1961)

Zahn, T.P.: Autonomic nervous system characteristics possibly related to a genetic predisposition to schizophrenia. Schizophrenia Bull. **3**, 49 (1977)

Zerbin-Rüdin, E.: Endogene Psychosen. In: Humangenetik. Bd. V/2. Becker, P.E. (Hrsg.). Stuttgart: Thieme 1967

Zerbin-Rüdin, E.: Zur Genetik der depressiven Erkrankungen. In: Das depressive Syndrom. Hippius, H., Selbach, H. (Hrsg.). München: Urban & Schwarzenberg 1969

Zerbin-Rüdin, E.: Genetische Aspekte der endogenen Psychosen. Fortschr. Neurol. Psychiatr. **39**, 459 (1971a)

Zerbin-Rüdin, E.: Das Anlage-Umwelt-Problem bei der Entstehung der Schizophrenie. Nervenarzt **42**, 613 (1971 b)
Zerbin-Rüdin, E.: Vererbung und Umwelt bei der Entstehung psychischer Störungen. Erträge der Forschung, Bd. 28. Darmstadt: Wissenschaftl. Buchgesellschaft 1974
Zerbin-Rüdin, E.: Psychiatrie, Morphologie und Verhaltensgenetik. Arch. Psychiatr. Nervenkr. **221**, 245 (1976)
Zerbin-Rüdin, E.: Genetische Aspekte des Suchtproblems. Suchtgefahren **23**, 1 (1977)
Zerbin-Rüdin, E.: Genetische Aspekte klinischer Störungen. In: Klinische Psychologie. Trends in Forschung und Praxis. Baumann, U. (Hrsg.). Bern-Stuttgart-Wien: Huber 1978
Zerbin-Rüdin, E.: Genetische Beratung bei psychiatrischen Erkrankungen. In: Therapie psychosomatischer Krankheiten in der Praxis. Wieck, H., Hillemacher, A. (Hrsg.). Erlangen: Perimed 1979
Zerssen, D. v.: Premorbid personality and affective psychoses. In: Handbook of studies on depression. Burrows, G.D. (ed.). Excerpta Med. (Human Genetics). Amsterdam-London-New York 1977
Zerssen, D. v., Koeller, D.-M.: Klinische Selbstbeurteilungs-Skalen (Ksb-S) aus dem Münchner Psychiatrischen Informations-System (PSYCHIS München). Weinheim: Beltz 1976

Konstitution

Von

D. v. Zerssen

Inhalt

A. Allgemeiner Teil 619
   I. Konstitution als Grundstruktur des Individuums 619
   II. Konstitutionsaufbau 622
   III. Abstraktionsstufen des Konstitutionsbegriffs 624
   IV. Konstitutionspathologie 627
   V. Konsequenzen für die klinische Arbeit 630
B. Spezieller Teil 632
   I. Allgemeine Konstitution 632
   II. Gruppenkonstitution 634
      1. Totalkonstitution 634
         a) Alterskonstitution 634
         b) Geschlechtskonstitution 642
         c) Rassische Konstitution 664
         d) Normale Varianten 665
         e) Abnorme Varianten 672
      2. Partialkonstitutionen 679
         a) Somatische Partialkonstitutionen 679
         b) Psychische Partialkonstitutionen 682
   III. Individuelle Konstitution 690
Literatur 692

A. Allgemeiner Teil
I. Konstitution als Grundstruktur des Individuums

Jeder individuelle Organismus steht in Wechselwirkung mit seiner belebten wie unbelebten Umwelt, wodurch diese und er selbst ständig verändert werden. Dabei erhält er aber – allen äußeren Einwirkungen zum Trotz – eine für ihn kennzeichnende *Grundstruktur* aufrecht. Wir bezeichnen sie als seine *Konstitution* (v. Zerssen, 1973b). Diese wird begrifflich abgehoben von der *Kondition* als dem *jeweiligen Zustand*, in dem sich der Organismus infolge wechselnder äußerer Einflüsse wie auch „spontaner" innerer Zustandsänderungen befindet (Szabó, 1938).

Zur Kondition eines höher entwickelten Lebewesens gehören u.a. der allgemeine Ernährungs- und Kräftezustand, Schlaf- bzw. Wachheit und deren Abstufungsgrade, Hunger, Durst, sexuelle Erregung, aber auch sog. Streß (v. Eiff, 1976; Henry u. Stephens, 1977) und aktuelle (akute wie chronische) krankhafte Zustände. Somit unterliegt die Kondition *per definitionem* einem ständigen und z.T. raschen Wechsel, wobei lediglich durch Konstanz der äußeren Reizbedingungen (Situation) u.U. ein relativer Dauerzustand bezüglich bestimmter Variablen (z.B. der Körperkraft bei entsprechendem Muskeltraining) entsteht.

Abb. 1 soll das Gesagte schematisch verdeutlichen. Reize aus der Umwelt (Merkwelt: v. UEXKÜLL, 1956), die zusammen die externe Reizsituation bilden (ENDLER, 1976), wirken auf den als innen gepunkteten Kreis dargestellten Organismus ein und verändern so seine aktuelle Kondition. Dies kann eine Reaktion auslösen, die ihrerseits die Umwelt (Wirkwelt: v. UEXKÜLL, 1956) beeinflußt. Es gibt aber auch von äußeren Reizen unabhängige aktive Handlungen, die auf die Umwelt einwirken. Die Auswirkungen solcher Aktionen, bzw. der Reizreaktionen des Organismus auf die Umwelt, bestehen ihrerseits in einer Veränderung der externen Reizsituation; zugleich erfolgt eine Rückmeldung der (Re-) Aktionen innerhalb des Organismus, die u.U. dessen Reizempfänglichkeit verändert (HASSENSTEIN, 1966). Diese internen Zustandsänderungen betreffen im allgemeinen nicht die als Kern des Schemas dargestellte Konstitution des Organismus, seine Grundbeschaffenheit. Sie sind aber – wie im Schema durch den senkrecht nach oben weisenden Pfeil angedeutet – von dieser abhängig. Die nach unten gerichtete kleinere Pfeilspitze zeigt an, daß in geringerem Maße auch die Konstitution durch Veränderungen der Kondition beeinflußbar ist.

Die Konstitution ist demnach keineswegs eine absolute, sondern eine – im Vergleich zur Kondition – *relative* Konstante (v. ZERSSEN, 1973a, 1977b). Weitgehend *konstant* bleibt die Erbsubstanz (das Genom); jedoch können sich auch an dieser regressive Veränderungen abspielen; man denke etwa an Chromosomenverlust, Chromosomenbrüche und andere Veränderungen an den Chromosomen durch Virusinfektionen sowie durch Alterungsprozesse (PELZ u. MIELER, 1972), die möglicherweise bei der Entstehung von Alterskrankheiten (z.B. seniler Demenz: NIELSEN, 1968) eine Rolle spielen. Im übrigen ist zu berücksichtigen,

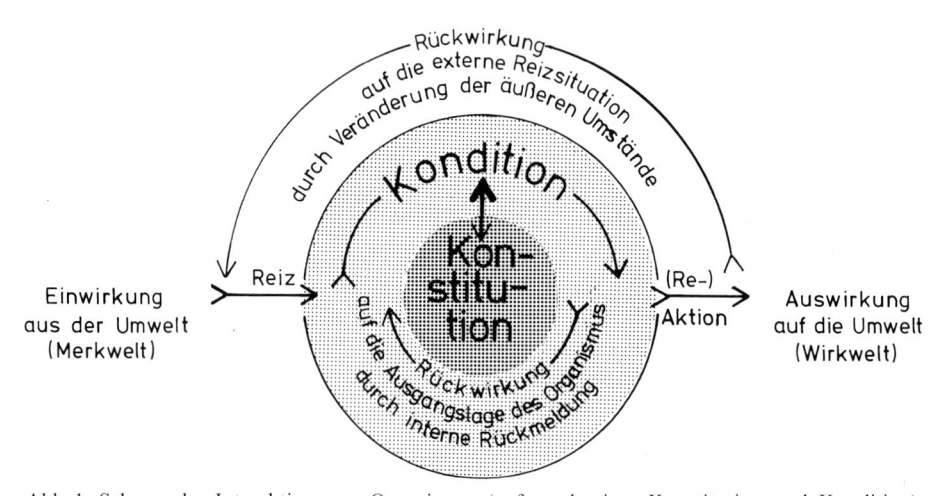

Abb. 1. Schema der Interaktion von Organismus (aufgrund seiner Konstitution und Kondition) und Umwelt (Merkwelt und Wirkwelt im Sinne v. UEXKÜLLS, 1956). Reizsituation = aktualisierter Anteil der Merkwelt. Ausgangslage = Zustand des Organismus bei Reizeinwirkung

daß die Konstanthaltung organismischer Strukturen im allgemeinen auf einem Fließgleichgewicht gegenläufiger Prozesse beruht (wie dem Stoffaustausch mit der Umwelt bzw. anabolen und katabolen Stoffwechselvorgängen: v. BERTALANFFY, 1932). Darüber hinaus können sukzessiv sich abspielende gegenläufige Prozesse eine endogene Periodik aufweisen, die ihrerseits durch weitgehende Konstanz ausgezeichnet ist. Diese endogene Periodizität ist u.U. erst nach Ausschaltung äußerer „Zeitgeber" nachzuweisen (wie in den Bunkerversuchen zur experimentellen Prüfung zirkadianer Phänomene: WEVER, 1979). Derartige Biorhythmen gehören demnach auch zur Grundstruktur des Organismus und sind somit als konstitutionelle Eigenschaften anzusprechen.

Daneben laufen in den Organismen – insbesondere höher differenzierten – Prozesse ab, die weitgehend irreversibel sind, wodurch die Grundstruktur selbst verändert wird. Es handelt sich dabei einmal um endogene, genetisch gesteuerte Entwicklungsprozesse evolutiver und involutiver Art, zum anderen um Auswirkungen äußerer Einflüsse, die nicht im Sinne der Homöostase ausgeglichen werden können. Die Konstitutionsentwicklung ist durch das Nebeneinander und Nacheinander von evolutiven und involutiven Prozessen gekennzeichnet, die sich bei allen höher differenzierten Organismen während des ganzen Lebens abspielen.

Dabei überwiegen am Lebensbeginn die evolutiven Prozesse (Wachstum und Differenzierungsvorgänge), während zum (physiologischen) Lebensende hin involutive (d.h. Rückbildungs-)Prozesse mehr und mehr in den Vordergrund treten. Dazwischen liegt gewöhnlich ein längerer Zeitabschnitt, in dem sich diese Vorgänge weitgehend die Waage halten, ohne daß es deshalb zu einem völligen Stillstand der Entwicklung käme. Trotzdem hebt man begrifflich im allgemeinen diesen Zeitabschnitt als „stationäre" Phase von der voraufgehenden Phase intensiven Wachstums ab (die beim Menschen mit der Adoleszenz endet: SCHWIDETZKY, 1970). Die evolutiven Prozesse werden zum Teil durch äußere Einwirkungen und durch Übung angeregt und/oder gefördert, umgekehrt durch das Fehlen solcher Einflüsse gehemmt (z.B. die Entwicklung verbaler Fähigkeiten des Menschen durch mangelndes Sprachtraining); andererseits werden involutive Prozesse teils durch relative Überbeanspruchung (Abnutzung), teils jedoch gerade durch fehlende Beanspruchung (Übungsmangel) gefördert (z.B. intellektueller Altersabbau in reizarmer Umgebung: LEHR, 1978).

Äußere Einwirkungen können – je nach ihrer Qualität (Reizform) und ihrer Quantität (Dauer und Stärke) sowie in Abhängigkeit vom Entwicklungsstand des Organismus und seiner momentanen Kondition – die Anpassungsmechanismen eines Organismus überfordern und zu irreparablen, die Konstitution verändernden Schäden oder gar zum Tode führen.

Umweltreize zeichnen sich nicht nur durch ihre physikochemischen Eigenschaften, sondern darüber hinaus durch ihren Informationsgehalt für den Organismus aus. Dieser und nicht etwa ihr Energiegehalt kann bei der Beeinflussung organismischer Vorgänge ganz im Vordergrund stehen. Das gilt auch für die Erzeugung irreversibler und damit konstitutionsbeeinflussender Veränderungen durch äußere Reize. Dadurch können Lebenserfahrungen einen direkten Einfluß auf die Konstitution ausüben, wie es für die „Prägung" von Instinktverhalten in sensiblen Phasen der Entwicklung bei verschiedenen Vogelarten nachgewiesen worden ist (HESS, 1975) und für eine Ausrichtung sexuellen (insbesondere sexuell devianten) Triebverhaltens beim Menschen durch einmalige – sexuell erregende – Reizeinwirkung diskutiert wird (MERKEL, 1972); allerdings dürften beim Menschen Lebenserfahrungen häufiger indirekt über eine Beeinflussung der Lebensweise auf die Konstitution einwirken (z.B. über die Entstehung eines chronischen Alkoholismus mit zum Teil irreversiblen Organschäden: FEUERLEIN, 1975; STEINBRECHER, 1975).

Unmittelbar wird die Konstitution im allgemeinen durch genetische Faktoren, die insbesondere bei den physiologischen Entwicklungsprozessen eine dominierende Rolle spielen, und/oder durch physische Einwirkungen aus der Umwelt – wie Nahrungsstoffe, Toxine, Strahlen u.dgl. – beeinflußt (MARTIN, 1966). Dabei hängt der Grad der Beeinflußbarkeit und das relative Gewicht, das der Lebenserfahrung in diesem Zusammenhang zukommt, in erheblichem Umfang von der phylogenetischen Entwicklungshöhe des Organismus ab. Die menschliche Konstitution steht im Vergleich mit der Konstitution auch hochentwickelter tierischer Organismen viel stärker unter dem unmittelbaren Einfluß der Lebenserfahrung (FORD u. BEACH, 1954). Dieser Einfluß ist insbesondere in den ersten Lebensjahren wirksam, wenn die Grundmuster des Verhaltens organisiert werden (THOMAE, 1959; SCOTT, 1962). Möglicherweise nimmt er im hohen Alter wieder zu, was durch die schon erwähnte Beschleunigung des intellektuellen Altersabbaus in reizarmer Umgebung nahegelegt wird. Demnach könnte die Regel gelten, daß der Einfluß der Lebenserfahrung von der Intensität evolutiver bzw. involutiver Prozesse in der Gesamtentwicklung eines Individuums abhängt.

Leider wird in der medizinischen Literatur – seit TANDLER (1914) und JULIUS BAUER (1924) – der Ausdruck „konstitutionell" immer wieder im Sinne von „genetisch bedingt" verwendet (CONRAD, 1963, 1967; HUBER, 1974). In dieser Fassung wäre er aber als Synonym eines eindeutig definierten Begriffes überflüssig – und damit auch der Ausdruck „Konstitution" (nämlich als Synonym für Erbanlage). Die hier verwendete weitere Fassung des Konstitutionsbegriffes verleiht ihm hingegen einen eigenen Stellenwert in der medizinischen Fachsprache und stimmt darüber hinaus vollkommen mit seiner Verwendung in der modernen anthropologischen Literatur überein (MARTIN, 1966; TANNER, 1977). So definiert KNUSSMANN (1968, S. 360) Konstitution als „*das relativ überdauernde, ganzheitliche Gefüge der körperlichen und seelischen Grundzüge des Individuums*". Nach SCHWIDETZKY (1970, S. 89) bezeichnet der Begriff „das gesamte Erscheinungs-, Funktions- und Leistungsgefüge eines Individuums in seiner *Erbbedingtheit* und *Umweltgeformtheit*. Das Hauptgewicht liegt dabei auf relativ dauerhaften Zügen (während flüchtige Modifikationen, z.B. Tonusveränderungen im Laufe des Tages, im allgemeinen außer Betracht bleiben) und auf den funktionell wichtigen Merkmalen, die die Reaktivität des Individuums beeinflussen". In ähnlichem Sinne äußern sich aber auch Mediziner wie z.B. CURTIUS (1959) oder KARL JASPERS (1973, S. 532f.). Sehr pronunziert betonen MAYER-GROSS et al. (1969, S. 75 u.a.) die Wandelbarkeit der Konstitution unter dem Einfluß äußerer Faktoren, wie überhaupt in der englischen Psychiatrie der Begriff überwiegend in dem hier dargestellten Sinne verwendet wird (REES, 1973).

II. Konstitutionsaufbau

Definitionsgemäß gehören zur Konstitution alle Merkmale eines Individuums, die seine Grundstruktur – nämlich „die relativ *umweltstabilen* und damit weitgehend *irreversiblen* und dementsprechend relativ *konstanten Anteile* des ...*Phänotypus*" – kennzeichnen (v. ZERSSEN, 1973a). In ihrer Gesamtheit ergeben diese sog. *Konstitutionsmerkmale* die psychophysische *Totalkonstitution*. Man kann die Konstitutionsmerkmale nach phänomenologischen Gesichtspunkten in bestimmte Bereiche gliedern, die jeweils als *Partialkonstitutionen* (MARTIN, 1966) Teilaspekte oder Komponenten der Totalkonstitution repräsentieren. Dabei darf freilich nicht vergessen werden, daß die Konstitution letztlich immer

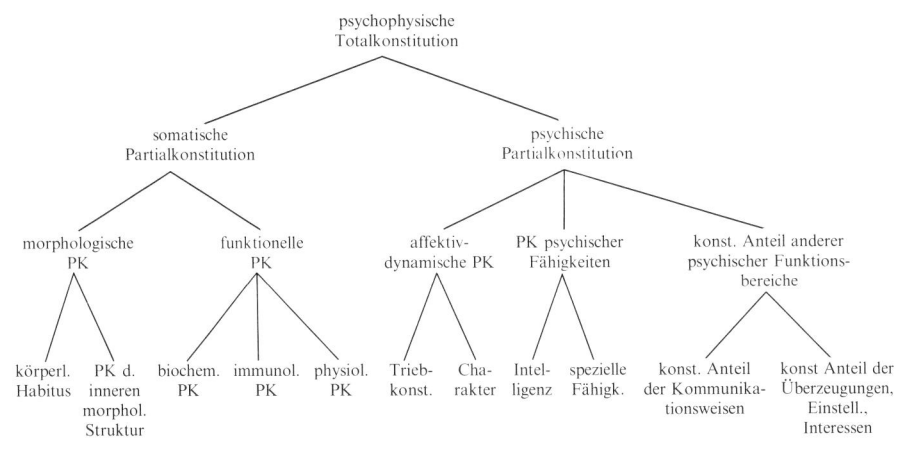

Abb. 2. Komponenten des Konstitutionsaufbaus (nach v. ZERSSEN, 1973a, erweitert)

ein Ganzes bildet, das nur im Interesse der Überschaubarkeit so dargestellt und untersucht wird, als setzte es sich aus Komponenten zusammen, die jede für sich existierten. Das ist bei der Betrachtung der Abb. 2 zu beachten, die den Aufbau der Konstitution aus einzelnen „Komponenten" – eben den Partialkonstitutionen – schematisch zur Darstellung bringt.

Es wird ohne weiteres einleuchten, daß die psychische Partialkonstitution von Hirnfunktionen abhängt, die zur somatischen Partialkonstitution zu rechnen sind. Auch ist die begriffliche Aufgliederung der somatischen Partialkonstitution nicht frei von Willkür. Dies wird besonders aus den Bezeichnungen in der untersten Reihe ersichtlich: Der körperliche Habitus – als das äußere Erscheinungsbild des Organismus – ist ja im Grunde nichts anderes als die Oberfläche seiner Binnenstruktur. Besonderheiten des Habitus gehen deshalb praktisch immer mit entsprechenden Besonderheiten der inneren morphologischen Struktur einher. Zu dieser inneren Struktur gehören der Bau der Organe, die Verteilung der Gewebe, der Aufbau der Zellen, die Zusammensetzung der Interzellularsubstanz, letztlich aber auch die Struktur der Moleküle, aus denen die Körpersubstanz zusammengesetzt ist. Die in diesem Schema getroffene Trennung von innerer morphologischer und biochemischer Partialkonstitution ist insofern nur bedingt gültig. Auch die immunologische und die physiologische Partialkonstitution lassen sich im Grunde nicht von ihrem morphologischen Substrat abstrahieren, wie es das Schema nahelegt.

Die Lebensfunktionen der somatischen Partialkonstitution *involvieren* – genau genommen – die rechts im Schema aufgeführten Komponenten der psychischen Partialkonstitution und treten nicht etwa sekundär mit ihnen zusammen, um so erst die leib-seelische Ganzheit der Totalkonstitution des Menschen zu bilden. Auch die Untergliederung der psychischen Partialkonstitution darf nicht darüber hinwegtäuschen, daß ihre verschiedenen „Komponenten" keine für sich existierenden Einheiten darstellen; sie sind vielmehr aus der Gesamtheit von relativ stabilen und damit weitgehend irreversiblen und konstanten Anteilen (s. oben) menschlichen Erlebens und Verhaltens begrifflich isoliert worden, um den Gegenstandsbereich überschaubar und einem methodischen Zugriff zugänglich zu machen. Nur unter diesem Gesichtspunkt erscheint es gerechtfertigt, die individuelle Gesamtverfassung elementar triebhafter Bedürfnisse als „Triebkonstitution" von der individuellen Struktur des Gefühls- und Willenslebens als dem „Charakter" abzutrennen und die Fähigkeiten so zu behandeln, als seien sie unabhängig von der affektiv-dynamischen Struktur eines Individuums vorhanden und entwickelten sich unabhängig von den Interessen und der Sprache eines Individuums.

Es mag verwundern, daß Sprache überhaupt einen konstitutionellen Anteil aufweisen soll, wie er in unserem Schema vorausgesetzt wird. Dieser muß aber postuliert werden, da Sprache und andere Kommunikationsweisen nur erlernt werden können, wenn eine entsprechende Lerndisposition vorhanden ist (LENNEBERG, 1972; CHOMSKY, 1976; s. auch PLOOGs Beitrag in diesem Band). Zudem übt die Muttersprache einen Einfluß auf die Entwicklung kognitiver Prozesse aus und kann auf diese Weise den Denkstil eines Menschen entscheidend mitbestimmen. Sie ist auch insofern – indirekt – am Konstitutionsaufbau beteiligt. Für die Berechtigung, ebenfalls bei Überzeugungen, Einstellungen und Interessen einen konstitutionellen Anteil anzunehmen, werden im Zusammenhang mit der Besprechung der Geschlechtskonstitution (s.S. 647) und der psychischen Partialkonstitutionen (s.S. 690) Argumente gebracht werden.

Die hier vorgenommene begriffliche Differenzierung orientiert sich im wesentlichen an den Gegenstandsbereichen etablierter wissenschaftlicher Disziplinen oder Arbeitsrichtungen. Tabelle 1 bringt eine Zuordnung der in Abb. 2 unten aufgeführten Partialkonstitutionen zu den wissenschaftlichen Disziplinen bzw. Arbeitsrichtungen, die sich vornehmlich mit ihnen beschäftigen, wobei krankhafte Konstitutionsanomalien und die für ihre Bearbeitung zuständigen Disziplinen ebenso unberücksichtigt bleiben wie jene, die sich mit den aufgeführten Partialkonstitutionen speziell unter dem Aspekt der Entwicklung befassen (wie Embryologie und Entwicklungspsychologie). Wegen der verschiedenartigen Aspekte, die bei der Beschäftigung mit der menschlichen Totalkonstitution zu berücksichtigen sind, ist ihre Erforschung eine typische Aufgabe interdisziplinärer Zusammenarbeit (TUCKER u. LESSA, 1940; v. ZERSSEN, 1976a).

III. Abstraktionsstufen des Konstitutionsbegriffs

In seiner abstraktesten Fassung bezieht sich der Konstitutionsbegriff auf das, was der Grundstruktur aller Individuen einer Art oder auch einer höheren systematischen Ordnung gemeinsam ist. In diesem Sinne kann man nicht nur von der *allgemeinen Konstitution* des Menschen oder des Schimpansen, sondern

Tabelle 1. Partialkonstitutionen als Objekte etablierter wissenschaftlicher Disziplinen oder Forschungsrichtungen

Partialkonstitution (PK)		Wissenschaftliche Disziplin
Somatische PK	Körperlicher Habitus	Körperbautypologie (als Forschungsgebiet von Anthropologie und Medizin)
	PK der inneren morphol. Struktur	Makroskop. u. mikroskop. Anatomie
	Biochemische PK	Biochemie
	Immunologische PK	Immunologie
	Physiologische PK	Physiologie
Psychische PK	Triebkonstitution	Sexualpsychologie, psychoanalytische Triebpsychologie
	Charakter	Persönlichkeitspsychologie, psychoanalytische Ichpsychologie
	Intelligenz/spez. Fähigkeiten	Intelligenzforschung
	Kommunikationsweisen[a]	Psychologische Kommunikationsforschung, Psycholinguistik
	Überzeugungen, Einstellungen, Interessen[a]	Einstellungs- und Interessenforschung

[a] konstitutioneller Anteil dieser Funktionsbereiche!

auch von der (allgemeinen) Konstitution der Primaten (PLOOG, 1964; COUNT, 1970) oder gar der Wirbeltiere sprechen. In dieser globalen Anwendung ist der Begriff logischerweise relativ merkmalsarm. Das Gegenstück bildet seine Anwendung auf ein konkretes Individuum. Er bezeichnet dann die *individuelle Konstitution* als das, was die Grundstruktur des betreffenden Individuums auszeichnet (CURTIUS, 1959).

Typische konstitutionelle Gemeinsamkeiten einer Gruppe von Individuen bezeichnet man als *Gruppenkonstitution*. Diese bildet den Gegenstand von *Konstitutionstypologien* (V. ZERSSEN, 1973a, b, 1977b). Die typologische Gliederung kann sich an verschiedenen Gesichtspunkten orientieren, bezieht sich aber immer auf das, was einer Gruppe von Individuen gemeinsam ist und sie von anderen Individuen unterscheidet, so daß innerhalb der Gruppe eine größere Ähnlichkeit zwischen den Individuen herrscht als zwischen diesen und anderen Individuen. Die Ähnlichkeit beschränkt sich allerdings gewöhnlich auf einen umschriebenen Merkmalsbereich und erlaubt – wegen der großen Variabilität der meisten in Betracht gezogenen Merkmale – keine scharfe Grenzziehung zwischen dem, was ähnlich und dem, was nicht mehr ähnlich ist. Man konstruiert deshalb gedanklich sog. *Typen*, die den Merkmalsbestand, auf dem die Ähnlichkeit bzw. Unähnlichkeit beruht, in vollkommener Ausprägung in sich vereinigen – ohne Rücksicht darauf, ob derart „typische" Merkmalskonstellationen in der Realität überhaupt vorkommen oder auch nur vorkommen können. Die Zuordnung konkreter Individuen zu einem solchen Typus erfolgt dann nach dem Grad ihrer Ähnlichkeit mit ihm (V. ZERSSEN, 1973a, b, 1977b).

Beim Vergleich verschiedener Individuen im zeitlichen Querschnitt findet man besonders eindrucksvolle Gemeinsamkeiten zwischen den Angehörigen verschiedener Altersstufen. Der Begriff *Alterskonstitution* (MARTIN, 1966) bezieht sich auf diese altersbedingten Gemeinsamkeiten. Gewöhnlich wird die „stationäre" Wachstumsphase des Erwachsenenalters von der voraufgehenden Phase intensiven Wachstums abgehoben. Diese läßt sich ihrerseits nach dem Gesichtspunkt der Ausprägung sekundärer Geschlechtsmerkmale und des Eintritts der Geschlechtsreife in Kindheit und Reifungsalter untergliedern. Die genannten Entwicklungsabschnitte können wiederum in weitere Abschnitte unterteilt werden, für die sich jeweils typische Gemeinsamkeiten angeben lassen. Eine Zuordnung von Individuen zu den unterschiedlichen Altersstufen kann deshalb mit einem relativ hohen Grad von Treffsicherheit auch ohne Kenntnis des Lebensalters aufgrund der für die verschiedenen Stufen typischen Merkmalskombinationen vorgenommen werden.

Noch eindeutiger gelingt – wenn man von seltenen Beispielen der Intersexualität (OVERZIER, 1961a; PRADER, 1978) absieht – die Zuordnung von Individuen nach dem *Geschlecht* allein anhand des Genitalbefundes. Doch dürfte von der Pubertät an in den meisten Fällen auch eine Zuordnung nach äußerlich sichtbaren sekundären Geschlechtsmerkmalen gelingen. Noch stärker als bei den Altersunterschieden wird allerdings in den meisten Kulturen der Geschlechtsunterschied durch Eigenarten von Haartracht, Schmuck und Kleidung unterstrichen. Einflüsse des sozialen Umfeldes wirken sich aber nicht nur auf geschlechtstypische Differenzen im äußeren Erscheinungsbild aus, sondern in noch stärkerem Maße auf Verhaltensunterschiede zwischen den Geschlechtern. Die Bestimmung der psychischen Geschlechtskonstitution ist dementsprechend wesentlich problematischer als die der entsprechenden somatischen Konstitution.

Aufgrund der anlagemäßigen *Bisexualität* des Menschen variiert die Ausprägung geschlechtstypischer somatischer wie psychischer Merkmale innerhalb eines Geschlechtes erheblich. Diesem Umstand trägt das Konzept der „*androgynen*" *Variation* (DRAPER, 1941) Rechnung, das sich auf die Merkmalsvariation zwischen den Extremen der geschlechtstypischen Ausprägung auf der einen Seite und der Ausprägung im gegengeschlechtlichen Sinne (bei verschiedenen Formen der Intersexualität) auf der anderen Seite bezieht (v. ZERSSEN, 1968, 1977b).

Eine andere Form der Gruppenkonstitution stellt die *rassische Konstitution* dar, womit Gemeinsamkeiten von Angehörigen größerer Fortpflanzungsgemeinschaften bezeichnet werden (SCHWIDETZKY, 1970). Auch bei der rassischen Konstitution fallen die Besonderheiten des körperlichen Habitus am stärksten auf und haben deshalb bis in neuere Zeit als Grundlage der Systematik menschlicher Rassen gedient. Erst in den letzten Jahrzehnten finden serologische Merkmale stärkere Beachtung, eignen sich aber allein nicht für die Diagnose der Rassenzugehörigkeit (SCHWIDETZKY, 1962). Bei solchen „Diagnosen" muß zudem immer berücksichtigt werden, daß die Aufhebung der Grenzen zwischen Fortpflanzungsgemeinschaften rassische Unterschiede verwischt und entsprechende Differenzierungen schwierig oder gar unmöglich macht.

Im Bereich der psychischen Konstitution stellen sich dem Versuch, echte Rasseneigentümlichkeiten nachzuweisen, auch beim Vergleich von Gruppen „reinrassiger" Individuen, besondere Schwierigkeiten entgegen; denn die Angehörigen verschiedener Rassen entstammen durchweg geographisch und bzw. oder durch Heiratsschranken innerhalb einer geographischen Region voneinander isolierten Populationen mit entsprechend unterschiedlichem kulturellem Hintergrund. Die Differenzierung von biologisch fundierten und soziokulturell bedingten psychischen Besonderheiten ist deshalb noch problematischer als bei den Geschlechtern. Daraus zu folgern, es gäbe überhaupt keine biologisch fundierten psychischen Rassenunterschiede, ist selbstverständlich wissenschaftlich nicht zulässig, geschieht aber heute häufig aus durchaus verständlichen politischen Motiven. Durch diese Politisierung wird eine wissenschaftliche Erforschung des ganzen Problemkreises zusätzlich erschwert (EYSENCK, 1975), so daß unser Kenntnisstand auf diesem Gebiet besonders dürftig ist.

Umfangreichere Forschungen als auf dem Gebiet der psychophysischen Rassenkonstitution sind über Typen der Totalkonstitution in Kollektiven gleicher Alters-, Geschlechts- und rassischer Zusammensetzung durchgeführt worden. Man ist dabei vorwiegend von der Typisierung der Variationen des körperlichen Habitus ausgegangen und hat erst sekundär nach Korrelaten dieser sog. *Körperbautypen* im Bereich der psychischen Partialkonstitution gesucht (v. ZERSSEN, 1976a). Am bekanntesten geworden sind die von KRETSCHMER (1977) beschriebenen Körperbauten der Pykniker, Leptosomen und Athletiker mit ihren *Korrelattypen* des zyklothymen, schizothymen und viskösen *Temperaments* sowie die Somatotypologie SHELDONS (SHELDON, 1949; v. ZERSSEN, 1973a, 1977b), die drei „Komponenten" des körperlichen Habitus (Endomorphie, Mesomorphie und Ektomorphie) mit drei Temperamentkomponenten (Viszerotonie, Somatotonie, Zerebrotonie) in Verbindung bringt. Diese und andere Konstitutionstypologien, die enge korrelative Beziehungen zwischen körperlichem Habitus und Temperament (als dem unmittelbar biologisch bedingten Anteil des Charakters) behaupten (SCHLEGEL, 1957; CONRAD, 1963), treten allerdings in ihrer wissenschaftlichen Bedeutung mehr und mehr in den Hintergrund, da die mit modernen objektivierenden Forschungsmethoden nachweisbaren psychomorphologischen Zusammenhänge durchweg gering sind und auch ihrer Art nach nur teilweise mit den ursprünglich mehr oder weniger intuitiv konzipierten Zusammenhängen in Einklang stehen (v. ZERSSEN, 1965a, b, 1966a, b, 1976a, 1977b).

Die älteren konstitutionstypologischen Systeme waren vor allem durch die Behauptung einer „Affinität" endogener Psychosen und anderer Formen aktueller psychischer Störungen zu den beschriebenen Körperbau- und Temperamentstypen von Interesse für die Psychiatrie (SHELDON, 1949; KRETSCHMER, 1977). Weniger Beachtung haben in diesem Fach hingegen die Beziehungen von *Anomalien des körperlichen Habitus* zu *abnormen Varianten der psychischen Partialkonstitution* gefunden, obwohl insbesondere die Zusammenhänge mit geistiger Behinderung gut gesichert sind und auch wohldefinierte Syndrome mit zumindest teilweise bekannter Ätiologie einschließen (v. ZERSSEN, 1976a). Diese Zusammenhänge gehören in den Bereich der *Konstitutionspathologie*, die in einem eigenen Abschnitt behandelt werden soll.

IV. Konstitutionspathologie

Den Gegenstand der Konstitutionspathologie bilden einerseits krankhafte Normabweichungen der Konstitution, die *Konstitutionsanomalien*, andererseits die *konstitutionelle Disposition* zu aktuellen krankhaften Störungen (CURTIUS, 1954). Bei den Anomalien handelt es sich um Normabweichungen der Konstitution selber, bei aktuellen krankhaften Störungen um prinzipiell reversible krankhafte Prozesse, welche die Kondition betreffen. Soweit krankhafte Veränderungen der Kondition nicht mehr rückbildungsfähig sind, sind sie als konstitutionell anzusprechen. Je nachdem, ob eine Störung von Entwicklungsprozessen vorgelegen hat, wodurch eine normale Merkmalsausprägung verhindert wurde, oder ob bereits normal ausgeprägte Konstitutionsmerkmale durch eine aktuelle krankhafte Störung sekundär alteriert worden sind, sollte man von *primären* oder von *sekundären Anomalien* sprechen.

Beispielsweise stellt die Verkümmerung der Extremitäten beim Dysmelie-Syndrom (WIEDEMANN et al., 1976) eine primäre körperbauliche Anomalie dar, während bei der Verstümmelung einer Extremität durch Verletzung eine sekundäre Anomalie vorliegt. Primäre Anomalien sind häufig – allerdings keineswegs immer – genetisch bedingt. Bei sekundären Anomalien verhält es sich umgekehrt. Ein Beispiel für eine nicht genetisch, sondern durch exogene Schädigung bedingte primäre (morphologische) Konstitutionsanomalie stellt das soeben erwähnte Dysmelie-Syndrom als Folgezustand einer Contergan-Einnahme der Mutter im ersten Trimenon der Schwangerschaft dar; Beispiele für genetisch bedingte sekundäre (funktionelle) Konstitutionsanomalien sind erbliche Formen des Diabetes mellitus (FROESCH u. ASSAL, 1978). Selbstverständlich liegen bei allen genetisch bedingten Anomalien bereits vor der klinischen Manifestation der Abnormität (in unserem Beispiel: des Kohlenhydratstoffwechsels) Normabweichungen vor, auch wenn sie mit den üblichen Methoden heute noch nicht nachweisbar sind. Teilweise dürfte es sich bei diesen klinisch latenten Normabweichungen um kompensierte Anomalien der Art handeln, wie sie nach Dekompensation zur klinisch manifesten Symptomatik führen; teilweise mögen auch die für die Anomalie verantwortlichen Gene erst in einem späteren Entwicklungsstadium aktiviert werden. Im letzten Falle läge primär nur eine Anomalie der betreffenden Gene vor.

Sekundäre Anomalien können als Folgezustände sowohl chronischer als auch akuter krankhafter Störungen entstehen. Die Abgrenzung chronischer Krankheitsprozesse von ihrem Wesen nach weitgehend irreversiblen konstitutionellen Anomalien kann allerdings schwierig sein. Die Grenzziehung ist insbesondere im Bereich krankhafter psychischer Normabweichungen problematisch (z.B. bei chronisch verlaufenden Neurosen und psychopathischen Entwicklungen), so daß häufig eine diagnostische Entscheidung nur mit Zurückhaltung getroffen werden kann oder ganz unterbleiben sollte. Es erscheint auch fraglich, wieweit das Gros aktueller krankhafter Störungen im somatischen wie im psychischen Bereich tatsächlich prinzipiell vollständig reversibel ist. Möglicherweise führen viele Erkrankungen, die folgenlos auszuheilen scheinen, doch zu klinisch nicht ohne weiteres erkennbaren Veränderungen der Konstitution. Diese Alterationen könnten sowohl in einer erhöhten Rezidivbereitschaft als auch in einer verminderten Anfälligkeit für die betreffenden oder auch andere Erkrankungen bestehen. So entwickelt sich eine Resistenz nach vielen Infektionskrankheiten. Die sog. Kinderkrankheiten hinterlassen sogar im allgemeinen eine lebenslange Immunität (HUMPHREY u. WHITE, 1971), die dann ein Konstitutionsmerkmal der betroffenen Individuen darstellt.

Mit den Begriffen *Anfälligkeit* und *Resistenz* ist die Disposition zu aktuellen krankhaften Störungen angesprochen (LETTERER, 1959). Unter Krankheitsdisposition versteht man den Grad der inneren Bereitschaft eines Organismus, krankhafte Störungen zu entwickeln. Diese Bereitschaft kann in Abhängigkeit von der Vitalität (v. ZERSSEN, 1973 b) *unspezifisch* vermindert bzw. (bei beeinträchtigter Vitalität) erhöht sein; häufiger kommt aber eine *spezifische* Verminderung bzw. Erhöhung der Disposition für bestimmte Krankheiten bzw. Krankheitsgruppen vor. Im engeren Sinne bezeichnet Disposition nur die erhöhte Krankheitsbereitschaft, während eine verminderte Krankheitsbereitschaft mit dem Begriff der (relativen oder absoluten) Resistenz belegt wird. Die (angeborene oder erworbene) *Immunität* ist *eine* Form der Resistenz.

Krankheitsdispositionen können ebenso wie die Resistenz angeboren oder erworben sein. Es gibt allerdings auch eine (vorübergehende) erworbene Resistenz, die angeboren ist, nämlich die auf der Übertragung mütterlicher Immunkörper beruhende Immunität gegenüber sog. Kinderkrankheiten, die gewöhnlich von der Geburt an über Monate erhalten bleibt (HUMPHREY u. WHITE, 1971). Im allgemeinen ist aber eine angeborene Resistenz genetisch bedingt und insofern schon konstitutionell. Eine erworbene Resistenz kann vorübergehender Natur sein oder lebenslang – unabhängig von den äußeren Lebensbedingungen – bestehen bleiben und somit konstitutionell sein. Entsprechendes gilt für Krankheitsdispositionen; allerdings können Resistenz und Disposition auch an bestimmte Entwicklungsphasen gebunden und dadurch Bestandteile der Alterskonstitution sein.

Außer der Disposition zur Entstehung sekundärer Konstitutionsanomalien, die ihrem Wesen nach selbst konstitutionell sind, gibt es eine konstitutionelle Disposition zu aktuellen krankhaften Störungen, die ihrerseits nicht zur Konstitution gehören, sondern lediglich krankhafte Veränderungen der aktuellen Kondition des Organismus darstellen. Die Verhältnisse lassen sich anhand der schematischen Darstellung der Interaktion von Organismus und Umwelt in Abb. 1 veranschaulichen. Die Einwirkung aus der Umwelt ist in diesem Zusammenhang lediglich als pathogene Situation zu interpretieren und der in den Organismus eindringende Reiz dementsprechend als schädigendes Agens zu betrachten. Dabei ist es gleichgültig, ob es sich um eine allein aufgrund ihrer physikochemischen Eigenschaften pathogen wirkende Noxe handelt (etwa einen Giftstoff) oder um einen Reiz bzw. eine Reizfolge, die durch ihren Informationsgehalt für das betroffene Individuum zu einem pathogenen Faktor wird (etwa bei einer „kränkenden" Äußerung, die neurotisch verarbeitet wird). Wieweit die Reizantwort des Individuums krankhaft ist, die im Schema durch einen vom Organismus ausgehenden Pfeil symbolisierte Reaktion also den Charakter eines Krankheitssymptoms annimmt, hängt einerseits vom momentanen Zustand des Individuums bei der Reizeinwirkung (seiner Kondition) ab; andererseits wird sie aber auch von der situationsunabhängigen Grundbeschaffenheit des Individuums (seiner

Konstitution) bestimmt, was durch den im Schema vom „Kern" in die „Schale" gerichteten Pfeil angedeutet wird. Die in entgegengesetzte Richtung weisende kleinere Pfeilspitze macht darauf aufmerksam, daß krankhafte Zustände u.U. ihrerseits auf die Konstitution einwirken, die Grundstruktur des Individuums also dauerhaft verändern können.

Das Schema macht verständlich, daß die Wahrscheinlichkeit für das Auftreten einer Erkrankung einerseits von konstitutioneller und konditioneller *Disposition*, andererseits aber von der *Exposition* des Organismus gegenüber den pathogenen Einwirkungen aus der Umwelt abhängt. Dies gilt für psychische Erkrankungen ebenso wie für somatische. Für die Entstehung der Disposition zu psychischen Erkrankungen spielt allerdings die individuelle *Lerngeschichte* eine besondere Rolle (KANFER u. PHILLIPS, 1975). Ebenfalls kommt bei vielen aktuellen psychischen Störungen pathogenen Situationen im *sozialen Umfeld* ein vergleichsweise starkes Gewicht zu. Soweit derartige dispositionelle und peristatische Faktoren bei somatischen Störungen in den Vordergrund treten, bezeichnet man diese als *psychosomatische Erkrankungen*. Der Thematik des Handbuches entsprechend werden die Beispiele im speziellen Teil dieser Darstellung aber im wesentlichen auf die Entstehung psychischer Krankheiten beschränkt bleiben und auch die Konstitutionsanomalien nur soweit behandeln, wie sie die psychische Partialkonstitution betreffen oder – bei Anomalien der Totalkonstitution – einbeziehen.

Häufig sind die inneren und äußeren Faktoren der Krankheitsentstehung und die Art ihres Zusammenwirkens im einzelnen nicht oder nicht genau bekannt; insbesondere ist dies bei Erkrankungen mit einer multikonditionellen Genese der Fall, bei denen kein Faktor als *conditio sine qua non* und damit als eigentliche Krankheitsursache anzusprechen ist. Man kann womöglich nur eine Reihe innerer und äußerer Faktoren angeben, die bei erkrankten Individuen häufiger als bei anderen nachzuweisen sind und deren Vorkommen bei (noch) nicht Erkrankten das Risiko einer späteren Erkrankung erhöht. Sie werden daher als *Risikofaktoren* bezeichnet (PFLANZ, 1973).

Man kann auch dann von Risikofaktoren sprechen, wenn *ein* pathogenes Agens als *conditio sine qua non* isoliert werden kann, aber allein nicht ausreicht, um die Krankheitsentstehung zu erklären. Dies gilt z.B. für den Alkohol, der zwar eine notwendige, aber nicht hinreichende Bedingung für die Entstehung eines Alkoholismus darstellt (FEUERLEIN, 1975). Risikofaktoren, die die Wahrscheinlichkeit dafür erhöhen, daß Alkohol in einer zur Abhängigkeit führenden Weise mißbraucht wird, betreffen einmal die Exposition (Leben in einem Weinanbaugebiet, Tätigkeit im Gaststättengewerbe etc.), zum anderen die Disposition, wobei konditionelle Faktoren (z.B. neurotische Konfliktspannungen) von konstitutionellen Faktoren (z.B. männliches Geschlecht) zu unterscheiden sind.

Solche Risikofaktoren können selbst echte Bedingungsfaktoren darstellen oder lediglich Indikatoren für das Vorliegen solcher Bedingungsfaktoren bilden. So können beispielsweise Merkmale, die sich gar nicht auf das Individuum selbst beziehen, als Indikatoren für dispositionelle Faktoren dienen, etwa Leben in einsamer Umgebung als Indikator für Mangel an sozialer Kommunikation und für Vereinsamungsgefühl, Alkoholismus bei Blutsverwandten als Indikator für eine in der genetischen Konstitution begründeten Krankheitsdisposition. Gerade das letzte Beispiel zeigt aber, daß Risikofaktoren im individuellen Falle einen sehr unterschiedlichen Stellenwert in der Ätiopathogenese einnehmen können: Alkoholismus bei (insbesondere mehreren und nahen) Blutsverwandten kann, muß aber nicht auf eine genetische Disposition zum Alkoholismus hinweisen. Im Einzelfall können die Trinkgewohnheiten der Angehörigen auch auf dem Wege sozialen Lernens übernommen worden sein – sie können jedoch auch abschreckend gewirkt und dadurch indirekt eine gewisse Schutzfunktion ausgeübt haben.

Bei ätiopathogenetischen Studien sollte grundsätzlich außer nach Risikofaktoren immer auch nach Faktoren gefahndet werden, die die Krankheitswahrscheinlichkeit *verringern* bzw. auf einen relativ günstigen Krankheitsverlauf hinweisen. Sie stellen manchmal, aber keineswegs regelmäßig, das Gegenteil der

Risikofaktoren dar (z.b. bei psychogenen Erkrankungen subjektiv positiv versus negativ gewertete Lebensereignisse oder das Vorhandensein einer Vertrauensperson in der Umgebung des Patienten versus soziale Isolierung). Über der Suche nach Risiko- und nach *Ausgleichsfaktoren* darf aber nicht vergessen werden, daß es letztlich darauf ankommt zu ergründen, wie das Krankheitsgeschehen mit diesen Faktoren verknüpft ist, ob z.b. Männer aufgrund biologischer Geschlechtsunterschiede oder aufgrund gesellschaftlich determinierter Verhaltenseigenschaften häufiger dem Alkohol verfallen als Frauen bzw. wieweit und auf welche Weise bei dieser geschlechtsabhängigen Krankheitsdisposition biologische und soziale Faktoren zusammenwirken.

V. Konsequenzen für die klinische Arbeit

Aus der Darstellung der Konstitutionspathologie ergeben sich folgende Konsequenzen für die praktisch-klinische Arbeit:

In der *Diagnostik* ist auf Konstitutionsanomalien zu achten und danach zu fragen, ob eine Kombination von Anomalien verschiedener Partialkonstitutionen vorliegt, die womöglich eine gemeinsame Ursache haben (wie bei vielen erblichen Syndromen bzw. chromosomalen Aberrationen, aber auch bei exogener Schädigung, insbesondere in frühen Entwicklungsabschnitten). Sodann ist zu prüfen, wieweit sich die festgestellten Anomalien nachteilig für das betroffene Individuum auswirken bzw. in Zukunft (z.B. unter besonderen Belastungen) auswirken könnten.

Bei den meisten Erkrankungen können – abgesehen von Konstitutionsanomalien – auch an sich normale konstitutionelle Eigentümlichkeiten (z.B. normale Persönlichkeitsvarianten; s. Kap. „Partialkonstitutionen", S. 684ff.) eine die Entstehung und den Verlauf günstig oder ungünstig beeinflussende Rolle spielen. Bei der *Prognostik* von Erkrankungen muß demnach der konstitutionelle Anteil am Zustandekommen und an der Unterhaltung bzw. Überwindung des Krankheitsgeschehens gebührend gewürdigt werden. Im allgemeinen trübt eine starke Beteiligung konstitutioneller Faktoren in der Ätiopathogenese die Prognose einer Erkrankung. Das Augenmerk muß aber auch auf solche konstitutionellen Faktoren gerichtet werden, die einen günstigen Einfluß auf den Krankheitsverlauf ausüben könnten, z.B. eine prämorbid ausgeglichene – „syntone" – Charakterstruktur auf den Verlauf einer schizophrenen Psychose (HUBER et al., 1978). Im übrigen können sich gewisse Konstitutionsanomalien durch eine starke Bindung an die Alterskonstitution im Laufe der Entwicklung ausgleichen. Dies gilt insbesondere für psychische Normabweichungen, z.B. eine „Neuropathie" (HARBAUER, 1976a), die sich schon beim Neugeborenen manifestieren, aber im Laufe der Entwicklung weitgehend zurückbilden kann. Dabei spielen äußere Einflüsse zweifellos eine beträchtliche Rolle, so daß gerade in früheren Entwicklungsstadien oft noch eine therapeutische Beeinflussung möglich ist.

Die Feststellung von Konstitutionsanomalien bzw. konstitutionellen Krankheitsbereitschaften schließt somit keineswegs die Möglichkeit gezielter *therapeutischer* Maßnahmen aus. Je nach Art der vorliegenden Anomalien bzw. Bereitschaften kommen verschiedenartige therapeutische Prinzipien zur Anwendung, von denen die wichtigsten hier aufgeführt seien. Bei morphologischen Anomalien (z.B. Mißbildungen und narbigen Defekten) besteht nicht selten die Möglichkeit der *operativen Korrektur* durch Resektion einer Fehlbildung bzw. eines narbigen Defektes oder durch einen plastischen Eingriff (wie den operativen Verschluß einer Hasenscharte). Das Ergebnis solcher Eingriffe kann auch für die psychische Entwicklung eines Individuums von entscheidender Bedeutung sein. Dies gilt insbesondere für die operative Korrektur genitaler Anomalien bei Intersexen, die möglichst noch vor Ausbildung der psychischen Geschlechtsidentifikation im zweiten/dritten Lebensjahr vorgenommen werden sollte (MONEY u. EHRHARDT, 1972).

Ein weiteres therapeutisches Prinzip besteht in der *Substitution* fehlender Körperteile durch Prothesen, wozu auch die Zahnprothetik zu rechnen ist. Bei Anomalien der biochemischen Partialkonstitution kommt evtl. eine pharmakologische Substitution in Frage, indem eine in unzureichender Menge gebildete körpereigene Substanz künstlich von außen zugeführt wird, wie bei der Substitutionstherapie des Insulinmangel-Diabetes. Umgekehrt gibt es die Möglichkeit einer pharmakologischen *Suppressions*therapie zur Unterdrückung einer konstitutionell erhöhten Produktion endogener Reize (z.B. bei der Epilepsie; s. unten) oder körpereigener Substanzen.

Bei der Behandlung des adrenogenitalen Syndroms werden beide therapeutischen Prinzipien (pharmakologische Substitution und Suppression) insofern miteinander kombiniert, als das von außen zugeführte Kortikoid-Präparat (z.B. Dexamethason) gleichzeitig das unzureichend gebildete Nebennierenrindenhormon (Cortisol) substituiert und die kompensatorische Hypersekretion des adrenokortikotropen Hypophysenhormons (ACTH) und damit – indirekt – auch die ACTH-bedingte Hypersekretion von adrenalen Androgenen supprimiert. Um eine pharmakologische Suppressionstherapie handelt es sich auch bei der medikamentösen Unterdrückung einer erhöhten zerebralen Anfallsbereitschaft durch die Dauereinstellung auf ein Antiepileptikum. Bei der Lithium-Prophylaxe affektiver Psychosen könnte es sich ebenfalls um die pharmakologische Suppressionstherapie einer konstitutionell erhöhten Krankheitsbereitschaft handeln. Allerdings ist über den Wirkungsmechanismus des Lithium sehr viel weniger bekannt als über den der Antiepileptika; darüber hinaus fehlt bei den affektiven Psychosen der Nachweis einer zerebralen Dysfunktion im freien Intervall, wie er für die meisten Formen der Epilepsie durch die Feststellung von Krampfpotentialen sowie unspezifischen Auffälligkeiten des Kurvenverlaufs im Elektroenzephalogramm (EEG) erbracht werden kann (KUGLER, 1966). Soweit diese EEG-Befunde nicht auf einen aktuellen Krankheitsprozeß (Hirntumor, Enzephalitis, Hypoglykämie bei insulinproduzierendem Inselzelladenom des Pankreas o.dgl.) zurückzuführen sind, muß man sie als Merkmale einer – primären oder sekundären (z.B. durch einen narbigen Defekt bedingten) – Konstitutionsanomalie der Hirnfunktion – also einer Abnormität der physiologischen Partialkonstitution – betrachten.

Besteht eine Stoffwechselanomalie darin, daß ein physiologischer Nahrungsbestandteil nicht oder nur unzureichend abgebaut werden kann (wie bei der Phenylketonurie), besteht die Möglichkeit, eine von den betreffenden Bestandteilen freie Diät zu verabfolgen (BICKEL u. KAISER-GRUBEL, 1971). Hierher ist auch die Einschränkung der Kohlenhydratzufuhr beim Diabetes mellitus zu rechnen. Im Prinzip handelt es sich um das Negativ der Substitutionstherapie.

Bei der *Kompensations*therapie handelt es sich um den Versuch, für die vorhandene Normabweichung einen Ausgleich durch die Mobilisierung von körpereigenen Reserven zu schaffen. In diesen Rahmen gehört auch die Übungstherapie, durch die beispielsweise irreversible Lähmungen u.U. funktionell weitgehend kompensiert werden können.

Die Übungstherapie leitet über zu *rehabilitativen* Maßnahmen, die bei krankhaften Konstitutionsanomalien von grundlegender Bedeutung sind und ebenfalls bei stark konstitutionsabhängigen, zur Chronifizierung neigenden Krankheiten eine bedeutsame Rolle spielen. Diese Maßnahmen dürfen sich nicht auf den häufig vergeblichen Versuch beschränken, einen vollen Funktionsausgleich der konstitutionellen Behinderung zu erreichen; vielmehr sind alle Möglichkeiten auszuschöpfen, die dazu beitragen, den Behinderten in das Leben in der Gemeinschaft zu reintegrieren, „wo er den besten Gebrauch von seinen Restfähigkeiten machen kann" (GOLDBERG, 1967). Scheitert eine Rehabilitation an der Schwere der Anomalie (z.B. bei hochgradiger Oligophrenie oder fortgeschrittener Demenz), so muß – wie bei unheilbaren, schweren Krankheitsprozessen – versucht werden, durch intensive *Pflege* das Schicksal des Patienten zu erleichtern.

Nicht zu vergessen sind auch die Möglichkeiten der *Prävention*, mögen sie auch noch so beschränkt sein. Eine primäre Prävention, die darauf abzielt, das Auftreten von Konstitutionsanomalien und konstitutionsabhängigen Krankheiten zu verhüten, wird in der genetischen Beratung versucht (FUHRMANN u. VOGEL, 1968; BERG, 1976). Durch sie wird jedoch allenfalls die Wahrscheinlichkeit für die Zeugung eines mit einer genetisch bedingten Konstitutionsanomalie behafteten Kindes reduziert. Durch intrauterine und perinatale Diagnostik im Rahmen von Schwangerenbetreuung und Geburtshilfe wird aber darüber hinaus die Möglichkeit frühzeitigen Eingreifens in einen gestörten Entwicklungsprozeß gegeben (EGGERS et al., 1976), was einer sekundären Prävention auf der Basis der Früherkennung gleichkommen kann. Auch im späteren Leben ist eine Prävention von (sekundären) Konstitutionsanomalien möglich, wenn die Entstehung von zur Defektbildung neigenden Krankheiten verhütet bzw. bei ausgebrochener Erkrankung alles getan wird, um eine möglichst weitgehende Remission zu erreichen.

Schließlich können umfassende *bevölkerungs-* und *gesundheitspolitische* Maßnahmen dazu verhelfen, Faktoren, die zur Entstehung von Konstitutionsanomalien führen oder beitragen, unter Kontrolle zu bringen. Dazu gehört das Verbot von Verwandtenehen zur Verhütung von (rezessiven) Erbkrankheiten, die Besteuerung von alkoholischen Getränken zur Einschränkung des Alkoholkonsums (ERNST, 1979) mit seinen u. U. konstitutionsschädigenden Konsequenzen (wie Leberzirrhose, alkoholische Demenz, Alkoholembryopathie) oder die Geburtenkontrolle sowie Verbesserung der Ernährungslage und der Hygiene in Entwicklungsländern zur Verhütung von Mangelernährung und Volksseuchen mit ihren oft bleibenden gesundheitlichen Folgeschäden.

B. Spezieller Teil

In diesem Abschnitt werden die im Allgemeinen Teil entwickelten Gesichtspunkte auf psychiatrische Probleme angewendet. Die Darstellung beinhaltet somit die Grundzüge einer psychiatrischen Konstitutionslehre.

I. Allgemeine Konstitution

Bei keiner anderen biologischen Spezies ist eine solche Fülle krankhafter Normabweichungen bekannt wie beim Menschen. Dies trifft in besonderem Maße auf sein Verhalten zu, welches – mit der stammesgeschichtlichen Zunahme von *Differenziertheit* und mit dem Gewinn von *Freiheitsgraden* (d.h. der geringeren Determiniertheit durch zeitlich vorausgehendes Verhalten und durch die momentane Umweltsituation) einhergehend – eine erhöhte *Störanfälligkeit* aufweist. Sie ist demnach in der artspezifischen (allgemeinen) Konstitution begründet, wird aber darüber hinaus noch durch selbstgeschaffene Umweltbedingungen – die menschliche Zivilisation – akzentuiert. Bestrebungen der Psychohygiene sind deswegen immer wieder auf Änderungen zivilisatorischer, insbesondere gesellschaftlicher Bedingungen gerichtet. Dabei wird freilich häufig außer acht gelassen, daß eine Optimierung äußerer Lebensbedingungen immer nur im Hinblick auf die Konstitution der Individuen, deren „Lebensqualität" verbessert werden soll, gelingen kann. Viele wohlgemeinte Bestrebungen zur Verbesserung dieser Qualität sind durch die unzureichende Berücksichtigung von konstitutionellen, in der Grundausstattung der Individuen liegenden Bedingungen zum Scheitern verurteilt.

Die psychische Störanfälligkeit des Menschen hängt einmal mit der auch gegenüber anderen Primaten weit fortgeschrittenen *Zerebralisation* zusammen (PLOOG, 1964; JUNG, 1967). Die Komplexität der zerebralen Organisation erhöht nicht nur die Vielfalt von Verhaltensweisen und Anpassungsmöglichkeiten, sondern auch die von Verhaltensstörungen und Fehlanpassungen. Die für den Aufbau zerebraler Strukturen erforderlichen Entwicklungsschritte sind so zahlreich und verteilen sich in der Ontogenese auf einen so langen Zeitraum, daß schon von daher die Wahrscheinlichkeit für das Auftreten von zerebralen Entwicklungsstörungen sehr viel größer ist als beim Aufbau einfacherer Strukturen; denn es ist sowohl die Zahl der für die Hirnentwicklung bedeutsamen *Gene* ungleich größer als bei anderen Spezies als auch der Zeitraum länger, in dem *exogene Faktoren* störend in diesen Ablauf eingreifen können. Darüber hinaus steht die Entwicklung des menschlichen Hirns viel stärker unter dem Einfluß individueller Lebenserfahrungen als bei anderen Arten. Der Komplexität der Reifungsgeschichte geht somit die Komplexität der *Lerngeschichte* parallel (KANFER u. PHILLIPS, 1975), so daß – außer den ihrer Natur nach körperlichen Schädigungsfaktoren – erfahrungsabhängige „Fehlprogrammierungen" des Verhaltens als Bedingungsfaktoren krankhafter Verhaltensauffälligkeiten eine entscheidende Rolle spielen können. Auch wenn es sich dabei überwiegend um prinzipiell reversible Normabweichungen handelt, die somit der Kondition und nicht der Konstitution zuzurechnen sind, schafft doch erst die Konstitution die Voraussetzungen dafür, daß die Erfahrung einen derartigen Einfluß auf die Verhaltensentwicklung und damit auch auf die Entwicklung von Verhaltensstörungen gewinnen kann.

Der Mensch ist nicht nur durch die Komplexität seiner zerebralen Organisation und die mit ihr verbundene lange Reifungs- und Lerngeschichte charakterisiert, sondern insbesondere auch durch sein Leben in sozialen Verbänden. Er ist seiner Konstitution nach als ein „ῷον πολιτικόν" (Aristoteles) angelegt und dadurch auf *soziale Kommunikation* und *Interaktion* angewiesen (COUNT, 1970; EIBL-EIBESFELDT, 1978; s. PLOOGS Beitrag in diesem Band). Diese Lebensweise hat eine der hohen Zerebralisation entsprechende Lebensform geschaffen, die menschliche Gemeinschaften grundsätzlich von allen tierischen unterscheidet: Es ist die auf einer Art „Selbstdomestikation" (LORENZ, 1943) beruhende

Zivilisation. Der Begriff wird hier in einem sehr allgemeinen Sinne und nicht nur als Lebensform industrialisierter Gesellschaften verstanden oder als rational-technologisches Gegenstück zur stärker emotional verankerten künstlerisch-schöpferischen Kultur aufgefaßt. Durch die Zivilisation ist der Mensch zwar nicht mehr so unmittelbar von der Natur abhängig wie alle anderen Lebewesen, hat sich aber durch eine künstliche Umwelt und durch eine starke Komplizierung und Anonymisierung sozialer Beziehungen auch eine Fülle *pathogener Lebensbedingungen* geschaffen, die zu Normabweichungen des Verhaltens führen können. Diese Faktoren reichen vom organisierten und öffentlich propagierten Alkoholangebot bis zum „Leistungsstreß" und seinem Gegenstück, der Langeweile.

Die Zivilisation bringt nicht nur eine Fülle pathogener Situationen hervor; sie reduziert auch den Einfluß der natürlichen Selektion. Dadurch werden die Überlebenschancen abnormer Varianten entsprechend erhöht. Das gilt auch für abnorme Varianten des Verhaltens. Analoge Varianten lassen sich zwar z.T. unter „Laborbedingungen" auch bei verschiedenen Tierarten – teils durch Züchtungsexperimente, teils durch exogene Schädigung – erzeugen (Fox, 1968), würden jedoch unter natürlichen Lebensbedingungen die Überlebenschance der betroffenen Individuen stark verringern und dadurch – zumindest über mehrere Generationen hinweg – eliminiert werden. Diese natürlichen Auslesebedingungen sind aber in menschlichen Gesellschaften – insbesondere den zivilisatorisch weit fortgeschrittenen – stark eingeschränkt. Das hat zweifellos mit zur großen Vielfalt von Verhaltensstörungen beim Menschen beigetragen. Die abnormen Varianten stellen aber definitionsgemäß eine Ausnahme dar und werden deshalb speziell bei der Besprechung der Gruppenkonstitution abgehandelt.

II. Gruppenkonstitution

Während die allgemeine Konstitution des Menschen durchgehend genetisch bestimmt ist, beruhen die konstitutionellen Gemeinsamkeiten bestimmter Gruppen von Menschen, die dem Begriff der Gruppenkonstitution zugrunde liegen, teils auf genetischen, teils auf nicht-genetischen Übereinstimmungen verschiedener Individuen. Sie können auf einzelne Partialkonstitutionen beschränkt sein, aber auch die Totalkonstitution betreffen.

1. Totalkonstitution

a) Alterskonstitution

Die über epochale und kulturelle Unterschiede hinweg nachweisbaren Gemeinsamkeiten von Angehörigen der gleichen Alters- (genauer gesagt Entwicklungs-)Stufe beruhen letztlich auf der sequentiellen Aktivierung von Genen sowie auf physikochemischen Gewebsalterationen, die sich – im Zusammenhang mit einem genetisch bedingten Nachlassen der Zellteilung – sowohl in den Körperzellen selber als auch besonders in der sie umgebenden Interzellularsubstanz abspielen (Bürger, 1960). Im höheren Lebensalter treten Funktionsstörungen durch abnorme DNA-Mutanten hinzu, die infolge zunehmender Insuffizienz zellulärer Repair-Mechanismen und einem Schwund der immunologischen Kompetenz nicht mehr eliminiert werden (Walford, 1974; Hildemann, 1978; s. auch Platt, 1976; Walter, 1978). Dadurch kommt es – auch ohne zusätzliche äußere Belastungen – mit der Zeit zum Untergang der Zellen und schließlich zum natürlichen Alterstod des Organismus (BRÜCKEL, 1975). Die Entwicklung vollzieht sich aber immer in der Auseinandersetzung mit der Umwelt (THOMPSON, 1968), und diese weist gerade beim Menschen alterstypische Unterschiede auf, die auf institutionalisierten Formen des Zusammenlebens und den mit ihnen verbundenen Forderungen, Förderungen und Einschränkungen beruhen. Das ist auch bei der ätiopathogenetischen Analyse der *Altersdisposition* für psychische Normabweichungen zu berücksichtigen. MAYER-GROSS et al. (1969) führen dazu aus: "As the individual develops, so his constitution constantly changes. Although the genetic equipment is always the same, at different times of his life a different constellation of genes is playing the critical role. The constitution is very different at the age of seven from what it is at seventeen, at forty-seven or seventy-seven. At these ages, also, the type of environmental factors which is important for further development will change. At any particular time, the reactions of an individual are the *compound result of a complexity of forces*" (S. 29f).

Daß beispielsweise Schulphobien mit der Zeit der Einschulung beginnen und im allgemeinen während der Grundschulzeit einen Manifestationsgipfel erreichen, hängt offenkundig mit den neuen institutionellen Anforderungen zusammen, die in dieser Zeit an das Kind gestellt werden. Die phobische Reaktionsweise ist andererseits – auch unabhängig von solchen Anforderungen – in der frühen bis mittleren Kindheit besonders ausgeprägt, wenngleich sich für sie keine eindeutige Bindung an eine bestimmte Entwicklungsstufe feststellen läßt. Immerhin werden andersartige neurotische Reaktionsweisen – wie die anankastische – offenbar in einem späteren Entwicklungsstadium angelegt als die phobische (NISSEN, 1976c).

Anstelle einer auf Vollständigkeit abzielenden Literaturübersicht über altersabhängige konstitutionelle Unterschiede in der Entwicklung psychischer Normabweichungen soll anhand der Tabelle 2 besprochen werden, welche psychischen Konstitutionsanomalien oder konstitutionsabhängigen psychischen Störungen sich in welchem Entwicklungsabschnitt am häufigsten erstmals manifestieren (s. auch V. BAEYER, 1977) und wodurch diese Entwicklungsabschnitte in anderer Hinsicht gekennzeichnet sind (s. auch THOMAE, 1959; MÖNKS et al., 1976).

Schon im Säuglingsalter können sich *psychische Konstitutionsanomalien* manifestieren. Von ihnen zeigt die als *Neuropathie* (HARBAUER, 1976a) bezeichnete allgemeine Nervosität die stärkste Bindung an die Alterskonstitution und damit eine vergleichsweise günstige Prognose.

Zeichen erhöhter nervöser Erregbarkeit machen sich in Form von häufigem Schreien, starker psychomotorischer Unruhe, Schreckhaftigkeit, Schlafstörungen und Schwierigkeiten bei der Nahrungsaufnahme oft schon frühzeitig bemerkbar, ohne daß dafür immer ungünstige Milieuverhältnisse anzuschuldigen wären. Die weitere Entwicklung dieser Anomalie hängt in starkem Umfange davon ab, wie die Umwelt – insbesondere die Mutter – auf die Symptome reagiert. Es kann sich ein Circulus vitiosus zwischen der erhöhten nervösen Erregbarkeit des Säuglings und hilfloser Verzweiflung seiner Mutter entwickeln und so eine Überwindung der Störung erschweren. Umgekehrt kann die Abschirmung des Säuglings gegenüber ihn belastenden Reizsituationen den weiteren Verlauf günstig beeinflussen. Möglicherweise liegt der Normabweichung häufig eine funktionelle Unreife zugrunde, die im Laufe der Entwicklung ausgeglichen wird; jedenfalls wäre es verfehlt, neuropathische Symptome als Vorboten einer psychopathischen Entwicklung in späteren Lebensjahren anzusehen, obwohl in einigen Fällen eine erhöhte nervöse Erregbarkeit auch unter keineswegs ungünstigen Umweltbedingungen bestehen bleibt. Insgesamt hängt aber die Prognose in starkem Umfange von Milieubedingungen ab.

Tabelle 2. Stufen der Konstitutionsentwicklung (nach v. ZERSSEN, 1977b, erweitert)

Entwicklungs-Stufe	Alter (Jahre)	Körperliche Merkmale	Psychische Merkmale	Psychiat. Erkrankungen (Gipfel d. Erstmanifest.)
Kindheit	0–10			
Säuglingsalter	0–1	Betonte Entwicklung von Kopf und Fettpolstern bei allgemein raschem Wachstum, primitive Motorik, Zahnen	Trieb- u. Affektbestimmtheit, Entwicklung von Wahrnehmung, präverbaler Kommunikation und sozialer Bindung	Neuropathie, Oligophrenie, infantiler Autismus,
Kleinkindalter	1–4	Aufrechter Gang, differenzierte Motorik, Beherrschung der Ausscheidungsfunktionen	Entwicklung von Denken, Sprache u. Ichbewußtsein, Identifikation mit der Geschlechtsrolle,	frühkindl. exogenes Psychosyndrom, Pavor nocturnus,
Vorschulalter	4–6	Betontes Längenwachstum bei allgemein verlangsamtem Wachstumstempo	Gruppenspiele, stärkere Verselbständigung, Leistungsmotivation, Aufgabenorientiertheit,	Enuresis, Stottern, Legasthenie,
Grundschulalter	6–10	Zahnwechsel, verstärktes Muskelwachstum	Fähigkeit zur Einordnung in eine Arbeitsgruppe	Nägelbeißen, Tics
Reifungsalter	10–18			
Vorpubertät	10–13	Ausbildung der sekundären Geschlechtsmerkmale, Wachstumsschub	Aktive Gruppenbildung, beginnende Ablösung vom Elternhaus, erhöhte sexuelle Stimulierbarkeit, Ausprägung d. sexuellen Orientierung, zunehmende sex. Aktivität, Abschluß der Intelligenzreifung	Psychopathie, Dissozialität, sex. Deviationen,
Pubertät	13–15	Geschlechtsreife, vorübergehende körperliche Disproportionierung		Anorexia nervosa, Zwangsneurose, Rauschdrogensucht
Adoleszenz	15–18	Ausklingen der Phase intensiven Wachstums		
Erwachsenenalter	18–			
Alter der körperl. Vollreife	18–45	Allmähliche Zunahme der Körperfülle („Pyknomorphierung") – bei ♀ Erlöschen der Fortpflanzungsfähigkeit –	Familiengründung, Stabilisierung der Sozialbeziehungen, soziale und berufliche Kompetenz	Schizophrene Psychosen, schizoaffekt. Psychosen, bipolare affekt. Psychosen, monopol. end. Depression
Involutionsalter	45–60			
Präsenium	60–70	Nachlassen d. körperl. Leistungsfähigkeit, Zahnverlust, zunehmender Verlust d. Hautturgors, Vermind. d. Körperhöhe, Rückbildung v. Muskulatur u. Fettgewebe	Nachlassen von sexueller Aktivität, Gedächtnisleistungen, seelischer Spannkraft und Flexibilität	Präsenile Demenz, arteriosklerot. Verwirrtheitszustände u. Demenz, senile Demenz
Senium	70–			

Anders liegen die Verhältnisse bei der *Oligophrenie*, also einer anlagebedingten oder früh erworbenen Behinderung der intellektuellen Entwicklung (HARBAUER, 1976b; INGALLS, 1978). Zwar können Milieueinflüsse eine solche Behinderung noch verstärken oder – zumindest in ihren Auswirkungen – abschwächen. Kompensieren lassen sie sich dadurch aber nicht, und auch eine spontane Rückbildung der Behinderung ist nicht zu erwarten; allerdings gibt es sog. *Spätentwickler*, die anfänglich den Eindruck von *Lernbehinderten* machen können. Die Gefahr einer Fehlbeurteilung besteht besonders dann, wenn man die Diagnose aufgrund verzögerter Funktionsreifung anhand von Normentabellen möglichst frühzeitig zu stellen versucht und dabei der Differentialdiagnose zwischen Lernbehinderung und lediglich verzögerter Entwicklung nicht genügend Beachtung schenkt.

Deshalb empfiehlt es sich, die diagnostische Entscheidung nicht schon im Säuglingsalter treffen zu wollen – es sei denn, daß ein hochgradiger Entwicklungsrückstand vorliegt oder sich andere (indirekte) Hinweise für eine Oligophrenie finden (charakteristische körperliche Dysplasien, sichere neurologische Zeichen, chromosomale Aberrationen, Stoffwechselanomalien). Im Falle einer Phenylketonurie kann durch eine Phenylalanin-freie Diät die Entstehung einer Oligophrenie u.U. verhindert bzw. – soweit eine solche schon besteht, sich aber noch im Anfangsstadium befindet – die weitere geistige Entwicklung günstig beeinflußt werden (BICKEL u. KAISER-GRUBEL, 1971).

Liegt bei der Oligophrenie vor allem eine gestörte Entwicklung von Denk- und Lernprozessen vor, so handelt es sich beim *infantilen Autismus* (NISSEN, 1976d; KEHRER, 1978) vornehmlich um eine Störung der Entwicklung von sozialer Perzeption mit spezifischer Beeinträchtigung von sprachlicher und nichtsprachlicher Kommunikation und sozialer Bindung. Wie bei der Oligophrenie scheinen für die Entstehung genetische Faktoren und exogene Hirnschäden in Frage zu kommen, während Milieueinflüsse nur eine modifizierende Rolle spielen dürften.

Die Störung macht sich gewöhnlich schon im Säuglingsalter bemerkbar, läßt sich aber erst im Kleinkindalter mit einiger Sicherheit diagnostizieren. Die Entwicklung ist im allgemeinen ungünstig und therapeutisch schwer zu beeinflussen. Immerhin können durch heilpädagogische Maßnahmen Sprachentwicklung und Sozialisation in begrenztem Umfang gefördert werden.

Je nach Lokalisation und Ausmaß führen *exogene Hirnschäden* bis ins mittlere und späte Kindesalter hinein zu grundsätzlich anderen Formen psychischer Störungen und Behinderungen als im späteren Lebensalter. Ausgedehnte Schädigungen – insbesondere des Cortex cerebri – führen zur Oligophrenie, während sich bei entsprechender Schädigung im späteren Leben eine Demenz entwickeln würde, die bereits eine entwickelte Intelligenz voraussetzt. Weniger gravierende Schäden äußern sich im frühen bis mittleren Kindesalter als *frühkindliches exogenes Psychosyndrom* (LEMPP, 1976), das erscheinungsbildlich deutlich vom *organischen Psychosyndrom* und der *organischen Wesensänderung* abgrenzbar ist, wie sie sich im *späteren Lebensalter* bei entsprechender Hirnschädigung zu entwickeln pflegen. Im hohen Lebensalter sind infolge der dann schon physiologischerweise eintretenden Abbauprozesse die entsprechenden Psychosyndrome vergleichsweise häufig; sie können sich aber bei exogener Schädigung in jedem Lebensalter etwa vom Grundschulalter an entwickeln.

Wie sich die Oligophrenie von der Demenz erscheinungsbildlich vor allem darin unterscheidet, daß bei ihr Störungen der Merkfähigkeit zurücktreten oder sogar gänzlich fehlen, so ist dieses Symptom auch beim frühkindlichen exogenen Psychosyndrom gegenüber dem organischen Psychosyndrom späterer Lebensjahre weniger ausgeprägt. Im Vordergrund der klinischen Bilder stehen vielmehr Aufmerksamkeits- und Konzentrationsstörungen, Hypermotilität und eine verminderte Impulskontrolle. Diese Erscheinungen können zwar persistieren, zeigen aber insgesamt eine bessere Rückbildungstendenz als organische Psychosyndrome späterer Jahre, insbesondere solche des höheren Lebensalters (MÜLLER, 1967).

Typische *exogene Psychosen* können bei entsprechender Schädigung schon im Kindesalter auftreten. Dabei dominiert aber die Bewußtseinsstörung, häufig verbunden mit epileptischen Anfällen. Floride psychotische Symptome treten demgegenüber zurück; vergleichsweise am häufigsten kommt es zum Auftreten von Delirien.

Psychotische Bilder ohne deutliche Bewußtseinstrübung sind hingegen sehr selten; bei sog. *Schizophrenien im Kindesalter* werden allerdings in einem höheren Prozentsatz als bei Erwachsenen deutliche Hinweise auf eine Hirnschädigung gefunden (neurologische Symptome, abnorme EEG-Muster, Ventrikelerweiterung), so daß die Frage entsteht, ob es sich hierbei nicht überwiegend um endomorphe Psychosen organischer Genese handelt (HANSON u. GOTTESMAN, 1976); zumindest erscheint eine starke Mitbeteiligung hirnorganischer Faktoren wahrscheinlich.

Der *Pavor nocturnus* – das nächtliche Aufschrecken aus dem Nachtschlaf, das sich bis zu panikartigen Zuständen steigern kann – stellt eine ganz von der Alterskonstitution geprägte Störung dar. Dies läßt sich auch von der *Enuresis* (HALLGREN, 1957) aussagen. Diese weist zudem – nach Familienuntersuchungen zu urteilen – eine deutliche hereditäre Komponente auf und ist somit – bei einem Teil der Fälle – offenbar auch in dieser Hinsicht konstitutionell verankert. Das gilt ebenfalls für das *Stottern* (ANDREWS et al., 1964).

Die *Legasthenie* (SCHENK-DANZINGER, 1978) ist überwiegend erblich bzw. (seltener) durch lokale Hirnschädigung bedingt. Ihr liegt zwar wahrscheinlich eine allgemeinere Form kognitiver Störung zugrunde; jedoch manifestiert diese sich erst in deutlicher Form beim Lesen und Schreiben. Ohne die entsprechenden Anforderungen würde die Störung – ebenso wie eine Rechenschwäche – wahrscheinlich unerkannt bleiben.

Dies weist auf die Möglichkeit hin, daß gewisse psychische Konstitutionsanomalien allein deshalb keine „Symptome" hervorrufen, weil sich diese nur unter bestimmten Umweltbedingungen manifestieren, denen ein Mensch nicht notwendigerweise ausgesetzt wird. Durch möglichst frühzeitig einsetzende spezielle Trainingsprogramme kann – zumindest intelligenteren – Legasthenikern häufig zu Leistungen im Lesen und Schreiben, die den normalen Anforderungen entsprechen, verholfen werden; eine gewisse Erschwerung dieser Leistungen dürfte aber auch bei so behandelten Fällen meist bestehen bleiben.

Im Unterschied zur Legasthenie bildet sich *Nägelbeißen* (NISSEN, 1976a) – eine zwar alterstypische, aber offenbar vorwiegend milieubedingte Störung, die durch Änderung des Milieus und psychotherapeutische Maßnahmen günstig zu beeinflussen ist – im allgemeinen auch ohne spezielle Maßnahmen schon vor oder während der Pubertät zurück. *Tics* (STRUNK, 1976) haben ebenfalls eine relativ günstige Prognose, sind aber nicht so stark an eine Altersstufe gebunden wie Nägelbeißen. In dem Maße, in dem an der Genese neben Milieufaktoren auch organische Faktoren beteiligt sind, wird die Prognose getrübt. Diese ist besonders ungünstig beim Gilles de la Tourette-Syndrom, bei dem generalisierte Tics mit Zwangsphänomenen kombiniert sind (STRUNK, 1976; SHAPIRO et al., 1978).

Psychische Auffälligkeiten im Kindesalter haben – von den genannten Ausnahmen abgesehen – im allgemeinen eine verhältnismäßig günstige Prognose (ROBINS, 1967). Sie bilden sich oft im Zuge des *puberalen Konstitutionswandels* zurück, ohne zwangsläufig anderen Störungen Platz zu machen. Dafür können im Reifungsalter neue und häufig andersartige Störungen entstehen. Ihre Wurzeln lassen sich zwar zumeist bis in die Kindheit zurückverfolgen, müssen aber selbst noch nicht den Charakter des Krankhaften getragen haben (v. BAEYER, 1977).

So kommt es oft erst im Reifungsalter zur Ausbildung von krankhaft abnormen Wesenszügen, die den Begriff der *Psychopathie* (WINOKUR u. CROWE, 1975) als einer pathologischen Variante der Charakterstruktur rechtfertigen, da sie im wesentlichen unverändert bis ins hohe Alter hinein bestehen bleiben. Sie können zwar in späten Lebensjahren abblassen (TÖLLE, 1966), verstärken sich aber nicht selten im Zusammenhang mit einer durch *Altersabbau* bedingten *Charakterveränderung*. Psychopathische Züge haben deshalb etwa von der Zeit der Vorpubertät an prognostische Bedeutung, während entsprechende Auffälligkeiten im Kindesalter kaum eine Vorhersage über die Charakterentwicklung im Erwachsenenalter erlauben (ROBINS, 1967). Die Diagnose einer Psychopathie sollte aber erst nach Abschluß der Reifungszeit gestellt werden, da bis dahin noch mit erheblichen Persönlichkeitsveränderungen gerechnet werden kann.

„Die habituelle Dauerhaftigkeit" der sich im Reifungsalter herausbildenden Charakterstruktur „schließt jedoch eine gewisse *Veränderbarkeit*, Schwankungen und *Wandlungen* im Laufe der Entwicklung und Entfaltung einer Persönlichkeit und in Abhängigkeit von peristatischen Faktoren, von Erfahrungen, Erlebnissen und Schicksalen keineswegs aus. Das Kriterium des Dauernden und Konstanten ist also zu relativieren. Bestimmte Persönlichkeiten und Persönlichkeitszüge sind dabei in verschiedenem Umfange wandlungsfähig und formbar" (HUBER, 1974; S. 222).

Bei der Entstehung verschiedener Formen von *Dissozialität* (ROBINS, 1966; NISSEN, 1976b) spielen peristatische Faktoren (GLUECK u. GLUECK, 1964) im allgemeinen eine größere Rolle als genetische (s. aber CLONINGER et al., 1978). Trotzdem tendieren sie zur Persistenz bis ins Erwachsenenalter (ROBINS, 1967), auch wenn sie im höheren Lebensalter gewöhnlich an Bedeutung verlieren. Ihre Entstehung hängt mit der Ablösung vom Elternhaus, der Hinwendung zu außerfamiliären Gruppen (insbesondere bei ungünstigen Milieuverhältnissen auch solchen von ausgesprochenem Bandencharakter), triebbedingten inneren Spannungen und schließlich mit der Intelligenzentwicklung zusammen, die erst in diesem Alter ein von außen schwer kontrollierbares Übertreten sozialer Verhaltensnormen ermöglicht.

Aus der puberalen *Umstrukturierung der Triebkonstitution* wird die Entstehung *sexueller Deviationen* gerade in diesem Entwicklungsabschnitt verständlich. Für die Entwicklung einzelner Formen der männlichen Homosexualität ist das Gewicht genetischer Faktoren besonders gut belegt (HESTON u. SHIELDS, 1968). Bei zahlreichen anderen Formen devianter Entwicklung des Sexualtriebs treten solche Faktoren gegenüber vorbestehenden exogenen Hirnschädigungen sowie prägenden Erlebnissen und anderen primär psychischen Einflüssen mehr in den Hintergrund.

Die Bindung der *Anorexia nervosa* (THOMÄ, 1961; VIGERSKY, 1977) an die Alterskonstitution ist besonders eindrucksvoll und hat der Erkrankung die Bezeichnung „Pubertätsmagersucht" eingetragen, obwohl der Manifestationsbeginn von der Vorpubertät bis ins frühe Erwachsenenalter hineinreicht. Im Unterschied zu vielen anderen Formen von *Pubertäts- und Adoleszenzkrisen* zeigt sie eine relativ ungünstige Prognose. Nach Abschluß der Adoleszenz kommt es allerdings häufig zu einem Syndromwandel, bei dem die Anorexie durch andere Formen einer Eßstörung bzw. durch ganz andersartige Verhaltensstörungen ersetzt wird oder ihnen gegenüber in den Hintergrund tritt. Vermutungen über primäre konstitutionelle Normabweichungen bei den Erkrankten erscheinen bisher nicht ausreichend gesichert. Reifungsangst mit Ablehnung der künftigen Geschlechtsrolle scheint im Zentrum der Pathogenese zu stehen.

Daß sich am Übergang von der Pubertät zur Adoleszenz *Zwangsneurosen* besonders häufig manifestieren, die dann meistens einen chronisch-progredienten oder -rezidivierenden Verlauf nehmen, läßt sich ebenfalls psychologisch mit altersspezifischen Ängsten erklären (Nissen, 1976c). Hier scheinen es vor allem Gewissensängste auf der Grundlage von Triebspannungen und ambivalenten Autonomiebestrebungen zu sein, die durch die Krankheitssymptomatik gebunden werden sollen. Die krankhafte Form der Angstbewältigung verhindert eine realitätsgerechte Auseinandersetzung mit den alterssspezifischen Problemen. Das verhindert die innere Reifung und eine adäquate äußere Anpassung, wodurch die Problematik konserviert und die Störung chronifiziert wird.

Abb. 3 zeigt in einer Darstellung von Nissen alterstypische Angstinhalte im Kindes- und Jugendalter. Es braucht wohl nicht hervorgehoben zu werden, daß diese *Ängste* weder allein aus der Alterskonstitution noch allein aus der alterstypischen Lebenssituation erwachsen, sondern nur durch deren Zusammenwirken zu erklären sind.

Es erscheint fraglich, ob die *Rauschdrogensucht* grundsätzlich in ähnlicher Weise wie die alterstypischen Angstinhalte aus einer solchen Interaktion von Alterskonstitution und alterstypischer Lebenssituation abgeleitet werden kann.

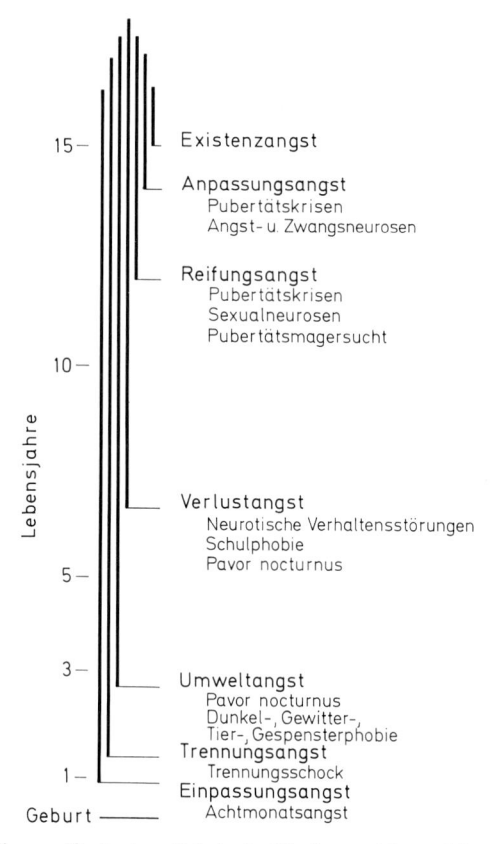

Abb. 3. Alters- und stadienspezifische Angstinhalte im Kindes- und Jugendalter (nach Nissen, 1976c)

Speziell auf die „Drogenwelle" (JANZ, 1977) trifft dieses Interaktionsmodell aber zweifellos zu: in der Alterskonstitution wurzelnde Autonomiestrebungen und eine durch sie bedingte Oppositionshaltung tradierten Wertvorstellungen gegenüber, eine mit dem „Anders-Sein-Wollen" einhergehende Tendenz zur Identifikation mit neuen Leitbildern, eine erhöhte Risikobereitschaft und andere Merkmale der Alterskonstitution von Adoleszenten und jungen Erwachsenen auf der einen Seite, alterstypische Rollenangebote einer pluralistischen Überflußgesellschaft, Verführung und Konformitätsdruck durch Altersgefährten und schließlich das Vorhandensein der Rauschdrogen in der „Szene" auf der anderen Seite.

Der Manifestationsbeginn von *Alkoholismus* (FEUERLEIN, 1975; SOLMS, 1975) und *Medikamentensucht* streut breit über das Alter der körperlichen Vollreife bis ins Involutionsalter hinein. Entsprechendes gilt für die meisten *Neurosen* des *Erwachsenenalters* (SCHULTE u. TÖLLE, 1977). Daß im *höheren Lebensalter* neurotische Störungen vornehmlich depressive und/oder hypochondrische Färbung zeigen (MÜLLER, 1967; MAYER-GROSS et al., 1969), wird allerdings nicht nur aus der durch Vereinsamung und Todeserwartung gekennzeichneten Lebenssituation, sondern auch durch altersbedingte Einbußen der psychischen Leistungsfähigkeit (RIEGEL, 1968) und durch körperliche Alterserscheinungen verständlich, die zu (depressiven) Versagenserlebnissen und (hypochondrischen) Befürchtungen um die körperliche Gesundheit führen.

Obwohl das Alter der körperlichen Vollreife entwicklungsbiologisch gesehen einen besonders stabilen Zustand charakterisiert und von der Entwicklungspsychologie sogar zumeist als eine Zeit, in der sich keine entscheidenden inneren Veränderungen abspielen, geradezu ausgeblendet worden ist (MÖNKS u. KNOERS, 1976), treten ausgerechnet in dieser „stationären" Phase am häufigsten körperlich nicht begründbare aktuelle psychische Störungen auf, darunter das Gros der *endogenen Psychosen*. Die bevorzugte Entstehung von Alkoholismus, Medikamentensucht und neurotischen Störungen im Erwachsenenalter ist möglicherweise in erster Linie durch die Lebenssituation in diesem Entwicklungsstadium zu erklären, u.a. durch die – im Vergleich zu Kindheit und Jugendzeit – größere Selbständigkeit und Verantwortung, mit der Möglichkeit des Scheiterns in Beruf, Partnerwahl, Ehe und Kindererziehung. Dagegen dürfte die *Altersbindung* der *endogenen Psychosen*, bei denen es sich um *genetische Dispositionskrankheiten* handelt, vorwiegend *konstitutionsbedingt* sein. Die Gründe hierfür sind allerdings weitgehend unbekannt.

Die *Unterformen der Schizophrenie* zeigen jeweils unterschiedliche Gipfel der Erstmanifestation (MAYER-GROSS et al., 1969). Hebephrene Formen beginnen am häufigsten zwischen dem 20. und 30. Lebensjahr, katatone um das 30. und paranoide Formen zwischen dem 30. und 40. Lebensjahr (ANGST et al., 1973). Ein Krankheitsbeginn in Adoleszenz oder sogar Pubertät ist bei der hebephrenen Form nicht selten, bei den anderen Formen die Ausnahme. Echte schizophrene Psychosen des Kindesalters (EGGERS, 1978) kommen nur in vergleichsweise wenigen Fällen vor (HANSON u. GOTTESMAN, 1976), während ein Krankheitsbeginn in der Involution bis ins höhere Lebensalter hinein in Form des sog. *Spätparanoids* gar nicht so selten ist; jedoch ist hier die Abgrenzung gegenüber andersartigen paranoiden Psychosen problematisch.

Die Erstmanifestation bipolarer *affektiver Psychosen* zeigt eine ähnliche Altersverteilung wie die paranoiden Formen der Schizophrenie, während der Erstmanifestationsgipfel monopolar verlaufender endogener Depressionen (unter

Einbeziehung von Involutionsmelancholie und Altersdepression) im Involutionsalter – also zwischen 40 und 50 Jahren – liegt (ANGST, 1966). Ein Krankheitsbeginn im Kindesalter ist bei affektiven Psychosen noch wesentlich seltener als bei schizophrenen Psychosen. In diesem Lebensalter diagnostizierte depressive bzw. manische Psychosen stellen sich im weiteren Verlauf zumeist als körperlich begründbare Psychosen oder atypisch beginnende Schizophrenien mit später deutlich werdender Defektbildung heraus.

Schizoaffektive Psychosen nehmen nicht nur bezüglich ihrer Symptomatik und Heredität, sondern auch bezüglich ihres Manifestationsalters eine Zwischenstellung zwischen den schizophrenen und den affektiven Psychosen ein (ANGST et al., 1976), während *rein paranoide Psychosen* eine ähnliche Altersverteilung zeigen wie rein depressiv verlaufende affektive Psychosen.

Im höheren Lebensalter treten *körperlich begründbare psychische Störungen*, die auf vaskulären und/oder primär zerebralen Altersveränderungen (wie bei präsenilen und senilen Demenzen) beruhen, in den Vordergrund (MÜLLER, 1967). Die Dynamik endogener Psychosen (BLEULER, 1972; CIOMPI u. MÜLLER, 1976), aber ebenfalls die vieler psychopathischer Persönlichkeitsabweichungen (TÖLLE, 1966) und chronifizierter neurotischer Störungen (ERNST et al., 1968) kann sich in diesem Alter zurückbilden. Auch geben nicht wenige Alkoholiker den Abusus auf bzw. schränken den Alkoholkonsum erheblich ein (HELGASON, 1964). Es kann aber ebenfalls – obwohl seltener – jeweils das Gegenteil eintreten; insbesondere können sich durch den Altersabbau einzelne Charakterzüge in so krasser Weise verstärken (MÜLLER, 1967), daß die Persönlichkeit ein psychopathisches Gepräge annimmt. Auch sollte die Beteiligung psychogener Faktoren bei der Entstehung krankhafter psychischer Normabweichungen im höheren Lebensalter nicht unterschätzt werden (MAYER-GROSS et al., 1969). Dies ist nicht zuletzt im Hinblick auf prophylaktische und therapeutische Maßnahmen stets zu bedenken.

Die Alterskonstitution läßt sich nur theoretisch, nicht aber praktisch streng von der rassischen und der Geschlechtskonstitution trennen; ferner müssen soziokulturelle Einflüsse stets berücksichtigt werden. So gelten die Altersangaben in Tabelle 2 speziell für Angehörige europider Rassen in modernen Industriegesellschaften und eher für das weibliche als für das männliche Geschlecht, bei dem insbesondere die konstitutionellen Veränderungen im Reifungsalter später einsetzen und auch später zum Abschluß kommen als beim weiblichen Geschlecht. Der seit dem letzten Jahrhundert weltweit zu verzeichnende Vorgang einer *Akzeleration* der menschlichen Entwicklung ist wahrscheinlich zivilisatorischen Einflüssen (vornehmlich einer eiweiß- und vitaminreicheren Ernährung) zuzuschreiben (TANNER, 1962; KNUSSMANN, 1968; SCHWIDETZKY, 1970). In besonders starkem Maße wird aber die psychische Konstitutionsentwicklung von zivilisatorischen Einflüssen im weitesten Sinne mitgeformt und nicht allein von der altersabhängigen Aktivierung verschiedener Gene bestimmt. Hier wie auch in anderem Zusammenhang läßt sich bezüglich menschlichen Verhaltens – in Abwandlung eines Wortes der Astrologen – sagen: Die Gene zwingen nicht, sie machen geneigt.

b) Geschlechtskonstitution

Wie alle sexuell differenzierten Organismen ist auch das menschliche Individuum *bisexuell* angelegt. Die *sexuelle Differenzierung* erfolgt in verschiedenen Stufen, insbesondere während der ersten Hälfte der intrauterinen Entwicklung (NEUMANN, 1977; WILSON, 1978) und im Reifungsalter (TANNER, 1962). Für die Entwicklung der psychischen Geschlechtskonstitution sind vor allem die ersten

Tabelle 3. Entwicklung der Sexualkonstitution bis zur Geschlechtsreife

Zeit	Somatische Partialkonstitution	Psychische Partialkonstitution
Befruchtung	Entstehung des Geschlechtschromosomensatzes	
Pränatale Entwicklungsperiode embryonal fetal	Keimdrüsendifferenzierung Geschlechtshormonproduktion (relevant: Androgenproduktion im fetalen Hoden!) Differenzierung der Geschlechtsorgane, sexuelle Differenzierung zerebraler (insbesondere hypothalamischer) Zentren, Herausbildung körperlicher	
Geburt	Größenunterschiede	
Kindheit		Auftreten geschlechtstypischer Verhaltensmerkmale Geschlechtsidentifikation Verstärkung geschlechtstypischer Verhaltensmerkmale
Reifungszeit	Hypothalam. Aktivierung der Hormonproduktion im Hypophysenvorderlappen (Gonadotropine), hypophysäre Aktivierung der Hormonproduktion in der Zona reticularis der Nebennierenrinde (Androgene) und in den Keimdrüsen (Androgene bzw. Östrogene und Gestagene), Wachstumsschub, Reifung der Keimdrüsen, Ausprägung der sekundären Geschlechtsmerkmale	Ausprägung des Geschlechtstriebes, weitere Verstärkung geschlechtstypischer Verhaltensmerkmale

Jahre der postpartalen Entwicklung und die Reifungszeit relevant (MONEY u. EHRHARDT, 1972; MONEY, 1978). Hierbei spielen soziokulturelle Einflüsse eine entscheidende Rolle, während die Entwicklung der körperlichen Geschlechtskonstitution (OUNSTED u. TAYLOR, 1972; WALTER, 1978) im wesentlichen genetisch gesteuert wird.

Die einzelnen *Entwicklungsstufen* der Geschlechtskonstitution sind in Tabelle 3 grob schematisch dargestellt.

Das Geschlecht eines Individuums wird bei der Empfängnis durch die väterliche Keimzelle festgelegt. Trägt diese in ihrem (haploiden) *Chromosomensatz* als Geschlechtschromosom ein X, das sich mit dem X-Chromosom des (ebenfalls haploiden) Chromosomensatzes der mütterlichen Keimzelle zur XX-Konstitution des (diploiden) Chromosomensatzes der Zygote verbindet, so entwickelt sich ein weiblicher Organismus; trägt die Samenzelle hingegen ein Y-Chromosom, so entwickelt sich (normalerweise) ein männlicher Organismus (PRADER, 1978).

Beim männlichen Embryo wandelt sich unter dem Einluß des Y-Chromosomes von der 7. Woche an die Medulla der primär sexuell indifferenten *Gonaden* in Testes um, während beim weiblichen Embryo die Umwandlung des Cortex der Gonaden in die Ovarien erst von der 10. Woche an erfolgt (MOORE, 1977; WILSON, 1978). Die weitere Genitalentwicklung steht unter dem Einfluß von *Wirkstoffen*, die in den sexuell differenzierten Gonaden gebildet werden. Die *Androgen*produktion in den männlichen Keimdrüsen führt zur männlichen Differenzierung der Geschlechtsorgane, einschließlich des äußeren *Genitale*. Ohne ihren Einfluß entwickelt sich die ursprünglich bisexuelle Anlage des Genitalapparates in weibliche Richtung (NEUMANN, 1977). Die Feminisierung des Organismus wird allerdings möglicherweise durch weibliche Geschlechtshormone aus den Ovarien noch verstärkt (TIMIRAS, 1971).

Später als die hormonale Differenzierung der – inneren und äußeren – Geschlechtsorgane vollzieht sich die *sexuelle Differenzierung* zerebraler, insbesondere *hypothalamischer Strukturen*. Die normalerweise in weibliche Richtung erfolgende Differenzierung wird bei männlichen Feten (wahrscheinlich während einer „sensiblen Phase" im zweiten Trimenon) durch *Androgeneinfluß* gehemmt, wodurch die Entwicklung eines zyklischen Ablaufes der Gonadotropin-Sekretion in der Pubertät unmöglich gemacht wird. Vermutlich werden auch beim Menschen im Anschluß an die Androgen-abhängige Beeinflussung hypothalamischer Strukturen, die für die spätere Steuerung der Gonadotropin-Sekretion verantwortlich sind, auch andere zerebrale (weitere hypothalamische sowie limbische) Strukturen beeinflußt, die an der Steuerung der psychosexuellen Entwicklung beteiligt sind (HUTT, 1978).

Das Ergebnis dieser komplizierten Entwicklungsvorgänge ist der morphologisch eindeutige Geschlechtsunterschied von Neugeborenen, der für die Zuweisung zum Geschlecht und die darauf gegründete erzieherische Beeinflussung und somit indirekt für die gesamte psychosexuelle Entwicklung von ausschlaggebender Bedeutung ist. Die hormonelle Beeinflussung zerebraler Strukturen in der Fetalperiode schafft darüber hinaus offenbar *Verhaltensdispositionen*, die an der Entstehung *psychischer Geschlechtsunterschiede* beteiligt sind. Diese sind allerdings teilweise durch einen Reifungsvorsprung weiblicher Individuen bedingt, der bei der Geburt einige Wochen, gegen Ende der Adoleszenz etwa zwei Jahre beträgt (TANNER, 1962; HUTT, 1978).

Mit Reifungsunterschieden der Geschlechter hängt es möglicherweise zusammen, daß männliche Neugeborene und junge Säuglinge motorisch unruhiger sind als weibliche; sie schreien auch mehr als diese und erwachen häufiger aus dem Schlaf (ARGANIAN, 1973). Mädchen lernen im allgemeinen früher laufen und sprechen und behalten in der verbalen Entwicklung einen deutlichen Vorsprung (HUTT, 1978). Einige Verhaltensdifferenzen sind aber weder durch Unterschiede im Reifegrad des zentralen Nervensystems noch durch erzieherische Einflüsse ausreichend zu erklären. So zeigt das explorative Verhalten von Knaben bereits im späten Säuglings- und frühen Kleinkindalter stärker expansive Züge als das von Mädchen. Unmutsäußerungen bis aggressiven Handlungen treten ebenfalls bei Knaben häufiger auf. Diese entwickeln auch mehr Initiative und neigen zu rauheren Umgangsformen als Mädchen, die ihrerseits anschmiegsamer und leichter lenkbar sind. Die genannten Unterschiede sind freilich im Vergleich zu den körperlichen Unterschieden gering und gelten nur für den statistischen Vergleich. Sie werden zudem beeinflußt durch Verhaltensvorbilder von älteren Angehörigen des gleichen Geschlechts und durch gesellschaftliche Einflüsse, die auch jene Vorbilder schon entscheidend geprägt haben. Dabei werden geschlechtsbezogene Unterschiede im Erziehungsstil nicht allein durch gesellschaftliche Stereotype von „männlichem" und „weiblichem" Verhalten (CHETWYND u. HARTNETT, 1978) bestimmt, sondern auch von offenbar primären Verhaltensunterschieden der Jungen und Mädchen provoziert.

Die *Identifikation* mit der *Geschlechtsrolle* erfolgt im wesentlichen erst von der zweiten Hälfte des zweiten Lebensjahres an bis ins dritte/vierte Lebensjahr hinein. Sie wird in erster Linie von der *Rollenzuweisung* und dem *Rollenangebot* und nicht von biologischen Faktoren bestimmt, obwohl diese möglicherweise einen *dispositionellen Hintergrund* bilden und nicht nur der prägenden Umwelt das Geschlecht signalisieren (MONEY u. EHRHARDT, 1972). Die Ausformung geschlechtstypischer Verhaltensweisen erfolgt auf dem Wege des *sozialen Lernens*, insbesondere durch operante Konditionierung und Lernen am Modell (BANDURA

u. WALTERS, 1963). Dabei kommt den Rollenspielen der Kinder besondere Bedeutung für die Verstärkung geschlechtstypischer Verhaltensmerkmale zu.

Mit Beginn der *Vorpubertät* gewinnen dann wieder *biologische Faktoren* eine stärkere Bedeutung für die *geschlechtstypische Verhaltensdifferenzierung*. Vor allem sind sie aber ausschlaggebend für die *somatische Geschlechtsentwicklung*, die teils mehr schubweise, teils mehr kontinuierlich bis ins Alter der körperlichen Vollreife hinein zu einem zunehmenden *Sexualdimorphismus* führt (TANNER, 1962).

Nach einem genetisch festgelegten Programm beginnt von jenen Anteilen des (ventro-medialen) Hypothalamus, der sich fetal in weiblicher bzw. männlicher Richtung differenziert hat, eine neurosekretorisch vermittelte Aktivierung des Hypophysenvorderlappens. Unbekannt sind allerdings vorläufig die Faktoren, die zur sog. *Adrenarche* führen. Bei dieser handelt es sich um eine partielle Aktivierung der Nebennierenrinde, die nun vermehrt Androgene (in wesentlich geringerer Menge auch Östrogene und Gestagene) bildet, welche zum Wachstumsschub und zur sekundären Körperbehaarung beitragen. Die der Adrenarche folgende Aktivierung der inkretorischen Funktion der Keimdrüsen ist der für die Pubertätsentwicklung entscheidende hormonale Faktor (SWERDLOFF u. RUBIN, 1978). Die zyklische Sekretion von follikelstimulierendem Hormon (FSH) und Luteinisierungshormon (LH) führt beim heranreifenden Mädchen zur *Menarche* und unterhält von da an den Menstruationszyklus, der erst gegen Ende der fünften Lebensdekade durch die Menopause abgelöst wird. Bis dahin reicht die *Geschlechtsreife*, wobei allerdings das Maximum der Fertilität um das 20. Lebensjahr herum liegt.

Bei Knaben schließt sich der Adrenarche die Keimdrüsenreifung unter dem Einfluß tonischer FSH- und LH-Sekretion an. Die Geschlechtsreife überdauert beim männlichen Geschlecht das Involutionsalter und erlischt gewöhnlich erst im Präsenium; aber auch die männliche Fertilität läßt, nachdem im dritten Dezennium ein Maximum erreicht wurde, allmählich nach.

Hand in Hand mit der einsetzenden Geschlechtsreife geht bei beiden Geschlechtern die Ausbildung der *sekundären Geschlechtsmerkmale*, auf die bei der Besprechung von Tabelle 4 näher eingegangen wird. Parallel zur körperlichen Umproportionierung vollzieht sich ein psychischer Strukturwandel, der insbesondere durch die Ausprägung des *Geschlechtstriebes* gekennzeichnet ist. Dieser wird offenbar vornehmlich durch Androgene (bei männlichen Jugendlichen in erster Linie durch das in den Hoden produzierte Testosteron, bei Mädchen – außer durch das hauptsächlich aus den Ovarien stammende Testosteron – durch Nebennierenrindenandrogene) aktiviert (MONEY u. EHRHARDT, 1972; MONEY, 1978). Seine spezifische Ausrichtung erfährt er aber durch frühere, vor allem mit der Geschlechtsidentifikation zusammenhängende und durch rezente Lebenserfahrungen; jedoch ist auch mit einer Abhängigkeit der sexuellen Trieborientierung von hormonellen Einflüssen auf die Differenzierung zerebraler Strukturen während der Fetalzeit zu rechnen. Möglicherweise sind diese Einflüsse allerdings für andere Formen psychischer Geschlechtsunterschiede, die nicht unmittelbar auf sexuelle Betätigung im engeren Sinne bezogen sind, bedeutsamer. Wie hoch dieser Einfluß auch zu veranschlagen ist, die geschlechtstypische Differenzierung der psychischen Partialkonstitution vollzieht sich auf jeden Fall im Reifungsalter und bleibt z.T. bis ins Senium erhalten.

Trotz dieser *Persistenz psychischer Geschlechtsunterschiede* dürfen diese nicht ohne weiteres der Konstitution zugerechnet werden, da ein nach Geschlecht differenziertes Rollenverständnis, das soziokulturell geprägt ist, den Menschen bis ins hohe Alter begleitet und dadurch Unterschiede im Erleben und Verhalten von Mann und Frau nicht nur hervorrufen, sondern auch aufrechterhalten kann. Dies gilt wahrscheinlich in besonderem Maße für geschlechtstypische Interessen, die mit der Arbeitsteilung der Geschlechter zusammenhängen bzw. von offenkundig stark kulturabhängigen

Tabelle 4. Beispiele konstitutioneller Geschlechtsunterschiede im Alter der körperlichen Vollreife (s. Tabelle 2)

Partialkonstitution (PK)	Mann	Frau
Körperlicher Habitus	Äußeres männliches Genitale, stärkere Körperbehaarung mit männlichem Typ der Schambehaarung, Bartwuchs, Neigung zur Glatzenbildung, größere Körperhöhe, robuste, zum Eckigen tendierende („athletische") Körperform mit betonter Extremitätenentwicklung, „Adamsapfel"	Äußeres weibliches Genitale, weibliche Brustentwicklung, weiblicher Typ der Schambehaarung, zarte, gerundete Körperform mit betonter Rumpfentwicklung, besonders in der Hüftregion
PK der inneren morphologischen Struktur	*Makroskopisch:* inneres männliches Genitale, stärkere Entwicklung von Muskulatur, Knochen- und Bindegewebe, männliche Beckenform	*Makroskopisch:* inneres weibliches Genitale, entwickeltes Brustdrüsengewebe, stärkere Entwicklung des Fettgewebes, insbesondere subkutan an Brust, Hüften, Nates und Oberschenkeln, weibliche Beckenform
	Mikroskopisch: spezifische Gewebsstruktur der Testes und der anderen Geschlechtsorgane, größere Zahl der Erythrozyten im Blut	*Mikroskopisch:* spezifische Gewebsstruktur der Ovarien und der anderen Geschlechtsorgane, Barrsche Körperchen in den Zellkernen, trommelschlegelartige Anhänger der segmentierten Leukozytenkerne im Blut
	XY-Konstitution der Geschlechtschromosomen in allen Zellkernen	XX-Konstitution der Geschlechtschromosomen in allen Zellkernen
Biochemische PK	Dominierende Testosteronproduktion in den Keimdrüsen	Dominierende, dabei zyklisch fluktuierende Östrogen- und Gestagenproduktion in den Keimdrüsen
Immunologische PK		Stärkere Tendenz zur Antikörperbildung
Physiologische PK	Spezifische Funktionsabläufe an den männlichen Geschlechtsorganen bei sexueller Erregung und beim Geschlechtsakt (u.a. Erektion u. Ejakulation), tiefere Stimmlage	Spezifische Funktionsabläufe an den weiblichen Geschlechtsorganen bei sexueller Erregung und beim Geschlechtsakt (u.a. Lubrikation der Scheidenschleimhaut u. Uteruskontraktionen), Menstruationszyklus, Empfängnis, Schwangerschaft, Wochenbett und Laktation
Triebkonstitution	Männlicher Sexualtrieb, erhöhte Aggressionsbereitschaft	Weiblicher Sexualtrieb
Charakter	„Androthymie": größere Aggressivität (s. oben), Expansivität u. Risikobereitschaft	„Gynäkothymie": größere Emotionalität, Anlehnungsbedürfnis und Fürsorglichkeit
Intelligenz/ spez. Fähigkeiten	Besseres räumliches Orientierungsvermögen	Größere Merkfähigkeit

Partialkonstitution (PK)	Mann	Frau
Kommunikationsweisen	Männliches Imponiergehabe	Weibliches Kokettieren
Überzeugungen, Einstellungen, Interessen	Männliche Identifikation, Kampfgeist (s. oben), stärkere Tendenz zum Einzelgängertum einerseits, zum Anschluß an extrafamiliäre Gemeinschaften andererseits, mehr sachbezogene (z.B. technische) Interessen	Weibliche Identifikation, stärkerer Familiensinn, mehr personenbezogene Interessen (z.B. Kinderpflege)

Ausgestaltungen des im engeren Sinne sexuellen Rollenverhaltens bestimmt werden (ROSENBLATT u. CUNNINGHAM, 1976). Untersuchungen an Intersexen zeigen aber, daß auch solche Interessen z.T. von biologischen Faktoren (nämlich dem Grad der fetalen Androgenisierung) abhängen und nicht ausschließlich vom sozialen Rollenangebot diktiert werden (MONEY u. EHRHARDT, 1972; EHRHARDT u. BAKER, 1974).

Die in Tabelle 4 dargestellte Übersicht über konstitutionelle Geschlechtsunterschiede im Alter der körperlichen Vollreife beschränkt sich auf einige markante Beispiele aus den in Abb. 2 (untere Reihe) angeführten Partialkonstitutionen. Dabei handelt es sich teils um nahezu absolute Unterschiede (wie die Konstitution der Geschlechtschromosomen und die primären Geschlechtsmerkmale, nämlich äußeres und inneres Genitale), die nur auf äußerst seltene Formen sexueller Zwischenstufen nicht mehr zutreffen, teils um relative Unterschiede, die sich nur aus einem statistischen Gruppenvergleich ergeben (wie Unterschiede der Fettverteilung und der Körperkraft sowie die meisten psychischen Geschlechtsunterschiede).

Daß die psychischen Geschlechtsunterschiede nur teilweise genetisch bedingt sind, vielmehr in hohem Maße von soziokulturellen Einflüssen abhängen (LLOYD u. ARCHER, 1976), wurde bereits hervorgehoben. Sie variieren dementsprechend erheblich zwischen verschiedenen Kulturen und auch innerhalb einer Kultur zwischen verschienen Epochen. Dabei können sich während der historischen Entwicklung einer Kultur psychische Geschlechtsunterschiede sowohl verstärken oder verwischen als auch strukturelle Veränderungen durchmachen. Diese historischen Veränderungen hängen weitgehend von sozioökonomischen Faktoren ab. Beispielsweise vollzieht sich in modernen Industrienationen unter dem Einfluß einer zunehmenden Entlastung der Frau von der Kinderpflege (infolge einer Einschränkung der Geburtenzahl durch systematische Anwendung empfängnisverhütender Mittel, technische Erleichterung der Haushaltsarbeit sowie Übernahme von Versorgungs- und Erziehungsaufgaben durch Kindergärten etc.) und vieler anderer Faktoren eine zunehmende Abschwächung von Geschlechtsunterschieden des Verhaltens. So hat seit Zunahme des Frauensports der Unterschied in sportlichen Höchstleistungen zwischen Männern und Frauen drastisch verringert. Er ist allerdings immer noch beträchtlich und dürfte schon infolge der physiologischerweise durchschnittlich größeren Körperkraft des Mannes auch in Zukunft nicht völlig aufzuheben sein. Entsprechendes gilt wahrscheinlich auch für zahlreiche ausgesprochen psychische Verhaltensunterschiede.

Die in der Tabelle aufgeführten *Beispiele* psychischer Geschlechtsunterschiede sind unter dem Aspekt ausgewählt, daß sie mit einiger Wahrscheinlichkeit einen echten „biologischen Kern" haben und sich dementsprechend voraussichtlich in allen menschlichen Populationen auf lange Sicht behaupten werden. Im einzelnen waren folgende Auswahlgesichtspunkte maßgebend:

1. Die Unterschiede sind überwiegend durch empirische, z.T. psychometrische Untersuchungen statistisch gesichert (GARAI u. SCHEINFELD, 1968; TERMAN u. MILES, 1968; MACCOBY u. JACKLIN, 1975; TAVRIS u. OFFIR, 1977).

2. Sie lassen sich in den meisten der daraufhin untersuchten menschlichen Gesellschaften verschiedener Zivilisationshöhe feststellen (D'ANDRADE, 1966; ROSENBLATT u. CUNNINGHAM, 1976).

3. Sie zeigen bei Intersexen (mit Ausnahme der Geschlechtsidentifikation) nicht allein eine Abhängigkeit von der Geschlechtszuweisung und der ihr entsprechenden Erziehung, sondern auch von biologischen Faktoren (insbesondere der fetalen „Androgenisierung"; MONEY u. EHRHARDT, 1972; EHRHARDT u. BAKER, 1974; MONEY, 1978).

4. Sie sind z.T. schon bei menschlichen Neugeborenen und jungen Säuglingen nachzuweisen, bei denen die Erziehung noch keinen entscheidend formenden Einfluß ausüben konnte (ARGANIAN, 1973).

5. Sie verstärken sich oder entstehen sogar erst in der Pubertät unter dem Einfluß der Geschlechtshormone, insbesondere der Androgene, und sind deshalb bei männlichen Frühkastraten im allgemeinen nur schwach ausgeprägt (BLEULER, 1964).

6. Sie entsprechen teilweise Geschlechtsunterschieden im Verhalten der Primaten (VAN GOODALL, 1968).

Daß fast alle menschlichen Kulturen gewisse, z.T. sogar weitgehende Übereinstimmungen im geschlechtstypischen Rollenverhalten hervorgebracht haben und daß dieses entsprechenden Verhaltensweisen der dem Menschen nächstverwandten Tierarten ähnelt, ohne daß dafür eine genetische Disposition verantwortlich sein sollte, erscheint wenig plausibel. Viele dieser Ähnlichkeiten geschlechtstypischen Verhaltens von Mensch und Tier sind freilich durch die unterschiedlichen Fortpflanzungsaufgaben und die durchweg größere Körperkraft männlicher Individuen bedingt. Wahrscheinlich hat jede Gesellschaft die genetisch vorgegebenen Verhaltensdispositionen im Hinblick auf ebenfalls biologisch vorgezeichnete Aufgaben bei der Kinderpflege, dem Nahrungserwerb und der kämpferischen Auseinandersetzung mit der Natur und mit anderen Menschengruppen jeweils auf ihre Art geformt und diese Ausformung zur gesellschaftlich verbindlichen Norm erhoben.

Für das Individuum können sich aus den so entstandenen normativen Forderungen der Gesellschaft Konflikte ergeben, soweit seine Disposition von diesem Grundschema erheblich abweicht – insbesondere dann, wenn unterschiedliche Erziehungsstile sowie widersprüchliche soziale Einflüsse die Anpassung an die vorgegebenen Normen erschweren, wie dies besonders in modernen Industriegesellschaften der Fall zu sein pflegt.

Innerhalb eines Geschlechtes variieren die typischerweise geschlechtsdifferent ausgebildeten Merkmale erheblich. Die Varianz innerhalb der Gruppe ist bei einigen von ihnen (vornehmlich, aber nicht ausschließlich bei psychischen) größer als die Varianz zwischen den Gruppen. Man kann dementsprechend Angehörige eines Geschlechtes nach dem Grad der Ausprägung geschlechtstypischer Merkmale in eine Rangreihe bringen, die vom Extrem einer geschlechtstypisch ausgeprägten zum Extrem einer dem Gegengeschlecht entsprechenden Merkmalskonfiguration (im Bereich der Intersexualität: OVERZIER, 1961a) reicht. Diese *androgyne Variation* (DRAPER, 1941; s. auch v. ZERSSEN, 1968; v. ZERSSEN, 1977b) wird in den nächsten Unterkapiteln im Zusammenhang mit den normalen Konstitutionstypen (s.S. 668ff.) bzw. den abnormen Varianten (s.S. 674ff.) abgehandelt werden.

Über der Beachtung der starken Merkmalsvarianz innerhalb eines Geschlechtes darf aber nicht vergessen werden, daß es sowohl im körperlichen wie im psychischen Bereich eine Reihe von Merkmalen gibt, für die keine Überlappung besteht. Zeugung und Empfängnis sind – auch im Falle eines echten Hermaphroditismus – beim menschlichen Individuum (im Unterschied zu einigen niederen Organismen) nicht beide möglich, sondern jeweils nur eines von beidem oder keines. Das Wissen darum begleitet den Menschen im allgemeinen spätestens vom Reifungsalter an und dürfte für sein Selbstverständnis von entscheidender Bedeutung sein.

Geschlechtsunterschiede bestehen auch im *Pathologischen* (HUTT, 1978; WALTER, 1978). Sie sind nur teilweise direkt konstitutionell bedingt; unter anderem hängen sie mit der unterschiedlichen Exposition der Geschlechter gegenüber äußeren Gefahrenmomenten (durch Krieg, Beruf, Straßenverkehr etc.) zusammen, die ihrerseits vom gesellschaftlichen Rollenangebot mitbestimmt wird (VESSEY, 1972).

Die statistischen Angaben, auf denen diese Darstellung fußt, entstammen Medizinalstatistiken aus verschiedenen Ländern (KATSCHNIG et al., 1975; MILAZZO-SAYRE, 1977; Bundesminister für Jugend etc., 1977; Japanisches Gesundheitsministerium, 1977), Übersichtsreferaten (SILVERMAN, 1968; DOHRENWEND u. DOHRENWEND, 1969; MAYO, 1976; PERRIS, 1976; LAUTER, 1977; SCHWAB u. SCHWAB, 1978) sowie wissenschaftlichen Originalarbeiten, die von der Ermittlung der Behandlungsinzidenz bzw. -prävalenz (SCHOTT, 1903; KIMURA, 1965; TASCHEV, 1965; SHEPHERD et al., 1966; KRAMER u. TAUBE, 1973; STRÖMGREN, 1973; WARHEIT et al., 1973; WEEKE et al., 1975; DIEBOLD et al., 1977) bis zu epidemiologischen Feldstudien (HELGASON, 1964; HAGNELL, 1970) und Familienuntersuchungen im Zusammenhang mit der Erforschung einzelner Krankheitsbilder (ANGST, 1966; PERRIS, 1966) reichen. Die Angaben beziehen sich dementsprechend auf verschiedene Länder und verschiedene Zeitabschnitte (seit Mitte des vorigen Jahrhunderts) und geben dadurch wahrscheinlich insgesamt ein annähernd zutreffendes Bild von den realen Verhältnissen. Zu seiner Überprüfung wird abschließend noch ein Vergleich mit einem nach allen psychiatrischen Unterdiagnosen der ICD (International Classification of Diseases; DEGKWITZ et al., 1975) aufgeschlüsseltes klinisches und poliklinisches Krankengut von Kindern, Jugendlichen und Erwachsenen vorgenommen, die in den vergangenen 12 Jahren am Max-Planck-Institut für Psychiatrie in München erstmals aufgenommen bzw. ambulant untersucht worden sind. Dies erscheint sinnvoll, weil eine derart weitgehende diagnostische Differenzierung im Zusammenhang mit epidemiologischen Fragestellungen im allgemeinen nicht bzw. nur für einzelne Krankheitsbilder vorgenommen wird, wodurch u.U. ausgeprägte Geschlechtsunterschiede innerhalb spezifischer Krankheitsgruppen verwischt werden können.

Eine *Geschlechtsdifferenz*, die durch Medizinalstatistiken aus verschiedenen Ländern mit unterschiedlicher Zivilisationshöhe und entsprechend unterschiedlicher Qualität der medizinischen Versorgung ausgewiesen wird, besteht in der höheren *Mortalität* männlicher Individuen. Diese Differenz findet sich postnatal in allen Lebensaltern, zeigt aber von der Geburt an eine fallende Tendenz (HUTT, 1978; WALTER, 1978). Die Annahme einer höheren Zahl männlicher zu weiblichen Konzeptionen (WALTER, 1978) wird durch Chromosomenanalysen des Gewebsmaterials von Frühaborten nicht gestützt (KAJII, 1973). Diese ergeben vielmehr ein leichtes Überwiegen weiblicher Früchte im Beginn der Gravidität. Durch eine höhere Zahl von weiblichen Frühaborten – die z.T. durch Chromosomenanomalien bedingt sind (BOUÉ u. BOUÉ, 1976) – kehrt sich die Geschlechtsproportion allmählich um, so daß die Zahl der Knabengeburten die der Mädchengeburten in allen daraufhin untersuchten Populationen übertrifft. In der Bundesrepublik Deutschland beträgt die Relation derzeit etwa 106 zu 100. Vom letzten Drittel der Gravidität an ist aber die Sterblichkeit männlicher Individuen größer als die der weiblichen. Postnatal verschiebt sich die Geschlechtsproportion kontinuierlich zum weiblichen Anteil hin, woraus im höheren Lebensalter schließlich ein Frauenüberschuß resultiert (Bundesminister für Jugend etc., 1977). Die Verschiebung der Geschlechtsproportion in Abhängigkeit vom Lebensalter wird durch epochale Ereignisse (wie die höhere Männersterblichkeit im Krieg) mitbestimmt, so daß Altersangaben zur Geschlechtsproportion u.U. mehr über unterschiedliche Expositions- als Konstitutionsfaktoren aussagen. Allerdings ist die höhere Lebenserwartung der Frauen nicht auf Epochen bzw. Gesellschaften mit kriegsbedingten Verschiebungen der Geschlechtsproportion beschränkt.

Der durchschnittlich höheren Mortalität des männlichen Geschlechts entspricht eine höhere *Morbidität* bezüglich vital bedrohlicher – insbesondere chronischer – körperlicher Erkrankungen. Nur bei Genitalkarzinomen und – in den Industrienationen (wahrscheinlich infolge stärkerer Fettsuchtneigung bei entsprechendem Nahrungsangebot: THEILE, 1977) – beim Diabetes (dieser Befund ist allerdings möglicherweise allein mit Unterschieden in den Ernährungsgewohnheiten zu erklären und somit letztlich soziokulturell bedingt) sowie bei einer Reihe seltener (sowie einiger harmloserer) Krankheiten überwiegen die Frauen, die zudem durch Komplikationen der Gestation zusätzlich gefährdet sind. Bis zum Eintreten der Geschlechtsreife kommen aber nahezu alle lebensbedrohlichen Erkrankungen häufiger beim männlichen als beim weiblichen Geschlecht vor. Dasselbe gilt für die meisten *Mißbildungen* (Bundesminister für Jugend etc., 1977). Diese gehen nicht selten mit *zerebralen Entwicklungsstörungen* einher, was zur größeren Häufigkeit von geistiger bzw. Lernbehinderung bei Knaben beiträgt (SANDBERG, 1976). Das Überwiegen der Mißbildungsrate bei Knaben reicht aber wohl kaum zur Erklärung ihres Überschusses an geistig bzw. Lernbehinderten aus, da sich ähnliche Geschlechtsproportionen wie bei der Oligophrenie auch bei solchen Formen *psychischer Konstitutionsanomalien* finden, bei denen die Mißbildungsrate wesentlich geringer ist (Neuropathie, infantiler Autismus, verzögerte Sprachentwicklung, Legasthenie, Rechenschwäche; HUTT, 1978).

Eine höhere Anfälligkeit des männlichen Gehirns gegenüber exogenen Schädigungen kommt in dem deutlichen Überwiegen der Knaben beim *frühkindlichen exogenen Psychosyndrom* zum Ausdruck (LEMPP, 1976). Freilich ist das männliche Geschlecht von der Kindheit an insgesamt vergleichsweise stärker unfallgefährdet (HUTT, 1978), was teils mit der – möglicherweise konstitutionell verankerten – stärkeren Ausprägung des Risikoverhaltens, teils aber mit stärkerer Exposition infolge unterschiedlicher Rollenverteilung zusammenhängt; so tragen Arbeits-, Verkehrs- und Sportunfälle zu dem deutlichen Überwiegen der Männer bei traumatischen Hirnschädigungen mit ihren psychischen Folgeerscheinungen (organische Psychosen, Wesensänderung, Demenz) bei. Insgesamt gleicht sich allerdings die zum männlichen Geschlecht hin verschobene Proportion der psychischen Morbidität etwa von der Pubertät an allmählich aus, wobei wahrscheinlich gesellschaftliche Faktoren eine wesentliche, wenn auch kaum die allein ausschlaggebende Rolle spielen dürften.

Im Kindesalter überwiegen auch bei den *psychoreaktiven Störungen* im allgemeinen die Knaben (NISSEN, 1976a), möglicherweise z.T. infolge ihrer konstitutionell erhöhten Irritierbarkeit, die schon beim Vergleich männlicher und weiblicher Säuglinge auffällt (ARGANIAN, 1973) und die sie offenbar auch gegenüber familiären Spannungen sensibilisiert (RUTTER, 1970). Lediglich bei ausgeprägt depressiven Syndromen überwiegen möglicherweise die Mädchen. Die meisten

Anomalien der Entwicklung von *Triebkonstitution* und *Charakter* (sexuelle Deviationen bzw. Psychopathien) herrschen aber beim männlichen Geschlecht vor, das somit von allen primären psychischen Konstitutionsanomalien stärker betroffen ist als das weibliche.

In der Ontogenese stellt die *Pubertätsmagersucht* (THOMÄ, 1961), die offenbar einen Protest gegen das Erwachsenenwerden und die Übernahme der spezifischen Geschlechtsrolle zum Ausdruck bringt, das erste psychiatrische Krankheitsbild dar, das beim weiblichen Geschlecht ungleich häufiger auftritt als beim männlichen (CRISP et al., 1977). Dies dürfte vornehmlich mit Problemen der Weiblichkeit (stärkere puberale körperliche Umgestaltung, Mutterschaft, Hausfrauenrolle) zusammenhängen, die in modernen Industriegesellschaften mit ihren Verlockungen eines ungebundenen Lebens und ihren vielseitigen Karriereangeboten zu geschlechtsspezifischen Rollenkonflikten führen können. Möglicherweise sind auch die andersartigen und komplizierteren hormonalen Pubertätsveränderungen des weiblichen Geschlechts für dessen starkes Überwiegen bei dieser Erkrankung mitverantwortlich.

Über die Geschlechtsverteilung psychiatrischer Erkrankungen im *Erwachsenenalter* gehen die Angaben in der Literatur erheblich auseinander, insbesondere bezüglich der Gesamtverteilung. Diese Widersprüche sind teils lokalen bzw. epochalen Faktoren zuzuschreiben, teils sind sie allerdings methodisch bedingt (DOHRENWEND u. DOHRENWEND, 1976).

Werden nur gravierende psychische Störungen gezählt, die der Umgebung auffallen, so überwiegen im allgemeinen die Männer; werden auch leichtere, vornehmlich subjektiv erlebte Störungen gezählt, so kommt es eher zu einem Überwiegen der Frauen. Werden bei der Ermittlung der Behandlungsinzidenz bzw. -prävalenz nur die Insassen großer Nervenkrankenhäuser als „psychiatrische Fälle" erfaßt, so überwiegen in einigen Ländern (z.B. den USA 1975: MILAZZO-SAYRE und Japan 1977: Japanisches Gesundheitsministerium) die Männer; rechnet man hingegen alle Fälle hinzu, die ambulante Einrichtungen (unter Einschluß niedergelassener Ärzte) wegen psychischer Störungen konsultieren, so kommt es gewöhnlich zu einer deutlichen Verschiebung der Geschlechtsproportion mit Überwiegen des weiblichen Anteils (DILLING u. WEYERER, 1978; s. auch KRAMER u. TAUBE, 1973). Entsprechende Unterschiede finden sich, wenn man bei epidemiologischen Feldstudien anstelle der früher häufig geübten Befragung von Gewährsleuten Direkterhebungen mit Fragebögen vornimmt (GOVE u. TUDOR, 1973; CLANCY u. GOVE, 1974). Auch hier kommt es durch die stärkere Erfassung subjektiv erlebter Beeinträchtigung zu einer Proportionsverschiebung zum weiblichen Anteil hin (VERBRUGGE, 1976; WARHEIT et al., 1973).

Wichtig ist zudem, wie weit *sozial* störendes Verhalten als Ausdruck *psychischer* Gestörtheit angesehen und dementsprechend in die Erhebungen einbezogen wird (ROBINS, 1966; MAZER, 1974). Während Dissozialität im Kindes- und Jugendalter im allgemeinen zum Verantwortungsbereich des (Kinder- und Jugend-) Psychiaters gerechnet wird und dadurch mit zum Überwiegen des männlichen Geschlechts in der Morbidität dieser Altersstufe beiträgt, wird sie im Erwachsenenalter nur selektiv unter gutachterlichen Aspekten als Gegenstand der Psychiatrie betrachtet und dementsprechend bei vielen epidemiologischen Erhebungen über Inzidenz und Prävalenz psychischer Störungen von Erwachsenen weitgehend ausgeblendet (DILLING u. WEYERER, 1978). Je nachdem, wie weit man – vom Kernbereich psychiatrischer Erkrankungen (Psychosen, Suchten, klassische Psychoneurosen etc.) ausgehend – in den Bereich regelwidrigen Sozialverhaltens einerseits (HASKELL u. YABLONSKY, 1974; KATSCHNIG u. STEINERT, 1977) bzw. aller Arten beeinträchtigten subjektiven Wohlbefindens andererseits vordringt (GOVE u. TUDOR, 1973; CLANCY u. GOVE, 1974), ergibt sich eine Proportionsverschiebung der psychiatrischen Gesamtmorbidität zum männlichen bzw. zum weiblichen Geschlecht hin. Mit der stärkeren Tendenz zu subjektiv erlebter Beeinträchtigung geht bei Frauen (jedenfalls in modernen Industrienationen) ein stärkeres Hilfesuchverhalten einher. Beide Erscheinungen zusammengenommen dürften die höhere Frequentierung medizinischer Einrichtungen durch Frauen weitgehend erklären. Hinzu kommt die höhere Lebenserwartung der Frauen und ihre geringere Chance, im Alter vom Ehepartner versorgt zu werden, wodurch sich im allgemeinen ein Überwiegen der Frauen bei den Alterskrankheiten ergibt.

Aus den genannten Gründen erscheint es wenig sinnvoll, bei einer Betrachtung der Geschlechtsdisposition zu psychischen Normabweichungen deren verschiedene Formen zu globalen Kategorien zusammenzufassen. Vielmehr muß eine möglichst weitgehende *diagnostische Aufschlüsselung* unter gleichzeitiger Berücksichtigung spezieller Selektionsfaktoren (wie Hilfesuchverhalten [MAZER, 1974], Überlebenschancen etc.) versucht werden.

In einer Untersuchung der psychiatrischen Morbidität der Bevölkerung von drei oberbayerischen Landkreisen mit insgesamt 424 442 Einwohnern ermittelten DILLING und WEYERER (1978) aufgrund der Patientendaten von niedergelassenen Nervenärzten und stationären psychiatrischen Einrichtungen eine *Behandlungsinzidenz* von 1 618 ($=3,8\,^0/_{00}$) und eine *Behandlungsprävalenz* von 3 788 ($=8,9\,^0/_{00}$) Fällen im Zeitraum von einem halben Jahr. Dabei überwog insgesamt jeweils das weibliche Geschlecht. Die Aufschlüsselung nach Diagnosen (Abb. 4) zeigt

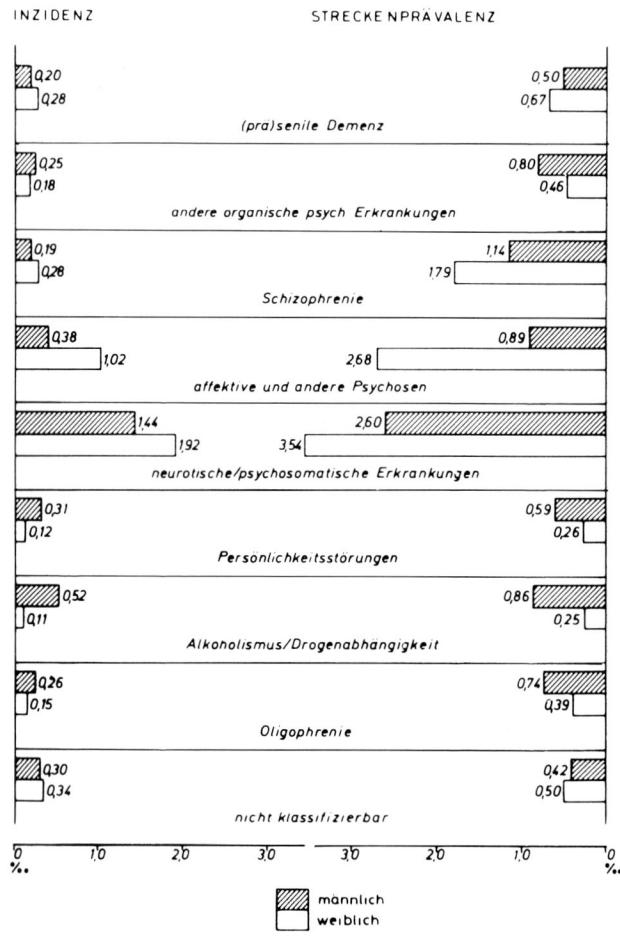

Abb. 4. Geschlechtsproportion der Behandlungsinzidenz und -prävalenz psychiatrischer Erkrankungen (nach DILLING u. WEYERER, 1978)

aber, daß diese Geschlechtsproportion fast ausschließlich auf das Konto der endogenen Psychosen sowie der neurotischen Störungen (einschließlich der als „psychosomatische Erkrankungen" bezeichneten Organneurosen) geht; sonst findet sich lediglich ein leichter Frauenüberschuß bei der (prä-) senilen Demenz und den nicht klassifizierbaren Störungen. Beim Alkoholismus (unter Einschluß der Drogenabhängigkeit), den Persönlichkeitsstörungen, der Oligophrenie und den körperlich begründbaren psychischen Störungen außer der (prä-) senilen Demenz überwiegen hingegen die Männer. Alle Unterschiede betreffen Inzidenz und Prävalenz, wenn auch in jeweils verschiedenem Ausmaß. Es ist klar, daß eine Gewichtung nach Schwere der Erkrankung und stationärer Behandlungsbedürftigkeit die Proportionen insgesamt zur männlichen Seite hin verlagern würde, da in der vorliegenden Statistik die neurotischen Störungen mit dem deutlichen Überwiegen der Frauen besonders stark zu Buche schlagen. Diese Verlagerung der Proportion zur männlichen Seite hin würde durch eine stärkere Einbeziehung psychisch auffälliger Straftäter noch akzentuiert werden.

Grundsätzlich ähnliche Verhältnisse wie bei der Ermittlung von Behandlungsinzidenz und Behandlungsprävalenz fanden die beiden Autoren[1] bei einer epidemiologischen *Feldstudie*, die in zwei Ortschaften der von ihnen untersuchten Region durchgeführt wurde. In einer repräsentativen Stichprobe von bisher 916 ausgewerteten Fällen im Alter ab 15 Jahren eruierten sie bei insgesamt fast 44% psychische Auffälligkeiten von Krankheitswert mit einem relativen Überwiegen der Frauen (rd. 46% gegenüber rd. 40% der Männer). Im wesentlichen gaben psychogene Störungen den Ausschlag für die Abweichung von einer prozentualen Gleichverteilung. Der Anteil der neurotischen und sog. psychosomatischen Störungen betrug bei den Frauen 31%, bei den Männern hingegen nur knapp 18%. Der ausgeprägteste Geschlechtsunterschied fand sich aber beim Alkoholismus (unter Einschluß der Drogenabhängigkeit) mit einem Anteil von 10,1% der Männer zu 0,2% der Frauen (was z.T. mit dem kleinstädtischen bzw. ländlichen Milieu zusammenhängen dürfte, da in modernen Großstädten ein derart krasser Geschlechtsunterschied beim Alkoholismus im allgemeinen nicht mehr besteht; FEUERLEIN, 1975; SOLMS, 1975). Die Geschlechtsverteilung der übrigen Diagnosen aus der – noch nicht abgeschlossenen – Feldstudie sollen wegen der relativ geringen Fallzahlen hier nicht im einzelnen besprochen werden. Der Richtung nach stimmen sie mit dem Ergebnis der an Behandlungsinstitutionen durchgeführten Untersuchung derselben Autoren sehr gut überein und belegen somit auch die Brauchbarkeit der an solchen Einrichtungen gewonnenen Daten für epidemiologische Zwecke. Allerdings müssen bei derartigen Erhebungen möglichst unterschiedliche – stationäre und ambulante – Einrichtungen berücksichtigt und deren spezielle Selektionsbedingungen in Rechnung gestellt werden.

Als Beispiel einer solchen Erhebung sei eine Auswertung über die Geschlechtsproportion in dem nach der ICD (International Classification of Diseases; DEGKWITZ et al., 1975) aufgeschlüsselten psychiatrischen Krankengut angeführt, das in den *ambulanten* bzw. *stationären* Einrichtungen der *Kinderpsychiatrischen* Abteilung und der Abteilungen für *Erwachsenenpsychiatrie* des Max-Planck-

---

[1] Den Autoren sei auch an dieser Stelle für die freundliche Überlassung noch nicht publizierten Zahlenmaterials gedankt.

Tabelle 5. Geschlechtsproportion psychiatrischer Erkrankungen bei Patienten des Max-Planck-Instituts für Psychiatrie, München. Erstkonsultationen bzw. Erstaufnahmen 1966-1977 (n = 22.742)

Diagnose nach ICD (8. Revision)		Kinderpsychiatrie						Erwachsenenpsychiatrie					
		Ambulant			Stationär			Ambulant			Stationär		
Code-Nr.	Kurzbezeichnung	n	%m	p(%)	n	%m	p(%)	n	%m	p(%)	n	%m	p(%)
290	*(Präs-) Senile Demenz*							56	45		13	62	
290.0	Senile Demenz							32	34				
290.1	Präsenile Demenz							17	59				
291	*Alkoholpsychosen*							297	71	*<0,1*	55	66	*<5,0*
291.0	Delirium tremens							153	77	*<0,1*	28	61	
291.1	Korsakow-Syndrom							53	70	*<1,0*			
291.2	Halluzinose							17	65		11	64	
291.4	Rausch							47	57				
292	*Psychosen b. intrakran. Infekt.*							19	42				
293	*Psychosen b. ander. Hirnkrh.*							453	39	*<0,1*	46	46	
293.0	Hirnarteriosklerose							330	34	*<0,1*	15	33	
293.1	And. cerebr. Durchbl.störungen							50	46		10	40	
293.5	Hirntraumen							23	74	*<5,0*			
294	*Psychosen b. and. körperl. Stör.*							206	49		67	48	
294.0	Endokrine Störungen							18	56				
294.1	Stoffwechselkrankheiten							30	33				
294.3	Intoxikationen (außer 291)							97	56		41	49	
295	*Schizophrenie*[a]	21	76	*<5,0*	12	50		731	46	*<5,0*	795	52	
295.0	Schizophrenia simplex							54	59		48	71	*<1,0*
295.1	Hebephrene Form							97	67	*<0,1*	127	68	*<0,1*
295.2	Katatone Form							23	52		32	53	
295.3	Paranoide Form							323	42	*<1,0*	347	52	
295.4	Akute Episode							31	19	*<0,1*	25	28	*<5,0*
295.5	Pseudoneurot. Schizophrenie							18	72		22	77	*<5,0*
295.6	Rest- bzw. Defektzustand							93	33	*<1,0*	82	43	

[a] Ohne 295.7

Diagnose nach ICD (8. Revision)		Kinderpsychiatrie						Erwachsenpsychiatrie					
		Ambulant			Stationär			Ambulant			Stationär		
Code-Nr.	Kurzbezeichnung	n	%m	p(%)	n	%m	p(%)	n	%m	p(%)	n	%m	p(%)
295.7	*Schizoaffektive Psychosen*							30	23	<1,0	99	27	<0,1
296	*Affektive Psychosen*							959	27	<0,1	519	35	<0,1
296.0	Involutionsdepression							367	20	<0,1	132	23	<0,1
296.1	Manie („monopolar")							34	53		64	47	
296.2	Monopolare Depression							440	30	<0,1	249	34	<0,1
296.3	Bipolare affektive Psychose							62	44		55	58	
297	*Paranoide Syndrome (außer 298.3)*							97	24	<0,1	69	32	<1,0
297.0	Paranoia							21	24	<5,0[b]	15	47	
297.1	Paranoide Involutionspsychose							48	21	<0,1	27	7	<0,1
298	*Andere Psychosen*							492	33	<0,1	53	38	<5,0
298.0	Reaktive depressive Psychose							425	33	<0,1	34	35	
298.1	Reaktiver Erregungszustand							28	18	<0,1			
298.3	Akute paranoide Reaktion							12	42		10	40	
299	*Nicht näher bez. Psychosen*							31	39				
300	*Neurosen*	41	56					4111	38	<0,1	1102	41	<0,1
300.0	Angstneurose	25	64					261	46		120	53	
300.1	Hysterische Neurose							276	25	<0,1	138	14	<0,1
300.2	Phobie							184	51		78	45	
300.3	Zwangsneurose							90	56		157	51	
300.4	Depressive Neurose							2424	32	<0,1	441	35	<0,1
300.5	Neurasthenie							130	40	<5,0	31	55	
300.6	Neurot. Depersonalisationssyndrom							10	40				
300.7	Hypochondrische Neurose							161	62	<1,0	42	67	<5,0
301	*Psychopathien*	16	63					867	46	5,0[b]	267	53	
301.0	Paranoide Persönlichkeit							13	54		10	50	
301.1	Thymopathische Persönlichkeit							51	49		13	46	
301.2	Schizoide Persönlichkeit							58	76	<0,1	39	77	<0,1

[b] Bei zweiseitiger Fragestellung. Richtung der Abweichung von der Zufallserwartung entgegen der Vorhersage!

656 D. v. Zerssen: Konstitution

Diagnose nach ICD (8. Revision)		Kinderpsychiatrie						Erwachsenenpsychiatrie					
		Ambulant			Stationär			Ambulant			Stationär		
Code-Nr.	Kurzbezeichnung	n	%m	p(%)	n	%m	p(%)	n	%m	p(%)	n	%m	p(%)
301.3	Erregbare Persönlichkeit							57	82	<0,1	17	65	
301.4	Anankastische Persönlichkeit							35	66	<5,0	23	70	<5,0
301.5	Hysterische Persönlichkeit							273	14	<0,1	71	14	<0,1
301.6	Asthenische Persönlichkeit							122	50	<1,0	34	62	
301.7	Antisoziale Persönlichkeit							41	73				
302	*Sexuelle Deviationen*							242	86	<0,1	33	91	<0,1
302.0	Homosexualität							83	87	<0,1			
302.2	Pädophilie							10	90	<5,0			
302.3	Transvestitismus							23	61				
302.4	Exhibitionismus							37	100	<0,1	13	100	<0,1
303	*Alkoholismus*							2563	68	<0,1	107	58	
303.0	Episodischer Mißbrauch							131	63	<1,0			
303.1	Gewohnheitsmäßiger Mißbrauch							556	80	<0,1	30	40	<1,0
303.2	Trunksucht							1759	65	<0,1	64	66	<5,0
304	*Medikamentenabhängigkeit*							723	40	<0,1	75	37	
304.0	Opium							152	59	<5,0	21	38	
304.1	Synthetische Morphine							63	41				
304.2	Barbiturate							39	28	<1,0			
304.3	Andere Hypnotika etc.							191	21	<0,1	20	30	
304.5	Cannabis							24	67				
304.6	Andere Stimulantien							24	33				
304.7	Halluzinogene							13	85	<5,0			
305	*Psychosomatische Störungen*	11	36		44	84	<0,1	1330	57	0,1	82	45	
305.0	Haut							18	56				
305.1	Bewegungsapparat							68	50		39	49	
305.2	Atmungsorgane							151	33	<0,1			
305.3	Herz- und Kreislaufsystem							160	58				
305.5	Magen-Darm-Trakt							193	38	<0,1	11	36	
305.6	Urogenitalsystem							692	69	<0,1			
306	*Besondere Symptome*	553	74	<0,1				223	47		145	32	<0,1

Spezieller Teil

Diagnose nach ICD (8. Revision)		Kinderpsychiatrie						Erwachsenenpsychiatrie					
		Ambulant			Stationär			Ambulant			Stationär		
Code-Nr.	Kurzbezeichnung	n	%m	p(%)	n	%m	p(%)	n	%m	p(%)	n	%m	p(%)
306.1	Spezielle Lernstörungen	107	80	<0,1									
306.2	Tic	31	94	<0,1				17	47				
306.3	Andere psychomot. Störungen	24	88	<0,1				16	75				
306.4	Schlafstörungen	21	62					24	67				
306.5	Eßstörungen	25	48		11	91	<1,0	66	12	<0,1	81	5	<0,1
306.6	Enuresis	106	73	<0,1									
306.7	Enkopresis	14	86	<1,0	10	90	<5,0						
306.8	Kopfschmerzen	15	80	<5,0				42	29	<1,0			
307	*Akute abnorme Reaktionen*							2617	30	<0,1	82	37	<1,0
308ᶜ	*Verhaltensstör. im Kindesalter*	1439	74	<0,1	144	72	<0,1	60	58		25	56	
308.2	Reifungskrisen	90	67	<1,0				21	52		16	50	
308.3	Asozialität/Verwahrlosung	44	73	<1,0				11	73				
308.4	Frühkindl. exog. Psychosyndrom	310	80	<0,1	37	92	<0,1						
308.5	Psychogene Verhaltensstörungen	815	72	<0,1	89	64	<1,0						
308.6	Psychogene Leistungsstörungen	161	74	<0,1									
309	*Organische Wesensänderung*	12	42					517	48		78	58	
309.0	Intrakran. Infektionen							17	59				
309.1	Intox. o. extrakran. Infekt.							61	56		13	46	
309.2	Hirnverletzungen							31	81	<0,1	17	88	<1,0
309.3	Kreislaufstörungen							232	48		11	64	
309.5	Stoffwechselstörungen etc.							39	36				
309.6	(Prä-) Sen. Hirnkrankheiten							70	40				
310–315	*Oligophrenien*	1072	61	<0,1	177	69	<0,1	172	62	<1,0	33	61	
310	Minderbegabung	490	62	<0,1	49	55		60	73	<0,1	10	70	
311	Leichter Schwachsinn	384	63	<0,1	78	85	<0,1	46	65	<5,0			
312	Deutlicher Schwachsinn	155	57		31	55		27	48		10	40	
313	Schwerer Schwachsinn	26	46		10	70							

ᶜ Mit hausinterner Untergliederung dieser Diagnosengruppe

ICD = International Classification of Diseases (no. 290–315); n = Fallzahl, wenn ≥10; %m = (abgerundeter) Prozentsatz der Knaben bzw. Männer; p(%) = Zufallswahrscheinlichkeit in Prozent nach dem Binomial- und/oder Chiquadrat-Test (je nach Fallzahl), bei Erwartungswert %m = 50; nur mindestens auf dem 5%- (1%- bzw. 0,1%-) Niveau signifikante Werte aufgeführt, bei einseitiger Fragestellung *unterstrichen*

Instituts für Psychiatrie (MPI-P) in München während eines 12jährigen Zeitraumes erfaßt worden ist (s. Tabelle 5). Es handelt sich um insgesamt 22742 Fälle, wobei nur *Erstkonsultationen* der ambulanten bzw. *Erstaufnahmen* der stationären Einrichtungen gezählt wurden. Jeder Fall ging nur mit der psychiatrischen Hauptdiagnose in die Auswertung ein. Für alle drei- und vierstelligen Diagnosenummern wurden die Fallzahl pro Einrichtung sowie die Geschlechtsproportion (als Prozentsatz der männlichen Patienten) und deren Abweichung von einer Gleichverteilung (je nach Fallzahl mit Hilfe des Binomialtests bzw. eines für den Vergleich von zwei Kategorien modifizierten Chi-Quadrat-Tests: PFANZAGL, 1974) berechnet, wobei für den angestrebten orientierenden Überblick einfachheitshalber ein Erwartungswert von 50% angesetzt wurde[2].

Das Institut ist räumlich einem großen Allgemeinkrankenhaus angegliedert, demgegenüber vertragliche Konsiliar- und Aufnahmeverpflichtungen bestehen, was sich besonders auf die Zusammensetzung der ambulanten Klientel der Erwachsenenpsychiatrie auswirkt. Die relativ geringe Bettenzahl zwingt zudem bei den stark forschungsorientierten Einrichtungen zu gewissen diagnostischen Eingrenzungen der stationären Aufnahmen. Insofern kann das Krankengut nicht als repräsentativ für die Verhältnisse in der Gesamtbevölkerung einer Großstadt und ihrer Umgebung, aus der die meisten Patienten stammen, oder des für diese Region zuständigen Nervenkrankenhauses angesehen werden. Am ehesten ist es noch mit dem stationären Krankengut einer Universitätsklinik vergleichbar. Eine Auswahl nach dem Geschlecht findet aber im allgemeinen nicht statt, es sei denn bei einzelnen Projekten oder aufgrund der begrenzten Bettenkapazität.

Die Übersicht beschränkt sich auf jene diagnostischen Kategorien, bei denen mindestens in einer der verglichenen Einrichtungen 10 oder mehr Fälle erfaßt wurden. Die anderen Kategorien sowie die nicht näher spezifizierten Untergruppen der ICD (*.8*, mit Ausnahme von *306.8*, und *.9*) sowie alle Angaben über Gruppengrößen unter 10 Fällen innerhalb einer der Einrichtungen sind nicht mit ausgedruckt. Bei den Wahrscheinlichkeiten werden nur mindestens auf dem 5%-Niveau signifikante Werte angeführt – sie sind bei einseitiger Fragestellung aufgrund klinisch und epidemiologisch begründeter Hypothesen über die Richtung der Abweichung von einer Gleichverteilung kursiv gesetzt. In zwei Fällen, in denen sich Abweichungen entgegen der Vorhersage fanden, wurde der Signifikanzwert für die zweiseitige Fragestellung ausgedruckt und mit einer entsprechenden Fußnote versehen. Von diesen beiden Ausnahmen abgesehen werden die Erwartungen aber durch die Daten weitgehend bestätigt.

So überwiegt im Krankengut der *Kinderpsychiatrie* fast durchweg das männliche Geschlecht. Das Gegenteil ist nur bei vereinzelten diagnostischen Kategorien des ambulanten Krankengutes zu finden und erreicht in keinem Fall das geforderte Signifikanzniveau von 5%. Beim schweren Schwachsinn (ICD-Nr. *313*) wird zudem die gefundene Abweichung zur weiblichen Seite hin durch eine entgegengesetzte Abweichung im stationären Krankengut ausgeglichen. Besonders ausgeprägt ist das Überwiegen des männlichen Geschlechts bei „besonderen Symptomen" (mehrere Untergruppen der Diagnosekategorie *306*), so bei speziellen Lernstörungen, Tics, Enuresis und Enkopresis, ferner bei Verhaltensstörungen (*308*), insbesondere beim frühkindlichen exogenen Psychosyndrom (*308.4*). Bei den Oligophrenien überwiegt zwar auch das männliche Geschlecht, erwartungsgemäß aber nicht so stark wie bei den vorgenannten Störungen und in statistisch signifikanter Ausprägung nur bei Minderbegabung und leichterem Schwachsinn (*310* und *311*).

---

[2] Genaugenommen müßte jeweils die altersentsprechende Geschlechtsproportion der Durchschnittsbevölkerung zugrunde gelegt werden, was die Auswertung enorm kompliziert, die Ergebnisse aber kaum entscheidend beeinflußt hätte.

Ein sehr viel differenzierteres Bild bieten die Geschlechtsproportionen der Krankheitsbilder *erwachsener* Patienten. Hier liegen – soweit die Fallzahlen für einen Vergleich ausreichen – ähnliche Abweichungen wie bei den Kindern und Jugendlichen nur bezüglich der *Oligophrenien (310–315)* und der *Sprachstörungen (306.0)* vor. Ein deutliches und statistisch signifikantes Überwiegen des männlichen Geschlechts findet sich erwartungsgemäß (HELGASON, 1964) auch bei *organischer Wesensänderung* und *organischen Psychosen nach Hirnverletzung (309.2 bzw. 293.5)*, beim *Alkoholismus (303)* und den *Alkoholpsychosen (291)*, den *sexuellen Deviationen (302)* und mehreren Unterformen der *Psychopathie (301)*, nämlich bei den schizoiden *(301.2)*, den erregbaren *(301.3)*, den anankastischen *(301.4)* und den antisozialen Persönlichkeiten *(301.7)*. Im Bereich *neurotisch-reaktiver Störungen (300* und *307)* besteht ein signifikantes Übergewicht der Männer nur bei der hypochondrischen Neurose *(300.7)* und im großen Formenkreis *endogener* bzw. *reaktiver Psychosen (295–298)* nur bei einigen Unterformen der Schizophrenie, und zwar speziell bei denen mit frühem Krankheitsbeginn, nämlich der hebephrenen Form *(295.1)*, der Schizophrenia simplex *(295.0)* und der pseudoneurotischen Schizophrenie *(295.5)*. Diese Abweichungen sind aufgrund der einschlägigen Literatur zu erwarten (bezüglich der Hebephrenie: MAYER-GROSS et al., 1969) oder stehen zumindest nicht im Widerspruch mit zahlreichen Literaturberichten (bezüglich Hypochondrie [ERNST et al., 1968] sowie einfacher und pseudoneurotischer Schizophrenie).

Daß bei sog. psychosomatischen Störungen im Bereich des Urogenitalsystems *(305.6)* im ambulanten Krankengut die Männer deutlich und signifikant überwiegen und infolge ihrer großen Fallzahl die Geschlechtsproportion in der Gesamtgruppe psychosomatischer Störungen *(305)* zur männlichen Seite hin verschieben, ist offenbar einem Selektionseffekt durch wissenschaftliche Projekte der Psychiatrischen Poliklinik über die Impotenz zuzuschreiben, die in der ICD unter *305.6* zu verschlüsseln ist. Ein anderer, der Erwartung direkt widersprechender Untersuchungsbefund im ambulanten Krankengut der Erwachsenenpsychiatrie ist offenbar ebenfalls selektionsbedingt. Es handelt sich um das (bei zweiseitiger Fragestellung auf dem 5%-Niveau signifikante) Überwiegen der Frauen bei den Psychopathien *(301)*, das durch die häufig gestellte Diagnose einer hysterischen Persönlichkeit *(301.5)* zustande kommt. Diese Diagnose überwiegt zwar im stationären Krankengut bei Frauen im selben Ausmaß. Die Diagnose wird hier aber vergleichsweise seltener gestellt, so daß insgesamt die Männer bei den Psychopathien vorherrschen. Es ist überaus wahrscheinlich, daß ein Selektionsfaktor durch die poliklinischen Konsiliarverpflichtungen in dem benachbarten Allgemeinkrankenhaus zu der vergleichsweise hohen Zahl von hysterischen Persönlichkeitsstörungen im ambulanten Krankengut geführt hat; denn diese Patientinnen nehmen erfahrungsgemäß häufig ärztliche Hilfe in den Disziplinen der somatischen Medizin in Anspruch, von wo aus dann wegen ihrer psychischen Auffälligkeit eine psychiatrische Untersuchung veranlaßt wird.

Das Überwiegen der Frauen bei den hysterischen Persönlichkeitsstörungen im ambulanten und stationären Krankengut entspricht im übrigen vollkommen der Erwartung (HELGASON, 1964); nur der relativ hohe Anteil dieser Fälle im ambulanten Krankengut und die daraus resultierende Verschiebung der Geschlechtsproportion zur weiblichen Seite in der Gesamtgruppe der Persönlichkeitsstörungen *(301)* ist offenbar selektionsbedingt. Das Beispiel zeigt, wie wichtig gerade bei der Analyse von Morbiditätsstatistiken aus Behandlungseinrichtungen die möglichst weitgehende diagnostische Aufschlüsselung des Krankengutes ist.

In der großen Rubrik „Besondere Symptome" *(306)* überwiegen die Patientinnen vornehmlich bei den *Eßstörungen*, die insbesondere im stationären Krankengut der Erwachsenenpsychiatrie vorwiegend Fälle von Anorexia nervosa betreffen. Dies ist zwar durch spezielle Forschungsinteressen mitbedingt, würde aber an sich keineswegs innerhalb dieses Krankheitsbildes zu einer bevorzugten Aufnahme weiblicher Patienten führen, da die Anorexia nervosa beim männlichen Geschlecht gerade wegen ihrer Seltenheit von besonderem wissenschaftlichen Interesse ist.

Daß die Frauen auch den größeren Anteil erwachsener Patienten mit Kopfschmerzen (*306.8*), ferner mit *akuten abnormen Reaktionen* (*307*) sowie mit verschiedenen *organneurotischen Syndromen* (*305.2* und *305.5*) stellen, ist nach fast allen einschlägigen klinischen und epidemiologischen Untersuchungen aus westlichen Industrienationen zu erwarten (HELGASON, 1964; KATSCHNIG u. STROTZKA, 1977; DILLING u. WEYERER, 1978). Dasselbe gilt für die *Medikamentenabhängigkeit* (*304*), die allerdings in epidemiologischen Untersuchungen oft mit dem Alkoholismus zusammengefaßt wird, so daß es zu einem scheinbaren Überwiegen der Männer kommt. Bei den Frauen sind es insbesondere die von Ärzten verordneten bzw. in Apotheken frei erhältlichen Schlaf-, Schmerz- und Beruhigungsmittel (*304.2* und *304.3*), die im Übermaß konsumiert werden, bei Männern hingegen eher die typischen „Schwarzmarktdrogen", zu denen auch die Halluzinogene (*304.7*) gehören (JANZ, 1977). Wie beim Alkoholismus sucht der Mann offenbar mehr den Rausch und scheut nicht die Illegalität bei der Beschaffung des Rauschmittels, während die Frau mehr die bloße Unterdrückung von Mißbefinden und vegetativen Störungen durch legal erhältliche Mittel erstrebt. Transkulturelle Vergleiche könnten dazu beitragen, die Rolle soziokultureller Faktoren bei der Entstehung geschlechtstypischen Suchtverhaltens genauer zu bestimmen, von der Rolle biologischer Dispositionsfaktoren abzugrenzen und die Interaktionen beider Faktorengruppen einer Analyse zugänglich zu machen. Wie Persönlichkeitsstörungen häufig die Grundlage für den Mißbrauch von Rauschdrogen bilden, so schaffen Neurosen im weitesten Sinne im allgemeinen die psychologischen Voraussetzungen für die Entstehung der Medikamentenabhängigkeit. Es nimmt daher nicht wunder, daß wie in den meisten einschlägigen Statistiken aus westlichen Industrienationen auch im Krankengut des MPI-P die Frauen den größten Anteil neurotischer Patienten stellen (HAGNELL, 1970; KATSCHNIG u. STROTZKA, 1977). Bemerkenswerterweise sind dafür aber im wesentlichen die beiden „typisch weiblichen" Neuroseformen – *hysterische Neurose* (*300.1*) und *neurotische Depression* (*300.4*) – verantwortlich.

Die Tatsache, daß außer der Zwangsneurose (*300.3*) auch die durch vorherrschende Angstsymptomatik gekennzeichneten Neuroseformen (*300.0* und *300.2*) eine ausgeglichene Geschlechtsrelation zeigen, läßt Zweifel daran aufkommen, daß das Vorherrschen hysterischer und depressiver Symptomatik bei Frauen allein gesellschaftlichen Geschlechtsstereotypen zuzuschreiben ist; gelten doch Frauen im allgemeinen als das ängstlichere Geschlecht, bei dem man deshalb auch eher geneigt ist, krankhafte Ängste zu tolerieren. Gerade das Fehlen des danach zu erwartenden Geschlechtsunterschiedes bei neurotisch bedingten Angstzuständen unterstreicht die Bedeutung, die dem Geschlecht bei der Entstehung der hysterischen und der depressiven Neurosen zukommt. Sie wird u.a. von dem starken Überwiegen des weiblichen Geschlechts bei den Suizidversuchen in allen darauf untersuchten Ländern reflektiert (STENGEL, 1969; BÖCKER, 1973), in dem offenbar die gleiche Tendenz demonstrativer Hilfsgkeit zum Ausdruck kommt, während gelungene Selbstmorde, die bei Männern deutlich häufiger vorkommen als bei Frauen (STENGEL, 1969; BÖCKER, 1973), eine stärker destruktive Note tragen, wie sie auch das nach außen gerichtete männliche Aggressionsverhalten kennzeichnet.

Es ist nicht von der Hand zu weisen, daß gesellschaftliche Einflüsse, zu denen u.a. die Idealisierung männlichen Kampfverhaltens gehört, die Entwicklung destruktiver Tendenzen beim männlichen Geschlecht stärker begünstigen als beim weiblichen und umgekehrt bei diesem die Tendenz zu demonstrativer Hilflosigkeit zu fördern vermögen, die schon bei Knaben sozial weniger erwünscht erscheint als bei Mädchen. Die stärkere Depressionsneigung der Frauen ist aber bemerkenswerterweise nicht auf neurotische Störungen beschränkt, sondern findet sich auch bei den endogenen Psychosen (SCHOTT, 1903; HELGASON, 1964; TASCHEV, 1965; ANGST, 1966; PERRIS, 1966; ADELSTEIN et al., 1968; ANGST u. PERRIS, 1968; SILVERMAN, 1968; DOHRENWEND u. DOHRENWEND, 1969; UCHTENHAGEN, 1975; WEEKE et al., 1975; PERRIS, 1976).

Das deutliche Überwiegen der Frauen bei den *affektiven Psychosen* (*296*) geht fast ausschließlich auf das Konto der monopolaren Depressionen (*296.2*), und zwar vornehmlich das ihrer Spätmanifestationsform, der Involutionsdepression (*296.0*). Bei frühem Krankheitsbeginn gehen zunächst monopolar verlaufende Depressionen nicht selten später noch in bipolare affektive Psychosen (*296.3*) über, bei denen die Geschlechtsproportion – auch nach Familienuntersuchungen – ausgeglichen ist. Allerdings scheint auch beim bipolaren Verlaufstyp affektiver Psychosen die Relation depressiver zu manischen bzw. hypomanischen Phasen bei Frauen stärker zum depressiven Anteil hin verschoben zu sein als bei Männern. Bei rein oder überwiegend manisch verlaufenden Psychosen verhält es sich hingegen eher umgekehrt (LEFF et al., 1976). Bei den *schizoaffektiven Psychosen* (*295.7*) mit ihrer oft ausgeprägten depressiven Symptomatik herrscht aber das weibliche Geschlecht ebenso deutlich vor wie in der Gesamtgruppe rein affektiver Psychosen (*296*) (KIMURA, 1965; MENTZOS, 1967; PERRIS, 1974). Das gleiche gilt für die als reaktiv bezeichneten depressiven Psychosen (*298.0*), bei denen es sich möglicherweise um endogene Depressionen mit deutlicher Auslösung durch Umweltereignisse handelt. Solche Ereignisse spielen offenbar in der Entstehung von depressiven Psychosen bei weiblichen eine größere Rolle als bei männlichen Patienten (SCHOTT, 1903; MATUSSEK et al., 1965; ANGST, 1966). Entsprechendes trifft offenbar auch auf andere Psychoseformen zu, so daß in der Gesamtgruppe *reaktiver Psychosen* (*298*) die Frauen deutlich überwiegen. In diese Gruppe könnten auch *akute Episoden* aus dem *schizophrenen Formenkreis* (*295.4*) gehören, die ebenfalls bei Frauen in größerer Häufigkeit auftreten als bei Männern.

Außer einer reaktiven Auslösung von Psychosen und einer depressiven Symptombildung kommt eine *paranoide Symptomatik* bei Frauen – zumindest vom Involutionsalter an (MAYER-GROSS et al., 1969) – wesentlich häufiger vor als bei Männern (*295.3* und *297*). Für die Paranoia (*297.0*) ist allerdings nach der Literatur eher mit einem Überwiegen der Männer zu rechnen (WINOKUR, 1977), so daß der signifikant höhere Anteil der Frauen in dieser Diagnosegruppe des poliklinischen Krankengutes überrascht. Die übrigen Verteilungen bei den paranoiden Psychosen (*295.3* und *297.1*) entsprechen aber der klinischen Erfahrung, die einen höheren Anteil von Frauen erwarten läßt. Je nachdem, ob die rein paranoiden Syndrome (*297*) und die schizoaffektiven Psychosen (*295.7*) zur Schizophrenie gerechnet werden oder nicht, ergibt sich bei dieser ein Überwiegen des weiblichen Geschlechts (HELGASON, 1964; UCHTENHAGEN, 1975; DILLING u. WEYERER, 1978) oder aber eine ausgeglichene Geschlechtsproportion (HUBER, 1974). Dies erklärt viele Diskrepanzen in den Ergebnissen epidemiologischer Untersuchungen (DOHRENWEND u. DOHRENWEND, 1969).

Abb. 5 soll der Veranschaulichung der unterschiedlichen Geschlechtsproportion bei verschiedenen psychiatrischen Erkrankungen dienen. Die angeführten

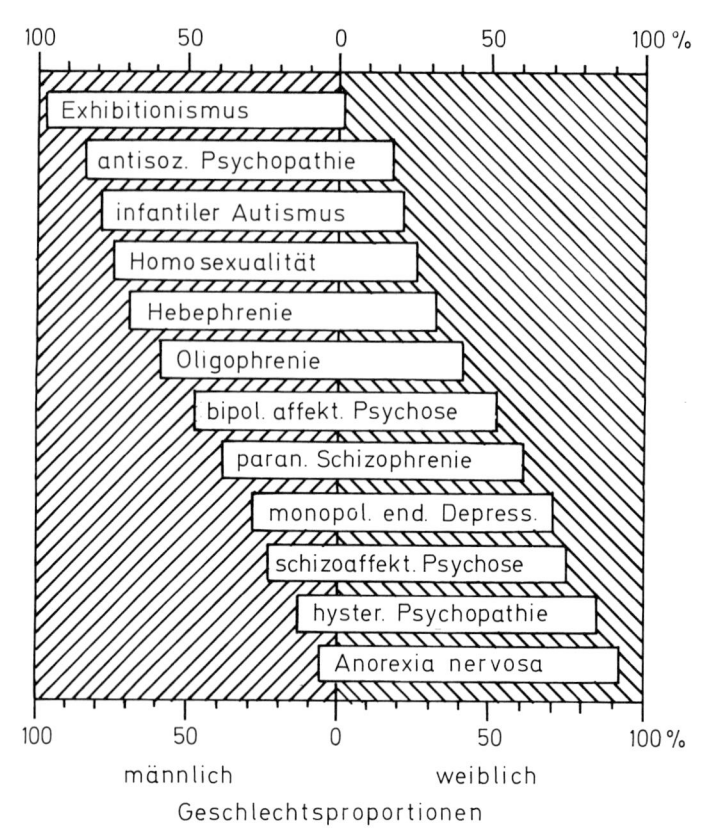

Abb. 5. Beispiele der Geschlechtsproportion von primären psychischen Konstitutionsanomalien und stark konstitutionsabhängigen aktuellen psychischen Krankheiten (Anorexia nervosa und endogene Psychosen). Grobe Schätzungen nach Literaturangaben und eigenen Untersuchungen (s. Tabelle 5)

Proportionen beruhen auf Schätzungen anhand von Daten aus Tabelle 5 und der im Text zitierten Literatur.

Eine eingehende *ätiopathogenetische Interpretation* der aufgewiesenen Geschlechtsunterschiede in Morbidität und Mortalität kann hier nicht gegeben werden. Sie müßte die verschiedenen Krankheitsbilder gesondert berücksichtigen und jeweils auf Untersuchungen Bezug nehmen, die in einem grundsätzlich andersartigen Kulturmilieu durchgeführt wurden. So sprechen epochale Verschiebungen der Geschlechtsproportion beim Alkoholismus (FEUERLEIN, 1975; SOLMS, 1975) für die Bedeutung gesellschaftlicher Faktoren. Das offenbar von historischen Einflüssen kaum berührte Überwiegen der Frauen bei depressiven Syndromen (SCHOTT, 1903) weist hingegen auf konstitutionelle Momente hin.

Allerdings wurde in Felduntersuchungen an nigerianischen Eingeborenen bei depressiven Störungen kein Geschlechtsunterschied gefunden (LEIGHTON et al., 1963; ORLEY u. WING, 1979). Es fehlen jedoch Anhaltspunkte für eine Gleichverteilung bei *endogenen* Depressionen. Bei diesen könnten hormonelle Faktoren im Spiel sein; denn im Greisenalter, wenn die hormonalen Unterschiede der Geschlechter nicht mehr so ausgeprägt sind wie im geschlechtsreifen Alter, kommt es anscheinend bei Männern häufiger zu Depressionen als bei Frauen (s. Abb. 6; SCHOTT, 1903). Möglicherweise

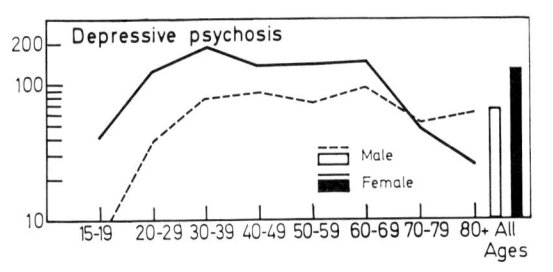

Abb. 6. Häufigkeitsverteilung der Inzidenz depressiver Psychosen bei Männern und Frauen in Abhängigkeit vom Lebensalter (aus ADELSTEIN et al., 1968)

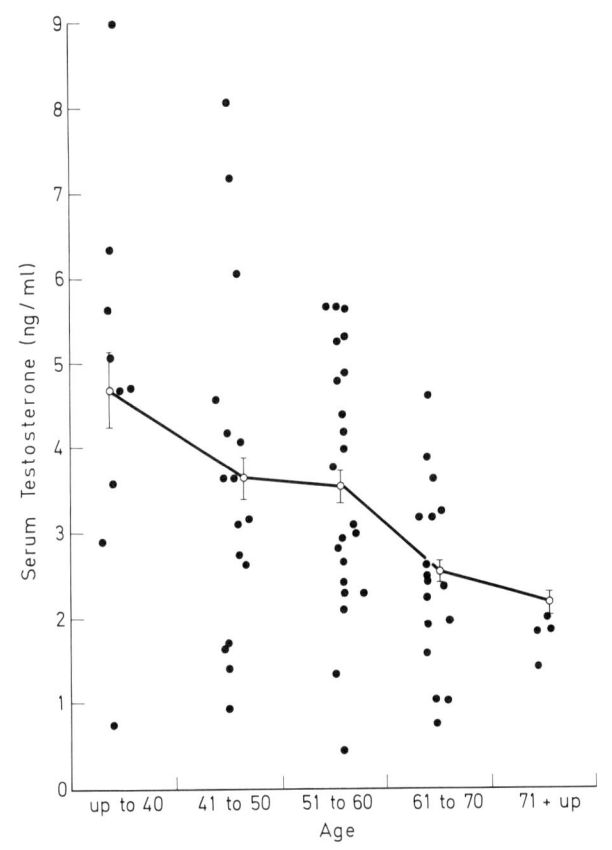

Abb. 7. Testosteron-Serumspiegel bei Männern in Abhängigkeit vom Lebensalter (aus ALBEAUX-FERNET et al., 1978)

üben die Androgene, deren Produktion beim Mann erst im höheren Lebensalter deutlich absinkt (s. Abb. 7), eine gewisse Schutzwirkung gegen die Entstehung depressiver Verstimmungen aus. Ihre Rolle als Antidepressiva (KLAIBER et al., 1976) ist allerdings umstritten. Auch muß ein depressionsfördernder Effekt der hormonalen Veränderungen bei geschlechtsreifen Frauen erwogen werden (POLLITT, 1977). Darüber hinaus sind gesellschaftlich bedingte bzw. mitbedingte Unterschiede der Geschlechterrollen bei der Interpretation der unterschiedlichen Depressionsanfälligkeit von Mann und Frau in Betracht zu ziehen. Ferner ist zu bedenken, daß keineswegs alle phänotypischen Geschlechtsunterschiede, die unmittelbar biologisch bedingt sind, hormonelle Faktoren zur Grundlage haben; vielmehr kann sich das Fehlen alleler Gene zum einen X-Chromosom des Mannes auch ohne Vermittlung der Geschlechtshormone positiv oder negativ auf die Manifestation von Konstitutionsmerkmalen bzw. konstitutionell verankerten Merkmalen der Kondition auswirken. Zu erwähnen sind in diesem Zusammenhang das deutliche Überwiegen des männlichen Geschlechts bei Erkrankungen mit rezessiv X-chromosomalem Erbgang (wie Hämophilie und verschiedene Formen der Farbblindheit) und das des weiblichen Geschlechts bei dominant X-chromosomal vererbten Krankheiten (wie hämolytische Anämie bei Glukose-6-Phosphat-Dehydrogenase-Mangel; LENZ, 1978). Hinweise auf einen dominant X-chromosomalen Erbgang wurden bei einem Teil bipolarer affektiver Psychosen durch „linkage"-Untersuchungen (mit Protanopie, Deuteranopie und der Xg-Blutgruppe) gefunden (MENDLEWICZ u. FLEISS, 1974). Die in Familienuntersuchungen ermittelte Gleichverteilung der Geschlechter, die sich auch aus unserer Analyse der Behandlungsprävalenz am Max-Planck-Institut für Psychiatrie in München (s. Tabelle 2) ergibt, läßt sich damit allerdings nicht ohne weiteres in Einklang bringen. Ein Interpretationsversuch dürfte beim derzeitigen Stand der Forschung noch verfrüht sein (GERSHON u. BUNNEY, 1977; KIDD u. WEISSMAN, 1978).

Von ebenso großem medizinischen Interesse wie die Geschlechtsunterschiede der Disposition zu psychischen Erkrankungen sind solche der Reagibilität gegenüber therapeutischen Maßnahmen. Dies betrifft sowohl die therapeutisch erwünschten Wirkungen als auch die unerwünschten Nebenwirkungen, z.B. der Psychopharmaka (GOLDBERG et al., 1966). In diesem Zusammenhang sei nur erwähnt, daß Neuroleptika bei Männern vergleichsweise häufiger initiale Dyskinesien, bei Frauen hingegen mehr parkinsonistische Symptome und eine Akathisie hervorrufen (SOVNER u. DIMASCIO, 1978).

c) Rassische Konstitution

Die rassische Konstitution ist zwar definitionsgemäß rein *genetisch* bestimmt. Da es aber im Bereich der psychischen Partialkonstitution keine rein genetisch bedingten Merkmale gibt, ist es kaum möglich, von psychischen Rassenmerkmalen zu sprechen. Soweit in psychometrischen Testuntersuchungen statistisch gesicherte Unterschiede zwischen Angehörigen verschiedener Rassen nachgewiesen wurden (LOEHLIN et al., 1975), ist oft schwer zu entscheiden, wie weit diese Differenzen tatsächlich auf genetische Faktoren zurückzuführen sind und wie weit sie auf verschiedenartigen Lebensgewohnheiten beruhen. Aus demselben Grunde ist es allerdings auch verfehlt, Populationsunterschiede in der psychiatrischen Morbidität ungeprüft allein auf Verschiedenheiten des soziokulturellen Milieus zu beziehen und rassische Faktoren gar nicht in Erwägung zu ziehen.

Auf jeden Fall scheinen einige mit psychischen Auffälligkeiten einhergehende genetische Syndrome und Chromosomenanomalien bei verschiedenen Rassen unterschiedlich häufig aufzutreten (s. z.B. NIELSEN, 1969).

Die akute intermittierende Porphyrie – ein autosomal-dominantes Erbleiden variabler Expressivität, zu dessen typischen Symptomen im akuten Schub psychische Alterationen bis zu schweren Psychosen gehören – findet sich in überdurchschnittlicher Häufigkeit in europiden Bevölkerungsgruppen Schwedens sowie – durch schwedische Emigranten bedingt – Australiens (DRUSCHKY, 1978).

Außer rassischen Unterschieden in der psychiatrischen Morbidität könnten auch solche in der Ansprechbarkeit auf psychotrope Substanzen bestehen. Beispielsweise ist bekannt, daß Angehörige mongolider Rassen eine besonders geringe Alkoholtoleranz aufweisen (WOLFF, 1972). Analoge Unterschiede könnten ebenfalls bezüglich der Psychopharmaka und ihrer Nebenwirkungen bestehen (GOLDBERG et al., 1966). Derartige Rassenmerkmale ließen sich methodisch sehr viel einfacher und sauberer erfassen als rassische Krankheitsdispositionen, die auf unterschiedlichen soziokulturellen Einflüssen beruhen bzw. durch unterschiedliche Exposition vorgetäuscht werden könnten.

d) Normale Varianten

Als Varianten bezeichnen wir in diesem Zusammenhang alle ausgeprägten Abweichungen der psychophysischen Totalkonstitution vom Durchschnitt einer nach Alter, Geschlecht und Rasse homogenen Population. Versuche, solche Varianten systematisch zu erfassen und typologisch zu ordnen, gehen bis in die Antike zurück (CIOCCO, 1936; TUCKER u. LESSA, 1940). Am bekanntesten geworden sind aber die in der ersten Hälfte dieses Jahrhunderts entwickelten *Typensysteme* von KRETSCHMER (1977) und von SHELDON (1949) (s. S. 626f.). Durch die Herstellung von Beziehungen zwischen *Normvarianten* des *Körperbaues* und mit diesen korrelierten *Temperamentseigentümlichkeiten* einerseits und der Inzidenz *endogener Psychosen* sowie verschiedener Formen normabweichenden – insbesondere kriminellen – Verhaltens andererseits haben diese Systeme einen starken Einfluß auf die psychiatrische Konstitutionsforschung ausgeübt. Dadurch haben sie zugleich die Beschäftigung mit anderen psychiatrisch relevanten Aspekten der Konstitution (Alter, Geschlecht, abnorme Varianten sowie vom Körperbau unabhängige Normvarianten einzelner Partialkonstitutionen) in den Hintergrund treten lassen.

Diese Einseitigkeit der Blickrichtung hat sich gerächt, nachdem die von KRETSCHMER und ebenfalls von SHELDON angenommenen *engen* Beziehungen zwischen Körperbautypen, Temperamentstypen und den Grundformen endogener Psychosen (affektive Psychosen, paranoide Psychosen und nicht-paranoide Schizophrenien) im wesentlichen auf Beobachtungs- und Interpretationsfehler zurückgeführt werden konnten (v. ZERSSEN, 1976a; s. unten). Anstatt sich nun verstärkt den bisher vernachlässigten Aspekten konstitutioneller Beziehungen zuzuwenden, hat man in der psychiatrischen Forschung das Interesse an Konstitutionsproblemen überhaupt weitgehend verloren. Untersuchungen auf diesem Gebiet werden nur noch vereinzelt und ohne größeren systematischen Zusammenhang durchgeführt, wogegen man sich seit dem Erscheinen von KRETSCHMERS „Körperbau und Charakter" (1921) mehrere Jahrzehnte hindurch intensiv mit Korrelationsstudien zu diesem speziellen Thema und besonders den Beziehungen zwischen Körperbau und Psychose beschäftigt hatte. Dabei waren freilich die typologischen Beurteilungen des Körperbaues und des Charakters sowie die psychopathologische Diagnostik zumeist vom selben Untersucher aufgrund subjektiver Einschätzungen vorgenommen worden, was zu einer systematischen Überschätzung der zwischen den verschiedenen Phänomenbereichen bestehenden Korrelationen geführt hat.

Darüber hinaus war gewöhnlich dem Altersfaktor nicht genügend Rechnung getragen worden. Man hatte übersehen, daß Patienten mit affektiven Psychosen im allgemeinen später erkranken und deshalb bei der psychiatrischen und der Körperbauuntersuchung im Schnitt ein höheres Alter erreicht hatten als schizophrene Patienten (REES, 1973; s. Abschnitt „Alterskonstitution", S. 641f.). Infolge der „relativen Pyknomorphierung" des körperlichen Habitus, die sich nach dem Abschluß der Phase intensiven Wachstums bis ins Präsenium vollzieht (s. Tabelle 2), erscheinen ältere Patienten ganz allgemein insgesamt pyknischer als jüngere – unabhängig davon, unter welcher Krankheit sie leiden mögen (v. ZERSSEN, 1969a).

Dieser Sachverhalt läßt sich mit anthropometrischen Daten belegen und ist bereits bei relativ kleinen Fallzahlen statistisch gegen den Zufall zu sichern. In ihm kommen die Umwandlungen des körperlichen Habitus zum Ausdruck, die in diesem Beitrag unter dem Begriff der Alterskonstitution (s. Tabelle 2) abgehandelt wurden. Solchen altersbedingten Veränderungen sind ebenfalls wohl im wesentlichen – wenn auch nicht ausschließlich (POLEDNAK, 1971; VERGHESE, 1978) – die Unterschiede im körperlichen Erscheinungsbild von paranoiden und nicht-paranoiden Schizophrenen zuzuschreiben. CONRADS (1967) Annahme, daß nicht die Grundform der Psychose, wohl aber die Verlaufsform vom Körperbautyp abhänge, beruht wahrscheinlich auf derselben Verkennung der gemeinsamen Alterskorrelation der Variablen, die auch KRETSCHMERS Annahme fundamentaler Körperbauunterschiede zwischen Patienten mit affektiven und schizophrenen Psychosen zugrunde lag; denn hebephrene Formen der Schizophrenie, bei denen man besonders häufig leptosomen Habitusformen begegnet, verlaufen nicht nur ungünstiger als paranoide Schizophrenien mit ihrem stärkeren Anteil an pyknischen Habitusformen; sie beginnen auch früher als diese (MAYER-GROSS et al., 1969).

Soweit überhaupt Unterschiede in der Verteilung normaler Varianten des körperlichen Habitus bei Haupt- oder Unterformen endogener Psychosen bestehen, treten sie in ihrer Ausprägung hinter den Unterschieden der Alters- und Geschlechtsverteilung stark zurück und sind somit für diagnostische und prognostische Zwecke unbrauchbar. Sie könnten trotzdem ein gewisses theoretisches Interesse beanspruchen, wenn ihre Ursachen bekannt wären. Hier schienen die von KRETSCHMER und später in z. T. anderer Form von SHELDON beschriebenen psychomorphologischen Beziehungen eine Brücke zu schlagen: Die *Psychosen* wurden als *Zerrformen normaler Persönlichkeitsvarianten* angesehen, die ihrerseits mit dem Körperbau korreliert sein sollten. Aber gerade diese psychomorphologischen Korrelationen sind bei Anwendung vorurteilsfreier Methoden zur Bestimmung von körperbaulichen Variationen einerseits und Variationen des Charakters andererseits statistisch nicht nachzuweisen bzw. quantitativ so gering (v. ZERSSEN, 1965a, b) und qualitativ z.T. andersartig (v. ZERSSEN, 1966a, b) als von KRETSCHMER bzw. SHELDON beschrieben, daß sie zur Erklärung von etwaigen Korrelationen zwischen Körperbau- und Psychosenform ungeeignet erscheinen (v. ZERSSEN, 1976a, 1977b).

Dieser Einwand gegen den konstitutionstypologischen Erklärungsansatz für die angebliche „Affinität" zwischen Körperbau- und Psychosenform wird auch durch psychometrische Vergleichsuntersuchungen an Patienten mit affektiven bzw. schizophrenen Psychosen gestützt. Faßt man mit KRETSCHMER das Temperament als denjenigen „Teil des Psychischen" auf, der „mit dem Körperbau in Beziehung steht" (KRETSCHMER, 1977, S. 347), so müßte sich dieses Korrelat des Körperbaus durch solche psychologischen Test-Items operationalisieren lassen, die signifikante Korrelationen mit Körperbaumerkmalen aufweisen. Eine auf diese Weise (anhand von Daten aus Untersuchungen an psychisch gesunden Probanden) konstruierte Selbstbeurteilungs-Skala differenzierte aber *nicht* zwischen Psychotikern des affektiven und solchen des schizophrenen Formenkreises (v. ZERSSEN, 1966a, b). Dabei soll doch nach KRETSCHMER die Psychose geradezu eine Zerrform der normalen Persönlichkeit darstellen, so daß die Unterschiede im psychotischen Zustand noch akzentuiert sein müßten.

Man könnte einwenden, psychotische Patienten seien zu angemessener Selbstbeurteilung ihrer Persönlichkeitszüge nicht imstande. Dagegen spricht aber, daß mit Hilfe von Skalen, deren Items nicht nach ihren Korrelationen mit Körperbaumerkmalen, sondern nach klinisch erarbeiteten Konzepten der prämorbiden Persönlichkeit von Psychotikern ausgesucht worden waren, statistisch gesicherte Unterschiede zwischen schizophrenen und affektpsychotischen Patienten selbst an kleinen, nach Alter, Geschlecht und verbaler Intelligenz einander entsprechenden Stichproben aufgewiesen werden konnten. Auf diese Untersuchungen wird im Zusammenhang mit der Besprechung psychischer Partialkonstitutionen eingegangen. Hier sei nur erwähnt, daß in einer unveröffentlichten psychomorphologischen Untersuchung an gesunden jungen Männern – von LASPE in Zusammenarbeit mit dem Autor durchgeführt – die für eine psychometrische Differenzierung zwischen Patienten mit schizophrenen und verschiedenen Formen affektiver Psychosen geeigneten Skalen keine signifikanten Korrelationen mit solchen somatometrisch bestimmten Körperbaumerkmalen erbracht haben, die eindeutig zwischen leptosomem und pyknischem Habitus differenzieren.

Im folgenden sollen die seit CONRADS Beitrag in der ersten Auflage dieses Handbuchs (1967) publizierten bzw. in seiner Darstellung noch nicht berücksichtigten Ergebnisse von *psychomorphologischen Korrelationsstudien* referiert werden, die sich auf die Totalkonstitution beziehen und zum Verständnis konstitutioneller Grundlagen psychischer Abnormitäten beitragen können. Sie lassen sich folgendermaßen zusammenfassen: *Faktorenanalytisch* (PAWLIK, 1968; GUILFORD, 1974; v. ZERSSEN, 1976a, 1977b) sind jeweils eigenständige Variationstendenzen für *umschriebene Merkmalskomplexe* aus dem *körperbaulichen*, dem *physiologischen*, dem *biochemischen* und dem *Persönlichkeitsbereich* nachweisbar (v. ZERSSEN, 1966b; MYRTEK, 1978). Darin stimmen die Ergebnisse von Untersuchungen an Menschen grundsätzlich mit denen an Hunden überein (BRACE, 1966). Insbesondere zeigen physiologische Variablen keineswegs engere Zusammenhänge mit Persönlichkeitsmerkmalen als die in der klassischen Konstitutionsforschung bevorzugten morphologischen Variablen (FAHRENBERG, 1967, 1977; v. ZERSSEN, 1966b; MYRTEK, 1978).

Auf der Ebene orthogonal rotierter Primärfaktoren ergeben sich gewöhnlich überhaupt keine gemeinsamen Faktoren für somatische und psychische Merkmale. Erst durch Sekundäranalysen nicht-orthogonal rotierter Primärfaktoren lassen sich schwache Beziehungen zwischen den verschiedenen Variablenbereichen nachweisen (MYRTEK, 1978). Solche Zusammenhänge sind gewöhnlich auch an der Struktur des ersten unrotierten Faktors einer Korrelationsmatrix psychischer und somatischer Merkmale ablesbar (v. ZERSSEN, 1966b). Auf diese und ähnliche Weise hat sich ein geringer, positiver Zusammenhang von Merkmalen körperbaulicher Robustheit mit Zügen eines sthenisch-vitalen, extravertierten und emotional stabilen Temperaments ergeben, außerdem ein schwach negativer mit der verbalen Intelligenz (v. ZERSSEN, 1966b). Darüber hinaus weist die Gesamtintelligenz eine schwach positive Beziehung zur allgemeinen Skelettentwicklung auf (s. unten). Zur Erleichterung der Übersicht sollen aber zunächst die verschiedenen, faktorenanalytisch differenzierbaren Variablenbereiche getrennt aufgeführt und erst dann miteinander in Beziehung gesetzt werden. Dabei wird davon abgesehen, daß die Ergebnisse von Faktorenanalysen – wie alle, auch intuitiv gewonnenen typologischen Strukturierungen einer Mannigfaltigkeit – stark von der Merkmalsauswahl und von der Art des Analyseverfahrens (Rotationskriterien etc.) abhängen. Die hier referierten Ergebnisse sind aber jedenfalls durch Kreuzvalidierung so weit abgesichert, daß sie nicht als bloße Kunstprodukte der Methodik eingestuft werden können.

Die *morphologischen Habitusvariationen* innerhalb von rassisch sowie nach Alter und Geschlecht homogenen Kollektiven lassen sich im wesentlichen auf die unterschiedliche Ausprägung von drei Komponenten beziehen, die ihrerseits weitgehend unabhängig voneinander variieren. Es sind dies die *allgemeine Skelettentwicklung*, deren unterschiedliche Ausprägung für Unterschiede der Körperlänge, der Beckenbreite und anderer Skelettmaße verantwortlich ist, die *Fettgewebsentwicklung*, die sich in Fettschichtdicken- sowie in Umfangsmaßen manifestiert und schließlich die „Muskularität" im Sinne von PARNELL (1958), die sich vornehmlich in der Dickenentwicklung von Muskeln und Gelenken äußert

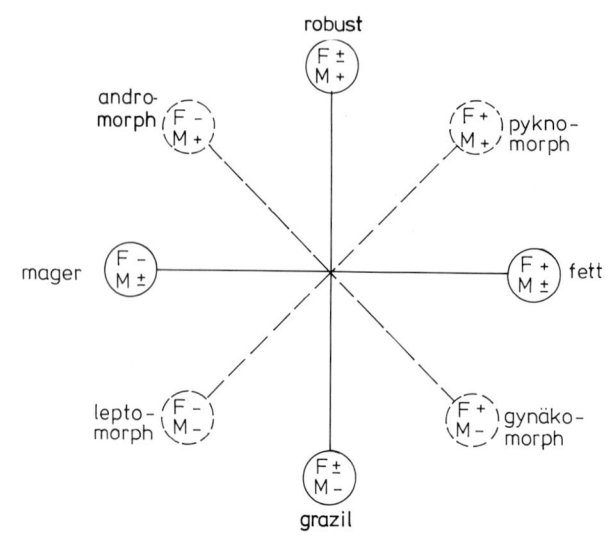

Abb. 8. Koordinatenkreuz zur Veranschaulichung der Dimensionen morphologischer Habitusvariationen, auf welche die biologisch bedeutsamsten Proportionsunterschiede in einem nach Alter, Geschlecht und Rasse homogenen Kollektiv geschlechtsreifer Individuen bezogen werden können (nach v. ZERSSEN, 1969a, modifiziert).
F = Fettgewebsentwicklung, M = „Muskularität" (Robustheit), + = starke Ausprägung, — = schwache Ausprägung, ± = mittlere Ausprägung, durchgezogene Linien = Bezugssystem vor Rotation, gestrichelte Linien = Bezugssystem nach Rotation

(v. ZERSSEN, 1966b; TANNER, 1977). Sie wirkt sich ebenfalls in der Breitenentwicklung des Brustkorbs und anderen Körpermaßen aus, weshalb man auch von *körperbaulicher Robustheit* sprechen kann (v. ZERSSEN, 1966a, b). Gleichsinnige bzw. gegensinnige Ausprägung der Muskularität und des Fettfaktors bestimmen im wesentlichen die Körperproportionen, die zur Konzeption von Körperbautypen angeregt haben (v. ZERSSEN, 1966b, 1969a). Dies wird durch die graphische Darstellung in Abb. 8 verdeutlicht, in der die beiden Komponenten als orthogonale Achsen eines Koordinatensystems repräsentiert sind. Die Winkelhalbierenden symbolisieren die durch gleichsinnige Entwicklung von Fett und Muskularität gekennzeichnete *leptopyknomorphe* bzw. die durch gegensinnige Ausprägung der Komponenten bedingte *androgynäkomorphe Variationsreihe,* deren *andromorphes Extrem* dem *athletischen Habitus* entspricht.

Daß die gegensinnige Ausprägung von Muskularität und Fettgewebsentwicklung etwas mit der Ausprägung männlicher (andromorpher) bzw. weiblicher (gynäkomorpher) Züge des körperlichen Habitus innerhalb eines Geschlechts zu tun hat, ergibt sich aus der unterschiedlichen Verteilung der Gewebskomponenten bei den Geschlechtern (TANNER, 1962), auf die in Tabelle 4 (unter „makroskopische Geschlechtsunterschiede der inneren morphologischen Struktur") bereits hingewiesen wurde. Ein Zusammenhang zwischen der Relation von Muskularität zu Fettgewebsentwicklung und dem Eindruck relativer Männlichkeit bzw. Weiblichkeit des Habitus sowie anderen Kriterien der Androgynäkomorphie ist darüber hinaus durch mehrere unabhängig voneinander durchgeführte faktorenanalytische Untersuchungen nachgewiesen worden (v. ZERSSEN, 1966b). Daß die gleichsinnig starke bzw. schwache Ausprägung von Muskularität und Fettgewebsentwicklung den Grad der relativen Körperfülle und damit die Stellung eines Individuums in der leptopyknomorphen Reihe bestimmt, dürfte unmittelbar einleuchten und ist zudem faktorenanalytisch ausreichend belegt. Ferner ist bekannt, daß im Alter der körperlichen Vollreife (s. Tabelle 2) die allgemeine Skelettentwicklung kaum noch zunimmt, wohl aber (jedenfalls anfänglich) die Robustheit und (fortschreitend) die Fettgewebsentwicklung. Das führt zu der bereits erwähnten „relativen Pyknomorphierung" des Habitus (v. ZERSSEN, 1969a, b).

Von den bisher daraufhin untersuchten *physiologischen und biochemischen Variablen* sind nur für die dynamometrisch bestimmte *Körperkraft* relativ enge Beziehungen zu Komponenten morphologischer Habitusvariationen aufgezeigt worden, und zwar sowohl zur *Muskularität* wie zur *allgemeinen Skelettentwicklung* (v. ZERSSEN, 1966b). Die übrigen physiologischen und biochemischen Merkmale variieren hingegen weitgehend unabhängig vom Körperbau, weisen aber untereinander z.T. relativ enge Zusammenhänge auf, die sich faktorenanalytisch in der Entstehung eigener Funktionsfaktoren niederschlagen (v. ZERSSEN, 1966b; FAHRENBERG, 1967; MYRTEK, 1978). Dabei handelt es sich allerdings offenbar überwiegend um „Zustands"-Faktoren, die mehr Information über die aktuelle Reaktionslage des Organismus (also über seine Kondition) als über ein relativ zeitkonstantes und umweltstabiles Funktionsgefüge (also über etwas Konstitutionelles) enthalten. Den klinisch konzipierten vegetativen Typen der Vagotonie, Sympathikotonie oder der allgemeinen vegetativen Labilität entsprechende Faktoren haben sich auch in Untersuchungen, die auf eine Objektivierung solcher Typen abzielten, nicht ergeben (v. ZERSSEN, 1966b; MYRTEK, 1978).

Immunologische Eigenschaften sind bisher faktorenanalytisch nicht untersucht worden. Dagegen gibt es eine Fülle faktorenanalytischer Untersuchungen von Persönlichkeitseigenschaften (PAWLIK, 1968; GUILFORD, 1974; BUSS u. PLOMIN, 1975), von denen einige für die Erforschung psychophysischer Zusammenhänge relevante Faktoren erbracht haben (v. ZERSSEN, 1976a, 1977b). Die betreffenden Analysen basieren durchweg auf Daten, die teils durch objektive Leistungstests, teils durch Selbsteinschätzungs-Skalen gewonnen wurden. Die Selbsteinschätzung bezog sich dabei teils auf Besonderheiten des Erlebens und Verhaltens im Sinne von Eigenarten des Charakters, teils auf Einstellungen und Interessen. Andere Datenquellen können unberücksichtigt bleiben, da sie entweder für die Erforschung psychomorphologischer Zusammenhänge ungeeignet sind (wie Interviewmethoden, deren Ergebnisse vom Anblick des untersuchten Probanden beeinflußt werden können) oder bisher nur wenige durch Kreuzvalidierung gesicherte, statistisch signifikante Beziehungen zu Körperbaumerkmalen ergeben haben (wie psychomotorische und Wahrnehmungstests).

Gemeinsame Faktorenanalysen von Tests zur Erfassung *intellektueller Leistungen* und von Selbsteinschätzungs-Skalen zur Erfassung von *Interessen* und von *charakterlichen Besonderheiten* haben übereinstimmend ergeben, daß die drei genannten Bereiche faktoriell voneinander weitgehend unabhängig sind und in sich wiederum faktoriell aufgegliedert werden können (v. ZERSSEN, 1966b). Dabei haben Interessentests bisher keine gesicherten korrelativen Beziehungen zum Körperbau ergeben.

Im Intelligenzbereich sind es vor allem die allgemeine Intelligenz als ein Faktor höherer Ordnung und gewisse verbale Intelligenzleistungen, für die psychomorphologische Zusammenhänge nachgewiesen werden konnten (PATERSON, 1930; v. ZERSSEN, 1966b; SCHWIDETZKY, 1971). Im charakterologischen Bereich ist die Sachlage etwas komplizierter. Sie soll deshalb anhand eines Schemas von Persönlichkeitsfaktoren (Abb. 9) verdeutlicht werden, in welchem der Komplexitätsgrad der Faktoren mit der Höhe ihrer räumlichen Anordnung zunimmt (v. ZERSSEN, 1977b). Unten links sind Teilkomponenten der Extraversion angegeben, wobei „Androthymie versus Gynäkothymie" geschlechtstypische Aspekte

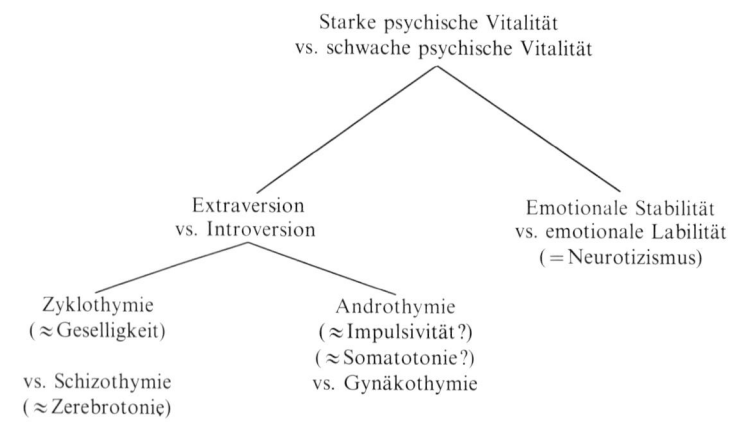

```
                    Starke psychische Vitalität
                   vs. schwache psychische Vitalität
                   ╱                              ╲
            Extraversion                    Emotionale Stabilität
           vs. Introversion                 vs. emotionale Labilität
          ╱             ╲                      ( = Neurotizismus)
   Zyklothymie        Androthymie
  (≈ Geselligkeit)   (≈ Impulsivität?)
                     (≈ Somatotonie?)
  vs. Schizothymie   vs. Gynäkothymie
  (≈ Zerebrotonie)
```

Abb. 9. Hierarchie von dimensionalen Extremtypen des Charakters, die (bei Männern) positiv – jeweils obere Zeile(n) – bzw. negativ – jeweils untere Zeile(n) – mit körperlicher Robustheit und umgekehrt mit körperlicher Grazilität korrelieren (nach v. ZERSSEN, 1977b, modifiziert)

der (bei Männern im Schnitt vergleichsweise stärker ausgeprägten) Extraversion kennzeichnet, während „Zyklothymie versus Schizothymie" weitgehend geschlechtsunabhängige Aspekte der Extraversion kennzeichnet (v. ZERSSEN, 1966b). Die von den beiden genannten Komponenten konstituierte Extraversion korreliert – nach zahlreichen Untersuchungen zu urteilen (GUILFORD, 1974) – schwach negativ mit „neurotischer Tendenz" (=Neurotizismus), was einer schwach positiven Korrelation mit emotionaler Stabilität entspricht. Die in dieser Korrelation zum Ausdruck kommende Gemeinsamkeit von Extraversion und emotionaler Stabilität bildet die Grundlage des von uns als „psychische Vitalität" bezeichneten Persönlichkeitsfaktors, der in mehreren unabhängigen Untersuchungen nachzuweisen war (v. ZERSSEN, 1966a, b; 1973b).

Die Komponenten der *psychischen Vitalität* korrelieren schwach positiv mit dem körperbaulichen Faktor der *Muskularität,* allerdings nur bei Männern, und auch bei diesen nur in der Größenordnung von r=0,2 (v. ZERSSEN, 1966a, b, 1976a, 1977b). Männer mit robustem Körperbau und entsprechend überdurchschnittlicher Muskelkraft tendieren demnach zu überdurchschnittlicher Ausprägung des Merkmalskomplexes psychischer Vitalität.

Ein Blick auf Abb. 8 läßt erkennen, daß die psychische Vitalität und ihre Komponenten außer zur Muskularität auch zur Pyknomorphie und zur Andromorphie gleichsinnige Beziehungen aufweisen müssen. Damit lassen sich nahezu alle statistisch gesicherten Ergebnisse psychomorphologischer Korrelationsstudien erklären, über die in der Literatur berichtet wird (v. ZERSSEN, 1976a, 1977b). Auch die negative Korrelation der Muskularität mit dem Ausmaß psychophysiologischer Streßreaktionen (in Form von Angstgefühlen und erhöhter Cortisolsekretion) in psychischen Belastungssituationen, die in mehreren Untersuchungen festgestellt wurde (BRIDGES, 1978), paßt in dieses Bild. Darüber hinaus macht es Beziehungen von körperbaulichen Normvarianten zu psychischen Verhaltensauffälligkeiten verständlich, die nicht durch den Altersfaktor vorgetäuscht werden.

So geht aus zahlreichen Untersuchungen hervor, daß *neurotische Männer* [und unter diesen insbesondere die von EYSENCK (1970) als Dysthymiker bezeichneten, zur Introversion neigenden Patienten mit einem neurasthenischen, depressiven oder Zwangs-Syndrom] eine Tendenz zu *körperbaulicher Grazilität* aufweisen

(PARNELL, 1958; EYSENCK, 1970). Umgekehrt findet man bei *jugendlichen Rechtsbrechern* ebenso wie bei *erwachsenen Kriminellen* eine Tendenz zu *körperbaulicher Robustheit* (SHELDON, 1949; GLUECK u. GLUECK, 1956; PARNELL, 1958; SELTZER, 1964; EYSENCK, 1977). Während allerdings bei den „dysthymen" Neurotikern offenbar alle Komponenten der psychischen Vitalität durchschnittlich schwach entwickelt sind, wie es bei verminderter körperbaulicher Robustheit zu erwarten ist, geht bei Kriminellen auf der charakterlichen Seite mit der stärkeren körperbaulichen Robustheit nur eine deutliche Ausprägung der Impulsivität – also einer Teilkomponente der Extraversion – einher (SCHALLING, 1978). Sie sind hingegen nicht übermäßig gesellig und zudem emotional weniger stabil, als es aufgrund der psychomorphologischen Korrelationen bei normalen Probanden zu erwarten wäre. Die Beziehungen zwischen Körperbau, Persönlichkeit und sozial deviantem Verhalten sind demnach zu komplex, als daß man sie allein von den psychomorphologischen Korrelationen herleiten könnte, die an Probanden mit unauffälligem Sozialverhalten nachgewiesen worden sind.

Möglicherweise haben alle hier besprochenen psychomorphologischen Beziehungen etwas mit verschiedenen Formen der Aggressionsverarbeitung zu tun, die bei körperbaulich robusten Männern eine mehr extrapunitive, bei körperbaulich grazilen eine mehr intrapunitive Note trägt. Körperliche Überlegenheit könnte bei robust gebauten, muskelstarken Knaben die Tendenz fördern, Aggressionen offen auszuleben; bei den ihnen körperlich unterlegenen, graziler gebauten, muskelschwächeren Rivalen würde hingegen häufiger eine Hemmung der Aggressionsabfuhr nach außen eintreten, die zu intrapunitiver Aggressionsverarbeitung disponiert. Neurotische Störungen wären dann die späte Frucht dieses sozialen Lernprozesses. In Abwandlung des bekannten Wortes von Sigmund FREUD, daß die Neurose das Negativ der Perversion sei, könnte man somit die Neurose als „Negativ der Kriminalität" bezeichnen (v. ZERSSEN, 1969b).

Auch die *verbale Intelligenz* weist eine Beziehung zur *körperbaulichen Robustheit* auf. Sie ist bei robust gebauten (LINDEGÅRD u. NYMAN, 1956; v. ZERSSEN, 1966b) (und somit auch bei pyknomorphen sowie bei andromorphen) Männern durchschnittlich etwas geringer als bei grazil gebauten (und somit auch leptomorphen und gynäkomorphen). Dies mag damit zusammenhängen, daß kräftig gebaute und entsprechend muskelstarke Knaben mehr auf die Tat als auf das Wort vertrauen, während es sich bei den körperlich schwächlichen gerade umgekehrt verhält. Eine solche Interpretation, die der sozialpsychologischen Interpretation psychomorphologischer Zusammenhänge im Bereich des Charakters entspricht, ist empirisch ebenso unzureichend belegt wie jene. Sie erscheint aber plausibel und läßt daran denken, daß psychomorphologische Zusammenhänge keineswegs ausschließlich auf einer Polyphänie der Gene beruhen müssen, mit der sie gewöhnlich erklärt werden (CONRAD, 1963; REES, 1973).

Ätiologisch ungeklärt ist letztlich auch die in zahlreichen Untersuchungen an Angehörigen verschiedener Rassen nachgewiesene *positive Korrelation* zwischen *Intelligenz* und *Körperhöhe* (als einem Teilaspekt der allgemeinen Skelettentwicklung) (PATERSON, 1930), die etwa in derselben Größenordnung liegt wie die zwischen körperbaulicher Robustheit und psychischer Vitalität. Möglicherweise führen schädigende Einflüsse während der Entwicklungszeit sowohl zu einer Verzögerung des Körperwachstums als auch zu einer Beeinträchtigung der zerebralen Entwicklung und auf diese Weise zu einer Minderung der Intelligenz. Die Tatsache, daß die Korrelation zwischen Körperhöhe und Intelligenz bei einem unter relativ primitiven Bedingungen lebenden Indianerstamm (den mexikanischen Otomi) deutlich ausgeprägter war (r ≥ 0,30) als bei europiden Bevölkerungsgruppen (r ≈ 0,10; SCHWIDETZKY, 1971) steht damit in Einklang; denn mit zunehmender Zivilisationshöhe werden Zahl und Ausmaß schädigender Einflüsse (Mangel- und Fehlernährung, schwere, langdauernde Infektionskrankheiten etc.) auf die psychophysische Konstitutionsentwicklung mehr und mehr eingeschränkt; zudem werden geistig Behinderte zunehmend in Sondereinrichtungen untergebracht und deshalb oft bei Untersuchungen der Durchschnittsbevölkerung gar nicht miterfaßt. Nachgewiesen ist allerdings auch bei Europiden, daß Oligophrene durchschnittlich im Wachstum zurückbleiben (WHEELER, 1929), was die klinische Bedeutung der korrelativen Beziehung zwischen Körperwachstum und Intelligenzentwicklung unterstreicht.

Ein Zusammenhang zwischen Körperbau und bestimmten Interessenrichtungen konnte bisher statistisch nicht belegt werden. Dies gilt auch für geschlechtstypische Interessen, die keinen Zusammenhang mit Kriterien körperbaulicher Androgynie aufweisen (v. ZERSSEN, 1966b). Sie variieren auch unabhängig von der als Androgynäkothymie bezeichneten Teilkomponente der Extraversion. Somit läßt sich das Konzept einer *psychophysischen Androgynie* im Bereich normaler konstitutioneller Variationen statistisch nicht untermauern (NETTER, 1970; v. ZERSSEN, 1977b). Die für alle *Transsexuellen* und einen Teil der *Homosexuellen* kennzeichnende Ausprägung von Interessen, die an sich für das andere Geschlecht typisch sind, hängt offenbar mit ihrem sexuellen Rollenverständnis und nicht mit einer Abweichung der psychophysischen Totalkonstitution zusammen. Dementsprechend fehlen auch sichere Hinweise auf das Vorliegen einer körperbaulichen Stigmatisierung von Transsexuellen und von Homosexuellen. Bei männlichen Homosexuellen konnte lediglich eine geringfügige Verminderung der Breitenentwicklung des Rumpfes nachgewiesen werden, die in derselben Größenordnung liegt wie bei Neurotikern (COPPEN, 1961) und wahrscheinlich – wie bei diesen – auf eine gewisse Grazilität des Körperbaus zu beziehen ist. Zudem geben neuere endokrinologische Untersuchungen Hinweise auf hormonelle Besonderheiten sowohl bei männlichen (DOERR et al., 1973, 1976) wie bei weiblichen (PAL, 1978) Homosexuellen, auf die bei der Besprechung von abnormen Varianten der psychischen Partialkonstitution (Triebkonstitution) eingegangen wird (s.S. 683). Dort kommen auch gegengeschlechtlich ausgeprägte Normvarianten von Einstellungen und Interessen bei in der Fetalzeit (und z.T. auch noch postpartal) androgenisierten Mädchen zur Sprache (s.S. 690).

e) Abnorme Varianten

Von abnormen Varianten der Totalkonstitution sprechen wir, wenn bei einem Individuum *mehrere* – somatische *und* psychische – *Partialkonstitutionen* deutliche *Normabweichungen* aufweisen. Dabei gilt die Regel, daß im Bereich der psychischen Partialkonstitution vornehmlich die Intelligenzentwicklung betroffen ist; bei stärkerer Beeinträchtigung derselben treten gewöhnlich Normabweichungen der Trieb- und Charakterentwicklung hinzu (BALTHAZAR u. STEVENS, 1975). Dabei spielen auch reaktive Momente (infolge einer Selbstwahrnehmung der körperlichen Stigmatisierung und der Erfahrung von Ablehnung oder Überfürsorglichkeit durch Personen der Umgebung) eine Rolle, ferner eine intelligenzbedingte Störung von Lernprozessen im Bereich triebhaften und affektiv-voluntativen Verhaltens. Es ist jedoch unwahrscheinlich, daß diese Faktoren allein für Normabweichungen der Triebkonstitution und des Charakters bei Oligophrenen im allgemeinen und solchen mit (multiplen) körperlichen Konstitutionsanomalien im besonderen verantwortlich gemacht werden können. Dies würde voraussetzen, daß sich eine gestörte Hirnentwicklung primär nur auf die intellektuelle Entwicklung nachteilig auszuwirken vermöchte, was schwer einzusehen wäre.

Man wird bei den verschiedenen Formen abnormer Varianten erst klären müssen, welcher Anteil der gestörten Trieb- und Charakterentwicklung biologischen und welcher Anteil psychoreaktiven Faktoren zuzuschreiben ist. Dabei hat man zu berücksichtigen, daß – statistisch gesehen – die Normabweichungen im Bereich der psychischen Partialkonstitution mit Zahl und Ausprägungsgrad der Normabweichungen im Bereich der somatischen Partialkonstitution zunehmen und daß sie insbesondere von deren Art abhängen. Verständlicherweise sind Mißbildungen am Kopf (SANDBERG, 1976), vor allem aber am Hirn selbst, sowie metabolische Störungen, die das Hirn betreffen bzw. einbeziehen, besonders eng mit psychischen Normabweichungen assoziiert. Diese Zusammenhänge von gestörter körperlicher und psychischer Konstitutionsentwicklung sind im klinischen Teil dieses Handbuchs eingehend dargestellt (DUPONT, Bd. II/2, S. 799–893). Abnorme Varianten der Geschlechtskonstitution werden zudem in BLEULERS Beitrag über endokrinologische Psychiatrie aus dem Jahre 1967 besprochen. Dort wird ferner auf abnorme Varianten des Entwicklungstempos eingegangen, wozu u.a. vorzeitige oder verspätete Geschlechtsreife (Pubertas praecox bzw. Pubertas tarda) und vorzeitige Vergreisung gehören; auch eine allgemein beschleunigte Entwicklung (Akzeleration) sowie das Steckenbleiben der Entwicklung in einer kindlich wirkenden körperlichen und psychischen Verfassung (Infantilismus) sind in diesem Zusammenhang zu erwähnen. Für die Entstehung neurotischer Konflikte sollen insbesondere „Teilretardationen" der Konstitutionsentwicklung (s. auch UNDEUTSCH, 1959) mit den daraus resultierenden Diskrepanzen unterschiedlich ausgereifter Persönlichkeitsanteile von Bedeutung sein (KRETSCHMER, 1959). Hier kann diese Problematik nur in groben Zügen umrissen und anhand einiger besonders instruktiver Beispiele verdeutlicht werden.

Die Häufigkeit *geistig Behinderter* in der Durchschnittsbevölkerung wird aufgrund epidemiologischer Untersuchungen auf etwa 4 pro Tausend der Bevölkerung geschätzt (INGALLS, 1978; LIEPMANN, 1979). Bei Kindern mit angeborenen *Mißbildungen* ist dieser Prozentsatz auf das 20fache erhöht (SANDBERG, 1976); läßt man Kinder mit isolierten Mißbildungen an Extremitäten bzw. vegetativen Organen unberücksichtigt, so verdoppelt sich der Prozentsatz nochmals. Umgekehrt findet man unter Oligophrenen – von dem schon erwähnten Minderwuchs abgesehen – gehäuft körperbauliche Normabweichungen bis zu schweren, oft multiplen Mißbildungen. Bei Körperbehinderten mit noch durchschnittlicher Gesamtintelligenz – insbesondere bei zerebralparetisch Geschädigten – finden sich häufig Beeinträchtigungen spezieller Fähigkeiten (STEINHAUSEN u. WEFERS, 1977), und in der Durchschnittsbevölkerung läßt sich eine schwach negative Korrelation zwischen körperbaulichen Dysplasien und dem Intelligenzniveau ermitteln (ANASTASI, 1965).

Viele der mit einer Beeinträchtigung der Intelligenz verbundenen multiplen Dysplasien bilden *charakteristische Syndrome* (HOLMES et al., 1972; HARBAUER, 1976b; WIEDEMANN et al., 1976), von denen der Kretinismus und der Mongolismus (Down-Syndrom) auch in Laienkreisen bekannt sind. Von den zahlreichen anderen, z.T. allerdings sehr seltenen Syndromen sind jedoch viele selbst den meisten Ärzten nicht vertraut, und eines der wahrscheinlich häufigsten – nämlich die sog. Alkohol-Embryopathie – ist sogar erst 1968 von LEMOINE et al. beschrieben und dann ab 1973 eingehender bearbeitet worden (JONES et al., 1973; BIERICH et al., 1976; MAJEWSKI et al., 1976).

Die Faktoren, welche die körperliche Gesamtentwicklung und mit ihr die Hirnentwicklung so stark beeinträchtigen, daß es zu multiplen Mißbildungen und zu Störungen der Intelligenz- sowie der Trieb- und Charakterentwicklung kommt, sind teils genetischer, teils nicht-genetischer Art. Bei den genetischen Faktoren spielen – außer abnormen Gen-Mutanten, wie sie auch bei isolierten Entwicklungsstörungen im Bereich einzelner Partialkonstitutionen vorkommen – numerische und strukturelle Chromosomenanomalien eine Rolle. Chromosomale Aberrationen führen praktisch immer zu einer Abnormität der psychophysischen Totalkonstitution (PELZ u. MIELER, 1972).

Als Beispiel einer *erblichen Form* abnormer Varianten sei das Laurence-Moon-Bardet-Biedl-Syndrom angeführt, ein seltenes, einfach autosomal-rezessives Erbleiden (WIEDEMANN et al., 1976). Es ist durch eine besonders vom 3./4. Lebensjahr an progressive Adipositas, Polydaktylie, hypogonadotropen Hypogenitalismus, Sehstörungen infolge retinaler Degeneration und anderer Anomalien des Sehapparates sowie eine geistige Entwicklungshemmung (gewöhnlich schwere Debilität bis Imbezillität) gekennzeichnet.

Von den abnormen Varianten infolge *chromosomaler Aberrationen* seien das *Down-Syndrom* (KOCH u. DE LA CRUZ, 1975), als Beispiel einer autosomal (durch Trisomie des Chromsoms 21) bedingten Konstitutionsanomalie, und das („echte") *Klinefelter-Syndrom* (NIELSEN, 1969; MURKEN, 1973), als Beispiel einer gonosomal bedingten Abnormität der Totalkonstitution, erwähnt. Das Klinefelter-Syndrom, das vornehmlich die Geschlechtskonstitution betrifft, beruht auf einer Polyploidie des Geschlechtschromosomensatzes mit (mindestens) zwei X- und (mindestens) einem Y-Chromosom (s.unten).

Die *Alkohol-Embryopathie* (BIERICH et al., 1976; MAJEWSKI et al., 1976) ist ein Beispiel für *exogen bedingte abnorme Varianten* der Totalkonstitution. Sie entsteht wahrscheinlich infolge des Übertritts von Alkohol in den embryonalen Kreislauf aus dem Blut chronisch alkoholisierter Mütter. Angeblich sollen mindestens ein Drittel der Kinder von chronischen Alkoholikerinnen das Syndrom in mehr oder weniger starker Ausprägung aufweisen. Das Vollbild (vgl. Abb. 10) besteht in einer oft schon bei Neugeborenen erkennbaren Wachstumsverzögerung, Mikrozephalie, kraniofacialer Dysmorphie mit Balkonstirn bzw. schmaler Stirn, Anomalien des äußeren Auges (Ptosis, Epikanthus), der Nase, die breit und kurz ist, des Kiefers (Retrogenie, Mikrognathie), des Mundes (schmales Oberlippenrot), nicht selten auch der Ohren, sowie – in wechselnder Häufigkeit und Ausprägung – Dysplasien an Extremitäten, Rumpf, äußerem Genitale und am Herzen. Beim Neugeborenen bestehen zudem häufig motorische Störungen (Tremor, wechselnder Muskeltonus) und eine hartnäckige Trinkschwäche. Besonders in den ersten zwei bis drei Lebensjahren fallen die Kinder durch eine ständige motorische Unruhe, starke Erregbarkeit und geringes Konzentrationsvermögen auf. Die Feinmotorik ist gestört, die intellektuelle Entwicklung verzögert. Vom dritten Lebensjahr an wird der Rückstand oft teilweise aufgeholt. Eine normale Intelligenz ist aber wohl nur bei den sog. Schwachformen des Syndroms erreichbar.

Die beiden folgenden Beispiele abnormer Varianten der Sexualkonstitution sollen die Schwierigkeiten bei der Interpretation psychomorphologischer Korrelationen demonstrieren. Sie beziehen sich auf relativ häufige Formen konstitutioneller Abnormität, die deshalb den meisten Ärzten in ihrer Tätigkeit beggenen, trotzdem aber sehr oft verkannt oder in ihrer Bedeutung für das betroffene Individuum unterschätzt werden. Es handelt sich einmal um das „echte" (d.h. Chroma-

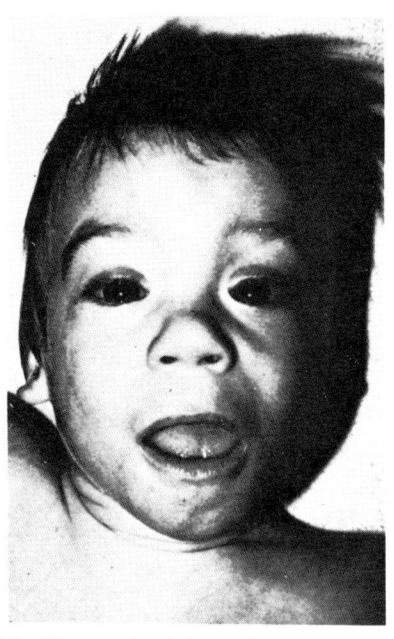

Abb. 10. Beispiel kraniofacialer Dysmorphie bei Alkoholembryopathie (aus BIERICH et al., 1976)

tin-positive) *Klinefelter-Syndrom*, das bei annähernd zwei von tausend Männern vorkommt (MURKEN, 1973), und den sog. *idiopathischen* (gewöhnlichen, konstitutionellen) *Hirsutismus*, einer virilen Form der Sekundärbehaarung, die bei einem noch höheren Anteil geschlechtsreifer Frauen ein für die Betreffenden störendes, oft sogar quälendes Ausmaß erreicht. Da es sich beim idiopathischen Hirsutismus um ein „graduelles Phänomen" handelt und sein Vorkommen stark populations- (insbesondere rassen-)abhängig ist, lassen sich genauere Zahlenangaben nicht machen (v. ZERSSEN et al., 1960).

Beide Formen einer abnormen Sexualkonstitution sind bei sorgfältiger körperlicher Untersuchung leicht zu erkennen; durch eingehende Exploration und ggf. zusätzliche psychologische Testuntersuchungen lassen sich ebenfalls häufig psychische Normabweichungen aufdecken. Bei oberflächlicher Untersuchung können aber die somatischen ebenso wie die psychischen Normabweichungen leicht übersehen werden.

In seiner häufigsten Form mit dem Karyotyp 47,XY bietet das *Klinefelter-Syndrom* im Alter der körperlichen Vollreife folgendes Bild (Literaturhinweise bei KOCH u. NEUHÄUSER, 1978):

Körperlicher Habitus: kleine, derbe Hoden und schwache Terminalbehaarung als konstanteste Merkmale; Gynäkomastie in fast der Hälfte der Fälle; häufig eunuchoider Hochwuchs mit Überlänge der Extremitäten, eher schwach entwickelter Muskulatur und – vom mittleren Lebensalter an – Neigung zu vermehrtem Fettansatz, besonders in der Hüftregion.

Innere morphologische Struktur: hyaline Tubulusdegeneration der Hoden mit Hyperplasie der Leydig-Zellen, Azoospermie; ferner Barrsche Kernkörperchen und trommelschlegelartige Anhänger an über 10% der segmentierten Leukozytenkerne (wie bei der normalen Frau durch das inaktivierte zweite X-Chromosom bedingt) als obligate Merkmale; schon im mittleren Lebensalter häufig Zeichen einer Osteoporose.

Biochemische Partialkonstitution: gewöhnlich leicht bis mäßig erniedrigter Testosteron- und deutlich erhöhter Gonadotropin-Spiegel im Blut.

Immunologische Partialkonstitution: möglicherweise verstärkte Tendenz zur Bildung von Autoimmunglobulinen.

Physiologische Partialkonstitution: Infertilität infolge der Azoospermie (obligat); Erektions- und Ejakulationsschwäche.

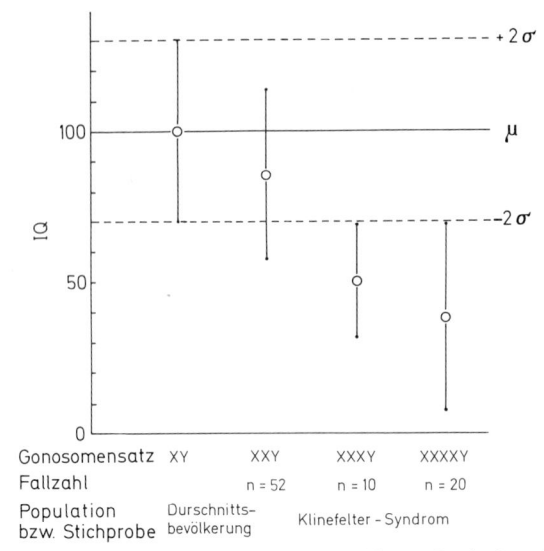

Abb. 11. Mittelwerte (Kreise) mit doppelter Standardabweichung (Punkte) und Normalbereichen (Verbindungslinien zwischen den Punkten) des Intelligenz-Quotienten (IQ) für die Durchschnittsbevölkerung und Männer mit einfachen numerischen Aberrationen des X-Chromosoms. Werte zusammengestellt von DOERING (1971). (Nach v. ZERSSEN, 1976a)

Triebkonstitution: sexuelle Triebschwäche und -unsicherheit mit Neigung zu deviantem Sexualverhalten (Homosexualität, Transvestitismus).

Charakter: Antriebsschwäche, Passivität, gesteigerte Ermüdbarkeit, geringe Frustrationstoleranz; vermehrt soziopathische Züge mit Neigung zu kriminellen Entgleisungen.

Intelligenz: gewöhnlich unterdurchschnittlich (niedrig-normal bis leicht-debil).

Spezielle Fähigkeiten und andere psychische Funktionsbereiche sind im allgemeinen nicht betroffen.

Die aufgeführten Besonderheiten der verschiedenen Partialkonstitutionen, die noch um weitere Details ergänzt werden könnten, lassen sich offenbar durchweg auf eine durch die Triploidie des Geschlechtschromosomensatzes bedingte Balancestörung genetischen Materials beziehen. Daß dies auch – zumindest teilweise – für die Abnormität im Bereich psychischer Partialkonstitutionen gilt, ist insbesondere für die Intelligenz durch den Vergleich mit anderen gonosomalen Aberrationen und vor allem durch den Vergleich verschiedener Varianten des Klinefelter-Syndroms erwiesen.

Abb. 11 zeigt die Abhängigkeit des psychometrisch bestimmten Intelligenzniveaus vom Grad der numerischen Aberration beim Klinefeter-Syndrom (v. ZERSSEN, 1976a): Beim Karyotyp 47,XXY ist es um knapp eine Standardabweichung gegenüber der Normalbevölkerung herabgesetzt; beim Karyotyp 48,XXXY beträgt das Ausmaß der Intelligenzminderung mehr als drei und beim Karyotyp 49,XXXXY sogar rund vier Standardabweichungen im Vergleich mit dem Bevölkerungsdurchschnitt. Die Einschränkung der Intelligenz nimmt also deutlich mit dem Ausmaß der numerischen Aberration zu. Ebenso verhält es sich mit Zahl und Ausmaß körperlicher Dysplasien. Bei einer chromosomalen Mosaikstruktur mit einem gewissen Anteil des normalen Karyotyps XY (d.h. 46/47,XY/XXY) ist der Grad der intellektuellen Beeinträchtigung anscheinend geringer als beim Karyotyp 47,XXY, bei Mosaiken mit zusätzlichen Extrachromosomen (47/48,XXY/XXYY oder 47/48,XXY/XXxY, wobei x ein X-Bruchstück kennzeichnet: REITALU, 1968) ist hingegen die Intelligenzminderung ausgeprägter als beim Karyotyp 47,XXY, aber keineswegs so kraß wie beim Karyotyp 48,XXXY (NOWAKOWSKI et al., 1967).

Die sexuelle Triebschwäche ist wahrscheinlich durch die mangelhafte Testosteronproduktion infolge des Hypogonadismus zu erklären, die auch für die spärliche Terminalbehaarung, den eunuchoiden Wuchs und die frühzeitig einsetzende Osteoporose verantwortlich zu machen ist. Die Neigung zu sexuell deviantem Verhalten könnte aus der sexuellen Triebschwäche in Verbindung mit soziopathischen Zügen herzuleiten sein. Die Entstehung solcher Züge ist aber ihrerseits wahrscheinlich nicht in erster Linie auf eine Balancestörung genetischen Materials bzw. den Hypogonadismus zu beziehen. Dafür spricht, daß sie sich vornehmlich bei Probanden finden, die aus einem ungünstigen Sozialmilieu stammen. Es ist deshalb zu vermuten, daß soziopathische Tendenzen durch das komplizierte Zusammenspiel von konstitutionell abnormer Persönlichkeitsentwicklung, intellektueller Minderbegabung, Selbstunsicherheit infolge mangelnder sexueller, intellektueller und sozialer Kompetenz und ungünstigen Umwelteinflüssen entstehen (ZÜBLIN, 1969; WITKIN et al., 1976). Antriebsschwäche, Passivität und leichte Ermüdbarkeit finden sich aber im Unterschied zu den soziopathischen Zügen auch bei Probanden aus sozial geordneten Verhältnissen, und zwar bereits in einem Alter, in dem – außer einer verzögerten Sprachentwicklung – noch keine Zeichen intellektueller Minderbegabung bemerkt werden und der körperliche Habitus ganz unauffällig ist (ZELLWEGER u. SIMPSON, 1977). Sie sind demnach offenbar unmittelbarer Ausdruck einer durch die Chromosomenanomalie als solche bedingten zerebralen Störung.

Die meisten Patienten mit mehr als 47 Chromosomen sind in Anstalten untergebracht, während nur etwa 1% der Probanden mit dem Karyotyp 47,XXY institutionalisiert sind. Relativ am häufigsten finden sie sich in Einrichtungen für Patienten mit leichtem Schwachsinn und Verhaltensstörungen (DOERING, 1971) – soweit derartige Spezialeinrichtungen existieren, wie es z.B. in Schweden der Fall ist. Außer unter den Oligophrenen sind unter stationären psychiatrischen Patienten solche mit einem Klinefelter-Syndrom vor allem unter den Psychopathen überrepräsentiert (NIELSEN, 1975). Eine erhöhte Morbidität für Epilepsie sowie für Psychosen aus dem schizophrenen Formenkreis wurde behauptet (HAMBERT, 1966), ist aber nicht unbestritten.

Die Diagnose des Syndroms gründet sich auf den Hodenbefund und den positiven Chromatinnachweis in den Zellen der Mundschleimhaut (als Barrsche Kernkörperchen) oder der Leukozyten (als trommelschlegelartige Anhänger von segmentierten Granulozytenkernen). Genaueren Aufschluß über die chromosomale Grundlage des Syndroms gibt eine Chromosomenanalyse. Im Kindesalter läßt sich die Diagnose nur aufgrund des Kerngeschlechtes bzw. des Chromosomenbefundes stellen. Die Prognose ist bezüglich der Fertilität infaust (es sei denn beim Karyotyp 46/47,XY/XXY), dagegen *quoad vitam* günstig: die Lebenserwartung ist gegenüber altersentsprechenden Männern ohne Chromosomenanomalie nicht herabgesetzt. Therapeutisch kann wegen der Potenzschwäche eine Testosteron-Behandlung angezeigt sein, die sich u.U. auch günstig auf Antrieb, Stimmungslage und – indirekt – auf das Selbstwertgefühl auswirkt. Durch langfristige Testosterongaben läßt sich die Entstehung einer Osteoporose verhüten. Die von vielen Patienten als sehr störend empfundene Gynäkomastie ist durch eine Hormonbehandlung nicht beeinflußbar; sie läßt sich nur durch plastische Operation beseitigen. Besonders wichtig ist in vielen Fällen eine psychologische Führung, verbunden mit rehabilitativen Maßnahmen zur Herstellung bzw. Stabilisierung sozialer Beziehungen und zur Verhütung häufigen Berufswechsels, der für viele Patienten charakteristisch ist.

Dem *Hirsutismus* der Frau (DEMISCH, 1977) liegt niemals eine Chromosomen-Anomalie zugrunde. Nach Ausschluß symptomatischer Formen (angeborenes adrenogenitales Syndrom, Androgen-produzierende Tumoren von Nebennierenrinde oder Ovar, Stein-Leventhal-Syndrom mit polyzystischen Ovarien, Therapie mit Steroidhormonen) kann ein idiopathischer Hirsutismus angenommen werden, der in der überwiegenden Mehrzahl der Fälle auf einem offenbar genetisch bedingten Androgenüberschuß beruht. Dieser entsteht vorwiegend im Ovar, z.T. auch in der Nebennierenrinde und in einigen Fällen wahrscheinlich auch durch Störungen des Hormonmetabolismus. Der Androgenüberschuß bewirkt auch andere Virilisierungszeichen als die abnorme Körperbehaarung (Akne, Kehlkopfvergrößerung, vorzeitige Knorpelverkalkung, Klitorishyperplasie, Uterushypoplasie u.a.; v. ZERSSEN et al., 1960). Die Triebkonstitution ist im allgemeinen nicht auffallend verändert. Auch die Intelligenz entspricht der Durchschnittsnorm. Einstellungen und Interessen sind nicht – wie beim adrenogenitalen Syndrom – zum Männlichen hin verschoben (starke Berufsbezogenheit, wenig Sinn

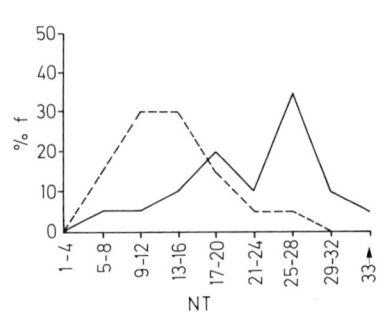

Abb. 12. Häufigkeitsverteilung der Skalenwerte für neurotische Tendenz (NT) aus dem MMQ (= Maudsley Medical Questionnaire, s. EYSENCK, 1953) bei Frauen mit *idiopathischem* Hirsutismus (n = 20) und einer gleichgroßen Kontrollgruppe

für die Beschäftigung mit kleinen Kindern etc.: (MONEY u. EHRHARDT, 1972; EHRHARDT u. BAKER, 1974); wohl aber bestehen häufig erhebliche emotionelle Störungen, bei denen die Frage aufkommt, wie weit sie Ausdruck einer konstitutionell bedingten Labilität sind, die ihrerseits durch die hormonelle Abnormität hervorgerufen wird.

Abb. 12 bietet einen Vergleich der Häufigkeitsverteilung von Punktwerten einer Selbstbeurteilungs-Skala zur Erfassung „neurotischer Tendenz" bei 20 Frauen mit idiopathischem Hirsutismus und der gleichen Anzahl altersentsprechender Frauen aus der Durchschnittsbevölkerung. Eingehende psychiatrisch-psychologische Fallstudien (MEYER u. v. ZERSSEN, 1960; MEYER, 1963) haben ergeben, daß offenbar die Entstehung einer virilen Behaarung im Alter der Geschlechtsreife für viele Frauen eine schwere seelische Belastung bedeutet und nicht selten zu einer Verunsicherung der Geschlechtsidentifikation, einer depressiven Grundstimmung sowie einer Tendenz zur sozialen Isolierung führt. Auffallend häufig gehen aber neurotische Störungen dem Auftreten der Behaarungsanomalie voraus. Sie entstehen im allgemeinen in alterstypischen Konfliktsituationen und sind schwerlich mit einer endogenen Überproduktion von androgenen Hormonen zu erklären; vielmehr scheint umgekehrt der mit neurotischen Konfliktreaktionen verbundene „Streß" bei entsprechend disponierten Frauen durch eine Aktivierung des Hypothalamus-Hypophysen-Nebennierenrinden-Systems einen vorbestehenden (genetisch bedingten) Hyperandrogenismus vorübergehend zu akzentuieren. Das kann die Entstehung einer virilen Behaarung fördern, wodurch dann psychoreaktive Störungen der oben beschriebenen Form in Gang gesetzt werden. Die resultierende psychophysische Korrelation (zwischen Hirsutismus und emotionellen Störungen) kommt demnach durch ein Zusammenwirken von psychosomatischen und psychoreaktiven Mechanismen zustande und ist wahrscheinlich nicht durch Hormonwirkungen auf körperliches Erscheinungsbild *und* Psyche bedingt.

Trotzdem kann – wenn die Diagnose nach Ausschluß eines symptomatischen Hirsutismus geklärt ist – eine Hormonbehandlung mit einem Antiandrogen (HAMMERSTEIN et al., 1975) in Kombination mit einem Östrogenpräparat (HOFFMANN et al., 1974), seltener mit einem Glukokortikoidpräparat – z.B. Dexamethason – in niedriger Dosierung zur Drosselung der Nebennierenrindenaktivität (ABRAHAM et al., 1976), auch psychologisch hilfreich sein; denn eine Verminderung der abnormen Behaarung (besonders des Gesichtes) bedeutet für viele Frauen auch eine seelische Entlastung. Allerdings ist die hormonelle Beeinflussung der Behaarungsanomalie oft unzureichend, so daß eine Epilation nicht zu umgehen ist, wenn die Behaarung als schwerer Makel erlebt wird. Vor allem sollte aber durch eine Gesprächstherapie versucht werden, den Frauen das Gefühl zu nehmen, durch die Behaarungsanomalie als Frauen entwertet zu sein und von anderen Menschen, insbesondere von Männern, abgelehnt zu werden (was tatsächlich im allgemeinen nicht der Fall ist – zumindest nicht in dem befürchteten Ausmaß). Zunächst muß man aber die Behaarungsanomalie als solche und ihren psychologischen Stellenwert erkannt haben. Viele der hirsuten Frauen verstehen es, durch (oft laienhafte, womöglich außerordentlich zeitaufwendige und kostspielige) Epilierungsmethoden ihre Behaarungsanomalie zu kaschieren, und genieren sich, selbst mit einem Arzt darüber zu sprechen. Dies ist der Grund, daß die Anomalie so häufig verkannt und in ihrer psychologischen Bedeutung für die betroffenen Frauen im allgemeinen unterschätzt wird.

2. Partialkonstitutionen

Die Partialkonstitutionen werden hier ausschließlich unter psychiatrischem Aspekt dargestellt. Dementsprechend wird auf normale und abnorme Varianten psychischer Partialkonstitutionen und auf solche Varianten somatischer Partialkonstitutionen eingegangen, für die ein Zusammenhang mit psychischen Normabweichungen durch empirische Untersuchungen nachgewiesen oder nahegelegt worden ist.

Tabelle 6 bringt Beispiele abnormer Varianten der verschiedenen Partialkonstitutionen, wobei nur bezüglich psychischer Konstitutionsanomalien Vollständigkeit angestrebt wurde. Körperliche Konstitutionsanomalien sind lediglich durch jeweils ein charakteristisches Beispiel repräsentiert.

a) Somatische Partialkonstitutionen

Körperlicher Habitus: Ohne Bezugnahme auf Persönlichkeitsfaktoren wurde die *Größenentwicklung* mit verschiedenen Formen psychischer Störungen in Verbindung gebracht. Außer bei Oligophrenen (WHEELER, 1929) wurde gelegentlich auch bei Schizophrenen bzw. bei Neurotikern eine geringgradig verminderte

Tabelle 6. Beispiele somatischer und psychischer Konstitutionsanomalien

Betroffene Partialkonstitution (PK)		Beispiele zugehöriger Anomalien
Somatische PK	Körperlicher Habitus	Dysmelie-Syndrom
	PK der inneren morphol. Struktur	Hydrocephalus internus
	Biochemische PK	Porphyrie
	Immunologische PK	Angeborener Immunkörpermangel
	Physiologische PK	Myotonia congenita Thomsen
Psychische PK	Triebkonstitution	Sex. Triebschwäche, Hypersexualität, sex. Perversionen[a]
	Charakter	Psychopathie, Wesensänderung[a] (organisch/epileptisch/schizophren)
	Intelligenz	Oligophrenie, organische Demenz[a]
	Spezielle Fähigkeiten	Legasthenie, Rechenschwäche
	Kommunikationsweisen[b]	Infantiler Autismus
	Überzeugungen, Einstellungen, Interessen[b]	Transsexualität

[a] weitgehend irreversible Formen
[b] konstitutioneller Anteil dieser Funktionsbereiche!

Körpergröße gefunden (SINGER et al., 1972; REES, 1973). Diese Befunde erscheinen allerdings unzureichend gesichert. Dasselbe gilt für ein angeblich vermehrtes Vorkommen körperbaulicher *Dysplasien* bei Schizophrenen (KRETSCHMER, 1977) und Neurotikern (WINTER, 1958/59), während ihre große Häufigkeit bei Oligophrenen völlig unbestritten ist (v. ROHDEN, 1926; ELSÄSSER, 1951). Auch bei Epileptikern kommen sie offenbar gehäuft vor (DELBRÜCK, 1926; v. ROHDEN, 1926; ELSÄSSER, 1951). Bei Schizophrenen scheinen es speziell Patienten mit frühem Beginn und ungünstigem Verlauf der Erkrankung (also vornehmlich Hebephrene) zu sein, bei denen Dysplasien etwas vermehrt zu verzeichnen sind. Bei Patienten mit paranoiden oder affektiven Psychosen sind Dysplasien dagegen nicht häufiger festzustellen als in der Durchschnittsbevölkerung (ELSÄSSER, 1951). Demnach korrelieren offenbar Zahl und Ausmaß der Dysplasien bei psychiatrischen Erkrankungen mit dem Gewicht, das (genetischen wie nichtgenetischen) Faktoren, die sich nachteilig auf zerebrale Reifungsvorgänge auswirken, in ihrer Ätiopathogenese zukommt.

Viele spezielle Dysplasieformen – wie das Dysmelie-Syndrom (extreme Verkürzung – insbesondere der oberen – Extremitäten, meist infolge Conterganeinnahme der Mutter im ersten Trimenon der Gravidität) – gehen in der Regel nicht mit Anomalien der psychischen Konstitution einher. Sie können allerdings die psychische Entwicklung infolge der sichtbaren körperlichen Verunstaltung bzw. mit ihr verbundener funktioneller Beeinträchtigungen nachteilig beeinflussen.

Innere morphologische Struktur: Hier werden nur solche Besonderheiten der inneren morphologischen Struktur in Betracht gezogen, die sich nicht auch im äußeren Erscheinungsbild manifestieren. Beziehungen derartiger morphologischer Eigenarten zu psychiatrischen Erkrankungen sind bisher für einige abnorme Varianten beschrieben worden. Beispielsweise wurde eine *Hyperostosis frontalis interna*, also eine nach außen nicht in Erscheinung tretende Verdickung der Schädelkalotte im Frontalbereich, in einem psychiatrischen bzw. neuropsychiatrischen Krankengut in einem höheren Prozentsatz gefunden als bei rein körperlich Kranken (WÅLINDER, 1977). Die Tatsache, daß psychiatrische Patienten mit einer solchen Dysplasie gegenüber altersentsprechenden Patienten ohne diese Anomalie häufiger eine Demenz aufweisen und daß ihre Geschwister signifikant seltener psychiatrisch erkranken, spricht dafür, daß exogene Schädigungsfaktoren für die Kombination psychischer Erkrankungen mit einer Hyperostosis frontalis interna verantwortlich zu machen sind – in ähnlicher Weise, wie dies für viele Kombinationen äußerlich sichtbarer Dysplasien mit psychischen Krankheiten anzunehmen ist. Ohne weiteres leuchtet diese Interpretation für die Kombination von psychiatrischen Erkrankungen mit einem *Hydrocephalus internus* ein. Sie findet sich bei Oligophrenien und organischen Demenzen, kommt aber auch beim Alkoholismus (FEUERLEIN u. HEYSE, 1970) und wahrscheinlich bei chronischem Mißbrauch von Schlaf- und Schmerzmitteln vor (v. ZERSSEN et al., 1970), ohne daß es bereits zur Ausbildung einer Demenz gekommen sein müßte.

Biochemische Partialkonstitution: Konstitutionelle Anomalien im biochemischen Bereich finden sich vor allem bei Oligophrenien und bei Demenzen (OMENN, 1976). Hier sind in erster Linie die *Speicherkrankheiten* infolge genetisch bedingter Enzymdefekte zu erwähnen.

Bei den akuten Krankheitsschüben der *intermittiereden Porphyrie* (s. Abschnitt „Rassische Konstitution", S. 664) handelt es sich um pathologische Veränderungen der aktuellen Kondition durch eine massive Anschoppung von Vorstufen der – durch einen enzymatischen Block (s. unten) gestörten – Hämsynthese (Delta-Aminolävulinsäure und Porphobilinogen; OMENN, 1976; DRUSCHKY, 1978). Diese bewirkt (außer der fast pathognomonischen Dunkelfärbung des Urins durch Oxydationsprodukte von Hämpräkursoren) zahlreiche, mehr oder weniger unspezifische Körpersymptome, wie Bauchkoliken, Tachykardie und Lähmungen infolge einer Polyneuropathie sowie eine Vielzahl psychischer Symptome und Syndrome. Diese reichen von leichten Verstimmungen bis zu floriden psychotischen Syndromen organischer Färbung mit wechselnden Graden von Bewußtseinstrübung, Störungen des Frischgedächtnisses und der Orientierung, hochgradiger Erregtheit, Verwirrtheit, Wahnideen, optischen und akustischen Halluzinationen. Den Schüben, die durch äußere Einflüsse (z.B. durch Barbiturateinnahme) ausgelöst werden können, liegt eine biochemische Konstitutionsanomalie – nämlich ein Mangel an Uroporphyrinogen I-Synthetase – zugrunde, die auch im symptomfreien Intervall nachweisbar ist, u.a. durch die vermehrte Ausscheidung der genannten Hämpräkursoren. Die häufigste Form ist erblich bedingt. Es gibt von dieser aber auch eine Phänokopie infolge chronischer Hepatopathie.

Konstitutionelle Anomalien des Biochemismus werden auch bei endogenen Psychosen vermutet, sind bisher aber nicht ausreichend belegt. Bemerkenswert erscheint der Befund einer reduzierten Aktivität der Monoamin-Oxydase (MAO) in den Blutplättchen von Patienten mit affektiven und solchen mit schizophrenen Psychosen (SULLIVAN et al., 1977), sowie von psychisch auffälligen Probanden aus der Durchschnittsbevölkerung, insbesondere solchen mit Suizidversuchen in der eigenen und/oder der Familienanamnese (BUCHSBAUM et al., 1976; MURPHY et al., 1976; BUCHSBAUM et al., 1977). Es erscheint daher nicht ausgeschlossen, daß eine niedrige MAO-Aktivität einen konstitutionellen Risikofaktor für psychische Störungen im allgemeinen und eine Suizidgefährdung im besonderen darstellt.

Ein spezieller Aspekt der biochemischen Partialkonstitution, nämlich die Verteilung exogen zugeführter Substanzen in den verschiedenen geweblichen Kompartimenten und ihre zeitlichen Veränderungen bildet den Gegenstand der Pharmakokinetik. Der Plasmaspiegel verschiedener Psychopharmaka und ihrer Metaboliten ist von besonderem Interesse für die psychiatrische Konstitutionsforschung. Ein auffallendes Ergebnis derartiger Untersuchungen ist die große interindividuelle Variabilität der Plasmaspiegel, die zu einem wesentlichen Anteil konstitutionell bedingt ist (OMENN u. MOTULSKY, 1976). Sie besitzt insofern klinische Relevanz, als es einen unteren Schwellenwert für die Wirksamkeit von Psychopharmaka gibt, der bei Anwendung einer Standarddosierung von einigen Patienten nicht erreicht wird.

Immunologische Partialkonstitution: Ein angeborener oder erworbener Immunkörpermangel (HUMPHREY u. WHITE, 1971) scheint nicht zu psychischen Störungen zu disponieren. Dagegen ist die Frage, ob die Bildung hirnspezifischer Autoimmunglobuline zur Entstehung endogener Psychosen, insbesondere solcher des schizophrenen Formenkreises führen könnte, seit Jahren immer wieder aufgeworfen und empirisch bearbeitet worden (HEATH, 1969; VARTANIAN et al., 1978). Überzeugende Befunde liegen bis heute nicht vor. Auch ist die Rolle solcher – gegen das eigene Hirngewebe gerichteter – Antikörper bei bestimmten Formen geistiger Behinderung (KIRMAN, 1975) und seniler Abbauprozesse (NAY, 1977) vorläufig ungeklärt. Autoimmunglobuline bei seniler Demenz sind möglicherweise als Folge und nicht als Ursache des zerebralen Abbaus zu betrachten.

Die Blutgruppenverteilung bei Patienten mit psychischen Störungen ist wiederholt unter der Hypothese eines manifestationsfördernden bzw. -hemmenden Einflusses der Blutgruppengene untersucht worden. Wegen der Widersprüchlichkeit der Befunde kann von einer Bestätigung oder Widerlegung dieser Hypothese vorläufig nicht die Rede sein (DIEBOLD, 1976). Entsprechendes gilt für Untersuchungen des HLA-Systems (HUMPHREY u. WHITE, 1971) bei endogenen Psychosen (RAFAELSEN et al., 1979).

Physiologische Partialkonstitution: Die Thomsensche *Myotonie* ist eine Funktionsanomalie der quergestreiften Muskulatur, die häufig mit einer allgemeinen Muskelhypertrophie einhergeht und insofern den körperlichen Habitus entscheidend prägen kann (BECKER, 1977). Dieser wirkt aber keineswegs abnorm; vielmehr besteht die eigentliche Anomalie in der myotonen Reaktionsweise der Muskulatur. Im Unterschied zur Dystrophia myotonica Curschmann-Steinert geht sie typischerweise nicht mit krankhaften Erscheinungen an anderen Organen unter Einschluß des Hirns sowie entsprechenden psychischen Veränderungen einher, weshalb man nicht von einer Anomalie der psychophysischen Totalkonstitution sprechen kann.

Ein physiologisches Konstitutionsmerkmal ist u.a. die Händigkeit, d.h. die bevorzugte Benutzung *einer* – zumeist der rechten – Hand. Diese periphere motorische Lateralisation korreliert mit der Sprachdominanz und anderen Formen funktioneller Hemisphären-Asymmetrie (DEEGENER, 1978), die ihrerseits mit einer Asymmetrie des *Planum temporale* der Großhirnhemisphäre (also einem Merkmal der morphologischen Partialkonstitution) korrelieren (GESCHWIND u. LEWITZKY, 1968). Die Frage, ob die Händigkeit angeboren oder erworben sei, ist wahrscheinlich falsch gestellt. Wie bei den meisten konstitutionellen Verhaltensmerkmalen ist vielmehr eine „Ergänzungsreihe" (FREUD, 1905/1968) von genetischer Disposition und persistatischen Faktoren anzunehmen. Die Wirksamkeit des erzieherischen Druckes zur Entwicklung der – in allen rezenten menschlichen Gesellschaften zur Norm erhobenen – Rechtshändigkeit kann sowohl durch eine ausgeprägte genetische Disposition zur Linkshändigkeit als auch durch eine (überwiegend) linkshirnig lokalisierte Schädigung zunichte gemacht werden.

Allein aus dem Befund einer Linkshändigkeit bei negativer Familienanamnese auf einen Hirnschaden zu schließen, wäre allerdings voreilig. Eine größere Häufung dieses Befundes bei hirnorganisch bedingter Verzögerung der sprachlichen Entwicklung kann jedoch als erwiesen gelten. Angaben über Beziehungen der Händigkeit zu psychischen Störungen, die sich erst im Erwachsenenalter manifestieren – wie verschiedene Formen endogener Psychosen (AST et al., 1976; METZIG et al., 1976; FLEMINGER et al., 1977) –, bedürfen hingegen weiterer Bestätigung.

Konstitutionelle *Normvarianten* und vor allem *abnorme Veränderungen* des *Elektroenzephalogramms* (EEG; KUGLER, 1966) finden sich nicht nur gehäuft bei Oligophrenie, organischer Demenz sowie organischer und epileptischer Wesensänderung, sondern auch bei anderen Formen psychischer Konstitutionsanomalien, insbesondere bei Psychopathien und bei Transsexualität (hier insbesondere in Form allgemeiner Spannungsverminderung und temporaler Thetawellen-Vermehrung; KOCKOTT u. NUSSELT, 1976; NUSSELT u. KOCKOTT, 1976). Ob die bei aktuellen psychischen Störungen (Neurosen, schizophrenen Psychosen) nachgewiesenen EEG-Veränderungen als konstitutionelle Indikatoren der Krankheitsdisposition zu betrachten sind oder ob es sich hierbei nur um Korrelate des Krankheitsgeschehens (also um Veränderungen der Kondition) handelt, ist vorläufig schwer zu entscheiden. Bei Schizophrenen scheint ihr Vorkommen negativ mit einer familiären Psychosenbelastung zu korrelieren, was auf die ätiopathogenetische Rolle hirnorganischer Schädigungen bei Psychosen von Patienten mit abnormen EEG-Befunden hinweisen könnte (HAYS, 1977).

b) Psychische Partialkonstitutionen

Triebkonstitution: Interindividuelle Unterschiede der Intensität und der spezifischen Ausrichtung menschlicher Triebe haben einen *konstitutionellen* und einen *konditionellen* Anteil (CHILTON, 1972). Aktuelles Triebverhalten ist zudem stark von *situativen* Einflüssen abhängig. Diese haben darüber hinaus einen bestimmenden Einfluß auf die Triebentwicklung, möglicherweise besonders in speziellen *sensiblen Phasen*, so daß man von *prägungsartigen Vorgängen* sprechen könnte. Das scheint jedenfalls für die *sexuelle Trieborientierung* zu gelten, die zumindest teilweise in demselben Entwicklungsabschnitt festgelegt wird wie die subjektive Geschlechtsidentifikation, nämlich zwischen dem zweiten und vierten Lebensjahr (FREUD, 1905/1968; MONEY u. EHRHARDT, 1972; s. Abschnitt „Geschlechtskonstitution", S. 664f.). Aber auch die Reifungszeit kann nochmals in besonderem Maße für prägende Einflüsse auf die sexuelle Triebentwicklung empfänglich machen. Daß sich in dieser Zeit die Mehrzahl sexueller Perversionen manifestiert, liegt allerdings wahrscheinlich daran, daß durch eine weitgehend hormonal bedingte Aktivierung sexueller Triebregungen deren Ausrichtung auf bestimmte Triebobjekte und Befriedigungsformen erst aktualisiert wird. Eine gewisse Vorprogrammierung liegt aber vermutlich schon vor. An ihr scheinen auch hormonelle Einflüsse während der Fetalzeit und – im Falle einer Fehlidentifikation – auch hirnorganische Schädigungen (besonders im Temporalbereich, s. oben) beteiligt zu sein (KOLÁŘSKÝ et al., 1967).

Durch Zwillingsuntersuchungen an *Homosexuellen* ist die Rolle genetischer Faktoren bei der Entstehung einzelner Formen dieser sexuellen Deviation belegt worden (HESTON u. SHIELDS, 1968); es läßt sich aber bisher nicht ausreichend beurteilen, wie weit die genetischen Einflüsse hormonal vermittelt werden. So wurde von amerikanischen Autoren (KOLODNY et al., 1971) ein erniedrigter Testosteron-Spiegel im Blut ausschließlich oder ganz überwiegend homosexueller Männer (Kinsey-Stufen 4 und 5) ermittelt – ein Befund, der von Untersuchern in der BRD nicht bestätigt werden konnte (DOERR et al., 1973, 1976). Diese fanden vielmehr eine vom Ausprägungsgrad der Homosexualität unabhängige Erhöhung von Dihydrotestosteron und dem Prozentanteil des freien Testosteron, aber auch von Östrogenen (Östron und Östradiol) sowie von luteinisierendem Hormon (LH), dessen vermehrte Sekretion aus dem Hypophysenvorderlappen den erhöhten Plasmaspiegel der anderen Hormone erklären könnte. Bei lesbischen Frauen wurden in einer Untersuchungsreihe erhöhte Testosteron-Werte festgestellt (PAL, 1978). Die sexuelle Orientierung könnte demnach u.a. von der Relation zwischen Östrogenen und Testosteronen im Blut abhängen. Hormonelle Behandlungsversuche bei Homosexuellen sprechen allerdings gegen eine solche Interpretation und lassen eher vermuten, daß vorbestehende Störungen im Hormongleichgewicht einen Einfluß auf die Triebentwicklung ausgeübt haben. Von einem gewissen Stadium der Entwicklung an dürfte sich die aktuelle Hormonsituation nicht mehr entscheidend auf die Triebausrichtung ausgewirkt haben. Dagegen führt Androgenmangel im allgemeinen zu sexueller Triebschwäche (BLEULER, 1964; MONEY, 1978). Es fehlt allerdings jeder Anhalt für die Annahme, daß die Mehrzahl quantitativer Normabweichungen der sexuellen Triebkonstitution auf diese Weise zu erklären ist.

Über konstitutionelle Faktoren bei nicht-sexuellen Triebanomalien ist vergleichsweise wenig bekannt. Es ist zwar nicht zu bezweifeln, daß eine *Hyperphagie* zur Fettsucht führen kann und daß es konstitutionelle Formen der Fettsucht gibt. Ob diese allerdings durch eine *konstitutionelle* Hyperphagie zustande kommen, ist vorläufig wohl kaum zu entscheiden (RIES, 1970). Immerhin gibt es gewisse Anhaltspunkte dafür, daß durch Überfütterung von Säuglingen eine Disposition zur Adipositas geschaffen wird, und zwar einmal durch die stark nahrungsabhängige Vermehrung von Fettzellen in den ersten Lebensmonaten und durch eine Art Prägung des Nahrungstriebes auf Überernährung (BOEHNCKE u. GERHARD, 1977). Diesem Vorgang könnte neurophysiologisch eine abnorme Sollwerteinstellung für das Sättigungsgefühl (in hypothalamischen bzw. limbischen Zentren) zugrunde liegen.

Charakter: Die charakterliche Eigenart eines Patienten ist von grundlegender Bedeutung für seine psychiatrische Beurteilung und Behandlung (MAYER-GROSS et al., 1969; FOULDS, 1965; v. ZERSSEN, 1977a). So lassen sich leichtere krankhafte Veränderungen oft nur auf dem Hintergrund einer genauen Kenntnis der *prämorbiden Charakterstruktur* richtig einschätzen. Charakterliche Besonderheiten können die Symptomatologie der Krankheit färben (wie im Falle der anankastischen Depression bei Zwangsstrukturen: VIDEBECH, 1975) oder durch die Erkrankung karikaturhaft übersteigert werden (z.B. bei arteriosklerotischen Abbauprozessen). Nach dem Abklingen eines akuten Krankheitsprozesses können *dauerhafte Persönlichkeitsveränderungen* zurückbleiben (wie bei schizophrenen oder organisch bedingten Formen der Persönlichkeitsveränderung). Die *Charakterstruktur* kann zudem – wie im Falle der Psychopathie – schon *primär* so *abnorm* sein, daß sie die Lebensbewältigung des Patienten auch ohne das Hinzutreten aktueller psychischer Störungen erheblich behindert und somit selber Krankheitswert besitzt. Insbesondere bei Oligophrenen können charakterlich bedingte Auffälligkeiten (z.B. Indolenz, Erethismus) das Zurechtkommen in einer normalen Umgebung zusätzlich erschweren (THOMAS u. CHESS, 1977) oder gar völlig unmöglich machen und dadurch zur Dauerhospitalisation führen, die aufgrund der Intelligenzminderung allein womöglich nicht erforderlich wäre.

Auch bei aktuellen psychischen Störungen stehen – primäre und sekundäre – charakterliche Normabweichungen mit sozialen Anpassungsstörungen, wie sie sich insbesondere bei Patienten aus dem schizophrenen Formenkreis finden, oft einer erfolgreichen Rehabilitation im Wege. Darüber hinaus wird die Kooperationsbereitschaft von Patienten mit aktuellen psychischen Störungen bei der Durchführung insbesondere langfristiger Therapien weitgehend von Persönlichkeitsfaktoren bestimmt, was beispielsweise bei der Indikationsstellung für psychoanalytische Behandlungen berücksichtigt werden muß. Schließlich hängt es auch weitgehend von Persönlichkeitsfaktoren ab, wie weit abnorme Belastungen (z.B. KZ-Haft; MATUSSEK, 1977) bewältigt werden bzw. zur Entstehung und Fixierung psychoreaktiver Störungen führen.

<small>Die Darstellung der hier angeschnittenen Probleme beschränkt sich im wesentlichen auf den Zusammenhang aktueller psychischer Störungen mit typischen Varianten prämorbider Charakterstrukturen. Es wird speziell auf solche Zusammenhänge eingegangen, die der klinischen Erfahrung entstammen (KRAEPELIN, 1909 u. 1913; KINKELIN, 1954; ARIETI, 1959; DIETRICH, 1961; ANGST, 1966; BUSS, 1966; FENICHEL, 1967; LEONHARD, 1968; MAYER-GROSS et al., 1969; KIELHOLZ, 1971; KRAUS, 1971; TELLENBACH, R., 1975; HAASE, 1976; TELLENBACH, H., 1976) und durch systematische Untersuchungen mit charakterologischen Selbst- und Fremdbeurteilungs-Skalen statistisch gesichert werden konnten. Untersuchungen mit Selbstbeurteilungs-Skalen werden nur insoweit berücksichtigt, als von den Patienten eine retrospektive Einschätzung von Verhaltensweisen und Einstellungen aus der Zeit *vor* Beginn der Erkrankung gefordert und das verbale Verständnis anhand eines entsprechenden</small>

Intelligenztests kontrolliert wurde oder aber die Erhebung nach Abklingen florider Krankheitserscheinungen erfolgte. Solche Untersuchungen wurden erst in jüngster Zeit aufgenommen, obwohl das Interesse an Zusammenhängen zwischen psychischen Störungen und den Eigenarten der prämorbiden Persönlichkeit bis in die Antike zurückreicht (BLANKENBURG, 1973) und JASPERS bereits in der ersten Auflage seiner „Allgemeinen Psychopathologie" (1913, S. 256) ausdrücklich auf das Fehlen genauerer statistischer Untersuchungen zu diesem Problemkreis aufmerksam gemacht hat.

Die Anwendung *objektivierender Untersuchungsverfahren* und *statistischer Datenanalysen* hat viele in der klinischen Literatur kontrovers dargestellte Beziehungen zwischen Charakterstruktur und krankhaften psychischen Störungen auf deskriptivem Niveau klären und dabei einige der gängigen Auffassungen eindeutig widerlegen können. Bestätigt wurde hingegen in neueren Untersuchungen (BRÄUTIGAM, 1974) das Bild der prämorbid *schizoiden Charakterstruktur* von *Schizophrenen*, wie es sich aus der psychiatrischen Literatur der letzten 100 Jahre ergibt (FRITSCH, 1976). Auch durch eine bezüglich Diagnose, Krankheitssymptomatik, Therapieform und familiärer Belastung mit Psychosen „blinde" Auswertung von Krankengeschichten hat sich diese Struktur deutlich von den Strukturen bei affektiven Psychosen abheben lassen (TELLENBACH, 1975). Die Schizoidie ist gekennzeichnet durch eine ausgeprägte Introversionsneigung und die von KRETSCHMER als „psychästhetische Proportion" bezeichnete Kombination von Überempfindlichkeit und kühler Distanz in den emotionalen Beziehungen (KRETSCHMER, 1977). Oft erschwert ein Hang zur Weltfremdheit die Anpassung an die Realität. Er ist mitbestimmend für die Interessen, die sich beispielsweise bei psychotisch erkrankten Studenten schon prämorbid auf die Wahl des Studienfaches ausgewirkt haben (VOGL, 1976): Überdurchschnittlich häufig erkranken Studenten der Kunstakademie sowie Studierende der Philosophie, der Theologie und der (theoretischen) Physik. Unterrepräsentiert sind hingegen Studierende der Zahnmedizin, der Betriebswirtschaft und des Ingenieurwesens (Technische Universität). Der Wunsch, die eigene Individualität in schöpferischer Tätigkeit zu verwirklichen oder letzte Geheimnisse des Daseins zu enträtseln, ist offenbar stärker entwickelt als die Tendenz zum Gelderwerb durch lebenspraktische Betätigung.

Schizoide Persönlichkeitszüge sind auch bei für Schizophrenie diskordanten eineiigen Zwillingen häufig konkordant (TIENARI, 1968), gewöhnlich sind sie aber beim jeweils erkrankten Paarling bereits prämorbid stärker ausgeprägt (STABENAU u. POLLIN, 1969). Ganz allgemein haben diese Persönlichkeitszüge die Tendenz, sich schon vor Beginn der Erstmanifestation psychotischer Symptomatik zu verstärken. Bei einer Schizophrenia simplex leiten sie oft unmerklich in die Psychose über, so daß sie von dieser nicht deutlich abzugrenzen sind (HUBER, 1974). Im Verlauf psychotischer Schübe pflegen sie bei allen Schizophrenieformen stärker hervorzutreten und können dann in dieser akzentuierten Form als Residuum der Erkrankung zurückbleiben. Da sie außerdem nicht allein bei manifest Erkrankten, sondern auch bei deren Blutsverwandten gehäuft zu finden sind, liegt der Verdacht nahe, daß sie Ausdruck derselben hereditären Faktoren sind, die der Psychose zugrunde liegen. Sie deshalb als eine Abortivform der Erkrankung anzusehen, erscheint aber wegen ihrer relativen Konstanz kaum gerechtfertigt; ist doch gerade ein Charakteristikum der Psychose ihr wechselvoller, überwiegend schubweiser Verlauf. Sie sind im übrigen zu unspezifisch, um bei nicht-erkrankten Probanden als Risikofaktoren für eine Schizophrenie gelten zu können – es sei denn, daß sich Psychosen unter den Blutsverwandten der Betreffenden finden. Bei den Erkrankten trübt das Vorliegen prämorboid schizoider Charakterzüge die Prognose (ASTRUP et al., 1962; HUBER et al., 1978), auch bezüglich des Ansprechens auf eine neuroleptische Behandlung. Wie weit sich die schizoide Struktur schizophrener Patienten durch somatische und/oder psychologische Behandlungsformen günstig beeinflussen läßt, ist nicht sicher bekannt.

Eine einheitliche Charakterisierung der prämorbiden Persönlichkeit von Patienten mit *affektiven Psychosen* – etwa im Sinne des zyklothymen Temperaments – ist nach neueren psychometrischen Untersuchungen nicht möglich (v. ZERSSEN, 1977a). Erst die vor KRAEPELIN übliche, von der Wernickeschen Schule beibehaltene und neuerdings vor allem von ANGST (1966) und von PERRIS (1966) wieder aufgegriffene Unterteilung nach der *Verlaufsform* läßt prämorbide Besonderheiten deutlich erkennen. Dabei müssen aus der Gruppe bipolarer Psychosen die überwiegend manisch verlaufenden Formen herausgehoben werden, um auch hier eine typische Merkmalskonstellation hervortreten zu lassen (v. ZERSSEN, 1977a). Während sich nämlich bei Patienten mit ausgesprochen zirkulären Verlaufsformen bisher – in Übereinstimmung mit älteren klinischen Untersuchungen von REISS (1910) und KRAEPELIN (1909 u. 1913) – psychometrisch keine eindeutigen Abweichungen der prämorbiden Persönlichkeitsstruktur vom Bevölkerungsdurchschnitt haben nachweisen lassen (HOFMANN, 1973; FREY, 1977), erscheint die Beziehung überwiegend *manisch* verlaufender Formen der Erkrankung zum „sanguinischen Temperament", die schon von ESQUIROL 1816 behauptet worden war, nach neueren Untersuchungen gesichert. Diese Persönlichkeitszüge wurden auch als „hypomanisch" bzw. „hyperthym" bezeichnet. Sie muten wie eine habituelle Form abgeschwächter Symptomatik der Erkrankung an und sind deshalb unter dem Begriff des *„Typus manicus"* zusammengefaßt worden (v. ZERSSEN, 1977a). Ähnlich wie schizoide Charakterzüge bei Schizophrenen verstärken sie sich manchmal schon vor Beginn der Erkrankung und bleiben u.U. zwischen den Krankheitsphasen in akzentuierter Form bestehen, so daß eine scharfe Abgrenzung von konstitutioneller Eigenart und aktueller krankhafter Veränderung derselben oft kaum zu treffen ist.

Die Übereinstimmung des „Typus manicus" mit dem zyklothymen Temperament betrifft nur dessen hypomanische Variante mit Eigenschaften wie einfallsreich, lebhaft, unbeschwert, unstet, risikofreudig, manchmal etwas überspannt, dabei kontaktfähig, aber stark egozentrisch und dominierend, nicht jedoch besonders anpassungsfähig und gemütlich-humorvoll. Im Unterschied zur Introversionsneigung des schizoiden Typus besteht beim „Typus manicus" eine ausgeprägte Extraversionsneigung. Sie findet offenbar auch in der Berufswahl (z.B. Schauspieler) ihren Niederschlag – ein Eindruck, der bisher allerdings noch nicht durch statistische Untersuchungen überprüft worden ist.

Wie im Falle schizophrener Psychosen scheint auch bei überwiegend manisch verlaufenden affektiven Psychosen eine gemeinsame Basis für die Entstehung von Charakterstruktur und Krankheit vorzuliegen, ohne daß diese sich näher spezifizieren ließe. Im Unterschied zur neuroleptischen Behandlung, die offenbar sowohl bei schizophrenen wie bei manischen Psychosen ausschließlich gegen die Krankheitssymptomatik gerichtet ist, scheint eine langfristige Lithiumanwendung die gemeinsame Basis von manischer Psychose und hypomanischer Persönlichkeitsstruktur zu beeinflussen; denn sie entfaltet nicht nur eine therapeutische und insbesondere prophylaktische Wirkung gegenüber den manischen Phasen, sondern vermag anscheinend auch den zur Ausgangspersönlichkeit gehörenden Antriebsüberschuß und die mit ihm verbundene erhöhte emotionelle Ansprechbarkeit zu dämpfen (BECH et al., 1976; BONETTI et al., 1977). Gerade daran scheitert aber manchmal die Intervallbehandlung mit Lithium; denn einige der Patienten fühlen sich durch sie in ihrer Erlebnisfähigkeit beeinträchtigt. Hinzu kommt, daß der dem „Typus manicus" eigene Mangel an vorausschauender Planung und konsequenter Lebensführung an sich schon die Bereitschaft zu langfristiger prophylaktischer Medikamenteneinnahme verringert, so daß u.U. lieber das Risiko eines Rezidivs in Kauf genommen als die ärztliche Verordnung regelmäßig befolgt wird.

Ganz anders verhalten sich in dieser Beziehung Patienten mit monopolar verlaufenden endogenen Depressionen.

Trotz mancher Gegensätzlichkeit zum „Typus manicus" erweckt das Charakterbild von monopolar Depressiven nicht den Eindruck einer abgeschwächten Dauerform der Erkrankung; vielmehr scheint diese einige der typischen Merkmale des „Typus melancholicus" geradezu in ihr Gegenteil zu verkehren (TELLENBACH, 1969): In gesunden Tagen sind die Patienten im allgemeinen besonders gewissenhaft, leistungsbetont, dabei – trotz einer ausgeprägten Tendenz, am Gewohnten, Althergebrachten festzuhalten – anpassungsbereit und zudem sehr anhänglich (JULIAN et al., 1963; METCALFE, 1968; v. ZERSSEN, 1969c, 1976b, 1977a; v. ZERSSEN et al., 1970; MARKERT, 1972; TELLENBACH, R., 1975; HAASE, 1976; TELLENBACH, H., 1976; FREY, 1977; PERRIS u. STRANDMAN, 1979; STRANDMAN, 1978). Sie sind dementsprechend meistens sehr beliebt in der Familie und ebenfalls am Arbeitsplatz, wo sie – im Unterschied zu Manikern – typischerweise eine Dauerstellung in abhängiger Position anstreben und gewöhnlich auch innehaben (TELLENBACH, 1976). In der Erkrankung dagegen vernachlässigen sich die sonst so ordentlichen Patienten oft, können sich schließlich zu keiner Leistung mehr aufraffen und kümmern sich nicht mehr um andere. Es gibt allerdings auch tendenzielle Gemeinsamkeiten von Persönlichkeitsstruktur und Krankheitssymptomatik, wie z.B. die starke Ausprägung des Gewissens, das in der Erkrankung übermächtig wird, was besonders in psychoanalytischen Theorien der Depressionsentstehung hervorgehoben wird (MENDELSON, 1974). Auf jeden Fall sind die Beziehungen zwischen Persönlichkeitsstruktur und Krankheitsbild komplizierter, als es beim „Typus manicus" offenbar der Fall ist.

Begriffe wie „subdepressives" oder „zyklothymes" Temperament erscheinen völlig ungeeignet, die prämorbide Persönlichkeitseigenart von monopolar Depressiven zu kennzeichnen (v. ZERSSEN, 1977a). Objektivierende Untersuchungen sprechen sogar dafür, daß diese Kranken schon vor Erkrankungsbeginn *weniger* zyklothym sind, als es dem Bevölkerungsdurchschnitt entspricht (v. ZERSSEN et al., 1970; EIBAND, 1979). Um so erstaunlicher ist es, daß auch ihre Struktur offenbar durch eine prophylaktische Lithiumanwendung in ihrer Ausprägung abgeschwächt wird; insbesondere scheinen sich gelegentlich Übergewissenhaftigkeit und perfektionistisches Leistungsstreben zurückzubilden (BAASTRUP, 1969; GLATZEL, 1974). Dies könnte dafür sprechen, daß – wie beim „Typus manicus" – die Daueranwendung von Lithium einen Einfluß auf die gemeinsame dispositionelle Basis von Persönlichkeitsstruktur und phasenhaften Krankheitsmanifestationen ausübt. Es muß aber auch erwogen werden, ob Lithium bei chronischer Anwendung in ganz unspezifischer Weise zu einer Nivellierung akzentuierter Persönlichkeitszüge führen kann, die nichts mit einer Disposition zu der im prophylaktischen Sinne beeinflußten Erkrankung zu tun haben. Bei akuter Lithium-Anwendung konnte anhand von Persönlichkeitsskalen (innerhalb von zwei Wochen) allerdings kein derartiger Einfluß ermittelt werden (JUDD et al., 1977); das schließt jedoch die Möglichkeit von Persönlichkeitsveränderungen bei langfristiger Anwendung des Lithium keineswegs aus.

Versuche, die *Entstehung depressiver Verstimmungsphasen* psychologisch aus der *Persönlichkeitsstruktur* der Erkrankten und der durch sie bestimmten Form der Verarbeitung aktueller Erlebnisse herzuleiten, können vorläufig nur als *Arbeitshypothesen* betrachtet werden. Charakterologische Untersuchungen an Patienten mit bipolaren affektiven Psychosen zeigen jedenfalls, daß der „Typus melancholicus" keineswegs eine *conditio sine qua non* für die Entstehung depressiver Phasen ist (EIBAND, 1979). Es muß allerdings damit gerechnet werden, daß sich in der prämorbiden Charakterstruktur von Patienten mit zirkulärer Verlaufsform affektiver Psychosen Züge des „Typus melancholicus" mit solchen des „Typus manicus" in einer Weise miteinander vermischen, daß sie psychometrisch-statistischen Untersuchungen bisher entgangen sind.

Ein Einfluß der depressiven Erkrankungsphasen auf die Persönlichkeitsstruktur ist bisher nicht überzeugend nachgewiesen worden, weder im Sinne einer Akzentuierung noch dem einer Abwandlung (etwa in Richtung auf eine chronisch depressive Gemütsverfassung). Das erleichtert die Rückkehr der Patienten in die gewohnten Verhältnisse und erklärt, daß es offenbar auch bei häufigen Rezidiven der Erkrankung selten zu gravierenden Veränderungen der sozialen Situation – Scheidung oder Auflösung eines Arbeitsverhältnisses – kommt.

Wegen der Spärlichkeit von Untersuchungsbefunden, die mit objektivierenden Methoden gewonnen wurden, muß auf die Besprechung der Charakterstruktur bei anderen Psychoseformen – z.B. beim sensitiven Beziehungswahn im Sinne KRETSCHMERS (1966) – verzichtet werden.

Klinische Untersuchungen zur Charakterstruktur von *Neurotikern* begannen um die Jahrhundertwende mit den Arbeiten des französischen Psychologen PIERRE JANET (1908). Sie wurden besonders von Psychoanalytikern fortgeführt und haben wesentlich zur Entwicklung der psychoanalytischen Theorie beigetragen (FENICHEL, 1967; JUNG, 1976). Die Beiträge anderer – darunter auch lerntheoretisch orientierter Autoren (wie z.B. EYSENCK, 1970) – basieren zumeist auf diesen älteren Untersuchungen. Trotz Divergenzen in Details stimmen die meisten Untersucher in der Auffassung überein, daß Symptomneurosen häufig auf dem Boden einer neurotisch geprägten Charakterstruktur erwachsen und daß die „Symptomwahl" von Besonderheiten der Charakterstruktur mitbestimmt wird, die auch unabhängig von einer neurotischen Disposition vorkommen. Beispiele sind die für Patienten mit zwangsneurotischer Symptomatik typische anankastische Struktur und die für Patienten mit hysterischer Symptomatik (Konversionssymptome, Dämmerzustände etc.) gewöhnlich als typisch geltende hysterische Struktur (JASPERS, 1973). Für neurotisch depressive Patienten wird im allgemeinen eine passiv-abhängige Charakterstruktur angenommen. Diese – in der psychoanalytischen Literatur auf „orale Fixierung" der Libido zurückgeführte – Struktureigentümlichkeit in Verbindung mit starker Ausprägung neurotischer Strukturmerkmale unterscheidet nach klinischem Eindruck die prämorbide Charakterstruktur neurotisch Depressiver vom prämorbid vorherrschenden „Typus melancholicus" endogen Depressiver mit monopolarem Krankheitsverlauf (v. ZERSSEN, 1977a).

Die klinisch gewonnenen Eindrücke von Beziehungen zwischen *Charakterstruktur* und *Symptomwahl* bei *Neurotikern* haben sich im großen und ganzen durch psychometrische Untersuchungen bestätigen lassen; allerdings ist die *Spezifität* dieser Beziehungen offenbar *geringer* als gewöhnlich vermutet. Die Übereinstimmungen in der Charakterstruktur von Patienten mit verschiedenen Neuroseformen sind größer als die zwischen ihnen bestehenden Unterschiede (KRAUSS, 1972). Auch ähneln diese Strukturen in mancher Hinsicht (innere Zwiespältigkeit, Kontaktscheu etc.) denen von schizophrenen Patienten. Die neurotisch Depressiven stehen strukturell einerseits dem „Typus melancholicus", andererseits der schizoiden Persönlichkeit nahe, wobei allerdings die Tendenz zu passiver Abhängigkeit besonders akzentuiert zu sein scheint (PAYKEL et al., 1976; EIBAND, 1979). In Abweichung von der gängigen Lehrmeinung, aber in Übereinstimmung mit Beobachtungen verschiedener Kliniker (BUSS, 1966), weisen Neurotiker mit hysterischer Krankheitssymptomatik im allgemeinen keine typisch hysterischen Strukturmerkmale auf (LADER u. SARTORIUS, 1968; KRAUSS, 1972). Solche Merkmale finden sich dagegen in deutlicher Ausprägung bei Patienten mit überwiegend monopolar verlaufenden endogenen Manien (EIBAND, 1979)!

Intelligenz/spezielle Fähigkeiten: Außer den Beziehungen aktueller psychischer Störungen zu Varianten der prämorbiden Charakterstruktur sind ihre Zusammenhänge mit Varianten der allgemeinen Intelligenz bzw. speziellen Fähigkeiten zu beachten.

So weisen bei für *Schizophrenie* diskordanten eineiigen Zwillingen die Indexfälle schon von der Kindheit an eine durchschnittlich geringere Intelligenz auf als die nicht erkrankten Paarlinge. Diese negative Korrelation zwischen Psychosenanfälligkeit und Intelligenz beruht offenbar auf nichtgenetischen Faktoren, die sich nachteilig auf die Intelligenzentwicklung auswirken und zugleich die Disposition zur psychotischen Dekompensation im späteren Lebensalter erhöhen. Umgekehrt verbessert bei Erkrankten eine hohe prämorbide Intelligenz die Prognose des Krankheitsverlaufs (HUBER et al., 1978). Bei den *affektiven Psychosen* scheint ein – wenn auch geringfügiger – Unterschied im Intelligenzniveau von Patienten mit monopolaren und solchen mit bipolaren (bzw. „monopolar" manischen) Verlaufsformen zu bestehen. Letztere weisen eine durchschnittlich etwas höhere verbale Intelligenz auf (EIBAND, 1979). Das könnte damit zusammenhängen, daß sie vergleichsweise häufig aus einem gehobenen Sozialmilieu stammen (WOODRUFF et al., 1971). Diese unterschiedliche Herkunft reflektiert möglicherweise den Einfluß, den die genetische Krankheitsdisposition innerhalb einer Familie auf konstitutionelle Faktoren ausübt, die für die soziale Bewährung von Bedeutung sind. Es könnte sich dabei um eine optimale Kombination von Zügen des „Typus manicus" mit solchen des „Typus melancholicus" (z.B. von Einfallsreichtum mit Zuverlässigkeit), wie sie im vorigen Abschnitt besprochen wurden, handeln.

Auch bei *Neurosen* finden sich Zusammenhänge zwischen klinischem Erscheinungsbild und Intelligenz; z.B. erzielen Patienten mit Zwangssymptomen eher überdurchschnittliche, Patienten mit hysterischer Symptomatik hingegen eher unterdurchschnittliche (verbale) Intelligenzleistungen (SLATER u. SLATER, 1944). Wie weit die Intelligenzentwicklung als solche die Symptomwahl mitbestimmt, ist unbekannt. Es könnte auch ein Einfluß neurosenspezifischer „Abwehrmechanismen" (FENICHEL, 1975) auf die Intelligenzentwicklung vorliegen, indem diese durch die für Zwangsneurotiker typische Tendenz zur Intellektualisierung gefördert, durch die für Patienten mit hysterischer Symptombildung typischen Abwehrformen der Verdrängung und Verleugnung hingegen gehemmt wird. Zu beachten ist ferner, daß eine genetisch oder durch exogene Schädigung bedingte Beeinträchtigung der intellektuellen Entwicklung zu emotionellen Problemen führen kann: Die Betreffenden werden womöglich von anderen zurückgesetzt und ausgenutzt bzw. leiden unter ihrer Unfähigkeit, Aufgaben in einer ihrer Altersnorm entsprechenden Weise zu bewältigen. Ähnliche Probleme können sich – besonders im Schulalter – beim Vorliegen umschriebener Leistungsstörungen (insbesondere einer Lese- und Rechtschreibeschwäche) ergeben.

Die klinischen Bilder primärer und sekundärer Beeinträchtigung intellektueller und anderer Fähigkeiten werden hier nur kurz erwähnt, da sie in entsprechenden Kapiteln der klinischen Bände dieses Handbuches ausführlich abgehandelt werden. Es handelt sich bei den primären Beeinträchtigungen um Entwicklungsstörungen wie *Oligophrenie* (HARBAUER, 1976b; INGALLS, 1978), *Legasthenie* (SCHENK-DANZINGER, 1978) und *Rechenschwäche* (WEINSCHENK, 1975), bei den sekundären dagegen um dauerhafte Folgezustände eines Abbaues bereits entwickelter Fähigkeiten, so bei irreversiblen Formen *organischer Demenz*. Ist ein solcher Leistungsverfall noch reversibel (wie beispielsweise im Anfangsstadium einer progressiven Paralyse), liegt definitionsgemäß noch keine (sekundäre) Konstitutionsanomalie vor. Die Frage, ob es bei ausgeprägten *schizophrenen Defektzuständen* (HUBER, 1974) zu einer irreversiblen Beeinträchtigung intellektueller Fähigkeiten oder nur zu einer unzureichenden Nutzung des an sich noch vorhandenen intellektuellen Potentials kommt, ist nicht ausreichend empirisch untersucht worden, um eine fundierte Antwort zu ermöglichen.

Kommunikationsweisen: Normvarianten der Kommunikationsweisen sind bisher zu wenig im Hinblick auf ihren konstitutionellen Anteil und seine Relevanz für die Entstehung oder spezifische Ausgestaltung aktueller psychischer Störungen bearbeitet worden, als daß es sich lohnen würde, sie an dieser Stelle zu besprechen. Hinzuweisen ist aber auf abnorme Varianten, deren eindrucksvollstes Beispiel der *infantile Autismus* darstellt (KEHRER, 1978).

Überzeugungen, Einstellungen und Interessen: Daß Überzeugungen, Einstellungen und Interessen einen konstitutionellen Anteil aufweisen, geht u.a. aus Untersuchungen an *fetal androgenisierten weiblichen Intersexen* hervor, die durch chirurgische Korrektur des Genitale in den ersten Lebensjahren und/oder eine kontinuierliche Hormonbehandlung im äußeren Erscheinungsbild von den Stigmen der Vermännlichung befreit bzw. vor einer entsprechenden Körperentwicklung bewahrt und die auch ihrem Geschlecht entsprechend erzogen worden sind. Sie zeigen im Vergleich mit ihren Altersgefährtinnen – außer einem manchmal auffallend *burschikosen Verhalten*, das unserer Einteilung der Partialkonstitutionen entsprechend dem Charakter zuzurechnen ist – ein vermehrtes *Interesse* an typisch männlichen Betätigungen (z.B. Kampfsport) und ein vermindertes Interesse an typisch weiblichen (je nach Alter Puppenspiele, Kosmetik u. dgl.; MONEY u. EHRHARDT, 1972; EHRHARDT u. BAKER, 1974).

Weitgehend irreversible Überzeugungen, Einstellungen und Interessen, die von der frühesten Kindheit an sozial „geprägt" werden, betreffen die Geschlechtsidentität und die mit ihr verbundene Übernahme geschlechtsdifferenter Rollenangebote. Dies wird durch Erfahrungen belegt, die an Intersexen gewonnen wurden. Die Geschlechtsidentität solcher Individuen entspricht im allgemeinen dem ihnen nach der Geburt zugewiesenen Geschlecht und nicht den Komponenten des somatischen Geschlechts (Geschlechtschromosomen, Keimdrüsen, Relation der männlichen und weiblichen Geschlechtshormone, inneres oder äußeres Genitale, sekundäre Geschlechtsmerkmale; ELLIS, 1945; MONEY et al., 1955; OVERZIER, 1961b). Auch die Entwicklung der Triebkonstitution vollzieht sich dabei gewöhnlich im Einklang mit der Geschlechtsidentität. Allerdings übt die puberale Androgenproduktion einen starken Einfluß auf die quantitative Ausprägung des Sexualtriebs aus.

Eine nach den bisher vorliegenden Untersuchungen auf den psychischen Bereich beschränkte Konstitutionsanomalie von Überzeugungen, Einstellungen und Interessen liegt bei der *Transsexualität* vor, die immer auch eine entsprechende Ausrichtung der sexuellen Trieborientierung einschließt, ohne primär von ihr bestimmt zu sein. Eine genetische oder milieutheoretische Erklärung für die Entstehung dieser psychischen Konstitutionsanomalie gibt es nicht. Es finden sich jedoch bei Transsexuellen gehäuft Normvarianten und abnorme Varianten elektroenzephalographischer Befunde (KOCKOTT u. NUSSELT, 1976; NUSSELT u. KOCKOTT, 1976), die durch exogene Hirnschäden bedingt sein könnten (KOLÁŘSKÝ et al., 1967). So ergeben sich auch hier – ähnlich wie bei der Homosexualität (s.oben) – Anhaltspunkte für einen Zusammenhang mit Besonderheiten der somatischen Konstitution. Eine isolierte Betrachtung der psychischen Konstitution wäre demnach bei einigen Triebanomalien schon heute verfehlt; bei anderen ist sie die notwendige Konsequenz mangelnder Kenntnis ihrer somatischen Korrelate. Die Aufdeckung solcher psychophysischer Zusammenhänge gehört zu den wichtigsten Aufgaben der Konstitutionsforschung.

III. Individuelle Konstitution

Infolge der großen *genetischen Variabilität* des Menschen (THOMPSON, 1968; CLARKE, 1975) und der Vielfalt von *äußeren Einflüssen* auf seine Konstitutionsentwicklung hat jedes Individuum eine einzigartige Konstitution, die u.a. seine Identifizierbarkeit ermöglicht (HUNGER u. LEOPOLD, 1978). Auch zwischen erbgleichen Zwillingen bestehen im allgemeinen bedeutsame konstitutionelle Unterschiede (BROWN et al., 1967; CLARIDGE et al., 1973), die u.a. in Manifestationsunterschieden konstitutionsbedingter Erkrankungen zum Ausdruck kommen (VERSCHUER, 1954).

So erkranken für Schizophrenie konkordante eineiige Zwillinge im allgemeinen nicht zur gleichen Zeit, wenn auch häufig in einem Abstand von nur wenigen Jahren. Sowohl die Symptomgestaltung wie die Verlaufscharakteristika weisen nicht selten individuelle Besonderheiten auf, die nicht ohne weiteres Unterschieden der Kondition oder der Exposition zugeschrieben werden können. Besonders eindrucksvoll läßt sich dies am Beispiel jener erbgleichen Vierlinge aufweisen, die alle an einer Psychose aus dem schizophrenen Formenkreis erkrankten, aber in Abständen bis zu einigen Jahren und unter jeweils anderen Symptom- und Verlaufsmustern (ROSENTHAL, 1963). Der früheste Beginn und ein besonders ungünstiger, chronischer Krankheitsverlauf fanden sich bei der Patientin, die sich von Geburt an durch geringeres Körpergewicht und später durch größere Inkongruenzen der Knochenreifung, durch verzögerte Sprachentwicklung, ausgeprägte Kontaktschwäche und geringere Intelligenzleistungen von den anderen unterschied. Daß hier kein zufälliger Zusammenhang vorliegt, wird durch Untersuchungen an für Schizophrenie diskordanten eineiigen Zwillingen belegt, nach denen sich bei dem erkrankten Paarling ebenfalls häufiger Hinweise auf eine beeinträchtigte körperliche und psychische Entwicklung finden (STABENAU u. POLLIN, 1969).

Derartige Untersuchungen zur *Gruppenkonstitution* (in diesem Fall von eineiigen, für Schizophrenie diskordanten Zwillingen) schaffen die Voraussetzung dafür, im Einzelfall Wahrscheinlichkeitsaussagen über Bedingungszusammenhänge sowie über zukünftige Entwicklungen und deren Beeinflußbarkeit zu machen, wie z.B. über die Rolle frühkindlicher Hirnschädigung für Entstehung, Verlauf und Therapierbarkeit einer schizophrenen Psychose. Je geringer die Kenntnis von Gruppenkonstitutionen ist bzw. je schwächer die an entsprechenden Gruppen nachgewiesenen Zusammenhänge sind, desto unsicherer wird die auf den Einzelfall bezogene Aussage. Zudem müssen verschiedene Gruppenkonstitutionen (Alterskonstitution, Geschlechtskonstitution etc.) in Betracht gezogen und die jeweilige Kondition berücksichtigt werden. Hinzu kommt die Vielfalt situativer Faktoren, die in die Betrachtung eingehen müssen (SARASON et al., 1975), um ein umfassendes Bild von dem betreffenden Individuum, von seinen Gefährdungen und Möglichkeiten gewinnen zu können. Über das hinaus, was das betreffende Individuum mit anderen gemeinsam hat, ist besonders darauf zu achten, was es von anderen unterscheidet, worin seine Einmaligkeit liegt (CURTIUS, 1959). Die *relative Konstanz individueller Merkmale* bzw. Merkmalskonstellationen unter wechselnden äußeren Umständen spricht dabei für ihre konstitutionelle Verankerung. Das gilt z.B. auch für die individuelle Reaktion auf Medikamente – von deren Pharmakokinetik bis zur Verträglichkeit bzw. Unverträglichkeit (infolge therapeutisch unerwünschter Nebenwirkungen; LADER et al., 1974). Dementsprechend gibt es für jeden Patienten ein eigenes Optimum der Medikation, das nicht allein von spezifischen Krankheitsfaktoren, sondern ebenfalls von seiner Grundbeschaffenheit, d.h. seiner Konstitution, bestimmt wird.

Der Arzt steht somit bei jedem seiner Kranken vor der – letztlich unlösbaren – Aufgabe, das Miteinander konstitutioneller, konditioneller und situativer Faktoren in der Genese krankhafter Normabweichungen zu erkennen und in seinem Behandlungsplan zu berücksichtigen. Die prinzipielle Unlösbarkeit dieser Aufgabe darf ihn aber keinesfalls dazu verführen, wesentliche Aspekte einfach auszublenden und sein Augenmerk einseitig auf konstitutionelle oder auf konditionelle bzw. situative Faktoren zu lenken. Es kommt vielmehr darauf an, eine möglichst repräsentative Auswahl relevanter Aspekte aus dem Gesamtspektrum von individuellen und Umweltvariablen zu treffen, die für das Krankheitsbild in Betracht kommen. Zu den für einen Patienten relevanten Umweltvariablen gehört immer auch der ihn untersuchende und behandelnde Arzt selber. Dies gilt nicht allein, aber in besonderem Maße für psychisch Kranke. Deshalb ist es für jeden Arzt, vornehmlich aber den Psychiater, wichtig, sich über die eigene Rolle in der therapeutischen Beziehung Klarheit zu verschaffen. Seine Interaktion mit dem Kranken wird nur aus der Reflexion über die Beiträge verständlich, die beide Partner aus ihrer Konstitution, Kondition und jeweiligen Situation heraus dazu leisten. Die Ausbildung zum Arzt – und nicht nur die zum Fachpsychotherapeuten – sollte die Grundlagen für ein solches Verständnis schaffen.

Literatur

Abraham, G. E., Maroulis, G.B., Buster, J.E., Chang, R.J., Marshall, J.R.: Effect of dexamethasone on serum cortisol and androgen levels in hirsute patients. Obstet. Gynecol. **47**, 395–402 (1976)

Adelstein, A.M., Downham, D.Y., Stein, Z., Susser, M.W.: The epidemiology of mental illness in an English city. Soc. Psychiat. **3**, 47–59 (1968)

Albeaux-Fernet, M., Bohler, C.C.S.-S., Karpas, A.E.: Testicular function in the aging male. In: Geriatric endocrinology. Greenblatt, R.B. (ed.), p. 201–216. New York: Raven Press 1978

Anastasi, A.: Differential psychology, 3rd ed. New York: Macmillan 1965

Andrews, G., Harris, M., Garside, R., Kay, D.: The syndrome of stuttering. London: Heinemann 1964

Angst, J.: Zur Ätiologie und Nosologie endogener depressiver Psychosen. Berlin, Heidelberg, New York: Springer 1966

Angst, J., Baastrup, P., Grof, P., Hippius, H., Poeldinger, W., Varga, E., Weis, P., Wyss, F.: Statistische Aspekte des Beginns und Verlaufs schizophrener Psychosen. In: Verlauf und Ausgang schizophrener Erkrankungen. Huber, G. (Hrsg.), S. 67–78. Stuttgart, New York: Schattauer 1973

Angst, J., Baastrup, C., Grof, P., Hippius, H., Poeldinger, W., Weis, P.: Zum Verlauf affektiver Psychosen. In: Multifaktorielle Probleme in der Medizin. Bochnik, H.J., Pittrich, W. (Hrsg.), S. 137–157. Wiesbaden: Akademische Verlagsgesellschaft 1976

Angst, J., Perris, C.: Zur Nosologie endogener Depressionen. Vergleich der Ergebnisse zweier Untersuchungen. Z. Gesamte Neurol. Psychiatr. **210**, 373–386 (1968)

Arganian, M.: Sex differences in early development. In: Individual differences in children. Westman, J.C. (ed.), p. 45–63. New York, London, Sydney: Wiley 1973

Arieti, S.: Manic-depressive psychosis. In: American handbook of psychiatry. Arieti, S. (ed.), Vol. I, p. 419–454. New York: Basic Books 1959

Ast, M., Rosenberg, S., Metzig, E.: Constitutional predisposition to central nervous system (CNS) disease determined by tests of lateral asymmetry. Neuropsychobiology **2**, 269–275 (1976)

Astrup, C., Fossum, A., Holmboe, R.: Prognosis in functional psychoses. Springfield/Ill.: Thomas 1962

Baastrup, P.C.: Practical clinical viewpoints regarding treatment with Lithium. Acta Psychiatr. Scand. Suppl. **207**, 12–18 (1969)

Baeyer, W.v.: Sozialpathologie der Entwicklungsphasen. In: Handbuch der Sozialmedizin. Blohmke, M., Ferber, C.v., Kisker, K.P., Schaefer, H. (Hrsg.), Bd.II, S. 447–472. Stuttgart: Enke 1977

Balthazar, E.E., Stevens, H.A.: Emotionally disturbed mentally retarded: A historical and contemporary perspective. Englewood Cliffs/N.Y.: Prentice-Hall 1975

Bandura, A., Walters, R.H.: Social learning and personality development. New York, Chicago, San Francisco: Holt, Rinehart & Winston 1963

Bauer, J.: Konstitutionelle Disposition zu inneren Krankheiten, 3. Aufl. Berlin: Springer 1924

Bech, P., Vendsborg, P.B., Rafaelsen, O.J.: Lithium maintenance treatment of manic-melancholic patients: its role in the daily routine. Acta Psychiatr. Scand. **53**, 70–81 (1976)

Becker, P.E., with contributions by Knussmann, R. and Kuhn, E.: Myotonia congenita and syndromes associated with myotonia. Stuttgart: Thieme 1977

Berg, J.M.: Genetics and genetic counseling. In: Mental retardation and developmental disabilities. Wortis, J. (ed.) p. 41–57. New York: Brunner/Mazel 1976

Bertalanffy, L.v.: Theoretische Biologie. Bd. 1. Berlin: Borntraeger 1932

Bickel, H., Kaiser-Grubel, S.: Über die Phenylketonurie. Psychometrische Erfolgsbeurteilung der phenylalaninarmen Diät bei phenylketonurischen Kindern. Dtsch. Med. Wochenschr. **96**, 1415–1423 (1971)

Bierich, J.R., Majewski, F., Michaelis, R., Tillner, I.: Über das embryo-fetale Alkoholsyndrom. Europ. J. Pediat. **121**, 155–177 (1976)

Blankenburg, W.: Persönlichkeit, prämorbide. In: Lexikon der Psychiatrie. Müller, C. (Hrsg.), S. 374–376. Berlin, Heidelberg, New York: Springer 1973

Bleuler, M.: Endokrinologische Psychiatrie. In: Psychiatrie der Gegenwart. Gruhle, H.W., Jung, R., Mayer-Gross, W., Müller, M. (Hrsg.), Bd. I/1B, S. 161–252. Berlin, Göttingen, Heidelberg: Springer 1964

Bleuler, M.: Die schizophrenen Geistesstörungen im Lichte langjähriger Kranken- und Familiengeschichten. Stuttgart: Thieme 1972

Böcker, F.: Suizide und Suizidversuche. Stuttgart: Thieme 1973

Boehncke, H., Gerhard, J.: Die Vernachlässigung des „unauffälligen" Neugeborenen als Ursache von Kommunikationsstörungen zwischen Mutter und Kind, vor allem von Anorexia nervosa und Fettsucht. Kinderarzt **8**, 35–42 (1977)

Bonetti, U., Johannson, F., Knorring, L.v., Perris, C., Strandman, E.: Prophylactic lithium and personality variables. An international collaborative study. Intern. Pharmacopsychiat. **12**, 14–19 (1977)

Boué, J.G., Boué, A.: Chromosomal anomalies in early spontaneous abortion. In: Developmental biology and pathology. Gropp, A., Benirschke, K. (eds.), p. 193–208. Berlin, Heidelberg, New York: Springer 1976

Brace, G.L.: Physique, physiology and behavior: An attempt to analyze a part of their roles in the canine biogram. Unpublished doctoral dissertation, Cambridge/Mass.: Harvard University 1962. (Cit. by Royce, 1966)

Bräutigam, W.: Untersuchungen zur Persönlichkeitsentwicklung im Vorfeld der Schizophrenie. Nervenarzt **45**, 298–304 (1974)

Bridges, P.K.: The biological basis of personality. In: Perspectives in endocrine psychobiology. Brambilla, F., Bridges, P.K., Endröczi, E., Heuser, G. (eds.), p. 479–502. London, New York, Sydney: Wiley 1978

Brown, A.M., Stafford, R.E., Vandenberg, S.G.: Twins: behavioral differences. Child Dev. **38**, 1055–1064 (1967)

Brückel, K.W.: Grundzüge der Geriatrie. München: Urban & Schwarzenberg 1975

Buchsbaum, M.S., Coursey, R.D., Murphy, D.L.: The biochemical high-risk paradigm: behavioral and familial correlates of low platelet monoamine oxidase activity. Science **194**, 339–341 (1976)

Buchsbaum, M.S., Haier, R.J., Murphy, D.L.: Suicide attempts, platelet monoamine oxidase and the average evoked response. Acta Psychiatr. Scand. **56**, 69–79 (1977)

Bürger, M.: Altern und Krankheit als Problem der Biomorphose, 4. Aufl. Leipzig: Thieme 1960

Bundesminister für Jugend, Familie und Gesundheit (Hrsg.): Daten des Gesundheitswesens, Ausgabe 1977. Kandel: Palatia-Druck Heitzer GmbH 1977

Buss, A.H.: Psychopathologic. New York, London, Sydney: Wiley 1966

Buss, A.H., Plomin, R.: A temperament theory of personality development. New York, London, Sydney: Wiley 1975

Chetwynd, J., Hartnett, O. (eds.): The sex role system. London, Henley, Boston: Routledge & Kegan Paul 1978

Chilton, B.: Psychosexual development in twins. J. Biosoc. Sci. **4**, 277–286 (1972)

Chomsky, N.: On the biological basis of language capacities. In: The neuropsychology of language. Rieber, R.W. (ed.), p. 1–24. New York-London: Plenum Press 1976

Ciocco, A.: The historical background of the modern study of constitution. Bull. Inst. Hist. Med. Johns Hopkins Univ. **4**, 23–38 (1936)

Ciompi, L., Müller, C.: Lebensweg und Alter der Schizophrenen. Berlin, Heidelberg, New York: Springer 1976
Clancy, K., Gove, W.: Sex differences in mental illness: an analysis of response bias in self-reports. Am. J. Sociol. **80**, 205–216 (1974)
Claridge, G., Canter, S., Hume, W.I.: Personality differences and biological variations: a study of twins. Oxford, New York, Toronto: Pergamon Press 1973
Clarke, B.: The causes of biological diversity. Sci. Am. **233**, 50–60 (1975)
Cloninger, C.R., Reich, T., Guze, S.B.: Genetic-enviromental interactions and antisocial behaviour. In: Psychopathic behaviour. Hare, R.D., Schalling, D. (eds.) p. 225–237. Chichester, New York, Brisbane: Wiley 1978
Conrad, K.: Der Konstitutionstypus, 2. Aufl. Berlin, Göttingen, Heidelberg: Springer 1963
Conrad, K.: Konstitution. In: Psychiatrie der Gegenwart. Gruhle, H.W., Jung, R., Mayer-Gross, W., Müller, M. (Hrsg.). Bd. I/1 A, S. 70–151. Berlin, Heidelberg, New York: Springer 1967
Coppen, A.J.: Body build of male homosexuals. In: Advances in psychosomatic medicine. Jores, A., Freyberger, H. (eds.) p. 154–160. New York: Brunner 1961
Count, E.W.: Das Bioprogramm. Frankfurt/M.: S. Fischer 1970
Crisp, A.H., Kalucy, R.S., Lacey, J.H., Harding, B.: The long-term prognosis in anorexia nervosa: some factors predictive of outcome. In: Anorexia nervosa. Vigersky, R.A. (ed.) p. 55–65. New York: Raven Press 1977
Curtius, F.: Konstitution. In: Handbuch der inneren Medizin. Bergmann, G.v., Frey, W., Schwiegk, H. (Hrsg.), 4. Aufl., Bd. VI/1, S. 1–337. Berlin, Göttingen, Heidelberg: Springer 1954
Curtius, F.: Individuum und Krankheit. Berlin, Göttingen, Heidelberg: Springer 1959
D'Andrade, R.G.: Sex differences and cultural institutions. In: The development of sex differences. Maccoby, E.E. (ed.), p. 173–204. Stanford/Cal.: Stanford University Press 1966
Deegener, G.: Beziehungen zwischen Händigkeit, Sprache und funktionaler Hemisphärenasymmetrie. Stuttgart: Enke 1978
Degkwitz, R., Helmchen, H., Kockott, G., Mombour, W. (Hrsg.): Diagnosenschlüssel und Glossar psychiatrischer Krankheiten. Deutsche Ausgabe der internationalen Klassifikation der WHO: ICD (ICD = International Classification of Diseases), 8. Revision, und des internationalen Glossars, 4. Aufl. Berlin, Heidelberg, New York: Springer 1975
Delbrück, H.: Über die körperliche Konstitution bei der genuinen Epilepsie. Arch. Psychiatr. Nervenkr. **77**, 555–572 (1926)
Demisch, K.: Hirsutismus – Diagnostik und Therapie. Dtsch. Arzt **13/14**, 54–63 (1977)
Diebold, K.: Zur Blutgruppenverteilung (AB0, Rh-Faktor, MNS) bei psychischen Störungen. Arch. Psychiatr. Nervenkr. **222**, 257–265 (1976)
Diebold, K., Arnold, E., Pfaff, W.: Statistische Untersuchungen nosologischer Parameter (Geschlechtsverteilung, Diagnostik, Ersterkrankungsalter) bei 120 endogen psychotischen Elter-Kind- und Geschwister-Paaren. Fortschr. Neurol. Psychiatr. **45**, 1–19 (1977)
Dietrich, H.: Analyse sozio-kultureller Faktoren bei depressiven Patientinnen. Confin. Psychiatr. **4**, 110–122 (1961)
Dilling, H., Weyerer, S.: Epidemiologie psychischer Störungen und psychiatrische Versorgung. München, Wien, Baltimore: Urban & Schwarzenberg 1978
Doering, W.: Intelligenz, Verhalten und Persönlichkeit chromatin-positiver Männer. Untersuchung an Hand der Literatur unter besonderer Berücksichtigung des Einflusses überzähliger X-Chromosomen auf die Intelligenz. Med. Diss., München 1971
Doerr, P., Kockott, G., Vogt, H.J., Pirke, K.M., Dittmar, F.: Plasma testosterone, estradiol, and semen analysis in male homosexuals. Arch. Gen. Psychiatry **29**, 829–833 (1973)
Doerr, P., Pirke, K.M., Kockott, G., Dittmar, F.: Further studies on sex hormones in male homosexuals. Arch. Gen. Psychiatry **33**, 611–614 (1976)
Dohrenwend, B.P., Dohrenwend, B.S.: Social status and psychological disorder: A causal inquiry. New York, London, Sydney: Wiley 1969
Dohrenwend, B.P., Dohrenwend, B.S.: Sex differences and psychiatric disorders. Am. J. Sociol. **81**, 1447–1454 (1976)
Draper, G.: The mosaic of androgyny maleness within female and femaleness within male. N. Engl. J. Med. **225**, 393–401 (1941)
Druschky, K.-F.: Die akute intermittierende Porphyrie. Stuttgart: Thieme 1978

Eggers, C.: Course and prognosis of childhood schizophrenia. J. Autism. Child. Schizophr. **8**, 21–36 (1978)

Eggers, H., Wagner, K.-D., Wigger, M.: Bedingungen und Störfaktoren der frühkindlichen Entwicklung. Stuttgart, New York: Fischer 1976

Ehrhardt, A.A., Baker, S.W.: Fetal androgens, human central nervous system differentiation and behaviour sex differences. In: Sex differences in bahaviour. Freedman, R.C., Richart, R.H., Van de Wiele, R.L. (eds.), p. 33–52. New York: Wiley & Sons 1974

Eiband, H.W.: Vergleichende Untersuchungen zur prämorbiden Persönlichkeit von Patienten mit verschiedenen Formen affektiver Störungen. Med. Diss., München 1979

Eibl-Eibesfeldt, I.: Grundriß der vergleichenden Verhaltensforschung, 5. Aufl. München: Piper 1978

Eiff, A.W.v. (Hrsg.): Seelische und körperliche Störungen durch Stress. Stuttgart, New York: Fischer 1976

Ellis, A.: The sexual psychology of human hermaphrodites. Psychosom. Med. **7**, 108–125 (1945)

Elsässer, G.: Körperbauuntersuchungen bei endogen Geisteskranken, sonstigen Anstaltsinsassen und Durchschnittspersonen. Z. menschl. Vererb.- u. Konstit.-Lehre **30**, 307–358 (1951)

Endler, N.S.: The case for person-situation interactions. In: Interactional psychology and personality. Endler, N.S., Magnusson, D. (eds.), p. 58–70. New York, London, Sydney: Wiley 1976

Ernst, K.: Eindämmung der Suchtkrankheiten: Nützen primärpräventive Gesetze? In: Die Psychiatrie-Enquête in internationaler Sicht. Kuhlenkampff, C., Picard, W. (Hrsg.), S. 72–87. Köln: Rheinland-Verlag 1979

Ernst, K., Kind, H., Rotach-Fuchs, M.: Ergebnisse der Verlaufsforschung bei Neurosen. Berlin, Heidelberg, New York: Springer 1968

Esquirol, J.E.D.: Von den Geisteskrankheiten. (Dtsch. Übers. von: Folie. In: Dictionnaire des Sciences Médicales **16**, 1816). Bern, Stuttgart: Huber 1968

Eysenck, H.J.: Fragebogen als Meßmittel der Persönlichkeit. Z. Exp. Angew. Psychol. **1**, 291–335 (1953)

Eysenck, H.J.: The structure of human personality, 3rd. ed. London: Methuen, New York: Macmillan 1970

Eysenck, H.J.: Die Ungleichheit der Menschen. (Dtsch. Übers. von: The inequality of man. London: Maurice Temple Smith 1973). München: List 1975

Eysenck, H.J.: Crime and personality, 3rd ed. London: Routledge & Kegan Paul 1977

Fahrenberg, J.: Psychophysiologische Persönlichkeitsforschung. Göttingen: Hogrefe 1967

Fahrenberg, J.: Physiological concepts in personality research. In: Handbook of modern personality theory. Cattell, R.B., Dreger, R.M. (eds.), p. 585–611. Washington, London: Hemisphere Publishing Corporation and New York, London, Sydney: Wiley 1977

Fenichel, O.: Perversionen, Psychosen, Charakterstörungen. Darmstadt: Wissenschaftliche Buchgesellschaft 1967

Fenichel, O.: Psychoanalytische Neurosenlehre. C. Psychoneurose, Mechanismen der Symptomausbildung und spezielle Neurosen. Olten, Freiburg/Br.: Walter 1975

Feuerlein, W.: Alkoholismus – Mißbrauch und Abhängigkeit. Stuttgart: Thieme 1975

Feuerlein, W., Heyse, H.: Die Weite der 3. Hirnkammer bei Alkoholikern. Arch. Psychiatr. Nervenkr. **213**, 78–85 (1970)

Fleminger, J.J., Dalton, R., Standage, K.F.: Handedness in psychiatric patients. Br. J. Psychiatry **131**, 448–452 (1977)

Ford, C.S., Beach, F.A.: Das Sexualverhalten von Mensch und Tier. (Dtsch. Übers. von: Patterns of sexual behavior. New York: Haper & Brothers 1951). Berlin: Colloquium 1954

Foulds, G.A., in collaboration with Caine, T.M., and with the assistance of Adams, A., Owen, A.: Personality and personal illness. London: Tavistock 1965

Fox, M.W. (ed.): Abnormal behavior in animals. Philadelphia, London, Toronto: Saunders 1968

Freud, S.: Drei Abhandlungen zur Sexualtheorie (1. Aufl. 1905), 4. Aufl. In: Gesammelte Werke, Bd. 5. Frankfurt/M.: Fischer 1968

Frey, R.: Die prämorbide Persönlichkeit von monopolar und bipolar Depressiven. Arch. Psychiatr. Nervenkr. **224**, 161–173 (1977)

Fritsch, W.: Die prämorbide Persönlichkeit der Schizophrenen in der Literatur der letzten hundert Jahre. Fortschr. Neurol. Psychiatr. **44**, 323–372 (1976)

Froesch, E.R., Assal, J.P.: Inselzellapparat, Stoffwechsel und Pathophysiologie des Diabetes mellitus.

In: Klinik der inneren Sekretion. Labhart, A. 3. Aufl., S. 695–731. Berlin, Heidelberg, New York: Springer 1978
Fuhrmann, W., Vogel, F.: Genetische Familienberatung. Berlin, Heidelberg, New York: Springer 1968
Garai, J.E., Scheinfeld, A.: Sex differences in mental and behavioral traits. Genet. Psychol. Monogr. **77**, 169–299 (1968)
Gershon, E.S., Bunney, W.E.: The question of X-linkage in bipolar manic-depressive illness. J. Psychiatr. Res. **13**, 99–117 (1977)
Geschwind, N., Lewitzky, W.: Left-right asymmetries in temporal speech region. Science **161**, 186–187 (1968)
Glatzel, J.: Kritische Anmerkungen zum „Typus melancholicus" Tellenbach. Arch. Psychiatr. Nervenkr. **219**, 197–206 (1974)
Glueck, S., Glueck, E.: Physique and delinquency. New York: Harper 1956
Glueck, S., Glueck, E.: Unraveling juvenile delinquency, 4th ed. Cambridge/Mass.: Harvard Univ. Press 1964
Goldberg, D.: Rehabilitation of the chronically mentally ill in England. Soc. Psychiatr. **2**, 1–13 (1967)
Goldberg, S.C., Schooler, N.R., Davidson, E.M., Kayce, M.M.: Sex and race differences in response to drug treatment among schizophrenics. Psychopharmacologia **9**, 31–47 (1966)
Goodall, J.L. van: The behaviour of free-living chimpanzees in the Gombe Stream reserve. Anim. Behav. Monogr. **1**, 161–311 (1968)
Gove, W.R., Tudor, J.F.: Adult sex roles and mental illness. Am. J. Sociol. **78**, 812–835 (1973)
Guilford, J.P.: Persönlichkeit, 6. Aufl. Weinheim: Beltz 1974
Haase, H.-J.: Depressionen. Entstehung-Erscheinung-Behandlung. Stuttgart, New York: Schattauer 1976
Hagnell, O.: The incidence and duration of episodes of mental illness in a total population. In: Psychiatric epidemiology. Hare, E.H., Wing, J.K. (eds.), p. 213–227. London, New York, Toronto: Oxford Univ. Press 1970
Hallgren, B.: Enuresis. A clinical and genetic study. Acta Psychiatr. Scand., Suppl. **114** ad vol. **32** (1957)
Hambert, G.: Males with positive sex chromatin. Göteborg: Elanders Boktryockeri Aktienbolag 1966
Hammerstein, J., Meckies, J. Leo-Rossberg, I., Moltz, L., Zielske, F.: Use of cyproterone acetate (CPA) in the treatment of acne, hirsutism and virilism. J. Steroid Biochem. **6**, 827–836 (1975)
Hanson, D.R., Gottesman, I.I.: The genetics, if any, of infantile autism and childhood schizophrenia. J. Autism. Child. Schizophr. **6**, 209–234 (1976)
Harbauer, H.: Neuropathie, psychopathische Entwicklung, vegetative Syndrome, Migräne. In: Lehrbuch der speziellen Kinder- und Jugendpsychiatrie, 3. Aufl. Harbauer, H., Lempp, R., Nissen, G., Strunk, P., S. 60–66. Berlin, Heidelberg, New York: Springer 1976a
Harbauer, H.: Oligophrenien und Demenzzustände. In: Lehrbuch der speziellen Kinder- und Jugendpsychiatrie, 3. Aufl. Harbauer, H., Lempp, R., Nissen, G., Strunk, P., S. 226–272. Berlin, Heidelberg, New York: Springer 1976b
Haskell, M.R., Yablonsky, L.: Crime and delinquency, 2nd ed. Chicago: Rand McNally College Pub. 1974
Hassenstein, B.: Kybernetik und biologische Forschung. In: Handbuch der Biologie. Gessner, F. (Hrsg.), Bd. I/2, S. 40–719. Frankfurt/M.: Athenaion 1966
Hays, P.: Electroencephalographic variants and genetic predisposition to schizophrenia. J. Neurol. Neurosurg. Psychiatry **40**, 753–755 (1977)
Heath, R.G.: Schizophrenia: evidence of a pathologic immune mechanism. In: Schizophrenia: Current concepts and research. Sankar, D.V.S. (ed.), p. 580–585. Hicksville/N.Y.: PJD Publications 1969
Helgason, T.: Epidemiology of mental disorders in Iceland. A psychiatric and demographic investigation of 5395 Icelanders. Acta Psychiatr. Scand., Suppl. **173** ad vol. **40** (1964)
Henry, J.P., Stephens, P.M.: Stress, health, and the social enviroment. Berlin, Heidelberg, New York: Springer 1977
Hess, E.H.: Prägung. Die frühkindliche Entwicklung von Verhaltensmustern bei Tier und Mensch. (Dtsch. Übers. von: Early experience and the developmental psychobiology of attachment. New York: Van Nostrand Reinhold Co. 1973). München: Kindler 1975

Heston, L.L., Shields, J.: Homosexuality in twins. A family study and a registry study. Arch. Gen. Psychiatry **18**, 149–160 (1968)
Hildemann, W.H.: Phylogenic and immunogenic aspects of aging. In: Genetic effects on aging. Bergsma, D., Harrison, D.E. (eds.), p. 97–107. New York: Liss 1978
Hoffmann, E., Meiers, H.G., Hubbes, A.: Wirkungen von Antikonzeptiva auf Alopecia androgenetica, Seborrhoea oleosa, Akne vulgaris und Hirsutismus. Dtsch. Med. Wochenschr. **99**, 2151–2157 (1974)
Hofmann, G.: Vergleichende Untersuchungen zur prämorbiden Persönlichkeit von Patienten mit bipolaren (manisch-depressiven) und solchen mit monopolar depressiven Psychosen. Med. Diss., München 1973
Holmes, L.B., Moser, H.W., Halldórsson, S., Mack, C., Pant, S.S., Matzilewich, B.: Mental retardation. An atlas of diseases with associated physical abnormalities. New York: Macmillan, and London: Collier-Macmillan 1972
Huber, G.: Psychiatrie. Stuttgart, New York: Schattauer 1974
Huber, G., Gross, G., Schüttler, R.: Schizophrenie. Berlin, Heidelberg, New York: Springer 1978
Humphrey, J.H., White, R.B.: Kurzes Lehrbuch der Immunologie. Hrsg. von Macher, E. (Dtsch. Übers. von: Immunology for students of medicine. Oxford: Blackwell 1970). Stuttgart: Thieme 1971
Hunger, H., Leopold, D. (Hrsg.): Identifikation. Berlin, Heidelberg, New York: Springer und Leipzig: Barth 1978
Hutt, C.: Biological bases of psychological sex differences. Am. J. Dis. Child. **132**, 170–177 (1978)
Ingalls, R.P.: Mental retardation. New York, Santa Barbara, Chichester: Wiley 1978
Janet, P.: Les obsessions et la psychasthénie. I-II. (1. Aufl. 1903), 2. Aufl. Paris: Felix Alcan 1908
Janz, H.W.: Epidemiologie süchtigen Verhaltens. In: Handbuch der Sozialmedizin. Blohmke, M., v. Ferber, C., Kisker, K.P., Schaefer, H. (Hrsg.), Bd. II, S. 328–374. Stuttgart: Enke 1977
Japanisches Gesundheitsministerium, Abt. f. seelische Gesundheit (Hrsg.): Die seelische Gesundheit unseres Volkes. Tokio 1977
Jaspers, K.: Allgemeine Psychopathologie (1. Aufl. 1913), 9. Aufl. Berlin, Heidelberg, New York: Springer 1973
Jones, K.L., Smith, D.W., Ulleland, C.N., Pythkowicz Streissguth, A.: Patterns of malformation in offspring of chronic alcoholic mothers. Lancet **1973**I, 1266–1271
Judd, L.L., Hubbard, B., Janowsky, D.S., Huey, L.Y., Attewell, P.A.: The effect of lithium carbonate on affect, mood, and personality of normal subjects. Arch. Gen. Psychiatry **34**, 346–351 (1977)
Julian, T., Metcalfe, M., Coppen, A.: Aspects of personality of depressive patients. Br. J. Psychiatry **115**, 587–592 (1963)
Jung, C.G.: Psychologische Typen (1. Aufl. 1921), 12. Aufl. Olten, Freiburg i. Br.: Walter 1976
Jung, R.: Neurophysiologie und Psychiatrie. In: Psychiatrie der Gegenwart. Gruhle, H.W., Jung, R., Mayer-Gross, W., Müller, M. (Hrsg.), Bd. I/1A, S. 325–928. Berlin-Göttingen, Heidelberg: Springer 1967
Kajii, T.: Chromosome anomalies in induced abortions. In: Les accidents chromosomiques de la reproduction. Chromosomal errors in relation to reproductive failure. Boué, A., Thibault, C. (eds.), p. 57–66. Paris: Institut National de la Santé et de la Recherche Médicale 1973
Kanfer, F.H., Phillips, J.S.: Lerntheoretische Grundlagen der Verhaltenstherapie. (Dtsch. Übers. von: Learning foundations of behavior therapy. New York, London, Sydney: Wiley 1970). München: Kindler 1975
Katschnig, H., Grumiller, I., Strobl, R.: Daten zur stationären psychiatrischen Versorgung Österreichs. Teil 1: Inzidenz, Teil 2: Prävalenz. Wien: Österreichisches Bundesinstitut für Gesundheitswesen 1975
Katschnig, H., Steinert, H.: Epidemiologie soziopathischer Handlungen. In: Handbuch der Sozialmedizin. Blohmke, M., v. Ferber, C., Kisker, K.P., Schaefer, H. (Hrsg.), Bd. II, S. 310–328. Stuttgart: Enke 1977
Katschnig, H., Strotzka, H.: Epidemiologie der Neurosen und psychosomatische Störungen. In: Handbuch der Sozialmedizin. Blohmke, M., v. Ferber, C., Kisker, K.P., Schaefer, H. (Hrsg.), Bd. II, S. 272–310. Stuttgart: Enke 1977
Kehrer, H.E. (Hrsg.): Kindlicher Autismus. Basel, München, Paris: Karger 1978

Kidd, K.K., Weissman, M.M.: Why do we not yet understand the genetics of affective disorders. In: Depression. Biology, Psychodynamics, and Treatment. Cole, J.O., Schatzberg, A.F., Frazier, S.H. (eds.), p. 107–121. New York, London: Plenum Press 1978

Kielholz, P.: Diagnose und Therapie der Depressionen für den Praktiker, 3. Aufl. München: Lehmanns 1971

Kimura, B.: Vergleichende Untersuchungen über depressive Erkrankungen in Japan und in Deutschland. Fortschr. Neurol. Psychiatr. **33**, 202–215 (1965)

Kinkelin, M.: Verlauf und Prognose des manisch-depressiven Irreseins. Schweiz. Arch. Neurol. Neurochir. Psychiatr. **73**, 100–146 (1954)

Kirman, B.H.: Clinical aspects. In: Mental retardation and developmental disabilities. Wortis, J. (ed.) vol. VII, p. 1–21. New York: Brunner/Mazel 1975

Klaiber, E.L., Broverman, D.M., Vogel, W., Kobayashi, Y.: The use of steroid hormones in depression. In: Psychotropic action of hormones. Itil, T.M., Laudahn, G., Herrmann, W.M. (eds.), p. 135–154. New York: Spectrum Publications 1976

Knussmann, R.: Entwicklung, Konstitution, Geschlecht. In: Humangenetik. Becker, P.E. (Hrsg.), Bd. I/1, S. 280–437. Stuttgart: Thieme 1968

Koch, G., Neuhäuser, G.: Das Klinefelter-Syndrom und seine Varianten XXY-XXXXY. Bibliographica Genetica Medica **10** (1978)

Koch, R., de la Cruz, F.F. (eds.): Down's syndrome (mongolism): Research, prevention and management. New York: Brunner/Mazel 1975

Kockott, G., Nusselt, L.: Zur Frage der cerebralen Dysfunktion bei der Transsexualität. Nervenarzt **47**, 310–318 (1976)

Kolářský, A., Freund, K., Machek, J., Polák, O.: Male sexual deviation. Association with early temporal lobe damage. Arch. Gen. Psychiatry **17**, 735–743 (1967)

Kolodny, R.C., Masters, W.H., Hendryx, J., Toro, G.: Plasma testosterone and semen analysis in male homosexuals. N. Engl. J. Med. **285**, 1170–1174 (1971)

Kraepelin, E.: Psychiatrie, 8. Aufl., Bd. 1 u. 3/II. Leipzig: Barth 1909 u. 1913

Kramer, M., Taube, C.A.: The role of a national statistics program in the planning of community psychiatric services in the United States. In: Roots of evaluations. Wing, J.K., Häfner, H. (eds.), p. 35–74. London, New York, Toronto: Oxford Univ. Press 1973

Kraus, A.: Der Typus melancholicus in östlicher und westlicher Forschung. Der japanische Beitrag M. Shimodas zur prämorbiden Persönlichkeit Manisch-Depressiver. Nervenarzt **42**, 481–483 (1971)

Krauss, W.: Objektivierende Untersuchungen zur prämorbiden Persönlichkeit von Neurotikern. Med. Diss., München 1972

Kretschmer, E.: Der sensitive Beziehungswahn (1. Aufl. 1918), 4. Aufl. Berlin, Heidelberg, New York: Springer 1966

Kretschmer, E.: Körperbau und Charakter (1. Aufl. 1921), 26. Aufl. von Kretschmer, W. Berlin, Heidelberg, New York: Springer 1977

Kretschmer, W.: Neurose und Konstitution. In: Handbuch der Neurosenlehre und Psychotherapie. Frankl, V.E., Gebsattel, E. v., Schultz, J.H. (Hrsg.), Bd. 2, S. 44–63. München, Berlin: Urban & Schwarzenberg 1959

Kugler, J.: Elektroencephalographie in Klinik und Praxis, 2. Aufl. Stuttgart: Thieme 1966

Lader, M., Kendell, R., Kasriel, J.: The genetic contribution to unwanted drug effects. Clin. Pharmacol. Ther. **16**, 343–347 (1974)

Lader, M., Sartorius, N.: Anxiety in patients with hysterical conversion symptoms. J. Neurol. Neurosurg. Psychiatry **31**, 490–495 (1968)

Lauter, H.: Epidemiologie der großen psychiatrischen Störungen. In: Handbuch der Sozialmedizin. Blohmke, M., v. Ferber, C., Kisker, K.P., Schaefer, H. (Hrsg.), Bd. II, S. 374–447. Stuttgart: Enke 1977

Leff, J.P., Fischer, M., Bertelsen, A.: A cross-national epidemilogical study of mania. Br. J. Psychiatry **129**, 428–437 (1976)

Leighton, A.H., Lambo, T.A., Hughes, C.C., Leighton, D.C., Murphy, J.M., Macklin, D.B.: Psychiatric disorder among the Yoruba. New York: Carnell Univ. Press 1963

Lehr, U.: Körperliche und geistige Aktivität – eine Voraussetzung für ein erfolgreiches Altern. Z. Gerontol. **11**, 290–299 (1978)

Lemoine, P., Haroussseau, H., Borteyru, J.-P., Menuet, J.-C.: Les enfants de parents alcooliques: anomalies observées, à propos de 127 cas. Arch. Franç. Pédiat. **25**, 830–831 (1968)

Lempp, R.: Organische Psychosyndrome. In: Lehrbuch der speziellen Kinder- und Jugendpsychiatrie, 3. Aufl. Harbauer, H., Lempp, R., Nissen, G., Strunk, P., S. 273–332. Berlin, Heidelberg, New York: Springer 1976

Lenneberg, E.H.: Biologische Grundlagen der Sprache. (Dtsch. Übers. von: Biological foundations of language. New York: Wiley 1967). Frankfurt/M.: Suhrkamp 1972

Lenz, W.: Medizinische Genetik, 4. Aufl. Stuttgart: Thieme 1978

Leonhard, K.: Aufteilung der endogenen Psychosen, 4. Aufl. Berlin: Akademie-Verlag 1968

Letterer, E. (Hrsg.): Allgemeine Pathologie. Stuttgart: Thieme 1959

Liepmann, M.C.: Geistig behinderte Kinder und Jugendliche. Bern, Stuttgart, Wien: Huber 1979

Lindegård, B., Nyman, G.E.: Interrelations between psychologic, somatologic, and endocrine dimensions. Lunds Universitets Årsskrift N.F. Avd. 2. Bd. 52, Nr. 9. Lund: Gleerup 1956

Lloyd, B., Archer, J. (eds.): Exploring sex differences. London, New York, San Francisco: Academic Press 1976

Loehlin, J.C., Lindzey, G., Spuhler, J.N.: Race differences in intelligence. San Francisco: Freeman 1975

Lorenz, K.: Die angeborenen Formen möglicher Erfahrung. Z. Tierpsychol. **5**, 235–409 (1943)

Maccoby, E.E., Jacklin, C.N.: The psychology of sex differences. Stanford/Cal.: Stanford Univ. Press and London: Oxford Univ. Press 1975

Majewski, F., Bierich, J.R., Löser, H., Michaelis, R., Leiber, B., Bettecken, F.: Zur Klinik und Pathogenese der Alkohol-Embryopathie. Münch. Med. Wochenschr. **118**, 1635–1642 (1976)

Markert, F.: Zur prämorbiden Persönlichkeitsstruktur endogen Depressiver: Ergebnisse vergleichender Testuntersuchungen durch Selbstbeurteilung nach Psychoseremission. Med. Diss., Frankfurt/M. 1972

Martin, R.: Lehrbuch der Anthropologie, 3. Aufl. von K. Saller. Bd. IV. Stuttgart: Fischer 1966

Matussek, P.: Bedrängnis und Bewältigung im Spiegel des Einzelschicksals. Individuelle Streßreaktion bei ehemaligen KZ-Häftlingen. Klin. Wochenschr. **55**, 869–876 (1977)

Matussek, P., Halbach, A., Troeger, U.: Endogene Depression. München, Berlin: Urban & Schwarzenberg 1965

Mayer-Gross, W., Slater, E., Roth, M. (Hrsg.): Clinical psychiatry, 3rd ed. London: Baillière, Tindall & Cassell 1969

Mayo, R.: Sex differences and psychopathology. In: Exploring sex differences. Lloyd, B., Archer, J. (eds.), p. 213–240. London, New York, San Francisco: Academic Press 1976

Mazer, M.: People in predicament: A study in psychiatric and psychosocial epidemiology. Soc. Psychiatry **9**, 85–90 (1974)

Mendelson, M.: Psychoanalytic concepts of depression, 2nd ed. Flushing/N.Y.: Spectrum Publication 1974

Mendlewicz, J., Fleiss, J.L.: Linkage studies with X-chromosome markers in bipolar (manic-depressive) and unipolar (depressive) illnesses. Biol. Psychiatry **9**, 261–294 (1974)

Mentzos, S.: Mischzustände und mischbildhafte phasische Psychosen. Stuttgart: Enke 1967

Merkel, C.: Prägung bei sexuellen Deviationen. Med. Diss., Kiel 1972

Metcalfe, M.: The personality of depressive patients: 1. Assessment of change. 2. Assessment of the premorbid personality. In: Recent developments in affective disorders. Coppen, A., Walk, A. (eds.), p. 97–104. Spec. Publ. No. 2 of the R.M.P.A. 1968

Metzig, E., Rosenberg, S., Ast, M., Krashen, S.D.: Bipolar manic-depressives and unipolar depressives distinguished by tests of lateral asymmetry. Biol. Psychiatry **11**, 313–322 (1976)

Meyer, A.-E.: Zur Endokrinologie und Psychologie intersexueller Frauen. Stuttgart: Enke 1963

Meyer, A.-E., Zerssen, D. v.: Psychological investigations in women with so-called idiopathic hirsutism. J. Psychosom. Res. **4**, 206–235 (1960)

Milazzo-Sayre, L.: Admission rates to state and county psychiatric hospitals by age, sex, and race, United States, 1975. Statistical Note No. 140. Rockville, Maryland: U.S. Department of Health, Education and Welfare 1977

Mönks, F.J., Knoers, A.M.P., unter Mitarbeit von Staay, F.J. van der: Entwicklungspsychologie. Stuttgart, Berlin, Köln: Kohlhammer 1976

Money, J.: Phylogeny and ontogeny in gender identity differentiation. In: Perspectives in endocrine psychobiology. Brambilla, F., Bridges, P.K., Endröczi, E., Heuser, G. (eds.), p. 467–478. London, New York, Sydney: Wiley 1978

Money, J., Ehrhardt, A.A.: Man and woman, boy and girl. Baltimore, London: Johns Hopkins Univ. Press 1972
Money, J., Hampson, J.G., Hampson, J.L.: An examination of some basic sexual concepts: the evidence of human hermaphroditism. Bull. Johns Hopkins Hosp. **97**, 301–319 (1955)
Moore, K.L.: The developing human, 2nd ed. Philadelphia, London, Toronto: Saunders 1977
Müller, C., unter Mitarbeit von Ciompi, L., Delachaux, A., Rabinowicz, T., Villa, J.L.: Alterspsychiatrie. Stuttgart: Thieme 1967
Murken, J.-D.: The XYY-syndrome and Klinefelter's syndrome. Stuttgart: Thieme 1973
Murphy, D.L., Wright, C., Buchsbaum, M., Nichols, A., Costa, J.L., Wyatt, R.J.: Platelet and plasma amine oxidase activity in 680 normals: sex and age differences and stability over time. Biochem. Med. **16**, 254–265 (1976)
Myrtek, M.: Psychophysiologische Konstitutionsforschung. Ein Beitrag zur Psychosomatik. Philos. Habil., Freiburg 1978
Nay, L.B.: Future perspectives in aging and dementia. In: Aging and dementia. Smith, W.L., Kinsbourne, M. (eds.), p. 203–215. New York: Spectrum Publications 1977
Netter, P.: Metrische Studien zur psychophysischen Geschlechtskonstitution. Med. Diss., Hamburg 1970
Neumann, F.: Hormonale Regulation der Sexualdifferenzierung bei Säugetieren. Vorlesungsreihe Schering, H. 3. Berlin, Bergkamen: Schering AG 1977
Nielsen, J.: Chromosomes in senile dementia. In: Senile dementia. Müller, C., Ciompi, L. (eds.), p. 59–62. Bern, Stuttgart: Huber 1968
Nielsen, J.: Klinefelter's syndrome and the XYY syndrome. Acta Psychiatr. Scand., Suppl. **209**, ad vol. **45** (1969)
Nielsen, J.: Chromosome examination of male patients in a psychiatric hospital. Br. J. Psychiatry **127**, 404–409 (1975)
Nissen, G.: Psychische Entwicklung und ihre Störungen. In: Lehrbuch der speziellen Kinder- und Jugendpsychiatrie, 3. Aufl. Harbauer, H., Lempp, R., Nissen, G., Strunk, P., S. 12–38. Berlin, Heidelberg, New York: Springer 1976a
Nissen, G.: Dissozialität und Verwahrlosung. In: Lehrbuch der speziellen Kinder- und Jugendpsychiatrie, 3. Aufl. Harbauer, H., Lempp, R., Nissen, G., Strunk, P., S. 82–94. Berlin, Heidelberg, New York: Springer 1976b
Nissen, G.: Psychogene Störungen mit vorwiegend psychischer Symptomatik. In: Lehrbuch der speziellen Kinder- und Jugendpsychiatrie, 3. Aufl. Harbauer, H., Lempp, R., Nissen, G., Strunk, P., S. 95–121. Berlin, Heidelberg, New York: Springer 1976c
Nissen, G.: Autistische Syndrome. In: Lehrbuch der speziellen Kinder- und Jugendpsychiatrie, 3. Aufl. Harbauer, H., Lempp, R., Nissen, G., Strunk, P., S. 380–392. Berlin, Heidelberg, New York: Springer 1976d
Nowakowski, H., Zerssen, D. v., Bergman, S., Reitalu, J.: Mosaikstruktur bei Patienten mit echtem Klinefelter-Syndrom und deren Relation zum Intelligenzdefekt. 12. Symposion der Deutschen Gesellschaft für Endokrinologie, S. 300–303. Berlin, Heidelberg, New York: Springer 1967
Nusselt, L., Kockott, G.: EEG-Befunde bei Transsexualität – ein Beitrag zur Pathogenese. Z. EEG-EMG **7**, 42–48 (1976)
Omenn, G.S.: Inborn errors of metabolism: Clues to understanding human behavioral disorders. Behav. Genet. **6**, 263–284 (1976)
Omenn, G.S., Motulsky, A.G.: Psychopharmacogenetics. In: Human behavior genetics. Kaplan, A.R. (ed.), p. 363–384. Springfield/Ill.: Thomas 1976
Orley, J., Wing, J.K.: Psychiatric disorders in two African villages. Arch. Gen. Psychiatry **36**, 513–520 (1979)
Ounsted, C., Taylor, D.C. (eds.): Gender differences: their ontogeny and significance. Edinburgh, London: Livingstone 1972
Overzier, C. (Hrsg.): Die Intersexualität. Stuttgart: Thieme 1961a
Overzier, C.: Hermaphroditismus verus. In: Die Intersexualität. Overzier, C. (Hrsg.), S. 188–240. Stuttgart: Thieme 1961b
Pal, S.B.: Hormonspiegel lesbischer Frauen. Sexualmedizin **7**, 386–387 (1978)
Parnell, R.W.: Behaviour and physique. London: Arnold 1958
Paterson, D.G.: Physique and intellect. Westport/C.T.: Greenwood Reprint of 1930
Pawlik, K.: Dimensionen des Verhaltens. Bern, Stuttgart: Huber 1968

Paykel, E.S., Klerman, G.L., Prusoff, B.A.: Personality and symptom pattern in depression. Br. J. Psychiatry **129**, 327–334 (1976)
Pelz, L., Mieler, W.: Klinische Zytogenetik. Stuttgart: Fischer 1972
Perris, C.: A study of bipolar (manic-depressive) and unipolar recurrent depressive psychoses. Acta Psychiat. Scand., Suppl. **194** ad vol. **42**, 68–82 (1966)
Perris, C.: A study of cycloid psychoses. Acta Psychiat. Scand., Suppl. **253**, 29–34 (1974)
Perris, C.: Frequency and hereditary aspects of depression. In: Depression: behavioral, biochemical, diagnostic and treatment concepts. Gallant, D.M., Simpson, G.M. (eds.), p. 75–107. New York: Spectrum Publications 1976
Perris, H., Strandman, E.: Psychogenic needs in depression. Arch. Psychiatr. Nervenkr. **227**, 97–107 (1979)
Pfanzagl, J.: Allgemeine Methodenlehre der Statistik. Bd. II, 4. Aufl. Berlin, New York: de Gruyter 1974
Pflanz, M.: Allgemeine Epidemiologie. Stuttgart: Thieme 1973
Platt, D.: Biologie des Alterns. Heidelberg: Quelle & Meyer 1976
Ploog, D.: Verhaltensforschung und Psychiatrie. In: Psychiatrie der Gegenwart. Gruhle, H.W., Jung, R., Mayer-Gross, W., Müller, M. (Hrsg.), Bd. I/1B, S. 291–443. Berlin, Göttingen, Heidelberg: Springer 1964
Polednak, A.P.: Body build of paranoid and non-paranoid schizophrenic males. Br. J. Psychiatry **119**, 191–192 (1971)
Pollitt, J.: Sex difference and the mind. Proc. Roy. Soc. Med. **70**, 145–148 (1977)
Prader, A.: Störungen der Geschlechtsdifferenzierung (Intersexualität). In: Labhart, A.: Klinik der inneren Sekretion, 3. Aufl., S. 654–688. Berlin, Heidelberg, New York: Springer 1978
Rafaelsen, O.J., Kramp, P.L., Shapiro, R.W.: HLA- and AB0-antigens in manic-melancholic disorders. In: Origin, prevention and treatment of affective disorders. Schou, M., Strömgren, E. (eds.), p. 155–161. London: Academic Press 1979
Rees, L.: Constitutional factors and abnormal behaviour. In: Handbook of abnormal psychology, 2nd ed. Eysenck, H.J. (ed.), p. 487–539. London: Pitman 1973
Reiss, E.: Konstitutionelle Verstimmung und manisch-depressives Irresein. Klinische Untersuchungen über den Zusammenhang von Veranlagung und Psychose. Z. ges. Neurol. Psychiat. **2**, 347–628 (1910)
Reitalu, J.: Chromosome studies in connection with sex chromosomal deviations in man. Hereditas **59**, 1–48 (1968)
Riegel, K.F.: Ergebnisse und Probleme der psychologischen Alternsforschung. In: Altern. Thomae, H., Lehr, U. (Hrsg.), S. 142–170. Frankfurt/M.: Akademische Verlagsgesellschaft 1968
Ries, W.: Fettsucht. Leipzig: Barth 1970
Robins, E.: Antisocial and dyssocial personality disorders. In: Comprehensive textbook of psychiatry. Freedman, A.M., Kaplan, H.I. (eds.), p. 951–958. Baltimore: Williams & Wilkins 1967
Robins, L.N.: Deviant children grown up. Baltimore: Williams & Wilkins 1966
Rohden, F. v.: Körperbauuntersuchungen an geisteskranken und gesunden Verbrechern. Arch. Psychiatr. Nervenkr. **77**, 151–163 (1926)
Rosenblatt, P.C., Cunningham, M.R.: Sex differences in cross-cultural perspectives. In: Exploring sex differences. Lloyd, B., Archer, J. (eds.), p. 71–94. London, New York, San Francisco: Academic Press 1976
Rosenthal, D. (ed.): The Genain quadruplets. New York, London: Basic Books 1963
Rutter, M.: Sex differences in children's responses to family stress. In: The child and his family. Anthony, E.J., Koupernik, C. (eds.), p. 165–196. New York, London, Sydney: Wiley 1970
Sandberg, S.: Psychiatric disorder in children with birth anomalies. A retrospective follow-up study. Acta Psychiatr. Scand. **54**, 1–16 (1976)
Sarason, I.G., Smith, R.E., Diener, E.: Personality research: Components of variance attributable to the person and the situation. J. Personal. Soc. Psychol. **32**, 199–204 (1975)
Schalling, D.: Psychopathy-related personality variables and the psychophysiology of socialization. In: Psychopathic behaviour. Hare, R.D., Schalling, D. (eds.), p. 85–106. Chichester, New York, Brisbane: Wiley 1978
Schenk-Danzinger, L.: Legasthenie. In: Handbuch der Psychologie. Gottschaldt, K., Lersch, P., Sander, F., Thomae, H. (Hrsg.). Bd. 8: Klinische Psychologie, 2. Halbbd. Pongratz, L.J. (Hrsg.), S. 2591–2625. Göttingen, Toronto, Zürich: Hogrefe 1978
Schlegel, W.S.: Körper und Seele. Stuttgart: Enke 1957

Schott, A.: Beitrag zur Lehre von der Melancholie. Arch. Psychiatr. Nervenkr. **36**, 819–862 (1903)
Schulte, W., Tölle, R.: Psychiatrie, 4. Aufl. Berlin, Heidelberg, New York: Springer 1977
Schwab, J.J., Schwab, M.E.: Sociocultural roots of mental illness. New York, London: Plenum Medical Book 1978
Schwidetzky, I.: Neuere Entwicklungen in der Rassenkunde des Menschen. In: Die neue Rassenkunde. Schwidetzky, I. (Hrsg.), S. 15–134. Stuttgart: Fischer 1962
Schwidetzky, I.: Konstitution. Rasse. Wachstum. In: Das Fischer Lexikon. Anthropologie, 3. Aufl. Heberer, G., Schwidetzky, I., Walter, H. (Hrsg.), S. 89–107, 187–215, 282–299. Frankfurt/M.: Fischer 1970
Schwidetzky, I.: Hauptprobleme der Anthropologie. Freiburg: Rombach 1971
Scott, J.P.: Critical periods in behavior developement. Science **138**, 949–957 (1962)
Seltzer, C.C.: A comparative study of the morphological characteristics of delinquents and nondelinquents. In: Unraveling juvenile delinquency. Glueck, S., Glueck, E. (eds.), p. 307–350. Cambridge/Mass.: Harvard Univ. Press 1964
Shapiro, A.K., Shapiro, E.S., Bruun, R.D., Sweet, R.D.: Gilles de la Tourette syndrome. New York: Raven Press 1978
Sheldon, W.H., with the collaboration of Hartl, E.M., McDermott, E.: Varieties of delinquent youth. New York: Harper 1949
Shepherd, M., Cooper, B., Brown, A.C., Kalton, G.: Psychiatric illness in general practice. London, New York, Toronto: Oxford Univ. Press 1966
Silverman, C.: The epidemiology of depression. Baltimore: Johns Hopkins Press 1968
Singer, K., Chang, P.T., Hsu, G.L.K.: Physique, personality and mental illness in the Southern Chinese. Br. J. Psychiatry **121**, 315–319 (1972)
Slater, E., Slater, P.: A heuristic theory of neurosis. In: Man, mind and heredity. Shields, J., Gottesman, I.I. (eds.), p. 216–227. Baltimore, London: Johns Hopkins Press 1971. Originally published in: J. Neurol. Psychiatry **7**, 49–55 (1944)
Solms, H.: Die Ausbreitung des Alkoholkonsums und des Alkoholismus. In: Sucht und Mißbrauch. Steinbrecher, W., Solms, H. (Hrsg.), 2. Aufl., S. III/3–III/41. Stuttgart: Thieme 1975
Sovner, R., DiMascio, A.: Extrapyramidal syndromes and other neurological side effects of psychotropic drugs. In: Psychopharmacology. Lipton, M.A., DiMascio, A., Killam, K.F. (eds.), p. 1021–1032. New York: Raven Press 1978
Stabenau, J.R., Pollin, W.: The pathogenesis of schizophrenia: II. Contributions from the NIMH study of 16 pairs of monozygotic twins discordant for schizophrenia. In: Schizophrenia: current concepts and research. Sankar, D.V.S. (ed.), p. 336–351. Hicksville/N.Y.: PJD Publications 1969
Steinbrecher, W.: Die klinischen Gesamtsyndrome bei Mißbrauch und Sucht unter besonderer Berücksichtigung intern-neurologischer Befunde. In: Sucht und Mißbrauch. Steinbrecher, W., Solms, H. (Hrsg.), 2. Aufl., S. IV/29–IV/133. Stuttgart: Thieme 1975
Steinhausen, H.-C., Wefers, D.: Körperbehinderte Kinder und Jugendliche. Weinheim, Basel: Beltz 1977
Stengel, E.: Selbstmord und Selbstmordversuch. (Dtsch. Übers. von: Suicide and attempted suicide. Harmondsworth: Penguin Books 1964). Frankfurt/M.: Fischer 1969
Strandman, E.: „Psychogenic needs" in patients with affective disorders. Acta Psychiatr. Scand. **58**, 16–29 (1978)
Strömgren, E.: Verlauf der Schizophrenien. In: Verlauf und Ausgang schizophrener Erkrankungen. Huber, H. (Hrsg.), S. 121–132. Stuttgart, New York: Schattauer 1973
Strunk, P.: Psychogene Störungen mit vorwiegend körperlicher Symptomatik. In: Lehrbuch der speziellen Kinder- und Jugendpsychiatrie. Harbauer, H., Lempp, R., Nissen, G., Strunk, P., 3. Aufl., S. 122–173. Berlin, Heidelberg, New York: Springer 1976
Sullivan, J., Stanfield, C.N., Dackis, C.: Platelet MAO activity in schizophrenia and other psychiatric illnesses. Am. J. Psychiatry **134**, 1098–1103 (1977)
Swerdloff, R.S., Rubin, T.: Psychological and endocrinological changes in puberty. In: Perspectives in endocrine psychobiology. Brambilla, F., Bridges, P.K., Endröczi, E., Heuser, G. (eds.), p. 287–308. London, New York, Sydney: Wiley 1978
Szabó, Z.: Vererbungswissenschaftliche Bestimmungen des Konstitutionsbegriffs. Z. Konstit.-Lehre **21**, 286–288 (1938)
Tandler, J.: Konstitution und Rassenhygiene. Z. angew. Anat. u. Konstit.-Lehre **1**, 11–26 (1914)

Tanner, J.M.: Wachstum und Reifung des Menschen. (Dtsch. Übers. von: Growth at adolescence. Oxford: Blackwell 1955). Stuttgart: Thieme 1962
Tanner, J.M.: Human growth and constitution. In: Human biology, 2nd. ed. Harrison, G.A., Weiner, J.S., Tanner, J.M., Barnicot, N.A. (eds.), p. 299–385. Oxford: Oxford Univ. Press 1977
Taschev, T.: Statistisches über die Melancholie. Fortschr. Neurol. Psychiatry **33**, 25–36 (1965)
Tavris, C., Offir, C.: The longest war. Sex differences in perspectives. New York, Chicago, San Francisco: Harcourt Brace Jovanovich 1977
Tellenbach, H.: Zur Freilegung des melancholischen Typus im Rahmen einer kinetischen Typologie. In: Das depressive Syndrom. Hippius, H., Selbach, H. (Hrsg.), S. 173–181. München, Berlin, Wien: Urban & Schwarzenberg 1969
Tellenbach, H.: Melancholie, 3. Aufl. Berlin, Heidelberg, New York: Springer 1976
Tellenbach, R.: Typologische Untersuchungen zur prämorbiden Persönlichkeit von Psychotikern unter besonderer Berücksichtigung Manisch-Depressiver. Confin. Psychiatr. **18**, 1–15 (1975)
Terman, L.M., Miles, C.C.: Sex and personality (1st print 1936). New York: Russell 1968
Theile, U.: Epidemiologie des Diabetes mellitus. In: Handbuch der Sozialmedizin. Blohmke, M., v. Ferber, C., Kisker, K.P., Schaefer, H. (Hrsg.), Bd. II, S. 146–154. Stuttgart: Enke 1977
Thomae, H.: Entwicklung und Prägung. In: Handbuch der Psychologie. Lersch, P., Sander, F., Thomae, H., Wilde, K. (Hrsg.), Bd. 3: Entwicklungspsychologie. Thomae, H. (Hrsg.), 2. Aufl., S. 240–311. Göttingen: Hogrefe 1959
Thomä, H.: Anorexia nervosa. Bern: Huber und Stuttgart: Klett 1961
Thomas, A., Chess, S.: Temperament and development. New York: Brunner/Mazel 1977
Thompson, W.R.: Development and the biophysical bases of personality. In: Handbook of personality theory and research. Borgatta, E.F., Lamberg, W.W. (eds.), p. 149–214. Chicago: Rand McNally 1968
Tienari, P.: Schizophrenia in monozygotic male twins. In: The transmission of schizophrenia. Rosenthal, D., Kety, S.S. (eds.), p. 27–36. Oxford, London, Edinburgh: Pergamon Press 1968
Timiras, P.E.: Estrogens as ‚organizers' of CNS function. In: Influences of hormones on the nervous system. Ford, D.H. (ed.), p. 242–254. Basel, München, Paris: Karger 1971
Tölle, R.: Katamnestische Untersuchungen zur Biographie abnormer Persönlichkeiten. Berlin, Heidelberg, New York: Springer 1966
Tucker, W.B., Lessa, W.A.: Man: a constitutional investigation. Quart. Rev. Biol. **15**, 265–289 und 411–455 (1940)
Uchtenhagen, A.: Psychische Störungen bei Frauen. Schweiz. Arch. Neurol. Neurochir. Psychiatr. **117**, 55–64 (1975)
Uexküll, J.v.: Bedeutungslehre (1. Aufl. 1921). Hamburg: Rowohlts Deutsche Enzyklopädie 1956
Undeutsch, U.: Das Verhältnis von körperlicher und seelischer Entwicklung. In: Handbuch der Psychologie. Lersch, P., Sander, F., Thomae, H., Wilde, K. (Hrsg.), Bd. 3: Entwicklungspsychologie. Thomae, H. (Hrsg.), 2. Aufl., S. 329–357. Göttingen: Hogrefe 1959
Vartanian, M.E., Kolyaskina, G.I., Lozovsky, D.V., Burbaeva, G.S., Ignatov, S.A.: Aspects of humoral and cellular immunity in schizophrenia. In: Birth defects: Original article series. Vol. XIV/5. Lerner, R.A., Bergsma, D. (eds.), p. 339–364. New York: Liss 1978
Verbrugge, L.M.: Sex differentials in morbidity and mortality in the United States. Soc. Biol. **23**, 275–296 (1976)
Verghese, A.: Relationship between body build and mental illness. Br. J. Psychiatry **132**, 12–15 (1978)
Verschuer, O. v.: Wirksame Faktoren im Leben der Menschen. Wiesbaden: Steiner 1954
Vessey, M.P.: Gender differences in the epidemiology of non-neurological disease. In: Gender differences: Their ontogeny and significance. Ounsted, C., Taylor, D.C. (eds.), p. 203–213. Edinburgh, London: Churchill Livingstone 1972
Videbech, T.: A study of genetic factors, childhood bereavement, and premorbid personality traits in patients with anancastic endogenous depression. Acta Psychiatr. Scand. **52**, 178–222 (1975)
Vigersky, R.A. (ed.): Anorexia nervosa. New York: Raven Press 1977
Vogl, G.: Studienfach und psychische Störungen bei Studenten. Med. Diss., München 1976
Walford, R.L.: Immunological theory of aging: current status. Fed. Proc. **33**, 2020–2027 (1974)
Walinder, J.: Hyperostosis frontalis interna and mental morbidity. Br. J. Psychiatry **131**, 155–159 (1977)

Walter, H.: Sexual- und Entwicklungsbiologie des Menschen. Stuttgart: Thieme 1978
Warheit, G.J., Holzer, C.E., Schwab, J.J.: An analysis of social class and racial differences in depressive symptomatology: a community study. J. Health Soc. Behav. **14**, 291–299 (1973)
Weeke, A., Bille, M., Videbech, T., Dupont, A., Juel-Nielsen, N.: Incidence of depressive syndromes in a Danish county. Acta Psychiatr. Scand. **51**, 28–41 (1975)
Weinschenk, C.: Rechenstörungen, 2. Aufl. Bern, Stuttgart, Wien: Huber 1975
Wever, R.A.: The circadian system of man. New York, Heidelberg, Berlin: Springer 1979
Wheeler, L.R.: A comparitive study of physical growth of dull children. J. Educ. Res. **20**, 273–282 (1929)
Wiedemann, H.-R., Grosse, F.-R., Dibbern, H.: Das charakteristische Syndrom. Blickdiagnose von Syndromen. Stuttgart, New York: Schattauer 1976
Wilson, J.D.: Sexual differentiation. Ann. Rev. Physiol. **40**, 279–306 (1978)
Winokur, G.: Delusional disorders (paranoia). Compr. Psychiatry **18**, 511–521 (1977)
Winokur, G., Crowe, R.R.: Personality disorders. In: Comprehensive textbook of psychiatry, 2nd ed. Freedman, A.M., Kaplan, H.I., Sadock, B.J. (eds.), vol. II, pp. 1279–1297. Baltimore: Williams & Wilkins 1975
Winter, E.: Über die Häufigkeit neurotischer Symptome bei „Gesunden". Z. Psychosom. Med. **5**, 153–167 (1958–59)
Witkin, H.A., Mednick, S.A., Schulsiner, F., Bakkestrøm, E., Christiansen, K.O., Goodenough, D.R., Hirschhorn, K., Lundsteen, C., Owen, D.R., Philip, J., Rubin, D.B., Stocking, M.: Criminality in XYY and XXY men. Science **193**, 547–555 (1976)
Wolff, P.H.: Ethnic differences in alcohol sensitivity. Science **175**, 448–451 (1972)
Woodruff, R.A. jr., Robins, L.N., Winokur, G., Reich, T.: Manic depressive illness and social achievement. Acta Psychiatr. Scand. **47**, 237–249 (1971)
Zellweger, H., Simpson, J.: Chromosomes of man. London: Heinemann Medical Books and Philadelphia: Lippincott 1977
Zerssen, D.v.: Biometrische Studien über „Körperbau und Charakter". Fortschr. Neurol. Psychiatr. **33**, 455–471 (1965a)
Zerssen, D.v.: Eine biometrische Überprüfung der Theorien von Sheldon über Zusammenhänge zwischen Körperbau und Temperament. Z. Exp. Angew. Psychol. **12**, 521–548 (1965b)
Zerssen, D.v.: Körperbau, Psychose und Persönlichkeit. Nervenarzt **37**, 52–59 (1966a)
Zerssen, D.v.: Körperbau, Persönlichkeit und seelisches Kranksein. Med. Habil., Heidelberg 1966b
Zerssen, D.v.: Habitus und Geschlecht. Homo **19**, 1–27 (1968)
Zerssen, D.v.: Methoden und Ergebnisse der biometrischen Konstitutionsforschung. In: Verhaltensforschung im Rahmen der Wissenschaften vom Menschen. Keiter, F. (Hrsg.), S. 44–55 und 233–235. Göttingen: Musterschmidt 1969a
Zerssen, D.v.: Comparative studies in the psychomorphological constitution of schizophrenics and other groups. In: Schizophrenia: Current concepts and research. Sankar, D.V.S. (ed.), p. 913–925. Hicksville/N.Y.: PJD Publications 1969b
Zerssen, D.v., unter Mitarbeit von Koeller, D.-M., Rey, E.-R.: Objektivierende Untersuchungen zur prämorbiden Persönlichkeit endogen Depressiver. In: Das depressive Syndrom. Hippius, H., Selbach, H. (Hrsg.), S. 183–205. München, Berlin, Wien: Urban & Schwarzenberg 1969c
Zerssen, D.v.: Methoden der Konstitutions- und Typenforschung. In: Enzyklopädie der geisteswissenschaftlichen Arbeitsmethoden. 9. Lfg.: Methoden der Anthropologie. Thiel, M. (Hrsg.), S. 35–143. München, Wien: Oldenbourg 1973a
Zerssen, D.v.: Konstitution. Konstitutionstypen. Typus. Vitalität. In: Lexikon der Psychiatrie. Müller, C. (Hrsg.), S. 307–310, 310–313, 540–542 u. 560–562. Berlin, Heidelberg, New York: Springer 1973b
Zerssen, D.v.: Physique and personality. In: Human behavior genetics. Kaplan, A.R. (ed.), p. 230–278. Springfield/Ill.: Thomas 1976a
Zerssen, D.v.: Der „Typus melancholicus" in psychometrischer Sicht. Z. Klin. Psychol. Psychother. **24**, 200–220 u. 305–316 (1976b)
Zerssen, D.v.: Premorbid personality and affective psychoses. In: Handbook of studies on depression. Burrows, G.D. (ed.), p. 79–103. Amsterdam, London, New York: Excerpta Medica 1977a
Zerssen, D.v.: Konstitutionstypologische Forschung. In: Die Psychologie des 20. Jahrhunderts. Strube, G. (Hrsg.), Bd. 5, S. 545–616. Zürich: Kindler 1977b
Zerssen, D.v., Fliege, K., Wolf, M.: Cerebral atrophy in drug addicts. Lancet **1970 I**, 313

Zerssen, D.v., Koeller, D.-M., Rey, E.-R.: Die prämorbide Persönlichkeit von endogen Depressiven. Eine Kreuzvalidierung früherer Untersuchungsergebnisse. Confin. Psychiatr. **13**, 156–179 (1970)

Zerssen, D.v., Meyer, A.-E., Ahrens, D.: Klinische, biochemische und psychologische Untersuchungen an Patientinnen mit gewöhnlichem Hirsutismus. Dtsch. Arch. Klin. Med. **206**, 334–360 (1960)

Züblin, W.: Chromosomale Aberrationen und Psyche. Basel, New York: Karger 1969

Auswahl wichtiger Neuerscheinungen zum Thema, die bei der Abfassung des Manuskripts nicht mehr berücksichtigt werden konnten:

Gomberg, E.S., Franks, V. (eds.): Gender and disordered behavior: Sex differences in psychopathology. New York: Brunner/Mazel 1979

Katzman, R. (ed.): Congenital and acquired cognitive disorders. New York: Raven Press 1979

Keller, H. (Hrsg.): Geschlechtsunterschiede. Psychologische und physiologische Grundlagen der Geschlechterdifferenzierung. Weinheim, Basel: Beltz 1979

Lenz, W.: Humangenetik in Psychologie und Psychiatrie. Heidelberg: Quelle und Meyer 1978

Lorenz, K.: Vergleichende Verhaltensforschung. Berlin, Heidelberg, New York: Springer 1978

Merz, F.: Lehrbuch der Differentiellen Psychologie, Bd. 3: Geschlechterunterschiede und ihre Entwicklung. Göttingen, Toronto, Zürich: Hogrefe 1979

Ohno, S.: Major sex-determining genes. Berlin, Heidelberg, New York: Springer 1979

Osborne, R.T., Noble, C.E., Weyl, N. (eds.): Human variation. New York: Academic Press 1978

Reid, W.H. (ed.): The psychopath: A comprehensive study of antisocial disorders and behaviors. New York: Brunner/Mazel 1978

Rubenstein, M., Burks, J.B.: Styles in interaction: Temperament in adult behavior. New York: Brunner/Mazel 1979

Rutter, M., Schopler, E.: Autism. New York: Plenum Press 1978

Schreiber, K. (Hrsg.): Die angeborenen Stoffwechselanomalien, 2. Aufl. Stuttgart: Thieme 1978

Willerman, L.: The psychology of individual and group differences. Reading (England): Freeman 1979

Deprivationsforschung und Psychiatrie

Von

P. Kempe und J. Gross

Inhalt

A. Einleitung 707
B. Deprivation im Kindesalter 709
   I. Geschichtliche Aspekte 709
   II. Methodische Aspekte 718
      1. Schwierigkeiten der Bedingungs- und Subjekt-Variablen-Kontrolle 718
      2. Die kindliche Entwicklung in der Interaktion mit seiner dinglichen wie menschlichen Umgebung 720
      3. Möglichkeiten und Probleme der Erfassung von Auswirkungen der Deprivation im Kindesalter mit unterschiedlichen Forschungsstrategien 722
   III. Auswirkungen der Deprivation im Kindesalter 726
      1. Einflüsse früher Trennung auf die Mutter-Kind-Beziehung 726
      2. Einflüsse früher Trennung auf die Vater-Kind-Beziehung 727
      3. Einflüsse auf das Kind 728
C. Experimentelle Deprivationsforschung an Erwachsenen 734
   I. Geschichtliche Aspekte 734
   II. Wirkungen der sensorischen und perzeptiven Deprivation auf erwachsene Versuchspersonen 735
   III. Klinische Anwendungsmöglichkeiten der Deprivation 738
      1. Diagnostischer Bereich 738
      2. Therapeutischer Bereich 740
D. Theorien zur Erklärung der Deprivationswirkungen 742
Literatur 745

A. Einleitung

Innerhalb einer Vielzahl von leider oft mit variierender Bedeutung gebrauchten Termini nimmt der aus dem angelsächsischen Sprachbereich stammende Begriff *Deprivation* eine zentrale Stellung ein. Er ist etwa mit Entbehrung, Mangel, Verlust synonym. Deprivation als Terminus höheren Allgemeinheitsgrades bezeichnet den *Zustand* von Individuen, der aus einer fortgesetzten Vorenthaltung hinreichender Befriedigung ihrer grundlegenden psychophysischen Bedürfnisse entsteht. Im engeren Sinne kann zwischen Privation und Deprivation unterschieden werden. Werden Kinder von Geburt an, bzw. vor der Ausbildung überdauernder Objektbeziehungen, von ihrer familiären Umgebung getrennt, so spricht man von *Privation*. Sie ist mit einem *Fehlen* adäquater Entwicklungsanreize von Beginn an gleichzusetzen. *Deprivation* entspricht dagegen einem *Verlust* solcher Bedingungen; dieser Begriff schließt also das subjektive Erlebsnis der Trennung bzw. der Entbehrung mit ein.

Menschen mit angeborener Blindheit z.B. sind gemäß der Definition einer Privation ausgesetzt, während später Erblindende eine Deprivation erleiden. Von maternaler Deprivation kann erst ab einem Alter von ca. 6 Monaten gesprochen werden. Erst dann nämlich hat das Kind stabile Objektrepräsentanzen entwickelt und kann klar zwischen der Mutter bzw. Ersatzmutter und anderen ihm fremden Personen unterscheiden (GERWITZ, 1961). Die Modalitäten solcher Trennungen lassen sich danach kategorisieren, ob es allein zu einer Trennung von der oder den Bezugsperson(en), zu einem Wechsel der gewohnten Umgebung allein oder aber zu Deprivationsbedingungen kommt, bei denen der Bezug der Kinder zu beiden Aspekten ihrer Umwelt mehr oder weniger vollständig unterbrochen wird.

Deprivation muß sowohl als *situations-* als auch wesentlich *individualspezifisch* determiniert angesehen werden. Sie ist das Resultat der jeweiligen Auseinandersetzung des Individuums mit den spezifischen, einschränkenden Umgebungsbedingungen, die mit der Befriedigung seiner Bedürfnisse unvereinbar sind, wobei auch die vorangehenden Stimulationsbedingungen berücksichtigt werden müssen.

Deprivation bedarf – wie sich aufgrund der bisherigen Forschungsresultate gezeigt hat – einer weiteren Spezifizierung, die idealerweise sowohl das *Ausmaß* als auch die *Art* der *Deprivationsbedingungen* kennzeichnet. Letzteres sollte nach unserer Ansicht durch Voranstellung von Adjektiven (z.B. ,,perzeptive Deprivation", ,,taktile Deprivation", ,,soziale Deprivation") erfolgen; komplexe Deprivationsbedingungen, die in den meisten Fällen vorliegen dürften, sollten durch Kennzeichnung ihrer verschiedenen Komponenten bestimmt werden. Darüber hinausgehende begriffliche Spezifizierungen sind sicher schwer praktikabel, doch sollte man sich im klaren darüber sein, daß die jeweilige Deprivation erst nach Bestimmung einer Reihe von Subjekt-Variablen hinreichend beschrieben ist. Angemerkt sei, daß in der Literatur der Begriff ,,Isolation" bzw. ,,Soziale Isolation" relativ verbreitet ist. Wir würden diese Termini gern durch ,,soziale Deprivation" ersetzt wissen.

Betrachtet man Untersuchungen zur *Deprivation im Kindesalter* und solche der *experimentellen Deprivation an Erwachsenen* von einem formalen Standpunkt aus, so fällt bei den ersteren die große Schwierigkeit der Bestimmung sowohl der Bedingungs- als auch der Subjekt-Variablen unmittelbar auf. Bei der letzteren dagegen liegt der Schwerpunkt der Spezifikation meist zu einseitig auf einer genauen Beschreibung der Deprivationsbedingungen, etwa der physikalischen Eigenschaften der Versuchsräume, der Meßbedingungen etc. Angesichts der großen, in den meisten Untersuchungen unaufgeklärt bleibenden interindividuellen Unterschiede ist es erstaunlich, wie wenig im letztgenannten Forschungsbereich bisher mit vorselegierten Versuchspersonengruppen experimentiert wurde.

Die Definition der *Deprivation als Zustand* ist vorteilhaft, weil sie u.E. den Blick in heilsamer Weise auf das Wesentliche lenkt: auf die erst aus der komplexen Wechselbeziehung zwischen dem Individuum mit seiner konstitutionellen wie erfahrungsbedingten Ausstattung und den spezifischen, einschränkenden Bedingungen resultierende und nur so erfaßbare Deprivationswirkung. Wir messen der Betonung eines solchen, auf die komplexe Wechselbeziehung ausgerichteten Konstruktes sowohl einen manche Vorstellungen korrigierenden, wie auch einen zu neuen Fragestellungen anregenden Einfluß zu und unterstützen damit die Ausführungen von LANGMEIER und MATĚJČEK (1977) bezüglich ihres Terminus „psychische Deprivation". Weniger glücklich halten wir demgegenüber das adjektiv „psychische", da es weder die Modalitäten in hinreichender Weise spezifiziert noch den Gesamtbereich der Deprivation – gerade im Säuglings- und Kleinkindalter – umfassen kann. Da bekannt ist, in welch starkem Maße hier taktile, kinästhetische, Wärme- und andere in den Bereich des Physischen gehende Reize eine Rolle spielen, müßte das Adjektiv auf „psychophysisch" erweitert werden und würde dann praktisch zur Spezifikation nichts mehr beitragen.

Wir glauben, daß eine solche Konstrukt-Definition auch partikularistischen Tendenzen entgegenwirken kann, die in diesem Forschungsbereich leider sehr ausgeprägt sind. Verschiedene Sektoren der Deprivationsforschung verselbständigten sich in der Vergangenheit in einer Weise, daß die Resultate aus dem einen Bereich aufhörten, die Ansätze in den anderen Sektoren zu beeinflussen. Je nach dem theoretischen Standort des Untersuchers und der jeweiligen spezifischen Ausrichtung der Untersuchung bestimmten Teilaspekte die Terminologie, so daß Sprachverwirrung und fehlende Übertragbarkeit der Untersuchungsresultate nicht selten die Folge waren. Bei allen, in diesem Teilbereich sicher notwendigen Spezifikationen wäre also ein gemeinsamer Bezug vor allem im Hinblick auf eine umfassende Theoriebildung dringend erforderlich.

Den diesbezüglich z.Z. sicher noch unbefriedigenden Erkenntnisstand berücksichtigend, werden wir versuchen, einen Abriß zu geben, der vor allem die aus psychiatrischer Sicht relevanten Aspekte der Deprivationsforschung in den Vordergrund rückt. Ausführlicher gehen wir auf die Befunde zur Deprivation im Kindesalter ein und beschränken die Darstellung der experimentellen Deprivationsforschung an Erwachsenen im wesentlichen auf die klinisch bedeutsamen Studien. Ergebnisse der Deprivationsforschung an Tieren werden wir nur in einigen Querverweisen berücksichtigen, da diese im Beitrag von PLOG ausführlicher behandelt werden. Einer Betrachtung, die historische Wurzeln der jeweiligen Forschungsbereiche aufzeigt, folgt eine Darstellung methodischer Aspekte sowie der einigermaßen konsolidierten Resultate. Abschließend werden Hinweise auf den Stand der gegenwärtigen Theoriediskussion gegeben.

B. Deprivation im Kindesalter

I. Geschichtliche Aspekte

Einen relativ hohen Bekanntheitsgrad hat der wohl erste Deprivationsversuch erlangt, der von dem Hohenstaufenkaiser Friedrich II. durchgeführt wurde. Diese frühe Auseinandersetzung mit dem Anlage/Umwelt-Problem verdankt seinen Aufmerksamkeitswert weder seiner Fragestellung noch seiner experimentellen Akribie, sondern vielmehr der inhumanen, absolutistischen Haltung, die dem Vorgehen zugrunde liegt, und dem fatalen Ausgang dieses „Experimentes". Friedrich II. ließ an Kindern eine umfassende und sehr lange dauernde Deprivation durchführen, um die „Ursprache des Menschen" zu ermitteln. Eine mittelalterliche Chronik aus dem Jahre 1268 beschreibt den Ausgang dieses „Deprivationsexperimentes" (zit. nach SCHMALOHR, 1968):

„Er wählte eine Anzahl verwaister Neugeborener aus und befahl ... den Ammen und Pflegerinnen, sie sollten den Kindern Milch geben, daß sie an den Brüsten säugen möchten, sie baden und waschen, aber in keiner Weise mit ihnen schöntun und mit ihnen sprechen. Er wollte nämlich erforschen, ob sie die hebräische Sprache sprächen, als die älteste, oder griechisch oder lateinisch oder aber die Sprache ihrer Eltern, die sie geboren hatten. Aber er mühte sich vergebens, weil die Kinder alle starben. Denn sie vermöchten nicht zu leben, ohne das Händepatschen und das fröhliche Gesichterschneiden und die Koseworte ihrer Ammen."

In der Folge wurde immer wieder von sogenannten „Experimenten der Natur" berichtet (z.B. COMENIUS, 1657; LINNÉ, 1774; WAGNER, 1794; BLUMENBACH, 1814; RAUBER, 1885). Es handelte sich um Kinder, die in früher Kindheit entliefen, ausgesetzt oder entführt wurden und in der Wildnis ohne oder nur mit ganz geringem Kontakt zur menschlichen Gesellschaft überlebten. Zum Teil sollen sie von wilden Tieren – vor allem Wölfen – großgezogen worden sein; ein Sachverhalt, der auch in Sagen Berücksichtigung fand. Im Jahre 1940 konnte der Amerikaner ZINGG eine Dokumentation über 31 solcher Fälle vorlegen. Eine ausführliche deutschsprachige Darstellung findet man in dem Buch *Die wilden Kinder* von MALSON et al. (1972).

Obgleich bis in die jüngste Vergangenheit immer wieder Berichte über Fälle verwilderter Kinder irgendwo in der Welt auftauchten und sie für eine Einschätzung der Plastizität menschlichen Verhaltens bedeutsam wären, weisen sie meist eine Reihe von Ungereimtheiten auf. Ungenauigkeiten in der Darstellung, Widersprüche und Hinweise auf Verfälschungen bedingen, daß ihre wissenschaftliche Brauchbarkeit in Frage gestellt werden muß (KOEHLER, 1952; PEIPER, 1958). Die Umstände, unter denen die Kinder in die Wildnis gelangten, die Bedingungen und die Dauer ihres Lebens in der Wildnis sind meist unklar und selbst die Umstände der Auffindung werden oft nicht hinreichend beschrieben (LANGMEIER und MATĚJČEK, 1977).

Den größten Bekanntheitsgrad – u.a. durch eine Verfilmung – haben die Erziehungsversuche des Arztes und Taubstummenlehrers ITARD an dem „wilden Knaben von Aveyron" erreicht. Ähnlich populär ist die Kontroverse über den Fall „Caspar Hauser", der im Jahre 1828, etwa 17jährig, in Nürnberg auftauchte und von ANSELM VON FEUERBACH untersucht und beschrieben wurde (*Caspar Hauser, Beispiel eines Verbrechens am Seelenleben des Menschen*, 1832). Eine umfangreiche Caspar-Hauser-Literatur, in der die vielen Ungereimtheiten auch dieses Falles immer wieder diskutiert und interpretiert werden, erstreckt sich bis in die Gegenwart (STUMPFE, 1969; LEONHARD, 1970).

Wesentlich besser dokumentiert und z.T. mit den Methoden heutiger Testpsychologie untersucht wurde eine Reihe von Kindern, die – meist von psychotischen oder überforderten Müttern – in den letzten 30 Jahren unter Bedingungen umfassender Deprivation versteckt gehalten und meist erst durch Zugriff der Sozialbehörden rehabilitativen, therapeutischen und erzieherischen Bemühungen zugeführt wurden. LANGMEIER und MATĚJČEK (1977) geben einen relativ umfassenden Überblick über Berichte von Kindern, die auf diese Weise depriviert wurden. Wir verweisen auf diese Darstellung, möchten aber hier einen kleinen Exkurs einfügen, um einige solcher Fälle zu schildern, die von den o. g. Autoren nicht beschrieben werden:

KÖTTGEN berichtete 1964 über einen Säugling, der wegen erheblicher Retardierung vorgestellt wurde. Es stellte sich heraus, daß seine Pflegemutter ihn durch Verdunkelung – möglicherweise auch durch Medikamente – weit über das übliche Maß hinaus schlafend gehalten hatte.

FREEDMAN und BROWN (1968) und FREEDMAN (1975) beschreiben ein Geschwisterpaar, das von seiner psychotischen Mutter von Geburt an bis zum Alter von vier bzw. sechs Jahren in fast vollständiger Deprivation gehalten wurde. Auf den ersten Blick glaubte man freundliche, zugängliche Kinder vor sich zu haben, doch es zeigte sich, daß die Kinder in ihren emotionalen Beziehungen völlig diffus waren. In ihrer „Zuneigung" machten sie keinerlei Unterschied zwischen fremden und ihnen vertrauten Personen. Anzeichen von Angst, Scheu oder Erstaunen konnten bei ihnen nicht festgestellt werden und auch für Körpergefühle schienen sie weitgehend unzugänglich zu sein. Bei Verletzungen zeigten sie keine Anzeichen von Schmerzempfindungen; sie aßen unkontrolliert und gierig, solange man ihnen etwas Eßbares vorsetzte. Als sie aus der ihnen vertrauten Umgebung und von ihren biologischen Eltern entfernt wurden, reagierten sie überhaupt nicht; auch nach einem $2^1/_2$jährigen Aufenthalt bei Pflegeeltern hatte sich die Unterschiedslosigkeit ihrer sozialen Kontaktnahme noch nicht verändert. Die Autoren beurteilen die Therapierbarkeit dieser frühen emotionalen Störungen und der fehlenden Differenzierung als sehr ungünstig.

KAGAN und KLEIN (1973) berichteten ebenfalls über ein von Geburt an beinahe vollständig depriviertes Geschwisterpaar. Eine Mutter, die sich der Versorgung ihrer Kinder nicht gewachsen fühlte, hatte deren Pflege ihrer damals achtjährigen Tochter überlassen. $2^1/_2$ bzw. $3^1/_2$ Jahre verbrachten die beiden Kinder 23 von 24 Stunden des Tages in einem Kinderbett, das in einer kleinen Kammer stand, und wurden nur zum Füttern herausgeholt. Völlig unterernährt, im Wachstum zurückgeblieben und psychisch schwer retardiert wurden sie von den Behörden in ein Krankenhaus eingeliefert und nach einem Monat einer Mittelklasse-Familie in Obhut gegeben, wo sie in Gesellschaft mehrerer kleinerer Kinder leben und spielen konnten. In der Folge wurden die beiden Mädchen mehrmals von den Autoren getestet und untersucht, wobei – zumindest bei dem jüngeren Mädchen – ein kontinuierlicher Anstieg der Intelligenzentwicklung beobachtet wurde, der immerhin soweit ging, daß dieses Kind in einer Reihe von Untertests durchschnittliche Leistungen erbringen konnte. Bei dem älteren Mädchen dagegen, das entsprechend länger depriviert gewesen war, erwies sich die Intelligenzentwicklung als nicht so günstig. Bedeutsam ist die Feststellung der Autoren, daß sich die beiden Mädchen z.Z. der letzten Untersuchung in ihrem interpersonalen Verhalten in keiner Weise mehr von dem der durchschnittlichen Jugendlichen ihrer ländlichen Umgebung unterschieden.

LANGMEIER und MATĚJČEK (1977) nehmen zu den von ihnen referierten sowie z. T. selbst beobachteten entsprechenden Kinderschicksalen Stellung. Sie meinen, daß bei den am schwersten betroffenen Kindern der Fortschritt ihrer Nachentwicklung sehr langsam und niemals vollkommen sei. Die von der Deprivation weniger betroffenen Kinder holten dagegen – nach anfänglich langsamen Fortschritten – ihre Rückstände in der Intelligenzentwicklung bald auf. Aber auch dort, wo sich die intellektuellen Fähigkeiten als weitgehend wiederherstellbar erwiesen hätten, seien gewöhnlich Störungen der Persönlichkeit zurückgeblieben. Nach anfänglich phobischem Verhalten zeigten sich solche Kinder später in ihren gefühlsmäßigen Beziehungen meist unbeständig und undifferenziert, wobei ihre Zudringlichkeit und Unersättlichkeit auffallend sei. Neben einer geringen Frustrationstoleranz und stürmischen Gefühlsausbrüchen sei besonders der moralische Überbau nur bruchstückhaft entwickelt.

Eine im gewissen Ausmaß hoffnungsvollere Prognose, die die *Wichtigkeit sofortiger rehabilitativer Bemühungen* unterstreicht, ergibt sich dagegen aufgrund der von KOLUCHOVÁ (1972, 1976) sowie von KAGAN und KLEIN (1973) beschriebenen Fälle.

Bei Betrachtung sowohl der ausgesetzten, wie auch der maximal deprivierten Kinder ist natürlich zu berücksichtigen, daß bei ihnen negative erbliche Belastungen relativ wahrscheinlich sind. Von psychisch gesunden Eltern wäre eine solche Behandlung ihrer Kinder wohl kaum zu erwarten.

Nach diesem Exkurs über einige der erschreckenden Einzelschicksale massiv und von frühester Kindheit an deprivierter Kinder, an denen das Ausmaß der durch Deprivation möglichen Schäden deutlich wurde, wenden wir uns wieder den historischen Entwicklungslinien dieses Forschungsbereiches zu. In den 40er Jahren traten amerikanische und englische Untersucher mit aufsehenerregenden Befunden über die Massenpflege in Kinderheimen an die Öffentlichkeit und lösten damit eine Flut wissenschaftlicher Untersuchungen über Deprivationsbedingungen in Säuglings- und Kleinkinderheimen aus.

Noch Mitte des 19. Jahrhunderts stellte die enorm hohe Sterblichkeit der in der Heimpflege versorgten Kinder das allergrößte Problem dar. Die Diskussion über Maßnahmen zur Abwendung dieser Zustände konzentrierte sich zunächst auf eine angemessene Ernährung; später standen strenge hygienische Maßnahmen im Vordergrund, um die wechselseitige Ansteckung der Kinder zu unterbinden. So konnte z.B. SCHLOSSMANN Anfang des 20. Jahrhunderts durch hygienische Maßnahmen innerhalb von 8 Jahren die Säuglingssterblichkeit in einem von ihm geleiteten Heim von 71,5% auf 17,3% senken. Aber nachdem die *Sterblichkeit* auf ein zuletzt recht geringes Maß reduziert worden war, traten um so stärker *körperliche Entwicklungsrückstände* zutage (z.B. SCHMIDT-KOLMER, 1963), und schließlich wurde auch das Problem der *seelischen Schädigungen* durch die Massenpflege erkannt.

Von Anbeginn an bestand in Deutschland eine Polarisierung der Lehrmeinung zum Problem der Massenpflege von Kleinkindern. Während SCHLOSSMANN – im Vertrauen auf seine spektakulären Erfolge bei der Senkung der Sterblichkeit – glaubte, daß auch die übrigen Probleme der Massenpflege zu beseitigen wären, hielt VON PFLAUNDLER die Massenpflege für „widernatürlich" und bezeichnete Säuglingsheime als „Pflegefabriken". SCHLOSSMANN realisierte ein nach seinen Vorstellungen vorbildliches Säuglingsheim, mußte aber schon bald einräumen, daß sich die mit viel Sorgfalt gepflegten und körperlich gesunden Kinder in dem Heim doch nicht so gut zu entwickeln schienen wie Kinder, die in ihren Familien blieben oder in Pflegefamilien großgezogen wurden. VON PFLAUNDLER führte in Verfolgung dieser Kontroverse schließlich die erste auf Beobachtungen gestützte Vergleichsuntersuchung zwischen Heim- und Familienkindern durch. Er verglich Heimkinder besserer Herkunft mit Familienkindern sozial niedriger stehender Eltern. Er konnte zeigen, daß die letzteren besser gediehen, geistig reger waren und sich auch kontaktfähiger erwiesen als die in der relativ guten Anstalt untergebrachten Kinder. Die Wahl seiner Vergleichsgruppen machte deutlich, daß schon VON PFLAUNDLER seine Argumentation vor allem gegen Einwände hereditärer Unterschiede zwischen Anstalts- und Familienkindern richten mußte.

Dieses in gewissem Umfang sicher richtige Gegenargument wird – insbesondere im deutschen Sprachbereich – bis heute gern herangezogen, um das Ausmaß einer Retardierung durch die Heimpflege zu relativieren. Offenbar eignet es sich vorzüglich, um die für die Pflegebedingungen in Kleinkinderheimen Verantwortlichen zu entlasten. Um diesem *Hereditätsargument* nachzugehen, möchten wir hier ein sicher einzigartiges „Experiment" – eine Spätfolge des Rassenwahns im Dritten Reich – anführen.

Unmittelbar nach Kriegsende stieß HELLBRÜGGE auf eine Reihe „auffallend hübscher Kleinkinder, die massive Retardierungen und emotionale Störungen aufwiesen". Es stellte sich heraus, daß es sich um Kinder handelte, die im Rahmen der NS-Organisation „Lebensborn" von ausgesucht erbgesunden und „rassisch-wertvollen" Frauen und Männern gezeugt und von Geburt an in den Lebensborn-Heimen aufgezogen worden waren. Es gelang ihm, insgesamt 70 der so in früher Kindheit deprivierten Jugendlichen im Alter von 17–23 Jahren ausfindig zu machen und 40 davon ausführlich zu testen. Bei der Schilderung der Untersuchungsbefunde möchten wir HELLBRÜGGE (1975) selbst zu Wort kommen lassen:

„Die 70 Kinder aus ausgesuchten Bevölkerungskreisen, deren Gesundheit und Herkunft durch Erbgesundheitszeugnisse bestätigt wurden, zeigten auf Grund der Berichte der Säuglingsheime bis zum dritten Lebensjahr deutliche Störungen in der statischen Entwicklung... Ein großer Teil der Kinder zeigte beträchtliche Störungen in der Sprachentwicklung... und bei fast allen wurden große Lernschwierigkeiten berichtet. In der Schule hatten sie fast doppelt so oft versagt wie die Kinder in der Vergleichsgruppe. Außerdem ergaben sich ernsthafte Erziehungsprobleme vor allem bei Kindern, die als Pflege- und Adoptivkinder später in normale häusliche Verhältnisse kamen. Bei einigen erwies sich eine Adoption sogar als unmöglich, sie wurden erneut ins Heim und schließlich in die Fürsorgeerziehung eingewiesen. Unter den 70 Jugendlichen waren 12 Fürsorgezöglinge! Zu ihren Erziehungspersonen hatten die Kinder entweder eine übertrieben starke Bindung oder ein äußerst gespanntes Verhältnis. Viele Kinder aus den Heimen waren überaus kontaktarm. Auch zeigten sie dreimal so häufig neurotische Symptome wie Kinder der Vergleichsgruppe. Ein nicht geringer Teil war bereits durch Asozialität, ja durch Kriminalität, aufgefallen. Streunen und Eigentumsdelikte waren in den Akten verzeichnet. Unter den neurotischen Anzeichen fielen Depressionen, Angst und Stottern auf. 5 der 70 Jugendlichen hatten im Alter von mehr als 17 Jahren noch Schwierigkeiten mit der Sauberkeit.... Die Jugendlichen, die ihre frühe Kindheit im Heim zugebracht hatten, besaßen allgemein einen erheblich niedrigeren durchschnittlichen Intelligenzquotienten, ihr Allgemeinwissen war wesentlich geringer als in der Vergleichsgruppe. Ihre Einstellung war wirklichkeitsfern, ihre Umweltbeziehungen gestört. Angst, Haltlosigkeit, Gefühlsarmut und Kontakthemmungen rundeten das Bild ab.... Gerade dieses Experiment zeigt deutlich, daß man das Versagen vieler Heimkinder im späteren Leben nicht in erster Linie ihrer Herkunft zuschreiben darf. Alle Erkenntnisse deuten vielmehr darauf hin, daß die Erlebnisse in der frühen Kindheit für die spätere Lebenstüchtigkeit oder -untüchtigkeit entscheidend sind."

Auch ein anderer Gesichtspunkt, die *Betonung hygienischer Maßnahmen*, stand und steht häufig auch heute noch der Einführung von Bedingungen entgegen, die eine Isolierung von Kindern und die damit verbundenen Deprivationsfolgen reduzieren würde. Einen Eindruck davon, wie schwierig es gerade zu Beginn der klinischen Deprivationsforschung war, gegenüber (übertriebenen) Hygieneforderungen zur Infektionsverhütung den Gesichtspunkt der Psychohygiene zum Tragen zu bringen, vermittelt die damals recht einflußreiche Arbeit *Einsamkeit bei Kindern* von BAKWIN (1942). In ihr werden die damaligen Zustände in den Kinderstationen der Krankenhäuser geschildert:

„Um die Gefahren der wechselseitigen Infektion zu vermeiden, wurden die großen offenen Stationen in kleine abgeschlossene Räume unterteilt, in denen maskiert und verhüllt arbeitende Schwestern und Ärzte sich so vorsichtig wie möglich bewegten, um keine Bakterien aufzuwirbeln. Den Eltern wird der Besuch strikt untersagt und die Kinder erhalten ein Minimum an Pflegekontakt.

> In der letzten Zeit wurden diese Anstrengungen zur Isolation verstärkt und kleine Behälter konstruiert, die es ermöglichen, das Kind so zu versorgen, daß es mit der menschlichen Hand nicht mehr in Berührung kommt.
> Gegenseitige Ansteckung stellt ohne Frage eine problematische Seite der Kinderpflege im Krankenhaus dar, es ist jedoch vernünftig zu fragen, ob die Maßnahmen, die Infektionen verhindern sollen, nicht für das Kind schädlich sind."

Er schildert dann als Symptome der im Krankenhaus versorgten Kinder, daß diese nicht zunehmen, weniger schlafen, seltener lachen oder lallen, apathisch und gleichgültig sind und kontrastiert damit ihr gutes Gedeihen, wenn sie nach Hause entlassen werden. BAKWIN macht die *psychologische Vernachlässigung im Krankenhaus* für diese Befunde verantwortlich; er glaubt, daß sie zu einem Abstumpfen der Kinder gegenüber emotionalen Reizen führt. Fieber- und Gewichtskurven vor und nach der Krankenhausentlassung, vor allem aber die gegenüber vergleichbaren Krankenhäusern in den Jahren 1930 bis 1940 deutlich stärker reduzierten Sterberaten in seinem, deswegen später berühmten Bellevue-Krankenhaus waren die entscheidenden Argumente. Überzeugend war vor allem die Tatsache, daß diese Mortalitätsreduktion erreicht werden konnte, obwohl in seinem Krankenhaus eine Reihe von Pflegemaßnahmen eingeführt worden waren, die nach damaligem Verständnis die so wichtigen hygienischen Vorkehrungen aufs stärkste gefährden mußten. So wurden die Schwestern angewiesen, vor allem die länger bleibenden Kinder so oft als möglich aufzunehmen, und auch die Assistenten hatten die Aufgabe, mit den Kindern in ihrer freien Zeit zu spielen. Schließlich wurden die Eltern der kranken Kinder aufgefordert, diese möglichst oft zu besuchen, sie auf den Arm zu nehmen und zärtlich mit ihnen zu sein.

BAKWINs Verständnis der kindlichen Bedürfnisse und seine Sicht der Mechanismen bei der Entstehung der Deprivationswirkungen muten – auch aus heutiger Sicht – so modern an, daß wir sie vor allem im Hinblick auf die Kontroversen der kommenden Jahrzehnte hier zitieren möchten:

> „Es ist deshalb nicht erstaunlich, daß das kleine Kind leidet, wenn es der Wärme und Sicherheit seiner Mutter oder Ersatzmutter beraubt wird. Es ist auch nicht verwunderlich, daß dieser Kontakt um so wichtiger erscheint, je jünger das Kind ist. Das kleine Kind ist bei der Befriedigung seiner psychologischen Bedürfnisse von seiner Umwelt ebenso abhängig wie bei seiner nahrungsmäßigen Versorgung. ... Es hat nur wenig Möglichkeit aus eigenen Resourcen zu schöpfen, wenn seine psychologischen Bedürfnisse depriviert werden. Dem Kind fehlt das geistige Rüstzeug, welches es den Erwachsenen und auch dem älteren Kind ermöglicht, über Zeiten der Einsamkeit mit Tagträumen oder Zukunftsplanungen hinwegzukommen."

BAKWIN stand damals mit seiner Meinung keinesfalls allein, er konnte sich auf die amerikanischen Autoren CHAPIN (1915), BRENNEMANN (1932) und LOWREY (1940) ebenso berufen wie auf die deutschen Autoren FREUD (1910) und STEINERT (1921) sowie den bekannten Pädiater CZERNY (1922). Angesichts dieser auch in Deutschland bereits so frühzeitig vorliegenden Einsichten, die in der Folge eine weitgehende Bestätigung in experimentellen Untersuchungen erfuhren, ist es erstaunlich, welche Widerstände z.B. gegenüber einer täglichen Besuchszeit oder aber dem „Rooming-in-Konzept" in Deutschland noch in den letzten Jahren bestanden und z.T. noch bestehen (BIERMANN und BIERMANN, 1973; FOLKERS, 1973).

Den maßgeblichsten Anstoß erhielt die Erforschung der Deprivation im Kindesalter aber durch die Untersuchungen der beiden Psychoanalytiker RENÉ

SPITZ und JOHN BOWLBY. SPITZ, der noch vor seiner Auswanderung nach Amerika mit den Entwicklungspsychologen der Wiener Schule (BÜHLER, HETZER, WOLF) zusammengearbeitet hatte, begann 1935 psychoanalytische Hypothesen zur Entwicklung in der frühen Kindheit, die vorher nur aus den retrospektiven Aussagen analysierter Erwachsener erschlossen worden waren, durch direkte Verhaltensbeobachtungen zu überprüfen. Die Wiener Testverfahren zur Bestimmung der Entwicklungsquotienten von Kindern, die bereits in Wien zu Vergleichsuntersuchungen zwischen Heim- und Familienkindern eingesetzt worden waren (z. B. DURFEE und WOLF, 1934), boten SPITZ willkommene Voraussetzungen für seine epochemachenden Untersuchungen an institutionalisierten Kindern. Es gelang ihm zudem, KATHARINA WOLF, die maßgeblichen Anteil an der Entwicklungsdiagnostik der Wiener Schule gehabt hatte, als Mitarbeiterin zu gewinnen. Über zwei Jahre hinweg untersuchten beide Forscher eine größere Kindergruppe, die vom dritten Lebensmonat an getrennt von ihren Müttern unter einwandfreien hygienischen Bedingungen in einem Waisenhaus lebte. Dieser stellten sie eine etwa gleich große Gruppe von Kindern gegenüber, die in der Kinderkrippe eines Frauengefängnisses von ihren Müttern (straffällige, ledige Frauen) versorgt wurde. Der zunächst eher überdurchschnittliche Entwicklungsquotient (EQ) der ersten Gruppe sank innerhalb eines Jahres um über 50 Punkte, während sich der durchschnittliche EQ der im Gefängnis von ihren Müttern betreuten Kinder geringfügig verbesserte. Um seine These zu belegen, daß dieses *Absinken der Entwicklungsquotienten als Folge der Entbehrung der mütterlichen Fürsorge* anzusehen sei, verglich SPITZ in Follow-up-Untersuchungen den Einfluß von Trennung und Wiedervereinigung mit den Müttern und konnte eindrucksvolle Resultate in Abhängigkeit von der Dauer der Trennung sichern. Wir stellen die Befunde durch Zusammenfügung zweier Tabellen aus der Arbeit von SPITZ (1972) dar:

Tabelle 1. Einfluß der Trennung von und Wiedervereinigung mit der Mutter auf den Entwicklungsquotienten in Abhängigkeit von der Dauer

Dauer der Trennung	Durchschnittliches Absinken durch Trennung in EQ-Punkten	Durchschnittliche Zunahme nach der Wiedervereinigung in EQ-Punkten
weniger als 3 Monate	−12,5	+25
3–4 Monate	−14	+13
4–5 Monate	−14	+12
über 5 Monate	−25	− 4

Während nach einer kurzfristigen Trennung von bis zu 3 Monaten ein deutliches Steigen des Entwicklungsquotienten zu verzeichnen war, fielen die Anstiege bei längerer Trennung nicht mehr so deutlich aus, und nach einer über 5 Monate dauernden Trennung schließlich konnte gar kein Anstieg mehr beobachtet werden. SPITZ führt diesen, durch den Entwicklungsquotienten abgebildeten geistigen Verfall auf die von ihm so benannte *anaklitische Depression* zurück, die er von der Depression Erwachsener unterscheidet. Zu seinen über 20 Jahre fortgeführten Untersuchungen nimmt er wie folgt Stellung:

„Bei der anaklitischen Depression tritt eine rasche Genesung ein, wenn man dem Kind innerhalb von 3–5 Monaten das Liebesobjekt wiedergibt. Wenn emotionale Störungen mit bleibenden Folgen eintreten, sind sie zu diesem Zeitpunkt nicht leicht zu erkennen. ... Wenn man jedoch Kindern im ersten Lebensjahr länger als 5 Monate alle Objektbeziehungen vorenthält, zeigen sich die Symptome eines zunehmend schweren Verfalls, der mindestens zum Teil irreversibel zu sein scheint." (SPITZ, 1972).

Aufgrund seiner umfangreichen Verhaltensbeobachtungen unterscheidet SPITZ zwischen vier Stufen der anaklitischen Depression, die etwa im Monatsabstand durchlaufen werden:

Erster Monat: Die Kinder werden weinerlich, anspruchsvoll und klammern sich an den Beobachter, sobald es ihnen gelungen ist, den Kontakt mit ihm herzustellen.

Zweiter Monat: Das Weinen geht oft in Schreien über. Es kommt zu Gewichtsverlusten. Der Entwicklungsquotient steigt nicht mehr.

Dritter Monat: Die Kinder verweigern den Kontakt. Sie liegen meistens in ihrem Bettchen auf dem Bauch – ein pathognomonisches Zeichen. Beginn der Schlaflosigkeit, weitere Gewichtsverluste. Es besteht eine Anfälligkeit für hinzutretende Erkrankungen und die motorische Verlangsamung wird allgemein. Erstes Auftreten des starren Gesichtsausdruckes.

Nach dem dritten Monat: Der starre Gesichtsausdruck wird zur Dauererscheinung. Das Weinen hört auf und wird durch Wimmern ersetzt. Die motorische Verlangsamung nimmt zu und mündet in Lethargie. Der Entwicklungsquotient fängt an zu sinken.

Eine länger als 5 Monate anhaltende Deprivation führt nach SPITZ (1972) zu einem noch schwereren Zustandsbild, das er mit dem Terminus *Hospitalismus* belegte. Weitere Verlangsamung, leerer, oft schwachsinniger Gesichtsausdruck, nachlassende Koordination der Augen und seltsame Bewegungen der Finger waren die Verhaltensauffälligkeiten, die SPITZ beobachtete. Der durchschnittliche Entwicklungsquotient dieser Kinder lag im Durchschnitt bei 45.

Über die Untersuchungen von SPITZ kann – leicht zugänglich – in der zuletzt 1972 erschienenen Monographie *Vom Säugling zum Kleinkind* nachgelesen werden.

Zu den Wegbereitern der Deprivationsforschung gehört auch W. GOLDFARB; er konnte im Jahre 1945 die Ergebnisse seiner ersten umfangreicheren Follow-up-Untersuchung in der Arbeit *Psychologische Privation in der Kindheit und nachfolgende Anpassung* vorlegen. In einer Zeitspanne bis zur Pubertät verglich er zwei Kindergruppen. Die Kinder der einen hatten seit ihrer frühesten Jugend in einer Pflegefamilie gelebt, während die Kinder der anderen Gruppe etwa bis zu ihrem dritten Lebensjahr in Heimen aufgewachsen und erst danach in Pflegefamilien großgezogen worden waren. Schwere Störungen der intellektuellen wie der emotionalen Entwicklung waren nach der Beobachtung von GOLDFARB die Folge der frühkindlichen Entbehrungen. Diese Störungen erwiesen sich im Verlauf weder im Milieu der Pflegefamilien noch in einer Spezialpflege mit psychologischer Therapie als reversibel. Nach seinen Aussagen kommt es zu einer Fixierung auf dem primitivsten Niveau der begrifflichen und emotionalen Entwicklung.

Aufgrund dieser frühen, die Öffentlichkeit relativ stark erschütternden Untersuchungsresultate kam es in der Folge – besonders im anglo-amerikanischen Raum – zu weitgehenden Verbesserungen der Pflege in den Säuglingsheimen. Vermutlich fielen deshalb die Resultate späterer Untersuchungen nicht mehr so kraß aus. Längst nicht mehr so viele Kinder wiesen Störungen auf, und vor allem Kinder mit der schwersten Symptomatik wurden wesentlich seltener gefunden. Mit den inzwischen entwickelten Untersuchungstechniken wurden in der Folge große Unterschiede zwischen Heimen festgestellt, es zeigte sich eine erhebliche Variabilität der in den Heimen realisierten Pflegebedingungen. Aufgrund der neueren Untersuchungen ergab sich dann auch ein insgesamt günstigeres Bild bezüglich der *Reversibilität* wie auch der Möglichkeiten der *Prävention* von Deprivationsfolgen in Kinderheimen.

Die wissenschaftliche Bearbeitung der Deprivation in der frühen Kindheit erhielt einen erneuten, bedeutsamen Impuls, als JOHN BOWLBY (1951) im Auftrag der Weltgesundheitsorganisation seine Monographie *Mütterliche Pflege und geistige Gesundheit* publizierte. Wohl kaum eine andere wissenschaftliche Publikation hat in einem solchen Ausmaß zu kontroversen Stellungnahmen geführt und so viele kritische Nachuntersuchungen angeregt wie diese auf psychoanalytischen Konzepten begründete Schrift. BOWLBY hielt es für die gesunde geistige Entwicklung eines Menschen für unabdingbar, daß dieser als Säugling und Kleinkind eine warme, enge und kontinuierliche Beziehung zu seiner Mutter erleben konnte. – BOWLBYS Schriften sind oft fehlinterpretiert worden, ihm wurde vor allem eine mystifizierende Betrachtung der mütterlichen Liebe nachgesagt, als sei es ihm nur auf einen gefühlsmäßigen Aspekt angekommen, der dem Kind ausschließlich von seiner Mutter selbst geboten werden könne. Auf der anderen Seite hat sich eine ganze Reihe von methodenkritischen Publikationen, die Schwächen in den von BOWLBY zitierten Arbeiten aufzeigten und auf unkontrollierte Verfälschungsmöglichkeiten und Widersprüche hinwiesen, als berechtigt erwiesen. Einschränkend ist bei solchen methodenkritischen Stellungnahmen aber zu berücksichtigen, daß es sich bei der Deprivation in der frühen Kindheit um einen wissenschaftlich relativ schwer zugänglichen Gegenstand handelt. Auch der heutige Stand des Problems ist noch weit davon entfernt, strengeren wissenschaftlich-methodischen Ansprüchen in allen Aspekten gerecht zu werden. BOWLBYS Verdienst besteht darin, daß er zum ersten Mal die verschiedenen Ansätze der Deprivationsforschung zu einer zusammenhängenden Argumentation zusammenfaßte. Seine Hauptschlußfolgerung, daß Deprivationserfahrungen in der frühen Kindheit schwerwiegende und lang anhaltende Entwicklungsschäden verursachen können, muß heute als überwiegend richtig angesehen werden, und eine ganze Reihe von seinen Beobachtungen haben sich – wenn auch mit einigen Modifikationen – als zutreffend erwiesen (RUTTER, 1972). Der von BOWLBY eingeführte Terminus „maternal deprivation" bewährte sich allerdings in seiner globalen Form nicht. Relativ bald wurde klar, daß „maternale Deprivation" eine ganze Anzahl unterschiedlicher Erfahrungen abdeckt, die besser getrennt beschrieben worden wären (AINSWORTH, 1962). Wie RUTTER (1972) bemerkt, verführte dieser Begriff häufig dazu, in unikausalem Denken einer Ursache ein Wirkungssyndrom zuzuordnen; er fordert daher, diesen zu allgemeinen Terminus aufzugeben.

Gegenüber der ungeheuren Vielzahl von anglo-amerikanischen Untersuchungen ist die Zahl der im deutschen Sprachraum durchgeführten Deprivationsstudien verschwindend gering geblieben, obwohl diese Fragestellung ursprünglich von hier ihren Ausgang nahm. Im wesentlichen ist der Leser auf die anglo-amerikanische Literatur angewiesen, wenn auch in der letzten Zeit einige Monographien in deutscher Sprache herauskamen. Nach der Monographie von SCHMALOHR, *Frühe Mutterentbehrung bei Mensch und Tier*, aus dem Jahre 1968 erschien *Mutterliebe und kindliche Entwicklung* von J. BOWLBY (1972) – fast 20 Jahre nach der Originalausgabe – und im Jahre 1977 das Buch von LANGMEYER und MATĚJČEK, *Psychische Deprivation im Kindesalter. Kinder ohne Liebe*. Auch die Publikationen von HELLBRÜGGE und PECHSTEIN vermitteln einen Einblick in den Forschungsbereich der Deprivation im Kindesalter, und sehr hilfreich sind die von BIERMANN zusammengetragenen internationalen Arbeiten aus diesem und verwandten Bereichen, die im Jahrbuch der Psychohygiene in deutscher Übersetzung erscheinen.

II. Methodische Aspekte

1. Schwierigkeiten der Bedingungs- und Subjekt-Variablen-Kontrolle

Bei Untersuchungen von Wirkungen der Deprivation im Kindesalter haben wir es mit dem Verhalten des sich entwickelnden, höchst differenzierten Lebewesens in seinem natürlichen – sich ebenfalls verändernden – Umgebungsbezug zu tun. Dies impliziert ganz erhebliche Schwierigkeiten nicht nur bei der Kontrolle der beteiligten Variablen, sondern auch und vor allem bei der Interpretation der resultierenden Veränderungen. Letztere gehen fast immer aus hochkomplexen Interaktionen hervor, für deren Existenz wir allenfalls erste – meist noch recht vage – Hinweise besitzen. Wenn wir auch in der Lage sind, eine ganze Reihe von Bedingungsvariablen zu benennen, die die frühkindliche Entwicklung beeinflussen, so ist ihre relative Bedeutsamkeit doch nur schwer bestimmbar. In Abhängigkeit von der verfolgten Forschungsstrategie wie auch der Art der Variablen kommt es zu einer unterschiedlichen metrischen Erfassung, was die vergleichende Bewertung verschiedener Forschungsresultate sehr erschwert. Wir stehen sicher noch am Beginn einer aus der Wechselbeziehung zwischen vergleichender Resultatsbetrachtung und daraus folgender Differenzierung der Konzepte stattfindenden Entwicklung, die zu einer schrittweisen Präzisierung der Fragestellungen und Methoden führt. Die Ausdifferenzierung des Begriffes Deprivation zeigt entsprechende Fortschritte, doch findet dieser Prozeß seine Begrenzung bzw. Behinderung in der Art, wie bei bestimmten Fragestellungen der metrische Zugang möglich ist. Betrachtet man z.B. die Untersuchungsresultate von RHEINGOLD (1960), nach denen institutionalisierte Kinder nur etwa ein Viertel der Zuwendung durchschnittlicher Familienkinder erhalten und dabei sechsmal so viele Bezugspersonen haben, oder die von MEIERHOFER (1973), die besagen, daß Kinder in Schweizer Heimen fast 23 von 24 Stunden sich selbst überlassen bleiben, so kann man sich – einmal ganz abgesehen von Unterschieden in der Qualität der Zuwendung – eine Vorstellung von der Bandbreite und

Komplexität fördernder bzw. behindernder Einflüsse machen, die in Vergleichsstudien allein schon innerhalb der Betreuungsmerkmale zu kontrollieren wären. Entsprechend müßten natürlich auch die Reizcharakteristika der jeweiligen Umgebungen berücksichtigt werden, in denen die Kinder aufwachsen. Mit Ausnahme der „Enrichment-Studien" (s. u.) erlauben die meisten Forschungsansätze jedoch nur einen relativ indirekten Zugang zur Erfassung dieser Variablen und müssen oft auf der Grundlage retrospektiver Angaben rekonstruiert werden.

Als weiterer, die experimentelle Aufklärung der Mutter-Kind-Interaktion erschwerender Faktor fällt die Tatsache ins Gewicht, daß Störungen und Einschränkungen dieser Interaktion mit Sicherheit ganz unterschiedliche Wirkungen haben, je nachdem zu welchem Zeitpunkt bzw. in welchem Stadium der individuellen Entwicklung des Kindes sie erfolgen. Wenn auch Übereinstimmung bezüglich einiger globaler Reaktionsunterschiede, wie z.B. der Reaktion auf Trennung vor bzw. nach dem 6. Lebensmonat besteht (THOMPSON, 1960; SCHAFFER und EMERSON, 1964; CASLER, 1968; YARROW, 1968, 1972), so ist die Altersabhängigkeit anderer Reaktionen empirisch noch zu wenig ergründet. Auch die Frage, in welchem Ausmaß „kritische Phasen" für spezifische Arten der sensorischen Stimulation differenzierbar sind, steht erst am Beginn ihrer Aufklärung.

In den meisten Studien müssen auch verfälschende Einflüsse durch unterschiedliche Selektivität in den Vergleichsgruppen hingenommen werden. So findet in Kinder- und Säuglingsheimen fast immer eine „Attraktivitätsselektion" statt. Jeweils die ansprechendsten, meist weniger gestörten Kinder werden von Adoptiveltern ausgesucht, und umgekehrt werden Kinder, die sich dann doch nicht in die Familie der Pflegeeltern einfügen können und Probleme machen, häufig wieder zurück ins Heim gegeben. Dieser Sortierungsprozeß führt sicher dazu, daß die im Heim verbleibende Restgruppe, die dann als längerfristig institutionalisierte Kinder in die Untersuchung eingehen, stärker gestört ist als dies bei unausgelesenen Stichproben der Fall wäre (CASLER, 1968).

Schließlich ist mit YARROW (1968) das bisher meist praktizierte Prinzip der isolierten Variation weniger Variablen in Frage zu stellen:

„Die Wirkung einer einzelnen Variable in einem hypothetischen Vakuum kann sehr unterschiedlich von der der gleichen Variable sein, wenn sie im Netzwerk mit anderen Variablen in komplexer Interaktion steht. ... Mit zunehmender Reifung der Verhaltenswissenschaften, glaube ich, werden wir die ungebührliche Bedeutung aufgeben, die wir der experimentellen Manipulation einiger weniger einfacher Variablen zumessen und der Entwicklung von Forschungsdesigns zunehmende Aufmerksamkeit zuwenden müssen, die eine kontrollierte Analyse komplexer Umgebungseinflüsse gestatten."

Bei skeptischerer Betrachtung bezüglich der Realisierbarkeit stimmen wir bezüglich der Richtung der erforderlichen Schritte mit YARROW (1968) überein, wenn er ausführt:

„Dieses unindirektionale Modell des Verständnisses der Mutter-Kind-Beziehungen sollte durch ein interaktionales ersetzt werden, das eine reziproke Wechselbeziehung zwischen dem Kind und seiner Umwelt – vor allem seiner menschlichen Umwelt – einbezieht. Das Kind antwortet nicht nur auf Reize, sondern ruft auch Reize von anderen Personen hervor, wie es auch seine Umgebung in unterschiedlicher Weise exploriert. Wir können nicht einfach einzelne Variable isolieren, sondern müssen alle nachfolgenden Erlebnisse beeinflußt denken von vorausgegangenen Erfahrungen, wobei die Erlebnisse zum Teil als vom Kind selbst determiniert angesehen werden müssen."

Dem Gedanken an eine experimentelle Verwirklichung solch extrem aufwendiger Forschungsdesigns, die zudem als Längsschnittstudie angelegt werden müßten, um die Dimension der kindlichen Entwicklung zu berücksichtigen, ist auch aus heutiger Sicht ein eher utopischer Charakter beizumessen. Wir wollen aber mit dieser – keineswegs vollständigen – Aufzählung von Problemen, die eine im experimentellen Sinn exakte Erfassung bestimmter Deprivationseffekte erschweren, jedoch nicht einem übertriebenen, an Idealforderungen orientierten, methodischen Skeptizismus das Wort reden. Eine solche Problematisierung war nur möglich vor dem Hintergrund einer Fülle von empirischen Untersuchungen, in denen – häufig in univariatem Ansatz – der Nachweis einzelner Effekte gelang. In der Folge werden wir eine Reihe solcher Resultate zusammentragen, die dieses komplexe, interaktionale Modell unter verschiedenen Aspekten erkennbar werden lassen.

2. Die kindliche Entwicklung in der Interaktion mit seiner dinglichen wie menschlichen Umgebung

Schon von Geburt an bestehen erhebliche interindividuelle Unterschiede, die den Kindern „ungleiche Startbedingungen" bezüglich der Verarbeitung normaler wie pathogener Umwelteinflüsse zuteilen. Das Ausmaß solcher konstitutionellen Unterschiede wird in letzter Zeit sowohl von lerntheoretischer wie auch von psychoanalytischer Seite stärker berücksichtigt (z.B. YARROW, 1972; SCHULTZ-HENCKE, 1965). Ob es sich bei solchen Reaktionsunterschieden wirklich immer um genuine Dispositionen handelt, oder ob sie zum Teil Resultate sehr früher Lernprozesse sind, ist nicht leicht zu entscheiden und hat aus pragmatischer Sicht nur begrenzte Bedeutung, denn nach Befunden von PAPOUŠEK (1975) finden solche Lernprozesse – bei großen Unterschieden in der Konditionierbarkeit – schon in den ersten Lebenstagen statt. Interessant ist, daß sich die frühkindliche Diskriminationsfähigkeit nach seinen Befunden keinesfalls monoton zunehmend entwickelt, sondern daß bereits innerhalb der ersten drei Monate auch Rückbildungsphasen erkennbar sind. Im Normalfall werden diese ersten Lernerfahrungen ganz entscheidend durch die Mutter bestimmt, denn sie konstituiert oder moderiert die ersten kinästhetischen, vestibulären, taktilen, akustischen und visuellen Umweltreize, die zu dem Kind gelangen.

Psychoanalytiker wie A. FREUD, SPITZ, MAHLER, WINNICOTT, BALINT und ERIKSON haben sich ausführlich mit diesen Einflüssen während der Phase einer frühen „extrauterinen Mutter-Kind-Symbiose" auseinandergesetzt und ihre grundlegende Bedeutung für den späteren Umweltbezug („Urvertrauen") herausgestellt. In ihrem, das Kind solcherart beeinflussenden Verhalten ist insbesondere die erstgebärende Mutter wiederum abhängig von einer ganzen Reihe von Umwelteinflüssen (KLAUS und KENNEL, 1973), und auch die Charakteristika des Kindes – Aussehen wie Verhalten – bestimmen ihre Zuwendungstendenzen in bedeutsamem Maße. Die Stellung in der Geschwisterreihe, das Ausmaß der Geburtskomplikationen, die Behaarung und das Geschlecht des Säuglings sind Faktoren, für die belegt werden konnte, daß sie die Interaktion der Mütter mit ihren Kindern beeinflussen (LEHR, 1978; CORTER und BOW, 1976). Sehr bald reagiert die Mutter aber auch in Abhängigkeit von dem Verhalten, das der Säugling ihr gegenüber zeigt (BELL, 1968, 1971; GRAHAM und GEORGE, 1972). OSOFSKY (1976) z.B. konnte konsistente Beziehungen zwischen Verhaltenscharakteristika von Neugeborenen und dem späteren Pflegeverhalten ihrer Mütter nachweisen. Die munteren, schnell reagierenden Kinder hatten in der Regel später Beziehungen größerer Interaktionsdichte mit ihren Müttern. Je ungestörter und effizienter diese frühe averbale Kommunikation erfolgt, die zu einer unmittelbaren, bedürfnisgerechten Versorgung des Kindes durch seine Mutter führt, desto befriedigender wird dann auch die Wechselbeziehung von der Mutter selbst erlebt. KLAUS und KENNEL (1973) sowie BARNETT et al. (1970) konnten z.B. zeigen, daß bedeutsame Unterschiede im Pflegeverhalten erstgebärender Mütter allein schon daraus resultieren, ob diesen ausführlicher oder eingeschränkter Kontakt zu ihren Kindern unmittelbar nach der Geburt gestattet wurde. Untersuchungen von RUBENSTEIN (1967) und BELL (1968) belegen andererseits, daß eine gesteigerte Aufmerksamkeit der Mütter für ihr Kind dessen exploratives Verhalten und seine frühe kognitive Entwicklung bedeutsam fördert.

Neben der Bedeutung, die der Mutter für die Ausbildung der Intentionalität zukommt, ist aber auch der fördernde bzw. bewahrende Einfluß der Mutter bzw. Ersatzmutter bei der Entfaltung der motorischen Fähigkeiten und ihrer Koordination sehr wichtig. So bedarf z.B. das eigeninitiative, explorative Verhalten des Kindes in seiner normalen, stimulationsreichen Umgebung, welches für die Ausbildung der grundlegenden visuellen Diskriminationsfähigkeit von erheblicher Bedeutung ist (SCHILDER, 1950; HELD, 1961), des aufmerksamen Schutzes und der Moderation durch eine Pflegeperson.

Der spezifisch menschliche und in seinen Wirkungen auffälligste fördernde Einfluß elterlicher Betreuungspersonen kommt schließlich im Stadium der Begriffsbildung und des Spracherwerbs zum Tragen. Ausmaß, Art und Klarheit der verbalen Interaktion mit dem Kind bestimmen seine sprachlichen Fortschritte und damit auch die Möglichkeiten zur Entwicklung der Denkfähigkeit. In späteren Phasen ist schließlich die im Rahmen der Sozialisation so wichtige Funktion der Eltern als „soziale Modelle" für die Übernahme von Normen und Werten zur Gewissens- und Selbstwertausbildung und zur sexuellen Identifikation zu nennen. Die Rolle des Vaters, die erst seit neuerer Zeit eine angemessenere Berücksichtigung erfährt, ist hier – vor allem für männliche Kinder – von besonderer Bedeutung (NASH, 1965; LEHR, 1978).

Aber nicht nur das Vorhandensein oder Fehlen solcher fördernden bzw. anregenden Einflüsse ist wichtig. Untersuchungen während und nach dem letzten Krieg haben vor allem die Schutzfunktion mütterlicher Fürsorge sehr drastisch deutlich gemacht. Entbehrungen, Gefährdungen und Traumata des Krieges oder der Flucht führten im wesentlichen nur dann nicht zu später nachweisbaren Schäden, wenn die Kinder während der Kriegswirren nicht von ihren Müttern getrennt worden waren (BRANDT, 1964; BURLINGHAM und FREUD, 1942).

Schwer erfaßbar, da mit anderen Einflüssen kontaminiert, sind Wirkungen von Erkrankungen, die in frühester Kindheit eine längerfristige Hospitalisierung erforderlich machten und das Kind dadurch von seiner fördernden Umgebung isolierten. Bekannt ist z.B. das häufigere Vorkommen emotionaler Störungen bei Kindern, die als Frühgeburten zur Welt kamen oder im Inkubator isoliert wurden (ROTHSCHILD, 1967). Auch sensorische Behinderungen des Kindes, die zum Teil nicht oder erst später entdeckt werden, stellen einen weiteren, die Interaktion der Eltern mit ihrem Kind bedeutsam einschränkenden Faktor dar.

So lassen sich bei tauben Kindern z.B. Entwicklungsrückstände auch bei der Identifizierung visueller Reize (STERRIT et al., 1966), Defizite der Begriffsbildung (NESS, 1964) und des Einfühlungsvermögens (RAINER und ALTSHULER, 1971) nachweisen. Persönlichkeitsstörungen, die auf die gestörte Interaktion zwischen Mutter und Kind zurückgeführt werden (LESSER und EASSER, 1972), können auch dann bestehen bleiben, wenn die Hörfähigkeit hergestellt wurde.

Besonders starke, die normale Interaktion der Kinder mit ihren Eltern behindernde oder störende Effekte sind natürlich bei Einschränkung der Sehfähigkeit gegeben (BURLINGHAM, 1964). Retardierungen ergeben sich z.B. bezüglich des Beginns eigeninitiativer Bewegungen (ADELSON und FRAIBERG, 1974), des Lächelns als Reaktion auf das Erkennen der Mutter (FREEDMAN, 1964) und in der Antizipation der mütterlichen Reaktion. CLANCY und McBRIDE (1975) weisen darauf hin, daß die Einschränkung der Interaktionsmöglichkeiten bei blinden Kindern viel weitgehender ist als bei tauben, und daß es vermutlich deshalb bei dieser Gruppe zu einem häufigeren Auftreten von Isolationssymptomen kommt (Ross et al., 1967; WILLIAMS, 1969; SMITH et al., 1969; FRAIBERG, 1964). Im Gegensatz zu den blind geborenen sind die von Geburt an tauben Kinder doch zu einer relativ normalen Körpersprache befähigt. Dagegen vermitteln blinde Kinder ihren Müttern häufig unklare, ja sogar oft gegenläufige Schlüsselreize, deren Folge Mißverständnisse und eine mangelnde Befriedigung der kindlichen Bedürfnisse sind. Nicht selten ist die Interaktion für Mütter mit blinden Kindern so wenig befriedigend, daß sie depressiv reagieren und dann erst recht in ihrer Interaktionsfähigkeit behindert sind (COLEMAN und PROVENCE, 1957; PATTON und GARDNER, 1962; CLANCY und McBRIDE, 1969).

3. Möglichkeiten und Probleme der Erfassung von Auswirkungen der Deprivation im Kindesalter mit unterschiedlichen Forschungsstrategien

In dieser Übersicht der wesentlichsten bisher angewandten Untersuchungsansätze wollen wir zeigen, daß jedem der methodischen Zugänge ein spezifischer – begrenzter – Stellenwert zukommt, und daß bei einer Beurteilung der Aussagekraft von Untersuchungsbefunden reflektiert werden muß, mit welchen relativen Stärken oder Schwächen die Daten aufgrund des angewandten Erhebungsverfahrens behaftet sind. Diese Betrachtung kann weder unabhängig vom Stand der theoretischen Diskussion noch von der Art der untersuchten Variablen erfolgen und hat zudem den Zeitbezug der Aussagen zu berücksichtigen. Gerade ein Vergleich von auf verschiedenem Wege gewonnenen Resultaten bietet die Chance, verfälschende Einflüsse zu erkennen bzw. zu eliminieren.

Generell kann festgestellt werden, daß die Erfassung von Langzeitwirkungen der Deprivation im Kindesalter ungleich schwieriger und aufwendiger ist als die von Kurzzeiteffekten, d.h. unmittelbaren Reaktionen der Kinder auf die einschränkenden Bedingungen. Dementsprechend different ist auch der derzeitige wissenschaftliche Erkenntnisstand. Während zu Kurzzeiteffekten der Deprivation bei Kindern relativ gut gesicherte Befunde vorliegen, sind die Resultate zu den Langzeitwirkungen noch Gegenstand sehr kontroverser Diskussionen.

In Abhängigkeit von der Qualität der verfügbaren Meßverfahren erscheinen auch die Resultate im Bereich intellektueller Leistung wesentlich gesicherter als solche, die den Bereich der Persönlichkeit und der sozialen Anpassung betreffen. Auch heute noch kann mit RUTTER (1972) festgestellt werden, daß individuelle Unterschiede bisher noch eine zu geringe Berücksichtigung erfahren haben.

Als den klassischen Forschungsansatz kann man die *begleitende Untersuchungstechnik* ansehen, wie sie die frühen Arbeiten von R. SPITZ kennzeichnet. In der Möglichkeit, durch teilnehmende Beobachtung das Verhalten der Kinder, ihre spezifischen Erfahrungen mit ihren Betreuungspersonen sowie die Charakteristika der Heimumgebung zu erfassen und auch Entwicklungstests durchzuführen, liegen die Stärken dieser Methode. Wegen des dabei notwendigen Aufwandes ist diese Technik vor allem für Studien mit kurzfristigem bis mittelfristigem Zeitbezug geeignet. Wenn hinreichend viele unabhängige Variablen erfaßt werden und deren Spektrum nicht zu schmal ist, kann man dies Verfahren als hypothesengenerierend einstufen. Insbesondere wenn Verlaufskennwerte aus der Zeit vor, während und nach der Deprivationsperiode verglichen werden und zuverlässige Meßverfahren zur Anwendung kommen, handelt es sich um einen sehr effizienten Meßansatz. Probleme bietet vor allem die Auswahl geeigneter Kontroll- bzw. Vergleichsgruppen, und es besteht die Gefahr eines Beobachter-Bias in Richtung der Hypothese. Kaum auszuschließen sind Verfälschungen durch die schon oben angeführte „Attraktivitätsselektion". Hereditäre Merkmale sowie prä- und postnatale Störungen fanden in Untersuchungen dieser Art bisher noch zu wenig Berücksichtigung.

Als Spezialfall der begleitenden Untersuchungstechnik sind die sogenannten „enrichment-Studien" anzusehen, die man auch als einen bestimmten Aspekt *experimenteller Isolationsstudien* einordnen könnte. Hierbei wird das Kontrollgruppenproblem dadurch umgangen, daß man in einem Heim Versuchsgruppen bildet, die nach Präwerten parallelisiert werden und einer davon als Behandlung z.B. eine anregende Betreuung bietet. Wenn gesichert ist, daß durch die zusätzliche Betreuung nicht gleichzeitig eine größere Vertrautheit mit den die Testuntersuchung durchführenden Untersuchern erzeugt und damit die zweite Messung verfälscht wird, können mit dieser Methode u.E. die genauesten und unter Präventionsgesichtspunkten relevantesten Befunde gesichert werden. Gerade in der letzten Zeit sind eine ganze Reihe solcher Untersuchungen mit wichtigen Resultaten durchgeführt worden (z.B. CASLER, 1965a, b; WHITE und LABARBA, 1976).

Unter rehabilitativem Gesichtspunkt bedeutsam sind Studien, in denen Kindern eine solche anregende Betreuung *nach* ihrem Heimaufenthalt geboten wird. In ihnen wird geprüft, ob durch solche Maßnahmen Entwicklungsrückstände oder -defizite aufgrund der vorausgegangenen Deprivationserfahrungen nachträglich noch ausgeglichen werden können. Bei diesem Vorgehen ist natürlich die Kontrolle der unabhängigen Variablen schon weniger genau; idealerweise müßte man das Ausmaß der durch die Deprivation im Einzelfall verursachten Retardierung kennen, um den Rehabilitationserfolg exakt abschätzen zu können.

Ein relativ ökonomisches und deshalb auch zum Nachweis von Langzeitwirkungen geeignetes Verfahren stellt die *Retrospektive Folgestudie* dar. Retrospektiv, z.B. aufgrund von Fürsorgeakten, wird bei diesem Vorgehen eine Gruppe von Kindern identifiziert, die während bestimmter Perioden ihres Lebens Deprivationsbedingungen (z.B. einem Heimaufenthalt) ausgesetzt war. Dieser wird eine Kontrollgruppe gegenübergestellt, die – mit Ausnahme der Heimunterbringung – unter sonst ähnlichen Lebensbedingungen aufwuchs. Die weitere Entwicklung der Kinder beider Gruppen kann nun unter kurz- oder längerfristigem Bezug verfolgt werden, wobei der Meßbereich möglichst breit angelegt sein sollte, um nicht wichtige Auswirkungen zu übersehen. Diese Vorgehensweise kennzeichnet vor allem die klassischen Untersuchungen von GOLDFARB.

Das Verfahren ist ökonomisch, indem es die Zeitperioden ausspart, in denen die einschränkenden Bedingungen wirksam waren, und je nach Fragestellung auch die Perioden überspringt, in denen Nachwirkungen nicht zu erwarten bzw. schon bekannt sind. Diese Ökonomie wird natürlich andererseits durch Ungenauigkeiten erkauft. Einmal stehen meist nur retrospektive Angaben über die Charakteristika der deprivierenden Bedingungen zur Verfügung, zum anderen kann meist nicht geklärt werden, ob nicht in den übersprungenen Perioden auch andere Einflüsse – die mit der Deprivation nichts zu tun haben – wirksam waren und die Resultate verfälschten. Abgesehen von der Gefahr von Zufallssignifikanzen innerhalb der vielen abhängigen Variablen, hängt die Aussagekraft der Befunde stark von der Qualität der Kontrollgruppe ab, und Probleme ergeben sich auch bei Ausschlußentscheidungen, deren Kriterien meist erst im Laufe der Erhebungen deutlich werden.

Wenn auch hypothetische Vorstellungen über den zu prüfenden Zeitbezug erforderlich sind, kann auch diesem Verfahren Erkundungscharakter, insbesondere bezüglich der Bereiche möglicher Schädigungen, zugesprochen werden.

Eine ganz andere Situation ist demgegenüber bei den *Retrospektiven Fallstudien* gegeben. Bei diesem Verfahren müssen eng umgrenzte und schon relativ verfestigte Hypothesen bereits vorliegen, wenn wissenschaftlich tragfähige Resultate ermittelt werden sollen. Hervorstechend ist andererseits die Ökonomie dieses Vorgehens, das kurz gekennzeichnet werden soll.

Eine Persönlichkeitsauffälligkeit bzw. ein bestimmtes Symptom, über dessen Entstehungsbedingungen bestimmte Hypothesen bestehen, wird an Erwachsenen festgestellt. Der Versuchsgruppe, die dieses Merkmal aufweist, wird eine Kontrollgruppe gegenübergestellt, die – bis auf das Fehlen gerade dieses Merkmals bzw. Symptoms – der ersten in möglichst vielen Aspekten, insbesondere den übrigen Lebensbedingungen, gleicht. Retrospektiv werden dann die spezifischen Lebensbedingungen in einer bestimmten frühen Periode für beide Gruppen rekonstruiert und miteinander verglichen. Wegen der Unschärfe der rekonstruierten Daten ist natürlich die Gefahr von Fehlklassifizierungen gegeben, die u.a. auch durch verfälschte Auskünfte der Probanden in Richtung der Hypothese ausfallen können. Sofern nicht „harte Belege" berücksichtigt werden, ist anzunehmen, daß gestörtere Erwachsene dazu tendieren, in stärkerem Ausmaß negative Einflüsse in ihre Kindheit zu projizieren. Wie bei den Retrospektiven Folgestudien entsteht auch hier das Problem, daß schwer abgeschätzt werden kann, ob nicht andere Einflüsse, die außerhalb der Betrachtung blieben, die eigentlich verursachenden Faktoren waren.

Eine Demonstration dieser Möglichkeit gelang RUTTER (1971). Er konnte zeigen, daß vorübergehende Trennungen kleiner Kinder von ihren Eltern nur dann zu späterem antisozialem Verhalten und Delinquenz führten, wenn diese Trennungen Familienunstimmigkeiten zur Ursache hatten. Trennungen aus anderen Gründen, z.B. in den Ferien oder durch eine Krankenhauseinweisung, bewirkten keine Erhöhung der späteren Antisozialität. Es ist also anzunehmen, daß die Trennungserfahrung nur ein kleiner Ausschnitt aus einer langen Kette schädigender Wirkungen in unharmonischen Familien war.

Andererseits besteht bezüglich der abhängigen Variablen die Gefahr, daß durch die Einengung auf ein Symptom eine artifizielle Auswahl aus einem Wirkungsmuster getroffen wird, dessen Gesamtbetrachtung relevanter gewesen wäre. Die Probleme dieser Vorgehensweise sind besonders an der Studie *44 jugendliche Diebe* von BOWLBY (1944, 1946) exemplifiziert worden.

Aus der vorangegangenen Methodendiskussion sollte erkennbar werden, daß die Kombination verschiedener Arten des Vorgehens, z.B. einer Retrospektiven Folgestudie mit einer nachfolgenden Retrospektiven Fallstudie, eine relativ ökonomische und dennoch aussagekräftige Art des Experimentierens darstellen kann.

Einen relevanten Stellenwert haben schließlich auch *Einzelfallbeschreibungen*, die in ihrer individuellen Ausrichtung eine recht genaue Darstellung der spezifischen Lebensumstände und Reaktionen der Kinder zulassen. Solche Schilderungen dienen einerseits der Veranschaulichung von Effekten, die mit den vorgenannten Verfahren gesichert wurden, sie können andererseits aber auch Anstöße geben, wenn bestimmte Hypothesen bisher nur zu generell geprüft wurden und einer weiteren Differenzierung bedürfen.

Ein gutes Beispiel solcher Kasuistiken ist die Arbeit von ROBERTSON und ROBERTSON (1971) über Kinder, die im Krankenhaus von ihren Eltern getrennt wurden.

Die einzige, überhaupt mögliche Vorgehensweise stellen solche Einzelfallschilderungen schließlich bei jenen seltenen Fällen maximaler Deprivation dar, bei denen Kinder z.B. von Geburt an wegen Immunschwäche isoliert gehalten werden müssen, oder von überforderten bzw. psychotischen Müttern von normalen Umweltreizen ferngehalten werden. Obwohl solche Fälle fast überall auf der Welt von Zeit zu Zeit bekannt werden, sind sie doch zu selten, als daß ein Forscher sich in standardisierter Weise ihrer Beschreibung widmen könnte. Ein sehr aussagekräftiges Beispiel einer solchen Einzelfallbeschreibung stellt die Studie von FREEDMAN (1975) dar.

Experimentelle Isolationsstudien im engeren Sinne, in denen kleinen Kindern über längere Zeit massive Einschränkungen des Umweltbezuges zugemutet werden müßten, verbieten sich aus ethischen Gründen. Analogieexperimente an Tieren, vor allem solche an Primaten, wie sie von HARLOW u. Mitarb. durchgeführt wurden, haben z.T. ganz erstaunliche Befunde ergeben, die auch Möglichkeiten der Therapie maximaler Störungen durch Isolation aufzeigen (SOUMI et al., 1972). Vorbehalte bezüglich einer Übertragbarkeit dieser Befunde auf den Menschen sind jedoch vor allem deshalb angebracht, weil dem Menschen ein ganz wesentlicher entwicklungsgeschichtlicher Vorsprung durch seinen Spracherwerb zu eigen ist.

Andererseits ist die enorme Ausweitung der wissenschaftlich gesicherten Erkenntnis, die im Breich der tierexperimentellen Deprivationsstudien aufgrund des einfallsreichen und folgerichtigen experimentellen Vorgehens vor allem der Gruppe von HARLOW (siehe HARLOW und HARLOW, 1971) in relativ kurzer Zeit möglich war und auch z.Z. noch anhält, sehr faszinierend. Eine sehr gute Übersicht über diesen Forschungsbereich, auf den wir hier nicht näher eingehen können, vermittelt BRONFENBRENNER (1971).

III. Auswirkungen der Deprivation im Kindesalter

Während den meisten frühen Untersuchungen ein einseitiges Wirkungsmodell zugrunde lag und typischerweise Einflüsse der „Mutter, als der wichtigsten Betreuungs- und Pflegeperson" auf Verhalten und Befinden des „total abhängigen Säuglings" erfaßt wurden, konzentrierten sich in den letzten Jahren einige Forscher auch auf den gegenläufigen Prozeß, und immer häufiger wird auch der Vater in die Betrachtung mit einbezogen. Wir wollen Resultate solcher Untersuchungen, bei denen zumeist das mütterliche Pflegeverhalten oder aber die Zuwendung des Vaters als abhängige Variable erfaßt werden, an den Beginn der folgenden Übersicht stellen.

1. Einflüsse früher Trennung auf die Mutter-Kind-Beziehung

Vorläufer dieser Betrachtungsweise waren Befunde der Verhaltensforschung an Haustieren, vor allem an Katzen und Ziegen. Muttertiere dieser Säuger zeigten markante und überdauernde Störungen ihres Brutpflegeverhaltens, wenn sie in einer „kritischen Phase" nach der Geburt durch Trennung an der Ausübung ihrer typischen Zuwendungsformen gehindert wurden (COLLINS, 1956; HERSCHER et al., 1958). Solche Muttertiere nahmen ihre Jungen nicht an, die Ausbildung der sonst typischen, spezifisch auf das eigene Junge ausgerichteten Verhaltensformen unterblieb.

Untersuchungen dieser Art am Menschen sollten vor allem Einflüsse aufklären, die mit einem Frühgeborenenschicksal oder aber sehr frühen, mit einer Trennung von der Mutter einhergehenden Erkrankung zusammenhing (BARNETT et al., 1970). Sie erbrachten aber auch Resultate, die im Zusammenhang mit der Diskussion um das „Rooming-in"-Programm sehr bedeutsam wurden (KLAUS und KENNEL, 1970, 1973; KLAUS et al., 1972; KENNEL et al., 1974).

Zeitraffer-Beobachtungen ließen erkennen, daß Mütter – ganz ähnlich wie die Muttertiere – mit typischen, stets in der gleichen Abfolge erscheinenden Zuwendungsformen reagierten, wenn ihnen ihr Kind kurz nach der Geburt gebracht wurde. Fingerspitzenberührungen, streichelndes Umfassen des kindlichen Körpers, vor allem aber „Auge zu Auge-Kontakte" spielen dabei eine große Rolle. Je nachdem, ob den Müttern derartige Frühkontakte ermöglicht („Enrichment") oder ob diese gemäß der zur Zeit der Untersuchung vorherrschenden Pflegepraxis unterbunden wurden, kam es nach den Beobachtungen der Autoren zu Unterschieden des nachfolgenden Bemutterungsverhaltens. Bemerkenswert ist vor allem die Relation zwischen dem geringen Umfang zusätzlichen Kontaktes einerseits und dem Ausmaß sowie der Persistenz der Wirkungen andererseits (KLAUS et al., 1972).

Von zwei relativ gut parallelisierten Versuchsgruppen erstgebärender Mütter erhielt die eine Gruppe nur den „Routine-Kontakt" zu ihren Kindern. Sie konnten gleich nach der Geburt einen kurzen Blick auf ihr Kind werfen, hatten nach sechs bis zwölf Stunden Kurzkontakt zur Identifikation und bekamen die Kinder tagsüber jeweils etwa 20 bis 30 Minuten zum Füttern. Der anderen Gruppe wurde ein „ausgedehnter Kontakt" ermöglicht. Innerhalb der ersten drei Stunden überließ man diese Neugeborenen ihren Müttern für ca. eine Stunde und auch an den drei folgenden Tagen erhielten diese Mütter ihre Kinder jeweils für etwa fünf Stunden. In einer ca. 30 Tage nach der Geburt erfolgenden Nachuntersuchung wurde das häusliche Bemutterungsverhalten erfragt und Verhaltensbeobachtungen unter zwei Standardbedingungen (ärztliche Untersuchung/Füttern der Kinder) durchgeführt. Zwischen beiden Gruppen ließen sich hochsignifikante Unterschiede in der erwarteten Richtung sichern. Die Mütter, denen ausgedehnter Kontakt zugestanden worden war, reagierten eher auf die Bedürfnisse ihrer Kinder, ließen sie seltener während des ersten Monats in der Obhut anderer, zeigten mehr Beschwichtigungsverhalten und Empfindsamkeit beim Weinen des Säuglings und verfolgten die ärztlichen Untersuchungen ihres Kindes mit größerem Interesse. Auch die Nachuntersuchungen dieser Mutter-Kind-Paare nach sechs Monaten und schließlich sogar nach einem Jahr ergaben entsprechende Resultate. Bemerkenswerterweise fanden die Autoren, daß die Kinder der Gruppe „ausgedehnter Kontakt" nach einem Jahr – vermutlich wegen der befriedigenderen Mutter-Kind-Interaktion – bedeutsam höhere Entwicklungsquotienten aufwiesen.

Wenn die Autoren ihre Bezeichnung „kritische Phase" auch nicht im Sinne einer einmaligen Prägung verstanden wissen wollen, so sehen sie doch die ersten Stunden und Tage nach der Geburt als eine hochbedeutsame Zeitspanne an und glauben, daß Kontakterlebnisse während dieser Periode das Verhältnis der Mutter zu ihrem Kind besonders nachhaltig beeinflussen. Eine drastische, wenn auch weniger beweiskräftige Bestätigung erhalten diese Beobachtungen durch Befunde bei Fällen der Kindesmißhandlung. Es ließ sich nachweisen, daß Mütter, die ihre Kinder mißhandelten oder ihre Mißhandlungen zuließen, in einem ganz erheblichen Anteil der Fälle (39%) kurz nach der Geburt von ihren Kindern getrennt worden waren (ELMER und GREGG, 1967; WESTON, 1968).

2. Einflüsse früher Trennung auf die Vater-Kind-Beziehung

Eine recht aufschlußreiche Studie zu diesem Bereich wurde schon relativ früh von STOLZ et al. (1954) publiziert. Eine Experimentalgruppe von Vätern, deren erste Kinder in der Zeit ihrer Abwesenheit (Kriegsdienst) geboren worden waren, wurde mit einer gematchten Kontrollgruppe verglichen, in der die Väter der Experimentalgruppe wieder bei ihren Familien waren. In die Experimentalgruppe wurden nur solche Väter aufgenommen, die während der Schwangerschaft und mindestens auch während des ersten Lebensjahres ihrer Kinder von ihren Familien getrennt waren. Interviews, Verhaltensbeobachtungen sowie projektive Spielsituationen gaben Aufschluß über das Verhältnis dieser Väter mit ihren Kindern. Es zeigte sich, daß die aus dem Krieg heimkehrenden Väter erhebliche Probleme bei der Übernahme ihrer Rolle als Familienoberhaupt zu überwinden hatten und daß ihre erstgeborenen Kinder ebenfalls schwer mit dieser Situation fertig wurden. Sie hatten sich damit auseinanderzusetzen, daß ein für sie fremder Mann in die Familie eindrang, die dominierende Position einnahm und die ihnen vertrauten Abläufe in der Familie durcheinanderbrachte. Die Kinder reagierten meist mit Scheu und Zurückhaltung, zeigten dem Vater gegenüber keine Zuneigung und wehrten seine Aufmerksamkeiten ab. Die Reaktionen der Väter auf diese Zurückweisung wiederum verschlimmerten meist die Situation und führten oft zu einer weitgehenden Entfremdung gegenüber den erstgeborenen Kindern. Diese Kinder waren meist stark an die Mutter fixiert und vor allem die Jungen zeigten Verhaltensauffälligkeiten, die mit ihrer gestörten männlichen Identifizierung zusammenhingen. Größere Ängstlichkeit, erhöhte Abhängigkeit von anderen Erwachsenen, weniger Geschick im Umgang mit Gleichaltrigen, ein höheres Maß an Feindseligkeit und andere Verhaltensprobleme unterschieden sie von den Kontrollkindern. Die Väter hatten mit Gefühlen der Unzulänglichkeit in ihrer Vaterrolle zu kämpfen und ärgerten sich vor allem über die „Unmännlichkeit" ihrer Söhne.

NASH (1965), nach dem wir diese Befunde referieren, glaubt, aufgrund dieser und anderer Resultate zur *paternalen Deprivation* auf eine „kritische Phase" der Entwicklung von Bindungen zwischen Vätern und ihren Kindern schließen zu können. Die kritische Zeit der Ausbildung solcher Bindungen, die er mit dem Phänomen der Prägung (LORENZ) in Verbindung bringt, nimmt er – analog zu entsprechenden Annahmen bezüglich der Mütter – ebenfalls recht früh an, die Zeit des Wirksamwerdens dieser Beziehung ordnet er allerdings der Vorschulperiode zu.

3. Einflüsse auf das Kind

Gemäß dem experimentell erfaßten Bezugszeitraum werden Deprivationswirkungen üblicherweise in kurz- oder langfristige Effekte unterteilt. Wir geben diese etwas künstliche Dichotomisierung auf, da fließende Übergänge zwischen beiden eher die Regel sind und die Zuordnung nur wenig mehr widerspiegelt als den methodischen Zugang. Man kann jedoch ohne Schwierigkeit zwischen einer *akuten Form* der Reaktion auf die Trennung des Kindes von seinen Bezugspersonen („akutes Verlassenheitssyndrom"/„despair-Syndrom") und *verschiedenen, sich eher chronisch entwickelnden Effekten* unterscheiden, die aus der einen oder anderen bzw. verschiedenen Arten der Deprivation resultieren.

Das akute Syndrom wurde in letzter Zeit vor allem durch die englischen Autoren ROBERTSEN und BOWLBY untersucht und sehr prägnant beschrieben, doch muß in diesem Zusammenhang auch an die frühen Beobachtungen von SPITZ zur „Anaklitischen Depression" (s.o.) erinnert werden. Eine gute deutschsprachige und praxisorientierte Darstellung findet man bei J. ROBERTSON (1974), *Kinder im Krankenhaus*, die wir hier zugrunde legen.

Innerhalb des akuten Syndroms unterscheidet man zwischen den drei Phasen *Protest, Verzweiflung* und *Verleugnung*, die von den Kindern in dieser Reihenfolge durchlebt werden. Die Beschreibung dieser Stadien vermittelt einen guten Einblick in die Dynamik, die sich bei der Auseinandersetzung der Kinder mit dem unterbrochenen Kontakt zu ihren Bezugspersonen ergibt.

Die Phase des *Protests*, die oft, aber keinesfalls immer, direkt nach der Trennung beginnt und sich über einige Stunden bis zu mehreren Tagen erstrecken kann, ist durch ein starkes Verlangen der Kinder nach ihren Müttern gekennzeichnet. Die Kinder setzen alle ihnen zur Verfügung stehenden Mittel ein, mit denen sie sonst immer das Erscheinen der Mutter bewirken konnten (Schreien, Weinen, Rütteln am Bett etc.). Sie achten aber gleichzeitig gespannt auf jedes Geräusch und jede Person, die sich als die verlorene Mutter entpuppen könnte. Kontaktversuche der Schwestern werden in diesem Stadium häufig zurückgewiesen.

In der darauf folgenden Phase der *Verzweiflung* sind die Kinder weniger unruhig, sie weinen monotoner und mit Unterbrechungen, ihr Verhalten drückt eine zunehmende Hoffnungslosigkeit aus. Sie wirken apathisch und verschlossen und scheinen in einem Stadium tiefer Trauer um die Mutter zu sein. Vom Pflegepersonal wird diese Phase oft als eine schon vollzogene Anpassung mißverstanden, da die Kinder im Vergleich zur Protestphase jetzt ruhiger und besser handhabbar sind. Besuche der Mütter während dieser Periode lassen Protestreaktionen beim Weggehen sofort wieder aufflammen – ein Grund dafür, warum häufig Besuche der Mütter vom Pflegepersonal mit gemischten Gefühlen betrachtet werden. Werden Kinder in dieser Phase nach Hause entlassen, so ist leicht erkennbar, daß ihr Gefühl der Sicherheit und des Vertrauens in ihre Mutter bereits gestört ist. Solche Kinder reagieren mit anklammerndem Verhalten und Ängstlichkeit, sobald die Mutter sie – und sei es auch nur kurzfristig – allein lassen will.

Müssen Kinder noch länger im Krankenhaus bleiben, so folgt häufig die Phase der *Verleugnung*. Die Kinder zeigen jetzt wieder mehr Interesse für ihre Umgebung, nehmen Befriedigungen an, die ihnen geboten werden. Sie spielen wieder und lächeln sogar. Dieses friedliche Bild ist aber keinesfalls als „glückliche Anpassung" zu verstehen, vielmehr hat das Kind – da es die Intensität seiner Verzweiflung nicht mehr ertragen konnte – die Gefühle zu seiner Mutter, ja das Bild der Mutter selbst verdrängt. Kinder in diesem Stadium erkennen ihre Mutter häufig kaum noch und weinen nicht mehr, wenn sie sich nach einem Besuch verabschiedet. Solche Verleugnungsprozesse können bei längerem Krankenhausaufenthalt sogar dann auftreten, wenn die Mutter täglich zu Besuch kommt. Ihr pathologischer Charakter wird auch ersichtlich, wenn die Kinder sich z.B. bei ihrer Entlassung weigern, mit der Mutter nach Hause zu gehen. Die Kinder tauen dann zu Hause nur langsam auf und finden – durch eine Phase der Unselbständigkeit und ängstlichen Anklammerung sowie exzessiver Forderungen an die Mutter hindurchgehend – nur langsam zu ihrem früheren Verhalten zurück. Typischerweise reagieren sie später mit Panik, wenn sie z.B. noch einmal im Krankenhaus vorgestellt werden sollen.

M. RUTTER (1972) macht auf eine Reihe von *modifizierenden Faktoren* aufmerksam, die mit der Auftretenswahrscheinlichkeit oder dem Ausprägungsgrad dieser akuten Reaktionsformen zusammenhängen. Eine wichtige Rolle spielt das *Alter* des Kindes. Das akute Syndrom tritt in der Zeit von 6 Monaten bis zu 4 Jahren besonders deutlich in Erscheinung, bei älteren Kindern sind solche Reaktionen weniger ausgeprägt. Der Entwicklungsstand von Säuglingen unter 6 Monaten läßt dagegen diese Reaktionsform noch gar nicht zu. Der Einfluß des *Geschlechts* scheint geringer zu sein, doch erwiesen sich in einigen Vergleichsuntersuchungen die männlichen Kinder als etwas anfälliger als die weiblichen. Deutlich ausgeprägt sind dagegen die Einflüsse *individueller Variabilität*. Bestimmte Verhaltensmerkmale, die vor der Trennung an den Kindern festgestellt wurden, waren bedeutsam verknüpft mit dem Ausmaß der akuten Reaktion auf die Krankenhausaufnahme. Kinder, die weniger leicht Kontakte anknüpfen konnten, sozial gehemmt bzw. aggressiv waren, zeigten die größten Schwierigkeiten (STACEY et al., 1970). Dementsprechend zeigten sich Kinder mit guten Beziehungen zu ihren Familien weniger durch solche Trennungen gestört als Kinder mit unbefriedigenden Familienbeziehungen (VERNON et al., 1965). Nach den Befunden der gleichen Autoren hängt der Einfluß *vorangegangener*

Trennungserfahrungen überwiegend davon ab, wie diese erlebt wurden. Kinder, die häufiger und gern bei Freunden oder Verwandten übernachtet hatten, zeigen unproblematischere Trennungsreaktionen, wenn einmal eine Hospitalisierung erforderlich wird. Dagegen war das Ausmaß der akuten Reaktion bei Kindern groß, die bereits unglückliche Trennungserfahrungen hinter sich hatten. Die Gestörtheit der Kinder durch eine Klinikaufnahme wird – das belegt eine ganze Reihe von Studien – entscheidend reduziert, wenn eine *Mitaufnahme der Mütter bzw. Geschwister* oder ein *häufiger Besuch der Eltern* möglich ist. Günstig wirkt sich ebenfalls aus, wenn Kinder während der Trennung in einer ihnen *vertrauten Umgebung* bleiben können.

Nach RUTTER (1972) lassen sich alle vorliegenden Resultate dahingehend interpretieren, daß der entscheidende Mechanismus bei der Auslösung des *akuten Syndroms* in einer *Störung der Familienbande* zu sehen ist.

Unter kurzfristigem wie längerfristigem Bezug sind verschiedene Formen der *Depression* mit Trennungserlebnissen in Verbindung gebracht worden, seien diese durch den Tod eines oder beider Eltern, durch die Auflösung der Familie oder durch eine Heimunterbringung der Kinder verursacht. So verglichen z.B. CAPLAN (1967) und CAPLAN und DOUGLAS (1969) Gruppen von neurotischen Kindern mit solchen, die eine depressive Symptomatik zeigten. Sie fanden, daß Trennungen längerer Dauer (>6 Monate) bei den depressiven Kindern wesentlich häufiger in der Zeit bis zum 8. Lebensjahr vorgekommen waren (45%, 51%) als bei den neurotischen (25%, 23%). Diese hochsignifikanten Unterschiede resultierten jedoch nur dann, wenn die Elternverluste mit einer Unterbringung in einer Pflegefamilie verbunden waren. Wenn die Kinder bei einem Elternteil bleiben konnten, trat dieser Effekt nicht auf. Anzumerken ist, daß das Ausmaß von Trennungserfahrungen auch in der neurotischen Gruppe gegenüber der normalen Inzidenzrate erhöht war.

Unter langfristigem Aspekt war die Studie von BROWN (1961) besonders einflußreich. Er untersuchte Patienten mit depressiven Reaktionen im Erwachsenenalter und ging dabei von der Annahme aus, daß Depressionen durch vorausgegangene Verluste ausgelöst werden, die mit schwerwiegenden Trennungserfahrungen in der Kindheit verknüpft sind. Die wesentliche Sensibilisierung nahm er also in der Kindheit an. Diesem Untersuchungsansatz schlossen sich – insbesondere in England – eine ganze Reihe anderer Untersucher an, doch sind die Befunde – vor allem wegen methodischer Schwierigkeiten bzgl. angemessener Kontrollgruppen – bis jetzt kontrovers geblieben. Die Arbeiten von BROWN (1961), DENNEHY (1966) sowie HILL und PRICE (1967) weisen eine bedeutsam erhöhte Inzidenz von Elternverlusten („Bereavement") in der Kindheit depressiver Patienten aus. Demgegenüber ergaben die Untersuchungen von MUNRO (1966), MUNRO und GRIFFITHS (1969) und BIRTCHNELL (1970) solche Unterschiede nur für Patienten mit schwerer Depression und GAY und TONGE (1967) fanden sie nur bei Patienten mit reaktiver Depression. Zwei Untersuchungen schließlich, in denen besondere Anstrengungen unternommen wurden, passende Kontrollgruppen (matched controls) zu finden, ergaben keine entsprechenden Unterschiede (ABRAHAMS und WHITLOCK, 1969; PITTS et al., 1965).

RUTTER (1972) sieht unter Bezug auf HILL (1972) vor allem die Adoleszenz als eine bedeutsame Periode für die Genese der Depression an. Er glaubt, daß ein Verlust der Eltern während dieser Periode besonders häufig in depressiver Symptomatik im Erwachsenenalter resultiert.

Mit einer Störung der Ausbildung von Bindungen – nicht mit ihrer Unterbrechung – wird dagegen das Symptom der *gefühlsarmen Psychopathie* („Affectionless Psychopathy", „Affectionless Character") in Verbindung gebracht. Man nimmt an, daß sich solche Bindungen etwa vom 6. Lebensmonat an entwickeln und bis etwa zum 3. Lebensjahr eine relativ sensible Phase für die Ausbildung solcher Beziehungen besteht (RUTTER, 1972). Werden Kleinkinder während dieser Zeit in Institutionen untergebracht, in denen nur wenig persönliche Interaktion stattfindet und die Routinepflege von häufig wechselndem Personal durchgeführt wird, so ist mit Störungen der Bindungsfähigkeit dieser Kinder zu rechnen. PRINGLE und BOSSIO (1960) untersuchten Kinder in Langzeitheimen und stellten fehlangepaßte einer Gruppe relativ stabiler Kinder gegenüber. Es zeigte sich, daß die gutangepaßten Kinder in der Regel bis über das 1. Lebensjahr hinaus bei ihren Müttern gelebt hatten und erst dann ins Heim eingewiesen worden waren. Im Gegensatz dazu war die andere Gruppe schon wesentlich früher ins Heim gekommen und hatte dementsprechend keine Gelegenheit zur Ausbildung von gefühlsmäßigen Bindungen gehabt. WOLKIND (1972), der psychiatrische Auffälligkeiten bei institutionalisierten Kindern untersuchte, fand, daß die Charakteristika wahlloser Freundlichkeit und sozialer Hemmungslosigkeit vor allem bei den Kindern vorkamen, die noch vor einem Lebensalter von 2 Jahren in die Heime gekommen waren.

Neuere Beobachtungen an einzelnen, in ihren Familien massiv deprivierten Kindern (FREEDMAN und BROWN, 1968; KAGAN und KLEIN, 1973; FREEDMAN, 1975; KOLUCHOVÁ, 1976) erlauben dagegen eine etwas optimistischere Einschätzung der Plastizität kindlicher Entwicklungsmöglichkeiten. Nur die von FREEDMAN wiederholt untersuchten Kinder, die bis zum 4. bzw. 6. Lebensjahr depriviert worden waren, zeigten die Symptomatik der gefühlsarmen Psychopathie in irreversibler Form. Demgegenüber konnten bei den vom 18. Lebensmonat bis zum 7. Lebensjahr deprivierten Zwillingen, die KOLUCHOVÁ in ihrer weiteren Entwicklung verfolgte, günstigere Resultate sowohl im Sozialverhalten wie auch in den intellektuellen Fähigkeiten festgestellt werden. Es bedarf aber sicher noch weiterer empirischer Belege, ehe über die Ausprägung und Erstreckung einer sensiblen Phase für die Entwicklung der Bindungsfähigkeit Verbindliches ausgesagt werden kann.

Auch das Bild einer *entwicklungsmäßigen Retardierung* ist unter dem Aspekt chronischer Einwirkung zu betrachten. Berücksichtigt man neuere Studien, die z.B. für Tageskrippen fordern, daß für 3 Säuglinge mindestens eine Pflegeperson zur Verfügung stehen sollte, um die kindliche Entwicklung nicht zu verzögern (FOWLER, 1975), so leuchtet unmittelbar ein, daß auch unter den heute herrschenden Bedingungen Entwicklungsverzögerungen zu erwarten sind, wenn Kinder längere Zeit in einem Krankenhaus oder Säuglingsheim verbleiben. Entsprechende Befunde aus dem europäischen Bereich berichten z.B. PECHSTEIN et al. (1972), MEIERHOFER (1973) und MATĚJČEK (1973). – Frühe motorische Funktionen werden noch am wenigsten, die der Wahrnehmung, der kognitiven und der Sprachfunktionen am meisten beeinträchtigt. Verzögerungen der Intelligenz- und Sprachentwicklung zeigen sich schon sehr früh und erfahren bei einem weiteren Verbleib im Heim eine stärkere Ausprägung (YARROW, 1972). Allerdings ergibt sich heute – je nach der Qualität der Heime – eine wesentlich größere Variabilität bezüglich der festgestellten Retardierungen. So fanden z.B. RHEINGOLD (1956, 1961) in Amerika und KLACKENBERG (1956) in Schweden bei ihren Heimstichproben Entwicklungsquotienten, die im normalen Bereich lagen. FLINT (1966) konnte durch die Einführung organisatorischer Verbesserungen und einer neuen Erziehungskonzeption recht günstige Resultate in einem kanadischen Heim erzielen, wobei allerdings die Erzieher:Kinder-Relation bei 1:1 (!) lag. Auch SCHAFFER (1965) wies nach, daß die Entwicklungsquotienten von Kindern in gut geführten Heimen, die sich durch einen hohen Grad sozialer Stimulation auszeichnen, nicht unterdurchschnittlich zu sein brauchen; Retardierungsbefunde fand er allerdings in Heimen mit geringer sozialer Stimulation.

„Enrichment-Studien" von RHEINGOLD (1965), RHEINGOLD et al. (1959), CASLER (1965a, b), WHITE (1967, 1971), KORNER und GROBSTEIN (1966), SAYEGH und DENNIS (1965) sowie SCHAFFER und EMERSON (1968) belegten, daß durch z.T. geringfügige zusätzliche taktile, verbale oder soziale Stimulation der Entwicklungsquotient von Heimkindern – zumindest kurzfristig – bedeutsam verbessert werden konnte. Und eine neuere völkerpsychologische Vergleichsstudie von KAGAN und KLEIN (1973) ergab, daß ein Ausgleich frühkindlicher Retardierung auch spontan erfolgen kann, wenn nur die entsprechenden Umweltreize für die Kinder erreichbar sind. Kinder von Eingeborenen aus Guatemala, die bis zum Alter von 15 Monaten in dunklen Hütten, fast ohne Stimulation gehalten wurden und danach massive Retardierungen aufwiesen, holten diese Rückstände wieder auf, als sie später Spielkontakte mit anderen Kindern aufnahmen und die Umgebung explorierten.

Bezüglich des *Alters* ist bei den Retardierungserscheinungen keine untere Grenze zu erkennen; schon im Alter von 2 Monaten wurden derartige Effekte belegt. Eine wichtige Rolle als *modifizierende Faktoren* spielen aber auch hier *individuelle Differenzen*. SCHAFFER (1966) konnte belegen, daß diejenigen Kinder im Verlauf eines Heimaufenthaltes die geringsten Abfälle im Entwicklungsquotienten zeigten, die vorher als die Aktivsten eingestuft worden waren. Die vorliegenden Studien weisen darauf hin, daß für das *Retardierungssyndrom* in erster Linie *Defizite der verschiedenen Arten sonst üblicher Stimulation* und ein *Mangel an Entwicklungsanreizen* verantwortlich zu machen sind.

Früher wurde noch eine Reihe weiterer Symptome in ursächlichem Zusammenhang mit einer Deprivation in der frühen Kindheit gesehen, doch zeigten neuere Untersuchungen, daß solche Wirkungen weder als deprivationsspezifisch anzusehen sind noch überwiegend auf fest mit Deprivationsbedingungen verknüpfte Faktoren zurückgehen. So ist *antisoziales Verhalten und Delinquenz* wesentlich enger mit gestörten, unharmonischen Familienbeziehungen verknüpft als mit einem Verlust oder der Trennung von den Eltern bzw. einem Elternteil. Es macht auch keinen wesentlichen Unterschied in der späteren Delinquenzrate, ob die gestörten Familienbeziehungen schließlich zu einer Auflösung der Familie und vollständiger parentaler Deprivation führen (RUTTER, 1971, 1972).

Enuresis kommt zwar bei vielen Kindern vor, die in Institutionen aufwachsen (STEIN und SUSSER, 1966, 1967; DOUGLAS, 1970), doch scheint dies nur zum Teil auf die im Heim herrschenden Bedingungen zurückzugehen, wesentlicher sind vermutlich Stressoren, die der Heimunterbringung vorausgingen (RUTTER, 1972). Wiederholte Krankenhausaufnahmen in den ersten 4 Lebensjahren – vor allem, wenn sie mit Schmerzen und operativen Eingriffen verbunden sind – stellen eine besonders häufig vorkommende ursächliche Konstellation dar (DOUGLAS und TURNER, 1970), aber auch eine Trennung oder Scheidung der Eltern oder der Tod eines Elternteils erhöhen die Inzidenzrate des Bettnässens bedeutsam (DOUGLAS, 1970).

Zwergwuchs („deprivation dwarfism"), der sich in bedeutsamen Verzögerungen des skelettalen und muskulären Wuchses sowie der sexuellen Reifung zeigt, wurde vor allem bei Kindern gefunden, die lange und extreme Deprivation durchgemacht hatten (PATTON und GARDNER, 1963; MONEY, 1977). Solche Kinder kommen aus schwer gestörten Familien, aber auch aus schlecht geführten Heimen, und es zeigt sich meist, daß sie zunehmen und wachsen, wenn sie in einer anderen Umgebung besser versorgt werden. Früher wurde angenommen, daß die wesentliche Ursache des Zwergwuchses in einer emotionalen Deprivation zu suchen sei (SILVER und FINKELSTEIN, 1967), also unabhängig von der nahrungsmäßigen Versorgung auftrete. Eine relativ frühe experimentelle Studie von WIDDOWSON (1951) legte dies nahe, da in einem Heim auch ein verbessertes Nahrungsangebot nicht zu Gewichtszunahmen führte, solange noch der alte, strenge und unsympathische Heimleiter anwesend war. Erst als ein freundlicherer Heimleiter die Kinder betreute, nahmen diese zu. RUTTER (1972) merkt zu dieser Studie an, daß darin zwar das aufgenommene Nahrungsangebot kontrolliert wurde, nicht jedoch die tatsächlich aufgenommene Nahrungsmenge; auch in dieser Studie könne eine Mangelernährung daher nicht ausgeschlossen werden. – Ein Experiment von WHITTEN et al. (1969) zeigte demgegenüber, daß die meisten der untersuchten zwergwüchsigen Kinder auch unter Deprivationsbedingungen zunahmen und wuchsen, wenn sie nur ausreichend kalorienreiche Nahrung zu sich nahmen. Die Autoren belegten, daß die Angaben von Eltern zwergwüchsiger Kinder über deren Nahrungsaufnahme häufig verfälscht sind. Sie veranlaßten die Mütter, ihren Kindern die Nahrungsmenge, welche sie als „regelmäßig verabreicht" angegeben hatten, im Beisein eines Beobachters zu füttern. Fast unmittelbar nach Einführung dieser Experimentalbedingung ließen sich bedeutsame Gewichtszunahmen bei den Kindern registrieren und schließlich bekannten die Mütter, daß ihre Kinder während dieser Periode mehr gegessen hätten als zuvor.

Mangelernährung ist wahrscheinlich ein wesentlicher Faktor, der häufig am Zustandekommen des Zwergwuchses beteiligt ist (RUTTER, 1972), doch haben andere Untersuchungen (POWELL et al., 1967; POWELL et al., 1973; BRASEL, 1973; BROWN, 1976) belegt, daß bei solchen Kindern auch endokrine Veränderungen bzw. ein Mangel des Wachstumshormons (ACTH) im Serum gefunden wird. Solange diese Kinder in ihrer deprivierenden Umgebung leben, weisen sie eine subnormale Ausschüttung dieses Hormons z.B. nach Stimulation mit Insulin auf, während sich diese Releasing-Funktion normalisiert, wenn die Kinder in eine normale Umgebung verbracht werden (GARDNER, 1977). – Schließlich dürfte bei nicht wenigen Fällen – vor allem mißhandelter Kinder – auch eine Schlafdeprivation, ebenfalls durch Unterdrückung der ACTH-Ausschüttung, am Zustandekommen des Zwergwuchses beteiligt sein.

C. Experimentelle Deprivationsforschung an Erwachsenen

In der Terminologie der experimentellen Deprivationsforschung wird im wesentlichen zwischen zwei Arten der Deprivation unterschieden:
a) *Sensorische Deprivation* bezeichnet eine möglichst weitgehende Reduktion der Intensität sensorischer Reize.
b) *Perzeptive Deprivation* bedeutet eine Reduktion oder Eliminierung des Informationsgehaltes sensorischer Reize, wobei deren Intensität etwa im normalen Bereich gehalten wird.

Versuchsanordnungen dieser Art beinhalten meist zusätzlich in mehr oder weniger ausgeprägter Form die Bedingungen der *Immobilisation* und der *sozialen Isolierung*. Wenn in einem oder mehreren Sinnesbereichen nur eine teilweise Einschränkung des sensorischen Zustroms gegeben ist, spricht man von *partieller Deprivation*.

Bei Versuchen mit sensorischer Deprivation befinden sich die Probanden meist in halbliegender Position in einem dunklen, schallisolierten Raum; perzeptive Deprivation wird durch Maskierung äußerer Reize – etwa durch „weißes Rauschen" und Milchglasabdeckung des Sichtfeldes erreicht. – Einen anschaulichen Überblick über die verschiedenen Techniken der experimentellen Deprivation und die dabei auftretenden methodischen Probleme gibt Rossi (1969).

Versuchsbedingungen mit totaler oder sehr weitgehender Deprivation werden benutzt, um weniger restriktive, aber wesentlich länger dauernde Einschränkungen, wie sie unter Alltagsbedingungen vorkommen, experimentell ökonomisch untersuchen zu können.

I. Geschichtliche Aspekte

Die ersten Untersuchungen mit sensorischer Deprivation (SD) an freiwilligen, erwachsenen Versuchspersonen wurde ab 1951 von der Forschungsgruppe um D.O. Hebb (W. Heron, W.H. Bexton, B.K. Doane, W. Mahatoo und T.H. Scott) an der McGill-Universität in Montreal/Kanada durchgeführt. Vorausgegangen waren Deprivationsuntersuchungen an Tieren, und aktuelle Anstöße waren damals neben theoretischen Interessen die Fragen nach den Mechanismen der sogenannten „Gehirnwäsche" und nach den Ursachen von Fehlverhalten, das bei Radarbeobachtern festgestellt worden war, die unter monotonen Umgebungsbedingungen arbeiten mußten. Der Begriff „Gehirnwäsche" stand für eine fiktive Methode, der die damals völlig unerklärlichen „Umerziehungserfolge" zugeschrieben wurden, welche amerikanische Kriegsgefangene in Korea zur (vorübergehenden) Aufgabe ihrer westlichen Wertvorstellungen veranlaßt hatten.

Die ersten Untersuchungen dieser Forschungsgruppe erbrachten eine solche Fülle von – vor allem unter psychiatrischen Aspekten – interessanten Befunden, daß in der Folge allein in Amerika 17 Forschungszentren mit dieser Methode zu experimentieren begannen. Starke Impulse erhielt die experimentelle Deprivationsforschung auch, als die Großmächte ihre bemannten Raumflüge vorbereiteten, da hier stark einschränkende Lebens- und Arbeitsbedingungen impliziert waren. – In Europa wurden SD-Fragestellungen nur sporadisch, meist unter klinisch-psychiatrischen Aspekten bearbeitet. Anwendungen, in denen sensorische Deprivation zur Vorbereitung oder Verstärkung psychotherapeutischer

Maßnahmen eingesetzt wird, traten erst in den letzten Jahren in den Vordergrund, wobei vor allem die Forschungsgruppe um P. SUEDFELD an der Universität von Britisch Columbien in Vancouver/Kanada zu nennen ist.

II. Wirkungen der sensorischen und perzeptiven Deprivation auf erwachsene Versuchspersonen

Obwohl es auch spezifische Kurzzeitwirkungen der Deprivation gibt (z.B. halluzinatorische Phänomene, Zeitverschätzungen), die schon nach wenigen Minuten einsetzen können, tritt die Mehrzahl der bisher gesicherten Effekte doch erst nach Zeiträumen von mehreren Stunden bis zu einigen Tagen auf. Meist handelt es sich um relativ flüchtige Effekte, die schon nach einer kurzen Latenz zwischen der SD-Periode und ihrer Messung nicht mehr nachweisbar sind. Versucht man Effekte der Deprivation mit längeren Testbatterien zu messen, hebt die Aktivierung durch die ersten Tests häufig Wirkungen auf, die durch die darauf folgenden Verfahren erfaßt werden sollen. Überdauernde Wirkungen (z.B. EEG-Veränderungen und Motivationsdefizite) wurden nur bei Experimenten extremer Dauer beobachtet. Sowohl bezüglich der Toleranz für Deprivation als auch bezüglich ihrer Wirkung auf einzelne Funktionsbereiche sind außerordentlich große *interindividuelle Unterschiede* festzustellen, deren Aufklärung bisher kaum gelungen ist. Die *Gefährlichkeit* des Experimentierens mit sensorischer Deprivation wird in der Öffentlichkeit häufig massiv überschätzt, obwohl dafür keine empirische Basis vorhanden ist. Es läßt sich klar belegen, daß die Methoden der sensorischen Deprivation eine im Vergleich mit pharmakologischen, aber auch psychotherapeutischen Einwirkungen extrem niedrige Komplikationsrate aufweist (0,03% entsprechend 1:3300, nach SUEDFELD, 1975). In der gesamten, bis heute erschienenen Literatur über Deprivationsexperimente findet sich nur eine Arbeit, in der von einer psychotherapiebedürftigen, vorübergehenden Entgleisung einer „gesunden" Versuchsperson berichtet wird (CURTIS und ZUCKERMAN, 1968). Dieser Bericht bezieht sich auf ein achtstündiges Deprivationsexperiment, in dem zusätzlich eine strikte Immobilisierung und eine eingeschränkte taktile Stimulation realisiert wurden. Die Reaktion dieses Probanden muß sicher auch im Zusammenhang mit seiner Persönlichkeit (MMPI: erhöhte Werte in Femininität, Psychopathie, Paranoia, Schizophrenie) und seiner Drogen-Anamnese (Marihuana, Halluzinogene, Sedativa, Tranquilizer) gesehen werden.

Halluzinatorische Phänomene und Wahrnehmungsveränderungen gehörten zu den Befunden, die in den 50er Jahren das meiste Aufsehen erregten. Im Lichte des heutigen Wissens haben diese Befunde viel von ihrer Dramatik eingebüßt. So umfassende Wahrnehmungsveränderungen, wie sie damals berichtet wurden, konnten meist nicht repliziert werden und den Halluzinationen kommt überwiegend die Qualität von *Pseudohalluzinationen* zu. Sie sind zudem strikt an die experimentellen Bedingungen gebunden. In einer Vielzahl von Untersuchungen wurde gefunden, daß halluzinatorische Phänomene (HP) unter Bedingungen der sensorischen Deprivation mit großer Intensität und Deutlichkeit erlebt werden, von einfachen Strukturen wie Lichtblitzen und geometrischen Formen bis zu hochkomplexen Szenen variieren und während relativ wacher Bewußtseinslagen auftreten.

Eine eigene Untersuchung (KEMPE, 1973; KEMPE und REIMER, 1976) ergab, daß unsere Versuchspersonen die HP zum weit überwiegenden Anteil als unwillentlich bzw. unkontrollierbar in bezug auf ihren Beginn (79%), ihren Inhalt (70%) und ihr Ende (66%) beurteilen. Mit zunehmender Komplexität wurden die HP häufiger als farbig, dreidimensional und bewegt gesehen sowie weiter in den Sehraum projiziert. Obwohl die HP am Ende des Experiments fast ausnahmslos als *nicht real* eingeschätzt wurden, benutzten die Versuchspersonen nach unseren Beobachtungen (Infrarot-Fernsehanlage) während der Erlebnisse doch häufig *äußere Realitätstestkriterien* (z.B. Hand-davor-Halten, Blinzeln, Vorbeugen etc.), um sich der Nichtrealität dieser Erscheinungen zu versichern. Dieses Realitätstestverhalten wurde in Abhängigkeit von der Komplexität der HP unterschiedlich häufig gezeigt (einfache: 50%, halbstrukturierte: 28%, komplexe: 14%). Dieser Unterschied dürfte seine Erklärung darin finden, daß hochstrukturierte HP oft individualspezifische Inhalte haben (z.B. „das Elternhaus"), die aufgrund *logischer Erwägungen* in der experimentellen Umgebung ausgeschlossen werden können. Vor allem die hochstrukturierten HP werden emotional positiv erlebt und als angenehme Abwechslung in der monotonen Umgebung angesehen.

Neben visuellen und akustischen HP berichtet ein erheblicher Anteil der Versuchspersonen unter SD-Bedingungen auch von *Körperschemaveränderungen.*

Unsere Untersuchung, die eine der wenigen systematisch angelegten Wiederholungsexperimente zu dieser Thematik darstellt, zeigte bedeutsame Veränderungen der Versuchsmotivation aufgrund der individuellen Erfahrungen, die unsere Versuchspersonen in der ersten experimentellen Sitzung mit den HP gemacht hatten. Die Tatsache, daß unsere Probanden die Realität ihrer Erscheinungen meist eindeutig ausschließen konnten, bedeutet natürlich nicht, daß dies auch der Fall ist, wenn Menschen nichtexperimentellen Deprivationsbedingungen ausgesetzt sind. In einer natürlichen Umgebung ist das Spektrum möglicher Inhalte ungleich größer, und häufig bestehen Erwartungshaltungen, die das Auftreten von HP wahrscheinlicher machen und gleichzeitig eher zu positiven Realitätsurteilen führen (GROSS et al., 1972). Solche Trugwahrnehmungen können – vor allem, wenn sie sich auf Inhalte beziehen, nach denen ein starkes Bedürfnis herrscht – sehr gefährlich werden. So kann man Berichten von Schiffbrüchigen, die sehr stark unter Durst litten, entnehmen, daß sich manche ihrer Kameraden erhoben und über die Bordwand kletterten, „um drüben in der Kneipe ein Bier zu holen". Erst durch die unerwartete Nässe wurden sie aus ihren Trugwahrnehmungen gerissen und ließen sich wieder auffischen.

Herrschen gleichartige, massive Bedürfnisse dieser Art bei mehreren Personen vor, so kann es zur Ausbildung sog. *kollektiver Halluzinationen* kommen (CRITCHLEY, 1943). Eindrucksvolle Beispiele solcher Trugwahrnehmungen finden sich nicht nur in den Berichten von Schiffbrüchigen (z.B. ANDERSON, 1942; BENNET, 1973), sondern wurden z.B. auch von Überlebenden bei Bergwerksunglücken erlebt (MENDE und PLOEGER, 1966; PLOEGER, 1968; COMER et al., 1967). Gerade aus den beiden erstgenannten Berichten wird deutlich, in welch schwer entwirrbarer Form es dabei zu einer Vermengung realer und irrealer Anteile im Halluzinationserleben kommen kann.

Auch *Beeinträchtigungen der kognitiven Leistungen* gehören zu den flüchtigen, unmittelbar an die experimentellen Bedingungen gebundenen Wirkungen. Oft wird von Versuchsteilnehmern schon nach relativ kurzer Zeit von Schwierigkeiten berichtet, sich zu konzentrieren, klar zu denken bzw. schlußfolgernde Denkschritte konsequent zu vollziehen. Nach Angaben der Probanden kommt es zu einem erhöhten, unkontrollierten und emotionsbezogenen Einfallsreichtum. In der psychoanalytischen Terminologie wird dieser Vorgang als Übergang von sekundärprozeßhaftem zu primärprozeßhaftem Denken beschrieben. In den psychologischen Tests schlägt sich dieser Effekt als Reduktion bei den Leistungen nieder, die komplexes Denken mit nicht vorgegebenen Lösungswegen und neuen Kombinationen erfordern (SUEDFELD, 1969a). Nicht gestört bzw. verbessert erwiesen sich demgegenüber Leistungen, die auf hochgeübten Denkakten beruhen und bei denen die Lösungswege vorgegeben sind.

Eine – vor allem unter theoretischen Aspekten – zentrale Bedeutung hat das unter monotonen Umgebungsbedingungen ausgelöste *Bedürfnis nach bedeutsamen, variablen Reizen ("Reizhunger")*, das von JONES (1969) am eingehendsten untersucht wurde. In Versuchsanordnungen, in denen die Probanden instrumentelles Verhalten zeigen mußten, um Reize bestimmter Art und Menge zugeführt zu erhalten, wurden folgende Befunde gesichert:
a) Die Antwortraten der Vpn sind eine monotone Funktion des Ausmaßes vorangegangener Deprivation.
b) Je mehr Information der „Belohnungsreiz" enthält und je bedeutsamer er für die Vp ist, desto mehr instrumentelles Verhalten wird gezeigt.
c) Dieses Bedürfnis nach Information ist homöostatisch; sowohl zu niedrige als auch zu hohe Reizpegel lösen eine Tendenz zur Wiederherstellung eines optimalen Niveaus aus.

Reizsucheverhalten dieser Art steht in Beziehung zu bestimmten Arten motorischen Verhaltens, die offenbar ebenfalls Eigenstimulationscharakter besitzen.

Im Zusammenhang mit den beiden letztangeführten Deprivationseffekten ist eine *Erhöhung der Suggestibilität* durch sensorische Deprivation zu sehen (SUEDFELD, 1972). Nach SUEDFELD führt der in der monotonen Umgebung entstehende Reizhunger dazu, daß sich die Probanden Beeinflussungsbotschaften – in Ermangelung anderer sinnvoller Informationen – auch dann bereitwillig anhören, wenn diese mit ihrem Wertsystem in Konflikt stehen. Zudem sei durch die sich unter Deprivationsbedingungen entwickelnde veränderte Bewußtseinslage eine differenzierte Beurteilung und damit mögliche Abwehr der Beeinflussungsbotschaft erschwert. Obwohl eine Reihe von Untersuchungen zumindest kurzfristige Beeinflussungseffekte wahrscheinlich machen, ist über deren Persistenz nur wenig bekannt, und eine neuere Untersuchung von SUEDFELD und IKARD (1974) ergab in kurz- wie längerfristigem Bezug keinen zusätzlichen Effekt durch Beeinflussungsbotschaften in einem Versuch zur Raucherentwöhnung. Untersuchungen des ersten Autors ergaben, daß eine Wechselwirkung zwischen der Subtilität der Beeinflussungsbotschaften und der Intelligenz der Probanden zustande kam. Je intelligenter die Probanden waren, desto weniger durchschaubar-einseitig durften die Botschaften formuliert sein, um Einstellungsveränderungen zu erzielen.

Unabhängig von der bisher sicher noch unzureichend erforschten Effektivität dieser Anwendung und der noch relativ ungeklärten Mechanismen, die solchen Effekten zugrunde liegen, sollte man sich der ethischen Ambivalenz dieses Ansatzes bewußt sein. Was in klinischen Applikationen (z.B. bei Alkohol-, Nikotin-, Drogen- oder Fettsüchtigen) therapeutisch sehr nützlich sein kann, könnte auch (z.B. von totalitären Regimen zur Umerziehung politischer Gegner) mißbräuchliche Anwendung finden.

In Langzeitexperimenten mit sensorischer Deprivation konnte die Arbeitsgruppe ZUBEK (1969) auch relativ persistierende *Effekte im Elektroenzephalogramm* belegen:
a) eine mit der Dauer der Deprivation zunehmende Verlangsamung im Alpha-Band und
b) eine Zunahme von Theta-Wellen im Temporalbereich.

Zehn Tage nach einem 14tägigen Deprivationsexperiment waren derartige Effekte noch nachweisbar und etwa gleichlang machten sich bei Versuchspersonen Motivationsverluste bemerkbar. Die sich solcherart zeigende *kortikale Desaktivierung* geht nach Befunden von BIASE und ZUCKERMAN (1967) mit einer *Erhöhung des autonomen Arousals* einher, wie sie u.a. in der psychogalvanischen Reaktion erkennbar wird.

Nach dieser Darstellung der unter klinischen Gesichtspunkten wesentlichsten Deprivationswirkungen wenden wir uns nun Anwendungsbezügen zu, denen unter diagnostischen und therapeutischen Gesichtspunkten psychiatrische Relevanz zukommt.

III. Klinische Anwendungsmöglichkeiten der Deprivation

1. Diagnostischer Bereich

Künstlich herbeigeführte Deprivationsbedingungen bieten Gelegenheit zur Veranschaulichung einer Reihe von *quasi-psychopathologischen Symptomen*. Im Selbstversuch hat der Psychiater die Möglichkeit, Erlebnis- und Verarbeitungsweisen, wie z.B. Halluzinationen, Körperschemaveränderungen, Depersonalisationserlebnisse und paranoide Verarbeitungsweisen – die er im täglichen Umgang mit psychiatrischen Patienten zu beurteilen hat, selbst aber kaum aus eigenem Erleben kennt – in einer dem klinischen Bild ähnlichen Form aus eigener Anschauung kennenzulernen. Nicht unwesentlich ist auch das Verständnis einer Reihe von psychotischen Entgleisungen und Störungen, zu denen der Psychiater häufig als Konsiliarius gerufen wird, durch Experimente mit sensorischer Deprivation gefördert worden.

Die *Simulation von klinischen Deprivationsbedingungen*, denen Patienten aufgrund ihrer Krankheit, ihrer Unterbringung oder der an ihnen durchgeführten therapeutischen Maßnahmen ausgesetzt sind, ist aus zwei Gründen bedeutsam:
a) Einerseits können aufgrund solcher Untersuchungen verbessernde Maßnahmen konzipiert und in ihrer Wirksamkeit erprobt werden,
b) andererseits kann man durch Aufklärung differentieller Wirkungsmechanismen z.B. solche Patienten identifizieren, die durch solche Bedingungen besonders stark beeinträchtigt werden.

Durch Untersuchungen an gesunden Versuchspersonen lassen sich so Erkenntnisse sammeln, die bei der Behandlung Kranker Berücksichtigung finden können.

In einem entsprechenden 6-Stunden-Deprivationsexperiment (KEMPE et al., 1977) hatten wir die Möglichkeit, simultan erfaßte subjektive Belastungsindikatoren, Abbruchverhalten und die als unabhängige Variablen eingehenden Merkmale der Persönlichkeit (Extremgruppenvergleich) aufeinander zu beziehen und erhielten so einen Einblick in die Wirkungsmechanismen, die der Toleranz unserer gesunden Versuchspersonen für die reizarmen Umgebungsbedingungen zugrunde lagen. Das als Toleranzkriterium dienende Abbruchverhalten spaltete die Gruppe wie folgt auf:
a) 25% der Probanden brachen den Versuch ab (ABB),
b) 50% spielten mit dem Gedanken an einen Abbruch (AAG) und
c) 25% gaben an, einen Versuchsabbruch nie in Erwägung gezogen zu haben (NAG).

Zur Prädiktion der solcherart bestimmten Deprivationstoleranz kann nach unseren Befunden ein zweistufig-hierarchisches Determinationsmodell aufgrund von Persönlichkeitskennwerten dienen. Im wesentlichen läßt die individuelle Ausprägung *habitueller Ängstlichkeit* eine Voraussage darauf zu, ob sich die Versuchspersonen unter den reizarmen Umgebungsbedingungen als subjektiv in stärkerem Maße belastet zeigen. Dieses Merkmal trennt hochbedeutsam die wenig tangierten Probanden der NAG-Gruppe von den sich als belastet darstellenden beiden anderen Gruppen. Letztere unterscheiden sich im subjektiven Bereich dadurch, daß die Abbrecher relativ schnell mit zunehmender Auslenkung in der Befindlichkeitsvariable „Verärgerung" reagieren, während die AAG-Gruppe längere Perioden auch stärkerer Belastung ohne bedeutsame Auslenkung dieser Variablen durchsteht und erst gegen Ende des Versuchs höhere Grade von „Verärgerung" zeigt. Das differente Verhalten dieser Gruppe wird jedoch nicht – wie zu erwarten gewesen wäre – durch das habituelle Persönlichkeitsmerkmal „aggressive Reizbarkeit" vorausgesagt, vielmehr besteht ein bedeutsamer Zusammenhang zur *habituellen „Risikobereitschaft"*. Risikobereite Probanden, die sich unter Deprivationsbedingungen belastet fühlten, reagierten also relativ schnell mit „Verärgerung" und brachen in der Folge den Versuch ab. Bemerkenswert ist, daß sich die drei nach ihrem Abbruchverhalten unterschiedenen Gruppen schon innerhalb der ersten zwei Stunden des Experiments relativ prägnant in den als Belastungsindikatoren dienenden Befindlichkeitsverläufen voneinander unterschieden.

SOLOMON (1967) führt folgende Krankheiten bzw. Behandlungsmethoden an, die ein erhebliches Ausmaß von Deprivation bedingen: neurologische Patienten in eisernen Lungen, kreislaufbedingte exogene Psychosen bei älteren dekompensierten Patienten, Arthritis-Patienten und chronische Invaliden, sogenannte „Black-Patch-Psychosen" bei Augenabdeckung nach Cataract-Operationen, Patienten im Gipsbett oder Streckverband, postoperative Isolation z.B. auf Intensivstationen, langdauernde Unterbringung in geschlossenen Stationen in der Psychiatrie und schließlich die soziale Isolation und Deprivation alter Menschen in Heimen. – Im deutschen Schrifttum finden sich dazu die Arbeiten von HAASE (1963) über alleinstehende Frauen und von JANZARIK (1973) über das sog. Kontaktmangelparanoid bei alleinlebenden alten Menschen.

Wenn die hier angeführten Behandlungsmaßnahmen zum Teil heute auch abgelöst bzw. verkürzt wurden, eröffnen sich doch insbesondere in der Intensivmedizin in zunehmendem Maße Bereiche, in denen analoge Bedingungen vorherrschen. Es muß auch darauf hingewiesen werden, daß Patienten, die in ihrer Sensorik eingeschränkt sind (Blinde, Schwerhörige bzw. Taube), durch solche Begleiteffekte therapeutischer Maßnahmen besonders schwer betroffen sind. Sprachbarrieren wirken sich ebenfalls verstärkend aus, wenn z.B. Gastarbeiter solchen therapeutischen Maßnahmen unterzogen werden müssen oder wenn ausländisches Personal Patienten unter solchen Bedingungen mitversorgt. Vor allem die fortschreitende Technisierung, Automation und Rationalisierung auf dem Gebiet der medizinischen Therapie bringt sicher eine Verstärkung derartiger psychisch negativ wirkender Faktoren mit sich.

Einen Überblick über Ansätze und Befunde dieser Art findet sich in dem Handbuchartikel *Clinical Sensory Deprivation* von C.W. JACKSON (1969). Wir möchten aber auch auf eine recht frühe deutsche Arbeit von JACOB (1949), *Der Erlebniswandel bei Späterblindeten*, hinweisen.

Individualdiagnostische Möglichkeiten bietet die Deprivation – verbunden mit sozialer Isolation – schließlich bei solchen Störungen, von denen man annimmt, daß sie sozial bzw. kommunikativ verankert sind (z.B. Stottern, Torticollis). Bei derartigen Untersuchungen wird erkennbar, in welchem Umfang die Störungen durch Aufhebung der sozialen Kontrolle reduzierbar sind (ŠVÁB et al., 1972), was Rückschlüsse auf ihre Heilbarkeit zuläßt.

2. Therapeutischer Bereich

Obwohl auf therapeutische Einsatzmöglichkeiten der Deprivation im Rahmen der Psychiatrie schon relativ früh hingewiesen wurde (z.B. AZIMA und CRAMER, 1956), haben solche Anwendungen bisher einen relativ bescheidenen Raum innerhalb der Deprivationsforschung eingenommen (KEMPE et al., 1974). Prinzipiell lassen sich drei verschiedene Ansätze unterscheiden:
a) Deprivation als eigenständige therapeutische Maßnahme,
b) Deprivation als Hilfsmittel zur Erzeugung therapeutisch notwendiger Einstellungsveränderungen,
c) Deprivation zur Vorbereitung bzw. Verstärkung einer der eingeführten psychotherapeutischen Techniken.

Untersuchungen zum ersten Ansatz wurden schon relativ früh aufgenommen, stagnierten dann aber Mitte der 60er Jahre, ohne eine hinreichende empirische Basis für eine wissenschaftliche Evaluation erreicht zu haben. Seit etwa 1970 traten demgegenüber Untersuchungen in den Vordergrund, die dem 2. und 3. Bereich zuzuordnen sind. Eine Monographie von P. SUEDFELD, *Therapeutic uses of reduced stimulation*, wird voraussichtlich 1980 erscheinen und eine detaillierte Übersicht über den derzeitigen Erkenntnisstand bieten.

Deprivation als eigenständige therapeutische Maßnahme – auch als „Anaclitische Therapie" bekannt – wurde vor allem von AZIMA und CRAMER (1956, 1957) in Kanada sowie von der Gruppe um ADAMS in den USA (z.B. COOPER et al., 1965) erprobt. Die zum Teil explorativen, zum Teil aber auch gut kontrollierten Studien belegen, daß bei psychiatrischen Patienten überdauernde positive Effekte nach Deprivation überwiegen. Symptomreduktion, Verbesserung des Selbstkonzeptes und ein weniger rigider Gebrauch von Abwehrmechanismen machten den Unterschied gegenüber der Kontrollgruppe aus. Die stärksten Verbesserungen schienen sich bei solchen Patienten einzustellen, die vorher am meisten gestört waren. – Es liegen allerdings auch Studien vor, in denen keine derartigen Verbesserungen beobachtet werden konnten (z.B. CLEVELAND et al., 1963), und es fehlen hinreichende katamnestische Untersuchungen.

Besondere Beachtung verdient sicher eine Studie von SCHECHTER et al. (1970), in der drei 5jährige autistische Knaben für Perioden von 40 bis zu 73 Tagen (!) depriviert wurden und mit ausgeprägten und anhaltenden Verhaltensverbesserungen reagierten. Während sie vor der Deprivationserfahrung den Kontakt mit den Eltern wie mit den Therapeuten vermieden, zeigten sie danach spontanes Annäherungsverhalten, suchten Zärtlichkeiten und stellten erheblich mehr Augenkontakt her. Sie adaptierten sich in der Folge recht gut an das Familienleben und konnten den Kindergarten besuchen. Angesichts der enorm langen Deprivationsperioden, denen die Kinder ausgesetzt wurden, ist die Mitteilung der Autoren wichtig, daß die Kinder positiv auf den Reizentzug reagierten und keine Anzeichen von Streß oder Angst erkennen ließen.

Auch der Ansatz, *Deprivation als Hilfsmittel zur Erzeugung von Einstellungsveränderungen* zu benutzen, wurde in mehreren Studien der Gruppe um ADAMS erkundet (z.B. ADAMS et al., 1972). Den Hauptanteil an der Erforschung dieser Anwendungsmöglichkeit aber hat P. SUEDFELD, der nach Übernahme des Lehrstuhls an der Universität von Britisch-Kolumbien in Kanada eine große Anzahl solcher Studien initiiert hat. Ausgehend von Untersuchungen zur Meinungsbeeinflussung unter Deprivationsbedingungen (SUEDFELD, 1963, 1964; SUEDFELD und VERNON, 1966) stellte SUEDFELD (1972) eine Zwei-Komponenten-Theorie der Einstellungsveränderung unter Deprivation auf (s.o.) und widmete sich in der letzten Zeit der Erprobung solcher Techniken mit Bezug auf zwei relativ gut quantifizierbare Zielsymptome, „Schlangenphobie" und „Rauchen mit Suchtcharakter". Besonders hervorzuheben ist eine Untersuchung, in der 72 starke Gewohnheitsraucher behandelt wurden (SUEFELD und IKARD, 1974). Zwei Experimentalgruppen (SD mit und ohne Antirauchinformation) wurden zwei Kontrollgruppen (Heimkontrollgruppe mit Antirauchinformation, unbehandelte Kontrollgruppe) gegenübergestellt. Beide Experimentalgruppen unterzogen sich einer 24stündigen sensorischen Deprivation, die mit einem ebensolangen Rauchverzicht gekoppelt war. Die therapeutische Wirksamkeit der beiden Experimentalbedingungen war im Vergleich zu der anderer Rauchertherapien überdurchschnittlich gut:
a) Unittelbar nach Behandlung lag die mittlere Reduktionsrate bei nahezu 100%,
b) nach einem Jahr betrug sie 52%, wobei 27% der Probanden noch abstinent waren und
c) von den nach 2 Jahren noch erreichbaren 18 Versuchspersonen waren immerhin noch 7 abstinent geblieben.

Entgegen der Erwartung hatte aber in diesem Experiment die Darbietung der Antirauchinformation keine bedeutsame Steigerung des therapeutischen Effektes zur Folge.

Wenn auch durch dieses Resultat die theoretischen Annahmen SUEDFELDS zunächst in Frage gestellt werden, kommt – weitere Replikationen vorausgesetzt – diesem therapeutischen Ansatz bezüglich seiner Effektivität ein hoher

Stellenwert zu, zumal Modifikationen für eine Reihe anderer Symptombereiche relativ leicht möglich erscheinen.

Noch verhältnismäßig wenig erprobt ist der Ansatz, *Deprivation zur Vorbereitung oder Verstärkung einer der eingeführten psychotherapeutischen Techniken* zu benutzen. In Anbetracht der Tatsache, daß sich schon FREUD Gedanken über die Auswirkungen sensorischer Einschränkungen auf die Ich-Funktionen gemacht hat, und das klassische psychoanalytische Setting eine Reihe von gemeinsamen Komponenten mit SD-Bedingungen hat (Liegen des Patienten, Therapeut außerhalb des Blickfelds, Verdunkelung, freie Assoziation), ist die Anregung, psychoanalytische Therapie in Kombination mit sensorischer Deprivation durchzuführen, sicher eine Erprobung wert (KUBZANSKY und LEIDERMAN, 1961). Schon in den Jahren 1961 bis 1967 haben GROSS und ŠVÁB (1969) nach Möglichkeiten einer Intensivierung therapeutischer Einflußnahme gesucht und die Möglichkeit einer zeitweiligen Verstärkung des Abhängigkeitsverhältnisses zwischen Patient und Therapeut durch sensorische Deprivation gesehen.

Die meisten Erfahrungen mit einer solchen Anwendung der sensorischen Deprivation sammelte die Gruppe um ADAMS (z.B. COOPER et al., 1975). Sie versuchten, die erhöhte Aufnahmebereitschaft für verbale Reize zu nutzen, um Widerstände im Verlauf der Therapie zu überwinden, erhöhte Einsicht und Selbstwahrnehmung zu vermitteln und den Prozeß der Persönlichkeitsänderung zu beschleunigen (ADAMS et al., 1966). Diese Gruppe behandelte zuletzt hypochondrische Patienten, indem – eingeschlossen in zwei therapeutische Sitzungen – $2^1/_2$ Stunden sensorische Deprivation appliziert wurde. Der erste therapeutische Kontakt diente dazu, das SD-Erlebnis vorzubereiten und zu strukturieren; in der sich an die Deprivation anschließenden Sitzung wurden demgegenüber soziale Rollen geübt und verstärkt, die dem schlecht angepaßten interpersonalen Verhalten entgegenstanden, welches die Patienten vorher gezeigt hatten. Eine Reduktion passiv-feindseligen Verhaltens und eine Abnahme der Arztbesuche in der Folge waren die Effekte, die nach 30 Tagen gesichert werden konnten.

Eine Kombination von sensorischer Deprivation mit der verhaltenstherapeutischen Desensibilisierungstechnik erprobten SUEDFELD und SMITH (1973) sowie SUEDFELD und BUCHANAN (1974) mit recht gutem Erfolg an Phobikern. Über eine entsprechende Erkundungsstudie in Deutschland berichteten vor kurzem auch SCHMIDTKE et al. (1977).

Insgesamt ist zu den therapeutischen Anwendungen der Deprivation zu bemerken, daß zwar alle drei Ansätze in bestimmtem Kontext erfolgversprechende Möglichkeiten erkennen lassen, daß aber bisher keiner von ihnen so weit entwickelt und empirisch überprüft worden ist, daß eine abschließende Bewertung möglich wäre. Obwohl in den letzten Jahren eine relative Zunahme der Forschungsbemühungen um therapeutische Nutzungsmöglichkeiten der Deprivation zu erkennen ist, finden wir es bedauerlich, daß solche Projekte bisher noch auf zu wenige Forschungsgruppen beschränkt blieben.

D. Theorien zur Erklärung der Deprivationswirkungen

Es gibt wenige Bereiche der Psychologie, in der eine ähnlich große Vielfalt konkurrierender Theoriekonzepte besteht, wie bei der Erklärung der Wirkungen, die *Deprivationen in früher Kindheit* zur Folge haben. Für nahezu alle gängigen Theorien des menschlichen und tierischen Verhaltens wurde in diesem Feld nach Belegen für die jeweiligen Annahmen gesucht. Diskussionen zwischen den Vertretern der konkurrierenden Erklärungsmodelle wurden zum Teil in überzogener Form geführt, wobei man sich nicht selten wechselseitig auf Positionen festlegte, die in dieser Form gar nicht vertreten worden waren. „Die verschiedenen theoretischen Ansätze beziehen sich jeweils nur auf bestimmte Teilaspekte eines sehr komplexen Geschehens, dessen vollständige Analyse vermittels einer einheitlichen Theorie heutzutage noch außerhalb der Möglichkeiten liegt", stellen LANGMEIER und MATĚJČEK (1977) zutreffend fest und versuchen, die einzelnen Erklärungsmodelle bestimmten differenten Bereichen der kindlichen Entwicklung zuzuordnen. Wenn auch einer solchen schwerpunktmäßigen, differentiellen Zuordnung in der Tendenz zuzustimmen ist, harmonisiert diese Darstellung den Stand der kontroversen Diskussion doch zu sehr und trägt dem Selbstverständnis und den zumindest implizit vertretenen Annahmen über die jeweiligen Geltungsbereiche der Erklärungsmodelle zu wenig Rechnung. Polemisch stellt RUTTER (1971) fest: „Unsere Theorien über die Bedeutsamkeit der Familie haben sich multipliziert und sind immer bestimmter und sicherer geworden, lange bevor wir eigentlich wußten, welches die Fakten sein würden, die die Theorien erklären sollten".

Ähnliche Schwierigkeiten, eine fruchtbare Wechselbeziehung zwischen induktiver Faktensammlung und deduktiver Hypothesenbildung zu erreichen, ergaben sich – wenn auch gerade in umgekehrter Richtung – auch bei der Erforschung von *Deprivationswirkungen an Erwachsenen*. Ein im Jahre 1959 in Amerika durchgeführtes Symposion hatte bezeichnenderweise den Titel „Facts in search of a theory". Im Jahre 1969 konstatiert ZUCKERMAN – zumindest für die zurückliegenden Jahre – noch den gleichen Tatbestand: „... die Befunde sind in der Zwischenzeit geometrisch angestiegen, während die Theorien statisch geblieben sind. Obwohl einige der Studien Relevanz für die eine oder die andere Theorie besitzen, wurden nur wenige Untersuchungen daraufhin geplant, den relativen Wert der Theorien zur Voraussage der Daten zu prüfen. Die experimentelle Deprivationsforschung ist immer noch eher induktiv als deduktiv und es wurde viel Zeit verschwendet, hinter irrelevanten Befunden herzujagen, wo es besser gewesen wäre, wichtigere theoretische Belange zu verfolgen".

In einer glücklicheren Lage ist demgegenüber die *experimentelle Deprivationsforschung an Tieren*, wo ethische Bedenken das Experimentieren nicht in dem Maße einschränkten, wie dies im Humanbereich der Fall ist. Zu verweisen ist hier auf die beispielhaften Experimentalserien der Gruppe um HARLOW (z.B. HARLOW und HARLOW, 1971) und die alle Tierspezies umfassende theoretische Übersicht von BRONFENBRENNER (1971).

Wir sehen uns außerstande, hier eine bewertende Gegenüberstellung der verschiedenen theoretischen Erklärungsmodelle vorzunehmen, dies ist beim gegenwärtigen Erkenntnisstand auch noch kaum in gesicherter Form möglich. Natürlich bestehen Unterschiede, inwieweit es den einzelnen theoretischen Positionen bisher gelungen ist, empirische Belege zu sammeln und inwieweit diese als spezifisch für das jeweilige Modell anzusehen sind, doch reichen solche Kriterien bei dem sehr unterschiedlichen Komplexitätsgrad der theoretischen

Annahmen zur Bewertung nicht aus. Wir beschränken uns deshalb darauf, dem interessierten Leser Hinweise zu geben, wo er relativ geschlossene Darstellungen der wichtigsten theoretischen Positionen findet, und werden nur einen neurophysiologisch orientierten Erklärungsansatz darstellen, der aufgrund empirischer Belege in allen drei Teilbereichen der Deprivationsforschung zu analogen, wenn auch noch unterschiedlich ausformulierten Annahmen führte.

Einen umfassenden Überblick über die im Brennpunkt der Diskussion stehenden *Theorien zur Deprivation in früher Kindheit* vermittelt AINSWORTH (1969). Sie stellt die *psychoanalytischen Ansätze* (Theorie der Ich-Entwicklung/Theorie der Objektbeziehungen) ebenso dar wie die *Theorien des sozialen Lernens* (Abhängigkeit als abgeleiteter Antrieb/Abhängigkeit als erlerntes Verhalten) und den *ethologisch orientierten Ansatz von* BOWLBY/AINSWORTH. Dieser Übersicht sind auch alle relevanten Primärquellen zu entnehmen, so daß sich diese Arbeit als Ausgangspunkt für eine theoretische Orientierung gut eignet. Zu verweisen ist darüber hinaus auf eine kürzlich erschienene Darstellung der letztgenannten Theorie von BOWLBY (1977a, b).

Die im Rahmen der *Deprivationsforschung an Erwachsenen* entstandenen Modelle lassen sich im wesentlichen auf die *neurophysiologischen,* die *informationstheoretischen* und die *psychologischen* Erklärungsansätze reduzieren, welche sozialpsychologische Aspekte des Experimentes in den Vordergrund stellen. Einen guten Einstieg dazu vermitteln die Kapitel von ZUCKERMAN (1969) und SUEDFELD (1969b).

Bei dem von uns angeführten neurophysiologischen Erklärungsmodell handelt es sich um die „Theorie des optimalen Stimulationsniveaus" von ZUCKERMAN (1969), die sich im Bereich der experimentellen Deprivationsforschung an Erwachsenen als relativ fruchtbar erwiesen hat. Diese Theorie stützt sich u.a. auf Annahmen von HEBB (1955), LINDSLEY (1961) und ist dem „Sensoristase-Modell" von SCHULTZ (1965) eng verwandt. Beide beruhen im wesentlichen auf folgenden Postulaten:

a) Das aktuelle Arousalniveau eines Individuums ist abhängig von der Art und Anzahl zuströmender Reize.
b) Stärke, Komplexität, Unvorhersagbarkeit, Inkongruenz und assoziierte Emotionen von Reizen wirken erhöhend.
c) Konstanz, Wiederholung und Bekanntheit wirken erniedrigend auf das Arousalniveau.
d) Jedes Individuum besitzt charakteristische optimale Stimulations- (OLS) und Arousal-Niveaus (OLA) für motorische und kognitive Leistungen wie für eine positive emotionale Gestimmtheit.
e) Diese individualspezifischen OLS und OLA variieren zusätzlich mit Faktoren wie z.B. Alter, vorausgegangenem Stimulationsniveau, Aufgabenanforderung und Tagesrhythmus.

Analoge Befunde sicherte FANTZ (1961) auch bei kleinen Kindern, die ihre Bevorzugung variabler, strukturierter und mehrdimensionaler Reize im Versuch ebenfalls durch operantes Verhalten erkennen ließen. Auch an Tieren konnte die „belohnende Wirkung" veränderter Stimulation nachgewiesen werden (BUTLER, 1961; ISAAC, 1962), und bereits 1960 kam man auch hier zur Konzeption eines „optimalen Stimulationsniveaus" (STEWART, 1960; WILSON, 1962). Unter

Bezug auf diese Befunde betrachtet z.B. CASLER (1968) die Situation institutionalisierter Kinder unter folgenden Annahmen:
a) Die meisten Heimkinder leben in einer Umgebung mit einem wenig variablen Reizangebot.
b) Wenn sich ein Reiz nicht verändert, verliert er schnell seine Fähigkeit zu stimulieren.
c) Ohne einen solchen aktivierenden Einfluß durch die retikuläre Formation wird das psychologische Funktionieren drastisch erschwert.

Sicher ist mit solchen Annahmen nur ein erstes, vorläufiges und noch sehr unvollständiges Gerüst geschaffen, doch passen eine Vielzahl auch lerntheoretischer Befunde zu diesen Annahmen (CASLER, 1968), und es bieten sich gute Ansätze zur Hypothesenbildung.

Betrachtet man die Entwicklung, die für den Gesamtbereich der Deprivationsforschung zu erkennen ist, so sind *Anzeichen einer Stagnation* nicht zu übersehen. Vor allem im Humanbereich ist die Diskrepanz zwischen dem experimentell Realisierbaren und dem aufgrund bisheriger begrenzter Einblicke notwendig erscheinenden Komplexitätsniveau der Versuchsanlage besonders groß. Neben dem fast unerschwinglichen Aufwand eines solchen Experimentierens wirkt sich auch das Fehlen angemessener statistischer Verfahren behindernd aus. Die Entwicklung ist zur Zeit eher dadurch gekennzeichnet, daß erprobte Vorgehensweisen in anderen – zum Teil periphereren – Bereichen eingesetzt werden, als daß Fortschritte oder gar Durchbrüche bei zentralen Fragestellungen erzielt werden.

Eine gerade unter theoretischen Gesichtspunkten sehr sinnvolle Bereicherung stellte in der experimentellen Deprivationsforschung z.B. die Einbeziehung der Bedingung „Überstimulation" in die Versuchspläne dar, doch blieben grundlagenorientierte Ansätze dieser Art bisher noch spärlich. Gegenwärtige Tendenzen des Wissenschaftsverständnisses stehen darüber hinaus – nicht nur in Deutschland – entsprechenden Anstrengungen in dieser Richtung entgegen, so daß die zukünftige Entwicklung nur schwer absehbar ist.

Literatur

Abrahams, M.J., Whitlock, F.A.: Childhood experience and depression. Br. J. Psychiatry **115**, 883 (1969)

Adams, H.B., Robertson, M.H., Cooper, G.D.: Sensory deprivation and personality change. J. Nerv. Ment. Dis. **143**, 256 (1966)

Adams, H.B., Cooper, G.D., Carrera, R.N.: Individual differences in behavioral reactions of psychiatric patients to brief partial sensory deprivation. Percept. Mot. Skills **34**, 199 (1972)

Adelson, E., Fraiberg, S.: Gross motor development in infants blind from birth. Child Dev. **45**, 114 (1974)

Ainsworth, M.D.: The effects of maternal deprivation: A review of findings and controversy in the context of research strategy. In: Deprivation of maternal care: A reassessment of its effects. Genf: WHO 1962

Ainsworth, M.D.: Object relations, dependency and attachment: A theoretical review of the infant-mother relationship. Child Dev. **40**, 969 (1969)

Anderson, E.W.: Abnormal mental states in survivors, with special reference to collective hallucinations. J. R. Nav. Med. Serv. **28**, 361 (1942)

Azima, H., Cramer, F.J.: Effects of partial perceptual isolation in mentally disturbed individuals. Dis. Nerv. Syst. **17**, 117 (1956)

Azima, H., Cramer, F.J.: Studies on perceptual isolation. Dis. Nerv. Syst. Monogr. Suppl. **18**, 80 (1957)
Bakwin, H.: Loneliness in infants. Am. J. Dis. Child **63**, 30 (1942)
Barnett, C., Leiderman, P., Grobstein, R., Klaus, M.: Neonatal separation: The maternal side of interactional deprivation. Pediatrics **45**, 197 (1970)
Bell, R.Q.: A reinterpretation of the direction of effects in studies of socialization. Psychol. Rev. **75**, 81 (1968)
Bell, R.Q.: Stimulus control of parent or caretaker behavior by offsprings. Dev. Psychobiol. **4**, 63 (1971)
Bennet, G.: Medical and psychological problems in the 1972 singlehanded transatlantic yacht race. Lancet **1973 II**, 747
Biase, D.V., Zuckerman, M.: Sex differences in stress response to total and partial sensory deprivation. Psychosom. Med. **29**, 380 (1967)
Biermann, G., Biermann, R.: Die Mutter-Kind-Situation in den Krankenhäusern der Bundesrepublik (Ergebnisse einer Umfrage). Jahrbuch der Psychohygiene **1**, 13 (1973)
Birtchnell, J.: Depression in relation to early and recent parent death. Br. J. Psychiatr. **116**, 299 (1970)
Blumenbach, J.F.: Handbuch der Naturgeschichte. 9. Ausg., Göttingen: 1814
Bowlby, J.: Forty-four juvenile thieves. Int. J. Psychoanal. **25**, 19 (1944)
Bowlby, J.: Forty-four juvenile thieves: their characters and home-life. Baillère: Tindall & Cox, 1946
Bowlby, J.: Maternal care and mental health. Genf: WHO 1951
Bowlby, J.: Can I leave my Baby? London: National Assoc. for Mental Health 1958
Bowlby, J.: Attachment and loss: I. attachment. London, New York: Hogarth Press 1969
Bowlby, J.: Mutterliebe und kindliche Entwicklung. München, Basel: Reinhard 1972
Bowlby, J.: The making and breaking of affectional bonds. I. Aetiology and psychopathology in the light of attachment theory. Br. J. Psychiatr. **130**, 201 (1977a)
Bowlby, J.: The making and breaking of affectional bonds. II. Some principles of psychotherapy. Br. J. Psychiatr. **130**, 421 (1977b)
Brandt, W.: Flüchtlingskinder. Wissenschaftliche Jugendkunde, Heft 6. München: Barth 1964
Brasel, J.A.: Review of findings in patients with emotional deprivation. In: Endocrine aspects of malnutrition – marasmus, kwashiorkor and psychosocial deprivation. Gardner, L.J., Amacher, P. (Hrsg.), S. 115. Santa Ynez 1973
Brennemann, J.: The infant ward. Am. J. Dis. Child **43**, 577 (1932)
Bronfenbrenner, U.: Early deprivation in mammals: A cross-species analysis. In: Early experience and behavior. Newton, G., Levine, S. (Hrsg.). Springfield: Thomas 1971
Brown, F.: Depression and childhood bereavement. J. Ment. Sci **107**, 754 (1961)
Brown, G.M.: Endocrine aspects of psychosocial dwarfism. In: Hormones, Behavior and Psychopathology. Sachar, E.J. (Hrsg.), S. 253. New York: 1976
Burlingham, D.: Hearing and its role in the development of the blind. Psychoanal. Study Child **19**, 95 (1964)
Burlingham, D., Freud, A.: Young children in war time: a year's work in a residential war nursery. London: Allen & Unwin 1942
Butler, R.A.: The responsiveness of rhesus monkeys to motion pictures. J. Gen. Psychol. **98**, 239 (1961)
Caplan, M.G.: Test correlates and family history of childhood depression. Unpubl. doctoral dissertation McGill Univ. 1967
Caplan, M.G., Douglas, V.J.: Incidence of parental loss in children with depressed mood. J. Child. Psychol. Psychiatry **10**, 225 (1969)
Casler, L.: The effects of extra tactile stimulation on a group of institutionalized infants. Genet. Psychol. Monogr. **71**, 137 (1965a)
Casler, L.: The effects of supplementary verbal stimulation on a group of institutionalized infants. J. Child Psychol. Psychiatry **6**, 19 (1965b)
Casler, L.: Perceptual deprivation in institutional settings. In: Early experience and behavior. Newton, G., Levine, S. (Hrsg.), Kap. 17. Springfield: Thomas 1968
Chapin, H.D.: Are institutions for infants necessary? J.A.M.A. **64**, 1 (1915)
Clancy, H., McBride, G.: The autistic process and its treatment. J. Child Psychol. Psychiatry **10**, 233 (1969)

Clancy, H., McBride, G.: The isolation syndrome in childhood. Dev. Med. Child. Neurol. **17**, 198 (1975)
Cleveland, S.E., Reitman, E.E., Bentinck, C.: Therapeutic effectiveness of sensory deprivation. Arch. Gen. Psychiatry **8**, 455 (1963)
Coleman, R.W., Provence, S.: Environmental retardation (hospitalism) in infants living in families. Pediatrics **19**, 285 (1957)
Collins, N.: The analysis of socialization in sheep and goats. Ecology **37**, 228 (1956)
Comenius, J.A.: The great didactic. London: Keating 1896 (Tschechische Originalausg. 1657)
Comer, N.L., Madow, L., Dixon, J.J.: Observations of sensory deprivation in a life-treatening situation. Am. J. Psychiatry **124**, 164 (1967)
Cooper, G.D., Adams, H.B., Cohen, L.D.: Personality changes after sensory deprivation. J. Nerv. Ment. Dis. **140**, 103 (1965)
Cooper, G.D., Adams, H.B., Dickinson, J.R., York, M.W.: Interviewer's role-playing and responses to sensory deprivation: A clinical demonstration. Percept. Mot. Skills **40**, 291 (1975)
Corter, C., Bow, J.: The mother's response to separation as a function of her infants sex and vocal distress. Child Dev. **47**, 872 (1976)
Critchley, M.: Shipwreck-survivors. A medical study. London: Churchill 1943
Curtis, G.C., Zuckerman, M.A.: Psychopathological reaction precipitated by sensory deprivation. Am. J. Psychiatry **125**, 255 (1968)
Czerny, A.: Der Arzt als Erzieher des Kindes. Bd. VI. Leipzig: Deuticke 1922
Dennehy, C.M.: Childhood bereavement and psychiatric illness. Br. J. Psychiatry **112**, 1049 (1966)
Douglas, J.W.B.: Broken families and child behaviour. J. R. Coll. Physicians Lond. **4**, 203 (1970)
Douglas, J.W.B., Turner, R.K.: The association of anxiety provoking events in early childhood with enuresis. Proc. Fifth Int. Sci. Meeting of Int. Epid. Assn. Sovremena Adinistracija, Belgrad, 1970
Durfee, H., Wolf, K.: Anstaltspflege und Entwicklung im ersten Lebensjahr. Zeitschr. f. Kinderforschung **42**, 273 (1934)
Elmer, E., Gregg, G.: Developmental characteristics of abused children. Pediatrics **40**, 596 (1967)
Fantz, R.L.: A method for studying depth perception in infants under 6 month of age. Psychol. Record. **11**, 27 (1961)
Feuerbach, A.J.P. von: Kaspar Hauser, Beispiel eines Verbrechens am Seelenleben des Menschen. Ansbach: Dollfuss 1832
Flint, B.: The child and the institution: a study of deprivation and recovery. Toronto: Univ. of Toronto Press 1966
Folkers, J.: Elterninitiative als Hilfe für Kinder im Krankenhaus. Jahrbuch der Psychohygiene **1**, p. 51 (1973)
Fowler, W.: How adult/child ratios influence infant-development. Interchange **6**, 17 (1975)
Fraiberg, S.: Studies in the ego development of the congenitally blind child. Psychoanal. Study Child **21**, 113 (1964)
Freedman, D.A.: Congenital and perinatal sensory deprivations: Their effect on the capacity to experience affect. Psychoanal. Q. **44**, 62 (1975)
Freedman, D.A., Brown, S.L.: On the role of coenesthetic stimulation in the development of psychic structure. Psychoanal. Q. **37**, 418 (1968)
Freedman, D.G. Smiling in blind infants and the issue of innate versus acquired. J. Child Psychol. Psychiatry **5**, 171 (1964)
Freud, W.: Über den Hospitalismus der Säuglinge. Ergeb. Inn. Med. Kinderheilkd. **6**, 333 (1910)
Gardener, L.J.: The endocrinology of abuse dwarfism. Am. J. Dis. Child. **131**, 505 (1977)
Gay, M.J., Tonge, W.L.: The late effects of loss of parents in childhood. Br. J. Psychiatry **113**, 753 (1967)
Gewirtz, J.L.: A learning analysis of the effects of normal stimulation, privation and deprivation on the acquisition of social motivation and attachment. In: Determinants of Human Behaviour. Foss, B.M. (Hrsg.), S. 213. London: Methuen 1961
Goldfarb, W.: Effects of psychological deprivation in infancy and subsequent stimulation. Am. J. Psychiatry **102**, 18 (1945)
Graham, P., George, S.: Childrens response to parental illness: individual differences. J. Psychosom. Res. **16**, 251 (1972)
Gross, J., Šváb, L.: Die experimentelle sensorische Deprivation als Modellsituation der psychotherapeutischen Beziehung. Nervenarzt **40**, 21 (1969)

Gross, J., Kempe, P., Reimer, Ch.: Wahn bei sensorischer Deprivation und Isolation. In: Wahn. Schulte, W., Toelle, R. (Hrsg.). Stuttgart: Thieme 1972

Haase, H.J.: Zum Verständnis paranoider und paranoid-halluzinatorischer Psychosen am Beispiel alleinstehender Frauen. Nervenarzt **34**, 315 (1963)

Harlow, H.F., Harlow, M.K.: Psychopathology in monkeys. In: Experimental psychopathology recent research and theory. Kimmel, H.D. (Hrsg.). New York, London: Academic Press 1971

Hebb, D.O.: Drives and the CNS (conceptual nervous system). Psychol. Rev. **62**, 243 (1955)

Held, R.: Exposure-history as a factor in maintaining stability of perception and coordination. J. Nerv. Ment. Dis. **132**, 26 (1961)

Hellbrügge, T.: Das sollten Eltern heute wissen. 3. Aufl. München: Kindler 1975

Hersher, L., Moore, A., Richmond, J.: Effects of postpartum separation of mother and kid on maternal care in the domestic goat. Science **128**, 1342 (1958)

Hill, O.W.: Childhood bereavement and adult psychiatric disturbance. J. Psychosom. Res. **16**, 357 (1972)

Hill, O.W., Price, J.S.: Childhood bereavement and adult depression. Br. J. Psychiatry **113**, 743 (1967)

Isaac, W.: Evidence for a sensory drive in monkeys. Psychol. Rep. **11**, 175 (1962)

Jackson, C.W.: Clinical sensory deprivation. In: Sensory deprivation, 15 years of research. Zubek, J.P. (Hrsg.). New York: Appleton, Meredith 1969

Jacob, H.J.: Der Erlebniswandel bei Späterblindeten. Abhandlungen für Psychiatrie, Psychologie, Psychopathologie und ihre Grenzgebiete. Band 1. Hamburg: Nölke 1949

Janzarik, W.: Über das Kontaktmangelparanoid des höheren Alters und den Syndromcharakter schizophrenen Krankseins. Nervenarzt **44**, 515 (1973)

Jones, A.: Stimulus-seeking behavior. In: Sensory deprivation, 15 years of research. Zubek, J.P. (Hrsg.). New York: Appleton, Meredith 1969

Kagan, G., Klein, R.E.: Cross cultural perspectives on early development. Am. Psychologist **28**, 947 (1973)

Kempe, P.: Bedingungen halluzinatorischer Phänomene bei Experimenten mit sensorischer Deprivation. Unpubl. Diss., Kiel: 1973

Kempe, P., Reimer, Ch.: Halluzinatorische Phänomene bei Reizentzug. Nervenarzt **47**, 701 (1976)

Kempe, P., Schönberger, J., Gross, J.: Sensorische Deprivation als Methode in der Psychiatrie. Nervenarzt **45**, 561 (1977)

Kempe, P., Closs, C., Andresen, B., Stemmler, G.: Aggression in einer reizverarmten Modellsituation und ihre physiologischen und biochemischen Korrelate. Unveröff. Abschlußbericht Sonderforschungsbereich 115, Projekt A7 Hamburg, Mai 1977

Kennel, J.H., Jerauld, R., Wolfe, H., Chesler, D., Kreger, N.C., McAlpine, W., Steffa, M., Klaus, M.H.: Maternal behavior one year after early and extended post-partum contact. Dev. Med. Child Neurol. **16**, 172 (1974)

Klackenberg, G.: Studies in maternal deprivation in infants homes. Acta Paediatr. Scand. **45**, 1 (1956)

Klaus, M.H., Kennel, J.: Mothers separated from their newborn infants. Pediatr. Clin. North Am. **17**, 1015 (1970)

Klaus, M.H., Kennel, J.H.: Auswirkungen früher Kontakte zwischen Mutter und Neugeborenem auf die spätere Mutter-Kind-Beziehung. In: Jahrbuch der Psychohygiene. Biermann, G. (Hrsg.), Bd. I. S. 100. München, Basel: Reinhardt 1973

Klaus, M.H., Jerauld, R., Kreger, N., McAlpine, W., Steffa, M., Kennel, J.: Maternal attachment: importance of the first post-partum days. New Engl. J. Med. **286**, 460 (1972)

Koehler, O.: „Wolfskinder", Affen im Haus und vergleichende Verhaltensforschung. Folia Phoniatr. (Basel) **4**, 29 (1952)

Köttgen, U.: Die Bedeutung der Reizverarmung, Monotonie, für die frühkindliche geistige Entwicklung. Z. Kinderheilkd. **91**, 247 (1964)

Koluchová, J.: Severe deprivation in twins. J. Child Psychol. Psychiatry **13**, 107 (1972)

Koluchová, J.: The further development of twins after severe and prolonged deprivation: a second report. J. of Child Psychol. Psychiatry **17**, 181 (1976)

Korner, A.F., Grobstein, R.: Visual alertness as related to soothing in neonates: implications for maternal stimulation at early deprivation. Child Dev. **37**, 867 (1966)

Kubzansky, E., Leiderman, P.H.: Sensory deprivation: an overview. In: Sensory deprivation. Solo-

mon, P., Kubzansky, P.E., Leiderman, P.H., Mendelson, J.H., Trumbull, R., Wexler, D. (Hrsg.). Cambridge, Mass.: Harvard Univ. Press 1961
Langmeier, L., Matějček, Z.: Psychische Deprivation im Kindesalter. Kinder ohne Liebe. München, Wien, Baltimore: Urban & Schwarzenberg 1977
Lehr, U.: Mutter-Kind-Beziehung im Wochenbett, Eltern-Kind-Beziehung in der ersten Lebenszeit. Vortrag am 23. 2. 1978, Kongreß für Fachärzte der Frauenheilkunde und Geburtshilfe, Mainz: 1978
Leonhard, K.: Kaspar Hauser und die moderne Kenntnis des Hospitalismus. Confin. Psychiatr. **13**, 213 (1970)
Lesser, S.R., Easser, B.R.: Personality differences in the perceptually handicapped. J. Am. Acad. Child Psychiatry **11**, 458 (1972)
Lindsley, D.B.: Common factors in sensory deprivation, sensory distortion and sensory overload. In: Sensory deprivation. Solomon, P. et al. (eds.), S. 174. Cambridge: Harvard University Press 1961
Linné, K. von: System der Natur. Bd. I., Nürnberg: Bauer 1774
Lowrey, L.G.: Personality distortion and early institutional care. Am. J. Orthopsychiatry **10**, 576 (1940)
Malson, L., Itard, J., Mannon, O.: Die wilden Kinder. Frankfurt/M.: Suhrkamp 1972
Matějček, Z.: Die langfristige Beobachtung der Entwicklung von Kleinkindern in Heimen in der CSSR. In: Jahrbuch der Psychohygiene. Biermann, G. (Hrsg.), Bd. I, S. 171, 1973
Meierhofer, M.: Entwicklungsprobleme bei sozial benachteiligten Kindern in den ersten Lebensjahren. In: Jahrbuch der Psychohygine. Biermann, G. (Hrsg.). Bd. I. München, Basel: Reinhardt 1973
Mende, W., Ploeger, A.: Das Verhalten und Erleben von Bergleuten in der Extrembelastung des Eingeschlossenseins. Nervenarzt **37**, 209 (1966)
Meyer, J.E.: Pers. Mitteilung 1978
Money, J.: The syndrome of abuse dwarfism (psychosocial dwarfism or reversible hyposomatotropism). Am. J. Dis. Child. **131**, 508 (1977)
Munro, A.: Parental deprivation in depressive patients. Br. J. Psychiatry **112**, 443 (1966)
Munro, A., Griffiths, A.B.: Some psychiatric non-sequelae of childhood bereavement. Br. J. Psychiatry **115**, 305 (1969)
Nash, J.: The father in contemporary culture and current psychological literature. Child Dev. **36**, 261 (1965)
Ness, M.L.: The deaf child's conception of physical causality. J. Abnorm. Soc. Psychol. **69**, 669 (1964)
Osofsky, J.D.: Neonatal characteristics and mother-infant interaction in two observational situations. Child Dev. **47**, 1138 (1976)
Papoušek, H.: Experimental studies of appetitional behavior in human newborns and infants. In: Early behavior, comparative and developmental approach. Stevenson, H.W., Hess, E.H., Rheingold, H.L. (Hrsg.). Huntington, New York: Krieger 1975
Patton, R.G., Gardner, L.J.: The influence of family environment on growth. The syndrome of maternal deprivation. Pediatrics **30**, 957 (1962)
Patton, R.G., Gardner, L.J.: Growth failure in maternal deprivation. Springfield: Thomas 1963
Pechstein, J., Siebenmorgen, E., Weitsch, D.: Verlorene Kinder? Die Massenpflege in Säuglingsheimen. Ein Appell an die Gesellschaft. München: Kösel 1972
Peiper, A.: Kaspar-Hauser-Kinder, verwilderte Kinder (Wolfskinder). Mediz. **36**, 1411 (1958)
Pitts, F.N., Meyer, J., Brooks, M., Winokur, G.: Adult psychiatric illness assessed for childhood parental loss and psychiatric illness in family members – a study of 748 patients and 250 controls. Am. J. Psychiatry **121** (Suppl. 1) i–x (1965)
Ploeger, A.: Persönlichkeitseigentümliche Angstabwehr durch psychogene Halluzinose: Die „Realangst-Halluzinose". Z. Psychother. Med. Psychol. **18**, 134 (1968)
Powell, G.F., Brasel, J.A., Raiti, S., Blizzard, R.M.: Emotional deprivation and growth retardation simulating idiopathic hypopituitarism: II. Endocrinologic evaluation of the syndrome. New Engl. J. Med. **276**, 1279 (1967)
Powell, G.F., Hopwood, N.J., Barratt, E.S.: Growth hormone studies before and during catch-up growth in a child with emotional deprivation and short stature. J. Clin. Endocrinol. Metab. **37**, 674 (1973)

Pringle, M.L.K., Bossio, V.: Early prolonged separations and emotional adjustment. J. Child Psychol. Psychiatry **1**, 37 (1960)
Rainer, J.D., Altshuler, K.Z.: A psychiatric programme for the deaf: experiences and implications. Am. J. Psychiatry **127**, 1527 (1971)
Rauber, A.: Homo sapiens ferus oder die Zustände der Verwilderten. Leipzig: Denicke 1885
Rheingold, H.L.: The measurement of maternal care. Child Dev. **31**, 565 (1960)
Rheingold, H.L.: The effect of environmental stimulation upon social and exploratory behaviour in the human infant. In: Determinants of Infant Behaviour. Foss, B.M. (Hrsg.), Bd. I. S. 273. London: Methuen 1961
Rheingold, H.L., Gewirtz, J., Ross, H.: Social conditioning of vocalization in the infant. Comp. Physiol. Psychol. **52**, 68 (1959)
Robertson, J.: Kinder im Krankenhaus. München, Basel: Reinhardt 1974
Robertson, J., Robertson, J.: Young children in brief separation. Psychoanal. Study Child **26**, 264 (1971)
Ross, J.R., Braen, B.B., Chapurt, R.: Patterns of change in disturbed blind children in residential treatment. Children **14**, 217 (1967)
Rossi, A.M.: General methodical considerations. In: Sensory deprivation, 15 years of research. Zubek, J.P. (Hrsg.). New York: Appleton, Meredith 1969
Rothschild, B.: Incubator isolation as a possible contributing factor to the high incidence of emotional disturbance among prematurely born persons. J. Genet. Psychol. **110**, 287 (1967)
Rubenstein, J.: Maternal attentiveness and subsequent exploratory behavior in the infant. Child Dev. **38**, 1089 (1967)
Rutter, M.: Parent-child separation: psychological effects on the children. J. Child Psychol. Psychiatry **12**, 233 (1971)
Rutter, M.: Maternal deprivation reassessed. London: Penguin 1972
Sayegh, Y., Dennis, W.: The effect of supplementary experiences upon behavioral development of infants in institutions. Child Dev. **36**, 81 (1965)
Schaffer, H.R.: Changes in developmental quotient under two conditions of maternal separation. Br. J. Soc. Clin. Psychol. **4**, 39 (1965)
Schaffer, H.R.: Activity level as a constitutional determinant of infantile reaction to deprivation. Child Dev. **37**, 595 (1966)
Schaffer, H.R., Emerson, P.E.: The development of social attachments in infancy. Monogr. Soc. Res. Child. Dev. Vol. 29, No. 94 (1964)
Schaffer, H.R., Emerson, P.E.: The effects of experimentally administered stimulation on developmental quotients of infants. Br. J. Soc. Clin. Psychol. **7**, 61 (1968)
Schechter, M.D., Shurley, J.T., Toussieng, P.W., Maier, W.J.: Autism Revisited. J. Okla. State Med. Assoc. **63**, 297 (1970)
Schilder, P.: The image and appearance of the human body. New York: Intern. Univ. Press 1950
Schmalohr, E.: Frühe Mutterentbehrung bei Mensch und Tier, Entwicklungspsychologische Studie zur Psychohygiene der frühen Kindheit. München, Basel: Reinhard 1968
Schmidt-Kolmer, E.: Der Einfluß der Lebensbedingungen auf die Entwicklung des Kindes im Vorschulalter. Berlin: Akademie 1963
Schmidtke, A., Schaller, S., Altherr, P.: Kontaktdesensitivierung nach sozialer Deprivation als therapeutische Möglichkeit bei Phobien, dargestellt am Beispiel einer generalisierten Schlangenphobie. Nervenarzt **48**, 77 (1977)
Schultz, D.P.: Sensory restriction: effects of behavior. New York: Academic Press 1965
Schultz-Hencke, H.: Lehrbuch der analytischen Psychotherapie. Stuttgart: Thieme 1965
Silver, H.K., Finkelstein, M.: Deprivation dwarfism. J. Pediatr. **70**, 317 (1967)
Smith, M.A., Chethick, M.S.W., Adelson, E.: Differential assessment of "blindisms." Am. J. Orthopsychiatry **39**, 807 (1969)
Spitz, R.A.: Vom Säugling zum Kleinkind. Naturgeschichte der Mutter-Kind-Beziehung im ersten Lebensjahr. Stuttgart: Klett 1972
Stacey, M., Dearden, R., Pill, R., Robinson, D.: Hospitals, children and their families. The report of a Pilot-Study. Boston: Routledge & Kegan 1970
Stein, Z.A., Susser, M.: Nocturnal enuresis as a phenomenon of institutions. Dev. Med. Child Neurol. **8**, 677 (1966)

Stein, Z.A., Susser, M.: Nocturnal enuresis as a phenomenon of institutions. Dev. Med. Child
Steinert, E.: Beiträge zur Frage des Hospitalismus und der Rolle der individuellen Pflege für das Gedeihen im Säuglingsalter. Z. Kinderheilkd. **28**, 255 (1921)
Sterritt, G.M., Camp, B.W., Lipman, B.S.: Efffects of early auditory deprivation upon auditory and visual information processing. Percept. Mot. Skills **23**, 123 (1966)
Stewart, J.: Reinforcing effects of light as a function of intensity and reinforcement schedule. J. Comp. Physiol. Psychol. **53**, 187 (1960)
Stolz, L.M.: Father relations of war-born children. Stanford: Stanford Univ. Press 1954
Stumpfe, K.D.: Der Fall Kaspar Hauser. Prax. Kinderpsychol. Kinderpsychiatr. **18**, 292 (1969)
Solomon, P.: Sensory deprivation. In: Comprehensive Textbook of Psychiatry. Freedman, A.M., Kaplan, H.I., Sadock, B.J. (eds.), S. 253. Baltimore: Williams & Wilkins 1967
Suedfeld, P.: Conceptual and environmental complexity as factors in attitude change. ONR Tech. Rept. 1963
Suedfeld, P.: Attitude manipulation in restricted environments: I. Conceptual structure and response to propaganda. J. Abnorm Soc. Psychol. **68**, 242 (1964)
Suedfeld, P.: Changes in intellectual performance and in susceptibility to influence. In: Sensory deprivation, 15 years of research. Zubek, J.P. (Hrsg.). New York: Appleton, Meredith 1969a
Suedfeld, P.: Theoretical Formulations II. In: Sensory deprivation, 15 years of research. Zubek, J.P. (Hrsg.). New York: Appleton, Meredith 1969b
Suedfeld, P.: Attitude manipulation in restricted environments: V. Theory and Research. Symposium paper, 20th Int. Congr. Psychol., Tokyo: 1972
Suedfeld, P.: The benefits of boredom: sensory deprivation reconsidered. Am. Sci. **63**, 60 (1975)
Suedfeld, P., Buchanan, E.: Sensory deprivation and autocontrolled aversive stimulation in the reduction of snake avoidance. Can. J. Behav. Sci./Rev. Can. Sci. Comp. **6**, 105 (1974)
Suedfeld, P., Ikard, F.: Use of sensory deprivation in facilitating the reduction of cigarette smoking. J. Consult. Clin. Psychol. **42**, 888 (1974)
Suedfeld, P., Smith, C.A.: Positive incentive value of phobic stimuli after brief sensory deprivation: Preliminary report. Percept. Mot. Skills **36**, 320 (1973)
Suedfeld, P., Vernon, J.: Attitude manipulation in restricted environments: II. Conceptual structure and the internalization of propaganda received as a reward for compliance. J. Pers. Soc. Psychol. **3**, 585 (1966)
Suomi, S.J., Harlow, H.F., McKinney, W.T.: Monkey psychiatrists. Am. J. Psychiatry **128**, 927 (1972)
Šváb, L., Gross, J., Lángová, J.: Stuttering and social isolation J. Nerv. Ment. Dis. **155**, 1 (1972)
Thompson, W.R.: Early environmental influences on behavioral development. Am. J. Orthopsychiatry **30**, 306 (1960)
Vernon, D.T.A., Foley, J.M., Sipowicz, R.R., Schulman, J.L.: The psychological responses of children to hospitalization and illness. Springfield: Thomas 1965
Wagner, J.M.: Beiträge zur Philosophischen Anthropologie, Psychologie und den damit verwandten Wissenschaften. Bd. I. Wien: Schaumburg 1794
Weston, J.: The pathology of child abuse. In: The battered child. Helfer, R., Kempe, C. (Hrsg.). Chicago: Univ. Chicago Press 1968
White, B.L.: An experimental approach to the effects of experience of early human behaviour. In: Minnesota Symposia on Child Psycholgy. Hill, J.P. (Hrsg.), Bd. I. Minneapolis: Minnesota Press 1967
White, B.L.: Human infants: experience and psychological development. Englewood Cliffs: Prentice-Hall 1971
White, J.L., Labarba, R.C.: The effects of tactile and kinesthetic stimulation on neonatal development in the premature infant. Dev. Psychobiol. **9**, 569 (1976)
Whitten, C.F., Pettit, M.G., Fischhoff, J.: Evidence that growth failure from maternal deprivation is secondary to undereating. J. Am. Med. Assoc. **209**, 1675 (1969)
Widdowson, E.M.: Mental contentment and physical growth. Lancet **1**, 1316 (1951)
Williams, C.: Behavior disorders in handicapped children. Dev. Med. Child Neurol. **10**, 736 (1969)
Wilson, J.J.: Photic reinforcement as a function of optimum level of stimulation. Psychol. rec. **12**, 17 (1962)
Wolkind, S.: Children in care: a psychiatric study. zit. nach Rutter, M.: Maternal deprivation reassessed. London: Penguin 1972

Yarrow, L.J.: The crucial nature of early experience. In: Environmental influences. Glass, D.C. (Hrsg.). New York: Rockefeller University Press and Russel Sage Foundation 1968
Yarrow, L.J.: Maternal Deprivation. In: The child, his psychological and cultural development. Comprehensive Textbook of Psychiatry Bd. I. Freedman, A.M., Kaplan, H. (Hrsg.). New York, Baltimore: Williams & Wilkins 1972
Zingg, R.M.: Feral man and extreme cases of isolation. Am. J. Psychol. **53**, 487 (1940)
Zubek, J.P., Physiological and biochemical Effects. In: Sensory deprivation, 15 years of research. Zubek, J.P. (Hrsg.). New York: Appleton, Meredith 1969
Zuckerman, M.: Theoretical Formulations I. In: Sensory deprivation, 15 years of research. Zubek, J.P. (Hrsg.). New York: Appleton, Meredith 1969

Neurophysiologie und Psychiatrie

Von

R. Jung

Inhalt

I. Einleitung	755
Neurophysiologie und Nachbardisziplinen	757
Psychiatrie und Neurophysiologie	762
II. Neurophysiologie und Psychiatrie in der Schichtstruktur der realen Welt	764
Neurophysiologie, Psychiatrie und Philosophie	765
Nicolai Hartmanns Kategorienlehre und Schichtprinzip	767
Psychiatrie und Neurophysiologie im Schichtenaufbau	768
Mißverständnisse der Schichtenlehren	772
Zwischenstellung der Biologie zwischen Anorganischem und Psychischem	773
Finalnexus und Kausalnexus	775
Tatsachenwissenschaft und Gesetzeswissenschaft	777
III. Psychologie und Neurophysiologie	779
Kausalbeziehung und Zweckmäßigkeit in Physiologie und Psychologie	779
Physiologische Psychologie	781
Experimentelle Psychologien und Neurophysiologie	786
IV. Tier und Mensch: Zoologische Verhaltensforschung, Neurophysiologie und Psychiatrie	796
Ethologie, Neurophysiologie und Psychologie	797
Unterschiede zwischen Mensch und Tier	802
Gemeinsamkeiten von Tier und Mensch	806
Umwelt und Kulturmilieu bei Tier und Mensch	808
Psychische Störungen bei Tieren	811
Neurophysiologie, Ethologie und Psychiatrie	811
Klinische Anwendung neurophysiologischer Befunde und tierpsychologischer Beobachtungen	812
Verhaltensbeobachtung und Introspektion als Ergänzungen der Neurophysiologie	814
Artefizielle Bedingungen der experimentellen Neurophysiologie und Verhaltensforschung	815
V. Neurophysiologische Grundlagen des Verhaltens: Neuronale Mechanismen der Sensomotorik	821
Analyse der Motorik als neurophysiologischer Beitrag zur Verhaltensforschung	822
Antizipierende Koordination in der Sensomotorik	825
Zielbewegung, Stützhaltung und Bewegungsentwurf	827
Cerebrale Bereitschaftspotentiale, Bewegungsentwurf und Rückmeldung	832
Langsame Hirnrindenpotentiale bei Bewegungsintention	832
Neurophysiologische Analyse komplexer motorischer Leistungen	835
Motorik, Trieb und Lernen	836
Cerebrale Systeme der Motorik	843
Wahrnehmung und Handlung	845
Mensch, Organismus und Maschine	848

VI. Technische Modelle des Nervensystems: Biokybernetik und Informationstheorie, Rechenmaschinen, Regelung und Reafferenz 851
  Kybernetik und Informationstheorie 852
  Digitale und analoge Rechenmaschinen im Vergleich mit dem Nervensystem 855
  Biologische Regelungen und Reafferenzprinzip 858
  Biologische Systeme und pathologische Syndrome in kybernetischer Betrachtung ... 860
  Kybernetische Modelle der Gehirnfunktionen 863
  Vorteile, Nachteile und Grenzen der Kybernetik 872
VII. Neurophysiologische Grundlagen der Hirnlokalisation und klinischen Hirnpathologie . 879
  Neurophysiologie und Hirnlokalisation 880
  Hirnreizungen beim Menschen und ihre psychischen Korrelationen 884
  Der Schichtenaufbau des Nervensystems 887
  Neurophysiologie und klinische Hirnpathologie 889
  Die Balken-Funktion als Informations-Transfer zwischen den Großhirn-Hemisphären . 890
  Hemisphärendifferenz und Dominanz 891
  Hirnpathologische Störungssyndrome und physiologische Funktionen 897
  Neurologische und physiologische Gesamtkonzeptionen der psychischen und cerebralen Funktionen 901
VIII. Objektive und subjektive Sinnesphysiologie: Neurophysiologie und Psychophysik des Sehens 906
  Subjektive und objektive Sinnesphysiologie 907
  Allgemeine Ergebnisse der subjektiven und objektiven Sinnesphysiologie 908
  Psychophysiologie und Neurophysiologie des Sehens 913
  Korrelationen von Neuronentätigkeit und Sehen 915
  Receptive und perceptive Felder 922
  Konturabstraktion, Orientierung und Klassifizierung 925
  Optische Halluzinationen, Eidetik und Diagramme bei Gesunden 930
  Experimentelle Halluzinationen 932
  Optische Halluzinationen bei Kranken ohne Psychose 933
IX. Neurophysiologie der Affekte und Triebe 937
  Cerebrale Auslösung von Affekten und Trieben im Tierexperiment 938
  Hirnlokalisation von Affekten und Trieben 943
  Allgemeine Triebphysiologie 945
  Ausdruck und soziale Mitteilung von Affekten und Trieben 948
  Triebstruktur und Konstitution 951
  Selbstreizung des Gehirns im Tierversuch 954
  Selbstreizung bei Tieren und Suchtverhalten bei Menschen 958
  Psychiatrische Anwendungen der Triebphysiologie 961
  Beziehungen von Affekten und Trieben zu „höheren" seelischen Funktionen 963
X. Bewußtsein und Aufmerksamkeit mit ihren physiologischen Bedingungen 968
  Bewußtsein, Aufmerksamkeit und Verhalten 969
  Bewußtseinsselektion und unbewußte Prozesse 972
  Kybernetische Theorien über Bewußtsein, Aufmerksamkeit und Sinnesinformationen . 975
  Neurophysiologische Untersuchungen über Weckeffekte und Aufmerksamkeit 976
  Funktionen der „unspezifischen" reticulo-thalamischen Hirnstammsysteme 977
  Hirnelektrische Befunde und Bewußtseinsstörungen bei Hypoxie und Narkose 981
  Neurophysiologie pathologischer Bewußtseinsstörungen bei Kranken 983
  Bewußtseinsstörungen und hirnelektrische Befunde 985
XI. Schlaf und Traum: Neurophysiologische und klinische Korrelationen 987
  Reiz- und Ausschaltungsexperimente zur Hirnlokalisation der Schlafregelung 989
  Biologie des Schlafes 990
  Verhalten und physiologische Symptome des Schlafes 993
  Elektrophysiologie des Schlafes 998
  Neuronentätigkeit im Schlaf 1004
  Biochemie und Stoffwechsel im Schlaf 1006
  Das Einschlafstadium als Übergang von Wach- und Schlafzustand 1007

Psychophysiologie des Träumens 1010
Neurophysiologie der Schlafstörungen und pathologischen Schlaf-Syndrome 1013
Psychosen, Schlaf und Traum 1018
Schlaf und Gedächtnis 1019
XII. Neurophysiologische Grundlagen von Lernen und Gedächtnis: Physiologie der bedingten Reaktionen 1023
Kurzzeitgedächtnis und Langzeitgedächtnis 1025
Die bedingte Reflexforschung und PAWLOWS Lehre 1027
Allgemeine Physiologie der bedingten Reaktionen 1030
Cerebrale Mechanismen der Konditionierung 1030
Allgemeine Physiologie von Lernen und Gedächtnis 1037
Gedächtnis und cerebrale Disposition, Wechselwirkung von Lernen, Instinkten, Affekten und Reflexen 1040
Physikalische Modelle des Gedächtnisses und Kybernetik 1044
Chemisch-makromolekulare Gedächtnishypothesen 1045
Gedächtnisstörungen und Hirnlokalisation 1047
XIII. Grundlagen des Elektrencephalogramms (EEG) 1050
Formen des menschlichen EEG 1051
Das EEG als Indicator cerebraler Störungen 1053
XIV. Schluß 1055
Neurophysiologische und psychiatrische Forschung 1056
Begrenzung naturwissenschaftlicher Forschung in der Psychiatrie 1061
Literatur 1068

I. Einleitung

„Wüßten wir auch Alles, was im Gehirn bei seiner Thätigkeit vorgeht, könnten wir alle chemischen, electrischen etc. Processe bis in ihr letztes Detail durchschauen – was nützte es? Alle Schwingungen und Vibrationen, alles Electrische und Mechanische ist doch immer noch kein Seelenzustand, kein Vorstellen. Wie es zu diesem werden kann – dies Rätsel wird wohl ungelöst bleiben bis ans Ende der Zeiten, und ich glaube, wenn heute ein Engel vom Himmel käme und uns Alles erklärte, unser Verstand wäre gar nicht fähig, es nur zu begreifen!"
W. GRIESINGER, Die Pathologie und Therapie der psychischen Krankheiten für Ärzte und Studierende. 2. Auflage 1861.

Von der Neurophysiologie zur Psychiatrie ist ein weiter Weg. Man kann auch mit Recht fragen, ob ein solcher Weg überhaupt existiert. Selbst wenn dies bejaht wird, bleibt es fraglich, ob er schon wissenschaftlich gangbar ist. Zwischen beiden Gebieten liegt die Kluft, die Somatisches und Psychisches trennt. Diese Kluft ist nicht durch physiologische Methoden zu überspringen. Ob ein naturwissenschaftlich fundierter Brückenbau möglich ist, erscheint ungewiß. Dabei kann offenbleiben, ob eine solche Kluft wirklich oder scheinbar ist. Scheinbar wäre sie, wenn eine leib-seelische Identität oder ein Kontinuum existierte und die Trennung vorgetäuscht ist durch die Grenzen des menschlichen Verstandes oder die Unfähigkeit des Gehirns, seine Tätigkeit zu erkennen. Aber auch dann bleibt eine *methodische Trennung:* Sie zeigt hier nur Psychisches, dort nur Somatisches. Pragmatisch denkende Biologen und Psychologen finden in ihrer Forschung allerdings zahlreiche *Korrelationen* zwischen Verhalten und introspektiver Beobachtung, zwischen cerebralen und psychischen Vorgängen. Solche Entsprechungen kennt auch der Neuropsychiater, der die psychischen Auswirkungen von Hirnerkrankungen und Medikamenten in der täglichen Praxis sieht.

Deshalb kann es für den Psychiater wertvoll sein, einiges über neurophysiologische Grundlagen des Verhaltens und der psychischen Funktionen zu erfahren und die hirnelektrischen Veränderungen zu kennen, die bei gewissen organischen Seelenstörungen vorkommen. Vielleicht ist es auch nützlich, diese Darstellung von einem Autor zu erhalten, der selbst in der Forschung den umgekehrten Weg, von der Psychiatrie zur Neurophysiologie, gegangen ist.

Was kann der Neurophysiologe über die Grundlagen psychischer Vorgänge oder psychiatrischer Symptome aussagen? Oder, behavioristisch formuliert, welche Befunde bringt die Neurophysiologie über somatisch-cerebrale Entsprechungen normaler und abnormer Verhaltensweisen? Vor einer Antwort auf diese Frage müssen zunächst einige negative Einschränkungen gemacht werden.

Die Neurophysiologie kann nichts zum Verstehen psychologischer und psychiatrischer Phänomene beitragen. Verstehen ist nur auf dem Wege über Seelisches möglich, durch sprachliche oder nicht-sprachliche Kommunikation. Über Ausdrucks- und Sprachfunktionen kann die Neurophysiologie aber weniger aussagen als zoologische Verhaltensstudien oder die menschliche Sprach- und Ausdrucksforschung. Der Neurophysiologe braucht vielmehr *selbst* seine sprachlichen und intellektuellen Funktionen, um Ordnung in die zahlreichen Einzeltatsachen zu bringen, die seine Forschung liefert. Obwohl Psychologen und Philosophen einen somatisch geregelten Unterbau des Seelischen annehmen, kann es auch nicht Aufgabe des Neurophysiologen sein, durch seine elektrophysiologischen Ableitungen oder neuropharmakologischen Experimente psychische Reaktionen und normale oder psychiatrisch-abnorme Verhaltensweisen zu erklären. Der Neurophysiologe kann nur einige gesetzmäßige Entsprechungen zwischen cerebralen Vorgängen und psychischen Phänomenen feststellen.

Auch der philosophische und weltanschaulich-religiöse Gegensatz von Monismus oder Dualismus der Seele und des Körpers kann für den Neurophysiologen unentschieden bleiben. Je nach der experimentellen Situation können monistische oder dualistische Theorien zweckmäßiger oder brauchbarer sein.

Selbst wenn wir bestimmte psychologisch faßbare Phänomene wie Aufmerksamkeit, Bewußtsein oder Affektivität in ihren neurophysiologischen Mechanismen oder biochemischen Vorgängen vollständig darstellen könnten, so würden sie uns damit nicht verständlicher. Die Zielstrebigkeit und Zweckmäßigkeit seelischer Phänomene bliebe ebenso rätselhaft. Das alte Bild, das schon vor 100 Jahren GRIESINGER [G 42] verwendet hat, ist auch heute noch treffend: Wenn ein Engel kommen würde, der uns die körperlichen Grundlagen psychischer Phänomene erklären wollte, wir würden ihn nicht verstehen. *Daher muß das psychophysische Problem als philosophische Aporie bei neurophysiologischen Untersuchungen ausgeklammert bleiben.* GRIESINGERS eigene Hypothese, die „Seele für die Summe aller Gehirnzustände zu erklären" und sein Postulat, daß Geisteskrankheiten Gehirnkrankheiten sind, wäre daher neurophysiologisch nicht zu beweisen. *Die Neurophysiologie beschränkt sich auf die Analyse kausaler Zusammenhänge und auf die Feststellung von Korrelationen zwischen physiologisch registrierbaren Vorgängen und psychologischen oder psychiatrischen Beobachtungen.* Diese Verbindung von körperlichen Funktionen mit kausalen Zusammenhängen und seelischen Vorgängen mit finaler Determinierung kann allerdings nur durch *kritisches und systematisches Denken* gewonnen werden. Die Neurophysiologie ist ein Zweig der Naturwissenschaften und arbeitet wie diese mit Experiment und Beobachtung, indem sie ihre Gesetze aus Zusammenhängen von experimentellen und beobachteten Tatsachen erschließt. Diese systematisch vorgehende *Gesetzesforschung der Neurophysiologie* unterscheidet sich grundsätzlich von der kasuistisch arbeitenden *Tatsachenforschung der klinischen Psychiatrie,* die ähnlich einer Geisteswissenschaft auf einzelne Aussagen, Erlebnisse und Individuen gerichtet ist (vgl. S. 777).

Was die Psychiatrie über diese Einzelphänomene hinaus an Gesetzmäßigkeiten kennt, sind entweder naturwissenschaftliche und psychologische Grundlagen oder systematische Klassifikationen oder reine Spekulationen.

Neurophysiologie und Nachbardisziplinen

Theorienbildung in der Neurophysiologie. Die Neurophysiologie beginnt ihre Experimente mit den Prinzipien der Kausalforschung in Physik und Chemie und analysiert damit zunächst die geordneten Strukturen des Nervensystems. Für die höchst integrierten Vorgänge des Gehirns verwendet sie die Verhaltensbeobachtung des intakten Organismus und psychologische Erkenntnisse. Die Theorienbildung der Neurophysiologie ist dementsprechend streng kausal nur für einzelne Funktionszusammenhänge. Bei komplexen Vorgängen braucht sie die Ergebnisse ihrer Nachbardisziplinen.

In einer Darstellung der allgemeinen Neurophysiologie [J 31] habe ich die Situation 1953 folgendermaßen bezeichnet: „Die physiologische Wissenschaft ist wie Physik und Chemie kausal orientiert, biologische Vorgänge erscheinen dagegen zielgerichtet, und unser Denken ist eindeutig final. Diese Verschiedenheit der Kategorien und Methoden erschwert eine einfache Darstellung, die zugleich exakt und verständlich sein soll. Wenn man aber die grundsätzlichen Verschiedenheiten dieser Kategorien im Methodischen eingesehen hat, so braucht man bei der Darstellung biologischer Zusammenhänge nicht allzu ängstlich die Verwendung psychologischer Bilder zu vermeiden. Komplizierte physiologische Sachverhalte lassen sich oft viel anschaulicher in psychologischer Sprache ausdrücken. Dies erscheint zwar methodisch verwerflich, ist aber didaktisch nützlich. Wenn wir uns darüber klar sind, daß das Leib-Seele-Problem als unlösbare philosophische Frage nicht hierher gehört, so dürften wir doch in der Physiologie wie in der Klinik psychische Vorgänge auch als *Indicator* für neurophysiologische Funktionen verwerten, ohne uns ins spekulative Gebiet zu verirren.

Theoretische Vorstellungen müssen in einer allgemeinen Neurophysiologie dann besprochen werden, wenn sie zu einer sinnvollen Verbindung verschiedener Einzeltatsachen beitragen. Denn es kann nicht Aufgabe dieser Darstellung sein, nur eine unverbindliche Aufzählung von Tatsachen zu bringen. Weniger die facta selbst, als ihre *Zusammenhänge* sind das wissenschaftlich Wichtige."

Trotz mancher praktischer Erfolge sind die Neurophysiologen in der allgemeinen Bewertung ihrer Ergebnisse meistens bescheidener als die Psychiater, Psychologen und Philosophen. Vor allem sind sie mißtrauisch gegen rein verbale Konstruktionen ohne experimentelle Kontrolle. Die Physiologie beansprucht nicht, „das Wesen des Menschen" oder das „Sein des Seienden" zu erkennen, wie die Physik nicht etwa das „Wesen der Schwerkraft" ergründet, sondern nur ihre *Wirkung* untersucht. *Wirkungen sind mit naturwissenschaftlichen Methoden meßbar.* Dies gilt nach HESS [H 65] auch für Psychisches. Die Physiologie versucht, aus mehrfach gesicherten Ergebnissen auf allgemeine *Naturgesetze* zu schließen. Dabei unterscheidet der Physiologe zwischen wichtigen und unwichtigen, zwischen statistisch gesicherten und zufälligen Befunden und ordnet die Spezialfälle unter allgemeingültige Gesetzmäßigkeiten. Aber eine „Wesenschau" überläßt er den Philosophen. Die Physiologie begnügt sich zunächst mit einer Darstellung objektiv faßbarer Vorgänge und ihrer experimentellen Verifizierung. Dieser folgt dann eine Korrelation mit anderen Funktionen und ihre Einordnung in biologische Zusammenhänge und Gesetze. Mit einer solchen objektiven Untersuchung von Einzelvorgängen und ihrer gesetzmäßigen Auswertung kann die Neurophysiologie auch ihren Teil zur Begründung subjektiver Phänomene und psychiatrischer Fragen beitragen, obwohl sie über das Psychische selbst nichts auszusagen hat.

Die Neurophysiologie ist nicht theorienfeindlich und treibt keine reine Tatsachenforschung, wenn sie die experimentellen Befunde in den Vordergrund stellt. Im Gegenteil, sie ist viel mehr *Gesetzeswissenschaft* als die vom Einzelfall ausgehende Psychiatrie. Es gibt viele Beispiele kühner und erfolgreicher Hypothesenbildung in der Physiologie des Nervensystems durch Auswertung weniger experimenteller Befunde. Die Hypothesen der Neurophysiologen sind allerdings meist kurzlebiger und korrekturbedürftiger als physikalische Theorien. Das liegt daran, daß unsere physiologischen Gleichungen zu viele Unbekannte enthalten, die eine eindeutige Lösung verhindern. Dennoch waren manche Hypothesen erfolgreich und erhielten den Wert einer Theorie, andere wurden bald experimentell widerlegt.

Bei *Auswertung neurophysiologischer Ergebnisse für den Menschen* stellt sich die Frage nach den allgemein-theoretischen Grundlagen. Drei extreme Thesen über das Wesen des Menschen stehen einander gegenüber: *„Der Mensch ist ein Tier",* sagen die Zoologen. *„Der Mensch ist eine automatische Rechenmaschine",* behaupten die Kybernetiker. *„Der Mensch ist Geist",* bleibt die These der Philosophen, auch wenn wir von dem platonisch-theologischen Zusatz, daß er eine unsterbliche Seele habe, absehen. Die Zoologen und Kybernetiker verlangen nun von der Neurophysiologie den Beweis für ihre Thesen durch experimentelle Untersuchungen der Gehirnmechanismen, die ihre Ähnlichkeit mit Tiergehirnen oder mit Automaten nachweisen sollen. Die Philosophen verzichten auf experimentelle Beweise, da sie ihre Thesen meistens a priori für richtig halten.

Man braucht weder Experimente noch Rechenmaschinen, um festzustellen, daß diese drei sich widersprechenden Thesen in ihrer absoluten Fassung falsch sein müssen. Dennoch steckt in allen drei Sätzen ein richtiger Kern: Der Mensch ist *auch* eine besondere und einzigartige Tierspecies, und sein Gehirn ist in Struktur und Funktion prinzipiell ähnlich dem der höheren Säugetiere. Das menschliche Gehirn arbeitet *auch* nach kybernetischen Prinzipien, ähnlich den Rechenmaschinen. Die menschliche Kultur entwickelt *auch* geistige Werte, die außerhalb des menschlichen Gehirns objektiv niedergelegt sind und die erst durch Lernen erworben werden. Aber der Mensch ist nicht *nur* ein Tier, ein Automat oder ein frei schwebender Geist, obwohl er von allen diesen etwas enthält.

Wenn wir die Neurophysiologie nicht ohne theoretische Grundlage behandeln wollen, so müssen wir uns im folgenden mit diesen drei widersprechenden Thesen auseinandersetzen. Bei der Besprechung der zoologischen Verhaltensforschung und der Kybernetik wäre zu zeigen, inwiefern die absoluten Thesen falsch sind, und wieweit in ihnen ein richtiger Grundgedanke steckt, der die Grenzen der einzelnen Forschungsmethoden und ihre Anwendung auf verschiedene Schichten der realen Welt bestimmt.

Beziehungen zur Verhaltensforschung und Kybernetik. Die in den letzten beiden Jahrzehnten entwickelte *zoologische Verhaltensforschung oder Ethologie* hat vielfältige Beziehungen zur Neurophysiologie und zur Psychiatrie. Die psychiatrisch relevanten Ergebnisse der Verhaltensforschung werden ausführlich mit einigen neurophysiologischen Entsprechungen an anderer Stelle dieses Werkes von PLOOG behandelt. Da die Ethologie eine Mittelstellung zwischen Neurophysiologie und Psychiatrie einnimmt, kann sie hier nicht übergangen werden. Überschneidungen mit PLOOGS Kapitel sind dabei nicht ganz zu vermeiden.

Neben den neurophysiologischen Grundlagen des angeborenen Verhaltens sind in den letzten Jahrzehnten auch die *physiologischen Bedingungen der Lern- und Gedächtnisfunktionen* untersucht worden. Seitdem PAWLOWS bedingte Reflexforschung [P 7] sich dieser erlernten Reaktion annahm, hat auch die Elektrophysiologie neue Beiträge gebracht. Die Verhaltensforschung hat einige Grenzen des Lernens aufgezeigt, und die Kybernetik hat mit den lernenden Maschinen diese Grenzen zur Technik erweitert.

Die Neurophysiologie der höheren Nerventätigkeit muß sich heute vor allem mit den modernen Richtungen der *Verhaltensforschung* und der *Kybernetik* auseinandersetzen. Dies gilt in erster Linie für solche neurophysiologischen Ergebnisse, die für die Psychiatrie interessant sind.

Tiere und Automaten zeigen besonders eindrucksvoll jeweils zwei verschiedene Seiten der integrierten Hirntätigkeit als Grundlagen seelischer Vorgänge: Die Tiere haben eine *Instinktdynamik,* mit der psychologisch *Affekte* und *Triebe* korrelieren. Die Rechenmaschinen betreiben ein *logisch-mathematisches Kalkül,* dem auf psychologischer Seite *Erkennen* und *rationales Denken* entsprechen. Trieb und Verstand charakterisieren gemeinsam den Menschen. Doch sind beide nicht für ihn allein spezifisch. Die Tiere zeigen in reichem Ausmaß das, was den Automaten fehlt, aber zu den Grundlagen menschlichen Seelenlebens gehört: Affekt, Trieb und Ausdruck. Die programmierbaren kybernetischen Apparate andererseits haben eine differenzierte, streng mathematisch-logische Form der Datenverarbeitung, die beim Tier wenig ausgebildet ist, aber beim Menschen rational das Denken und Verhalten steuert. *Gemeinsam* ist Menschen, programmierten Automaten und höheren Tieren *Gedächtnis und Lernen*. Die Lernfähigkeit ist beim Menschen auf das Höchste und Umfassendste ausgebildet, aber gewisse Vorstufen und Modelle können wir auch bei Tieren und Maschinen studieren.

Instinkt und Lernen. Durch die Lern- und Verhaltensforschung wurde der uralte Streit um die Bedeutung von Anlage und Umwelt wieder aktuell, der in der Philosophie seit KANT obsolet geworden ist und dessen die Psychiater schon längst überdrüssig waren. Die alte Frage "nature or nurture" wird in der Diskussion zwischen LORENZ [L 39] und TINBERGEN [T 8] als Erforschern angeborenen Verhaltens einerseits und LEHRMAN [L 10] als Verteidiger erlernter Reaktionen andererseits wieder lebendig [R 32]. Da wir beim Menschen keinen „Kaspar-Hauser-Versuch" machen können, der bei Tieren angeborene Erbkoordinationen ohne Umwelteinwirkung klar nachweist, ist es schwer, „reines" angeborenes Instinktverhalten des Menschen darzustellen und unmöglich, es experimentell zu demonstrieren. Noch unmöglicher ist es aber, „reines" Lernen anzunehmen. *Lernen wird nur durch eine äußerst differenzierte physiologisch-anatomische Struktur des Gehirns ermöglicht und erwächst auf der Grundlage angeborenen Verhaltens.* Die zentralnervöse Funktionsstruktur aber ist wiederum *vererbt* wie bestimmte Instinktvorgänge und Erbkoordinationen, die vom ZNS gesteuert werden. Dem klinischen Psychiater und einsichtigen Psychotherapeuten ist es längst selbstverständlich, daß beides, *Anlage und Erfahrung*, miteinander eng verflochten ist und menschliches *Instinkt- und Triebverhalten durch Erlebnisse, soziale Bedingungen und Lernvorgänge erheblich verändert wird.*

Am menschlichen Triebverhalten ist dies leicht einsichtig zu machen. Niemand wird bestreiten, daß die *Nahrungsaufnahme* eine bei allen auch dem Menschen, instinktiv vorgebildete Triebhandlung ist. Und dennoch, welche Vielfalt von Eß-Sitten haben die Menschen entwickelt. Man braucht nur an das mühsame Erlernen gesitteten Essens zu denken, das wir unseren Kindern beibringen, um zu verstehen, welche Bedeutung erlerntes Verhalten für die Verwirklichung menschlicher Triebhandlungen im sozialen Leben gewinnt. Instinkt- und triebgesteuert ist zweifellos auch das *Sexualverhalten*. Dennoch, vom altindischen Kamasutram bis zu modernen Ehebüchern hat es nicht an Versuchen gefehlt, diese Triebfunktionen zu variieren und erlernbar zu machen. Die schöne Literatur mit ihren für jede Generation und Gesellschaftsform neu geschriebenen Liebesromanen, von der Sprechstunde des Psychotherapeuten ganz zu schweigen, ist ein beredtes Zeugnis für die vielfältige Abhängigkeit der Erotik von Erfahrung und sozialem Milieu.

Trotz dieser engen Wechselwirkung von Triebanlage und Erfahrung ist ihre Trennung für die Forschung notwendig. Für die Neurophysiologie ist die Abgrenzung von angeborenem Instinktverhalten und erlernten Reaktionen deshalb von Bedeutung, weil die Erforschung dieser Verhaltens- und Reaktionsweisen grundsätzlich *verschiedene Methoden* verlangt.

Bereits *in der phylogenetischen Reihe aufwärts* von den niederen Wirbeltieren bis zu den Primaten *gewinnt Erfahrung und Lernen eine zunehmende Bedeutung für das Verhalten*. Daß beim Menschen das erfahrungsgesteuerte Handeln triebhaftes Verhalten überformt, ist demnach auch vom biologischen Standpunkt aus verständlich.

Eine neuroanatomische Parallele zur zunehmenden Bedeutung erlernten Verhaltens ist offenbar die auch in der phylogenetischen Reihe progressive *Entwicklung der Großhirnrinde* und die starke Ausbildung ihres ungeheuer differenzierten Assoziationsapparates beim Menschen. Diese Parallele wurde früher vielleicht zu sehr betont, aber in den letzten Jahrzehnten mit ihrem vorwiegenden Interesse an subcorticalen Hirnregionen auch ungebührlich vernachlässigt. Die Einseitigkeit beider Lehren, der corticozentrischen und der subcorticozentrischen soll hier vermieden werden. Die neuere Forschung hat auch auf dem Gebiet der bedingten Reflexe durch neurophysiologische Experimente gezeigt, daß bei allen diesen *erlernten Vorgängen subcorticale Mechanismen mitspielen* [A 25, G 2]. Das ist nicht verwunderlich, wenn wir uns das Verhalten niederer Tiere ansehen, die schon sehr bemerkenswerte Lernvorgänge zeigen, obwohl sie fast keine Hirnrinde haben. Jeder Aquarienliebhaber kann dies an seinen Fischen sehen. Andererseits ist die Rolle des Großhirns für die differenzierten menschlichen Gedächtnisleistungen unbestritten, da großhirnlose Menschen und höhere Säuger ohne Cortex nichts lernen. Die von psychiatrischen Klinikern, vor allem von GAMPER [G 5a, 6] schon seit 1926 hervorgehobene Bedeutung des Rhinencephalon und seiner subcorticalen Verbindungen mit dem Corpus mamillare für die Merkfähigkeit und Emotionalität ist jetzt auch von Neurophysiologen mit gutem Erfolg experimentell untersucht worden (vgl. S. 944).

Methodologische Trennung und biologische Zusammenhänge. Die Psychiatrie nimmt von anderen Forschungsrichtungen und aus den Grenzgebieten jeweils das, was für sie *brauchbar* ist. Brauchbar sind andere Ergebnisse aber nur, wenn sie mit methodologischer Kritik verwendet werden. Die Verbindung verschiedener Forschungsrichtungen hat drei Gefahren: 1. Inadäquate Übernahme. 2. Unkritische Verallgemeinerung. 3. Unsachliche Überwertung einzelner Methoden mit Ablehnung anderer. Kritiklose Übernahme und Verallgemeinerung heterogener Ergebnisse anderer Spezialgebiete kann schädlicher sein als einseitige Spezialforschung, die nur ihren Weg verfolgt und die Verbindungen zu den Nachbargebieten vernachlässigt. Denn andere Forscher werden diese Verbindungswege bald finden und die praktischen Anwendungen ziehen. Die 3. Gefahr einer aus Vorurteilen erfolgenden Ablehnung einzelner Forschungsrichtungen mit Überwertung anderer zeigt die verbreitete Geringschätzung der „veralteten" experimentellen Psychologie und „Assoziationspsychologie" und die Überschätzung der „Ganzheitspsychologie". Die experimentelle Psychologie des 19. Jahrhunderts ist mit der Fechnerschen Psychophysik [F 4] auch heute noch lebendig und kann uns die notwendigen subjektiven Korrelate der objektiven Sinnesphysiologie liefern, welche die modernen Methoden der Neurophysiologie erst sinnvoll und für den Menschen anwendbar machen.

Schwierigkeiten einer zu strengen methodologischen Beschränkung und scharfen Trennung von naturwissenschaftich-erklärender und psychologisch-verstehender Betrachtungsweise, die von DILTHEY und JASPERS [J 13] zuerst gefordert wurde, ergeben sich für den Neurophysiologen dann, wenn er von einer speziell methodischen zu einer *synthetischen* Betrachtung kommen will. Allein synthetische Korrelationen können für die Psychiatrie brauchbar sein. Im biologischen Bereich ist eine finale Betrachtung nicht sinnlos und eine psychologische Terminologie nicht immer unpassend. Zwar versucht der Physiologe alle Vorgänge soweit möglich kausal und physikalisch-chemisch zu erklären. Doch kann er in der Darstellung zweckmäßiger Regulationen körperlicher Vorgänge, die CANNON "The wisdom of the body" nannte [C 3], auch im somatischen Bereich psychologische Termini nicht entbehren. Wie auf S. 797 begründet, wird man sie, um anschaulich und verständlich zu bleiben, mindestens als Metapher verwenden.

Die Gegenüberstellung kausalgesetzlicher und sinngesetzlicher Vorgänge, die Trennung von Erklären und Verstehen im Sinne von KARL JASPERS, der empirische Dualismus KURT SCHNEIDERS, alle diese Grenzbestimmungen mögen notwendig sein. *Aber sie dürfen für die Forschung kein Hindernis bedeuten, biologische und neurophysiologische Zusammenhänge mit psychischen Vorgängen verständlich darzustellen.* Es ist sicher kein Zufall, daß naturwissenschaftlich eingestellte Neurophysiologen wie SHERRINGTON [S 33] und HESS [H 65] immer wieder das Grenzgebiet des Psychischen berühren und in ihren synthetischen Arbeiten allgemeine Begriffe wie Integration oder Ordnung in den Vordergrund stellen. SHERRINGTON hat eine streng dualistische Einstellung bis in seine letzten Schriften [S 33] beibehalten. HESS verwendet dagegen in seiner Psychologie aus biologischer Sicht eine monistische Betrachtung des Psychischen [H 65].

Psychiatrie und Neurophysiologie

Anregungen der Psychiatrie für die Neurophysiologie. In der *historischen Entwicklung* sind Neurophysiologie und Psychiatrie eng verbunden. Man sollte nicht vergessen, daß *die Neurophysiologie wesentliche und entscheidende Impulse aus der Psychiatrie erhalten hat*. Hirnelektrische Ableitungen beim Menschen und die Konzeptionen der subcorticalen Bewußtseinssteuerung, die zur Physiologie des thalamoreticulären Systems führten, sind zuerst von psychiatrischen Klinikern entwickelt worden.

Es ist sicher kein Zufall, daß die klinisch wichtigste neurophysiologische Untersuchungsmethode, das *Elektrencephalogramm* (EEG) beim Menschen von einem *Psychiater,* HANS BERGER, entdeckt und erst viel später von physiologischen Forschern nach einer Periode größter Skepsis und Zurückhaltung übernommen und experimentell fundiert wurde.

Viele moderne neurophysiologische Vorstellungen über die Regulation von Aufmerksamkeit und Bewußtsein durch Hirnstammechanismen gehen zurück auf *klinische* Beobachtungen der Neuropsychiatrie. Psychiater wie REICHARDT [R 8, 9], KÜPPERS [K 59] und KLEIST [K 17] oder Neurologen wie VON ECONOMO [E 7, 8] haben in den Jahren 1917–1934 nach vielfältigen klinischen Erfahrungen die Regulation des Bewußtseins und des Schlafes durch median gelegene Zwischen- und Mittelhirnzentren postuliert. Später kam die experimentelle Neurophysiologie, von Tierversuchen ausgehend, zu ähnlichen Vorstellungen: HESS tat den ersten Schritt 1929/44 durch seine Thalamusreizversuche mit Schlafeffekt [H 49, 59], MORISON und DEMPSEY [M 56] haben 1942 ihre Thalamusreize mit Cortexableitungen und MORUZZI und MAGOUN [M 66] 1949 ihre hirnelektrischen Ableitungen mit Reticularisreizungen so präzisiert, daß man die thalamo-reticulären Strukturen des Zwischen- und Mittelhirns als Substrat dieser Regulationsfunktionen bestimmen konnte. Seit 1960 hat die Neuropharmakologie und die

Entdeckung spezifischer synaptischer Transmitter in subcorticalen Systemen (Abb. 35) die Hirnstammwirkungen auf den Cortex wieder kompliziert [J 18, 19].

Begrenzte Anwendungen der Neurophysiologie in der Psychiatrie. *Die praktische Bedeutung neurophysiologischer Methoden für die eigentliche Psychiatrie der Psychosen ist gering.* Daß EEG-Registrierungen nicht viel Positives für die Psychiatrie bringen, war schon eine Enttäuschung für HANS BERGER. Das EEG kann zur Diagnose der endogenen Psychosen nichts beitragen und nur organische Hirnveränderungen und epileptische Störungen anzeigen. Die psychiatrische Bedeutung des EEG beschränkt sich im wesentlichen auf die Epilepsie und ihre Grenzgebiete und auf Erkennung und Ausschluß hirnorganischer Störungen. So wenig das EEG in der eigentlichen Psychiatrie über die Hirnmechanismen von Psychosen aussagt, soviel ist doch über das EEG bei Psychosen geschrieben worden. Auch die in den letzten Jahren von verschiedener Seite aufgenommenen Untersuchungen über direkte Hirnableitungen mit implantierten Elektroden sind großenteils an Geisteskranken durchgeführt worden.

Von theoretischer Bedeutung ist die experimentelle Neurophysiologie vor allem für die Erforschung der Sinnesfunktionen, der Aufmerksamkeit, des Bewußtseins, der Affekte und Triebe. Schon BERGERS erste EEG-Untersuchungen [B 25, 26] hatten festgestellt, daß Bewußtseins- und Aufmerksamkeitsänderungen mit EEG-Veränderungen einhergehen. EEG-Formen des Schlafes und der Bewußtseinsstörungen können zwar verschieden sein, aber die Regel bleibt auch heute noch gültig, daß bei deutlich gestörtem Bewußtsein – sei es auf physiologischer oder pathologischer Grundlage – auch das EEG verändert ist [J 27, 37]. Nachdem schon 1935 GIBBS u.Mitarb. [G 21] bei verschiedenen Bewußtseinsstörungen des Menschen charakteristische EEG-Veränderungen beschrieben haben, sind tierexperimentelle Untersuchungen über das sog. unspezifische Aktivierungs-System des Hirnstamms ein mächtiger Anstoß für die Forschung geworden (vgl. S. 976). Dazu kamen Hirnreizversuche mit Auslösung von Affekten und Trieben (vgl. S. 938).

Im folgenden werden einige Grundlagen der Neurophysiologie mit möglichen psychologischen Korrelationen und psychiatrischen Anwendungen dargestellt. Neben Ergebnissen der objektiven Sinnesphysiologie, die Ergänzungen und Bestätigungen der Psychophysik des 19. Jahrhunderts mit modernen objektiven Registriermethoden brachten, behandeln wir biologische Aspekte der Psychologie, die Koordination von Hirnrinde und Hirnstamm bei Mensch und Tier, und die Physiologie von Bewußtsein und Schlaf. Die Lernphysiologie sowie einige neurophysiologische Ergänzungen der Ethologie und Reflexforschung werden kurz besprochen.

Wie läßt sich die verwirrende Vielseitigkeit unserer ärztlich-psychiatrischen Beziehungen einfach darstellen, und wie ist die Rolle der Neurophysiologie und der naturwissenschaftlichen Forschung darin einzuordnen? Ich glaube, dies wird am besten durch das *Schichtenprinzip* verständlich.

Zusammenfassung

Beziehungen und Unterschiede von Psychiatrie und Neurophysiologie sind charakterisiert durch eine *methodische Trennung*, die auf der einen Seite nur

Psychisches, auf der anderen Seite nur Somatisches zeigt. Dennoch finden sich zahlreiche *Korrelationen* zwischen Verhalten und Erleben und zwischen cerebralen und psychischen Vorgängen. Die psychiatrische Praxis zeigt diese Beziehungen zwischen Gehirntätigkeit und seelischen Vorgängen durch psychische Auswirkungen von Hirnerkrankungen und Medikamenten. Die Neurophysiologie kann nichts zum Verstehen psychologischer und psychiatrischer Phänomene beitragen, aber einige psycho-physiologische Bedingungen und Entsprechungen erforschen. Auch das Leib-Seele-Problem muß als philosophische Aporie ausgeklammert werden. Neurophysiologische Untersuchungen beschränken sich auf Analysen kausaler Zusammenhänge und für den Psychiater auf Beobachtungen von physiologisch-psychologischen Korrelationen. Theorienbildungen sind heuristische Hilfen für die Anwendung von neuen Methoden und die Erkennung von Zusammenhängen. Die Neurophysiologie ist keine Tatsachenwissenschaft, sondern eine *Gesetzeswissenschaft,* die Tierexperimente und Beobachtungen bei Menschen in Theoriensystemen zu vereinigen sucht. Extreme Thesen über das Wesen des Menschen, der biologisch als „Tier", kybernetisch als „Rechenmaschine" oder philosophisch als „Geist" aufgefaßt wird, sind Vereinfachungen von beschränkter Gültigkeit. Mit Einschränkung brauchbar sind sie bei Tieren für Parallelen von Affekten, Trieben und Lernen, bei Rechenmaschinen für logisch-mathematisches Kalkül und in der menschlichen Kulturwelt für geistige Werte. Angeborene Fähigkeiten und durch Lernen erworbene Erfahrung sind jeweils eng verflochten. Psychiatrie und Neurophysiologie können sich gegenseitig anregen. Neurophysiologische Methoden liefern praktisch-diagnostische Anwendungen in der Neuropsychiatrie.

II. Neurophysiologie und Psychiatrie in der Schichtstruktur der realen Welt

> „Nun bildet die Mannigfaltigkeit der Formen offenbar ein Stufenreich, dessen Rangordnung im groben wohlbekannt ist: Ding, Pflanze, Tier, Mensch, Gemeinschaft – und vielleicht noch einiges mehr."
> N. HARTMANN: Neue Wege der Ontologie, 1946.

> „Die durchgehend kausal geordnete Welt ist also kein Hindernis für die Teleologie des Wollens und der Handlung, sondern geradezu deren unerläßliche Vorbedingung."
> N. HARTMANN: Diesseits von Idealismus und Realismus, 1924.

Vor der Besprechung spezieller neurophysiologischer Fragen erscheint es sinnvoll, zu überlegen, an welchem Ort die Forschung in Klinik und Laboratorium einsetzt. Die Neurophysiologie beschränkt sich auf ein eng umschriebenes Gebiet der Biologie. Die Psychiatrie bewegt sich dagegen in verschiedenen Grenzgebieten zur allgemeinen Medizin, zur Naturforschung, zur Psychologie, zur Rechtswissenschaft bis zu den einzelnen Geisteswissenschaften.

Die Verhältnisse sind am besten mit der *Schichtstruktur der realen Welt und der sie bearbeitenden Wissenschaften* darzustellen. Nach NICOLAI HARTMANNS philosophisch konzipierten Schicht-Dependenzen und ihren kategorialen Gesetzen soll im folgenden ein schematischer Abriß gegeben werden (Abb. 1). „Von den exakten Wissensgebieten der anorganischen Natur heben sich durch einen klaren Grenzstrich die biologischen ab; diesen folgt die Psychologie mit ihren Nebenzweigen, von der sich ihrerseits wieder die eigentlichen Geisteswissenschaften nach Gegenstand und Methode scheiden" (N. HARTMANN [H 12] 1946). Ähnlich hat schon seit 1874 der französische Philosoph BOUTROUX [B 53a, 53b] ein hierarchisches Schichtungsprinzip für die Naturgesetze in verschiedenen Ebenen postuliert, indem er von der Logik über die Mathematik, die Mechanik, Physik, Chemie, Biologie und Psychologie zur Soziologie aufsteigt. Eine Abhängigkeit von niederen Schichten und ihre Überformung in der vitalen Schicht lehrte auch CLAUDE BERNARD, der sagte, das Lebendige gehorche zwar den mechanischen Gesetzen, aber gebe dem Mechanischen eine Richtung, die ohne das Leben nicht eingeschlagen würde [B 41].

Neurophysiologie, Psychiatrie und Philosophie

Psychiatrie und Neurophysiologie nehmen aus der Philosophie nur das, was für sie brauchbar ist. Die Neurophysiologie hat schon früh Anregungen und Ordnungsprinzipien von der Philosophie erhalten. HELMHOLTZ [H 27] begründete seine Sinnesphysiologie auf KANTS Erkenntnistheorie, aber bestritt die primäre Existenz der Raumkategorie, da räumliche Wahrnehmungen aus Sinneserfahrungen erworben werden. Sein Schüler VON KRIES war ebenfalls ein kritischer Kantianer, wie seine Schrift über KANT [K 52] und sein großes Buch über die Logik bezeugen. KANT selbst war seit seiner Himmelstheorie immer naturwissenschaftlich und psychologisch interessiert geblieben. Seine „Kritik der Urteilskraft" [K 5] ist in ihrem naturwissenschaftlichen Teil noch heute für Biologen und Physiologen richtungsweisend. Daher ist es charakteristisch, daß NICOLAI HARTMANN bei seiner ersten Berührung mit den Naturwissenschaften [H 10] aus dem Neu-Kantianismus der Marburger Schule kam und sich in seiner Kategorienlehre auch auf KANT stützt.

Während NICOLAI HARTMANNS Philosophie und ihre Schichtenlehre das naturwissenschaftliche Weltbild glücklich ergänzt, kann die später in der Psychiatrie vorherrschende Existenzphilosophie in der von HEIDEGGER [H 23] begründeten Form vielleicht einige psychologisch-psychiatrische Untersuchungen anregen, aber einer naturwissenschaftlich-physiologischen Forschung wenig geben. Zwar erkennt auch HEIDEGGER an, daß die moderne Naturwissenschaft Regeln und Gesetze entdeckt, aber in der Naturwissenschaft geht das Denken andere Wege als in HEIDEGGERS Existenzphilosophie. Wir suchen nicht das Sein des Seienden, sondern das Gesetzmäßige des Besonderen. So bleibt die Existenzphilosophie auch für die wissenschaftliche Psychiatrie nur von begrenztem Wert. Allgemeine Deutungen psychiatrischer Phänomene durch philosophische Existenzialien können nicht mit bestimmten Prinzipien der Naturwissenschaft korreliert werden, obwohl dies mehrfach versucht wurde [K 60]. Solche philosophischen Interpretationen scheitern an der Reichhaltigkeit der Natur wie an den individuellen Besonderheiten psychotischer Erlebnisformen und ihren verschiedenen somatischen Bedingungen.

Die Angst, die HEIDEGGER eine Grundbefindlichkeit des Daseins nennt und an der er die Existenzialien des menschlichen Daseins ableitet, ist für den naturwissenschaftlich eingestellten Forscher nur eines von mehreren vitalen Gefühlen, dem keine spezielle Bedeutung für den Menschen zukommt. Offenbar haben auch Tiere Angst, wahrscheinlich sogar häufiger und stärker als Menschen. Der

Biologe kann daher in der Angst keine spezifisch menschliche Befindlichkeit erkennen. Angst entsteht auch beim Menschen unter sehr verschiedenen Bedingungen, sowohl freisteigend oder reaktiv bei Gesunden wie unter abnormen Bedingungen bei Kranken. Experimentell ist Angst bei der psychiatrischen Schockbehandlung durch grobe äußere Einwirkungen auf die Hirntätigkeit, durch Pharmaka oder elektrische Reizung auszulösen [J 28]. Als pathologisches Phänomen erscheint sie vor allem bei der epileptischen Aura [W 15] zusammen mit konvulsiven Entladungen bestimmter Hirnteile. Daß die *Sorge* im Gegensatz zur Angst eine spezifisch *menschliche* Grundbefindlichkeit ist, darin wird auch der biologisch eingestellte Naturforscher und Psychiater mit der Philosophie übereinstimmen.

Philosophie kann nicht aprioristisch den Gang der Naturwissenschaft leiten. Kurt Schneider hat einmal gesagt, es habe wenig Sinn, mit Theorien und Denkmöglichkeiten gegen die geschlossenen Türen somatischer Forschungsergebnisse anzurennen, wenn diese Türen nur von der anderen Seite zu öffnen sind [S 12a]. Ergebnisse neuer Methoden sind nicht voraussehbar, auch wenn man ihre Grenzen a priori annähernd voraussagen mag. Noch vor 50 Jahren schien es unmöglich, die Hirnrindentätigkeit beim Menschen physiologisch zu registrieren. Ein Jahr später hatte Berger [B 24] die Methode des Elektrencephalogramms entwickelt, welche die elektrische Aktivität der Hirnrinde mit ihren Veränderungen im Schlafen und Wachen aufzeichnet. Wiederum 20 Jahre später gelang es, von einzelnen Nervenzellen der Hirnrinde abzuleiten [J 52]. Wir dürfen deshalb hoffen, daß methodische Fortschritte auch die Gesetzmäßigkeiten der Neuronenphysiologie des Gehirns weiter klären werden. Allerdings können brauchbare Ergebnisse nur durch methodische Beschränkung in Einzeluntersuchungen erhalten werden.

Die im folgenden entwickelten Gedanken über die Beziehungen von Neurophysiologie und Psychiatrie geben nur eine *Ordnung möglicher Problemrichtungen*, keine Erklärungen und keine vollständigen Bilder. Sie können bestenfalls *Anregungen* bringen. Wenn uns klar wird, was wir noch *nicht* wissen, dann zeichnen sich Richtlinien und Wege für notwendige Untersuchungen ab. Methodische Besinnung und Beschränkung bewahrt davor, Unverständliches und Nichterklärbares verstehen und erklären zu wollen. Sie lehrt uns auch, mit offenen Augen Forschungsprobleme von anderen Disziplinen her zu betrachten. In einer übersichtlichen Ordnung sehen wir nicht nur persönliche Denkbefriedigung für den einzelnen, sondern auch methodische Notwendigkeit für die Wissenschaft. Neues kann aber nicht aus methodologischer Betrachtung kommen. Entscheidend sind erst positive Ergebnisse.

Richtige wissenschaftliche Einsichten sind durch Philosophie weder zu begründen noch zu widerlegen. Die Philosophie würde damit eine Metabasis begehen. Wenn Philosophie nach Kant aber bedeutet, seine Grenzen erkennen, dann hat sie auch in wissenschaftlichen Erörterungen ihren Platz. Allerdings nützen weder aprioristische Grundlegungen, noch dogmatische Feststellungen, noch dialektische Auseinandersetzungen: Wahrheit ist nicht wissenschaftlich, vielleicht philosophisch zu erfassen. Richtigkeiten stellen wir wissenschaftlich fest. Wenn wir uns kantisch ausdrücken dürfen: Ideen und Kategorien der Philosophie sind uns lediglich *Schemata,* die wir in der Erfahrungswissenschaft anwenden. Sie sind wissenschaftlich nur heuristische Prinzipien oder, um wiederum Kant zu variieren, *Analogien der Erfahrung* [K 4]. Obwohl Philosophie nicht die Ergebnisse der Naturwissenschaften begründen oder widerlegen kann, so vermag sie doch zu ihrer *Deutung* und *Ordnung* beizutragen.

Nicolai Hartmanns Kategorienlehre und Schichtprinzip

Bei NICOLAI HARTMANN [H 10–14] arbeitet die Philosophie auf einem breiten Grunde der *Erfahrung* und setzt auch die Ergebnisse der Naturwissenschaften voraus. Unter Vermeidung spekulativer Konstruktionen „diesseits von Idealismus und Realismus" werden im Anschluß an KANT zunächst die Grenzen der Erkenntnis und die Gesetze apriorischer Ansicht und möglicher Erfahrung bestimmt. Dann wird eine Synthese neuer ontologischer Kategorien mit einer *Darstellung der realen Welt in ihrer Schichtstruktur* gegeben. Denn Erkenntnisprinzipien sind zugleich Seinsprinzipien [H 11, 12].

Für HARTMANN sind Kategorien allgemeine Prinzipien des Seienden. Sie sind das unverstandene Selbstverständliche an allen Dingen, mit dem sich die Philosophie befaßt. Jedes Phänomengebiet hat seine eigenen, unvertauschbaren Kategorien. Für sie gelten bestimmte *kategoriale Gesetze.* Es gibt kategoriale Stufen im Aufbau der realen Welt und Schichten der Struktur des Körperlichen und Seelischen. Die unteren, einfachen und gebundenen Schichten tragen die höheren, differenzierteren und freieren. Eine kategoriales Grundgesetz besagt, daß höhere Gesetzlichkeit, trotz ihrer Bewegungsfreiheit über der niederen, doch bedingter, abhängiger und damit „schwächer" ist als diese. Derart überschichtet verhalten sich auch Kausalgesetz und finale Zweckmäßigkeit. Physik, Biologie und Psychologie sind die Grundwissenschaften der *drei Schichten des Anorganischen, Vitalen und Psychischen.* Jedes Gebiet hat seine eigenen Kategorien.

Auf der Grundlage anorganischer, physikalisch-chemisch faßbarer Vorgänge baut sich die nächste *organische Schicht des Biologischen* auf. Während die anorganische Natur außer chemischen Unterschieden keine individuellen Besonderheiten kennt, entsteht bei den Lebensvorgängen eine *komplexe Variation der Individuen und Arten mit verschiedenen Stufen der Entwicklung,* die eigenen Gesetzmäßigkeiten und Zielen folgen. Diese Sonderung ist in unserem Schema durch Unterbrechungen der Linie bezeichnet (Abb. 1). In der biologischen

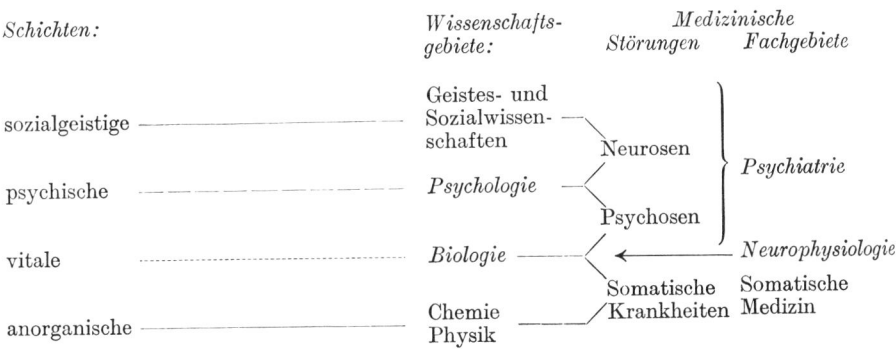

Schichten:		Wissenschafts-gebiete:	Medizinische	
			Störungen	Fachgebiete
sozialgeistige	————————	Geistes- und Sozialwissenschaften	Neurosen	} Psychiatrie
psychische	– – – – – – –	*Psychologie*	Psychosen	
vitale	··············	*Biologie*	←	*Neurophysiologie*
			Somatische	Somatische
anorganische	————————	Chemie Physik	Krankheiten	Medizin

Abb. 1. Schichtenschema der realen Welt mit Einordnung der psychiatrischen und neurophysiologischen Forschung. Die Aufgaben der Psychiatrie reichen über mehrere Schichten von den somatisch bedingten Hirnkrankheiten über die genuinen Psychosen mit ihren Wechselwirkungen vitaler und psychischer Vorgänge bis zu den Konflikten der seelischen und sozialen Schichten bei den Neurosen. Die Psychiatrie hat damit Beziehungen zu den verschiedensten Wissenschaften von der Biologie über die Psychologie zur Soziologie. Die *Neurophysiologie* als Teil der Biologie erforscht die Hirntätigkeit allein in der vitalen Schicht und verwendet die Phänomene der höheren psychischen Schicht nur als *Indicator* für Funktionszustände des Gehirns

Schicht gelten zwar auch die Gesetze der physikalisch-chemischen niederen Schicht, doch gibt es neue Gesetzmäßigkeiten, die als zielgerichtete Anpassungen auf der unteren Ebene des Anorganischen nicht bekannt sind. Allerdings dient die biologische Zweckmäßigkeit nach KANT [K 5] nur scheinbaren Zwecken, die auf uns unbekannten Naturgesetzen beruhen.

Auf einer wiederum „höheren" Ebene oberhalb der biologischen Funktionen liegt die beim Menschen über Handeln und Denken entscheidende *psychische Schicht*. In dieser sind *individuelle Besonderheiten* viel stärker ausgeprägt als in der organischen Schicht und ihre *finale Ausrichtung* wird eindeutig. Im Schema wird die stärkere individuelle Sonderung durch einzelne Striche in größeren Abständen angedeutet.

Über dieser psychischen Schicht ist noch eine höhere *geistig-soziale Schicht* anzunehmen. Für diese gelten neue *kollektive Gesetzmäßigkeiten*, die wiederum die individuelle Sonderung überbauen und für die gesamte menschliche Gesellschaft von Bedeutung sind: Es ist die Sphäre der sozialen Kommunikationen, der *geistigen, ethischen und religiösen Werte*, die für die Menschheit gemeinsam gelten und mit denen sich die Geisteswissenschaften beschäftigen. „Sie transzendieren das Bewußtsein des Einzelnen" [H 12]. *Jede dieser Schichten hat ihre eigene Gesetzmäßigkeit und ihre Besonderheit, aber die höhere Schicht ist abhängig von der niederen:* Die niederen Schichten begründen die höheren und sind daher „stärker" als diese. Die *höhere Schicht kann nicht ohne die niedere bestehen, wohl aber die niedere ohne die höhere.* Physikalisch-chemische Vorgänge können ohne biologische oder seelische Einwirkung ablaufen. Psychische Vorgänge sind aber nicht möglich ohne Grundlagen physikalisch-chemischer Veränderungen und biologischer Funktionen. Allerdings sind die höheren Ebenen in ihrer Form und Eigenart *nicht nur* von den niederen Schichten bestimmt, sie haben bei größerer Differenziertheit ihre *eigenen Gesetze*. Jede höhere Schicht hat trotz ihrer Abhängigkeit von den niederen doch den Gewinn größerer *Freiheitsgrade*. Aber kausale Gesetze, die in den niederen Schichten allein herrschend sind, gelten auch für die höheren als Fundierung ihrer eigenen Gesetzlichkeit.

Psychiatrie und Neurophysiologie im Schichtenaufbau

Nach dem Schema der Abb. 1 ist es klar, daß die *Aufgabe der Psychiatrie über mehrere Schichten reicht*, da psychische Störungen durch die verschiedensten Veränderungen auf diesen Ebenen bedingt sein können. *Die Neurophysiologie ist dagegen auf die beiden unteren Schichten begrenzt*. Sie arbeitet mit physikalisch-chemischen Methoden in einem eng begrenzten Gebiet der Biologie des Nervensystems.

Der *Ort* der verschiedenen Störungen, welche die Psychiatrie beschäftigen, ist mit der Schichtenlehre leicht verständlich zu machen. Er kann bei *somatisch bedingten Hirnkrankheiten*, etwa Vergiftungen, traumatischen oder symptomatischen Psychosen vorwiegend im Bereich der physikalisch-chemischen und biologischen Wechselbeziehungen liegen. Die eigentlichen *Geisteskrankheiten* sind im höheren Bereich der Wechselwirkung von biologischen und psychologischen Vorgängen zu suchen. Die meisten *„Neurosen"*, die Konfliktsituationen zwischen Individuum und Gemeinschaft darstellen, spielen sich in den höchsten psychologischen und geistig-sozialen Schichten ab. Da wiederum Psychosen tief in die Beziehungen von Individuum und Gemeinschaft eingreifen, ist hier eine sekundäre Auswirkung von Störungen der niederen Schichten auf die höheren anzunehmen. Die endogenen Psychosen sind aber nicht, wie eine das soziale Moment überbewertende Psychiatrie lehrt, aus Konflikten zwischen den sozialen und psychischen Schichten erklärbar. Wer diesen Schichtenaufbau und ihre Gesetze verstanden hat, dem erscheint der Streit um die Frage überflüssig, ob das Leben „nur" ein physikalisch-chemischer Vorgang sei oder das Seelische im Grunde ein körperlicher Vorgang.

Lebensvorgänge haben ihre eigenen Gesetze, die nicht den physikalisch-chemischen Prozessen zukommen, auf denen das Leben beruht. Seelische Phänomene sind zwar von biologischen Vorgängen abhängig, haben aber wiederum eigene Gesetze. Trotz solcher Autonomie sind alle oberen ohne die unteren Schichten nicht möglich.

Somato-psychische und psycho-somatische Wechselwirkung. In der Wechselwirkung der organischen und psychischen Schicht sieht man auch die *Grenzen der psychosomatischen Beeinflussung*. Nehmen wir als Beispiel körperlich-seelischer Beziehung etwa Herztätigkeit und Psyche: Seelische Vorgänge können zwar die Herztätigkeit beeinflussen, beschleunigen oder verlangsamen, vielleicht sogar über vegetative Nerven funktionelle Durchblutungsstörungen hervorrufen. Aber die psychische Einwirkung geht nicht so weit, daß das Herz durch seelischen Einfluß zu schlagen aufhört. Sonst könnten schwer Depressive, die sich den Tod wünschen, ohne körperliche Einwirkung sterben. *Die höheren Schichten sind also schwach gegenüber den niederen.* Umgekehrt führt aber ein somatisch oder physisch bedingter Herzstillstand zum sofortigen Erlöschen der psychischen Funktionen. *Die niedere Schicht ist hier stärker als die höhere,* weil sie deren Grundlage ist. Ferner geht jede psychische Einwirkung auf den Körper nur über die Gesetzmäßigkeiten der organischen Funktionen, meist über das vegetative Nervensystem.

Aus diesen Wechselwirkungen und dem Ort ihrer Effekte ergeben sich auch gewisse Indikationen und *Grenzen der Therapie* (vgl. S. 771). Eine somatische Behandlung setzt an den stärkeren niederen Schichten ein, mit physikalischen Mitteln wie beim Elektroschock oder chemischen Einwirkungen wie bei der Pharmakotherapie. Ihre Wirkungen sind daher tiefgreifender als die der Psychotherapie. Psychotherapie ist gegenüber körperlichen Vorgängen ohnmächtig, beschränkt sich auf seelische Einwirkungen und kann auch soziale Gesetzmäßigkeiten nicht ändern. Alle sog. „psychosomatischen" Wirkungen finden ihre Grenzen an biologischen Ordnungen und naturwissenschaftlichen Gesetzen, die sie nicht verändern können. Die *somato-psychischen* Störungen dagegen, die pathologischen Einwirkungen des Körperlichen auf die Psyche, gehen von der stärkeren unteren Schicht aus, beeinflussen aber kausal auch die höhere Schicht und sind deshalb vorwiegend somatisch und nur zusätzlich psychisch zu behandeln.

Psychiatrische Konsequenzen der Schichtenlehre. In der praktischen Psychiatrie wird man immer die verschiedensten im Einzelfalle zusammenkommenden Störungen körperlicher, seelischer und sozialer Natur berücksichtigen müssen. Dies gibt der Psychiatrie ihre große Ausdehnung und ihren anregenden Kontakt mit vielen anderen Wissenschaften, aber es bedingt auch ihre wissenschaftliche

Gefährdung. Hier können wir nur exakt bleiben bei klarer begrifflicher Trennung der verschiedenen Faktoren und einer strengen Fassung des Krankheitsbegriffs. Das gilt vor allem für die *Trennung von Erlebnisreaktionen und echten Psychosen* als einer der wichtigsten Erkenntnisse der neueren Psychiatrie. Ein Ehekonflikt ist ein psychischer und Umweltkonflikt, aber keine Geisteskrankheit. Eine Rentenneurose ist Ausdruck des Rentenbegehrens und deren sozialer Bedingtheit. Aber eine paranoische Schizophrenie, die Ehekonflikte verursacht oder zur Rentenquerulanz führt, oder eine Depression, auch wenn sie durch Milieuwechsel ausgelöst wurde, bleibt doch eine Krankheit, die im Organisch-Biologischen wurzelt und entsprechend zu behandeln ist.

Die Unterschiede der verschiedenen Schichten sind daher sowohl von theoretischer wie von praktischer Bedeutung. In der klinischen Praxis sind die Störungen in den einzelnen Ebenen sehr verschieden zu bewerten. Sie müssen, wie die deutsche Psychiatrie – im Gegensatz zur angelsächsischen "dynamic psychiatry" ohne Diagnosenstellung – immer gefordert hat, diagnostisch möglichst weit geklärt werden, um ärztlich handeln zu können. Ein Ehekonflikt kann z.B. rein als Milieustörung oder zwischenmenschliches Problem auf psychoneurotischer Grundlage erwachsen, er kann aber auch durch eine Geisteskrankheit oder durch eine körperliche Erkrankung bedingt sein. Eine diagnostisch und therapeutisch gleich wichtige Aufgabe ist zunächst die Erkennung pathologischer Verhältnisse in den *niederen* Schichten. Erst nach Ausschluß solcher elementaren somatischen Störungen ist eine rein seelische Behandlung der Konflikte in „höheren" Schichten medizinisch gerechtfertigt.

Wenn die Konfliktsituationen der Neurosen bis in die sublimsten menschlichen Werte mit ethischen und religiösen Bindungen hineinreichen, so liegen sie auf einer höheren Ebene, die wir naturwissenschaftlich nicht beeinflussen und neurophysiologisch nicht erklären können. Aber wenn ähnliche Konflikte auf dem Boden einer somatischen Störung, etwa einer Depression oder Schizophrenie erwachsen, wird eine Behandlung der körperlichen Störung notwendig. Zur somatischen Therapie, etwa einer Pharmakotherapie oder Schockbehandlung, kann dann auch die Neurophysiologie etwas beitragen.

Wir haben die psychiatrischen Konsequenzen der Hartmannschen Kategorienlehre 1947 am Beispiel der Schocktherapie besprochen [J 28]. Es sei erlaubt, einiges davon zu wiederholen und mit Ergänzungen und Auslassungen zu variieren:

Betrachten wir die Schockbehandlung mit Anwendung der kategorialen Gesetze, so gewinnen wir manche Einsichten. Aus dem Ansatz NICOLAI HARTMANNS wird klar, daß *körperliche Behandlung* der niederen tragenden Schichten *wirkungsvoller sein wird als seelische Beeinflussung,* wenn Geisteskrankheit auf körperlichen Störungen beruht. Dagegen wird somatische Therapie bei rein seelischen Konfliktreaktionen unangemessen bleiben. Daß alle Krankheiten und damit auch die Geisteskrankheiten körperlich sein müssen, ist in der modernen Psychiatrie weitgehend anerkannt. KURT SCHNEIDER [S 15] hat diese Tatsache mehrfach in aller Klarheit formuliert und die Abgrenzung gegen nicht krankhafte seelische Erlebnisreaktionen und Charaktervariationen herausgearbeitet. Die Hoffnungslosigkeit einer reinen Psychotherapie der Psychosen beruht auf der Ohnmacht höherer Kategorien, in die Gesetze der niederen einzugreifen. Die seelische Wirksamkeit der körperlichen Beeinflussung durch Psychopharmaka oder Schocktherapie ist ebenso wie das Auftreten psychischer Störungen nach somatischen Erkrankungen als Abhängigkeit der höheren seelischen Schichten von den grundlegenden niederen körperlich-vitalen zu deuten.

In der allgemeinen Biologie hat MAX HARTMANN die Prinzipien NICOLAI HARTMANNs systematisch verwendet [H 8]. In der Pathopsychologie hat KURT SCHNEIDER [S 13] die kategorialen Gesetze N. HARTMANNs mit dem Aufbau des Trieb- und Willenslebens in Parallele gesetzt. Andere ältere Schichtenlehren, wie die JACKSONS [J 1] in der Neurologie und JANETS [J 5] in der Psychopathologie, in denen ein ähnlicher Gedankenkern steckt, beruhen auf evolutionstheoretischen Konzeptionen des 19. Jahrhunderts. Sie sind nicht bis zu allen Konsequenzen durchgeführt worden wie das Schichtenprinzip N. HARTMANNs. Die psychologische Schichtenlehre ROTHACKERS [R 33] ist ein Beispiel für weitere Bemühungen in dieser Richtung.

Die Darlegungen NICOLAI HARTMANNs stimmen überein mit den in der Psychiatrie [S 12, 15] und Hirnforschung [V 11] seit langem geforderten Verfahren, *verschiedene wissenschaftliche Methoden an einer Problemstellung anzusetzen*. Es ist ein Fehler, nur lösbare Probleme für wissenschaftlich zu halten. Oft müssen wir uns begnügen, in der Beschreibung die Phänomene zu wahren.

Mit dem Ineinandergreifen und dem Gefüge der Methoden kann wissenschaftliche Erkenntnis in ihren natürlichen Grenzen fortschreiten. Prinzipien sind nicht absolut gültig. Theoretisch und als abstrakte Postulate können sie auf beliebige Gebiete ausgedehnt werden. Sie sind nur mit dem *Konkreten,* in dem viele Prinzipien zusammengewachsen sind, sinnvoll. Einzelne Prinzipien sind nur Teilbedingungen, niemals voller Seinsgrund. Das Allgemeine und Prinzipielle hat keine Wertvorzüge vor dem Konkreten [H 11]. *Wirklich Wertvolles ist konkret, individuell und begrenzt.* In dieser Feststellung ist auch die *Schwierigkeit allgemein psychologischer und psychiatrischer Forschung* begründet, da sie immer mit *Individuen* zu tun hat und doch *Allgemeines* aussagen will.

Für wissenschaftliche Untersuchungen gibt es nur das „Arbeiten aus der Mitte", in manchen Fällen auch „von unten herauf". Die obersten Kategorien sind wegen ihrer außerordentlichen Kompliziertheit, die untersten wegen ihrer Einfachheit undurchsichtig. Daraus ergibt sich für uns: *Die höchsten Stufen des Persönlichen und des Individuellen können wissenschaftlich nicht vollständig erfaßt werden.*

Mit dem Verzicht, das Persönliche und Individuelle wissenschaftlich zu fassen, gelangen wir zu ähnlichen Gedanken von KARL JASPERS [J 13]. Er stellt fest, daß die rohen Kategorien der Psychopathologie nicht in den Grund des Menschen dringen. Er wendet sich aus methodischen Gründen gegen die Anwendung ontologischer Methoden in der Psychologie, die sich oft durch unbemerkte Philosophie überwältigen läßt. Das Sprechen von Existenz und Transzendenz trübt die wissenschaftliche Psychopathologie. Trotz dieser kritischen Einstellung anerkennt auch JASPERS die Existenzerhellung als Antrieb verstehender Psychologie und billigt der Daseinsontologie den Wert einer Theorie zu. Wir müssen uns nur vor Scheinverstehen hüten. Körperliches ist nicht zu verstehen, nur zu erklären. Vitales ist Unaufhellbares, Unverstehbares, Existenz ist hell-werdendes Unverstandenes. Auf JASPERS' eigene Existenzphilosophie können wir an dieser Stelle nicht näher eingehen. Das, was er „Transzendenz" nennt, die freie Entscheidung und Gestaltung des Lebens, ist offenbar eine Grundbedingung individuellen Seins, die bei den Geisteskrankheiten gestört ist. Wie aber solche Störungen durch körperliche Eingriffe bedingt und verändert werden, das kann Philosophie nicht erklären.

Mißverständnisse der Schichtenlehren

So klar der Stufenbau der verschiedenen Schichten mit ihrer gegenseitigen Abhängigkeit ist, so wenig wird er doch in der Naturforschung und Geisteswissenschaft beachtet. Nicht nur in der Psychologie, sondern auch in der Psychiatrie werden die kategorialen Grenzen wegen der weiten Ausdehnung psychiatrischer Untersuchungen und Anwendungen oft übersehen. Es werden ohne Begründung „autonome" seelische Vorgänge angenommen, wo es sich offenbar um körperlich gebundene Funktionen handelt.

Ob Psychiater und Psychologen, die von der „Autonomie des Seelischen" reden, den „reinen Geist", das „Dasein" oder die „geistige Welt" behandeln, wirklich an eine vom Körperlichen unabhängige Seele glauben, wie Spiritisten an Geister, habe ich allerdings nie ganz herausfinden können. Ich denke, einige geben sich nur den Anschein aus Freude am Paradox oder um die Somatiker zu ärgern. Die Mehrzahl der Forscher behandelt seelische Vorgänge und geisteswissenschaftliche Fragen zwar mit Anerkennung ihrer somatisch-biologischen Grundlagen, aber ohne diese zu erwähnen. Mit Recht, denn ein dauernder Rückbezug auf die niederen Schichten wäre unnötig umständlich und würde den Blick für die spezifischen Gesetze der höheren Schichten trüben. Darum kann man auch Psychiatrie treiben, ohne viel von Neurophysiologie zu wissen.

Dennoch: die Freiheit der höheren Schichten ist begrenzt. „Sie hat ‚keinen Spielraum im Niederen', wohl aber ‚über' ihm" [H 12]. Bei aller philosophischen Hochschätzung des Geistes und menschlicher Freiheit ist die Einsicht in die Gebundenheit, das Ergänzungsbedürfnis, die Unselbständigkeit und das Fehlen einer abgeschlossenen Ganzheit des menschlichen Wesens auch von Philosophen wie LITT [L 31] besonders betont worden. Mit NICOLAI HARTMANN wird dabei anerkannt, daß die Freiheit nur durch Gebundenheit an die Naturgesetze möglich wird und daß die von der Geisteswissenschaft mit Recht hochbewertete Entwicklung der *Sprache* in ihrer semantischen Funktion zur Auswechselbarkeit und *Zweideutigkeit der Erkenntnis führen kann* [L 31].

Obwohl N. HARTMANN einmal sagt: „Das Seelenleben ist keine Überformung des leiblichen Lebens", hat er doch die Leibgebundenheit des Geistes immer wieder betont: „Der Geist ist und bleibt leibgebunden, er kommt nur im organischen Wesen vor, ruht auf dessen Leben auf, lebt von seinen Kräften: Und da das organische Leben der materiellen Welt angehört und in ihren Energieumsatz eingefügt dasteht, so ist es mittelbar auch von ihr getragen" [H 12].

Ein häufiges Mißverständnis der Hartmannschen Kategorienlehre muß noch erwähnt werden: Die „Unabhängigkeit" der niederen Schichten von den höheren gilt nur für die Gesetzmäßigkeiten dieser niederen Schichten, aber nicht für jede Form der Beeinflussung. *Ein Eingreifen aus höheren Schichten in die niederen ist durchaus möglich. Es geschieht mit dem Kausalgesetz, nicht ihm entgegen* [H 12]. Die *höheren Schichten können die niederen „überformen"*, aber nicht um-

formen, und müssen sich an die grundlegenden Gesetze der niederen Schichten anpassen. Obwohl menschlicher Einfluß und zielgerichtetes Handeln in Naturereignisse eingreifen kann, so ist dies eben *nur nach Kenntnis der Naturgesetze,* durch Anpassung an diese und mit Befolgung der Kausalgesetze der Natur möglich.

Die Geisteswissenschaftler und Philosophen, welche die Macht des Geistes und seine Freiheit verteidigen, übersehen oft diese Grenzen. Sie benutzen auch keine guten Argumente, wenn sie auf die Beherrschung der Natur durch den Menschen hinweisen, die eben nur durch die Leistungen der Naturwissenschaften mit Berücksichtigung ihrer Gesetzmäßigkeiten möglich wird.

Zwischenstellung der Biologie zwischen Anorganischem und Psychischem

Die Neurophysiologie ist eine Teildisziplin der Biologie. Das Feld der Biologie liegt zwischen den Wissenschaften vom Anorganischen und Psychischen. Weder die streng mathematisch faßbaren Gesetze und voraussagbaren Ereignisse der Physik und Chemie, noch die nicht berechenbaren, individuell-variablen und schwer voraussehbaren geistig-seelischen Phänomene, deren vielfältige Bedingungen auch nicht annähernd wissenschaftlich erfaßt werden können, passen zur Biologie. Die Biologie (von der die Physiologie einen Teil darstellt) hat neben Beobachtung und Beschreibung der zahlreichen Variationen des Lebendigen vor allem die Aufgabe, *gesetzmäßig wiederholte Vorgänge* in ihren Mechanismen zu studieren, und erhält damit vorwiegend den Charakter einer Gesetzeswissenschaft. Die Neurophysiologie fordert daher mit Recht, zumindest einen Teil der biologischen Eigenschaften des Nervensystems auf physikalisch-chemische Gesetze zurückzuführen. Damit ist aber nicht alles getan. Vielmehr muß die Physiologie auch die *spezifisch-biologischen Gesetzmäßigkeiten höherer Ordnung* untersuchen, die nicht physikalisch-chemisch erklärbar sind, obwohl sie durch Physik und Chemie fundiert werden.

Kategoriale Unbestimmtheit der biologisch-vitalen Schicht. In der allgemeinen Biologie und in allen Naturphilosophien – von KANTs regulativem Prinzip und seiner „Zweckmäßigkeit ohne Zweck" bis zu NICOLAI HARTMANNs Philosophie der Natur [H 13] und seinem „nexus organicus" – sieht man eine gewisse Verlegenheit, die spezifischen Kategorien des Lebendigen zu definieren, für die weder der Kausalnexus allein zureichend ist, noch der Finalnexus wirklich paßt. Auch N. HARTMANN [H 13] gibt, entgegen seiner sonstigen Bestimmtheit, nur Ansätze: Er leitet den „nexus organicus" vom Selektionsprinzip und der *Evolution* ab. Er läßt den Gang des biologischen und des psychischen Geschehens in seinen Einzelheiten immer noch kausal ablaufen, obwohl im Triebleben der Tiere schon vor der psychischen Schicht ein Finalnexus mit zielstrebigem Verhalten hinzukommt.

N. HARTMANNs Ansatz zur Überwindung des kartesianischen Dualismus in der gemeinsamen Dimension der Zeit als kategorialem Grund von Außen- und Innenwelt – sowohl für die „extensio" als Substanz der Dinge wie der „cogitatio" als Substanz der Innenwelt – ist nicht bis zum Ende durchgeführt und wohl auch nicht durchführbar.

Nach HARTMANN ist das Seelische direkt gegeben, das Dingliche gleichfalls. Zwischen beiden steht das Lebendige. Die Gesetze und Zusammenhänge der Lebewesen sind in ihrer Eigenart weder kausal noch teleologisch vollständig zu erfassen. Daraus ergibt sich die ontologische *Unmöglichkeit von Teleologismus und psychologischer Deutung der Lebensprozesse*: Damit würde die niedere Schicht des Lebens von der höheren des Bewußtseins abhängig. Mechanistische Erklärung der Lebensprozesse arbeitet zwar mit unzureichendem Instrument, leistet aber mehr, weil sie die kategorialen Seinsgesetze nicht auf den Kopf stellt. Die angemessene kategoriale Bestimmung der Lebensprozesse in ihrer Eigenheit ist noch nicht klar herausgearbeitet.

Auch die Versuche biologischer Forscher, eine *theoretische Biologie* zu begründen [B 42, H 9, U 1], haben keine allgemeingültige Definition der biologischen Schicht ergeben. Sie gehen aus von der Irreversibilität der Lebensvorgänge (EHRENBERG [E 10]), von der Umweltrelation der Organismen (UEXKÜLL [U 1]) oder „belebten Organismen als Dingen der Außenwelt im Raum" (BERTALANFFY [B 42]) oder lehnen sich wie MAX HARTMANN [H 8] an NICOLAI HARTMANNS Schichtenlehre an und begründen die Biologie mit der lebenden Zelle [H 9]. HESS bezeichnet biologische Funktionen als *erfolgsbezogen* und erstrebt eine Verbindung mit der Psychologie [H 65]. Zur Erklärung verwendet er wie N. HARTMANN die lange phylogenetische Entwicklung. Das schon von MACH diskutierte Ökonomieprinzip, das AVENARIUS [A 38] in seiner „Philosophie als Denken der Welt gemäß dem Prinzip des kleinsten Kraftmaßes" zu einer gemeinsamen Grundlage philosophischer, psychologischer und biologischer Weltbetrachtung erweitert hat, erlaubt keine Definition und Abgrenzung der Lebensprozesse. GRANIT hat neuerdings die Notwendigkeit teleologischen Denkens in der Biologie betont [G 34], aber auch keine überzeugende Definition des Lebendigen gegeben.

Gefühle und Triebe als biologisch-seelische Grenzphänomene. HARTMANNS Schichtenlehre enthält eine *Einengung der seelischen zugunsten der geistig-sozialen Schicht*. Dies hängt wahrscheinlich mit der schwierigen Abgrenzung und Definition der biologischen Schicht zusammen. Was HARTMANN als seelische Schicht bezeichnet, das Reich der Gefühle und Triebe, ist offenbar nicht für den Menschen spezifisch, sondern findet sich auch bei Tieren. Das Affekt- und Triebleben, das die Erfolgsbezogenheit biologischer Vorgänge besonders deutlich macht, kann auch als differenzierter Teil der biologischen Schicht aufgefaßt werden. Wie weit NICOLAI HARTMANN solche „psychischen" Phänomene, die auch im Tierreich als Triebe durchaus zielgerichtet sind, also einen Finalnexus enthalten, noch zur vital-biologischen Sphäre zählt, muß offen bleiben. Es sind offenbar Grenzphänomene der vitalen und seelischen Schichten, die *zwischen Biologie und Psychologie* liegen. Zielgerichtete Triebmotivationen des Verhaltens sind ebenso wie psychischer Ausdruck in Wahrnehmung und Bewegung schwer von biologischen Mechanismen abgrenzbar. *Man könnte daher die psychische Schicht auch als besondere Erlebnisform der vitalen Schicht einordnen* und damit die aristotelische Entelechie des Lebens umkehren. Wenn man aber die Schichteneinteilung nicht als scharf abgegrenzte Stufen, sondern als sich gegenseitig überformende Bereiche erfaßt, deren differenzierte Formen aus den niederen jeweils in die höheren Schichten eindringen, macht die Unterscheidung der vitalen und psychischen Schichten keine Schwierigkeit. Wegen methodischer Verschiedenheiten der Erfahrung psychischer und vitaler Phänomene bleibt es zweckmäßig, beide Schichten voneinander abzugrenzen und die biologischen und psychologischen Wissenschaften als eigenen Bereich zu erhalten. Vitale und seelische Funktionen regeln über den rein kausalen Zusammenhang hinaus erfolgsbezogene gezielte Handlungen der lebenden Organismen.

KURT SCHNEIDER [S 14] erklärt den relativ geringen Einfluß NICOLAI HARTMANNS auf die Psychiatrie und Psychologie durch seine Verkleinerung der seelischen Schicht gegenüber der geistigen. Der geringe Einfluß in der Psychiatrie blieb, obwohl HARTMANNS Philosophie auf naturwissenschaftlichen Kenntnissen basiert oder vielleicht gerade deshalb. Wahrscheinlich hat die mangelnde Beachtung der Philosophie HARTMANNS in der Psychiatrie und der größere Einfluß der existenzphilosophischen Richtungen noch eine andere Ursache: Viele Psychiater haben eine Abneigung gegen präzises naturwissenschaftliches Denken und gegen exakte Definitionen, aber eine Freude an pseudophilosophischer Dunkelheit, an literarischen Worten mit vielfältiger Bedeutung bis zu einem unkontrollierten und unkontrollierbaren Gerede, das der neueren Psychiatrie so verhängnisvoll wurde. Es ist bezeichnend, daß diejenigen Psychiater, die kurze Darstellungen und Klarheit der Definition bevorzugen, wie GRUHLE und KURT SCHNEIDER, im scharfen Gegensatz zu dieser pseudophilosophischen Psychiatrie stehen. N. HARTMANNS Kategorienlehre hatte dennoch wenig psychiatrische Resonanz [B 2]. Obwohl K. SCHNEIDER das Schichtenprinzip für das Verhältnis vom Trieb und Willen verwendet, hat er die Unterscheidung von vitalen und seelischen Gefühlen nicht ausdrücklich auf HARTMANNS Schichten bezogen [S 13, 15].

Finalnexus und Kausalnexus

Begrenzung der Finalität durch Kausalität. Kausale Beziehungen gelten für die gesamte reale Welt. Nicht nur die niederen Schichten des Anorganischen, sondern auch die lebenden Organismen, die seelischen Vorgänge und geistigsozialen Beziehungen sind nach N. HARTMANN kausal geordnet [H 11]. Den Unfug „akausaler" Beziehungen kann die Wissenschaft dem Spiritismus und der Astrologie überlassen. Der Finalnexus der Zweckbestimmung schließt den Kausalnexus der Verursachung nicht aus. Vielmehr ist *kausale Ordnung die Vorbedingung für zweckhaftes Handeln* [H 12]. Jede Freiheit der höheren Schichten ist auch durch kausale Beziehungen begrenzt. „Freiheit" des menschlichen Wollens ist nur möglich durch Anpassung an die Natur. Kausale Gesetze bedingen nicht nur die Ohnmacht des Geistes gegenüber der Materie, sondern ermöglichen auch eine gewisse Beherrschung der Materie durch Kenntnis der kausalen Naturgesetze. Allerdings kennen wir zahlreiche kausale Bedingungen der höheren Schichten meistens nicht genügend. Unkenntnis von Ursachen bedeutet aber nicht fehlende Ursachen. Wenn eine Änderung der Umwelt durch zielgerichtetes Handeln möglich ist, so geschieht dies nur unter Berücksichtigung kausaler Beziehungen. N. HARTMANN formuliert dies klar: „Der Menschengeist kann auf mannigfache Weise die Einzelgebilde oder die lokalen Verhältnisse der Natur umgestalten, und zwar je einfacher deren Gesetzlichkeit ist, um so mehr. Aber er kann auf keine Weise ihre Gesetze selbst umgestalten" [H 12]. Der menschliche Geist bleibt in seiner Macht begrenzt. Struktur und Gesetzlichkeit der niederen Schichten kann er nicht verändern. Die kategorialen Gesetze bestreiten nicht eine Gestaltung der niederen Schichten durch die höheren, aber diese ist nur möglich innerhalb der Grenzen, welche die materiellen Gesetze der niederen Schichten zulassen. *Es gibt keine Herrschaft des Geistes über die Materie: „Sein Herrschen beruht auf seinem Gehorchen"* sagt N. HARTMANN treffend. Geistige Beeinflussung wird nur ermöglicht durch die Fähigkeit, „die eigene Gesetzlichkeit dieser Kräfte zu verstehen und sich in seinem technischen Schaffen seinerseits ihnen anzupassen". Beherrschen kann der Mensch die Natur „stets nur soweit, als er ihre Gesetze befolgt". *Der Geist schreibt nur die Zwecke vor, „die er mit der Naturkraft als gegebenem Mittel verfolgt ... Aber er kann das nur, sofern er ihre Eigenart respektiert* ... Denn gegen Zwecke verhalten sich die Naturkräfte gleichgültig. Sie selbst verfolgen keine Zwecke, darum lassen sie sich als Mittel fremder Zwecke gebrauchen" [H 12].

Heterogonie der Zweck- und Zielhandlung und mehrfache kausale Bedingtheit. Die Schwäche der oberen Schichten mit ihrer finalen Determinierung und die Stärke der niederen mit ihrem Kausalnexus, der bis zur höchsten Ebene reicht, zeigt sich noch in einem fast gesetzmäßigen Phänomen der *Abweichung vom Zweck*. Final geplante Prozesse führen oft *nicht* zu dem gesetzten Ziel und erreichen nicht den gewünschten Zweck. Vielmehr haben ihre Zweckmotive im Erfolg andersartige „Nebenwirkungen", die in unvorhergesehener, sogar der determinierenden Tendenz entgegengesetzter Richtung verlaufen können. WUNDT [W 33] nannte dies die *„Heterogonie der Zwecke"*. Er meinte damit unbeabsichtigte kausale Wirkungen, die durch final geplante Prozesse angestoßen werden und dann ihren eigenen Weg nehmen. WUNDT sah darin ein Gesetz der Wirkungen, die zu neuen Motivreihen und Korrekturen der Zwecksetzung führen [W 33]. Solche kausalen „Nebenwirkungen" werden desto häufiger zur Hauptwirkung, je komplexer die Struktur und je höher die Schicht ist. Diese andersartige Entwicklung intendierter Einwirkungen ist vor allem in der Soziologie, der Politik und Gesetzgebung wohl bekannt. Sie spielt auch im psychologischen und zwischenmenschlichen Kommunikationsbereich eine große Rolle, wie in der Erziehung und Psychotherapie und gilt auch im Grenzgebiet der Biologie.

Diese Unvorhersehbarkeit des Endeffekts einer Zweckhandlung ergibt sich aus der komplexen *Wechselwirkung vieler kausaler Bedingungen*. Gewöhnlich sehen wir nur die letzten dieser Bedingungen, und die Mehrzahl bleibt unbekannt. Obwohl auch die wissenschaftliche Forschung nur wenige dieser Kombinationen ermittelt, ist es doch nicht nötig, auf den Kausalnexus zu verzichten und wie VERWORN eine „konditionale Weltanschauung" zu postulieren [V 6]. Übrigens beklagt VERWORN schon 1912 die Massenproduktion der Wissenschaft und vergleicht die logarithmische Kurve der menschlichen Geistesentwicklung seit dem 19. Jahrhundert mit einem Tumorwachstum: „... so wächst beängstigend die Zahl der wissenschaftlichen Publikationen. Sollte der wissenschaftlichen Forschung das Schicksal des Tumors und der geistigen Kultur schließlich das Ende des Organismus beschieden sein? Oder läßt dieses drohende Geschick sich durch die Kunst kluger Ärzte abwenden?" – „Sollte unser Gehirn schließlich zu eng werden für diese unabsehbare Entwicklung?"

Er fordert schon damals Regulationen und Korrekturmittel, bessere Verwertung und rationellere Organisation der wissenschaftlichen Arbeit. Wenn er die nach 60 Jahren weiter angewachsene heutige wissenschaftliche Produktion sehen könnte, würde VERWORN noch mehr über die mangelnde Kenntnis und Verwertung wissenschaftlicher Arbeiten klagen und mit noch größerem Recht verlangen, daß Spezialuntersuchungen nur aus dem planvollen Zusammenhang der „großen Probleme" und allgemeiner Fragestellungen bearbeitet werden sollen. Aber er würde wie alle Planwissenschaftler in der Heterogonie der Zweckhandlungen bald seine Grenzen finden.

Die Heterogonie der Zweckhandlungen erfährt der Neurophysiologe bei seinen Experimenten oft genug. Viele scheinbar gut geplante Versuche mißlingen, nicht wegen „Tücke des Objekts", sondern weil zu viele unbekannte Kausalfaktoren mitspielen, die nicht alle vorauszusehen waren. Daher die Forderung zu möglichster Vereinfachung der Versuchsanordnung und zur Ausschaltung anderer störender Faktoren im neurophysiologischen Experiment.

Zeitparadox der Zweckdetermination. Nicht nur Philosophen und Psychologen, sondern auch manche medizinische und naturwissenschaftliche Autoren überschätzen den teleologischen Standpunkt und den Finalnexus, wenn sie ihn auch für eine *rückläufige* Determination in Anspruch nehmen, so bei WEIZÄCKER [W 18], bei TEILHARD DE CHARDIN [T 1] und bei AUERSPERG [A 37]. Nach den Dependenzgesetzen NICOLAI HARTMANNS [H 11] widersprechen die Zwecksetzungen des Finalnexus nicht der durchgängigen Gültigkeit des Kausalnexus, der überhaupt erst Ziel- und Zweckvorgänge ermöglicht. Die Zielbestimmung für die Zukunft ist nicht eine reale Umkehr der Zeitfolge, sondern nur eine imaginäre.

Teleologische Betrachtungen erscheinen nur wie zeitliche Umkehrungen biologischer Prozesse, wenn man vergißt, daß Vorwegnahme und Erwartung künftiger Ereignisse *allein in der Vorstellung* als einem inneren Umweltmodell, nicht in der realen Welt stattfindet. Solche Antizipationen in einem vorgestellten Umweltbild sind biologisch und psychologisch für alle Trieb- und Zielhandlungen notwendig. Eine *Antizipation* späterer Ereignisse ist nicht nur beim menschlichen Denken, sondern auch in einfacher Form bei Tieren anzunehmen: Eine jagende Katze, die vor einem Mauseloch lauert, *erwartet* das Beutetier und bereitet sich auf den Sprung vor. Beim Menschen sind auch hirnelektrische Korrelate solcher Vorbereitungsprozesse mit WALTERS Erwartungswelle und KORNHUBERS Bereitschaftspotential objektiv registrierbar (s. S. 832). Alle willkürlich gesteuerten Zielbewegungen bedürfen neben der auf die Zukunft gerichteten Zielvorstellung auch einer kontinuierlichen Kontrolle und erlernten Übung, die im Handlungsentwurf und Intentionsprozeß mit ähnlichen hirnelektrischen Korrelaten koordiniert werden [J 57], wie Abb. 763 zeigt. Ein Schema der psychologischen und physiologischen Vorgänge bei Zielbewegungen gibt Abb. 766 C.

Tatsachenwissenschaft und Gesetzeswissenschaft

Der Gegensatz geisteswissenschaftlicher und naturwissenschaftlicher Einstellung bringt eine fruchtbare Spannung in unser Fach mit der Anregung, die Phänomene von verschiedensten Aspekten her zu betrachten und wissenschaftlich anzugehen. Gehen wir aus von DILTHEYS, WINDELBANDS, RICKERTS und CARL STUMPFS überzeugender Darstellung der Prinzipien von Geisteswissenschaft und Naturwissenschaft [S 56], so können wir diesen Antagonismus auch im psychiatrischen Gebiet besser verstehen. Ein verbreitetes Mißverständnis ist die Überwertung der Einzeltatsache und des Einzelbefundes in der Naturforschung. Nicht die Naturwissenschaften, sondern die *Geisteswissenschaften sind „Tatsachenwissenschaften"*, in der die einmalige Tatsache, sei sie geschichtlicher oder individueller Art, sei sie ein Kunstwerk, ein Vertrag oder ein Geburtsdatum oder eine Archivnotiz, entscheidend ist. *Naturwissenschaft hingegen ist Gesetzes-*

wissenschaft, in der die einmalige Tatsache allein wenig bedeutet. Die bestbeobachtete Tatsache wird ein belangloser Einzelbefund, wenn sie ohne *Zusammenhang* mit anderen bekannten Tatsachen bleibt oder wenn sie nur längst bekannten Gesetzmäßigkeiten entspricht, die keiner Bestätigung durch Einzelbeobachtungen mehr bedürfen.

Seit KANT sind sich Philosophie und Wissenschaft darüber einig, daß der Mensch und seine Forschung die Totalität der Bedingungen von Natur- und Lebensvorgängen niemals erfassen kann [K 5]. Die Wissenschaft kann nur eine Aufklärung von *Teilaspekten* geben und muß die zahlreichen Lücken mit Hypothesen ausfüllen. Für bestimmte psychiatrische Fragen sind einzelne neurophysiologische Aspekte der Gehirnfunktionen und ihrer Störungen wichtig, andere können als unwesentlich vernachlässigt werden. Neurophysiologische Untersuchungen haben psychiatrisch relevante Teilaspekte für das Gebiet der Epilepsie und der organischen Psychosen ergeben, sowie psychophysiologische Korrelationen für bestimmte normale Regulationen des Wach-Schlafrhythmus, der Aufmerksamkeits- und Bewußtseinsvorgänge, der Affekte und Triebe und der Wahrnehmung.

Für die Fragen des Geltungsbereichs physiologischer Methoden und Erkenntnisse erscheint es nützlich, zunächst das Verhältnis von Psychologie und Physiologie und dann die Parallelen und Unterschiede von Hirnfunktionen und Verhalten bei Menschen und Tieren darzustellen.

Zusammenfassung

Das Verhältnis von Neurophysiologie und Psychiatrie ist am besten mit der Schichtstruktur der realen Welt und entsprechender Ordnung ihrer Wissenschaften zu verstehen. Nach NICOLAI HARTMANNS Kategorienlehre wird ein *Schema der anorganischen, vitalen, psychischen und sozial-geistigen Schichten* gegeben: Die somatische Medizin wirkt in den unteren physikalisch-chemischen und biologischen Schichten, die Neurophysiologie erforscht mit der Neurobiologie die biologisch-vitale Schicht mit ihren physikalisch-chemischen Grundlagen und die Psychiatrie behandelt die Störungen der vitalen und psychischen Schichten (Psychosen) und der psychisch-sozial-kulturellen Schichten (Neurosen). Die Zwischenstellung der vitalen Schicht und der Biologie zwischen den anorganischen und psychischen Schichten ist kategorial unbestimmt. Kausale Bestimmungen allein gelten in der anorganischen Schicht, in der psychischen Schicht bestimmen vorwiegend finale Ziele den Ablauf. In der vitalen Schicht gelten beide, kausale und finale Gesetze, durch Ziel- und Zweckhandlungen lebender Organismen.

Eine kausal geordnete Welt ist Vorbedingung für die Zweckrichtung des Wollens und der Handlung, da Ziele und Zwecke nicht gegen, sondern nur *mit* dem Kausalzusammenhang zu erreichen sind. Die unteren Schichten sind „stärker" als die höheren. Durch ihre Abhängigkeit von vielen kausalen Faktoren ist auch die Unsicherheit finaler Planung bedingt: kausal bestimmte Prozesse können ihren eigenen Weg gehen und so die Überwertung des Zweck- und Zielbegriffs in biologisch-psychischem und sozialen Bereich verhindern. Dem entspricht WUNDTS „Heterogonie der Zwecke".

III. Psychologie und Neurophysiologie

> „Erkenntnisprinzipien ... sind zugleich Gegenstandsprinzipien."
> NICOLAI HARTMANN: Diesseits von Idealismus und Realismus, 1924.
>
> „Ist es also nicht durchschaubar, wie physiologische Prozesse auf seelische und diese wiederum auf sie einwirken können, so ist das kein Grund, den Wirkungszusammenhang als solchen abzulehnen."
> NICOLAI HARTMANN: Neue Wege der Ontologie, 1946.

In einer Darstellung neurophysiologischer Grundlagen der Psychiatrie müssen auch die Beziehungen zur Psychologie besprochen werden. Bei den unterschiedlichen Aspekten der verschiedenen psychologischen Richtungen ist dies nur fragmentarisch mit Stichworten möglich, wenn wir uns auf das biologisch Relevante beschränken. Nicht nur die Psychophysik und Psychophysiologie oder die experimentelle Psychologie, auch die heute oft vergessene Würzburger Schule, der Behaviorismus und die Gestaltpsychologie, die Ganzheitspsychologie und sogar philosophische Richtungen der Phänomenologie und des Existentialismus oder einige psychologische Einsichten der Psychoanalyse können für die Neurophysiologie Hinweise auf zentralnervöse Ordnungsprinzipien geben. Solche Korrelationen sind allerdings nur von begrenzter Gültigkeit.

Psychologische Termini bedeuten für den Neurophysiologen wie für den Verhaltensforscher oft nur *Abbreviaturen, die komplexe und integrierte intrazentrale Vorgänge oder äußere Verhaltensweisen verständlich machen und prägnant kennzeichnen, ohne jedoch exakte naturwissenschaftliche Präzision zu erreichen.* Dabei wird meistens vorausgesetzt, daß psychische Vorgänge die inneren Aspekte neurophysiologischer Mechanismen und äußeren Verhaltens darstellen. Eine weitere Voraussetzung einer solchen pragmatischen Verwendung psychologischer Metapher in der Neurophysiologie ist die von KANT vertretene und von N. HARTMANN klar formulierte *Koexistenz kausaler und teleologischer Gesetzlichkeiten in einer identischen Welt* [H 12]. Dagegen hat POPPER [P 31, 32] einen dualistischen „Interaktionismus" seelischer und körperlicher Prozesse vorgeschlagen vgl. S. 791).

Kausalbeziehung und Zweckmäßigkeit in Physiologie und Psychologie

Physiologische und psychologische Verfahren und Deutungen. *Kausale und teleologische Deutungen schließen sich nicht gegenseitig aus, sondern ergänzen sich auf verschiedenen Ebenen.* Dies ergibt sich aus der oben besprochenen Ontologie NICOLAI HARTMANNS [H 11] (vgl. S. 767). *Naturwissenschaftlich-physiologische Deutungen* (etwa als Reflexe oder Reaktionen des Organismus auf äußere Reize oder als innere Regulationen und „Automatismen" zentralnervöser Tätigkeit) und *psychophysische Deutungen* als von „psychischen" Vorgängen begleitete oder durch sie bestimmte Ordnungen sind bei fast allen Lebensäußerungen möglich. Bei einfachen biologischen Vorgängen wird die physikalisch-chemische und physiologische Erklärung meistens genügen, bei komplexen Entwicklungen kann man psychologische Darstellungen meist nicht entbehren, wenn das Ganze „verständlich" werden soll. Verständlich werden solche komplexen Vorgänge erst durch *Anschaulichkeit*.

Tatsächlich vereinfachen psychologische Termini die Darstellung komplizierter biologischer Systemzusammenhänge erheblich, weil sie die unübersehbaren physiologischen Einzelmechanismen in klare Vorstellungen und einfache *Bilder* zusammenfassen. Für die Physiologie bleibt diese psychologische Beschreibung allerdings immer nur ein Bild, eine *Metapher*. Solche Metaphern sind, wie eingangs dargestellt, nicht nur für das menschliche Denken und Handeln, sondern auch für das Verständnis komplexen tierischen Verhaltens unentbehrlich. Sie werden auch von Physiologen verwendet, um funktionelle Zusammenhänge und ihre biologische Bedeutung darzustellen (vgl. S. 971). Notwendig sind solche psychologischen Bilder und Vorstellungen für die physiologische und psychiatrische Forschung, wenn man beide Aspekte verstehen und sich nicht in einem unübersehbaren Labyrinth neurophysiologischer Einzelmechanismen verirren will. Man kann beide Aspekte allerdings nicht simultan sehen und untersuchen, sondern nur nacheinander entweder den einen oder den anderen methodischen Weg gehen. Diese Beschränkung erschwert die Verständigung zwischen Physiologie und Psychologie. Sie schließt aber Korrelationen zwischen beiden nicht aus.

Die methodische Beschränkung einer getrennten Untersuchung somatisch-physiologischer und seelisch-psychologischer Vorgänge bedeutet keinen Zweifel an der Koexistenz und Koordination beider im lebenden Organismus. Sie widerlegt auch nicht eine mögliche reale *Identität* jenseits der Phänomene. Der Streit um das Vorhandensein unbewußter psychischer Vorgänge erscheint vom neurophysiologischen Standpunkt aus unnötig: *Unbewußte Mechanismen sind physiologische Vorgänge,* die nur unter bestimmten Bedingungen und für beschränkte Zeit, durch den Scheinwerfer der Aufmerksamkeit erhellt, bewußt werden können [J 36]. Nach K. JASPERS' [J 13] Bild treten diese Vorgänge als Akteure kurzzeitig jeweils auf die Bühne des Bewußtseins, die eine beschränkte Kapazität hat und nur das jeweils Aktuelle und Bedeutungsvolle für die Regulation des bewußten Verhaltens aufnimmt. *Damit erhält auch der alte Begriff, der ,,Enge des Bewußtseins" einen physiologischen und einen psychologischen Sinn* (vgl. S. 972).

Auf die in der ersten Auflage 1967 gegebene kurze Charakteristik der verschiedenen psychologischen Forschungsrichtungen in ihrer Beziehung zur Neurophysiologie kann ich hier verzichten. Nachdem der vorangehende Band I/1 die heute aktuellen und psychiatrisch relevanten psychologischen Richtungen mit der klinischen Neuropsychologie ausführlich darstellt, verweise ich auf diese Beiträge von HEIMANN [H 24], FAHRENBERG [F 2] und ASSAL-HECAEN [A 35].

In der klinischen Pathopsychologie ist das Interesse an methodologischen Grundlagen und der psychopathologischen Diagnostik im Sinne KURT SCHNEIDERS [S 12, 13] nach ihrer Blüte in den 20er Jahren heute zurückgegangen und JASPERS' strenge Zweiteilung von Verstehen und Erklären wurde unter dem Einfluß der Psychoanalyse, die alles Seelische konstruktiv-dogmatisch zu erklären versucht, verwischt. Die Psychophysik hat sich verselbständigt und wurde zu einer Spezialwissenschaft der subjektiven Sinnesphysiologie, die im Kapitel VIII kurz besprochen wird. Sie bildet mit ihren messenden Quantifizierungen eine Brücke zur objektiven Sinnesphysiologie [J 45].

Physiologische Psychologie

Psychophysik. FECHNER hat die Psychophysik als messendes psychologisches Verfahren der subjektiven Sinnesphysiologie vor 100 Jahren begründet [F 4]. Die psychophysischen Methoden versuchen, die *Antworten des Organismus auf bestimmte quantifizierte Sinnesreize messend zu erfassen.* Sie benutzen dazu die menschliche Sinneswahrnehmung als feinsten Indicator und schalten die Störungen und Fehler statistisch aus (mittlerer Fehler FECHNERS). Trotz der subjektiven Natur der Sinnesempfindung erhält man beim Menschen damit quantitativ zuverlässigere Ergebnisse als durch Verhaltensreaktionen nach Sinnesreizen beim Tier, die durch andere unkontrollierbare (äußere oder endogene) Faktoren beeinflußt werden können. Im sinnesphysiologischen Experiment beim Menschen kann man solche störenden Faktoren durch adäquate Einstellung eher ausschalten, oder, wenn sie doch auftreten, auch introspektiv als Fehlerquelle erkennen.

In dem 1860 erschienenen Buch „Elemente der Psychophysik" hat FECHNER neben zahlreichen originellen sinnesphysiologischen Beobachtungen sein *psychophysisches Gesetz* einer logarithmischen Beziehung zwischen Reizstärke und Empfindung begründet. Es wird seitdem Weber-Fechnersches oder *Fechnersches Gesetz* genannt (vgl. S. 908). Ferner hat FECHNER eine Reihe von *psychophysischen Axiomen* aufgestellt, die G.E. MÜLLER [M 77] noch schärfer formulierte und die neuerdings von METZGER [M 39] in Zusammenhang mit der objektiven Sinnesphysiologie besprochen wurden. Der Hiatus zwischen psychologischer und physiologischer Forschung, den METZGER in der anschaulichen psychischen Kontinuität als Gegensatz zur physiologischen Diskontinuität sieht [M 39], ist in den praktischen Ergebnissen der Sinnesphysiologie nicht so groß, und beide sind nicht so unvereinbar wie es in der Theorie erscheint. Man kann z.B. diskontinuierliche Aktionspotentiale des Sehsystems durchaus mit entsprechenden Intensitätsänderungen der Helligkeitswahrnehmung korrelieren (vgl. S. 915, Abb. 23). Eine technische Parallele gibt es beim Übergang eines digitalen in ein analoges Informationsmuster der Kybernetik (vgl. S. 855).

Ähnlich liegen die Verhältnisse im akustischen Sinnesbereich. Die Diskontinuität der Schallwellen, die bei niederen Frequenzen noch taktil als Schwingung wahrgenommen werden kann, verschmilzt in der auditiven Wahrnehmung zu der Kontinuität des Tones. Nur bei Intensitätsunterschieden (bei Unterbrechung des Schalles, bei Schwebungen benachbarter Frequenzen oder der Taktbetonung einer Melodie) erscheinen diskontinuierliche Sinnesphänomene.

Alle diese Sinnesinformationen werden physiologisch nur durch eine diskontinuierliche Abfolge von Nervenaktionspotentialen von den Sinnesorganen zum Gehirn fortgeleitet, oder wie der Techniker sagt, als *Impulsfrequenzmodulation* geleitet und codiert. Im Gehirn werden diese Impulsfolgen durch Zwischenschaltung langsamer Vorgänge integriert. Wenn diese Informationen von einer Hirnregion zur anderen geleitet werden, werden sie wiederum in einzelne Nervenaktionspotentiale aufgelöst. Welcher Art die langsamen Zwischenvorgänge sind, die bei der Integration der Nervenaktionsströme mitwirken, ist noch nicht bekannt. Man nimmt chemisch-humorale Prozesse an, wie bei den Überträgerstoffen der Synapsen [E 5].

FECHNER arbeitete mit der Methode der *Unterschiedsschwelle,* der kleinsten, „eben merklichen Unterschiede" der Sinneswahrnehmung (just noticeable difference: j.n.d. der angelsächsischen Literatur) für die Stärke der Empfindung. Wegen der adaptationsbedingten Schwellenänderung führt diese Methode des sukzessiven Vergleichs (gewissermaßen das minimum separabile der Empfindungsintensität im zeitlichen Ablauf) zu manchen Ungenauigkeiten. Das Fechnersche Gesetz ist daher oft angegriffen worden. Dennoch gelten diese logarithmischen Beziehungen für fast alle Sinnesreaktionen, vor allem auch in der objektiven Sinnesphysiologie mit hinreichender Genauigkeit im mittleren Intensitätsbereich. Man kann sie auch so formulieren, daß die Unterschiedsschwelle jeweils ein konstanter Bruchteil der vorangehenden Reizintensität ist. Wahrscheinlich bezeichnet STEVENS' *Potenzfunktion* verschiedene Sinnesmodalitäten besser.

Ein neuer Protest von STEVENS [S 52] gegen das „Dogma" des Fechnerschen Gesetzes und die Unterschiedsschwellenmethode betont mit Recht die erheblichen Verschiedenheiten der Exponenten bei verschiedenen Sinnesqualitäten und Reizarten. Doch benutzt STEVENS auch subjektive Schätzungen numerischer Sinnesintensitäten und findet lineare Korrelationen von Reiz und Empfindung nur mit doppelt logarithmischer Skala seiner „power function". Seine Darstellung bedeutet für den Physiologen nicht eine Widerlegung der vielfach bestätigten logarithmischen Beziehungen von Reiz und Sinneserregung. STEVENS' Methode der subjektiven Skalierung gibt jedoch gute Möglichkeiten der Quantifizierung von Wahrnehmungen [D 31].

Die Verschiedenheit der Exponenten der Unterschiedsschwelle bei verschiedenen Sinnesqualitäten ist wohl auch eine Ursache für das vergebliche Bemühen, *die* psychische Einheit zu finden. Die Empfindung ist komplexer als nur ein Meßindicator und hat im physikalischen Reiz keine funktionale Entsprechung. Daher ist die Formulierung einer exakten Beziehung Reiz-Empfindung ohnehin eine Abstraktion. Das psychophysische Problem eines funktionellen Zusammenhangs beider Größen ist nicht mit einer mathematischen Zuordnung zu lösen.

Nachdem die psychophysische Forschungsrichtung zunächst übertriebene Hoffnungen auf die Meßbarkeit seelischer Phänomene enttäuscht hatte, wurde sie in der deutschen Psychologie zugunsten der gestaltspsychologischen Richtung zu sehr vernachlässigt. Bis etwa 1925 wurde sie noch von physiologischer Seite gepflegt und als Grenzgebiet zwischen Psychologie und Physiologie durch v. KRIES [K 51] auch erkenntnistheoretisch unterbaut. In der deutschen Psychologie wurde seit den letzten Schriften G.E. MÜLLERS [M 79, 80] die psychophysische Forschung von der Gestaltpsychologie abgelöst und dann durch die Testpsychologie verdrängt. Doch haben die angelsächsischen Psychologen die Psychophysik auch in den letzten Jahrzehnten experimentell weiter gefördert. Heute besteht begründete Aussicht, psychophysische Ergebnisse mit der objektiven Sinnesphysiologie durch naturwissenschaftlich-technische Registriermethoden an Receptionsorganen, afferenten Nerven und Hirnzentren exakt zu begründen.

Psychophysiologie. Die physiologische Psychologie hat eine doppelte Wurzel. Sie entwickelte sich 1. aus FECHNERS psychophysischer Richtung der Sinnesphysiologie, 2. aus WUNDTS Anwendung physiologischer Methoden zur objektiven Registrierung körperlicher Begleitvorgänge psychischer Phänomene. WUNDT hatte als Schüler von HELMHOLTZ auch LUDWIGS objektive Registriermethoden im Tierversuch kennengelernt und sie dann beim Menschen angewandt. So bringt der erste Band von WUNDTS physiologischer Psychologie fast allein neuroanatomische und neurophysiologische Daten. Da die objektive Sinnesphysiologie mit der Registrierung von Sinnesorganen damals noch wenig entwickelt war, erfaßten die Psychophysiologen neben motorischen Reaktionen vor allem vegetative Begleitvorgänge, zunächst die vasomotorischen Reaktionen im Plethysmogramm, später den galvanischen Hautreflex. Eine kurze Übersicht über die ältere Literatur findet sich bei BERGER 1937 [B 28]. Die Hoffnung WUNDTs und seiner Schule, entgegengesetzte Reaktionen bei Lust und Unlust, Erregung und Ruhe, Spannung und Lösung zu finden, erfüllte sich nicht. Man fand nur allgemeine vegetative Begleiterscheinungen bei verschiedenen affektiven Erregungen und Aufmerksamkeitsänderungen. Auch die zahlreichen anderen Methoden, wie Messungen der Reaktionszeiten, brachten trotz der jahrelangen Bemühungen KRAEPELINs und seiner Schüler, die in den Bänden seiner psychologischen Arbeiten [K 46] niedergelegt sind, nur wenige Ergebnisse, die für die Psychiatrie von praktischem Interesse waren. Doch waren KRAEPELINs Experimente über die psychophysiologischen Wirkungen von Arzneimitteln grundlegend für die moderne Psychopharmakologie. Nach längerer Pause sind diese Versuche erst in den letzten Jahren systematisch wieder aufgenommen worden (vgl. in ds. Band). KRAEPELIN war Schüler WUNDTs und wurde von ihm zur experimentellen Psychophysiologie angeregt, bevor er die klinische Psychiatrie neu gestaltete.

Der experimentellen Psychologie WUNDTs gingen spekulative Entwürfe voraus, welche die mathematische und physiologische Begründung zunächst nur postulierten: HERBARTs „Psychologie als Wissenschaft, neu gegründet auf Erfahrung, Metaphysik und Mathematik", 1824/25 und LOTZEs „Medizinische Psychologie" 1852. Die Bezeichnung *„Physiologische Psychologie"* wurde von LOTZE 1852 in diesem Buche [L 43] eingeführt und gegen die alte animistische Psychologie abgegrenzt. LOTZE postulierte eine „Physiologie der Seele", blieb aber doch skeptisch gegenüber der allgemeinen Gültigkeit physiologischer Entdeckungen, die „eine durchschnittliche Lebensdauer von etwa vier Jahren haben" [L 43]. In der Sinnesphysiologie hat er zwar kaum experimentiert, doch hat er sie durch seine *Konzeption der „Lokalzeichen"* stark beeinflußt: „... so muß jede Erregung vermöge des Punktes im Nervensystem, an welchem sie stattfindet, eine eigenthümliche Färbung erhalten, die wir mit dem Namen ihres *Lokalzeichens* belegen wollen" [L 43]. Die moderne Psychophysiologie ist mit ihren historischen Wurzeln in Bd. I/1 von FAHRENBERG ausführlich dargestellt, so daß ich hier darauf verzichte.

Psychologie im biologischen Aspekt. Von der Biologie sind psychologische Fragen unter sehr verschiedenen Aspekten behandelt worden. Am Ende des 19. Jahrhunderts waren es evolutionistische Gesichtspunkte der Entstehung und Arterhaltungsfunktion von Instinkten oder sinnesphysiologische Untersuchungen. Die Tierpsychologie und vergleichende Verhaltensforschung, die in den letzten Jahrzehnten im Vordergrund stand, wird an anderer Stelle besprochen (S. 797).

Von physiologischer Seite hat W.R. HESS eine Zusammenfassung von Hirnphysiologie und Psychologie versucht. Für HESS [H 65] kann psychisches Geschehen nicht durch energetische Konzeptionen erfaßt werden, sondern nur als *Ordnung* eines Kräftegefüges, die „den gemeinschaftlichen Nenner von neuronalem und psychischem Geschehen darstellt". Diese Ordnung kann sich in Kraft und Stoff manifestieren, ist aber weder Materie noch Energie, sondern wird nur repräsentiert in der Hirnorganisation und in psychischen Vorgängen. Der Begriff der *„psychischen Kraft"* ist sowohl auf Grund neurophysiologischer Experimente durch W.R. HESS wie früher schon von psychologischer und psychophysiologischer Seite aus der Konzeption der „psychischen Energie" entwickelt worden [L 7, 8]. Auch HEAD und andere Neurologen verwendeten energetische Konzeptionen [H 18].

„Psychische Kraft" und „psychische Energie". Die energetische Betrachtung blieb rein spekulativ wie bei C.G. JUNG [J 24] BERGER [B 23], hoffte, die psychische Energie aus der chemischen Energie des Hirnstoffwechsels nach Abzug der Wärmeproduktion und elektrischen Energie des Gehirns extrapolieren zu können. In seiner psychologischen Konzeption bezeichnet ROHRACHER [R 21] alle Trieb-, Willens-, Interessen- und Gefühlsfunktionen als „psychische Kräfte" und trennt sie von anderen psychischen Funktionen, wie Wahrnehmung, Denken, Vorstellung, Gedächtnis, auf welche die psychischen Kräfte wirken. Beide, der Neurophysiologe HESS und der Psychologe ROHRACHER, sehen darin „echte" Kräfte, deren Wirken wir sowohl in der Selbstbeobachtung erleben, wie im Verhalten beobachten können. „Sie sind die *einzigen* Kräfte in der Natur, von denen wir unmittelbare Kenntnis haben" (ROHRACHER [R 22]). Obwohl die neurophysiologischen Korrelate solcher Kräfte noch nicht genügend geklärt sind, kann ihr Vorhandensein nicht bezweifelt werden. Die Auswirkungen dieser Kräfte können durch einfache physikalische Effekte wie die elektrische Hirnreizung beeinflußt werden [P 9–17].

Die Natur psychischer Kräfte ist unbekannt und wird auch von HESS offengelassen [H 65]. Im Gegensatz zu dem Begriff der „psychischen Energie", der nur bei Korrelation mit echten energetischen Umwandlungen im ZNS sinnvoll wird, – wie bei BERGERS Postulaten – bedarf die *Annahme psychischer Kräfte nicht eines Rückgriffs auf noch unbekannte physiologische Prozesse.* Doch kann sie manche Parallelen zu physiologischen Erfahrungen liefern. Das in der Neurophysiologie häufige Phänomen eines relativen Gleichgewichts reziproker Systeme kann auch für psychische Kräfte angewandt werden. Der moderne Informationsbegriff kann vielleicht die energetischen Schwierigkeiten der Wirkungen psychischer Kräfte überwinden.

Utopie einer physiologischen Erklärung psychologischer Phänomene. Es ist aufschlußreich und nützlich, in einem aktuellen Forschungsgebiet an alte theoretische Versuche früherer Generationen zu erinnern, die in der gleichen Richtung tendieren. Moderne neurophysiologische Bestrebungen, Korrelationen mit psychophysischen Befunden herzustellen, finden wie in der Sinnesphysiologie ihre Vorläufer am Ende des 19. Jahrhunderts. Obwohl die Hirnphysiologie sich damals auf Reiz- und Ausschaltungsexperimente beschränkte, sind schon ähnliche psychophysiologische Konzeptionen vor mehr als einem halben Jahrhundert unter dem Eindruck der hirnanatomischen Entdeckungen der 90er Jahre auf der Basis der Neuronentheorie geäußert worden.

Es ist wohl kein Zufall, daß es psychologisch interessierte Mediziner und Physiologen waren, die damals eine Darstellung neuronaler Grundlagen psychischer Funktionen versuchten. Die Erfolge der Neuronentheorie in Anatomie, Physiologie und Neurologie schienen psychologische und psychiatrische Anwendungen zu rechtfertigen.

Die ersten derartigen Neuronenschemata psychischer Funktionen stammen von EXNER und von FREUD. Der Wiener Physiologe SIGMUND EXNER hat 1894 einige wesentliche Prinzipien der neuronalen Grundlagen psychischer Vorgänge erkannt und wie in Abb. 2 schematisch dargestellt [E 29]. FREUD [F 28] machte 1895 entsprechende theoretische Entwürfe.

Nachdem wir heute über die Physiologie des zentralen Nervensystems wesentlich mehr wissen als 1894 beim Erscheinen von EXNERS „Physiologischer Erklärung der psychischen Erscheinungen" [E 29] gibt es auch jetzt noch keine Psychophysiologie, die seelische Vorgänge in physiologischer Sprache darstellt. EXNER hat die ersten klaren Neuronenschemata mitgeteilt, die eine bahnende und hemmende Funktion der Aufmerksamkeitsvorgänge und eine zentrale Grundlage der Instinkt- und Affektvorgänge zu begründen versuchen (Abb. 2). Trotz vieler

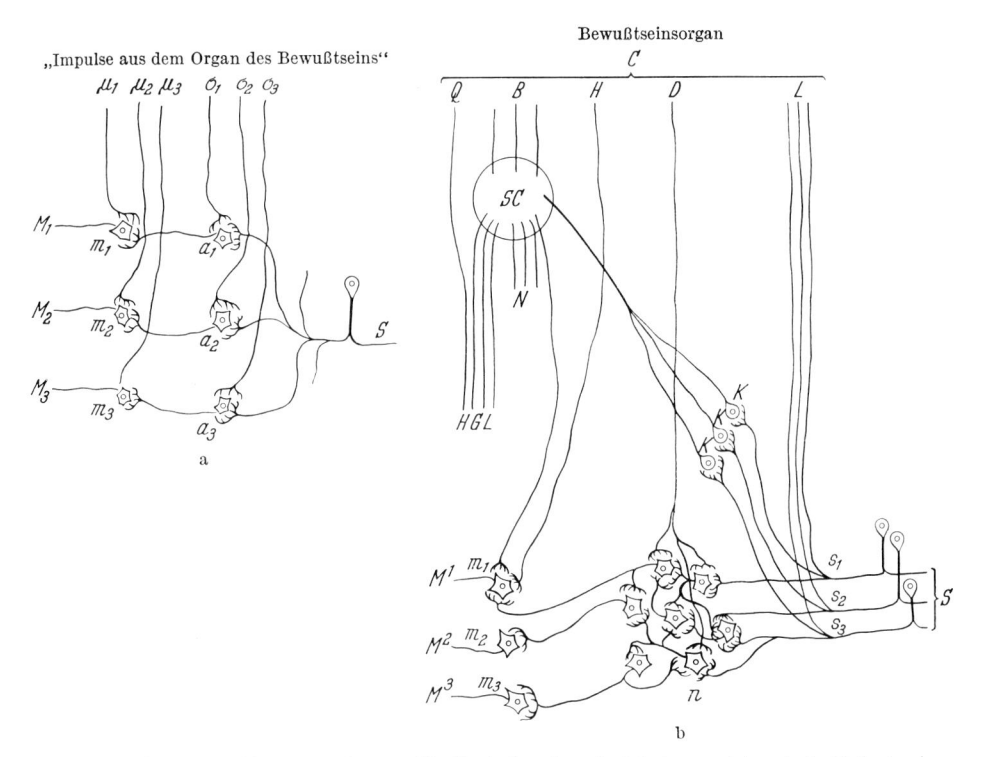

Abb. 2a u. b. EXNERS Neuronenschemata für die Aufmerksamkeitsbahnung (a) und die Unlustreaktionen bei Schmerzreizen (b). Nach EXNER [E 29] 1894. a zeigt in einem vereinfachten Schema, daß EXNER neben einer motorischen Bahnung an den Motoneuronen (m, 1–3) bereits eine zentrale Bahnung an den sensiblen Schaltzellen der Zwischenneurone (a, 1–3) postulierte, wie sie erst 60 Jahre später festgestellt wurde. b EXNERS Konzeption eines „Unlustzentrums" in Verbindung mit Schmerzreceptoren der Peripherie und effektorischen Fasern zu inneren Organen (Herz, Gefäße, Lungen) und der Körpermuskulatur. Die motorische Koordination auf spinaler Ebene dient zur Organisation von Abwehrbewegungen. EXNERS Erklärung lautet: „Schema des Unlustcentrums, C. Organ des Bewußtseins, S. sensorische, M. motorische Rückenmarksfasern, s. Teilungsstellen der sensorischen Fasern, m. motorische Ganglienzellen, n. Rückenmarkszentrum, k. Summationszentren, SC die Summe der Centren für die Muskeln der Abwehrbewegung, zu welchen Muskeln die Bahnen N führen. Mit diesen Centren hängen weiter zusammen gewisse zu dem Herzen, den Gefäßen und den Lungen gehende Fasern (H, G, L). Von den letztgenannten Gebilden führen sensorische Fasern (Q) zu dem Organe des Bewußtseins, das weiterhin durch die Bahnen B, H, D und L von den Vorgängen in den subcorticalen Zentren Nachricht bekommt"

neuer Befunde über neurophysiologische Grundlagen von Aufmerksamkeit, Instinkt- und Affektvorgängen wird aber auch jetzt bei besserer Kenntnis der neuronalen Mechanismen kaum jemand so optimistisch sein, das von EXNER bezeichnete psychophysiologische Programm zu erfüllen:

"Das nachstehende Werk stellt sich die Aufgabe, die Erklärbarkeit der psychischen Erscheinungen zu erweisen. – Unter einer Erklärung der psychischen Erscheinungen verstehe ich eine Zurückführung derselben auf uns anderweitig bekannte physiologische Vorgänge im Zentralnervensystem. – Ich betrachte es also als meine Aufgabe, die wichtigsten psychischen Erscheinungen auf die Abstufungen von Erregungszuständen der Nerven und Nervenzentren, demnach alles, was uns im Bewußtsein als Mannigfaltigkeit erscheint, auch quantitative Verhältnisse und auf die Verschiedenheit der zentralen Verbindungen von sonst wesentlich gleichartigen Nerven und Zentren zurückzuführen."

Nachdem auch EXNER zugegeben hat, daß seine Begründungen weitgehend hypothetisch sind, bleibt eine solche vollständige Rückführung seelischen Lebens auf physiologische Prozesse heute und vermutlich auch in der Zukunft selbst bei detaillierter und bester Kenntnis der Neurophysiologie und Kybernetik ein unerfüllbares Postulat.

Das soll keinen Zweifel daran ausdrücken, daß diese seelischen Vorgänge durch physiologische Neuronenprozesse bedingt sind. Wir werden aber jeweils die integrierten Endleistungen des Gehirns in ihren psychologisch-introspektiven oder ihren verhaltensmäßig äußeren Aspekten besser verstehen, als wir die ihnen zugrunde liegenden Koordinationsleistungen der Milliarden von Neuronen darstellen können.

Experimentelle Psychologien und Neurophysiologie

Ein Teil der experimentellen Psychologien wurde bereits mit der Psychophysik und Psychophysiologie besprochen. Hier sollen nur noch einige allgemeine Aspekte vom Standpunkt der Neurophysiologie dargestellt werden.

WUNDT und seine Schule. Es war in Deutschland üblich geworden, die experimentelle Psychologie, die mit WUNDT das Psychische als Naturphänomen auffaßte und naturwissenschaftliche Methoden in die Psychologie einführte, in unzulässiger Simplifizierung als „Assoziationspsychologie" zu bezeichnen. Man pflegte sie mit einem Ton der Verachtung als längst obsolet abzulehnen, oder sie gar mit der alten Vermögenspsychologie zusammenzuwerfen, die schon von HERBART und WUNDT ad absurdum geführt wurde. Nach dieser abschätzigen Beurteilung könnte man annehmen, daß die experimentelle Psychologie nichts anderes geleistet hätte, als seelische Phänomene durch Assoziationen zu erklären. In Wirklichkeit bildete diese psychologische Richtung die *Synthese der exakten empirischen Sinnesphysiologie des 19. Jahrhunderts mit einer gründlich durchdachten erkenntnistheoretischen Fundierung,* in der Begriffe psychischer Kausalität und Methoden finaler und kausaler Naturbetrachtung vereinigt wurden [W 33]. Dazu kam der pragmatische Verzicht WUNDTs auf metaphysische Zusammenhangsfragen von Körper und Seele, durch die frühere Psychologen auf spekulative Abwege geführt wurden.

In den experimentellen Arbeiten WUNDTs und seiner Lehre steckt auch viel neurophysiologisch Interessantes, ebenso wie in den gründlichen und meist sehr langen Schriften G.E. MÜLLERs und seiner Schüler. Von WUNDT angeregt wurden z.B. die ersten exakten Registrierungen der menschlichen Augenbewegungen von STRATTON [S 53]. G.E. MÜLLER hat neben seiner Ausarbeitung von FECHNERs psychophysischen Axiomen (Unterscheidung psychonomer und apsychonomer Prozesse) und seinen Studien über Gedächtnis und Zahlen-Diagramme [M 78] mit verschiedenen psycho-physischen Untersuchungen moderne Erkenntnisse der Neurophysiologie vorweggenommen: MÜLLERs Untersuchungen über die statischen Variationen der subjektiven Vertikalen haben eine Konvergenz optischer und vestibulärer Afferenzen vorausgesagt und seine theoretischen Postulate über das Farbensehen und die Farbenblindheit [M 80] sind neuerdings durch die Befunde SVAETICHINs an der Retina elektrophysiologisch verifiziert worden [S 57–62].

Zwar hat sich WUNDT nicht mit allen seinen allgemeinen Ansichten durchsetzen können. Seine Suche nach psychischen „Elementen" ist mit Recht kritisiert worden. Sein Prinzip, vom Elementaren zum Komplexen fortzuschreiten und nur einfache Vorgänge zu quantifizieren, ist durch die Erfolge der Testpsychologie und Persönlichkeitsforschung widerlegt, die unbekümmert um theoretische Bedenken auch Intelligenz und Triebstruktur meßbar erfaßte. WUNDTs „Koexistenz" psychischer und physischer Vorgänge ist ein gemilderter psychophysischer Parallelismus mit der empirischen Feststellung einer unvollständig nachweisbaren Entsprechung physiologischer und psychologischer Forschungsergebnisse [W 33, 34]. Sehr modern erscheint uns heute WUNDTs Bestreben, entgegen einer rein rationalen Psychologie emotionale Vorgänge und Triebe hoch zu bewerten, um die affektiven Grundlagen und die Gesamtheit des Seelischen zu erfassen. WUNDT hat mehrfach die inneren *Zusammenhänge aller seelischen Funktionen* betont und sich nicht auf eine Elementarpsychologie beschränkt: Psychische Elemente oder einfache Empfindungen sind „immer erst Produkte einer psychologischen Abstraktion ..., weil sie in Wirklichkeit nur in Verbindungen vorkommen" [W 33]. WUNDTs Konzeption der Willensvorgänge führt zur modernen Lehre der Motivationen.

WUNDTs „Voluntarismus" ist allerdings in Mißkredit gekommen. Doch steckt in seiner weiten Fassung des Wilensbegriffes, wenn man ihn auf biologische Trieb- und Zielvorgänge ausdehnt, wie dies WUNDT versucht hat, doch ein sehr brauchbarer Kern. Die moderne Verhaltensforschung hat gezeigt, daß tierische Organismen mit angeborenen Instinkten zweckvolle und zielgerichtete Handlungen durchführen, ohne oder nur mit geringer Erfahrungskomponente und ohne daß ein „Lernen" vorausging. Zwar kann jeder kausale Zusammenhang in unserem Denken teleologisch verwendet werden, indem unsere Vorstellung das Endergebnis vorwegnimmt. *Auf einer solchen denkenden Vorwegnahme beruht auch jede naturwissenschaftlich-experimentelle Forschungsmethode.* Das notwendig *teleologische Denken* des Forschers *dient der Untersuchung kausaler Zusammenhänge* (vgl. S. 775). Zweckvoll ist aber in Wirklichkeit nicht der biologisch-physikalisch-chemische Mechanismus, sondern nur die *zielgerichtete* Willenshandlung. WUNDT hat offenbar recht, wenn er diese Zweckvorgänge nicht nur als rückwärts gekehrte Kausalbetrachtung, sondern als vorwärts gerichtete Bedingung des tierischen Handelns sieht. Eine solche Anerkennung von Zweckhandlungen im psychischen und Verhaltensbereich ist nicht mit dem teleologisch-animistischen Prinzip der Entelechie des ARISTOTELES oder universeller organischer Zweckmäßigkeit als Werk einer vorausberechnenden Intelligenz oder mit SCHOPENHAUERs unbewußtem allgemeinem Willensprinzip zu verwechseln. Trieb, Wille und Zweckmotiv werden jeweils nur für *individuelle* Handlungen angenommen, soweit sie noch nicht kausal-mechanisch erklärt werden können. *Zweckmotiv und Zweckerfolg brauchen sich aber nicht zu decken* (vgl. S. 776).

Es ist in der experimentellen Psychologie ähnlich wie in anderen Naturwissenschaften: Als Einzeltatsachen sind auch die exaktesten empirischen Befunde wissenschaftlich wertlos, wenn sie nicht in den Zusammenhang begrifflicher Ordnung gebracht werden (vgl. S. 778). *Naturwissenschaftliches Erkennen ist vor allem Ordnung und Verbindung gesetzmäßiger Vorgänge,* die auf Grund des Kausalprinzips ablaufen. Auf den schwierigen Begriff und die Begründung der psychischen Kausalität, der uns auch bei den Entsprechungen neurophysiologischer und psychischer Phänomene immer wieder begegnet, können wir hier nicht eingehen. Die Annahme einer psychischen Kausalität wird dadurch erleichtert, daß, wie WUNDT sagt, „die kausale Beziehung selbst in der inneren Wahrnehmung gegeben ist". In der Naturwissenschaft muß sie dagegen immer erst indirekt erschlossen werden: *Psychische Kausalität und erlebte Kausalzusammenhänge sind anschaulich, physische Kausalzusammenhänge sind begrifflich erschlossen.* Gerade diese Anschaulichkeit erleichtert aber die Betrachtung komplexer psychischer Zusammenhänge in der Psychologie und Psychiatrie, während wir in der Neurophysiologie anschauliche Regeln erst mühsam aus einzelnen Experimenten in speziellen Mechanismen ableiten müssen. Psychisch erleben wir die ganze Integration der neuronalen Prozesse „von innen", physiologisch können wir nur einzelne Teile „von außen" feststellen. Auch in der Sinnesphysiologie profitieren wir von dieser unmittelbaren Anschaulichkeit. Es liegt daher nicht nur in der historischen Entwicklung, sondern auch im Wesen der Sinnesvorgänge selbst, daß die sinnesphysiologischen Gesetzmäßigkeiten zuerst im subjektiven Versuch und erst später in ihrem neurophysiologischen Mechanismus erforscht wurden (vgl. S. 907).

Begrenztheit der experimentellen Psychologie und Neurophysiologie. Die Schwierigkeiten einer psychiatrischen Anwendung der experimentellen Psychologie liegen ähnlich wie bei der experimentellen Neurophysiologie in der Begrenzung auf die einschränkenden Bedingungen des Laboratoriumsversuchs. In der Neurophysiologie sind nur beim Menschen erhaltene Ergebnisse für Psychologie und Psychiatrie direkt verwendbar. Die Resultate von Tierversuchen können nur vorsichtig zu wertende Analogien bringen oder allgemeine Gesetzmäßigkeiten des Nervensystems darstellen, deren psychiatrische Bedeutung gering ist.

In der Psychologie ist der Mensch zwar Forschungsobjekt, doch werden die psychologischen Ergebnisse eingeschränkt nicht nur durch die Begrenztheit der experimentellen Bedingungen, sondern auch durch die *psychologische Rückwirkung der Prüfungssituation oder der Selbstbeobachtung.* Dem entspricht die Überlegenheit einer lebendigen psychiatrischen Exploration, die alle wesentlichen Situationen und Umweltfaktoren berücksichtigen kann, gegenüber schematischen psychologischen Testmethoden. Daher kann auch die klinische Psychologie ebenso wie die Neurophysiologie nur eine Ergänzung der Klinik, aber nicht ihre echte Grundlage sein.

„Würzburger Schule". Die *Würzburger Psychologen* KÜLPE, BÜHLER und ihre Mitarbeiter haben die *Selbstbeobachtung mit dem Experiment vereint* und damit neue Einsichten in Denkpsychologie und Dynamik des Vorstellungsablaufs gewonnen [B 70]. Die aktive, intendierte Komponente des Denkprozesses wurde mit der determinierenden Tendenz herausgearbeitet. In Widerlegung der Skepsis, mit der WUNDT die Würzburger Bestrebungen aufnahm, hat diese Methode einer Kombination von Versuchsleiter und Beobachter sowohl gewisse Einseitigkeiten des reinen Reaktions- und Verhaltensexperiments wie die Fehlspekulationen unkontrollierter Introspektion überwunden. Sie hat auch die engsten Beziehungen zur psychiatrischen Exploration psychopathologischer Phänomene, die ebenfalls beides, *Selbstschilderung und Verhaltensbeobachtung,* vereint. Nur der tierexperimentellen Neurophysiologie ist die Introspektion verschlossen. Doch kann eine ähnliche doppelte (sprachliche und objektiv registrierende) Erfassung des „Innen" und „Außen" in der klinischen Neurophysiologie beim Menschen verwendet werden, etwa bei der Darstellung psychischer und hirnelektrischer Veränderungen des kleinen epileptischen Anfalls [J 26]. Zwar erscheint es wenig aussichtsvoll, die formalen Vorgänge der Denkprozesse neurophysiologisch aufzuklären, doch fand W. KÖHLER Parallelen zielgerichteten Handelns bei höheren Affen [K 29], die nach ähnlichen Denkgesetzen abzulaufen scheinen, wie sie KÜLPE, BÜHLER und SELZ [S 220] festgestellt haben. Ob die Steuerung solcher Denk-Vorgänge später einmal mit physiologischen Gesetzmäßigkeiten der Antriebs- und Aufmerksamkeitsregulierung in verschiedenen Sinnesgebieten korreliert werden kann, muß offen bleiben. Neurophysiologisch registrierbar sind bisher nur hirnelektrische Korrelate der Aufmerksamkeit [B 25, J 36], der Reizerwartung [W 10], der Bewegungsbereitschaft [K 43] und der Zielbewegungskontrolle [G 43, 44]. Beispiele zeigen Abb. 11 und 43 (vgl. S. 832).

Gestaltpsychologie. In den letzten Jahrzehnten ist die *Psychologie der Gestaltwahrnehmung* in der von WERTHEIMER und W. KÖHLER [K 32] entwickelten Form zusammen mit der Ganzheitspsychologie auch in die Neurologie und Psychiatrie eingedrungen. GOLDSTEIN [G 29] hat sie für seine Konzeptionen der Hirnverletzungsfolgen angewandt und CONRAD verwendet vor allem den Begriff der „Vorgestalt", den der Psychologe SANDER aus tachistoskopischen Untersuchungen entwickelte, für die Aphasielehre und Hirnpathologie [C 9, 10].

CONRADs Vorgestalt bezeichnet ähnlich wie die Prägnanztendenz in der Gestaltpsychologie eine diffuse Qualität des Angemutetseins, die zu einer gestaltlichen Präzisierung drängt, aber bei hirnpathologischen Störungen eine bewußte Präzision nicht erreicht. Wir haben in einer Diskussion mit CONRAD hervorgehoben, daß eine solche Vorgestaltung mehr im Bereich der unbewußten und neurophysiologischen Integrationsmechanismen zu suchen ist [J 29]. Bewußtes Wahrnehmen oder Vorstellen ist beim Gesunden bereits weitgehend gestaltet [C 11]. Nur im Traum und bei hirnpathologischen Störungen erscheinen unpräzisere, oft affektabhängige, unvollkommen gestaltete Vorgänge. In der *vorbewußten Sphäre* der Phantasie oder des Traumes überwiegt aber oft gerade die *bildhaft gestaltete eidetische Schau* über das unanschaulich diffuse Gefühlserlebnis. Besonders wertvoll sind gewisse Einsichten der Gestaltpsychologie für die *Sinnesphysiologie.* Neurophysiologische Gestaltungsprozesse sind von den Gestaltpsychologen bereits früh postuliert worden. Wenn sie im einzelnen auch noch nicht physiologisch faßbar sind, so ergeben sich doch, wie im sinnesphysiologischen Kapitel (vgl. S. 929) dargestellt, erste Ansätze für neurophysiologische Parallelen. Dennoch bleibt die Gestaltpsychologie wie andere Psychologien relativ unabhängig von der Neurophysiologie. METZGER [M 38] sagt daher 1936: „Mit unserer Wahrnehmungslehre beugen wir uns nicht vor der Physiologie, sondern wir geben ihr Aufgaben." Zweifellos ist eine solche Forschungsbeziehung und Aufgabestellung aber nicht einseitig von der Psychologie zur Physiologie gerichtet, sondern *wechselseitige Anregung beider Fächer*. Auch die Psychologie darf es nicht ablehnen, Aufgaben von der Neurophysiologie zu übernehmen.

Reflexologie und Lernpsychologie. Die von PAWLOW [P 7], BECHTEREW [B 19] und amerikanischen Behavioristen [T 5, W 12] begründete Lernphysiologie hat einen großen Einfluß sowohl auf die physiologische, wie auf die psychologische Forschung gehabt. Einige physiologische Korrelationen werden im Kapitel über die bedingten Reflexe besprochen (vgl. S. 1027).

Behaviorismus. Die von WATSON begründete behavioristische Forschungsrichtung [W 12], die sich auf Analysen des Verhaltens beschränkt und die Introspektion ablehnt, hat die amerikanische Psychologie stark beeinflußt. Durch WATSONS Analyse des kindlichen Lernens und der Entstehung neurotischer Verhaltensweisen gegenüber der Umwelt ist auch die Psychiatrie angesprochen worden. Schließlich wurde die Verhaltensforschung bei Tieren, der auch nur behavioristische Kriterien zur Verfügung stehen, durch WATSON und seine Schüler angeregt, vor allem durch SKINNER [S 35]. Der Behaviorismus hat ein berechtigtes Mißtrauen gegenüber den oft affektiv gefärbten Erkenntnissen der Introspektion begründet. Ihr Hauptverdienst liegt in der Anregung experimenteller Verhaltensuntersuchungen. Doch geht diese Forschungsrichtung zu weit, wenn sie aus dogmatischen Erwägungen auf unsere wichtigste psychologische Erkenntnisquelle der unmittelbaren inneren Anschauung verzichtet. Ihre umständliche Terminologie, die sich aus dem Verzicht auf direkte psychische Zustandsbeschreibungen ergibt, ist ein unnötiger Ballast. Sie beläßt den Psychologen auf demselben Stand wie den Ethologen bei der Verhaltensforschung an Tieren. Trotz dieser Einseitigkeit gab der Behaviorismus auch Anregungen für die Neurophysiologie durch die Entwicklung von HULLS Lerntheorie und ihrer experimentellen Anwendungen. In einer sehr gemilderten Form ist auch HEBBS Psychologie [H 21] behavioristisch oder pseudobehavioristisch. Wenn HEBB die kognitiven Prozesse als höhere Formen des Verhaltens bezeichnet und seelische Vorgänge mit zur Analyse des Verhaltens verwendet, so ist dies kein reiner Behaviorismus mehr.

Geisteswissenschaftliche Psychologien. Die geisteswissenschaftliche Psychologie DILTHEYS mit ihrer strengen Unterscheidung psychologischen Verstehens und naturwissenschaftlichen Erklärens, die von JASPERS mit großem Erfolg in die Psychiatrie eingeführt wurde, bringt der Neurophysiologie nicht mehr als methodologische Besinnung. Die nüchtern beschreibende und ordnende psychologische Phänomenologie von KARL JASPERS [J 13] läßt mit dessen einprägsamen Bildern für die Funktion des Bewußtseins vielleicht einige neurophysiologische Anwendungen zu (vgl. S. 971).

Am wenigsten Beziehung hat die Neurophysiologie zur „Wesensschau" der *Phänomenologen* und *Existentialisten*. *Entgegen* den Intentionen ihrer philosophischen Begründer Husserl und Heidegger, die den „Psychologismus" bekämpften, hat die Phänomenologie und Existenzphilosophie doch zu psychologischen und psychiatrischen Anwendungen geführt. Der Neurophysiologe kann damit nicht viel anfangen.

Psychoanalyse. Auf die zahlreichen Versuche, psychoanalytische und tiefenpsychologische Vorstellungen in ein neurophysiologisches Gewand zu kleiden, können wir hier nicht eingehen. Sie reichen von Freuds Neuronenhypothese [F 27] von 1895 (S. 603) und seinem Postulat quantitativer Libidomechanik über den Begriff der psychischen Energie C.G. Jungs [J 24] bis zu hirnanatomischen Konstruktionen des Symbolwerts bestimmter Hirnteile [R 34]. Sie enden in Versuchen einer modernen Hirnmythologie, neben Bewußtsein und Aufmerksamkeit auch das unbewußte „Es" in die Reticularis des Hirnstamms oder das limbische System zu lokalisieren [M 13], und in psychosomatischen Konstruktionen über Objektbilder des Sexualtriebs im Schläfenlappen [O 11]. Das „Ich" wird dann nach den jeweiligen Konzeptionen der Zeit im Cortex oder in der Reticularis lokalisiert. All das sind Spekulationen ohne objektives neurophysiologisches Korrelat.

Gehirn und Selbst bei Popper und Eccles. Eine neue *dualistische Konzeption von Gehirn und Bewußtsein* haben Popper und Eccles, 1977 mit ihrem Buch "The Self and its Brain" [P 32] vorgeschlagen. Sie postulieren eine Wechselwirkung von Körper und Seele als *„interactionism"* und greifen damit auf Descartes zurück. Bei strenger Trennung von Materie und Geist wird die für Descartes' Theorie fatale Frage nach dem Sitz der Seele vermieden, da dem Gehirn als „liaison brain" eine Eigentätigkeit zugestanden wird, die eine Entwicklung des psychischen Selbst ermöglicht. Die Theorie berücksichtigt zwar alle modernen Ergebnisse der Hirnforschung, aber unterscheidet mit ihrer Welt 2 und 3 den seelischen und kulturellen Bereich von den körperlichen Mechanismen. Im Gegensatz zu dem bei Naturwissenschaftlern verbreiteten monistischen Glauben, daß Psychisches und Somatisches nur zwei verschiedene Aspekte der gleichen Person und ihrer Hirntätigkeit sind, werden Seele und Gehirn als *Interaktion zweier Einheiten* aufgefaßt.

Popper geht aus von seinem früheren Schema dreier verschiedener Welten [P 31], die in Tabelle 1 schematisch dargestellt sind: 1. *materielle Welt*, 2. *individuelles Selbst* und 3. *Kulturwelt* der Menschheit. In der Kulturwelt 3 ist alles verarbeitete Wissen der Menschengeschichte enthalten, das auch in objektiver Form als Literatur, Geistes- und Naturwissenschaft und Technik existiert. Es wird als Bildung vom einzelnen Menschen erworben und daher auch im Gedächtnis cerebral gespeichert, ist aber materiell auch in Welt 1 enthalten, wird in Bibliotheken dokumentiert und in Schulen und Universitäten gelehrt usw.

Der Dualismus der beiden Autoren postuliert, daß die Erlebniseinheit des Bewußtseins nicht als Hirnmechanismus zu verstehen ist, sondern mit dem Bewußtsein selbst geschaffen wird oder – wie Eccles sich ausdrückt – als „selfconscious mind" oder „self" in jedem Menschen mit der Kindesentwicklung entsteht. Der Körper- und Hirnmechanismus ist also nicht wie bei Descartes nur von der in der Epiphyse als Kommandozentrale gedachten spirituellen *Seele* (anima der Scholastiker) gesteuert, sondern hat selbst seinen Anteil an der Reifung und Differenzierung des menschlichen „Selbst". Dieses Selbst führt jedoch ein

Tabelle 1. POPPERs Welten 1, 2 und 3. Nach POPPER und ECCLES (1977) [P 32] und ECCLES (1978) [E 5c]. *Welt 1* ist die materielle belebte und unbelebte Welt. *Welt 2* ist das bewußte Selbst. *Welt 3* entspricht den menschlichen Kulturwerten. Welt 1 enthält auch die vom Menschen geschaffenen Kulturwerte, soweit sie objektiv als Material der Kulturwelt 3 wie in Büchern, Bildern usw., nach einem Lernprozeß auch im Gehirn gespeichert und über die Wahrnehmung indirekt zugänglich sind. Cerebral sind sie als Gedächtnisspeicher vorhanden und dort direkt abrufbar. Alle Wechselwirkungen der Welten 2 und 3 gehen daher jeweils immer über die materielle Welt 1

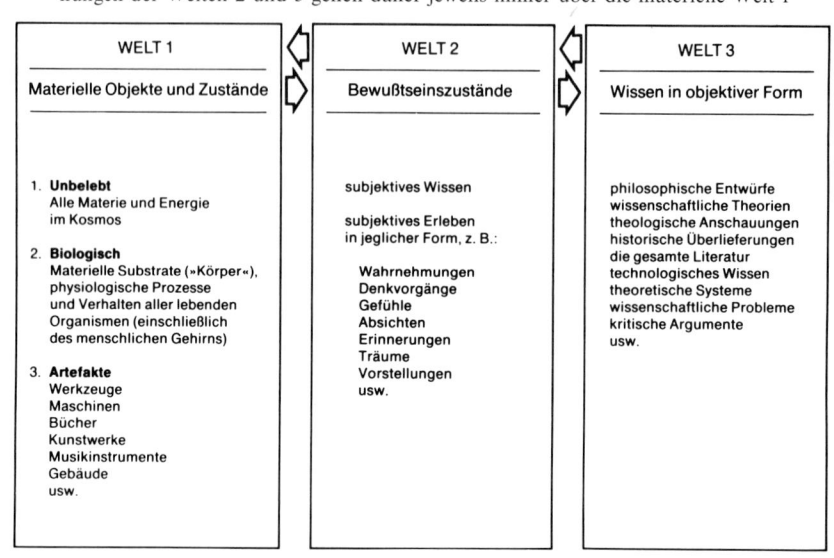

WELT 1	WELT 2	WELT 3
Materielle Objekte und Zustände	Bewußtseinszustände	Wissen in objektiver Form
1. **Unbelebt** Alle Materie und Energie im Kosmos 2. **Biologisch** Materielle Substrate (»Körper«), physiologische Prozesse und Verhalten aller lebenden Organismen (einschließlich des menschlichen Gehirns) 3. **Artefakte** Werkzeuge Maschinen Bücher Kunstwerke Musikinstrumente Gebäude usw.	subjektives Wissen subjektives Erleben in jeglicher Form, z. B.: Wahrnehmungen Denkvorgänge Gefühle Absichten Erinnerungen Träume Vorstellungen usw.	philosophische Entwürfe wissenschaftliche Theorien theologische Anschauungen historische Überlieferungen die gesamte Literatur technologisches Wissen theoretische Systeme wissenschaftliche Probleme kritische Argumente usw.

Eigenleben und ist nicht nur ein anderer Aspekt der neuronalen Mechanismen „seines" Gehirns, wie es die monistische Konzeption postuliert. Die Einheitlichkeit und Kontinuität des Bewußtseins, die wir als Erlebnisselektion der Wahrnehmung aus den zahlreichen Sinnesmeldungen deuten und die einen sehr begrenzten Informationseingang von etwa 16 bit/sec hat (vgl. S. 975), soll nach ECCLES nicht eine neurophysiologische Synthese, sondern eine spezielle integrierende Funktion des Selbstbewußtseins sein. Das Selbst bezieht seine Information aus dem Verbindungsgehirn der „liaison brain" und spielt auf diesem wie auf einem Musikinstrument [P 32]. Aber wie diese Welt 2, das bewußte Selbst mit den differenzierten Hirnmechanismen zusammenhängt, bleibt auch bei dieser Konzeption unklar. Zwar zieht ECCLES für sein Verbindungshirn neuere Konzeptionen der modularen Ordnung heran, aber auch wenn er sagt, daß mit 2 Millionen „moduls" im Cortex alle Erlebnisse eines langen Lebens verarbeitet und als Muster (pattern) gespeichert werden können, bleibt ihre Projektion ins Bewußtsein ungeklärt. ECCLES' Schema der Abb. 4 läßt offen, wie die über dem Gehirn schwebende Welt 2 ihre Verbindungspfeile zu den Hirnmechanismen betätigt. In ECCLES' deutscher Übersicht über seine Theorien [E 5c] erscheint die dualistische Konzeption stärker simplifiziert als in dem Buch mit POPPER, in dem die verschiedenen Leib-Seele-Theorien von der Antike bis zur modernen Zeit ausführlich diskutiert werden [P 32]. POPPER gibt auch zu, daß ein monistisches Konzept später einmal annehmbar sein kann, aber er hält dies für nicht wahrscheinlich. Die *Koexistenz von finalem Denken und relativer Willensfreiheit*

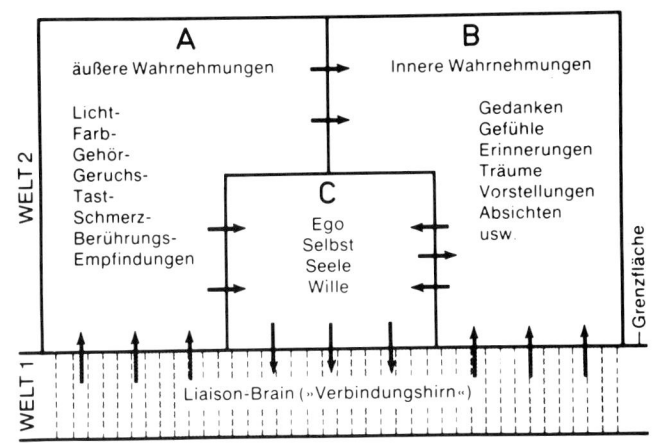

Abb. 3. ECCLES' Informationsfluß-Schema zwischen Gehirn und Bewußtsein. Nach ECCLES (1978) [P 32, E 5c].
A: Äußere Wahrnehmungen über die Sinnesorgane.
B: Die Vorstellungen werden zusammen mit dem Denken von ECCLES als „innere Wahrnehmung" zusammengefaßt, die mit den Sinneswahrnehmungen koordiniert werden und als Gedächtnisspeicher im Verbindungsgehirn deponiert sind.
C: Der Kern des bewußten und wollenden Selbst kommuniziert zwar im Gehirn mit seinen Wahrnehmungskomponenten, aber mit der Außenwelt nur indirekt über das Verbindungshirn und seine moduläre Struktur, die als senkrechte Kolumnen schematisiert sind

in einer kausal determinierten Welt ist einfacher und deutlicher mit N. HARTMANNS *Schichtprinzip* [H 11] auszudrücken, das von POPPER nicht beachtet und zitiert wird. Die Abhängigkeit der oberen seelischen von den unteren biologisch-physikalischen Schichten und ihre begrenzte Freiheit bezeichnet klarer die *Grenzen* der seelischen Handlungsführung und der Willensfreiheit in der realen Welt. POPPERS Weltkonzept wäre mit HARTMANNS Dependenzgesetz etwa so zu formulieren: *Das Selbst der Welt 2 ist nur dann relativ frei für Willensentscheidungen, wenn es dem Gesetz der Welt 1 gehorcht und die Kenntnisse dazu aus dem Wissen der Kulturwelt 3 schöpft.* Auch in der Welt 3 haben sich eigene soziale Regeln entwickelt, die von dem Selbst der Welt 2 bei seinen Konzepten zu beachten sind.

Aus diesem Überblick über neurophysiologische Aspekte der verschiedenen Psychologien wird klar, daß beide Wissenschaften, die psychologische wie die neurophysiologische Forschung, zwar ihre eigenen Gesetze haben, aber in gegenseitiger Anregung und Wechselwirkung stehen. *Die Psychologie hat Zugänge zu den höchstintegrierten Leistungen des Gehirns, welche die Neurophysiologie nur in einigen Elementarvorgängen erfassen kann.* Beide Disziplinen können neue Erkenntnisse gewinnen, wenn sie Korrelationen mit den Ergebnissen des anderen Faches beachten. So gering die Bedeutung der psychophysiologischen Forschung noch für die praktische Psychiatrie ist, so vielversprechend sind ihre Ergebnisse für die Neurophysiologie der cerebralen Koordinationsvorgänge.

Die Psychologie kann nur in begrenztem Umfange Anregungen aus der Neurophysiologie erhalten, und umgekehrt die Physiologie von der Psychologie

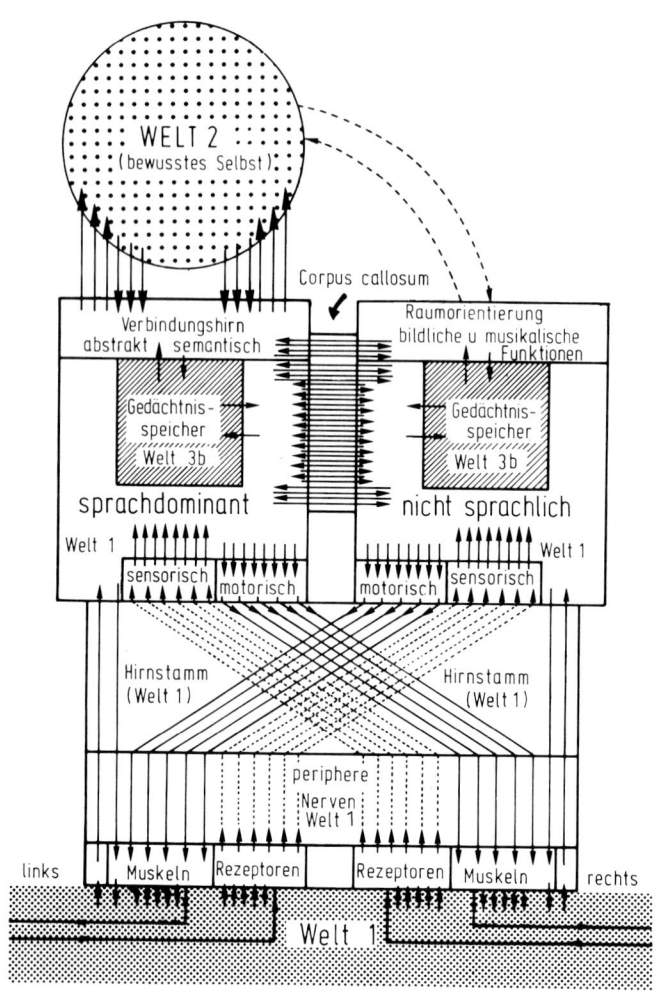

Abb. 4. Eccles' Schema der Welten 1–3 mit dem Impulsfluß von und zur Außenwelt über das Gehirn. Nach Popper und Eccles (1977) [P 32] und Eccles (1978) [E 5c]. Afferente Sinnesmeldungen laufen über die Receptoren zu beiden Großhirnhemisphären und efferente Impulse zurück zur Muskulatur mit der Aktivität der Organismen in der Umwelt.

Die vorwiegend gekreuzten Bahnverbindungen zu und von den Großhirnhemisphären werden durch Balkenimpulse über das Corpus callosum koordiniert. Das bewußte Selbst, Welt 2, wirkt entsprechend der Sprachlokalisation vorwiegend über die linke Hemisphäre des Verbindungshirns. Außenwelt und auch andere Menschen gehören zu Welt 1, die nur über das Verbindungshirn auf die Welt 2, das bewußte Selbst, einwirken kann. Die kulturelle *Welt 3* ist nur als Gedächtnisspeicher im individuellen Gehirn vorhanden, aber außerdem als objektiver Kulturvorrat der Menschheit auch in Welt 1 mit allen zivilisatorischen Organisationen, Bibliotheken usw. deponiert. Die Kulturwelt 3 ist, also wiederum für das Selbst nur über Welt 1 zu erreichen, indirekt über Sinnesmeldungen der objektiven Kulturprodukte und direkt über den Gedächtnisspeicher, der trotz subjektiver Zugänglichkeit auch somatisch im Gehirn deponiert ist

nur wenige Ergebnisse integrierter Endleistungen als Indicatoren für ihre Forschung verwenden. Neurophysiologisch exakt zu untersuchen sind Korrelate oder Grundlagen von solchen psychischen Phänomenen und Leistungen, die entweder *Reaktionen auf äußere Reize* sind, oder die als *„endogene" Vorgänge mit objektiv faßbaren körperlichen Begleiterscheinungen* einhergehen. Vor allem geeignet sind *quantifizierbare* psychische Phänomene, wie sie vorwiegend in der Wahrnehmung auftreten. Unter besonderen Bedingungen können auch Affekte und Triebe oder triebbedingte „Stimmungen" bei Tieren quantativ untersucht werden, wie von Holst [H 84] gezeigt hat. Nicht korrelierbar mit physiologischen Vorgängen sind primäre psychische Qualitäten. Zur Zeit bieten die folgenden psychischen Phänomene gute Voraussetzungen für eine neurophysiologische Analyse: Wahrnehmungsphänomene (S. 906) Motivations- und Triebvorgänge (S. 937), Bewußtseinsveränderungen und Schlaf (S. 968 und 987), Lernen und Gedächtnis (S. 1023). Schließlich können auch interindividuelle Kommunikationen und Informationen, die bis jetzt nur wenig neurophysiologisch bearbeitet sind, wahrscheinlich durch kybernetische Untersuchungen noch besser gefördert werden (vgl. Kapitel VI).

Bevor wir diese speziellen Korrelationen darstellen, soll die Situation der experimentellen Neurophysiologie und des Tierversuchs mit der Vergleichbarkeit von Tieren und Menschen besprochen werden.

Zusammenfassung

Psychologie und Neurophysiologie sind durch ihre verschiedenen Methoden und deren adäquate Anwendung auf zwei Schichten der menschlichen Lebensäußerungen charakterisiert. Die Abhängigkeit der „höheren" psychischen Schicht von den niederen vitalen Prozessen entspricht einer *Koexistenz kausaler Mechanismen und finaler Prozesse in einer identischen Welt*. Monistische oder dualistische Konzeptionen der Gehirn-Seele-Beziehung können ebenso wie Poppers Drei-Welten-Schema je nach der Fragestellung physiologisch brauchbar sein. Psychologische Termini geben den Neurophysiologen und Verhaltensforschern nützliche Abkürzungen für komplexe Hirnfunktionen und zielbestimmte Verhaltensweisen und können diese prägnant kennzeichnen. Einige physiologische Korrelationen von Psychologie und Psychophysik werden mit allgemeinen Konzeptionen der psychischen Kraft und psychischen Energie besprochen. Obwohl deren physiologische Grundlagen noch unklar bleiben, können alle quantitativ-psychologischen *Methoden der Skalierung und psychophysischen Sinnesmessungen* mit neurophysiologischen Registrierungen korreliert werden. Die Utopie rein physiologischer Erklärungen psychischer Phänomene wird am Beispiel der Neuronen-Schemata Exners und Freuds dargestellt. Die Psychologie kann auch integrierte Hirnleistungen in Wahrnehmung, Planung und Handlung erfassen, während die Neurophysiologie nur einige ihrer Elementarvorgänge darstellt. In Poppers und Eccles' Schema (materielle Welt 1, bewußte Welt 2 und kulturelle Welt 3) gehen alle Beziehungen über die materielle Welt 1 und ihr „Verbindungsgehirn". Das „Selbst" der Welt 2 kann aber nach N. Hartmann nur selbständig handeln, wenn es den materiellen Gesetzen (Welt 1) gehorcht und das Wissen der Kulturwelt 3 (über den Gedächtnisspeicher) berücksichtigt.

IV. Tier und Mensch: Zoologische Verhaltensforschung, Neurophysiologie und Psychiatrie

„... alles dieses kann nur dann ... eingesehen werden, wenn wir nicht wie bisher ... den Menschen im Thiere suchen, sondern wenn wir von unten herauf anfangen und das einfachere Thier im zusammengesetzten Menschen endlich wieder entdecken."

J.W. GOETHE: Vorträge über die drey ersten Capitel des Entwurfs einer allgemeinen Einleitung in die vergleichende Anatomie, ausgehend von der Osteologie, 1796

„Thierische Triebe wecken und entwickeln die geistigen. Thierische Empfindungen begleiten die geistigen ... Die Thätigkeiten des Körpers entsprechen den Thätigkeiten des Geistes. Geistige Lust hat jederzeit eine thierische Lust, geistige Unlust jederzeit eine thierische Unlust zur Begleiterin."

F. SCHILLER: Versuch über den Zusammenhang der thierischen Natur des Menschen mit seiner geistigen. 1780.

Die Neurophysiologie gewinnt ihre Ergebnisse vorwiegend aus dem *Tierversuch*. Die beim Menschen anwendbaren physiologischen Methoden sind in ihrem wissenschaftlichen Erkenntniswert sehr begrenzt und ihre Zulässigkeit ist beschränkt, vor allem auch durch ethische Rücksichten. Alle physiologischen und experimentellen Methoden, die mit Eingriffen am Gehirn verbunden sind oder Schädigungen hinterlassen können, sind dem gesunden Menschen nicht zumutbar: Sowohl „Kaspar-Hauser-Versuche" strenger frühkindlicher Isolierung wie direkte Elektrodenapplikationen im Hirngewebe können bleibende Schäden verursachen und müssen daher unterbleiben. Die Isolierung würde die psychische Entwicklung hemmen, und die direkten Ableitungen könnten die Hirnsubstanz schädigen. Direkte Hirnableitungen sind nur bei Kranken durchzuführen, bei denen eine medizinische Indikation für solche Eingriffe besteht. So ist die Neurophysiologie für die Grundlagenforschung auf *Analogieschlüsse aus dem Tierversuch* angewiesen, wenn sie nicht überhaupt darauf verzichten will, etwas über neurophysiologische Entsprechungen psychischer Phänomene auszusagen. Ein vor allem den Psychiater interessierender direkter Vergleich subjektiven Erlebens mit objektiven Leistungen des ZNS ist auf wenige Beobachtungen beim Menschen und auf Analogien beim Tier beschränkt. Es ist deshalb unvermeidbar, kurz auf *Gemeinsamkeiten und Unterschiede von Tier und Mensch* einzugehen.

Daß, wie die Tierarten untereinander, so auch der Mensch von ihnen allen erheblich verschieden ist, bedarf keiner Ausführung. Es ist nur die Frage, ob es sich wirklich um so grundsätzliche Unterschiede handelt, daß jeder Vergleich unmöglich wird, wie manche Philosophen und Geisteswissenschaftler annehmen. *Den Neurophysiologen interessiert vor allem das, was Mensch und Tier gemeinsam haben.* Deshalb wird seine Forschung am erfolgreichsten sein, wenn er sich auf solche gemeinsamen Funktionen beschränkt. Wenn wir im folgenden vereinfachend von „Mensch" und „Tier" sprechen oder Eigenschaften „des" Menschen und „der" Tiere anführen, so sollen weder Artmerkmale noch individuelle oder Altersunterschiede übersehen werden. Es sollen nur menschliche Arteigenschaften erwähnt werden, die ihn von Tieren unterscheiden, wie auch solche, die er mit ihnen gemeinsam hat. Die zoologische Verhaltensforschung (Ethologie) hat sich mit diesen allgemeinen Fragen mehr beschäftigt als die Neurophysiologie. PLOOGS Kapitel in diesem Band gibt eine ausführliche Übersicht der Soziobiologie von Affen und Menschen.

Ethologie, Neurophysiologie und Psychologie

Die Ethologie oder Verhaltensforschung nimmt eine Mittelstellung zwischen neurophysiologischer und psychologischer Forschung ein. *Komplexe Regulationen des Nervensystems sind in ihrem Verhaltensaspekt einfacher zu beschreiben als in ihren neuronalen Mechanismen.* Wiederum sind bestimmte *Verhaltensreaktionen einfacher zu verstehen, wenn man sie in psychologischer Sprache darstellt.* Daher die Bezeichnung „Tierpsychologie" für die zoologische Verhaltensforschung. Die Gefahr einer anthropomorphen Deutung ist dabei geringer als das Risiko der Unverständlichkeit und Umständlichkeit. Psychologische Termini sind in Kauf zu nehmen, wenn man die Beschreibung von Ausdruck und Verhalten kurz und verständlich machen will. „Wutreaktion", „Demuthaltung", „Triumphgeschrei" sind solche psychologischen Abbreviaturen der Verhaltensforschung für sonst nur sehr umständlich zu beschreibende motorische Entäußerungen mit Affektcharakter. Wie es unzweckmäßig wäre, Verhaltensreaktionen von Tier und Mensch (etwa auf die Wahrnehmung eines Artgenossen) neurophysiologisch mit der komplexen Koordination von Erregung und Hemmung aller daran beteiligten Sinnes- und Neuronensysteme zu beschreiben, ebenso unsinnig wäre es, rein behavioristisch einen psychologischen Wahrnehmungsvorgang nur durch die von Sinnesreizen ausgelösten motorischen und mimischen Begleiterscheinungen des Verhaltens zu beschreiben. Wenn wir den integrierten Wahrnehmungsvorgang selbst introspektiv erkennen und sprachlich beschreiben können, genügt meist eine kurze psychologische Bezeichnung. Da dies aber nur bei Menschen möglich ist, wird man sich beim Tier auf eine Verhaltens*deutung* beschränken, der gewisse Unsicherheiten anhaften. Um die Verhaltensbeobachtungen verständlich zu machen, können wir ebenso wie für die Neurophysiologie komplexer integrierter Vorgänge psychologische Termini nicht entbehren. In diesem Sinn gibt es auch eine wissenschaftliche „Tierpsychologie", die über die reine Verhaltensbeschreibung hinausgeht und nicht populärer Anthropomorphismus ist, wie er an BREHM und anderen älteren Zoologen oft gerügt wurde.

Die verschiedenen Positionen des Physiologen, Ethologen und Psychologen bei der Untersuchung von Tier und Mensch hat ROEDER [R 20] in einem *Schema* klar zusammengefaßt (Abb. 5). Der *Physiologe* (Ph) versucht, die Einzelmechanismen des tierischen Verhaltens zu analysieren, indem er mit seinen Methoden Teile des Nervensystems ausschaltet, reizt oder unter bestimmten Bedingungen von einzelnen Strukturen ableitet. Er kann dies meist nur unter sehr eingeschränkten artefiziellen Bedingungen tun, die bis zur Narkose des Versuchstieres reichen und daher nicht gleichzeitig das normale Verhalten des ganzen Tieres untersuchen. Der *Ethologe* (E) beobachtet das ganze Tier in natürlicher oder

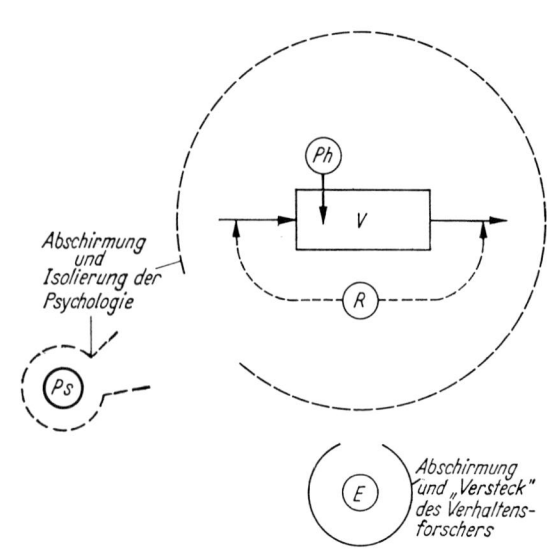

Abb. 5. Schema neurophysiologischer, ethologischer und psychologischer Forschung am Nervensystem. Modifiziert nach ROEDER, 1961 [R 25]. *V* bezeichnet das *Versuchsobjekt* (Tier oder Mensch). Die *Physiologen* (*Ph*) dringen in das Nervensystem ein, indem sie Teile ausschalten, reizen oder elektrische Phänomene ableiten. Sie beschränken sich damit auf *Einzelmechanismen*. Die *Reiz-Reaktionsforscher* (*R*) stehen zwischen den Neurophysiologen (*Ph*) und Ethologen (*E*), indem sie durch afferente Reize Reflexe und Reaktionen auslösen und auch am ganzen Tier komplizierte Lernvorgänge und bedingte Reaktionen erforschen. Die *Ethologen* (*E*) begnügen sich als Verhaltensforscher mit der Beobachtung des intakten Tieres in natürlicher oder künstlicher Umgebung und verstecken sich, um die Tiere nicht zu stören. Die *Psychologen* verwenden für sich und die Versuchsperson eine doppelte Abschirmung gegen störende Einflüsse, benutzen mehr oder weniger künstlich vereinfachte Situationen und beschränken sich auf sprachliche Kommunikationen oder verhaltensanalytische Beobachtungen

künstlicher Umgebung, indem er sich von der übrigen Welt abschirmt. Aber da seine Zeit begrenzt ist, wird er zur Lösung bestimmter Fragestellungen auch nicht auf künstliche Reize und eingeschränkte Bedingungen verzichten können. Die physiologisch ausgerichteten Reaktions-Ethologen (R) untersuchen, ebenso wie die Konditionierungs-Forscher, bestimmte Reiz- und Reaktionsbeziehungen, die durch Rückmeldung beeinflußt und beschränkt werden. Der *Psychologe* (Ps) setzt sich selbst ebenso wie das Versuchstier oder die Versuchsperson in eine Abschirmung, die er mit Hilfe verbaler Kommunikation oder auch durch Verhaltensanalyse durchdringt. Er benutzt ebenfalls künstliche Versuchsbedingungen zur Untersuchung komplexer Vorgänge und ihrer Erlebnisseite.

Alle Methoden, Beobachtungen und Experimente müssen Einschränkung und Begrenzung auf wenige Fragestellungen und Versuchsbedingungen in Kauf nehmen, wenn sie wissenschaftlich brauchbare Ergebnisse bringen sollen. Aus dieser Begrenztheit der experimentellen Verhaltensforschung ergibt sich die Notwendigkeit ihrer *Ergänzung durch psychologische Methoden*.

Psychologische Terminologie und Verhaltensbeschreibung. Die Verwendung psychologischer Termini und Betrachtungsweisen hat den Vorteil leichter Verständlichkeit und unmittelbarer Erfassung von Ganzheitsqualitäten. Die Warnung der Verhaltensforscher und Physiologen vor dem „Psychologisieren" ist zwar berechtigt, doch darf ein Verzicht auf psychologische Termini nicht zu umständlicher und unverständlicher Darstellung führen. Was wir psychologisch mit einem treffenden Wort bezeichnen und sofort verstehen, ist durch Verhaltensbeschreibung nur sehr viel umständlicher darzustellen.

Wenn man nach einer Gruppenbeobachtung von Affen auf Grund eines oft wiederholten freundlichen Verhaltens eines Tieres oder mehrfachen aggressiven Verhaltens zu einem dritten kurz sagt, daß der Affe A den Affen B „gern hat" und den Affen C „nicht mag", so ist dies eine unmittelbar verständliche, für den Verhaltensforscher aber unexakte Bezeichnung. Wenn man beschreibt und zählt, wie oft A bei B Hautpflege übt oder Hautkontakte ausführt, oder C androht, angreift oder ihm Imponierverhalten zeigt, so erhält man eine quantitative Grundlage exakter Verhaltensbeobachtung. Diese verlangt einen größeren Zeitaufwand und längere Beschreibung mit indirekter Erfassung psychologisch evidenter affektiver Beziehungen. Wenn man dazu noch versuchen wollte, die Aktivierung und Hemmung der verschiedenen cerebralen Mechanismen, die zu diesem Verhalten führen, darzustellen, so würde ein so komplexes und konfuses Bild entstehen, daß niemand diese neurophysiologischen Zusammenhänge verstehen würde, selbst wenn sie in allen Einzelheiten genau bekannt wären.

Verhaltensforschung (Ethologie) bei Tier und Mensch. Schon bei der Verwendung psychologischer Termini in der Ethologie beginnen die Schwierigkeiten einer Anwendung auf das menschliche Verhalten. „Auch der Mensch ist ein Tier" sagen TINBERGEN und andere Verhaltensforscher mit Recht, aber jeder weiß, daß damit über die Besonderheiten des menschlichen Verhaltens noch nichts ausgesagt ist. Der Mensch „ist eine beachtliche und in vieler Hinsicht einzige Art, aber ein Tier ist er doch ... So ist es nur natürlich, daß der Zoologe bei seinem ethologischen Studium nicht vor dem Menschen haltmacht", meint TINBERGEN 1953 [T 8]. Es ist charakteristisch, daß die einzige wirklich naturwissenschaftliche Studie über das menschliche Sexualverhalten von Zoologen (KINSEY u.Mitarb.) durchgeführt wurde [K 15].

TINBERGEN glaubt an eine *Vermittlerrolle der Verhaltensforschung zwischen Physiologie und Psychologie.* Er erwartet eine Verschmelzung der Ethologie mit der Neurophysiologie und widerspricht falschen Vorstellungen über die Grenze zur Psychologie: „Wer in objektiver Forschungsweise von Stufe zu Stufe die hierarchische Leiter erklimmt, von den Reflexen oder Automatismen zur Lokomotion, von ihr zum nächsthöheren Niveau der Instinktbewegung und so fort, müsse an eine Grenze kommen, wo die Warnungstafel: »Objektive Forschung verboten: nur für Psychologen!« ihm Halt gebiete. Es ist grundlegend wichtig, in solchen Vorstellungen den Selbstbetrug zu erkennen. So lange die Neurophysiologen ihre Aufmerksamkeit allein auf niedere Stufen richteten, war tatsächlich der Abstand zwischen den Interessengebieten der Physiologie und Psychologie so groß, daß man die Existenz der Grenzschranke irgendwo im Niemandsland weder beweisen noch widerlegen konnte. Aber die Neurophysiologie hat höhere und immer höhere Stufen in ihren Arbeitsbereich miteinbezogen; die Psychologie beginnt auch die Instinktstufe mitzubeachten. Die *Ethologie* hat mittenninne Fuß gefaßt: ihre tiefsten Stufen behandelt sie gemeinsam mit den *Physiologen,* auf ihren höchsten begegnet sie den *Psychologen*. Und eines der ersten Ergebnisse solchen Einanderfindens und Sichbegegnens ist die Erkenntnis, daß die besagte *Schranke nicht existiert*. Die Denkweise der Neurologie und der Verhaltensforschung ist die gleiche, beide werden immer enger zusammenarbeiten und endlich zu einer Wissenschaft verschmelzen. Psychologie im engsten Sinne als die Wissenschaft vom Subjektiven wird stets als selbständige, unabhängige Disziplin neben der Ethologie stehen. Die höheren Stufen nervöser Leistungen können *beide* Wissenschaften untersuchen, *ohne je in Konflikt* zu geraten; jede von beiden wird einen der beiden Aspekte des jeweils Untersuchten enthüllen."

„Als Forscher sind wir gezwungen, die *Dualität* unseres Denkens als Gegebenheit hinzunehmen. Tun wir das, so können wir menschliches Verhalten objektiv untersuchen, ohne Gefahr zu laufen, in unverzeihlicher Engstirnigkeit den Wert der anderen Denkweise zu bezweifeln. Mit anderen Worten: beiderlei Daten, die aus *Introspektion* und die aus *objektiver Forschung,* sind Tatsachen. Wird der Futtersuchtrieb erregt, so spürt das Subjekt Hunger, und währenddessen arbeiten seine neuronalen Mechanismen. Wer diese Mechanismen entdeckt, entdeckt gewiß nicht, daß es keinen Hunger gäbe.

Die andere Möglichkeit wäre die, die Ausdrucksweisen der Umgangssprache nicht nur als hinreichende Beschreibung des subjektiv Empfundenen, sondern zugleich auch als Kürzel für den entsprechenden physiologischen Vorgang zu gebrauchen. Aber dann kommt der Ethologe immer zu spät; denn der Psychologe hat diese Ausdrücke längst mit Beschlag belegt, mit subjektiver Bedeutung beladen, und selbst, wenn der Ethologe sich ihrer unter der ausdrücklichen Verwahrung bedient, er gebrauche sie rein deskriptiv, so klagt der Psychologe ihn an, er überschreite seine Grenzen; ja man wirft ihm vor, er habe durch sein Verwenden subjektiver Begriffe die Unmöglichkeit objektiven Verhaltensforschens bewiesen (vgl. z.B. BIERENS DE HAAN, 1947). Daher ist größte Vorsicht geraten, solange das Mißverstehen von Ziel und Umfang beider Wissenschaften anhält" (TINBERGEN [T 8]).

Instinkt und Trieb bei Tier und Mensch. Wir können hier nicht den von Zoologen und Verhaltensforschern vielfach und verschieden definierten *Instinktbegriff* in seinen verschiedenen Bedeutungen diskutieren. Weder die Ausweitung dieses Begriffs bei den Neurologen v. MONAKOW und MOURGUE [M 51], die bei Mensch und Tier arterhaltende, sexuelle und soziale Instinkte und beim Menschen sogar „religiöse Instinkte" annehmen, noch die Überbetonung der erlernten Funktionen in der angelsächsischen Psychologie und der russischen bedingten Reflexforschung mit der Vernachlässigung der Instinkte erscheint zweckmäßig: Denn offenbar ist Lernen erst auf dem Boden angeborener zentralnervöser Koordinationen und ihrer Instinktmanifestierung mit erblichen Auslösemechanismen möglich. Daher läßt sich eine scharfe Gegenüberstellung von erlerntem Verhalten als „höheren" Regulationen und Instinktverhalten als niederen Regulationen praktisch nicht durchführen. Für neurophysiologische Untersuchungen kann man *Triebe und Instinkte weitgehend identifizieren*. Dies entspricht allerdings nicht ganz dem Sprachgebrauch der Ethologen: LORENZ [L 37] beschränkt den Instinkt auf seine *Verhaltensseite,* die Instinktbewegung. Diese wird durch äußere Reize über den *angeborenen Auslösemechanismus (AAM)* oder durch innere Reize (Hormone) in Gang gesetzt oder entsteht automatisch im „Leerlauf" ohne erkennbaren Reiz. Dabei wirken äußere und innere Reize zusammen (vgl. S. 947). Auch menschliche Triebhandlungen sind, ähnlich wie es CRAIG [C 12] für das tierische Instinktverhalten klar dargestellt hat, aus suchendem *Appetenzverhalten* und trieblösender *Endhandlung* (consummatory action) zusammengesetzt. Die Appetenzkomponente entspricht bei uns einem mehr oder weniger bewußten „psychischen" Äquivalent des *Triebes*. Die Endhandlung kann zwar als physiologischer Vorgang mit reflektorischem oder automatischem Ablauf aufgefaßt werden, geht aber mit dem bewußten Erlebnis der *Befriedigung* einher. Aus dieser beim Menschen deutlichen und sprachlich zu bezeichnenden „psychischen" Äquivalenz kann nicht eine Sonderstellung menschlicher Triebe abgeleitet werden. Eine Vergleichbarkeit ist nicht nur phylogenetisch sondern auch neurophysiologisch und ethologisch zu postulieren.

Instinktbewegungen und Verhalten der Tiere. Nach WHITMAN und LORENZ beruhen die Instinktbewegungen auf angeborener, erblich fixierter Grundlage (im Englischen auch "fixed patterns" genannt). Diese angeborenen Muster der Instinktbewegungen werden auf dem Boden einer triebbedingten zentralnervösen „Stimmung" (Hunger, Sexualtrieb) aktiviert und durch äußere Reize über den Mechanismus eines angeborenen Schemas ausgelöst. Der *angeborene Auslösermechanismus* (AAM, früher von LORENZ [L 36–38] als „angeborenes Schema" bezeichnet) ist ein erblich fixierter Automatismus des Zentralnervensystems, der meist arteigen ist und mehr oder weniger spezifisch auf bestimmte *Signale von Sinnesreizen* (Auslöser) reagiert. Die meist sehr einfachen Signalreize der Auslöser passen zum angeborenen Schema wie der Schlüssel zum Schloß. Nach dieser Auslösung läuft die Instinktbewegung fast automatisch ab. Reflektorische Mechanismen können den weiteren Ablauf u.a. in Form von Taxien sichern und steuern. Die angeborene Instinktbewegung wird dann bei richtiger Auslösung und Steuerung zur situationsgemäßen „*Instinkthandlung*". Bei starker Kumulierung der Triebkomponente können Instinktbewegungen aber auch *ohne* adäquate Auslösung im „*Leerlauf*" entstehen (LORENZ [L 37, 39]). Vielleicht können auch menschliche Ausdrucksphänomene wie das Weinen und Lachen auf solche angeborenen Mechanismen zurückgeführt werden. Sicher vorgebildet und als angeborenes Schema beim Menschen wie bei Tieren vorhanden ist das „Kindchenschema", das bestimmte Verhaltensweisen der Fürsorge, Zärtlichkeit und Pflege auslöst [L 38, 42]. Hier kann die vergleichende Verhaltensforschung eine Brücke schlagen zwischen der Neurophysiologie und der Trieb- und Gefühlspsychologie. Triebhandlungen des Menschen können ebenso wie Instinkthandlungen der Tiere, wenn der Trieb nicht befriedigt wird, schließlich im *Leerlauf* vor sich gehen und auch beim Menschen ohne Beteiligung des Willens ablaufen. Das Daumenlutschen des Säuglings und wohl auch das Zigarettenrauchen des Erwachsenen sind vielleicht Ersatzhandlungen oraler Triebmechanismen. Deutlicher wird die Triebgrundlage noch in der sexuellen Sphäre: Die nächtlichen Pollutionen bei unbefriedigtem Sexualtrieb sind ein allgemein bekanntes Beispiel eines solchen Leerlaufs. Sie entstehen offenbar nach den normalen Erektionen, die jeder gesunde Mann im Traumstadium allnächtlich hat (vgl. S. 996 u. Abb. 38). Von den normalen Triebhandlungen und ihrem Leerlauf lassen sich Beziehungen zu den abnormen Verhaltensweisen der Neurosen herstellen, bei denen neben Triebabweichungen Automatisierung und Gewohnheitsbildung eine

Rolle spielen (vgl. S. 813 u. 964). Die experimentellen Untersuchungen über Affekt- und Triebhandlungen werden auf S. 938 besprochen.

Bei Hemmung oder Verhinderung einer Instinkthandlung kann eine andere als „*Übersprung*" auftreten. Diese hier zunächst sinnlose Bewegung kann sekundär für den Partner oder die Gemeinschaft der Artgenossen eine Bedeutung erhalten, indem vermutlich auf dem Wege der Selektion die Übersprungshandlung sozialen Mitteilungswert gewinnt. Wenn bei einem solchen Bedeutungswandel des Übersprungs in eine soziale Auslösefunktion die ursprüngliche Bewegungsfolge verändert und besonders auffällig wird, spricht die Verhaltensforschung von *Ritualisierung* [H 98, T 8].

Beim Menschen sind solche, oft auch ritualisierten Übersprungshandlungen ebenfalls zu beobachten, meist in Form von Verlegenheitsbewegungen. Gewisse Ausdrucksbewegungen wie Lachen, Weinen und Gähnen könnten so auch soziale Bedeutung gewonnen haben. Sie zeigen Freude, Trauer oder Ermüdung der Umgebung an und „stecken an". Genauere Vorstellungen über die neurophysiologischen Grundlagen der Aktivierung, Hemmung und Enthemmung dieser Phänomene haben wir noch nicht. Der modernen Verhaltensforschung ging die Umweltlehre UEXKÜLLs [U 1] voraus. UEXKÜLL hat bereits ähnliche Konzeptionen vorausgenommen, die den angeborenen Auslösermechanismen mit ihren Schlüsselreizen von LORENZ in der Ethologie entsprechen. Doch hat UEXKÜLL sie vitalistisch und subjektivistisch interpretiert, indem er *Merkwelt* und *Wirkwelt* des einzelnen Tieres mit einer individuellen „Umwelt" koordiniert, die sich von der objektiven Umwelt unterscheidet.

Die Stellung der Verhaltensforschung zur Neurophysiologie und zu anderen Nachbarwissenschaften, dem Behaviorismus, der Psychologie und der Philosophie hat LORENZ in seiner Harvey-Lecture [L 41] übersichtlich dargestellt. Er betont die Grenzen der quantifizierbaren Forschung und die Notwendigkeit, daß Gemessenes und Gezähltes zunächst richtig gesehen werden müssen, um vergleichen, unterscheiden und zählen zu können.

Ähnliche Prinzipien gelten auch für die Klinik. Auch hier müssen Beobachtung und Beschreibung einzelner Fälle und Syndrome mit Hervorhebung des Wesentlichen und systematische Ordnung erst der Messung und Zählung vorausgehen, wenn die quantifizierende Arbeit der Laboratoriumsforschung sinnvoll angewendet werden soll.

Unterschiede zwischen Mensch und Tier

Die Vergleichbarkeit tierischer Verhaltensweisen mit dem menschlichen Verhalten, Sprechen und Denken wird von zwei verschiedenen Seiten bestritten: 1. von der philosophischen Anthropologie und 2. von der physiologischen Forschung über die bedingten Reflexe:

Die philosophisch ausgerichtete verstehende Psychologie und Phänomenologie postuliert eine absolute Sonderstellung des Menschen und bestreitet jede Vergleichbarkeit mit dem Tier. Selbst aus der Physiologie kommende Vertreter dieser Richtung, wie BUYTENDIJK [B 77], verteidigen noch den Standpunkt der idealistischen Philosophie des 19. Jahrhunderts, daß der Mensch „inkarnierter

Geist" sei [B 78]. Die soziale Kommunikation der Tiere wird nur als Stimmungsausdruck gewertet und die Vergleichbarkeit mit dem menschlichen Sprechen abgelehnt. Ähnlichkeiten physiologischer Mechanismen werden gering eingeschätzt. Die Gegensätze werden, wie O. KOEHLER [K 27, 28] kritisch hervorgehoben hat, in überspitzten Antithesen dargestellt.

Von physiologischer und biologischer Seite wird eine fast ebenso scharfe Gegenüberstellung von Tier und Mensch durch PAWLOW [P 7] und seine Schule [R 6] vertreten: Obwohl diese Richtung der bedingten Reflexforschung auf Verhaltenskriterien beruht, sieht sie in der menschlichen *Sprache* eine grundsätzlich neue und qualitativ verschiedene *„Funktion des 2. Signalsystems"*, das nur dem Menschen zukommt (vgl. S. 1029). Während die körperlichen Bauunterschiede zwischen uns und Menschenaffen gewiß nicht größer sind als die zwischen diesen und niederen Affen, liegt der Hauptunterschied in der Sprache und den menschlichen Kulturleistungen, die wir aus dem, was wir mit Tieren gemeinsam haben, durch die Sprache aufgebaut haben.

Homo faber: Werkzeugherstellung als spezifisch menschliche Eigenschaft. Seitdem die Paläanthropologie die Werkzeugherstellung als Haupt-Kriterium der Menschheitsentwicklung erkannt hat, ist die Anfertigung von Werkzeugen und ihr systematischer Gebrauch als typisches Merkmal der menschlichen Kultur selbstverständlich geworden. Die menschliche Werkzeugtechnik und ihre Geschichte vom einfachen Steinbeil bis zur komplizierten Maschine ist oft dargestellt und dem gelegentlichen, unsystematischen oder instinktgebundenen Werkzeuggebrauch der Tiere gegenübergestellt worden. Die wenig differenzierte Verwendung von vorhandenen Werkzeugen bei höheren Affen [K 24, 29] ist viel primitiver. Die erstaunlichen Leistungen der Tiere, die ohne Werkzeuge ihre Nester und Höhlen bauen [F 31], zeigen auch die prinzipiellen Unterschiede zur kulturtradierten und mathematisch berechnenden Technik der Menschen.

GEHLEN hat den Menschen ein „biologisches Mangelwesen" genannt, das viele Eigenschaften aus Entbehrung und Not entwickelt habe [G 15]. Doch ist die Entwicklung neuer Fertigkeiten und Sozialformen aus der Not nicht für den Menschen spezifisch, sondern ein allgemein biologisches Phänomen der Selektion. Es leuchtet ein, daß Feuer, Werkzeuggebrauch und Kleidung mit anderen Verstandesleistungen beim Menschen in der Not der Eiszeit entwickelt wurden, um gewisse biologische Mängel auszugleichen. Die geringe Behaarung des Menschen ist nach DARWIN durch geschlechtliche Zuchtwahl entstanden [D 1]. Nachdem der Urmensch gewissermaßen sein Haarkleid dem erotischen Vergnügen geopfert hatte, mußte er in der Eiszeit aus Fellen eine künstliche Haar- und Tuchbekleidung herstellen, um die Kälte überleben zu können. *Die Entwicklung der Hirnfunktionen und der Handfertigkeit wurde eine biologische Notwendigkeit.* Doch übertreffen diese und zahlreiche andere Formen des menschlichen Verhaltens, wie die Jagd mit Waffen, das Ernten und Zubereiten der Pflanzennahrung oder die geplante gesellschaftliche Arbeitsteilung schon bei primitiven Menschen alle von Tieren jemals erreichten Stufen erlernter und sozialer Funktionen. Überlebenschancen hatte nicht der einzelne, sondern nur der zur Gruppe und *organisierten Gemeinschaft* zusammengeschlossene Urmensch. Soziale Eigenschaften hatten damit einen positiven Selektionswert. Diese früh entwickelten sozialen Besonderheiten des Menschen, die für Psychologie und Psychiatrie von großer Bedeutung sind, können nicht mit neurophysiologischen Methoden untersucht werden.

Sprache und Kultur. Sicher *verschieden* vom Tier ist der Mensch durch seine *Sprache* und alle dadurch bedingten speziellen menschlichen *Kulturleistungen*. Erst die Sprache ermöglichte Schriften, Zahlensysteme und andere symbolische Abstraktionen realer oder psychischer Vorgänge. Damit konnte die menschliche Kultur und Wissenschaft unabhängig von persönlicher Tradition entwickelt und objektiv weitergegeben werden. Damit entwickelte sich das, was POPPER [P 31, 32] die „Welt 3" genannt hat (vgl. S. 791 und Abb. 3). Die objektive, in Schrift und Kulturtradition deponierte Welt 3 wurde viel reichhaltiger als die im einzelnen Individuum repräsentierte und damit nicht nur von der beschränkten Merkfähigkeit des vermittelnden Menschen und den möglichen Verfälschungen durch subjektive Wiedergabe abhängig. *Die begrenzten Leistungen eines Gehirns konnten* durch die literarischen Hilfsmittel der Kultur *vergrößert und vervielfältigt werden*. Dennoch werden alle diese kulturellen Werte erst ermöglicht durch die *Lernfunktionen des menschlichen Gehirns*. Auch die wertvollste Bibliothek ist wertlos ohne einen Menschen, der die Sprachen der Bücher versteht und der daran Interesse hat, die in Schriften aufgespeicherten geistigen Werte zu lesen und daraus zu lernen. Alle diese objektiven Leistungen der Kultur finden ihren Sinn nur in der sprachlichen Vermittlung über den denkenden Menschen und seine Hirnfunktionen. Die objektive „extracerebrale" Speicherung von Wissensstoff in der Schrift ist per se unverständlich. Wir müssen sie erst *lesen lernen*, wie Sprache und Schrift vergangener Epochen erst enträtselt werden müssen.

Verschieden von den Tieren sind die Menschen auch durch ihr besseres *rationales Einsichts- und Abstraktionsvermögen* und die dadurch ermöglichte relative Befreiung vom Zwang der Instinkte. Die so gewonnene Freiheit mit *Beherrschung und Beschränkung von Trieben und Affekten* in relativer individueller Handlungsfreiheit wird aber wieder erkauft durch *stärkere soziale Bindungen*.

Die *Sonderstellung des Menschen* ist bekanntlich neben der aufrechten Haltung und dem freien Gebrauch der Hand für Werkzeuge vor allem durch die *Gehirnentwicklung* und die damit ermöglichte *Sprachfähigkeit* bedingt. Seit HERDER [H 31] ist dies von Geistes- und Naturwissenschaften gleichermaßen anerkannt. Man sollte annehmen, daß neben der Neuroanatomie auch die Neurophysiologie zur Aufklärung der menschlichen Hirndifferenzierung beitragen könnte. Doch lehren uns neurophysiologische Untersuchungen des menschlichen Gehirns nicht mehr über artspezifische Hirnfunktionen des Menschen als die Anatomie. ADRIANs alter Hinweis [A 9] auf die Ähnlichkeit seines eigenen EEG mit den Ganglienrhythmen eines Wasserkäfers (Abb. 6) zeigt eindrucksvoll, wie allgemein verbreitet und unspezifisch diese rhythmischen Hirnwellen sind. Das EEG beim Tiefschlaf mit langsamen Wellen, das den Menschen vom Carnivoren unterscheidet, ist nach neueren Untersuchungen von CAVENESS [C 6] dem des Makakenaffen sehr ähnlich. Obwohl neben diesen allgemeinen Ähnlichkeiten auch deutliche persönliche Unterschiede und Eigenheiten der Hirnwellen bestehen, sagen diese weder etwas über die Leistungen der betreffenden Gehirne und Individuen, noch über ihre Artspezifität aus. Die wissenschaftliche Erfassung individueller Leistungen und allgemeiner, aber artspezifischer menschlicher Qualitäten in der Entwicklung der Sprache und des Denkens gehört – von bei

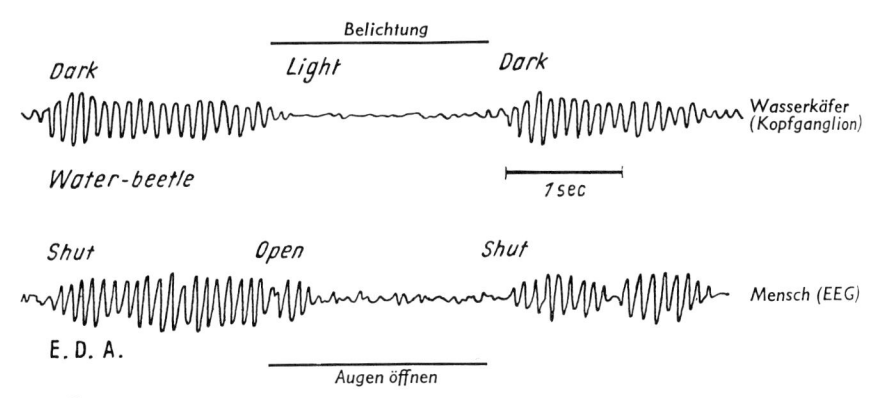

Abb. 6. Ähnliche Hirnrhythmen aus dem menschlichen Gehirn und dem Kopfganglion eines Wasserkäfers. Nach ADRIAN u. MATTHEWS, 1935 [A 9]. Die untere Kurve eines Nobelpreisträgers (E.D.A.) zeigt sehr ähnliche α-Wellen wie die obere Kurve des Käfers. Blockierung der α-Wellen durch Lichtreize ist in beiden Fällen ähnlich. Die Abbildung soll zeigen, daß es sich bei den EEG-Wellen trotz zahlreicher individueller und Artverschiedenheiten um Grundeigenschaften zentralnervöser Strukturen handelt

Tieren vergleichbaren Vorstufen abgesehen – in den Bereich der Kulturwissenschaften. Aber weder diese noch die Psychologie können die schöpferischen Leistungen des Menschen erklären. Erst recht kann die Neurophysiologie dazu nichts beitragen.

Einsicht, Triebbeherrschung und nicht-vitale Bedürfnisse. Das auch Tieren eigene sensorische Abstraktionsvermögen wird durch die Sprache in eigenartiger und folgenschwerer Weise erweitert. Verschieden von den Tieren sind die Menschen ferner durch ihr *rationales Einsichtsvermögen,* das auch von der Sprache fundiert wird. Dadurch befreit sich der Mensch bis zu einem gewissen Grade vom Zwang der Instinkte. Die so gewonnene Freiheit mit *Beherrschung von Trieben und Affekten* in relativer individueller Handlungsfreiheit wird jeweils eingeschränkt durch stärkere soziale Rücksichten als sie bei sozialen Tieren bestehen. Dies ist durch eine für den Menschen typische, langdauernde Lernausbildung begründet, durch die er seine Stellung in der menschlichen Gemeinschaft erwirbt.

Ein evidenter, aber wenig beachteter Unterschied von Mensch und Tier ist neben der Eigenentwicklung von Sprache und Denken auch die *relative Unabhängigkeit des geistigen Lebens von vitalen Bedürfnissen beim Menschen.* Dies zeigt sich in einer *erhöhten Bedeutung von erworbenen geistigen Bedürfnissen des Menschen* gegenüber den biologischen Trieben, die bis zu einer reziproken Beeinflussung gehen kann, wie im mönchischen Leben. Solche nicht-vitalen Strebungen manifestieren sich in den *moralischen Werten* und im Phänomen des *Gewissens.* Auf ihre positive und negative Rolle für die Entstehung von Neurosen und ihre Situationsabhängigkeit hat KORNHUBER in seiner Gefangenschaftspsychologie hingewiesen [K 38]. Über die cerebralen und physiologischen Grundlagen solcher geistigen Bedürfnisse, die notwendig auch ein somatisches Korrelat haben müssen, wissen wir nichts.

Spezifisch menschlich sind also nur rationales, planendes Denken für die Zukunft, sprachlich-unanschauliche Abstraktionsfähigkeit und produktive Abbildungsfähigkeit als Darstellung der Kunst im weitesten Sinne.

Wenn die moderne Psychologie heute dazu neigt, Stimmung, Gefühl und Gestaltvorgänge der Wahrnehmung höher zu werten, so wählt sie damit gerade *nicht* spezifisch-menschliche seelische Funktionen aus. Was Tieren offenbar fehlt, ist die Fähigkeit, von der momentanen Stimmung zu abstrahieren. Allerdings ist dies auch vielen Menschen nicht immer möglich, und affektive Antriebe müssen immer wieder eingreifen und anregen. „Reines" Denken ohne emotionale Antriebe und soziale Kontakte verliert sich in unverbindlicher Spekulation und wird unproduktiv. Rein affektiv gesteuertes Denken dagegen verläuft in engen emotionalen Kreisen, wie der Psychiater es am deutlichsten bei der Depression erlebt.

Mutter-Kind-Kontakt. HASSENSTEIN hat die Beziehungen von Mutter und Kind bei Mensch und Säugern verglichen und einen langdauernden Kontakt von Mutter und Kind beim Menschen als notwendige Bedingung für eine gesunde Entwicklung postuliert [H 15]. Allerdings hat der Mensch wegen der viel länger dauernden menschlichen Kindheit und der dann folgenden Ausbildungsphase über 2 Jahrzehnte eine Sonderstellung auch gegenüber den anderen höheren Primaten. Parallelen der Mutterbindung von Menschen und Tieren sind daher mit größter Vorsicht zu bewerten. Auch die Verhaltensregulationen durch hormonelle Einflüsse sind offenbar sehr verschieden. Wenn eine Rattenmutter ihr Kind nur dann annimmt, wenn sie es in der ersten Stunde nach der Geburt gesehen hat und sonst als Fremdtier behandelt, so kann man dies natürlich nicht auf die menschliche Mutter übertragen. Sicher ist es für die optimale Entwicklung eines Kindes gut, wenn der Säugling so weit wie möglich von der eigenen Mutter gepflegt und ernährt wird. Doch sprechen jahrhundertelang befolgte Sitten der Ammenernährung mit früher Trennung von der eigenen Mutter dagegen, daß früh unterbrochener körperlicher und Pflege-Kontakt beim Säugling ernsthafte Dauerschäden der Mutter-Kind-Beziehung verursacht. Auch dies ist wahrscheinlich während der längeren kindlichen Entwicklung kompensierbar.

Gemeinsamkeiten von Tier und Mensch

Menschen haben mit höheren Säugetieren und anderen Tieren, wenn auch natürlich immer artverschieden, folgende Eigenschaften gemeinsam: *Die einzelnen Sinne und ihre Verwendung für die Raumorientierung und Verhaltenssteuerung, die vitalen Triebe und Affekte mit ihrem Ausdruck und einer Skala von Stimmungen, ferner Lernvermögen, Gedächtnis und ein unbenanntes Denken, sowie den Wechsel von Schlafen und Wachen.*

Intelligenz ohne Sprache bei Tieren und Menschen. W. KÖHLER hat durch seine Schimpansenuntersuchungen gezeigt, daß Menschenaffen zu Intelligenzleistungen mit Werkzeugen fähig sind, die *Einsicht* und selbsterfundene *neue Kombinationen* und nicht nur Erlerntes oder bedingte Reflexe enthalten [K 29]. KLÜVER hat ähnlichen Werkzeuggebrauch und einsichtiges Lernen bei Java-Affen nachgewiesen [K 24]. Dies ist von der Pawlowschen Schule bestritten worden. Nach PAWLOWS Lehre, daß die Sprache als „zweites Signalsystem" Vorbedingung für Abstraktion und Ideation ist, dürfen die sprachlosen Schimpansen auch keine eigenen Ideen haben. PAWLOWS Theorie haben VATSURO und RAZRAN [R 6] durch neue Schimpansenversuche mit Werkzeugen zu stützen versucht: Diese Affen benutzten ihre Werkzeuge nur in der *erlernten* Weise ihrer bedingten Reflexe, blieben aber unfähig, sie durch Abstraktion und Kombination für andere Zwecke zu verwenden. RAZRANS Schimpanse benutzte einen bestimmten Becher nur, wie er es gelernt hatte, zum Löschen einer Flamme, die den Zugang zu den Früchten versperrte, aber nicht wie einen anderen Becher zum Schöpfen von Wasser, um sich abzukühlen. Immerhin zeigte derselbe Affe doch sehr gute eigene Leistungen für den Übergang von einem Floß auf das andere mit Hilfe eines Bambusstockes. KOHTS' vergleichende Entwicklungsstudien an Kindern von Menschen und Schimpansen [K 4, 5] ergaben zwar ähnliche emotionale Ausdrucksformen und Mimik, aber stärkere ungezügelte Affektivität bei Schimpansenkindern und besseres Lernen bei Menschenkindern.

Die Fähigkeit *sprachlosen Denkens* bei Tieren wurde vor allem von O. KOEHLER betont. Er spricht von „unbenanntem Denken" bei Tieren, das Gemeinsamkeiten mit menschlichem sprachlosem Denken aufweist [K 26, 27]. Das durch Dressurversuche nachgewiesene unbenannte Zahlendenken enthält sukzessives Abhandeln gesehener oder gehörter Anzahlen, Abstraktion in Anordnung, Größe und Form der Einheiten einer gesehenen Menge und ermöglicht auch heteromodale Übertragungen. Das simultane Sehen und sukzessive Abhandeln reicht je nach der Methode oder Tierart (bei äußerster Erschwerung der Versuchsbedingungen) bis zu den Zahlen 5 oder 8. Ohne rechnerische Schulausbildung bleibt auch das Hantieren mit Zahlen etwa bei unkultivierten Völkern in ähnlich niederen Bereichen, die nur sprachlich überschritten werden können.

Unbenanntes Denken hat nicht nur der Säugling vor Erwerb der Sprache. Es spielt auch beim Kind mit seinem vorwiegend *eidetisch-anschaulichen Denken* eine große Rolle und ist sogar beim Erwachsenen bei *allen anschaulichen und bildhaften Vorstellungen,* vor allem auch bei den Leistungen der *bildenden Kunst* von größerer Bedeutung als sprachliches Denken. Wohl wegen dieser vorsprachlichen Struktur wird dieses produktive anschauliche Denken von einigen Forschern, wie KUBIE [K 53] als „Vorbewußtes" (preconscious) bezeichnet (vgl. S. 973). Besser wäre die Bezeichnung *vorsprachlich.*

Beobachtungen bei gesunden Menschen und bei Kranken mit Aphasien zeigen, daß zwar die meisten Abstraktionsprozesse sprachlich vermittelt werden, daß aber erhebliche *Diskrepanzen zwischen Sprachleistungen und Intelligenzleistungen* bestehen. Gutes Sprachvermögen bedeutet nicht besseres Abstraktionsvermögen und beides ist sogar oft reziprok ausgebildet: Gute Sprecher sind oft schlechte Denker und umgekehrt. Vom Sprachlichen unabhängig sind ferner die durch visuelle Vorgänge unterstützten Kombinations- und Abstraktionsleistungen und rein mathematische Abstraktionen.

Sprachlose Ausdruckskommunikation bei Tieren. Da wir über das subjektive tierische Erleben nichts wissen und nichts erfahren können, ist der Streit müßig, ob auch Tiere ein Bewußtsein haben oder nicht. Jedenfalls *verhalten* sich die höheren Tiere so, *als ob* sie Gefühls- und Trieberlebnisse hätten oder sogar willensähnlich unter mehreren Möglichkeiten wählen könnten. Ähnlich wie es beim Menschen eine *sprachlose Verständigung durch die Beobachtung von Mimik und Verhalten* gibt, können wir auch beim Tier ohne sprachliche Kommunikation allein nach dem Ausdrucksverhalten manche Korrelationen erkennen, die wir bei uns selbst sicher als „psychisch" bezeichnen würden. Oft können wir nach solchem „einfühlenden" Ausdruckserkennen tierisches Verhalten voraussagen, ohne den Vorwurf anthropomorpher Illusionen fürchten zu müssen. Umgekehrt können Tiere aus dem menschlichen Verhalten vieles „erkennen" und ihr eigenes Verhalten danach einrichten. Die „Freude" eines Hundes bei der Begrüßung seines Herrn können wir unmittelbar miterleben. Auch der Hund reagiert ebenso deutlich auf eine veränderte Stimmung, eine freudige Zuwendung oder verärgerte Ablehnung beim Menschen.

Ausdrucksverhalten ist trotz erheblicher individueller und Artverschiedenheiten Menschen und Tieren gemeinsam. Bei den Tieren ohne Sprache ist es zu einer hohen Perfektion und zu Mitteilungen von großem Informationswert entwickelt worden. Diese von DARWIN [D 2] studierten „expressions of emotions" sind vorwiegend angeboren und artcharakteristisch, doch ist deren Mitteilungsfunktion nicht nur artspezifisch, sondern auch zwischen den Arten wirksam.

Ausdrucksverhalten ist nur sinnvoll als Wechselwirkung verschiedener Organismen, wenn die *Bedeutung des Ausdrucks anderen Individuen erkennbar ist*. Die Ausdrucksbewegung hat daher *soziale Funktionen*. Die Ethologie hat gezeigt, daß manche Verhaltensweisen aus sozial sinnvollen Ausdrucksbewegungen zu sinnlosen Übersprungsbewegungen werden oder zu artspezifisch veränderter Bedeutung sich entwickeln können. Daher hat die Schlußfolgerung aus dem Ausdrucksverhalten natürlich ihre großen Fehlerquellen, die nur zum Teil durch Erfahrung korrigiert werden können. Doch ist erstaunlich, wie gut auch verschiedene Tierarten, etwa ein Raubtier und ein Nagetier oder gar verschiedene Tierklassen, etwa eine Schlange und ein Mungo, sich in Verhalten und Ausdruck erkennen und aufeinander einstellen [B 77].

Es liegt nahe, darin eine biologische Vorstufe dessen zu sehen, was wir beim Menschen *psychisches Einfühlungsvermögen* nennen. In der Psychiatrie verwenden wir eine ähnliche aus dem Verhalten abgeleitete Einfühlung oder eine mangelnde Einfühlbarkeit auch für die Diagnose: Aus Mimik und Verhalten eines Schizophrenen, der uns mit einer charakteristischen zögernden und unbeteiligten Bewegung die Hand gibt, können wir oft unmittelbarer auf die Diagnose schließen als nach einer längeren Exploration, bei der dieser Kranke seine sprachlichen Fertigkeiten verwendet, um psychotische Symptome zu negieren. Allerdings kann auch dieses Negieren diagnostisch wegweisend sein. Kennzeichnend ist aber wiederum vor allem das *Ausdrucksverhalten* des Kranken bei dieser Negation. Über schizophrenen Ausdruck und Vergleiche mit mimischer Kommunikation bei Affen s. PLOOG in diesem Band.

Umwelt und Kulturmilieu bei Tier und Mensch

Der Mensch ist mit dem von ihm selbst geschaffenen sozialen und kulturellen Milieu mindestens ebenso eng verbunden, wie das Tier mit seiner naturgegebenen Umwelt, an die es sich im Laufe der Entwicklung angepaßt hat. Nur ist das

Milieu des Menschen durch seine eigene Arbeit entstanden und von ihm aktiv verändert worden, während das Tier passiv von der Umwelt abhängig bleibt. Die Tiere sind offenbar noch enger an ihre Umwelt gebunden und in ihren Reaktionsmöglichkeiten auf diese beschränkt als die Menschen, obwohl UEXKÜLL auch bei uns solche Umweltbeschränkungen beschrieben hat [U 1]. Die Anpassung des Menschen bezieht sich großenteils auf die von der menschlichen Gesellschaft entwickelten und wandelbaren soziologischen Bedingungen. Soziales Verhalten im Tierreich ist von anderer Art, da es vorwiegend auf starres Instinktverhalten zurückgeht und die Plastizität des Erlernten wenig Einfluß hat. *Das selbst geschaffene soziale Milieu gehört in anderer Weise zum Menschen als zur Biene der Stock und zur Spinne das Netz.*

Soziale Anregungen von Sprache und Denken beim Menschen. Bei der Sprache ist klar, daß sie nur aus der *Wechselwirkung mehrerer Individuen* entstehen konnte. Bei der Intelligenz ist dies weniger deutlich, aber auch eine hervorragende Intelligenz gerät auf Irrwege, wenn sie autistisch wird und Korrekturen durch andere ablehnt. Die Erfahrung zeigt, daß „reines Denken" wissenschaftlich wenig produktiv ist und zur Konstruktion spekulativer Denkgebäude führt, die empirischer Nachprüfung nicht standhalten. Dagegen ist *das durch Mitteilung und Diskussion lebendig erhaltene und durch andere Menschen, durch Tatsachen und Experimente korrigierte Denken* weitaus fruchtbarer. Reine Spekulation führt zu unlebendigen Denksystemen, reine Gefühlskommunikation zur Dichtung. Mit beiden kann die Wissenschaft nichts anfangen. Emotionaler Kontakt, den auch das Tier kennt, führt zu einem Gemeinschaftsgefühl zwischen Menschen und auch zwischen Tier und Mensch (Hund und Herr, Katze und Kind). Aber er bringt wenig wissenschaftliche Erkenntnisse.

Die Unterschiede von tierischem und menschlichem Verhalten betreffen vorwiegend die rationale und abstrahierende, vorausberechnende Seite des menschlichen Lebens, über die der Neurophysiologe nichts aussagen kann. Die emotionale Einstellung auf die Umwelt ist zwar auch beim Menschen differenzierter, aber im Prinzip ähnlich wie beim Tier. Auch Lernvorgänge und Gedächtnis unterscheiden sich beim Menschen vorwiegend durch ihre Differenziertheit von den Gedächtnisleistungen höherer Tiere (vgl. S. 1026). Nach dem Verhalten ist anzunehmen, daß Angst, Furcht, Verlegenheit, einfache Schamreaktionen wie alle Sympathie- und Antipathie-Vorgänge auch bei Tieren vorkommen (vgl. S. 807). Spezifisch menschlich scheint nur die lang *vorausdenkende Sorge* zu sein, die auch ohne aktuellen Anlaß durch spontane, produktive abstrahierende Denkvorgänge genährt wird. Es ist daher auch biologisch einsichtig, wenn von philosophischer Seite die Sorge zu den „Grundbefindlichkeiten" des Menschen gerechnet wird [H 23].

Soziale Ordnungen im Tierreich. Die bei Tieren vorkommenden Sozialordnungen sind erheblich von denen des Menschen verschieden. Sie können eher als Karikaturen der menschlichen Ordnungen dienen, wie sie die Fabel schon seit Urzeiten verwendet. Die Staatenbildung der Evertebraten, die bei den Insekten am stärksten differenziert ist, beruht offenbar auf angeborenen Instinktvorgängen und wird kaum durch Lernen und Erfahrung modifiziert, obwohl das Verhalten der Einzelinsekten dieser Staatenvölker erfahrungsgesteuert sein kann. Ähnliche starre, genetisch determinierte Staatenbildungen fehlen bei den höheren

Tieren. Die kleineren sozialen Einheiten, die bei Säugern als Herden- und Rudelbildung häufig vorkommen, haben eine ausgeprägte *soziale Rangordnung*, die vor allem von SCHENKEL [S 4] bei Wölfen genauer studiert wurde. Diese soziale Ordnung beruht, ähnlich wie beim Menschen, auf *erlerntem* und bedingtem Verhalten.

Einige Ansätze zum Studium und zur Beeinflussung der Volksstruktur sind bei Rattenvölkern [S 50] und Affenvölkern [K 64, P 56] gemacht worden, die menschlichen Sozialstrukturen am ehesten verwandt erscheinen. Hier bleibt der vergleichenden Soziologie, Psychologie und Neurophysiologie ein großes Feld sozialer Verhaltensforschung.

Eindrucksvolle Parallelen zur menschlichen Sozialordnung bieten die Beobachtungen von STEINIGER [S 50] an Wanderratten. Sie zeigen die große Breite des sozialen Verhaltens dieser lissencephalen Tiere: Bildung von Rudeln aus Familien, Entwicklung örtlicher Traditionen und Spezialisierungen besonderer Jagd- und Tötungsarten, Aufhebung der Rangordnung in der überindividuellen Einheit des Rudels, Variationen von Paarbildung und Rudelbildung, Revierkämpfe auf Leben und Tod mit Ausrottung der schwächeren Gegner. Dagegen sind die Affenhorden bestimmter Makakenarten offenbar wesentlich friedlicher.

Mensch und Tier gemeinsam ist eine auf Artgenossen gerichtete „*intraspezifische*" *Aggression*, deren biologische Bedeutung für die Revierabgrenzung, Lösung der Familienbindung und die Ausbreitung der Art von LORENZ hervorgehoben wurde [L 42]. Im menschlichen Leben findet man ähnliche rational nicht begründbare Aggressionen, die sich mit einem Distanzbestreben vor allem auf Familienangehörige und Verwandte richten und die vielleicht auf einen entsprechenden Instinktmechanismus zurückzuführen sind (vgl. S. 947).

Verhaltenstraditionen bei Affen. Die großen Unterschiede sozialen Verhaltens bei verschiedenen, auch derselben Gattung angehörigen Affenarten [K 64] sind eine Warnung gegen zu frühe Deutungen als angeborene Verhaltensmuster und Vergleiche mit menschlichem Sozialverhalten. Das von PLOOG [P 25] genau studierte exhibitionistische Imponiergehabe männlicher Totenkopfaffen, das auch zur Grußzeremonie werden kann, scheint artspezifisch und ritualisiert zu sein. *Erlernte Verhaltenstraditionen* japanischer Affen sind für das menschliche Sozialleben besonders interessant, da diese Tradition über mehrere Generationen weitergegeben werden kann [K 10]. Dieses von den Eltern oder anderen Gruppenmitgliedern imitierte Waschverhalten unterscheidet sich von dem anderer Affensippen derselben Art. Es ist also erlernt und *sippenspezifisch* und ähnelt menschlichen Sitten, die für einzelne Volksgruppen charakteristisch sind.

Ebenso wie innerhalb einer Tierart Rassen, Varietäten und Konstitutionen unterscheidbar sind, so auch beim Menschen. Ferner gibt es bei Tieren *Variationen und Veränderungen des Trieblebens*, die den Charaktervariationen mit psychopathischen Trieb- und Gefühlsanomalien beim Menschen entsprechen. Sie sind bei domestizierten Tieren wie Pferden und Hunden besonders gut zu beobachten. Ähnlich wie beim Menschen sind es sowohl vorwiegend angeborene Trieb- und Verhaltensvariationen entsprechend der Psychopathie [K 55] wie durch Umwelterfahrungen erworbene Veränderungen, die den Neurosen ähneln. Derartige Veränderungen sind auch als experimentelle Neurosen bei Tieren ausgiebig studiert worden [A 22, G 7, L 22, M 24, P 7].

Psychische Störungen bei Tieren

Experimentelle Neurosen bei Tieren. PAWLOW [P 7] hat zuerst bei seinen Versuchen über bedingte Reflexe bei Hunden experimentelle Neurosen beobachtet. Ähnliche abnorme Reaktionen und neuroseähnliche Einstellungen wurden dann von LIDDELL vor allem bei Schafen systematisch untersucht [A 22, G 7, L 22]. MASSERMANS Untersuchungen an Katzen [M 24], die durch plötzliches Anblasen bei der Nahrungsaufnahme „neurotisiert" waren, wurden systematisch zu einer psychobiologischen Neurosentheorie ausgebaut [M 25, 26].

Neurophysiologie, Ethologie und Psychiatrie

Die zoologische Verhaltensforschung und tierexperimentelle Neurophysiologie kann zur Psychiatrie nicht nur durch Versuche über experimentelle Neurosen beitragen. Ihre wichtigsten Beiträge liegen in der *Grundlagenforschung*. Wenn nicht voreilig von speziellen Eigenschaften einzelner Tierarten Schlüsse auf den Menschen gezogen und umgekehrt, wenn anthropomorphe Deutungen tierischen Verhaltens vermieden werden, können Ethologie und Neurophysiologie ebenso bedeutsame Beiträge zur psychiatrischen Forschung liefern wie Psychologie oder Neuroanatomie.

Die scharfe cartesianische Zweiteilung, die nur den Menschen Erlebens-, Entscheidungs- und Denkfähigkeit, den Tieren, auch in ihren höchstentwickelten Species aber nur automatische Mechanismen zugebilligt hat, war schon im 17. Jahrhundert bestritten und ist von der modernen Biologie oft widerlegt worden. Nach dem viel zitierten Wort PASCALS, der doch sicher die geistige Natur des Menschen nicht unterschätzt, ist auch der Mensch *beides*, Automat und Geist und vereinigt Instinkt und Erfahrung. Er verbindet vitale Mechanismen des ZNS, die für alle höheren Tiere gültig sind, mit einem differenzierten seelischen Erleben, das größtenteils sprachlich ausdrucksfähig ist.

Psychiatrie und Ethologie. War es noch vor wenigen Jahren notwendig, in der Psychiatrie auf die zahlreichen Parallelen mit der Verhaltensforschung hinzuweisen und darauf aufmerksam zu machen, daß die Ergebnisse dieser Forschungsrichtung neue Einblicke in die Anomalien des neurotischen und psychotischen Verhaltens ermöglichen, so muß man heute schon beinahe umgekehrt vor einer kritiklosen Übernahme warnen. Die Grenzen der Ethologie und Psychiatrie hat PLOOG bereits klar bezeichnet [P 25]. Die *Gefahr, daß Mißverständnisse und Schwierigkeiten durch Übernahme ethologischer Termini in klinisch-psychiatrisches Gebiet entstehen*, ist nicht gering. Sie muß klar erkannt, und kritiklose Konjekturen und unbemerkte Äquivokationen müssen vermieden werden. Seitdem die Ergebnisse der Ethologie ausführlich von physiologischer und klinischer Seite diskutiert worden sind, hätte man eine Klärung der verschiedenen Standpunkte erwarten können. Statt dessen findet man jetzt nicht selten eine unkritische und bedenkenlose Übernahme der Begriffe der Verhaltensforschung auf Gebiete, für die sie nicht geschaffen waren. Daher sollten auch die methodischen Grenzen wieder mehr betont werden. *Was die Verhaltensforschung untersucht, sind nicht psychologisch sinnvolle Zusammenhänge, sondern vorgebildete Mechanismen, deren neurophysiologische Grundlage noch nicht bekannt ist.* Im Sinne von JASPERS sind es zwar *kausale* und nicht verständliche Zusammenhänge, doch können wir den kausalen Mechanismus im einzelnen nicht bestimmen. Dennoch wird man die mit Instinkthandlungen vergleichbaren menschlichen Verhaltensweisen besser wie physiologische „*Mechanismen*" untersuchen oder mit KRETSCHMER [K 49] „Schablonen" nennen, um sie klar von *psychologisch verständlichen Reaktionen abzutrennen*. Wie bei allen biologischen Vorgängen ist ihre scheinbare „*Zweckmäßigkeit*" *eng begrenzt und nur für den* „*Normalfall*" *gültig. Außerhalb solcher begrenzten Bedingungen können diese Mechanismen zu unzweckmäßigen und sinnlosen Störungen führen*. Instinktive, biologisch „zweckmäßige" Verhaltensformen können so unter veränderten Umständen zur „neurotischen" Anomalie oder gar zum krankhaften Symptom werden. Dies zeigen auch die sog. Kinderfehler.

Kinderfehler und Instinkthandlungen. Bisher wurde bei den sog. Kinderfehlern zu wenig beachtet, daß einige abnorme Gewohnheiten und triebhafte Verhaltensweisen, z.B. Nägelkauen oder Daumenlutschen, zunächst als natürliche, *biologisch sinnvolle Trieb- und Instinkthandlungen* entstanden waren, die nur im Kulturmilieu überflüssig wurden. Das Abkauen der Nägelränder war offenbar eine zweckmäßige Begrenzung des Nagelwachstums, das der zivilisierte Erwachsene durch Nägelschneiden korrigiert. Bei Urmenschen und den frühen Steinzeitmenschen, die sicher keine Scheren hatten, war das Abbeißen der Nägel also eine sinnvolle Instinktbewegung, die einem natürlichen Trieb entspricht. Bei Kleinkindern kann das Nägelbeißen daher als zweckmäßige Regulation beginnen, die dann durch Erziehungsmaßnahmen unterdrückt wird. Ähnliches gilt für das Fingerlutschen der Kinder als natürliche Ersatzhandlung des Nahrungstriebes. Da die Nahrungsaufnahme des Säuglings durch Brustsaugen erfolgt, erscheint es verständlich, daß ein gesunder Säugling einen Saug- und Lutschtrieb hat und bei Hunger zwischen der Brusternährung an seinem Daumen saugt. Beides, Daumenlutschen und Nägelkauen, kann auch als Übersprungshandlung bei verschiedenen Triebstauungen auftreten und wird dann bei emotional labilen Kindern eine schwer zu beeinflussende Gewohnheit. Das Fingerlutschen wie das Gähnen ist eine vom *Hirnstamm* koordinierte Instinktbewegung, da GAMPERS Mittelhirnwesen, ein Kind ohne Großhirn, lutschen und gähnen konnte [G 4, 5].

Die Beziehung der Verhaltensforschung und tierexperimentellen Neurophysiologie zur Psychiatrie ist um so geringer, je weiter die betreffende Tierart in der phylogenetischen Reihe vom Menschen entfernt ist, je spezialisiertere Merkmale sie hat und je mehr sich die Gehirnstruktur der Art vom Menschen unterscheidet. Daher sind die Parallelen mit den sozialen Insekten, die seit FABRES und FORELS Ameisenuntersuchungen [F 1, 22] auch in der Psychiatrie oft erwähnt werden, sehr begrenzt. Bei den Insekten sind starre Instinkthandlungen viel bedeutungsvoller und modifizierbare Lernvorgänge spielen eine geringere Rolle. Beim Menschen ist das Verhältnis umgekehrt.

Klinische Anwendung neurophysiologischer Befunde und tierpsychologischer Beobachtungen

Die Ergebnisse der Neurophysiologie können mehr zur Symptomerklärung der organischen Nervenkrankheiten beitragen, die Beobachtungen der Instinkt- und Verhaltensforschung sind von größerem Interesse für die Symptomatologie der Psychosen und Neurosen.

Die experimentelle Neurophysiologie liefert zwar einige exakte Grundlagen für Funktionsweisen und Funktionsstörungen des Nervensystems, doch liegt die tierexperimentelle Forschung schon methodisch dem klinischen Denken so fern, daß sich nur wenige Beziehungen zur Psychiatrie entwickelt haben. *Für die psychiatrische Klinik wird die Neurophysiologie erst interessant, wenn sie mit der Verhaltensforschung bei Tieren verbunden wird.*

Die Ergebnisse zoologischer Verhaltensuntersuchungen sind in ihrer Anwendung beschränkt: Viele Befunde gelten nur für spezielle Tierarten und ihre artspezifischen Verhaltensweisen, und eine Verallgemeinerung ist nicht möglich, erst recht nicht eine Übertragung auf den Menschen. Dennoch erscheinen manche klinischen Beobachtungen parallel mit den Ergebnissen der zoologischen Verhaltensforschung unter einem neuen biologischen Gesichtspunkt. Einzelne der klinischen Symptome verlieren damit den Aspekt pathologischer Kuriositäten, sie können besser eingeordnet und einem wissenschaftlichen Verständnis nähergerückt werden.

Der Beitrag PLOOGs in diesem Band bringt eine systematische Bearbeitung der psychiatrisch relevanten Ergebnisse der Verhaltensforschung. Die folgende Tabelle soll einige Parallelen zwischen beiden Gebieten darstellen.

Tabelle 2. Mögliche Parallelen zwischen den Ergebnissen der Verhaltensforschung bei Tieren und psychiatrischen Beobachtungen beim Menschen

Verhaltensphysiologische Beobachtungen	Klinisch-psychiatrische Symptome
Wechselwirkung und Exclusion verschiedener Triebe und Affekte	Affektive Verdrängung und neurotische Triebverschiebung
Überlagerung verschiedener Affektäußerungen	Emotionale Besetzung und Vermischung. „Inadäquate" und „ambivalente" Gefühle
Elektrische Selbstreizung und ihre suchtähnliche Fortsetzung	Selbstauslösung photogener Epilepsien. Süchtiges Verhalten
Hormonelle Steuerung des Verhaltens	Psychische Veränderungen und Delikte in der Pubertät, Menstruation und Gravidität
Instinkthandlungen und Übersprungsvorgänge. Bedeutungswandel durch Ritualisierung	Impulshandlungen und Zwangsritual
Gewöhnungs- und Prägungsvorgänge. Automatisierung erlernter und dressierter Handlungen	Neurotische Bindung, Fixierung und Automatisierung. Perversionen. Psychotische Beeinflussungserlebnisse
Soziale Rangstufen und ihre Störungen in tierischen Gemeinschaften	Soziale Konfliktsituationen und ihre neurotische Verarbeitung

Spezifisch-menschliche und vital-tierische Anteile bei Neurosen und Psychosen. Gegen den Vergleich von Verhaltensstörungen bei Tieren mit den Neurosen beim Menschen wird eingewendet, daß bei Tieren nicht die seelischen Konfliktsituationen aufträten, die menschliche Neurosen kennzeichnen. Man bezweifelt also, daß die Tiere ihre Neurosen als Konflikte erleben und nimmt an, daß bei den experimentellen Neurosen der Tiere nur sekundäre affektive und Verhaltensstörungen auftreten, die zwar bei menschlichen Neurosen vorkommen, aber nicht ihr Wesen ausmachen. Diese Unterschiede sind aber ebenso akademisch-theoretisch und unbeweisbar wie andere Unterscheidungen menschlicher und tierischer „Psyche". Alle diese Differenzierungen arbeiten mit einem unbekannten Faktor, nämlich einem etwaigen Bewußtseinsvorgang bei Tieren. Nur was Tiere mit ihren Sinnen unterscheiden und was sie lernen, ist objektiv feststellbar.

Auf gesichertem Boden bewegen wir uns im Bereich des Verhaltens bei Tieren und im Bereich der Sprache bei Menschen. Es ist daher nur logisch, wenn PAWLOW [P 4–7] mit Ethologen, Neurophysiologen und Philosophen den entscheidenden Fortschritt des Menschen im Sprachlichen erblickt, dem sog. 2. Signalsystem der Pawlowschen Lehre als der notwendigen Voraussetzung aller spezifisch-menschlichen Leistungen und einer wichtigen Bedingung ihrer Störungen.

Die Einwirkungen der sozialen Umwelt, ihre verhaltensmodifizierenden und erzieherischen Effekte sind kaum zu überschätzen. Zahlreiche soziale Muster der Kultur, ihre zivilisatorischen und edukatorischen Einflüsse verändern die angeborenen Formen menschlichen Verhaltens und menschlicher Geistestätigkeit. Ein im Kaspar-Hauser-Versuch isoliert aufgezogener Mensch würde viele spezifisch-menschliche Eigenschaften nicht entwickeln können [E 6].

Verhaltensbeobachtung und Introspektion als Ergänzungen der Neurophysiologie

Der mit Tierexperimenten beschäftigte Neurophysiologe kann nur durch *Beobachtung des Verhaltens* seiner Versuchstiere solche Reaktionen und Veränderungen erkennen, die beim Menschen komplexen, psychologisch faßbaren Vorgängen entsprechen. Bei Tieren bleibt die Verhaltensbeobachtung der einzige Zugang zum „Psychischen". Beim Menschen können wir weitere sprachliche Informationen über die „inneren" Aspekte psychischer Vorgänge erhalten. Diese dem reinen Verhaltensforscher verdächtige *Introspektion* bildet trotz ihres subjektiven Charakters eine wertvolle Ergänzung der Neurophysiologie.

Beobachtung von Verhalten und Ausdruck ist nicht nur in der Tierpsychologie, sondern auch *beim Menschen* in der praktischen Alltagspsychologie von größter Bedeutung. So wichtig die Verhaltensbeobachtung im täglichen Leben ist, in dem wir aus Blick, Gesichtsausdruck und Haltung eines Menschen oft mehr schließen als aus seinen sprachlichen Äußerungen, so ist doch behavioristische Ausdrucksbeschreibung einseitig und unverständlich oder mehrdeutig. Sinnvoll wird sie erst in Verbindung mit psychischem Erleben.

Psychologisch-introspektive Methoden in der Neurophysiologie grundsätzlich unberücksichtigt zu lassen, wäre eine sinnlose petitio principii, wenn wir eine Korrelation von Neurophysiologie und Psychiatrie überhaupt für möglich halten. In der Sinnesphysiologie kommen wir nur durch Vergleich introspektiver Erfahrungen mit neurophysiologischen Ergebnissen weiter (vgl. S. 907).

Zwar wird man zunächst nur einfache, *formale* Korrelationen zwischen Neurophysiologie, Psychologie und Psychiatrie feststellen und von allem Inhaltlichen absehen. Die formalen Grundlagen psychischer Phänomene wie Aufmerksamkeit und Bewußtsein, zeigen engere Beziehungen zu neurophysiologischen Befunden und zum Elektrencephalogramm (vgl. S. 968).

Artefizielle Bedingungen der experimentellen Neurophysiologie und Verhaltensforschung

Die Neurophysiologie kann nicht, wie die Verhaltensforschung, vorwiegend mit einfacher Beobachtung arbeiten. Sie benötigt das *Experiment* mit rationeller Planung und theoretischer Grundlage. Jedes Experiment bedeutet einen aktiven *Eingriff in die natürlichen Zusammenhänge* und dadurch auch eine Störung. Naturfremde Eingriffe braucht auch die experimentelle Verhaltensforschung, die mit ihren Atrappenversuchen in der normalen Umwelt nicht vorkommende Kunstformen oder mit dem Kaspar-Hauser-Versuch eine unnatürliche Isolierung verwendet. Zwar bleibt beim Verhaltensexperiment das Zentralnervensystem wenigstens äußerlich intakt, doch können Reaktionen und Entwicklung des Gehirns dadurch beeinflußt werden. Man kann aus dem Verhaltensversuch nur *indirekt* auf zentrale Funktionen schließen. Die Neurophysiologie versucht dagegen, das Nervensystem *direkt* anzugehen. Selbst die schonendsten Formen neurophysiologischer Methoden, wie Ableitungen von elektrischen Erscheinungen an Gehirn und Nerven oder Reflexuntersuchungen schaffen unnatürliche, vom normalen Milieu entfernte Bedingungen. Alle anderen neurophysiologischen Methoden, wie direkte Ableitungen von bestimmten Hirnregionen oder einzelnen Neuronen (Abb. 7e, f), Reizexperimente (Abb. 7h) und Ausschaltungsversuche am Gehirn (Abb. 7a, b) sind mit erheblichen Eingriffen in das Nervensystem verbunden. Auch PAWLOWS Methode der bedingten Reflexe, die am intakten Tier arbeitet, erzeugt unnatürliche Umweltveränderungen eines artefiziellen Milieus (Abb. 7c, d). Der Hesssche Reizversuch am freien Tier, der eine dem natürlichen Zustand möglichst ähnliche Bewegungsfreiheit anstrebt, wird ebenfalls in einer von der Umwelt des Tieres weit entfernten Laboratoriumssituation durchgeführt (Abb. 7h).

Man muß sich über diese verschiedenen Bedingungen der neurophysiologischen Laboratoriumsforschung klar sein, wenn man die Beziehungen von Neurophysiologie und Psychiatrie bespricht. Wie in der Psychiatrie das Klinik- und Anstaltsmilieu großen Einfluß auf das Verhalten des Geisteskranken hat, so beeinflußt und begrenzt das Laboratoriumsmilieu die Ergebnisse der Neurophysiologie. Physiologisches Experiment und psychiatrische Exploration scheinen zunächst unvereinbar. *Physiologisches Experiment und ärztliches Gespräch schließen sich gegenseitig aus.* Nicht nur nach dem Sinn der Kommunikation und der Art und Einstellung der Partner, auch in der äußeren Umweltrelation sind beide grundverschieden. Zwar werden in beiden Fällen Fragen gestellt, zu denen eine Antwort gesucht wird, doch in völlig andersartiger Umwelt. Der Gegensatz zwischen der Situation des Laboratoriumstieres im neurophysiologischen Experiment und des Kranken bei der psychiatrischen Exploration zeigt schon äußerlich die methodische Verschiedenheit und die Unvergleichbarkeit der physiologischen und psychiatrischen Forschung. Das psychiatrische Gespräch oder die freie Assoziation der Psychoanalyse könnten eher mit Testuntersuchungen oder einfachen Verhaltensbeobachtungen von Tieren verglichen werden.

Abb. 7 zeigt *verschiedene Situationen des Tierversuchs bei der neurophysiologischen Forschung*. Ein Blick auf dieses Bild läßt erkennen, wie wenig solche eingreifenden Experimente mit der psychiatrischen Untersuchung beim Menschen verglichen werden können.

a

b

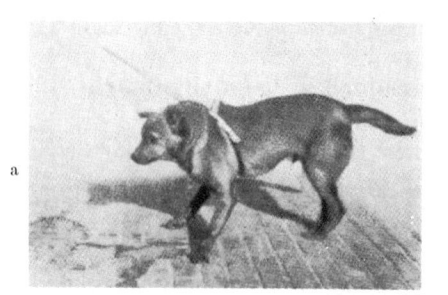

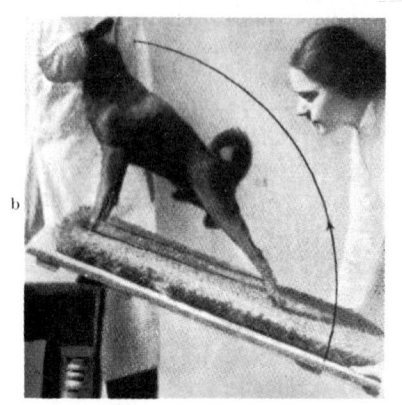

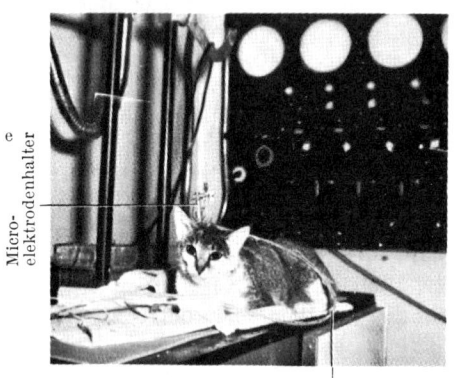

c

d

Micro-
elektrodenhalter

Zuleitung

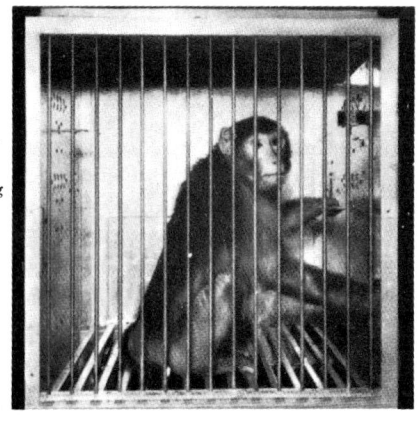

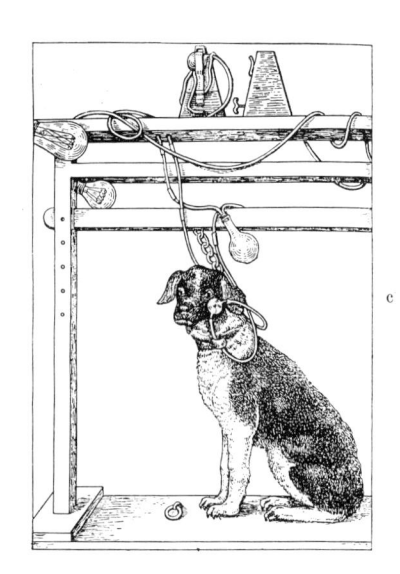

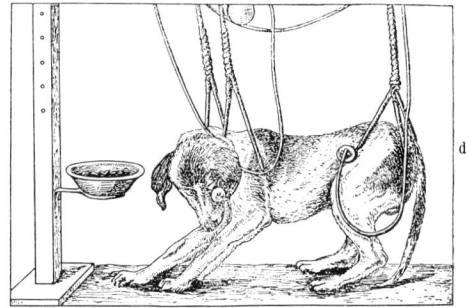

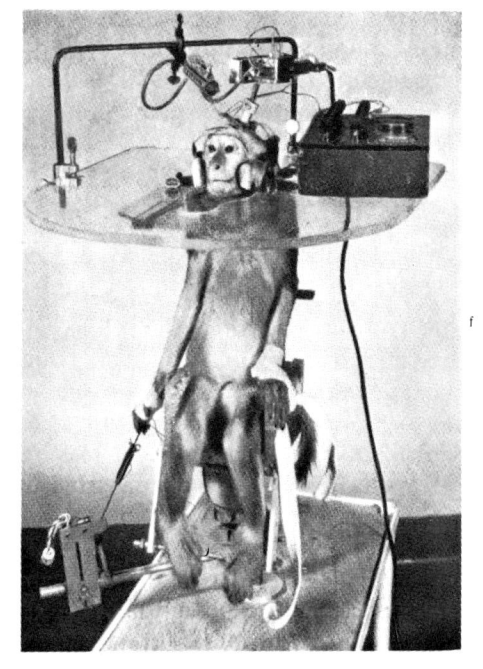

e

f

g

Tier und Mensch: Zoologische Verhaltensforschung, Neurophysiologie und Psychiatrie   817

h

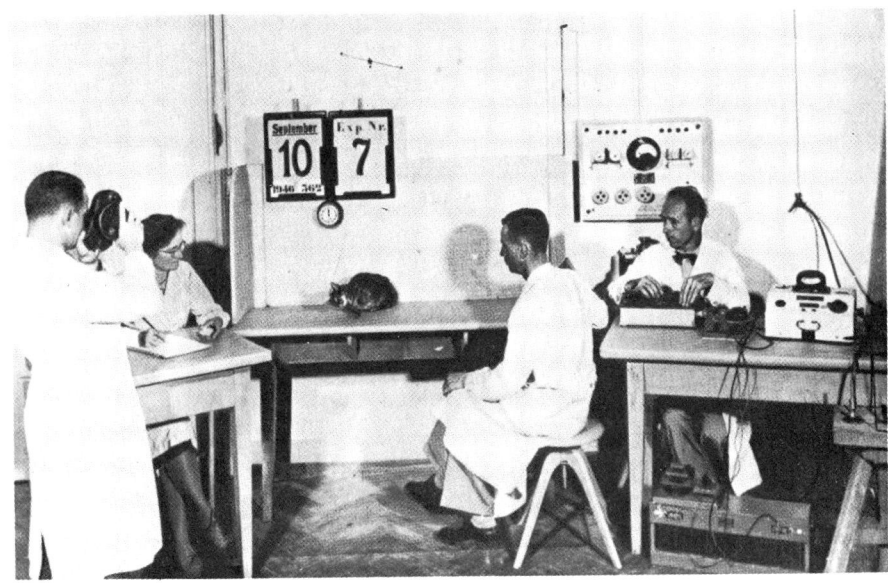

Abb. 7a–h. Versuchstiere in verschiedenen Situationen neurophysiologischer Untersuchungen: Ausschaltungsexperimente (a, b), Bedingte Reflexuntersuchungen (c, d), Mikroableitungen für Schlaf (e) und bedingte Reaktionen (f), Neuropharmakologisches Experiment (g), Reizversuch an der freien Katze nach HESS (h)
a) Großhirnloser Hund an der Leine
b) Kleinhirnloser Hund mit Kopfkappe bei der Stemmbeinreaktion. a, b nach RADEMAKER (1931) [R 1]
c) Pawlowscher Hund mit Speichelfistel im Gestell zur Untersuchung der bedingten Reflexe. Die elektrischen Lampen und Metronome sind die Reizgeber. Die Schläuche gehen zur Absaugflasche für die Messung der Speichelsekretion
d) Schlafender Hund im Pawlowschen Gestell. Die unnatürliche Stellung entsteht durch die Seilfixierung der Extremitäten. c, d nach PAWLOW (1926) [P 7]
e) Mikroelektrodenableitungen mit Schlafuntersuchungen an der freien Katze. Hinter dem Tier die für die Sicht der Katze abdeckbaren Beobachtungsröhren der elektrischen Hirnvorgänge. Auf dem Kopf befestigt ist der Elektrodenhalter
f) Mikroableitungen beim Affen im bedingten Reflexversuch. Das Tier hat die Aufgabe, bei bestimmten Reizen mit der rechten Hand einen Hebel zu ziehen. Währenddessen werden die Nervenzellentladungen der motorischen Rinde registriert. Nach RICCI et al. (1957) [R 14]
g) Affe im Käfig bei der Bedienung des Hebels, der zu einem automatischen Zählgerät führt. Untersuchungen über Neuropharmaka nach BRADY (1959) [B 55]
h) Tierexperiment an der frei laufenden Katze im Laboratorium von W.R. HESS. Vor und während der Reizung wird die Katze beobachtet und gefilmt. Gleichzeitig werden die Ergebnisse protokolliert

Während der reine Verhaltensforscher die Tiere in deren natürlichen Umgebung aus einem Versteck beobachtet, untersucht die experimentelle Forschung nur gewisse *Teilaspekte des Verhaltens* (behavior segments) und experimentiert mit *erlernten Vorgängen und bedingten Reflexen* (operant behavior mit der in USA sehr verbreiteten Skinner box und operant conditioning). Unter noch unphysiologischeren Verhältnissen leben die für elektrophysiologische Kontrollen tage- und wochenlang in einem speziellen Stuhl fixierten Affen (Abb. 7f). Aber auch Affen, die im Testkäfig ihre Tasten drücken und damit Zuckerstücke verdienen oder drohende elektrische Schläge abwehren (Abb.7g), sind kaum mit dem natürlichen Verhalten des wilden Tieres zu vergleichen. Die mehr oder weniger stereotypen Handlungen dieser Tiere im Käfigmilieu werden durch Zeitmesser, magnetische Zähler und automatische Rechenmaschinen aufgezeichnet, die im Nebenraum ihr kontinuierliches Ticken ertönen lassen. Auch unter nicht-experimentellen Bedingungen der Gefangenschaft im Zoologischen Garten werden offenbar eintönig wiederholte Handlungen begünstigt. Jeder Zoobesucher kennt gewisse Stereotypien und Verhaltensanomalien, die gefangene Tiere im Käfig entwickeln (vgl. Diskussion der Selbstreizungsversuche, S. 955). Neben dem Milieu ist die *Art der Versuchstiere* von großer Bedeutung für die Ethologie und Neurophysiologie.

Bei der *Auswahl des Versuchstieres* in der Neurophysiologie und Verhaltensforschung sind die großen Artverschiedenheiten in Verhalten und Hirnstruktur der Säugetiere zu beachten. Tiere der gleichen Art können in einzelnen Funktionen den menschlichen sehr ähnlich, in anderen sehr verschieden sein. Je nach dem Untersuchungsziel sind auch in ihrer Hirnstruktur ähnliche, domestizierte Raubtiere wie Hund und Katze verschieden geeignet. Der sozial angepaßte, ursprünglich in Rudeln lebende *Hund* ist für Lernversuche viel besser brauchbar als die Katze und ist daher das bevorzugte Versuchstier der bedingten Reflexforschung. Die individuell eingestellte, sozial wenig anpassungsfähige *Katze* mit ihren starken Instinktreaktionen eignet sich weniger für Lernversuche, doch hat sie eine differenzierte Motorik, schläft gerne und zeigt sehr ausgeprägte Affektäußerungen. Sie wird daher von den Neurophysiologen mehr für die Untersuchung der Motorik und allgemein-neurophysiologischer Eigenschaften der Affekt- und Trieb- und Wachregulationen verwendet. *Affen,* außer den Menschenaffen ebenfalls Herdentiere, mit dem Menschen ähnlicher Großhirnstruktur sind die geeignetsten Versuchstiere für höhere corticale Funktionen und Lernversuche. Es ist wohl kein Zufall, daß Katzen bevorzugte Versuchstiere in der anglo-europäischen, Hunde in der russischen und Affen in der amerikanischen Neurophysiologie sind.

Wenn man bedenkt, daß die Mehrzahl der neurophysiologischen Untersuchungen höherer Hirnfunktionen an nur drei Tiergattungen – *Katze, Hund* und *Makakusaffe* – durchgeführt wurden, so wird auch darin ein weiter Abstand zur Ethologie deutlich.

Verbindung von Verhaltensbeobachtungen und neurophysiologischen Experimenten. Für die Untersuchung komplexer Triebstrukturen, erlernter Handlungsfolgen und ihrer sozialen Auswirkungen war die ethologische Beobachtung intakter Tiere in mehr oder weniger natürlicher Umgebung bisher die einzig brauchbare Methode. Deshalb haben Neurophysiologen schon früh versucht, Verhaltensstudien mit ihren Experimenten über cerebrale Einzelmechanismen zu verbinden, doch blieb es zunächst bei vereinzelten Ausschaltungsversuchen nach Dressuren und bedingten Reaktionen. Die erste systematische Kombination von Hirnreizungen mit Verhaltensanalysen verdanken wir Hess [H 51–63] mit cerebralen Reizversuchen an der freien Katze und ihrer Filmauswertung 1932–1948. Die Versuchstechnik von Hess bringt für einzelne Tiere klare Ergebnisse (Abb. 7h). Sie kann noch durch Veränderungen des Milieus und durch Atrappendarbietungen für die Untersuchung von Trieben und Affekten erweitert

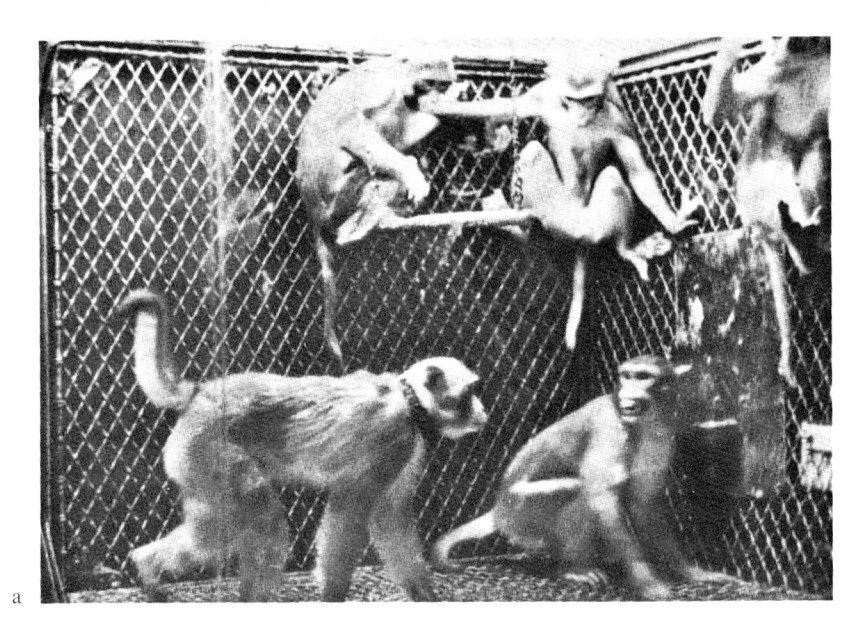

Tier und Mensch: Zoologische Verhaltensforschung, Neurophysiologie und Psychiatrie 819

Abb. 8a u. b. Soziale Aggression und ihre Ausbreitung bei Affen im zentralen Reizversuch. Nach DELGADO [D 12]
a) Der linke vordere Affe wurde drahtlos im zentralen Höhlengrau unterhalb des oberen Vierhügels gereizt und beginnt danach einen gerichteten Angriff auf die übrigen Affen der Kolonie. Der Angriff richtet sich immer zuerst gegen den Affen, mit dem er verfeindet ist, niemals gegen einen Freund
b) Kurz darauf beginnt auch die „Freundin" des großen Affen, der in a) gereizt wurde, die übrigen Koloniemitglieder anzugreifen, und zeigt damit eine soziale Ausbreitung der elektrisch ausgelösten Aggression

werden (HUNSPERGER, v. HOLST, vgl. Abb. 27), aber findet ihre Grenze bei sozialen Verhaltensweisen.

Da den Psychiater neben Triebmechanismen vor allem *Wechselwirkungen von Individuum und Gemeinschaft* interessieren, wäre es wünschenswert, neurophysiologische Untersuchungen über soziale Auswirkungen cerebraler Reizungen auch bei Tiergruppen durchzuführen. Dies war bis vor kurzem aus methodischen Gründen noch unmöglich, ist aber in den letzten Jahren von DELGADO bei Affenkolonien zu einem exakt auswertbaren Verfahren entwickelt worden [D 12, 13]. Kleinste subcutan eingebaute Empfänger und intracerebrale Elektroden ermöglichen drahtlose Hirnreizung an mehreren frei beweglichen Affen und eine beliebige isolierte Reizung einzelner Tiere der Gruppe. Bei vorheriger Kenntnis der sozialen Rangordnung und der affektiven Beziehungen der verschiedenen Individuen der Affengemeinschaft lassen sich dann auch reizbedingte interindividuelle Wechselwirkungen mit Filmanalyse und Auswertung quantitativ untersuchen. Reaktionen anderer Affen auf Verhaltensänderungen des gereizten Tieres geben weitere Hinweise auf feinere Signale von Triebanregungen, die dem menschlichen Beobachter und der Filmanalyse entgehen. DELGADO berichtet über sexuelle Auswirkungen einer Thalamusreizung, die nur durch das verstärkte Kopulationsverhalten der Männchen in der Gruppe zu erkennen waren. DELGADOs Methode zeigt auch soziale Auswirkungen der Hirnreizung mit gemeinsamem Aggressionsverhalten befreundeter Tiere (Abb. 8).

Eine andere Form der Hirnreizung in einer sozialen Gruppe von Affen [D 13, 14] ergab eine weitere interessante Beziehung zum Lernen und zur Rangordnung: Affen der niederen Ranggruppe lernten es, durch Hebeldruck das leitende α-Tier durch Caudatum-Reizung zu hemmen. Bei dieser Reizung blickten die rangniederen Affen den gehemmten „Boß" ungeniert an, obwohl sie dies sonst nicht zu tun wagten.

Zusammenfassung

Einige Ergebnisse der zoologischen Verhaltensforschung können mit neurophysiologischen und psychiatrischen Befunden in Verbindung gebracht werden. Die Neurophysiologie gewinnt ihre Ergebnisse vorwiegend aus Tierversuchen, und Übertragungen auf den Menschen sind nur mit Einschränkungen, Beachtung der Artunterschiede und Berücksichtigung ähnlicher Befunde am menschlichen Nervensystem möglich. Die Stellung der Verhaltensforschung zur Neurophysiologie und Psychologie wird mit ROEDERs Schema anschaulich gemacht und die Beziehungen von Introspektion und objektiver Forschung dargestellt. *Die Verhaltensforschung hat eine Vermittlerrolle zwischen Physiologie und Psychologie.* Die Unterschiede von Mensch und Tier sind bei gleicher biologischer Grundlage durch die *Sonderstellung des Menschen mit Sprache und Kultur* bedingt. Spezifisch menschlich sind rational planendes Zukunftsdenken, sprachliche Abstraktion, geistige Bedürfnisse und produktive Kunstleistungen. Den höheren *Tieren und Menschen gemeinsam* sind Raumorientierung, Triebe und Affekte, Lernvermögen, Gedächtnis, Wechsel von Schlafen und Wachen. Eine Verhaltenssteuerung durch äußere Einwirkungen, Triebe und Lernen gibt es daher bei Tier und Mensch; bei Menschen ist sie durch *geistige Bedürfnisse und Kul-*

tureinflüsse überbaut und verfeinert. Die Sonderentwicklung von Sprache und Schrift ist Vorbedingung für spezifisch-menschliches Verhalten und Entwicklung von Werten, die POPPER als *Welt 3* bezeichnet. Die künstlichen Laboratoriumsbedingungen der experimentellen Neurophysiologie, die nur Teilaspekte des Verhaltens erforscht, werden zur klinischen Exploration kontrastiert. Physiologisches Experiment und ärztliches Gespräch schließen sich gegenseitig aus. Die Möglichkeiten von telemetrischen Verhaltensexperimenten bei Affengruppen über soziale Aggressionsausbreitung sind begrenzt.

V. Neurophysiologische Grundlagen des Verhaltens: Neuronale Mechanismen der Sensomotorik

„Hierauf gründet sich nun die Befugniß ... alle Producte und Ereignisse der Natur, selbst die zweckmäßigsten, soweit mechanisch zu erklären, als es immer in unserem Vermögen ... steht."
I. KANT, Kritik der Urtheilskraft, 1790.

«Comment les esprits animaux sont produits dans le cerveau. ... car ce que je nomme ici des esprits ne sont que des corps, et ils n'ont point d'autre propriété sinon que ce sont des corps très-petits et qui se meuvent très-vite ... il en entre quelques-uns dans les cavités du cerveau, il en sort aussi quelques autres par les pores qui sont en sa substance, lesquels pores les conduisent dans les nerfs, et de là dans les muscles, au moyen de quoi il meuvent le corps en toutes les diverses façons qu'il peut être mû. Comment se font les mouvements des muscles. Car la seule cause de tous les mouvements des membres est que quelques muscles s'accourcissent et que leurs opposés s'allongent ...; et la seule cause qui fait qu'un muscle s'accourcit plutot que son opposé, est qu'il vient tant soit peu plus d'esprit du cerveau vers lui que vers l'autre.»
R. DESCARTES, Les passions de l'âme, 1649.

Wer die Motorik von Tieren und Menschen, die zielsicheren, eleganten Bewegungen einer springenden Katze oder die komplizierte Fingerarbeit eines Klavierspielers beobachtet, dem erscheint es wenig aussichtsreich, diese äußerst zweckmäßigen Koordinationsleistungen in einzelne neuronale Mechanismen aufzulösen. Und doch ist dies Aufgabe der Neurophysiologie.

Einen ersten spekulativen Deutungsversuch, das Verhalten rein mechanistisch als Maschine zu erklären, machte DESCARTES vor 300 Jahren. Er ließ in der «bête machine» und im Menschen die Nervenimpulse als «esprits animaux» vom Gehirn bis zu den Muskeln verlaufen. Wenn man DESCARTES' Vorstellungen von der «machina quae corpus constituit» ihres barocken Mantels entkleidet, und statt «esprits animaux» Nervenimpulse sagt, statt «corps tres-petits» Ionen, die durch die Poren der Neurone und Nervenmembranen wandern, so kann man sie in eine moderne wissenschaftliche Sprache übersetzen. Aber auch dann bleibt noch ein weiter Weg bis zu den «passions de l'âme», die DESCARTES erklären wollte, und die den Psychiater vor allem interessieren. Die Elementarprozesse der Ionenpermeabilität an den Nerven-Membranen sind noch zu weit von den integrierten cerebralen Funktionen entfernt und deshalb für die Psychiatrie uninteressant. Diese Einschränkung gilt nicht für die Funktionen einzelner Neurone, die hier besprochen werden müssen. Denn an einer einzigen Nervenzelle läßt sich bereits eine komplexe Wechselwirkung von Erregung und Hemmung mit einer Integration verschiedener Sinnesmeldungen darstellen, die neurophysiologische Grundlagen der Motorik und des Verhaltens bilden.

In den letzten 30 Jahren haben sich viele Forscher um neurophysiologische Analysen der Motorik bemüht. Solche Untersuchungen sind früher vor allem durch mechanische Registrierungen, in den letzten Jahren mehr durch elektrophysiologische Methoden gefördert worden. Die ersten geschlossenen Darstellungen stammen von SHERRINGTON [S 32, C 14] für die spinale Reflexphysiologie, von P. HOFFMANN [H 74] für die Eigenreflexe des Menschen und von WACHOLDER [W 1] für die menschliche Willkürmotorik. Alle diese Untersuchungen begnügten sich mit der Registrierung *peripherer* Vorgänge der Muskulatur, meist mit myographischen oder elektromyographischen Methoden, die beide nur indirekte Schlüsse auf die Gehirnvorgänge zulassen. Die *cerebralen* Koordinationen der Motorik sind erst in den letzten Jahrzehnten durch systematische Reizversuche und einzelne Neuronableitungen weiter aufgeklärt worden.

Analysen der Motorik und ihre theoretischen Ausarbeitungen sind die wichtigsten Beiträge der Neurophysiologie zur Verhaltensforschung.

Analyse der Motorik als neurophysiologischer Beitrag zur Verhaltensforschung

Die Verhaltensforschung beruht auf der Beobachtung *motorischer Äußerungen*. Die Motorik bildet beim Tier sowohl für spontanes Ausdrucksverhalten wie für experimentelle Lernversuche oder Erforschung der bedingten Reflexe den einzigen Zugang zur sog. höheren Nerventätigkeit. Wegen der fehlenden Sprachinformation können wir etwaige „psychische" Vorgänge beim Tier nur im Ausdruck äußeren motorischen Verhaltens und nicht, wie beim Menschen, „von innen" durch Selbstbeobachtung und sprachliche Mitteilung untersuchen. Die Neurophysiologie kann zur Verhaltensforschung zunächst durch *Analyse motorischer Mechanismen beitragen*.

Bereits an der vorwiegend „unbewußt" arbeitenden *extrapyramidalen Motorik* sind so zahlreiche Apparate des Gehirns und Rückenmarks beteiligt, daß schon die einfachsten Vorgänge motorischen Verhaltens, wie Fortbewegung und Gleichgewichtsregulation ein komplexes Wechselspiel sensorisch-sensibler Afferenzen mit zentralen Automatismen und motorischer Efferenz zeigen (vgl. Abb. 9). Noch komplizierter liegen die Verhältnisse bei der *Willkürmotorik*, die nur auf der Grundlage unwillkürlicher Bewegungs-, Haltungs- und Stützregulationen und erlernter Vorgänge möglich ist und deren corticale Startimpulse über die Pyramidenbahn auch das Kleinhirn und extrapyramidale Mechanismen beteiligen [J 47, 56]. Neben der willkürlichen und unwillkürlichen Körpermotorik sind affektive Ausdrucksbewegungen und Mimik und schließlich auch die *Sprache* motorische Entäußerungen, die eng mit psychischen Vorgängen verbunden sind. Die Funktionen der extrapyramidalen Körpermotorik sind bereits so kompliziert, daß eine physiologische Analyse der höheren motorischen Leistungen, wie der Sprache, wenig Hoffnung auf eine neurophysiologische Klärung komplexer Verhaltensweisen bringt.

Die mit dem Triebverhalten eng verbundene *affektive Motorik* und *Mimik*, die der *Psychomotorik* zugrunde liegt, erscheint einer physiologischen Erforschung zugänglicher, weil sie beim Tier experimentell untersucht werden kann. Bevor wir die trieb- und affekt-bedingte Motorik besprechen, die durch das Triebziel antizipierend gesteuert wird (vgl. S. 838), sollen noch sensomotorische Mechanismen und gewisse Antizipationen in der Regulation der Stütz- und Willkürmotorik dargestellt werden.

Neuronenphysiologie und Verhalten. Für das Verhältnis von Neurophysiologie und Verhaltensforschung gelten ähnliche allgemeine Regeln wie für die Beziehungen von objektiver Sinnesphysiologie und psychologischer Wahrnehmungslehre. Wir können neurophysiologisch nur einige *Grundlagen einfacher Verhaltensvorgänge* untersuchen, aber nicht den gesamten Mechanismus einer Verhaltensweise in neurophysiologischer Sprache beschreiben. Eine Darstellung aller neuronalen Mechanismen solcher Verhaltensvorgänge würde dann so lang und umständlich, daß wir sie nicht mehr verstehen könnten. Beschreibungen derselben Vorgänge in psychologischer oder Verhaltensterminologie, die meistens Sinn und Ziel erkennen lassen, bleiben dagegen leichter verständlich und anschaulich. Wenn wir eine einfache aktive *Kopfwendung* in ihren komplizierten Wechselwirkungen der Willküraktion mit Labyrinth- und Halsreflexen in ihren Neuronenmechanismen darstellen wollten, brauchten wir mehrere Seiten und zahlreiche erklärende Abbildungen und Schemata. Eine solche Einzelanalyse dieser motorischen Vorgänge ist von MAGNUS und RADEMAKER durch Ausschaltungsversuche [M 17, R 1] und von DUENSING und SCHAEFER durch Neuronenableitungen im Hirnstamm [D 37] durchgeführt worden. Die Kompliziertheit der neurophysiologischen Mechanismen, die differenzierten Verhaltensweisen zugrunde liegen, läßt es hoffnungslos erscheinen, sie annähernd vollständig als neuronale Vorgänge darzustellen.

Da sehr viele zentralnervöse Strukturen und Regulationen bei einer einfachen Bewegung, etwa dem Laufen eines Tieres, zusammenspielen, erscheint es wenig sinnvoll, alle neuronalen Mechanismen speziellen tierischen Verhaltens bei Kampf, Flucht, Orientierung, Paarung oder Brutpflege im Detail zu analysieren und zu beschreiben. Man kann nur vereinfachte *Schemata der beteiligten Neuronenverbindungen* mit Prinzipschaltungen abbilden, wie sie Abb. 9 für die Blickmotorik zeigt. Ferner kann man die Prinzipien der zielgesteuerten Handlung mit ihrer psychologischen und physiologischen Regulation schematisch darstellen wie in Abb. 14C.

Leichter mit der Verhaltensforschung zu korrelieren sind neurophysiologische Untersuchungen auf höherer Ebene, auf der die *Integration dieser Verhaltensweisen* stattfindet. So zeigen HESS' Reizversuche im Zwischenhirn von Katzen und v. HOLSTs Hühnerexperimente, daß relativ *komplexe motorische Leistungen* wie Dreh- und Wendebewegungen oder sogar affektive Verhaltensweisen der Wut, Abwehr oder Flucht und des Schlafes *durch cerebrale Reize ausgelöst werden können* (vgl. S. 940, Abb. 8 u. 27).

Psychologische und biologische Betrachtung der Motorik. Eine psychologische Darstellung der Willkürmotorik (zum Unterschied von physiologischen Untersuchungen der einzelnen Funktionen des ZNS, die psychische Willensvorgänge begründen) gibt LEWIN 1926 in seiner Analyse der Willenshandlung [L 15a]. Hier muß man auch Zweck und Sinn des Handelns berücksichtigen und mit Trieb und Willen auch das Bewußtsein, das selbst die reine Verhaltensanalyse beim Menschen nicht ausschalten darf. *Psychische Intentionen* und willkürliches Handeln, wie psychologische Begriffe überhaupt, sind *auf Ziel und Leistung gerichtet und nicht auf den Handlungsablauf.* Mechanismus und Ablauf der Handlung sind nur *physiologisch* zu erfassende, vorwiegend unbewußt ablaufende Vorgänge. Bei *biologischer* Betrachtung wird jedoch *beides,* Zielerfolg und Handlungsablauf kombiniert. Die Regelungen beider führen dann zur Biokybernetik. Hier kann intentionales, automatisches und reflektorisches Handeln nicht so scharf getrennt werden wie es der Physiologe wünscht. Beim Menschen kann man jedoch einige hirnelektrische Korrelate der Handlungsbereitschaft und Zielkontrolle registrieren (S. 833 und Abb. 11).

Sensomotorische Koordination. Der Begriff der *Sensomotorik* ist seit seiner Prägung durch EXNERS „Sensomobilität" [E 29] zunächst vorwiegend für Reflexvorgänge verwendet worden [H 75, 76]. Dann wurde er unter dem Einfluß der Gestaltpsychologie mehr spekulativ für v. WEIZSÄCKERS „Gestaltkreis" [W 18] und GOLDSTEINS organische Ganzheitsbetrachtung [G 29] ausgewertet. Neuere experimentelle Ergebnisse und physikalisch-mathematische Modelle über Regelvorgänge des Nervensystems führen in die gleiche Richtung und bringen biokybernetische Theorien für Wahrnehmung und Bewegung. Sie werden mit den langsamen Hirnpotentialen vor und während der Bewegung (S. 833) und der Kybernetik besprochen (s.S. 858).

Neurophysiologische Befunde über *sensomotorische Regulationen der Bewegung* [H 56, J 58] und über die *rückläufige Beeinflussung sensorischer Meldungen* bei verschiedenem Verhalten zum Umwelt [H 38], bei Aufmerksamkeit [H 2, 38] und Gewöhnung [H 36, B 50] und bei experimenteller elektrischer Reizung [H 37, 65] haben die enge Verbindung von Sensibilität und Motorik auch in ihren Einzelmechanismen weiter aufgeklärt. Neben der *Konvergenz afferenter Sinnesmeldungen an motorischen Neuronen* gibt es auch eine *efferente Kontrolle der Sinnesafferenzen* die verschiedene Prinzipien verwendet: direkte Innervation der peripheren afferenten Strukturen wie die γ-Innervation der Muskelspindeln, Innervation der Pupille und der Mittelohrmuskeln, periphere Endigungen efferenter Fasern an Receptorstrukturen des Innenohres [E 18], zentrale Beeinflussung von Rückmeldungsvorgängen der motorischen Neurone (Renshaw-Mechanismus [E 2]) und von sensiblen Hemmungsvorgängen mit Kontrasteffekt (präsynaptische Hemmung [E 5]) auf spinaler Ebene, Konvergenz corticaler Impulse an den Relaiskernen der Hinterstrangssensibilität [H 1] und an Neuronen des reticulären Systems, die wiederum komplexe Verhaltensmechanismen steuern. Danach ist es klar, daß auch die *angeborenen Instinktvorgänge,* deren Erb-Koordinationen als „fixed patterns" zu verlaufen scheinen, *während ihres ganzen Ablaufs unter sensomotorischer Kontrolle stehen.* Dies ist schon deshalb notwendig, weil die meisten Instinkthandlungen auf ein *„Ziel"* oder einen *Partner* gerichtet sind.

Bei jedem Verhalten arbeiten afferente Sinnesmeldungen und efferente Regulationen eng zusammen und dies erfordert eine differenzierte geregelte Koordination, an der die verschiedensten Strukturen des ZNS teilnehmen.

Antizipierende Koordination in der Sensomotorik

Im Gegensatz zu den automatischen Rhythmen sind alle anderen Bewegungsfunktionen *zielgerichtet.* Bereits die Analyse einfacher motorischer Leistungen weist auf ein für die Psychomotorik wichtiges Prinzip: Nicht nur die motorischen Handlungen des Triebverhaltens (Nahrungssuche und -aufnahme, sexuelles Verhalten) sind zielgerichtet, sondern auch einfache motorische Koordinationen: Die Bewegungen des Blickes, des Ganges, des Sprunges oder des Werfens, die meist einer Stützmotorik bedürfen, enthalten eine *sensomotorische Antizipation* [J 58]. Diese vorwegnehmende Funktion der motorischen Koordination und ihre Vorbereitung ist nicht auf die Willkür- und Zielmotorik beschränkt.

Eine sensorisch gesteuerte Zielbewegung ist auch die *Blickmotorik,* bei der die stützende Komponente nur eine geringe Rolle spielt. Exakte Daten haben wir für die optomotorischen Reaktionen der Augeneinstellung, der Kopf- und Körpermotorik auf Umwelt- und Eigenbewegungen. Vor allem der *optokinetische Nystagmus* und sein neuronales Substrat im optisch-vestibulären System des Cortex und des Hirnstammes, ist genauer untersucht [J 33, D 30, 31].

Blickmotorik. Die Blickbewegungen sind eng mit der Aufmerksamkeitsrichtung und der Bewegungsantizipation korreliert. Augenbewegungen werden sensorisch durch zwei Sinnesorgane, das *Auge* und den *Vestibularapparat,* bei Eigen- und Umweltbewegungen gesteuert. Der Vestibularapparat hat mit seinen 3 Bogengängen einen klaren Aufbau in *drei Raumebenen.* Das Auge wird von 3 Muskelpaaren in diesen Raumkoordinaten bewegt: horizontal, vertikal und rotierend. Die Blickmotorik kann so mit der Körpermotorik im dreidimensionalen Raum koordiniert werden. Das zentrale Substrat dieser optisch-vestibulären Koordination liegt im Hirnstamm zwischen Vestibularis- und Augenmuskelkernen, vorwiegend in der *Formatio reticularis.* Abbildung 9 zeigt die Zentren und Bahnen dieses optisch-vestibulären Systems, dessen neuronale Mechanismen in den letzten Jahrzehnten sehr genau erforscht wurden. *Die antizipierende Funktion der Augenbewegungen liegt in der Vorwegnahme der somatomotorischen Zielbewegung.* Bevor wir etwas ergreifen, wenden wir den Blick zu dem Objekt hin und orientieren uns damit über die räumliche Situation. Übergeordnet über die optisch-vestibulären Hirnstammregulationen der Blickbewegungen ist die *parietale Hirnrinde.* Im parietalen Feld 7 haben MOUNTCASTLE u.Mitarb. [M 73, L 44] spezifische, durch die gerichtete Aufmerksamkeit aktivierte Neurone gefunden, nachdem wir schon theoretisch Fixationsneurone und Blickfolgeneurone im Cortex postuliert hatten [J 45]. Die parietalen Rindenfelder 5 und 7 steuern mit diesen funktionsspezifischen Neuronen die optische Aufmerksamkeit und das Greifen im Nahraum mit gerichteten Blickbewegungen.

Die visuell-optomotorische Kontrolle ist vielseitiger und selektiver als die vestibuläre. *Die vestibulären und proprioceptiven Informationen sind für die Stützmotorik prävalent* gegenüber den optischen. Dagegen ist *für die Optomotorik die visuelle Information prävalent* und die vestibuläre nur eine korrigierende

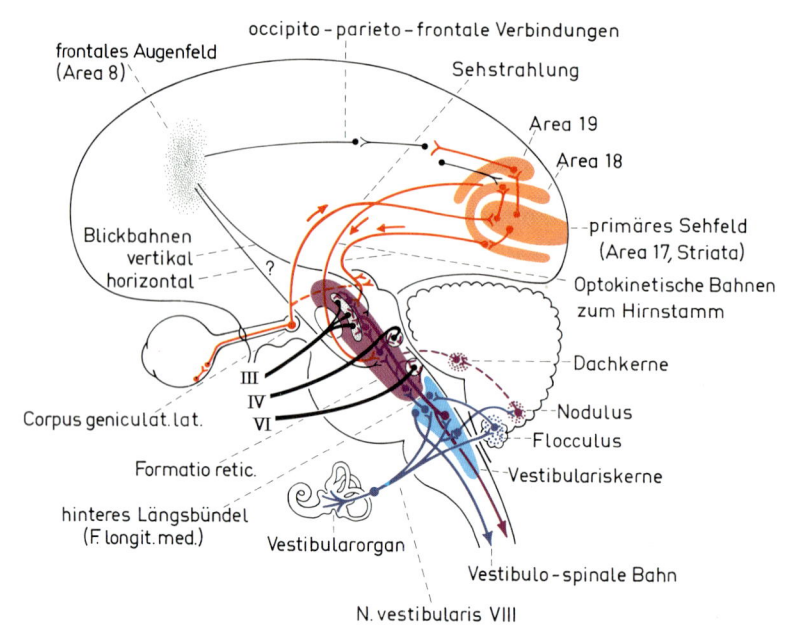

Abb. 9. Schema der Zentren und Bahnen der optisch-vestibulären Regelung der Blickmotorik. Modifiziert nach JUNG (1953 und 1978) [J 33, 49]. Das vestibuläre System ist *blau,* das optische System *rot* bezeichnet. Die Koordination beider Systeme für die Augenbewegungen und für die Regulation der Körpermotorik in der Substantia reticularis ist *violett.* Die willkürliche Blickregulation mit frontalen Augenfeldern und Parietalregion und die Motoneurone der Augenmuskelnerven sind schwarz. Die violetten Kerngebiete in Mittelhirn und Brücke sind die *Formatio reticularis,* deren paramediane Anteile („pontines Blickzentrum") die Blickbewegungen zur homolateralen Seite steuern. Eine schnelle Leitung von Vestibulariskernen zu den Augenmuskelkernen über zwei Neurone läuft über das hintere Längsbündel (F. longit. med.) für vestibulo-oculäre Reflexe. Eine Nebenschaltung über das Kleinhirn bilden Flocculus, Nodulus und Dachkerne. Die frontalen Augenfelder erhalten corticale Sehinformationen über die Parietal- und Temporalrinde und subcorticale Meldungen über Augenbewegungen aus dem Mittelhirn wahrscheinlich mit doppelläufigen Bahnen. Die occipito-temporo-frontalen und ponto-neocerebellaren Bahnen wurden weggelassen und die Kreuzungsverhältnisse nicht berücksichtigt

und modulierende Komponente bei beschleunigten Eigenbewegungen des Kopfes [J 40, D 29]. Die antizipierende Komponente bei den Augenbewegungen ist vor allem durch die gerichtete *Aufmerksamkeit* bedingt, die beim Menschen auch in ihrer willkürlichen Steuerung untersucht werden kann. Bei Willkürbewegungen geht dementsprechend die Augenbewegung der Kopf- und Körperwendung voraus, was als visuelle Sicherung biologisch sinnvoll ist. Bei vestibulären Bewegungen ist die Reihenfolge dagegen Körper-Kopf-Auge [J 33]. Dies ist wiederum verständlich, weil die Erhaltung des Körpergleichgewichts auch für die Augenbewegungen grundlegend ist: wenn der Körper fällt, ist optomotorische Regulation zwecklos.

Das biologisch bedeutungsvolle *Bewegungssehen* enthält schon bei niederen Tierformen neben der Bewegungsanpassung an Umweltveränderungen (Kompensation der Luft- und Wasserströmung bei Insekten und Fischen) auch ein Formerkennen bewegter Objekte und spezielle mit dem Triebverhalten koordinierte Reaktionen: *Vorausberechnung und Auswertung der Objektgeschwindigkeit und Koordination mit der eigenen Bewegung* (Beutefang mit „Vorhalten" oder Ausweichen und Flucht vor dem feindlichen Angriff). Die komplizierteren Verhaltensweisen der visuell gesteuerten Motorik sind neuronal noch nicht erklärbar. Bereits relativ einfache Reaktionen auf bewegte Beute bei Insekten wie der Fangschlag der Mantis benötigten komplizierte kybernetische Modelle [M 49].

Zielbewegung, Stützhaltung und Bewegungsentwurf

Zielmotorik und Stützmotorik. Nachdem man schon früher die *Wechselwirkung von Haltung und Bewegung* zu verstehen versuchte, entwickelte W.R. HESS ein klares Konzept ihrer Funktionen. HESS [H 66] bezeichnet die *Haltung als Handlungsbereitschaft* und Ausgangsstellung für aktive Bewegungen des wachen Organismus. Mit ihrer Muskeltonisierung ist die *Stützhaltung* notwendiger Unterbau und „*aktive Stabilisierung eines dynamischen Gleichgewichtes*". HESS [H 57, 66] unterscheidet nach physiologischen Verhaltensanalysen die *Zielmotorik* („teleokinetische Motilität") *und Stützmotorik* („ereismatische Motilität") als zwei sich ergänzende Bewegungskoordinationen. Die auch als Haltung bezeichnete Stützinnervation ist damit eine notwendige Vorbedingung jeder Zielaktion, die dieser vorangeht und ihr bis zum Abschluß koordiniert bleibt.

Ein lebendes Modell der menschlichen Ziel- und Stützmotorik zeigt Abb. 10 nach einer Filmaufnahme von HESS [H 57]. Es ist eine anschauliche Demonstration für die *Notwendigkeit statischer Regulationen bei dynamischen Bewegungen mit ihren Kräften und Gegenkräften.* Diese Kräfte werden im Modell durch drei Personen repräsentiert, die bei der Zielaktion eines Menschen verschiedenen Teilen seines Muskel-Skeletapparates entsprechen. Beim Menschen mit seiner aufrechten Haltung wird die Stützmotorik noch mehr als bei anderen Landtieren zur *Kompensation von Schwerkraftwirkungen* eingesetzt.

Stützmotorik als Vorbereitung und Kontrolle der Zielbewegung. Zum Gelingen einer gezielten Aktion muß die *Stützmotorik frühzeitig aktiviert werden.* HESS' Modellversuch in Abb. 10 zeigt die Abhängigkeit der Bewegung von der *Haltungsvorbereitung* und damit ein Primat der Haltung für die Bewegungsbereitschaft. In der realen Anwendung dieses Modells auf den Bewegungsapparat *eines* Menschen kann man den „*Träger*" mit Skelet und schwerkraftkompensierender Muskulatur, den „*Stützer*" mit der Halteinnervation rumpfnaher Muskeln in Schulter und Becken identifizieren und den „*Springer*" mit der dynamisch-ballistischen Muskelaktion. Träger und Stützapparate müssen *vor* der Zielbewegung antizipatorisch aktiviert werden, um die physikalischen Begleitkräfte rechtzeitig zu kompensieren. Auch hier kommen reine Reflexe zu spät oder sind unzureichend, wenn sie nicht vorher mit der Bewegungsbereitschaft gebahnt werden.

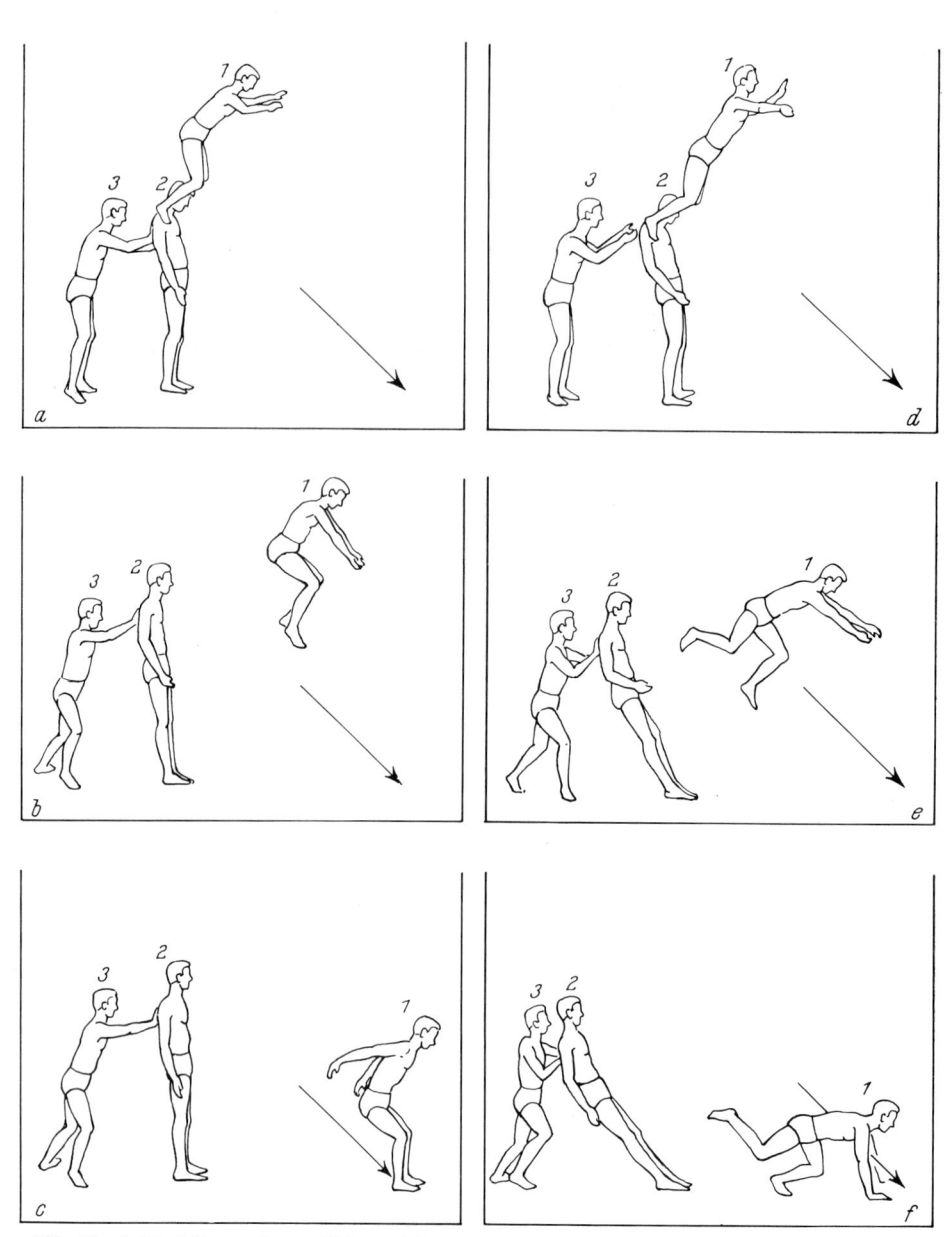

Abb. 10a–f. Modellversuch zur Ziel- und Stützmotorik: Nach HESS teleokinetische Zielbewegung und ereismatischer Rückhalt (Umrißzeichnungen aus einem Film von HESS [H 57] 1943, nach JUNG u. HASSLER [J 58] 1960). Durch 3 Personen werden die Kräfte und Gegenkräfte einer gezielten Willkürbewegung mit dem Rückhalt „unwillkürlicher" Halte- und Stützmotorik dargestellt: Der *„teleokinetische"* Springer (*1*) kann nur mit Hilfe der *„ereismatischen"* Träger (*2*) und Stützer (*3*) sein Ziel erreichen: (a–c) *Der Sprung gelingt zum bezeichneten Ziel* (Pfeil), wenn der richtige Rückhalt gegeben wird und der Träger über den Moment des Sprungs orientiert und *vorbereitet* ist. (d–f) *Derselbe Sprung mißlingt ohne vorbereiteten Rückhalt.* Der unvorbereitete und ungestützte Träger fällt beim Absprung rückwärts und muß als Nothilfe durch die 3. Halteperson aufgefangen werden. Der Sprung von *f* wird zu kurz und der Springer fällt, weil die Rückhaltefunktion seiner Absprungbasis ungenügend war. Allgemeine Prinzipien der Stützmotorik als Grundlagen der Zielbewegung sind demnach: *Bereitschaft und Anpassung der* Rückhaltefunktionen: 2. und 3. Mann müssen den Moment des Sprungs *wissen,* Gewicht und Absprungkraft *fühlen,* und sich an die dadurch bedingten Haltungsveränderungen *anpassen.* Ohne diese Hilfsmechanismen ist jede Zielbewegung unmöglich. Die Filmbilder sind 1965 von HESS [H 66] mit einer physikalischen Analyse sensomotorischer Leistungen reproduziert worden

HESS' Bild erklärt, warum neben einer dauernden *statischen Stütze* (passiv-mechanisch durch den Skelet- und Bandapparat und aktiv durch Muskelinnervation) frühere aktive Koordinationen notwendig sind: *Vor* der Bewegung erfolgt eine *antizipatorische Haltungsbereitschaft* durch vorbereitende Innervation von entfernten Muskelgruppen als Basis für die gezielte Endhandlung. *Während der Bewegung müssen sensible Meldungen des Bewegungsmoments und der Gegenkräfte des Rückstoßes* zur Kompensation eingesetzt werden. Eine *Regelung aller motorischen Kräfte,* auch der vom bewegenden Glied entfernten erzielt Anpassung an neue Lagen bei verschiedenen Haltungsveränderungen. Ohne diese Vorbedingungen muß die Zielbewegung, wie in Abb. 10 d–f, mißlingen. Die Stützmotorik erweist sich damit als *zeitlich vorangehendes Primat der Haltung vor der gezielten Bewegung* [D 28, H 56, 66].

Folgende neurophysiologische Mechanismen können diese *Koordination von Stütz- und Zielmotorik* vermitteln:
1. *Vorprogrammierung der Bewegungs- und Haltungsaktivierung* in zeitlicher Abfolge mit vorangehender Bereitstellung der Haltemuskulatur vor der zielgesteuerten Bewegung.
2. *Allgemeine Bereitschaftsaktivierung proprioceptiver Kontrollen durch Gammaerregung der Muskelspindeln.* Dabei werden nicht nur die primär innervierten Muskeln, sondern auch entfernte und kontralaterale Muskelspindelapparate fusimotorisch aktiviert, um spätere *Rückstoßwirkungen* der Zielbewegung auf die Körperhaltung aufzufangen und spinal zu kompensieren.
3. *Kontinuierliche Steuerung und Regelung der Bewegung und Haltung* mit Anpassung an unvorhergesehene Widerstände und veränderte Bewegungsentwürfe. Neben dem motorischen Cortex und dem Kleinhirn sind auch neuronale Regelkreise extrapyramidaler Zentren an diesen Kontrollen beteiligt.

Alle diese Mechanismen erhalten erst durch Übung und Lernen, offenbar in Zusammenarbeit von Großhirnrinde und Kleinhirn, volle Wirksamkeit (vgl. S. 838).

Zeitliche Antizipation der Stützmotorik. Die *tonische Vorinnervation der Stützmuskeln* betrifft bei Armbewegungen neben der Schulter auch die Rumpfmuskulatur. Dies ist am Beispiel einer *Wurfbewegung* leicht zu sehen. Vor dem Werfen muß die Bein- und Rumpfhaltung stabilisiert, Körper und Arm zurückgedreht werden und erst nach dieser vorbereitenden Haltungsinnervation kann die dynamische ballistische Wurfbewegung erfolgreich ausgeführt werden (Abb. 12 A). Hinweise auf die tonische stützmotorische Bewegungsvorbereitung geben elektromyographische Ableitungen von Rumpf- und Extremitätenmuskeln: *vor* einer Armbewegung werden bereits die Haltungsmuskeln von Schulter und Rumpf aktiviert (Abb. 12 C).

Zielmotorik, Werkzeuggebrauch und Spiel. Im menschlichen Kulturmilieu gibt es zahlreiche spezifische motorische Leistungen in Handwerk, Musik und Sport, die Werkzeuge, Instrumente oder Fahrzeuge verwenden. Solche Leistungen sind charakteristisch für den Menschen, den *homo faber,* da Tiere, selbst höhere Affen nicht oder nur gelegentlich, aber nie systematisch Werkzeuge verwenden. Erstaunliche Bewegungsleistungen höchster Präzision, die dauernder Übung bedürfen, zeigen sich beim Spielen von Musikinstrumenten, über die es bisher nur wenige physiologische Studien gibt [T 11a]. Handwerkstätigkeiten und auch Sportleistungen wie das Ballspiel sind *durch Übung und Ausbildung erworbene Fertigkeiten*. Scheinbar einfache Leistungen, z.B. ein gezielter Ballwurf, benötigen exakt gesteuerte und komplizierte Bewegungsfolgen. Man kann sie nur mit einigen Koordinationsprinzipien anschaulich darstellen, aber noch nicht physiologisch erklären. Wie der Mensch diese Übung durch sportliches Training für den Wettkampf erwirbt, so das Tier durch Spielen für Beutefang und Kampf. Offenbar liegt der *biologische Zweck des Spiels* bei Tier und Mensch in einer Übung komplizierter Handlungsfolgen im Wechselspiel mit Partnern und Gegnern. Bei allen diesen Leistungen im Spiel und Kampf werden die Triebbewegungen mit erlernten Handlungsfolgen und angeborenen elementaren Hirnmechanismen koordiniert.

Planung, Regelung und Flexibilität. Die *Realisierung des Bewegungsentwurfs* kann sich nicht nur auf zeitlich fixierte Innervationsfolgen von Stütz- und Zielmotorik mit fester Vorprogrammierung beschränken, sondern verlangt eine *flexible Planung der motorischen Handlung,* die auf veränderte Umweltsituationen einstellbar ist. Psychologisch entspricht die primäre Bewegungsintention einer Erwartung und Voraussicht der Subjekt-Umweltrelation, die als *Einstellung* (englisch „set") bezeichnet wird. Kybernetisch ist es ein Modellprogramm mit *Steuerung und Regelung* der Bewegung. Jede unvorhergesehene Änderung der Umweltbedingung *stört* den programmierten Bewegungsablauf. Nach der klassischen Lehre, die HOFFMANN als Beziehung von Willen und Reflex [H 76] bezeichnete, wird die Störung durch *reflektorische Mechanismen* kompensiert. Schon die tägliche Erfahrung des Fehltritts einer falsch eingeschätzten Treppenzahl, die trotz Reflexkontrolle zum Hinfallen führen kann, zeigt aber die *Grenzen der reinen Reflexkontrolle,* deren Bedeutung früher überbewertet wurde. Wenn wir einen als schwer erwarteten Gegenstand aufheben, der sich als leicht herausstellt und umgekehrt, so muß die Stütz- und Zielbewegung neu eingestellt werden. Diese Steuerung geschieht nicht nur spinal-reflektorisch, sondern über Hirnrinde und Kleinhirn (vgl. S. 845).

Solche Erfahrungen, die Analyse von rhythmischen Gang- und Sprungbewegungen [M 37a, 37b] sowie die noch komplizierteren Wechselwirkungen verschiedener Personen bei Spiel und Sport zeigen die Notwendigkeit einer den Reflexen vorangehenden *Bereitschaftsinnervation und einer Modulation der Vorprogrammierung durch kontinuierlich regulierte Einstellungen,* die veränderte Umweltsituationen nach Meldungen zahlreicher Sinnesorgane berücksichtigen. Diese Einstellung auf eine wechselnde Umwelt und auf den Bewegungpartner in Spiel und Kampf ist besser psychologisch als neurophysiologisch zu beschreiben, da nur wenige Einzelmechanismen der meist multisensorischen Regulationen bekannt sind.

Intersensorische Transformationen des Bewegungsentwurfs. Ähnlich wie die Sinneswahrnehmung wird auch die Motorik *multisensorisch kontrolliert,* und die gleiche Handlung kann, einmal von einer Sinnesmodalität ausgelöst, auch von anderen Sinnen gesteuert werden, nachdem ein Programm vorliegt. Es ist noch nicht geklärt, wie diese intersensorische Transposition zwischen verschiedenen Sinnen abläuft. Offenbar werden, wie beim bilateralen Transfer zwischen den Großhirnhemisphären über den Balken, *cortico-corticale* Verbindungen und *multisensorische Konvergenzen* zwischen verschiedenen Sinnesmodalitäten auch zur Bewegungssssteuerung verwendet. Multisensorische Neurone wurden in verschiedenen Rindenfeldern gefunden [J 59]. Sie sind wahrscheinlich für Konditionierungs- und Lernvorgänge von Bedeutung. Zwischen optischen, akustischen und taktilen Wahrnehmungen und Bewegungskontrollen besteht offenbar ein reger Informationstransfer, dessen Einbau in die Motorik noch zu untersuchen ist.

Nach schweren Ausfällen einzelner Sinne kann diese multisensorische Transformation sehr effektiv entwickelt werden. Beim Blinden wird z.B. die fehlende optisch-räumliche Orientierung durch taktile und akustische Wahrnehmungen kompensiert, die ein Abschätzen von Hindernissen ermöglichen.

Eine gute Demonstration, wie *optisch* erlernte und im Schreibvorgang auch *sensomotorisch* verwendete Gestalten ohne besondere Übung rein *taktil* erkannt werden, ist das *Zahlenschreiben auf die Haut*. Jeder Neurologe verwendet diese Hautschrift als Test und erwartet, daß ein Gesunder mit leichter Berührung auf die Haut geschriebene Zahlen erkennt, obwohl er die Hautschriftwahrnehmung niemals vorher geübt hat und die Zahlenform bisher nur *gesehen* oder mit der Hand *geschrieben* wurde. Die umgekehrte Transformation von der Handschrift zum Lesen und Schreiben ist bei Taubstummen möglich. Das erstaunlichste Beispiel räumlicher Wahrnehmung über die Haut mit taktiler Transformation in die Sensomotorik ist die *blinde und taube* HELEN KELLER [K 12]. Sie erlernte *Lesen und Schreiben* nur über *taktile Hautschrift*: Ihre Lehrerin ließ sie zunächst ihre Puppe fühlen und schrieb dazu das Wort „doll" auf die Hautoberfläche der Hand. Auf diese Weise lernte HELEN KELLER ohne Auge und Ohr immer neue Worte und Bedeutungen erkennen und schließlich mit normaler Schrift auf Papier schreiben.

Handlungsbereitschaft, Willkürmotorik, erledigte und unerledigte Handlungen. Wenn man nach physiologischen Grundlagen der Willkürhandlung sucht, so wird man von einfachen Situationen *motorischer Bereitschaft* ausgehen. Die modernen automatischen Auswerte-Rechenmaschinen (Computer) erlauben es, zeitlich korrelierte elektrische Begleitphänomene des Gehirns vor, während und nach Willkürbewegungen aus zufälligen Veränderungen auszusieben. Mit einfacheren Methoden hat BATES [B 9] zuerst 1951 die Beziehung von Willkürbewegungen und α-Wellen des EEG untersucht. Neben statistischen Korrelationen des Bewegungsbeginns mit α-Wellen fand er ein kleines längeres Hirnpotential nach der Willkürhandlung. WALTER, KORNHUBER und ihre Mitarbeiter haben ähnliche Versuche mit modernen Computermethoden gemacht (Abb. 11). Konstant ist bei diesen Befunden der *plötzliche positive Potentialumschlag bei Erledigung der Handlung*. Solche Methoden werden es vielleicht ermöglichen, neurophysiologische Grundlagen für die Handlungsbereitschaft der Willkürmotorik und die eigenartigen langdauernden Veränderungen im ZNS bei der Willensintention und bei *unerledigten Handlungen* zu erfassen. Außer den Aufschubhandlungen (delayed responses) im Verhaltensexperiment bei Affen [B 11] sind Probleme der Handlungserledigung vorwiegend psychologisch bearbeitet worden: FREUDS Abreaktion mit ihrer affektiven Entladung [F 30] oder LEWINS Feldpsychologie [L 16–18] bringen vielleicht Ansätze für neurophysiologische Korrelationen. Die psychologischen Theorien beziehen sich meist auf die Fortdauer emotionaler Spannungen. Sie betonen damit zu sehr die Affektseite und zu wenig mögliche physiologische Mechanismen, die der Handlungsbereitschaft, dem Willensentschluß und dem Fortwirken unerledigter Handlungen zugrunde liegen können. Vielleicht gelingt es mit Weiterentwicklung der oben genannten Methoden, auch langfristige und kompliziertere Bedingungen der Handlungsbereitschaft neurophysiologisch zu erfassen und mit LEWINS Feldkonzeptionen von Trieb und Willen zu korrelieren. Auch kybernetische Modelldarstellungen dieser Mechanismen wären möglich, nachdem psychologische Befunde [Z 1] erste Hinweise gaben.

Cerebrale Bereitschaftspotentiale, Bewegungsentwurf und Rückmeldung

Bereitschaftspotentiale und Willkürmotorik.

Wenn man physiologische Grundlagen des Bewegungsentwurfs bei Willkürhandlungen untersuchen will, so wird man zunächst bei einfachen Bewegungen nach Korrelaten motorischer Bereitschaft im Gehirn suchen. Die modernen automatischen Auswerte-Rechenmaschinen (Computer) erlauben es, zeitlich korrelierte *elektrische Begleitphänomene des Gehirns vor, während und nach Willkürbewegungen* aus zufälligen Veränderungen auszusieben, die im *Electrencephalogramm* (EEG) enthalten sind. Beim Menschen fanden KORNHUBER und DEECKE [K 43] mit Elektroden auf der Kopfhaut kleine *negative Potentialverschiebungen über der parietalen, motorischen und frontalen Hirnrinde bei Handlungsbereitschaft* vor Willkür-Aktionen mit folgender positiver Verschiebung. Die negativen und positiven Gleichspannungen sind bei einseitiger Bewegung stärker über der kontralateralen Zentralregion (Abb. 5). Sie können weiter in verschiedene Komponenten zerlegt werden, von denen das kürzere „motor potential" über dem kontralateralen motorischen Cortex auftritt [D 10, K 41]. Bei bedingten Reaktionen durch Kombination von Sinnesreizen beschrieb WALTER eine entsprechende oberflächennegative Potentialverschiebung vorwiegend bilateral frontal, die nach dem ersten konditionierenden Reiz auftrat und die er *„Erwartungswelle" (expectancy wave)* nannte [W 10], da sie mit einer Erwartungseinstellung auf den zweiten Reiz korreliert war. Konstant ist in allen diesen Registrierungen das *oberflächennegative Hirnpotential während der Bereitschaft zur Willkürbewegung* (mit freigewähltem Zeitpunkt) *oder zur reizsignalisierten Reaktionsbewegung* (bei konditionierter Zeitbestimmung). Konstant ist ferner bei beiden, dem Bereitschaftspotential und der Erwartungswelle, der plötzliche *positive Potentialumschlag nach Erledigung der Handlung*.

Langsame Hirnrindenpotentiale bei Bewegungsintention

Corticale, langsame Potentiale über dem motorischen, parietalen und frontalen Cortex sind beim Menschen *vor* kurzdauernden Bewegungen und *während* längerer Zielbewegungen als hirnelektrische Äquivalente intentionaler und gesteuerter Motorik ableitbar. Diese langsamen Spannungsverschiebungen werden bei den üblichen EEG-Ableitungen vernachlässigt oder durch kurze Zeitkonstanten physikalisch ausgeschaltet. Umgekehrt werden bei diesen Registrierungen die kurzdauernden rhythmischen Hirnpotentiale (Alphawellen usw.) des EEG als zufällig statistisch ausgeschaltet, so daß nur konstante *bewegungskorrelierte* Hirnpotentiale sichtbar bleiben.

Vorbereitungs- und Zielbewegungspotentiale. Hirnelektrische Begleiterscheinungen willkürlicher Bewegungen können beim Menschen nur global durch Hirnpotentialableitungen vom Schädel erfaßt, aber nicht wie beim wachen Tier (Abb. 13) direkt am Cortex und dessen Neuronen [E 25–27] registriert werden. Cerebrale Korrelate der Vorbereitung von reaktiven, durch Sinnesreize ausgelösten „bedingten" Reaktionen und Willkürbewegungen sind langsame, negative Potentialverschiebungen über beiden Frontoparietalregionen, die bis zu einer Sekunde *der Bewegung vorausgehen*. Sie wurden von WALTER bei Konditionierung mit Doppelreizen *Erwartungswelle* [W 10] oder *„contingent negative variation"* (CNV) genannt (Abb. 11 A). Ähnliche, dem eigenen Willensentschluß korrelierte Potentiale die *ohne* Sinnesreize auftreten, hat KORNHUBER vor Willkürbe-

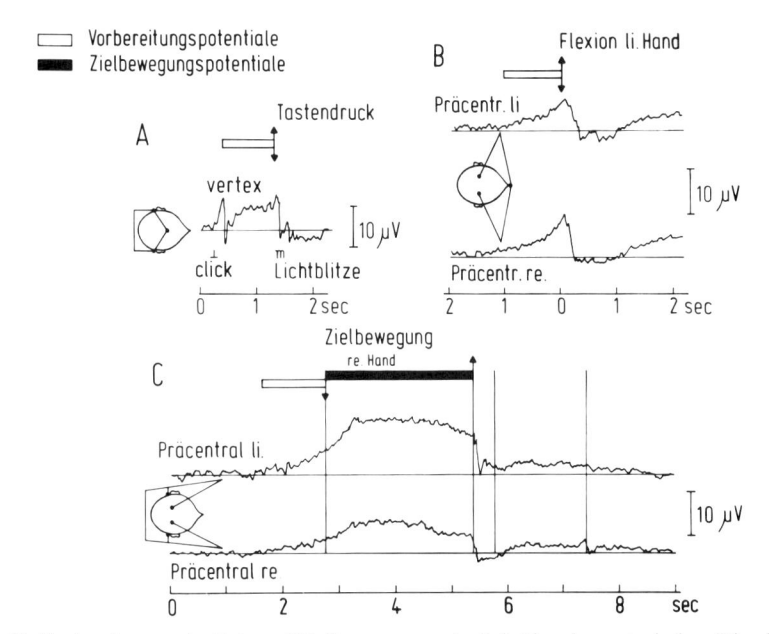

Abb. 11. Vorbereitungspotentiale und Zielbewegungspotentiale über der motorischen Hirnrinde beim Menschen vor und nach Willkürbewegungen.
A: Erwartungspotentiale nach WALTER (1964/65) [W 10].
B: Bereitschaftspotentiale nach KORNHUBER und DEECKE (1965) [K 43].
C: Zielbewegungspotentiale nach GRÜNEWALD-ZUBERBIER u. Mitarb. (1978) [G 43, 44]. Die Originalkurven wurden für eine einheitliche Verstärkung gleicher 10µV-Eichung umgezeichnet.

Alle mit *Bewegungsintention* korrelierten corticalen Spannungsverschiebungen sind über dem Cortex jeweils *oberflächennegativ* gegen Ohrableitungen sowohl die *vor* der Bewegung erscheinenden *Erwartungs- und Bereitschaftspotentiale* (AB) und die *während* der richtungs-kontrollierten Handlung ablaufenden *Zielbewegungspotentiale* (C). Oberflächenpositive Potentiale erscheinen erst mit Intentionsende: Bei Einsetzen kurzer Bewegungen (A Tastendruck, B Handbeugung) werden die Vorbereitungspotentiale durch eine positive Potentialverschiebung beendet. Diese Beendigung durch die Bewegung gilt für WALTERS konditionierte, durch Sinnesreiz in Erwartung des zweiten Reizes ausgelösten „expectancy waves" oder CNV (A) und die durch freien Willensentschluß induzierten Bereitschaftspotentiale KORNHUBERS (B). Dagegen werden die Zielbewegungspotentiale (C) noch während der Bewegung größer und enden erst *nach Erreichen des Zieles* mit positiver Potentialverschiebung

wegungen als *Bereitschaftspotentiale* [K 43] bezeichnet (Abb. 11 B). Diese *vor* Bewegungen auftretenden Negativierungen entsprechen dem *Bewegungsentwurf* und werden mit dem Beginn der Bewegung durch eine positive Potentialverschiebung beendet, die KORNHUBER und DEECKE als Reafferenz deuten [K 43]. Im Gegensatz zu diesem raschen Ende der Vorbereitungspotentiale findet man *während* sensorisch kontrollierter Zielbewegungen eine Vergrößerung und Verstärkung des vorbereitenden Bereitschaftspotentials, die bis zum Erreichen des Zieles andauern (Abb. 11 C). Wir haben diese größeren negativen Potentialverschiebungen, die während intendierter und aufmerksamer Kontrolle von gezielten Handlungen auftreten, daher mit GRÜNEWALD *Zielbewegungspotentiale* genannt [G 43, 44].

Es gibt also *drei Arten* von langdauernden corticalen Spannungsverschiebungen, die in Abb. 11 dargestellt sind und alle eine *elektronegative* Potentialverschiebung über der Cortexoberfläche zeigen.

A) Die sensorisch ausgelöste „Erwartungswelle" WALTERS (expectancy wave) [W 10], die in Konditionierungsversuchen nach dem Warnreiz in Erwartung des 2. Reizes bilateral auftritt und durch Tastendruck beendet wird (Abb. 11 A). Sie wird jetzt meist „contigent negative variation (CNV)" genannt.

B) *Bereitschaftspotentiale* von KORNHUBER und DEECKE [K 43], die *vor* kurzdauernden Willkürbewegungen beiderseits etwa 1 sec vor der Bewegung beginnen, bei Bewegungsausführung dagegen mit Positivierung enden. Negative und positive Potentialverschiebungen sind jeweils über der kontralateralen rechten Präzentralregion größer als in der linken homolateralen, während parietal und frontal keine oder nur sehr geringe Seitendifferenzen auftreten. Abb. 11 B zeigt das negative Potential vor und das positive nach willkürlichen kurzen Handflexionen mit Rückwärts- und Vorwärtsanalyse vom Zeitpunkt Null (Beginn des Fingerbeugerelektromyogramms).

C) *Zielbewegungspotentiale* von GRÜNEWALD-ZUBERBIER u. Mitarb. [G 43, 44], die *während* kontrollierter Zielbewegungen der rechten Hand auftreten und größer als das Bereitschaftspotential sind sowie oft doppelte Amplituden erreichen (Abb. 11 C). Sie dauern im Gegensatz zu A) und B) mehrere Sekunden an bis das *Ziel* unter visueller Kontrolle erreicht wird (Pfeil nach oben). Auch hier sind die Potentiale präzentral kontralateral zur Bewegungsseite größer als homolateral, doch können parietal auch größere homolaterale Spannungsverschiebungen auftreten.

Gemeinsam ist diesen drei Vorgängen eine *Intention zur Bewegung mit gerichteter Aufmerksamkeitsspannung*. Diese Intention wird bei den Konditionierungsversuchen (A) durch ankündigende Sinnesreize ausgelöst und bei Erscheinen des erwarteten zweiten Reizes beendet, bei den rein willkürlichen kurzen Bewegungen (B) und längeren kontrollierten Zielbewegungen (C) hält die negative Potentialverschiebung über der Hirnrinde so lange an, wie die Bewegungsintention oder die Zielbewegungskontrolle dauert. Unterteilungen dieser Potentiale, die ein kurzdauerndes „Motor potential" vorwiegend über der kontralateralen Präzentralregion unterscheiden [D 10], sind von geringerem Interesse und ihre Deutung zum Teil umstritten.

Diese oberflächennegativen Potentialverschiebungen können Korrelate von Intentionsprozessen bei *Vorbereitung und Kontrolle von Willkürhandlungen* sein.

Die Ähnlichkeit dieser langsamen negativen Hirnpotentiale, die ihr Maximum jeweils über der Scheitelregion haben und präzentral kontralateral zum bewegten Glied etwas größer sind, zeigt Abb. 11 mit drei Beispielen verschiedener Autoren: A Erwartungswelle, B Bereitschaftspotential und C Zielbewegungspotential. Alle diese oberflächennegativen Potentiale über den vorderen Großhirnregionen dauern solange wie die *Bewegungsintention und Zielkontrolle*. Psychologische Korrelate solcher Negativierungen sind daher durch den Willen gesteuerte *Handlungsintentionen*. Dagegen entspricht die *positive* Potentialverschiebung am Ende jeweils der Ausführungsmeldung und *Erledigung der Handlung*, also einer Löschung des Intentionsprozesses, die vielleicht auch durch reafferente Rückmeldung aus der Peripherie unterstützt wird. Solche hirnelektrische Äquivalente von zielgerichteten und zweckvollen Intentionen und ihrer Ausführungskontrolle sind vorläufig nur grobe globale Zeichen simultaner cerebraler Vorgänge, sagen aber noch nichts über spezifische neuronale Korrelationen der Willensprozesse und des programmierten Handlungsentwurfs.

Neurophysiologische Analyse komplexer motorischer Leistungen

Spontanmotorik und Reflexe. Seit MAREY im 19. Jahrhundert den menschlichen Gang mit photographischer Registrierung durch Leuchtpunkte an bestimmten Körperstellen analysierte [M 37a], sind koordinierte Bewegungen zunächst durch Filmaufnahmen registriert worden. Dann folgte die Elektromyographie. Entsprechende kinematographische und elektromyographische Untersuchungen wurden auch für die abnorme Motorik verschiedener Hyperkinesen seit langem durchgeführt. Doch sind die Ergebnisse bisher nur wenig mit neurophysiologischer Fragestellung ausgewertet worden. Die beste Darstellung der Motorik mit Analyse der mechanischen und elektromyographischen Vorgänge ist auch heute noch die Monographie von WACHHOLDER [W 1]. Die neurophysiologische Forschung beschränkte sich zunächst mit SHERRINGTON und HOFFMANN auf die Reflexforschung, deren Ergebnisse mehr für die Neurologie als für die Psychiatrie von Interesse waren. Seitdem die Überwertung der Reflexlehre, die das gesamte Nervensystem nach dem Reflexschema erklären wollte, als Irrtum erkannt ist, wurde auch die Spontanmotorik genauer untersucht. SHERRINGTON selbst kannte die Grenzen des Reflexbegriffs genau. Er nannte den reinen Reflex eine physiologische Fiktion. Reflexe sind nur Teilmechanismen von Regelkreisen.

Telemetrische Bewegungsanalyse beim Menschen. Neue methodische Möglichkeiten der Bewegungsuntersuchung brachte die Telemetrie mit drahtloser Übertragung von freilaufenden Tieren und Menschen. Nachdem telemetrische Ableitungen von Muskel- und Hirnpotentialen zunächst bei Katzen und Affen (Abb. 8) begonnen wurden, haben wir mehrfache Registrierungen von Muskelaktionsströmen für menschliche Sportleistungen zur Untersuchung des motorischen Lernens verwendet [J 57]. Abbildung 12 zeigt Beispiele solcher Untersuchungen beim Kugelstoßen und Werfen, die auch Wechselwirkungen von Seitendominanz und Seitenpräferenz durch Training demonstrieren (vgl. S. 840). Trainingseffekte sind nicht nur eine Kraftsteigerung durch Muskelhypertrophie. Die im Training durch Übung erreichte Geschicklichkeit und Leistungssteigerung beruht vielmehr auf einer *optimalen Bewegungskoordination des ganzen Körpers* mit erlernter zeitlicher Abfolge bestimmter Muskelaktivierungen. Beim rechtsseitigen Stoß und Wurf des Rechtshänders werden *beide* Körperseiten in die Bewegungsordnung einbezogen, nicht nur die seitendominant innervierten Muskeln. Der trainierte Sportler stößt und wirft in einer geregelten Innervationsfolge fast aller Körpermuskeln von Rumpf, Beinen und Armen, die der finalen Extension des stoßenden Armes vorausgeht (Abb. 12 A a, b). Der Untrainierte (Abb. 12 B) stößt und wirft dagegen vorwiegend mit einem Arm. Daher ist der Schub seiner Körpermitbewegung viel geringer als beim Trainierten und die Mitinnervation des kontralateralen Armes fehlt (Abb. 12 D). Auch die *Leistung* steigt entsprechend der optimalen Ordnung der Gesamtinnervation, so daß Stoß- und Wurfweiten bei Hochtrainierten etwa zwei- bis dreifach größer sind als bei Ungeübten [J 57]. Diese Unterschiede sind zum Teil durch die verschiedene Schubkraft der energie-übertragenden Masse zu erklären: Der Trainierte stößt mit der ganzen Körpermasse, der Ungeübte mehr mit dem Arm, der weniger als 5% der Körpermasse ausmacht. Die durch Übung erworbenen Bewegungsprogramme sind für die Leistung und für die *Präzision* der Bewegung entscheidender als angeborene Seitendominanzen beim Rechtshänder. Daher kann auch ein rechtsschreibender Linkshänder mit entsprechender Übung rechts besser schreiben als links.

Motorik, Trieb und Lernen

Wenn man das Zusammenspiel der zahlreichen sensomotorischen Einzelmechanismen verstehen will, so muß man zunächst einige Prinzipien von *Trieb- und Zielhandlungen* kennen, bevor man ihre Beziehungen zu den cerebralen Systemordnungen darstellen kann. Unser Wissen über dieses Gefüge von Hirnstrukturen und Triebmechanismen ist heute noch sehr unvollständig, aber für eine Theorie der Bewegungsphysiologie sind diese biologisch-psychologischen Beziehungen bedeutungsvoll.

Abb. 12. Übungseffekte der Motorik beim Kugelstoßen: Bewegungsabfolge eines hochtrainierten Sportlers (A) und einer ungeübten Frau (B) mit telemetrischen *Elektromyogrammen* (EMG) von beiden Oberarmen beim trainierten Rechtsstoß (C) und untrainierten Linksstoß (D). Nach JUNG und DIETZ (1976) [J 57]

A: Der *Hochtrainierte* stößt die Kugel nach Bewegungsvorbereitung aus einer rückgedrehten Stellung (a), so daß die gesamte Körpermuskulatur mit Rumpf-, Bein- und Armkoordination in geordneter Abfolge aktiviert wird (b). Aus gebeugter Armhaltung erfolgt die terminale Armextension rechts erst in der letzten Abstoßphase (c) mit Beugung des linken Armes. Das lose Gürtelband zeigt die Richtung der Schubkraft des Rumpfes nach vorn und oben. Kugelstoßweite 15 m.

B: Die *untrainierte Frau* stößt die Kugel vorwiegend durch Armextension rechts bei geringer Mitarbeit von Rumpf und kontralateralem Arm. Die Beinarbeit beschränkt sich auf anfängliche Kniebeugung (a) und leichte Streckung links mit Abheben des rückgestellten rechten Beines. Kugelstoßweite 3,7 m.

C u. D: Typische *EMG-Innervationsmuster beider Oberarmmuskeln* beim trainierten Kugelstoß rechts (C) und untrainierten Linksstoß (D). C Die Tricepsaktivierung der finalen Armextension rechts entspricht etwa der kontralateraler Muskeln mit Anbeugung des linken Armes und Bicepsaktivierung. Die Schubkraft entsteht vorwiegend durch Rumpf- und Beinbewegung mit bremsender reziproker Bicepsaktivierung nach Kugelstoß rechts.

D: Der *ungeübte Linksstoß* erfolgt vorwiegend durch Armextension mit Tricepsaktivierung links, und die Mitarbeit der übrigen Armmuskeln und des rechten Armes fehlt im Gegensatz zu C

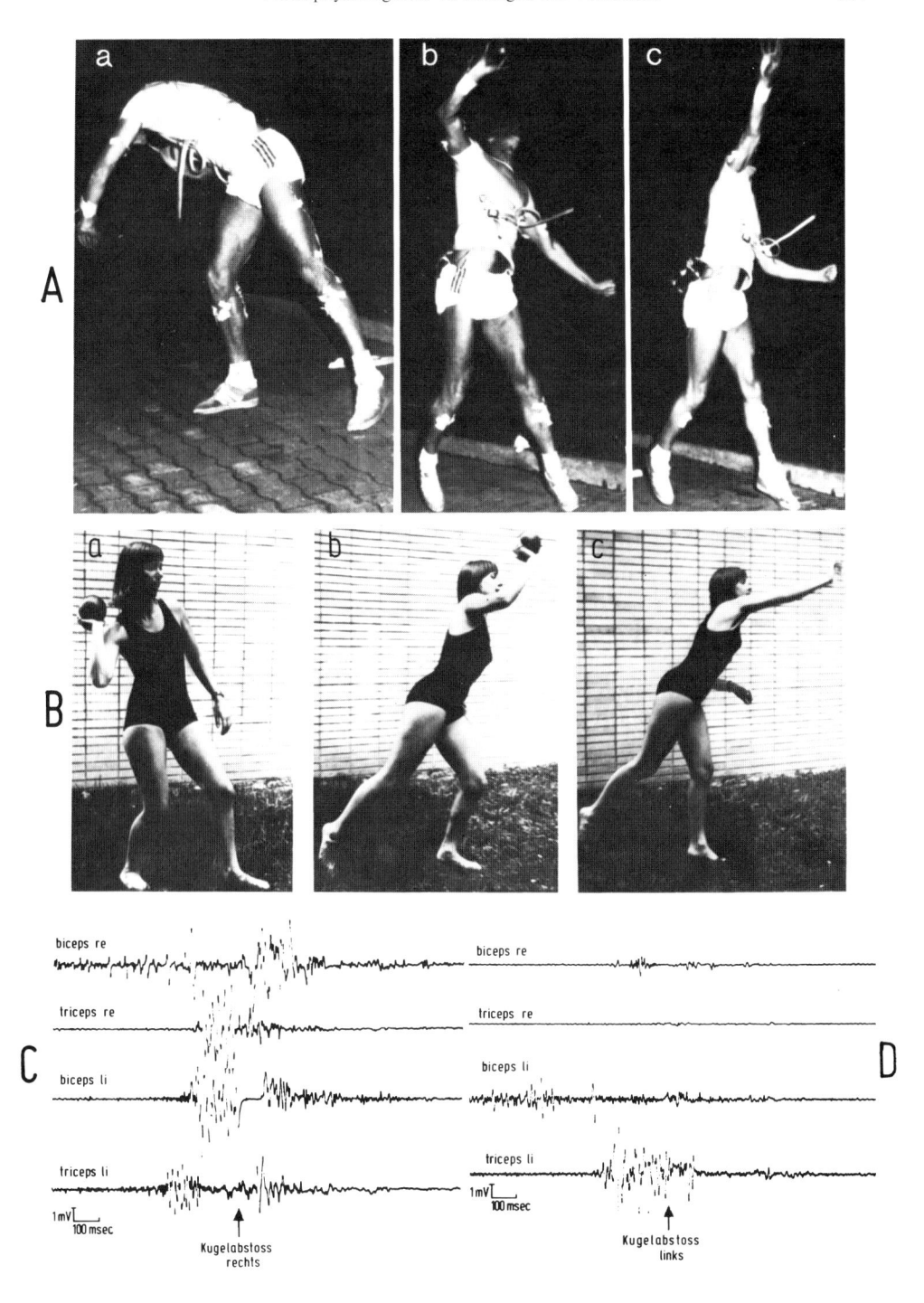

Neurophysiologische Grundlagen des Verhaltens   837

biceps re

triceps re

biceps li

triceps li

1mV
100 msec

↑ Kugelabstoss rechts

biceps re

triceps re

biceps li

triceps li

1mV
100 msec

↑ Kugelabstoss links

Trieb und Willen als Bewegungsmotive. Im Gegensatz zu Reflexen, die nur durch äußere Sinnesreize ausgelöst werden, entstehen biologisch bedeutsame Bewegungen *„spontan"* im Organismus selbst. Triebe, Instinkte und Willensentschlüsse können allgemein als innere *Bewegungsmotivationen* zusammengefaßt werden, die dann auf äußere Ziele gerichtet werden. *Der Trieb sucht und der Wille bestimmt sein Ziel.* Das Zusammenwirken von Instinkten, Trieben und Willensvorgängen wird von psychologischer Seite meist als *Selektion des Willens* aufgefaßt. Die Willenswahl soll bestimmte psychische oder besser psychisch-vitale Kräfte und Triebautomatismen bahnen oder hemmen. Entsprechende selektive Hemmungs- und Bahnungsprozesse sind wahrscheinlich auch als neurophysiologische Mechanismen an höheren Bewegungsleistungen beteiligt, selbst wenn deren Zielsteuerung von Sinneswahrnehmungen abhängig ist.

Willenshandlung als Wahl mit Ziel- und Zeitsetzung. Die in der Willenspsychologie entwickelte Lehre, daß der Wille ein *Wahlvorgang* ist, der aus Trieben und Affektmotivierungen auswählt, bringt für die Physiologie der Willkürbewegung einige Hinweise auf die Selektionsprozesse der Aufmerksamkeit. Zwar ist auch die Willensmotorik auf eine Wahl der strukturell und funktional gegebenen sensomotorischen Mechanismen angewiesen, aber der Wille kann mehr als das: Er hat eine selektive *Zielbestimmung* und eine relativ freie Entscheidung über den *Zeitpunkt der Aktion.*

Der Mensch kann zweifellos eine Zielbewegung „willkürlich" beginnen und ausführen, ohne auf Triebe oder Emotionen angewiesen zu sein. Er kann das *Willensziel setzen und Zeit und Tempo der Aktion selbst bestimmen.* Wenn wir einen Gegenstand ergreifen oder anblicken, so ist zwar eine Sinneswahrnehmung für die Raumlokalisation beteiligt, aber die aktive Aufmerksamkeit kann sowohl die Wahrnehmung wie die Aktion steuern: Die *Aufmerksamkeitshinwendung wählt und sucht bestimmte Ziele* in der Außenwelt und das Verhaltenskorrelat dieser sensorisch-motorischen Auswahlprozesse sind *Orientierung und Zuwendung von Kopf und Augen.* Diese aktive Selektionsfunktion von Aufmerksamkeit und Bewußtsein kann mit dem Bild des Scheinwerfers verstanden werden (Abb. 32). Die neurophysiologischen Grundlagen sind noch umstritten. Nachdem HESS [H 62] und MAGOUN [M 18] eine Steuerung durch subcorticale Mechanismen in Thalamus und Reticularis für die Aktivierung von Bewußtsein, Aufmerksamkeit und Schlaf annahmen und DELL [D 16, 17] Regelungen zwischen Cortex und Hirnstamm mit reziproker Beeinflussung feststellte, ist die Theorie eines zentral regulierenden thalamoreticulären Systems wieder zweifelhaft und durch den Nachweis verschiedener monoaminhaltiger Neuronensysteme im Hirnstamm (Abb. 35) komplizierter geworden. Ein „Willenszentrum", das alle Intentionen von Wahrnehmung und Handlung steuert, hat noch niemand gefunden, und man kann nur vermuten, daß Beziehungen zum cerebralen Substrat der Triebe und Instinkte bestehen.

Sensomotorisches Lernen und Programmierung. Alle motorischen Handlungen bedürfen nicht nur der sensorischen Kontrolle, sondern auch einer *Übung durch Lernen.* Die neurophysiologischen Mechanismen des sensomotorischen Lernens sind noch ebenso unklar wie alle anderen Lernprozesse. Allgemein wird zwar eine Synapsenbahnung als Gedächtnisgrundlage angenommen, aber wie das Erlernte fixiert, über Jahrzehnte konstant gespeichert und im Gedächtnis für komplizierte Erregungs- und Hemmungsmuster verfügbar bleiben kann, ist auch nach modernen chemisch-molekularbiologischen Gedächtnishypothesen unbekannt. Auch die bedingte Reflexforschung hat die Gedächtnismechanismen nicht klären können. Lernen ist vor allem für die menschliche Motorik von großer Bedeutung.

Programmierung der Motorik. Der *sensomotorische Lernprozeß* wird oft mit einer Computerprogrammierung verglichen. Obwohl Neuronenschaltungen anders arbeiten als Rechenmaschinen, kann dieser Vergleich für die Differenzierung des motorischen Lernens in verschiedenen Schichten nützlich sein. Alle sensomotorischen Systeme sind an *programmierten Bewegungen* beteiligt, doch sind die Programmschaltungen unterschiedlich modulierbar. Beim *Reflex* ist die Programmierung starr und auf angeborene Schaltverbindungen beschränkt. Die Auslösung dieser *festen Programmschaltungen* der Reflexe geschieht durch Sinnesafferenzen, die mit dem „Reflexbogen" einen bestimmten Neuronmechanismus in Gang setzen. Die Neuronverbindungen der spinalen Reflexe sind zwar durch Bahnung und Hemmung modulierbar, aber werden durch Lernprozesse kaum beeinflußt. Dagegen sind die *cerebralen* sensomotorischen Strukturen viel plastischer und *durch Übung und Lernen modifizierbar.* Wenn das Pyramidensystem zumindest bei Primaten und beim Menschen durch Direktleitung vom motorischen Cortex mit nur einer Synapse über die Vorderhornzellen Bewegungen startet, einzelne Muskelgruppen „willkürlich" aktiviert und erlernte Bewegungen steuert, so ist dies nicht mit einer starren monosynaptischen Reflexschaltung zu vergleichen: vielmehr geht eine komplizierte *Vorprogrammierung dem pyramidalen Startsignal voraus,* das für die Zielhandlung *erst nach einem Bewegungsentwurf mit Aktivierung der Stützmotorik* über spinale, extrapyramidale und cerebellare Regelungen gegeben wird. Das *extrapyramidale System* steht mit zahlreichen *Automatismen* zwischen der Reflexmotorik und der Willkürmotorik. Daher sind extrapyramidale Störungssymptome nicht Lähmungen, sondern meist abnorme unwillkürliche Bewegungen. Die Zielhandlungen werden durch diese unkontrollierbaren Hyperkinesen behindert. Der Parkinsontremor verlangsamt alle Willkürhandlungen auf Frequenzen unterhalb der Tremorrate. Ein Ausfall automatischer Mitbewegungen entsteht vor allem bei der Parkinsonakinese. In den Bewegungsprogrammen des extrapyramidalen Systems gibt es, wie bei Reflex- und Instinktbewegungen, vorgebildete „fixed patterns", deren Koordinationen durch Sinnesreize ausgelöst und durch Triebe aktiviert oder gehemmt werden. Solche *Triebprogramme* können wiederum in die rasche Startaktion des Pyramidensystems eingreifen. Auch das von *Gedächtnisprogrammen* für Willkürhandlungen aus anderen Rindenfeldern gesteuerte Pyramidensystem führt nicht nur diese Programme aus, sondern *moduliert* sie je nach der aktuellen Situation. Diese *kontrollierten Programmierungen* sind Funktionen des Kleinhirns und seines Kurzzeitgedächtnisses. Zusammen mit peripheren und cerebellaren Regelungen kann sich die Neuronentätigkeit des motorischen Cortex zweckmäßig an die wechselnden Bedingungen der Umwelt anpassen.

Großhirn und Kleinhirn als Lernorgane. PAWLOWS Lehre, daß Lernen und bedingte Reflexe Funktionen der *Großhirnrinde* sind [P7], ist nur cum grano salis richtig. Einfache bedingte Reflexe können noch bei großhirnlosen Tieren erworben werden. Klinische Erfahrungen über Apraxien als Störungen erlernter Handlungsfolgen bei Großhirnbalkenläsionen sprechen zwar ebenfalls für die Rolle des Cortex, aber wie bei allen Bewegungen sind Hirnstamm- und Kleinhirnmechanismen auch beim motorischen Lernen beteiligt. Wahrscheinlich ist neben der Großhirnrinde vor allem das *Kleinhirn* für das motorische Lernen entscheidend. Allerdings ist die cerebellare Funktion bei erlernten Bewegungen bisher nur theoretisch postuliert und durch klinische Erfahrungen gestützt, aber experimentell noch wenig begründet. Vielleicht lassen sich experimentelle Beweise aus den Untersuchungen THACHS [T 3] entwickeln, der den Kleinhirnhemisphären (Neocerebellum) die *Bewegungsprogrammierung*, dem Kleinhirnwurm und dem übrigen Paläocerebellum vorwiegend *Bewegungskontrolle* zuschreibt [T 3]. Erlernte Programme und Kontrollen wären dann am Kleinhirn getrennt zu untersuchen. Beides ist aber offenbar eine gemeinsame Leistung der Großhirn- und Kleinhirnkoordination.

Motorisches Lernen. Obwohl man seit Jahrhunderten weiß, daß Übung und Training Vorbedingungen differenzierter Bewegungsleistungen sind, wurde das Studium des motorischen Lernens bei Menschen bisher sehr vernachlässigt. Alle motorischen Leistungen beim Menschen brauchen erlernte Bewegungsfolgen. Diese sind besonders gut bei Sportleistungen zu untersuchen. Telemetrische Registrierungen der Muskelpotentiale beim Ballwerfen und Kugelstoßen mit Vergleich der dominanten geübten mit der nicht-dominanten ungeübten Seite zeigten einen überwiegenden Einfluß des Trainings auf ein optimales Bewegungsprogramm [J 57]. So wurde auch die Beziehung zur angeborenen Seitendominanz und erlernten Seitenpräferenz beim Werfen und Stoßen des Menschen analysiert. Bei allen menschlichen Bewegungsleistungen sind *Seitendominanz* und *Seitenpräferenz* zu unterscheiden (vgl. S. 893).

Bei differenzierten Bewegungen ist eine *bilaterale Koordination* Bedingung optimaler Leistung: Abb. 12 zeigt Beispiele geübter und ungeübter Versuchspersonen beim Kugelstoßen: A, B trainierte und untrainierte Versuchspersonen, C gute Seitenkoordination beim geübten Kugelstoß rechts, D fehlende Mitarbeit der kontralateralen Seite beim ungeübten Kugelstoß links, obwohl der rechte Arm dominant ist. Die Trainingseffekte betreffen also *beide* Körperseiten unabhängig von der Seitendominanz. Beim Stoß und Wurf des nichttrainierten Armes (links beim Rechtshänder und beidseitig beim total Ungeübten) fehlt die Koordination des kontralateralen Armes, obwohl dieser vorwiegend von der dominanten Großhirnhemisphäre innerviert wird.

Daß nicht angeborene Hemisphärendominanz, sondern beide Körperseiten betreffende Übungen für optimale Leistungen entscheidend sind, ergibt sich aus vier konstanten Ergebnissen dieser Untersuchungen: 1) optimale Stoß- und Wurfweiten mit bilateralen Innervationsmustern bei Trainierten, 2) fehlende Mitarbeit des rechten (dominanten) Armes beim Linksstoß und Linkswurf des rechts Trainierten, 3) minimale Rechts-Links-Differenz bei Untrainierten und 4) die Unabhängigkeit von Seitendominanz und Seitenpräferenz.

Motorisches Lernen verwendet zunächst vorhandene Programmierungen in verschiedenen spinalen und cerebralen Schichten, um dann *neue Programme* zu entwickeln. Primär bewußte und willkürlich gesteuerte Bewegungen werden durch Übung sekundär zu unbewußten *automatisierten Bewegungsfolgen*.

Psychomotorik und Willkürmotorik. Als Psychomotorik im weiteren Sinne pflegt man beim Menschen alle Bewegungserscheinungen zu bezeichnen, die eng mit seelischen Vorgängen verknüpft sind, sowohl unwillkürliche Ausdrucksbewegungen emotionaler Vorgänge wie mehr oder weniger bewußte intentionale Aufmerksamkeits- und Hinwendungsbewegungen. Meistens wird die Beziehung aber auf die *affektive Ausdrucksmotorik und Mimik* beschränkt, die weitgehend unbewußt und *nicht intendiert* abläuft.

Emotionaler Ausdruck in der Motorik. Affektive Psychomotorik haben zweifellos auch *Tiere* bei ihrem Ausdrucksverhalten [D 2]. Solche affektiven Ausdrucksbewegungen können im zentralen Reizversuch leicht ausgelöst werden, wie später im Kapitel der affektiven und Triebmechanismen besprochen wird (vgl. S. 938). Die einzelnen neuronalen Mechanismen der affektiven Psychomotorik sind aber nur unvollständig bekannt. Ausdrucksphänomene des Verhaltens sind bei Tieren von der Ethologie sehr genau beobachtet und experimentell untersucht. Ausdrucksbewegungen spielen auch in der Alltagspsychologie des menschlichen Lebens wie in der psychiatrischen Diagnostik oft eine größere Rolle als sprachliche Äußerungen: Blick, Gesichtsausdruck oder Haltung eines Kranken können für eine psychiatrische Diagnose entscheidend sein. Über die neurophysiologischen Grundlagen dieses charakteristischen Verhaltens des *emotionalen Ausdrucks* wissen wir aber meist nichts. Auch Tiere sind für den Blick von Menschen, Artgenossen oder Feinden besonders empfindlich. In speziellen sozialen Situationen vermeiden Tiere oft einen direkten Blickkontakt, obwohl die Aufmerksamkeit auf den nicht-fixierten Partner gerichtet sein kann.

Intentionale Hinwendungsbewegungen sind bei Tieren bekannt und z.T. experimentell untersucht, sowohl als Reaktionen auf äußere Reize vor bedingten Reflexen (*Orientierungsreflexe* PAWLOWS) wie als cerebral ausgelöste Effekte im zentralen Reizversuch (richtungsspezifische Bewegungen, HESS). Die Verbindung der neuronalen Strukturen mit dem reticulären und extrapyramidalen System, die solche Hinwendungen steuern, wird im Kapitel über Aufmerksamkeit und Bewußtsein besprochen. Bei Tieren gibt es bei den niederen bis zu den höheren Formen eine zunehmend differenzierte Reihe von quasi-reflektorischen Mechanismen, die *Tropismen* oder *Taxien* genannt werden [L 32] und die man noch nicht zur Psychomotorik rechnen kann. Sie steuern Instinkthandlungen und sind vielleicht Vorstufen psychomotorischer Hinwendungsbewegungen. Die *optokinetischen Reaktionen* sind ein Teil des motorischen Verhaltens der Aufmerksamkeitsregulierung. Auch alle *abnormen Adversiv-Effekte* bei epileptischen und torsionsdystonischen Störungen mit gerichteter Wendung von Kopf und Augen, die von den verschiedensten corticalen und subcorticalen Hirnteilen auslösbar sind, können als isolierte Hinwendungsbewegungen aufgefaßt werden. Sie sind häufige Symptome bei Herd- und Anfallskrankheiten des Gehirns und werden teils durch Enthemmung niederer motorischer Zentren, teils durch Gleichgewichtsstörungen symmetrischer Strukturen oder als Reizsymptome mit epileptischen Entladungen ausgelöst.

Die *affektive Ausdrucksmotorik* ist bekanntlich vor allem bei Erkrankungen des extrapyramidalmotorischen Systems gestört: Verminderung beim Parkinsonsyndrom, Verstärkung bei Chorea und Athetose. Neurophysiologisch ist aber über diese Korrelation von *Affekt*, Ausdruck und Stammganglienfunktion wenig bekannt. Wir wissen nur von Einzelneuronableitungen, daß Caudatum und Putamen Afferenzen von verschiedenen Sinnesreceptoren erhalten [A 18].

Rechts- und Linkshändigkeit in der menschlichen Motorik. Alle Menschen haben für differenzierte und geübte Handbewegungen eine eindeutige *Seitendominanz,* die bei 80–90% der Gesunden die *rechte* Seite betrifft. Höhere Affen haben dagegen eine etwa gleiche Verteilung der Rechts- und Linksbevorzugung ihrer Hände. Die Rechtshändigkeit und die bessere Übungsfähigkeit der linken motorischen Rinde entspricht der Sprachdifferenzierung in der linken Großhirnhemisphäre. Bei *Rechtshändern liegen die „Sprachzentren" in der linken frontotemporo-parietalen Großhirnrinde.* Linkshänder haben etwa zur Hälfte ihre Sprachregion in der rechten, zur anderen Hälfte in der linken Großhirnhemisphäre. Wie die linke Hemisphäre für Sprache und Händigkeit spezialisiert und dominant ist, so ist die andere Großhirnhemisphäre, bei Rechtshändern also die rechte, für Funktionen der räumlichen und zeitlichen Orientierung spezialisiert. Man sollte daher nicht allgemein die linke Hemisphäre als „dominant" bezeichnen, sondern nur als *sprachdominant.* Die Hemisphären-Dominanz betrifft vorwiegend *erlernte* Funktionen.

Bei Kindern sind noch Umstellungen der Sprachfunktion auf die rechte Hemisphäre möglich, wenn linksseitige Hirnläsionen auftreten. Bei Erwachsenen sind solche Übernahmen einer Funktion durch die gegenseitige Hemisphäre kaum mehr möglich, weil nach langjähriger Lernerfahrung die Großhirnrinde sich für bestimmte Funktionen der Motorik und Sprache differenziert hat und diese Programmschaltungen lokalisatorisch fixiert sind.

Entsprechend dem spiegelsymmetrischen Bau des menschlichen Körpers sind auch die *Bewegungen links und rechts bevorzugt spiegelbildlich.* Man sieht dies auch beim Gehen, bei den automatischen Mitbewegungen der Arme oder bei beidseitig koordinierten Bewegungen. Linkshänder tendieren daher auch zur Spiegelschrift mit der linken Hand, z. B. Leonardo da Vinci. *Diagonale Schraffierungen beim Zeichnen* werden von Rechtshändern von rechts oben nach links unten (////) ausgeführt, von Linkshändern von links oben nach rechts unten (\\\\). Linkshändige Zeichner sind an diesen Schraffierungen zu erkennen. Diese Strichlagentendenz kann nur durch Umwendung der Handhaltung und Schraffieren von oben umgekehrt werden. Die Seitenbetonung des Beines ist weniger konstant als bei der Arm- und Sprachfunktion. Auch wenn der Linkshänder gelernt hat, rechts zu schreiben, benutzt er die linke Hand für differenzierte und mit Kraft koordinierte Bewegungen, z. B. beim Werfen eines Steines.

Sprechen und erlernte Fertigkeiten. Eine spezifisch menschliche Form der Willkürbewegung ist die *Sprache.* Sprechen wird *erlernt* und durch Nachahmung erworben. Welche Sprache erlernt wird, ist zunächst nur von der Sprachumwelt der ersten Lebensjahre abhängig. Individuelle und Rassencharakteristika spielen eine geringe Rolle: ein europäisches Neugeborenes, in einer chinesischen Familie aufgezogen, wird nur chinesisch sprechen, ein Chinesenbaby, in einer deutschen Familie aufgenommen, wird dagegen deutsch lernen.

Die Mechanismen des Sprechens, die zum zum Teil bekannt sind, werden kurz im Teil VII besprochen. Sprechen ist eine sensomotorische Fertigkeit, die dauernde Übung braucht. Trotz Beteiligung vieler cerebraler Strukturen am Sprechvorgang ist die *Lokalisation der „Sprachzentren"* in der „dominanten" frontotemporo-parietalen Großhirnrinde erstaunlich eng umschrieben. Diese corticale Lokalisation betrifft aber nur höhere Funktionen des Sprachverständnisses und des Sprechentwurfes. Sonst sind am motorischen Sprechakt auch

Stammganglien, Kleinhirn und Oblongata beteiligt. Die Kehlkopf-, Mund- und Zungenmuskeln bilden körpereigene „Werkzeuge" der Sprache. Dementsprechend sind im *sensomotorischen Cortex* auch *Lippe, Zunge und Kehlkopf* als Sprechorgane und die *Hände* als Organ anderer erlernter Fertigkeiten besonders ausgedehnt vertreten (s. PENFIELDS Schemata [P 17]).

Erlernte Fertigkeiten, englisch „skill", werden durch Übung erworben und sind beim Menschen meist mit *Werkzeuggebrauch* verbunden. Zwar sind an Fertigkeitsbewegungen verschiedene Hirnregionen und spinale Neuronensysteme beteiligt, doch bilden im menschlichen Gehirn Großhirnrinde und Kleinhirn die führenden Substrate dieser erlernten Feinbewegungen. Das Kleinhirn arbeitet bei motorischen Lernvorgängen und ihrer sensomotorischen Kontrolle eng mit der Großhirnrinde zusammen [E 5a, 6].

Cerebrale Systeme der Motorik

Das klassische Konzept der cerebralen Motorik bezeichnet die *motorische Hirnrinde* und Pyramidenbahn als System der Willkürmotorik, die extrapyramidalen *Stammganglien* als automatisches Kontrollsystem für Muskeltonus und Triebbewegungen und das *Kleinhirn* als sensorisch geregeltes Rückmeldesystem. Das sind schematische Vereinfachungen, aber sie enthalten einen richtigen Kern. Zwar arbeiten die drei Systeme immer koordiniert zusammen, doch bestehen *System-Präferenzen* für bestimmte Bewegungsarten. Die vorwiegend pyramidale Steuerung der Hand- und Fingerbewegungen ist bei Affe und Mensch gesichert, die Startfunktion für automatisch geregelte Laufbewegungen gut begründet. Die extrapyramidale und cerebellare Kontrolle des Muskeltonus wurde beim Menschen durch stereotaktische Eingriffe quasi-experimentell nachgewiesen. Nachdem die Arbeitsweise des Kleinhirns durch Hemmungsfunktion der Purkinje-Zellen von ECCLES u. Mitarb. [E 6a] geklärt wurde, ist die cerebellare Koordination mit den extrapyramidalen Kernen und dem motorischen Cortex untersucht worden [J 4]. Damit wurden die Kontrollfunktionen des Großhirns, Hirnstamms und Kleinhirns aufgeklärt. Doch bleibt eine neuronale Systemtheorie der Bewegungssteuerung und Bewegungskontrolle noch eine Aufgabe der Zukunft.

Bewegung, Verhalten und Neuronentätigkeit. Wenn man von den Einzelelementen ausgeht, kann man zwar die Funktion des ganzen Nervensystems noch nicht erfassen, aber wie einzelne Individuen und bestimmte Eigenschaften einzelner Menschen auch für das Verhalten von Massen bedeutsam sind, so muß man für das Verständnis neurophysiologischer Gesetzmäßigkeiten die Neuronenphysiologie kennen. Sie muß in allen den Schichten des ZNS untersucht werden, die für diese Leistung repräsentativ sind.

Die Bedeutung eines einzelnen Neurons für die gesamte Hirnfunktion wird mit einem schon von ADRIAN gebrauchten Bild verständlich: Bei demokratischen Abstimmungen kann zwar der einzelne Wähler mit nur einer Stimme den Wahlausgang nicht bestimmen; dennoch trägt auch diese Einzelstimme zum Gesamtergebnis bei und allgemeine Gesetze und Motivationen, die für den einzelnen gelten, beeinflussen auch den Wahlausgang von Millionen von Stimmen.

Mikrophysiologie corticaler Nervenzellen. Die *Funktionsgesetze der Nervenzellen* sind seit 1951 durch Mikroelektrodenforschung elektrophysiologisch geklärt worden, nachdem ECCLES die synaptischen und Membranvorgänge an der einzelnen Nervenzelle registrieren konnte. Diese *intracellulären Ableitungen* von spinalen Motoneuronen durch ECCLES [E 2, 5] und seine Schule brachten den entscheidenden Beweis für die Gültigkeit der Neuronenlehre, der Membrantheorie, der synaptischen Erregung und Hemmung an der Nervenzelle, des Alles-oder-Nichts-Gesetzes und der fortgeleiteten Entladung.

Die *Mikrophysiologie des Gehirns* begnügte sich zunächst mit *extra*cellulären Ableitungen im Tierversuch [J 34, M 70]. Die Neurone der Sehrinde [J 39, 52] der Substantia reticularis [M 62, 63], des Thalamus [M 71, 76] und der motorischen Hirnrinde [P 21, E 23–27] wurden systematisch untersucht. An allen diesen Strukturen zeigte sich eine unerwartet große Konvergenz von verschiedenen Afferenzen. 1956 ist es PHILLIPS [P 21] gelungen, auch von Riesenpyramidenzellen des Cortex *intra*celluläre Ableitungen zu erhalten. EVARTS hat seit 1966 Neuronableitungen im motorischen Cortex beim wachen Affen mit erlernten und quasi-willkürlich gesteuerten Bewegungen durchgeführt [E 24–27]. Abb. 13 zeigt Beispiele solcher Registrierungen bei erlernten und freien Bewegungen von zur Pyramidenbahn projizierenden Zellen des Motorcortex.

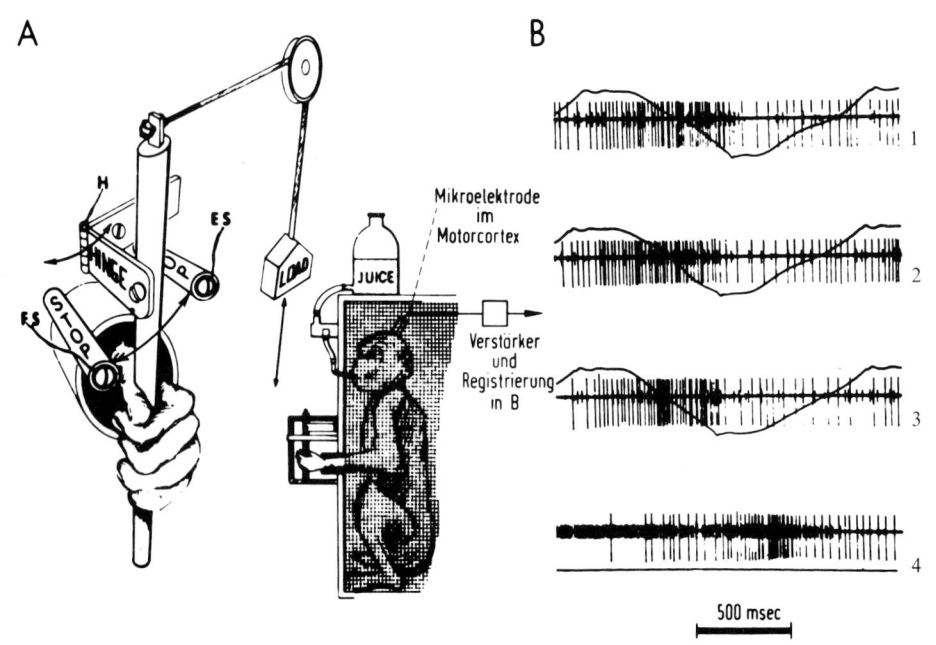

Abb. 13. EVARTS Versuchsmethodik zur Registrierung corticaler Pyramidenzellentladungen bei willkürlich gesteuerten Bewegungen wacher Affen. Nach EVARTS (1967) [E 24].
A: Der im Käfig sitzende Rhesusaffe greift einen außerhalb angebrachten Stab, der mit der Hand hin- und herbewegt wird und durch Gewichte (load) verschieden belastet werden kann. Die Stabbewegungen nach links und rechts sollen gegen einen federnden Widerstand mit bestimmtem Intervall und Geschwindigkeit zwischen zwei Anschlägen (↔) (stop) erfolgen. Bei richtiger Zeitdauer wird der Affe durch Orangensaft (juice) belohnt.
B: Pyramidenzellentladungen im kontralateralen motorischen Cortex werden über eine implantierte Mikroelektrode mit den mechanischen Stabbewegungen registriert. In den oberen drei Reihen 1–3 Aktivierung eines kleinen und großen Pyramidenneurons bei Stabbewegung nach links (Kurve nach unten) und verminderte Entladung bei Rechtsbewegung. In der untersten Ableitung 4 erfolgt eine *freie Schulter-Armbewegung* ohne Stab mit verschiedener Koordination beider Neurone: Das kleine Neuron wird zuerst stark, das große erst später und geringer aktiviert, im Gegensatz zu der gemeinsamen Entladung bei der gesteuerten Willkürbewegung 1–3

Das Kleinhirn als sensomotorische Rechenmaschine. Cerebellare Regulationen der Motorik sind zwar seit langem durch Ausschaltungsversuche und neurologische Studien der Kleinhirnataxie untersucht worden, doch wurden die neuronalen Einzelmechanismen und ihre Programmschaltungen erst im letzten Jahrzehnt geklärt. Die komplizierten, aber anatomisch exakt definierten Neuronenschaltungen sind in der ganzen Kleinhirnrinde prinzipiell gleichartig und haben im Gegensatz zur Großhirnrinde keine spezifischen Feldunterschiede. Die Funktion des Kleinhirns wurde daher von ECCLES als Computerschaltung bezeichnet. Vorher waren von SNIDER u. Mitarb. die Projektionen verschiedener Sinnessysteme und verschiedener Großhirnregionen [S 35a] und von MORUZZI die paläocerebellaren Hemmungssysteme [M 61a] geklärt worden. HASSLER [J 58] hat die Koordination des Kleinhirns mit Hirnstamm und Großhirn in Rückmeldungskreisen dargestellt, die auch das pyramidale System und die Ponskerne einschließen. Alte Vorstellungen von rein proprioceptiven und vestibulären Kleinhirnafferenzen entsprechend SHERRINGTONS Bezeichnung des Kleinhirns als „Kopfganglion der Proprioceptivität", waren schon durch SNIDER angezweifelt worden, als er optische und akustische Projektionen im Kleinhirn feststellte [S 35a]. Alle Efferenzen der Kleinhirnrinde laufen über Purkinje-Neurone, die nur *Hemmungssynapsen* haben.

Die *Hemmungsfunktionen des Kleinhirns* für die Bewegungsmodulation wurden von ECCLES mit der Tätigkeit eines *Bildhauers* verglichen, der aus einem groben Steinblock die Feinheiten der Form durch *Wegnehmen* herausarbeitet [E 5a]. Das Kleinhirn reguliert mit den Hemmungsimpulsen der Purkinje-Axone durch Weghemmung überschüssiger grober Innervationen die Feinheit unserer Bewegungen. Wie ein Bildhauer die Oberfläche einer Skulptur modelliert, so moduliert die cerebellare Hemmungsefferenz je nach der aktuellen Konstellation die pyramidalen und exrapyramidalen Impulsströme mit dem Ergebnis einer glatten angepaßten Bewegungsfolge. Durch erlernte sensomotorische Schaltungen des Kleinhirns können eingeübte Handlungsfolgen bereits *vorprogrammiert* werden. Nach THACHS [T 3] letzten Untersuchungen regelt das phylogenetisch ältere Paläocerebellum die Motorik vorwiegend *während* der Bewegung, dagegen liefert das mit der Großhirnrinde verschaltete Neocerebellum schon Programmierungen *vor* der Bewegung.

Wahrnehmung und Handlung

Beim Verhalten von Tier und Mensch sind *Wahrnehmen und Handeln eng verbunden*. Auch subjektiv erleben wir Sinneseindrücke und Aktion als *einheitlich*. Bei diesen Wechselwirkungen von Sinnesafferenz und Motorik kann jeweils ein passives Wahrnehmungs- oder ein aktives Handlungserlebnis subjektiv im Vordergrund stehen. Das erste erkennt man am besten beim Sehen mit Blickbewegungen: Die aktive Hinwendung mit Blickzielbewegung und Fixation geht der Detailwahrnehmung voraus, ohne daß wir uns einer motorischen Aktion bewußt sind. Umgekehrt erleben wir eine Greifbewegung als aktive Handlung, ohne die visuellen Vorbereitungen und die kontinuierlichen sensorischen Kontrollen zu beachten. Ein Schema der physiologischen und psychischen Vorgänge bei der aufmerksamkeitsgesteuerten Willenshandlung gibt Abb. 14 C. Sinnesmeldungen regeln und steuern alle Willkürbewegungen. Die afferenten Meldungen aus verschiedenen Sinnesorganen sind neurophysiologisch sehr gut untersucht (vgl. Kapitel VIII). Die Informationsverarbeitung der Wahrnehmung von den

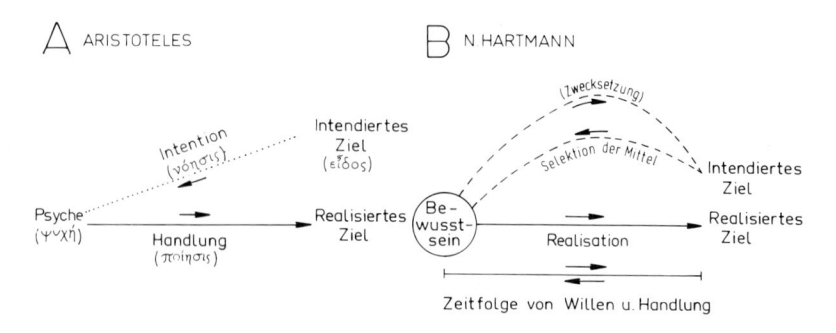

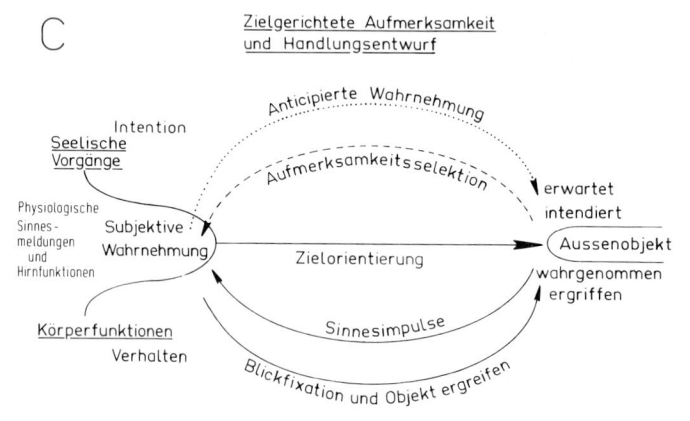

Abb. 14. Konzepte willensgesteuerter Zielhandlungen seit ARISTOTELES. A, B: Psychische Abläufe mit Antizipation und Rückwirkung der Zielintention nach NICOLAI HARTMANN (1951) [H 14]. *C:* Psychische und physiologische Korrelate einer programmierten Zielhandlung. (Eigenes Schema.). A: ARISTOTELES beschrieb die Willensantizipation (noesis) für eine Zielvorstellung (eidos). Das intendierte Zielbild der zweckgesteuerten Aktion bewirkt rückläufig die Vorbereitung der Handlung (poiesis), die dann das Ziel realisieren kann.

B: HARTMANN differenzierte das aristotelische Konzept in 2 Stufen: 1. finale Zwecksetzung mit Wechselwirkung von Wille und Vorstellung unter zeitlicher Vorwegnahme des angestrebten Zieles und 2. intendierte Mittelwahl. Beide gehen der realisierten Handlung *voraus* und die intentionale Zielvorstellung antizipiert entgegen dem Zeitfluß die spätere Handlung. Die Zeitfolge von Willen und Handlung verläuft daher scheinbar umgekehrt (Pfeile ⇄).

C: *Aufmerksamkeitsrichtung und Bewegungsentwurf* einer Zielhandlung ist oben für psychische und unten für somatische Funktionen dargestellt, links mit dem planenden Organismus, rechts mit dem intendierten Außenobjekt. Oben erscheint deutlicher als in HARTMANNs Schema B auch die Antizipation der Wahrnehmung mit Erwartungshaltung und psychischem Regelkreis durch Auswahlfunktion der Aufmerksamkeit

Receptoren bis zu den corticalen Sinnesfeldern ist im Tierexperiment und auch nach evozierten Potentialen beim Menschen objektiv erfaßbar. Weniger weiß man über die intentionale und motorische Seite der Trieb- und Willkürbewegungen. Seit MAREY [M 22a, b] beim Menschen die Bewegungsbilder beim Laufen und Springen registrierte und seit man im letzten Jahrzehnt auch die Muskelkoordinationen beim Laufen, Werfen und Stoßen telemetrisch erfassen konnte, wurden die Innervationsmuster einer Analyse zugänglich. Die cerebralen Korrelate der Willkürhandlung sind ebenfalls durch hirnelektrische Studien über Bereitschafts- und Zielbewegungspotentiale des Menschen registrierbar geworden (Abb. 11). Beim Menschen beschränken sich diese Ableitungen noch auf Massenpotentiale ohne neuronale Registrierungen. Bei Affen wurden auch Einzelneuronableitungen aus der motorischen Hirnrinde von quasi-willkürlichen erlernten Bewegungen registriert und mit Muskelpotentialen korreliert. Abb. 13 zeigt ein Beispiel von EVARTS' Affen-Experimenten mit Registrierung von Pyramidenneuronen des motorischen Cortex bei optisch und sensorisch gesteuerten Handbewegungen.

Zielintention, Antizipation und Willensentschluß. Schon im Altertum hat ARISTOTELES in seiner Metaphysik eine Korrelation von gedanklicher Voraussicht und intendiertem Bewegungsziel postuliert. Er nannte diese planende Antizipation *noesis,* das bildmäßig vorgestellte und intendierte Ziel *eidos* und die Zielbewegung selbst *kinesis.* NICOLAI HARTMANN hat 1951 [H 14] diese alte aristotelische Konzeption schematisch dargestellt (Abb. 14 A) und durch ein eigenes zweites Schema (Abb. 14 B) ergänzt. Diese Bilder sollten die Zweckbestimmung des Willensvorgangs, die zeitliche Vorwegnahme des Zieles in der Vorstellung und die Freiheit der Anschauungszeit mit der Zukunftsplanung erläutern. *Die bewußte Vorstellung nimmt vor dem Willensakt und der Handlung das angestrebte Ziel zeitlich vorweg.* Diese *Antizipation des Willens* verläuft in scheinbarer Paradoxie des umgekehrten Zeitablaufs der Handlung. Solche anschaulichen Schemata vereinfachen zwar die komplexen psychischen und physiologischen Vorgänge, können aber für die Analyse der Intentionsprozesse und ihrer hirnelektrischen Korrelate bei zielgerichteten Bewegungen nützlich sein. Die physiologischen und psychologischen Korrelate gezielter Handlungen in der Umwelt sind sehr viel komplizierter, aber im Prinzip einer Analyse zugänglich. Abb. 14 C zeigt oben die Bedingungen der zielgerichteten Aufmerksamkeit und des Handlungsentwurfs im intentional-psychischen Bereich und unten die somatischen Mechanismen der Wahrnehmung und Handlung mit Verhaltenskorrelationen. Oben ist in C wie bei ARISTOTELES und HARTMANN die gezielte *Intention,* die in der Vorstellung zukünftige Wahrnehmungen erwartet und das Ziel planend vorwegnimmt, durch Doppelpfeile symbolisiert. Die vorbereitende Aufmerksamkeit hat wie HARTMANNs Mittelwahl linksgerichtete Pfeile. Die Ausführung und ihre im realen Zeitfluß ablaufenden Mechanismen haben rechtsgerichtete Pfeile. Im unteren Teil bringen die Sinnesmeldungen eine afferente Regelung für efferente Blickfixation und Objektergreifen und bilden so einen somatischen Regelkreis. Beide, psychische Vorgänge der Innenwelt und physiologische Körperfunktionen brauchen ein *Umweltmodell* und Reafferenz (vgl. S. 859). In Wechselwirkung von Innen- und Außenwelt führen Modellprogramme, steuernde Intentionen und regelnde Sinnesmeldungen zur gezielten Wahrnehmung und Handlung. Beim Sehen ist gezielte *Aufmerksamkeit mit Blickbewegungen verbunden* und optisch-vestibulär reguliert (vgl. das physiologische Schema der cerebralen Blickmotorik Abb. 9). Die Sehwahrnehmung wird jeweils mit den Blickbewegungen koordiniert. Dies ist beim Bewegungssehen und optokinetischen Nystagmus besonders deutlich und quantitativ untersucht [D 30, 31]. Die Reafferenz stammt beim Sehen aus der Retina, bei Zielbewegungen vorwiegend aus Muskel- und Gelenk-Proprioceptoren und Hautafferenzen, die unsere Gliedbewegungen steuern. Doch bedeuten diese reafferenten Meldungen *während* der Bewegung mit ihren „feed-back"-Regelungen durch die in C unten links gerichteten Pfeile nicht eine zeitliche Antizipation wie bei der „noesis" des ARISTOTELES und der Mittelwahl bei HARTMANN (Abb. 14A, B), sondern nur kontinuierliche Rückmeldungen, die positiv oder negativ sein können und damit die Bewegung *bahnen, hemmen* und *zielsteuern.* Der Willensbildung ähnliche *Vorwegnahmen eines Zieles* mit mehr oder weniger bewußter oder bildhafter Vorstellung haben jedoch die *Affekte und Triebe,* die auch bei Tieren das Verhalten motivieren und daher physiologische Mechanismen haben müssen. Solche emotionalen Motivationsprozesse überlagern sich auch mit den bewußten Zielhandlungen. Motivation und Aufmerksamkeit verstärken die Bereitschafts- und Erwartungspotentiale [K 43, W 10] als hirnelektrische Korrelate der Intention (vgl. S. 834, Abb. 11 und 43).

Wille ist Wahl zwischen verschiedenen Antrieben und Handlungsmustern. Die Willkürhandlung überformt mit Ziel- und Zeitsetzung das Instinkt- und Lernverhalten in einer höheren Schicht, ist aber in der Durchführung auf Mechanismen und Regelungen der „niederen" Motorik angewiesen. Triebverhalten und Willkürmotorik entstehen aus ähnlichen Bewegungsmotivationen. Ihre Bewegungsprogramme sind durch Lernen und Sinnesmeldungen modulierbar.

Intention, Zweckhandlung und Umweltmodell. Die inneren Vorgänge der gezielten Willkürhandlung sind zunächst nur philosophisch und psychologisch genauer analysiert worden. Das Erstreben vorgestellter Ziele, das Vorausdenken eines noch unwirklichen Zweckes und die Freiheit der Anschauungszeit wurden von ARISTOTELES bis NICOLAI HARTMANN [H 14] klar formuliert. Dazu kamen in den letzten 50 Jahren auch biologische und kybernetische Konzepte innerer Modellbildung, die das philosophisch schon über 2000 Jahre alte Problem der Ziel- und Willenshandlung einer physiologischen Betrachtung näherbringen.

Seit UEXKÜLL in der Biologie [U 1] und CRAIK in der Biokybernetik [C 13] wurde die Wechselwirkung von Organismus und Umwelt durch ein *Umweltmodell* erklärt. Philosophen und Psychologen hatten sich meist auf die bewußtseinsimmanenten Vorgänge der Willensbildung und des Entschlusses „in mente" beschränkt. Neue Gesichtspunkte brachten moderne kybernetische Konstruktionen, die mit der Programmierung von Rechenmaschinen und Regelkreisen technische Modelle entwickelten (vgl. S. 853). Eine anschauliche Darstellung alter und neuer Lösungsversuche der Willensintention und der Zweck- und Zielhandlung seit ARISTOTELES gibt Abb. 14 A–C. Das dritte Schema C ist nur ein vorläufiger Versuch, die Korrelationen der psychischen Intention und der somatischen Funktionen mit neurophysiologischen Mechanismen sensomotorischer Regelkreise anschaulich zu machen. Die langsamen Hirnpotentiale bei Vorbereitung und Kontrolle von Willenshandlungen bringen Hinweise auf cerebrale Korrelationen der Bereitschaft, Intention und Ausführung von Zielhandlungen.

Mensch, Organismus und Maschine

Ein Maschinenvergleich. Ordnung und Abfolge der Bewegungsmechanismen können durch einen bildhaften Vergleich veranschaulicht werden [J 57]. Wenn man die Koordination der Motorik mit einem *Automobil* und seiner Steuerung und Schaltung durch den Fahrer vergleicht, wird auch das Schichtverhältnis der höheren (übergeordnet corticalen) Intentionen und der niederen (untergeordnet automatischen) Mechanismen der Bewegung klarer. Beim Auto ist ein *Fahrer* für die Zielbewegung notwendig. Aktionen und Sinnesmeldungen des Autofahrers können höhere intentionale Komponenten der Willkürhandlung und ihre Abhängigkeit von der Wahrnehmung anschaulicher darstellen als eine Computerautomatik, obwohl beide nach ähnlichen Prinzipien arbeiten. In einer mechanisch-elektronisch zielgesteuerten Flugzeug- oder Raumfahrtautomatik ist zwar der gesamte Ablauf der Motorik mathematisch erfaßbar, aber weniger anschaulich.

Die Erfahrung zeigt, daß auch bei solchen vollautomatisch gesteuerten Fahrzeugen nur einprogrammierte Kontrollen gut funktionieren, daß aber bei neuen, unvorhergesehenen Ereignissen die menschliche Pilotenentscheidung notwendig ist, während sie bei Eingreifen in automatisierte Mechanismen durch Fehlmeldungen überforderter Sinnesorgane (z. B. Otolithen bei großer Flugbeschleunigung) eher stört. Das gilt auch fürs Autofahren.

Dem Start jeder Bewegung muß eine *Vorbereitung und Bereitschaftsaktivierung* vorangehen, wie beim Auto der Motor eine gewisse Umdrehungsgeschwindigkeit noch im ausgekuppelten Zustand haben muß, bevor der Wagen abfahren kann. Die mechanische *Bewegungsbereitschaft* wäre daher zu vergleichen mit dem Anlassen und der Vorbeschleunigung des Motors. Die Gangschaltung und Richtungsorientierung mit dem ersten Ausrichten der Steuerung bedarf der übergeordneten Fahrerinitiative, die der Intention und Vorprogrammierung einer Zielbewegung entspricht. Nur nach programmierter Zielbestimmung kann die Einzelausführung der Willkürbewegung den niederen sensomotorischen Mechanismen überlassen werden. Erst *nach* dieser Ziel- und Bereitschaftsvorbereitung erfolgt der eigentliche *Bewegungsstart* durch die Kupplung von Motor und Getriebe. Dieses *Einkuppeln* ist daher dem *Willkürstart* über die Pyramidenbahn vergleichbar.

Die Fahrleistungen des Autos sind von *zwei Kontrollfunktionen* abhängig, die beide geregelt sind, während nur die zweite zielgesteuert ist. Die *erste* ist die *mechanische Konstruktion* und ihre Automatik, die bei der menschlichen Bewegung den vorgebildeten Strukturmechanismen des sensomotorischen Bewegungsapparats und ihrer Koordination und inneren Kontrolle entsprechen. Die *zweite* ist die Fahrtsteuerung nach einem *Zielprogramm*, das an die jeweiligen Außenbedingungen angepaßt wird. Nur diese äußere Zielsteuerung wird durch den Fahrer verwirklicht, der sich aber für die inneren Regelungen auf zahlreiche eingebaute Automatismen der mechanisch-energetischen Prozesse verläßt. Die Kontrollen der Fahrleistung enthalten also *übergeordnete Steuerungen des Fahrers* und *untergeordnete Regelungen des Apparats*. Für die Zielprogrammsteuerung werden die *Sinnesorgane des Fahrers,* besonders die Augen benötigt, die auch die Ausführung laufend kontrollieren, während die innere Kontrolle der Benzinzufuhr, der Kühlung, des Differentials usw. automatisch abläuft. Die äußere Steuerung ist im lebenden Organismus vorwiegend von exteroceptiven Sinnen kontrolliert, während die innere Kontrolle mehr den proprioceptiven Regelungen der Motorik vergleichbar ist.

Fahrer und Maschine. Die *Willkürhandlung* ist nur in ihrer Vorbereitung und Zielsteuerung einer Fahrerleistung vergleichbar, aber in der *Ausführung* großenteils *automatisch* von der niederen Sensomotorik kontrolliert wie die Maschine. Auch *Triebhandlungen,* soweit sie zielgesteuert sind, bedürfen eines Fahrerprogramms, selbst wenn sie angeborene Instinktbewegungen sind, die von einem Schlüsselreiz ausgelöst, scheinbar automatisch ablaufen. Die Grenze zwischen Fahrerleistung und Apparatkontrolle liegt für die Willkür- und Triebhandlung auf verschiedenem Niveau, wie auch das Auto unterschiedliche Automatik haben kann. Die Triebbewegung verwendet weitgehend automatisierte Mechanismen. Die mit präziser Augenkontrolle durchgeführte Willkürbewegung entspricht mehr einem Fahren mit Kupplung ohne Gangschaltungsautomatik, kann aber durch Lernen in einen mehr automatisierten Ablauf übergeführt werden. Der Fahrer des Autos entscheidet in bestimmten Situationen über das Einschalten der *Bremse.* Deren Bedienung wird bei überraschenden Ereignissen allein von Sinnesmeldungen ausgelöst, aber ist sonst beim Halten am Ziel auch programmiert.

Der *Fahrer,* der über Betätigung von Kupplung, Gaspedal oder Bremse entscheidet, kann mit dem motorcortex und *höheren corticalen Strukturen* verglichen werden. Hier werden Willkürbewegungen geplant und mit dem cerebralen sensomotorischen Apparat programmiert. Vom Cortex und seinen multisensorischen Informationen wird auch die Zielsteuerung überwacht und der Bewegungsentwurf moduliert. Der *motorische Cortex* leitet mit der Pyramidenbahn den Bewegungsbefehl zu den Motoneuronen: Erstens startet er die Bewegung durch Einschalten der *„Kupplung".* Zweitens bestimmt er *Kraft* und *Geschwindigkeit* schon durch eine vorprogrammierte Impulsrate der intendierten Bewegung, wie der Autofahrer durch „Gasgeben". *Drittens regelt er* diese Impulsgebung in Agonisten und Antagonisten der spinalen Motoneurone je nach den erwarteten oder angetroffenen peripheren Widerständen, ähnlich wie der Fahrer beim Bergfahren nicht nur die Gasgebung sondern auch die Gangschaltung der Steigung der Straße anpaßt.

Arbeitsteilung und Zusammenspiel der linken und rechten Großhirnhemisphäre und beider Pyramidenbahnen für doppelseitige Bewegungen und Sprache sind mit diesem Bild nur unvollkommen zu erfassen, wohl aber die beidseitige Bewegungsbereitschaft und die Hemmungs- und Ausgleichsfunktionen verschiedener Schichten mit inneren Kontrollen. Wenn ein Auto aus einer Parklücke herausgefahren werden soll, so muß das Lenkrad *vorher* in der Bewegungsrichtung eingestellt und die Kupplung bei laufendem Motor bedient werden. Ähnlich muß vor einer Zielbewegung die Stützmotorik aktiviert und die richtige *Ausgangsposition* hergestellt werden, d.h. der Bewegungsentwurf und sein cerebrales Korrelat der Bereitschaftspotentiale werden in beiden Großhirnhälften vorbereitet.

Wie alle Vergleiche hinken, so hat auch diese Maschinenmetapher für die Motorik ihre Grenzen. Doch illustriert das Bild neben der Cortex- und Pyramidentätigkeit mit der Kupplungsfunktion der Willkürmotorik auch die Notwendigkeit einer Bewegungsvorbereitung durch höhere Steuerungen und der fortlaufenden Regelung durch untergeordnete Mechanismen.

Grenzen der Bewegungsphysiologie beim Menschen. Obwohl die Neuronentladungen einzelner motorischer Einheiten seit ADRIAN und BRONK [A 8a] schon über 50 Jahre beim Menschen objektiv erfaßbar sind, können die Hirnvorgänge unserer motorischen Systeme noch nicht direkt registriert werden. *Unser Wissen über cerebrale Mechanismen der menschlichen Bewegung wurde nur durch Analogieschlüsse aus neuronalen Befunden des Tierversuchs gewonnen.* Daher sind wir noch weit davon entfernt, die motorischen Leistungen des Menschen neuronal zu erklären. Diese Einschränkung gilt nicht nur für komplexe und präzise Handlungsfolgen in Handwerk, Sport, Spiel und Musik, sondern auch für einfache Bewegungskoordinationen. Wir beginnen erst jetzt die Reihenfolge der Muskelinnervationen und das Zusammenwirken der Ziel- und Stützmotorik beim Greifen, Werfen, Laufen und Springen telemetrisch zu registrieren (Abb. 12 C, D). Vorläufig ist für die Erfassung integrierter Bewegungsmuster die Verhaltensanalyse unentbehrlich.

Zusammenfassung

Neurophysiologische Grundlagen des Verhaltens sind sensomotorische Mechanismen. Im Bewegungsentwurf der Ziel- und Willkürbewegung sind psychische Intentionen und neurobiologische Triebvorgänge eng verbunden.

Ziel- und Stützmotorik sind koordiniert und werden im Bewegungsentwurf vorprogrammiert: das cerebral vorbereitete *Bewegungsprogramm* muß *vor* der Zielbewegung eine stützende Ausgangsposition herstellen. Elektrophysiologische

Korrelate des Bewegungsentwurfs im Großhirn sind KORNHUBERS *Bereitschaftspotentiale vor Willküraktionen*. Korrelate gezielter Bewegungskontrolle sind die *Zielbewegungspotentiale während der Aktion*. Beide sind cerebrale Korrelate der *Bewegungsintention*. Die Bewegungskontrolle arbeitet mit peripheren Regelungen und zentralen Steuerungs- und Rückmeldungskreisen, die Rückenmark, Großhirn, Kleinhirn und Stammganglien beteiligen. Der Motorcortex startet und steuert beim Menschen und höheren Primaten über die Pyramidenbahn die Willkürbewegungen, die dann durch periphere Rückmeldungen an veränderte Außenveränderungen angepaßt werden. Die *Willkürhandlung* steuert bereitliegende cerebrospinale Programmschaltungen. *Wille ist Wahl* zwischen verschiedenen Antrieben und Handlungsmustern. Die Willkürhandlung überformt mit Ziel- und Zeitsetzung das Instinkt- und Lernverhalten in einer höheren Schicht, ist aber in der Durchführung auf Mechanismen und Regelungen der „niederen" Motorik angewiesen. Vorbereitung, Start und Steuerung der Willkürbewegung wird mit Anlassen, Einkuppeln und Steuern eines Autos durch den *Fahrer* verglichen. Die Bewegungsausführung wird dagegen mit Rückmeldungen und Kontrollen automatisch geregelt, wie bei einer *Maschine*.

Triebverhalten und Willkürmotorik entstehen aus ähnlichen Bewegungsmotivationen. Ihre Bewegungsprogramme sind durch Lernen und Sinnesmeldungen modulierbar. *Motorisches Lernen* verwendet zunächst vorhandene Programmierungen in verschiedenen spinalen und cerebralen Schichten, um dann neue Programme zu entwickeln. Primär bewußte und willkürlich gesteuerte Bewegungen werden durch *Übung* sekundär zu unbewußten automatisierten Bewegungsfolgen.

VI. Technische Modelle des Nervensystems: Biokybernetik und Informationstheorie, Rechenmaschinen, Regelung und Reafferenz

> "Thought models or parallels reality, its essential feature being not 'the mind', 'the self', but symbolism of the kind which is familiar to us in mechanical devices which aid thought and calculation, ... In this way the organism carries in its head not only a map of external events but a small-scale model of external reality and of its own possible actions."
>
> E.D. ADRIAN: The Physical Background of Perception, 1947.

DESCARTES hatte seine Maschinentheorie des Organismus noch auf die Sensomotorik beschränkt und das Denken streng davon abgetrennt. Aber schon seit PASCAL und LEIBNIZ im 17. Jahrhundert die ersten Rechenmaschinen bauten, galten solche Apparate als Modelle für logische Abstraktionsvorgänge und mathematisches Denken. Selbst biologisch eingestellte Physiologen wie ADRIAN haben *Parallelen des Denkens und symbolischer geistiger Tätigkeit mit mechanischen Rechenmaschinen* für möglich gehalten [A 8]. Die neuesten Fortschritte der elektronischen Computer-Technik und ihrer informationstheoretischen Grundlagen haben uns die außerordentliche Leistungsfähigkeit dieser Apparate gezeigt, die man sich vor drei Jahrzehnten noch nicht vorstellen konnte. So ist es verständlich, daß Biologie und Physiologie moderne Entwicklungen und Anregungen der *Kybernetik und Informationstheorie* dankbar ergriffen haben. Denn biologische Prozesse sind geregelte und gesteuerte Vorgänge, und die Informationsübertragung im Organismus und seinem Gehirn ähnelt wenigstens im Prinzip der Nachrichtentechnik.

Das binäre Prinzip, das alle Zahlen durch die beiden Zeichen 1 und 0 ausdrücken kann, und zur Codierung von digitalen Rechenmaschinen dient, wurde vor 300 Jahren von LEIBNIZ 1679 theoretisch entwickelt und 1703/5 in der Pariser Akademie publiziert [L 11]. Es dauerte dann 240 Jahre, bis es praktisch für die Rechenmaschinen verwendet wurde.

Die eindrucksvollen Leistungen der modernen Nachrichtenübermittlung und automatischen Zeichenerkennung haben zu oft phantastischen Vorstellungen über die Leistungsfähigkeit sog. „Elektronengehirne" und über „Bewußtseinsvorgänge" in solchen Maschinen geführt. Auch wenn man derartige Spekulationen ablehnt, so sind doch die kybernetischen Maschinen, die Modelle und Symbole der Umwelt entwickeln und Lernvorgänge imitieren, von großer Bedeutung für die Physiologie und Psychologie. Sie geben damit auch Anregungen für die Psychiatrie.

Kybernetik und Informationstheorie

Nachrichtentechnik, Regeltechnik und Informationstheorie haben in glücklicher Ergänzung neue Möglichkeiten für die Erforschung und Erklärung der komplizierten Nachrichtenverarbeitung des Nervensystems gegeben. Die *Nachrichten-Technik* liefert uns *Modelle* für die neurophysiologisch schwer zu erfassenden Vorgänge der Datenspeicherung, Datenverarbeitung und Erkennungsleistung im Organismus, deren Endergebnisse in den psychischen Phänomenen des Gedächtnisses, der Wahrnehmung und des Denkens zutage treten. Die von SHANNON [S 29] entwickelte *Informationstheorie* gibt uns die Möglichkeit, komplizierte Informationsverhältnisse, wie sie im Organismus vorliegen, mathematisch auszudrücken und schwierige semantische Fragen *quantitativ zu erfassen*. Die menschlichen Leistungen des Sprechens und Lesens, deren Analyse für den Neurophysiologen zu kompliziert ist, können so mit kybernetischen Methoden angegangen werden [K 57]. Die Elektrophysiologie, die mit ihren Methoden nur wenige einzelne Neurone aus den Milliarden der Nervenzellen des Gehirns oder uncharakteristische Masseneffekte registrieren kann, wird daher durch die Kybernetik und Informationstheorie wirksam ergänzt.

Bei dem heute verbreiteten Optimismus, der von der Kybernetik die Lösung der schwierigsten Probleme in Biologie, Psychologie und Soziologie erwartet, ist es aber notwendig, auch *Grenzen und Mißverständnisse der kybernetischen Betrachtung* in der Neurophysiologie und Psychologie zu erwähnen. Obwohl die automatischen Rechenmaschinen (englisch „computer") das Gehirn durch Schnelligkeit und Präzision übertreffen, bleiben die Leistungen des lebenden Gehirns in vieler Hinsicht den Leistungen der Automaten überlegen.

Definition der Kybernetik. Der von WIENER 1948 in seinem Buch [W 22] geprägte Terminus *Cybernetics (Steuerungslehre)* wurde als Oberbegriff für diejenigen Forschungsrichtungen eingeführt, die *gemeinsame Funktionsprinzipien in Technik und Biologie* behandeln, und *technische Modelle von lebenden Organismen* herstellen. Als „*Kybernetik*" werden alle biologischen Anwendungen der Regeltechnik, Nachrichtentechnik und Rechenmaschinenkunde bezeichnet. In der Neurophysiologie nennt man die aus informationstheoretischen, mathematischen und biologischen Prinzipien entwickelten *Modellkonstruktionen des Nervensystems* Biokybernetik. In der Biologie spricht man allgemein zum Unterschied von der Nachrichtentechnik statt von „Kybernetik" besser von *biologischer Kommunikationsforschung*.

In Amerika wurde diese Richtung von SHANNON [S 27–29] und WIENER [W 22–24] theoretisch begründet und zunächst von MCCULLOCH [M 33–36], ROSENBLITH [R 25] und ihren zahlreichen Schülern praktisch angewendet, in England von WALTER [W 6, 7], ASHBY [A 34], BARLOW [B 7], MACKAY [M 3–5, 8], in Deutschland von WAGNER [W 4], v. HOLST [H 79, 82], MITTELSTAEDT [M 48, 49], HASSENSTEIN [H 15] in der Physiologie und Zoologie, von KÜPFMÜLLER [K 57], REICHARDT [R 10, 11], STEINBUCH [S 45–49], MEYER-EPPLER [M 41], OPPELT [O 9] u.a. in der Technik und Biophysik vertreten.

Regelung und Steuerung. *Regelung* ist eine automatische Anpassung durch Meßfühler mit selbsttätiger Einstellung durch einen eigenen *Rückmeldungskreis* zum Regler. *Steuerung* ist eine rückwirkungsfreie Einstellung eines Sollwertes. Zum Beispiel wird eine Ölheizung ohne Thermostat durch eine bestimmte Ölzu-

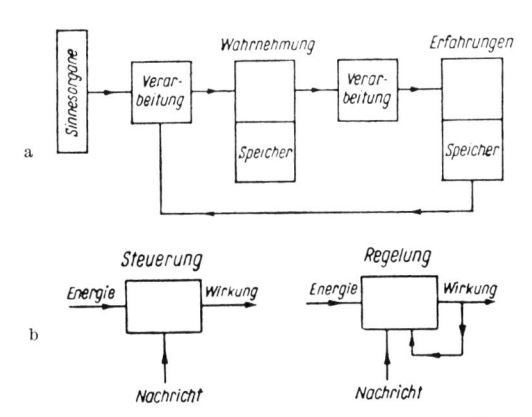

Abb. 15a u. b. Kybernetische Blockschemata der Nachrichtenverarbeitungen mit Steuerung und Regelung. Nach KÜPFMÜLLER (1962) [K 57]. a) *Blockschema einer Rückkopplung bei der Nachrichtenverarbeitung des Organismus:* Aus den Meldungen der Sinnesorgane (links) werden durch zentrale Verarbeitung Wahrnehmungen gewonnen, die durch das Gedächtnis gespeichert werden. Durch weitere Verarbeitung der Wahrnehmung werden komplexe Erfahrungen gesammelt und ebenfalls gespeichert. Aus dem Erfahrungsspeicher des Gedächtnisses zeigen die unteren Pfeile Rückkopplungen mit Sinnesmeldungen. Sie dienen der geordneten Wahrnehmung und Erkennung von Sinnesinformationen. b) *Prinzipien der Steuerung und Regelung.* Bei den Steuerungsvorgängen wirkt die Nachricht, sei es direkt von den Sinnesorganen oder aus ihrer Verarbeitung rückkopplungsfrei auf den Energiefluß und seine Wirkung. Bei Regelungsvorgängen wirkt die Nachricht mit Rückkopplung über die erzielte Wirkung wieder auf den Energiefluß der Nachrichtenverarbeitung zurück. Diese Regelungskreise enthalten Rückkopplungen zwischen der Auswirkung und dem Energiefluß der Nachrichtenübertragung. Sie arbeiten mit einem Vergleich zwischen Istwert und Sollwert (vgl. Abb. 16)

fuhr rückwirkungsfrei *gesteuert,* oder nach Einstellung auf einen bestimmten Temperaturwert durch Thermostaten *geregelt* und so indirekt die Ölzufuhr mit der Wärmeproduktion im Energieumsatz reguliert. In politischen Systemen überwiegt in einer Diktatur die Steuerung, in einer Demokratie die Regelung. Die demokratische Regelung verwendet zahlreiche Rückwirkungen der unteren Stellen, die autoritäre Steuerung bestimmt vor allem ein Soll und vermeidet, soweit möglich, Rückmeldungen der ausführenden Organe. In Abb. 15b ist das Prinzip der Regelung und Steuerung schematisch dargestellt. Das Schema eines Regelkreises mit den normierten Fachworten der Kybernetik zeigt Abb. 16 nach HASSENSTEIN [H 15]. Die Regeltheoretiker unterscheiden *Steuerungsmechanismen in offenen Systemen* und *Regelungsmechanismen in geschlossenen Systemen mit Regelkreisen.* Beide enthalten meist Maschen- und Kettenschaltungen.

Mit solchen kybernetischen Vorstellungen könnte man vieles in der Neurophysiologie durch informationstechnische Begriffe bezeichnen. Denn zur *biologischen Steuerung und Regelung* gehört die Übertragung und Verarbeitung der Nachrichten von den Sinnesorganen über das Nervensystem zu den ausführenden Organen, d.h. die Übertragung der Meßwerte von den *Meßfühlern (Receptoren)* des Organismus über eine *Leitung (Nerven)* zum *Regler (ZNS), Stellglied* und *Organ (Effektoren).* Schließlich gibt es in der Technik Apparate zur *automatischen Zeichenerkennung,* die von der spezialisierten Nachrichtentechnik entwickelt wurden, aber ihre biologischen Vorbilder des Lesens und Erkennens noch

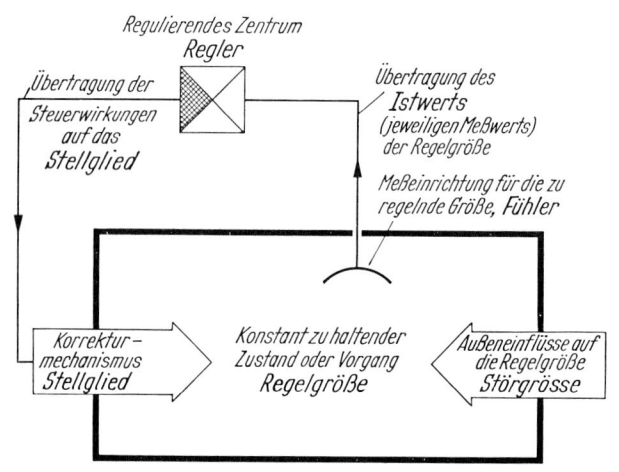

Abb. 16. Schematische Darstellung eines Regelmechanismus in technischen und biologischen Regulationen. Nach HASSENSTEIN [H 15]. In dem Blockschema sind die typischen kybernetischen Termini durch größeren Druck hervorgehoben: Regler, Stellglied, Regelgröße und Störgröße, Istwert oder Sollwert, Fühler. Die Einzelmechanismen dieser Regulationen sind in verschiedenen Strukturen unterschiedlich. Das Blockschema zeigt nur das Prinzip eines solchen kybernetischen Regelkreises, für den verschiedene Modelle und biologische Lösungen möglich sind. Fühler sind im Organismus meistens Receptoren für innere und äußere Sinnesinformationen. Störungen kommen sowohl von der Außenwelt wie aus dem Organismus selbst. Regler und Stellglieder sind die verschiedensten biologischen Koordinationen, in der Neurophysiologie vorwiegend cerebrale und spinale Neuronenapparate

nicht erreicht haben [S 47]. Solche Apparate sind nicht nach lebenden Modellen gebaut, sondern werden nach rein technischen Prinzipien entwickelt (S. 863).

Regel- und Steuervorgänge gibt es in jedem Lebewesen und in jeder Zelle. Offenbar handelt es sich bei der biologischen Regelung um ein Grundprinzip zur *Erhaltung konstanter Milieubedingungen gegenüber inneren und äußeren Störfaktoren.* Verschiedene Regel- und Steuer-Mechanismen im Organismus sind oft eng miteinander verbunden und im einzelnen schwer erkennbar. Deshalb muß diese Anwendung technischer Prinzipien auf biologische Objekte mit großer Vorsicht geschehen. *Die Analogien des geregelten biologischen Organismus mit regeltechnischen Apparaten dürfen nicht dazu führen, daß man kybernetische Gesichtspunkte einfach auf Lebewesen und ihre Hirnfunktionen anwendet, ohne deren physiologische Mechanismen zu kennen.* Die Wärmeregulation eines Organismus unterscheidet sich wesentlich von einer auf konstante Raumtemperatur geregelten Ölheizung. Das Gehirn ist sehr verschieden von einer Rechenmaschine. Für den Physiologen ist die von der Kybernetik angestrebte mathematische Durchdringung der Biologie, Psychologie und Soziologie allgemein zu begrüßen. Bei speziellen Entwicklungen fehlen aber meistens noch entsprechende biologische Informationsdaten. Natürlich dürfen mathematische, regeltechnische und informationstheoretische Anwendungen auf den Organismus nicht nach hypothetischen Annahmen oder ungenügenden und inkonstanten biologischen Meßwerten durchgeführt werden.

Die in den letzten Jahren rasch anschwellende *Literatur über Kybernetik und Informationsverarbeitung* ist schon jetzt immens. Angeregt durch die Erfolge der Nachrichtentechnik, der Rechenmaschinen und der automatisch regulierten Apparate, sowie durch die Raumschiffahrt haben zahlreiche Symposien [C 6a, F 16a, G 15a, R 11a, W 24a] stattgefunden, auf denen Biologen und Physiologen mit Nachrichtentechnikern und Mathematikern diskutiert haben. Die Termini der Technik wurden normiert und großenteils auch von biologischer Seite übernommen [H 15]. Doch haben viele Neologismen für die biologischen Anwendungen und Modelle das Gebiet wieder unübersichtlich gemacht. Sie haben die Verständigung eher erschwert als erleichtert. Man spricht, außer von Kybernetik und Informationsverarbeitung am besten von *Kommunikationsforschung* (communication sciences). Weniger zweckmäßig sind neue Namen wie „neurodynamics" [R 24], „bionics" [W 2], „biosimulation", „artificial intelligence" [M 85] usw. Wenn man der Sache auf den Grund geht, findet man darin oft nur wenig überzeugende Analogien mit dem lebenden Organismus.

Digitale und analoge Rechenmaschinen im Vergleich mit dem Nervensystem

Die beiden Prinzipien der mathematischen Technik, nach denen die komplizierten Rechenmaschinen aufgebaut sind, können hier nicht im einzelnen dargelegt werden. Man unterscheidet *digitale* Maschinen, die nach dem binären Prinzip einer *Alles-oder-Nichts-Erregung* mit *1 oder 0, ja oder nein,* arbeiten und *analoge* Maschinen, die ohne Einzelimpulse mit *kontinuierlichen Funktionen* arbeiten. Bei digitalen Maschinen kann man die Information in „bit" *(binary digit)* messen. *Das bit ist die mathematische Einheit der Nachrichtenmenge* als erforderliche *Zahl von Ja-Nein-Entscheidungen,* um ein bestimmtes Symbol aus einer Gesamtzahl von Symbolen auszuwählen. Die *Messung des Nachrichtenflusses in bit/sec* ist auf die Informationsleitung im Nervensystem mit ihren Alles-oder-Nichts-Impulsen übertragen und auf die verschiedenen Sinnesorgane, die Zahl ihrer Receptoren und Nervenfasern und die Neurone des Gehirns angewandt worden (Abb. 33) sowie auf die Sprache, und auf kompliziertere Wahrnehmungsvorgänge wie das Lesen. Für einzelne Buchstaben des Alphabets wird eine Information von etwa 4 bit angenommen [K 57]. Je nach der Darbietungszeit ergeben sich dann verschiedene Nachrichtenmengen und eine maximale Lesegeschwindigkeit von 43 bit/sec. Die Aufnahmefähigkeit der Sinnesmeldungen von Auge und Ohr wird auf etwa 40 bit/sec geschätzt, während der maximale Nachrichtenfluß (Informationskapazität) des Auges viel größer ist (etwa 10^8 bit/sec). Eine gute, allgemein verständliche Darstellung findet man bei KÜPFMÜLLER [K 57], von dem auch Abb. 15 stammt. Es lag sehr nahe, die Ähnlichkeit der digitalen Ja-Nein-Entscheidung mit der *Alles-oder-Nichts-Erregung der Neurone* zu vergleichen, wie es WIENER [W 22] und MCCULLOCH [M 33] getan haben. Dieser Vergleich führte aber fälschlicherweise zu einer Identifizierung beider [M 35]. Oft wird vergessen, daß *die binär-digitalen Maschinen in prinzipiell anderer Weise ihre Ja-Nein-Entscheidung auf streng begrenzte Intervalle codieren, während im Nervensystem offenbar nur mittlere Impulsfrequenzen für die Sinnesinformationen bedeutungsvoll, die Einzelintervalle aber sehr variabel sind.* GRÜSSER [G 47] hat diese Verschiedenheiten am Beispiel des Sehsystems und seiner Neuronentätigkeit klar dargestellt. Die daraus abgeleitete Informationskapazität einzelner Nervenzellen wurde allerdings von BARLOW [B 8a] bestritten.

Die digitalen binären Rechenmaschinen arbeiten ähnlich arithmetischen Zahlenoperationen der Potenzrechnung mit einzelnen Impulsen, deren jeder in Zweierpotenzen gezählt wird ($2^0 = 1$, 2^1, $2^2 = 4$, $2^1 + 2^0 = 3$ usw.). Sie erreichen daher eine hohe Genauigkeit über 8 Dezimalstellen und machen nur geringe Fehler. Dagegen arbeitet der 2. Typ der *Analog-Rechenmaschinen* mit *kontinuierlichen Funktionen,* die den berechneten Werten nur „analog" sind, ohne daß einzelne Impulse als 0 oder 1 gezählt werden, z.B. werden bestimmte Werte durch eine elektrische Spannung oder Spannungsänderung dargestellt. Die Rechengenauigkeit der Analogmaschinen ist daher geringer. Ähnlich arbeitet auch der messende Physiker, der Skaleninstrumente benutzt, oder der Biologe, wenn er Veränderungen im Organismus mit physikalischen oder chemischen Vorgängen erklärt. Jedes Zeigermeßinstrument mit einer Skala wäre ein einfaches Modell einer Analogmaschine oder auch ein Rechenschieber, dessen logarithmische Skala ein Kontinuum darstellt. Die elektronischen Analogmaschinen arbeiten mit Röhren oder Transistoren, ähnlich den Verstärkern in Radioapparaten. Das Analogprinzip kann auch für komplizierte Apparaturen und Lernmatrizen verwendet werden [S 48]. Ferner sind beide Prinzipien, Digital- und Analogrechner zu kombinieren. Da die Arbeitsweise des Nervensystems mehr Ähnlichkeit mit einer analogen als mit einer digitalen Rechenmaschine hat, sind die *Analog-Apparate für Modelle des Nervensystems geeigneter als die digitalen Maschinen.*

Nach dem ersten Enthusiasmus MCCULLOCHS für das Gehirn als digitalem Computer [M 33—36] hat MACKAY diese Parallele von Nervensystem und Rechenmaschine widerlegt und 1952 mit MCCULLOCH die schlechtere Information eines rein digitalen Mechanismus der Neuronentätigkeit festgestellt [M 8]. Dennoch blieb die Meinung sehr verbreitet, daß die Nervenfasern digital arbeiten würden und nur Nervenzelle und Synapsen ein Analogsystem darstellen [R 25]. Doch hat auch die Nervenfaser eine kontinuierliche Frequenzskala von Entladungen, deren einzelne Impulse an bestimmten Synapsen mit chemischer Übertragung integriert werden. Selbst wenn die Axone digital arbeiten würden, wäre bei synaptischer Integrierung keine digitale Übertragung im Nervensystem mehr möglich. Ungeklärt ist noch die Frage, ob neben der Frequenz der Impulse die von Technikern wegen ihrer Unregelmäßigkeit als *Impulsrate* bezeichnet wird, auch das einzelne Impuls*intervall* von Bedeutung ist. Dies wäre bei bestimmten synaptischen Konstellationen möglich, ist aber nur in dem zeitlich sehr präzise arbeitenden akustischen System wahrscheinlich, weniger im optischen System. Daher ist es nur sicher, daß die „Codierung" neuronaler Informationen mit einer Pulsfrequenzmodulation erfolgt, aber ungewiß, ob dem Impulsintervall die von MacKay und McCulloch [M 8] postulierte Bedeutung zukommt.

Mißverständnisse zwischen Biologie und Kybernetik. Die *Informationstheorie* hat nicht nur messende Methoden und Theorien für die Nachrichtentechnik, sondern auch theoretische Grundlagen für die Informationsvermittlung im biologischen Bereich geschaffen. Die Anwendung einer solchen quantitativen Theorie, die Informationsgehalt und Informationskapazität biologischer Vorgänge mathematisch darstellen läßt, ist bis jetzt in der Biologie begrenzt. Sie beschränkt sich auf die Untersuchung der Leistungsfähigkeit informativer Leitungssysteme. Darüber hinaus will die *Kybernetik* im weiteren Sinne die Regelung und Steuerung im lebenden Organismus und in sozialen Systemen untersuchen. Sie will damit auch zur Erklärung psychischer Vorgänge beitragen. Durch den unterschiedlichen Sprachgebrauch dieser verschiedenen Gebiete ergibt sich manche Schwierigkeit, die nur durch die fast utopische Forderung einer gemeinsamen Terminologie beseitigt werden könnte. Daher haben kritische Autoren wie Quastler [Q 1] schon früh davor gewarnt, die Begriffe der Informationstheorie ohne weiteres in die Biologie zu übertragen. Offenbar hat schon Shannon selbst die Ausweitung seiner Informationstheorie in Biologie und Psychologie mit Skepsis betrachtet und zur Entwicklung eigener adäquater Theorien geraten.

Die Terminologie der Regellehre und Informationstheorie entspricht meist nicht dem physiologischen Sprachgebrauch und noch weniger dem psychologischen. Mißverständnisse und Äquivokationen in grundlegenden Fragen sind die Folge. Ein typisches Beispiel ist die Gleichsetzung der digitalen Codes der Rechenmaschinen mit der Alles-oder-Nichts-Entladung der Neurone [M 35]. Auch sonst bedeuten die gleichen Worte in Technik und Biologie verschiedenes: Die Techniker verwenden den Begriff „Signal" meist für physikalische Vorgänge bis zu den Nervenimpulsen, aber nicht für die Information selbst. In der Physiologie wird der Signalbegriff meist in viel weiterem Sinne gebraucht und weniger scharf begrenzt. Im Englischen spricht man bei allen Sinnesmeldungen und Nervenimpulsen von „signals". Bei Pawlows Signalsystemen wird „Signal" auch für komplexe Information und ihre differenzierte sprachliche Verarbeitung verwendet [P 4, 7]. Ein häufiges Mißverstehen entsteht daraus, daß Techniker manche biologischen Vorgänge oder Resultate physiologischer Experimente ohne Rücksicht auf ihre große Variabilität wie feste mathematische Grundlagen behandeln und daraus eine „mathematische Biophysik" aufbauen. Noch schlimmer sind kybernetische Ausarbeitungen unrichtiger physiologischer Hypothesen.

Die Quantifizierung der Informationsbeziehung durch die Kybernetik ist vor allem für die Wahrnehmungsphysiologie und die Aufmerksamkeitsselektion von

Nutzen. Ein Beispiel zeigt Abb. 33. Doch führt es nicht weiter, wenn man Funktionen des lebenden Organismus mit technischen Ausdrücken belegt und einfach das Sinnesorgan einen Nachrichtenwandler, das Gedächtnis einen Informationsspeicher oder das Lernen eine Programmierung nennt.

Biologische Regelungen und Reafferenzprinzip

Vorkybernetische Modellvorstellungen des Nervensystems. Über der modernen wissenschaftlichen Welle der elektronischen Technik mit ihrer Anwendung der Regeltechnik auf das Nervensystem wird oft vergessen, daß Regelprinzipien und mechanische Modelle bereits früher von Physiologen benutzt wurden, um die Zusammenfassung von Sensibilität und Motorik in der geordneten Leistung darzustellen. CANNON hat mit seiner *Homeostase* bereits ähnliche biologische Prinzipien der Regeltechnik für den Organismus verwendet [C 3]. WAGNER diskutierte 1925 als erster Regelvorgänge in der Motorik [W 3]. W.R. HESS gab 1934/35 in 2 Darstellungen über Lokalisation und Plastizität und den Zentrenbegriff [H 53, 54] *Modellschemata zentraler Koordinationsvorgänge* und führte sie 1941 am Beispiel der Augenbewegungen mit räumlichen Modellen der zentralen Innervationsschaltungen weiter aus [H 55]. 1948/49 haben wir mit TÖNNIES das Prinzip der *Rückmeldung* im ZNS entwickelt [T 9, 11]. Schließlich haben v.

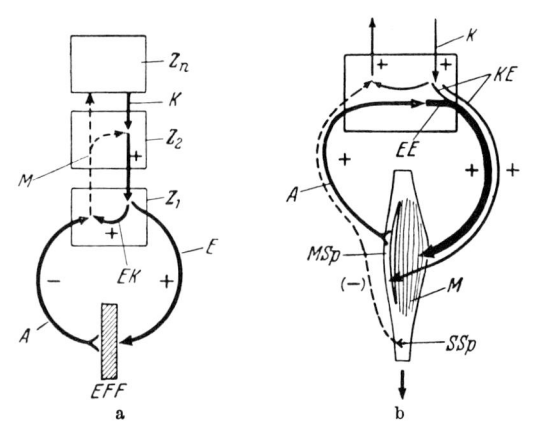

Abb. 17a u. b. Reafferenzprinzip nach v. HOLST [H 79, 82]. a) Ein niederes Zentrum Z_1 versorgt einen Effektor motorisch und sensibel. Andere Zentren Z_2–Z_n sind übergeordnet. Kommandoimpulse der oberen Zentren veranlassen eine efferente Impulsfolge E, die einen zentralen Aktivitätsrückstand, ähnlich der Tönniesschen Rückmeldung, hinterläßt. Die efferenten Impulse lösen über periphere Receptoren afferente Impulse aus, die den Erfolg in das Zentrum melden und normalerweise die Efferenzkopie annullieren. Die Efferenzkopie wird ausgelöscht, wenn sie mit der Meldung genau übereinstimmt. Zusätzliche afferente Impulse (Exafferenz) ergeben als Differenz der Efferenzkopie eine zu den höheren Zentren laufende Meldung. Zn übergeordnete Zentren, K Kommando, Z_1, Z_2 untere Zentren, M Meldungen zu übergeordneten Zentren (Rapporte), E efferente Impulse, A afferente Impulse (Reafferenz), EFF Effektor. b) *Reafferenz und Eigenreflex*. Ein durch Kommandoimpulse K gespannter Muskel (M) erhält durch Dehnung und Eigenreflexe mit der parallel geschalteten Muskelspindel zusätzliche efferente Impulse. Die in Serie geschalteten Sehnenreceptoren SSp erzeugen bei zu starker Muskelspannung eine Eigenhemmung entsprechend den Versuchen GRANITS

HOLST und MITTELSTAEDT 1950 zunächst unabhängig von der Kybernetik ihr *Reafferenzprinzip* aus biologischen und sinnesphysiologischen Daten abgeleitet [H 79, 82].

HESS [H 56] weist darauf hin, daß die *Raumvorstellung zur Motorik in einer Parallelschaltung* stehen muß, ähnlich wie dies später die Kybernetiker für innere Modelle der Außenwelt formuliert haben. Als allgemein wichtiges Prinzip der Organisation des ZNS gilt sowohl für die Physiologie wie für die Kybernetik, *daß alle innervatorisch möglichen Varianten im Gehirn bereits strukturmäßig vorgebildet sind.* Die morphologische Struktur des Gehirns ist eine Grundlage der physiologischen Ordnung. *Die Mannigfaltigkeit und Veränderlichkeit cerebraler Funktionen läßt sich sehr wohl mit der Funktionsspezifität seiner Elemente vereinigen.* Das ZNS zeigt eine *differenzierte, aber durchaus festgefügte Organisation, in der die plastischen variablen Reaktionen bereits als mögliche Struktur-Verbindungen angelegt sind, jedoch nur unter besonderen Bedingungen benutzt werden.*

Wir sehen mit HESS [H 56] in der organisierten Funktionsstruktur des Zentralnervensystems die Grundlage seiner Ordnung. Die periphere Rückleitung des „negative feed back" entspricht der alten Propriozeptivität, auf der HESS [H 56] seine Funktionsschemata aufgebaut hat. Die Verbindung dieser peripheren negativen Rückkopplung mit der Eigentätigkeit des Zentralnervensystems ist in seinem Einzelmechanismus von WIENER [W 22] und McCULLOCH [M 35] noch nicht genügend klargestellt worden. Die Zusammenarbeit mit der zentralen Rückmeldung, deren Bedeutung TÖNNIES 1949 begründet hat [T 9], blieb offen. Diesen Schritt haben erst v. HOLST und MITTELSTAEDT.

v. HOLSTs Reafferenzprinzip. Das *Reafferenzprinzip verbindet die zentrale Rückmeldung mit einer peripheren Rückleitung.* VON HOLST nennt die im Zentralnervensystem zurückbleibende Aktivitätsänderung nach einer efferenten Impulsfolge *Efferenzkopie.* Die weitere Verwertung und Verarbeitung dieser Efferenzkopie ist nach v. HOLST die eigentliche Leistung der zentralen Koordination nach dem Reafferenzprinzip [H 79]. Der Grundgedanke ist in Abb. 17 schematisch dargestellt. Wenn ein niederes Zentrum, etwa angeregt durch ein Kommando aus übergeordneten Zentren, einen Impulsstrom in das periphere Erfolgsorgan (Effektor) sendet, so wird im Zentralnervensystem eine Registrierung dieser *zentralen* efferenten Impulse zurückbehalten *(Efferenzkopie)* [H 82]. Von den sensiblen Endorganen der Peripherie wird wiederum eine afferente Meldung der durch den efferenten Impuls ausgelösten *peripheren* Zustandsänderung in das Zentralnervensystem zurückgesandt *(Reafferenz).* Entspricht diese *Reafferenz dem beabsichtigten peripheren Effekt des efferenten Impulsstromes, so löschen sich Efferenzkopie und Reafferenz gegenseitig aus* (+ und − im Schema). Es wird keine weitere Meldung in die oberen Zentren geschickt, denn die periphere Reafferenz hat die gleiche Größe wie die Efferenzkopie. Der Ausgleich wird allein von den niederen Zentren vorgenommen und braucht daher nicht gemeldet zu werden. Anders wird dies, wenn der efferente Impulsstrom auf Widerstand und Veränderungen der Umgebung stößt, etwa bei einer motorischen Leistung: Finden wir beim Heben eines Gegenstandes diesen unvermutet schwer, so müssen wir die motorische Innervation der von den peripheren Receptoren gemeldeten Schwere anpassen. In diesem Fall kommen zu der Reafferenz der beabsichtigten Zustandsänderung neue afferente Impulse hinzu, die nicht direkte Folge der

Efferenz sind, sondern auch durch äußere Einwirkungen entstehen. Diese nennt v. HOLST *Exafferenz*. Solche von außen kommenden Impulse sind in der Efferenzkopie nicht vorgesehen, es entsteht daher nicht mehr eine einfache Auslöschung der im Zentralorgan verbliebenen Efferenzkopie: Zunächst erfolgt bei plötzlicher Dehnung der Muskulatur ein rascher *reflektorischer Ausgleich* durch den Hoffmannschen Eigenreflex, der bekanntlich nur über 2 Neurone geleitet wird und eine Synapse enthält [H 74]. Diese reflektorische Regelung, die nach v. HOLST ohne Mitwirkung einer Efferenzkopie vor sich geht, genügt aber nur für einen momentanen Ausgleich. Bei durch Außenweltveränderungen komplizierter Bewegung muß die der Exafferenz entsprechende Differenz zwischen efferenten und afferenten Impulsen *als Sinneswahrnehmung in die oberen Zentren gemeldet werden,* eventuell unter Zwischenschaltung niederer Koordinationszentren (Z_2). In diesen oder in den höheren Zentren wird dann *eine erneute Änderung der Kommandoimpulse hervorgerufen, die sich den neuen Gegebenheiten anpaßt.* Der unerwartet schwere Gegenstand wird jetzt mit dem entsprechenden Kraftaufwand gehoben. Das ganze System arbeitet also mit *Selbstregulation und Anpassung an veränderte Bedingungen der Außenwelt entsprechend der Regeltechnik.*

Bisher wurde eine „Efferenzkopie" der motorischen Entladungen, z.B. der Augenmuskelinnervation physiologisch noch nicht nachgewiesen. So konnte das Reafferenzprinzip v. HOLSTs auf den unteren Ebenen der Sensomotorik in den letzten 20 Jahren noch nicht verifiziert werden. Für die Erklärung der *Raumkonstanz der Sehdinge* erscheint MACKAYS Rückbewertungskonzept (re-evaluation, matching) einfacher und brauchbarer [M 7]. Wir erwarten eine Umweltkonstanz und setzen die Stabilität der Umwelt voraus, wenn wir unseren Blick auf verschiedene Objekte richten. Eine Bewegung wird nur wahrgenommen, wenn eine langsame Blickfolgebewegung einem bewegten Objekt folgt oder retinale Bildverschiebungen bei Blickfixation oder bei zurückbleibender Blickfolge auftreten [D 31].

Biologische Systeme und pathologische Syndrome in kybernetischer Betrachtung

Biologische Regelvorgänge gibt es in allen Teilen des Körpers, nicht nur im Nervensystem. Auch in der Nervenzelle, in den Wechselwirkungen der Fermente und Hormone, wie in den Neuronenverbänden sind Regelmechanismen am Werke und schließlich auch zwischen dem Zentralnervensystem und den endokrinen Systemen. Eine kurze Übersicht über diese *intracellulären Regelungen von biochemischen und Stoffwechselvorgängen,* die uns hier nicht beschäftigen, findet man bei HOLZER [H 85]. Von größerem Interesse für die Psychiatrie sind Wechselwirkungen zwischen dem *Hypothalamus und den Hormonregulationen,* die SZENTAGOTHAI nach kybernetischen Prinzipien dargestellt hat (Abb. 18).

Das hypothalamisch-endokrine Regelsystem. Bereits im Wechselspiel der verschiedenen Hormone war ein Regelprinzip erkennbar: Die Hormonproduktion und ihre Anregung durch übergeordnete endokrine Vorgänge wurde gebremst, sobald dieses Hormon in größerer Menge ausgeschüttet oder dem Körper zugeführt wurde. Es ist wahrscheinlich, daß die bisher weitgehend rätselhafte Wechselwirkung von Hormon und ZNS nach einem Regelprinzip arbeitet.

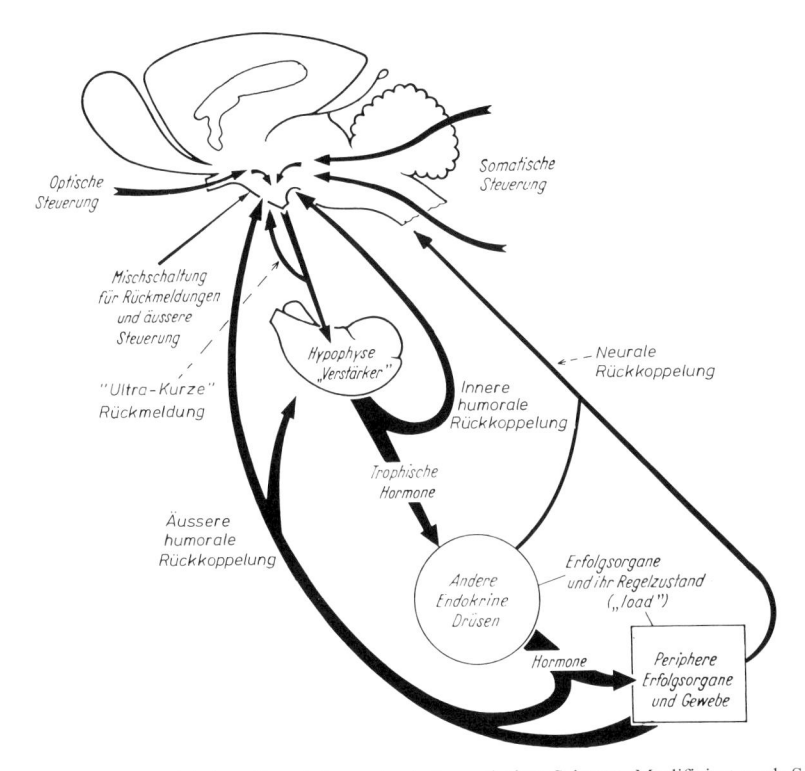

Abb. 18. Die neuro-endokrinen Regulationen im kybernetischen Schema. Modifiziert nach SZENTA-
GOTHAI u.Mitarb. (1962) [S 65]. Im Hypothalamus treffen alle Regulationen in einer Mischschaltung
zusammen. Die wichtigste efferente Bahn wirkt durch die Neurosekretion von den Neuronen selbst
hormonproduzierend. Von der Hypophyse geht eine innere Rückmeldung, von den übrigen Hormonen eine äußere Rückmeldung zum Hypothalamus zurück. Alle gegenseitigen Beeinflussungen sind
vorwiegend bremsende Regulationen mit negativer Rückkopplung (negative feed back). Über die
peripheren Erfolgsorgane, die Sinnesorgane, das Kleinhirn und afferente Bahnen können weitere
somatische Steuerungen in den Regelmechanismus eingreifen

SZENTAGOTHAI u.Mitarb. [S 65] haben ein kybernetisches Schema dieser endo-
krin-nervösen Regelfunktion entwickelt. Abb. 18 zeigt das Prinzip dieses Regelsystems, nach dem der Hypothalamus als Mischschaltung von Rückmeldungsme-
chanismen und äußeren Kontrollen durch verschiedene Afferenzen arbeitet, entsprechend dem „negative feed back" bei zentralnervösen und peripheren Regulationen. Wie bei neuronalen Regelmechanismen werden auch im endokrinen
System äußere und innere Regelkreise und äußere Kontrollmechanismen unterschieden. Die äußeren Regler melden Hormonwirkungen an peripheren Organen
und Geweben, die inneren Regler sind nach neuroendokrinologischen Ergebnissen der letzten Jahre sehr komplizierte Wechselwirkungen von sog. Releaser-
Faktoren des Hypothalamus. Ihre Receptorfunktionen sind für die Sexualhormone geschlechtsspezifisch und in der frühen Ontogenese in den gleichen Hirnstrukturen bestimmt (vgl. PLOOG in diesem Band). Entsprechende Receptorwir-
kungen gibt es für die Temperaturregulation bei starker Erwärmung oder Käl-

teeinwirkung oder die Wasserregulation mit äußeren Regelkreisen durch Osmoreceptoren. Auch eine diffuse Licht-Dunkel-Afferenz der endokrin-vegetativen Funktionen ist nach Erfahrungen im Polarwinter diskutiert worden. Wie jedoch gestaltete optische Reize, die sicher bei den Sexualfunktionen eine Rolle spielen, auf das System einwirken sollen, bleibt noch völlig rätselhaft.

Ansätze für neurophysiologische Untersuchungen geben die Befunde von SAWYER über länger dauernde hirnelektrische Veränderungen bei sexueller Aktivität [S 2, 3], obwohl die offenbar auch hier beteiligten endokrinen Mechanismen noch unklar sind.

Positive Rückkopplung und Circulus vitiosus in der Neuropsychiatrie. Während die negative Rückmeldung (negative feedback) im Organismus wie in der Maschine eine Stabilisierung hervorruft, so bewirkt jede *positive Rückkopplung* (positive feedback = Rückkopplung im engeren Sinne) *Instabilität*. Solche vermehrten positiven Rückkopplungen führen zum *Circulus vitiosus*. Bei einem Radioapparat hören wir eine abnorme positive Rückkopplung als lautes Störgeräusch. Im lebenden Nervensystem ist das extremste Beispiel positiver Rückkopplung die *epileptische Krampfentladung*. Im Gegensatz zu SELBACH [S 22] sehen wir im epileptischen Anfall nicht eine abnorm starke überschießende Gegenregulation, sondern ein *Versagen* der normalen Regelungen und Rückmeldungen [J 31]. Beim Gesunden werden die geordneten, der Situation angemessenen Funktionen des Gehirns durch negative Rückmeldungen um ein mittleres Erregungsniveau geregelt, auf dem sich Erregungs- und Hemmungsvorgänge etwa die Waage halten [J 62].

Doch ist die positive Rückkopplung nicht immer eine abnorme Funktion im Organismus. Bei gewissen Affekt- und Triebmechanismen kann positive feedback offenbar eine wichtige *Antriebsfunktion* sein (vgl. S. 951). Bei vielen Regelungen ist, kybernetisch gesprochen, eine *Mischung von negativen und positiven Rückkopplungen* beteiligt. Erst nach Ausfall oder Verminderung von negativen Rückmeldungen der Hemmungen und Bremsungen überwiegt die positive Rückkopplung und es kann eine epileptische Entladung auftreten [J 62]. Durch die verschiedensten Einwirkungen, elektrische, chemische, pharmakologische Reize oder durch pathologische Zerstörungen mit Ausfall hemmender Strukturen können solche Verminderungen der negativen Rückmeldung entstehen, die dann der positiven Rückkopplung freie Bahn geben. Nicht nur bei der Epilepsie mit ihren verschiedenen Syndromen vom generalisierten Anfall bis zu den lokalisierten epileptischen Entladungen, sondern wahrscheinlich auch bei zahlreichen anderen krankhaften Störungen des Nervensystems kann ein solcher Circulus vitiosus auftreten. Im einzelnen sind diese Regelungen und falschen Zirkel noch nicht genügend erforscht.

Bei den *Suchten*, deren Rückkopplungsmechanismen mit der Selbstreizung auf S. 959 besprochen werden, ist ein Circulus vitiosus schon vor dem Einbruch der Kybernetik in der Biologie diskutiert worden. Es ist wahrscheinlich, daß noch verschiedene andere psychotische und neurotische Symptome als Circulus vitiosus mit verstärkter positiver Rückkopplung erklärt werden, ohne daß echte epileptische Entladungen auftreten.

Eine allgemeine *regeltechnische Deutung der Neurosen* hat MCCULLOCH [M 32, 35] vorgeschlagen: Er erklärt den neurotischen Mechanismus als Umwandlung des normalen negativen feed back unserer zentralnervösen Regulationen in eine positive Rückkopplung. Solche groben regeltechnischen Mechanismen können die äußerst fein differenzierten Zusammenhänge neurotischer Vorgänge noch nicht erklären. Immerhin erscheint es möglich, daß mit einer besseren Kenntnis neuronaler Mechanismen der Affekte und Triebe und ihrer Beeinflussung durch Lernen und bedingte Reflexe auch kybernetische Erklärungen einzelner neurotischer Vorgänge gewonnen werden. Diese würden allerdings den psychotherapeutischen Weg einer verständlichen Auflösung der Neurosen nicht überflüssig machen, sondern nur ergänzen.

Kybernetische Gesichtspunkte für die *schizophrene Informationsverarbeitung* hat ELKES 1961 in seinem Versuch neurophysiologischer Korrelationen der schizophrenen Denkstörungen [E 15] verwendet: Das "schizophrenic disorder as a disturbance of information processing" sei eine Störung höherer Auswertungen und Vergleiche neuer mit gespeicherten Informationen, die später zu koordinierten Mustern aufgebaut würden. Das menschliche Gehirn wird als chemisch arbeitendes Informationsorgan bezeichnet.

Die Anwendung kybernetischer Prinzipien für hochdifferenzierte Funktionen und Störungen des Nervensystems bleibt heute noch problematisch. Erfolgreicher waren zunächst einfache technische Modelle des Nervensystems.

Kybernetische Modelle der Gehirnfunktionen

Aus der Vielzahl technischer Modelle des Nervensystems geben wir im folgenden einige Beispiele, die für den Neurophysiologen und Psychiater von Interesse sind.

Technische Modelle für bedingte Reflexe. Für die Bahnungsvorgänge bei bedingten Reflexen wurden schon früh technische Modelle entwickelt, die ähnliche Leistungen boten. GOZZANO u. Mitarb. [G 31] konstruierten eine einfache Schaltung als elektronisches Modell für bedingte Reflexe. WALTER [W 6, 7] entwickelte ein vollkommeneres Modell eines einfachen künstlichen Organismus, der mit optischen, taktilen und akustischen Receptoren arbeitete und primitive Lern- und Gedächtnisleistungen zeigte. Zahlreiche neuere kybernetische Modelle wie STEINBUCHS Lernmatrizen leisten noch wesentlich mehr (vgl. S. 864). Ein bekanntes Beispiel rein mechanisch-mathematischer Konstruktion von Hirnfunktionen ist ASHBYS "*Design for a brain*" [A 34]. Es setzt sich zum Ziel, die Adaptations- und Lernfähigkeit des Organismus und seine homeostatischen Regulationen im Sinne CANNONS auf rein technischer und mathematischer Basis zu erklären. Der von ASHBY postulierte und konstruierte „Homeostat" entspricht einem gut ausregulierten System von großer Stabilität. ASHBY selbst betont, daß er zur Ruhe kommt, wenn alle äußeren Störungen ausgeglichen sind. Er hat kein anderes Ziel als eine solche *Adaptation gegenüber der Umwelt*. Daß dies beim Gehirn anders ist und für die biologische Struktur nicht genügt, ist klar. Diese Einschränkung gilt leider für fast alle neueren, von technischer Seite entwickelten „Elektronengehirne", die meistens ohne Kenntnis des Nervensystems konstruiert sind und daher auch kein Modell für das Gehirn darstellen können.

WALTERs „Schildkröte" als einfaches Modell eines Organismus. Das von W.G. WALTER [W 6] entwickelte Tiermodell (Machina docilis oder Machina speculatrix) mit drei Receptoren für optische, taktile und akustische Reize – wegen seiner Form und langsamen Beweglichkeit kurz „Schildkröte" genannt – zeigt mit seinen einfachen elektrischen Schaltungen bereits bedingte Reaktionen und einfache „Gedächtnis"leistungen. Durch mehrfache Reizkombinationen verschiedener Receptoren werden neue Erregungskreise geschlossen, ähnlich den bedingten Reflexen. Die Leistungen verschiedener Modelle dieser „Schildkröte" und ihre Parallelen mit dem Verhalten von Organismen sind von WALTER ausführlich dargestellt [W 6, 7] und in verschiedenen kybernetischen Schriften oft wiederholt worden. Werden mehrere solche Modelle der „Machina docilis" zusammengebracht, so daß Lichtreize des einen Modells auf die Receptoren des anderen einwirken können, so ergeben sich ziemlich komplizierte Wechselwirkungen zwischen verschiedenen „Schildkröten".

STEINBUCHs Lernmatrizen als wahrnehmende, abstrahierende und lernende Automaten. Lernende Automaten werden heute vielfach gebaut. Ein besonders einfaches und leistungsfähiges kybernetisches Modell von Lernvorgängen hat STEINBUCH mit seiner *„Lernmatrix"* [S 45] erfunden, die erlernte Zuordnung zwischen bestimmten „Eigenschaften" und „Bedeutungen" in einem elektromagnetischen Schaltsystem ermöglicht. Das Prinzip wird wie folgt dargestellt. *Senkrechte Linien* bezeichnen verschiedene *Eigenschaften* eines bestimmten Bildmusters, jede der waagerechten Linien jeweils eine bestimmte „*Bedeutung*" des Musters (Buchstabe, Wort, Wortbedeutung, Zusammenhang). Nach dem binärdigitalen Prinzip wird mit 1 oder 0 ein Strom oder kein Strom (in einem Bild etwa hell oder dunkel eines bestimmten Punktes entsprechend) in die senkrechten Leitungen gegeben, wo sie magnetisch bestimmte *Veränderungen des Leitwertes zu den waagerechten Leitungen in der „Lernphase" des Apparates verursachen*. In der „Kannphase" kann die Matrix dann sowohl das einer bestimmten „Bedeutung" entsprechende Muster anzeigen, wie aus einem angebotenen Muster dessen „Bedeutung" bestimmen.

Für die Neurophysiologie ist interessant, daß die weitere Ausarbeitung dieser Matrizen für eine Gestalterkennung und Abstraktion bestimmter Grundformen eine *Beweglichkeit des optischen Receptorapparates* verlangt, wie er auch an den Augen der lebenden Organismen vorhanden ist und die Kontrastbildung fördert (unwillkürliche Augenunruhe und andere Augenbewegungen). Eine interessante Parallele zum lebenden Organismus ist ferner die *Selbstkorrektur* solcher Schaltungen, die mit zunehmender Zahl der Eingänge auch eine Zunahme der Kompensationsmöglichkeiten defekter Leitungen ermöglicht [S 47].

Neue Konstruktionen der Lernmatrix in Dipolschaltung, die STEINBUCH in der 3. Auflage seines Buches beschreibt, können noch weitere Modelle der Außenwelt kybernetisch realisieren. Sie können ferner Unterscheidungen zwischen wesentlichen und unwesentlichen Informationen durchführen. STEINBUCH nennt dies eine „Bewertungsschaltung", die gewissermaßen Zensuren der Information „gut" oder „schlecht" gibt.

Invarianz der Wahrnehmung als kybernetisches Problem. Die biologischen Funktionen der Sinnesverarbeitung im Nervensystem haben eine erstaunlich hohe Unabhängigkeit der Gestaltwahrnehmung von äußeren Veränderungen der Perspektive, der Variation und Abwandlung einzelner Objekte erreicht. Wir erkennen einen Tisch in der verschiedensten Projektion perspektivischer Verzerrung oder in den verschiedensten Stilarten der Gotik, des Barock und des Rokoko immer sofort als Tisch. Ein Automat kann das noch nicht. Ob Lernmatrizen auch einige Grundphänomene der Gestaltpsychologie, wie das Prägnanzerkennen unvollkommener Gestalten und die Invarianz von Gestalten aus verschiedener Perspektive apparativ imitieren können, bleibt abzuwaren. Eine technische Invarianzbildung ist heute nur in sehr unvollkommener Weise möglich und in den Berechnungen REICHARTS [R 11] und den Lernmatrizen STEINBUCHS [S 48] nur als Möglichkeit angedeutet. Bisher ist nicht bekannt, ob im Nervensystem das Gestalterkennen mit Prägnanz- und Invarianzbildung nach entsprechenden Prinzipien abläuft.

Selektion und Informationsverlust. Spezifizierung und Integration der Information. Jede Informationsverarbeitung im Organismus ist mit Auswahl- und Integrationsvorgängen verbunden. Aus dem gesamten Angebot einlaufender Sinnesmeldungen wird jeweils das für die innere und äußere Konstellation Passende und mit früher Erlerntem Zusammengehörige ausgewählt. Diese Informationsverarbeitung ist daher eng mit einer *Selektion* durch *Aufmerksamkeit, Bewußtsein und Gedächtnisvorgänge* verbunden. STEINBUCHS und FRANKS Wahrnehmungs- und Bewußtseinsschema [S 48] gibt eine klare Darstellung dieser Selektion (Abb. 33). Dort wird der gesamte Eingang von Sinnesinformationen auf eine Größe von 10^{11} bit/s geschätzt, der in den cerebralen Projektionszentren ankommende Informationsstrom auf 10^7 bit/s, die für das Bewußtsein selektionierten Wahrnehmungsprozesse dagegen nur auf 16 bit/s. Der jeweilige Informationsgewinn der mit Aufmerksamkeit ins Bewußtsein aufgenommenen spezifischen Sinnesmeldungen ist daher mit einem sehr großen Informations*verlust* für alle übrigen Sinnesmeldungen verbunden. Es handelt sich nicht nur um einen reinen Auswahlprozeß mit Ausschaltung anderer Sinnesmodalitäten, sondern auch um eine *Spezialisierung und Integration von Sinnesdaten mit multisensorischer Verarbeitung*. Dazu kommen neue Informationen aus dem *Gedächtnisspeicher* für kognitive Leistungen, die frühere Wahrnehmungen zum Wiedererkennen aktivieren.

Im kybernetischen Schema von STEINBUCH und FRANK [S 48] wird die Lernmatrix als Modell solcher „Perceptoren" und zur Definition eines abstrakten Perceptionsbegriffes verwendet. In der Auswertung der Lernmatrix würde die Einheit des identifizierten Objekts erscheinen und verschiedene Einheiten würden durch Invariantenbildung zu Klassen zusammengefaßt werden.

Beschränkung kybernetischer Hirnmodelle. Der Optimismus, der manche Techniker glauben läßt, die cerebralen Vorgänge in komplexen Neuronensystemen durch Anwendung der modernen Rechenmaschinentechnik nachahmen zu können, ist bisher nicht genügend begründet. Solche Darstellungen von „Elektronengehirnen" oder „Gehirnschaltungen" schaffen Erwartungen, die sich nicht erfüllen lassen. Sie haben wie eine schlechte Reklame der guten Sache der Kybernetik geschadet.

Vorteile der genannten unkomplizierten Modelle sind ihre *einfachen Prinzipschaltungen*. Sie entsprechen gewissen logisch-elementaren Grundlagen von Gehirnfunktionen, ohne in Einzelheiten die komplexen neuronalen Schaltungen des Gehirns nachzuahmen. WALTERS Schildkröte verwendet je *ein* Element für die Licht- und Schallrezeption, während der Organismus Millionen von Receptoren und Nervenfasern für diese Sinne besitzt. Solche Modelle beanspruchen nicht, wie zahlreiche spätere, oft sehr komplizierte Modellschaltungen für Wahrnehmung, Motorik und Gedächtnis, spezielle Neuronensysteme des Nervensystems darzustellen. Zu einem solchen komplexen Modell würden gehören: 1. ein sehr großer Aufwand an Schaltelementen, 2. eine exakte anatomisch-physiologische Kenntnis der beteiligten Neuronensysteme, die heute noch dem Neurophysiologen und erst recht dem Techniker fehlen, 3. eine genaue Korrelation der zeitlichen und räumlichen Verhältnisse von Erregungs- und Hemmungsfunktionen sowie der Reizparameter und Verbindungen der Einzelelemente in Nervensystem und Modell. Diese Bedingungen heute schon zu erfüllen, ist eine utopische Forderung.

Die meisten Nachrichtentechniker sind sich über die Unterschiede von Maschine und Gehirn im klaren. Sie wissen, daß auch die besten automatischen Rechenmaschinen kein „Elektronengehirn" sind und den Informationsgehalt, den man hineingibt, nicht vermehren oder zu neuen Ideen und Programmen entwickeln können. Diese Maschinen können Informationen speichern und ordnen, indem sie zuverlässiger und schneller rechnen als ihre Erbauer. Damit wird die Informationsmenge, die man durch die Shannonsche Theorie heute viel besser messen kann, ähnlich wie bei einem Abstraktionsprozeß vermindert. Die Leistung dieser Maschinen, die oft „artificial intelligence" genannt wird, ist *verschieden von der menschlichen Intelligenz*. Nur wer schnelles Rechnen mit Intelligenz gleichsetzen würde, könnte den Computer intelligent nennen. Das wichtigste Kriterium der Intelligenz, die Fähigkeit, *neue* Wege des Denkens zu finden, können sie nicht erfüllen. *Die Leistung dieser Maschinen ist ganz auf ihre Programmsteuerung angewiesen.* Man muß viel Intelligenz aufwenden, um ein gutes Programm für einen komplizierten Computer zu machen, und ihn damit für eine Aufgabenlösung verwenden zu können. Was dann herauskommt, sind wiederum nur bei intelligenter Anwendung brauchbare Resultate. Ohne Auswertung durch den menschlichen Geist sind diese Maschinen ebenso tot und unwirksam wie andere Speicherformen menschlicher Werke. Ein Buch muß gelesen und verstanden werden, wenn sein geistiger Gehalt wirksam werden soll, sonst ist es mit schwarzen Zeichen bedrucktes Papier. Ein Computer muß programmiert werden. Allerdings muß auch der Mensch viel lernen, um eine im Leben brauchbare Person zu werden. Vielleicht liegt darin eine gewisse Parallele mit der Programmierung von Rechenmaschinen.

Wertvolle Leistungen der modernen Rechenmaschinen sind 1. *Zeitersparnis*, 2. geordnete *Hervorhebung von einzelnen Signalen* aus einem statistisch ungeordneten Hintergrund und 3. *exaktere Simultanverarbeitung komplexer Zusammenhänge* mit weniger Fehlern. Durch schnellere Arbeit kann die Maschine in Sekunden und Minuten die mühsame Auswertung von Stunden und Jahren abkürzen. *Aber die Maschine kann nicht wesentlich mehr leisten, als ein Mensch bei größerem Zeitaufwand mit Papier und Bleistift auch sonst errechnen könnte.* Die durch den Computer ermöglichte Erfassung und Verarbeitung von Signalen hat eine entfernte Ähnlichkeit mit der intelligenten Erkennung von Wesen und Bedeutung komplexer Wahrnehmungen durch frühere Erfahrungen. Der Apparat ist aber der menschlichen Intelligenz in der Anwendungsbreite erheblich unterlegen und nur für gewisse, sehr begrenzte, Aufgaben „besser" als diese. Beispiele für solche

Spezialistenleistungen sind etwa die für bestimmte Spiele konstruierten Automaten, die ihre Erbauer im Mühle- oder Schachspielen besiegen. Wenn man aber Maschinen bauen wollte, die relativ einfache menschliche Leistungen in der Verarbeitung komplexer rasch wechselnder Situationen imitieren sollten, etwa die Führung eines Fahrzeuges im Straßenverkehr, so müßte man einen außerordentlich großen Aufwand nicht nur an Material, sondern auch an menschlicher Intelligenz hineinstecken, die dem Ergebnis nicht adäquat wäre. Die Neurone unseres Gehirns sind nicht nur viel zahlreicher als die Elemente der Rechenmaschinen, sondern auch in ihrer geordneten Leistung und ihrem Wirkungsgrad für die Verarbeitung psychischer Phänomene, mit denen es Psychologie und Psychiatrie zu tun haben, adäquater und leistungsfähiger als der beste Computer. Kurz gesagt: Natürliche menschliche Gehirne sind besser, vielseitiger, leichter und „billiger" als Rechenmaschinen, vor allem aber anpassungsfähiger an unsere Welt. Automaten sind jeweils nur für wenige Spezialaufgaben brauchbar.

Eine allgemeine Übersicht über Regelprozesse bei psychischen Vorgängen und über Parallelen kybernetischer und psychologischer Betrachtung gibt ROHRACHER [R 22]. Anwendungen der Kybernetik und ihrer Regelprinzipien auf normale und pathologische psychische Funktionen bespricht SELBACH [S 21] mit seinen schon früher entwickelten Regelvorstellungen des ZNS. SELBACH nimmt für grundlegende psychische Funktionen der Affekte, Triebe und Wahrnehmungsvorgänge Regelvorgänge mit periodischen Änderungen an. Er beschränkt solche Regulationen nicht nur auf die unbewußten Vorgänge, die Stimmung und Antrieb beeinflussen, sondern postuliert auch für die höheren, beim Menschen besonders entwickelten Leistungen bestimmte Regelvorgänge. Ausführlich diskutiert ist das Für und Wider kybernetischer Deutungen psychischer Vorgänge bei STEINBUCH [S 47]. So wertvoll STEINBUCHS Lernmatrizen als Modelle technischer Gedächtnis- und Abstraktionsvorgänge sind, so wird doch die Neurophysiologie STEINBUCHS allgemeine Konzeptionen über die physikalische Natur geistiger Vorgänge noch nicht als experimentell nachprüfbare Hypothesen annehmen können. Der Neurophysiologe wird daher noch ebenso zurückhaltend in den allgemeinen Korrelationen mit psychischen Vorgängen sein wie der Psychiater, nur aus verschiedenen Gründen. Die Psychiatrie vermißt noch praktische Anwendungen kybernetischer Vorstellungen, der Neurophysiologie fehlt die experimentelle Basis für psychophysiologische Korrelationen bei den Automaten ebenso wie bei den Versuchstieren.

Nur die Vereinfachung der Bewußtseinsfrage durch die Kybernetik bringt der Neurophysiologie einigen Nutzen. Für den Kybernetiker ist Bewußtsein gleichbedeutend mit einem aus den Gesamtinformationen abstrahierten *Modellbild der Außenwelt*. Ein solches Modell kann sowohl in Rechenmaschinen oder Automaten wie im Gehirn entwickelt werden. Wenn dies so ist, dann ergeben sich damit neue Möglichkeiten der *Quantifizierung* von Bewußtseinsvorgängen durch den Nachrichtenfluß (vgl. S. 975 u. Abb. 33). Seit CRAIK (1943) ist das Parallelmodell äußerer Vorgänge im Gehirn die leitende Vorstellung der Kybernetik [C 13].

Vereinfachung des Leib-Seele-Problems und der Bewußtseinsfrage durch die Kybernetik. Die Neurophysiologie vereinfacht – wie meist auch die Neuropsychiatrie – das Leib-Seele-Problem durch die Einengung auf eine Gehirn-Seele-

Beziehung. Die Kybernetik vereinfacht das Bewußtseinsproblem, indem sie Bewußtsein mit einem codierten *Abbild der Außenwelt* gleichsetzt. Ähnliche Bestrebungen gab es schon früher in dem philosophischen Identitätsglauben.

Die von SPINOZA bis FECHNER [F 4] durch Philosophen und Psychologen vertretene Identitätslehre, nach der theologisch Gott und Natur, philosophisch Idee und Materie, psychologisch Seele und Leib nur verschiedene Aspekte der *gleichen* Substanz seien, gewissermaßen ein „Innen" und „Außen" desselben Dinges, ist auch heute sehr verbreitet. Sie führt – vielleicht mit Ausnahme der gestaltpsychologischen Beschränkung der Isomorphielehre – zu einer wissenschaftlich nicht beweisbaren Allbeseelung, zum Hylozoismus. Die Leib-Seele-Unterscheidung wäre demnach ein Scheinproblem. Die Identitätslehre kann aber die verschiedene Differenzierung und die sehr speziellen Bedingungen der Bewußtseinsphänomene, die nur bei geordneter Hirntätigkeit erscheinen [J 37], nicht erklären.

Die Kybernetik macht sich die Lösung der Bewußtseinsfrage noch leichter, indem sie erklärt, daß Bewußtsein kein Problem, sondern Informationsverarbeitung sei. Viele Kybernetiker schreiben ihren Maschinenmodellen bei genügender Kompliziertheit eine Art „Bewußtsein" zu, wenn sie nur ein *codiertes Modellbild der Außenwelt* enthalten [W 16]. STEINBUCH [S 47] begnügt sich zunächst mit der Feststellung, daß Bewußtsein und geistige Funktionen „Aufnahme, Verarbeitung, Speicherung und Abgabe von Informationen" seien, die im Organismus nicht prinzipiell anders als in der Maschine ablaufen. Damit sei zur Klärung des Bewußtseins keine weitere Voraussetzung als eine entsprechende Kompliziertheit der Maschinen notwendig. Wenn man sie fragen könnte, würde eine solche Rechenmaschine von sich behaupten, ein Bewußtsein zu haben, sobald sie sich ein *Modell der Umwelt* erworben habe [S 47]. Dies ist eine ebenso unbeweisbare Annahme wie die des Bewußtseins von Tieren, aber auch eine viel unwahrscheinlichere.

Brauchbar wird die kybernetische Konzeption nur dann, wenn man vom subjektiven Aspekt des Bewußtseins absieht und nur den Informationswert betrachtet. Kurz gesagt, *das innere Modell oder Bild der realen Welt, das kybernetische Maschinen in ihrem speziellen Code herstellen können, bedeutet eine eigene Form der Nachrichtenverarbeitung und Speicherung, die relativ unabhängig von der Außenwelt werden kann.* Es erscheint aber nicht überzeugend, in dieser Abgelöstheit von der Außenwelt mit STEINBUCH bereits ein Kriterium des Bewußtseins zu sehen. Der Unterschied zwischen subjektivem Bewußtsein und automatischer Informationsspeicherung kann nicht nur auf den verschiedenen Standpunkt des Beobachters reduziert werden. Die Enge des Bewußtseins wird durch selektive Begrenzung des Nachrichtenflusses auf 16–20 bit/s dargestellt (Abb. 33, S. 975).

Es ist möglich, daß diese Vorstellungen für manche kybernetischen und neurophysiologischen Untersuchungen eine nützliche Vereinfachung und eine brauchbare *Arbeitshypothese* darstellen.

Für den Psychiater, Psychologen und Geisteswissenschaftler kann diese Hypothese von doppeltem *Nutzen* sein: Erstens kann sie die von dem speziellen Material der Maschine unabhängige *logische Allgemeingültigkeit* in der Natur solcher Modelle demonstrieren, zweitens kann sie die verschiedene *Entstehung* eines solchen kybernetischen Bewußtseinsmodells mit seiner *Abhängigkeit von der Außenweltinformation* bei mehr oder weniger kompliziertem und automatisiertem Bedeutungerkennen darstellen. Für den Biologen ist sie ein brauchbares Modell für das Postulat eines „quasi-Bewußtseins" der Tiere: Umweltadäquates Verhalten von Tieren in bestimmten Situationen zeigt, daß sie innere Modelle oder „Bilder" der Außenwelt besitzen und danach handeln. Dies Umweltmodell zeigt offenbar mit zunehmender Vereinfachung des Nervensystems in der absteigenden Tierreihe auch einfachere Formen, geringere Variationen und verminderten Informationsgehalt in den Hirnsystemen der einzelnen Tierklassen [B 34–39].

Mancher Forscher sieht in dieser Konzeption bereits eine geniale Vereinfachung oder eine „Lösung" des Leib-Seele-Problems. Er meint damit eine Ausschaltung unnötiger Problematik. Der Neurophysiologe, der die Kompliziertheit von Bau und Funktion des Gehirns kennt und der Psychiater, dem die außerordentliche Differenzierung seelischer Vorgänge und ihre große Nuancenbildung bewußt ist, wird diese Modellhypothese des Bewußtseins zu den so viel zitierten „schrecklichen Vereinfachungen" rechnen. Damit ist aber nicht ausgeschlossen, daß solche Simplifizierungen, so schrecklich sie zunächst erscheinen, für bestimmte Fragen doch *nützlich und brauchbar* sein können.

Bewußtsein ist wahrscheinlich *mehr* als ein Modell der Außenwelt oder ein Hilfsmittel der Orientierung. Wenigstens beim Menschen rechnen wir neben Wachheit und Orientierung zu den spezifischen Bewußtseinsphänomenen auch Ich-Bewußtsein, Besinnung und Reflexion. Diese wiederum werden angetrieben durch Affekte, Triebe und soziale Bedürfnisse als Motivationen. Bei Tieren wissen wir von einem reflexiven Ich-Bewußtsein noch weniger als von den Antrieben, dem Situationsbewußtsein und der Repräsentanz der Außenwelt, die wir aus dem Verhalten erschließen können. Auch bei den kompliziertesten Maschinen sind keinerlei Anzeichen für derartige Vorgänge erkennbar, weder für Affekte, Triebe, Motivationen, noch für Ich-Bewußtsein und Reflexion. Es ist zumindest äußerst unwahrscheinlich, daß auch der beste Automat über sich selbst und seine Reaktionen nachdenkt oder Affekte und Triebe besitzt, die ihn dazu anregen würden. Hier führt also die Vereinfachung des Bewußtseinsproblems in der Kybernetik nicht weiter. Die Verwendung kybernetischer Bewußtseinsmodelle für die Psychologie und Psychiatrie ist damit sehr begrenzt.

Ein „kybernetisches Gehirn" ist eine Utopie. Bis heute ist es für die Kybernetik eine unerreichbare Aufgabe, auch nur relativ einfache Gehirne mit einigen tausend Neuronen zu imitieren, wie sie in den Insektenganglien vorkommen. Der Bau eines Katzengehirns, um vom Menschen noch nicht zu sprechen, mit seinen vielen Millionen von Neuronen, liegt für die Technik heute in unerreichbarer Ferne. Wenn die Kybernetik also die Schaltungsvorgänge bei relativ einfach gebauten Hirnen von Tieren noch nicht nachbauen kann und wir über die „psychischen" Erlebnisse von Tieren nichts wissen und nichts wissen können, wäre es doch ein hoffnungsloses Beginnen, auch nur das Hirn eines Esels durch Schaltungen herzustellen. Warum sollte man überhaupt die immensen Kosten aufwenden, um hirnähnliche Automaten herzustellen, welche die Natur mit viel besserer Funktionsweise gewissermaßen gratis liefert?

Vorläufig sind gehirnähnliche Schaltungen der Kybernetik nur zweckvoll für Bedingungen, in denen ein lebender Organismus nicht existieren kann, z.B. bei der Raumschiffahrt. Da man diese Apparate wesentlich unempfindlicher für

Beschleunigungen, Temperaturschwankungen und Strahlenschäden machen kann als einen lebenden Organismus, bietet die Kybernetik für diese Fragen wesentliche Vorteile, obwohl sie auf kleinem Raum weit hinter den Leistungen des lebenden Gehirns zurückbleibt. Da es beim Raumschiff, ähnlich wie beim Organismus, auf Reduktion von Ausdehnung und Gewicht ankommt, sind auch in der Astronautik *Geräte mit kleinsten Schaltelementen* erforderlich. Dafür ist das menschliche Gehirn ein technisch unerreichbares Vorbild, weil es in einem Schädelraum von etwas über einem Liter mit einem Gewicht von $1^1/_2$ kg über 100 Milliarden Neurone als Schalteinheiten enthält. Hier bleibt also die Technik gegenüber dem biologischen Organismus noch zurück. Wieweit die modernen Mikroschaltungen Besseres leisten, bleibt abzuwarten. Der Natur ist es nicht nur gelungen, im lebenden Gehirn solche neuronalen Schaltungen auf kleinstem Raum zu bauen, sondern sie auch durch Fortpflanzung und Vererbung in großen Mengen zu *reproduzieren*.

Maschinen-Bewußtsein und Leib-Seele-Problem. Selbst wenn es möglich wäre, kybernetisch ein Gehirn nachzubauen, so würde dies für die somato-psychischen Zusammenhänge nicht weiterführen. Alle kybernetischen Erklärungen seelischer Phänomene haben dieselben Schwierigkeiten wie die physiologisch-biologischen Erklärungen. *Ein Maschinen-Bewußtseins-Problem ist nicht einfacher zu lösen als ein Leib-Seele-Problem.* Die subjektive Empfindung ist mit elektrischen Schaltungen ebensowenig zu verstehen, wie mit neuronalen Verbindungen. Die Informationstheorie hat die gleichen Schwierigkeiten für die Decodierung ihrer Nachrichten im Nervensystem.

Die kybernetischen Apparate zeigen nur, wie kompliziert die Konstruktion einer Maschine sein muß, wenn sie eine gehirnähnliche Informationsverarbeitung leisten soll. Dies könnte als Parallele für die Beobachtung gelten, daß *psychische Vorgänge nur als Funktion einer sehr differenzierten komplexen Organisation des Gehirns möglich sind* und bei Störungen dieser Funktion oder nach Vernichtung des Substrates ausfallen.

Nur *Identitätslehre und Isomorphismus* scheinen hier einen bequemen, aber nicht befriedigenden Ausweg aus dem Leib-Seele-Dilemma zu geben. Mit dem Isomorphismus können wir aber noch nicht verstehen, wie psychische und Sinnesqualitäten durch materielle Vorgänge entstehen. Warum wir die Wellenlänge von 600 mµ als rote Farbe sehen, ist nicht erklärbar. Dies wird sogar von extremen Vertretern der kybernetischen Bewußtseinsthese wie WEIDEL [W 16] zugegeben, die auch den Rechenmaschinen ein Bewußtsein zubilligen. Wir wissen nicht einmal, ob die subjektive Rotqualität, die andere Menschen sehen, bei gleichem Reiz dieselbe ist wie unser eigenes Rot.

Die von FECHNER [F 4], G.E. MÜLLER [M 77] bis zu METZGER [M 38] vertretene und von KÖHLER [K 31] erneut formulierte *Isomorphismus* neuronaler und psychischer Phänomene vermeidet lediglich eine Schwierigkeit der Informations-Theorie: Bei Annahme informativer Codierung und Decodierung für die Informationsübertragung im ZNS wäre eine Art „Homunculus" an der Endstätte des Informationswegs zu postulieren, der den neuronalen „Code" des Informationsflusses *dechiffriert* und in subjektive Empfindungen umsetzt. Dieser Homunculus wird nur bei Annahme einer isomorphen Repräsentation der Außenwelt im Gehirn unnötig.

Ausdruckslosigkeit und Affektleere der kybernetischen Maschine. Ein banaler, aber wenig beachteter Unterschied von Organismus und Automat ist die fehlende Ausdrucksfähigkeit der Maschinen. Im biologischen Bereich, vor allem bei den höheren Säugetieren, gibt es eine ungewöhnlich reiche Skala von Ausdrucksbewegungen und ihrer sozialen Auswertung. Bei höheren Säugern, vor allem bei Affen, ist die lebhafte Augenmotorik, Mimik und Gestik mit dem unmittelbaren Ausdruck der Affektlage auch für den Menschen erkennbar. Man darf annehmen, daß bei den Automaten nicht nur der Ausdruck von Affekten und Trieben fehlt, sondern auch diese selbst. Beides, Trieb und Affekt, sind aber für uns ein wesentlicher Teil des Seelischen, den wir auch mit den Tieren gemeinsam haben. Es gibt keinen Anhalt dafür, daß eine kybernetische Maschine etwas wie Trauer oder Freude, Sympathie oder Abneigung hat, auch wenn sie es nicht ausdrücken kann. Das bedeutet eine wesentliche Beschränkung etwaiger sozialer Kommunikationen, selbst wenn man eine solche in einer künstlichen Population von „Robotern" erzeugen wollte. Wenn schon die Bürokratie in einer komplizierten sozialen Organisation beim Menschen persönliche Sympathieregungen verdrängt, so wird man in einer Gruppe von Menschen kaum positive oder negative Affekte erwarten können. Solche Gefühls- und Triebvorgänge sind auch unabhängig von einem etwaigen Ausdrucksvermögen. Es ist weniger der mangelnde Ausdruck, der uns die Maschinen tot erscheinen läßt, als Mangel an Affektivität und Eigenantrieb. Zwar wäre es technisch denkbar, daß man dem Automaten gewisse Ausdrucksmöglichkeiten über innere Zustände gäbe, etwa sprachliche Äußerungen darüber, daß ihm zu heiß wird. Der Automat könnte dann etwa ein Magnetband einschalten, das im Lautsprecher tönt: „Mir ist warm, mir ist warm, kühlt mich ab, kühlt mich ab." Selbst wenn ein solcher Automat dann etwas über seinen Zustand aussagen könnte, würde dies noch keine Vorstufe eines Zustandsgefühles, einer Motivation oder eines Ichbewußtseins darstellen. Man könnte allerdings affektähnliche Mechanismen auch in Maschinen einbauen, doch würden diese mehr stören als nützen.

Automat und Mensch. Während STEINBUCH eine Generalisierung der Kybernetik für Maschine und lebenden Organismus anstrebt [S 47], und die gleiche physikalische Terminologie empfiehlt, sind andere Nachrichtentechniker wie KÜPFMÜLLER [K 57] vorsichtiger. Nach OPPELT steht der technische Automat zwischen Materie und lebendem Wesen [O 9]. Automaten haben, wie Organismen, Materiestruktur und Informationsverarbeitung in sich vereinigt, aber sind wahrscheinlich nicht zu echter Wahrnehmung fähig und offenbar ohne Selbstbewußtsein. Hier liegt eine *Grenze zwischen Mensch und Maschine, die einen weiteren Abstand bezeichnet als zwischen Mensch und Tier*. Tiere haben zumindest ähnliche Triebe und Affekte, die bei Automaten fehlen. Als Denkmodell für menschliches Verhalten sind Automaten insoweit brauchbar, als sie den Signalfluß und die Informationsverarbeitung der Sinnesorgane mit ihrer „Verdatung" darstellen, wie lebende Wesen auch eine Rückmeldung haben, also über prinzipiell, aber nicht strukturell ähnliche „feedback"-Mechanismen verfügen und räumliche und zeitliche Signalmuster verarbeiten. Doch überwiegen die Verschiedenheiten auch bei ähnlichen Prinzipien der Informationsverarbeitung von Organismen und Maschinen. Ich glaube nicht wie OPPELT [O 9], daß autogenes Training und Meditationsvorgänge mit solchen Automaten darstellbar sind und man für klinisch-psychiatrische Fragen aus ihrem Studium viel lernen kann. Nützlich können biokybernetische Programme vor allem für die *Quantifizierung* von Wahrnehmungs- und Lernvorgängen und für die Darstellung der Bewußtseinsselektion sein, wie sie STEINBUCH und FRANCK abgebildet haben (Abb. 33, S. 875).

Vorteile, Nachteile und Grenzen der Kybernetik

Zweifellos bedeuten kybernetische Methoden im weitesten Sinne durch Systematisierung der wissenschaftlichen Information und durch Beschleunigung der Datenverarbeitung einen großen Fortschritt und eine wertvolle Hilfe für die Forschung. Die Kybernetik ist mit diesen nützlichen Leistungen vorwiegend eine *Hilfsmethode* verschiedener Wissenschaften. Ihre allgemeine Gültigkeit bleibt beschränkt. Die Technik kann der Biologie nicht helfen, wenn sie in der Entwicklung von Rechenmaschinen nur einen Selbstzweck sieht. Die Computerapparate haben ihre eigenen technischen Gesetzmäßigkeiten.

Nutzen der Kybernetik für die Biologie. Kybernetik und Informationstheorie können für die Neurophysiologie dann von Nutzen sein, wenn sie eine *mathematische Behandlung* ihrer Resultate ermöglichen. Für eine solche mathematische Bearbeitung fehlen uns aber noch die entsprechenden exakten neurophysiologischen Grundlagen. Selbst für einfache Vorgänge wie die laterale Hemmung der visuellen Neurone ist die mathematische Bearbeitung sehr kompliziert. Darum bleiben die kybernetischen und informationstheoretischen Ansätze der Neurophysiologie zunächst mathematisch noch ungenutzt.

Brauchbarkeit einfacher Neuronmodelle. Es ist bereits ein erheblicher technisch-physikalischer Aufwand mit zahlreichen mathematischen Formeln notwendig, um ein elektrophysikalisches Modell einfacher biologischer Strukturen herzustellen, wie HODGKIN und HUXLEYS Modell der Zellmembran einer Nervenfaser des Tintenfisches [H 73]. Wenn man diesen großen Aufwand für eine Nervenfaser ohne Synapse bedenkt, so scheint es nicht sehr hoffnungsvoll, die vielen Milliarden, in sehr komplexen Synapsenschaltungen miteinander verbundenen Neurone unseres Gehirns mathematisch und physikalisch zu erfassen, selbst wenn man die Einzelneurone mit vereinfachten Schaltelementen darstellt.

Für den Neurophysiologen ergibt sich die weitere Schwierigkeit, daß unsere anatomischen und physiologischen Kenntnisse über neuronale Schaltungen im Gehirn noch sehr unvollkommen sind, und daß in den bisherigen Modellen zahlreiche Vereinfachungen und Schematisierungen vorgenommen wurden, um sie verständlich zu machen. *Daher sind alle unsere „einfachen" Neuronenschemata* z.B. über das visuelle System (Abb. 23), die Koordination der Augenbewegungen (Abb. 11) oder die Körpermotorik (Abb. 7) *mehr oder weniger „falsch" und unvollständig*. Alle diese Schemata erfüllen zunächst nur didaktische Zwecke der *Veranschaulichung einfacher Ordnungen* mit neuronalen Regelkreisen und Serienschaltungen der Elemente.

Das biologische Prinzip der Parallelschaltung Tausender von Receptoren und Fasern ist damit ebensowenig darzustellen wie in kybernetischen Modellen. Die Schemata geben aber einige Hinweise auf die strenge *Ordnung cerebraler Neuronenschaltungen*. Sie zeigen, daß eine rein statistische Behandlung der Hirnelemente nicht die allgemeinen Gesetze des Gehirns oder bestimmter Hirnteile aufklären kann, wie dies etwa für die ungeordneten Molekülhaufen von Gasen durch den Physiker BOLTZMANN mit Erfolg durchgeführt wurde. Die biologischen Gesetze der Neuronenkoordination wären eher mit *Strukturformeln* für chemische Reaktionen zu vergleichen, die es erlauben, mit Papier und Bleistift neue Verbindungen als Übergänge einer molekularen Ordnung in eine andere darzustellen und vorauszusagen. Die Grenzen dieser Methoden in der makromolekularen Chemie der Eiweißkörper mit ihren Ketten Tausender von Aminosäuren sind evident und geben uns Hinweise für entsprechende Grenzen kybernetischer Modelle des Gehirns. *Kybernetische Modelle können dann von großem Nutzen sein, wenn sie wie chemische Strukturformeln anschauliche Bilder oder praktisch brauchbare Hypothesen über Zusammenhänge und Reaktionen geben, mit denen man Voraussagen über Neuronenkoordinationen machen kann, die experimentell prüfbar sind.*

Allerdings muß man sich klarmachen, daß ein naturwissenschaftlich exaktes Verständnis der Interaktion neuronaler Systeme letztlich nur durch sehr *abstrakte Vereinfachungen auf mathematischer Grundlage* möglich sein wird. Bis jetzt haben die Mathematiker aber den Neurophysiologen noch keine allgemein befriedigende Adaptation mathematischer Theorien für neuronale Systeme liefern können. Durch die Informationstheorie sind jedoch Techniker und physikalisch-mathematische Grundlagenforscher auf biologische Probleme aufmerksam gemacht worden. Es ist wahrscheinlich eine Frage der Zeit, bis es gelingt, einige Teilgebiete der neuronalen Funktionskomplexe in mathematischen Formulierungen zusammenzufassen. Der experimentelle Biologe muß sich vielleicht darauf einrichten, ähnlich wie der Experimentalphysiker, ohne anschauliche Vergegenwärtigung des erforschten Objekts nur die Position eines Kontrollorgans mit messender Funktion zu übernehmen. Die Neuropsychiatrie kann für manche Probleme der Hirnpathologie, wie die *Aphasie- und Agnosieforschung,* einigen Nutzen aus Fragestellungen der Informationstheorie, der Regeltechnik und der Linguistik ziehen.

Verzicht auf Anschaulichkeit in der Kybernetik. Ein wesentlicher Unterschied zwischen der klassischen Physiologie und der modernen Kybernetik liegt weniger in der technisch-mathematischen Methodik kybernetischer Modelle, als in dem kybernetischen *Verzicht auf Anschaulichkeit.* Darin unterscheiden sich die errechneten Ergebnisse der Kybernetik auch von den anschaulichen Modellen v. Holstscher Regelmechanismen. Die modernen mathematischen Methoden führen in der kybernetischen Physiologie, ähnlich wie in der theoretischen Physik notwendig zu unanschaulichen Berechnungen, deren Ergebnisse nicht mehr psychologisch verstehbar sind. Erklärende Methoden und Ergebnisse der Physiologie waren bisher meistens anschaulich und damit auch für komplexe Funktionen des Nervensystems verständlich. Wieweit die moderne Physiologie mit der zunehmenden Anwendung mathematisch-technischer Methoden und Automaten bei der Analyse komplizierter Prozesse des Gehirns diesen Bereich der Anschaulichkeit verlassen muß, wird die Zukunft zeigen. Vielleicht müssen die in der anschaulichen Forschung erzogenen und an bildmäßig darstellbare Ereignisse gewöhnten Neurophysiologen diese grundsätzlich andere kybernetisch-rechnerische Betrachtungsweise einer jüngeren Generation überlassen.

Vorteile und Nutzungsgrenzen der Rechenmaschinen. Ein rein *methodischer Nutzen* für die Biologie liegt in der Verwendung von elektronischen Rechenmaschinen für die Auswertung physiologischer Experimente.

Die vorteilhaften Leistungen von Computer-Apparaten sind:

1. Zeitersparnis für die Auswertung von Daten,
2. erheblich vermehrte Kapazität in der Bearbeitung großer Zahlenmengen,
3. geringere Fehlerwahrscheinlichkeit bei komplizierten Rechnungen.

Rechenmaschinen und andere kybernetische Apparaturen sind in der Schnelligkeit und Kapazität der Datenverarbeitung dem menschlichen Gehirn überlegen. Doch sind sie den Leistungen unseres Gehirns hoffnungslos unterlegen bei allen Arbeiten, die Urteil und höhere Intelligenz erfordern. Darum ist das für die Forschung heute so dringliche Problem einer Literaturverarbeitung und Informationsordnung der in fast geometrischer Progression zunehmenden wissenschaftlichen Publikationen kaum durch technische Methoden zu lösen. Die Maschine kann vielleicht schematisch dargestellte Ergebnisse ordnen und vergleichen, aber sie kann sie noch *nicht bewerten*. Neue Entwicklungen der Lernmatrizen STEINBUCHs erstreben allerdings auch maschinelle Bewertungen (vgl. S. 864). Diese sind aber von echten Werturteilen noch weit entfernt.

Die Beurteilung, ob eine Arbeit gut oder schlecht, zuverlässig oder zweifelhaft und nach Methode und Persönlichkeit des Forschers unsicher ist, bleibt eine Sache menschlicher Erfahrung und eine geistige Leistung. Die Bemühung um solche Urteile können wir nicht an Rechenmaschinen abgeben. Auch wenn uns diese Maschinen manche Routinearbeit in der Auswertung von Experimenten abnehmen können und dem menschlichen Gehirn Zeit für produktivere Arbeit ersparen, so bleibt die Notwendigkeit, unser in seiner Leistung begrenztes Gehirn für Aufnahme, Verständnis und Wertung wissenschaftlicher Informationen zu verwenden.

Die Maschinen werden uns sehr bald mehr Daten liefern, als wir geistig verarbeiten können. Eine solche Überfülle unverstandener Daten und Ergebnisse kann trotz guter Sortierungsarbeit der Forschung nur wenig nützen. Verständnis und objektives Urteil werden uns die Rechenmaschinen kaum erleichtern. Auch der moderne Forscher muß die Mühe des Begriffs und das Risiko der Bewertung auf sich nehmen: Die damit verbundenen Nachteile subjektiver Voreingenommenheit, affektiver Beschränkung und erworbener Vorurteile, mit denen die menschliche Tätigkeit belastet ist, sind mit in Kauf zu nehmen. Solche subjektiven Begrenzungen werden unsere geistige Freiheit weniger einengen als kybernetische Postulate, die als Wertbestimmungen mißverstanden oder als gültige Wahrheiten angenommen werden.

Begrenzte Anwendung technischer Automaten. Zwei Arten von Apparaten der Technik und Kybernetik sind zu unterscheiden: *a) Automaten,* die von der Technik für Funktionen entwickelt wurden, die biologischen Leistungen ähnlich sind, ohne den Anspruch einer Nachahmung dieser physiologischen Funktionen zu machen und *b) Modelle,* die diese biologischen Funktionen imitieren („simulieren" nach dem technischen Sprachgebrauch). Bei den komplizierten Automaten und Modellen handelt es sich nicht nur um die einmalige Registrierung eines Bildes, die technisch auf einfache Weise möglich ist, sondern um die *Auswertung* von Bildern und komplexen Vorgängen. Hier hat auch die Zuverlässigkeit, Sicherheit und Leistungsfähigkeit der Maschinen ihre Grenzen. *Die Leistungsfähigkeit der Automaten ist auf ein sehr enges Gebiet begrenzt.* Die Leistungen der Organismen sind zwar auch an bestimmte Umwelten angepaßt, umfassen aber einen sehr viel größeren Bereich dieser Umwelt.

Die Automatentechnik ist für den Forscher nur eine wertvolle Hilfe zur Erleichterung und Beschleunigung der wissenschaftlichen Arbeit. Wenn in der Raumschiffahrt etwa ein genaues Bild der anderen Mondseite oder der Oberfläche eines Planeten gewonnen und übermittelt werden soll, so macht dies eine photographische Kamera und eine Fernsehübertragung besser und zuverlässiger als menschliche Augen und Gehirne, die auf die Wahrnehmung bewegter und dauernd veränderter Umwelt eingestellt und im Weltraum nicht lebensfähig sind. Wenn es auf die Messung magnetischer Felder ankommt, so können nur Apparate und automatische Auswertungsgeräte verwendet werden, da der Organismus kein Sinnesorgan für magnetische Wellen hat. Wenn die optische Aufnahme und Auswertung bewegter und dauernd veränderter Objekte erforderlich ist, so baut die Fernsehtechnik Apparaturen, die dem menschlichen Auge bewegte Bilder vorführen können. Solche Apparate erscheinen kompliziert und benötigen viel Raum. Dennoch sind sie äußerst einfach im Vergleich zum menschlichen Gehirn, das auf kleinstem Raum Milliarden von Schaltelementen enthält.

Schwierigkeiten biologischer Anwendungen der Regeltechnik. Obwohl biologische Systeme ähnliche Regel- und Steuerungsvorgänge zeigen, wie die technisch-mathematischen Modelle, ist es bereits bei den maschinenartig reagierenden Insekten mit einfacher gebautem Nervensystem schwierig, ihre Reaktionen durch technische Schaltungen oder mathematische Gleichungen nachzubilden. MITTELSTAEDT [M 48] hat bei Besprechung von Regeltheorie und Verhaltensanalyse 1961 betont, daß auch die beste Imitation eines biologischen Prozesses durch technische Modelle und mathematische Gleichungssysteme den Verhaltensforscher nicht zufriedenstellen kann.

Die Höchstleistungen des Gehirns der Säugetiere und des Menschen mit ihrer differenzierten Struktur und Funktion sind die erstaunlichsten Erfindungen der Naturentwicklung. Diese lebenden Naturwunder sind von der Technik noch unerreicht und können nicht durch Maschinen imitiert werden. Doch bleibt das Gehirn an bestimmte Bedingungen des organischen Lebens und der Stoffwechselvorgänge gebunden, von denen wiederum die Maschine unabhängig ist.

Die Regelvorgänge der Organismen werden auch seit dem Erscheinen von WIENERS „Kybernetik" mit rein *biologischen Methoden* und *physiologischen Fragestellungen* erforscht. Sonst führt die kybernetische Technik der „Biosimulation" nur auf biologische Abwege. Ihr Anspruch, lebendige Vorgänge im Nervensystem zu imitieren oder wie die Amerikaner sagen, zu „simulieren", wird dann zu dem, was wir in der Medizin Simulation nennen: Zur Vortäuschung von nicht vorhandenen Symptomen einer Krankheit.

Das beste moderne Beispiel kybernetischer Regelkreise, die Gammaregulation der Muskelspindeln, ist nicht durch regeltechnische Postulate, sondern durch *neurophysiologische Experimente* entdeckt und erforscht worden [G 33, S 37]. Die Einordnung in das Regelprinzip erfolgte später, nachdem gewisse Postulate der Kybernetiker als nicht zutreffend korrigiert wurden. VON HOLSTs Modellschema der Reafferenz (Abb. 17) wurde auf rein biologischer Grundlage gedanklich entwickelt und gab ein zutreffenderes Bild der sensomotorischen Koordination als kybernetische Konstruktionen.

So *wertvoll diese Modellvorstellungen als Arbeitshypothesen sein können, so wenig dürfen sie zu technischen Dogmen für die Physiologie werden.* Wie jede andere Hypothese müssen sie jeweils mit der Entdeckung neuer Befunde und Gesetzmäßigkeiten verändert und an die derzeitigen Ergebnisse der Wissenschaft angepaßt werden. Kybernetische Modelle sind für den Physiologen nichts anderes als vereinfachende *Schemata, die ein physiologisches Experiment vorbereiten. Ob sie brauchbar sind, zeigt erst der Versuch am lebenden Organismus.* Ob solche kybernetischen Schemata allgemein gültig sind, kann erst durch Synthese zahlreicher physiologischer Versuchsergebnisse mit der Verhaltensbeobachtung und mit psychologischen Erkenntnissen wahrscheinlich gemacht werden.

Grenzen technisch-mathematischer Kybernetik. Wie alle Modelle biologischer Vorgänge entsprechen kybernetische Apparaturen für praktische Zwecke vereinfachten Hypothesen über spezielle Funktionen, die gewisse neuronale Regulationsvorgänge darstellen und anschaulich machen sollen. *Sie haben gegenüber anderen allgemeinen Hypothesen den Vorteil, daß man mit ihnen besser experimentieren und in Formeln rechnen kann.* Kybernetische Modelle sind exakter prüfbar als verbale Hypothesen. Sie haben gezeigt, daß es bei Hirnmodellen weniger auf materielle und energetische Parallelen als auf bestimmte *Informationsbeziehungen* ankommt.

Eine Gefahr der technischen Kybernetik liegt darin, daß man die Unterschiede von Modell und biologischer Struktur vergißt und eine mathematische Biophysik von Utopien treibt, die mit dem lebenden Organismus nichts mehr zu tun hat. Die meisten mathematischen Theorien des Nervensystems, die in den biophysikalischen Veröffentlichungen über Computermodelle seit 1950 erschienen sind, blieben biologisch und physiologisch wertlos.

Dieses *Versagen* der ersten mathematischen Kybernetik beruht erstens auf der *Unbrauchbarkeit des digitalen Prinzips in der Neurophysiologie,* zweitens auf *quantitativen Differenzen von Rechenmaschine und Gehirn,* und drittens auf der *unterschiedlichen Einstellung von Technikern und Biologen.*

Manche vereinfachten Formulierungen der Nachrichtentechnik müssen die Kritik nicht nur des Neurophysiologen, sondern auch des Psychologen hervorrufen. Ein Beispiel mag das zeigen:

„Was wir an geistigen Funktionen beobachten, sind Aufnahme, Verarbeitung, Speicherung und Abgabe von Informationen. Auf gar keinen Fall scheint es mir wahrscheinlich oder gar bewiesen, daß zur Erklärung geistiger Funktionen irgendwelche Voraussetzungen gemacht werden müssen, welche über die normale Physik hinausgehen" [S 47].

Diese von STEINBUCH in „Automat und Mensch" vertretene These erscheint dem Physiologen angreifbar, weil nicht einmal die komplexen chemischen Vorgänge des Organismus Berücksichtigung finden, und sind dem Psychologen verdächtig, weil die hochintegrierten seelischen Funktionen mit physikalischen Methoden nicht untersucht werden können. Die Schwäche einer solchen rein physikalischen Erklärung vitaler und psychischer Prozesse wird deutlich, wenn man sie nach dem Schichtenprinzip betrachtet (vgl. S. 767 und Abb. 1).

KEIDEL hat die Grenzen der Regelungslehre in der Biologie zusammenfassend behandelt [K 11]. Er übernimmt die Gesetze der Regeltechnik uneingeschränkt nur für die vegetativen Funktionen und die niedere Motorik. KEIDEL warnt ebenso wie SHANNON selbst und QUASTLER [Q 1] vor einer zu weiten Ausdehnung der Informationstheorie auf den Menschen. Er sieht die Grenzen ihrer Anwendung in der Welt menschlicher Werte, in den Qualitäten des Seelischen sowie in individuellen Besonderheiten der Persönlichkeit, die nicht informationstheoretisch erfaßt werden können.

Es kann der Kybernetik nur schaden, wenn sie sich in der Hierarchie der Wissenschaften auf eine zu hohe Stufe stellt und eine Führungsrolle beansprucht. Man kann sie auch nicht als Synthese der Fachwissenschaften bezeichnen. Die Kybernetik ist nicht die Königin, sondern die *Dienerin der anderen Wissenschaften*. Man könnte sie auch eine *Dolmetscherin* nennen, die Informationen aus den verschiedenen Sprachen der Einzelwissenschaften übermittelt. Als solche kann sie eine nützliche *Vermittlerrolle* spielen.

Rechenmaschine und Gehirnleistungsfähigkeit. Der lebende Organismus ist zwar gegenüber den kybernetischen Maschinen durch kompliziertere und langsamere Erregungen und Leitungsvorgänge der biologischen Membranen benachteiligt. Aber unser Gehirn kann diesen Zeitverlust durch größere Zahlen und geringeren Raumbedarf der Nervenzellen, sowie durch vielseitige und komplexere Leistungen seines Neuronenapparates wettmachen. Die Leistungen der Rechenmaschinen werden daher vom Gehirn durch Vielseitigkeit und bessere Anpassung an eine variable Umwelt übertroffen.

Die moderne Technik macht uns Hoffnung, daß mit Vervollkommnung der Schaltungen auf kleinstem Raum auch der bisherige große Aufwand an Umfang und Gewicht dieser Maschinen verkleinert würde, und daß mit den modernsten Mikromethoden Schaltelemente auf Bruchteile von Millimetern kombiniert werden könnten, die den geringen Größenordnungen der Nervenzellen nahe kommen. Man fragt sich aber: Lohnt sich ein solcher Aufwand für einen cerebralen Homunculus? Macht es die Natur nicht besser und billiger? Offenbar wäre es ein hoffnungsloses Beginnen und ein ungerechtfertigter Kostenaufwand, einen kybernetischen Roboter mit Milliarden von Schaltelementen herzustellen, der ähnliche Leistungen wie die 100 Milliarden Nervenzellen des Gehirns vollbringen soll. Die zu erwartenden Reparaturen und die Störungssuche in solchen elektronischen Gehirnen wäre noch schwieriger und würde wiederum viele intelligente, geduldige und spezialisierte menschliche Gehirne benötigen.

Jeder weiß, daß auf dem natürlichen Wege der biologischen Fortpflanzung durch die Befruchtung einer einzigen Eizelle im mütterlichen Organismus ein normales leistungsfähiges Gehirn heranwächst, das bessere und originellere Kombinationen macht als ein Computer. Ferner ist klar, daß beim Menschen Belehrung und Erziehung wesentlich vollkommnere und vielseitigere Intelligenzleistungen fördern können als Programmierungen der Rechenmaschinen, die nur wenige einseitig spezialisierte Funktionen haben. Daher erscheinen die Bestrebungen mancher kybernetischer Techniker, mit riesigen Kosten gehirnähnliche Großautomaten zu produzieren, weder von der theoretischen noch von der praktischen Seite her berechtigt. Sie wären höchstens für extreme Bedingungen gerechtfertigt, in denen ein Mensch nicht leben kann, etwa für die interstellare Raumschiffahrt.

Die Überlegenheit der lebendigen Sinneswahrnehmung und ihrer Informationscodierung über die künstlichen Systeme der Nachrichtenübertragung und Kybernetik kann ich nicht besser ausdrücken als mit Worten, die HELMHOLTZ schon vor über 100 Jahren verwendet hat [H 28]. In seinem Vortrag über die Theorie des Sehens 1868 hat HELMHOLTZ schon manche modernen Prinzipien der Informationscodierung klar gesehen. Obwohl er die Zahl der Opticusfasern noch um das Vierfache zu klein schätzt [B 67], hat er die Reichhaltigkeit unserer Sinneswahrnehmung im Vergleich zur Schriftsprache eindrucksvoll geschildert:

„Die elementaren Zeichen unserer Sprache sind nur 24 Buchstaben, und wie außerordentlich mannigfaltigen Sinn können wir durch deren Combination ausdrücken und einander mittheilen! Nun bedenke man im Vergleich damit den ungeheuren Reichthum der elementaren Zeichen, die der Sehnervenapparat geben kann. Man kann die Zahl der Sehnervenfasern auf 250000 schätzen. Jede derselben ist unzählig vieler verschiedener Grade der Empfindungen von einer oder drei verschiedenen Grundfarben fähig. Dadurch ist natürlich ein unendlich viel reicheres System von Combinationen herzustellen, als mit den wenigen Buchstaben, wozu dann noch die Möglichkeit schnellsten Wechsels in den Bildern des Gesichtes kommt. So dürfen wir uns nicht wundern, wenn die Sprache unserer Sinne uns so außerordentlich viel feiner abgestufte und reicher individualisierte Nachrichten zuführt, als die der Worte."

Solange man noch nicht weiß, ob im lebenden Organismus den kybernetischen Modellen ähnliche Strukturen und Verbindungen überhaupt existieren, hat es wenig Sinn, schon vorzeitige Lösungen anzugeben. TEUBER [T 2a] hat diese Situation noch treffender formuliert: *Die Kybernetik will bereits Antworten auf etwas geben, für das die Biologie noch keine präzisen Fragen formuliert hat.* Es ist klar, daß solche vorfabrizierten Antworten auf unformulierte Fragen auch in die Irre führen können.

Niemand kann wissen und voraussagen, welche neuen Methoden und technischen Hilfsmittel die Forschung noch entwickeln wird. Viele skeptische Prognosen für die Wissenschaft sind durch neue Entdeckungen rasch widerlegt worden. Es ist eine mißliche Sache, in der Naturwissenschaft endgültige Grenzen der Erkenntnis zu behaupten; denn heute Unmögliches kann morgen durch eine methodische Neuerung erreicht sein. Jetzt noch unübersteigbar scheinende Grenzen können wenige Jahre später verschwunden sein.

Unsere kritische Besinnung auf Grenzen kybernetischer Methoden in der Biologie soll kein skeptisches Ignorabimus aussprechen. Sie soll nur die *zentrale Stellung des physiologischen Experiments in der Erforschung biologischer Regelmechanismen* betonen und auf die Schwierigkeiten einer rein technischen Betrachtung in der Biologie hinweisen. Kybernetische Vorstellungen und Methoden der Kommunikationsforschung können dem physiologischen Experiment und der klinischen Praxis eine wertvolle Hilfe sein. Doch sollten übertriebene Erwartungen korrigiert und auf ihr richtiges Maß zurückgeführt werden. Die Ordnungen des organismischen Lebens können durch die Rechenmaschinentechnik allein nicht erklärt oder ersetzt werden. Wir müssen wissen, wie schwierig, unzweckmäßig und teuer es wäre, die für ihre Umwelt optimal angepaßten lebenden Organismen durch technische Konstruktionen zu ersetzen.

Zusammenfassung

Nachrichtentechnik, Regeltechnik und Informationstheorie ergänzen als *Biokybernetik* die Erforschung des Nervensystems. Technische Automaten und Rechenmaschinen sind allgemeine *Modelle für Regelung und Steuerung im Nervensystem,* aber ihre Mechanismen sind sehr verschieden von der Gehirntätigkeit. Die Meßeinheit der Information *bit* (Nachrichtenmenge als Zahl von Ja-Nein-Entscheidungen) ermöglicht quantitative Messungen des Nachrichtenflusses und Wahrnehmungsgehaltes auch im lebenden Organismus. Computermodelle der Gehirnfunktionen, Maschinen mit durch Receptoren gesteuerten Bewegungen und lernende Automaten können mit sensomotorischen Regelungen und logischen Denkprozessen verglichen werden, sind aber keine „Elektronengehirne". Vorteile und Nutzungsgrenzen der Rechenmaschinen und Grenzen der Kybernetik mit ihren Anwendungen für die Bewußtseinsselektion und Leib-Seele-Probleme werden besprochen. Regelungen durch negative Rückmeldung und Aktivierung durch positive Rückkoppelung gibt es sowohl bei Maschinen wie im lebenden Organismus. Das lebende Gehirn arbeitet mit seinen Neuronen zwar langsamer als elektronische Rechenmaschinen, aber die cerebrale Ordnung ist komplizierter und übertrifft durch Vielseitigkeit und bessere Anpassung an eine variable Umwelt auch die besten Computer.

Kybernetische Ansätze sind nur biologisch brauchbar, wenn sie Antworten auf präzise neurophysiologische Fragen geben. Erst das physiologische Experiment kann über die Brauchbarkeit biokybernetischer Modelle entscheiden.

VII. Neurophysiologische Grundlagen der Hirnlokalisation und klinischen Hirnpathologie

> "A great part part of our clinical knowledge is nothing else than anatomical and physiological; pathology is only the third element of a clinical problem ... To locate a lesion in any centre is an anatomical proceeding. All about nervous discharges, the amounts and rates of those discharges and the degrees of resistance encountered by nerve impulses in cases of diseases of the nervous system is as much abnormal physiology as consideration of these things in healthy people is normal physiology ... The pathological process (abnormal nutrition) is that which, directly or indirectly, *leads* to abnormal functional (that is, abnormal physiological) states."
>
> J.H. JACKSON: On post-epileptic states. A contribution to the comparative study of insanities, 1888/89.

Bei der Hirnlokalisation berühren sich Anatomie und Physiologie mit ihren Methoden besonders eng. Manche physiologischen Methoden dienen einer anatomischen Lokalisation. Das gilt für die cerebralen Reizversuche seit FRITSCH und HITZIG (1870) bis zu den modernen stereotaktischen Methoden. Neben der seit über 100 Jahren verwendeten elektrischen Reizung sind auch die neueren

Registrierungen cerebraler Aktionspotentiale nach lokalisierten peripheren Reizen (evoked potentials) in erster Linie zur anatomischen Lokalisation ausgewertet worden. Physiologisch brauchbare Ergebnisse haben die Ableitungen mit Mikroelektroden gebracht, die nach peripheren Reizen eine weite Ausbreitung und eindrucksvolle Konvergenz verschiedener Sinnesmodalitäten gezeigt haben [J 59]. Nachdem die Konvergenz an einzelnen corticalen Neuronen bereits im Motorik-Kapitel dargestellt wurde, bespreche ich im folgenden allgemeine Fragen der Hirnlokalisation und der klinischen Hirnpathologie.

Die spezifisch menschlichen Leistungen des Sprechens, der geplanten Handlungen, der Werkzeugherstellung und der symbolischen Zeichenerkennung von Schrift und Sprache sind in ihren zentralen Mechanismen noch zu wenig mit neurophysiologischen Methoden untersucht. Außer einigen Innervationsstudien über das Sprechen sind die neuronalen Grundlagen dieser Leistungen im Gehirn noch unbekannt. Lediglich neurologische Erfahrungen bei Herderkrankungen des Großhirns geben einige Hinweise für die Lokalisation der corticalen Zentren dieser differenzierten Funktionen. Wenn man bedenkt, wie komplex bereits die neuronalen Schaltungen einfacher motorischer Leistungen der Augenmotorik oder des Ganges sind, die in Kapitel V besprochen wurden, erscheint es zunächst wenig aussichtsreich, schon heute die neuronalen Grundlagen des Sprechens, Erkennens und Handelns zu untersuchen. Im folgenden sollen einige physiologische Grundlagen der hirnpathologischen Forschung auf Grund von *Tierexperimenten* besprochen werden, insbesondere die Aufklärung der Balkenfunktion. Ferner werden einige Ergebnisse der Cortexreizungen PENFIELDS mit ihren psychischen Korrelationen beim Menschen dargestellt. Es ist zu hoffen, daß kybernetische Methoden der automatischen Zeichenerkennung und der Informationstheorie einige logische Grundprinzipien entwickeln werden, die später eine exaktere neurophysiologische Untersuchung der Aphasien, Agnosien und apraktischen Syndrome ermöglichen.

Neurophysiologie und Hirnlokalisation

Die Schwäche der alten Hirnanatomie und Hirnpathologie liegt in ihrem Mangel an physiologischer Korrelation und funktioneller Begründung. Ihre Forschung beschränkte sich auf morphologische Befunde. Die Lehre der Hirnarchitektonik von den Rindenfeldern als einzelnen „Organen" blieb ein hypothetisches Postulat. Selbst da, wo die architektonische Begrenzung durch Reizversuche begründet wurde, wie bei VOGT [V 10] und FULTON [F 34], handelte es sich nicht um echte Funktionsanalysen, sondern um unphysiologische elektrische Reize. Bei physiologischer Analyse von Sinnesreizen und evoked potentials oder Neuronableitungen aus der Hirnrinde sieht die Verteilung der Sinnesmodalitäten wesentlich anders aus als in der Architektonik der primären Sinnesfelder. Es zeigt sich eine viel weitere Ausbreitung der afferenten Impulse aus den einzelnen Projektionsfeldern und damit auch eine Konvergenz verschiedener Sinnesmodalitäten [J 59]. Bisher sind nur die einfachsten corticalen Funktionen des Sehsystems [H 87, J 39] und der motorischen Rinde [J 11] in ihren neuronalen Mechanismen aus dem Tierversuch bekannt. Eine Analyse differenzierter corticaler Leistungen beim Menschen wie Sprechen und Lesen ist noch nicht möglich.

Erregungsbegrenzung und neuronale Ordnung als Basis der Hirnlokalisation.
Die Notwendigkeit einer Erregungsbegrenzung im Nervensystem ist auch die physiologische Grundlage des Lokalisationsprinzips [J 31]. Volle Aktivität ist im Gehirn nur sinnvoll, wenn sie wenige *Teile* in einer geregelten *Ordnung* betrifft. Das Alles-oder-Nichts-Gesetz gilt nur für die kleinsten neuronalen Einheiten innerhalb solcher Teilabschnitte des ZNS, aber es betrifft nicht diese Hirnteile selbst, weder Rindenfelder noch Kerne. Erst recht gilt es nicht für das ganze Gehirn. Totale aktive Erregung würde einen epileptischen Anfall und völlige Erschöpfung zur Folge haben. In der Ordnung des Nervensystems beschränken sich die Erregungsvorgänge in ökonomischer Weise. Bei allen geordneten Hirnfunktionen, seien es Instinkt- oder Lernprozesse, wird diffuse Irradiation mit zunehmender Übung auf selektive und zweckmäßige *Teilaktivierung* begrenzt.

Daß die Erregungen im Nervensystem sich nicht unbegrenzt ausbreiten können, sondern mit bestimmter Ordnung und zeitlicher Abfolge in verschalteten neuronalen Mustern ablaufen müssen, ergibt sich aus allen physiologischen Erfahrungen. Die Untersuchung der elementaren Synapsenfunktionen, die Hemmungsvorgänge an einzelnen Neuronen und einfachen Reflexen und die kompliziertesten neuronalen Koordinationsvorgänge zeigen eine solche Erregungsbegrenzung. Die geordnete Funktion des Nervensystems verlangt eine zeitliche und eine räumlich-lokalisatorische Erregungsbeschränkung. Innerhalb der morphologischen Struktur und ihrer relativ festen zentralen Ordnung sind die verschiedensten Schaltungen möglich. Die zahlreichen Kombinationen, die sich aus Millionen von Neuronen als Einzelelemente ergeben, ermöglichen wiederum neue Konstellationen der neuronalen Erregung und Hemmung, wie sie bei Lernprozessen oder den spontanen Leistungen einsichtiger Verhaltensweisen und der Intelligenz zu fordern sind. Alle nicht-lokalisierten, sich grenzenlos auf das ganze Gehirn ausbreitenden ungehemmten Erregungen sind pathologische Vorgänge epileptischer Entladung. Die normale neuronale Ordnung zeigt neben Integration und Konvergenz ein Überwiegen von *Hemmungsvorgängen*.

Psychologisch zeigen *Aufmerksamkeit* und *Bewußtsein* eine entsprechende Begrenzung und Selektion. Bewußtsein ist eine sinnvolle Auswahlfunktion für begrenzte Erlebnisinhalte (S. 971, Abb. 32 u. 33). Die *Enge des Bewußtseins* beschränkt sich notwendig auf Ausschnitte des seelischen Gesamts in einer bestimmten Ordnung. *Ordnung verlangt Beschränkung*. Wie die physiologische Koordination der Sensomotorik nur bestimmte, der Situation adäquate Erregungsmuster aktiviert und andere hemmt, so sind geordnete psychische Abläufe nur durch Begrenzung auf bestimmte jeweils aktuelle Bewußtseinsinhalte mit Hemmung möglich. In dieser Begrenzung mit gegenseitiger Hemmung liegt der physiologische Sinn aller Lokalisationslehren. Im *Wettstreit verschiedener Erregungsvorgänge* wird jeweils die aktuelle und zweckmäßige neuronale Kombination gefördert, alle anderen werden gehemmt.

Wenn nicht jeweils nur wenige Neuronensysteme die Führung übernähmen, würde ein allgemeines Chaos durcheinanderlaufender Erregungen entstehen. Adäquates Verhalten und Bewußtsein ist offenbar nur möglich durch *geordnete Auswahl, Lokalisation und Koordination der neuronalen Prozesse im Gehirn*.

Pawlow [P 4] hat 1926 ein gutes neurophysiologisches Bild für die Selektionsfunktion des Gehirns und die wechselnde Lokalisation von Bewußtseinsvorgängen gegeben. Wenn das Gehirn durch die Schädelkapsel sichtbar und die bewußtseinsregulierte Aktivität als Helligkeit erkennbar wäre, so würde man nach PAWLOW folgendes Bild sehen: Über die Großhirnhemisphäre läuft ein dauernd bewegter Lichtpunkt, der in Größe und Form wechselt, von einem dunkleren Kontrastschatten der Hemmung umgeben ist und der einmal hier, einmal dort länger oder kürzer verweilt und dann wieder auf andere Stellen überspringt. Wenn man eine solche in ihren Bezügen wechselnde Bewußtseinsfunktion des Gehirns mit Aktivierung und Hemmung der verschiedensten Sinnes- und Gedächtnisvorgänge im Cortex annimmt, müßte sie auch von einer zentralen Stelle reguliert werden. Ein solches „Zentrum" der Bewußtseinsregulation wurde auf Grund klinischer Erfahrung zunächst allgemein im Hirnstamm vermutet [K 17, R 8] und dann nach physiologischen Experimenten im intralaminären Thalamus und der Formatio reticularis lokalisiert [D 11, M 19].

Schon im 19. Jahrhundert haben Physiologen mit FLOURENS [F 15] eine einheitliche Funktion der gesamten Hirnrinde postuliert, als Gegensatz zur anatomischen Hirnlokalisation und Phrenologie GALLS und zur Vermögenspsychologie. Dann hat die Entwicklung der corticalen Reiz- und Ausschaltungsexperimente durch HITZIG [H 71] und FERRIER [F 7] wieder die Lokalisations- und Zentrenlehre in den Vordergrund gestellt.

Theoretische Diskussionen über das Lokalisationsprinzip sind seitdem nach weiteren klinischen und experimentellen Erfahrungen oft wiederholt worden. Meist wurden ähnliche Argumente mit jeweils neuen Beispielen aus der aktuellen Forschung für und gegen die Lokalisation gebracht, die wenig zur Klärung beitrugen. Für den Physiologen kann es keinen Zweifel geben, daß Lokalisation und Begrenzung ebenso notwendig zu den Grundprinzipien des Nervensystems gehören, wie Erregungsausbreitung und Koordination der verschiedensten Hirnregionen zu einheitlicher und umweltadäquater Leistung (vgl. S. 889).

Neuere Methoden der Neurophysiologie in der Lokalisationsforschung. Die Neurophysiologie hat in den letzten Jahrzehnten die funktionellen Grundlagen der Hirnanatomie, die früher nur auf den klassischen Reiz- und Ausschaltungsmethoden beruhten, nach vier Richtungen erweitert:

1. Entwicklung der Hirnreizung ohne Narkose. a) Reizung subcorticaler Strukturen am freilaufenden Tier (HESS [H 51]), b) neurochirurgische Reizuntersuchungen beim Menschen am Cortex (PENFIELD [P 17]) und im Zwischenhirn (SPIEGEL [S 43], RIECHERT [R 17, 18], HASSLER [H 17] u.a.).

2. Ausbau und Ergänzung der cerebralen Ausschaltungen durch systematische Lernversuche und Verhaltensbeobachtungen. Damit gelang vor allem die Aufklärung der Balkenfunktion durch SPERRY [S 40] und MYERS [M 92].

3. Elektrophysiologische Lokalisationsforschung im Gehirn. Mit Makroelektroden wurde zunächst die afferente Impulsverteilung am Cortex und in subcorticalen Kernen durch Registrierung der „evoked potentials" in Narkose untersucht (ADRIAN [A 7], WOOLSEY [W 32] und viele andere). Dann wurden mit Hilfe von automatisch-statistischen Methoden entsprechende Untersuchungen im menschlichen EEG erfolgreich durchgeführt (DAWSON [D 7, 8]). Diese brachten durch moderne Computer neue Ergebnisse zur Willkürbewegung (KORNHUBER [K 43]) und zur Erwartung bedingter Sinnesreize (WALTER [W 10]). Die sog. physiologische Neuronographie mit dem Studium der Ausbreitung von Krampfentladungen nach lokaler Strychninisierung durch DUSSER DE BARENNE, MCCULLOCH u. Mitarb. [D 39] hat ebenfalls zur funktionellen Ergänzung der Anatomie beigetragen.

4. Mikrophysiologie des Gehirns. Durch *Mikroelektroden* wurden einzelne Hirnregionen mit ihrer neuronalen Tätigkeit analysiert und die Erregungsmuster nach afferenter Reizung studiert.

Hirnreizung ohne Narkose. Die alten Experimente der klassischen Reizphysiologie von FRITSCH und HITZIG [F 32, H 71] bis zu VOGT [V 10] wurden im akuten Versuch meist in tiefer Narkose durchgeführt und hatten nur kleine Teile des Cortex nach den motorischen Reaktionen als elektrisch erregbar festgestellt. Seit 3 Jahrzehnten haben drei Forschungsrichtungen dieses Gebiet erweitert und auch die nicht-motorischen Hirnregionen der Untersuchung zugänglich gemacht:

1. Die hirnelektrische Forschung hat durch das EEG die objektive Registrierung der cerebralen Reizeffekte im Gehirn selbst ermöglicht. Dadurch wurden alle Hirnregionen dem Reizexperiment zugänglich und die Ausbreitung der Reizwirkungen konnte unabhängig von den motorischen Effekten genau untersucht werden.

2. Reizexperimente an frei beweglichen Tieren hatten ohne Narkose durch implantierte Elektroden genauere Korrelationen mit Verhaltensbeobachtungen ermöglicht. So erweiterte der Ausbau des Reizexperiments beim unnarkotisierten Tier die wenigen elektrisch erregbaren Rindenteile der alten Versuche und ergab motorische und Verhaltenseffekte in einem viel größeren Teil der Hirnrinde und der subcorticalen Regionen. Die heute schon klassischen Reizversuche von HESS im Zwischen- und Mittelhirn mit Verhaltensbeobachtung des Tieres ergaben die Aktivierung zahlreicher spezialisierter Verhaltensweisen, Affekt- und Triebhandlungen bei verschieden lokalisierter Reizung [H 51–63]. Die Ergebnisse werden zusammen mit ähnlichen Versuchen v. HOLSTS bei Hühnern [H 84] im Kapitel der Affekte und Triebe besprochen und sind auch bei PLOOG in diesem Werk dargestellt (Band I, 1 B, S. 370).

3. Die systematischen Cortexreizversuche von FOERSTER [F 18] und PENFIELD [P 8–17] am Menschen bei neurochirurgischen Operationen, über deren Wirkungen der nicht-narkotisierte Patient berichten konnte, haben die bei Tieren festgestellten Reizkarten des Cortex wesentlich erweitert. Sie ergaben eine weitere corticale Ausdehnung der motorischen und sensiblen Reizeffekte mit verschiedenen Schwellen und psychischen Reaktionen. Komplexe seelische Erlebnisse als Reizeffekte wurden allerdings fast nur bei Epileptikern gefunden [P 14, 16].

Sensomotorik und cerebrale Somatotopik. Die *somatotopische Repräsentation in den sensiblen und motorischen Regionen der Großhirnrinde entspricht der Ausbildung und dem differenzierten Gebrauch der Werkzeugorgane des Körpers bei den verschiedenen Tierarten.* Die Extremitäten und vor allem Hand und Fuß, aber auch Kopf und Schwanz sind um so stärker vertreten, je größer ihre sensomotorische Differenzierung ist: Beim Waschbär, bei den meisten Affen und beim Menschen sind die Handregion, bei Affen mit Greifschwanz die Schwanzregion besonders entwickelt [W 32]. Bei Tier und Mensch sind die *oralen Funktionen* stark vertreten. Beim Menschen haben sie durch die *Sprache* eine Sonderentwicklung erfahren. Daher nimmt beim Menschen der Kehlkopf mit Zunge und Mund einen großen Teil der unteren motorischen Region ein [P 17].

Beispiele für subcorticale somatotopische Anordnungen im Thalamus des Menschen brachte HASSLER nach stereotaktischen Reizversuchen in der ersten Auflage dieses Bandes [siehe auch H 17].

Cortexreizungen und Lernvorgänge. DOTYS Versuche über bedingte Reflexe bei Rindenreizung wurden mit peripheren Reizen kombiniert. Es gelang DOTY, verschiedene bedingte Reaktionen bei corticalen und subcorticalen Reizen unterschiedlicher Lokalisation auszulösen [D 32–34]. Trotz großer Ausdehnung wirksamer Reizstellen im ganzen Gehirn reagierten Katzen und Affen bei verschiedenen Reizstellen unterschiedlich. Die Reizschwelle war für solche bedingten Reaktionen auffallend niedrig [D 34]. Elektrische Auslösung von früheren Erlebnissen, die erlernt und im Gedächtnis deponiert waren, beschreibt PENFIELD nach Schläfenlappenreizung beim Menschen [P 9, 13].

Hirnreizungen beim Menschen und ihre psychischen Korrelationen

Cortexreizung, psychische Symptome und Hemisphärendifferenz. Nachdem schon JACKSON [J 1] die fokale Epilepsie und ihre Auraphänomene für die Lokalisation im Cortex des Menschen verwendet hatte, brachte die systematische Cortexreizung in der Neurochirurgie eine exaktere und quasi-experimentelle Ausarbeitung der Rindenlokalisation. FOERSTERS Cortexreizversuche bei hirnchirurgischen Operationen in Lokalanaesthesie [F 18, 20] ergaben zuerst deutliche Korrelationen von Auraerlebnissen, sensibel-sensorischen und motorischen Symptomen mit lokalisierten Rindenreizungen. In der Occipitalregion fanden FOERSTER und PENFIELD [F 20, P 17] optische Halluzinationen nach Reizung der paravisuellen Regionen (Brodmanns areae 18, 19) im Gegensatz zu elementaren Photismen nach Reizen der primären Sehregion (area 17). Unterschiede der dominanten und nicht-dominanten Hemisphäre wurden von FOERSTER weniger beachtet, da er vorwiegend die Reizeffekte motorischer und sensibler Felder untersuchte.

PENFIELD hat die Cortexreizung bei zahlreichen Kranken, vorwiegend mit Epilepsie, systematisch auch mit ihren psychischen Symptomen studiert [P 8–17]. Er hat diese Ergebnisse mit seiner allgemeinen Konzeption der Cortexfunktionen und ihrer Steuerung durch das „centrencephale System" des Hirnstamms zu einer Theorie der Gedächtnisfunktionen ausgearbeitet (vgl. S. 886). Durch elektrische Reizung der Sprachregionen und Vergleich von Schläfenlappenepilepsien der rechten und linken Großhirnseite wurden auch die *Funktionen der dominanten und nicht-dominanten Hemisphäre* untersucht.

Cortexreizung und Sprache. In den klassischen Sprachregionen von BROCA und WERNICKE frontal und temporal, ebenso wie im Angularisgebiet ergibt Reizung nur eine aphasische *Sprachhemmung* (aphasic arrest). Reizung der motorischen und sensiblen Regionen des Mund- und Kehlkopfareals am Fuß beider Zentralregionen und der parasagittalen Supplementärarea ergibt *Vokalisation* mit rhythmischem oder kontinuierlichem Schreiben und artikulatorische Sprachhemmung (vocalization, speech arrest). Die parasagittale Supplementärarea kann nach PENFIELD auch aphasische, nicht nur artikulatorische Sprachhemmung hervorrufen, wenn die dominante Seite gereizt wird [P 17]. Dies entspricht klinischen Erfahrungen bei parasagittalen Meningeomen, die oft aphasische Symptome machen, obwohl sie weit von den fronto-temporalen Sprachregionen entfernt sind.

Elektrische Reizungen der motorischen und sensorischen Sprachregionen der dominanten Seite ergaben immer eine *Störung* der Sprachfunktion *(aphasic arrest)*. *Unartikulierte Vokalisationen* (meist längerdauernde Schreie) fanden sich nach Reizung der unteren motorischen und der supplementär-motorischen Regionen *beider* Hemisphären, frontal oft rhythmisch unterbrochen. Aphasische Sprachhemmung ist nur von der *dominanten* Hemisphäre auslösbar. Eine Übersicht über die verschiedenen Reizeffekte auf die Sprachfunktion von der dominanten Hemisphäre zeigt Abb. 19. Es findet sich vorwiegend *Sprachhemmung*. Der „aphasic arrest" kann in der parieto-temporalen Sprachregion eine echte aphasische *Wortfindungsstörung* sein: Der Patient zeigt dann während der Cortexreizung keine völlige Blockierung der Sprache, sondern beginnt wie ein amnestisch Aphasischer zu sagen: „Dies ist ein ..." ohne das Wort aussprechen zu können, oder spricht falsche, paraphasische Worte.

Cortexreizung und Wahrnehmung. Mit PEROT hat PENFIELD seine Erfahrungen über die *komplexen akustischen und optischen Erlebnisse nach Rindenreizung* dargestellt [P 16]. Es sind vorwiegend Sprachhalluzinationen, aber auch andere akustische Erinnerungen wie Musik und kombinierte akustische und optische Halluzinationen bei Epilepsien. Die Reizpunkte lagen für die *Spracherlebnisse* und andere Hörerinnerungen vorwiegend in der ersten Temporalwindung neben

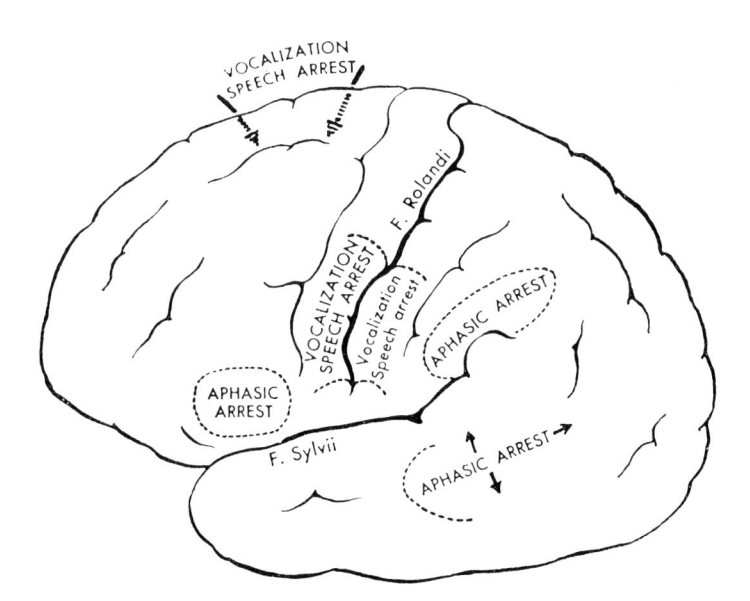

Abb. 19. Rindenareale der dominanten Hemisphäre, deren Reizung beim Menschen Sprachstörung oder Vokalisierung auslöst. Nach PENFIELD und RASMUSSEN (1950) [P 17]. Vokalisierung und Sprachhemmung (speech arrest) kann von *beiden* Hemisphären, Aphasie (aphasic arrest) nur von der *dominanten* Seite ausgelöst werden

dem eigentlichen akustischen Projektionsfeld der Heschlschen Querwindung, einige auch weiter medial am Übergang zur Insel. Meistens waren es bekannte *Stimmen.* Die *optischen, szenenhaften Bilder* konnten in der gleichen Temporalregion, häufiger aber im temporal-occipitalen Übergangsgebiet ausgelöst werden, die *kombinierten optisch-akustischen Szenen* nur im Temporallappen. Optische Szenen wurden wesentlich häufiger von der nicht-dominanten Seite ausgelöst, akustische und kombinierte Erlebnisse etwas häufiger von der dominanten Seite. In der eigentlichen Sprachregion der dominanten Hemisphäre konnten derartige Erlebnisse niemals ausgelöst werden, wohl aber von symmetrischen Cortexregionen der nicht-dominanten Seite.

Die beteiligten Cortexregionen zwischen Hör- und Sehrinde werden von PENFIELD „interpretive cortex" genannt, weil die Erlebnisse sowohl Erinnerungen wie Interpretationen alter und gegenwärtiger psychischer Inhalte sind. Sie unterscheiden sich deutlich von elementaren, optischen und akustischen Halluzinationen bei Reizung der Sinnesprojektionsfelder. Da Excision der entsprechenden Rindenfelder die Erinnerung nicht ausschaltet, postuliert PENFIELD eine Aktivierung anders lokalisierter Erinnerungen durch bestimmte neuronale Verbindungen. Für die Sprachhalluzinationen erscheint eine *indirekte Aktivierung der Sprachregion durch geordnete Impulse aus anderen Rindenfeldern,* die durch den elektrischen Reiz indirekt angeregt wurden, wahrscheinlicher als direkte Reizeffekte, denn derartige Wirkungen fehlen bei direkter Reizung der Sprachzentren, die nur Sprachhemmung auslöst. PENFIELD glaubt, daß eine *Funktion des Schläfenlappens* die „comparative interpretation", eine *vergleichende Einordnung von Wahrnehmungen* ist: Die Wahrnehmungen würden dort analysiert und die Komponenten der Sinnesmeldungen mit Gedächtniserlebnissen verglichen. Nach dieser vergleichenden Analyse sollen die Wahrnehmungen einem „centrencephalen" Bewußtseinssubstrat vermittelt und dann ihrer Bedeutung gemäß ins Gedächtnis eingeordnet werden [M 84].

Im Gegensatz zu PENFIELDS Aurauntersuchungen fand BALDWIN [B 1] bei Hirnreizungen eine weniger deutliche Bevorzugung des nicht-dominanten rechten Temporallappens. Seine Temporalreizungen mit Tiefenelektroden ergaben komplexe „psychische" Reaktionen aus *beiden* Schläfenlappen [B 1].

Genauere *Quantifizierungen der elektrischen Cortex-Reizung beim Menschen* und Korrelationen mit der bewußten Empfindungsschwelle haben LIBET u. Mitarb. [L 21] durchgeführt. Im Gegensatz zu Hautreizungen der Receptoren und peripheren Nerven, die schon nach 2–3 Einzelimpulsen eine Empfindung auslösen, brauchen die sensiblen Rindenfelder *vielfach wiederholte Reize* mit einer Reizseriendauer von 0,5–1 sec für subjektive Empfindungen. Ein Einfluß von Weckreizen mit Alphablockierung auf die Wahrnehmungsschwelle corticaler Reize war nicht festzustellen.

Intracerebrale und stereotaktische Hirnreizungen bei Menschen. Zahlreiche neuere Untersuchungen über lokalisierte *subcorticale Hirnreizungen* und ihre psychischen Effekte mit *intracerebralen Elektroden* bei Epilepsie und anderen Erkrankungen sind in einem 1960 erschienenen Symposion zusammengestellt [R 4]. Die Untersuchungen von DELGADO [D 15], BALDWIN [B 1], BICKFORD [B 43] wurden mit hirnelektrischen Ableitungen kontrolliert. BICKFORD [B 43] beobachtete nach subcorticaler Reizung bilaterale wiederholte Bewegungskomplexe, die situationsbeeinflußt und willkürähnlich waren, und vom Patienten nicht als durch Reizung erzwungen erlebt wurden.

SEM-JACOBSEN [S 23] berichtet auch über Selbstreizungen und ihre emotionalen Begleiterscheinungen (vgl. S. 958). Bei Reizung im Temporallappen ergaben sich ähnliche Befunde wie bei PENFIELDS intraoperativen Reizungen. Obwohl eine direkte Sprachproduktion durch elektrische Reize nicht nachgewiesen ist, konnten viele Patienten über ihre Erlebnisse während oder kurz nach der Reizung berichten. Sprachlich-akustische Halluzinationen und komplexe szenenhafte Halluzinationen wurden mehrfach berichtet. MAHL u. Mitarb. [M 21] fanden bei psychopathologischen Studien elektrischer Hirnreizungen einen Einfluß der jeweiligen Situation und der Sphäre des aktuellen Vorstellungsinhalts auf die reizbedingten Erlebnisse.

Aus diesen und früheren Untersuchungen PENFIELDS geht hervor, daß *komplexe psychische Phänomene durch Cortexreizung vorwiegend bei Epileptikern ausgelöst werden* können. Obwohl die Reizeffekte nicht immer der klinischen Aura entsprechen, handelt es sich z.T. doch um *experimentell ausgelöste epileptische Aura-Phänomene*. Deshalb muß die Beziehung dieser Phänomene mit normalen Hirnmechanismen vorsichtig geschehen. Die durch Hirnreizung ausgelösten Erlebnisse werden von den Patienten oft mit Träumen verglichen, ähnlich den produktiven temporalen Dämmerattacken.

Die *elektrische Cortexreizung,* die eine geregelte, sehr komplexe neuronale Struktur verändert, ist *eine Störung normaler Koordinationen und nicht die Reproduktion eines physiologischen Vorganges*. Dies wird am deutlichsten bei Reizung der Sprachregion, die das *negative Symptom einer Sprachhemmung,* aber keine positiven Sprachleistungen auslöst (Abb. 19). Der elektrische Cortexreiz als Störung normaler Funktionen der Hirnrinde kann auch bremsende, *hemmende Gegenreaktionen* auslösen, die ein normales Erregungsgleichgewicht herzustellen versuchen [J 62].

Bildlich gesprochen ist der elektrische Reiz der Hirnrinde nach TÖNNIES (1949) eher mit einem Blitzschlag in eine Telefonzentrale zu vergleichen [T 9]. Er wird die geregelten Verbindungen einer solchen Zentrale zunächst stören. Wenn der Cortexreiz dennoch positive Symptome und seelische Erlebnisäquivalente auslöst, so geschieht dies wahrscheinlich durch Vermittlung anderer Strukturen, deren geordnete Funktionen durch die Reizung enthemmt werden.

Der Schichtenaufbau des Nervensystems

Eine charakteristische Eigenschaft unseres Nervensystems ist der *Schichtenaufbau* oder, wie man nicht ganz zutreffend sagt, die *hierarchische Struktur des ZNS*. Die Ordnung der verschiedenen Schichten (levels der angelsächsischen Literatur) ist nicht nur morphologisch begründet, sondern steht auch in physiologischer Korrelation zur zentralnervösen Koordination. Ferner finden sich ähnliche Schichtdependenzen, wie sie N. HARTMANN für den Aufbau der anorganischen und organischen Welt dargestellt hat (vgl. S. 767): Von den peripheren Receptoren und Nerven, den „niederen" spinalen Kerngebieten bis zu den „höchsten" Strukturen des Großhirns ist jede Schicht für die nächsthöhere fundierend. Die oberen Schichten sind ohne die Grundlage der unteren nicht funktionsfähig. Dennoch haben die oberen Schichten ihre eigene Gesetzlichkeit und wesentlich mehr Freiheitsgrade. Die nach oben gesandten Meldungen sind bereits durch die Koordinationsarbeit der unteren Schichten *integriert,* sie gelangen dann *seligiert* und *kontrolliert* in die höheren Zentren, wo sie je nach ihrer Wichtigkeit entweder nur registriert oder weiter ausgewählt und verarbeitet werden, um neue Befehle wieder von oben nach unten zu geben. Ähnlich wie in einem komplizierten Verwaltungsapparat viele Kleinarbeit bereits von den unteren Organen ausgeführt wird und die oberen Stellen nur die allgemeinen Richtlinien geben, so arbeiten auch die verschiedenen Schichten des Nervensystems, nur mit einem wesentlichen *Unterschied:* Der Personalbestand an Neuronen wird nicht wie in einer Hierarchie von unten nach oben kleiner, sondern größer. Oben im Cortex sitzt nicht ein Papst oder Monarch, sondern ein großes Parlament, das die Entscheidungen trifft. Das *Nervensystem arbeitet nicht wie eine Monarchie, sondern wie eine Demokratie* [J 31]. Auf der höchsten Ebene findet sich vor allem bei den Säugern und beim Menschen keine Spitze mit nur wenigen entscheidenden Stellen, sondern ein ungewöhnlich *ausgedehnter Koordinationsapparat mit den Strukturen und Funktionen der sehr differenzierten Hirnrinde,* die sich den einfacheren Integrationsorganen des Hirnstamms überlagert. Beim Menschen werden dem Cortex sehr viele Vorgänge gemeldet, die bei niederen Tieren nur in den Hirnstammzentren verarbeitet werden. Der Cortex leistet daher nochmals eine erhebliche Kleinarbeit, die sich aber mehr in der Wahrnehmung psychischer Vorstellungs- und Wahlfunktionen und in potentiellen Vorentwürfen und Denkmöglichkeiten ausdrückt als in Bewegung und Handlung, die mit Hilfe unterer Apparate ausgeführt werden.

Es ist nicht ohne Zwang möglich, Struktur und Funktion des Gehirns mit den Prinzipien menschlicher Sozialordnungen, hierarchischer oder demokratischer Organisation zu vergleichen. Diese Prinzipien entsprechen mehr einem extremen und pathologischen Verhalten. Totalitäre Prinzipien der absoluten Unterordnung und der fehlenden peripheren Regulation sind nur im epileptischen Anfall rein ausgeprägt: Hier beherrschen maximale Entladungen der Großhirnstrukturen alle anderen neuronalen Vorgänge und verhindern die normale Koordination ihrer differenzierten Teilfunktionen. Extreme demokratische Freiheit, in der die verschiedensten Instanzen mitreden und nebeneinander und auch entgegengesetzt entscheiden können und in der eine straffe Führung fehlt, kann zur Anarchie führen und ist dann in dem inadäquaten Verhalten Schizophrener repräsentiert. Rein hierarchische Unterordnung unter eine für dauernd bestimmte einzelne Führung gibt es im ZNS nicht. Die oberste Instanz im Cortex und Subcortex wechselt und arbeitet ähnlich einigen parlamentarischen Prinzipien mit wechselndem „Personal" der Neuronensysteme über eine gesetzlich geregelte Stufung der einzelnen Schichten des ZNS.

Zwar finden sich dieselben Elementarstrukturen, Nervenzelle, Axone und Synapsen, sowohl in den einfachsten wie in den kompliziertesten Strukturen des Nervensystems. Ähnliche elektrische Erregungen und sie begründende Stoffwechselvorgänge laufen in peripheren Nerven wie in der Hirnrinde ab. Dennoch, trotz dieser Ähnlichkeit der Elementarvorgänge gelten doch *verschiedene* Gesetze für die einzelnen Ebenen, denn die höheren Schichten sind viel komplizierter. Die oberen Schichten sind allerdings ohne die Grundlage der niederen nicht funktionsfähig und sind insofern abhängig von der Arbeit der unteren Schichten. Dennoch haben sie ihre *Eigengesetzlichkeit und mehr Freiheit der Entscheidung.*

Die *Wechselwirkung der verschiedenen Schichten* ist sehr kompliziert. Man kann sie zwar schematisch auf die beiden Vorgänge der Bahnung und Hemmung zurückführen. Seit JACKSON [J 1] nimmt man vor allem an, daß die höheren

Schichten die niederen zügeln und hemmen. Das ist nur zum Teil richtig. Man kann damit erklären, warum bei Ausschaltung höherer Funktionen eine Aktivierung einfacher Mechanismen im Nervensystem auftritt, wie etwa die Reflexsteigerung nach Ausschaltung der Pyramidenbahn. Es ist aber sicher nicht so, daß die höheren Schichten die niederen nur durch Wegfall einer Dauerhemmung beeinflussen. Von oben kann eine direkte Steuerung und Anregung für die unteren Strukturen ausgehen, die vielleicht mit kybernetischen Regeln genauer untersucht werden kann.

Die höheren Schichten können wie gesagt nur funktionsfähig sein, wenn die niederen richtig arbeiten. Ähnlich verhält es sich mit der Abhängigkeit des Nervensystems von den nicht-nervösen Körperfunktionen, die es dirigiert, so daß z.B. ein Ausfall der Durchblutung jede Tätigkeit des Nervensystems ausschaltet.

Neurophysiologie und klinische Hirnpathologie

Die höheren Großhirnfunktionen wurden seit den 100 Jahre alten Aphasiebeobachtungen BROCAS zunächst nur durch klinische Erfahrungen der menschlichen Hirnpathologie erforscht. Die experimentelle Neurophysiologie hat zunächst nur durch Reiz- und Ausschaltungsversuche bei Tieren dazu beigetragen. Sie gab mit FRITSCH und HITZIGS [F 32] Entdeckung des motorischen Cortex durch Reizexperimente beim Hund 1870 einen mächtigen Anstoß für die Erforschung der Großhirnlokalisation und hat durch MUNKS Ausschaltungsversuche auch die Agnosieforschung angeregt, doch blieb die klinische Beobachtung beim Menschen mit ihren Vor- und Nachteilen einer Kasuistik die wichtigste Quelle der Hirnpathologie. Die experimentelle Neurophysiologie hat im letzten Jahrzehnt als einzige große Leistung die Erkenntnis der Balkenfunktionen gebracht, die durch klinische Untersuchungen nicht aufgeklärt werden konnten (vgl. S. 890). Die Grenzen der klassischen Methoden des Reiz- und Ausschaltungsexperiments bei Tieren sind auch durch neue Erkenntnisse der Elektrophysiologie für hirnpathologische Untersuchung nur wenig erweitert worden, obwohl wir über die Koordination der neuronalen Funktionen im Cortex heute sehr viel mehr wissen als noch vor 1–2 Jahrzehnten.

Hirnelektrische Koordination beider Großhirnhemisphären und verschiedener Hirnregionen. Die elektrische Hirntätigkeit, die mit dem EEG bei Tier und Mensch ableitbar ist, zeigt trotz lokaler Verschiedenheiten ähnliche und *synchronisierte Grundrhythmen der Großhirnrinde,* die beim Menschen dem α-Rhythmus entsprechen. *Die α-Wellen über beiden Großhirnhemisphären sind rechts und links in ihrer Phasenrichtung meist übereinstimmend,* am stärksten in der Frontalregion, weniger konstant mit einzelnen Phasendifferenzen in der Occipitalregion [H 91].

Die synchronisierten elektrischen Hirnpotentiale sind elektrophysiologische Zeichen für die *Zusammenarbeit verschiedener Hirnrindenregionen,* die Regeln der relativen Koordination VON HOLSTS folgen [J 27]. Die rhythmischen Hirnwellen des EEG sind wahrscheinlich Korrelate metabolischer Regulationen, die von differenzierter und lokalspezifischer Neuronentätigkeit unterschieden sind.

Heute wird meistens eine gemeinsame Aktivierung und Rhythmisierung des Cortex durch subcorticale Hirnteile, vor allem durch den Thalamus, angenommen. Dies hat mit dem Begriff des centrencephalen Systems und mit der „unspezifischen" Formatio reticularis zu neuen Systemkonzeptionen geführt (vgl. S. 978).

Hirnlokalisation erlernter Funktionen und Altersentwicklung. Die Lehre der älteren Hirnpathologie über die corticale Lokalisation erlernter Reaktionen und Sprachleistungen wurde in den letzten 50 Jahren in ihrem Wert oft angezweifelt. Die guten Kompensationsleistungen, mit denen vor allem ein jugendliches Gehirn Ausfälle des „Sprachzentrums" ausgleicht, wurden allgemein für die Plastizität und gegen die Lokalisationslehre verwendet. Doch zeigt der Gegensatz kompensierbarer und nicht kompensierbarer Ausfälle in verschiedenen Lebensaltern nur an, daß eine *feste Lokalisation erlernter Leistungen erst mit der Altersentwicklung allmählich erworben wird*. Dies ist jetzt experimentell im Tierversuch nachgewiesen: Neue Untersuchungen über Frontalhirnläsionen an Affen verschiedenen Lebensalters durch HARLOW u.Mitarb. [H 3] haben die Lokalisation erlernter Leistungen im Frontalhirn als Funktion des Lebensalters mit der Methode der aufgeschobenen Reaktion genauer studiert.

Dieselben frontalen Hirnläsionen ergaben bei neugeborenen Affen keine Störung, bei 5 Monate alten Affen leichte Störungen und bei 1–2jährigen Tieren schwere und dauernde Ausfälle in der Erlernung aufgeschobener Reaktionen. Diese Untersuchungen sind nicht nur wichtig für die erworbene Lokalisation erlernter Funktionen im Laufe der Altersentwicklung, sondern auch für die Frage der *Kompensation*. Sie können mit den Erfahrungen bei menschlichen Aphasien verglichen werden, wenn man die längerdauernde Lernperiode der Menschen berücksichtigt und von der einseitigen Hemisphärendominanz der Sprachzentren absieht. Gute Kompensationen der Rindenläsionen von Sprachgebieten im Kindesalter und bleibende Ausfälle der gleichen Läsionen bei älteren Menschen entsprächen einer etwa *10–20mal längeren plastischen Lernperiode des menschlichen Gehirns gegenüber den Affen.*

Die Balken-Funktion als Informations-Transfer zwischen den Großhirn-Hemisphären

Die mächtigste und faserreichste Bahnverbindung des menschlichen Gehirns ist der *Balken,* der als Commissur beide Großhirn-Hemisphären verbindet. Doch wußte man bis vor wenigen Jahren fast nichts über die Funktion dieser Commissur. Nachdem schon seit 100 Jahren die Dominanz der linken Hemisphäre für die Sprachfunktion beim Rechtshänder bekannt war und seit 60 Jahren eine Beteiligung des Balkens bei den apraktischen Störungen diskutiert wurde, blieb die physiologische Bedeutung des Corpus callosum doch ein Rätsel. Erst die Tierexperimente von SPERRY und MYERS klärten mit *kombinierter Chiasma- und Balken-Durchtrennung* (split brain) die Transferfunktionen des Balkens, der mit etwa 200 Millionen Nervenfasern Informationen von einer Hemisphäre zur anderen trägt [G 14, M 86–92, S 40, 42].

Transferfunktionen des Balkens. Die „split brain"-Experimente wurden folgendermaßen durchgeführt: Die Versuchstiere konnten nach Durchtrennung der Chiasmakreuzung optische Informationen von einem Auge nur in die gleichseitige Großhirn-Hemisphäre leiten. Dennoch waren sie bei Dressurversuchen mit intaktem Balken noch fähig, Objekte, die sie mit einem Auge kennengelernt hatten, mit dem anderen wiederzuerkennen. Nach Balken-Durchschneidung war dieser Transfer nicht mehr möglich. Das vom anderen Auge noch nie gesehene Bild mußte also mit seinem physiologischen Informationsgehalt und seiner Dressurbedeutung für die Futterwahl durch den Balken in die andere Hemisphäre transferiert worden sein. Ebenso zeigte sich, daß Affen nach erlernter stereognostischer Tasterkennung bestimmter Objekte mit einer Hand dieselben Gegenstände bei intaktem Balken mit der anderen Hand wieder erkennen konnten, da die Meldungen offenbar sofort transferiert wurden, daß aber nach Balken-Durchschneidung dieser Transfer nicht mehr gelang.

Frühere Versuche, beim Menschen nach partiellen Balkendurchtrennungen wesentliche Störungen nachzuweisen, waren vergeblich. Erst in den letzten 15 Jahren haben SPERRY u. Mitarb. an *Patienten mit totalen Balkendurchschneidungen* systematische Studien über Transferfunktionen und Hemisphärendominanz durchgeführt. Die Sprachdominanz des linken und die nicht-sprachlichen Funktionen des rechten Großhirns konnten mit verschiedener Reizexposition im linken und rechten Gesichtsfeld exakt nachgewiesen werden [E 6, S 40, 42]. [S 41] Mit dieser Methodik konnten auch die dominanten Funktionen der rechten und linken Großhirnhemisphären genauer untersucht werden, als dies beim Gesunden oder Patienten mit anderen Großhirnherden möglich ist [E 6].

Im Gegensatz zur Transferfunktion mit ihren massiven Faserverbindungen des Balkens ist die anatomisch-physiologische Grundlage der *Hemisphären-Dominanz* ungeklärt. Die in der dominanten Rolle einer Hemisphäre für die menschliche Sprache zum Ausdruck kommende *Hemisphärendifferenz,* die verschiedene Funktion der linken und rechten Großhirnrindenfelder, beruhen vorwiegend auf *erlernten* Funktionsänderungen. Ihre strukturelle Grundlage ist noch ebenso unbekannt wie das Substrat von Lernen und Gedächtnisfunktionen allgemein. Beide Großhirnhemisphären sind etwa gleich groß, fast genau gleichartig gebaut und enthalten die gleichen cytoarchitektonischen Felder. In der dominanten Hemisphäre sind Brodmanns Felder 22 und 44 wichtig für die Sprachfunktion. In der nicht-dominanten Hemisphäre haben dieselben Rindenfelder aber offenbar andere Funktionen, da die Sprache bei ihrer Läsion nicht gestört wird. Ähnliches muß man bei den höheren Affen annehmen, bei denen entsprechende architektonische Rindenfelder der menschlichen „Sprachregionen" gut entwickelt sind, ohne daß der Affe je sprechen lernt.

Man kann sich vorstellen, daß mit dem Transfer jeweils ein Spiegelbild der von den Sinnesorganen gemeldeten Wahrnehmung einer Körperseite auf die andere Hemisphäre übertragen wird. Dies zeigt sich besonders deutlich bei Linkshändern, die rechts schreiben gelernt haben und dann leicht mit der linken Hand in Spiegelschrift schreiben, wie LEONARDO DA VINCI [J 48].

Hemisphärendifferenz und Dominanz

Die merkwürdige Tatsache, daß die anatomisch fast identischen spiegelbildlich symmetrisch gebauten Großhirnhemisphären beim Menschen außer der Vertretung der kontralateralen Körperhälfte auch ganz *verschiedene integrative Funktionen* haben, verlangt eine *physiologische* Erklärung, die uns allerdings bis heute noch fehlt. Die Anatomie hilft uns hier nicht weiter, obwohl die Neuropathologie diese auffallende Seitendifferenz bei der Aphasie entdeckt hat. Zwar hat GESCHWIND 1974 eine stärkere Entwicklung des linken Planum temporale bei Rechtshändern als Grundlage der Sprachlokalisation festgestellt [G 18], doch wird von vielen Anatomen eine solche Asymmetrie als Ursache der Sprachdominanz des linken Großhirns bestritten.

Sprache und Händigkeit wird von der „*dominanten*", beim Rechtshänder der *linken* Hemisphäre koordiniert, in deren temporo-frontaler Hirnrinde die viel diskutierten Sprachzentren liegen. Dagegen werden räumlich-zeitliche Regulationen und Koordinationen vorwiegend von der „*nicht-dominanten*" meist *rechten* Hemisphäre und deren parieto-occipitaler Rinde gesteuert. Da bei Linkshändern meistens, aber nicht immer, die rechte Hemisphäre für die Sprachfunktionen maßgebend ist, richtet man sich für die Dominanzbestimmung mangels anderer Kriterien nach der Händigkeit. Die Bezeichnung „Dominanz" ist aber nur für bestimmte mit der Sprache verbundene Leistungen, mit Lesen und Schreiben, zutreffend, dagegen nicht für andere wichtige Funktionen, die ebenfalls von großer Bedeutung sind wie die Praxis und Orientierungsfunktionen: *Für die räumlich-zeitliche Integration ist offenbar die rechte Hemisphäre führend.* Man kann auch nicht sagen, daß die sog. dominante Hemisphäre vorwiegend erlernte Funktionen, wie Sprache, Lesen und Schreiben steuert, denn auch räumlich-zeitliche Vorgänge sind zumindest großenteils erworbene und erlernte Funktionen, die durch das Gedächtnis ermöglicht werden.

Die anatomisch identischen, spiegelbildlichen Großhirnhemisphären haben jeweils enge Commissur-Verbindungen durch die Balkenfasern, deren Transfer-Funktionen durch tierexperimentelle Untersuchungen von SPERRY [M 92, S 39] und MYERS [M 87] entdeckt wurden (s. 890).

Für die komplexen erlernten Funktionen von Sprache, Lesen und Schreiben scheinen aber diese Transferinformationen der gegenseitigen Hemisphäre nicht auszureichen. Sie werden offenbar nur in der frühen Kindheit und beim ersten Schreib- und Leseerwerb mitverwendet. Ein Rest dieser Transferfunktion zeigt sich in der Neigung, mit der nicht dominanten Hand spiegelbildlich zu schreiben und in dem Wiederauftreten einer primär erlernten Schreibform (Deutsche Schrift) bei manchen Aphasikern, die mit der linken Hand schreiben wollen [Z 3].

Wenn wir der Einfachheit halber von „Linksdominanz" und „Rechtsdominanz" sprechen, so ist dies für Großhirn und Händigkeit beim *Rechtshänder* gemeint, bei dem im allgemeinen die linke Hemisphäre für die Sprachfunktion dominant ist.

Linksdominanz der Sprache im menschlichen Gehirn. Experimentelle und physiologische Untersuchungen zur Hemisphärendominanz sind dadurch erschwert, daß eine dem Menschen entsprechende Linksdominanz, die offenbar mit der Sprachentwicklung und Rechtshändigkeit zusammenhängt, bei Tieren nicht bekannt ist. Bei Katzen und Affen gibt es zwar eine Prävalenz der Geschicklichkeit auf der linken oder rechten Körperseite, aber keine überwiegende Hemisphärendominanz wie bei der menschlichen Rechtshändigkeit. Die Beziehungen von Händigkeit und Sprachlokalisation sind beim Menschen nur statistisch nachgewiesen, aber noch nicht in ihrer Entstehung geklärt. Obwohl dies bisher nicht an größeren Zahlen von Tieren untersucht zu sein scheint, ist die Rechts- und Linksbevorzugung der Hände bei Affen etwa gleich häufig. Auch wenn Affen und Katzen eine Bevorzugung der einen oder anderen Extremität mit besserer Übung zeigen, so fehlt doch eine überwiegende Beziehung zu einer Seite und zu einer bestimmten Hemisphäre. Obwohl die sprachliche Linksdominanz mit erlernten Funktionen verbunden ist und anatomisch keine Unterschiede zwischen rechter und linker Hemisphäre nachweisbar sind, scheinen doch genetische Faktoren eine Rolle zu spielen. Dafür sprechen Beobachtungen über familiäres Vorkommen der Linkshändigkeit.

Seitendominanz und Seitenpräferenz. Nach Untersuchungen motorischer Leistungen bei Rechts- und Linkshändern haben wir vorgeschlagen, eine *angeborene Seitendominanz* von einer durch Übung *erworbenen Seitenpräferenz* zu unterscheiden [J 48]. Beim Rechtshänder sind Rechtsdominanz und Rechtspräferenz identisch. Der *Linkshänder,* dem eine linksseitige Dominanz angeboren ist, erwirbt dagegen, wenn er in der Schule rechts schreiben lernt, eine spezifische *Rechtsseitenpräferenz nur für das Schreiben* mit der rechten Hand. Für feinere Bewegungsleistungen (Zeichnen u.a.) benutzt er aber weiter die bei ihm dominante linke Hand. Diese linke Hand ist dann seitendominant und seitenpräferent für alle anderen erlernten Handlungen wie Zeichnen, Schrauben, Nähen, und die meisten linkshändigen Maler bevorzugen für Zeichnen und Malen die linksdominante Hand, auch wenn sie rechts schreiben [J 48]. Die linke Hand ist dann auch für das Zeichen seitendominant und seitenpräferent wie beim Rechtshänder die rechte. Sowohl Rechts- wie Linkshänder zeigen die besten motorischen Leistungen jeweils für alle spezifisch *geübten* Handlungen der bevorzugten und seitenpräferenten Hand. Diese Seitenpräferenz entspricht beim Rechtshänder in der Regel der Seitendominanz. Eine Seitenpräferenz kann aber beim Linkshänder für spezielle erlernte Handlungen, wie Schreiben, von der Linksdominanz unabhängig werden.

Ein Symposion über die Beziehung beider Großhirnhemisphären und die Hemisphärendominanz [M 72] zeigte, daß *bei Tieren einschließlich höherer Affen keine Seitendominanz nachgewiesen ist.* Affen zeigen nur *Seitenpräferenzen.* Die Hemisphärendominanz scheint also ein spezifisch *menschliches* Merkmal zu sein, das eng mit der Entwicklung der *Sprache* verbunden ist. Die erlernte Sprache wird bekanntlich allein durch die sprachliche Umgebung des Kindes bestimmt. Ein kleines Kind, gleich welcher menschlichen Rasse, lernt chinesisch, russisch, deutsch oder englisch, je nach dem sprachlichen Milieu, in dem es aufwächst. Aber kein Affe hat bisher in einem solchen Milieu sprechen gelernt, und die taubstummenähnliche Gestensprache, die einigen Schimpansen beigebracht wurde [G 8], ist nicht mit dem Reichtum menschlicher Sprache zu vergleichen.

Obwohl also angeborene Faktoren für das Erlernen einer speziellen Sprache keine Bedeutung haben, muß doch eine artspezifische angeborene Disposition beim Menschen das Erlernen der Sprache und die Hemisphärendominanz ermöglichen.

Die Lokalisation erlernter Sprachfunktionen ist in den ersten Lebensjahren noch weitgehend plastisch, und erst nach dem Schulalter entsteht beim Menschen eine lokalisatorische Fixierung und mangelnde Kompensation durch die andere Hemisphäre. Tierexperimentelle Erfahrungen über erworbene Lokalisation und

Fixierung von Lernvorgängen bleiben zunächst die einzige experimentelle Parallele zur Sprachlokalisation. Ob Untersuchungen über aufgeschobene Reaktionen als vereinfachte Modelle der Sprachlokalisation zu verwenden sind, muß vorläufig offen bleiben.

Außer den experimentellen Untersuchungen über die Balkenfunktion hat die Neurophysiologie zur hirnpathologischen Forschung der höheren corticalen Funktionen noch nicht viel beigetragen. Das Phänomen der cerebralen Dominanz ist in seiner physiologischen Bedeutung ungeklärt. Sicher erscheint nur, daß man nicht eine Hemisphäre allgemein als dominant bezeichnen kann, sondern nur für spezielle Funktionen. *Die linke Hemisphäre ist beim Rechtshänder und selten auch beim Linkshänder für die Sprachfunktionen, für Lesen und Rechnen dominant. Die rechte Hemisphäre ist dagegen dominant für räumliche und andere gnostische Funktionen sowie für bestimmte Handlungsfolgen.* POETZLS Vergleich der linken Hemisphäre mit Komponist und Orchester und der rechten Hemisphäre mit dem Dirigenten ist allerdings nur cum grano salis gültig.

Zur Aphasieforschung haben weder Rindenreizungen noch EEG-Ableitungen viel beitragen können. PENFIELDS *Rindenreizungen* [P 18] in verschiedenen Sprachregionen haben nur eine *Unterbrechung des Sprechens* auslösen können (Abb. 19). Eine solche negative Funktionsstörung war bei einer differenzierten Funktion wie der Sprache zu erwarten, da der grobe elektrische Reiz hier nur blockierend auf die koordinatorischen Sprachintegrationsvorgänge wirken kann. Reizungen in der Umgebung der Sprachregion konnten ungeformte Vokalisationen auslösen. Neue Reizversuche bei zweisprachigen Patienten von OLJEMAN sprechen für leichte lokalisatorische Verschiedenheiten der früh und spät erlernten Sprachen im Broca- und Wernicke-Areal.

EEG-Befunde bei Aphasien. Hirnelektrische Untersuchungen ergeben bei Aphasien keine spezifischen Resultate. Man sieht lediglich mehr oder weniger ausgeprägte Herdbefunde über dem dominanten Schläfenlappen. Solche Herdbefunde wie die auch bei Gefäßinsulten oft sehr deutlichen temporalen Delta-Foci bleiben auffallend lange erhalten, auch wenn die Aphasie sich bessert. Niemals kann man allein auf Grund des EEG auf eine Aphasie schließen. Man kann sie höchstens bei temporalen Herden der dominanten Hemisphäre vermuten. Nur selten ist es gelungen, bei temporalen Epilepsien mit vorübergehender Aphasie ein EEG abzuleiten. EEG-Befunde im aphasischen Anfall zeigten Herde, die mehr an der temporalen Konvexität lokalisiert waren als die meist basaltemporalen Herde der temporalen Epilepsie ohne Aphasie.

Im übrigen ergeben diese *EEG-Ableitungen* bei Anfällen mit aphasischen Erscheinungen nur die für temporale Epilepsie typischen steilen Wellen, die nicht immer temporal lokalisiert sind. Nur eine von BRAIN [B 58] mitgeteilte Untersuchung von SPILLANE ergab eine lokalisatorische Differenzierung bei solchen Aphasie-Anfällen: fronto-temporal bei expressiver, temporo-parietal bei rezeptiver Sprachstörung. Ein aphasischer Anfall mit rhythmischen fokalen Krampfspitzen der linken Broca-Region bei unverändertem EEG der rechten Seite wurde von JASPER abgeleitet und von PENFIELD und RASMUSSEN [P 17] abgebildet. Trotz motorischer Sprachhemmung war das Denken im Anfall erhalten. Abb. 20 zeigt einen motorisch-aphasischen Anfall bei einer traumatischen Epilepsie. Der Patient blieb während des Anfalls bewußtseinsklar mit erhaltenem

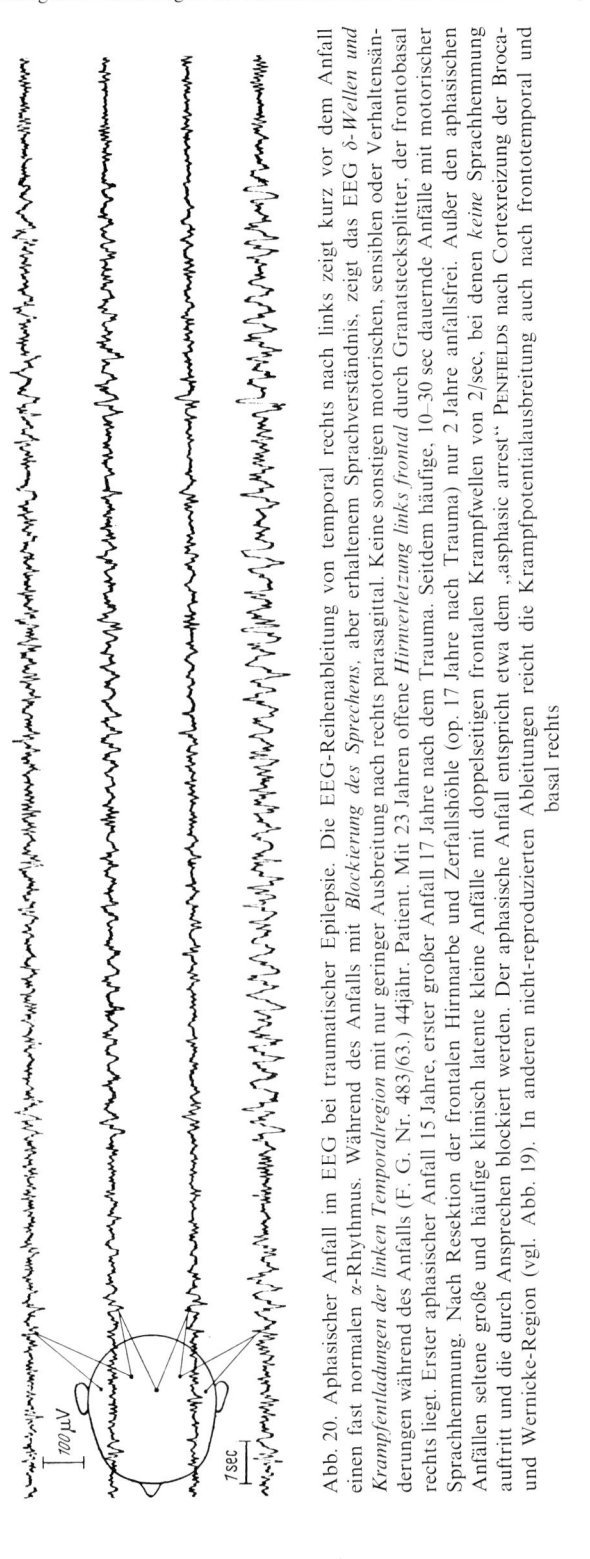

Abb. 20. Aphasischer Anfall im EEG bei traumatischer Epilepsie. Die EEG-Reihenableitung von temporal rechts nach links zeigt kurz vor dem Anfall einen fast normalen α-Rhythmus. Während des Anfalls mit *Blockierung des Sprechens*, aber erhaltenem Sprachverständnis, zeigt das EEG δ-*Wellen und Krampfentladungen der linken Temporalregion* mit nur geringer Ausbreitung nach rechts parasagittal. Keine sonstigen motorischen, sensiblen oder Verhaltensänderungen während des Anfalls (F. G. Nr. 483/63.) 44jähr. Patient. Mit 23 Jahren offene *Hirnverletzung links frontal* durch Granatsteckesplitter, der frontobasal rechts liegt. Erster aphasischer Anfall 15 Jahre, erster großer Anfall 17 Jahre nach dem Trauma. Seitdem häufige, 10–30 sec dauernde Anfälle mit motorischer Sprachhemmung. Nach Resektion der frontalen Hirnnarbe und Zerfallshöhle (op. 17 Jahre nach Trauma) nur 2 Jahre anfallsfrei. Außer den aphasischen Anfällen seltene große und häufige klinisch latente kleine Anfälle mit doppelseitigen frontalen Krampfwellen von 2/sec, bei denen *keine* Sprachhemmung auftritt und die durch Ansprechen blockiert werden. Der aphasische Anfall entspricht etwa dem „asphasic arrest" PENFIELDS nach Cortexreizung der Broca- und Wernicke-Region (vgl. Abb. 19). In anderen nicht-reproduzierten Ableitungen reicht die Krampfpotentialausbreitung auch nach frontotemporal und basal rechts

Sprachverständnis, aber konnte während der Krampfpotentiale links temporal nicht sprechen. Ähnliche Anfälle mit Sprachblockierung haben wir auch bei parasagittalen Meningeomen ohne temporalen Krampffocus gesehen. Sie entsprechen vielleicht der Sprachblockierung nach Reizung von PENFIELDS Supplementärarea. Die Beispiele zeigen, daß Herdlokalisation im EEG und Aphasietyp des Anfalls nicht immer übereinstimmen. Doch zeigen die EEG-Befunde bei Aphasie jeweils gute Korrelationen mit der dominanten Hemisphäre.

Sprache ist sinnesphysiologisch wie alle komplexen akustischen Reizmuster mehr durch *zeitliche Folgen sukzessiver Reize* als durch simultane Wahrnehmungsprozesse charakterisiert. *Zeitliche Integration und Ordnung* ist daher eine wichtige physiologische Vorbedingung des Sprachverständnisses und des Sprechens. Die von MONAKOW [M 51] in seinen letzten Schriften betonte „chronogene Lokalisation" cerebraler Funktionen bezeichnete allgemeine Grundlagen solcher zeitlich geordneten Hirnvorgänge. Neuere Tendenzen der Sprachforschung besprechen PLOOG in diesem Band und ASSAL und HECAEN [A 35].

Sprache als erlernte und auswechselbare semantische Funktion. Die Schwierigkeiten neurophysiologischer Sprachuntersuchungen mit der inadäquaten Anwendung biologischer Methoden in der Sprach- und Aphasieforschung liegen im semantischen Wesen der Sprache selbst. Die verschiedenen Sprachen, die Auswechselbarkeit der Worte und Zeichen, die in den einzelnen Sprachen mit unterschiedlichen Symbolen denselben Gegenstand bezeichnen, und die Abhängigkeit der Spracherlernung vom Sozialmilieu erschweren die naturwissenschaftliche Erfassung. Sie beschränken die Anwendung physiologischer Methoden auf phonetische Probleme, auf den Sprechakt und die groben cerebralen Störungen des Sprechens. Variabilitäten der Sprache, um von den Variationen des „Geistes" nicht zu reden, sind von anderer Art als etwa die genetischen Variationen der Arten, deren naturwissenschaftliche Klärung bereits große Schwierigkeiten macht.

Eine negative Seite der Sprache mit ihrer erlernten und willkürlichen Beherrschung ist ferner, daß sie nicht nur zur echten Mitteilung, sondern auch zur falschen Propaganda und Lüge verwendet werden kann. Dennoch ist die Sprache in allen Wissenschaften von größter Bedeutung, weil außer mathematischen Formeln, graphischen Kurven und Abbildungen, die andere Symbolfunktionen verwenden, fast alle Forschungsergebnisse sprachlich mitgeteilt werden müssen. So hat die Sprache auch starken Einfluß auf die Darstellung wissenschaftlicher Ergebnisse. Die Macht der Sprache wirkt besonders stark in der Psychiatrie, wie auch die unterschiedlichen psychiatrischen Entwicklungen verschiedener Sprachgebiete zeigen. Wenn man die semantische Natur und Auswechselbarkeit der Sprachzeichen beachtet, kann man am besten eine Überwertung sprachlicher Äquivokationen und verbaler Deutungen vermeiden, die unter dem Einfluß moderner philosophischer Strömungen auf die Psychiatrie übergegriffen hat.

Sprachdeprivation. Eine durch mangelnde Sprachkommunikation verhinderte Entwicklung des Sprechens ist vor allem bei Taubstummen studiert worden. Bei normal hörenden Menschen wurde seit Kaspar Hauser eine völlige Sprachdeprivation in den ersten Lebensjahren bis zur Pubertät nur bei einem Mädchen in Amerika beobachtet und von Linguisten studiert [C 20, 21]. Das von einem psychotischen Vater eingesperrte Kind hatte vor dem 13. Lebensjahr keine menschliche Sprache gehört und konnte dann erst mühsam das Sprechen erlernen [E 6, C 20, 21]. Nach 5jährigem Sprechunterricht lagen Sprachverständnis und Sprachleistung weit unterhalb denen eines gesunden Kindes. CURTISS glaubt, daß die später erlernte Sprache mehr von der rechten Hirnhälfte koordiniert wird [C 20, 21], da die linksseitigen Sprachzentren durch Nichtgebrauch funktionell atrophierten, nachdem das Sprechen erst nach der Pubertät und nicht in der kritischen Periode der ersten Kindheit erlernt wurde.

Hirnpathologische Störungssyndrome und physiologische Funktionen

Lokalisation von Läsionen und Funktionssubstraten. Trotz großer Variabilität zeigen die verschiedenen höheren hirnpathologischen *Störungssyndrome* der Aphasien, Apraxien und Agnosien doch bestimmte, durch systematische Untersuchungen erfaßbare neurologische Symptomenkomplexe. Dagegen erscheinen die physiologischen Mechanismen der zugrunde liegenden *normalen Funktionen* des Sprechens, des Handelns und Erkennens so kompliziert, daß es noch nicht möglich ist, sie in neurophysiologischer Sprache auszudrücken. Es ist relativ einfach, eine Artikulationsstörung durch Nachsprechen schwieriger Worte zu prüfen, aber äußerst schwierig und meistens unmöglich, den gestörten Sprachmechanismus physiologisch zu definieren. Daher kann die Neurophysiologie zur Hirnpathologie höherer corticaler Funktionsstörungen nicht viel beitragen.

Ein ungelöstes, und vielleicht unlösbares Problem ist die *Korrelation von Läsion und Funktion.* Durch JACKSON [J 1] und v. MONAKOW [M 50] ist die Problematik einer Funktionslokalisation bei anatomisch exakter Lokalisation der Hirnläsion mit ihren Ausfallsymptomen bereits klar erkannt und dargestellt worden. Leider wurde die Schwierigkeit dieser Frage aber von den naiven neurologischen „Lokalisatoren" nicht genügend beachtet. Das *Schichtenprinzip* JACKSONS, nach dem bei Ausfällen „höherer" Hirnstrukturen die „unteren" Zentren in ihrer Funktion *enthemmt* werden und dadurch die positiven Symptome einer neurologischen Erkrankung erzeugen, gilt auch nur cum grano salis. Ferner gilt die Enthemmung nicht nur für untergeordnete, sondern auch für gleichgeordnete Schichten.

Dominanzfunktionen der Großhirnhemisphären. Da neurophysiologische Befunde vorläufig nicht weiterführen, muß die Funktionsdifferenzierung der beiden Hemisphären zunächst weiter mit klinischen und anatomischen Mitteln betrieben werden.

Das Kapitel von ASSAL und HECAEN in Bd. I/1 berichtet über den neuesten Stand der neurpsychologischen Forschung. Die Autoren empfehlen, von *funktioneller Hemisphären*asymmetrie, statt von Dominanz zu sprechen. Wenn man *Sprachendominanz* für die linken und *Orientierungsdominanz* für die rechten Hirnregionen sagt, sind Mißverständnisse eher auszuschließen.

Da bei optisch-räumlichen Störungen vorwiegend Herde der *rechten* Hemisphäre gefunden werden, bestimmte Erkennungs- und Handlungsfolgen ebenfalls mehr durch rechtsseitige Großhirnläsionen gestört werden und die physiognomische Agnosie als visuelle Erkennungsstörung individueller Züge auch häufiger bei rechtsseitigen Läsionen entsteht, nimmt HECAEN für rechte Hemisphäre als übergeordnete Funktion Individuationsprozesse an, die sowohl Erkennen wie

Handeln betreffen. Er spricht von „Apractagnosie" als dominanter Störung der rechten Hemisphäre [H 22].

Zweifellos sind die Leistungen der rechten, meist als „nicht-dominant" bezeichneten Großhirnhemisphäre in der älteren Hirnpathologie bis zu KLEIST unterschätzt worden. Die auffallenderen Störungen der Sprachfunktionen wurden überwertet und die diskreteren Symptome bei rechtsseitigen Herden weniger beachtet. Optisch-räumliche Störungen bei rechtsseitigen Hirnläsionen waren zwar seit JACKSON [J 1] bekannt und schon von REICHARDT u.a. mit der rechten Parietalregion in Verbindung gebracht worden. doch hat die durch Aphasie-Befunde begründete Lehre von der Linksdominanz alle Konzeptionen zugunsten einer leitenden Funktion der linken Hemisphäre beeinflußt.

Parietale Rechtsdominanz der Raumorientierung und Linksneglekt. Die parietalen Rindenfelder 5 und 7 steuern beim *Affen* auch die visuelle Aufmerksamkeit mit den Blickbewegungen beim Greifen [M 75]. Diese Rindenfelder enthalten nach MOUNTCASTLES Experimenten [M 73, L 44] Fixationsneurone und Blickfolgeneurone, die wir 1973 postuliert hatten [J 45], ohne ihre Lokalisation zu kennen. Diese Steuerung der Aufmerksamkeitsrichtung beim Affen betrifft vorwiegend den Greifarm der Gegenseite, ohne daß eine Seitendominanz der Raumorientierung erkennbar ist. Beim *Menschen* findet man jedoch im Gegensatz zur Sprachdominanz der linken Großhirnhemisphäre eine Raumdominanz der *rechten* Parietalrinde.

Die rechte Parietalregion ist beim rechtshändigen Menschen für die Raumorientierung relativ dominant, wie hirnpathologische Erfahrungen zeigen. Ein neurophysiologisch interessantes Syndrom bei parietalen Herden ist der *kontralaterale Neglekt,* eine Störung der gerichteten Aufmerksamkeit zur gegenseitigen Sehwelt. Schwere Ausfälle sind vorwiegend bei *rechtsseitigen Parietalläsionen zur linken Seite* beschrieben. Dieser *Linksneglekt* betrifft nicht nur die visuelle Aufmerksamkeit und Wahrnehmung, sondern auch das zielgerichtete Handeln nach der Gegenseite, selbst wenn keine Apraxie vorliegt. Patienten mit Linksneglekt vernachlässigen beim Zeichnen die linke Seite mit Weglassen der Grenzkonturen und der Detailstrukturen dieser Seite. Das Zifferblatt einer Uhr wird z.B. nur auf der rechten Seite mit Zahlen gefüllt. Die Kompensation des Linksneglekts geschieht meist langsam und kann viele Monate dauern. Ein besonders eindrucksvolles Beispiel zeigen die Selbstporträts nach einer rechts-parietalen Hirnläsion eines Malers (Abb. 21). Anfangs zeichnete der Kranke bei seinen Selbstporträts, die er zwei Monate nach dem Gefäßinsult wieder begann, nur die rechte Gesichtshälfte und ließ die linke Malfläche frei. Mit halbjähriger geduldiger Übung nach mehreren links unvollständigen Bildern (b–e) gelang es ihm erst 9 Monate nach der Läsion, sein vollständiges Selbstbildnis zu malen (Abb. 21f). Die genauere Betrachtung zeigt auch in diesem Bild noch linksseitige Ungenauigkeiten, die besonders am Auge und der Brille deutlich sind. Auch bei dem Maler CORINTH, bei dem eine linksseitige Handparese zurückblieb, dauerte die Kompensation mehrere Monate, andere Maler kompensierten den Linksneglekt rascher [J 46]. Da solche schweren Neglektsyndrome häufiger nach links bei rechtsseitigen Parietalherden als nach rechts bei linksseitigen Läsionen vorkommen, ist anzunehmen, daß die nicht-sprachdominante, rechte Parietalregion bei Rechtshändern für die Raumorientierung wichtiger ist als die linke.

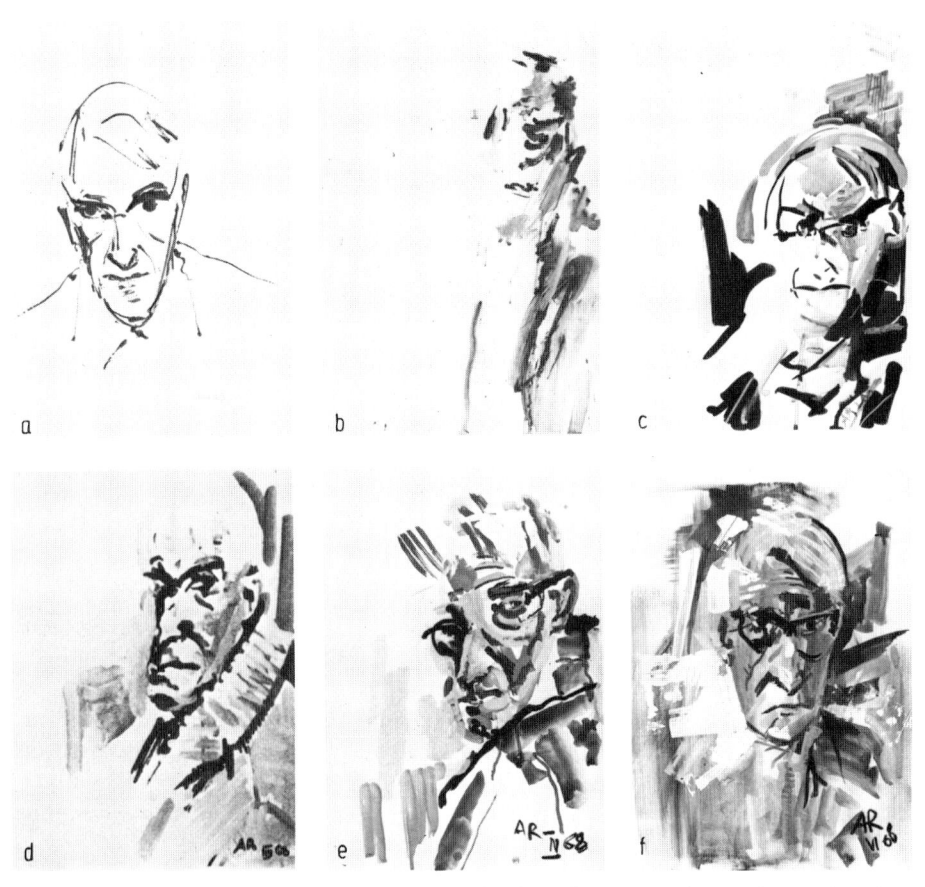

Abb. 1a–f. Linksseitenneglekt und seine Kompensation in Selbstporträts eines Malers nach rechtsseitigem parietalem Gefäßinsult. Nach JUNG (1974) [J 46]. Der 75jährige Maler A. RÄDERSCHEIDT versuchte nach seiner Parietalläsion rechts (Okt. 1967) durch wiederholte Selbstporträts die Maldefekte der linken Seite auszugleichen.

a Selbstbildnis 1965 2 Jahre *vor* der Erkrankung.
b 2 Monate nach Insult, erster Malversuch im Dezember 1967. Die linke Bildhälfte bleibt leer, nur wenige Pinselstriche versuchen, die rechte Gesichtshälfte mit Ohr, Auge und Schulter darzustellen: Dabei malt er oft über die Grenze der Malpappe hinaus nach rechts auf das Holz der Staffelei.
c $3^{1}/_{2}$ *Monate* nach Insult noch deutlicher Linksneglekt. Der Kopf wird verzerrt in die rechte Bildhälfte gesetzt ohne linke untere Gesichtsgrenze mit wenigen ungestalteten Pinselstrichen in der linken Bildhälfte.
d 5 Monate nach Insult bessere Strukturen der rechten Gesichtshälfte, aber Fehlen der linken mit einigen gestaltlosen Pinselstrichen.
e 6 Monate nach Insult noch bessere Darstellung der rechten Gesichtshälfte, aber Verlagerung des linken Auges nach unten und fehlende Außengrenzen am linken Kopf.
f 9 Monate nach dem Insult im Juni 1968 gelingt dem Maler nach $^{1}/_{2}$jährigem Bemühen ein gestaltetes Gesicht mit Seitenasymmetrien und unscharfer Darstellung der linken Gesichtshälfte besonders des Auges und der Brille links

Enthemmung. Innerhalb einer Schicht auf derselben Funktionsebene sind zwei Entstehungsbedingungen von Enthemmungserscheinungen bekannt. Erstens können nach HESS [H 56] bei symmetrisch-antagonistisch geschalteten, tonisierten bilateralen Strukturen *kontralaterale* Substrate eines doppelseitig gezügelten oder tonisierten Funktionskomplexes nach Läsion einer Seite überwiegen. Beide symmetrischen Substrate repräsentieren Kräfte, die normalerweise im Gleichgewicht sind. Bei Ausfall einer Seite überwiegt die andere je nach ihrer Funktion mit einseitiger Erregung oder Hemmung. Dies ist besonders im vestibulären System mit dem kontralateralen Nystagmus bei Ausfall eines Labyrinthes oder eines Vestibulariskernes deutlich [J 33].

Zweitens können auch unvollständige Läsionen Enthemmungs- und Krampferscheinungen *in der lädierten Struktur selbst* hervorrufen. Die Mehrzahl der epileptischen Phänomene entsteht aus solchen ungehemmten Teilfunktionen bei partiellem Ausfall koordinierender und bremsender Mechanismen. Diese Art der Enthemmung wird meist als *Reizsymptom* bezeichnet. Neurophysiologisch sind solche Reizsymptome durch Gleichgewichtsverschiebungen der neuronalen Koordination zu erklären. Wahrscheinlich handelt es sich um eine überwiegende Ausschaltung neuronaler Hemmungsmechanismen, die bei reziproker Schaltung in enger räumlicher Nachbarschaft mit den aktivierten Neuronen liegen.

Zentrenbegriff. Eine kurze Bemerkung noch zu dem in den letzten Jahrzehnten so viel geschmähten Terminus „Zentrum": Wenn man ihn im Sinne von WINTERSTEIN [W 28] und HESS [H 64] verwendet, ist gegen den Gebrauch des Wortes „Zentrum" in der Neurophysiologie kein ernsthafter Einwand möglich. „Zentrum" ist damit einfach eine Abbreviatur für *Ort und Substrat einer zentralnervösen Koordinationsleistung.*

Zentrenlehre und Funktionsspezifität. Die Erkenntnis, daß eine *erworbene und erlernte Funktion wie die Sprache durch einseitige lokalisierte Herde im frontotemporalen Cortex verlorengehen kann,* war für die Neurologen des 19. Jahrhunderts so eindrucksvoll, daß eine Funktionslokalisation ohne Bedenken akzeptiert wurde. Nach klinischen Erfahrungen ist es wahrscheinlich, daß spezielle Neuronensysteme in umschriebenen Hirnregionen für die *erlernten* Funktionen des Sprechens, Lesens und Schreibens von Bedeutung sind und daß diese Neuronensysteme im Sinne der Zentrenlehre solche erlernten Leistungen steuern. Denn nach lokalisierten Verletzungen dominanter Großhirnstrukturen entstehen regelmäßig schwere und zum Teil irreversible Störungen dieser erworbenen Funktionen. Bei aller Problematik eines Rückschlusses von Funktionsstörungen auf normale Funktionen kann sich der Physiologe nicht auf die Feststellung beschränken, diese Leistungen würden nur durch Läsion solcher Hirnregionen gestört, aber nicht von ihnen gesteuert.

Eine Leugnung der Funktionsspezifität bestimmter Hirnregionen widerspräche den Prinzipien der Ordnung und der Erregungsbegrenzung im ZNS. Es ist daher nicht nur erlaubt, sondern auch notwendig, die hirnpathologischen Werkzeugstörungen mit lokalisierten Hirnrindenläsionen zu korrelieren. Alle Versuche, diese Werkzeugstörungen der Sprache, Gnosis und Praxis auf eine einheitliche „Grundstörung" zurückzuführen, sind mißlungen. Seit PIERRE MARIE unter dem Eindruck der häufigen Demenz seiner senilen Aphasiker die Bedeutung des Intelligenzabbaus bei aphasischen Patienten betont hat, sind doch alle Bestrebungen, die Sprachstörungen wieder in den alten, schlecht abgrenzbaren Komplex der Demenz zurückzuführen, nicht von Erfolg gewesen. Ganzheitsbestrebungen in der Leistungsanalyse mit den Begriffen von GOLDSTEINS „kategorialer Störung" [G 29], WEIZSÄCKERS [W 18] „Funktionswandel" oder CONRADS [C 9] „Vorgestalt" waren nicht geeignet, die speziellen und spezifischen Ausfälle der corticalen Werkzeugstörungen zu erklären. Richtig ist bei diesen Konzeptionen nur, daß *auch lokalisierte Herde meistens eine allgemeine Leistungsminderung zur Folge haben,* entsprechend dem klinischen Begriff der „Hirnleistungsschwäche". Doch kann eine allgemeine Leistungsminderung nie die speziellen Funktionsausfälle erklären. In manchen Fällen kann eine allgemeine Hirnleistungsschwäche die spezifischen Funktionsstörungen verschleiern, in anderen durch mangelnde Kompensation gewisse Funktionsausfälle stärker hervortreten lassen.

Diese Verteidigung des Lokalisationsprinzips im ZNS soll natürlich nicht alte Verirrungen der Lokalisationslehre entschuldigen, die bis zur Lokalisierung einzelner Worte oder Buchstaben im Gehirn reichten. Solche schematischen Vorstellungen wurden nicht von Physiologen entwickelt. Die Physiologie ist gewohnt, funktionelle Ordnungen zu untersuchen, die *mehrere* Strukturen verbinden. Schon das EEG mit seiner ausgedehnten Koordination des Alpha-Rhythmus in verschiedenen Hirnregionen zeigt eindrucksvoll die *Zusammenarbeit* vieler Rindenfelder und die Abhängigkeit vom Subcortex. *Hier bilden Strukturgrenzen nicht Funktionsgrenzen, sondern Funktionsverbindungen.* Dies zeigen die Einzelneuronbefunde noch besser, wenn sie an der Nervenzelle als niederster Einheit Konvergenz verschiedener Afferenzen nachweisen [K 39]. Neurophysiologische Bestrebungen, solche Funktionsverbindungen durch *Systemkonzeptionen* zu erfassen, werden auf S. 902 besprochen.

Wie nach cerebralen Reizversuchen nicht einzelne Muskeln in der motorischen Region lokalisiert vertreten sind, sondern gewisse Bewegungsrepräsentationen und ihre afferente Konvergenz, so müssen die höheren Koordinationszentren einen viel komplexeren Aufbau haben: Hier findet sich ein geordnetes Netz konvergierender Substrate vieler Funktionen mit durch Lernen erworbenen Informationsverbindungen, mit Bahnung und Hemmung multipler Leitungen. Dann hat auch der Begriff der „Leitung" cerebraler Erregungen seinen guten Sinn, ebenso wie der zu Unrecht geschmähte Begriff des „Zentrums".

Bei manchen hirnpathologischen Syndromen, wie der reinen Alexie, erscheint es jedenfalls zulässig, die Störung der Leseleistung durch eine *„Leitungsstörung"* zwischen optischen und sprachlichen „Zentren" zu erklären. Die klassischen Konzeptionen apraktischer Leitungsstörungen sind in den letzten Jahren durch GESCHWIND wieder erneuert worden. Er nennt die Leitungsunterbrechungen zwischen integrierenden Hirnzentren „disconnection syndromes" [G 17].

Neurologische und physiologische Gesamtkonzeptionen der psychischen und cerebralen Funktionen

Synthetische Betrachtungen der psychischen Hirnfunktionen sind nur von wenigen Neurologen und Psychologen gegeben worden. Nach der klassischen „Hirnpathologie" von KLEIST [K 17] 1934 bringt die Monographie von SCHLESINGER [S 8] 1962 eine Übersicht über die Beziehungen von psychischen Funktionen und cerebralen Störungen sowie über die neuere Literatur. Dazu kommt in den letzten Jahren noch das *Modulprinzip* der Koordination von Funktionseinheiten, die nach dem technischen Baukastenprinzip in der Hirnrinde angeordnet sind und nach übergeordneten Funktionsordnungen aktiviert werden. Darstellungen dieser „modulären Ordnung" des Großhirns findet man bei MOUNTCASTLE [M 74], ECCLES [P 32] und SZENTAGOTHAI [S 63, 64].

KLEISTs Hirnpathologie und die Neurophysiologie. Die notwendige physiologische Ergänzung der hirnpathologischen Forschung wird deutlich in dem Werk KLEISTs [K 17]. Die Größe von KLEISTs Werk liegt in der systematischen Vollständigkeit der anatomischen Lokalisation und der allesumfassenden Einordnung, seine Schwäche in der methodischen Einseitigkeit und physiologisch unbegründeten Funktionskorrelation mit den Brodmannschen Rindenfeldern. Damals gab es nur VOGTs Reizexperimente [V 10]. Heute, ein Vierteljahrhundert später, haben HUBEL und WIESEL einige physiologische Korrelationen von Rindenfeldern mit neuronalen Funktionen für die Sehrindenfelder entdeckt [H 87, 88].

Die höheren Funktionsstörungen bei Erkrankungen der Hirnrinde bezeichnet KLEIST als „hirnpathologische" und „psychopathologische" Symptome. Zu den letzteren rechnet er schon die Agnosien und Aphasien als Störungen komplexer Funktionen, an denen Gedächtnisphänomene teilhaben und die damit dem Kern unserer seelischen Verfassung näher stehen [K 18].

Solche Zuordnungen können heuristisch fruchtbar sein, aber auch zu Grenzverwischungen führen, besonders da die von JACKSON geforderte Differenzierung von positiven und negativen Symptomen und die Unterscheidung von Symptom und Funktion nicht genügend scharf durchgeführt wird. Dies ist von THIELE [T 4] und LANGE [L 1] in Koreferaten zu KLEISTs Lehre klar dargestellt worden.

SCHLESINGERs Hirnkonzeption. In einer originellen Monographie über die höheren Hirnfunktionen und ihre klinischen Störungen diskutiert SCHLESINGER die cerebralen Grundlagen des emotionalen Lebens, des Denkens und der Motorik mit kybernetischen Mechanismen [S 8]. Er verwendet andere Gesichtspunkte als KLEISTs areale Gliederung psychischer Funktionen. SCHLESINGER geht von folgenden Positionen aus: Er vergleicht das Nervensystem mit einem *Analogrechner,* also einem Datenverarbeitungsapparat. Dieser soll Umweltvorgänge als korrespondierende Informationsprozesse (simulacra) widerspiegeln. Die Verarbeitung dieser Umweltbilder kann neue, in dem Neben- und Nacheinander der primären Daten nicht enthaltene Kombinationen gewinnen. Solche biologischen Computer sollen der Auswertung und Beantwortung bestimmter Reizkonstellationen dienen.

Auf dieser theoretischen Basis aufbauend, hat SCHLESINGER in seinem Buche versucht, die organischen Grundlagen der Psychologie und Psychiatrie zusammen mit den neurologischen Störungen der höheren corticalen Funktionen darzustellen. Er gibt eine unkonventionelle Ordnung mit der Dreiteilung Affektivität, Denken und Fertigkeiten. Im Rahmen der *Affektivität (affectivity)* bespricht er diencephale und rhinencephale Störungen, Neurosen und Frontalhirnstörungen. Beim *Denken (thought)* behandelt er Unter- und Überbegabungen, Schwachsinn und Genie und diskutiert ausführlich kybernetische Vorstellungen über „Elektronengehirne". Bei den *Fertigkeiten (skill)* werden zunächst extrapyramidale und pyramidale Bewegungsregulationen und die Integration der feineren Bewegungen in beiden Hemisphären besprochen, dann die agnostischen, apraktischen und aphasischen Störungen und in einem Appendix die hirnphysiologischen Quellen der Kunst und die Bedeutung der Übung und Affektivität für künstlerische Leistungen dargestellt.

Physiologische Gesamtkonzeptionen. Bereits vor den modernen Erfahrungen über die Beeinflussung der Großhirnfunktionen durch thalamo-reticuläre Strukturen, die zu neuen Systemkonzeptionen führten, haben LASHLEY [L 4] und W.R. HESS [H 64] vom physiologischen Standpunkt Hirnfunktionen und Verhalten in Beziehung gesetzt. HESS geht aus von der Wechselwirkung vegetativer und animaler Funktionen und vom Schlaf. In seiner letzten Darstellung [H 65] *„Psychologie aus physiologischer Sicht"* gibt HESS eine kurze Übersicht über die cerebralen Grundlagen des Psychischen vom Standpunkt des Neurophysiologen (vgl. S. 783). LASHLEYS antilokalisatorische Einstellung hat Physiologen und Psychologen stark beeinflußt und muß daher besprochen werden. LASHLEY stützte sich vor allem auf Labyrinthversuche bei Ratten mit verschiedenen Cortexläsionen, die mit Ausnahme der Sehrinde keine wesentlichen Unterschiede zeigten. Weniger die Lokalisation als die Menge der entfernten Hirnsubstanz beeinflußte das Verhalten. Ähnliche Folgerungen zogen WOLFF u. Mitarb. [C 23] aus der Untersuchung neurochirurgisch operierter Menschen mit verschieden großem Hirnsubstanzverlust unterschiedlicher Lokalisation. LASHLEY postulierte eine cerebrale „Massentätigkeit", bei der verschiedene Cortexregionen ähnlich oder gleichwertig sein können (equipotentiality).

LASHLEYS Konzeption der cerebralen „mass action" [L 3] war nicht als ungeordnete Totalerregung gemeint. Trotz seiner Konzeption der Äquipotentialität gibt LASHLEY zu, daß eine *spezifische Funktion* zumindest in den Projektionsfeldern des Cortex vorhanden ist. Er schließt corticale Lokalisation daher nicht völlig aus. Für das Formensehen hatte LASHLEY nach seinen Rattenversuchen eine lokalisierte Funktion der Sehrinde zugegeben. Die Schwäche der klassischen Lokalisationslehre wurde von LASHLEY klar gesehen. Sie kann nicht erklären, wie die spezialisierten Teile des Cortex *koordiniert* werden und die psychische und Verhaltensintegration des Organismus zustande kommt. Eine solche *Koordination und Integration verschiedener Funktionen* und Strukturen ist aber für ein geordnetes Verhalten ebenso notwendig *wie spezialisierte Funktionen mit Arbeitsteilung in verschiedenen Abschnitten des Gehirns,* die auch von LASHLEY nicht völlig bestritten wurden. "No one today can seriously believe that the different parts of the cerebral cortex all have the same functions or can entertain for a moment the proposition that because the mind is a unit the brain must also act as a unit."

Nach LASHLEYS Ansicht könnte allerdings dasselbe corticale Feld einmal als hochdifferenziertes System, ein anderes Mal gewissermaßen als amorphe Masse wirken. Bei Labyrinthversuchen ist die Ratte in ihrer Raumlokalisation weitgehend unabhängig vom Sehen, obwohl bei Menschen und höheren Tierformen räumliche Orientierung vorwiegend optisch ist. Blinde und sehende Ratten unterschieden sich kaum in ihren Labyrinthleistungen [D 3]. Dennoch soll der *visuelle Cortex* nach LASHLEY für diese Funktion von besonderer Bedeutung sein [L 2, 4]. Doch zeigen LASHLEYS Hirnkarten, daß die Läsionen über die

Sehrinde nach vorn in *parietale Felder* reichen. Es ist daher wahrscheinlich, daß die von LASHLEY der Sehrinde zugewiesene Steuerungsfunktion im Labyrinthversuch mehr durch vordere Nachbarfelder geleistet wird. Diese würden bei der Katze dem Gyrus suprasylvius, bei Affen und Menschen den *parietalen* und *temporalen* Rindenfeldern entsprechen, in denen multisensorische Afferenzen verarbeitet werden und die visuelle Aufmerksamkeit gesteuert wird [M 73]. LASHLEYS Konzeptionen sind auch durch neuere Systemauffassungen der Hirnleistungen zu modifizieren, zu denen LASHLEY auf einem Symposion nur kurz Stellung genommen hat [L 5]. Diese anatomisch-physiologischen Systemtheorien wurden aus neurophysiologischen Befunden über „unspezifische" Hirnstammfunktionen entwickelt.

Neurophysiologie zentraler Systemorganisation. Seit der Entdeckung der Weckfunktionen des reticulären Systems und ihrer Korrelation mit der Abflachung des EEG durch MORUZZI und MAGOUN [M 19, 66] 1949 ist eine neue Form des Systemdenkens in der Neurophysiologie und Neuroanatomie entstanden. Bestimmte Hirnregionen des Hirnstamms und der phylogenetisch alten „rhinencephalen" Rinde, die anatomisch lange bekannt, aber physiologisch wenig untersucht waren, wurden zu allgemeinen Funktionssystemen zusammengefaßt: Die ponto-mesencephale Reticularis und der intralaminäre Thalamus wurden funktionell zum *„thalamoreticulären System"*. Ammonshorn, Mandelkern, Cingulum und ihre Verbindungen zum Septum, Zwischen-, Mittelhirn wurden zum *„limbischen System"*. Ohne bestimmte anatomische Abgrenzung von diesen, z.T. sich überschneidend mit dem thalamo-reticulären System hat PENFIELD das *centrencephale System* aufgestellt. Manche dieser Systemkonzeptionen gehen schon auf alte *klinische Konzeptionen* zurück: Die anatomisch noch ungenau definierte alte Lokalisation von Bewußtseinsvorgängen im Hirnstamm und Thalamus durch REICHARDT [R 8], KÜPPERS [K 59] und KLEIST [K 17] würde etwa dem reticulo-thalamischen System entsprechen. Das *„Innenhirn"* von KLEIST [K 18], in dem er vegetative und Triebfunktionen lokalisierte, kann etwa mit dem limbischen System und Rhinencephalon gleichgesetzt werden. Das vorwiegend nach klinischen Erfahrungen und Cortexreizungen definierte Centrencephalon von PENFIELD entspräche etwa dem reticulo-thalamischen System und seinen noch ungeklärten Verbindungen zum Cortex (vgl. S. 977). Zwischen diesen Konzeptionen lag das anatomisch abgeleitete Postulat von PAPEZ, der dem Neuronenkreis zwischen Ammonshorn, Cingulum und Zwischenhirn eine besondere Funktion für die Regulation der Affekte zusprach [P 1]. MACLEAN unterteilte das limbische System in je ein Substrat, das der Arterhaltung und ein anderes, das der Selbsterhaltung dienen sollte [M 12]. Neuere Versuche, das limbische System mit Motivation und Gedächtnisfunktionen zu korrelieren, bringen KORNHUBER (1973) [K 42] und ECCLES (1979) [E 5c, P 32]. Im Kapitel IX über Affekte und Triebe und X und XI über Bewußtsein und Schlaf werden neurophysiologische Korrelationen dieser Systemkonzeptionen dargestellt.

Lokalisations- und Ganzheitslehren als koordinierte Prinzipien des ZNS. Der Gegensatz von Ganzheits- und Lokalisationslehren ist ein Scheinproblem, dessen Antagonismus in der Neurologie und Aphasielehre zu viel unnötigem Streit geführt hat. Die Mißverständnisse der wissenschaftlichen Diskussion entstanden meist durch die mangelhafte Unterscheidung zwischen lokalisierten Läsionen und der Lokalisation von Funktionen, zu denen auch zahlreiche andere Strukturen des ZNS und der Peripherie gehören. In der Psychiatrie war die extrem lokalistisch eingestellte Forschung seit dem Mißerfolg von WERNICKES Lokalisation psychischer Funktionen im Cortex [W 20], der begrenzten Anwendbarkeit von KLEISTS Hirnpathologie [K 17], und den Versuchen, die Symptome der Encephalitis epidemica durch Lokalisation von Antrieb und Affekt im Hirnstamm zu erklären [B 51, T 3], zum Stillstand gekommen, bis sie in den letzten Jahren durch physiologische Untersuchungen über Regulationen von Bewußtsein und Aufmerksamkeit im thalamo-reticulären System des Hirnstamms wieder erneut aktuell wurde (vgl. Kapitel X, S. 968). Trotz aller Kompensations- und Restitutionsphänomene und der erstaunlichen Anpassungsfähigkeit des Nervensystems an Läsionen sieht auch der Neuropsychiater bei der Untersuchung organischer Hirnerkrankungen sehr bald die Grenzen dieser Kompensation und die Bedeutung bleibender Funktionsdefekte nach lokalisierten Hirnläsionen. Die gemeinsame Anwendung von Lokalisations- und Ganzheitstheorien im Gehirn wird verständlich, wenn man ihre physiologischen Grundlagen kennt. *Die physiologische Basis der Lokalisationslehre ist die Notwendigkeit der Erregungsbegrenzung im Gehirn* [J 29], *die Differenzierung und Begrenzung der Informationen verlangt. Die Funktionsgrundlage der Ganzheitslehren ist die notwendige Ausbreitung von Informationen im ZNS und ihre geordnete Integration zum Verhalten des Einzelorganismus.* Wenn das Ganzheitsprinzip sinnvoll sein soll, so kann es nur *Ordnung und Selektion* von Reiz und Erregung bedeuten, nicht Totalerregung oder undifferenzierte Irradiation. *Ganzheitsleistungen enthalten als geordnete Integrationen und Selektionen daher auch lokalisierte und differenzierte Teilfunktionen und sind deshalb nur auf der Basis des Lokalisationsprinzips möglich.*

Zusammenfassung

Die anatomisch orientierte Hirnpathologie betonte am Ende des 19. Jahrhunderts nach Entdeckung der Sprachzentren das *Lokalisationsprinzip* der Hirnfunktionen, hatte aber mit den Reiz- und Ausschaltungsmethoden nur auf die Motorik beschränkte physiologische Ergebnisse. Erst elektrobiologische Untersuchungen der letzten Jahrzehnte brachten physiologische Korrelate der Hirnlokalisation für die Projektionen der Sinnesafferenzen. Neurophysiologische Grundlage des Lokalisationsprinzips ist die Notwendigkeit einer Erregungsbegrenzung im Nervensystem mit geordneter Koordination spezialisierter Hirnstrukturen und gegenseitiger Hemmung. Ganzheitslehren verlangen eine Integration einzelner Teilfunktionen und damit auch eine Anerkennung des Lokalisationsprinzips.

Einseitige Großhirnhemisphärendominanz gibt es nur beim Menschen. Die Sprache wird als erlernte Funktion von einer Großhirnhälfte koordiniert und ist durch Leitungsunterbrechungen dieser Seite störbar. Beim Rechtshänder ist die *linke* Großhirnhemisphäre für *Sprache, Lesen und Rechnen* dominant. Die *rechte* Hemisphäre ist dagegen besonders in der Parietalregion dominant für *räumliche Orientierungsleistungen*. Der Linksseitenneglekt bei rechtsseitigen Parietalherden und seine Kompensation wird an Selbstbildnissen eines Malers demonstriert. In der Motorik ist angeborene *Seitendominanz* von durch Übung erworbener *Seitenpräferenz* zu unterscheiden.

Ergebnisse und Grenzen der Cortexreizung beim Menschen und ihrer psychischen Korrelate werden mit PENFIELDS Reizeffekten in den Sprachregionen und der Temporalrinde besprochen. Der *Informationstransfer zwischen beiden Großhirnhemisphären* wird mit der *Balkenfunktion* und der Seitendominanz dargestellt. Die Beziehungen und Unterschiede von hirnpathologischen Syndromen und physiologischen Funktionen werden mit JACKSONS Prinzipien, KLEISTS Hirnpathologie, SCHLESINGERS Hirnkonzeption und LASHLEYS antilokalistischer Massenaktion besprochen.

VIII. Objektive und subjektive Sinnesphysiologie: Neurophysiologie und Psychophysik des Sehens

> „Nempe nihil est in intellectu quod non fuerit in sensu, nisi ipse intellectus."
> G.W. LEIBNIZ, Brief an BIERLING 1709.

> „Das Höchste wäre: zu begreifen, daß alles Factische schon Theorie ist. Die Bläue des Himmels offenbart uns das Grundgesetz der Chromatik. Man suche nur nichts hinter den Phänomenen; sie selbst sind die Lehre."
> J.W. GOETHE, Über Naturwissenschaft im Allgemeinen, einzelne Betrachtungen und Aphorismen (posthum 1833).

Die sensualistischen Theorien der tabula rasa, die das gesamte seelische Leben aus Sinneswahrnehmungen und Erfahrungen ableiteten, sind zwar unhaltbar, doch darf die Bedeutung der Wahrnehmung für psychische Vorgänge deshalb nicht unterschätzt werden. Wenn LEIBNIZ in seiner obigen Korrektur des empiristischen Sensualismus von LOCKE den Verstand selbst mit seinen Funktionen und mit DESCARTES' „eingeborenen Ideen" der Sinneswahrnehmung voranstellte, so meinte er damit die anlagebedingten Fähigkeiten. Ähnlich wird auch der Neurophysiologe die vorgegebenen Strukturen und Funktionsgesetze der Sinnesorgane und des Gehirns zur Grundlage einer wissenschaftlichen Sinnesforschung machen. Wenn er nicht eine reine Reflex-Reaktionsforschung oder eine abstrakte Sinnespsychologie treiben will, so muß er *beide* Seiten, die objektiven cerebralen Mechanismen und die subjektive Wahrnehmung beachten. Für den Physiologen entsprechen die angeborenen Strukturen des Nervensystems mit ihren neuronalen Verbindungen dem a priori Gegebenen, dagegen die durch äußere Reize angeregten Informationen der Sinnesorgane und ihre zentralen Verarbeitungen dem empirisch Erworbenen. Daher hat auch KANTS Erkenntniskritik und seine Synthese von rational-aprioristischen mit anschaulich-sinnesbedingten psychischen Funktionen die Sinnesphysiologie des 19. Jahrhunderts stark beeinflußt. Obwohl HELMHOLTZ [H 27] die empirisch erworbene Natur der Raumvorstellung betonte und KANTS aprioristische Lehre von der Raumkategorie ablehnte, blieb die Sinnesforschung bis v. KRIES [K 51, 52] kantianisch. HELMHOLTZ' skeptische Ansicht, daß die Sinnesfunktionen nur „Zeichen" der Außenwelt geben, wirkt in veränderter, realistischer Form mit der Signallehre

PAWLOWs weiter [P 7]. Die Gestaltpsychologie erkannte dann wieder den Bild- und Gestaltcharakter zentraler Wahrnehmungsmuster und erneuerte den Apriorismus KANTS. Die moderne Sinnesphysiologie hat schließlich eine Synthese psychophysischer und physiologischer Vorgänge ermöglicht: Die von FECHNER [F 4] geschaffene messende Psychophysik der Sinne und die von ADRIAN [A 4-8] begründete moderne Elektrophysiologie der Receptorfunktionen brachten weitgehende Parallelen von Neurophysiologie und Psychologie, obwohl auch hier noch viele Aporien blieben [J 39].

Das *sinnesphysiologische Experiment* ist in erster Linie geeignet, ein echter „Vermittler von Subjekt und Objekt" in GOETHES Sinne zu werden. Allerdings ist GOETHES Mahnung, die Phänomene selbst zu sehen und nichts „hinter" ihnen zu suchen, nur psychologisch richtig, aber *physiologisch falsch*. Dennoch hat die Sinnesphysiologie mit einem reinen Studium der Phänomene begonnen. Die Sinneserscheinungen unserer Wahrnehmungswelt zeigen reproduzierte Abbilder der Umwelt mit großer Klarheit und Überzeugungskraft, sie lassen aber nicht erkennen, wie diese Endergebnisse physiologisch zustande kommen. Die physiologischen *Mechanismen* der anschaulichen Sinnesphänomene sind erst in mühsamer Einzelarbeit durch naturwissenschaftliche Methoden zu erforschen.

Die Sinnesforschung ist ein gutes Modell für das Verhältnis von Neurophysiologie und Psychologie, weil sie mit beiden Methoden subjektiver Beobachtung und objektiver Registrierung, arbeitet. Die Sinnesphysiologie hat damit gezeigt, daß zahlreiche Wahrnehmungsphänomene, die man früher als rein „psychisch" ansah, in ihren neurophysiologischen Korrelaten exakt physikalisch registrierbar sind.

Subjektive und objektive Sinnesphysiologie

Außer der speziellen Untersuchung physikalischer und morphologischer Eigenschaften der Sinnesorgane, die hier nicht interessiert, gibt es zwei Hauptforschungsrichtungen: 1. Die *subjektive Sinnesphysiologie* schließt aus dem Vergleich von Reiz und Empfindung auf zwischen beiden liegende Sinnesfunktionen. 2. Die *objektive Sinnesphysiologie* untersucht den physiologischen Mechanismus der Sinne durch direkte Registrierung der Vorgänge an Sinnesreceptoren, ihren Nerven und ihren Zentren im Gehirn. Nur durch die zweite Methode können wir die zwischen Reiz und Wahrnehmung liegenden Einzelmechanismen analysieren.

Die subjektive Psychophysiologie der Sinnesleistungen wurde von 1802–1865 durch YOUNG, PURKINJE, JOHANNES MÜLLER, WEBER, FECHNER, HELMHOLTZ und HERING begründet. Sie hat sich rasch zu größter Höhe entwickelt, indem sie die subjektive Empfindung beim Menschen nach klar definierten physikalischen Reizen beobachtete und soweit wie möglich messend erfaßte (*Psychophysik* FECHNERS [F 4], S. 908). Neben der Entdeckung einiger, für verschiedene Sinnesmodalitäten geltender Regeln wurde vor allem die Physiologie des Sehens mit diesen Methoden zu hoher Differenzierung und Exaktheit geführt: die wichtigsten sinnesphysiologischen Gesetzmäßigkeiten des Simultankontrastes, des Sukzessivkontrastes, der optisch-vestibulären Koordination, der binocularen Koordination, des Wettstreites der Sehfelder sowie der Konstanz der Sehdinge wurden entdeckt und in ihrer funktionellen Bedeutung erkannt. Eine gute Übersicht gibt BORING [B 54].

Die objektive Neurophysiologie der Sinnesfunktionen ist seit 1926 von E.D. ADRIAN begründet worden, nachdem es ihm gelang, Aktionspotentiale einzelner sensibler Nervenfasern zu registrieren. Diese mikrophysiologischen Methoden wurden zunächst von ADRIAN und ZOTTERMAN [A 4-6] für die peripheren Nerven der Hautsensibilität verwendet, dann von HARTLINE [H 4, 5] und GRANIT [G 26, 32] für die Retina und von uns für die Sehrinde [J 34, 52] entwickelt. Dazu kamen mikrophysiologische Untersuchungen auf allen Ebenen des somatosensiblen [M 70, 71] und des akustischen Systems [K 8, 10, R 25].

Allgemeine Ergebnisse der subjektiven und objektiven Sinnesphysiologie

Reiz und Empfindung in der psychophysischen Sinnesforschung. Die *subjektive Erforschung der Sinnesvorgänge*, ausgehend von Beobachtungen der Empfindung und Wahrnehmung, die mit bestimmten physikalischen Sinnesreizen verglichen wurden, hat die ersten Regeln und Gesetzmäßigkeiten der Sinnesphysiologie mit diesen Methoden gewonnen. JOHANNES MÜLLER formulierte 1826 sein Gesetz der *spezifischen Sinnesenergie* [M 82]. Es besagt, daß verschiedene Sinnesorgane, gleichgültig wie sie gereizt werden, jeweils eine für sie spezifische Empfindung und Sinnesqualität hervorrufen. DUBOIS-REYMOND hat für das Müllersche Gesetz folgendes Bild gegeben: Wenn es möglich wäre, den Sehnerven mit dem Hörnerven auszutauschen, so würden wir den Donner sehen und den Blitz hören. Es handelt sich also um ein *Gesetz des unabänderlichen Erfolges,* wie HERMANN später formuliert hat. Dieser Erfolg ist abhängig von den *zentralen Verbindungen der Sinnesafferenzen* mit bestimmten Hirnregionen. Die Spezifität der Hautsinne wurde erst seit 1883 durch BLIX, GOLDSCHEIDER und VON FREY an den Sinnespunkten der Haut genauer untersucht, konnte aber noch nicht mit den anatomischen Verschiedenheiten der Hautreceptoren korreliert werden. Eine moderne Handbuchdarstellung gibt IGGO [I 1].

E.H. WEBER [W 14] und G.TH. FECHNER [F 4] entdeckten durch quantitative und Schwellenuntersuchungen der Sinne die logarithmische Beziehung von Reiz und Empfindung, das sog. *Weber-Fechnersche Gesetz: Die Stärke der Empfindung steigt mit dem Logarithmus der Reizstärke.* Obwohl es bei verschiedenen Sinnesqualitäten manche Abweichungen von dieser Regel gibt, hat sich doch die logarithmische Beziehung in der objektiven Sinnesphysiologie bestätigt. Für die subjektive Schätzung der Empfindungsstärke und der sensomotorischen Wahrnehmungsfunktionen mit Augenbewegungen und Kraftaufwendung hat sich dagegen STEVENS' *Potenzfunktion* besonders bewährt [S 52]. Diese Potenzformel wurde zuerst von PLATEAU für Sehversuche vorgeschlagen [P 23].

Der *Gegensatz von Sinnesqualität und physikalischer Reizbedingung* hat zu unnötigen Streitigkeiten und Mißverständnissen zwischen Physikern, Psychologen und Philosophen geführt. Mißverständnisse entstanden meistens aus einer Übertragung der subjektiv richtig beobachteten und beschriebenen Sinnesphänomene auf physikalische Gesetzmäßigkeiten, wie bei GOETHES Streit gegen NEWTON. HERING und seine Schüler haben versucht, diese Mißverständnisse durch eine eigene Terminologie für die *Sehqualitäten* und einen „*exakten Subjektivismus*" in der Sinnesphysiologie [T 12] auszuschalten. Neuerdings hat SCHRÖDINGER [S 17] als Physiker bei diesen Reiz-Wahrnehmungsgegensätzen, die sich vom Altertum bis in die moderne Physik fortsetzen, eine vermittelnde Stellung gegenüber der Sinnesphysiologie eingenommen: Die sinnliche Wahrnehmung sagt zwar nichts über den objektiven physikalischen Vorgang. Dennoch sind unsere physikalischen Theorien und Vorstellungen durch Informationen der Sinneswahrnehmung gewonnen und diese Vorstellungen werden wiederum durch experimentelle physikalische Tatsachen und unanschauliche mathematische Ableitungen verändert. Naturwissenschaftliche Theorien ermöglichen so eine Synthese von Beobachtung und Experiment in der Sinnesphysiologie und Physik.

Reiz und Reizeffekte in der neurophysiologischen Sinnesforschung. Die objektive Registrierung der Sinnesvorgänge begann in der Peripherie. Mit elektrophysiologischen Methoden wurden von ADRIAN [A 4, 5] und ZOTTERMAN [A 10, Z 4, 5] die *Erregungen der peripheren Sinnesreceptoren durch ihre Signale in den sensiblen Nerven* und deren Leitung zum ZNS registriert.

Im Prinzip findet sich bei allen Sinnesorganen ein ähnlicher Mechanismus der Receptorenerregung, wie er auf Abb. 22 nach ADRIAN schematisch dargestellt ist. Ein mehr oder weniger kontinuierlicher Reizvorgang wird durch den Receptor des Sinnesorgans in eine diskontinuierliche Impulsfolge umgewandelt, die eine mit der Stärke des Reizes zunehmende Frequenz aufweist. Diese Impulsfolge wird über den Sinnesnerven ins Zentralnervensystem gemeldet und hier über mehrere Synapsen umgeschaltet. Als Endergebnis erscheint wiederum eine kontinuierliche Empfindung im Bewußtsein, die allerdings nur annähernd dem Außenreiz entspricht (Abb. 23). Die unterste Schwelle des Minimum perceptibile findet ihre Grenze an der Brownschen Molekularbewegung.

Wie uns die objektive Sinnesphysiologie gelehrt hat, zeigen die Erregungen der verschiedenen Sinnesorgane gewisse gemeinsame Prinzipien der Erregungsleitung mit rhythmischen Impulsen in einzelnen Nervenfasern. Auch die höchst spezialisierten Sinnesorgane arbeiten mit ihren Einzelelementen ähnlich wie die einfachsten Receptoren. Daher kann man, wie SHERRINGTON [S 32] schon früher betont hat, die Leistungen der hochdifferenzierten Sinnesorgane im Prinzip auf die Tätigkeit der einfachen zurückführen: Das Auge würde dann wie ein System

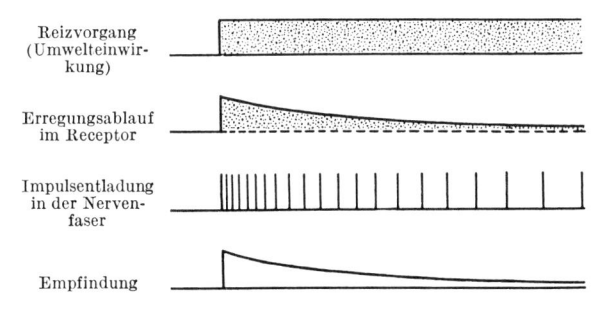

Abb. 22. Beziehung zwischen Reiz, Receptorenerregung, Nervenfaserentladung und Empfindung. Nach ADRIAN (1928) [A 5]. Schema der Druckreceptoren der Haut. Der kontinuierliche Reiz eines Druckes auf die Haut erzeugt einen durch *Adaptation* langsam abklingenden Erregungsprozeß im sensiblen Endorgan (Receptor). Dementsprechend sendet der Receptor eine allmählich langsamer werdende Impulsentladung durch seine Nervenfaser in das Zentralnervensystem. Dort entsteht eine Empfindung, deren Stärke etwa der Frequenz der Nervenfaserentladung entspricht

spezialisierter Warmreceptoren oder das Ohr wie eine Gruppe spezialisierter Tastreceptoren mit sehr komplizierter Koordination arbeiten. Wenn man diese Gemeinsamkeiten der verschiedenen Sinne im Auge behält, so kann man sehr wohl an Beispielen von Spezialsinnen die allgemeinen sinnesphysiologischen Gesetzmäßigkeiten darstellen.

Nach v. KRIES' allgemeiner Sinnesphysiologie [K 51] hat RENQVIST-REENPÄÄ versucht, sehr allgemeine Grundlagen der Sinnesphysiologie mit Beziehungen zur Logistik und Erkenntnistheorie darzustellen [R 12]. Mit Recht betont RENQVIST die *Abstraktionsvorgänge* bei der Sinneswahrnehmung. Seine verschiedenen Stufen der Klassenbildung bleiben aber hypothetisch ebenso wie sein Vergleich mit Gleichheitsrelationen der Logistik CARNAPS und mit dem Formalismus HILBERTS.

Wiederbelebung und Ergänzung der Psychophysik durch die Neurophysiologie. Neue objektive Methoden der Elektrophysiologie haben die Psychophysik und Sinnesforschung des 19. Jahrhunderts wieder zu frischem Leben erweckt, vor allem in angelsächsischen Ländern. Die ersten Pioniere der objektiven Sinnesphysiologie gingen bei ihren Experimentplanungen von der subjektiven Sinneswahrnehmung aus. ADRIAN [A 5] und ZOTTERMAN [Z 4, 5] verwendeten ihre Ergebnisse am peripheren Nerven für die physiologische Erklärung der Hautsinne, HARTLINE verglich seine Neuronregistrierungen vom Auge mit dem menschlichen Sehen [H 4–6], obwohl er sich immer mehr auf das primitive Auge des Limulus [H 4–6] beschränkte.

Neurophysiologie und die Psychophysik ergänzen sich gegenseitig. Auch heute, nachdem wir viel mehr über die neuronalen Mechanismen der Sinnesvorgänge wissen als im 19. Jahrhundert, gilt noch HERINGS bescheidener Ausspruch: Der Sinnesphysiologe ist gewöhnt, „zu den Empfindungen als den Zeigern der Uhr seine Zuflucht zu nehmen, so oft der weitere Einblick in den Gang des Räderwerks ihm versagt" bleibt [H 34]. Wenn wir diesen „Uhrzeiger" der subjektiven Wahrnehmung in der psychophysischen Forschung als Indicator für objektive neurophysiologische Prozesse des neuralen „Räderwerks" verwenden, so besteht begründete Hoffnung, auch einen gemeinsamen Weg mit der objektiven Sinnesphysiologie zu finden, der die Wahrnehmungsgrundlage psychischer Vorgänge mit neuronalen Mechanismen korreliert [J 39]. Die ideale Forderung, neuronale Vorgänge und Sinneswahrnehmung gleichzeitig an derselben menschlichen Versuchsperson zu untersuchen ist allerdings noch unerfüllbar. Meistens müssen wir uns mit Analogien und Korrelationen aus *Tierversuchen* begnügen. Nur ganz wenige Untersuchungen einzelner afferenter Nervenentladungen sind beim *Menschen* durchgeführt worden.

Ableitungen von Sinnesnerven beim Menschen. Elektrische Registrierungen von Sinnesnervenfasern aus Receptoren der Hautsinne, der Seh-, Gehör-, Gleichgewichts-, Geschmacks- und Geruchsorgane und ihrer zentralen Projektionen im Gehirn wurden zunächst bei *Tieren* erhalten. Sie zeigten bereits weitgehende Korrelationen mit den Ergebnissen der subjektiven Sinnesuntersuchungen beim Menschen. Die Korrelationen subjektiver und objektiver Sinnesphysiologie waren daher zunächst Übertragungen vom Tierversuch auf den Menschen. Den Tierexperimenten entsprechende Ableitungen von Einzelstrukturen menschlicher Sinnesorgane stießen zunächst auf große methodische Schwierigkeiten. Zunächst gelangen beim *Menschen* nur Ableitungen der elektrischen Potentiale der gesamten Netzhaut (Elektroretinogramm) [M 83], der Hautnerven [E 12, D 9] und der oberflächlich gelegenen sensiblen und sensorischen Hirnrindenregionen [C 7, D 7, 8] im EEG. Sie brachten zwar einige Ergebnisse über die Leitungszeiten der Nerven vom Sinnesorgan zum Cortex beim Menschen [D 7, M 52] aber nur geringe Beziehungen zur subjektiven Sinnesphysiologie.

Nervenableitungen in situ. Die ersten Untersuchungen von EICHLER [E 12] über den Vergleich subjektiver Empfindung und percutaner Registrierung der *Potentiale menschlicher Nerven durch die Haut,* und mit verbesserter Technik wiederholte Versuche von DAWSON [D 9] zeigten nur wenige Korrelationen für die inadäquate elektrische Reizung. Erst seit 1961 ist es gelungen, die Aktionspotentiale in situ von den menschlichen Fingernerven bei *adäquater mechanischer Reizung* der Nagelreceptoren zu registrieren [S 20]. Exakte Untersuchungen über einzelne Neurone der menschlichen Sinnessysteme sind bisher auch nur an Hautnerven gelungen.

Einzelfaserregistrierungen von menschlichen Hautnerven. HENSEL und BOMAN [H 29, 30] haben 1959/60 die ersten Aktionsstromableitungen von einzelnen Nervenfasern des Menschen im Selbstversuch vorgenommen und mit den Sinnesempfindungen bei gleichen Reizen verglichen.

Die Schwelle für die Auslösung eines Einzelimpulses entsprach etwa der einer subjektiven Berührungsempfindung. Bei größerer Reizstärke und entsprechend verstärkter Druckempfindung konnten einzelne Receptoren mit ihren Fasern sehr hohe Entladungsfrequenzen (bis zu 330/s) erreichen. Die deutliche Übereinstimmung von subjektiver und objektiver Schwelle der Druckempfindung ist die erste exakte Korrelation von subjektiver und objektiver Sinnesphysiologie von Einzelelementen beim Menschen, die an der *gleichen Versuchsperson* erhalten wurde. Allerdings war streng simultane Prüfung von Empfindung und Impulsableitung noch nicht möglich, weil die Hautnerven durchschnitten wurden und die subjektive Kontrolle daher vorangehen mußte.

Das erstaunliche Ergebnis HENSELS, daß die subjektive Schwelle der Haarreceptoren bei bestimmter Winkeldeformation der Haare mit der Auslösung eines einzelnen Impulses in den afferenten Nervenfasern identisch ist, darf nicht verallgemeinert werden. Daraus folgt nicht, daß jeder einzelne Nervenimpuls vom Receptor zur Hirnrinde gemeldet wird, sondern nur, daß dies prinzipiell möglich ist.

Subjektive Sinnesphysiologie und Tierexperiment. Außer den genannten Ergebnissen HENSELS an menschlichen Hautnerven [H 30] und Ableitungen ZOTTERMANS von Geschmacksnerven der Chorda tympani [B 53] gibt es noch keine parallelen Untersuchungen von Sinnesempfindungen und Entladungen der Sinnesnerven, die beide an der gleichen menschlichen Versuchsperson durchgeführt sind. Die Korrelationen beschränken sich im übrigen auf Tierversuche: bei Katzen, Affen und anderen Laboratoriumstieren, die dem Menschen ähnliche Sinnesvorgänge haben, werden von Receptoren, Nervenfasern und Neuronen des Sinnesorgans und ihrer zentralen Projektion die Erregungsvorgänge nach bestimmten Reizen registriert; diese werden dann mit den beim Menschen unter entsprechenden Bedingungen erhaltenen Sinnesempfindungen verglichen [J 39]. In den letzten Jahren haben sich viele Parallelen zwischen den vorwiegend tierexperimentellen Befunden der objektiven Sinnesphysiologie und den subjektiven psychophysischen Beobachtungen am Menschen gezeigt, so daß wir heute schon zahlreiche *Korrelationen zwischen Sinnesphänomenen und neuronalen Mechanismen* aufstellen können (Tabelle 4, S. 917). Diese Korrelationen beziehen sich natürlich zunächst nur auf relativ *einfache* Sinnesphänomene, sie zeigen aber, wie weit man mit den heute verfügbaren elektrophysiologischen Methoden in die Welt der Sinne eindringen kann.

Gemeinsames Ziel psychophysischer und tierexperimenteller Methoden. Trotz methodischer Unterschiede und verschiedener Objekte haben subjektive und objektive Sinnesphysiologie bei Tier und Mensch doch das gleiche Ziel: Die Aufklärung der Sinnesvorgänge. HERING hat früher einmal das Bild gebraucht, daß psychologische und physiologisch-experimentelle Methoden wie ein Tunnelbau von zwei entgegengesetzten Seiten in das unbekannte Gebiet der Sinnesfunktionen eindringen. Zwar glauben viele, daß diese beiden Tunnelbauten sich nie treffen können und einander verfehlen müssen, doch kann es für beide Teile nur von Vorteil sein, auf die Klopfarbeit der anderen Tunnelmannschaft zu hören und sich danach auszurichten. Die Korrelationen und Parallelen zwischen beiden Forschungsrichtungen zeigen, daß ein anderes Bild den Tatsachen noch besser gerecht wird: Nicht entgegengerichteter, sondern *paralleler Wegebau,* bei dem sich beide Methoden, die subjektive und die objektive gegenseitig korrigieren und anregen können, verspricht die besten Resultate. Wenn die subjektive und die objektive Forschung einen *doppelten* Weg in das Gebiet der Sinnesfunktionen bahnt, so wird trotz zeitlicher und methodisch bedingter Verschiebungen im Bau dieser Wege doch ein gemeinsames Vorgehen ermöglicht. *Koordinierung subjektiver und objektiver Methoden ist die Via regia der Sinnesphysiologie für Untersuchung und Erkennung der Sinnesleistungen* [J 39]. Nur bei gegenseitiger Anregung und Kontrolle subjektiver und objektiver Methoden sind gesicherte neue Erkenntnisse möglich. Die direkte Anschaulichkeit der subjektiven Empfindungen macht uns die Ergebnisse der objektiven Methoden verständlich. Die psychologischen Befunde sind hier mehr als Bilder und Metaphern physiologischer Vorgänge. Sie geben uns nicht nur eine Illustration sondern eine direkte anschauliche *Integration und Zusammenfassung der Sinnesleistungen.* Zwar gelangen wir niemals aus der geschlossenen Kette physikalisch-physiologischer Prozesse in den Bereich des Psychologischen. Eine solche Transzendenz hat auch HERING nicht angenommen und er hat immer einen dualistischen Standpunkt vertreten. In seinem letzten posthumen Buch über den Lichtsinn [H 32] zeigte er durch sein Gleichnis vom Spiegel, daß es ebenso unmöglich ist, eine Umwandlung physischer Vorgänge in psychische zu erfassen, wie das scheinbar hinter der Spiegelfläche befindliche Bild zu ergreifen. Dennoch erleichtern uns die subjektiv-anschaulichen Sinnesphänomene das Verständnis der meist unanschaulichen, nur begrifflich oder mathematisch erfaßbaren Teilprozesse der objektiven Sinnesphysiologie. *Psychophysische Erkenntnisse nützen dem Physiologen selbst dann, wenn sie nur virtuelle Spiegelbilder realer Vorgänge sein sollten, die uns in einer imaginären Welt erscheinen, zu der physiologische Methoden keinen Zugang haben.*

Nur bei einfacher Versuchsanordnung können wir klare Resultate und Korrelationen erwarten. Daß aber auch bei Anwendung einfacher Methoden auf komplexe Verhältnisse des Konturen- und Farbensehens dieselben Gesetze gelten können, haben BAUMGARTNER [B 13] und HURVICH [H 96] gezeigt: BAUMGART-

NER [B 14, 15] fand in der objektiven Neuronenphysiologie die gleichen Regeln, die für das subjektive Kontrastsehen gelten. L. und M. HURVICH [H 96] deduzierten vom subjektiv-sinnesphysiologischen Versuch Gesetzmäßigkeiten der Gegenfarben, deren objektive Grundlage durch Weiterentwicklung von SVAETICHINS [S 57, 62] und DE VALOIS' [V 1–5] Versuchen zu finden sein wird.

Am weitesten entwickelt sind die Parallelen der subjektiven Sinnesphysiologie mit objektiven Registrierungen an den *Neuronen des Sehsystems*. Durch Registrierung von einzelnen Fasern und Nervenzellen in Retina, Geniculatum und visuellem Cortex der Katze konnten zahlreiche Parallelen mit sinnesphysiologischen Befunden beim Menschen festgestellt werden. Die in Tabelle 4 (S. 917) genannten 19 Seh-Phänomene zeigten die besten Entsprechungen von subjektiver Empfindung beim Menschen mit Neuronentladungen bei der Katze [J 39].

Psychophysiologie und Neurophysiologie des Sehens

Dominanz des Sehsystems in der Sinnesafferenz. Wenn sich die folgende Darstellung der Sinnesphysiologie auf das Sehsystem beschränkt, so geschieht dies nicht nur, weil ich das visuelle System aus eigener Arbeit am besten kenne, sondern auch wegen der großen Bedeutung des Sehens für den Menschen und die höheren Säuger. Auch andere Darstellungen der modernen Sinnesphysiologie, wie GRANITs Buch [G 26] oder TEUBERs Handbuchbeitrag [T 2] gehen vom visuellen System aus, ähnlich wie schon die subjektive Sinnesphysiologie im neunzehnten Jahrhundert und die Gestaltpsychologie in den letzten Dezennien [K 32, M 38]. *Nicht nur nach der subjektiven Wahrnehmung oder dem objektiven Verhalten, sondern auch nach der Zahl der Sinnesafferenzen ist der Mensch vorwiegend ein „Sehtier".* Der Mensch hat etwa 200 Millionen Photoreceptoren und 2 Millionen Sehnervenfasern [B 67]. Nach Zählungen und Schätzungen der verschiedenen Sinnesafferenzen stammen von allen afferenten Nervenfasern etwa $1/3$ aus dem optischen System [G 33]. Diese *Dominanz des visuellen Systems* ist keine spezifisch menschliche Eigenschaft, sondern gilt ebenso für die meisten Primaten und die anderen höheren Säugetiere.

Viele Grundphänomene des Sehens und optische Täuschungen waren schon seit Jahrhunderten bekannt. Doch wurden sie meist nur als Einzelphänomene beschrieben, als Kuriositäten betrachtet oder vorzeitig in ein spekulatives System gebracht. Ein solches physikalisch unbegründetes und psychologisch motiviertes System ist GOETHEs Farbenlehre, die mit ihrer rein phänomenologischen Betrachtung gegen physikalische und physiologische Analyse gerichtet war, aber doch von einem physikalischen Versuch ausging: dem Tyndall-Phänomen der Farben trüber Medien. Erst die von YOUNG, PURKINJE, HELMHOLTZ, HERING und FECHNER im 19. Jahrhundert begründete Sehphysiologie hat zu klaren psychophysischen Ergebnissen geführt. Fast 100 Jahre vergingen, bis die Elektrophysiologie in den vierziger bis fünfziger Jahren des 20. Jahrhunderts entsprechende objektivsinnesphysiologische Korrelate des visuellen Systems feststellen konnte [G 32, H 5, J 39].

Der wissenschaftliche Streit über die physiologische oder psychologische Deutung der subjektiven Sehphänomene, über Empirismus oder Nativismus zwischen HELMHOLTZ, V. KRIES und ihrer Schule auf der einen und HERING,

MACH und ihren Schülern auf der anderen Seite ist nicht nur von wissenschaftshistorischem, sondern auch von psychologisch-psychiatrischem Interesse. Die erbitterten wissenschaftlichen Streitigkeiten der einzelnen Autoren können heute nach den Ergebnissen der objektiven Sinnesphysiologie besser verstanden und ausgeglichen werden. *Trotz schärfster Polemik zwischen* HELMHOLTZ [H 26] *und* HERING [H 34] *haben sich gerade ihre beiden Forschungsrichtungen in idealer Weise ergänzt,* wie ein „Kampf der Teile" im lebenden Organismus schließlich zur harmonischen Einheit führt.

WUNDTS und HELMHOLTZ' psychologische Formulierungen haben mit der Anerkennung „unbewußter Schlüsse" zunächst physiologische Erklärungen der Kontrastphänomene behindert, die MACH [M 1, 2] und HERING [H 32, 34] seit 1865 entwickelten. Ungünstig für HERINGS Lehren waren andererseits seine stoffwechselphysiologischen Deutungen der Assimilation und Dissimilation. Doch wirkten HERINGS Konzeptionen von 2 antagonistischen Prozessen anregend auf die allgemeine Neurophysiologie bis zur reziproken Innervation von SHERRINGTON [S 32].

Das *Primat der physiologischen Regulationen* gegenüber der psychologischen Erfahrung geht daraus hervor, daß sie nach HERINGS Worten *„schon beim Erwerb dieser Erfahrungen in Funktion sind und diese Erfahrungen erst mit ermöglichen"* [H 32]. Das Sehen ist nach HERING eine physiologisch gesteuerte Sinnesleistung des Organismus, die bereits im Auge selbst für das Kontrastsehen und die komplizierten zentralen Vorgänge koordiniert wird. HERINGS Auffassung vermeidet die unnötig scharfe und physiologisch unzweckmäßige Trennung von Empfindung und Wahrnehmung und die künstliche Isolierung einfacher Empfindungen, die nach der Helmholtz-Wundtschen Lehre schon „vor" der Wahrnehmung vorhanden sein sollen.

In der *Farbenlehre* postuliert HELMHOLTZ in der nach YOUNG weiter entwikkelten *Dreifarbentheorie* als „Grundfarben" rot, grün und violett, für die 3 verschiedene Receptorbahnen angenommen wurden. HERING vertrat dagegen eine *Gegenfarbentheorie,* die im Grunde auch eine Dreifarbenlehre darstellt, da jeweils *3 Paare von antagonistischen Gegenfarben, schwarz-weiß, rot-grün, gelb-blau,* verwendet werden [H 32]. Daher ist v. KRIES' Bezeichnung „Vierfarbenlehre" unter Weglassung des Schwarz-Weiß-Paares mißverständlich. Die *erste Konzeption der Gegenfarben* ist älter. Sie wurde schon von LEONARDO DA VINCI um 1500 ausgesprochen. Eine spätere Formulierung stammt von SCHOPENHAUER, der in seiner Dissertation 1816 bereits *drei Farbenpaare*: schwarz/weiß, rot/grün, blau/gelb annahm und sie als „eine in zwei sich bedingende, sich suchende und zur Wiedervereinigung strebende Hälften zerfallende Tätigkeit des Sehorgans" beschrieb. Er versuchte sie dann der Geotheschen Farbenlehre anzugleichen. Nach HERING sind die Gegenfarben nicht komplementär, sondern echt antagonistisch: „Sie ergänzen sich nicht zu weiß, sondern lassen dieses nur rein hervortreten, weil sie als Antagonisten sich gegenseitig ihre Wirkung unmöglich machen."

Am besten paßt zu allen Befunden eine *Synthese der Helmholtzschen und Heringschen Vorstellungen mit ihrer Begrenzung auf bestimmte Teile des Sehsystems.* Dies hat v. KRIES zuerst in seiner *Zonentheorie* 1911 versucht [K 50], später ähnlich auch JUDD [J 23]. Für die peripheren Vorgänge nimmt er die Helmholtzschen Komponenten, für die zentralen („terminaler Farbensinn" zum

Unterschied vom zentralen Gesichtsfeld der Fovea) die Heringschen Gegenfarben an. Heute kann man die bei v. KRIES noch unsichere Grenze zwischen beiden Zonen klarer bestimmen: HELMHOLTZ *gilt nur für die Receptoren der Retina und ihre photochemischen Prozesse,* HERING *für die neuronalen Vorgänge nach der ersten Synapse der Receptoren.*

Korrelationen von Neuronentätigkeit und Sehen

Im Gegensatz zu der frühen und erfolgreichen Entwicklung der subjektiven Sehphysiologie brachte die objektive Sinnesphysiologie zunächst kaum brauchbare Korrelationen mit dem menschlichen Sehen. Das schon 1865 durch HOLMGREN [H 77] entdeckte *Elektroretinogramm* (ERG) hat nur wenig zum Verständnis des Sehvorganges beigetragen, da diese Massenableitung elektrischer Phänomene des Auges keine Auskunft über die beteiligten Strukturen und einzelnen Neuronerregungen gibt.

Dieser wenig befriedigende Stand der objektiven Sehphysiologie änderte sich mit einem Schlag, als die *mikrophysiologischen Methoden* eingeführt wurden: Seit HARTLINE 1932 am Limulusauge und 1938 am Froschauge [H 4] von einzelnen Opticusfasern ableitete und die Dunkelaktivierung der off-Neurone entdeckte, GRANIT ab 1940 retinale Neuronabteilungen entwickelte [G 32], und in unserem Laboratorium seit 1952 auch die Tätigkeit einzelner Nervenzellen der Sehrinde registriert werden konnte [J 34, 52, B 15, 16], ergaben sich zahlreiche Parallelen zwischen Neuronentätigkeit und Sehen.

Nachdem diese Korrelationen an anderer Stelle [J 39, 42] dargestellt sind, seien im folgenden die wichtigsten Befunde mit einer Tabelle über Beziehungen subjektiver und objektiver Sinnesphysiologie und einem Schema zusammengefaßt: Tabelle 4 und Abb. 23 beschränken sich auf das *Hell-Dunkel-Sehen.*

Dualitätsprinzip neuronaler Hell- und Dunkelmeldung. Die Physiologie der Hell- und Dunkelwahrnehmung ist am besten durch ein Dualitätsschema mit zwei reziprok arbeitenden antagonistischen Neuronensystemen zu verstehen, die „heller" und „dunkler" melden. Diese gegensätzlich geschalteten Nervenzellsysteme, die von der Retina über den lateralen Kniekörper zur Sehrinde leiten, wurden mit ihren retinalen Schaltungen und ihrer rezeptiven Feldorganisation bereits kurz charakterisiert: Ein *lichtaktiviertes Hellsystem* der on-Zentrum-Neurone, das wir *B-System* nennen, meldet relative Helligkeit als Kontrast zur Umgebung oder zur vorangehenden Belichtung. Ein *lichtgehemmtes Dunkelsystem* der off-Zentrum-Neurone, das *D-System,* meldet relative Dunkelheit durch verminderte oder kontrastierte Lichtreize; im Extremfall des Licht-Dunkelkontrastes führt es zur Schwarzempfindung. Die Bezeichnung ist im Deutschen und Englischen leicht verständlich, da die Neurone des *B*-Systems *B*elichtung oder Helligkeit (*B*rightness) und das *D*-System *D*unkelheit (*D*arkness) signalisieren. Diese entgegengesetzte Information wird durch die *antagonistische Organisation der rezeptiven Felder* gewonnen, die KUFFLER entdeckt hat [K 61].

Ein konstanter Informationswert *„Heller"* für alle B-Neurone und *„Dunkler"* für alle D-Neurone ergab sich übereinstimmend aus den Untersuchungen von KUFFLER u. Mitarb. [B 8b, K 61] mit Zweiteilung retinaler on-center- und off-center-Neurone wie aus den Kontrastlichtuntersuchungen von BAUMGARTNER [B 14, 15]. Durch gleichzeitige Registrierung von B- und D-Neuronen im visuellen Cortex der Katze ist die reziprok-antagonistische Entladungsfolge dieser Neurone bei Licht- und Dunkel-Reizen auch in der Sehrinde nachgewiesen (Abb. 23). Bei fehlenden Lichtreizen zeigen beide Neuronsysteme eine unregelmäßige Ruheentladung, deren Frequenz im D-System ein wenig höher liegt (Abb. 23, Eigengrau). Diese *Ruheentladung* ist charakteristisch für alle visuellen Neurone des Auges und der unteren zentralen Sehstrukturen.

Das B- und D-System und seine Hell-Dunkel-Information. *Alle im Feldzentrum lichtaktivierten Neurone bilden das B-System* (on-Zentrum-Neurone in Retina und Geniculatum und B-Neurone des Cortex), da sie unter allen uns bekannten Bedingungen durch Lichtinkremente in ihrem Feldzentrum oder Kontrastlicht gegenüber dem Umfeld erregt werden. *Alle im Feldzentrum durch Lichtdekremente* (Verdunkelung auch relativ gegenüber dem Umfeld) *aktivierten Neurone gehören zum D-System* (off-Zentrum-Neurone von Retina und Geniculatum, D- und E-Neurone des Cortex). Diese *Informationskonstanz der beiden reziproken B- und D-Neuronensysteme* erklärt die neuronale Grundlage des Hell-Dunkel-Sehens unter den verschiedensten Bedingungen diffuser und kontrastgestalteter Lichtreize. Abb. 23 zeigt, wie das jeweilige Überwiegen der reziprok verschalteten beiden Systeme mit der subjektiven Hell- und Dunkelempfindung korreliert. Dies gilt für fehlenden Lichtreiz, für Belichtung mit folgendem Sukzessivkontrast und für den Simultankontrast.

Das B-System der on-Zentrum-Neurone wird durch Belichtung im Feldzentrum (Licht an, light-on oder Kontrastlicht) aktiviert und durch Belichtung im Umfeld gehemmt. Das D-System der off-Zentrum-Neurone wird nach Licht aus (light off), im Feldzentrum und durch Belichtung des Umfeldes aktiviert, die durch Kontrast das Feldzentrum relativ zum Umfeld verdunkelt. Dies sind die physiologischen Grundlagen des *Simultankontrastes,* durch den wir helle Flächen gegen dunkleren Grund heller und umgekehrt dunkle Flächen gegen helleren Grund schwärzer sehen. Tabelle 3 zeigt die neuronalen Korrelate der simultanen und sukzessiven Hell- und Dunkelinformation.

Tabelle 3. Hell- und Dunkelinformation der Sehwahrnehmung und der Neuronensysteme B und D

Subjektives Hell-Dunkelsehen	Neuronale Korrelate
„Heller" als die Umgebung (räumlich-simultan), als die vorangehende Empfindung (zeitlich-sukzessiv).	*Lokale B-Aktivierung der on-Zentrum-Neurone* mit reziproker Hemmung des D-Systems und lateraler Umfeldhemmung des B-Systems in Retina, Geniculatum und Sehrinde.
„Dunkler" als die Umgebung (simultan), als die vorangehende Empfindung (sukzessiv).	*Lokale D-Aktivierung der off-Zentrum-Neurone* mit reziproker Hemmung des B-Systems und lateraler Lichtaktivierung des D-Systems in Retina, Geniculatum und Sehrinde.

Das B- und D-System informiert also jeweils über *kontrastbedingte Helligkeit und Dunkelheit,* die relativ zum räumlichen Umfeld (Simultankontrast) oder zur zeitlichen Abfolge der Retinabelichtung (Sukzessivkontrast) z.B. durch Augenbewegungen geändert werden. Tabelle 4 zeigt die zahlreichen Entsprechungen zwischen Hell-Dunkelsehen und Neuronentätigkeit des B- und D-Systems.

Tabelle 4. Korrelationen von subjektiven Phänomenen des Hell-Dunkel-Sehens und neuronalen Vorgängen. Auf der Neuronenseite ist das Substrat, in dem das Phänomen neurophysiologisch nachgewiesen ist, durch einen Buchstaben in Klammer bezeichnet: R für *Retina*, G für *Geniculatum* und Co für *Cortex*. Wenn keine Artbezeichnung verwendet wurde, handelt es sich um Untersuchungen bei Katzen. Modifiziert nach JUNG [J 39]

Subjektives Sehen	Neuronale Korrelate in Retina (R), Geniculatum (G) oder visuellem Cortex (Co)
Eigengrau	Ruhe-Entladung von B- und D-System (R, G, Co) mit überwiegender D-Aktivität
Bewegungen im Eigengrau	Circulating neuronal activity (G)
Relative Helligkeit	B-Aktivierung, D-Hemmung [B-(on-center) Überwiegen in R, G, Co]
Relative Dunkelheit	D-Aktivierung, B-Hemmung [D-(off center) Überwiegen in R, G, Co]
Weber-Fechner-Beziehung der Helligkeitszunahme	Logarithmische Zunahme der B-Entladungen bei vermehrter Bleuchtungsstärke G, Co
Charpentier-Intervall (bande noire)	Entladungspause des B-Systems nach Primärentladung mit on-Entladung des D-Systems
Sukzessivkontrast (kurze Nachbilder und Dunkelintervalle)	Periodisch alternierende B- und D-Aktivierung und -Hemmung
Simultankontrast und Kontur	Lateral inhibition (R, G, Co). Maximale Kontur-Aktivierung des B- und D-Systems mit Umkehr im Hell- und Dunkelfeld
Zentrale Aussparung im Hermann-Gitter	Kleinere rezeptive Feldzentren in der Macula (14–24 µ ~ 50 Zapfen) (Mensch)
Geringe binoculare Helligkeitssummation und Fechner-Paradox	Vorwiegend monoculare Verschaltung des B- und D-Systems von Retina über Geniculatum bis Cortex
Binocularer Wettstreit	Gegenseitige Hemmung monocularer Impulse (G, Co)
Flimmerfusion (CFF)	Maximale neuronale CFF corticaler Neurone
Brücke- und Bartley-Effekt	Maximale B-Entladung bei mittlerer Flimmerfrequenz (R, Co)
Ähnliche monoculare und binoculare CFF	Vorwiegend monoculare neuronale CFF corticaler Neurone mit geringer binocularer Beeinflussung oder Hemmung
Lokaladaptation (bis zum Eigengrau)	Angleichung der B- oder D-Entladungen bei längeren Licht- oder Dunkelreizen bis zur Ruheentladung (R, G, Co)
Subjektive Lichterscheinungen bei Weck- und Schreckreizen (Weckblitz, Schreckblitz)	Unspezifische Aktivierung corticaler Neurone, vorwiegend des B-Systems
Aufmerksamkeitssteuerung des Sehens	Konvergenz retinaler und thalamo-reticulärer Impulse an corticalen Neuronen
Höhere CFF bei Wachheit und Aufmerksamkeit als bei Ermüdung	Erhöhung der neuronalen CFF durch thalamo-reticuläre Reize
Hell- und Dunkelempfindung bei anodischer und kathodischer galvanischer Retinareizung	Umgekehrte Beeinflussung der on-off-Entladung des retinalen B- und D-Systems bei Umpolung der Retina-Polarisation

Neuronale Entsprechungen der Hell-Dunkel-Wahrnehmungen. Vergleicht man verschiedene subjektive Wahrnehmungen des Hell-Dunkelsehens beim Menschen mit den objektiven Befunden der B- und D-Entladungen der Katze, so findet man zahlreiche eindrucksvolle Parallelen, die in Abb. 23 und Tabelle 4 zusammengefaßt sind.

Charakteristiken und Spezialleistungen von Nervenzellen der Sehrinde. Corticale Neurone höherer Ordnung sind im Gegensatz zu Geniculatumzellen oft *binocular* erregbar. Auch im Cortex findet sich aber noch eine *monoculare Dominanz* vieler Neurone, die nicht nur in Area 17, sondern auch in Area 18 und 19 beibehalten wird [H 88]. Dies paßt zu der für räumliches Sehen notwendigen Unterscheidung der Ortswerte beider Augen, zu subjektiven Phänomenen der Fusion und zum Doppeltsehen bei Abweichung beider Augenachsen. Auch das stereoskopische Sehen ist neuronal untersucht [B 45, 48a, P 20a]. Unsere erste Einteilung der Neuronenreaktionen auf diffuse Lichtreize in die Klassen A–E (Abb. 23) ist durch HUBEL und WIESELs Untersuchungen über die Feldorganisation der Cortexneurone überholt [B 66, H 87, 88].

Zusammengefaßt unterscheiden sich die visuellen Neurone der Area 17 von den retinalen und geniculären Neuronen durch folgende Besonderheiten: 1. Stärkere Adaptation mit kürzeren phasischen Lichtreaktionen der Cortexneurone. 2. Größere Verschiedenheit neuronaler Reaktionstypen im Cortex. 3. Frequenzuntersetzung mit langsamerer Entladungsrate corticaler Neurone. 4. Binoculare Koordination und Spezifizierung der rezeptiven Felder in der Sehrinde. 5. Topologische Orientierung gleicher Achsenrichtung rezeptiver Felder in einzelnen Zellsäulen der Sehrinde. 6. Umwandlung einfacher Hell-Dunkelmeldungen des B- und D-Systems in Neuronantworten mit spezialisierten Informationen (Kontur-, Richtungs- und Bewegungsmeldungen und Stereoeffekt). 7. Corticocorticale Verbindungen der Sehrindenneurone mit paravisuellen und kontralateralen Rindenfeldern. 8. Stärkere Konvergenz spezifischer und unspezifischer Afferenzen.

Abb. 23. Schema der subjektiven und objektiven Phänomene des Hell-Dunkel-Sehens. Modifiziert nach JUNG (1961) [J 39]. *Oben* die *Lichtempfindung beim Menschen, unten* die entsprechende *Neuronentätigkeit bei der Katze.* Das neuronale Korrelat wird auf *zwei reziproke Neuronensysteme B und D* mit konstantem Informationswert vereinfacht: Das *B-System gibt Hellinformation* durch die B-Neurone und die seltenen E-Neurone mit on-Zentren (on-off B). Das *D-System gibt Dunkelinformation* durch die D-Neurone und häufigen E-Neurone mit off-Zentren (on-off D). Lichtreiz 500 Lux am helladaptierten Auge. *Links* sind in *zeitlicher* Reihenfolge der Abszisse dargestellt: Eigengrau, Licht- und Dunkeleffekte mit Sukzessivkontrast der Nachbilder. Darunter die verschiedenen Reaktionstypen der corticalen Neurone. Das *Überwiegen des B-Systems* über das D-System (Verhältnis B/(B+D) > 0,5) entspricht der *Hellempfindung,* das *Überwiegen des D-Systems* (Verhältnis D/(B+D) > 0,5) der *Dunkelempfindung.* Im *Eigengrau* ohne Lichtreiz entsteht kein Ausgleich, sondern ein Überwiegen des D-Systems (vgl. Tab. S. 917). *Rechts* bildet die *räumliche* Anordnung des *Simultankontrastfeldes* die Abszisse in Sehwinkelgraden. Der *zeitliche* Ablauf der Erregung ist darunter senkrecht in den reziprok-antagonistischen Neuronensystemen B und D für die verschiedene Lage des Rezeptivfeldes im Kontrastbereich bei „Licht-an" und „Licht-aus" dargestellt. Der neuronale Grenzkontrast korreliert nach BAUMGARTNER [B 14, 15] jeweils mit der Summe der Neuronenentladungen in der ersten halben Sekunde nach Licht-an. Die verschiedene Intensität der B-Entladung entspricht etwa der Hellempfindung im Kontrastfeld

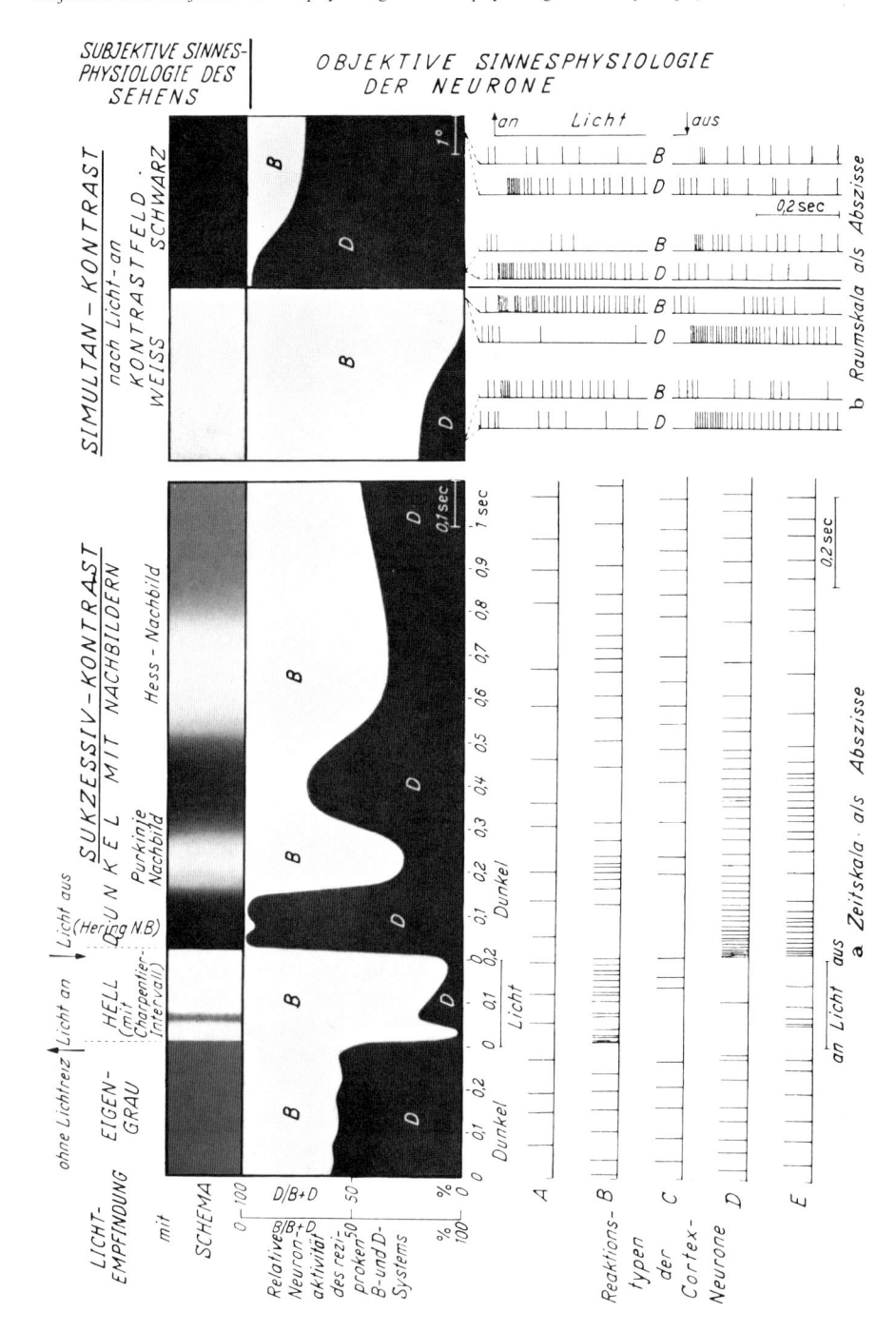

Objektive und subjektive Sinnesphysiologie: Neurophysiologie und Psychophysik des Sehens 919

Die *neuronalen Reaktionen der paravisuellen Felder* Area 18 und 19 wurden von HUBEL und WIESEL [H 88] mit geformten Lichtreizen untersucht: In Area 18 sind häufiger als in Area 17 Neurone mit „komplexen" rezeptiven Feldern, die auf gerichtete Konturen und lineare Lichtreize unabhängig davon antworten, wo der Reiz im rezeptiven Feld gegeben wird. Als neuen Zelltypus von Area 18 und 19 fanden HUBEL und WIESEL „hyperkomplexe" Neurone, die ebenfalls durch bestimmt gerichtete lineare Muster oder helle oder dunkle Konturen aktiviert werden, aber selektiv nur dann antworten, wenn dieses Reizmuster eine bestimmte Länge hat. Sogenannte „hyperkomplexe Neurone höherer Ordnung" reagieren selektiv auf zwei verschieden gerichtete, in ihrer Länge begrenzte hellere oder dunklere Konturen, die etwa senkrecht zueinander stehen. Die beiden Reizformen dieser „dualen" Neurone können zusammen eine Ecke oder einen *Winkel* bilden.

In den corticalen Neuronschaltungen werden flächenhafte Hell-Dunkelmeldungen wie beim Umrißzeichnen zu Grenzkonturen abstrahiert (vgl. S. 925). Diese Konturen werden in höheren Neuronen der visuellen und paravisuellen Rindenfelder weiter verarbeitet: 1. als Signale für bestimmt orientierte und gestaltete *Formen* und 2. als Meldungen richtungsspezifischer *Bewegungen*. Diese integrierten Informationen werden mit binocular-stereoskopischen Koordinationen und mit Augen- und Umweltbewegungssignalen verrechnet. Die Sehrinde leistet sowohl eine Integration wie eine Analyse der Neuronmeldungen aus Retina und Geniculatum. Mit den para- und perivisuellen Feldern bildet der Cortex einen kybernetischen Apparat von Neuronschaltungen für die Nachrichtenverarbeitung und Speicherung von Sehwahrnehmungen.

Neuronales Kontur-, Form- und Tiefensehen. Wie ein komplexes Bild in der neuronalen Verarbeitung der Sehrinde entsteht, können wir bisher noch nicht erklären. Man kann zwar für die Konturmeldungen der „simple neurons" von HUBEL und WIESEL [H 87] eine der Strichzeichnung ähnliche Umrißstruktur mit Abstraktion auf die linearen Formgrenzen als corticale Bildprojektion annehmen (Abb. 25 b, d). Doch sind solche richtungsorientierten Linien und Winkel, die von einzelnen Neuronpopulationen gemeldet werden, natürlich noch kein volles Umweltbild, wie wir es mit Licht, Schatten, Farben und Tiefenwahrnehmung sehen. Eine von CREUTZFELDT und NOTHDURFT [C 18] neuerdings vorgeschlagene Deutung, daß die komplexen Zellen den Ort bewegter Reize, die einfachen nur Konturgrenzen melden, erklärt noch nicht das Form- und Bewegungssehen. Auch der physiologische Mechanismus der Raumkonstanz der Umweltwahrnehmung bei Augenbewegungen, die sowohl die Netzhautbilder wie die corticalen Migränephosphene [J 50] mit dem Blick verschieben, ist noch umstritten. Neuronale Korrelate des binocularen Tiefensehens durch Querdisparation beider Netzhautbilder [B 45] wurden auch in den Sehrindenfeldern 17 und 18 bei Affen registriert [H 88a, P 28], aber wie die Fusion mit den Augenbewegungen reguliert wird, ist noch ungeklärt.

Die corticale Neuronentransformation in den Sehfeldern verläuft offenbar in mehrfachen Umschaltungen mit verschiedenen *Stufen abwechselnder Spezialisierung und Generalisierung.* Während die „einfachen" Felder HUBEL und WIESELS auf bestimmt orientierte Kontrastgrenzen an definierten Gesichtsfeldstellen reagieren, zeigen „komplexe" Felder eine gewisse Generalisation ihrer Reaktion, da die Lokalisation der Kontrastgrenze weniger kritisch wird. „Hyperkomplexe" Felder dagegen führen wieder zu einer Spezialisierung der Information, da sie lediglich orientierte Kontrastlinien bestimmter Länge anzeigen [H 87]. Die visuellen Cortexfelder leisten daher nicht nur zunehmende Generalisierungen der Sinnesinformationen, sondern vor allem auch Spezifizierungen, die auf das Gestalterkennen vorbereiten.

Obwohl Seherfahrung und Lernen zweifellos die höheren visuellen Neuronschaltungen erheblich verändert, sind die elementaren neuronalen Schaltungen der rezeptiven Felder in Area 17 angeboren. Ihre Funktion wird dann durch den Sehvorgang angeregt und mit höheren Transformationen differenziert. WIESEL und HUBEL [W 24b] konnten die kongenitale Anlage der Felderschaltung an neugeborenen Katzen ohne Seherfahrung feststellen und zeigen, daß nach monocularem Ausschluß des Formensehens in den ersten Lebensmonaten diese neuronalen Mechanismen ausfallen, ähnlich wie bei der menschlichen Amblyopie.

Die genannten neuronalen Korrelationen genügen vielleicht zur Widerlegung des psychologischen Einwands, daß die Neurophysiologen mit ihren Ableitungen von Einzelelementen eine atomistische Forschung treiben, die nichts mit dem eigentlichen Sehen zu tun hat. Zwar ist es richtig, daß die Registrierung einzelner Neurone nur eine sehr begrenzte Auswahl der Millionen funktionierender Nervenzellen eines geordneten Systems geben kann. Diese Auswahl bringt aber mehr als zufällige Resultate, wenn die registrierten Neuronenpopulationen repräsentativ gesammelt und ihre Funktionen in gut geplanten Experimenten analysiert werden. Die Mikrophysiologie hat mehr brauchbare Korrelate des Sehens geliefert als die Elektrophysiologie mit Makroelektroden. Nur durch Mikroelektrodenuntersuchungen an einzelnen Neuronen war es möglich, gewisse Grundmechanismen neuronaler Koordination in dem regulierten komplexen System des Cortex aufzudecken. Um seine Experimente richtig zu planen, braucht der Neurophysiologe die Vorarbeit und theoretische Basis der subjektiven Sinnesphysiologie. Die psychophysiologische Untersuchung des Sehens ist der neurophysiologischen Analyse um mehr als 100 Jahre vorausgegangen (S. 907). Diese alten subjektiv-sinnesphysiologischen Erfahrungen können auch heute bei neurophysiologischen Experimenten Richtung und Weg zeigen.

Alle subjektiv-sinnesphysiologischen Erscheinungen des Sehens sind als ganzes Phänomen unmittelbar *anschaulich,* wenn auch zeitlich weniger exakt bestimmbar. Die objektiven Registrierungen neuronaler Vorgänge sind zwar zeitlich völlig exakt zu messen, aber *unanschauliche* Teilausschnitte komplexer Vorgänge und müssen durch Analysen und Auszählungen erst indirekt erschlossen werden. Diese *Verschiedenheit anschaulicher subjektiver Sinnesphänomene und indirekt erschlossener objektiver Registrierungen* machen die gegenseitige Ergänzung beider Untersuchungsmethoden der Sinnesfunktionen notwendig und fruchtbar.

Der Neurophysiologe kann und darf nicht auf die anschaulichen Ergebnisse des subjektiven Sehens verzichten, wenn er gut geplante Experimente machen und sich nicht in Einzelheiten verlieren will. Ebensowenig darf der Psychologe physiologische und kausal erklärbare Vorgänge außer acht lassen, die seine begrifflichen Kriterien kontrollieren und korrigieren. Einseitige Untersuchungen, die nur die subjektiven oder objektiven Aspekte der Sinnesfunktionen ohne Rücksicht auf die Ergebnisse des anderen Forschungsgebietes verwenden, führen entweder zu uninteressanten und unverständlichen Einzelergebnissen neurophysiologischer Registrierungen oder zu phantasievollen, somatisch nicht begründbaren psychologischen Postulaten. Diese Seitenwege enden daher früher oder später in einer wissenschaftlichen Wildnis, entweder in zusammenhanglosen, trockenen Tatsachen oder in üppig wuchernder Spekulation. Nur die gemeinsam gebahnten Wege der psychophysischen und neurophysiologischen Forschung führen aus dieser Wildnis heraus zu koordinierter Erforschung der Sinnesleistungen bei Mensch und Tier.

Receptive und perceptive Felder

Objektive Feldmessung und subjektive Feldschätzung. Analog der direkten Messung receptiver Felder einer Nervenzelle kann man auch beim menschlichen Sehen entsprechende Felder *indirekt* bestimmen, indem man die subjektiven Effekte von Kontrastmustern untersucht, die den Reizbedingungen im Tierversuch entsprechen (Abb. 24). Offenbar ist die Wahrnehmung ein integriertes Endergebnis koordinierter Organisation von Nervenzellpopulationen, die noch das Grundprinzip der rezeptiven Felder erkennen läßt. Um objektive Messungen an Neuronen und subjektive Ergebnisse des menschlichen Sehens auch terminologisch klar zu trennen, haben wir vorgeschlagen, *zwei* verschiedene Bezeichnungen zu verwenden und *receptive und perceptive Felder* zu unterscheiden [J 61 a]. Sie werden wie folgt definiert: **Receptive Felder** sind die räumlichen Projektionen visueller Neurone aus solchen Netzhautarealen, deren Reizung spezifische neuronale Entladungen auslöst. Sie werden *objektiv* gemessen durch Nervenzellregistrierungen nach lokalen Kontrastlichtreizen der Umwelt auf das Retinaprojektionsgebiet visueller Neurone. **Perceptive Felder** sind räumlich begrenzte Sehphänomene, deren Ausdehnung analog der receptiven Feldorganisation im Gesichtsfeld als Helligkeitskontrast sichtbar wird. Ihr Durchmesser wird *subjektiv* durch Kontrastmuster beim Menschen psychophysisch geschätzt [J 61 a, S 43 a].

Die receptiven Felder bestimmen den *retinalen Ortswert der Receptormeldungen* einzelner Sinneszellen, die perceptiven Felder die entsprechende *Ortslokalisation in einer Umweltprojektion* der Sinneswahrnehmung. Beides entspricht dem

---

Abb. 24. Kontrasteffekte des Hermann-Gitters auf perceptive Felder beim Menschen und receptive Felder im Tierversuch: Optische Reizung mit dem gleichen Gittermuster erzeugt subjektiv und objektiv entsprechende Wirkungen, die im menschlichen Sehen anschaulich sichtbar (A), im Sehsystem der Katze neuronal registrierbar sind (C) (nach JUNG und SPILLMANN [J 61a]).
A Subjektive Kontrastwirkungen nach HERMANN [H 35] *und* BAUMGARTNER [B 13]. Man sieht in den Kreuzungsarealen graue Flecke, die bei fovealer Fixation verschwinden. Dies erklärt sich durch verschiedene Belichtung und Größe perceptiver Felder: Wenn das Feldzentrum etwa der Streifenbreite entspricht, wird das Umfeld in den Kreuzungen mehr belichtet und das Feldzentrum durch laterale Hemmung (−) vermindert aktiviert (+). Es erscheint daher dunkler als in den Streifen (++).

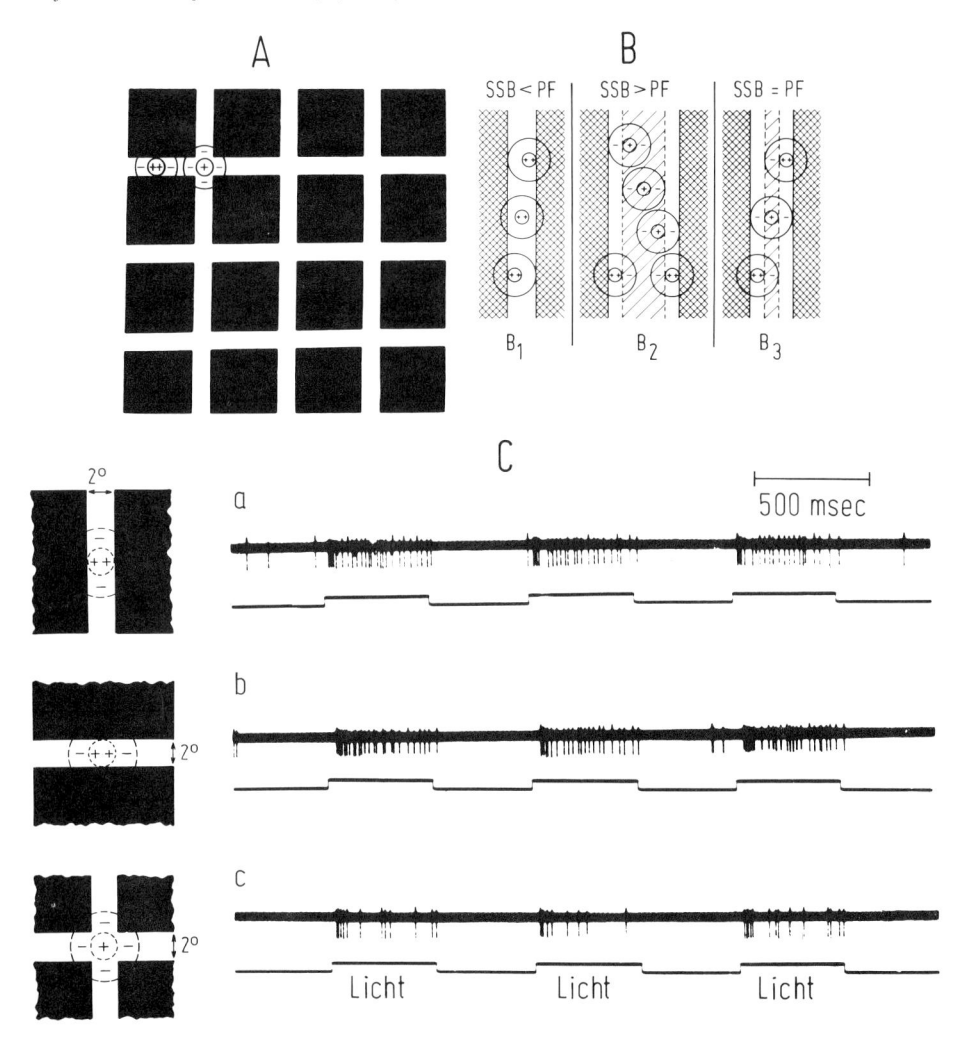

B Größenbeziehungen der perceptiven Felder (PF) und des Sehwinkels der Streifenbreite (SSB).
Entsprechend dem Augenabstand des Gitters wird die Streifenprojektion auf die Retina und ihre perceptiven Felder kleiner oder größer. Wenn die Streifen kleiner als das perceptive Feld ist (B 1), wird die laterale Umfeldhemmung immer durch Abdecken des Umfeldes vermindert und das Feldzentrum mehr aktiviert (++). Wenn der Sehwinkel der Streifenbreite größer (B 2) oder gleich (B 3) dem Durchmesser des perceptiven Feldes ist, erscheint ein graues Band in der Mitte der hellen Streifen, weil der Grenzkontrast nur in den Randfeldern die Umfeldhemmung vermindert. Man sieht die grauen Bänder, wenn man den Augenabstand des Gitters A zwischen 50 bis 10 cm variiert.
C Objektive Lichtantworten eines hellmeldenden B-Neurons der Katzensehrinde. (Registrierung von BAUMGARTNER u. Mitarb.)
Bei verschiedener Projektion des Hermann-Gitters auf das receptive Feld entspricht die Neuronentladung etwa der subjektiven Helligkeit in A. Bei Projektion auf die Kreuzung (c) ist die Neuronaktivierung um etwa die Hälfte geringer als in den senkrechten und waagerechten Streifen (a und b). Die abgeleitete Nervenzelle der Area 17 hatte ein rundes receptives Feld von 6° Durchmesser, das 20° lateral von der retinalen Area centralis lokalisiert war

"Lokalzeichen", das seit LOTZE jeder Sinnesnachricht zugesprochen wird. Seine Ortslokalisation in der realen Umwelt ermöglicht die Einordnung in ein räumliches Umweltmodell der Wahrnehmung.

Analogien perceptiver Felder und neuronaler Organisation. Der Vergleich receptiver und perceptiver Felder bildet eine Brücke zwischen der Neurophysiologie und der Psychophysik, obwohl die Umwandlung von visuellen Neuronenentladungen in eine Sehwahrnehmung noch nicht erklärbar ist. Zwar ist das receptive Feld eine einfache Raumprojektion des retinalen Reizfeldes, von dem eine Sinneszelle beeinflußt wird, und das perceptive Feld die subjektive Raumprojektion nach komplexen neuronalen Wechselwirkungen in Zellpopulationen auf verschiedenen Ebenen des Sehsystems. Dennoch zeigt der Vergleich zwischen Einzelneuronregistrierungen bei Tieren und Kontrastphänomenen beim menschlichen Sehen entsprechende elementare Gesetze neuronaler Erregung und Hemmung, die sich ähnlich wie in der Retina offenbar auch in höheren Sehstrukturen auswirken und schließlich subjektiv die menschliche Sehwahrnehmung bestimmen. Beide, receptive und perceptive Felder sind nach dem gleichen, von KUFFLER entdeckten Prinzip der antagonistischen *Zentrum-Umfeld-Verschaltung* organisiert.

BAUMGARTNER [B 13] hat zuerst 1960 erkannt, daß das Kontrastsehen des von HERMANN 1870 beschriebenen Gitters [H 35] analoge *Größenbestimmungen receptiver Felder beim Menschen* ermöglicht [S 43a]. Abb. 24 zeigt am Beispiel des *Hermann-Gitters*, wie in A die Organisation perceptiver Felder subjektive Kontrasttäuschungen durch Umfeldhemmung erklären kann und wie in C durch Neuronenentladungen nach gleicher Reizung im Tierversuch ein analoges objektives Korrelat der receptiven Feldorganisation registrierbar ist. Beide sind durch laterale Hemmung bei Belichtung des receptiven und perceptiven Umfelds zu erklären.

Die reziproken Verschaltungen der hell- und dunkelmeldenden beiden Neuronensysteme B und D können durch entsprechende Hermann-Gitter in schwarz und weiß anschaulich gemacht werden. Sie zeigen ähnliche Gittertäuschungen für den Kontrast von *weißen Gittern auf schwarzem Grund* und *schwarzen Gittern auf weißem Grund*. Daraus ergibt sich, daß die Kontrastphänomene in *beiden* Untersystemen, dem hellmeldenden B- und dunkelmeldenden D-System, nach ähnlichen Prinzipien verschaltet werden. Beide Kontrastmuster zeigen an den Kreuzungen mit größerer Exposition des Umfeldes eine Verminderung der spezifischen Information „weiß" und „schwarz" in Richtung auf *grau*. Dem entspricht *verminderte Helligkeit für B und verminderte Dunkelheit für D*. Dies korreliert mit einer spezifischen *Feldzentrumsinformation des B-Systems für weiß und des D-Systems für schwarz*.

Natürlich sind neuronale Tierexperimente von der menschlichen Wahrnehmung nicht nur in der Registriermethode, sondern auch in der Komplexität der Ergebnisse verschieden. Einzelneuronableitungen bei Tieren geben nur kleine Ausschnitte aus der komplizierten Organisation des Sehsystems. Diese Ausschnitte können aber, wenn sie systematisch nach ihrer Bedeutung für Hell- und Dunkelmeldung ausgewertet werden, durch die antagonistische Feldorganisation und durch reziproke Erregung und Hemmung von zwei neuronalen Untersystemen (Abb. 23) alle wesentlichen Phänomene des Hell-Dunkel-Sehens erklären. Daraus ergibt sich, daß trotz methodischer Grenzen am Einzelneuron, in der neuronalen Massenfunktion und beim subjektiven Sehen *analoge Prinzipien* wirksam sind. Neben den zahlreichen Parallelen von Sehen und Neuronenaktivierung der Tabelle 4 gibt das Hermann-Gitter das anschaulichste Beispiel für funktionelle Korrelationen der Sehsysteme von Mensch und Katze.

Größenzunahme perceptiver und receptiver Felder in der Retinaperipherie. Subjektive und objektive Methoden zeigen prinzipiell gleiche Korrelationen der Felddurchmesser mit der Netzhautexzentricität. Man kann mit dem Hermann-Gitter, wie SPILLMANN seit 1964 gezeigt hat, auch die *lineare Größenzunahme perceptiver Felder mit der retinalen Exzentrizität* in der Netzhaut psychophysisch messen [S 43a]. Dies entspricht FISCHERS gesetzmäßiger Beziehung zwischen Empfindlichkeit, Größe und Lage receptiver Felder in der Katzenretina. Ähnliche Korrelationen bestehen auch mit der Receptor- und Ganglienzelldichte in der menschlichen Netzhaut. Beim Menschen zeigt der Größendurchmesser der receptiven Felder von der Fovea zur Peripherie nur im ersten parafovealen Bereich einen steileren Anstieg. Ab 10° neben der Fovea zur Peripherie ist er flacher als der ebenfalls lineare Anstieg der Feldgrößen mit zunehmender Exzentrizität bei der Katze.

Konturabstraktion, Orientierung und Klassifizierung

Visueller Grenzkontrast, Kontur und Zeichnung. Die wesentlichen Informationen über die optische Welt erhalten wir nicht aus der Wahrnehmung heller und dunkler oder farbiger Flächenreize, sondern von ihren *Grenzen*, also den *Flächenkonturen*. Zur Erklärung und Veranschaulichung wollen wir wiederum von den komplizierteren Verhältnissen der bunten Farben und ihrer Kontrasterscheinungen in den Gegenfarben gelb-blau und grün-rot absehen und uns auf den *Schwarz-Weiß-Kontrast* beschränken. Dann läßt sich nach den neurophysiologischen Kontrastuntersuchungen verstehen, warum Grenzkonturen viel besser wahrgenommen werden als Flächen. BAUMGARTNERS Untersuchungen an einzelnen Neuronen [B 14, 15] haben deutlich gezeigt, daß die stärkste Neuronentladung jeweils von den receptiven Feldern der Konturen im Grenzkontrast ausgeht (Abb. 23 rechts). BARLOW [B 7, 8] betonte, daß es sich bei den Kontrastphänomenen um eine zweckmäßige Codierung der visuellen Signale mit einer Verminderung von Redundanz handelt, wie sie die Informationstheorie fordert. Durch übereinanderkopierte positive und negative Bilder, entsprechend Abb. 25b, zeigte BARLOW, daß bei einem Ausgleich der Flächenhelligkeiten in einem gleichmäßigen Grau mit einem Rest von Konturen nur wenig Information verloren geht. Ähnlich können bei stärkerer Lokaladaptation nach längerer Fixation oder unter der Prismenbrille die Farb- und Helligkeitsunterschiede der Flächen verblassen, aber noch einzelne Konturen erhalten bleiben.

Die corticalen Neuronensysteme arbeiten ähnlich abstrahierend wie ein Künstler beim Zeichnen. Die Zeichnung leistet eine dem Simultankontrast entsprechende Vereinfachung und Abstraktion flächenhafter Bilder auf die Konturen. Schon Kinder stellen in ihren ersten primitiven Zeichnungen die Körper*umrisse* dar, ohne etwas von Fläche, Linie oder Kontur zu wissen. Diese *Konturendarstellung* wird in den graphischen Künsten zu besonderer Höhe entwickelt. Durch *Zeichnung*

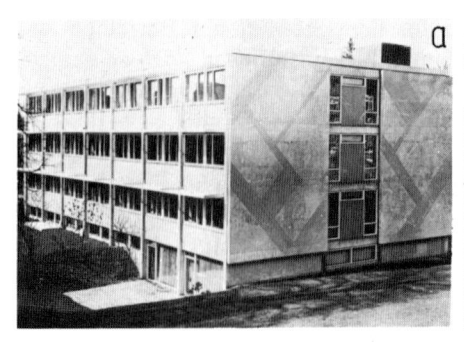

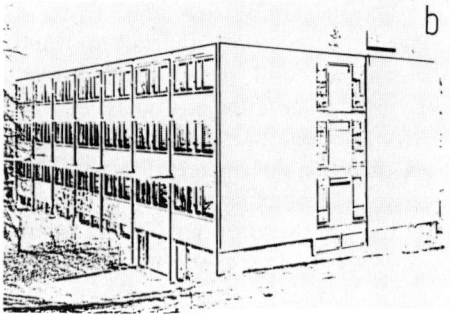

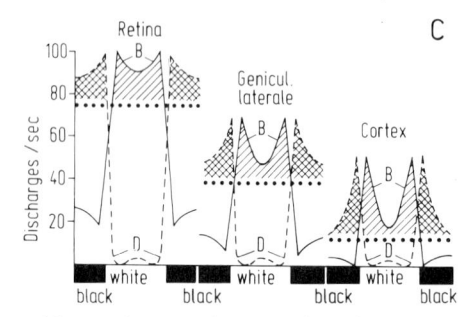

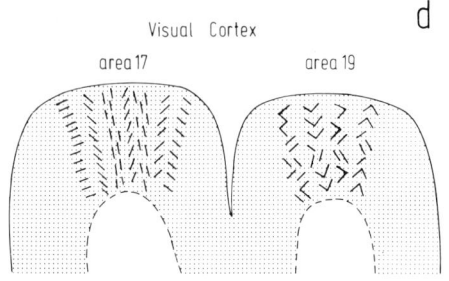

Abb. 25a–d. Konturbetonung des Sehsystems: Verwandlung des Flächenbildes in eine Linienzeichnung (a–c nach JUNG und BAUMGARTNER, 1965 [J 53]) und Ordnung der Konturdetektoren der Sehrinde (d modifiziert nach HUBEL und WIESEL, 1963 u. 1965 [H 87, 88]).
a–b Imitation der Konturbildung durch verschobene photographische Positiv-Negativ-Kopien nach BARLOW. *a* Photographie *mit flächenhaften Helldunkelstufen und Halbtönen entsprechend etwa dem Netzhautbild. b* Konturbild *in Schwarzweiß entsprechend der corticalen Neuronenabstraktion d im Gehirn (Sehrinde).*
c Zunehmende Kontrastverstärkung der Neuronenmeldungen vom Auge über das Geniculatum laterale bis zur Hirnrinde, in der eine Konturabstraktion *auf den Grenzkontrast erfolgt. Die Unterschiede zwischen diffuser Flächenbelichtung und Verdunkelung sind schraffiert für das hellmeldende B-System und kreuzschraffiert für das dunkelmeldende D-System. Die Entladungsrate bei diffuser Reizung (...) wird vom Auge bis zur Sehrinde geringer, während die Differenz zwischen diffuser und Kontrastlichtreizung zunimmt.*
d Schema der Nervenzellsäulen in der Sehrinde, die Liniengrenzen und Winkel in einer Richtung melden. Die einzelnen Zellsäulen werden jeweils durch charakteristisch orientierte Konturen in verschiedenen Winkeln zur Horizontalen spezifisch gereizt. Das gesehene Umweltbild kann so in lineare Konturen für verschiedene Richtungen zerlegt werden (vgl. b). Die „einfachen" Neurone im Feld 17 reagieren auf jede Linie gleicher Orientierung, gewisse „hyperkomplexe" Neurone im Feld 19 nur auf begrenzte *Kontraste bestimmter Länge und Winkelneigung* [H 88]

Abb. 26a u. b. Flächenbild und Umrißzeichnung als Beispiel für Konturabstraktion und Vereinfachung im Sehsystem. *a* Bild eines römischen Gebäudekomplexes mit Darstellung der Flächen und Lichtwerte [S. Sabina und S. Alessio, Museo di Roma, *Ölbild* von F. ROESLER (durch freundliche Vermittlung von Dr. CALLIERI, Rom)]. *b* Umrißzeichnung von *a* im römischen Skizzenbuch von INGRES 1810 (*Bleistiftzeichnung* Ingres-Museum). Die Zeichnung gibt alle wesentlichen Teile mit Ausnahme des zufälligen Vordergrundes klar und präzise wieder, obwohl sie auf jede flächenhafte Darstellung und auf Belichtungseffekte verzichtet. Zur Angleichung an *a* wurden linke und untere Teile der Zeichnung nicht reproduziert. (Nr. 96 Abb. 62 in H. NAEF: Ingres Rom. Zürich: Manesse 1962)

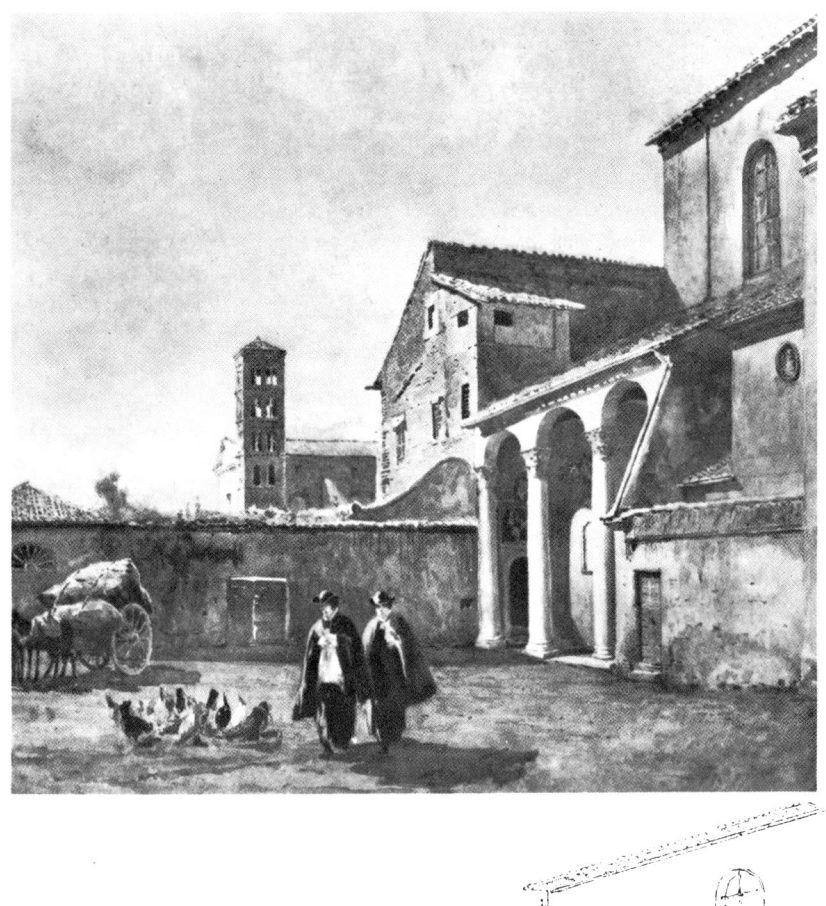

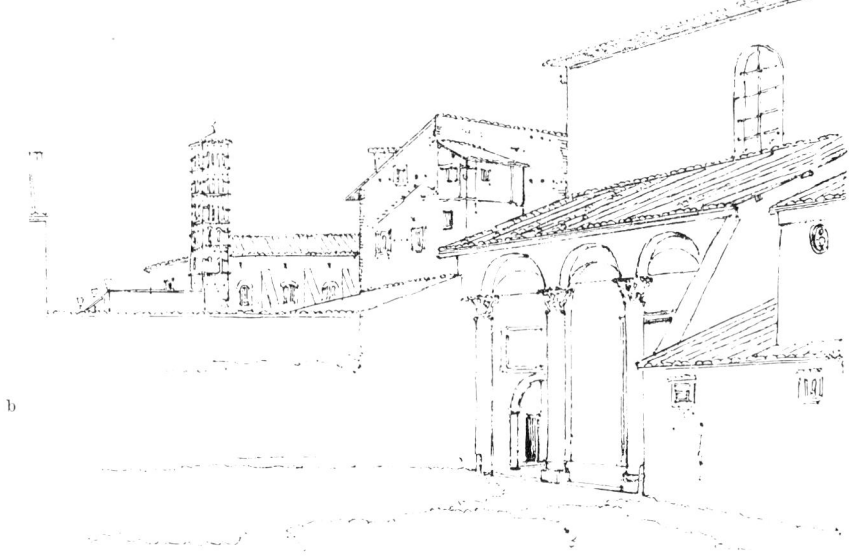

a

b

der Grenzkonturen gelingt es dem Künstler, Gebäude und Landschaften oft klarer darzustellen, als es die Photographie mit ihrer flächenartigen Reproduktion vermag. Abb. 26b zeigt an einem Beispiel, wie ein hervorragender Meister der Linie, INGRES, einen Gebäudeaspekt schärfer und prägnanter erfassen kann als das photographische Bild oder die mit Farbflächen arbeitende Malerei. Eine gute Zeichnung gibt die Gestalt eines Gegenstandes meist deutlicher wieder als ein getreues Flächenabbild. Die Zeichnung betont mit der Kontur also den *Gestaltcharakter* des Dargestellten. Physiologisch wird die Kontur durch neuronale Kontrastvorgänge ermöglicht [B 14, 15]. Man kann daher annehmen, daß in der weiteren Verarbeitung der Kontrastmeldungen im corticalen Neuronensystem eine *echte Gestaltinformation* aus dem neuronalen Korrelat des Konturensehens entwickelt wird.

Beziehungen der neuronalen Konturabstraktion zu zeichnerischen Formdarstellungen wurden an anderer Stelle [J 44, 46] besprochen. Der Zeichnungsvorgang verläuft von der Konturlinie zum Bild *zeitlich invers* gegen den Abstraktionsvorgang des Sehens, der wie in Abb. 25a–c vom Gesamtbild zum Umriß führt: Der Zeichner beginnt mit einfachen Linien von Umrißformen, die erst später durch Schraffur und Lavierung für Licht, Schatten und Raumillusion ergänzt werden. Je nach dem künstlerischen Stil versucht der Zeichner auch, reine Konturen abzuschwächen, aufzulockern oder zu deformieren [J 44]. Obwohl der Maler auch von den Gesetzen des Sehens abhängig ist, hat er doch eine größere Freiheit künstlerischer Gestaltung.

Pathologische Störungen dieser zeichnerischen Leistungen und der Bildsymmetrie durch Linksneglekt nach rechtsseitigen parietalen Hirnläsionen (Abb. 21) zeigen, daß auch Hirnregionen außerhalb der occipitalen Sehrindenfelder an der visuellen Aufmerksamkeit und der Bildordnung beteiligt sind [J 46].

Orientierungsleistungen, Raum- und Bewegungswahrnehmung. Die *Orientierung in Raum und Zeit* ist eine Spezialfunktion multisensorischer Aufmerksamkeit, die auch bei Nichtsäugern und wirbellosen Tieren in erstaunlicher Weise entwickelt und mit dem Instinktverhalten koordiniert ist. Die Sonnenorientierung der Bienen und der sprachähnlichen Kommunikation eines Honigziels, die v. FRISCH entdeckt hat [F 31], über die Ultraschallortung der Fledermäuse bis zu den Interkontinentalreisen der Zugvögel sind Beispiele tierischer Orientierungsleistungen, die meistens von mehreren Sinnesmodalitäten gesteuert werden. Für die Sehorientierung ist vor allem die optisch-vestibuläre Koordination zwischen *Auge und Labyrinth* von Bedeutung, deren Prinzipschaltungen beim Menschen Abb. 9 zeigt. Die psychophysischen Untersuchungen über optisch-vestibuläre Koordinationen und die Regulation von Augen- und Körperbewegungen beim Menschen haben DICHGANS und BRANDT [D 30] zusammengefaßt.

Gemeinsam ist allen Orientierungsleistungen von Tieren und Menschen eine *Motivationsauslösung,* die den Antrieb gibt und eine genetische Determination der Orientierungsmechanismen, deren Programmierung an variable Umweltbedingungen durch Lernprozesse angepaßt wird. Eine vergleichende Übersicht über die Orientierungsleistungen der Tiere gibt LINDAUER [L 26]. Wechselwirkungen von Eigenbewegung und Objektbewegung sind in der Wahrnehmung relativ einfach zu beschreiben, aber beruhen auf physiologisch sehr komplexen Koordinationen multisensorischer Meldungen, die wahrscheinlich von parietalen Rindenfeldern gesteuert werden [M 75]. Bewegungstäuschungen ergeben Hinweise auf die physiologischen Mechanismen. Bisher sind alle allgemeinen Erklärungen der *Raumkonstanz der Wahrnehmung* wie v. HOLSTS *Reafferenztheorie* [H 79] und MACKAYS *matching hypothesis* [M 7] physiologisch noch nicht bewiesen. Für v. HOLSTS Postulat einer Efferenzkopie gibt es noch kein physiologisches Korrelat. MACKAYS Stabilitätserklärung ist einleuchtender, da er als „*Nullhypothese*" die Stabilität der optischen Umwelt voraussetzt, so daß nur unerwartete Veränderungen als Bewegungen wahrgenommen werden. So könnten sowohl Augenfolgebewegung mit konstantem Retina-Bild wie Retina-Bildwanderungen bei Augenfixierung richtig als Bewegungen verrechnet und in der Wahrnehmung ausgewertet werden. Die von HERING [H 31a, 34] so genannte Raumkonstanz der Wahrnehmung ist in ihren Einzelmechanismen zwar viel untersucht, aber noch nicht aufgeklärt.

Die optisch-vestibuläre Koordination ist für die neurologische Diagnostik wichtiger als für die Psychiatrie. Psychiatrisch interessant ist die vielfach gesicherte Beobachtung, daß in besonnenen *Dämmerzuständen* auch komplizierte Orientierungshandlungen mit richtiger Verfügung über gedächtnisfixierte Ortskenntnisse ausgeführt werden können, obwohl sie völlig amnesiert werden. Wie das Gehirn bei Ausschaltung der Gedächtnisfixierung diese erstaunlichen Orientierungsleistungen durchführen kann, ist noch ungeklärt.

Die *Auswahlkriterien der Wahrnehmung* aus dem großen Angebot von Sinnesmeldungen durch die Aufmerksamkeit sind nicht nur trieb- und affektbedingt, sondern vor allem auch *erlernt*. Die Selektion bedeutungsvoller und neuer Wahrnehmungen dient der Sicherung der Umweltbeziehungen, wie GIBSON überzeugend dargestellt hat [G 27, 28]. Symbolische Bedeutungen sind vorwiegend erlernt, können aber mit angeborenen Mechanismen kombiniert sein [G 27].

Abstraktion und Klassifizierung benötigen auch Erfahrung, Lernen und Gedächtnis, deren neurophysiologische Grundlagen noch wenig geklärt sind. Neuronale Mechanismen bedingter Reflexe, wie sie JASPER u.Mitarb. in der motorischen Rinde registriert haben [J 11, 12], sind im visuellen Cortex noch nicht für verschiedene Gestaltreize untersucht worden. Die bedingten Reaktionen werden seit PAWLOW durch zeitliche *Assoziationen und Konvergenzen verschiedener Sinnesmodalitäten* erforscht.

Die Prozesse der Abstraktion und Klassifizierung sind noch mit modernen kybernetischen Methoden und Modellen zu untersuchen. CRAIK [C 13] hat 1943 zuerst auf die *innere Modellbildung der Umwelt im Nervensystem* hingewiesen. Solche Modellvorgänge sind in den letzten 20 Jahren neurophysiologisch leider noch nicht genügend erforscht worden. Hier können nur exakte Experimente an den Neuronensystemen der höheren Sinneszentren weiterführen. Abstrakt konstruierte kybernetische Modelle sind in großer Zahl denkbar, aber nur dann brauchbar, wenn sie auf Grund physiologischer Befunde entwickelt wurden (vgl. S. 877).

Motivation, Intention und Wahrnehmung. Schon frühe psychologische Versuche der Würzburger Schule von KÜLPE u.Mitarb. [K 56] mit tachistoskopischer Technik haben gezeigt, wie bedeutsam *Aufgabe, Einstellung* und *Abstraktion* bei der Wahrnehmung ist. In der theoretischen Psychologie und Phänomenologie ist der aktive Anteil der Einstellung (englisch „set") auch als *intentionale* Komponente der Wahrnehmung bezeichnet worden. In der neuen amerikanischen Forschung ist der Einfluß der *Motivation* als intermodaler Richtungs- und Wertungsfaktor vor allem von ALLPORT [A 20], BRUNER [B 68 a] und POSTMAN [P 33] untersucht worden.

Psychiatrisch interessant sind einige *Parallelen mit psychotisch-affektiven Störungen,* da Umgestaltungen der Wahrnehmung und Erinnerung durch affektive Projektion schon bei Gesunden vorkommen und bei Frauen noch durch normale hormonelle Umstellungen der Menstruation und Schwangerschaft begünstigt werden. Wenn man weiß, daß schon bei Geistesgesunden erhebliche Wahrnehmungsverfälschungen auftreten, die unter affektiver Spannung bis zu wahnhaften Erlebnissen reichen, so wird man bei Kranken für paranoische Veränderungen der Wahrnehmung ähnliche Mechanismen vermuten können.

Die alte Parallele von psychotischen Wahnwahrnehmungen und Sinnestäuschungen mit hypnagogen und traumhaften Wahrnehmungsstörungen kann nur bei den symptomatischen Psychosen durch Ähnlichkeiten des Schlaf-EEG und des Traumschlafes begründet werden (vgl. S. 1018).

Zu den Bemühungen der Psychopathologie, einen grundsätzlichen qualitativen Unterschied zwischen psychotischer Wahnwahrnehmung und wahnhaften Deutungen bei Gesunden festzustellen, kann die Neurophysiologie nichts beitragen. Quantitative Unterschiede mit spezieller Aktivierung der gleichen physiologischen Mechanismen, welche die hypnagogen und Traumphänomene auslösen, wären ebenso möglich: Psychotischer Wahn und wahnhafte Deutungen bei Gesunden könnten ähnliche cerebrale Grundlagen haben. Experimentell beim Menschen untersucht sind bisher nur die umgekehrten Vorgänge, nämlich die Einflüsse von affektiv ansprechenden Wahrnehmungen auf vegetative Reaktionen und auf die Pupille.

Beeinflussung vegetativer Reaktionen durch den Wahrnehmungsinhalt. Daß *Sinn, Inhalt und Bedeutung von Wahrnehmungen* nicht nur psychologische Wirkungen haben, sondern auch somatische vegetative Reaktionen beeinflussen, ist seit langem bekannt. Seit C.G. JUNG und L. BINSWANGER den galvanischen Hautreflex beim Assoziationsversuch studierten [B 44, P 19], sind vor allem akustische Wahrnehmungen mit Registrierung vegetativer Reaktionen untersucht worden. Bei optischen Reizen ist ein Einfluß der Bildbedeutung auf die Pupillenreaktion erkennbar. Eine neuere Untersuchung von HESS und POLT [H 41] über die *Pupillenerweiterung bei verschiedenartigen Bildern* zeigte deutliche individuelle und Geschlechtsunterschiede: Babybilder machten bei Frauen starke, bei Männern keine oder geringe Pupillenerweiterung, Landschaftsbilder lösten nur geringe Pupillenerweiterung aus, oder bei Frauen sogar Verengung. Aktbilder ergaben jeweils die stärksten Reaktionen bei dem entgegengesetzten Geschlecht.

Optische Halluzinationen, Eidetik und Diagramme bei Gesunden

Optische Halluzinationen sind häufige Phänomene bei allen Gesunden. Jeder Mensch kennt die Halluzinationen des Traumes. Auch die mehr elementaren, bruchstückhaften, hypnagogen Halluzinationen vor dem Einschlafen sind wahrscheinlich bei allen Menschen vorhanden, werden aber nicht immer beachtet und erinnert. Im Wachzustand haben die meisten Gesunden nur optische Vorstellungen ohne Halluzinationscharakter. Lebhaftere und leibhafte Bilder kommen nur bei eidetischer Veranlagung vor. Sie können experimentell als Kristallvisionen und bei sensorischer Isolierung ausgelöst werden (vgl. S. 932). Die Eidetik ist bei Jugendlichen häufig und wird mit zunehmendem Alter seltener. Die neurophysiologische Grundlage der Traumhalluzinationen wird im Kapitel X behandelt. Psychopathologische Bemühungen, echte Halluzinationen und Pseudohalluzinationen zu unterscheiden [J 13], können hier unberücksichtigt bleiben.

Optische Halluzinationen und Eidetik. Die seit langer Zeit zur Auslösung von Illusionen und Halluzinationen verwendete Methode der *Kristallvisionen* ist neurophysiologisch noch nicht geklärt. Die seit dem Altertum bekannten Illusionen und gestalteten Halluzinationen bei Fixierung blanker Flächen oder Körper (Spiegel, flüssigkeitsgefüllte Gefäße, Schuster-Kugel) im Dunkel sind nur von psychologischer Seite genauer studiert worden. JANET benutzte sie zuerst zur Untersuchung für experimentelle Visionen. MCDOUGAL [M 37] verglich sie mit sensorischen Automatismen, die ähnlich den Traumbildern, durch unbewußte Tendenzen in das Bewußtsein eindringen. BENDER [B 20a] studierte mit einer hinter der Kristallkugel dargebotenen Testmaske die Beziehung zur Eidetik. Von seinen meist aus dem Rheinland stammenden Versuchspersonen zeigten etwa $1/5$ beim Erstversuch lebhafte Kristallvisionen, meist bewegte filmartige Szenen, zum Teil vergessene Kindheitserinnerungen. Farben waren selten, automatisches Lesen kam gelegentlich vor. Suggestionsvorgänge spielen auch eine Rolle.

Die Diagramme. Die von GALTON [G 3] als *number-forms* zuerst beschriebenen visualisierten Zahlendiagramme sind *räumlich und meistens farbig erscheinende Schemata der Zahlenreihen und der Zeitperioden* (Jahre, Monate), welche als lebhafte optische Bilder das Zählen, Rechnen sowie die Zeitvorstellungen begleiten. Sie wurden von G.E. MÜLLER genauer studiert [M 78]. LEONHARD hat, ohne auf diese älteren Untersuchungen einzugehen, die Verwendung von Diagrammen und Zahlenbildern beim Rechnen in einer Gruppe von Intellektuellen untersucht [L 14]. Über den hirnphysiologischen Mechanismus wissen wir nichts. Veränderungen der Diagramme nach Hirnläsionen sind nur selten gefunden worden [S 38]. GALTON hat schon das Vorkommen ähnlicher Diagramme in der gleichen Familie beschrieben und eine „hereditary tendency" angenommen [G 3]. Das familiäre Vorkommen spricht für eine spezifische *Anlage zu räumlicher Visualisierung* als Grundlage der Diagramme. Es ist wahrscheinlich, daß auf dieser hereditären Grundlage mit dem Erlernen von Zahl- und Zeitbegriffen die spezielle Form der Diagramme als kybernetische Programmierung eines vorhandenen cerebralen Substrates in der Kindheit *erworben und fixiert* wird. Offenbar kann die Form der Diagramme bei diesem Programmierungsprozeß auch *emotional beeinflußt* werden. Dafür spricht die Hervorhebung, Erhellung und Verlängerung bestimmter für Kinder affektiv bedeutsamer Zeiten wie Geburtstag oder Weihnachten in den Jahresdiagrammen. Einzelne Zahlen können auch angenehme oder unangenehme Gefühlstöne haben.

Die Monographie von AHLENSTIEL [A 12] bringt eine zusammenfassende Darstellung über die optischen Trugwahrnehmungen bei Gesunden im Wach- und Schlafzustand. Sie reichen von den Nachbildern und eidetischen Visualisierungsvorgängen ohne äußere Sinnesreize, die bei Blinden genauer studiert sind [J 2], über geometrische Halluzinationen bis zu den vorwiegend im Traum vorkommenden allegorischen und symbolischen Phänomenen.

Experimentelle Halluzinationen

Toxische Halluzinationen. Die seit den Mescalin-Versuchen von BERINGER [B 34] und MAYER-GROSS [M 31] oft beschriebenen optischen Halluzinationen durch psychotomimetische Pharmaka sind nicht ausführlich zu besprechen, da ihre neurophysiologische Grundlage noch wenig geklärt ist. KLÜVER [K 23] gibt eine systematische Übersicht und betont die Formkonstanz und Geometrisierung im Frühstadium des Mescalinrauschs. Diese oft rechtwinkligen oder netzartigen Strukturen optischer Halluzinationen sind vielleicht als Desintegrierung und *Visualisierung von isoliert und enthemmt aktivierten rezeptiven Feldorganisationen in corticalen Neuronenverbänden* erklärbar. Es ist wahrscheinlich, daß solche toxischen Halluzinationen *Enthemmungen vorgebildeter Hirnmechanismen* sind, da die Reihenfolge ihres Auftretens ähnlich ist wie bei anderen nicht-toxischen Halluzinationen. Die ohne Pharmaka nach sensorischer Isolierung und Immobilisierung entstehenden optischen Halluzinationen haben die gleiche Reihenfolge ihrer Entwicklung wie nach Mescalin, LSD oder anderen Halluzinogenen: Zuerst erscheinen geometrisch geformte Trugbilder, dann komplexere Szenen optischer Halluzinationen zusammen mit affektiven Veränderungen (vgl. S. 933).

EEG-Untersuchungen während halluzinatorischer Zustände haben noch nicht zu klaren Ergebnissen geführt. Klinische Ähnlichkeiten mit den traumhaften Sinnestäuschungen bei der temporalen Epilepsie sind im EEG nicht zu verifizieren. Hirnelektrische Veränderungen sind besser bei den hypnagogen Halluzinationen des Einschlafstadiums festzustellen sowie bei optischen Sinnestäuschungen des Traumes (vgl. S. 1010). Diese unspezifischen EEG-Veränderungen, die mit Bewußtseinsänderungen einhergehen, geben noch keine Hinweise auf neuronale Mechanismen.

Halluzinationen bei Gesunden nach sensorischer Isolierung (sensory deprivation). Die von HEBB und seiner Forschungsgruppe, insbesondere von HERON systematisch durchgeführten Isolierungsversuche sind sowohl von psychiatrischem wie von physiologischem Interesse.

Die Isolierungsversuche benutzten drei verschiedene Methoden: 1. Radikale Minderung aller sensiblen und sensorischen Reize im warmen Bad und mit Masken nach LILLY u.a. 2. Verminderung geformter und gestalteter Sinnesreize, optisch durch Brillen mit diffusem homogenem Licht und haptisch proprioceptiv mit partieller Immobilisierung der Arme und behandschuhten Händen (HERON u.Mitarb. [H 39, 40]). 3. Monotonisierung der Reize ohne wesentliche Intensitätsminderung mit Beschränkung des Gesichtsfeldes und monotonem Geräuschhintergrund.

Alle diese Halluzinationen werden zwar oft mit dem Traum verglichen, unterscheiden sich aber von diesem durch regelmäßiges Vorangehen elementarer, bruchstückhafter Sinneserscheinungen, die dem Traum selbst fehlen und nur beim Einschlafen als hypnagoge Halluzinationen vorkommen. Auch die Halluzinationen bei Mescalinvergiftung und anderen Psychodrogen zeigen eine entsprechende Reihenfolge. Die *zeitliche Abfolge von elementaren zu komplexen, szenenhaften Bildern* kann man daher als *typisch für alle experimentellen Halluzinationen* ansehen: Beginn mit einfachen geometrischen Figuren, oft verbunden mit einer Aufhellung des Sehfeldes, dann isolierte Objekte bei homogenem Hintergrund und schließlich komplexe zusammenhängende Szenen, bei denen Einzelheiten durch gerichtete Aufmerksamkeit und Augenbewegungen genau betrachtet werden konnten. Die Halluzinationen bei sensorischer Isolierung waren wenig vom Willen zu beeinflussen und immer sehr lebhaft, meist bewegt, zum Teil auch in unnatürlicher Weise, etwa Teile von Landschaften, die sich in umgekehrter Richtung bewegten.

Die Latenzzeit bis zum Auftreten der Halluzinationen war bei Isolierungsversuchen sehr unterschiedlich zwischen 20 min und 70 Std. Optische Halluzinationen waren am besten und langdauerndsten unter der Brille mit diffusem Licht. Durch Verdunkelung wurden sie nur vorübergehend verstärkt, verschwanden dann aber nach 2 Std und konnten durch belichtete Brillen wieder hervorgerufen werden. Eine zusammenfassende Darstellung und Diskussion der Isolationsversuche beim Menschen durch verschiedene Autoren und Fachrichtungen ist 1961 in einem Symposion [S 36a] erschienen. Neben den Wahrnehmungsveränderungen wurden bei den Isolierungsversuchen vor allem ausgeprägte *affektive und Verhaltensstörungen* beobachtet. Reizhunger und imperative Aktionsbereitschaft traten besonders bei LILLYs Versuchen mit stärkerer sensibler Isolierung bereits nach kürzerer Zeit auf. Auch diese Erfahrungen sprechen für eine enge Verbindung der Wahrnehmung mit affektiven und motorischen Funktionen. Durch *Testuntersuchungen* wurden die psychischen Veränderungen während der Isolierung noch genauer zu erfassen versucht.

Die kognitiven Störungen der Testleistungen waren schon in den ersten Stunden der Isolierung erkennbar, ohne wesentliche Verschlechterung nach 12 und 48 Std, obwohl die subjektiven Denkstörungen eine weitere Zunahme mit längerer Isolierung zeigten.

Die Testuntersuchungen und die introspektiv festgestellten Störungen scheinen uns ebenso wie die EEG-Veränderungen für einen *partiellen oder abortiven Einschlafmechanismus* mit hypnagogen Bildern während der Isolierung zu sprechen. Ferner geben diese Versuche Hinweise auf ähnliche Mechanismen, die wahrscheinlich zu den *halluzinatorischen Psychosen in Einzelhaft* führen. Die Ähnlichkeit mit gewissen toxischen Halluzinationen nach Mescalinvergiftung läßt daran denken, daß solche partiellen Schlafmechanismen auch bei anderen symptomatischen Psychosen mit optischem Halluzinieren wirksam werden.

Optische Halluzinationen bei Kranken ohne Psychose

Reizung und Ausschaltung verschiedener visueller Strukturen. Pathologische Erfahrungen beim Menschen mit Erkrankungen des Sehsystems haben vorwiegend die Lokalisation der Strukturen des Gesichtsfeldes aufgeklärt. Über die Funktionen des Sehsystems lehrten uns weder die elementaren Halluzinationen bei Augenkrankheiten [U 2] noch die komplexen Sinnestäuschungen bei Hirnerkrankungen Wesentliches. Hirnpathologische Erfahrungen haben daher nur wenig zur Sehphysiologie beigetragen. Neuronale Korrelationen waren daraus nicht ableitbar. Elektrische *Reizungen* [F 20, P 17, U 4] *der optischen Rindenfelder 17, 18 und 19 bei Hirnoperationen* zeigten einige Verschiedenheiten der ausgelösten Halluzinationen, die in Area 17 elementarer waren als in den anderen Feldern. Doch waren komplexe optische Halluzinationen und Erinnerungsbilder noch besser von der Temporalregion auslösbar [P 16]. Die Entstehung der hemianopischen Halluzinationen und ihre Beziehung zu subcorticalen Hirnregionen ist noch nicht geklärt, ebensowenig die bei Mittelhirnläsionen auftretende ,,hallucinose pedonculaire", die man vielleicht mit Funktionsänderungen des unspezifischen reticulären Systems in Verbindung bringen kann.

Die einfachen geometrischen Trugbilder bei neurologischen Störungen, wie die *Flimmerskotome der Migräne* wurden mit der ,,spreading depression" am geschädigten Cortex von Tieren verglichen [M 46]. Selbstbeobachtungen bei Migränephosphenen beweisen den Einfluß von Blickbewegungen und vestibulären Reizen auf corticale Erregungsfoci des Sehfelds 17 [J 50]. Die Größe der Flimmerfiguren wächst von der Fovea zur Peripherie entsprechend den perceptiven Feldern und ihrer Säulenordnung [R 15, J 50].

Von besonderem Interesse sind die optischen Halluzinationen nach Augenverlust und längerer Augenverdunkelung, obwohl auch diese Syndrome noch nicht neurophysiologisch untersucht sind.

Optische Halluzinationen bei längerer Augenverdunkelung und Blindheit. Seit JOHANNES MÜLLERS Beschreibung der phantastischen Gesichtserscheinungen gesunder Eidetiker bei Augenschluß [M 81] und UHTHOFFS Studien über die Gesichtstäuschungen der Blinden und Augenkranken [U 2] sind zahlreiche klinische und psychologische, aber wenige physiologische und anatomische Untersuchungen über diese Phänomene durchgeführt worden. Es ist nach klinischen Erfahrungen anzunehmen, daß die initialen Gesichtstäuschungen bei peripherer Erblindung *retinal*, die optischen Reizerscheinungen bei Hirnerkrankungen und Epilepsie *cerebral* ausgelöst werden, und daß bei der Migräne beides vorkommt. Dazu kommt als weiterer Faktor die sensorische Isolierung. Nicht selten sind *halluzinatorische Episoden nach Kataraktoperationen* mit längerer Augenabdeckung [F 16, G 46].

Veränderungen der Visualisierung und optische Halluzinationen bei Blinden sind von JACOB [J 2] bei Späterblindeten sorgfältig untersucht worden. Wie weit es sich aber um eine Eigenleistung der Sehzentren mit vollständiger Isolierung des zentralen optischen Systems von den peripheren Afferenzen handelt, ist noch nicht genügend geklärt.

Einige Beobachtungen bei diesen Späterblindeten sind auch für den Neurophysiologen interessant. Sie sprechen für ein Erhaltenbleiben der *affektiven Beeinflußbarkeit* und der *Aufmerksamkeitskontrolle,* die man vielleicht als reticulär-thalamischen Einfluß auf den Cortex deuten kann. Photismen und Lichtblitze bei affektiver Erregung hat JACOB [J 2] bei zahlreichen Blinden beschrieben. Die Lichtphänomene sind stärker als der Schreckblitz des Gesunden. Im Gegensatz zu diesen häufigen Elementarphänomenen werden szenische Halluzinationen nach akuten Affekten bei Blinden nicht beschrieben [J 2]. Willkürliche Aufmerksamkeit läßt die optischen Halluzinationen oft verschwinden.

Das Substrat des *veränderten Eigengrau,* das bei Totalerblindeten nach initialem Schwarzsehen meist als frontal gerichtete "Nebelwand" geschildert wird [J 2], ist nach beiderseitiger Retinazerstörung offenbar rein cerebral lokalisiert.

Leider fehlen anatomische Kontrolluntersuchungen darüber, ob Halluzinationen, Nebelsehen, optische Bewegungsillusionen, hypnagoge und Traumbilder auch nach völliger *Atrophie* des primären optischen Systems vom Auge bis zum Geniculatum möglich sind. Ungeklärt ist auch, wie weit diese visuellen Phänomene durch geringe ungestaltete restliche Afferenzen aus der Retina gefördert oder vermindert werden. Wahrscheinlich sind die Halluzinationen seltener bei total Erblindeten. Das spräche gegen ein sensorisches Isolierungssymptom in den zentralen Sehstrukturen. Zur Klärung dieser Fragen können sorgfältige Fallbeobachtungen mit anatomischen Untersuchungen bei Blinden wahrscheinlich mehr beitragen als neurophysiologische Experimente.

Wie weit Beziehungen der Blindenhalluzinationen und sensorische Isolierungserscheinungen zu einer eidetischen Anlage bestehen, ist noch ungeklärt. Schon GALTON [G 3] hat bei sich selbst beschrieben, daß seine eidetischen Bilder in der Isolierung und bei Ausschaltung sensorischer Reize stärker hervortreten. Doch können eidetische Phänomene auch durch bestimmte optische Reize wie im Kristallversuch gebahnt werden (vgl. S. 931).

Mögliche neurophysiologische Grundlagen der Halluzinationen. Eine neurophysiologische Theorie der Halluzinationen kann heute noch nicht gegeben werden. Einerseits wissen wir noch zu wenig über die physiologischen und pathologischen cerebralen Veränderungen bei experimentellen Halluzinationen mit Ausnahme der Untersuchungen über das Traum-EEG (vgl. S. 1010) und das EEG bei sensorischer Isolierung. Andererseits ist die Neuronenphysiologie normaler und abnormer Wahrnehmungsvorgänge nur bei Tieren exakt untersucht, bei denen wir zwar die receptorischen Vorgänge steuern, aber nichts über subjektive Wahrnehmung oder Halluzinationen wissen können. Nach den Verhaltensreaktionen der Tiere ist von mehreren Forschern angenommen worden, daß subcorticale Reizungen Halluzinationen hervorrufen [H 81, 84]. Bei Thalamusreizung am Menschen sind Halluzinationen selten [H 72]. Nach Cortexreizung wurden sie bei Epileptikern ähnlich einer Aura beschrieben [P 17]. Optische szenenhafte Trugwahrnehmungen wurden auch nach Thalamusausschaltungen beobachtet.

EVARTS' Versuch einer neurophysiologischen Theorie der Halluzinationen [E 22a], verwendet neben allgemeinen Konzeptionen und PENFIELDS Reizversuchen am Cortex zunächst nur den Schlafmechanismus als Erklärung. EVARTS postuliert eine dauernde Hemmung des corticalen Neuronensystems im Wachzustand und eine *Enthemmung im Schlaf.* Im tiefen Schlaf wäre die Enthemmung so stark, daß eine gestaltete Aktivität nicht mehr auftreten könne. Die neuronalen Koordinationsprozesse, die den Halluzinationen und normalen Vorstellungen zugrunde liegen, sind aber wahrscheinlich zu komplex, um sie durch einfache Vorgänge der Hemmung und Enthemmung erklären zu können. Wahrscheinlich wirkt die bei fehlenden Lichtreizen vermehrte "Dunkelentladung" der Retina zentral hemmend [A 28a, J 42].

Bisher kann man nach neurophysiologischen Daten nur vermuten, daß eine Aktivierung von Wahrnehmungen, Vorstellungen oder Erinnerungen, bis zu traumähnlichen halluzinatorischen Vorgängen durch aktivierende Hirnstammsysteme oder spezifische synaptische Transmitter erfolgt. Offenbar handelt es sich um eine *subcorticale Beeinflussung der corticalen Funktionen in solchen Hirnrindenfeldern, die auch bei der direkten Wahrnehmung beteiligt sind.* Eine unspezifische Aktivierung visueller Neurone mit Konvergenz spezifisch-optischer Afferenzen ist sicher nachgewiesen [A 17, C 15]. Ferner erfolgt eine Aktivierung dieser Neurone der Sehrinde im Schlaf [E 22], obwohl die genaueren Beziehungen zu den Traumstadien neuronal noch wenig untersucht sind. Wenn der Schlaf in seinen verschiedenen Stadien aber durch den Hirnstamm gesteuert wird (vgl. S. 989), so ist es wahrscheinlich, daß auch die *hypnagogen Halluzinationen* des Einschlafstadiums wie die *Traumhalluzinationen* mit ihren verschiedenen affektiven Komponenten subcortical ausgelöst werden. Beim Traum könnten die regelmäßig gefundenen raschen Augenbewegungen mit bewegten Traumbildern und die rhythmischen Ammonshornwellen mit der Affektkomponente der Traumhalluzinationen in Verbindung gebracht werden. Genauere Vorstellungen über den physiologischen Mechanismus der optischen Bildaktivierung gibt es noch nicht. Wie räumlich-zeitlich relativ geordnete und affektiv gesteuerte sensorische Muster dabei entstehen, ist unbekannt.

Zusammenfassung

Sinneswahrnehmungen liefern die Information über Umwelt und Innenwelt für psychische Inhalte und das Verhalten. Die *subjektive Sinnesphysiologie,* die sich im 19. Jahrhundert zu großer Höhe entwickelt hat, vergleicht äußere Reize und Sinnesempfindungen. Die *objektive Sinnesphysiologie,* 1926 durch ADRIANS Registrierungen von einzelnen afferenten Fasern begründet, registriert die Mechanismen der Informationsverarbeitung von Sinnesmeldungen. Sie ergänzt und erweitert damit die subjektive Sinnesphysiologie. Die psychophysische Weber-Fechner-Relation, der Anstieg der Empfindungsstärke mit dem Logarithmus der Reizstärke, gilt mit Einschränkungen für subjektive und objektive Sinnesnachrichten. Auch STEVENS' Potenzfunktion ist für Empfindungsschätzungen gut verwendbar. An Beispielen des *Sehsystems* werden die Beziehungen subjektiver und objektiver Sinnesphysiologie demonstriert, die gute Korrelationen für einfache Sehwahrnehmungen zeigen. Das Sehsystem leistet von der Retina bis zur Sehrinde eine *Konturabstraktion* flächenhafter Bilder zu Umrissen, ähnlich wie ein Zeichner komplexe Gestalten auf ihre Konturen reduziert. Der Zeichner eines Bildes arbeitet jedoch von der Konturlinie zum Bild zeitlich invers gegen die Konturabstraktion des Sehsystems. Optische *Halluzinationen* können bei Gesunden im Traum, nach sensorischer Isolierung oder Intoxikationen, bei Kranken nach Hirnläsionen auftreten. Die Formen der Migräne-Phosphene und gewisser toxischer Halluzinationen machen cerebrale Strukturcharakteristika sichtbar, doch sind sie in ihrem neurophysiologischen Mechanismus noch nicht erklärbar.

IX. Neurophysiologie der Affekte und Triebe

„ᾧ δ' αἴσθησις ὑπάρχει, τούτῳ ἡδονή τε καὶ λύπη καὶ τὸ ἡδύ τε καὶ λυπρόν, οἷς δε' ταῦτα, καὶ ἡ ἐπιθυμία · τοῦ γὰρ ἡδέος ὄρεξις αὕτη."

(Wo aber Sinnesempfindung vorhanden ist, da erscheint auch das Gefühl von Lust und Unlust, von Angenehmem und Unangenehmem. Wer aber dies alles hat, der hat auch Begierde; denn diese selbst ist Streben nach dem Angenehmen).

ARISTOTELES: Περὶ Ψυχῆς (Über die Seele, Buch II, Kap. 3). Um 330 v. Chr.

„Ein rein triebhafter Mensch wäre noch kein Mensch, ein rein bewußter Mensch wäre kein Mensch mehr. Zwischen beiden Polen treibt der menschliche Mensch hin und her."

K. SCHNEIDER: Klinische Psychopathologie, 1959

Man braucht nicht ARISTOTELES und EPIKUR für den Nachweis, daß *Affekte und Triebe an fast allen psychischen Erscheinungen beteiligt sind* und von der Wahrnehmung über das Denken bis zum Handlungsentschluß eine Rolle spielen. Schon die Alltagserfahrung zeigt uns, daß bereits Sinneswahrnehmungen oft mit *Lust oder Unlust* verbunden sind. Bei anderen Erlebnisformen ist dies noch deutlicher. Affekte und Triebe müssen zusammen behandelt werden, da eine scharfe Trennung psychologisch und physiologisch schwierig ist. *Alle Affekte haben eine Triebkomponente, alle Triebe erzeugen Affekte.* Eine Trennung der Trieb-Affekt-Gruppe von Wahrnehmungs-, Denk- und Lernvorgängen gelingt leichter, obwohl eine Triebdynamik auch hier beteiligt ist. Schon in der Antike wurde klar, daß weder das stoische Ideal der Affektfreiheit noch der epikureische Hedonismus allgemeingültige Regeln geben, und daß emotionale und triebhafte Motive nur Teilvorgänge des seelischen Lebens sind. Seit FREUD wird viel diskutiert, wie weit unbewußte Vorgänge an Trieben und Affekten beteiligt sind. *Unbewußtes bedeutet für uns aber Physiologisches.* Die Neurophysiologie hat in den letzten Jahren die Hirnmechanismen der Affekt- und Triebvorgänge systematisch untersucht. Vorher hatte die Psychophysiologie durch WUNDT [W 33] und seine Schule um die Jahrhundertwende körperliche Begleiterscheinungen von Lust und Unlust beim Menschen beschrieben, doch waren die Ergebnisse, die sich vor allem auf vegetative Effekte bezogen, nicht sehr aufschlußreich. Auch die tierexperimentelle Forschung begnügte sich zunächst mit wenigen vereinzelten Beobachtungen: Die Affektäußerungen der Tiere ohne Cortex wurden von GOLTZ [G 30], CANNON [C 2] und BARD [B 3] in Ausschaltungsexperimenten beschrieben, die cerebralen Mechanismen der affektiven Abwehrreaktionen entdeckte W.R. HESS nach lokalisierter Zwischenhirnreizung [H 67]. Diese Befunde waren Ausgangspositionen der weiteren Forschung über cerebrale Grundlagen der Triebvorgänge.

Affekte und Triebe sind bei Tieren und Menschen die stärksten Motivationen des Verhaltens und des psychischen Lebens. Daher wurde sie auch als Ursache neurotischer und psychotischer Störungen von allen psychiatrischen Schulen hoch bewertet und in ihren verständlichen Zusammenhängen untersucht. Es wäre aber unzweckmäßig, sich nur mit psychologisch-phänomenologischen Studien über Gefühle und Triebe zu begnügen, oder eine hypothetische psychoanalytische „Triebdynamik" zu betreiben, ohne ihre cerebralen Mechanismen zu beachten. *Wenn etwas über somatische Grundlagen und Mechanismen von Affekten und Trieben erfahrbar ist, so wird dies offenbar auch für die Psychiatrie von Nutzen sein.* Solche neurophysiologischen Untersuchungen können durchaus bestehen neben allen anderen Deutungen von Trieben und Affekten in der Psychologie, Ethologie und Psychotherapie. Allerdings bleiben die physiologischen Ergebnisse auf die Affekt- und Trieb*mechanismen* beschränkt. Der Neurophysiologe kann nicht wie der Ethologe die soziale Rolle der Triebe erforschen, die oft zu Widersprüchen individueller und gesellschaftlicher Ordnungen führt und vielen neurotischen Störungen zugrunde liegt. Er kann auch nicht wie der Psychologe die allgemeine Bedeutung der Affekte und Triebe im menschlichen Leben oder in der Krankengeschichte behandeln oder gar ihre eindrucksvolle Darstellung in Biographie und Dichtung. Schilderungen tragischer Triebkonflikte mit Schicksal und Schuld, die auch bei größter Einsicht und vernünftiger Überlegung kein Entrinnen zulassen, sind jahrhundertelang die anschaulichsten Grundlagen für die Triebpsychologie gewesen, deren Anwendungen bis zu manchen psychiatrischen Konfliktsituationen reichen. Der neurophysiologischen Forschung entziehen sich auch alle ethologischen und ethisch-religiösen Trieb-Interpretationen als Wurzeln des Bösen im Menschen. Selbst psychoanalytisch-tiefenpsychologische Deutungen der Triebe als unbewußte Mächte schlagen noch keine Brücke zur Physiologie. Unsere Darstellung geht daher aus von einigen *experimentellen Grundlagen und cerebralen Mechanismen des Affekt- und Trieblebens*. Im Anschluß an das IV. Kapitel sollen die Triebmechanismen dargestellt werden, die wir mit den Tieren gemeinsam haben und die psychiatrische Anwendungen zulassen.

Experimentelle Untersuchungen über intracerebrale Reize am frei beweglichen Tier und die Technik der Selbstreizversuche haben die Triebphysiologie sehr gefördert. Damit haben sie auch einige psychiatrisch interessante Ergebnisse über die Triebdynamik, über Parallelen zum Suchtverhalten und über hirnlokalisatorische Substrate neuropharmakologischer Wirkungen gebracht.

Gegenüber diesen Ergebnissen der tierexperimentellen Forschung hat die intracerebrale Reizung und Ableitung beim Menschen, abgesehen von ihrer in manchen Fällen ethisch zweifelhaften Rechtfertigung, vorwiegend neurologisch relevante Resultate (S. 884) und nur wenige psychiatrisch anwendbare Ergebnisse gebracht, die auf S. 958 besprochen werden.

Cerebrale Auslösung von Affekten und Trieben im Tierexperiment

Die neurophysiologische Erforschung von Trieb- und Affektverhalten wurde nach den alten Ausschaltungsversuchen [B 3, G 30] erst durch die modernen Methoden der intracerebralen Reizung ermöglicht. Sie beginnen mit den Pionieruntersuchungen von HESS [H 44–51] über *Zwischenhirnreizungen bei der frei beweglichen Katze*. Diese Experimente konnten in bestimmten Regionen des Hypothalamus und Thalamus typische Affektentladungen und andere instinktiv vorgebildete Verhaltensweisen auslösen (affektive Abwehrreaktionen vgl. S. 940,

Schlaf S. 989). Die Untersuchungen von HESS wurden in der 1. Auflage von PLOOG mit Abbildungen ausführlicher dargestellt (S. 368, I/1 B). Die Reizung mit implantierten Elektroden am sonst intakten Tier ist heute ein viel bearbeitetes Gebiet der physiologischen Verhaltensforschung. Die Reizuntersuchungen von HESS wurden durch Ausschaltungsexperimente, anatomische Kontrollen und funktionelle Lokalisationsversuche ergänzt. Abschließend hat HESS noch die Korrelationen der physiologischen mit psychologischen Deutungen besprochen [H 65].

Ähnliche Untersuchungen durch v. HOLST u.Mitarb. [H 80, 84] über *Hirnstammreizungen bei Hühnern* verzichten zwar auf lokalisatorische Auswertungen, bringen dafür aber eine noch weitergehende *funktionelle Ordnung in das Wirkungsgefüge der Triebe*.

Neurophysiologische Untersuchungen über Hunger und Durst. Unter den elementaren Trieben sind Hunger und Durst am besten physiologisch untersucht. Die Ergebnisse zeigen, wie kompliziert die Regulationen scheinbar so einfacher Triebe sind und welche Wechselwirkungen zentraler und peripher-nervöser, vegetativer und hormoneller Faktoren bestehen.

Beim *Nahrungstrieb* wurde die Beziehung des *Hungergefühls* zu den periodischen Magenkontraktionen von CANNON u.Mitarb. [C 2] beim Menschen studiert und die Signalisierung des Hungers in dem bekannten Magenknurren registriert. Dann folgten Untersuchungen über die Beziehung zum hormonell regulierten Blutzuckerspiegel und über den Hunger bei Hypoglykämie nach Insulingabe, deren extreme Formen auch in der Psychiatrie durch die Insulinbehandlung wohlbekannt sind. Schließlich wurden die *zentralen Substrate des Nahrungstriebes im Zwischenhirn* mit einem „Freßzentrum" im ventrolateralen Hypothalamus [A 21] lokalisiert. Ein zu diesem reziprokes „Sättigungszentrum" [B 65] wurde ebenfalls gefunden. Nach Zerstörung des letzteren zeigten die Versuchstiere eine unkontrollierte Nahrungsaufnahme mit starkem Fettansatz. Beziehungen zur Körpertemperaturregulierung und zum Blutzuckerniveau wurden festgestellt [B 65].

Ähnliche Untersuchungen über den *Durst* mit lokalen Reizungen des Hypothalamus von ANDERSSON [A 23] und seinen Mitarbeitern zeigten eine etwas andere Hirnlokalisation im medialen Hypothalamus (N. paraventricularis und supraopticus), wo man schon früher nach Befunden beim Diabetes insipidus [G 13] Beziehungen zur Neurosekretion und zum Hypophysenhinterlappen angenommen hatte [S 65].

Daß auch der sehr elementare Nahrungstrieb mit den speziellen Richtungen des Appetits durch *erlernte* Vorgänge verändert und beeinflußt wird, ist seit PAWLOW [P 5–7] experimentell gesichert. Die *bedingten Reflexe der vegetativen Speichelsekretion* zeigen solche durch Lernen modifizierte Affekte und Triebmechanismen sehr deutlich [P 7].

Sexuelle Triebmechanismen, ihre Mehrdeutigkeit und Irradiation. Die Zwischenhirnreizversuche und Verhaltensbeobachtungen von PLOOG, MACLEAN u.Mitarb. [M 15] ergaben im präoptischen Gebiet oberhalb des C. mammillare und im Bereich des Viq d'Azyrschen Bündels regelmäßig *Erektionseffekte*. Bei größeren Reizstärken oder bei geringen Elektrodenverschiebungen wurden in der Nachbarschaft andere Affektäußerungen, vor allem Angstschreie, ausgelöst.

Bei diesen Totenkopfaffen haben Erektionen nicht nur sexuelle Bedeutung, sondern sind auch ritualisiertes *Imponierverhalten*, vor allem gegenüber gleichgeschlechtlichen Artgenossen in der Gruppe. Der sexuelle Orgasmus wurde auch hirnelektrisch untersucht [M 67, S 2]. Die drei Triebreaktionen *Aggression, Flucht* und *Sexualverhalten* stehen in einem gewissen Antagonismus, doch sind Irradiationen von einem zum anderen möglich. Diese *Irradiation sexueller und anderer affektiver und Triebmechanismen* scheint bei Tieren ausgeprägter zu sein als beim Menschen. Bei Hengsten werden unspezifische Erektionen bei verschiedenen asexuellen Erregungen beobachtet. Beim Menschen ist unspezifische Auslösung von Erektionen ohne sexuellen Reiz nach KINSEY [K 15] vor allem bei Kindern und Jugendlichen häufig. Auch bei Neurotischen wird dies oft beobachtet, vielleicht als Zeichen mangelnder Ausreifung der Sexualfunktionen. Auch wenn man nicht an FREUDS Deutungen fixierter polymorpher infantiler Sexualwünsche glaubt, erscheint diese durch neurophysiologische und Verhaltensexperimente gesicherte *Mehrdeutigkeit* sexueller Mechanismen von psychiatrischer Bedeutung.

Wutaffekte und Aggressionstrieb. Die *affektive Abwehrreaktion*, die HESS bei Katzen im caudalen Hypothalamus durch elektrische Reizung auslöste, zeigt alle Kriterien der Wut und Aggression dieser Tiere. Je nach der Umweltsituation richtet die Katze ihre Wut gegen andere Tiere oder Menschen im typischen Angriffsverhalten. Sie nimmt eine Drohstellung ein. Ob diese in Abwehr, Angriff oder Flucht übergeht, wird durch die Außenreize bestimmt. HESS schließt aus dem Verhalten auf ein inneres Erlebnis der Bedrohung und „gereizte Stimmung". Bei vorzeitiger Beendigung des Reizes kommt die Katze vor einem etwaigen Angriff nach Manifestierung des Wutverhaltens wieder zur Ruhe. Die von HESS bestimmten Kerngebiete des Hypothalamus sind nur Teile eines größeren Systems von Trieb-Regulationen für Abwehr, Angriff und Flucht, die nach HUNSPERGER vom zentralen Höhlengrau des Mittelhirns über den Hypothalamus bis zum basalen Schläfenlappen reichen (s.S. 944).

Angriff und Flucht im zentralen Reizversuch. Die von HESS beschriebene affektive Abwehrreaktion nach Zwischenhirnreizung kann zu *Angriffs- oder Fluchtverhalten* führen. Nach HUNSPERGERS Untersuchungen [F 6, H 93–95] sind Angriff und Flucht bei der Katze von nahe beieinanderliegenden Regionen des *zentralen Höhlengraus im Mittel- und Zwischenhirn* auszulösen: Angriffsverhalten war häufiger von den zentralen, Fluchtverhalten mehr von den Randgebieten mit gegenseitiger Überlagerung auszulösen. Bei gleichzeitiger Reizung der Angriffs- und Fluchtregion zeigte sich eine *Verstärkung des Angriffsverhaltens und eine Verzögerung des Fluchtverhaltens* [H 95]. Die Reizergebnisse waren auch durch *Sinnesreize* von Attrappen (ausgestopfte Katzen oder Hunde) weiter zu beeinflussen. Flucht wird auch durch spezielle *Umweltkonstellationen* begünstigt, die ein rasches Verstecken ermöglichen. Angriff oder Flucht werden als alternative Reaktionen des Selbstschutzes aufgefaßt, die durch koordinierte Hirnstrukturen gesteuert werden. Diese Experimente geben wichtige Hinweise auf gegenseitige Beeinflussungen verschiedener Triebhandlungen und der Wahrnehmung. Sie wurden schon von HESS und MEYER [H 68] diskutiert, aber noch nicht durch simultane Reizung verschiedener Triebsubstrate untersucht. Erst v. HOLST [H 83] hat solche systematischen Mehrfachreizungen durchgeführt.

Tierexperimente über Wechselwirkung verschiedener Triebvorgänge. Die gegenseitige Beeinflussung elektrisch ausgelösten Triebverhaltens und die Veränderungen ihrer Reizschwelle in der Kombination verschiedener Verhaltensweisen haben v. HOLST und ST. PAUL [H 84] an dem für stereotype Instinktvorgänge besonders geeigneten *Huhn* ausführlicher untersucht. Einige Beispiele der sensorischen Steuerung und zentralen Anpassung und *Umstimmung* durch elektrische Hirnreizungen sind in Abb. 27 dargestellt.

Die Experimente v. HOLSTS zeigen, daß physiologische Begriffe wie Schwelle und Adaptation auch auf Triebe und komplexe Verhaltensmuster anwendbar sind. Neurophysiologisch und verhaltensphysiologisch besonders wichtig und psychiatrisch interessant ist die *gegenseitige Beeinflussung von Stimmungen und Trieben*, die aus dem Verhalten des Huhnes abgelesen werden kann. Einer experimentellen Klärung zugänglich ist auch die *Triebmodifikation durch äußere Sinnesreize*, wie die Auslösung des Bodenfeind-Verhaltens der gereizten Henne (Abb. 27). Hier ist auch die *Umkehr von Angriffs- und Fluchtverhalten* deutlich erkennbar, die im Leben der Tiere eine große Rolle spielt. HUNSPERGER hat Angriff und Flucht nach zentraler Reizung bei der Katze noch genauer untersucht (F 5, 6, H 95).

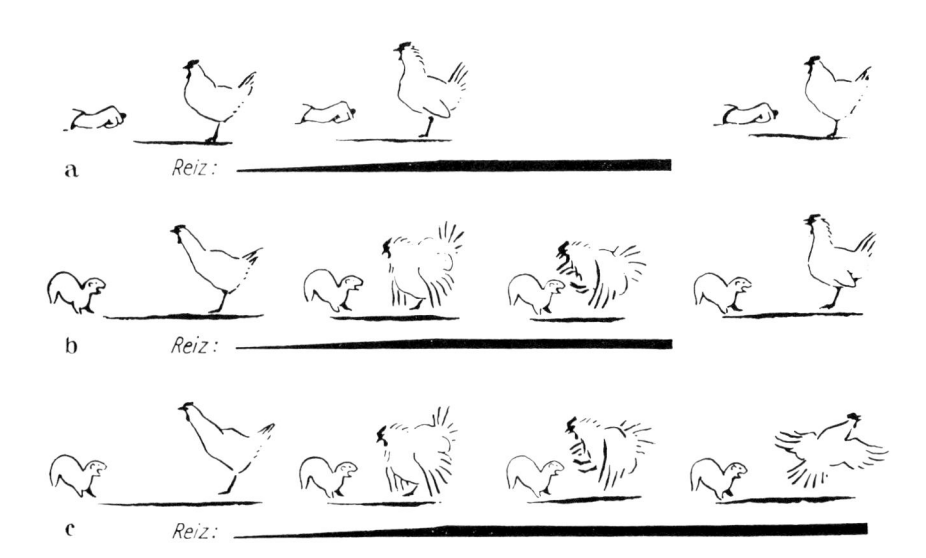

Abb. 27a–c. Zentrale Auslösung und visuelle Steuerung von Angriffs- und Fluchtverhalten beim Huhn nach Zwischenhirnreizung. Nach v. HOLST und ST. PAUL (1960) [H 84]. a) *Zwischenhirnreizung ohne Feind*. Das Bodenfeind-Verhalten der gereizten Henne bei cerebraler Reizung ohne natürliche Gegner und Vorzeigen einer menschlichen Hand besteht nur in leichter Unruhe mit Drohen. b) *Gleiche Reizung mit Feind* (ausgestopfter Iltis) *ergibt Angriffshandlungen*. Die Iltis-Attrappe wird ohne Reizung nur aufmerksam betrachtet. Während der Reizung entsteht Bedrohung und Angriff. Danach noch leichte Unruhe mit Drohen. c) *Noch längere Reizung verwandelt den Angriff in* Flucht. Schematische Zeichnungen nach Filmaufnahmen. Die elektrische Zwischenhirnreizung entspricht der zunehmend dicker werdenden *Linie*, die unter den in zeitlicher Folge von links nach rechts folgenden Verhaltensskizzen eingezeichnet ist

Soziale Folgen cerebraler Triebreizung. Untersuchungen von DELGADO bei Makakus-Affen [D 12] ergaben ebenfalls Wut und Aggression oder affektive Abwehr bei Reizung des zentralen Höhlengraus, ähnlich HUNSPERGERs Befunden bei der Katze. Durch moderne Methoden drahtloser intracerebraler Reizung konnte DELGADO [D 12, 13] bei Gruppen sozial organisierter Makaken Trieb- und Instinkthandlungen mit kollektiven Reaktionen auslösen (Abb. 8). Bei diesen Affen traten die *sozialen Auswirkungen mit Gruppenausbreitung künstlich erregter Aggressionen* deutlich hervor. Die durch den cerebralen Reiz ausgelösten Angriffshandlungen oder „antisozialen" Instinkte berücksichtigen *individuelle Beziehungen des gereizten Tieres in der Affengesellschaft:* Sie richten sich vorwiegend gegen solche Tiere, die auch ohne Reizung als „feindlich" gelten, aber nicht gegen „befreundete" Tiere der Affengruppe. Diese soziale Ausbreitung mit bevorzugter Angriffsrichtung auf bestimmte Gegner und Mitbeteiligung befreundeter Affen, die dem aggressiven Tier beistehen, ist in Abb. 8 auf S. 819 dargestellt. DELGADO fand, daß auch das Sexualverhalten durch Hirnreizung beeinflußt werden kann. Reizungen im dorsalen Thalamus weiblicher Affen ohne sichtbare Verhaltensänderung des gereizten Tieres induzierten dennoch ein verändertes Verhalten der männlichen, nicht-gereizten Käfiggenossen, für die das gereizte Weibchen plötzlich sexuell anziehend wurde.

Affen als Modelle des Affektverhaltens. Den unverhüllten Ausdruck von Affekten und Trieben zeigen viele Affen noch besser als Menschen. Besonders in Einzelfamilien lebende Menschenaffen wären noch geeigneter zum Studium des Affektverhaltens und seiner physiologischen Grundlagen als kollektiv lebende Makakus-Affen, Hunde oder Wölfe, die mehr soziale Triebregulationen, deren Hemmungsmechanismen und Rituale erkennen lassen. Leider gibt es nur wenige ethologische Affektstudien und fast keine neurophysiologischen Untersuchungen bei anthropoiden Affen. Das Verhalten solcher Affen, besonders der Schimpansen, ist offenbar mehr von Affekten und Trieben als von sozialen und erlernten Regeln beherrscht. Sie zeigen im motorischen Ausdruck und im vegetativen System massive Auswirkungen der Affekte, starke Affektmimik, deutliche Piloarrektion bei Wut, aktivierte Darmtätigkeit mit Entleerungen bei Angst usw. Dies ermöglicht dem Ethologen und Physiologen die Erkennung und Registrierung vegetativer und motorischer Begleiterscheinungen der Affekte und Triebe. Das Verhalten solcher Affen entspricht dem von extrem affektgeladenen und vegetativ labilen Menschen. Kurz, psychiatrisch gesprochen, verhalten sich die *Schimpansen ähnlich triebhaften, gefühlslabilen und reizbaren menschlichen Psychopathen.*

Bei guter Ausbildung von Hirnrinde und Lernfähigkeit wird das Verhalten aller Affen, die in Familien oder Herden leben, sowohl durch angeborene Affekte und Triebe gesteuert wie durch erworbene Bedürfnisse, Gruppeneinflüsse und Lernvorgänge verändert. Affen zeigen deutlich die Grenzen von Instinkt und Lernen (S. 1041) und sind damit auch für die Untersuchung der *Wechselwirkungen von erlerntem und affektivem Einzel- und Gruppenverhalten* geeignet (Abb. 8).

Die Triebentladungen bei Hunger, Sexualtrieb, Nachkommenschutz und Kampftrieb mit Angriff, Verteidigung, Kopulation oder Flucht führen bei Affen zu ähnlichen *sozialen Auswirkungen und Konflikten* wie beim Menschen. Bei verschiedenen Völkern der gleichen japanischen Affenart sind auch bestimmte ethnologische Unterschiede beobachtet worden, die mit kulturellen Volkssitten beim Menschen verglichen werden können. So ergibt sich die Möglichkeit, gruppenspezifische und soziale Triebkonflikte durch Verhaltensbeobachtungen und Tierexperimente mit Hirnreizungen zu untersuchen.

Hirnlokalisation von Affekten und Trieben

Nachdem schon die ersten Studien über großhirnlose Hunde [G 30] Erhaltenbleiben oder Steigerung des Affektverhaltens gezeigt hatten, war man geneigt, im Hirnstamm das Substrat der Affekte zu suchen. Die Beobachtungen BARDS [B 4–6] über enthemmte Wutreaktionen großhirnloser Tiere (*sham rage*) und die Entdeckung von HESS und BRÜGGER [H 67], daß durch Zwischenhirnreizung bei Katzen eine *affektive Abwehrreaktion* ausgelöst werden kann, die dem Wutverhalten normaler Katzen entspricht, ermöglichten hirnlokalisatorische Deutungen der Triebe und Affekte. Die durch Zwischenhirnreizung auslösbare Abwehrreaktion entspricht äußerlich dem natürlichen Aggressionsverhalten und ist offenbar eine echte, instinktiv vorgebildete Koordinationsleistung des ganzen Organismus.

Hirnstamm-Mechanismen. Sowohl nach tierexperimentellen Befunden wie nach klinischen Beobachtungen werden *Hypothalamus und Thalamus* als cerebrale Regulationsstellen von Affekten und Stimmungen angesehen. KLEIST [K 17] bezeichnete 1934 nach Erfahrungen bei Hirnverletzten das Zwischenhirn, speziell den Hypothalamus als „Zentrale der Affekt- und Trieberregbarkeit", die unter Kontrolle des Orbitalhirns steht. FOERSTER und GAGEL [F 19] beschrieben 1935 manische Symptome bei Operation eines suprasellären Tumors und mechanischer Reizung des Hypothalamus. Über intracerebrale elektrische Reizungen im Hypothalamus beim Menschen ist wenig bekannt, da es keine klinischen Indikationen für diese gibt.

Das von BERINGER [B 36] beschriebene periodische Alternieren von Antriebssteigerung mit manischen Symptomen und Antriebsminderung mit depressiver Verstimmung nach einer Encephalitis ist anatomisch nicht als Zwischenhirnerkrankung gesichert. Dasselbe gilt für die von AKERT und HESS [A 16] bei einem Hypophysentumor beschriebenen affektiven Verwirrtheits- und Erregungszustände mit Bewußtseinsstörungen. Die oft diskutierte Zwischenhirnbeteiligung bei temporaler Epilepsie ist noch unklar. Es ist nicht bekannt, ob bei den seltenen Dämmerattacken mit Aggressionshandlungen, die mi den Mandelkernreizungen HUNSPERGERS bei Katzen [F 5, 6] zu vergleichen wären, der Hypothalamus mehr beteiligt ist als bei anderen Dämmerattacken. Nach HUNSPERGERS Befunden könnte es sich auch um abnorme Entladungen im zentralen Höhlengrau des Mittelhirns handeln. Welche Hirnregionen bei deliranten Zuständen und symptomatischen Psychosen mit affektiver Erregung vorwiegend betroffen sind, ist beim Menschen noch nicht genügend neurophysiologisch untersucht. Ich hätte bedenken, die akutenexogenen Reaktionsformen BONHOEFFERS mit den ergotropen Effekten nach Hypothalamusreizung gleichzusetzen, wie dies AKERT und HESS [A 16] vorschlagen.

Das limbische System des Rhinencephalons. Alte hirnpathologische und neuroanatomische Erfahrungen sprachen für eine *Bedeutung des sog. Rhinencephalons,* *der phylogenetisch alten Cortexstrukturen des basalen Schläfenlappens für die Affektivität.* Cytoarchitektonische Befunde zeigten ihre ausgedehnte Entwicklung und Differenzierung beim Menschen. KLEIST [K 17] sah 1934 in diesem „Innenhirn" eine Repräsentation von Funktionen des Nahrungs- und Sexualtriebs und enteroceptiver Wahrnehmungen und Gefühle. PAPEZ [P 1] postulierte 1939 einen „*neuronal circuit for emotions*" zwischen Ammonshorn, Fornix, vorderem Thalamus und Cingulum, GRÜNTHAL [G 45] ein Aktivierungssystem im Ammonshorn. MACLEAN [M 9, 10] bezeichnet das Rhinencephalon mit seinen Verbindungen als *limbisches System,* das die Triebe reguliert.

Alle diese Postulate erhielten eine tierexperimentelle Grundlage, als KLÜVER und BUCY 1939 die schweren *Verhaltensstörungen bei Affen nach beidseitigen Temporallappenläsionen* beschrieben (orale Tendenzen mit Freß-Sucht, enthemmtes, wahl- und objektloses Sexualverhalten, agnostische und amnestische Störungen, verminderte Aggressivität bei relativ erhaltener „Intelligenz mit Werkzeuggebrauch") und durch Ausfall des Rhinencephalons erklärten [K 25]. Seitdem sind die Beziehungen des rhinencephalen oder limbischen Systems zu *psychisch-affektiven Störungen* und zum Sexualverhalten besonders beachtet worden.

Doch ist bisher nur ein typischer Fall von vollständigem Klüver-Bucy-Syndrom beim Menschen beschrieben worden (TERZIAN u.Mitarb. [T 1a]). Sexuelle Enthemmung nach Temporalläsionen ist beim Menschen sehr selten. Viel häufiger ist bei temporaler Epilepsie eine Verminderung des Sexualtriebs [G 10a].

Isolierte Allocortex- und Amygdalaläsionen zeigen geringere Störungen bei Affe und Mensch als große doppelseitige Temporallappenläsionen. ORBACH u.Mitarb. [O 10] fanden bei Testuntersuchungen nach isolierter Resektion des Allocortex mit dem Mandelkern weniger schwere Störungen des affektiven Verhaltens als KLÜVER und BUCY [K 24] bei ihren Affen mit vollständiger temporaler Lobektomie, aber konstantere kognitive Störungen.

Von AKERT u.Mitarb. [A 15] wurde neuerdings festgestellt, daß das Klüver-Bucy-Syndrom auch ohne Schädigung des Rhinencephalons durch Läsionen des *neocorticalen* Assoziationscortex im Schläfenlappen hervorgerufen werden kann. Allerdings waren in einem Teil ihrer Affen auch Mandelkernläsionen vorhanden. Vor allem waren die afferenten Fasern zum Amygdalum und der pyriformen Rinde zum Cingulum und Uncinatus-System geschädigt.

Zwischenhirn und Riechhirn als koordinierte Substrate emotionaler Vorgänge. Nachdem zunächst das Zwischenhirn mit Thalamus und Hypothalamus als Substrat affektiver Mechanismen angesehen wurde, ist seit KLÜBERS und BUCYS Untersuchungen [K 25] und PAPEZs Hypothesen [P 1] die Hirnlokalisation affektiver Funktionen vorwiegend am Rhinencephalon oder limbischen System untersucht und diskutiert worden. Erst FERNANDEZ MOLINA und HUNSPERGER haben die anatomisch wahrscheinliche Zusammenarbeit von Temporalhirn und Zwischenhirn auch physiologisch geklärt [F 5, 6]. Bestimmte Kerngebiete des Amygdalums beeinflussen die affektiven Abwehrreaktionen mit Wut- und Fluchtverhalten, die nach Reizen im caudalen Hypothalamus entstehen.

Die Untersuchungen über die im limbischen System lokalisierten Affekt- und Instinkthandlungen werden in PLOOGS Beitrag ausführlich dargestellt. Die von MACLEAN postulierten beiden Funktionskreise *Septum, Ammonshorn und Cingulum* (septum circle) werden für das *Sexualverhalten* und für affektive und instinktive Grundlagen der Arterhaltung in Anspruch genommen, die Neuronenkreise von *Mandelkern und frontotemporalem Cortex* (amygdaloid circle) für das *Nahrungs- und Kampfverhalten* als Grundlagen der Selbsterhaltung des Individuums [M 10, 12, 14].

Subcorticale Reizversuche beim Menschen mit Aktivierung von Affekt- und Triebmechanismen [B 60] sind neuerdings bei stereotaktischen Operationen durchgeführt worden [H 17] und in der ersten Auflage dieses Werkes von HASSLER besprochen. Solche stereotaktischen Stammhirnreizungen im menschlichen Zwischenhirn sind aus verständlichen Gründen noch nicht systematisch genug, um sie für eine hirnlokalisatorische Erklärung der Affekte verwenden zu können.

Allgemeine Triebphysiologie

Ordnung der Triebe. Eine allgemeine terminologische Ordnung der Triebeinteilung ist für den Physiologen deshalb von Interesse, weil er danach seine Untersuchungen klarer auf einzelne Triebmechanismen einengen kann. Nahrungstrieb und Sexualtrieb sind als spezifisch allgemein anerkannt. Eindeutige Bestimmungen ergeben sich zunächst aus dem *Verhalten*, dann aus den konkreten *Triebzielen* und der *Triebbefriedigung*, doch erscheinen theoretisch abstrakte Zielrichtungen als zweifelhafte anthropomorphe Konstruktionen für den sog. „Selbsterhaltungstrieb" oder einen „Arterhaltungstrieb". Sicher gibt es Hunger, Durst, Reinigungstrieb, die alle der Selbsterhaltung dienen, doch kann man daraus keinen gemeinsamen Trieb der Erhaltung des Individuums machen. Sicher gibt es einen Geschlechtstrieb, aber ob es einen Trieb zur Arterhaltung gibt, zu dem auch die der Selbsterhaltung dienenden Triebwirkungen beitragen müßten, erscheint sehr zweifelhaft. Noch unwahrscheinlicher erscheint dem Biologen der „Todestrieb" der Psychoanalyse.

Neben den *Nahrungs- und Sexualtrieben* werden andere triebhafte Instinkte oft vernachlässigt, obwohl auch sie von größter biologischer Bedeutung sind. 4 weitere Gruppen von angeborenen Verhaltensweisen kann man grob vereinfachend als Triebe bezeichnen und mit menschlichen Strebungen und Bedürfnissen vergleichen: *Aggressionstrieb, Fluchttrieb, Putztrieb* und *Sammeltrieb* sind im Tierreich allgemein verbreitet und auch beim Menschen mit ihren psychologischen und psychiatrischen Auswirkungen zu studieren. Offenbar besteht auch ein instinktiver Trieb zur Besetzung und Verteidigung des heimatlichen Territoriums. Obwohl die Bezeichnung *Territorialinstinkt* nicht allgemein verwendet wird, ist dieser Trieb doch bei allen höheren Tieren sehr ausgeprägt. Er bestimmt nach Besetzung eines eigenen „Reviers", das als Umwelt weit über Nest oder Höhle hinausreicht, auch das Sexualverhalten und die Familiengründung mit einem gemeinsamen Territorium. Eindringen anderer Artgenossen in das Territorium führt zu seiner Verteidigung durch heftige Gegenangriffe. Es handelt sich offenbar um einen allgemein verbreiteten *Heimattrieb*, der vielleicht biologische Grundlage des Heimatgefühls und der Vaterlandsliebe beim Menschen ist.

Beim *Aggressionstrieb* sind weniger die Jagd- und Angriffshandlungen der Raubtiere von psychologisch-psychiatrischem Interesse als vielmehr die *Aggressionen innerhalb derselben Species*, die bei allen sozialen Tieren vorkommen, bei denen persönliche Bindungen, sei es für die Gruppe oder das Paar, stark entwickelt sind. LORENZ hat diese „intraspezifische Aggression" in ihrer biologischen Bedeutung für die Ausbreitung der Arten und ihre allgemeinen Konsequenzen dargestellt [L 42] (vgl. S. 947).

Der *Fluchttrieb,* dessen psychologisch-introspektive Seite die *Angst* ist, wirkt für alle frei lebenden Tiere, nicht nur die Gejagten, sondern auch die Jagenden, lebensrettend und arterhaltend. Beim Menschen zeigt er sich in den verschiedenen Formen unbegründeter oder ungenügend motivierter Angst. Mitigierte Formen dieser Angst mit Fluchttendenz sind wahrscheinlich auch die menschliche Schüchternheit bis zum „Lampenfieber" der Schauspieler.

Der *Putztrieb* zur systematischen *Körperpflege* ist vor allem bei den Säugern und Vögeln für die Erhaltung ihres Haar- oder Federkleides lebenswichtig. Beim Menschen in zivilisierten Verhältnissen hat der Putztrieb durch Kleidung, Wohnung und Hygiene seine biologische Bedeutung verloren. Er zeigt sich noch im Übersprung als Verlegenheitshandlung (Kopfkratzen, Hautreiben) oder in sozial verwandeltem Luxurieren, vor allem bei Frauen. Diese nicht-vitalen Auswirkungen des Putztriebes sind bestenfalls indirekt durch Beeinflussung der Sexualwahl von arterhaltender Bedeutung. Um so größer ist die *Luxusentwicklung des Putztriebes* in der menschlichen Kultur, in der er durch Mode und Kunst schöne, aber auch seltsame oder groteske Blüten treibt. Eine ebenfalls sozial stark verwandelte Triebentwicklung zeigt der *Sammeltrieb* mit seinen verschiedenen Objekt- und Kulturformen und seinem Luxurieren bei Briefmarken- und Kunstsammlern.

Übersprung von Trieben und Instinkten. In bestimmten Umweltsituationen kann ein bedrohter Vogel statt anzugreifen oder zu flüchten, wie es der Situation angemessen wäre, sich im „Übersprung" putzen oder Nestbaubewegungen machen oder sogar in Schlafstellung gehen. Dieses Ausweichen von einer „intendierten" in eine andere Verhaltensweise ist ein sehr verbreitetes Phänomen. Wenn bei häufiger Verhinderung einer Instinkthandlung eine andere als Übersprung regelmäßig auftritt, so kann diese *zunächst sinnlose Bewegung sekundär* für den Partner oder die Gemeinschaft eine gewisse *Bedeutung erhalten.* Sobald die Artgenossen auf solche Übersprungsbewegungen reagieren und diese Reaktion arterhaltend wirkt, kann auf dem Wege der Selektion ein sinnvoller Zusammenhang zwischen Übersprunghandlungen und sozialen Beziehungen der Individuen untereinander entstehen. Wenn sich die Übersprunghandlung mit dieser sozialen Auslöserfunktion verändert, so wird dies von der Verhaltensforschung *Ritualisierung* genannt (S. 802).

Auch im menschlichen Verhalten sind solche Übersprungsbewegungen in Form der *Verlegenheitsbewegungen* häufig. Ferner könnten manche Ausdrucksbewegungen, deren Zweck zunächst nicht ohne weiteres einsichtig ist, auf dem Wege der Ritualisierung entstanden sein, etwa das Lachen oder Weinen oder auch das Gähnen, das die Ermüdung der Umgebung anzeigt und dann „ansteckend" wirkt. Noch größere Bedeutung hat der Übersprung wahrscheinlich für abnorme Reaktionen bei der Entstehung von „Neurosen", psychogenen Tics und anderen hysterischen Mechanismen, vielleicht auch für manche psychotischen Verhaltensweisen mit scheinbar sinnlosen Handlungen oder Wahngedanken (vgl. S. 813).

Arteigene Aggression und Aggressionshemmung bei Tier und Mensch. In seinem 1963 erschienenen Buch [L 42] behandelt LORENZ ausführlich verschiedene Verhaltensformen des Angriffstriebes innerhalb der Arten und mögliche Anwendungen auf menschliche Verhältnisse. Er erinnert daran, daß DARWINS „struggle for life" weniger zwischen unterschiedlichen Tierarten, als *innerhalb derselben Art* zum Überleben des Tüchtigsten führte. Die *„intrapezifische Aggression"* gegen den Artgenossen ist ein biologisch zweckmäßiger Vorgang zur Ausbreitung der Arten mit gleichmäßiger Verteilung der Reviere. Angriffstrieb und Kampf dienen nicht nur wie bei DARWIN zur Herauszüchtung der Stärkeren oder bei Herdentieren zur Selektion der sozial Nützlicheren und der angriffslustigen Herdenverteidiger. Die arteigene Aggression ist am „mächtigsten" bei den in kleinen Familien oder einzeln lebenden Tieren. Bei diesen ist sie auch mit stärkeren individuellen Bindungen und mit Treueverhalten zu bestimmten Artgenossen korreliert, die bei Herdentieren mit geringerer Aggression oft fehlen. Ob dies mehr als Koinzidenzen sind und bestimmte kausale Beziehungen zwischen Aggression und emotionaler Bindung bestehen, wie LORENZ annimmt, mag offen bleiben. Für menschliche Aggressionen ist bekannt, daß die abgeschwächten verbalen Formen im engeren Familienkreis und bei Frauen wenig durch persönliche Bindungen gehemmt werden.

Beim Menschen postuliert LORENZ [L 42] zur Erklärung der kollektiven Angriffstriebe spezifische Selektionsprozesse während der Frühsteinzeit mit starker Aggression der Urmenschen durch Kriege von kleinen Sippengenossenschaften. Kollektive Aggression kann auch in milderer Form, wie beim „Hassen" der Vögel zum biologisch wichtigen Kennenlernen von Feindgestalten führen und damit Lernvorgänge bahnen. Das „Böse" der Aggressionstriebe kann auch „gute" biologische Wirkungen haben.

Gegenseitige Hemmungen der verschiedenen Triebe mildern die negativen Folgen der intraspezifischen Aggression oder verwandeln sie in positive Werte. Der Einfluß von Lernvorgängen zeigt sich auch im Laufe der Stammesentwicklung durch Ausbildung von ritualisierten Verhaltensformen. Mit der als *Ritualisierung* bezeichneten Ausdruckswirkung von Instinktbewegungen auf Artgenossen [H 98] entsteht vor allem soziale Hemmung. Wie ungewohnte Handlungen oder Beobachtungen bei manchen Menschen Angst und Gehemmtsein erzeugen, so können auch bei Tieren affektiv veränderte Instinkthandlungen und ihre Wahrnehmung mit *Hemmungsmechanismen* verbunden sein. Die Demutstellung des im Kampf mit Artgleichen unterlegenen Tieres, die bei Wölfen und Hunden besonders ausgebildet ist, bewirkt mächtige affektive Hemmungen gegen tödliche Aggressionshandlungen. Solche *Triebhemmungen bei Tieren* sind vor allem von psychiatrischem Interesse. LORENZ bringt in seinem Buch [L 42] zahlreiche Beispiele mit Parallelen zum menschlichen Verhalten. Die Triebhemmungen wurden bisher von der Ethologie genauer erforscht als von der Physiologie.

Die Auslösung der ethologisch studierten Aggressionshemmungen geschieht nach LORENZ [L 42] vorwiegend über das Sehen, z.B. bei der Demutshaltung und dem Kindchenschema [L 38] – oder über den Geruch, z.B. bei weiblichen Artgenossen. Charakteristische Körperhaltungen des Gegners oder bestimmte Körperformen der Jungtiere oder spezifische Gerüche bewirken als sensorische Auslöser diese Angriffshemmungen mit angeborener Grundlage.

Noch weniger wissen wir über die Neurophysiologie *erworbener Hemmungen*. Hier findet sich eine komplexe Verflechtung erinnerter Bilder und angeborener Mechanismen. Diese im einzelnen unbekannte Wechselwirkung von Instinkt- und Gedächtnisvorgängen mit der Ritualisierung hat wahrscheinlich im Laufe der Stammesentwicklung zu neuen Instinkten und Trieben geführt. Durch Ritualisierung neu entstandene Instinktbewegungen können auch *Kopien anderer Triebhandlungen* sein. Sie erinnern an gewisse *Symbolbildungen* in der menschlichen Kultur, wie LORENZ ausführlich dargestellt hat [L 38, 42].

Ausdruck und soziale Mitteilung von Affekten und Trieben

Affektausdruck. Bei Tieren und Menschen sind Affekte und Triebe durch ihre körperlichen und mimischen Begleiterscheinungen schon äußerlich erkennbar. Diese Ausdrucksfunktion vermittelt ihre soziale Bedeutung in der Gemeinschaft. *Emotionale Ausdrucksvorgänge sind die „Sprachen" der Gefühle und Triebe.* Schon BELL [B 20] hat 1806/44 gesagt: "Expression is to passion what language is to thought." Die Bedeutung des Affektausdrucks bei Tier und Mensch wurde schon in Kapitel IV dargestellt (S. 808).

Körperliche Begleiterscheinungen emotionaler Vorgänge wurden durch die klassische Psychophysiologie untersucht. Nach DARWINS Ausdrucksstudien [D 2] und MOSSOS Registrierungen von Atmung und Plethysmogramm bei Affekt-Vorgängen [M 68] wurden vor allem die galvanischen Hautreflexe, das Pupillenspiel und die Haut- und Hirntemperatur aufgezeichnet. Weder für die menschliche Psychologie oder die tierische Verhaltensforschung noch für die klinische Psychiatrie haben diese Untersuchungen vegetativer Begleiterscheinungen große Bedeutung erlangt. Nachdem sich herausstellte, daß die sog. vasomotorische „Volumstarre" im Plethysmogramm der Katatonen eine sekundäre, wärmeregulatorische Folge ihrer Immobilität war, die nach Erwärmen verschwand [J 54] und die Pupillenstörung der Katatonie keine diagnostische Bedeutung hatte, war das psychiatrische Interesse an diesen Methoden stark zurückgegangen. Übersichten finden sich in BERGERS älteren Büchern [B 21–23] und seinem Handbuchbeitrag 1937 [B 28]. HESS' Pupillenbefunde [H 43] sind auf S. 930 beschrieben.

Nachdem wir 1939 eine Apparatur zur gleichzeitigen Registrierung des EEG mit vegetativen und animalen Funktionen des ZNS angegeben [J 25] und für die Begleiterscheinungen des kleinen epileptischen Anfalls verwendet haben [J 26], sind solche polygraphischen Registrierungen in den letzten Jahren wieder häufiger zu psychophysiologischen Untersuchungen verwendet worden [F 2]. Doch brachten diese Methoden bisher für die Psychiatrie wenig brauchbare Ergebnisse. Ich verzichte daher auf einen genaueren Bericht und verweise auf die regelmäßig erscheinenden Newsletters der amerikanischen Psychophysiologie-Gesellschaft und FAHRENBERGS Beitrag [F 2].

Der zuverlässigste Indicator für Affekte und Triebe bleibt die *Körpermotorik* und damit die Verhaltensbeobachtung und ihre Registrierung im Film.

Cerebrale Reizversuche zeigen ebenso wie natürliche Kämpfe der Tiere plötzliche Übergänge zwischen *Abwehr, Aggression und Flucht*. Solche Wechselwirkungen zwischen Angreifen und Fliehen entsprechen in psychologischer Terminologie den Beziehungen von *Wut* und *Angst*, die auch durch Umweltsituationen verändert werden. Bei ausweglosen Situation, wenn ein Tier in einer Raumecke nicht entkommen kann, entsteht auch aus der Angst HEDIGERS ,,Kritische Reaktion" [H 22a]: die Umwandlung von der ,,ängstlichen" Flucht zum Angriff mit dem ,,Mut der Verzweiflung". In der *Mimik* der Tiere und ihrer *Bereitschaftshaltung* sind diese verschiedenen ,,Stimmungen" des Kampfes oft schon früher ausgedrückt als in dem folgenden Endverhalten. Dies zeigen mimische Ausdrucksbilder am Hundekopf von LORENZ [L 42] besonders deutlich (Abb. 28). Sie erlauben eine Voraussage des kommenden *Angriffs bei reiner Wut* (g) oder der folgenden *Flucht bei Angst* (c). Bei Mischungen beider (i) erfolgt Angriff oder Flucht jeweils etwa gleich häufig [L 40]. Der Affektausdruck macht so bei Tier und Mensch gewisse Motivationen vor den eigentlichen Triebhand-

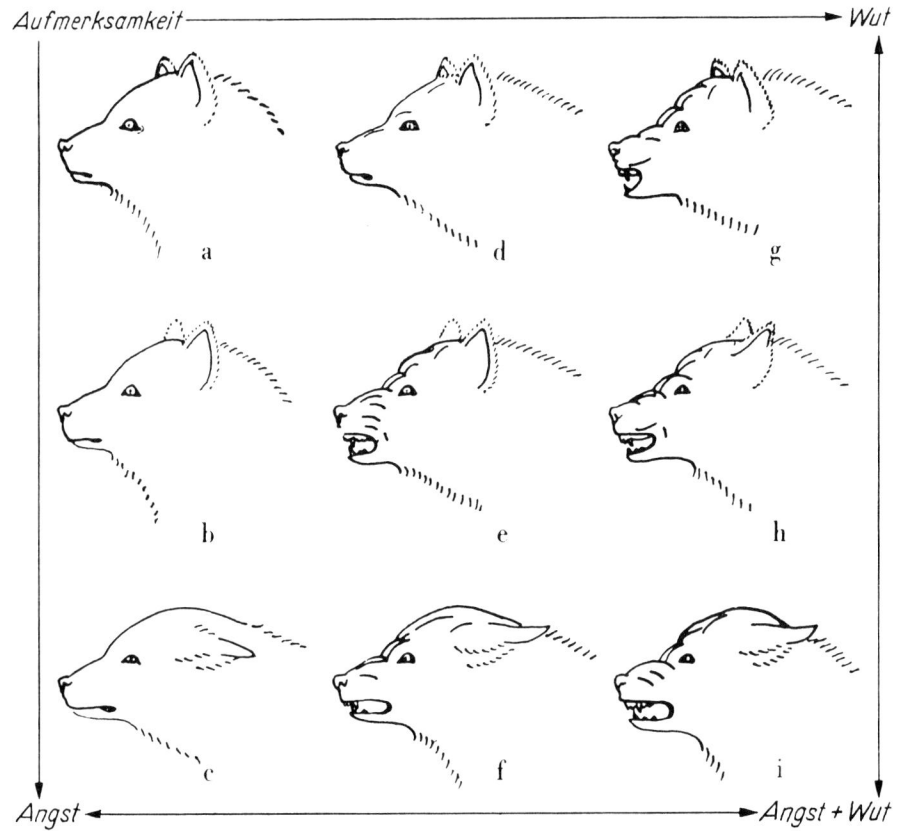

Abb. 28a–i. Affekt-Ausdruck von Angst und Wut mit ihrer Mischung beim Hund. Nach LORENZ (1953) [L 40] mit ergänzter Beschriftung. Vom Ausdruck aufmerksamer Beobachtung links oben (*a*) wächst nach rechts der Wutaffekt (*g*), nach unten die Angst (*c*). Rechts unten Mischung von Angst und Wut (*i*). Im *Verhalten* des Tieres führt die Wut zur Aggression, die Angst zur Flucht. Bei *Mischung* beider Affekte wird das Verhalten je nach der Umweltsituation zur Flucht *oder* zum Angriff gesteuert. Nach dem mimischen Ausdruck kann man mit Wahrscheinlichkeit das folgende Verhalten des Tieres voraussagen

lungen erkennbar. Diese Ausdruckswahrnehmung ist für das Verhalten und Überleben der Tiere von großer biologischer Wichtigkeit.

Von KRETSCHMER [K 49] wurde im Anschluß an die Instinktforschung der Begriff „motorische Schablone" geprägt und für psychomotorische Störungen bei Psychosen verwendet. Damit sollte eine Korrelation zwischen tierischen Instinkten und menschlichen Verhaltensschablonen ermöglicht werden, deren phylogenetische, ontogenetische und hirnphysiologische Zusammenhänge noch zu erforschen sind. Die psychiatrische Anwendung dieser Korrelationen hat allerdings gewisse Grenzen. *Hinter derselben motorischen Schablone können verschiedene psychische Inhalte und Motivationen stehen*, die erst psychopathologisch zu untersuchen sind. Ferner können motorische Schablonen als negative oder positive Symptome erscheinen. Es ist sowohl möglich, daß normale Automatismen bei neuropsychiatrischen Störungen ausfallen, wie daß onto- und phylogenetisch ältere Hirnstamm-Mechanismen bei cerebralen Abbauvorgängen wieder zum Vorschein kommen, wie Saugreflexe, Greifreflexe, Kopfbewegungen, wie beim Brustsuchen der Säuglinge [B 44a, P 35]. Umgekehrt verläuft die Entwicklung in der Ontogenese, z.B. beim Schreckverhalten des Säuglings gehen generalisierte Zuckungen in lokalisierte Reaktionen des Gesichts über [W 25, 26]. Das Zusammenschrecken wird beim Erwachsenen dann wieder durch Hirnerkrankungen enthemmt [S 55].

Quantifizierung von Triebvorgängen. Quantitative Untersuchungen des Triebverhaltens sind von LORENZ [L 39] mit seinem hydrodynamischen Modell postuliert und durch v. HOLST an labyrinthoperierten Fischen durchgeführt worden [H 78]. v. HOLSTs „Messung von Stimmungen" ist aber von diesem Sonderfall noch nicht auf höhere Arten anwendbar. Die schwierige Messung von Affekten, Trieben und Motivationen erschwert die objektive Untersuchung neurophysiologischer Korrelate. Die vegetativen Begleiterscheinungen mit ihrer wechselnden Irradiation und großen individuellen Variabilität erlauben keine gute Quantifizierung. Das Ausdrucksverhalten ist nur begrenzt zählbar und meßbar. Die Verhaltensforscher verwendeten zunächst *Auszählungen wiederholter Affekt- und Triebhandlungen* als Maß der Triebstärke. Die elektrische Reizung, mit der HESS und v. HOLST [H 63, 83] Triebhandlungen im Gehirn auslösten, ist zwar exakt zu dosieren und zu messen, ergibt aber mit intracerebralen Elektroden lokalisatorisch sehr verschiedene Resultate. Es bleibt ein Unsicherheitsfaktor, welche von den multiplen und komplexen Hirnstrukturen jeweils gereizt wurde. Bei fehlender anatomischer Kontrolle ist eine quantitative Korrelation zwischen Hirnreizung und Verhalten (v. HOLST, Abb. 26) begrenzt. Eine einfache Methodik zur *Messung des Hungertriebs* hat FREEMAN 1959 angegeben [F 24]: Er registriert mechanisch die Intensität, mit der eine hungrige Katze dem Futter zustrebt, über eine Haltevorrichtung, die am Thorax angebracht wird. Diese mechanische Meßmethode wurde für die Korrelation von Verhalten und hirnelektrischen Veränderungen verwendet [F 25, 26].

Neurophysiologische Grundlagen des Antriebs. Nach den Konzeptionen von MAGOUN [M 19], BREMER [B 64] und zahlreichen anderen Forschern [J 8, L 27], die sich mit der Physiologie des reticulären Systems beschäftigt haben, wird das *„aufsteigende Aktivierungssystem" der Formatio reticularis im Hirnstamm nicht nur für die Wachheit, sondern auch für den Antrieb des Cortex in Anspruch* *genommen* (recticular activating system s.S. 977). Die Untersuchungen der letzten Jahre haben allerdings gezeigt, daß diese Konzeption einer reticulären Antriebsaktivierung des Cortex zu einfach ist. Nach DELL u.Mitarb. [D 17, H 89] besteht eine *reziproke Hemmungsfunktion zwischen Reticularis und Cortex*, und neuropharmakologische Studien über synaptische Transmitter zeigten verschiedene aufsteigende Systeme, die für Schlafregulation und emotionale Steuerung bedeutsam sind (vgl. S. 980 und Abb. 35).

Antrieb und positive Rückkoppelung im Triebleben. Die meisten Regulationen des Nervensystems wirken homeostatisch, haben also entsprechend den kybernetischen Vorstellungen eine *negative* Rückkoppelung und damit eine Tendenz zum *Ausgleich*. Doch haben gerade die Triebe einen umgekehrten *Aktivierungseffekt*, der das System nicht zur Ruhe kommen läßt, also eine *positive* Rückkoppelung. *Die Triebe bilden daher wichtige Elemente der allgemeinen Antriebsfunktion.* Es ist allerdings noch nicht klar, ob „Antrieb" eine eigene physiologische Funktion ist, die sich selbst unterhält und nur von den Trieben und den wachheitsregulierenden Hirnsystemen angeregt wird, oder ob allein das Zusammenwirken der Triebe im Wachzustand bereits als Antriebskraft genügt und die sog. psychische Energie darstellt.

Die zoologische Verhaltensforschung hat weniger den allgemeinen Antrieb studiert als spezielle Instinktmechanismen, welche antriebsfördernd wirken. Im ethologischen Aspekt könnte man den Antrieb sogar als *Summe der verschiedenen Instinkte oder Triebe* bezeichnen, die nach LORENZ einen eigenen automatischen Ablauf haben, der auch ohne äußere Schlüsselreize im „Leerlauf" zur Instinktaktivierung führt (s.S. 801). Zu den speziellen Trieben kommt noch das *Wachsein* als antriebsfördernde Funktion, oder, wenn man so will, als allgemeine Vorbedingung des Antriebs hinzu. Nur im Wachzustand können Triebe und Gefühle zu wohlgeordneten Leistungen des Denkens und Handelns führen. Im Schlaf erzeugen sie lediglich bruchstückhafte Erlebnisse als Träume, in denen Affekte und Triebe ein unkoordiniertes, der realen Welt nicht adäquates Eigenleben führen. Für eine partielle Beteiligung des den Wachzustand regulierenden „reticular activating system" im Traum spricht das ähnliche flache EEG bei Traum und Aufmerksamkeit (s.S. 970 u. 1010).

Triebstruktur und Konstitution

KRETSCHMER [K 48] und andere Konstitutionsforscher haben ausführlich die eindrucksvollsten Korrelationen zwischen Körperbau und Temperament beschrieben. Körperbau, Temperament und *Triebstruktur* werden meist als parallele Entsprechungen angesehen, oder es wird dem Körperbau die primäre Rolle zugewiesen. Zu wenig bekannt ist aber, daß *primäre Eigenarten des Affekt- und Trieblebens* auch *sekundäre körperliche Veränderungen verursachen können*.

Triebdominanzen und Konstitutionen. Bei den Korrelationen, welche die Konstitutionsforschung zwischen psychischen Eigenschaften und Körperbau gefunden hat, wird die Triebkomponente zu wenig beachtet. Doch zeigt schon die tägliche Erfahrung, daß *Trieb und Triebbeherrschung* sich auch somatisch auswirken können. *Bestimmte Triebdominanzen haben selbst einen formenden Einfluß auf die Körperkonstitution.* Dominierende Triebe und Bedürfnisse als „psychische" Eigenschaften cerebraler Genese fördern eine somatische Veränderung in der gleichen Konstitutionsrichtung, sind also kausal wirksam, vielleicht in Form eines Circulus vitiosus.

Der vermehrte *Nahrungstrieb des Pyknikers* führt zu größerer Eßlust und fördert damit den Fettansatz, der erst im Erwachsenenalter erworben wird. Der vermehrte *Bewegungstrieb des Athletikers* zusammen mit seiner Perseverationsneigung begünstigt oft wiederholte sportliche Übung und damit die Hypertrophie seiner Muskulatur. Die geringere Ausbildung und bessere Kontrolle dieser beiden Triebe erklärt die *motorische Sparsamkeit und den verminderten Essensgenuß des Asthenikers* und damit auch seine schwache Ausbildung von Muskulatur und Fettansatz. Wer kennt nicht den pyknischen Gourmand, der uns bei der gemeinsamen Mahlzeit eben versichert, daß er äußerst knappe Diät halte und doch mit sichtlichem Genuß die fette Sauce über seinen Teller ausbreitet. Während er mit größtem Behagen diese calorienreiche Speise verzehrt, sieht man den daneben sitzenden Astheniker mit deutlich geringerem Appetit in dem gleichen Essen mit der Gabel stochern. Wer solche Beobachtungen macht, wird auch ohne statistische Untersuchungen über Calorienverbrauch und Körperbewegung überzeugt sein, daß der *Appetit als Symptom des Nahrungstriebes, das Muskeltraining als Folge des Bewegungstriebes und das Bedürfnis, beide Triebe zu reduzieren, den Körperbau der drei Konstitutionstypen beeinflußt.*

Der Pykniker ißt gern. Wenn er uns dennoch immer wieder versichert, er esse wenig, so gilt diese Einschränkung vielleicht für die Quantität, aber nicht für die Qualität der Nahrung und den Caloriengehalt hochwertiger Nährstoffe. Obwohl eine solche, in kultivierter gastronomischer Form sich äußernde Freude am Essen von der Freßsucht bei organischen Hirnerkrankungen deutlich verschieden ist, wird man doch neurophysiologische Grundlagen in den zentralen Repräsentationen des Triebverhaltens annehmen dürfen. Es ist auch möglich, daß diese Funktionsgrundlagen einer erfahrungsgesteuerten psychologischen Modifizierung zugänglich sind. Dennoch setzt sich die konstitutionsbestimmte Triebstruktur oft mit überraschender Penetranz durch.

Triebregulation und Verhalten. Die Dominanz bestimmter Triebe bei verschiedenen Konstitutionen ist schon in *Ausdruck* und *Haltung* erkennbar. Dies zeigen besonders deutlich typische Bilder von SHELDON (Abb. 29) mit ihren Meßwerten der Konstitutionsanteile [S 30].

Sekundäre physiologische Regulationen finden sich bei anderen konstitutionellen Eigentümlichkeiten des Verhaltens, die nur z.T. triebbedingt oder psychologischen Ursprungs sind. Im wesentlichen sind es echte *somatisch-physiologische Regulationsbedürfnisse,* wie die Neigung des rasch überhitzten Pyknikers und des körperlich aktiven Athletikers zur Entblößung und die Tendenz des Leptosomen zur geschlossenen, warmen Kleidung, die den physiologischen *Bedürfnissen der Wärmeregulation* parallel gehen. Im sozial-psychologischen Aspekt werden sie oft anders gedeutet, und es wird dem Verhalten ein Ausdruckscharakter unterlegt. Triebbedingt ist wahrscheinlich auch das größere *Schlafbedürfnis* mancher Athletiker, vielleicht auch Folge ihrer größeren motorischen Aktivität. SHELDON [S 30, 31] sieht in diesen und anderen extremen Verhaltenskriterien der Konstitutionstypen charakteristische Eigenschaften: Die geringe Neigung des Leptosomen zum Leben im Freien und sein Rückzug auf das geschlossene

a (Typ 117) b (Typ 136)

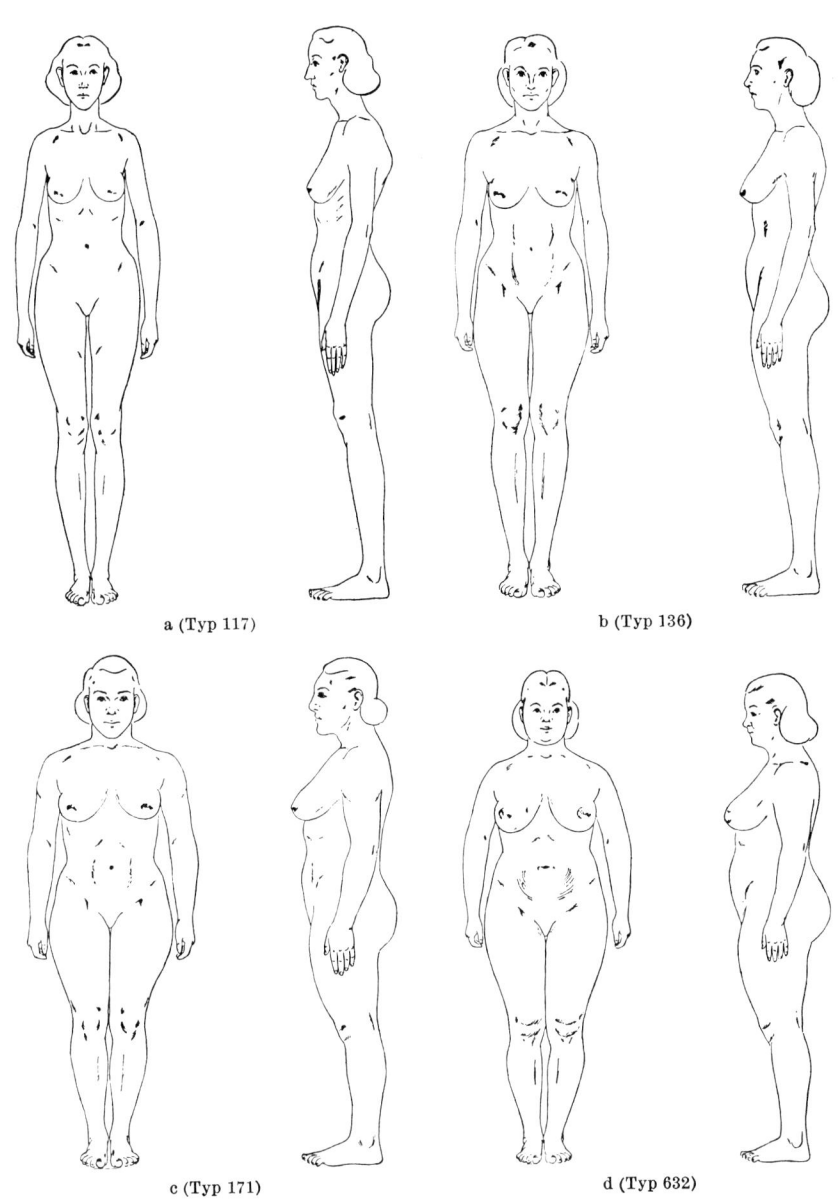

c (Typ 171) d (Typ 632)

Abb. 29a–d. Weibliche Konstitutionstypen mit verschiedener Triebdominanz in Ausdruck und Körperhaltung. Nach SHELDON (1940) [S 30]. Die Zahlen von 1–7 bezeichnen den Grad der drei Komponenten: *1. Zahl endomorph* (~pyknisch), *2. Zahl mesomorph* (~athletisch), *3. Zahl ektomorph* (~asthenisch). *a* Rein *asthenisch-ektomorpher Typ* (117) mit vermindertem Bewegungs- und Nahrungstrieb; entspannte Haltung und geringe Ausprägung von Kiefern, Leib und Muskulatur. Magerkeit als Folge verminderter Eßlust. *b* Vorwiegend *ektomorpher Typ mit mesomorpher* Komponente (136) zeigt etwas straffere Haltung und Muskelaktivität. *c* Rein *mesomorph-athletischer Typ* (171) mit straffer Haltung und aktiver Muskelspannung in Bereitschaft zu motorischen Aktionen als Ausdruck des Bewegungstriebes. *d* Vorwiegend *endomorph-pyknischer Typ* (632) mit ruhigerer Haltung, weichen Konturen und stärkerer Leibentwicklung als Ausdruck und Folge vermehrten Nahrungstriebes

Zimmer oder die umgekehrte „claustrophobe" Abneigung des athletischen „Somatotonen" gegen den geschlossenen Raum sind häufige, aber nicht gesetzmäßige Korrelationen. Vielleicht sind es auch mehr oder weniger zweckmäßige Regulationen von Triebdominanzen.

Manche *überschießenden Regulationen* im Gebiet der Affekte und vegetativen Funktionen bei den verschiedenen Konstitutionstypen sind vielleicht ursprünglich zweckmäßig. Die verstärkte affektive Anregung der Magen-Darm-Funktionen und die affektive Empfindlichkeit des Pyknikers wirkt offenbar seinen häufigen Obstipationen entgegen. Die vermehrte Blutdrucksenkung nach Schmerz und Angst bei Athletikern kompensiert die vermehrte Kreislaufbelastung seiner verstärkten Motorik, führt allerdings auch nicht selten zum Kollaps. Die raschere Verarbeitung von Außensituationen beim Leptosomen kompensiert seine emotionale Indifferenz. Das Abwechslungsbedürfnis des Leptosomen kann teils Vorbedingung für seine intellektuelle Aktivität, teils Kompensation seiner geringen affektiven Ansprechbarkeit sein. Die späte oder fehlende psychische Sättigung des Athletikers und Epileptoiden verhindert raschen Wechsel der Umwelteinstellung und echten „esprit". Emotionale Perseveration und längerdauernde affekt- und triebbedingte Verstimmungen ohne Willenssteuerung und ohne äußeren Anlaß sind bei athletischen und pyknischen Konstitutionen häufiger. Solche komplexen Wechselwirkungen konstitutioneller, affektiver und intellektueller Funktionen bleiben in ihren cerebralen Mechanismen noch ungeklärt.

Vom neurophysiologischen Standpunkt aus kann man zunächst nur vermuten, daß in der Triebstruktur ein gemeinsames Bindeglied zwischen körperlichen und psychischen Eigenschaften der Konstitutionstypen liegt.

Einzelne psychische Eigenschaften und Verhaltenskriterien bestimmter Konstitutionstypen haben wahrscheinlich auch neurophysiologische Korrelate. Der Trieb zu oft wiederholter Körperbewegung bei geringer Variation des Denkens und das unelastische Verhalten vieler Athletiker, das bis zur Perseveration reicht, könnte durch ähnliche verlangsamte und sich selbst unterhaltende cerebrale Vorgänge bedingt sein wie sie in stärkerer und pathologischer Ausprägung bei gewissen Epilepsien, endokrinen und Hirnerkrankungen auch im EEG erkennbar sind. Bei solchen „enechetischen" Athletikern findet man häufiger einen langsamen α-Rhythmus oder konstitutionelle „Dysrhythmie". Die umgekehrte Eigenart mancher Asthenikern und Pykniker mit raschem Wechsel des Denkablaufs, früher psychischer Sättigung und Abwechslungsbedürfnis, das bei gewissen Asthenikern bis zur Sprunghaftigkeit geht, könnte mit rascheren cerebralen Erregungsvorgängen einhergehen. Doch sind höher frequente EEG-Wellen zwar bei Hyperthyreosen oder Intoxikationen, aber nicht bei diesen Konstitutionstypen zu finden. Offenbar ist das EEG kein geeigneter Indikator für diese Funktionen. Da „reine" Konstitutionstypen Ausnahmen sind und wenig charakteristische Mischtypen in allen Populationen überwiegen, sind exakte Untersuchungen schwer durchführbar. Die Neurophysiologie kann daher zur Konstitutionsforschung noch nicht viel beitragen. Über die ersten Eindrücke LEMERES [L 12], daß Pykniker häufiger große α-Wellen und Astheniker mehr flache EEGs haben, sind spätere Untersucher nicht wesentlich hinausgekommen.

Selbstreizung des Gehirns im Tierversuch

Die von OLDS und MILNER 1954 eingeführte Methode der „self stimulation" bei Tieren [O 8], die eine neue Anwendung der Hessschen Reiztechnik darstellt, hat zu interessanten Einblicken in die Triebphysiologie geführt [O 5]. Zunächst wurde eine kontinuierliche Selbstreizung bei Ratten mit Dauerelektroden im *Septum* des Vorderhirns [O 8], dann in zahlreichen anderen Hirnregionen entdeckt. Diese verlängerten triebartigen Handlungen der Tiere, die ihr eigenes

Gehirn stundenlang reizten, wurden von OLDS und MILNER [O 8] als „*positive reinforcement*" bezeichnet, entsprechend der positiven Rückkopplung in der Kybernetik. Sie ergaben die ersten experimentellen Beweise für eine *positive Rückkoppelung von triebähnlichen Mechanismen im Gehirn*. Nach den systematischen Versuchen von OLDS an Ratten wurden ähnliche Beobachtungen auch an Katzen, Delphinen [L 25], Affen [B 56, L 24] und schließlich auch bei Menschen [S 23] gemacht.

Wenn man bei Ratten dünne Drahtelektroden im Gehirn einheilen ließ und den Tieren dann die Möglichkeit gab, durch einen Hebeldruck mit der Pfote einen Strom zu schließen, der bestimmte Hirnregionen elektrisch reizte, so machten sie von dieser zunächst zufällig gefundenen Reizung eifrig Gebrauch. Bei bestimmten Elektrodenlokalisationen im Hypothalamus, Septum und Riechhirn taten die Tiere schließlich nichts anderes, als den Hebel der Hirnreizung zu drücken (Abb. 30).

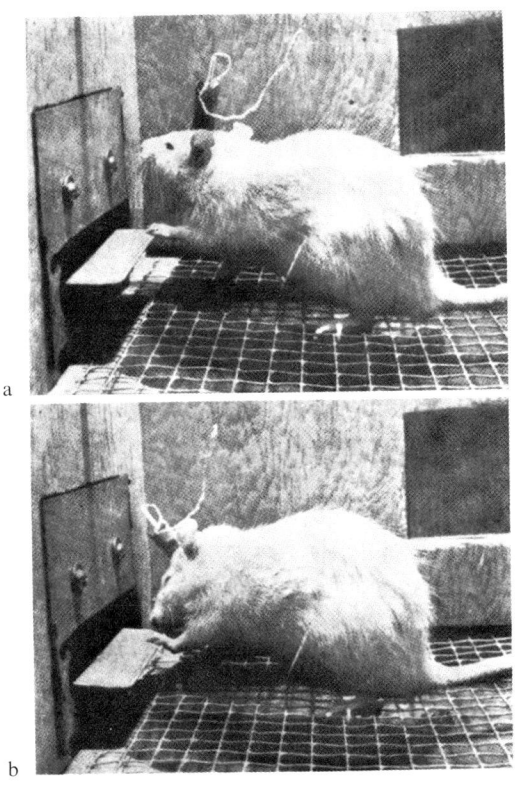

Abb. 30 a u. b. Ratte bei der Selbstreizung. Nach OLDS [O 3] Sci. Am. (1956). *a* Beginn der Selbstreizung mit Aufsuchen des Hebels. *b* Reaktion auf den Selbstreiz mit leichter Kopfdeviation. Die Reizdauer der schwachen Sinusströme von weniger als 1 mA liegt unter 1 sec. Er wird durch jeden Hebeldruck nur einmal ausgelöst, so daß für jeden neuen Reiz ein weiterer Hebeldruck benötigt wird. Wenn die Elektrode in Hirnstellen mit positiver Rückkoppelung lokalisiert ist, wie im Hypothalamus, reizt sich die Ratte bis zu 5000mal in der Stunde wie in *b*

Schon die ersten Versuche von OLDS zeigten, daß *Ratten eine selbst ausgelöste elektrische Hirnreizung der normalen Triebbefriedigung durch Futter vorzogen* (Abb. 31).

Zunächst seien die *Ergebnisse der Selbstreizversuche von* OLDS *bei Ratten* besprochen. Ein früherer Bericht über OLDS' erste Versuchsserien [O 5] wird damit erweitert und ergänzt.

Hirnlokalisation. *Positive Effekte,* die zu einer Wiederholung der Selbstreizung führten, waren bei OLDS' Ratten vor allem im *Rhinencephalon, Hypothalamus* und *basalen Mittelhirn* lokalisiert. *Abschreckende Effekte* zeigten sich vorwiegend in der *Mittelhirnhaube* und einigen benachbarten Gebieten von Thalamus und Hypothalamus. Ein Maximum des positiven Effektes bis zu 7000 Selbstreizungen in der Stunde ergab sich im *Nucleus interpeduncularis* des basalen Mittelhirns. Im caudalen Hypothalamus oberhalb der Corpora mammillaria zeigten die Höchstreizzahlen oft bis zu 5000/Std, im vorderen Hypothalamus nur noch 400 bis 1100/Std, im präoptischen Gebiet weniger, bis zu 200/Std. *Je weiter die Elektroden nach vorne in die Cortex-Regionen kamen, desto geringer war der Belohnungseffekt.* Dagegen fanden sich *fehlende Sättigungseffekte vorwiegend im Zwischenhirn und basalen Schläfenlappen.*

Wechselbeziehung zwischen Selbstreizung und normalen Triebmechanismen. Da die elektrische Hirnreizung einer realen Belohnung glich oder noch stärkere Effekte hatte, glaubt OLDS, daß der elektrische Strom solche Nervenzellen erregt, die normalerweise im bedingten Reflexversuch triebverstärkende Mechanismen leiten und wie Futter oder Sexualobjekte wirken. Labyrinthversuche zeigten, daß die Tiere den elektrischen Reiz wirklich suchten, dafür Hindernisse überwanden und für den Reiz meist schneller rannten als für Futter. Sie nahmen auch Schmerzreize auf sich, um zu den erstrebten Hirnreizen zu gelangen. *Der Trieb zur Selbstreizung war in der Überwindung von Hindernissen bei manchen Tieren um das Doppelte stärker als der Hungertrieb nach 24stündigem Fasten.* Eintägiger Hunger ist also schwächer als der Selbstreiztrieb.

Allgemeine Beziehungen zur Triebphysiologie. Reizwirkungen auf die *trieblösende Endhandlung* (consummatory behavior) ergaben folgendes: Wenn die Tiere nach Belieben fressen konnten, zeigten sie bei Reizung im hinteren ventralen Hypothalamus mit lateraler Elektrodenanlage vermehrtes Fressen, mit medialer Elektrodenanlage vermindertes Fressen. Die laterale Lokalisation ergab meist eine außerordentlich hohe Zahl spontaner Selbstreizungen. Die mediale Lokalisation, die den Hunger verminderte, ergab geringere Zahlen von Selbstreizung. Hungereffekte wurden aber auch im Vorderhirn gefunden. Triebwirkung und Belohnungseffekt bei Selbstreizung sind jedenfalls nicht einfach korreliert.

Die elektrischen Selbstreize wirken bei der Ratte ähnlich wie echte Belohnungen, die eine Triebbefriedigung bringen. Der elektrische Reiz wirkt lange Zeit gleichartig, doch kann die Appetenz des Tieres für die Selbstreizung an Hirnstellen, die mit Futterbelohnung interferieren, bei wechselndem Hunger steigen oder fallen. Sättigungseffekte fehlen im Zwischenhirn, sind dagegen in Endhirnstrukturen erkennbar. In bestimmten Hirnregionen besteht eine Beeinflussung der Selbstreizung durch Wechselwirkung mit normalen Triebmechanismen. Hunger und Sexualhormone können auch reziprok wirken und eine vorübergehende Vermehrung oder Verminderung der Selbstreizung auslösen. Die Selbstreizung kann wahrscheinlich gewisse Triebbefriedigungsakte ersetzen, obwohl sie keine Sättigung erzeugt und offenbar nicht zur Triebbefriedigung selbst führt.

OLDS' Folgerungen aus seinen Selbstreizungsexperimenten. Zusammenfassend schließt OLDS aus seinen Versuchen folgendes:

1. Das neuronale Substrat für den primären Belohnungseffekt der Selbstreizung (reward effect, approach behaviour) ist verschieden von dem Substrat des primären Straffeffektes (punishing effect, avoidance behaviour).

2. Trotz dieser relativen Unabhängigkeit der Belohnungs- und Straffeffekte besteht wahrscheinlich eine gegenseitige Hemmung zwischen beiden Systemen; Belohnung vermindert die Schmerzempfindlichkeit für Straffeffekte und Bestrafung mindert den Belohnungseffekt.

3. Das neuronale Substrat primärer Belohnungseffekte der Selbstreizung ist in mediobasalen Hirnregionen lokalisiert und reicht vom Mittelhirn über den Hypothalamus zum medialen Thalamus und von dort bis in die subcorticalen und corticalen „rhinencephalen" Strukturen.

4. Die primären Belohnungssysteme (reward systems) sind in verschiedene Triebbefriedigungssysteme mit Beziehungen zu Hunger und Sexualtrieb gegliedert.

5. Da die neuronalen Strukturen dieser Systeme eine verschiedene Empfindlichkeit für unterschiedliche chemische Stoffe haben, bestehe die Hoffnung, später einmal diese Triebbefriedigungssysteme bei Verhaltensstörungen pharmakologisch kontrollieren zu können.

Selbstreizung bei Affen, Delphinen und Menschen. Nach den ersten Experimenten von OLDS bei Ratten wurden Selbstreizungsversuche auch bei Tieren mit höher entwickelter Hirnstruktur und sogar bei Menschen vorgenommen und mit experimentellen Reizen kombiniert.

Bei *Affen* [L 24] und *Delphinen* [L 25] fand LILLY ein „Start-System" und ein „Stop-System" in verschiedenen cerebralen Strukturen, die anatomisch noch nicht genau definiert sind. Durch Reizung des Start-Systems wird Selbstreizung ausgelöst und unterhalten, entsprechend einer Belohnung. Reizung des Stop-Systems wirkt abschreckend, entsprechend einer Bestrafung. Bei Delphinen lösten im Gegensatz zu den Affen die „Start"- oder „Stop"-Reize oft eine Vokalisierung aus, entsprechend der differenzierten, vorwiegend im Ultraschallgebiet ablaufenden „Sprache" dieser Tiere. Die akustischen Äußerungen waren komplexer bei Reizung positiver Startzonen. Einige Delphine konnten auch dazu gebracht werden, durch spezifische Geräusche die von ihnen gesuchte Hirnreizung auszulösen. Delphine konnten ferner die starken reflexartigen Fluchtreaktionen, die bei Reizung negativer Stopzonen auftreten, besser unterdrücken und hemmen als Affen. LILLY und MILLER [L 25] schlossen daraus, daß die Delphine gegenüber den Affen schneller lernen, eine bessere Kontrolle über ihr subcorticales Modifikationssystem besitzen und zu sprachähnlichen Vokalisationen fähig sind, mit denen sie den Wunsch zur positiven Reizung oder zum Abstellen negativer Reizeffekte ausdrücken.

Über Selbstreizungsversuche bei *Menschen* sind bisher noch keine genaueren Studien veröffentlicht, insbesondere fehlen exakte Untersuchungen und Schilderungen der bei der Reizung auftretenden subjektiven Sensationen und Stimmungsänderungen, die vor allen von Interesse wären. Da es sich meistens um

Geisteskranke oder Epileptiker handelte, ist der Aussagewert für physiologische und normalpsychologische Fragen sehr begrenzt. Aus einigen Diskussionsbemerkungen von OLDS [O 4] über Untersuchungen von SEM-JACOBSEN mit Fremd- und Selbstreizungen bei Schizophrenen und Epileptikern mit intracerebralen Elektroden geht folgendes hervor: *„Angenehme" Empfindungen*, in 2 Fällen auch mit sexueller Färbung, konnten beim Menschen vom *ventralen Hypothalamus* ausgelöst werden. Die Reizeffekte waren z.T. mit *Lachen* verbunden. Oberhalb dieser Region erzeugte derselbe Reiz *Schmerz* mit sehr unangenehmen Sensationen. Weitere Mitteilungen von SEM-JACOBSEN [S 23] sind psychopathologisch noch zu wenig ausgearbeitet, da Schilderungen psychotischer Patienten über ihre Selbstreizungserlebnisse ungenügend waren. Die Hirnlokalisation der verschiedenen Punkte ist nicht eindeutig geklärt, da sie nur nach Röntgenbildern vorgenommen wurden. *Die stärksten affektiven Wirkungen wurden nahe der Mittellinie in Diencephalon und Mesencephalon beobachtet.* Dort konnten beim Menschen sowohl Freude und euphorisches Lachen wie Angstzustände ausgelöst werden.

Selbstreizung bei Tieren und Suchtverhalten bei Menschen

Süchtiges Verhalten ist ein psychiatrisches Syndrom, das meist mit affektiven und Triebstörungen, unerledigten Konflikten oder sekundär mit somatischen Veränderungen durch das Suchtmittel erklärt wird. Daß ein Mensch seine Intelligenz und sein bewußtes Handeln nur darauf verwendet, um sich in einen Zustand toxischer Bewußtseinsstörung zu versetzen und seine Interessen schließlich ganz auf diese Sucht einengt, ist sicher ein bemerkenswertes Beispiel abnormer menschlicher Motivation. Ähnliche einseitige Motivationsstörungen finden sich auch bei den sexuellen Perversionen. Wenn sich ähnlich motiviertes Verhalten auch im Tierversuch *ohne* pharmakologisch-chemische Einwirkungen nachweisen ließe, so würde dies von neurophysiologischem und klinischem Interesse sein. Damit würde auch die von KORNHUBER [K 40] diskutierte positive Trieb-Rückkoppelung wahrscheinlicher.

Die Gewöhnung und *körperliche Abhängigkeit* (physical dependence) *von dem Suchtmittel,* die in den letzten Jahren besonders genau studiert wurde, kann das süchtige Verhalten allein nicht erklären. Bei den verschiedenen Mitteln ist die Gewöhnung sehr unterschiedlich, und schließlich gibt es suchtähnliches Verhalten auch *ohne Pharmaka* wie bei manchen sexuellen Perversionen und bei den seltenen selbst-provozierten photogenen Epilepsien [E 11]. Im Tierexperiment gibt es ein solches *Modell suchtähnlichen Verhaltens ohne toxische Einwirkungen* bei den *Selbstreizexperimenten*. Besonders bemerkenswert und für die abnorme Triebphysiologie von Bedeutung sind schließlich Beobachtungen von *Menschen,* bei denen das *Selbstreizsyndrom mit sexuellen Perversionen verbunden ist*.

Epileptische Anfallssucht, Selbstreizung und sexuelle Triebhandlungen. Aus der klinischen Erfahrung ergibt sich eine deutliche Parallele der Selbstreizung mit dem seltenen Syndrom der *Anfallssucht bei photogener Epilepsie* [E 11]. Es handelt sich um Epilepsien mit vorwiegend kleinen Anfällen, meistens Kinder oder Jugendliche, die zufällig entdeckt haben, daß Flackerlicht ihre Anfälle auslöst. Die Kranken rufen dann diese kleinen Anfälle, die mit Bewußtseinsstörungen und euphorischen affektiven Zuständen einhergehen, willkürlich hervor, indem sie in helle Lichtquellen (meist die Sonne) blicken und durch Bewegung der gespreizten Finger Flimmerreize erzeugen. In einem unserer Fälle, der über 32 Jahre ärztlich beobachtet und von EHRET und SCHNEIDER [E 11] beschrieben wurde, führten die durch Selbstreizung mit Licht erzeugten Anfallszustände zu sexueller Erregung (Abb. 31). Nach solchen Selbstreizungen mit photogenen Anfällen kam es mehrfach zu Sexualdelikten an Kindern. Die Tendenz, diese Anfälle bei sich selbst hervorzurufen, war so überwältigend, daß der Patient alles andere vernachlässigte und über viele Stunden die Anfallsauslösung fortlaufend mit mehrfacher Masturbation betrieb, wenn er nicht gestört wurde [E 11]. Psychisch und verhaltensmäßig war der Patient völlig auf die Anfallsauslösung und den damit erzielten Lustgewinn eingeengt. Er ähnelte damit anderen Süchtigen und den Selbstreiztieren.

Da OLDS [O 4] bei Selbstreizexperimenten seiner männlichen Ratten mit positivem Belohnungseffekt oft Erektionen beobachtete, ist die Parallele der Selbstreizung der Tiere mit der von EHRET und SCHNEIDER beschriebenen Auslösung kleiner Anfälle beim Menschen in dieser Hinsicht fast vollständig. Auch die langdauernde Fortführung der Anfallsauslösung mit sexueller Stimmung ohne Endhandlung und Trieblösung als „Vorlust" entspricht den Tierversuchen, bei denen jede „consummatory action" fehlte. Der Kranke unterschied sich

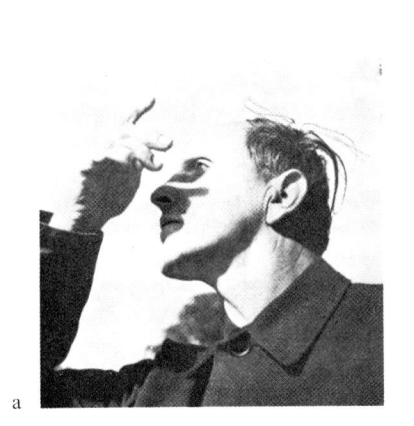

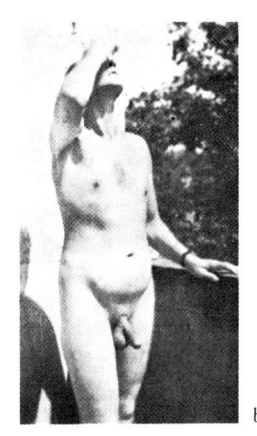

Abb. 31 a u. b. Photogene Epilepsie mit suchtartiger Selbstauslösung kleiner Anfälle und sexueller Erregung. Nach EHRET und SCHNEIDER (1961) [E 11]. *a* Absence nach „Fächeln" mit der rechten Hand, das im Sonnenlicht zu intermittierenden Lichtreizen führt. Während der Absence (5–40 s) wird das Fächeln kurz unterbrochen, die Hand bleibt erhoben. Augenzuckungen nach oben, selten Myoklonien. *b* Nach 3 min Fächeln bei starker Sonnenbestrahlung und mehrfachen kurzen petits maux beginnende Erektion. Der 45jährige Patient hat seit 32 Jahren Petit mal-Anfälle und betreibt seit 20 Jahren die aktive Selbstauslösung kleiner Anfälle bei Sonnenlicht. Nach mehrfacher Anfallsauslösung entsteht regelmäßig sexuelle Erregung, in der häufig Sexualdelikte begangen wurden, welche zur Internierung führten. Im EEG der atypischen petits maux multiple Krampfspitzen und polyphasische spike-wave-Gruppen von 3–5 sec

aber darin, daß er nach $^1/_4$–1stündigen Intervallen durch Masturbation oder sadistische Aggressionen eine Triebentladung mit Orgasmus auslöste und nach einer Pause die Anfallprovokation wieder aufnahm [E 11]. Solche Reaktionen sexueller Entladung sind bei Tieren mit Selbstreizung bisher nicht bekannt. Eine Parallele sind vielleicht die von MACLEAN 1957 berichteten genitalen Stimulationen bei Katzen nach elektrischer oder chemischer Reizung des Ammonshorns [M 11]. Ammonshornkrämpfe wurden auch von MACLEAN und PLOOG [M 15] bei ihren Zwischenhirnreizungen mit Erektionseffekt beobachtet.

Derartige Kranke mit Selbstauslösung von Anfällen sind seltene Ausnahmen. In der epileptischen Aura ist Angst das häufigste Symptom, eine Glückaura ist dagegen sehr selten [W 15]. Wenn die Hirnregionen mit positiven Effekten beim Menschen so ausgedehnt wären, wie bei OLDS' Ratten und das ganze Rhinencephalon betreffen würden, in dem epileptische Entladungen häufig sind, sollte man erwarten, daß auch entsprechende positive Sensationen bei der menschlichen Epilepsie häufiger vorkommen, was sicher nicht der Fall ist.

Elektrische Selbstreizsucht. Bei Schmerzkranken mit den neuerdings zur cerebralen Schmerzbeeinflussung intrakraniell applizierten Reizelektroden im Centrum medianum des Thalamus, die vom Patienten selbst an- und abgestellt werden, können ähnliche *Selbstreizsuchten* auftreten, wie sie bei Tieren beobachtet wurden. Manche Patienten, die ihre Schmerzen durch cerebrale Reizung bessern können, werden dann „*reiz-süchtig*", besonders wenn sie vorher medikament-süchtig waren. Solche Kranken verlieren normale Bedürfnisse und Antriebe, bleiben im Bett und reizen sich täglich in kurzen Zeitabständen mit dem Reizgerät. Ähnlich wie die transcutane und spinale Reizung leichte Paraesthesien und ein Indifferenzgefühl gegenüber dem Schmerz erzeugt, führt die cerebrale Reizung zu einem angenehmen Gefühlszustand oder traumartigen Erlebnissen, die der Patient anstrebt. Ob dabei ähnliche neurochemische Vorgänge durch Freisetzung von Endorphinen und Peptiden ausgelöst werden wie bei Morphingabe, ist noch nicht geklärt. Biokybernetisch sind alle diese suchtartigen Wiederholungen, auch bei Triebhandlungen und Perversionen, *positive Rückkoppelungen,* seien sie physikalischer, biochemischer oder emotionaler Natur.

Unterschiede von Selbstreizung und Sucht. Begünstigend für langdauernde Selbstreizungsserien der Tiere ist die schon genannte Milieuwirkung der Käfigisolierung, die durch den Mangel an ablenkenden Reizen offenbar zu dem abnormen Verhalten beiträgt. Von echten Suchten unterscheidet sich das Verhalten der Selbstreizungstiere durch die kontinuierliche Reizung mit Fehlen eines auch nur vorübergehenden Sättigungseffektes. Bei allen Suchten besteht sonst ein regelmäßiger *Wechsel* zwischen dem vermehrten Trieb zu dem Suchtmittel und einer folgenden, allerdings oft unvollständigen Triebbefriedigung, die nach Einnahme des Mittels oder Durchführung der erstrebten Handlung eintritt und Sättigungspausen hervorruft. Wenn man von einzelnen Extremen suchtartigen Verhaltens absieht, fehlen beim Menschen Suchten, die wie Selbstreizungen im Zwischenhirn zu einer über Stunden und Tage ununterbrochenen *Serie* von Triebhandlungen führen. Ferner sind die Bedingungen für das Auftreten von Suchten und Perversionen beim Menschen sicher viel komplizierter als die sehr einfache Situation der Selbstreizung im Tierversuch.

Psychiatrische Anwendung der Triebsphysiologie

Affekt- und Antriebsstörungen nach Hirnläsionen. Nach seinen Untersuchungen über enthemmte Affekte der "sham rage" [B 3, 4] hat BARD mit MOUNTCASTLE [B 6] *vermehrte Angriffslust* bei Katzen und Temporalhirnläsionen an Mandelkern und Ammonshorn beschrieben. SCHREINER und KLING [S 16] u.a. fanden nach Mandelkernläsionen von Katzen *enthemmtes Sexualverhalten* bei vermehrter Zahmheit, ähnlich wie es KLÜVER und BUCY [K 25] bei größeren Schläfenlappenläsionen von Affen mitteilten (vgl. S. 944).

Störungen des Antriebs sind nach klinisch-neuropathologischen Erfahrungen am Menschen vor allem bei *Stirnverletzungen und Zwischenhirnläsionen* beschrieben worden [B 35, 36]. Doch können auch *hormonelle Störungen* bei der Hypothyreose, bei Hypophysentumoren und anderen endokrinen Erkrankungen schwere Antriebsstörungen hervorrufen (vgl. BLEULER, Bd. I/1 B). Die hirnphysiologischen Grundlagen dieser hormonellen Antriebsstörungen sind noch nicht genügend bekannt.

Pathologisches Affektverhalten beim Menschen nach Hirnreizungen und Hirnläsionen. Außer der reaktiven Affektlabilität nach Hirnläsionen und beim neurasthenischen Syndrom gibt es auch beim Menschen rein automatisch ablaufendes, affektives Ausdrucksverhalten, z.B. in der Aura epileptischer Anfälle. Von HASSLER und RIECHERT [H 17] ist nach *Thalamusreizung* und Koagulation zwanghaftes *Lachen* beschrieben worden. Es wurde bei bestimmten Patienten regelmäßig durch elektrische Reizung des vorderen Thalamuskernes ausgelöst und war meist mit einem entsprechenden Gefühl der Heiterkeit verbunden. Nach Ausschaltung dieses Kerngebietes fand sich aber kein Ausfall des Lachens, sondern nur eine *kontralaterale mimische Facialisparese* bei lachenden Gesichtsbewegungen. Dies ist bisher die einzige Beobachtung über Affektauslösung nach elektrischer Reizung beim Menschen, die mit neurophysiologischen Methoden untersucht wurde.

Durch viele klinische Beobachtungen bekannt ist das *Zwangslachen* und *Zwangsweinen* bei verschiedenen Hirnerkrankungen [M 23, P 26]. Besonders häufig sind diese Zwangsaffekte bei Thalamusherden, bei der Pseudobulbär-Paralyse und bei der amyotrophen Lateralsklerose. Bei dieser letzten Systemerkrankung könnte vielleicht auch das anatomische Substrat dieser Enthemmungsphänomene gefunden werden. Doch hat bisher niemand die Hirnstammgebiete oberhalb des Mittelhirns bei dieser Krankheit genauer untersucht, um etwaige Kernatrophien im Thalamus festzustellen. Das Affektverhalten großhirnloser Menschen kann vielleicht zunächst in der vorläufigen Lokalisation helfen. Es kann zeigen, welche Hirnstammstrukturen als niederste Substrate eines Affektgeschehens notwendig und unentbehrlich sind. GAMPERS Mittelhirnwesen konnte weinen, gähnen, saugen und Finger lutschen, aber nicht lachen [G 4]. Man kann daher annehmen, daß „Zentren" dieser instinktiven Affekthandlungen außer dem Lachen in Hirnstammstrukturen unterhalb des Zwischenhirns liegen.

Trieb und Triebinterpretation bei Gesunden und Kranken. Es ist eine merkwürdige, aber unbezweifelbare Beobachtung, daß Menschen ihre spezifisch-menschliche Intelligenz und ihre Sprachfunktionen dazu benutzen, um ihren „tierischen" Bedürfnissen und Trieben zur Befriedigung zu verhelfen. Verändert wird nur die *Interpretation* des Triebgeschehens. Die vitale Grundlage wird dabei oft verschleiert und zu geistigen Werten „sublimiert" oder auch offen manifestiert. Diese Unterordnung der geistigen unter die vitalen triebhaften Funktionen entspricht N. HARTMANNs Vorstellung von der „Stärke" der niederen Schichten (s.S. 767). Sie zeigt, daß im Gefüge von Trieb, Willen und Einsicht zwar ein hierarchischer Aufbau vorliegt, aber nicht notwendig die „höhere" geistige Einsicht die „niederen" vitalen Triebe beherrscht. Körperliche, vitale und geistige Funktionen zeigen trotz gewisser Schichtdependenzen und Überformungen doch die verschiedensten Abhängigkeiten voneinander. Je nach der Konstellation kann die eine oder andere Schicht dominieren. Gerade in der Psychiatrie findet man die besten Beispiele für die Macht von Affekten und Trieben über Intellekt und Willen. Hier liegt eine Grenze psychologischen Verstehens und psychoanalytischen Erklärens. Sie gibt die Berechtigung, diese bei Tier und Mensch prinzipiell ähnlichen Funktionen auch somatisch-neurophysiologisch zu untersuchen. Manche emotional-triebhaften und instinktartigen Funktionsabläufe, die sich auch gegen den Willen und gegen bessere Einsicht durchsetzen, sind eben *nicht* spezifisch menschliche Eigenschaften. Wir haben sie mit den Tieren gemeinsam, ebenso wie die Sinneswahrnehmungen. Der Mensch hat nur den Vorteil, daß er diese psychischen Vorgänge sprachlich ausdrücken und interpretieren kann. Offenbar ist auch unsere Selbstbeobachtung besser. Neurotische und psychotische Menschen benutzen ihre psychischen Fähigkeiten auch dazu, gestörte Funktionen der tieferen Schichten zu beobachten und zu interpretieren wie bei Zwangsneurosen, bei Depressiven oder Schizophrenen. Eine andere mehr traumähnliche und passive Weise der Beobachtung abnormer seelischer Vorgänge mit bildartigem Ablauf und symbolischer Verarbeitung von Affekten und Trieben findet man bei den symptomatischen Psychosen.

Psychische und physiologische Mechanismen der Neurosen. Die psychiatrischen und psychotherapeutischen Definitionen der Neurose verwenden bei aller Verschiedenartigkeit der Begriffe doch immer psychologische und soziale Gesichtspunkte, über die der Neurophysiologe nichts aussagen kann. Weder die Kriterien des subjektiven Leidens oder der Störung des sozialen Kontakts, noch die von FREUD betonte Minderung der Leistungs- und Genußfähigkeit in der Neurose sind physiologisch faßbar. Die Neurophysiologie könnte nur zu möglichen *cerebralen Mechanismen neurotischen Verhaltens* mit ihren Trieb- und Lernkomponenten etwas beitragen. In Übereinstimmung mit psychotherapeutischen Theorien ist anzunehmen, daß bestimmte affektive und Triebmechanismen beim neurotischen Verhalten einseitig und auf Kosten anderer hervortreten oder verdrängt werden, und daß abnorme neurotische Verhaltensweisen durch Gewöhnung und Lernprozesse fixiert werden. Der *Lernfaktor* entspricht dem klinischen Begriff der psychischen Fixierung des neurotischen Verhaltens und der introspektiv erkennbaren Dominanz bestimmter Erinnerungen und Erlebnisse in den Komplexen der Neurose. Dieser Lernfaktor kann im bedingten Reflexversuch experimentell untersucht werden, wie es PAWLOW [P 7], MASSERMAN [M 24] u.a. getan haben. Der *Triebfaktor,* der im Freudschen „Es" mehr oder weniger somatisch aufgefaßt wird, ist der neurophysiologischen und Verhaltensforschung ebenfalls experimentell zugänglich. Der neurophysiologische Mechanismus dieser Lernvorgänge ist aber noch weitgehend ungeklärt. Daher sind die Ergebnisse der physiologischen Forschung zur Genese der Neurosen heute noch sehr gering. Dies schließt nicht aus, daß bei besserer Kenntnis physiologischer Grundlagen der Triebmechanismen und Lernvorgänge in fernerer Zukunft auch Beiträge der Neurophysiologie zur Neurosenforschung möglich sind.

Beziehungen von Affekten und Trieben zu „höheren" seelischen Funktionen

Affekte geben bekanntlich dem blassen Gedanken die frische emotionale Färbung. Triebe und Instinkte liefern rationalen Strebungen den lebendigen Antrieb. Alle diese seelischen Funktionen werden für die sozialen Ordnungen verwendet. Wenn eine Korrelation von Neurophysiologie und Psychiatrie möglich ist, so wird sie am ehesten auf dem Gebiet des emotionalen und Instinktlebens durchführbar sein. Deshalb muß noch einiges über das Verhältnis der Triebe zu „höheren" seelischen Leistungen, insbesondere über die Beziehungen zum Wollen und zu sozialen Ordnungen gesagt werden.

Triebe und Lernen. Auf die Beziehungen zwischen Trieb, Affekt und Lernen können wir hier nicht eingehen. Einiges wird im Kapitel über Lernen und Gedächtnis dargestellt (S. 1042). Erwähnt sei hier nur das Neugierverhalten und der *Explorationstrieb* der Affen, der zur lernenden Orientierung über die Umwelt führt und PAWLOWS *Orientierungsreflex,* der durch Aufmerksamkeitsverhalten bedingtes Lernen vorbereitet [P 7].

Neben diesen triebähnlichen Vorbedingungen und Motivationen des Lernens gibt es noch durch Erfahrung *erworbene Bedürfnisse* und *erlernte Strebungen,* denen zum Teil einfachere Triebe zugrunde liegen. Solche erlernten Strebungen oder erworbene Affekte auf bestimmte Reize können als Motivationen positiv gerichtet sein (Zuneigung) oder negativ (Abneigung, Furcht). Positive Bedürfnisse haben im Kulturmilieu beim Menschen als *Interessen* große Bedeutung, da sie mehr auf geistige Werte gerichtet sind. Erlernte Triebhandlungen und erworbene Bedürfnisse werden in der experimentellen Psychologie allgemein „learnable drives" genannt [M 42].

Affektive Bahnung und Blockierung der Sprach- und Denkleistungen. Die bahnende und blockierende Wirkung des Affekts auf erlernte Funktionen ist beim Menschen besonders deutlich bei differenzierten Denk- und Sprachvorgängen und Intelligenzleistungen erkennbar. Durch Freude, Sympathie oder auch mäßigen Ärger beflügelt, sprechen oder schreiben wir besser und eindrucksvoller. Durch Verlegenheit, Trauer und Antipathie, aber auch durch übermäßige Freude fühlen wir uns im Denken und sprachlichen Ausdruck gehemmt. Wie eine solche emotionale Einwirkung auf die differenziertesten, sprachlichen und intellektuellen Vorgänge zu deuten ist, kann man sich neurophysiologisch noch nicht vorstellen.

Affektive Perseveration und sprachliche Redundanz. Stärke und Irradiation der Affekt- und Triebvorgänge auf Verhalten und Denken wirkt sich beim Menschen auch sprachlich aus und führt zur *Wiederholung* und zu *redundanter Information.* Wie ein triebgesteuertes Tier immer von neuem das Triebziel auf verschiedenen Umwegen zu erreichen sucht, bewirkt ein affektbeladener Trieb auch beim Menschen wiederholte Handlungen. Beim sprachbereiten Menschen kommt es zu gehäuftem Wiederholen des *verbalen Affektausdrucks* mit verschiedenen Variationen, in denen der gleiche Inhalt sprachlich formuliert werden kann. Diese sprachlichen Abwandlungen der Ausdruckswiederholung entsprechen der „Redundanz" in der Kybernetik. Höhere psychische Störungen zeigen diese sprachliche Redundanz und Wiederholung des Affektausdrucks am deutlichsten bei *Manien* und *agitierten Depressionen*. Bei grob organischen Hirnerkrankungen findet man gleichförmigere Perseverationen der Sprache oder Wiederholung gleicher automatisierter Affektentladungen ohne sprachlichen Affektausdruck (z.B. Zwangslachen und Zwangsweinen bei Hirnatherosklerose und Bulbärparalyse).

Triebunterdrückung in der sozialen Gemeinschaft. Bereits die Sozialordnungen der *Tiere* verlangen eine Zügelung individueller Triebe und Affekte. Die Verhaltensforscher haben diese soziale Triebunterdrückung in den verschiedenen Rangordnungen der gesellig lebenden Tiere sehr genau untersucht und beschrieben. In unserer Zivilisation ist die durch soziale Bindungen vorgeschriebene *Beherrschung der Triebe und Unterdrückung affektiver Äußerungen* besonders ausgeprägt. Diese Verdrängung der Affektivität hat im abendländisch-christlichen, im buddhistischen und chinesischen Kulturkreis ihre größte Ausdehnung erreicht. Jedenfalls ist sie sehr viel stärker als in der Antike. Wir haben keine Dyonysien und Bacchanalien mehr. Bewußte emotionale Frigidität ist ein Kennzeichen unserer Kultur. Da die einzige ungehemmte Trieb- und Affektentladung, die dem Erwachsenen im modernen Leben erlaubt ist, sich nur unter gewissen Vorbedingungen als sexuelles Verhalten äußern kann, das unsere Kultur auf die Einehe beschränkt, sind die affektiven Äußerungsmöglichkeiten notwendig begrenzt. FREUDS Psychoanalyse [F 30] mit ihrem Versuch, die Trieb- und Affektdynamik nicht hirnphysiologisch, sondern in psychologischer Sprache zu erklären, kam vielleicht deshalb zu ihrer pansexuellen Deutung, nachdem die Prüderie des 19. Jahrhunderts andere Formen erotischer Beziehungen aus früheren Kulturzeiten verschüttet hatte. Neurophysiologisch sind alle psychologischen Trieb- und Verdrängungstheorien, obwohl sie manches verständlich machen können, unbefriedigend. Denn über die physiologische Triebdynamik können sie, wie auch FREUD selbst zugab, nichts aussagen [F 30].

Alle Affekte und Triebe erzeugen eine *egozentrische Einstellung,* die im psychiatrischen Bereich überspitzt bei den affektiven Psychosen erscheint. Sowohl bei der Manie wie bei der Depression ist diese Egozentrik deutlich, wenn auch in ganz verschiedener Richtung: Im manischen Antrieb erscheint eine *aktive* Überwertung des Ich mit Rücksichtslosigkeit gegenüber anderen, in der Depression eine *passive* Icheinstellung mit eigenbezüglichen Schuldvorstellungen und Rückzug auf depressive Ideen, die um die eigene Person kreisen. Psychopathologisch wird dieser affektive Eigenbezug oft zu wenig beachtet.

Über neurophysiologische Grundlagen weiß man nichts. Nur als Parallele zu der weiten Ausstrahlung der Affektveränderungen erscheint auch im hirnelektrischen Bild bei verschiedenen affektiven Erregungen eine deutliche allgemeine Aktivierung. Diese beginnt meist mit flachem EEG, dann folgt eine Vermehrung der α- und Zwischenwellen, die einen von der Außenwelt abgewendeten Ruhezustand mit Entspannung einleitet. Ob die bei Manisch-Depressiven im Gegensatz zu Schizophrenen meist deutlicher ausgeprägten großen α-Wellen des Ruhe-EEG mit der Affektivität korreliert sind, ist unbekannt.

Körperschönheit, abstrakte Körperformen und biologisches Triebverhalten. DARWIN [D 1] hat als erster die auffallenden Farben und Formen im Haar- und Federkleid und die Bevorzugung „schöner" Körperformen bei Tieren und Menschen als Selektionsprozeß der geschlechtlichen Zuchtwahl erklärt. Beim Menschen ist trotz KANTS Definition des Schönen als „interesseloses Wohlgefallen" [K 5] auch ein *vitales Interesse* mit Affekt- und Triebkomponenten bei manchen Werken der bildenden Kunst beteiligt. Die Häufigkeit der weiblichen Aktdarstellung in der Skulptur entspricht der erotischen Bevorzugung des schönen Körpers in der geschlechtlichen Selektion. Bei der sexuellen Zuchtwahl der Tiere wird das Verhalten durch solche Wahrnehmungen beeinflußt, die unserem menschlichen ästhetischen Empfinden ähneln: Über die *visuelle Anregung des Instinktverhaltens und des Sexualtriebs* hat die Zuchtwahl vor allem bei Vögeln zu der Entwicklung spezieller Formen des Federkleides und zu Nestbauten [F 31a] geführt, die auch dem Menschen „schön" erscheinen. Beim Menschen ist wahrscheinlich das längere Kopfhaar und die verminderte Körperbehaarung der Frauen durch sexuelle Zuchtwahl entstanden [D 1].

Selektion der Willensentscheidung und Triebe. Noch wichtiger als die Hemmungsfunktion der Triebunterdrückung für das Verhalten ist die Selektionsfunktion, die man psychologisch meist als *Willensentscheidung* bezeichnet. Wie es schon bei Tieren eine Triebunterdrückung durch erlernte und soziale Einwirkungen gibt, so entsteht auch durch Erfahrung und Erziehung eine *erlernte Selektion bestimmter Triebvorgänge.* Zwar ist die Macht dieser Willensselektion geringer als die Wucht der Antriebe, doch hat die Willensentscheidung ein Mehr an Freiheitsgraden in der Auswahl. Die psychologische Formulierung „Wille ist Wahl", hat wahrscheinlich auch eine physiologische Grundlage, deren Mechanismus allerdings noch unbekannt ist. Für die Selektion der verschiedenen Triebe und Antriebsfunktionen, die beim Menschen als Willen bezeichnet wird, haben sich vorwiegend Psychologen und Philosophen interessiert. Die sog. „Freiheit des Willens" wurde dabei meist überschätzt. Daß es keine absolute Willensfreiheit geben kann, ist für den Biologen, der die Macht der Triebfunktionen kennt, selbstverständlich, doch muß auch er anerkennen, daß die Willensvorgänge größere Freiheiten und vielseitigere Wahlmöglichkeiten haben als die jeweils nur in *einer* Richtung strebenden Triebe.

Instinkt, Trieb und Willen. THIELES treffende Formulierungen „Der Wille *setzt* sich sein Objekt, der Trieb ... sucht sein Objekt, der ziel- und richtungslose ‚blinde' Drang *findet* sein Objekt" [T 3] reichen über ihre pathopsychologische Ableitung von postencephalitischen Drangzuständen hinaus bis in die biologische Verhaltensbeobachtung. Sie zeigen zwar Unterschiede im Objektbezug, aber auch Gemeinsamkeiten der Antriebsfunktion von Drang, Trieb und Willen mit Beeinflussung durch Instinktvorgänge und gemeinsame sensorische und motorische Strecken. Beim höheren tierischen Instinkt- und Triebverhalten findet man nur graduelle Unterschiede, aber keine grundsätzlichen Gegensätze zu menschlichen Drang-, Trieb- und Willenshandlungen. Bei Tieren gibt es Handlungen, die einer menschlichen Willenswahl ähneln: Ein „Wille" im weiteren Sinne ist daher schon früh, von SCHOPENHAUER bis zu WUNDT, auch im vitalen Bereich anerkannt worden. Die Zielrichtung von Trieben kann ebenso wie das Willensziel bei Tier und Mensch durch Erfahrung, innere Modellbildungen und soziale Einflüsse verändert werden. Wenn ein Wolf im natürlichen Rudel entgegen seinen primären Trieben sich sozial verhält oder wenn ein gut erzogener Hund lernt, in bestimmten Situationen entgegen seinen Triebwünschen zu handeln, ohne daß äußerer Zwang einwirkt, so kann dies mit menschlicher Willenswahl verglichen werden. Wahrscheinlich sind in beiden Fällen neurophysiologisch ähnliche cerebrale Mechanismen wirksam. Nicht nur bei dem durch v. HOLST untersuchten Wettstreit verschiedener durch Hirnreizung ausgelöster Triebe [H 83], sondern auch bei der sozialen Unterdrückung spontaner individueller Triebregungen sind ähnliche antagonistische Hemmungsmechanismen im Gehirn anzunehmen.

Emotionale triebgesteuerte Wahl und rationale Willensentscheidung. Eine ähnliche künstliche Zweiteilung wie bei Instinkt und Erfahrung wird oft auch für emotionale und rationale seelische Vorgänge verwendet. Beides, Gefühl und Überlegung, ergänzt sich ebenso gut wie Instinkt und Lernen. Die von ROUSSEAU bis zur Psychoanalyse oft vertretene These, daß alles Unglück unserer rationalen Kultur aus der Veränderung „natürlicher" Umweltbedingungen und aus der zivilisatorisch notwendigen Unterdrückung von Affekten und Trieben entstehen solle, hat noch nie von der Überlegenheit des Triebhaften überzeugen können. Bei aller Anerkennung der großen Bedeutung des Emotionalen für das menschliche Leben und seine Antriebe wäre es unsinnig, die *Überlegenheit rationaler Entscheidungsfähigkeit bei komplexen Konstellationen der Umwelt oder Innenwelt* zu übersehen. Überall dort, wo Abwägen mehrerer Möglichkeiten und kompliziertere Entscheidungen mit echter Zukunftsplanung notwendig sind, versagt eine rein affektive oder triebgesteuerte Wahl, die nur wenige Freiheitsgrade hat. *Emotionale Wahl ist nur für einfach determinierte Ja- oder Nein-Entscheidungen brauchbar und blind für andere Möglichkeiten.* Noch mehr versagt die emotionale Regulation bei pathologischen oder abnormen Bedingungen in Psychose und Neurose. Selbst wenn man zugibt, daß viele scheinbar rationale Entscheidungen auch beim Gesunden triebgesteuert sind, ist es doch nicht erforderlich, dem Trieb jeweils das Primat zuzusprechen. Mancher wird fragen, was das alles mit neurophysiologischen Grundlagen der Psychiatrie zu tun hat. Die Antwort ist: Affekte und Triebe können durch Hirnerkrankungen enthemmt, ausgelöst und verändert werden, sie können, wenigstens z.T., naturwissenschaftlich erforscht werden. Emotionale und Triebvorgänge können experimentell durch neurophysiologische, endokrinologische, pharmakologische oder biochemische Einwirkungen verändert und beeinflußt werden [B 18a, E 16, O 5]. Für das rationale Denken und die Willensentscheidung bedeuten solche somatischen Affekt- und Triebänderungen allerdings meist negative Beeinflussungen einer Störung. Diese Störungen entstehen also sekundär über Triebe und Affekte, durch die wiederum die Denkvorgänge verändert werden. Doch kommen nicht nur solche Störungen, sondern auch die positiven *Antriebe* des Denkens und Wollens offenbar vorwiegend aus der Triebsphäre.

Koordination von Triebverhalten, Willen und Einsicht. Schon bei Tieren wird das Triebverhalten durch zahlreiche äußere Reize gesteuert, durch erlernte Reaktionen und soziale Bindungen beherrscht und in seiner Manifestation verändert. Trotz dieser vielfältigen Beeinflussungen bleibt das tierische Verhalten einheitlich und meist harmonisch. Angeborene Instinkte und erlernte Reaktionen werden geordnet zusammengefügt und zu *integrierten Verhaltensweisen* verschmolzen. Ähnlich entwickelt sich beim Menschen eine *Einheit von Bewußtsein und Verhalten,* die oft weniger treffend „Ganzheit" genannt wird. Wie diese individuelle Einheit physiologisch aus angeborenen und erlernten Koordinationen entsteht, ist unbekannt.

Die wichtigste Aufgabe des Menschen, sich durch Einsicht und Willen in die Gemeinschaft einzuordnen und sein Triebverhalten mit bewußter Überlegung harmonisch zu vereinen, würde auch dann eine geistige Entscheidung bleiben, wenn wir die cerebralen Mechanismen dieser Regulationen genau kennen und beherrschen könnten. Dennoch geschieht die höhere Einsicht auf einer vitalen Grundlage.

Neurophysiologischen Untersuchungen zugänglich sind bisher nur einige Lernvorgänge mit den bedingten Reaktionen (S. 1027) und ihre Auswirkungen auf Triebverhalten und soziale Regulationen. Die Störungen im Verhältnis von Trieb und Einsicht bei Psychopathen und Psychosen sind damit noch nicht in Parallele zu setzen.

Zur Integration von Einsicht und Trieb, zur rationalen und affektiven Einordnung in die soziale Umwelt verwendet der Mensch die Funktionen von Bewußtsein und Aufmerksamkeit, über deren cerebrale Grundlagen neuere hirnphysiologische Untersuchungen uns einiges gelehrt haben.

Zusammenfassung

Affekte und Triebe sind bei Tieren und Menschen die stärksten Verhaltensmotivationen, so daß ihre somatischen Grundlagen auch psychiatrisches Interesse gewinnen. Psychologische, physiologische und Verhaltensaspekte von Affekt, Trieb und Antrieb werden besprochen. Triebverhalten und Instinktbewegungen können im Tierexperiment durch lokale *Hirnreizungen* ausgelöst werden vorwiegend *im Zwischenhirn und limbischen System,* wo auch nach Erfahrungen der menschlichen Pathologie bei Affekt- und Triebstörungen Herdveränderungen vorkommen. Nur die elementaren Affekt- und Triebvorgänge haben bei Menschen und höheren Säugern ähnliche Hirnkorrelate. Die von LORENZ betonten arteigenen Aggressionen und Aggressionshemmungen sind bei den einzelnen Tierarten unterschiedlich und zeigen neben Parallelen erhebliche Unterschiede zum menschlichen Aggressionsverhalten. Abnorme emotionale Labilität beim Menschen kann mit dem ungebremsten Affektverhalten gesunder Schimpansen verglichen werden. Triebe und Affekte beruhen auf cerebralen Mechanismen, die auch durch hormonelle Vorgänge und somatische oder seelische Bedürfnisse gesteuert werden. Zu wenig beachtet sind Korrelationen von *Triebstruktur und Konstitutionstyp:* vermehrter Nahrungstrieb beim Pykniker, Bewegungstrieb beim Athleten und motorische Sparsamkeit beim Astheniker begünstigen das Manifestwerden dieser Konstitutionen. Periodische Aktivierungen des Affekt- und Trieblebens sind von cerebralen und endokrinen Regelfunktionen abhängig.

Einige Ergebnisse der *Selbstreizung des Gehirns* im Tierversuch zeigen Parallelen zum Suchtverhalten mit positiver Rückkoppelung, die sich bei Mensch und Tier der metabolisch-körperlichen Abhängigkeit vom Suchtmittel überlagert.

Die Triebunterdrückung des Individuums in der sozialen Gemeinschaft ist auch bei gesellig lebenden Tieren eine soziale Anpassung. Der sprachliche Ausdruck von Affekten und Trieben ermöglicht beim Menschen ungleich differenziertere Signale als bei den Ausdrucksbewegungen der Tiere. Die Koordination von Triebverhalten, Willen und Einsicht beim Menschen kann noch nicht in ihren neurophysiologischen Grundlagen untersucht werden.

X. Bewußtsein und Aufmerksamkeit ihren physiologischen Bedingungen

> "Consciousness is not an unvarying independent entity. Consciousness arises during activity of some of those of our highest nervous arrangements by which the correspondence of the organism with its environment is being effected. As this correspondence is continually changing, the nervous arrangements concerned are continually different. Our present consciousness is, psychologically speaking, the present relation betwixt the subject and the object, or, anatomico-physiologically speaking, it arises during the present adjustment of the organism to its environment."
>
> J.H. JACKSON: On the scientific and empirical investigation of epilepsies, 1876.

> «..., toutes les combinaisons se formeraient par suite de l'automatisme du moi subliminal, mais seules, celles qui seraient intéressantes pénétreraient dans le champ de la conscience. Et cela est encore très mystérieux. Quelle est la cause qui fait que, parmi les mille produits de notre activité inconsciente, il y en a qui sont appelés à franchir le seuil, tandis que d'autres restent en deçà?»
>
> H. POINCARÉ: Science et Methode, 1909.

Was kann die Neurophysiologie zu den komplizierten Problemen der Bewußtseinsregulation beitragen? Kritische Köpfe werden antworten: Nichts. Tierexperimente können keine Bewußtseinsphänomene erfassen, und die simultane Beobachtung von Bewußtseinsvorgängen mit physiologischen Registrierungen beim Menschen ist in ihrem Wert zweifelhaft. Dennoch hat die Neurophysiologie in den letzten Jahrzehnten kaum ein Gebiet so viel bearbeitet wie die Regulation von Aufmerksamkeit und Bewußtsein und ihre experimentellen Bedingungen. Diese Untersuchungen haben auch einige psychiatrisch interessante Ergebnisse und Analogien gebracht. Allerdings muß man allzu optimistischen Darstellungen widersprechen, die den Eindruck erwecken, als ob Bewußtsein und Aufmerksamkeit in bestimmten Hirnstammregionen lokalisiert und durch aufsteigende Funktionsverbindungen der Formatio reticularis mit ihrer Beeinflussung des Cortex geklärt wären.

Korrelationen bewußten Erlebens und neurophysiologischer Vorgänge sind nur *beim Menschen* zu untersuchen. Dennoch müssen für die Erforschung hirnphysiologischer Mechanismen der Bewußtseinsregulation auch *experimentelle Ergebnisse bei Tieren* berücksichtigt werden. Diese betreffen allerdings vorwiegend unbewußte *Vorbedingungen* für die Selektionsprozesse der Aufmerksamkeit und des Bewußtseins zur Steuerung des *Verhaltens*.

Bewußtsein, Aufmerksamkeit und Verhalten

Verhaltenskriterien des Bewußtseins bei Mensch und Tier. Da die Neurophysiologie zur Untersuchung von Aufmerksamkeit und Bewußtsein tierexperimentelle Grundlagen benötigt, sind einige Kriterien des Bewußtseins bei Tier und Mensch zu besprechen. Bewußtsein ist für den Neurophysiologen nicht nur durch den subjektiven Aspekt bestimmt, sondern auch eine übergeordnete Selektion aktueller Verhaltensregulationen für komplexe Beziehungen zwischen höheren Organismen und Umwelt. Diese Regulation geschieht durch *Modelle der Außenwelt*, die der Organismus aus Sinnesdaten gewinnt [C 13]. Solche Modellvorstellungen hat die Kybernetik für Bewußtsein und Gedächtnis entwickelt (S. 975). Mit rein introspektiv-verbalen Bewußtseinsbestimmungen begnügen sich heute nur noch die Philosophen. Die experimentelle Psychologie und die Psychiatrie brauchen neben sprachlicher Auskunft über Bewußtseinsvorgänge zusätzliche *Verhaltensbeobachtungen* und möglichst auch objektive Registrierungen hirnelektrischer Vorgänge. Allerdings ist eine subjektive Beobachtung mit objektiver Registrierung körperlicher Begleiterscheinungen des Bewußtseins selbst beim Menschen nur beschränkt möglich, weil *Registrierung und Beobachtung den Ablauf der Bewußtseinsvorgänge stört*. Beim Menschen kann die Sprache einiges über Bewußtseinsinhalte aussagen. Dagegen sind wir *beim Tier allein auf eine Beobachtung und Registrierung des Verhaltens angewiesen*. Man wird auch beim Menschen durch das Verhalten mit motorischen Tests (etwa regelmäßige Signalisierung [F 9, 12] oder Schreibversuche [K 45, P 34]) den Bewußtseinszustand und die Kommunikation mit der Umwelt graphisch kontrollieren. Klinische und experimentelle Erfahrungen ergänzen die mit Verhaltensbeobachtung und hirnelektrischen Untersuchungen gewonnenen Ergebnisse. Sie zeigen, daß Bewußtsein eine *Hirnfunktion* ist und daß es auch durch lokalisierte Tätigkeitsänderungen, Schädigungen und Erkrankungen des Gehirns verändert werden kann.

In periodischem Wechsel sind bei Mensch und Tier zwei verschiedene Verhaltensweisen schon äußerlich erkennbar, die offenbar mit *normalen physiologischen Bewußtseinsveränderungen* verbunden sind:

1. *Wachsein* (wakefulness, alertness, awareness, vigilance), das durch Zuwendung der Sinnesfunktonen zur Umwelt, aktive Aufmerksamkeit und erhaltene Reaktionsfähigkeit, meist auch durch vermehrten Muskeltonus, aktive Motorik und zielgerichtetes Handeln charakterisiert ist.

2. *Schlaf* mit Abwendung von der Umwelt, geschlossenen Augen, fehlender Aufmerksamkeit und gestörter Reaktionsfähigkeit, aber erhaltener Weckbarkeit durch Sinnesreize, Verminderung des statischen Muskeltonus und passive Motorik. Nach *Erwecken* (arousal) aus dem Schlaf wird das wache Verhalten wieder hergestellt.

Was wir beim Tier als *abnorme* Wachheitsstörung durch Anoxie, Narkose oder anderes beobachten, entspricht etwa dem menschlichen Verhalten bei anoxischen, narkotischen oder komatösen Bewußtseinsstörungen. Trotz theoretischer Bedenken erscheint es daher berechtigt, die hirnelektrischen Korrelate dieser Zustände bei Mensch und Tier zu vergleichen.

Einschränkend ist zu sagen, daß Wachsein nur eine *Vorbedingung* für das Bewußtsein ist und daß die Korrelationen zwischen Elektroencephalogramm

(EEG) und psychologisch faßbaren Bewußtseinsveränderungen nicht einfach sind. Abgesehen von der großen Mannigfaltigkeit wechselnder Bewußtseinsinhalte zeigen auch die formalen Bedingungen des bewußten Erlebens vielseitige Aspekte, die nicht mit EEG-Veränderungen korreliert werden können. Selbstverständlich bestehen keine Beziehungen zwischen Bewußtseinsinhalten und EEG, eine naive Erwartung, über die schon BERGER gespottet hat.

Nachdem BERGER bei seinen ersten EEG-Ableitungen 1930 feststellte, daß Aufmerksamkeit die α-Wellen blockierte [B 25], fand er in den nächsten Jahren bei Untersuchung von Schlaf [B 26], Narkose [B 26, 30] und Anoxie [B 29] einige Veränderungen des EEG bei Bewußtseinsstörungen. BERGER postulierte eine Regulation des EEG durch subcorticale Hirnteile, insbesondere den Thalamus [B 27]. Diese rein theoretischen Vorstellungen sind dann durch tierexperimentelle Untersuchungen der letzten Jahre in ihren hirnphysiologischen Mechanismen genauer begründet worden. Eine Übertragung der Untersuchungen bei Tieren auf Veränderungen beim Menschen ist zwar nur mit Einschränkungen möglich. Doch soll im folgenden versucht werden, eine Übersicht über die tierexperimentellen Grundlagen und über hirnelektrische Befunde bei Bewußtseinsveränderungen des Menschen zu geben.

Bewußtsein und Aufmerksamkeit ist beim Menschen durch Wahrnehmung von Reizen, sprachliche Verständigung und Reaktionsfähigkeit annäherungsweise zu erfassen. Doch geben psychologische oder Verhaltensuntersuchungen keine Auskunft über neurophysiologische Mechanismen, die der Regulation von Bewußtsein und Wahrnehmung zugrunde liegen. Bewußtsein kann besser durch *Bilder und Metaphern* illustriert als definiert werden.

Metaphern der Bewußtseins- und Aufmerksamkeitsvorgänge. Wie an anderer Stelle 1954 dargestellt [J 36], bezeichnen wir für derartige Untersuchungen das *Bewußtsein als selektive Funktion des Wachzustandes, die das aktuelle psychische Erleben begrenzt und seine Inhalte unter den zahlreichen potentiell-psychischen Phänomenen des Unbewußten und Vorbewußten auswählt.* Die *Aufmerksamkeit* ist eine Hilfsfunktion der bewußten Wahrnehmung und wird mit einem *Scheinwerfer* verglichen [J 36, W 15]. Der Scheinwerfer der Aufmerksamkeit beleuchtet einzelne Vorgänge im dunklen, unbewußten Feld der inneren und äußeren Welt (Abb. 32). Durch diese Beleuchtung werden bestimmte seelische Inhalte für das Bewußtsein ausgewählt [J 36, M 40]. Durch klinisch-neurologische Erfahrungen erscheint es genügend begründet, daß Bewußtsein und Aufmerksamkeit *Funktionen des Gehirns* sind. Unbewußte cerebrale Vorgänge oder Vorbedingungen formaler Bewußtseinsregulationen können als somatische neurophysiologische Vorgänge erfaßt werden, während es unsicher bleibt, ob auch echte Korrelate von Bewußtseinsinhalten unter den registrierten neuronalen Prozessen sind. Solche Bewußtseinskorrelate bleiben neurophysiologischen und Verhaltens-Untersuchungen bei Tieren verborgen und müssen daher aus hirnelektrischen *Analogien des Tierversuchs mit EEG-Ableitungen beim Menschen erschlossen werden*.

Die *Koordination von Bewußtsein und Aufmerksamkeit* ist in dem schematischen Diagramm der Abb. 32 metaphorisch dargestellt. Sie zeigt die selektive Funktion von Aufmerksamkeit und Bewußtsein als Erhellungs- und Auswahlwirkung eines Scheinwerferlichts: Der bewegliche Scheinwerfer der Aufmerksamkeit kann sich auf Teile der „inneren" Welt wie auf Einzelheiten der „äußeren"

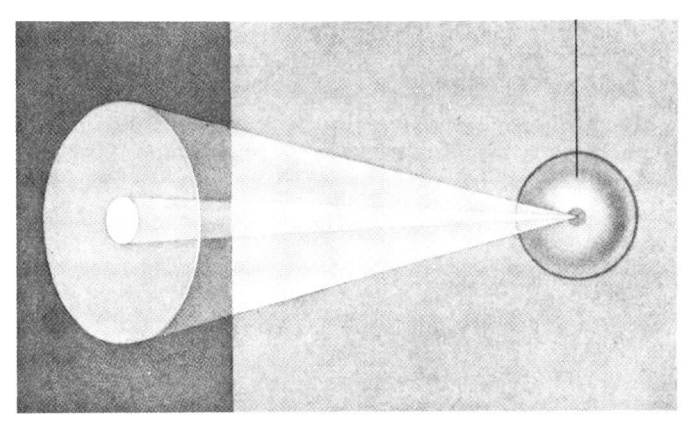

Abb. 32. Bildschema der selektiven Funktion von Bewußtsein und Aufmerksamkeit als Scheinwerfer. Nach JUNG (1954) [J 36]. Der Lichtkegel des beweglichen Scheinwerfers der Aufmerksamkeit beleuchtet einzelne Teile der Innen- und Außenwelt und wählt dadurch bestimmte seelische Inhalte für das Bewußtsein aus. Der Scheinwerfer kann auf verschiedene Bewußtseinsinhalte oder Wahrnehmungsobjekte der Außenwelt gerichtet werden. Er hat veränderliche Blenden, durch die konzentrierte Einengung oder diffuse Weite der Aufmerksamkeit und des Bewußtseins entstehen. Eine weniger stark beleuchtete Randsphäre umgibt den hell beschienenen zentralen Focus der Aufmerksamkeit. Dem aktiven Scheinwerfer der Aufmerksamkeit dieses Bildes entsprechen im Bewußtseinsschema der Kybernetik mehr passive selektive Filterwirkungen des Informationsflusses für afferente Meldungen (Abb. 33)

Welt richten. Die Beleuchtung und *Selektion innerer und äußerer Erlebnisinhalte* geschieht meistens *koordiniert,* indem ein zur Außenwelt-Wahrnehmung passender innerer Sektor von Erinnerungen erhellt wird. Der durch den Scheinwerfer hell und klar beschienene zentrale Sektor bildet den Focus, der wenig beleuchtete äußere Rand das *Umfeld* inneren Erlebens und äußerer Wahrnehmung. Beides wäre etwa in WUNDTS „Apperception" erhalten. Der unscharf beleuchtete Rand entspricht etwa dem, was BÜHLER [B 70] und SCHILDER [S 5] die „Sphäre" genannt haben. Der Scheinwerfer der Aufmerksamkeit kann auch selektiv die Außen- oder Innenwelt bevorzugen: Er richtet sich entweder auf bestimmte Objekte oder Sinnesorgane und ihre Projektion der *Außenwelt (äußere Aufmerksamkeit)* und kann sich dabei auch zu diffuser Belichtung eines großen Feldes erweitern, oder das Scheinwerferlicht konzentriert sich vorwiegend auf einzelne Gebiete des *inneren Erlebens (innere Aufmerksamkeit, Konzentration)* [J 36].

Die Konzentration auf innere Erlebnisse wird auch als *Meditation* bezeichnet und ist durch bestimmte religiöse Techniken entwickelt worden. Ähnliche Methoden werden auch psychotherapeutisch im „autogenen Training" von I.H. SCHULTZ [S 18] verwendet. Die Aufmerksamkeitsrichtung kann in Kombination mehrerer Sinnesqualitäten auf einzelne äußere Objekte oder innere Vorstellungen gewendet werden und sie *selektiv* erhellen, oder eine weite Umwelt oder Innenwelt (Kontemplation) *diffus* mit geringerer Helligkeit umfassen. Die Aufmerksamkeit ist meist ein *aktiver* Prozeß, wird aber in pathologischen Fällen wie bei der epileptischen Aura auch zur *passiven* Faszination [W 15].

Diese Metapher des Scheinwerfers hat ihre Grenzen, da sie nicht die dynamische Seite, den „Bewußtseinsstrom", den „stream of thought" von JAMES [J 4] bezeichnen kann. Das zuerst von HERING [H 33] und KARL JASPERS [J 13] verwendete Bild der *Bühne des Bewußtseins* illustriert diesen Strom verschiedener Bewußtseinsinhalte besser: Dauernd wechselnde Bühnenszenen mit Auftreten verschiedener „Schauspieler" bewußten Denkens und Fühlens vermitteln eine gewisse Kontinuität des Denkstromes. HERING hat 1870 mit dem Bühnenbild zuerst die *Beziehungen zum Gedächtnis und Unbewußten* diskutiert: „Leicht erkennt man bei näherer Betrachtung, daß das Gedächtnis nicht eigentlich als ein Vermögen des Bewußten, sondern vielmehr des Unbewußten anzusehen ist. Was mir gestern bewußt war und heute wieder bewußt wird, wo war es von gestern auf heute? Es dauerte als Bewußtes nicht fort, und doch kehrte es wieder. Nur flüchtig betreten die Vorstellungen die Bühne des Bewußtseins, um bald wieder hinter den Kulissen zu verschwinden und andern Platz zu machen. Nur auf der Bühne selbst sind die Vorstellungen, wie der Schauspieler nur auf der Bühne König ist. Aber als was leben sie hinter der Bühne fort?" [H 33].

Unbewußte Funktionen agieren *hinter* der Bühne mit dem Gedächtnis. Die Regie der Bühne führen die Antriebsfunktionen, Affekte, Triebe und Motivationen. Der Scheinwerfer der Aufmerksamkeit beleuchtet selektiv diese von anderen Kräften bewegten Akteure, aber kann sie nicht selbst in ihrer Aktion beeinflussen. Der Scheinwerfer kann weit und diffus die ganze Bühne beleuchten oder auf einen Spieler sehr hell und scharf konzentriert sein [M 40, W 15]. Die nichtbeleuchteten oder hinter der Bühne verborgenen Akteure sind physiologische, aber *potentiell psychische Prozesse*.

Der Zuschauer sieht nur die sinnvollen Vorgänge auf der Bühne, wie der Psychologe sinnvolle psychische Leistungen untersucht. Neurophysiologische Mechanismen bleiben für den Beobachter eines lebenden Organismus wie die Regie und Bühnentechnik des Theaters im Verborgenen. Sie können nur in ihren zweckmäßigen *Wirkungen* erkannt werden. Der Neurophysiologe muß daher *hinter der Bühne* arbeiten und seine Tätigkeit zunächst auf die Registrierung einzelner Korrelate der Bewußtseinsfunktionen beschränken. Solche Einzelfunktionen sind *unbewußte* Prozesse.

Bewußtseinsselektion und unbewußte Prozesse

Enge des Bewußtseins. Alle Bewußtseinsbestimmungen und Bewußtseinsbilder von HERINGS Bühne bis zu PAWLOWS wanderndem Lichtpunkt stimmen darin überein, daß jeweils das Bewußtsein nur eine sehr beschränkte *Auswahl* aus den gesamten potentiellen psychischen Phänomenen darstellt, die dann notwendig unbewußt sind. Bereits im 3. Kapitel wurden Parallelen neurophysiologischer Befunde mit dieser Bewußtseinsselektion erwähnt, die in der älteren Psychologie *„Enge des Bewußtseins"* genannt wird: Aus der Vielzahl der im Gehirn ablaufenden physiologischen Vorgänge, die mit geordneten neuronalen Entladungen verbunden sind, werden jeweils einzelne ausgewählt, die durch die Aufmerksamkeitsbahnung als aktuell hervorgehoben werden. Die speziellen neurophysiologischen Kriterien dieser Aufmerksamkeitsbahnung sind unbekannt. Die „unspezifische Aktivierung" aus dem reticulären System ist zu diffus über den Cortex ausgebreitet, um eine selektive Funktion zu erklären. JASPER hat deshalb angenommen, daß die höheren thalamischen Strukturen des unspezifischen Systems speziell die *Aufmerksamkeitsrichtung* regulieren [J 8, 9]. Direkte Beweise für diese Annahme gibt es noch nicht. Sie paßt aber gut zu allgemeinen und kybernetischen Schemata der Aufmerksamkeits- und Bewußtseinsvorgänge (Abb. 32 u. 33).

Unklar ist noch die Beziehung der Aufmerksamkeit zu Antrieb, Trieben und Affekten und ihrer selektiven Aktivierung bestimmter, aus dem Gedächtnis erweckter Vorstellungen und Verhaltensweisen. Psychologie, Psychoanalyse und Verhaltensforschung sind zwar darin einig, daß eine sehr wirkungsvolle Bahnung der Aufmerksamkeit von Trieben und Affekten ausgeht, doch haben Hirnreizungsversuche mit Aktivierung von Triebhandlungen den neuronalen Mechanismus noch nicht klären können. Emotionale Antriebe beteiligen sich zwar auch an höheren Bewußtseinsregulationen, doch beeinflussen sie noch stärker bestimmte vorbewußte Funktionen. Eine positive Symbolfunktion solcher vorbewußter Prozesse ist neuerdings von KUBIE [K 53] betont worden.

Vorbewußtes, Unbewußtes und potentiell Psychisches. Nach KUBIE [K 53, 54] kommt der Strom psychischer Prozesse nie ganz zu Bewußtsein, weder im Wachzustand noch im Schlaf. KUBIE nennt solche von ihm noch als „psychisch" aufgefaßten Prozesse „Vorbewußtsein" (*preconciousness*). Er sieht in diesem Vorbewußtsein "a direct and inevitable product of the primary and most universal function of conditioning" (in PAWLOWS Sinn). Das Vorbewußte soll vier Eigenschaften haben, die aber für den Neurophysiologen nichts Charakteristisches darstellen, sondern ganz *allgemeine Eigenschaften aller zentral-nervösen Prozesse* sind: 1. multiple Eingänge mit multiplen Verbindungen, 2. integrative Prozesse mit koordinierten Signalen, von denen nur ein kleiner Teil bewußt wird, 3. multiple Ausgänge, 4. Regulationsmechanismen mit Rückkopplungskontrolle (feed back).

Der Fluß des Bewußten erhält nach KUBIE *symbolische Prozesse aus dem Vorbewußten*, die vor allem zwischen Schlafen und Wachen und im Traum von Bedeutung sind [K 53]. Diese bildartigen Symbolprozesse treten in deliranten Zuständen, vor allem auch unter pharmakologischer Einwirkung stärker hervor.

KUBIES Auffassung von Bewußtsein und Vorbewußtsein paßt trotz seiner Überwertung des Vorbewußten zu unserem Bild einer selektiven Auswahl aus dem großen Strom potentiell psychischer Vorgänge. Wir meinen allerdings, daß die Mehrzahl dieser Prozesse als physiologische Vorgänge zunächst *unbewußt* bleiben und erst durch Zuwendung und Aufmerksamkeit ins Bewußtsein gerückt und erhellt werden (Abb. 32). KUBIES *Vorbewußtsein entspricht also unseren potentiell psychischen Prozessen*, die unter der „Schwelle" des Bewußtseins im Unbewußten wirken [J 36].

Antrieb, Wille, Aufmerksamkeit und Bewußtsein. Aufmerksamkeit und Wachbewußtsein bedürfen eines *Antriebes*. Die Antriebsfunktion und ihre Abgrenzung von Affekten und Trieben ist weder psychologisch noch physiologisch geklärt (vgl. S. 951). Auch die Verhaltensforschung hat mit der Instinktmotivation und ihren hormonellen Anregungen nur wenige Beiträge zur Antriebsregelung gebracht und sich mit allgemeinen Vergleichen und Metaphern begnügt, wie dem Energiereservoir für das Instinktverhalten von LORENZ [L 39].

Antrieb ist eine wichtige Eigenschaft der menschlichen Persönlichkeit. Dieser Antrieb wurde beim Menschen in seiner höheren Koordinationsleistung und Steuerung des Denkens und Verhaltens ungenügend untersucht. Daher gibt es bisher keine gute Definition und auch kein klares Verhaltenskriterium der Antriebsfunktionen, die meistens verkannt werden, wenn man sie allein nach *Eigenantrieb* und *Fremdantrieb* differenziert. Man erfaßt damit nur einfache, *niedere Antriebe*. Was beim Tier als Antrieb bezeichnet und im Verhalten erkennbar wird, sind oft nur motorische Manifestationen von Triebwirkungen, vor allem des Bewegungstriebes.

Der Antriebsmangel bei menschlichen Frontalläsionen imponiert als Fehlen allgemeiner menschlicher Antriebe und Erlöschen früher vorhandener Interessen und ist oft verbunden mit EEG-Veränderungen und einer Minderung affektiver und Triebäußerungen. Doch ist Antrieb offenbar mehr als die Summe der einzelnen Triebe und Affekte. Antrieb ist auch mehr als allgemeine Aktivierung, mehr als die Stromquelle seelischer Funktionen.

Der menschliche Antrieb erscheint als höhere integrative, systematisierende und steuernde Funktion, die mehr der Selektion des Willens ähnelt. Die Willenswahl kennt eine Vielzahl von Trieben und läßt nur wenige auf lange Sicht planmäßig zur Wirkung kommen. Eine entsprechende zeitliche Planung auf entfernte Ziele enthält auch der menschliche Antrieb. Dazu kommt eine relative *Konstanz der Motivation,* die sich auf *erlernte* Zusammenhänge und Interessen richtet. Die Antriebsfunktionen erhalten somit enge Beziehungen zu den Selektionsvorgängen von Gedächtnis, Aufmerksamkeit und Bewußtsein.

Selektion und Abschirmung als Funktionen von Aufmerksamkeit und Bewußtsein. Die offenbar wichtigste Funktion der Bewußtseinsregulierung ist eine *Auswahl der situationsgemäßen, bedeutungsvollen Vorstellungen und Wahrnehmungen zur Koordination adäquaten Verhaltens.* Diese Selektion ist schon in der Sinneswahrnehmung als bahnende Aufmerksamkeitsfunktion deutlich, die nur bestimmte adäquate Meldungen unter den zahlreichen Afferenzen der Sinnesorgane ins Bewußtsein treten oder auf das Verhalten einwirken läßt. Je nachdem, ob Aktivierung oder Abschirmung als Aufmerksamkeitsfunktion in den Vordergrund gestellt wird, kann man verschiedene Bilder für diese Bewußtseinsselektion verwenden. In den kybernetischen Bewußtseinsentwürfen (Abb. 33) wird diese Funktion mehr als *Abschirmung* zur Ausschaltung allzu vieler sich anbietender Informationen der Sinnesreceptoren dargestellt, deren Auswertung nur wenige bedeutungsvolle Meldungen aussiebt. Neben solchen passiven Abschirmungen unpassender Informationen ist aber auch eine *aktive Bahnung* passender, „interessanter" Wahrnehmungen und bedeutungsvoller Vorstellungsinhalte anzunehmen, ähnlich EXNERS neuronaler Bahnung (Abb. 2a) und WUNDTs Apperzeption [W 33]. Eine solche aktivierende Bahnung liegt neurophysiologisch unserem Bild des *Scheinwerfers von Aufmerksamkeit und Bewußtsein* zugrunde (Abb. 32). Etwas Ähnliches meinten wohl schon die antiken Vorstellungen des ARISTOTELES, die beim Sehen eine Art Belichtung der Außenwelt durch das Auge postulierten, oder die neueren Vergleiche PAWLOWS [P 7] mit wandernden Lichtpunkten des Bewußtseins im Gehirn. In der Bahnung und Aktivierung bestimmter Wahrnehmungen, Vorstellungen und Gefühlszustände ist stillschweigend eingeschlossen eine Abschirmung und Ausschaltung vieler anderer psychischer Inhalte mit *Hemmung* neuronaler Prozesse, die neben der gebahnten Scheinwerferprojektion im Dunkeln außerhalb des Bewußtseins bleiben.

Für diese selektive Bahnung und Hemmung haben experimentelle und kybernetische Forschungsergebnisse mehr *konkrete Modelle* geliefert: Die Neurophysiologie des aufsteigenden reticulo-thalamischen Systems und die Bewußtseinsmodelle der Kybernetik müssen daher im folgenden dargestellt werden.

Kybernetische Theorien über Bewußtsein, Aufmerksamkeit und Sinnesinformationen

Wahrnehmungsselektion und Bewußtsein. Die kybernetischen Vorstellungen von Sinnesafferenz, Aufmerksamkeit und Bewußtsein stimmen gut mit den neurophysiologisch und psychologisch entwickelten Bewußtseinskonzeptionen überein. Die Biokybernetik betont allerdings zum Unterschied von der aktiven Aufmerksamkeitsbahnung der Neurophysiologie mehr die Filterfunktion der cerebralen Funktionen und stellt Aufmerksamkeit und Bewußtsein daher als *Abschirmungsvorgänge* dar. Dies ergibt sich aus der Abb. 33 nach STEINBUCH

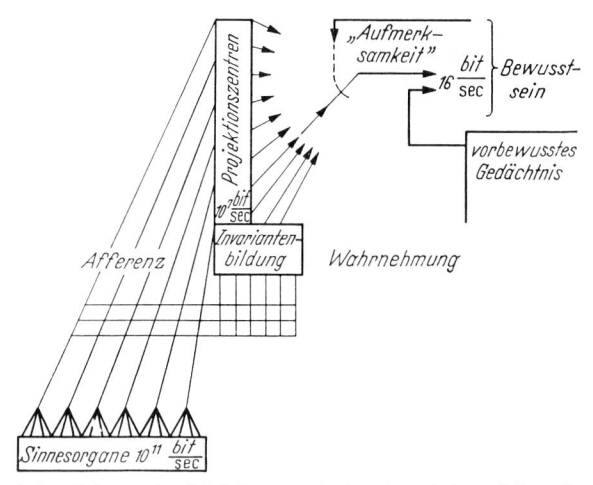

Abb. 33. Kybernetisches Schema der Selektion von Aufmerksamkeit und Bewußtsein im Wahrnehmungsprozeß. Nach STEINBUCH und FRANK (1962) [S 48]. Die Originalbezeichnungen „Perzeption" und „Apperzeption" wurden durch *Afferenz* und *Wahrnehmung* ersetzt. Aus dem großen Informationsangebot, das die Sinnesorgane dauernd in das ZNS melden, werden durch Integration, Selektion und Koordination mit gespeicherten Informationen bestimmte *aktuelle Sinnesmeldungen ausgewählt* und ins Bewußtsein gebracht. Die *Menge der Information* wird nach quantitativen Berechnungen der Informationstheorie in *bit pro Sekunde* bezeichnet (vgl. S. 438): Der gesamte Informationsstrom aus verschiedenen Sinnesorganen von etwa 100 Billionen bit/sec wird in peripheren Teilen reduziert, so daß nur etwa *10 Millionen bit/sec in das Gehirn* und seine Projektionszentren gelangen. Diese werden mit gespeicherten Informationen und ihren abstrahierten Gestalten durch Invariantenbildung klassifiziert und durch die *Aufmerksamkeit,* die hier als Abschirmung gekennzeichnet ist, ausgewählt. Zusammen mit weiteren Gedächtnisinhalten kommt nur ein sehr *kleiner Informationsstrom von 16 bit/sec* im Bewußtsein an. Die *Enge des Bewußtseins und der Wahrnehmung* wird durch Reduktion der zahlreichen von außen auf die Sinnesorgane einwirkenden Reize quantitativ deutlich gemacht

und FRANK [S 48], welche die Phasen des Wahrnehmungsprozesses nach der Informationstheorie quantitativ darzustellen versucht und WUNDTs alte Trennung von Perzeption und Apperzeption verwendet. Neurophysiologisch sprechen wir statt dessen von *Afferenz* und *Wahrnehmung*. Das Bild bezeichnet vor allem die starken *Selektionsprozesse der Informationsverarbeitung,* die von den Sinnesmeldungen bis zur bewußten Wahrnehmung ablaufen.

Zunächst seligieren schon die Sinnesorgane selbst, gemäß den ihnen adäquaten und spezifischen Reizqualitäten gewisse Merkmale der Außenwelt. Das Auge z.B. ist aus dem großen Bereich der elektromagnetischen Schwingungen nur für den kleinen Wellenbezirk sichtbaren Lichtes der Spektralfarben zwischen 400 und 750 mµ Wellenlänge empfindlich. Die Wärmereceptoren sprechen auf noch langwelligere Ultrarotschwingungen an, das Ohr nur auf mechanische Schwingungen usw.

Die von den zahlreichen Receptoren der Sinnesorgane aufgenommene Informationsmenge ist wesentlich größer als ihre Leitungskanäle in den afferenten Fasern zum ZNS melden können. Im Auge werden die Erregungen von etwa 100 Millionen Receptoren (Stäbchen und Zapfen) auf etwa 1 Million Opticusfasern weitergeleitet. Ein Teil dieser Information wird daher schon *peripher verarbeitet und integriert*. Eine weitere Einengung geschieht durch Zusammenfassung in Gestalten und Begriffen mit Invariantenbildung. Alle diese Vorselektionen sind offenbar neurophysiologische Regulationsprozesse, die *außerhalb des Bewußtseins* ablaufen. Wenn sie durch technische Apparaturen imitiert werden können, so sagt dies noch nichts über das Bewußtwerden der Wahrnehmung und erst recht nichts über das Ichbewußtsein. Der eigentliche Erkennungsvorgang der ,,Apperception" entsteht durch Mithilfe von Gedächtnisinhalten von *früheren* Informationen und Erfahrungen. STEINBUCH [S 45] vergleicht daher seine nicht-digitale *Lernmatrix* mit einem Organismus und bezeichnet beide als Perceptor [S 48]. Dazu ist einschränkend zu sagen, daß die Invariantenbildung bisher noch nicht mathematisch und technisch gelöst ist. Ein ähnliches Schema der Sinnesafferenzen von 10^7 bit/s mit Bewußtseinsreduktion auf 20 bit/s und der motorischen Efferenz von 50 bit/s hat KÜPFMÜLLER 1971 gegeben [K 58].

Neurophysiologische Untersuchungen über Weckeffekte und Aufmerksamkeit

BERGER hat 1930 bei seinen ersten hirnelektrischen Untersuchungen am menschlichen Elektroencephalogramm (EEG) bereits das Verschwinden der α-Wellen mit Abflachung und vermehrten kleinen β-Wellen zur Konzentration der Aufmerksamkeit in Beziehung gesetzt [B 25]. Diese EEG-Abflachung wurde dann auch bei den verschiedensten tierexperimentellen Untersuchungen mit Hirnstromableitungen vom Cortex und Subcortex gefunden. Der Mechanismus dieser Abflachung wurde von ADRIAN als Desynchronisierung und differenzierte Tätigkeit des Cortex gedeutet [A 9]. Später wurde die EEG-Abflachung meist als *Weckreaktion* (arousal) bezeichnet. BERGER [B 30] nannte diesen EEG-Typus ,,aktives EEG", im Gegensatz zum passiven EEG bei Ruhe und Entspannung, in dem α-Wellen überwiegen. Die Steuerung dieser in verschiedenen Hirnregionen nach Sinnesreizen und am freien Tier auch spontan bei Aufmerksamkeitshinwendung und Orientierung auftretenden EEG-Abflachungen blieb noch offen, nachdem eine umgekehrte Synchronisierung bei denselben Reizen im Ammonshorn gefunden wurde [J 60]. Erst die Untersuchungen von MORUZZI und MAGOUN (1949) entdeckten die zentrale Rolle der Formatio reticularis des Mittelhirns für diese Arousal-Effekte [M 66]. Vorher hatten schon MORISON und DEMPSEY ausgedehnte Reizeffekte mit rekrutierenden Wellen in beiden Großhirnhemisphären nach Reizung medialer Thalamuskerne gefunden [D 26, 27, M 56]. Diese intralaminären Thalamuskerne, die nach Rindenläsionen erhalten bleiben, wurden dann mit der F. reticularis von Mittelhirn und Brücke zu einen unspezifischen thalamo-retikulären System zusammengefaßt (vgl. S. 978). Es ist üblich geworden, allgemein die Reizeffekte solcher zentraler Hirnstammstrukturen mit einer Weckreaktion gleichzusetzen, obwohl ähnliche EEG-Formen auch in bestimmten sog. paradoxen Schlafstadien (vgl. S. 1010) vorkommen.

Die Weckreaktionen im Großhirn (Isocortex und Allocortex). Die Weckreaktion (arousal) zeigt im Isocortex, Thalamus und Striatum eine gleichartige Abflachung mit schnellen Wellen, die meist als „Desynchronisierung" beschrieben wird. Sie entspricht dem von BERGER [B 25–30] im menschlichen EEG beschriebenen, „aktiven EEG" mit Verschwinden der α-Wellen und vermehrten β-Wellen.

Eine besondere Form der Weckreaktion, die durch verschiedenartige Sinnesreize ausgelöst werden kann, haben wir 1938 mit KORNMÜLLER im *Allocortex* (Ammonshorn, Subiculum und Area entorhinalis) beschrieben [J 60]: Gleichzeitig mit der Abflachung der Hirnwellen im Isocortex, Striatum und Thalamus zeigen die *Ammonsformationen* und einige mit ihnen verbundene Zwischenhirnstrukturen eine rhythmische Aktivierung mittelfrequenter Wellen von 4–6/sec [A 2, G 36, P 20]. Mikroelektrodenableitungen ergaben gruppierte Neuronenentladungen und Pausen mit diesen Wellen [E 19–21, G 41].

Die rhythmischen Ammonshornwellen der ϑ-Frequenz erscheinen bei Ableitungen mit implantierten Elektroden von Hunden, Katzen und Kaninchen bei spontaner Aktivität des Tiers, wenn es Artgenossen oder Feinde sieht, oder in der ersten Orientierungssituation der bedingten Reflexe [A 2] sowie in bestimmten paradoxen Schlafstadien [G 37, J 41, S 34].

Funktionen der „unspezifischen" reticulo-thalamischen Hirnstammsysteme

Wie in der Einleitung erwähnt, wurden die in der deutschen Neuropsychiatrie durch VON ECONOMO, 1917, REICHARDT, 1919 und KLEIST, 1924 entwickelten Vorstellungen über eine Regulation von Bewußtsein und Schlaf in subcorticalen Hirnteilen später durch Tierexperimente genauer präzisiert: 1929–1949 haben die Reizversuche von W.R. HESS [H 49–63] und 1941–1950 die hirnelektrischen Ableitungen von MORISON und DEMPSEY [D 26, M 56] und MORUZZI und MAGOUN [M 18, 66] thalamo-retikuläre Einwirkungen auf den Cortex nachgewiesen und als *Regulationsfunktionen der zentralen Kerngebiete von Zwischenhirn und Mittelhirn* (medianer Thalamus und Substantia reticularis) gedeutet. Dieses *unspezifische Regulationssystem der Formatio reticularis,* die nach HERRICK [H 41] bei niederen Wirbeltieren auch das höchstorganisierte Zentrum zur Steuerung des Verhaltens darstellt, wurde 1950–1960 das beliebteste Forschungsobjekt der

Neurophysiologen. MAGOUNs Benennung "nonspecific reticular activation system" vermeidet zwar eine Vermischung von physiologischen und psychologischen Begriffen, bezeichnet aber auch als unspezifisches retikuläres Aktivierungssystem nicht ganz die Substrate und Funktionen dieser Hirnstammzentren. Das reticulo-thalamische System leistet offenbar *mehr* als nur eine Aktivierung: auch die „Passivierung" des Schlafes wird von ihm gesteuert. Ferner ist eine spezielle Richtung der Aufmerksamkeit auf einzelne Objekte und Sinnesgebiete keine „unspezifische" Funktion und nicht allein eine Wirkung aufsteigender Verbindungen zum Cortex, sondern auch Resultat reziproker Wechselwirkung verschiedener Teile des reticulo-thalamischen Systems und von Cortex und Hirnstamm [D 19, H 89, 90] (vgl. S. 979). JASPER und DROOGLEEVER-FORTUYN [J 10] haben auch klinische Parallelen mit der Petit mal-Epilepsie aus intrathalamischen Reizversuchen abgeleitet, die von INGVAR [I 2] allerdings nicht voll bestätigt wurden. PENFIELD postulierte nach Cortexreizungen beim Menschen ein *centrencephales System* im Hirnstamm, das Bewußtseins- und Gedächtnismechanismen steuert (vgl. S. 886). Nicht nur Regulationen von Aufmerksamkeit, Bewußtsein und Schlaf mit der Regelung afferenter Systeme oder die Auslösung pathologisch-epileptischer Bewußtseinsstörungen und Erinnerungen, auch die Triebsteuerung des Verhaltens wurde mit mehr oder weniger großer Vorsicht im reticulo-thalamischen System und für die affektiven Komponenten in dem damit verbundenen limbischen System des Archicortex [G 40, M 9, 10] lokalisiert (vgl. S. 940 u. 944).

Neue Gesichtspunkte über *extraneuronale Einflüsse des unspezifischen Hirnstammsystems auf die Hirnrinde* brachten Untersuchungen von INGVAR am *isolierten Cortex* [I 2]. Auch nach völliger Durchtrennung der Verbindung zwischen Reticularis und Cortex zeigt die isolierte Hirnrinde eine Veränderung ihrer elektrischen Tätigkeit nach Reticularisreizen mit längerer Latenz und zusammen mit einer Gefäßerweiterung. Eine *humorale Übertragung* dieser Wirkung, die nach Barbitursäuregabe verschwindet, ist äußerst wahrscheinlich, obwohl die dafür verantwortlichen Stoffe noch nicht geklärt sind.

Obwohl die Anatomie der reticulo-cortico-reticulären Verbindungen noch ungeklärt ist, kann an der physiologischen Realität einer komplizierten Wechselwirkung nicht gezweifelt werden. Wichtig sind vor allem die Vorstellungen von DELL u. Mitarb. [D 17, H 89] über die cortico-reticulären Hemmungswirkungen. Sie zeigen ein Regelsystem mit vorwiegender Hemmung vom Cortex auf die Reticularis. Bei Ausfall des Cortex wird die Reticularis enthemmt. Entsprechend den Vorstellungen von HESS [H 48, 60] über die Beziehungen psychischer und vegetativer Funktionen gibt es auch Korrelationen humoraler Vorgänge (CO_2- und Adrenalingehalt des Blutes [D 18]) mit vegetativen Afferenzen in der Reticularis (Abb. 34, nach DELL). Es ist allerdings noch nicht geklärt, wie und wo neben indirekter Beeinflussung über die Chemoceptoren auch direkt das Adrenalin auf die Reticularis einwirkt und ob dies über die noradrenergen Neuronensysteme geschieht.

Psychologische Konzeptionen von Aufmerksamkeit und Wachbewußtsein entsprechen im Verhaltensaspekt einer *Aktionsbereitschaft und Reaktionsfähigkeit,* in hirnelektrischen Befunden einer α-Blockierung oder dem „aktiven EEG" BERGERS [B 30]. Es ist daher kein Zufall, daß die vom zentralen Reizversuch mit Verhaltensbeobachtung ausgehenden Forscher wie HESS [H 59, 64] und Elek-

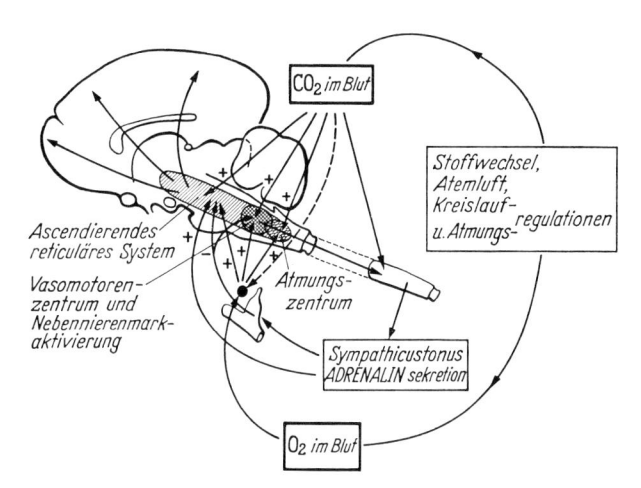

Abb. 34. Das reticuläre Hirnstammsystem und seine vegetativen und humoralen Regulationen mit den Ergebnissen von DELL u.Mitarb. [B 52, D 18]. Nach JUNG (1958) [J 38]. Das „unspezifische" reticuläre System regelt die Tätigkeit der Hirnrinde mit Wachen und Schlafen (aufsteigende Pfeile zum Cortex) wie die spinale motorische und vegetative Innervation (Pfeil zum Rückenmark). Die Afferenzen der Reticularis kommen aus allen Receptoren des Körpers und im Oblongataanteil werden vorwiegend humoral-vegetative Funktionen reguliert. Das *Atmungszentrum* der caudalen Formatio reticularis ist, wie lange bekannt, CO_2-empfindlich. Ob die Adrenalinwirkung direkt oder über die Chemoreceptoren und Pressoreceptoren am Carotissinus verläuft, ist noch nicht geklärt. Das „milieu interier" des Körpers beeinflußt mit CO_2, O_2 und Adrenalin das reticuläre System und damit indirekt mit seinen ascendierenden Teilen auch Thalamus, Cortex und Verhalten. Die Atmung ist mit der Schlaf-Wach-Regulierung verbunden. Sympathicusaktivität und Innervation der Nebenniere sind, wie der untere rechte Block zeigt, in diese Regelkreise einbezogen

trophysiologen wie MORUZZI und MAGOUN [M 19] auf verschiedenen Wegen zu einer ähnlichen Auffassung über die funktionelle Bedeutung des thalamoreticulären Hirnstammsystems gelangen, die mit psychologischen Erfahrungen übereinstimmt.

Eine Synthese der Ansichten von HESS [H 61, 64], BREMER [B 63], MAGOUN [M 19] und DELL [D 17] kann etwa wie folgt formuliert werden: Nur die *koordinierte* Tätigkeit des intralaminären Thalamus und der F. reticularis zusammen mit humoralen Funktionen, ascendierenden Verbindungen und afferenten spezifischen Sinneserregungen kann die elektrobiologische und funktionelle Erhaltung des Wachzustandes erreichen. Eine zweckvolle subcorticale Steuerung der Cortexfunktionen ist nicht durch „diffuse" Aktivierung möglich, sondern nur durch *selektive* Koordinationen, die milieuadäquat geregelt sein müssen und die wir im einzelnen noch nicht kennen. Die Nervenzellen der F. reticularis erhalten eine Konvergenz zahlreicher verschiedener sensorischer Afferenzen [M 62, R 28]. Dies entspricht schon alten Konzeptionen der Reticularis als „Centrum receptorium" [K 35]. Diese „klassischen" Lehren von der Reticularisfunktion sind im letzten Jahrzehnt durch die Entdeckung verschiedener zum Großhirn aufsteigender Transmittersysteme von neurochemischer Seite weiterentwickelt und für die Schlafforschung differenziert worden.

Monoaminerge und cholinerge Neuronensysteme des Hirnstamms. Die einfache Vorstellung, daß das aufsteigende reticuläre System als Ganzes die Großhirntätigkeit aktiviert oder bremst, mußte wesentlich modifiziert werden, nachdem seit 1962 neurochemisch verschiedene ascendierende Neuronensysteme mit charakteristischen synaptischen Transmittern nachgewiesen wurden. Ferner fand man neben schon früher bekannten Neurotransmittern im Hirnstamm und Rückenmark Peptide ähnlich der Substanz P mit Morphin-ähnlichen Eigenschaften, die für die Schmerzwahrnehmung und hypophysär-hypothalamischen Funktionen bedeutungsvoll waren. Diese Untersuchungen der letzten 15 Jahre sind für die Katecholamine zwar vorwiegend an Ratten und Katzen, nicht an höheren Primaten durchgeführt worden, doch ist anzunehmen, daß sie mit gewissen Einschränkungen auch beim Menschen gültig sind. Der zentrale Hirnstamm enthält *drei monoaminerge und zwei cholinerge Neuronensysteme* mit diffuser Einwirkung auf Cortex und Stammganglien:

1) ein noradrenerges System mit *Noradrenalin* als synaptischem Überträger,
2) ein dopaminerges System mit *Dopamin* als Überträger,
3) ein serotonerges System mit *Serotonin* (5-Hydroxytryptamin) als Überträger,
4) ein cholinerges reticuläres und
5) ein cholinerges limbisches Neuronsystem, beide mit *Acetylcholin* als Transmitter.

Das aufsteigende reticuläre Aktivierungssystem wurde als cholinerg erkannt, mit Acetylcholin als Transmitter. Auch im limbischen System wurden cholinerge Neurone gefunden, deren Zusammenhang mit den anderen Acetylcholin-haltigen Systemen noch nicht geklärt ist. Alle diese Neuronensysteme sind auch an dem periodischen Ablauf des Nachtschlafes und seiner verschiedenen Phasen beteiligt, wie JOUVET gezeigt hat [J 19]. Lokalisation und Verbindungen der monoaminergen Hirnstammsysteme sind in Abb. 35 dargestellt.

Die Nervenzellen dieser Systeme finden sich in kleinen umschriebenen Gruppen oder verstreut im Hirnstamm von der Oblongata bis zum Zwischenhirn vorwiegend in der *Formatio reticularis,* der *Raphe* und den pigmenthaltigen Kernen des *Locus coeruleus* und der *Substantia nigra.* Die Anatomie dieser Systeme ist hier nicht zu besprechen. Alle diese Neuronensysteme sind an den Wirkungen der *Psychopharmaka* beteiligt und daher auch für die Psychiatrie interessant.

Beim Menschen hat das von der Substantia nigra zum Striatum aufsteigende *Dopamin-System* vorwiegend motorische Funktionen und ist mit seinem Ausfall beim Parkinson-Sydrom und dessen Kompensation durch L-Dopa wichtig. Zwischenhirnneurone mit Dopamin-Überträgern sind wahrscheinlich mehr mit neuroendokrinen Vorgängen korreliert und beim Menschen noch wenig untersucht. Die *Serotoninneurone* sind zum Teil absteigend reticulospinal oder aufsteigend zum Zwischenhirn, zum Ammonshorn und Allocortex und zu den isocorticalen Feldern des Neocortex. Die *cholinergen Systeme* entsprechen vorwiegend dem klassischen Aktivierungssystem der Reticularis. Die Funktionen der Acetylcholinhaltigen Nervenzellen des Ammonshorns sind noch wenig geklärt. Gemeinsam ist allen diesen Neuronensystemen ihre *diffuse Projektion vom Hirnstamm zum Großhirn* mit langen Axonen aus großen Nervenzellen. Eine Übersicht gibt die

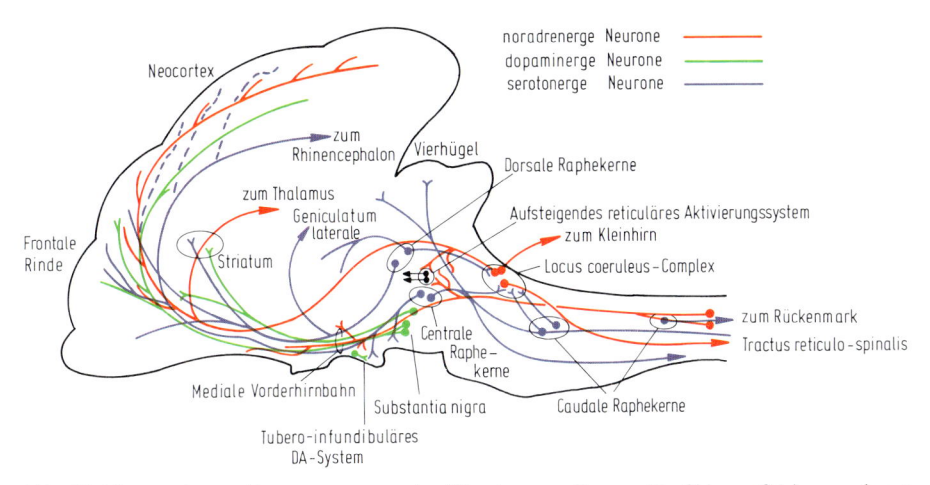

Abb. 35. Monoaminerge Neuronensysteme des Hirnstamms, die zum Großhirn aufsteigen und zum Rückenmark absteigen. Modifiziert nach JOUVET (1972) [J 19].
Die nach Befunden bei der Katze in medialen Teilen von Brücke und Oblongata und in der Nigra lokalisierten Zellkörper haben *Dopamin (grün)*, *Noradrenalin (rot)* und *Serotonin (blau)* als axonale Transmitter. Diese monoaminergen Neuronensysteme regulieren den motorischen Antrieb und die verschiedenen Schlafstadien und mit caudalen, absteigenden Bahnen den Muskeltonus. Das serotonerge *Raphe-System* (blau) hat 2 Teile: die Neurone der caudalen Raphe haben ihre Synapsen im Coeruleus und der caudalen Reticularis, von wo noradrenerge Neurone nach caudal und cranial verlaufen. Die Serotonin-haltigen Neurone der cranialen Raphe ascendieren zum Großhirn und Striatum und regulieren vorwiegend den synchronisierten Tiefschlaf. Im noradrenergen Locus coeruleus entstehen auch Kleinhirnprojektionen. Die dopaminergen Neurone (grün) stammen vorwiegend aus der Substantia nigra und projizieren in das Striatum und zur Großhirnrinde.
Außer den Monoamin-Systemen gibt es auch cholinerge aufsteigende Neuronensysteme, vorwiegend in der Reticularis zum Cortex. Diese vor allem bei Ratten und Katzen untersuchten Neuronensysteme haben bei Menschen und anderen Primaten wahrscheinlich ähnliche Funktionen, sind aber im einzelnen noch nicht geklärt

Abb. 35 nach JOUVET. Außer für die Schlaffunktionen und die extrapyramidalen Wirkungen der nigro-striatalen Dopamin-Verbindungen kann man beim Menschen über die Funktion noch nicht viel aussagen.

Die monoaminergen Systeme werden anatomisch vorwiegend mit histochemischen Fluorescenz-Methoden dargestellt und neurochemisch und neuropharmakologisch im Tierexperiment erforscht. Die Psychopharmakologie versucht, solche experimentellen Befunde mit klinischen Erfahrungen der medikamentösen Psychosentherapie zu vereinigen. Dieses Forschungsgebiet ist noch weitgehend im Fluß und wird mit seinen therapeutischen Korrelationen an anderer Stelle dieses Werkes besprochen.

Hirnelektrische Befunde und Bewußtseinsstörungen bei Hypoxie und Narkose

Der Schlaf, das Muster aller normalphysiologischen Bewußtseinsstörungen, wird mit seinen hirnelektrischen Veränderungen und den pathologischen Schlafsyndromen ausführlich im folgenden Kapitel behandelt (S. 987). Für die Klinik interessant sind vor allem EEG-Befunde bei abnormen *künstlich induzierten Bewußtseinsverlusten durch Hypoxie und Narkotica*. Bewußtseinsstörungen bei cerebralem Sauerstoffmangel und bei Narkose haben Beziehungen zu klinischen Anfallssyndromen. Ohnmachten oder synkopale Anfälle sind wohl cerebrale Hypoxien durch Mangeldurchblutung. Ähnlich wie bei Bewußtseinsstörungen nach experimenteller Hypoxie durch O_2-Minderung in der Atemluft zeigt das EEG der Synkope große, langsame Wellen (Abb. 36).

EEG und Hypoxie im Tierexperiment. Hypoxie und Anoxie des Gehirns erzeugen konstante und zeitlich gut abgrenzbare Bewußtseinsstörungen. Die Hypoxieveränderungen des EEG sind am genauesten untersucht, sowohl im Tierversuch mit Makroelektroden [G 1] und an einzelnen Neuronen [B 17, C 17], wie beim Menschen mit Kontrolle des Bewußtseinszustandes und der Willkürmotorik [K 6, 7, 45]. Die Anoxie ist auch deshalb ein wichtiges Modell, weil sie die Abhängigkeit des Bewußtseins und EEG vom aeroben Stoffwechsel und O_2-Verbrauch des Gehirns beweist.

Im Tierversuch war während des beim Menschen zum Bewußtseinsverlust führenden EEG-Stadiums der Hypoxie mit langsamen Wellen nur noch die Hälfte der registrierten Neurone tätig [C 17]. Man könnte daher annehmen, daß für die Aufrechterhaltung des Bewußtseins mehr als 50% der corticalen Neurone entladen müssen.

EEG und Neuronenentladungen bei Narkose im Tierexperiment. Die narkotische Bewußtseinsstörung ist mit experimenteller Konstanz bei Tier und Mensch auslösbar und hirnelektrisch genau untersucht. Seit ADRIAN und MATTHEWS 1934 hirnelektrische Veränderungen bei Narkosemitteln (Äther und Barbiturica) fanden, sind zahlreiche tierexperimentelle Arbeiten über den Einfluß verschiedener Anaesthetica erschienen, die hier nicht alle zu besprechen sind. Zusammenfassende Berichte gaben BRAZIER [B 59] und SCHNEIDER u.Mitarb. [S 10, 11].

Bei Mikroableitungen in Barbitursäurenarkose fanden CREUTZFELDT u.Mitarb. [J 55] nach einem inkonstanten Excitationsstadium mit kurzdauernder Beschleunigung neuronale Gruppenentladungen und *zunehmende Verlangsamung der Entladungsfrequenz corticaler Neurone mit wachsender Narkosetiefe* bis zu längerer Entladungsruhe in tiefer Narkose. Wenn die Verlangsamung durchschnittlich auf etwa ein Drittel der Entladungsfrequenz der Neurone im Wachzustand gesunken ist, sind auch alle Zeichen des Bewußtseinsverlustes oder Schlafes vorhanden. Auch hier findet sich also eine relativ einfache Beziehung der Neuronentladungen mit Bewußtseinsstörungen.

Hypoxieveränderungen im EEG des Menschen. Seitdem BERGER [B 29] 1934 den ersten Hypoxieversuch mit Sackatmung und EEG-Ableitung bei einem Assistenten mitteilte, und eine Vergrößerung und Verlangsamung der Hirnwellen bis 3/sec in der hypoxämischen Bewußtlosigkeit fand, sind die O_2-Mangelveränderungen des EEG beim Menschen genau studiert worden. Da ein zusammenfassender Bericht über Hypoxie und EEG an anderer Stelle [J 35] gegeben wurde, bespreche ich im folgenden nur einige Studien über Bewußtsein und EEG bei Hypoxieveränderungen.

Die erste EEG-Untersuchung mit Beobachtung und Registrierung des Bewußtseinszustandes durch Signalgabe der Versuchsperson bei N_2-Atmung ist von GIBBS, DAVIS und LENNOX [G 21] 1935 kurz mitgeteilt worden. Sie fanden große langsame δ-Wellen während des Bewußtseinsverlustes. Genauere Hypoxieversuche mit Signal- oder Schreibkontrollen wurden von KORNMÜLLER, PALME u.Mitarb. [K 45]; PRAST und NOELL [P 34] und KASAMATSU [K 6, 7] durchgeführt.

KASAMATSU [K 6] arbeitete mit reiner N_2-Atmung, die anderen Autoren mit 7% O_2. Die Ergebnisse beider Versuchsserien sind etwas verschieden. Bei *reiner Anoxie mit N_2* entsteht der Bewußtseinsverlust sehr plötzlich wenige Sekunden nach dem Übergang schneller Wellen in das δ-Stadium des EEG, wie bereits GIBBS u.Mitarb. [G 21] festgestellt hatten. Die Wiederkehr des Bewußtseins geschieht ebenfalls plötzlich genau zu der Zeit, wenn die δ-Wellen im EEG verschwinden [K 6]. Bei *Hypoxie mit 7% O_2* [K 45, P 34] erscheinen die Bewußtseinsstörungen später, manchmal weniger plötzlich nach vorangehenden Störungen im Schreibversuch (kritische Schwelle [K 45]) weniger konstant mit bestimmten EEG-Veränderungen gekoppelt und durch Anpassung gemildert. Die Zeit bis zur kritischen Schwelle kann von 3–30 min interindividuell variieren.

Narkoseveränderungen im EEG des Menschen. BERGER [B 26, 30] hat 1931 und 1933 zuerst EEG-Veränderungen bei Chloroform- und Barbituratnarkose beschrieben. Nach Chloroform fand er im Excitationsstadium eine kurzdauernde Vergrößerung, später eine Verlangsamung und Abflachung der α-Wellen, nach Barbituraten eine längerdauernde Vergrößerung mit Gruppenbildung und späterer Verlangsamung. 1937 haben GIBBS u.Mitarb. große, langsame δ-Wellen in der tiefen Barbiturat- und Äthernarkose beschrieben, und die EEG-Veränderungen durch Pharmaka, die Bewußtseinsstörungen hervorrufen, genauer dargestellt [G 25]. Systematische Untersuchungen über das menschliche EEG in Narkose durch zahlreiche Autoren führten zu praktischen Anwendungen des EEG als Indicator der Narkosetiefe zur Überwachung der chirurgischen Anaesthesie, die hier nicht zu besprechen sind. Sie wurden durch TÖNNIES' EISA-Methode noch genauer quantifiziert [T 10].

Weckreaktionen des EEG mit K-Komplex sind in den ersten und mittleren Stadien der Narkose noch erhalten. Bei tiefer Narkose sind auch nach starken Reizen keine sicheren EEG-Veränderungen mehr erkennbar. Die periodischen Unterbrechungen zwischen den black-out-Perioden der Barbituratnarkose mit kurzen Gruppen steiler Wellen werden von SCHNEIDER und THOMALSKE mit dem K-Komplex des physiologischen Schlafes verglichen [S 11].

Neurophysiologie pathologischer Bewußtseinsstörungen bei Kranken

Störungen des Wachzustandes und EEG-Verlangsamung nach Hirnläsionen bei Tier und Mensch. Experimentell sieht man bei Katzen, Hunden und Affen im Verhalten und im EEG schwere *Wachheitsstörungen mit komaähnlichen pathologischen Schlafzuständen,* vor allem nach Läsionen in der Mittelhirnhaube. MAGOUN u.Mitarb. [L 28, 29] haben durch lokalisierte Zerstörung der Formatio reticularis tegmenti gezeigt, daß dies nicht eine Folge der Unterbrechung afferenter Bahnen ist, wie BREMER [B 62] zur Erklärung des Schlafverhaltens beim „cerveau isolé" nach Mittelhirnschnitt angenommen hatte. Isolierte Läsionen der Afferenzen im Mittelhirn ohne Reticularisschädigung haben keinen Schlafeffekt. Es wird daher angenommen, daß die Mittelhirnhaubenherde zum Großhirn aufsteigende Verbindungen der F. reticularis selbst unterbrechen (ascending reticular system MAGOUNs [M 19]). Zwar gibt es auch beim Menschen ähnliche Bewußtseinsstörungen nach Mittelhirnherden, doch sind sie oft von kürzerer Dauer. Längerdauernde, schwere Bewußtseinsstörungen und entsprechende EEG-Veränderungen mit langsamen Wellen sind beim Menschen häufiger nach doppelseitigen Zwischenhirn- und Großhirnherden *oberhalb* des Mittelhirns.

Einfluß von Aufmerksamkeit und Sinnesreizen bei Synkopen und petits maux. Die *synkopalen Ohnmachten* sind von neurophysiologischem Interesse, weil sie durch orthostatische Belastung oder Schmerzreize ausgelöst und dann genauer untersucht werden können. Wenig bekannt und psychiatrisch interessant ist eine *Reaktionsfähigkeit mit völliger Amnesie,* die während der synkopalen Bewußtseinsstörung vorkommt und die manchen epileptischen Dämmerzuständen ähnelt. Auch bei Ohnmachten können einfache verbale Kommandos befolgt werden, obwohl keine Erinnerung zurückbleibt [J 35, 36]. Ein Beispiel zeigt Abb. 36 mit Augenöffnen nach Anruf und Abflachung des EEG. Es handelt sich offenbar um ein unvollständiges „arousal" des Gehirns mit reizbedingter

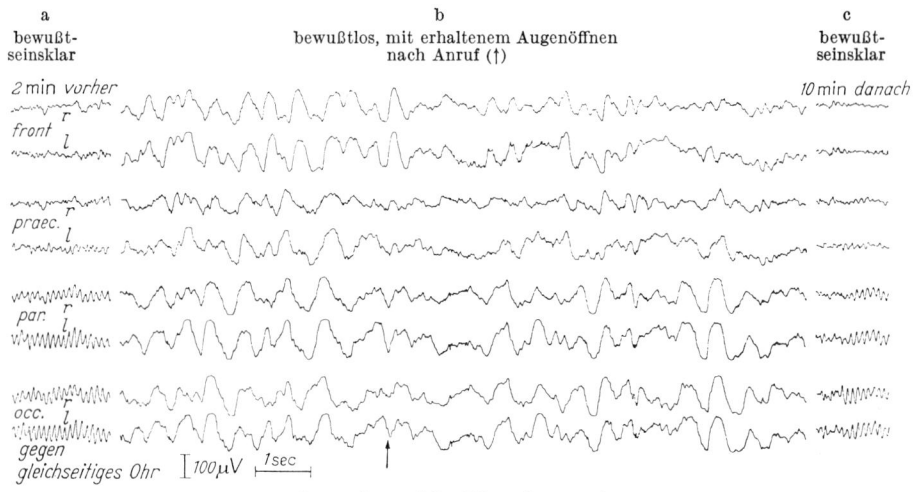

Abb. 36 a–c. EEG bei synkopaler Bewußtseinsstörung mit erhaltener Reaktion auf Ansprechen und späterer Amnesie. Nach JUNG (1954) [J 35]. Bei dem Pfeil (↑) wurde „Augen öffnen" befohlen und ausgeführt. Während dieses arousal-Effekts wird das EEG flacher. Vor dem Anfall normales EEG mit ausgeprägtem occipitoparietalem α-Rhythmus (*a*). Der Anfall beginnt plötzlich innerhalb 1 sec mit Verschwinden der unregelmäßig und langsamer werdenden α-Wellen und Auftreten großer, langsamer, unregelmäßiger δ-Wellen über allen Hirnregionen (*b*). Bei Ansprechen im Beginn des Anfalls (↑) noch geringe Reaktion mit Augenöffnen und teilweiser Blockierung der langsamen Wellen und späterer Amnesie. Dauer der Ohnmacht 50 sec. Nach 25 sec verschwinden die δ-Wellen allmählich. Nach einem flachen EEG mit Zwischenwellen (nicht abgebildet) und vorübergehender Verlangsamung des α-Rhythmus von 9,5 auf 8/sec in der 2. min, ist das EEG in der 3. bis 10. min wieder normalisiert (*c*). Der Blutdruck betrug vorher 140/80, konnte während des Anfalls nicht gemessen werden und war 3 min nach dem Anfall bei bereits wieder normalem EEG noch 80/50, stieg dann über 95/60 und nach Veritol auf 100/60. (24jährige Frau mit Kreislauflabilität und seltenen Ohnmachtsanfällen. Nr. 324/52)

Veränderung der Aufmerksamkeitsrichtung. Selbstbeobachtungen von Patienten zeigen, daß willkürliche *Konzentration und veränderte Aufmerksamkeitsrichtung Ohnmachten verzögern* und verhindern können.

Eine Verhinderung oder *Verzögerung epileptischer Anfallsvorgänge durch Konzentration und Anspannung der Aufmerksamkeit* ist ebenfalls bekannt. LENNOX und GIBBS haben 1936 zuerst beobachtet, daß kleine Anfälle durch konzentrierte Aufmerksamkeit verhindert werden können [L 13]. Wir konnten dies bestätigen und 1939 den Einfluß von Sinnesreizen auf die petits maux quasi-experimentell untersuchen [J 26]. Auch im petit mal-Status mit kontinuierlichen „spikes and waves" wirken sensible Reize verschiedenster Modalität vorübergehend blockierend auf die Krampfpotentiale, können aber den Status nicht völlig unterbrechen [J 36]. Kürzere petits maux werden durch Sinnesreize mit totalem Anfallsstop beendet. Nach der ersten Sekunde eines kleinen Anfalls können die Krampfpotentiale (spikes and waves) durch starke Sinnesreize (besonders akustische und Schmerzreize) blockiert werden [J 26, 36]. *Im Gegensatz zur Anfallsauslösung durch rhythmische diffuse Lichtreize (Flackerlicht) haben akustische und Schmerzreize im Anfall einen Weckeffekt und wirken anfallshemmend.* Auch große Anfälle mit fokalem Beginn können manchmal durch starke Sinnesreize oder aktive Konzentration des Patienten verzögert und blockiert werden. Die Kranken erleben dies als Abwendung von der Aura und als aktive Richtungsänderung der Aufmerksamkeit auf andere Bewußtseinsinhalte außerhalb des Auraerlebens. Die Aufmerksamkeitsfesselung und Faszination durch die Aura wird durch solche bewußte aktive Aufmerksamkeitsveränderung durchbrochen [W 15].

Wahrscheinlich entsprechen die den Bewußtseinsverlust verhindernden physiologischen Mechanismen der Aufmerksamkeitsbahnung sowohl bei Synkopen wie beim petit mal einer Aktivierung des unspezifischen thalamo-retikulären Systems. Doch bleibt noch unklar, ob die Synkopen und kleinen Anfälle auch durch Funktionsumstellungen dieses Systems ausgelöst werden.

Bewußtseinsstörungen und hirnelektrische Befunde

Überblickt man die Korrelationen zwischen Bewußtseinsstörungen und EEG-Veränderungen, so erscheinen folgende Punkte bemerkenswert [J 37]:

1. Die EEG-Formen bei verschiedenartigen Bewußtseinsstörungen des Schlafs, der Anoxie, der Narkose und der Epilepsie sind sehr unterschiedlich. Dies entspricht der Ansicht früherer Untersucher, die keine allgemein gültigen Regeln für das EEG bei Bewußtseinsveränderungen des Menschen gefunden haben [J 6]. *Dennoch zeigen fast alle Bewußtseinsstörungen auch deutliche EEG-Veränderungen.* Diese Regel erlaubt noch nicht die umgekehrte Folgerung, aus dem EEG allein den Bewußtseinszustand zu bestimmen.

2. Die Abhängigkeit der corticalen EEG-Veränderungen von subcorticalen spezifischen und unspezifischen Afferenzen ist nach Tierexperimenten und Beobachtungen bei stereotaktischen Reizen am Menschen wahrscheinlich, aber im Einzelmechanismus noch nicht geklärt.

3. Trotz der Vielgestaltigkeit der EEG-Formen bei Bewußtseinsänderungen zeigen Mikroelektrodenuntersuchungen im Tierversuch bei solchen experimentellen Hirnfunktionsstörungen, die beim Menschen einem konstanten Be-

wußtseinsverlust entsprechen, gewisse gesetzmäßige Veränderungen: Bei Anoxie und Narkose entsteht eine erhebliche Verminderung, beim epileptischen Anfall dagegen eine Vermehrung der durchschnittlichen Neuronentladungen des Cortex.

Aus diesen und anderen Beobachtungen ist zu schließen, daß *Bewußtseinsphänomene nur bei einem mittleren Aktivitätszustand wohlgeordneter Neuronentätigkeit der Hirnrinde unter subcorticaler Kontrolle möglich sind.* Das subcorticale reticulo-thalamische Aktivierungssystem zeigt neben einer *diffusen* und humoralen Beeinflussung des Cortex mit allgemeinem Weckeffekt auch *partielle* Veränderungen über bestimmten Hirnregionen und eine Koordination von spezifischen und unspezifischen Afferenzen. Mögliche Parallelen mit psychologischen Vorstellungen über die Polarität des Bewußtseins [Z 6] und die Unterscheidung von allgemeiner Aufmerksamkeit und gerichteter Konzentration [M 40] bieten sich an. Doch ist die Kluft zwischen experimentellen EEG-Befunden und psychologischen Beobachtungen noch so groß, daß eine Korrelation zur Zeit noch nicht genügend begründet werden kann.

Obwohl das Bewußtsein psychologisch gesehen ein „Ganzes" mit einheitlicher Ordnung darstellt, sind neurophysiologisch sehr verschiedene neuronale Prozesse an der Bewußtseinsregulation beteiligt. Es ist daher unwahrscheinlich, daß diese Prozesse nur zweidimensional mit der Polarität Wachsein und Schlaf reguliert werden. Innerhalb der Bewußtseinsänderungen des Schlafes gibt es bereits unterschiedliche cyclische Abläufe der Schlaftiefe und Traumstadien im EEG (Abb. 37 u. 39). Einschlaf- und Traumphasen zeigen eine gegensätzliche Beteiligung der Affektivität, während die Gedächtnisfixierung bei beiden sehr gering ist. So nimmt es nicht wunder, daß auch psychotische Bewußtseinsstörungen sehr verschiedener Art und Amnesierung auftreten können, die nicht allein am Kriterium der Bewußtseinstrübung bestimmbar sind. Die Benommenheit eines bewußtseinsgetrübten Tumorkranken oder die Antriebs- und Erlebnisleere eines schweren Frontalhirndefektes sind nicht nur psychopathologisch verschieden von der Halluzinose einer toxischen Psychose. Auch elektrophysiologisch zeigen sie unterschiedliche EEG-Veränderungen, die nicht ohne weiteres mit der Polarität von Schlafen und Wachen zu erfassen sind. Zwischen beiden liegt der *Traumschlaf* mit charakteristischen neurophysiologischen Befunden. Daher bleiben Schlaf- und Traumstadien die wichtigsten Modelle und physiologischen Parallelen abnormer und psychotischer Bewußtseinsänderungen. Da die Neurophysiologie im letzten Jahrzehnt zahlreiche neue Befunde über Schlaf und Traum gebracht hat, sind diese im folgenden mit ihren normalen und pathologischen Veränderungen darzustellen.

Zusammenfassung

Aufmerksamkeit und Bewußtsein sind psychische Vorgänge, deren neurophysiologische Korrelate in den letzten Jahrzehnten erforscht wurden. Die Enge des Bewußtseins und die Selektion der Aufmerksamkeit können mit einem Scheinwerfer verglichen werden, der aktuelle Inhalte aus dem dunklen, unbewußten Feld der Innen- und Außenwelt beleuchtet (Abb. 32). Kybernetische Schemata der Informationsreduktion des Bewußtseins (Abb. 33) ermöglichen eine

Quantifizierung: Aus dem großen afferenten Informationsfluß des Sinnesorgans von etwa 100 Billionen bit/s werden trotz zusätzlicher Aktivierung von Gedächtnisinhalten im Erkennungsprozeß *nur 16–20 bit/s bewußt.* Die mögliche Aktivierung von Aufmerksamkeit und Bewußtsein durch vom Hirnstamm zur Hirnrinde aufsteigende Neuronverbindungen wird mit der Konzeption des reticulären Aktivierungssystems und verschiedenen Neuronensystemen mit spezifischen synaptischen Überträgern besprochen. Die alte Konzeption eines zum Cortex aufsteigenden reticulo-thalamischen Systems war zu einfach. Neben physiologischen und neurochemischen Wechselwirkungen von Cortex und Hirnstamm sind auch komplexere Einwirkungen der Psychopharmaka auf verschiedene Neurotransmittersysteme zu berücksichtigen. Unter den *monoaminergen Neuronensystemen* regulieren die ascendierenden Neurone mit Serotonin und Noradrenalin als Überträger die Schlafperiodik (Abb. 35).

XI. Schlaf und Traum: Neurophysiologische und klinische Korrelationen

„Wir schlafen nicht ..., weil unsere Hirnzentren arbeitsunfähig geworden sind, wir schlafen, damit sie es nicht werden."
H. WINTERSTEIN: Schlaf und Traum, 1932.

„El sueno de la razon produce monstruos."
F. GOYA, Caprichos Nr. 43, 1797.

Der Schlaf ist neurophysiologisch, psychologisch und psychiatrisch gleich interessant: Für die Neurophysiologie ist die Schlafveränderung der Hirnfunktionen ein allen höheren Tieren gemeinsames Phänomen, das durch hirnelektrische Ableitungen objektiv registriert werden kann und das die Erholungsbedürftigkeit des Gehirns demonstriert. In der Biologie ist der Schlaf Teilerscheinung der Tag- und Nachtperiodik und des Wechsels von Aktivität und Ruhe. Für die Psychologie sind Schlaf, Traum und Einschlaferleben Modelle für normale Bewußtseinsveränderungen bei Gesunden. In der Psychotherapie werden Traumerlebnisse seit FREUD zur Neurosen-Analyse verwendet. Für alle Ärzte und Psychiater sind Schlafstörungen praktisch wichtige Symptome, die den Kliniker täglich beschäftigen. Schlafstörungen sind nicht nur das Achsensymptom der Depression, sondern auch bei anderen Psychosen und Neurosen oder bei organischen Hirnerkrankungen häufig und von diagnostischem wie therapeutischem Interesse. Künstlicher Schlafentzug kann bei Mensch und Tier schwere psychische und Verhaltensstörungen bis zu psychotischen Phänomenen hervorrufen. Die Neurophysiologie des Schlafes muß daher als Grundlage dieser Hirnfunktionsveränderungen ausführlich besprochen werden.

Schlaf und Traum zeigen Koordinationen von somatisch-vegetativen und psychischen Funktionen, die sowohl äußerlich im Verhalten des ganzen Organismus wie introspektiv als Abschaltung von der Umwelt erkennbar sind. Verhaltensaspekte des Schlafes und subjektive Schilderungen der Träume sind seit Jahrhunderten bekannt, doch wurde die Neurophysiologie des Schlafes erst in den letzten 30 Jahren genauer studiert, nachdem neuropathologische Erfahrungen bei der Encephalitis ECONOMO 1917 auf eine Hirnstammlokalisation schlafregulierender Zentren hingewiesen hatten [E 7, 8]. Die Reizexperimente von W.R. HESS, die im X. Kapitel besprochenen Untersuchungen über das unspezifische Hirnstammsystem und EEG-Untersuchungen beim Menschen haben die lange von der Physiologie vernachlässigten Schlaf- und Wachregulationen zu einem aktuellen und viel bearbeiteten Forschungsgebiet gemacht. Zahlreiche Ergebnisse der tierexperimentellen Grundlagenforschung und der Schlafregistrierung beim Menschen sind von klinischem Interesse. Ihre Bedeutung für die allgemeine Neurophysiologie und Psychiatrie wird im folgenden dargestellt.

Hirnelektrische Veränderungen des Schlaf-EEG bei Gesunden ergeben Ähnlichkeiten mit dem EEG bei pathologischen Bewußtseinsstörungen, die bei den symptomatischen Psychosen auch klinisch einem partiellen Schlaf- und Traumzustand verglichen wurden [C 11]. Das EEG ermöglicht es, cerebrale Vorgänge beim physiologischen Schlaf und bei pathologischen Bewußtseinsstörungen exakt zu untersuchen und ihre verschiedenen hirnelektrischen Formen zu unterscheiden. Genauere objektive Untersuchungen über den Schlaf und seine Störungen bei verschiedenen psychiatrischen Krankheitsbildern sind allerdings erst im Beginn. Die folgenden allgemeinen Ausführungen über die Physiologie von Schlaf und Traum benutzen eine frühere Zusammenfassung [J 41] und ergänzen sie in psychologischer und psychiatrischer Hinsicht.

In den letzten Jahren sind neben vielen Schlafsymposien [A 14, B 18, F 10, H 7, J 18, 19, J 21, K 33, 34, W 31] verschiedene zusammenfassende Berichte über den Schlaf und seine Störungen mit ausführlichen Literaturangaben erschienen: KLEITMANs Monographie in einer ergänzten 2. Auflage [K 20] gibt einen Gesamtüberblick bis 1963. OSWALDs Buch [O 12] berücksichtigt ausführlicher die psychologische und Traumliteratur, HARTMANNs populäre Schrift mehr die Psychiatrie [H 7], KOELLAS [K 33, 34] und ein eigener Bericht [J 41] mehr die Elektrophysiologie. Die Beiträge von MORUZZI [M 65] und JOUVET [J 19] bringen alles Wesentliche über die Neurophysiologie und Neurochemie des Schlafes bis 1971.

Wie in der Großhirnpathologie gingen auch bei der Schlafforschung klinische Erfahrungen und hirnlokalisatorische Untersuchungen den neurophysiologischen Experimenten und ihren psychiatrischen Anwendungen voraus. Die Schlafkrankheit und die Encephalitis epidemica haben während der hirnpathologischen Ära der Psychiatrie größere Aufmerksamkeit gefunden als die eigentlichen psychiatrischen Schlafstörungen. Ein Zusammenhang der Schlafregulation mit subcorticalen Funktionen erschien danach neurologisch sehr wahrscheinlich. Einen mächtigen Impuls erhielt die physiologische Schlafforschung durch die *diencephalen Reizversuche* von W.R. Hess, der im medianen Thalamus eine *hypnogene Zone* fand und sie nach vorangehenden theoretischen Erwägungen [H 48] mit einer vegetativen Beeinflussung des Cortex in Verbindung brachte [H 52].

Reiz- und Ausschaltungsexperimente zur Hirnlokalisation der Schlafregelung

Nachdem Ausschaltungsexperimente im Hirnstamm nur Komazustände erzeugten, die vom natürlichen Schlaf verschieden waren, ermöglichten Reizexperimente von Hess [H 49, 50, 59] und hirnelektrische Untersuchungen eine physiologische Klärung der Schlafmechanismen, die in systematischen Studien auch nach lokalisatorischen Gesichtspunkten weitergeführt wurden.

Tierversuche über Schlafauslösung. Die ersten klaren experimentellen Befunde über die Neurophysiologie des Schlafes ergaben 1929–1944 die *Reizversuche von W.R. Hess im medialen Thalamus* [H 49, 59], die allen Untersuchungen über subcorticale Regulationssysteme der Cortexfunktionen für Aufmerksamkeit und Bewußtsein vorangingen (vgl. S. 976). Hess zeigte bei der Katze, daß *niederfrequente Reize im medialen Thalamus Schlaf auslösten* und daß dieser Reizeffekt nach Verhaltenskriterien dem natürlichen Schlaf entsprach. Ähnliche Inaktivierungsaffekte bei Caudatumreizung waren vom echten Schlaf zu unterscheiden [A 14a]. Die subcorticalen Hirnteile der Schlafregelung beschränken sich nicht auf das Zwischenhirn und orale Mittelhirn, wie man zunächst nach neurologischen Erfahrungen bei der Encephalitis lethargica annahm.

Untersuchungen von Jouvet [J 15, 16, 17, 20], Moruzzi u.Mitarb. [B 10, M 16, 64, R 27] ergaben, daß auch *rhombencephale Reticulariskerne* der Brücke und Oblongata bestimmte Schlafstadien und den Muskeltonus beeinflussen. Traumstadien des Menschen mit EEG-Abflachung und der paradoxen Schlafphase der Tiere wurde von Jouvet als „rhombencephaler Schlaf" gedeutet. Auch der synchronisierte Tiefschlaf mit großen langsamen EEG-Wellen wurde tierexperimentell durch Reizung im unteren Hirnstamm ausgelöst. Hemmungseffekte nach Reizung der unteren Oblongata zeigten sich in langsamen schlafähnlichen Rhythmen des EEG im Großhirn [M 64].

Unspezifische hypnogene Effekte wurden durch Reizung sehr unterschiedlicher peripherer und zentraler Nervenstrukturen erhalten. Elektrische Reize verschiedener Hirnregionen ergaben hypnogene Effekte auch *außerhalb des thalamischen Schlafzentrums* von Hess. Schlaf-Effekte waren nur auslösbar, wenn *langsame Reizfrequenzen* verwendet wurden. Reizungen in folgenden Hirnteilen konnten Schlaf bei Katzen erzeugen: in der von Hess [H 61] so genannten trophotropen Zone des *vorderen Hypothalamus* [C 8] mit der *lateralen präoptischen Region, im C. mammillare* und *Ammonshorn* [P 2, 3] und in der *medialen Reticularis der unteren Oblongata* nahe der descendierenden Hemmungsregion Magouns [M 20] und der ascendierenden Hemmungsregion Moruzzis [M 64]. Schließlich kann auch niederfrequente Reizung peripherer *Hautnerven* Schlaf auslösen [P 29, 30], wie man es von rhythmischen Sinnesreizen seit langem weiß. Monnier postuliert eine antagonistisch reziproke Struktur der Schlafregulation innerhalb des unspezifischen Systems mit einer aktivierenden reticulothalamocorticalen und einer dämpfenden intralaminären thalamocorticalen Komponente [M 53].

Zwei 1972 erschienene Übersichten über den Schlaf von Moruzzi über die Physiologie [M 65] und von Jouvet über die Neurochemie [J 19] bringen auch allgemeine Schlafkonzeptionen.

MORUZZI deutet den Schlaf als triebhafte *Instinkthandlung*, die auf einem tieferen biologischen Niveau gegenüber Affekten und Nahrungstrieb steht. Wie andere Instinkte hat der Schlaftrieb eine appetitive Phase und eine Sättigungsphase, und beide Schlaftypen, der *„synchronisierte" mit langsamen EEG-Wellen* und der *„desynchronisierte" REM-Schlaf mit raschen Augenbewegungen*, induzieren sich gegenseitig. MORUZZI postuliert für alle diese Regulationen eine reticuläre physiologische Inaktivierung, die mit Weckreizen reversibel ist. Unbeeinflußbar durch Weckreize ist nur die pathologische Inaktivierung im Koma.

JOUVET postuliert, daß die Dauer des Wachzustandes den Erholungsvorgang des Schlafes mit langsamen Wellen bestimmt und daß dieser wiederum den REM-Schlaf induziert. Er trennt scharf den Schlaf mit langsamen Wellen und den „paradoxen" REM-Schlaf. Nur der synchronisierte Schlaf soll ein echter Erholungsprozeß sein. Der biologische Zweck des REM-Schlafes, der etwa $1/10$ der Wachzeit dauern soll, ist nach JOUVET ein genotypisch bestimmter Hirnprozeß, der Instinkthandlungen bahnt, die sich auch subjektiv in Traumbildern äußern können. Der Traumschlaf wäre dann nicht nur, wie wir vorgeschlagen haben, eine innere affektive Abreaktion [J 43], sondern ein spontaner, cerebraler Übungsvorgang für biologisch determinierte Instinktkoordinationen [J 19, M 65].

Biologie des Schlafes

Schlafverhalten und Schlaffunktion. HESS kennzeichnet den Schlaf als *aktiven biologischen Vorgang*, der nicht negativ durch Ausschaltung eines aktivierenden Systems erklärt werden kann [H 52, 59, 62]. Nach Vergleich des Schlafes mit anderen vegetativen und Triebvorgängen erklärt HESS die im Schlaf zu beobachtenden Hemmungserscheinungen als positive Funktionskoordination.

Für einen aktiven Vorgang sprechen außer der Erholungswirkung auch verschiedene Begleitsymptome des Schlafes, der tonische Augenschluß, die Pupillenverengung und die verschiedenen Schlafstellungen, die je nach Milieusituation und Tierart wechseln. Corticale Hemmungen, die im Schlaf auftreten und die PAWLOW bei seiner Schlaftheorie in den Vordergrund stellt [P 7], sind nicht Ausschaltungen der Cortexfunktionen. Sowohl neurophysiologische wie psychologische Beobachtungen sprechen für eine Fortführung differenzierter corticaler Prozesse im Schlaf: *1.* die gegenüber dem Wachzustand nicht verminderten corticalen Neuronenentladungen, die im Schlaf nur veränderte Muster zeigen [C 16], *2.* die seit BURDACH [B 72] bekannte Wirksamkeit spezifischer Weckreize, die von der Lautstärke unabhängig nach ihrem Bedeutungscharakter wirken, und *3.* die im Traum ablaufenden psychischen Vorgänge, die zwar meistens vergessen werden, aber auch das Wacherleben beeinflussen können.

Der Bewußtseinsverlust des Schlafes erscheint nicht sinnlos wie eine Ohnmacht oder ein epileptischer Anfall, sondern wird *vorbereitet* durch Aufsuchen und Auswahl des Schlafortes, durch individuelle und artverschiedene Schlafstellungen. *Während des Schlafzustandes bleiben bestimmte* lebenswichtige *motorische Funktionen erhalten:* auf schwankendem Ast schlafende Vögel regulieren weiter ihr Gleichgewicht, ebenso wie schlafende Fische durch leichte Flossenbewegungen ihre normale Stellung im Wasser regulieren. Schlafende Menschen zeigen noch *adäquate Anpassungen der Körperhaltung an die Umgebungsbedingungen.* Ein Gesunder fällt im Schlaf fast nie aus dem schmalsten Bett, obwohl zahlreiche unbewußte Bewegungen und Lageänderungen während der Nacht vorkommen. Eine von der bewußten Wahrnehmung unabhängige sensomotorische Verhaltensregulation mit Anpassung an die jeweilige Situation muß daher auch im Schlaf erhalten bleiben.

Die *Weckwirksamkeit spezifischer bedeutungsvoller Sinnesreize im Schlaf* ist nicht nur beim Menschen beobachtet, sondern findet sich auch bei Tieren, sowohl bei Wildtieren, für die eine spezifische Weckbarkeit durch Feindgeräusche lebensnotwendig ist, wie auch bei Haustieren.

Die Erholungsfunktion des Schlafes ist zwar in ihrem Mechanismus unbekannt, aber jedem aus eigener Erfahrung und nach Verhaltensbeobachtungen klar. In der Ermüdung sind sowohl körperliche wie geistige Leistungen erschwert, nach dem Schlaf sind sie erleichtert. Die experimentell-psychologisch festgestellten Differenzen der Leistungen in der Ermüdung und nach dem Schlaf sind zwar nicht sehr erheblich. Doch liegt das daran, daß der Schlaf *protektiv* wirkt und schon *vor* Absinken zur Leistungsunfähigkeit eintritt [W 27].

Periodischer Ablauf des Nachtschlafes. Neben der großen Tagesperiodik von Schlafen und Wachen, die als physiologische Uhr bei Mensch und Tier mit anderen periodischen Funktionsänderungen gekoppelt ist, gibt es auch kürzere periodische Cyclen von Wachheit und Schlaf. Diese kürzeren Perioden ähneln den kurz dauernden Schlaf-Wachperioden des menschlichen Säuglings im ersten Lebensjahr und finden sich beim Erwachsenen nur im cyclischen Schlafverlauf mit Wechsel von Tiefschlaf und Traumperioden. Schlaftiefenbestimmungen und Untersuchungen über Schlaf-EEG und Augenbewegungen zeigen übereinstimmend *cyclische Perioden, die sich 3–5mal während der Nacht wiederholen* (Abb. 37, 41). Auf der Höhe dieser Cyclen erscheint eine Abflachung des EEG, ähnlich dem B-Stadium im ersten Einschlafen. Im Gegensatz zum B-Stadium, in dem langsame Augenbewegungen auftreten [K 63], zeigt diese spätere EEG-Abflachung rasche Augenbewegungen, aber meist nur geringe Körperbewegungen. Wenn man die Schlafenden in dieser Zeit weckt, berichten die meisten Versuchspersonen von *Träumen* [D 23–25]. Die Traumperioden scheinen etwas regelmäßiger zu wechseln als die übrigen EEG-Stadien des Schlafes (vgl. Abb. 37).

Die Untersuchungen von KLEITMAN [K 20] u.Mitarb. [A 31, 32] über Augenbewegungen im Schlaf und Traum beim Menschen und die tierexperimentellen Ergebnisse über das „paradoxe" EEG-Stadium des Schlafes und seine Verbindung mit Augenunruhe (vgl. S. 1010) ergeben auch interessante Hinweise auf periodische subcorticale Funktionsänderungen im Schlaf, da die Augenkoordination vorwiegend subcortical gesteuert wird.

Schlafdauer. Die Schlafdauer variiert bei verschiedenen Arten und auch beim Menschen intraindividuell und interindividuell erheblich. Bei Erwachsenen ist ein *Durchschnitt* von 7–8 Std Schlaf im 24-Stundencyclus immer wieder gefunden worden, mit relativ häufigen Variationen zwischen 5 und 10 Std. Im *Säuglingsalter* ist die Schlafdauer mehr als verdoppelt, aber beim Neugeborenen noch auf mehrere kürzere Perioden über Tag und Nacht verteilt. Im ersten Lebensjahr wird mit Änderung der Ernährungsweise auch der Schlaf mehr auf die Nachtzeit mit kürzerem Tagschlaf (6–3 Std) und längerem Nachtschlaf (8–10 Std) verlagert

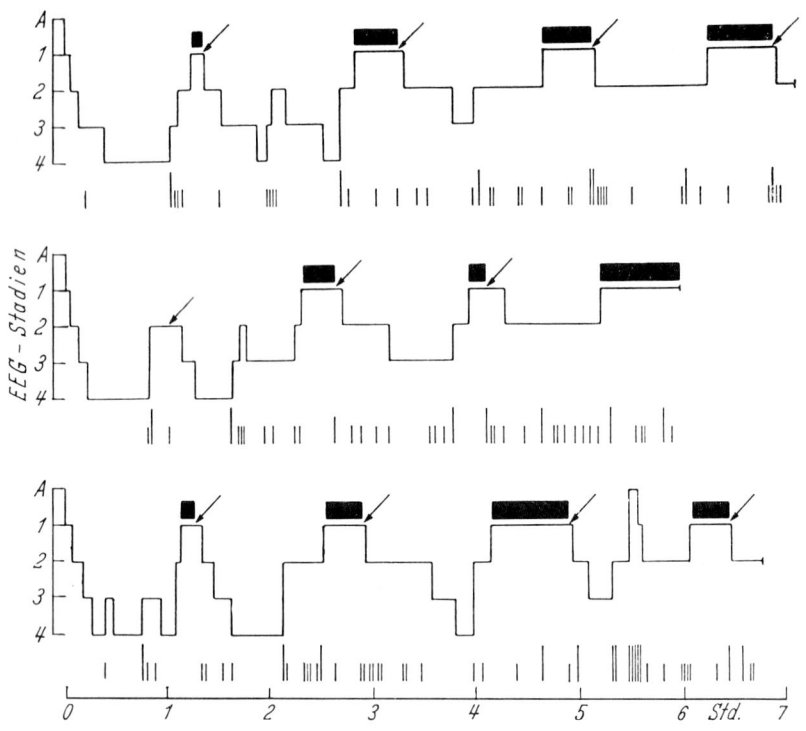

Abb. 37. Cyclischer Ablauf des Schlafes mit Traumstadien, charakterisiert durch rasche Augenbewegungen (■) und flaches EEG. Nach DEMENT und KLEITMAN (1957) [D 25]. Cyclen der Schlafstadien während dreier Nächte bei demselben Gesunden. Die EEG-Stadien werden durch die kontinuierliche Linie angezeigt und sind nach KLEITMANS Einteilung mit Nummern von 1-4 angegeben, die etwa den Stadien B-E von LOOMIS entsprechen: A entspricht dem Wach-EEG, 2 sowohl dem B-Stadium wie dem Traumstadium REM der neueren Literatur: In den Traumstadien entsteht für einige Minuten bis zu einer Stunde ein flaches EEG ähnlich dem B-Stadium, zusammen mit *raschen Augenbewegungen* (dicke schwarze Blöcke). Die untersten vertikalen Striche bezeichnen Körperbewegungen (lang: Lageänderung, kurz: kleinere Bewegungen). Die Pfeile bezeichnen das Ende einer cyclischen EEG-Periode nach dem Traumstadium und den Beginn der nächsten

[K 21]. Die gesamte Schlafdauer für einen Tag-Nacht-Cyclus soll von 18 Std beim Neugeborenen über 10 in der Pubertät auf 5-6 in höherem Alter sich langsam vermindern. Die durchschnittliche Schlafdauer erscheint weitgehend unabhängig von äußeren Bedingungen. Nachtschlaf oder Tagschlaf bei Nachtarbeit hat etwa gleiche Dauer. Auch unter extremen Bedingungen mit *fehlendem Tag-Nachtwechsel in Polargebieten* und auf verschiedene Stunden unregelmäßig verteilten Schlafzeiten ergaben systematische Schlafdauermessungen erstaunlich konstante Zeiten: Wenn der Schlaf bei wenigen zeitlich begrenzten Tätigkeiten nach Belieben gewählt werden konnte und zum Teil nur kurze mehrfache Perioden in 24 Std betraf, war das Endergebnis doch im Durchschnitt konstant, zwischen 7 und 8 Std [K 22, L 19]. Wenn auch einige Menschen im Winter etwas länger schliefen, so war dies wahrscheinlich ein „Luxuskonsum" an Schlaf. Die Kälte hatte keinen sicheren Einfluß, doch waren soziale Faktoren eher wirksam [L 19].

Schlafmangel, Übermüdung und Schlafentzug. Über totalen Schlafentzug bestehen sehr widersprechende Ansichten. Bei Tieren ist Schlafentzug meist mit starker Bewegungsbeanspruchung untersucht worden, so daß die beschriebenen, oft tödlichen Folgen des Schlafentzugs zum Teil durch extreme motorische Erschöpfung und Nebennierenschädigung zu erklären sind. Beim *Menschen* hat freiwillige Schlaflosigkeit, die bis zu vier Tagen durchgehalten wurde, ohne motorische Beanspruchung zwar zahlreiche psychische Veränderungen mit Halluzinationen und kurzen Teilschlafzuständen hervorgerufen, aber keine faßbaren körperlichen Schädigungen oder Nachwirkungen [B 32] außer epileptischen Manifestationen bei besonders disponierten Personen. In dem folgenden Endschlaf erfolgt eine gute Erholung mit Verschwinden der Symptome des Schlafentzuges. Biochemische Untersuchungen über Schlafentzug, die für die Frage der „Hypnotoxine" besonders wichtig wären, fehlen bisher. Anatomische Befunde über Verminderung der Nissl-Substanz in corticalen Nervenzellen nach Schlafentzug bei Hunden [L 6] sind durch motorische Beanspruchung schwer auswertbar.

Bei Übermüdung und kurzdauerndem Schlafmangel mit verspätetem Einschlafen ist die *Selbstwahrnehmung kurzer Schlafperioden stark vermindert*. EEG-Untersuchungen zeigen, daß Übermüdete zwar rasch und kurz in tiefere Schlafstadien C, D und E geraten [G 48]. Wenn sie spontan oder nach Außenreizen daraus erwachen, bestreiten sie aber meistens, geschlafen zu haben, obwohl das EEG eindeutige Schlafkurven zeigte [B 48]. Die psychischen und EEG-Veränderungen nach Schlafentzug werden auf S. 1002 besprochen.

Verhalten und physiologische Symptome des Schlafes

Reaktionsfähigkeit im Schlaf. Zahlreiche Beobachtungen zeigen, daß Sinnesreize im Schlaf verarbeitet und zum Teil beantwortet werden. Im EEG finden sich dabei meistens die verschiedenen Typen einer Weckreaktion, die in den einzelnen Schlafstadien verschieden sind, von der α-Aktivierung im leichten Schlaf des B- und C-Stadiums bis zum K-Komplex im C-, D- und E-Stadium und einer kurzen Abflachung der langsamen Wellen im E-Stadium. FISCHGOLD und SCHWARTZ haben 1961 die *Reaktionsfähigkeit auf einfache Sinnesreize in verschiedenen Schlafstadien* untersucht: Lichtblitze sollten mit einer kurzen motorischen Reaktion (Doppelsignalisierung) ohne sprachliche Leistungen beantwortet werden [F 12]. Ihre Versuchspersonen reagierten im Wachzustand immer richtig, im A-Stadium diffuser α-Aktivität mit vereinzelten fehlenden oder falschen Antworten, im B-Stadium mit mehr falschen, aber meist noch erhaltenen Reaktionen, im C-Stadium nur noch mit $1/3$ richtiger Antworten. Im tieferen Schlaf des D-Stadiums wurden keine Reize mehr beantwortet. Trotz fehlender motorischer Reaktionen wurden im C-D und E-Stadium auf die gleichen Reize meist noch deutliche hirnelektrische Antworten mit K-Komplex oder α-Aktivierung registriert.

Weckeffekte und *Reaktionen auf bedeutungsvolle Sinnesreize* im Schlaf sind biologisch wichtige Funktionen und vor allem bei Tieren lebensnotwendig. Eine Differenzierung von Sinnesreizen mit verschiedenem Weckeffekt ist nicht nur bei Wildtieren, sondern auch bei Haustieren zu beobachten: Ein Hund kennt den Schritt der Hausbewohner auch im Schlaf und regt sich nicht, wenn sie eintreten. Dagegen weckt jeder fremde Schritt den Hund sofort und bringt ihn zum Bellen. Hunde schlafen während eines lebhaften menschlichen Gesprächs im gleichen Zimmer, aber spitzen die Ohren, sobald man sie nur leise beim Namen ruft. Solche differenzierten Wahrnehmungen im Schlaf sind also allgemeingültige biologische Vorgänge und aktive Erkennungsleistungen des schlafenden ZNS bei Tier und Mensch.

Seit BURDACH 1830 darauf hingewiesen hat, daß die Wirksamkeit von Weckreizen weniger von der Lautstärke als von ihrem Bedeutungscharakter abhängt [B 72], sind solche Beobachtungen oft gemacht und an vielen Beispielen illustriert worden. Eine Mutter wird sofort durch leises Weinen eines Kindes, aber nicht durch lauten Verkehrslärm wach. Da Weckwirkungen beim Menschen vor allem durch sprachliche Kommunikation stattfinden und besonders auf den eigenen Namensanruf gerichtet sind, kann man eine erhaltene Funktion der corticalen Sprachzentren im Schlaf annehmen.

Periphere Funktionsänderungen im Schlaf. Periphere Schlafsymptome sind offenbar sekundär durch die Funktionsumstellung des ZNS und Vegetativum bedingt: Der *Augenschluß,* die *Pupillenverengung* und die *Schlafhaltung* sind aktive, die *Muskeltonusminderung,* das *Verschwinden der Eigenreflexe,* die *Blutdruckminderung* und die *Dilatation der Hautgefäße,* vielleicht auch die *Erektionen,* sind mehr passive, hemmende Änderungen der peripheren Funktionen. Folge der Schlafhemmung sind auch die *Hautwiderstandsvermehrung* (verminderte Schweißsekretion) und die *alveoläre CO_2-Vermehrung* (verminderte Atemtiefe), die einen ähnlichen Verlauf beim Schlafenden haben können. Die Areflexie im Schlaf ist nur zum Teil Folge der verminderten Grundinnervation der Muskulatur während der Schlafatonie (vgl. S. 995). Die vegetativen Reflexe der Vasomotorik und die galvanischen Hautreflexe bleiben im Schlaf erhalten oder sind sogar stärker ausgeprägt, wenn sie im Wachzustand durch Gewöhnung vermindert waren [J 36]. Periodische Tag-Nacht-Rhythmen verschiedener Organfunktionen wie der Leber sind in ihrer Beziehung zu tagesrhythmischen endokrinen Funktionen, zum Schlaf und zu den cerebralen Veränderungen noch nicht geklärt.

Schlaf und Atmung. Seit langem ist bekannt, daß die Atmungsventilation im Schlaf geringer ist als im Wachzustand und daß eine CO_2-Vermehrung des Blutes entsteht. Auch bei Gesunden können im Schlaf Atempausen von mehreren Sekunden auftreten. BÜLOW [B 71] hat die Atmungsveränderungen im Schlafen und Wachen genauer mit CO_2-Analysen und CO_2-Reizen untersucht. Er fand einen engen *Parallelismus zwischen Wachheitsgrad* (gemessen am EEG), *Atmungsaktivität und CO_2-Empfindlichkeit.* Selbst kurze Verminderungen der Wachheit mit EEG-Abflachung und Verlangsamung von wenigen Sekunden können bereits Atemventilationsminderungen hervorrufen. Diese Untersuchungen wie andere Erfahrungen sprechen für eine *enge Verbindung der Hirnstammstrukturen, die Wachheit und Atmung regulieren,* also der F. reticularis von Oblongata, Pons und Mittelhirn.

Eine extreme Variation oder Karikatur der verminderten CO_2-Empfindlichkeit mit periodischen Atempausen des normalen Schlafes findet sich beim Pickwick-Syndrom: Die CO_2-Empfindlichkeit ist schon im Wachen vermindert. Daher entstehen kurze Atemstillstände mit Einschlafen bereits aus dem vollen Wachzustand. Während des Nachtschlafes erscheinen längere Atempausen mit schwerer Cyanose (vgl. S. 1016).

Körpermotorik und Schlaf. Neben den oben erwähnten unbewußten Regulationen der Körperstellung und den unwillkürlichen Augenbewegungen gibt es im Schlaf charakteristische motorische Haltungsänderungen mit großen individuellen Variationen. Relativ konstant und zum Teil Gewohnheitsfolge, zum Teil genetisch bedingt sind die individuell verschiedenen *Schlafstellungen und Schlafhaltungen.* Sie sind bei eineiigen Zwillingen konkordant und bei zweieiigen meist verschieden. Andere motorische Begleiterscheinungen des Schlafes sind charakteristisch für bestimmte Schlafstadien: Die *Einschlafzuckungen* erscheinen mit dem ersten B-Stadium des Schlaf-EEG. Sie werden meistens nicht bemerkt, doch können sie bei unruhigem Einschlafen auch zu kurzem Erwachen und sensiblen Mißempfindungen führen.

Tonusverlust und Areflexie im Schlaf. Die Muskelatonie im Schlaf ist allgemein bekannt und auch dem Laien als „Einnicken" des Kopfes beim sitzenden Einschlafen geläufig. Auch das Verschwinden der Eigenreflexe wurde als Begleiterscheinung dieser Muskelatonie aufgefaßt. Maximale Muskelatonie entsteht im paradoxen Schlaf des Traumstadiums [J 15–17]. Neue Versuche von POMPEIANO, GASSEL u.Mitarb. [G 9, 19] an Katzen zeigten eine echte *descendierende Hemmung aus der unteren Reticularis* während des Schlafes. Danach ist es wahrscheinlich, daß die raschen Augenbewegungen und vielleicht auch die unregelmäßigen Zuckungen der Gesichtsmuskeln, die im Traumstadium beobachtet werden, in Neuronensystemen der bulbären Reticularis entstehen, die mit den Vestibulariskernen verbunden sind. Der verminderte Muskeltonus des paradoxen Schlafes kann bei vierbeinigen Tieren vor allem in der Nackenmuskulatur registriert werden. Beim Menschen ist die Entspannung der Nackenmuskulatur bekanntlich schon im B-Stadium bei leichtem Einschlafen Sitzender durch Vornüberfallen des Kopfes zu erkennen. Im menschlichen Schlaf mit Rückenlage ist die Tonusminderung des Traumstadiums besser von der vorderen Halsmuskulatur zu registrieren [J 3].

Pupillen und Augenbewegungen im Schlaf. Die *Pupillenverengerung Schlafender* ist seit 200 Jahren bekannt, seitdem FONTANA 1765 die Miose im Schlaf untersucht hat [F 21]. Diese Schlafmiose ist bei Mensch und Tier sehr konstant und auch bei BREMERs Präparationen des cerveau isolé und encéphale isolé mit verschiedenem Schlafverhalten erkennbar [B 61]. Sie wurde von HESS für seine Theorie des Schlafes als trophotroper Funktion verwendet [H 52]. Untersuchungen der Pupillenweite in verschiedenen Schlafphasen und während rascher Augenbewegungen im paradoxen Schlaf von MORUZZI u.Mitarb. [B 40] mit einem Pupillenfenster bei der Katze zeigten, daß auch blinde Katzen eine starke Schlafmiose, sowohl im Schlaf mit langsamen Wellen wie im paradoxen Schlafstadium haben. Leichte Weckreize erzeugten deutliche Pupillenerweiterungen, auch wenn das EEG keine arousal-Abflachung erkennen ließ. *Die raschen Augenbewegungen* im paradoxen „desynchronisierten" Schlafstadium waren immer mit phasischer *Pupillenerweiterung* verbunden. Neben den konjugierten raschen Augenbewegungen fanden sich bei der Katze auch asymmetrische dissoziierte Stellungen beider Augen [B 40].

Unwillkürliche Augenbewegungen Schlafender wurden zuerst beim Menschen von RAEHLMANN und WITKOWSKI 1874 als konjugiert oder dissoziiert beschrieben [R 3]. Sie blieben lange unbeachtet, bis ASERINSKY, KLEITMAN [A 31, 32] und DEMENT [D 24, 25] 1955–1957 die *raschen Augenbewegungen* als typisch für das Traumstadium erkannten und sie von den langsamen Deviationen abgrenzten. Seitdem gehört die Registrierung von Augenbewegungen zur neurophysiologischen Schlafuntersuchung bei Mensch und Tier, weil sie zur Charakteristik der Schlafstadien beiträgt und ein Erkennen des Traumstadiums erleichtert (vgl. Abb. 37).

Langsame und rasche Augenbewegungen im Schlaf. Bei gleichzeitiger Registrierung von EEG und Augenmotorik im Schlaf fanden ASERINSKY, DEMENT und KLEITMAN [A 31, D 24] *zwei Arten unwillkürlicher Augenbewegungen*: 1. *Langsame* rhythmische Deviationen sind fast immer horizontal gerichtet und erscheinen vor allem im Schlafbeginn und bei Körperbewegungen während des Schlafes. In Tiefschlafstadien fehlen diese langsamen Augenbewegungen, die auch in Perioden von etwa halbstündigen Abständen auftreten. 2. *Rasche* Augenbewegungen (ähnlich den Fixationsbewegungen im Wachzustand) erscheinen im Schlaf nur in bestimmten Perioden mit längeren, meist ein- bis mehrstündigen Abständen (Abb. 37). Sie sind oft horizontal, aber nicht selten auch vertikal gerichtet. Perioden rascher Augenbewegungen dauern bis zu 20 min und sind mit Steigerung der Pulsfrequenz und der Atmung verbunden sowie mit einem *flachen* EEG und verminderter Körpermotorik, mit Ausnahme gelegentlicher Gliedzuckungen oder Grimassen. Systematische Weckversuche ergaben keine Beziehung der langsamen Augenbewegungen zu Traumvorgängen, doch erscheinen sie im Einschlafstadium B zusammen mit hypnagogen Halluzinationen [K 63]. Nach Erwecken und Befragen der Versuchspersonen konnten *rasche Augenbewegungen fast immer mit Träumen korreliert werden*. KLEITMAN glaubt, daß es sich um *Folgebewegungen der Augen bei optischen Traumhalluzinationen* handelt.

Periodische Erektionen im Schlaf. Die bei Männern beobachteten periodischen Erektionen im Schlaf wurden zunächst ohne EEG-Kontrollen untersucht [O 1, 2]. Es handelt sich um mehrfache, in 1–2stündigen Perioden wiederholte Erektionen, die nicht zu Pollutionen führen. Sie wurden zunächst nur an wenigen Gesunden registriert, so daß die Häufigkeit des Vorkommens, die individuellen Variationen und mögliche Beziehungen zur sexuellen Abstinenz, zu Trauminhalten und bestimmten EEG-Stadien noch unbekannt waren. OHLMEYER u.Mitarb. [O 1, 2] bezeichnen diese Erektionen ausdrücklich als periodische Vorgänge. Da der cyclische Verlauf des Nachtschlafes bei diesen Befunden noch unbekannt war, blieben die Beziehungen zu Traumphasen noch nicht geklärt.

FISHER u.Mitarb. [F 13] haben 1965 OHLMEYERS Befunde mit polygraphischer Methodik bestätigt und eine enge *zeitliche Verbindung der periodischen Erektionen mit dem Traumstadium REM* festgestellt: Die Erektion beginnt mit der EEG-Abflachung und den raschen Augenbewegungen des paradoxen Traumstadiums oder einige Minuten vor dieser EEG-Veränderung (Abb. 38). Erektionen dauern meistens ebenso lang wie das REM-Stadium im EEG, manchmal auch länger, selten kürzer, wenn man nicht die volle Erektion, sondern die partielle Penisvergrößerung mitrechnet. Bei 95% aller Traumstadien wurden zeitlich kor-

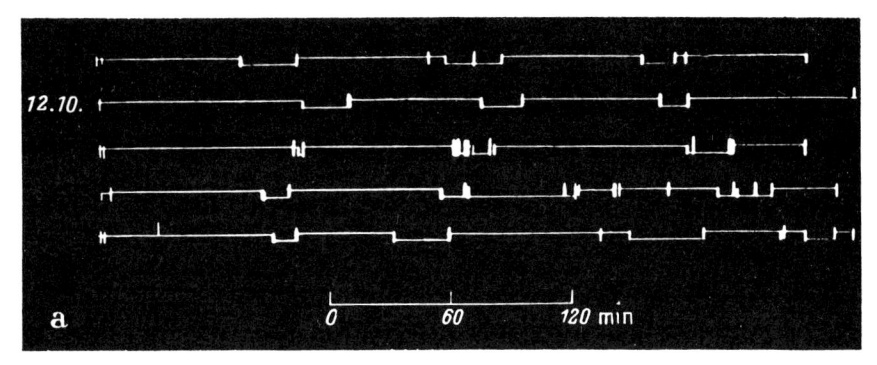

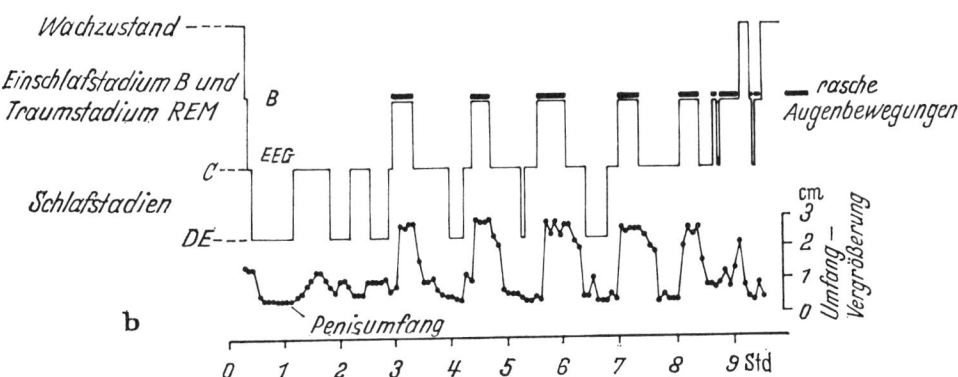

Abb. 38. Gleichlaufende Periodik der Traumstadien und der Erektionen im Nachtschlaf beim Mann. *a* Periodische Erektionen eines Mannes in 5 aufeinanderfolgenden Nächten nach OHLMEYER u.Mitarb. (1944) [O 2]. Die Untersuchungen wurden noch nicht mit EEG-Kontrollen verbunden, zeigten aber etwa die gleiche Zeitperiodik wie sie später für die Traumstadien festgestellt wurde (vgl. Abb. 37). Die mechanisch registrierten Erektionen sind die Ausschläge des Kymographions nach unten. *b Gleichzeitige Registrierung von EEG, raschen Augenbewegungen und Penisumfang* nach FISHER u.Mitarb. (1965) [F 13]. Die Erektionen beginnen etwa gleichzeitig mit dem Traumstadium REM und den raschen Augenbewegungen und überdauern meistens dieses Stadium noch einige Minuten. Im Einschlafstadium B, das im EEG eine ähnliche Abflachung wie das Traumstadium zeigt, fehlt die Erektion und im ersten Tiefschlaf entsteht eine Penisverkleinerung. Die vertikale Skala der letzten Kurve bezeichnet mit 0 den Umfang des erschlafften Penis und mißt nur die bei der Erektion auftretende Vergrößerung

relierte Erektionen registriert. Bei 17 Männern mittleren Lebensalters wurden keine Erektionen in anderen Schlafstadien gefunden, außer im B-Stadium. *Die Erektionen waren unabhängig von sexueller Abstinenz oder Befriedigung.* Als Erklärung werden u.a. diskutiert: vermehrte Erregung des limbischen Systems, unspezifische Irradiation von Instinkt- und Triebentladungen. Eine Beziehung zum Trauminhalt wurde oft vermißt, so daß die Autoren eine primäre *physiologische Ursache* und nicht eine Begleiterscheinung sexueller Traumvorstellungen annehmen. Bemerkenswert war jedoch eine negative Beziehung zu Trauminhalten, da *bei ängstlichen Träumen Erektionshemmungen* auftraten [F 13]. Neuere Studien [J 22] bestätigten FISHERs Befunde.

Es gibt abnorme *Steigerungen der Traumerektionen:* Bei längerer Dauer solcher Erektionen mit Weckeffekt kommen Patienten wegen dieser Symptome manchmal zum Arzt und die Erektionen werden als pathologischer Priapismus angesehen. Man kann die Patienten beruhigen, daß es sich nur um stärkere Ausprägung normaler Begleiterscheinungen des Schlafes handelt, die keine pathologische Bedeutung haben. Es ist noch wenig untersucht, aber wahrscheinlich, daß entsprechende lokale sexuelle Reizerscheinungen auch bei Frauen vorkommen. Wegen der geringen Größe des homologen Organs sind sie beim weiblichen Geschlecht bisher nicht registriert worden.

Elektrophysiologie des Schlafes

Im folgenden werden einige hirnelektrische Charakteristika des Schlafes bei Mensch und Tier besprochen. Untersuchungen über das *Elektrencephalogramm* (EEG) beim Menschen haben zwar unsere Vorstellungen über die Schlaffunktion in den letzten 30 Jahren sehr erweitert, doch beschränken sich die menschlichen EEG-Befunde auf die Hirnrinde der Konvexität, also den Isocortex. Subcorticale oder allocorticale Hirnpotentiale und Entladungen einzelner Neurone im Schlaf sind fast nur tierexperimentell untersucht, da beim Menschen nur wenige Beobachtungen über subcorticale Ableitungen vorliegen. Wir sind daher, wie auch sonst in der Neurophysiologie, auf Analogieschlüsse aus Tierversuchen angewiesen. Die elektrophysiologisch am besten untersuchten Katzen, Hunde und Affen schlafen ähnlich wie der Mensch. Bei diesen und anderen Säugern sind außer den verschiedenen typischen Schlafstadien auch die physiologischen Begleiterscheinungen der menschlichen Traumstadien nachgewiesen. Wir können zwar nicht wissen, ob auch Tiere Traumerlebnisse haben, ihr Verhalten spricht aber zumindest für Ähnliches. Da wir hier nicht psychische Inhalte, sondern cerebrale Mechanismen zu besprechen haben, mag der Analogieschluß von Tier- und Menschenbefunden bei der Schlafforschung wie in der Sinnesphysiologie und Triebphysiologie erlaubt sein.

EEG und Schlaf beim Menschen. Seitdem BERGER [B 26] 1931 zuerst EEG-Veränderungen im Schlaf feststellte, ist das Schlaf-EEG vor allem beim Menschen sehr genau untersucht worden. Die Schlafveränderungen des EEG, die bei jedem Gesunden allnächtlich auftreten und vor allem in einer Verlangsamung und Vergrößerung der Hirnwellen bestehen, unterscheiden sich stärker vom normalen Wach-EEG als das EEG bei vielen pathologischen Hirnerkrankungen. GIBBS, DAVIS und LENNOX [G 21] beschrieben 1935 zuerst langsame δ-Wellen im Schlaf-EEG, und LOOMIS u.Mitarb. [L 33–35] haben 1936–1938 eine genaue Untersuchung des Schlaf-EEG durchgeführt und verschiedene Schlafstadien A bis E unterschieden. F. und E. GIBBS haben dann Variationen des Schlaf-EEG in verschiedenen Altersstufen [G 22] und die pathologischen Veränderungen bei Hirnkrankheiten und Epilepsie [G 23] systematisch untersucht. Seit LOOMIS unterscheidet man die *EEG-Stadien A, B, C, D und E,* die vom Wachzustand mit Ermüdung (A) über das Einschlafen (B) und den leichten Schlaf (C) bis zum Tiefschlaf (D, E) reichen. Abb. 39 zeigt diese EEG-Stadien bei einem gesunden Erwachsenen. Ihr periodischer Ablauf wird durch flache EEG mit Augenbewegungen unterbrochen; die Traumstadien des paradoxen Schlafes werden jetzt meistens *REM-Stadium* genannt. Obwohl KLEITMAN [D 25, K 20] und andere

[R 7] unterschiedliche Bezeichnungen der Schlafstadien nach Nummern bevorzugen, ist es zweckmäßig, bei der alten Terminologie von LOOMIS zu bleiben. *Die einzelnen Schlafstadien können spontan und unter dem Einfluß äußerer Reize innerhalb kurzer Zeit wechseln.* Kurzzeitige Veränderungen des EEG bei spontanen Körperbewegungen und Schnarchen können auch entstehen, wenn ein Schläfer sich selbst durch lautes Schnarchen, das als akustischer Reiz wirkt, in ein leichteres Schlafstadium oder zum Erwachen bringt (z.B. von E in C oder von C in A).

Das Traumstadium des EEG (paradoxer Schlaf, REM-Stadium) entspricht nach den Untersuchungen von DEMENT [D 23–25] und KLEITMAN [K 19, 20] und den Befunden FISCHGOLDS [F 12] einem von LOOMIS weniger beachteten *Schlaftypus mit flachem EEG*, das *mit raschen Augenbewegungen einhergeht* (vgl. S. 1010). Dieses Traumstadium REM ähnelt dem *B-Stadium* LOOMIS, tritt aber nicht wie dieses kurz nach dem Einschlafen, sondern periodisch während des tiefen Nachtschlafes auf, entsprechend dem „paradoxen Schlaf" der Tiere (vgl. Abb. 37 u. 41).

Weckeffekte des EEG beim Menschen. Die Weckreaktionen des EEG sind verschieden, je nach dem Schlafstadium. Bei Ermüdung und im leichten Schlaf des B- und C-Stadiums geht meistens zunächst eine α-*Aktivierung* der α-Blockierung des arousal-EEG voran. In mittleren und tieferen Schlafstadien erscheint der von LOOMIS [D 6, L 35] beschriebene *K-Komplex*, eine große langsame Potentialschwankung mit einem Maximum parietal, auf der sich meist *a*-Wellen überlagern. Alle diese Phänomene sind verschiedene Formen einer *Bereitschaftsaktivierung des Cortex:* Die Aktivierung des EEG durchläuft in verschiedenen Zuständen corticaler Tätigkeit gewisse Stadien in bestimmter Richtung: von großen langsamen Wellen (Schlaf-EEG) über mittlere Rhythmen (α-EEG, BERGERS passives EEG) bis zu kleinen frequenten Schwankungen (β-EEG, BERGERS aktives EEG, arousal-EEG). Diesen Weckeffekten im EEG folgen dann die vegetativen Reaktionen des galvanischen Hautreflexes und der Vasomotorik [J 36] als weitere „ergotrope" Phänomene.

Wir haben die EEG-Veränderungen bei Schlaf und Weckreizen 1939/41 mit den Hessschen Konzeptionen der *ergotropen und trophotropen Beeinflussung des Cortex* in Parallele gesetzt [J 27]: Der *ergotropen Richtung* entsprechen auf der *psychologischen* Seite aktives Verhalten, Aufmerksamkeit, Hinwendung zur Außenwelt und Konzentration und die *elektrophysiologischen* EEG-Kriterien, Beschleunigung, Verkleinerung und verminderte Synchronisierung der Hirnwellen. Umgekehrt entsprechen der *trophotropen Richtung: psychologisch* passives Verhalten, Abwendung von der Außenwelt, Bewußtseinsverminderung bis zum Schlaf und *elektrophysiologisch* Verlangsamung, Vergrößerung und rhythmische Synchronisierung der Hirnwellen. Die physiologischen Mechanismen dieser vom Hirnstamm induzierten Cortexveränderungen sind durch Interaktion verschiedener aufsteigender Neurosysteme mit monoaminergen synaptischen Transmittern kompliziert (vgl. Abb. 35).

Die langsamen Wellen der Hirnpotentiale sind wahrscheinlich Ausdruck überwiegender Hemmungsvorgänge der cerebralen Strukturen. WALTER hat diese Schutz- und Hemmungsfunktion der langsamen Wellen poetischer ausgedrückt, indem er – wie FREUD vom Traum – von diesen Wellen als den „*Wächtern des Schlafes*" spricht [W 7].

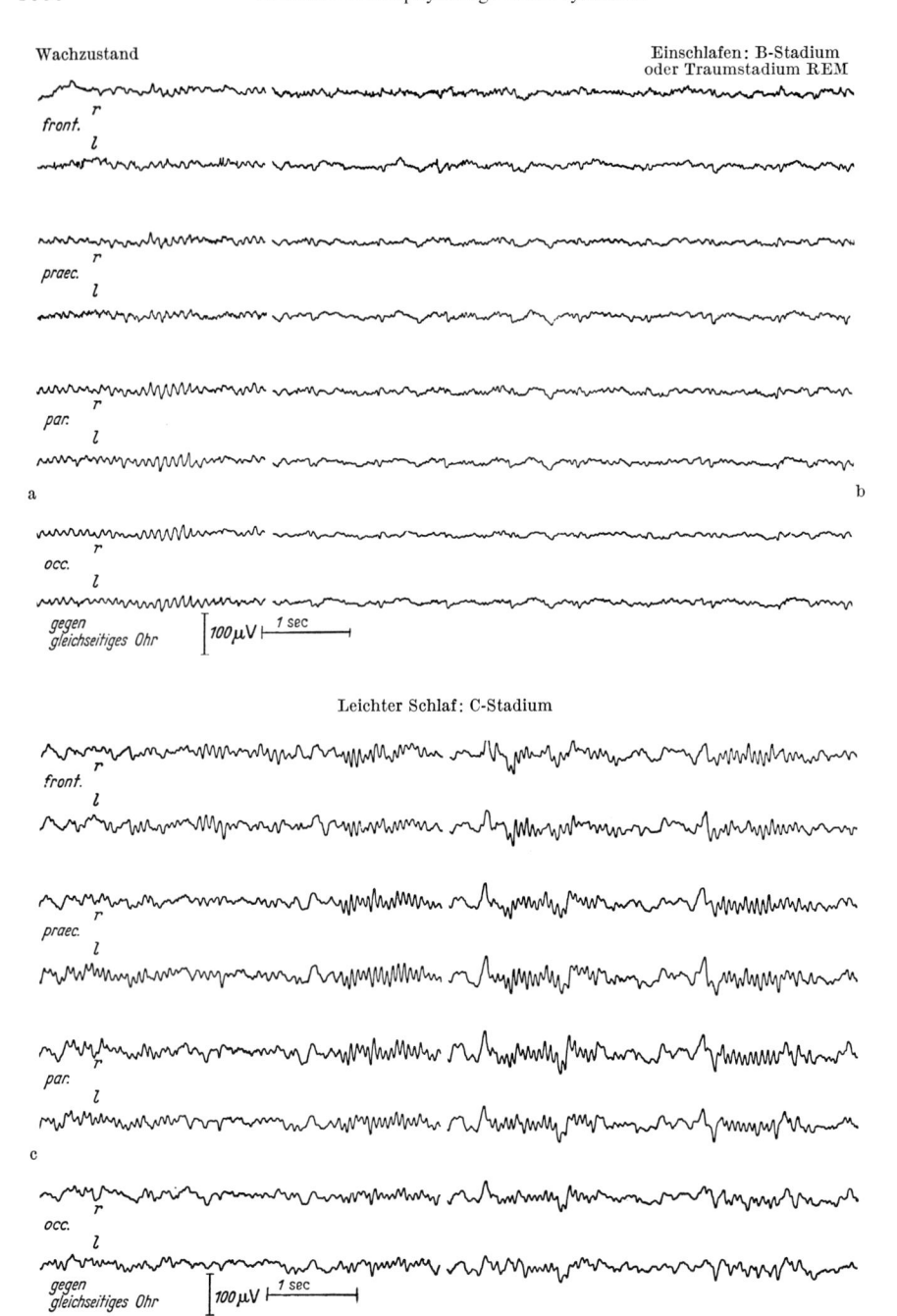

Abb. 39a–e. Das EEG der verschiedenen Schlafstadien beim Gesunden (nach Jung, 1953 [J 32]). Wachzustand: A, Schlafstadien B–E nach der Definition von Loomis u.Mitarb. [L 33, 34]. *a* Im Wachzustand periodische α-Wellen. *b* Nach dem Einschlafen B-Stadium: flaches EEG mit uncharakteristischen kleinen Wellen wechselnder Frequenz. Ein ähnliches EEG zeigt das *Traumstadium* in dem noch rasche Augenbewegungen dazu kommen. *c* Leichter Schlaf des C-Stadiums: typische

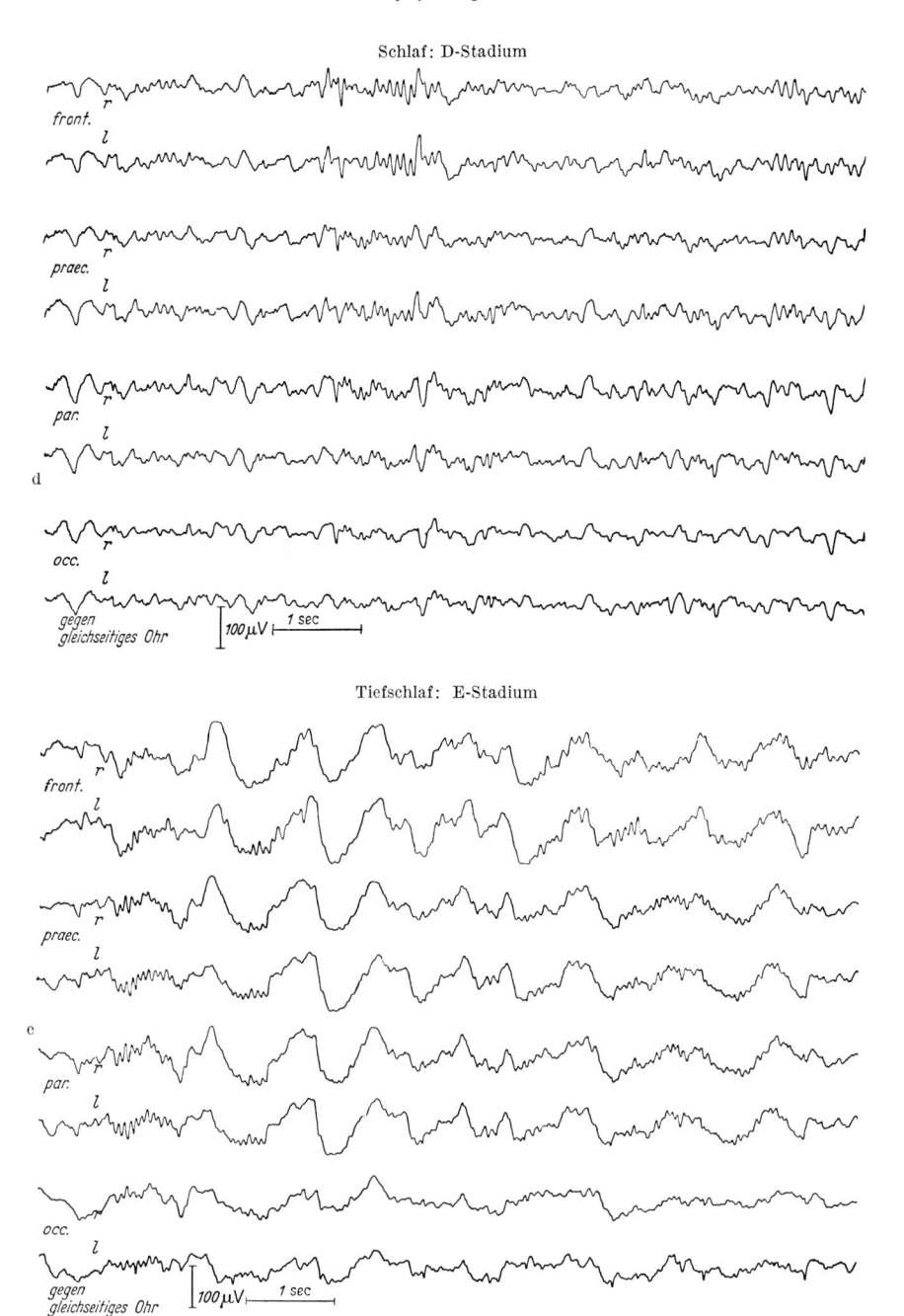

Schlafspindeln um 14/s mit größter Amplitude präzentral. Allmählich zunehmende kleine Zwischen- und δ-Wellen. *d* Mittlerer Schlaf im D-Stadium. Größere δ-Wellen um 3/sec und einzelne steile Wellen. Kleinere Schlafspindeln mit langsamer Frequenz von 12–13/sec. *e* Tiefschlaf im E-Stadium mit großen langsamen δ-Wellen von 0,6–1/sec und seltenen Schlafspindeln beim Übergang vom D-Stadium (29jähriger gesunder Mann)

Schlaf-EEG und Altersentwicklung. Die Veränderungen des *Schlaf-EEG in verschiedenen Altersstufen* sind bei F. und E. GIBBS systematisch ausgewertet und mit zahlreichen typischen Beispielen abgebildet [G 22]. Beim Säugling sind die Schlafperioden kürzer und die Grenzen von Einschlafen und Aufwachen schwerer zu bestimmen, da bereits das Wach-EEG des Säuglings langsame Wellen enthält. Bei älteren Kindern ist die Grenze gegen konvulsive Potentiale von Epileptikern, die auch im Schlaf aktiviert werden [G 22, 23] ebenfalls schwer erkennbar. Die im Einschlaf-EEG von Kindern zwischen zwei und acht Jahren häufigen Perioden langsamer δ-Wellen ähneln den Krampfwellen der Petit mal-Epilepsie und dürfen nicht mit ihnen verwechselt werden, ebensowenig die großen steilen Wellen, die bei älteren Kindern präzentral und parietal erscheinen (parietal humps GIBBS). Die Schlaf-EEG-Untersuchungen wurden von DREYFUS-BRISAC u. Mitarb. [D 36] noch auf Frühgeburten ausgedehnt. Sie haben die Entwicklung des Schlaf-EEG bei Frühgeburten und Säuglingen in einem übersichtlichen Schema 1957 dargestellt [D 36] und besonders deutliche Veränderungen im achten Monat nach der Konzeption und im dritten Monat des Säuglingsalters gefunden. Eine ähnliche Altersentwicklung des Schlaf-EEG fand CAVENESS [C 6] bei *Macacus-Affen*. Allerdings verläuft die Reifung zum Schlaftyp des Erwachsenen beim Affen rascher als beim Menschen. Die altersspezifischen Schlafstörungen bei Kindern werden mit ihren EEG-Korrelationen auf S. 1017 besprochen.

K-Komplex und Wahrnehmungsbereitschaft. Der K-Komplex ist eine in tiefen Schlafstadien auftretende EEG-Veränderung mit Gleichspannungskomponente, die oft, aber nicht immer als Reaktion nach Weckreizen auftritt. Beim K-Komplex erscheint zunächst eine längere elektronegative Potentialverschiebung mit maximaler Amplitude parietal und dann eine Gruppe von α-Wellen über dem gesamten Cortex. Er entspricht daher einer kurzen Periode verminderter Schlaftiefe, die aber subjektiv nicht zum Erwachen führt. Schon als LOOMIS u. Mitarb. [D 6, L 35] den K-Komplex des Schlaf-EEG nach akustischen Reizen beschrieben, bemerkten sie, daß entsprechende EEG-Muster auch ohne äußere Reize im Schlaf *spontan* auftraten. Dieses spontane Auftreten wurde aber bisher wenig beachtet und meist als Weckreaktion auf unbemerkte und im Versuch unbeabsichtigte innere oder äußere Sinnesreize oder als Schlafschutz [W 7] erklärt. VETTER und BÖKER [V 9] haben WALTERS Vorstellung, daß der K-Komplex ein Wächter des Schlafes sei, durch genauere Reiz-Reaktionsversuche als *Wahrnehmungsbereitschaft* präzisiert. Die spontanen K-Komplexe traten bei den beschriebenen Versuchspersonen in Abständen von etwa 1 min auf. Sie werden als *biologischer Schutzmechanismus* gedeutet, durch den der Schlafende periodisch wieder mit der Umwelt in Kontakt kommt. Bei gleichzeitig im selben Raum schlafenden Personen treten sie nicht synchron auf, sind also nicht durch äußere Reize, sondern höchstens durch innere Periodik zu erklären. Da der K-Komplex im Schlaf die *Bereitschaft zu Wahrnehmungen* verbessert, kann er mit der Erwartungswelle G. WALTERS und dem Bereitschaftspotential KORNHUBERS [K 43] im Wach-EEG verglichen werden (vgl. Abb. 11).

Schlafentzug und EEG. Es gibt verschiedene neuere Untersuchungen über *Schlafentzug* mit EEG-Kontrolle. Die ersten Beobachtungen von BLAKE und GERARD [B 47] 1937 mit 60stündigem Schlafentzug zeigten bereits bei leichter Entspannung ein rascheres Einschlafen mit großen langsamen Wellen. Ähnliches fanden GRÜTTNER und BONKALO [G 48] und TYLER u.Mitarb. [T 13, 14]: Längerdauernde EEG-Veränderungen fanden sich erst nach 50stündigem Schlafentzug mit langsamen δ-Wellen-Perioden (Mikroschlaf) und frequenten β-Wellen beim forcierten Wachzustand, der oft mit Halluzinationen und Wahnerlebnissen einhergeht [M 61, R 19].

RODIN u.Mitarb. [R 19] fanden mit langdauerndem Schlafentzug bis zu 120 Std neben dem Verschwinden von α-Wellen nach längerer Schlafkarenz und dem raschen Auftreten von langsamen Wellen auch vereinzelte abnorme *konvulsive Potentiale* und größere Lichtantworten bei Flimmerlichtreizung. Nach Weckmitteln wurde bei einer von 16 Versuchspersonen ein epileptischer Anfall ausgelöst, bei drei Versuchspersonen spikes und waves im EEG, ähnlich wie beim Petit-mal. Diese ungewöhnlich starken EEG-Anomalien und eine vermehrte Reaktion auf Megimid nach Schlafentzug entsprechen klinischen Beobachtungen über vermehrte Krampfbereitschaft von Epileptikern und latenten Epileptikern bei Schlafentzug.

Im ersten Nachtschlaf nach Schlafentzug von 4 Tagen zeigte das EEG nach BERGER und OSWALD [B 32] wesentlich *mehr langsame Wellen der Tiefschlafstadien und wesentlich kürzere Traumperioden*, die nach den raschen Augenbewegungen bestimmt wurden: Normal waren 6% Tiefschlaf mit langsamen Wellen, 22,5% Traumperioden mit raschen Augenbewegungen; nach Schlafentzug dagegen 26% Tiefschlaf, 7% Traumperioden. In der 2. Nacht des Erholungsschlafes wurden die Traumzeiten etwas länger als im Durchschnitt bei denselben Versuchspersonen.

Gleichspannungsänderung des Cortex im Schlaf. CASPERS [C 4] u.Mitarb. [C 5] fanden bei Ratten mit implantierten Elektroden, daß *mit oder vor dem Einschlafen eine oberflächenpositive Verschiebung der epicorticalen Gleichspannung* eintritt (Abb. 40), die während des Schlafes mit der Schlaftiefe wechselt. Nach *Weckrei-*

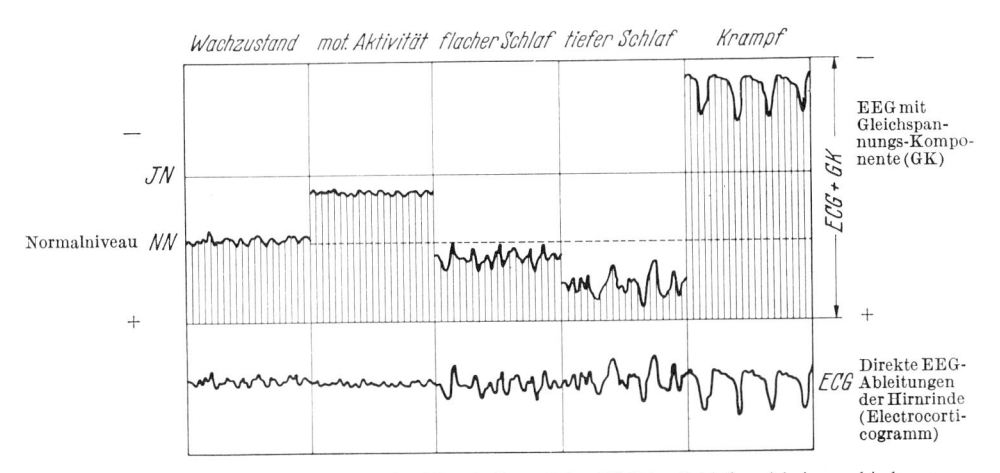

Abb. 40. Gleichspannungsänderungen der Hirnrinde und des EEG im Schlaf und bei verschiedenen Aktivitätszuständen Schema nach CASPERS und SCHULZER (1959) [C 5]. Im Wachzustand zeigt das Gleichspannungsniveau den Normalzustand NN (gestrichelte Linie). Im Schlaf verschiebt sich das Niveau nach der positiven, bei motorischer Aktivität und arousal nach der negativen Seite. Die Amplitude der EEG-Potentiale (Electrocorticogramm EGG und Gleichspannung GK) wird bei Verschiebung in beide Richtungen größer und tendiert zur Mittellage

zen findet sich umgekehrt eine oberflächen*negative* Gleichspannungsverschiebung [A 28]. Dieser entspricht wahrscheinlich die negative Komponente des „*K-Komplexes*" im menschlichen Schlaf-EEG. Ähnliche kleinere Gleichspannungsänderungen zeigt im Wachzustand die Erwartungswelle WALTERS [W 10] und das Bereitschaftspotential KORNHUBERS (vgl. S. 833). Es wird angenommen, daß diese corticalen Dauerpotentiale durch das unspezifische System reguliert werden, da nach Reizung von Thalamus und Reticularis ähnlich negative Gleichspannungsänderungen beobachtet wurden [A 28]. Entsprechende systematische Untersuchungen von Gleichspannungsänderungen im Schlaf bei Katzen und höheren Tieren liegen noch nicht vor, sind aber in Zusammenhang mit bedingten Reflexuntersuchungen [R 36] begonnen worden. Eine negative Gleichspannungsänderung zeigt sich im paradoxen Schlaf [K 9].

Es scheint eine allgemeine Regel zu sein, daß *oberflächennegative Gleichspannungen des Cortex mit Bereitschaftshaltung* und „arousal" korreliert sind, *oberflächenpositive dagegen mit Entspannung, Passivität und schließlich auch mit Schlaf.* Ausnahmen sind nur die großen oberflächennegativen Potentiale bei petit mal-Epilepsie [J 26] (vgl. S. 1035).

Neuronentätigkeit im Schlaf

Mikrophysiologie des Schlafes. Trotz der zahlreichen EEG-Untersuchungen über den Schlaf gibt es nur wenige *Mikroelektrodenuntersuchungen über Schlafen und Wachen.* Diese zeigen entgegen der Erwartung einer verminderten Neuronentätigkeit des Cortex im Schlaf bei Katzen eine auffallend lebhafte Entladung der Neurone sowohl im motorischen Cortex wie in der Sehrinde. Die Durchschnittsfrequenz ist im Wachen und Schlafzustand oft nur wenig verschieden und durch Weckreize werden einige Neurone aktiviert, andere gehemmt (C 16). Dies ist bei differenzierter Tätigkeit eines Neuronenkollektivs zu erwarten. Im Hirnstamm zeigen Reticularisneurone im paradoxen Schlaf vermehrte rasche Entladungen [H 97], wahrscheinlich eine Enthemmung.

Neuronale Aktivität im Cortex. Deutliche Unterschiede zwischen Schlaf und Wachen zeigt das *Entladungsmuster* der Cortex-Neurone: Die mehr oder weniger kontinuierlichen und mit unregelmäßiger, zum Teil auch reizabhängiger Aktivierung und Hemmung begleiteten Einzelentladungen der „wachen" Neurone werden im Schlaf in eine *periodische Gruppenentladung mit längeren Pausen* zwischen den Gruppen verändert. Diese Gruppenentladungen erscheinen etwa zu gleicher Zeit in benachbarten Neuronen, aber in verschiedenen Rindenarealen in unterschiedlicher Weise: Im sensomotorischen Cortex mit niederer Entladungsfrequenz meistens mit den Schlafspindeln des EEG, im visuellen Cortex dagegen mit hoher spike-Frequenz zwischen den Spindeln. An der freien Katze mit implantierten Mikroelektroden werden im natürlichen Schlaf in unregelmäßigen Abfolgen einzelne „spikes" der corticalen Nervenzellen nach Einschlafen in Gruppenentladungen mit mehr oder weniger hochfrequenten „bursts" verwandelt, die durch längere Pausen getrennt sind [H 86, V 8]. Ähnliche periodische Gruppen geringerer Frequenz haben Neurone des motorischen Cortex [C 16, E 23]. Diese gruppierten Neuronentladungen zeigen in ihrer Durchschnittsfrequenz gegenüber dem Wachzustand meistens keine wesentliche Verminderung, oft sogar höhere Durchschnittsfrequenz. Doch kann die Entladungsfrequenz durch Weckreize noch weiter gesteigert werden. EVARTS [E 22] fand, daß die Neurone in der Sehrinde während des Schlafes gegenüber dem Wachzustand vermehrt tätig sind. Mikroableitungen zeigen, daß im natürlichen Schlaf die Neurone des Cortex veränderte Entladungsmuster mit periodischer Aktivität zeigen.

Man kann aber nicht feststellen, ob andere Neurone, die in den Ableitungen nicht erscheinen, während des Schlafes inaktiv sind. Eine neuronale Entladungsruhe wie in tiefer Narkose besteht jedenfalls auch während des Tiefschlafes nicht.

Neuronale Schlafveränderungen im Subcortex. Bei der schlafenden Katze findet man ähnliche periodische Gruppenentladungen wie im Cortex nur im Thalamus, aber nicht in der mesencephalen Reticularis [S 7]. HUTTENLOCHER [H 97] zeigte, daß Mittelhirnneurone der Katze erheblich *schneller als im Wachzustand* (bis zur 40fachen Frequenz) entladen können. In der mesencephalen Reticularis finden sich aber auch Neurone, die beim Schlaf mit langsamen Wellen schwächer entladen und im Wachzustand beschleunigt werden. VERZEANO und NEGISHI [V 7, 8] fanden im Schlaf eine stärkere Synchronisierung der Neurone im Geniculatum und in den Reticularkernen des Thalamus mit Gruppenentladungen und langsam kreisender Erregung. Ähnliche periodische Entladungen sind in verschiedenen Zwischenhirnregionen, vor allem im Thalamus bei Barbituratnarkose, nachgewiesen [S 7]. Auch die Vestibulariskernneurone zeigen deutliche Veränderungen im Schlafen und Wachen [B 46].

Neuronale Weckreaktionen. Schon die ersten Beobachtungen an Neuronen der Pyramidenbahn durch WHITLOCK, ARDUINI und MORUZZI [W 21] 1953 zeigten, daß gewisse Neurone durch Weckreize häufig *gehemmt* werden. Doch haben wir 1957 auch neuronale *Aktivierungen* während des flachen aurousal-EEG an Neuronen des motorischen Cortex beschrieben [J 55]. Untersuchungen mit CREUTZFELDT [C 16] über mehrfache Neuronableitungen des motorischen Cortex der Katze zeigten ein *verschiedenes Weckverhalten der Neurone je nach ihrer Grundfrequenz:* Die „schnellen" Neurone, die während des Schlafes eine Frequenz von mehr als 9/s hatten, wurden durch Weckreize meistens weiter beschleunigt. Die „langsamen" Neurone mit niederen Entladungsfrequenzen im Schlaf wurden beim „arousal" meistens verlangsamt. Ähnliches hat auch EVARTS im visuellen Cortex gefunden [E 22].

Cerebrale Schlafregulation und Schlaffunktion. Der Schlaf ist nicht nur fehlende Wachaktivierung oder Abschaltung afferenter Impulse. Schlaf entsteht durch eine *aktive Leistung hypogener Mechanismen,* die vorwiegend vom *medialen Thalamus gesteuert* werden, aber – zum Teil antagonistisch-reziprok – auch von tieferen Teilen des *reticulären Systems in Mittelhirn, Pons und Oblongata,* jeweils in Zusammenarbeit mit höheren Strukturen, wie dem Caudatum und dem Cortex.

EEG-Registrierungen und Mikroelektrodenuntersuchungen zeigen ebenso wie die Verhaltensforschung und die Traumstadien, daß der Schlaf nicht ein passiver Zustand corticaler Inaktivität ist, sondern als eine *koordinierte Funktion cerebraler Regulationen* abläuft, die mit bestimmten neuronalen Hemmungs- und Erregungsvorgängen des Cortex verbunden ist. Die Schlafkoordination der

Hirnrinde wird durch subcorticale Strukturen geregelt. Cortex und Subcortex stehen in einer dynamischen Wechselwirkung für eine Restitutionsfunktion der höheren Hirntätigkeit; d.h. Schlaf hat eine *Erholungsfunktion*.

Biochemie und Stoffwechsel im Schlaf

Synaptische Überträgerstoffe und Schlafregulation. Biochemische und neuronale Transmitterveränderungen im Schlaf sind erst seit einem Jahrzehnt genauer untersucht worden. Die heute sehr aktuelle Neurochemie des Schlafes wird hier nicht behandelt, da dieses Gebiet noch sehr im Fluß ist: Zahlreiche neue Aspekte haben sich erst in den letzten 10 Jahren ergeben, und die vorwiegend bei niederen Säugern (Ratten) gefundenen schlafregulierenden Systeme des Hirnstammes müssen erst in ihrer Gültigkeit für den Menschen erwiesen werden. Eine aktuelle Übersicht über die Neurochemie des Schlafes bis 1971 gibt der Artikel von JOUVET [J 19]. Für eine geschlossene Darstellung dieses Gebietes ist die Zeit noch nicht reif.

In den letzten 20 Jahren haben schwedische und österreichische Forschungsgruppen von CARLSSON, HILLARP und HORNYKIEWICZ durch biochemische Analysen und fluorescierende Färbemethoden chemische Überträgerstoffe des Hirnstamms und der Stammganglien darstellen können, die das Großhirn beeinflussen. Diese Entdeckungen von FUXE, DAHLSTRÖM, UNGERSTEDT, HORNYKIEWICZ, BIRKMAYER, BERNHEIMER u.Mitarb. führten zu neuen Entwicklungen der Neurochemie und Neuropharmakologie, welche die hier darzustellende Neurophysiologie ergänzen [J 19]. Die neurochemischen Befunde wurden anatomisch unterbaut durch den Nachweis von aufsteigenden Neuronensystemen des Hirnstamms, die *spezifische Überträgerstoffe* (Transmitter) an den Kontaktstellen der Nervenzellen (Synapsen) freisetzen und durch ihre Monoamintransmitter – vorwiegend *Noradrenalin, Serotonin* und *Dopamin* – die verschiedenen Schlafperioden steuern (S. 980 u. Abb. 35). Die globale Funktionskonzeption der Formatio reticularis, die nach den Untersuchungen der 50er Jahre vor allem für die Regulierung von Wachheit und Bewußtsein diskutiert wurde, war damit zu ergänzen und zu korrigieren. Es wird Aufgabe zukünftiger Forschung sein, die im letzten Jahrzehnt entdeckten Neuronensysteme mit synaptischen Überträgern der Monoamine und des Acetylcholins, die vom Hirnstamm zum Großhirn projizieren und Veränderungen des Wachseins, des Antriebes und bestimmte Schlafstadien auslösen, mit den elektrophysiologischen, psychischen und Verhaltensuntersuchungen zu korrelieren.

Neurochemische Mechanismen der Schlafregulation im Hirnstamm sind nach JOUVET [J 19] verschiedene, zum Großhirn aufsteigende Neuronensysteme mit verschiedenen synaptischen Transmittern (Abb. 35). Die *serotonergen* Neuronensysteme sollen vorwiegend den *Erholungsschlaf* mit langsamen EEG-Wellen auslösen. Die *noradrenergen* Neuronensysteme können sowohl Weckwirkungen haben als auch sekundär den *REM-Schlaf* induzieren. Andererseits kann auch der Serotonin-induzierte Tiefschlaf den Mechanismus des REM-Schlafes in Gang setzen. Auch das *dopaminerge* System, das die Nigra vorwiegend mit dem Striatum verbindet und den motorischen Antrieb regelt, soll an der Schlaf-Wachregulation beteiligt sein. Eine Übersicht über drei monoaminerge Neuronensysteme, für Noradrenalin, Dopamin und Serotonin als Überträger gibt Abb. 35. Die

Zusammenarbeit dieser Transmitter mit den Actylcholin-Neuronen der cholinergen Hirnstammsysteme der oralen F. reticularis ist noch umstritten. JOUVETS Postulat, daß der synchronisierte Schlaf mit langsamen EEG-Wellen eine molekulare Erholungswirkung auf die Rindenzellen hat und der paradoxe REM-Schlaf Instinktmechanismen bahnt und übt, ist eine interessante aber noch unbewiesene Hypothese.

Schlaf und Hirnstoffwechsel. Das unklarste Kapitel der Schlafphysiologie sind die bisher nur vermuteten Stoffwechselveränderungen. Wenn der Schlaf ein Erholungsvorgang ist, so sollte man erwarten, daß im Schlaf auch Stoffwechselumstellungen gegenüber dem Wachzustand eintreten. Über diese metabolischen oder chemischen Veränderungen weiß man aber noch wenig.

Nach den vorliegenden Daten ist anzunehmen, daß *weder Durchblutung noch O_2-Verbrauch des Gehirns wesentliche Veränderungen während des Schlafes zeigen.* KETY [K 14, M 22] fand die Hirndurchblutung im Schlaf unverändert oder leicht erhöht, obwohl bei Weckreaktionen mit Blutdrucksteigerung im Tierversuch auch noch stärkere Durchblutungsvermehrungen festgestellt wurden [I 3]. Da auch hirnelektrische Ableitungen nur Formveränderungen der langsamen Potentiale, aber keine wesentliche Verminderung der Neuronentladungen zeigen, ist wahrscheinlich, daß der *Energiestoffwechsel des Gehirns während des Schlafes nicht wesentlich verändert ist.* Man wird daher nicht erwarten, Veränderungen des ATP und anderer energiereicher Phosphate zu finden. Die Schlafveränderungen der cerebralen Funktionen mit der Ausschaltung des Bewußtseins und der Änderung der Körperstatik und Motorik sind vielmehr Koordinationsumstellungen der Neurone und vielleicht auch der Glia. WÖHLISCHS Vorstellung [W 29], daß die vermehrte Aktivität des wachen Nervensystems eine Energieschuld auf sich nimmt, und diese einer echten Sauerstoffschuld entspricht, die während des Schlafes abgetragen wird, ist unbewiesen und unwahrscheinlich. Es scheint danach wenig aussichtsreich, nach biochemischen Umstellungen des Energiestoffwechsels im Schlaf zu suchen. Eher sind *Veränderungen des fermentativen Zellstoffwechsels und Strukturstoffwechsels* zu erwarten, vielleicht auch Änderungen in der Synthese der Desoxyribonucleinsäuren (DNS) oder Ribonucleinsäuren (RNS) der Zellkerne oder periodische Schwankungen des Stofftransports und der Bluthirnschranke in *Gliazellen.*

Das Einschlafstadium als Übergang von Wach- und Schlafzustand

Psychische und elektrophysiologische Einschlafveränderungen und Vorschlafstadien. DAVIS u.Mitarb. haben schon 1937 bei ihren Einschlafstudien [D 4, 5] enge *Korrelationen zwischen subjektiven Bewußtseinsänderungen und B-Stadium des EEG* exakt beschrieben. Ihre Versuchspersonen konnten vor dem eigentlichen Schlaf auftretende kurze Phasen von Wachheitsminderung einige Sekunden danach signalisieren. Diese Signale korrelierten gut mit der Abflachung des occipitalen α-Rhythmus, zum Teil auch mit langsameren Wellen in der Scheitelregion. In ihrer zweiten Arbeit [D 5] haben DAVIS u.Mitarb. die Beschreibungen der Einschlafphänomene, des „floating" ergänzt und versucht, sie vom echten Schlaf abzugrenzen. Sie bezeichnen die α-Verlangsamung als 4. Stadium der Einschlafveränderungen, durch die sie die Stadien A und B unterteilen, unterscheiden aber nicht scharf zwischen hypnagogen Halluzinationen und „dreaming", da das echte Traumstadium mit flachem EEG damals noch nicht bekannt war. Diese Untersuchungen wurden von KUHLO und LEHMANN [K 63] erweitert: Sie fanden, daß eine α-Verlangsamung schon bei sehr kurzdauernden Bewußtseinsschwankungen von 1–3 s auftreten kann und brachten eine bessere Abgrenzung zwischen hypnagogen Halluzinationen und Träumen. Diese kurzen Einschlafstadien werden von den meisten Versuchspersonen noch nicht als „Schlaf", sondern als „Wegbleiben", „Nicht-Da-Sein", „Abwesend-sein", „Einschlafbilder" und ähnliches bezeichnet.

Hypnagoge Halluzinationen, phantastische Gesichtserscheinungen und Träume. Die Psychologie des Einschlafens mit hypnagogen Halluzinationen ist seit JOHANNES MÜLLER 1826 und MAURY 1957 sorgfältig beschrieben und in ihren Beziehungen zu psychopathologischen Phänomenen oft diskutiert worden [M 27, 28, M 81]. Seit DAVIS [D 5] fehlten aber exakte Korrelationen mit EEG-Registrierung und Differenzierung vom Traumerleben. Dies haben KUHLO und LEHMANN [K 62, 63] bei Gesunden mit Kontrollen des EEG und der Augenbewegungen durchgeführt. Die Tabelle auf S. 1009 gibt eine Übersicht ihrer Ergebnisse. Bei EEG-Kontrollen ergab sich auch eine deutliche *Unterscheidung zwischen den seltenen „phantastischen Gesichtserscheinungen"* J. MÜLLERS *und hypnagogen Halluzinationen* im engeren Sinne [K 63]: Die phantastischen Gesichtserscheinungen entstehen *vor* dem Einschlafen mit einem Wach-EEG und sind lebhafte Bilder, die oft mit szenenhaftem Ablauf und häufig mit emotionaler Spannung einhergehen. Diese fehlen dagegen bei den elementaren, flüchtigen, blassen hypnagogen Sinnestäuschungen. Übergänge sind wahrscheinlich möglich und schon von J. MÜLLER beschrieben [M 81].

Die hypnagogen Einschlafbilder werden oft mit Traumbildern verglichen. Dennoch sind *hypnagoge Halluzinationen durch einen ungeordneten, flüchtigen, bruchstückhaften elementaren Charakter und das Fehlen affektiver Besetzung und subjektiver Aktivität vom Traum zu unterscheiden* [K 63]. Fortlaufend gestaltete Zusammenhänge und Handlungen fehlen beim Einschlafen, szenenhafte Darstellungen sind selten, im Gegensatz zum echten Traum. Die während hypnagoger Halluzinationen auftretenden *Augenbewegungen* sind langsame, mehr oder weniger rhythmische, horizontale Pendeldeviationen [K 63]. Dagegen erscheinen in den Traumstadien sehr unregelmäßige rasche fixationsähnliche Augenbewegungen in allen Richtungen [A 31, D 23, K 19, 20], die auf S. 996 beschrieben wurden.

Die Weckschwelle ist im Traumstadium erhöht, beim Einschlafen und während der hypnagogen Halluzinationen dagegen niedrig. Bei etwa einem Viertel von KUHLO und LEHMANNs Versuchspersonen fehlten hypnagoge Halluzinationen auch bei Weckversuchen. Die Beobachtungsfähigkeit für die kurzen Bewußtseinsveränderungen des Einschlafstadiums ist individuell sehr verschieden. Bei solchen Personen, die einen ausgeprägten kontinuierlichen α-Rhythmus hatten, konnten bereits kurze α-Pausen von 1–3 sec und Verlangsamung des α-Rhythmus von 10% durch die subjektive Beobachtung signalisiert werden [K 63].

Korrelation neurophysiologischer und psychischer Schlafsymptome. Nach vergleichenden Studien über EEG, Einschlafstadien und Träumen haben KUHLO und LEHMANN eine Übersicht psychischer und physiologischer Schlafphänomene gegeben, die in Tabelle 5 dargestellt ist.

Tabelle 5. Schema der neurophysiologischen und psychologischen Korrelationen in Wach- und Schlafstadien nach KUHLO und LEHMANN [K 63]. Die objektiven Befunde für EEG und Augenbewegungen sind in allen Schlafstadien exakt untersucht. Die subjektive psychologische Analyse ist dagegen nur im Schlafstadium B gut kontrolliert, aber wegen der mangelnden Selbstwahrnehmung in den tieferen Schlafstadien C, D und E zum Teil hypothetisch. Die gestrichelte Kurve der Affektstärke kann für diese Schlafstadien nur damit begründet werden, daß bei den seltenen Traumerlebnissen im C- und D-Stadium ebenfalls, ähnlich wie im Traumstadium, eine emotionale Besetzung erkennbar war, niemals dagegen bei hypnagogen Halluzinationen, die sich dadurch von phantastischen Gesichtserscheinungen in der Vorschlafphase unterscheiden (vgl. S. 1008).

Die Schlafstadien B, C, D und E von LOOMIS, DAVIS u.Mitarb. (D 5, L 34] entsprechen den Nummern 1–4 von KLEITMAN [K 19], das Traumstadium entspricht dem paradoxen Schlaf, dem Stadium REM der amerikanischen Literatur [D 25, R 7] und AB mo von FISCHGOLD [F 12]

	Wachzustand		Schlafstadien		
EEG-Stadien	arousal	A	B	C D E	Traumstadium „paradoxes" Stadium REM
EEG-Muster	flach	Alpha	verlangsamt abgeflacht Zwischen-W.	Spindeln Delta-W. K-Kompl.	niedrig unregelmäßig
Aufmerksamkeit	aktiv, vorwiegend nach außen gerichtet (offene Augen)	diffus, vorwiegend nach innen gewendet (geschlossene Augen)	fluktuierend, vermindert	fehlend	passiv von Traumbildern angezogen
Wahrnehmung und Vorstellung	Zieldenken	partielle gesteuerte Vorstellung freie Assoziationen	ungesteuerte Vorstellung Visualisierung. Hypnag. Halluzinationen Sinneselemente spontane Bilder	Szenen u. Traumfragmente	Träume mit gestalteten Handlungen
Ordnungsgrad der psychischen Inhalte	geordnet		ungeordnet		oneiroide Traumordnung
Erinnerbarkeit psychischer Inhalte	selektiv	gut	flüchtig oder fehlend	fehlend	partiell selektiv oder fehlend
Affektstärke					
Aktivitätsbewußtsein	aktiv	nachlassend	passiv		?
Situative Orientierung	real	real	dissoziiert oder fehlend	fehlend	irreal
Weckschwelle					
Augenbewegungen	willkürlich	unwillkürlich, seltene kleine Deviationen	rhythmische langsame, große horizontale Pendeldeviationen	keine	unregelmäßige rasche Augenbewegungen in allen Richtungen

Psychophysiologie des Träumens

Die paradoxen Schlafphasen als Traumperioden. Psychische Vorgänge laufen während der Schlafunterbrechung in veränderter Form weiter und sind seit alten Zeiten als Träume viel beachtet und verschieden gewertet worden. Die cerebralen Korrelate des Traumes bleiben lange unklar. Erst DEMENT und KLEITMAN [D 24, 25] konnten 1957 bestimmte periodische Schlafstadien mit flachem EEG und raschen Augenbewegungen dem Traumstadium zuordnen. DEMENT fand dann ähnliche EEG-Stadien mit solchen raschen Augenbewegungen auch bei Katzen [D 21]. Dieses Schlafstadium wurde bei den verschiedensten Tierarten festgestellt und als paradoxer Schlaf bezeichnet (vgl. S. 991). Die tierexperimentellen Untersuchungen über den paradoxen Schlaf ergänzten die EEG-Untersuchungen über die Traumstadien beim Menschen. Veränderungen in tieferen Hirnregionen während des paradoxen Schlafes sind uns daher zunächst nur bei Tieren bekannt. Die Analogien mit dem menschlichen Traumstadium sind so groß, daß keine Bedenken bestehen, auch diese Tierversuche zur Deutung der cerebralen Veränderungen im menschlichen Traumstadium heranzuziehen.

Neurophysiologische Korrelate des Träumens. Die Untersuchungen der letzten Jahre über das „paradoxe" Schlafstadium mit flachem EEG und raschen unwillkürlichen Augenbewegungen ergaben beim Menschen eine gute Korrelation dieser Schlafstadien mit Träumen. KLEITMAN, DEMENT u.Mitarb. [D 24, 25] beschrieben zuerst klare Korrelationen von Träumen mit *raschen Augenbewegungen* in bestimmten Schlafperioden. Diese raschen Augenbewegungen findet man jeweils mit einem *flachen EEG*, in späteren Schlafperioden 3–6mal während eines Nachtschlafes. Das EEG ist in diesem „paradoxen" Schlafstadium sehr ähnlich dem B-Stadium (stage 1 KLEITMANS) beim Einschlafen. Vom B-Stadium unterscheidet sich das Traumstadium nicht durch das EEG, sondern durch diese raschen Augenbewegungen, die auch für die Bezeichnung des „paradoxen" Schlafes verwendet werden: "rapid eye movements" = REM-stage der angelsächsischen Literatur. Im B-Stadium des Gesunden entstehen nur langsame rhythmische Augendeviationen, aber keine raschen Augenbewegungen. Diese erscheinen erst später, wenn die Tiefschlafstadien D und E in periodischem Wechsel von paradoxen Schlafstadien abgelöst werden (Abb. 38). *Wenn die Schläfer in diesem „paradoxen" Stadium geweckt werden, berichten sie meistens über Träume.*

Nach etwa 1 Std des ersten Tiefschlafes (C–E) erscheint oft eine kurze Periode mit flachem EEG entsprechend dem B-Stadium, die meistens *nicht* mit Augenbewegungen und Träumen verbunden ist. *Rasche Augenbewegungen sind daher ein besseres neurophysiologisches Kriterium für Träume als die EEG-Muster.* Sobald die raschen Augenbewegungen auftraten, verminderten sich auch Muskeltonus und unwillkürliche Körperbewegungen. Ein vermehrtes Wiedereinsetzen der Körperbewegungen im Schlaf entsteht nach Beendigung des Augenbewegungsstadiums.

Die Traumstadien der *"rapid eye movement periods"* (REM), verbunden mit Abflachung des EEG, die den langsamen Wellen des C-, D- oder E-Stadiums folgen (Abb. 41), erscheinen 3–6mal in der Nacht und haben eine zunehmende Dauer von durchschnittlich 9–34 min. Jeweils nach einer Periode des Tiefschlafs

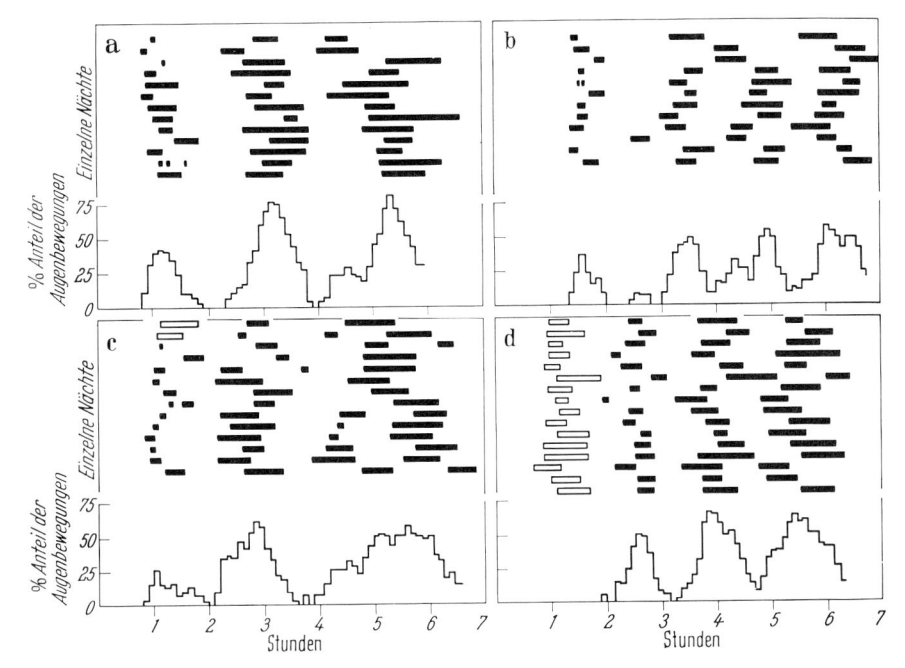

Abb. 41 a–d. Traumstadien mit raschen Augenbewegungen im Nachtschlaf von 4 verschiedenen Personen (a–d). Nach DEMENT und KLEITMAN (1957) [D 25]. Die schwarzen Blöcke oben bezeichnen die Dauer der raschen Augenbewegungen während der Traumstadien in verschiedenen Nächten. Jede horizontale Linie entspricht einer Nacht. Die offenen Rechtecke bezeichnen das C-Stadium des ersten Schlafcyclus. Unten sind Histogramme und Augenbewegungsperioden in % für die gesamten Nächte angegeben, die das Durchschnittsauftreten der Traumcyclen in etwa 2stündigen Intervallen bei jedem Individuum besonders deutlich zeigen

mit EEG-Stadium D und E entstehen in Abständen von 1–3 Std die typischen Cyclen mit Augenbewegungen und flachem EEG.

Die Deutung KLEITMANS, daß die raschen Augenbewegungen das *Verfolgen von Traumbildern* ermöglichen [K 19], ist noch umstritten. Für diese Deutung spricht der Befund von BERGER u. Mitarb. [B 31], daß bei Blinden rasche Augenbewegungen nur auftreten, wenn visuelle Bildvorstellungen und Traumhalluzinationen vorhanden sind, daß dagegen bei kongenital Blinden und älteren Blinden ohne visuelle Vorstellungen Augenbewegungen meist fehlen. Gegen Zusammenhänge mit cortical lokalisierten Sehbildern sprechen Befunde JOUVETS [J 17], daß rasche Augenbewegungen im paradoxen Schlaf auch bei Katzen ohne Hirnrinde erhalten bleiben und die Ergebnisse von BERLUCCHI u. Mitarb. [B 40], daß neugeborene Katzen ohne Seherfahrung die gleichen raschen Augenbewegungen haben.

Die zahlreichen experimentellen Versuche über die Beeinflussung von Traumbildern können hier nicht besprochen werden. Neurophysiologisch interessant, aber durch spätere Untersuchungen nicht genügend bestätigt, sind PÖTZLS Experimente über Auslösung von Traumbildern durch im Wachzustand nicht klar erkannte tachistoskopische Reize [P 27]. Eine Diskussion dieser und anderer experimenteller Untersuchungen einschließlich der Mescalin-Halluzinationen findet man bei KLÜVER [K 23]. Alle psychologischen Traumstudien sind durch die Amnesierung erschwert und bleiben in ihren Ergebnissen vieldeutig.

Traumentzug. DEMENT hat bei gesunden jungen Versuchspersonen die Traumperioden mit EEG-Kontrollen jeweils durch Weckreize unterbrochen. Er fand, daß nach einem solchen Traumentzug die Traumphasen in den nächsten Nächten verlängert waren und daß die Versuchspersonen Angst, Reizbarkeit und Konzentrationsstörungen zeigten. Meistens fand sich auch ein vermehrter Hunger in den Tagen nach Traumentzug. Diese Veränderungen verschwanden, sobald wieder ununterbrochene Traumzeiten eintraten. Durch Kontrollen mit Weckreizen in anderen Schlafstadien wurde sichergestellt, daß die Veränderungen nicht unspezifische Weckeffekte waren. DEMENT schließt aus diesen Untersuchungen, daß eine bestimmte Traumzeit für den gesunden Menschen notwendig ist [D 22].

Träume als affektive Abreaktionen mit Amnesierung. Nach physiologischen und psychologischen Befunden ist anzunehmen, daß jeder Gesunde allnächtlich in 3–5 Traumstadien mehr oder weniger visualisierte Abreaktionen von Triebspannungen durchmacht, aber sie *völlig amnesiert*. Eine Ausnahme bilden nur die wenigen Träume, die bei raschem Erwachen erinnert werden. Solche *affektiven Abreaktionen mit Amnesierung* erscheinen im Traum automatisch und sind weitgehend unabhängig von bewußtem Erleben und Umwelt. Der träumende Schläfer erhält seine Triebentladungen gewissermaßen „gratis" ohne Verhaltenskonsequenzen und neue Umweltkonflikte. Daß sowohl angenehme wie unangenehme Affekte dabei beteiligt sind, ergibt sich aus dem Trauminhalt. Wenn manche Personen unangenehme ängstliche Träume öfter erinnern, so sind auch diese Erinnerungen offenbar Ausnahmen unter den häufigeren, völlig amnesierten ähnlichen Angstträumen.

Die Traumstadien erscheinen damit physiologisch als zweckmäßige und für den sozialen Kontakt unschädliche, intracerebrale Manifestationen der Affekt- und Triebmechanismen, die in periodischer Folge während des Nachtschlafes erscheinen. Ob sie bewußt erlebt und erinnert werden, ist damit sekundär. Die oben erwähnten Experimente DEMENTS über den Traumentzug (durch frühzeitiges Wecken im paradoxen Schlafstadium) sprechen für unbewußte, affektive Traummechanismen, obwohl sie keinen Beweis für die Zweckmäßigkeit des Traumgeschehens bilden. Die verlängerten und früh auftretenden atypischen Traumstadien, die bei Narkolepsien im Nachtschlaf erscheinen, und die mit einer vermehrten affektiven Labilität der Narkoleptiker verbunden sind, zeigen die *beschränkte Wirksamkeit der Traummechanismen für eine Stabilisierung des Affekt- und Trieblebens*. Narkolepsien haben trotz ihrer verlängerten Traumstadien meistens eine vermehrte emotionale Labilität. Ob diese wiederum verlängerten REM-Schlaf auslöst, ist unbekannt.

Beim Menschen sprechen Beobachtungen über die Menstruations- und Pollutionsträume für hormonelle Einwirkungen auf Traummechanismen und Trauminhalte. Ob diese Beeinflussungen direkte Hormonwirkungen auf das limbische System sind, die nach hirnelektrischen Befunden diskutiert wurden, bleibt vorläufig offen.

Bei Nahrungsmangel enthält der Trauminhalt vorwiegend Bilder des Eßtriebes. Man kann daher annehmen, daß bei allgemeiner Aktivierung von Triebspannungen im Traumstadium jeweils unterschiedliche affektive Abreaktionen von Trieben entstehen können.

Psychoanalytische Traumdeutungen und Neurophysiologie. Obwohl hirnelektrische Befunde nichts über seelische Inhalte aussagen können, stimmen doch Psychoanalyse und Neurophysiologie darin überein, daß Affekte und cerebrale Triebmechanismen am Traumgeschehen beteiligt sind. Es wäre aber eine unzulässige Verallgemeinerung, wenn man Träume nur als Affekt- und Triebwirkungen im Schlaf auffassen wollte, oder sie wie FREUD [F 29] nur sexuell deuten würde.

Wie immer ist es leichter, psychologisch verständliche Vorgänge in Träume zu projizieren, auch wenn sie sinnlos erscheinen, oder durch Herausgreifen einzelner Symbolbeziehungen einen Traum zu deuten, als ihn physiologisch zu erklären. *Dennoch impliziert der psychoanalytische Rückgriff auf das Unbewußte damit auch nicht-seelische, neurophysiologische Prozesse.* Die Rolle von Sinnesreizen und Organstörungen ist zwar für die Traumentstehung weniger wichtig als man früher glaubte, aber doch sichergestellt und experimentell prüfbar. Exakte Nachprüfung psychotherapeutischer Traumdeutungen ist aber meistens nicht möglich. Die Zusammenhänge sind entweder evident oder nicht. Deshalb kann der Psychotherapeut viel unbeschwerter Traumdeutungen vorschlagen, als der Neurophysiologe das Traumgeschehen erklären kann. Dem Physiologen glaubt man nur nach experimentellen Nachweisen, die mehrfach gesichert sein sollen. Für den Psychotherapeuten genügt im Einzelfalle der Glaube seines Patienten. Es würde die Analyse auch nicht weiterführen, wenn wir durch EEG-Untersuchungen wüßten, ob die berichteten Träume im ersten oder letzten Traumstadium auftraten, ob sie mit flachem EEG oder Schlafspindeln verbunden und ob Tagträume mit einem Wach-EEG korreliert sind.

Man sieht aus allen Untersuchungen mit objektiver Registrierung, wie *unzuverlässig die Traumerinnerung ist.* Die bei der Psychotherapie verwendeten Träume betreffen wahrscheinlich nur eine kleine Selektion von Morgenträumen und vielleicht auch von Affektträumen mit Weckwirkung. Bei der Unklarheit und Unsicherheit der Traumerinnerung muß man damit rechnen, daß viele Traumberichte verändert und ausgeschmückt wiedergegeben werden.

Neurophysiologie der Schlafstörungen und pathologischen Schlaf-Syndrome

Die neurophysiologischen Schlafuntersuchungen bringen auch manche klinisch wichtigen Anregungen. Schlafstörungen waren bis zur Entdeckung des EEG eines der unsichersten Kapitel klinischer Forschung, da meist nur subjektive Angaben von Patienten vorlagen. Es fehlten exakte Untersuchungen und klare Kriterien über Schlaftiefe, Schlafdauer, Weckwirkung, periodische Schlafzeiten und Halbwachen bei psychiatrisch Kranken. Ältere Schlaf- und Weckuntersuchungen wurden nur bei wenigen gesunden Versuchspersonen durchgeführt. Außer einzelnen Neurasthenikern wurden keine pathologischen Schlafstörungen untersucht. Diese unbefriedigende Situation änderte sich auch nicht, als nach FREUDS Traumbuch [F 29] 1900 eine sehr ausgedehnte Beschäftigung der Psychotherapie mit dem Traum einsetzte. Da Traumerinnerungen unsicher und oft verfälscht sind und sich, wie oben beschrieben, meist auf wenige Morgenträume oder auf Träume mit kurz darauf folgendem Erwachen beschränken, blieb die Traumforschung mehr Spekulation und Symboldeutung als Wissenschaft. Auch exakte deskriptive Bemühungen um die Schlaf- und Traumforschung durch französische Untersucher im 19. Jahrhundert [M 27, 28] und durch HOCHE [H 72] waren wegen der geringen Zahl der Selbstbeobachter und mangels objektiver Registrierungen für den Physiologen unbefriedigend. Erst die oben beschriebenen EEG-Studien über die Periodik des Schlafes und die typischen Traumstadien mit flachem EEG und Augenbewegungen ermöglichten objektive Untersuchungsmethoden in der Schlaf- und Traumforschung.

Die neurasthenischen Schlafstörungen (chronische Schlaflosigkeit). Diese in der allgemeinen Praxis häufigste chronische Schlafstörung ist nach EEG-Untersuchungen [K 13, S 19] keine „Schlaflosigkeit". Der Glaube an fehlenden Schlaf entsteht bei diesen Patienten durch eine *niedrige Weckschwelle* und vermehrte subjektive Beachtung der normalen Schlafperiodik mit *affektiver Überbewertung kurzer Wachperioden*. Eine *erniedrigte Weckschwelle* führt zu kurzem Erwachen durch unbedeutende Sinnesreize (Glockenschlag, Verkehrslärm), die der Gesunde nicht beachtet. Die affektive Besetzung bedingt vermehrte Beachtung und Verlängerung von normalen kurzen Wachperioden des Nachtschlafes.

Ohne scharfe Grenze zeigt die chronisch-neurasthenische „Schlaflosigkeit" Übergänge zu zwei *passageren* physiologischen Schlafstörungen, die meistens nur kurzdauernd bei den meisten Gesunden auftreten: 1. verzögertes Einschlafen und leichtere Erweckbarkeit bei Erregung, Furcht und Sorge, 2. äußerlich bedingte Unregelmäßigkeiten des Schlafrhythmus durch vermehrte Weckreize, Nachtdienst, Überarbeitung oder Reisen mit Verschiebung der Tag-Nacht-Grenze.

Wer diese Störungen genauer beobachtet und hoch bewertet, glaubt, ebenso wie die chronisch „Schlaflosen", sehr wenig oder nicht geschlafen zu haben. Dennoch zeigen Kontrollen mit dem EEG, daß *Schlafdauer und Periodik des Nachtschlafes bei der neurasthenischen „Schlaflosigkeit" nur wenig verändert sind:* Beim Vergleich von angeblich völlig „Schlaflosen" mit gesunden Kontrollen gleichen Alters findet man nur eine längere Einschlaflatenz mit etwas längeren Wachphasen, aber etwa gleiche Schlafdauer [K 13, S 19]. Das EEG mit voller nächtlicher Registrierung beweist, daß auch solche Neurastheniker, die fest glauben, nicht geschlafen zu haben, *mehrfach in der Nacht einen Tiefschlaf erreichen,* wie man schon immer nach häufigem Schnarchen vermutet hat. Der „Schlaflose" kann also ziemlich tief schlafen, obwohl er es nicht weiß und meist energisch bestreitet. *Die Dauer der Schlaflosigkeit wird von dem Patienten, der „jede Stunde schlagen hört", überschätzt, da er die Schlafperioden zwischen den Wachperioden nach weckenden Reizen nicht bemerkt.* Umgekehrt bemerkt der Gesunde nicht die kurzen Wachzeiten, die bei Geräuschen oder nach Traumstadien den Schlaf kurz unterbrechen. Die Häufigkeit solcher Wachzeiten mit wiederkehrenden α-Wellen zeigt jede kontinuierliche EEG-Registrierung des Nachtschlafes bei Gesunden. Die mehrgipflige Schlaftiefenkurve, die nach alten Weckuntersuchungen charakteristisch für Neurastheniker sein sollte [E 17], ist nach den neueren EEG-Registrierungen eine normale Folge der Schlafperiodik, die auch alle bisher untersuchten Gesunden mit gutem Schlaf hatten. Wirklicher Schlafmangel würde bei den Patienten nur dann auftreten, wenn sie aus Ungeduld über verzögerten Schlaf längere Zeit Licht machen, lesen oder aufstehen. Man wird deshalb von solchen Schlafunterbrechungen abraten, auch dem „Schlaflosen" entspannte Bettruhe empfehlen und möglichst wenig Schlafmittel verschreiben. Günstige Wirkungen von Schlafmedikamenten sind wahrscheinlich rascheres Einschlafen und erhöhte Weckschwellen. Beides läßt sich vielleicht auch durch Psychotherapie erreichen.

Die depressive Schlafstörung. Gestörter Nachtschlaf ist ein Achsensymptom der Depression [J 30]. Die depressive Schlafstörung ist häufiger und konstanter als andere somatische Begleiterscheinungen der Depression, wie Obstipation und Appetitmangel oder sogar als psychische Melancholiesymptome wie Antriebsminderung, Hemmung, hypochondrische Ideen oder Schuldgefühle. Sie ist oft mit vermehrter Ermüdbarkeit am Tage verbunden, aber nicht nur sekundäre psychische Folge der Verstimmung. Doch gibt es auch seltene *Depressionen mit vermehrter Schlafneigung* und längerem Nachtschlaf. Die Beziehungen zwischen Depression und Schlafregulation sind offenbar sehr komplex, da auch kurzer Schlafentzug depressive Verstimmungen bessern kann [F 8]. Wahrscheinlich sind die vom Hirnstamm zum Großhirn aufsteigenden Systeme mit verschiedenen synaptischen Transmittern für Schlaf- und Stimmungsregulation durch unterschiedliche Psychopharmaka beeinflußbar.

Die depressive Insomnie ist schwerer als die neurasthenische Schlafstörung. *Depressive haben längerdauernde nächtliche Wachperioden von mehrstündiger Dauer, die zu echtem Schlafmangel führen:* Hirnelektrische Registrierungen des Nachtschlafs von OSWALD u.Mitarb. [O 14] zeigen bis zu $4^1/_2$ Std kontinuierliche Wach-EEG-Perioden bei Depressionen, während bei Gesunden nächtliche Wach-EEG-Perioden fast nie über $^1/_2$ Std dauern und bald von Schlafperioden des B-, C- und D-Stadiums abgelöst werden.

Nach OSWALD u.Mitarb. [O 14] bewirkte die Barbituratbehandlung neben kürzeren Wachperioden vor allem in den frühen Morgenstunden auch Verkürzungen der Traumstadien mit raschen Augenbewegungen. Die Registrierung der Körperbewegungen zeigte bei Depressiven nur in den Traumstadien, während derer sich Gesunde wenig bewegen eine stärkere Körpermotilität. Wie Thymoleptica die depressiven Schlafstörungen verändern, ist noch wenig untersucht. Von physiologischem Interesse wäre die Wirkung von Monoaminooxydasehemmern auf die monoaminhaltigen Neuronensysteme des Hirnstamms und des Ammonhorns.

VAN REY und WISSFELD [R 13], fanden ähnliche Schlaf-EEGs wie OSWALD mit langen Wachperioden bis zu 3 Std Dauer, alternierend mit durchschnittlicher Schlaftiefe bei einzelnen Depressiven. Häufiger zeigten ihre depressiven Patienten einen *flachen Schlafverlauf mit rascher Fluktuation zwischen Wachsein und leichten Schlafstadien*.

Die Narkolepsie. Die *Schlafanfälle* unterscheiden sich im EEG kaum vom normalen Schlaf. Der affektive Tonusverlust oder die *Kataplexie* zeigt kurze Abflachung der α-Wellen [J 7]. Im Liegen kann auch beim kataplektischen Anfall ein Schlaf-EEG entstehen [H 44]. Die *Wachanfälle*, ein verzögertes motorisches Erwachen mit traumhaften Erlebnissen wurden im EEG selten genau untersucht. Folgender stark vereinfachter Vergleich von Normalschlaf und Narkolepsie erscheint neurophysiologisch erlaubt: *Der Schlafanfall entspricht Schlafstadien mit langsamen Wellen (C, D), die Kataplexie ähnelt mehr dem Traumstadium (REM).*

Der *Nachtschlaf des Narkoleptikers* unterscheidet sich vom normalen Nachtschlaf: Untersuchungen von RECHTSCHAFFEN u.Mitarb. [R 7] 1963 über kontinuierliche Registrierungen des Nachtschlaf-EEGs der Narkoleptiker mit Augenbewegungen zeigten *vorzeitig auftretende Traumstadien anstelle des normalen B-Stadiums,* weniger langsame δ-Wellen und häufigere α-Wellen über der vorderen Schädelhälfte und stärkere motorische Unruhe. Dieses frühe Traumstadium paßt zu der klinischen Erfahrung, daß Narkoleptiker oft über abendliche Einschlafstörungen mit optischen Halluzinationen und traumähnlichen Zuständen klagen. Offenbar haben viele Narkolepsien schon beim abendlichen Einschlafen *vorzeitige Traumstadien,* die sich von den hypnagogen Halluzinationen auch subjektiv durch eine komplexe Erlebnisweise und ihre affektive Betonung unterscheiden. Psychopathologisch finden sich Übergänge zu den phantastischen Gesichtserscheinungen JOHANNES MÜLLERS [M 81], die im halbwachen Zustand ohne äußere Schlafzeichen und ohne den Tonusverlust des Schlafes auftreten. RECHTSCHAFFEN u.Mitarb. [R 7] deuten die frühen Traumstadien der Narkoleptischen im Anschluß an JOUVETS „rhombencephalen Schlaf" [J 15] als vorzeitiges Ausklinken von *pontin-reticulären Schlafmechanismen.* Offenbar besteht bei der *Narkolepsie mit Kataplexie* eine stärkere *Dissoziation zwischen dem niederen und höheren reticulären System.* Das relative Überwiegen des einen oder anderen Systems würde dann die Symptomatologie bestimmen: Bei Dominanz diencephaler Schlafmechanismen wären *Schlafanfälle* das häufigste und führende Symptom, bei Enthemmung der pontinen Reticularis würden die selteneren *kataplektischen Zustände* entstehen.

Das Pickwick-Syndrom. Diese Form der periodischen Hypersomnie wurde früher verkannt und als atypische Narkolepsie angesehen. Erst Untersuchungen amerikanischer Autoren [A 36, B 75] haben die Kombination von *Adipositas, alveolärer Hypoventilation (mit* CO_2*-Vermehrung im Blut), Cyanose und mehrfachem, kurzen Einschlafen mit periodischen Atempausen* klar beschrieben. Der Name stammt aus DICKENS Roman „Pickwick papers", der einen „fat boy" beschreibt, der solche periodischen Schlafzustände zeigte. Durch die Schwere dieser Atemstörungen mit längeren Atempausen und tiefer Cyanose unterscheiden sich solche Patienten von Narkoleptikern. Patienten mit Pickwick-Syndrom berichten im Gegensatz zu Narkoleptikern nicht über auffällige hypnagoge Halluzinationen beim Einschlafen oder über Dissoziationsphänomene wie „Wachanfälle". Auch affektiver Tonusverlust wurde nie beobachtet. Das *EEG der Pickwick-Patienten* zeigt schon am Tage *gleichzeitig mit einer Apnoe Abflachungen entsprechend dem B-Stadium.* Ohne Atmungsbeobachtung oder -registrierung kann das EEG kaum von den kurzen Einschlafzuständen der Narkoleptiker oder übermüdeter Gesunder unterschieden werden [G 16, K 62].

Die Atemstörungen sind besonders beim *Nachtschlaf* verstärkt mit bis zu 40 sec dauernden Atempausen, tiefer Cyanose und dann folgenden einzelnen tiefen schnarchenden Atemzügen. Die Nachtschlafregistrierungen wurden erst neuerdings von KUHLO [J 61, K 62] systematisiert und zeigten durch diese Atempausen und Fehlen langer, früher Traumstadien deutliche Unterschiede gegenüber der Narkolepsie. Von internistischer Seite wurden vor allem die cardio-vasculären Störungen mit O_2-Minderung und CO_2-Vermehrung in der Alveolarluft und im Blut untersucht [B 75, D 35, G 16].

Die *Therapie durch Entfettung* bessert zwar diese Hypoventilation und das Einschlafen am Tage wird seltener, die Atmungspausen werden kürzer, doch bleibt der abnorme Nachtschlaf mit kurzer Apnoe erhalten.

Periodische Schlafzustände (Kleine-Levin-Syndrom). Dieses zuerst von KLEINE [K 16] 1925 in der Kleistschen Klinik und LEVIN [L 15] 1936 erneut beschriebene Syndrom der periodischen Schlafzustände findet sich fast nur bei jungen Männern nach der Pubertät. Es handelt sich um *mehrtägige Schlafzustände,* die mit kurzen Pausen und verschiedener Tiefe bis zu Wochen andauern. Sie können als einmalige Episode erscheinen oder mehrfach, um im späteren Alter zu verschwinden. Zwischen diesen Schlafperioden sind die Kranken unauffällig. Während der Schlafperioden sind sie für kurze Zeit erweckbar und zeigen oft vermehrten *Hunger mit Polyphagie und Verstimmungen* [C 19]. Hypnagoge Halluzinationen mit partiellen Schlafzuständen kommen gelegentlich vor, doch fehlen typische Narkolepsieanfälle. Oft entstehen im Schlaf oder Halbwachzustand besonders am Ende der Schlafperiode *sexuelle Erregungszustände,* die zu vermehrter Masturbation führen. Die Schlafperioden werden oft durch Infekte eingeleitet, doch ist deren Zusammenhang mit den Schlafzuständen ungeklärt. Der Blutzucker ist meist etwas erniedrigt, aber es besteht keine schwere Hypoglykämie. Eine endokrine Genese ist oft diskutiert, aber nie nachgewiesen worden. Das EEG entspricht dem natürlichen Schlafzustand [R 26].

Somnambule Schlafsyndrome. *Pavor nocturnus* ist eine häufige, Schlafwandeln eine seltene Schlafstörung bei Kindern. Auch diese Syndrome sind als partielle Schlafzustände zu deuten, die aber entgegengesetzt zur Kataplexie ein *motorisches Erwachen mit psychischem Schlaf* darstellen: Der Schlafwandler bewegt sich unbewußt mit guter motorischer Koordination und ist nach dem Wecken für seine somnambulen Handlungen amnestisch, ähnlich wie ein Epileptiker im Dämmerzustand. Der Schlafwandler zeigt im EEG die Kennzeichen des Tiefschlafes [J 3a]. Dagegen scheint der Pavor nocturnus mehr dem Traumschlaf verwandt. Obwohl Nachtwandeln meist als neurotische Störung angesehen wird und wie andere Schlafstörungen auch durch psychische Konflikte gebahnt werden kann, ist eine organische Grundlage, sei es durch Besonderheiten der kindlichen Hirntätigkeit oder hereditär familiäre Disposition wahrscheinlich. Fließende Übergänge bestehen offenbar vom Pavor auch zum „unruhigen Schlaf" mancher Gesunder mit „Alpdruck" und lebhaften Angstträumen, die zum Aufschreien und Sprechen im Schlaf führen. In solchen Fällen tritt das Symptom bei Erwachsenen nur vorübergehend in einer ungelösten Konfliktsituation auf.

Das EEG von Kindern mit Pavor nocturnus ist entweder normal oder zeigt im Wachzustand vermehrte Dysrhythmien, vor allem temporal, die aber schwer von den normalen Variationen des kindlichen EEG und der cerebralen Reifung zu unterscheiden sind. Das Schlaf-EEG ist noch wenig untersucht und kann normal sein oder selten Anomalien, wie die von GIBBS [G 24] beschriebenen 14 und 6/sec positiven Spitzen, zeigen. Noch seltener finden sich epileptische Zeichen im EEG. *EEG-Befunde während somnambuler Zustände* zeigten, daß die somnambulen Episoden nicht im Traumstadium, sondern im Tiefschlaf mit langsamen Delta-Wellen auftreten.

GASTAUT teilt die verschiedenen nicht-epileptischen Schlafepisoden in drei Klassen: 1. *Integrierte Automatismen,* bei denen der Schlaf unverändert weiterläuft, wie *Einschlafzuckungen, automatisches Kauen, Jactatio capitis.* 2. *Inerrante Episoden,* die in ein leichteres Schlafstadium überleiten, aber nicht zum Erwachen führen: *Schlafsprechen, automatische Gesten, somnambule Handlungen und Enuresis.* 3. *Aberrante Episoden,* die den Schlaf mit Erwachen unterbrechen: *Alpdruck mit schweren Angstzuständen* und vegetativen Entladungen, *Schlaftrunkenheit.* In der dritten Gruppe fanden sich niemals echte Träume, sondern nur nachträgliche ad hoc-Erklärungen der Angstzustände [G 10a].

Psychosen, Schlaf und Traum

Einschlafdenken, Traum und psychiatrische Symptomatologie. *Parallelen von Traum und Psychose* sind schon seit DESCARTES von GRIESINGER [G 42], MOREAU DE LA TOUR [M 54], MAURY [M 28] vor allem im 19. Jahrhundert mit ihren psychologischen Beziehungen oft diskutiert worden. Ähnlichkeiten hypnagoger und traumhafter Halluzinationen bei Gesunden mit dem Halluzinieren bei deliranten und oneiroiden Psychosen (MAYER-GROSS u.a.) und bei Hirnstammencephalitiden wurden zunächst ohne EEG-Untersuchungen beschrieben [C 11, M 29, 30]. CARL SCHNEIDER [S 9] hat nach introspektiven Beobachtungen Parallelen des dissoziierten Einschlafdenkens mit schizophrenen Denkstörungen diskutiert und CONRAD [C 11] hat die Beziehungen von Wahn und Traum behandelt (vgl. S. 1019). Seit FREUD [F 29] ist die Traumanalyse zu einer wichtigen Methode der Psychotherapie geworden. Alle diese Entwicklungen verliefen ohne Kenntnis der physiologischen Grundlagen von Traum und Schlaf, die erst durch das EEG gefördert wurden.

Die *Beziehungen von Schlaf und Psychose* bei der *Depression* sind noch ungeklärt. Die Schlafstörung als Achsensyndrom der Depression wird durch die Schockbehandlung beseitigt, indem die epileptische Entladung einen Erholungsschlaf erzwingt [C 14a]. Andererseits kann verkürzter Schlaf auch depressive Stimmungen günstig beeinflussen [F 8], während Schlafmittel allein ohne Thymoleptica wenig wirksam sind.

Symptomatische Psychosen und partielle Schlafmechanismen: Delir und Traum. Bei symptomatischen und epileptischen Psychosen, insbesondere bei den deliranten Syndromen ist die klinisch eindrucksvolle Parallele mit dem Traumerleben seit dem vorigen Jahrhundert psychopathologisch begründet worden. Wenn epileptische Dämmerattacken als traumhaft geschildert werden (dreamy states JACKSONS) oder „neurologische" Schlafstörungen wie die narkoleptischen Teilsyndrome der Kataplexie und des Tonusverlustes durch partielle dissoziierte Schlafzustände erklärt werden, so sind auch für das *Delir partielle physiologische und psychische Schlafmechanismen des Traumes* in Erwägung zu ziehen. Ähnlich dem Traumerleben zeigen auch die Delirien vorwiegend visuelle Sinnesphänomene mit bewegten optischen Halluzinationen und häufige Traumaffekte wie Angst und Spannung. Zwar erscheint das motorische Verhalten des Deliranten mit Tremor, unstetem Blick und Bewegungsunruhe der Ruhe des Schlafes gerade entgegengesetzt zu sein. Doch ist daran zu erinnern, daß die „Traumstadien" des Schlafes bei Mensch und Tier neben schnellerem Puls und aktivierter oder unregelmäßiger Atmung auch durch vermehrte rasche Augenbewegungen, Zukkungen der Gesichtsmuskulatur, also auch durch eine relative Bewegungsunruhe charakterisiert sind. Das delirante Fehlen der normalen Schlafruhe ist besonders beim Alkoholdelir deutlich, dessen tagelange Unruhe meistens von einem Terminalschlaf abgelöst wird. Im Gegensatz zu den Entziehungsdelirien nach Barbiturat- und Meprobamatabusus, die meist epilepsieähnliche EEG-Veränderungen mit langsamen Wellen zeigen, findet man beim Alkoholdelir auch flache oder fast normale EEGs ohne langsame Wellen, die erst später oder terminal mit dem Schlaf auftreten. Da auch die Traumstadien des menschlichen Schlafes mit flachem EEG ohne langsame Wellen einhergehen (vgl. S. 1010), würde das Alkoholdelir im EEG sogar dem Traum ähnlicher sein als andere Delirformen mit epileptischen Erscheinungen. Nur bei manchen Formen der temporalen Epilepsie, ihren Dämmerattacken und „dreamy states", könnte man in den rhythmischen Krampfentladungen des basalen Schläfenlappens eine unsichere hirnelektrische Ähnlichkeit mit den beim Tier festgestellten vergrößerten Ammonshornrhythmen des „paradoxen" Schlafes der Traumstadien [G 36, S 34] sehen.

C. FISHER hat psychopathologische und psychoanalytische Folgerungen aus der modernen Schlafforschung und aus eigenen Registrierungen der Traumphasen dargestellt [F 12a]. Neuropharmakologische Beobachtungen über Verkürzungen der Traumphasen nach bestimmten Medikamenten werden für eine Deutung der *Entziehungspsychosen* verwendet: Da Barbiturate, Alkohol und Weckmittel wie Dexedrin die Traumphasen verkürzen und Entziehungspsychosen nach Medikamentabusus auslösen, werden diese Psychosen als *Einbruch der Traumphase in den Wachzustand* erklärt. Ob dies auch für halluzinierende Schizophrene gilt, muß zunächst offen bleiben.

Anwendungen auf schizophrene Störungen. CARL SCHNEIDERS Vergleiche von Einschlaferleben und Schizophrenie haben mehr die Unterschiede als die Gemeinsamkeiten beider herausgestellt und keine neurophysiologischen Folgerungen ermöglicht [S 9]. CONRAD [C 11] hat *Wahn und Traumerleben* verglichen und angenommen, daß ein gleichartiges physiologisches Geschehen beidem zugrunde liege, das im Schlaf auf physiologische, im Wahn auf pathologische Mechanismen zurückgehe. Die katathymen paranoiden Mechanismen sollen sich „zum echten Wahn verhalten wie der Wachtraum zum Schlaftraum": Obwohl der Inhalt von Traum und Psychose durch emotionale Vorgänge und frühe Erlebnisse mitbedingt wird, bleibt doch der physiologische Zustand des Schlafes die eigentliche Ursache des Traumes und nicht die psychogene Inhaltsdeterminierung aus der Erfüllung von Wünschen und Ängsten. Für Beziehungen zum psychotischen Wahn sind die Beobachtungen wichtig, daß Wahnerlebnisse bei Menschen nach mehrtägigem Schlafentzug regelmäßig vorkommen [B 32, O 13]. Diese kurzen paranoiden Erlebnisse beim Schlafentzug sind im Gegensatz zum psychotischen Wahn meist flüchtig. Sie werden später nicht emotional fixiert und oft vergessen.

Schlaf und Gedächtnis

Schlafamnesie und Gedächtnisfixierung. Eine fehlende Erinnerung ist charakteristisch für den Schlaf, auch für die Traumstadien und die Schlafpausen. Ob diese Schlafamnesie mit einer Gedächtniserholung oder mit etwaigen amnestischen Fixierungsvorgängen während des Schlafes zusammenhängt, ist noch nicht bewiesen aber wahrscheinlich. Die Erinnerungsfähigkeit wird von der Ermüdung über das Einschlafstadium bis zum Tiefschlaf zunehmend schlechter und eine Amnesie ist für den Nachtschlaf die Regel. Ausnahmen sind stärkere und bedeutungsvolle Weckreize, gelegentlich erinnerte hypnagoge Halluzinationen, eindrucksvolle Träume oder affektiv bedingte Einschlafstörungen oder längere Schlafunterbrechungen. Die Schlafamnesie bewirkt offenbar auch das Vergessen kurzer Schlafpausen. Selbst stärkere Affekt- und Triebentladungen von Träumen werden meistens völlig amnesiert, wenn sie nicht durch Wecken im Traumstadium unmittelbar exploriert werden. Das Vergessen dieser Träume und nächtlichen Schlafpausen zeigt, daß weder das B- oder Traumstadium (mit flachem EEG, ähnlich dem „arousal") noch die Schlafpausen mit α-Wellen dem Tages-Wachzustand mit Bewußtseinsklarheit und guter Erinnerung gleichzusetzen sind. Es bleibt offen, ob der einzige im EEG faßbare Unterschied (geringe Verlangsamung der α-Wellen gegenüber dem Wachzustand) mit der Störung der Gedächtnisfunktionen korreliert ist. Ähnlicher dem Wachzustand sind die Schlafunterbrechungen bei neurasthenischer „Schlaflosigkeit", die durch affektive Bahnung besser erinnert werden als ähnliche Schlafpausen bei Gesunden. Im Gegensatz zur Merkfähigkeitsstörung während des Schlafes werden jeweils vor dem Schlaf erworbene Gedächtnisinhalte durch Schlafvorgänge nicht beeinträchtigt, sondern eher in ihrer Erhaltung verbessert und im Gedächtnis fixiert.

Durch psychologische Experimente über Lernvorgänge vor und nach dem Schlaf wurde mehrfach bestätigt, daß Schlafen die Fixierung von Gedächtnisvorgängen begünstigt. PLOOG [P 24] hat daher angenommen, daß die physiologischen *Schlafvorgänge zur Konsolidierung der Gedächtnisprozesse beitragen*. Dies geschieht, obwohl, oder gerade *weil* während des Schlafes Lernen und Gedächtnis *ausgeschaltet* sind. Über die physiologischen Mechanismen dieser Schlafkonsolidierung von Gedächtnisinhalten wissen wir noch ebensowenig wie über die Grundlagen des Gedächtnisses allgemein. JOUVET hat eine spezielle Funktion der paradoxen Schlafphasen für die Gedächtnisvorgänge angenommen und während der Traumstadien eine Informationsspeicherung molekularer Prozesse mit Übung von Instinkt-Koordinationen vermutet [J 17, 19]. Wahrscheinlicher ist eine Beteiligung *aller* Schlafstadien an einer *Gedächtnisfixierung vorangehend erworbener Erinnerungen*. Ob der integrierte Erholungsschlaf mit langsamen EEG-Wellen oder der dissoziierte Traumschlaf mit flachem EEG jeweils an der Gedächtniskonsolidierung stärker beteiligt sind, ist noch unbekannt.

Amnesierung des Schlaferlebens und amnestische Syndrome. Typisch für alle psychischen Schlafphänomene, von den hypnagogen Bildern bis zu den Träumen ist ihre mangelnde Erinnerung. *Die Merkfähigkeit für neue Erlebnisse und echte Lernfunktionen sind im Schlaf weitgehend ausgeschaltet.* Nur baldiges Erwachen kann Reste der Schlaferlebnisse bewahren. „Lernen im Schlaf" ist eine contradictio in adjecto. Alle modernen Schlaf- und Traumuntersuchungen mit kombinierten psychologischen und neurophysiologischen Methoden zeigen rasches *Vergessen* des Einschlaf- und Traumerlebens. Die Ursachen dieser Amnesierung sind noch nicht geklärt, scheinen aber mit den elektrophysiologischen Begleiterscheinungen des Schlaf-EEG ebenso korreliert wie amnestische Syndrome der traumatischen Psychosen mit Allgemeinveränderungen des EEG. Bei der geringen Ordnung mit mangelnder Klarheit und Bewußtseinshelle des Einschlaf- und Traumerlebens ist auch eine geordnete Erinnerung erschwert. Daß vorwiegend affektiv verstärkte Trauminhalte erinnert werden, könnte durch Weckwirkung solcher emotionaler Träume erklärt werden. Affektiv indifferente Einschlaferlebnisse sind meistens nur durch Weckversuche unmittelbar nach dem Erleben zu erfahren, bevor sie dem Vergessen anheim fallen.

Ähnliche hirnelektrische Veränderungen im Schlaf und bei pathologischen Bewußtseinsstörungen lassen auch ähnliche physiologische Prozesse bei normalen und pathologischen Merkstörungen vermuten. Ob die Verlangsamung der EEG-Wellen oder die Gleichspannungsverschiebungen für die Amnesierungsvorgänge wichtiger sind, ist noch unbekannt. Vermutlich ist beides mit biochemischen Umstellungen verbunden. Allerdings sind die EEG-Formen bereits im Schlaf recht verschieden, doch gilt die Regel, daß die *Erinnerung um so schlechter ist, je mehr das EEG langsame Wellen zeigt.* Ähnlich korreliert die Intensität traumatischer amnestischer Syndrome mit der Ausprägung und Rückbildung pathologischer Allgemeinveränderungen und langsamen Wellen im EEG. Delirien und Halluzinosen mit flachem EEG haben bessere Erinnerungsfähigkeit für die Psychose.

Die seit FREUD bevorzugte Erklärung der Traumamnesierung durch Verdrängung ist offenbar zu einseitig und nicht für pathologische Amnesiesyndrome gültig. Obwohl gezielte Verdrängung *ein* Faktor des Vergessens sein kann, ist ein anderer viel wichtigerer die *fehlende Ordnung* der Erlebensweisen, die sich auch in hirnelektrischen Veränderungen zeigt. Deshalb wird der Neurophysiologe affektive oder zensurierte Verdrängungsamnesierungen nicht als allgemeine Grundlage des Vergessens anerkennen; denn er kann nur Korrelationen amnestischer Zustände mit Hirnfunktionsänderungen und EEG-Störungen feststellen, aber nicht mit affektiven Entladungen oder erlernten Zensurbestimmungen. Die Amnesierung ist für die emotional indifferenten gleichgültigen Einschlafbilder mindestens ebenso stark wie für emotional beladene Traumbilder. Die EEG-Muster sind bei beiden Zuständen (B-Stadium und paradoxer Schlaf) fast identisch. Den übrigen Schlafstadien ähnliche EEG-Veränderungen mit langsamen Wellen entsprechen bei Gesunden und Kranken psychische Befunde verminderter Merkfähigkeit und Bewußtseinsklarheit. Fehlende Verarbeitung und mangelnde Ordnungsfunktion der Erlebniszusammenhänge sind auch psychologische Bedingungen mancher Amnesierungsvorgänge, die wenigstens teilweise mit neurophysiologischen Kriterien verminderter Hirnpotentialfrequenz korrelieren. Ähnliches gilt vermutlich für die frühkindliche Amnesie. Vorbedingung für ein gut funktionierendes Gedächtnis komplexer Zusammenhänge ist außer einem wachen Gehirn eine *Ordnung und Systematisierung der Erfahrung.* Diese kann nur bei klarem Bewußtsein und nach längerer Verarbeitung der Lernprozesse aufgebaut werden, aber nicht im Schlaf. Im Traum auftretende Erinnerungen an längst vergangene Erlebnisse sind meistens stark modifiziert.

Schlaf, Bewußtseinskontinuität und Gedächtnis. W. JAMES' [J 4] Bezeichnungen "stream of thought" und "stream of consciousness" sollten die dynamische Funktionsverbindung der Bewußtseinsinhalte hervorheben. Aber auch dieser Bewußtseinsstrom fließt nicht gleichmäßig und dauernd: Der *Schlaf* unterbricht den kontinuierlichen Ablauf der Bewußtseinsvorgänge. Dennoch, trotz dieser häufigen normalen Perioden von Bewußtlosigkeit hat unser Bewußtsein eine *Kontinuität* in der Zeit, die durch unbewußte physiologische Prozesse garantiert sein müßte. Die Verbindung zwischen dem Wachbewußtsein verschiedener Tage über den Schlaf hinaus ist das *Gedächtnis,* obwohl die Merkfähigkeit im Schlaf stark vermindert ist. Die relative Stabilität dieser Gedächtnisfunktion gegenüber den erheblichen hirnelektrischen Veränderungen im Wach- und Schlafzustand ist eines der Argumente für die Substanzhypothesen des Gedächtnisses. HERING [H 33] hat diese *Brückenfunktion* der mnestischen Vorgänge über das Unbewußte sehr eindrucksvoll bezeichnet: „Zwischen dem, der ich heute bin, und dem, der ich gestern war, liegt eine Kluft der Bewußtlosigkeit, der Schlaf der Nacht, und nur das Gedächtnis spannt eine Brücke zwischen meinem Heute und meinem Gestern". „So liegt das einende Band, welches die einzelnen Phänomene unseres Bewußtseins verbindet, im Unbewußten: und da wir von diesem nichts wissen, als was uns die Untersuchung der Materie aussagt, da mit einem Worte für die rein empirische Betrachtung Unbewußtes und Materie dasselbe sein muß, so kann der Physiologe mit vollem Recht das Gedächtnis im weiteren Sinne des Wortes als ein Vermögen der Hirnsubstanz bezeichnen, dessen Äußerungen zwar zum großen Teil zugleich ins Bewußtsein fallen, zum anderen und nicht minder wesentlichen Teil aber als bloße materielle Prozesse unbewußt ablaufen."

Die Lern- und Gedächtnisvorgänge müssen daher als wichtigste biologische und psychologische Verbindungsfunktionen noch mit ihren neurophysiologischen Grundlagen dargestellt werden.

Zusammenfassung

Der *Schlaf* als normale Bewußtseinsveränderung ist neurophysiologisch, psychologisch und psychiatrisch von gleichgroßem Interesse. Die Schlafstadien können objektiv hirnelektrisch und polygraphisch registriert, Traum und Einschlaferleben subjektiv nur bruchstückhaft erfaßt werden. Der menschliche Nachtschlaf hat einen periodischen Ablauf mit 3–5 Cyclen der *synchronisierten EEG-Schlaf-Stadien* (C–E) und des *„paradoxen" Traumstadiums* (REM) mit flachem EEG und raschen Augenbewegungen. Die *zwei Schlafarten* unterscheiden sich hirnelektrisch, biologisch und psychologisch: *1) Der integrierte Erholungsschlaf* zeigt ein synchronisiertes EEG mit langsamen Wellen, Atmungs- und Pulsverlangsamung und totaler Amnesie. *2) Der dissoziierte „paradoxe" Traumschlaf (REM-Schlaf)* ist durch desynchronisiertes EEG (ähnlich dem Wachzustand), rasche Augenbewegungen, unregelmäßige Atmung, Pupillenerweiterung, Erektion und nur partielle Amnesierung charakterisiert, hat aber auch eine erhöhte Weckschwelle. Der Erholungsschlaf C–E entspricht einer rein trophotropen Einstellung nach HESS, der REM-Schlaf einer Mischung von trophotroper Erholung und ergotroper Aktivierung. Die Neurochemie des Schlafes und die Beziehungen zum Hirnstoffwechsel und zu den zum Cortex aufsteigenden Hirnstammneuronensystemen mit den synpatischen Transmittern Serotonin, Dopamin und Acetylcholin sind bisher vorwiegend bei Ratten untersucht, und ihre Gültigkeit für den menschlichen Schlaf bleibt noch hypothetisch.

Abnorme Schlafsyndrome sind die neurasthenischen Schlafstörungen mit verlängertem Einschlafen und vermehrten Schlafpausen, aber etwa normaler Gesamtschlafdauer, die depressiven Schlafstörungen mit mehrstündigen Wachperioden, die Narkolepsie mit Schlafanfällen, Kataplexie mit frühen REM-Stadien kurz nach dem Einschlafen und das Pickwick-Syndrom mit Adipositas, Hypoventilation und längeren Atempausen. Die periodischen Schlafzustände des Kleine-Levin-Syndroms entsprechen im EEG dem natürlichen Schlaf.

Die somnambulen Schlafsyndrome sind Pavor nocturnus und Schlafwandeln. Schlafwandeln entsteht im Tiefschlaf mit langsamen EEG-Wellen. Parallelen der symptomatischen Psychosen mit den REM-Stadien sind vor allem beim Delir erkennbar.

Die *Schlaf-Amnesie* erlaubt nur wenige partielle Erinnerungen erlebter Trauminhalte, die meist aus dem Morgenschlaf stammen oder nach affektbedingtem Erwachen behalten werden. Da Träume in der Regel vergessen werden, können sie, wie das REM-Stadium allgemein, auch als unbewußte affektive und instinktive Abreaktionen ohne Verhaltenskonsequenzen gedeutet werden, deren Amnesie zweckmäßig ist.

XII. Neurophysiologische Grundlagen von Lernen und Gedächtnis: Physiologie der bedingten Reaktionen

„So steht schließlich jedes organische Wesen der Gegenwart vor uns als ein Produkt des unbewußten Gedächtnisses der organisierten Materie, welche immer wachsend und immer sich teilend, immer neuen Stoff assimilierend und andern der anorganischen Welt zurückgebend, immer Neues in ihr Gedächtnis aufnehmend, um es wieder und wieder zu reproduzieren, reicher und immer reicher sich gestaltete, je länger sie lebte."

E. Hering: Über das Gedächtnis als eine allgemeine Funktion der organisierten Materie, 1870.

«A celui qui aborde sans idée préconçue, sur le terrain des faits, l'antique problème des rapports de l'âme et du corps, ce problème apparaît bien vite comme se resserrant autour de la question de la mémoire, et même plus spécialement de la mémoire des mots: c'est de là, sans aucun doute que devra partir la lumière capable d'éclairer les côtés plus obscurs du problème.»

H. Bergson: Matière et Mémoire, 1896.

Das Gedächtnis dient der Informationsspeicherung und ist Vorbedingung dauerhafter Veränderungen der Hirnfunktionen, des Verhaltens und Erlebens. Übung, Lernen und Gedächtnis sind beim Menschen und bei allen höheren Tieren nachweisbar und einer experimentellen Prüfung zugänglich.

Lernvorgänge und Gedächtnisprozesse bilden die menschliche *Sprache* und durch Wahrnehmungsverarbeitung, Erkennen, Erinnerung und Übung die Grundlagen für alle *Umweltbeeinflussungen*. Milieueinflüsse im weitesten Sinn wirken plastisch formend auf Verhalten und Denken des Menschen. *Umweltanpassung, Erziehung, Sprache und Bildung sind daher auch Gedächtnisfunktionen.* Alle höheren psychischen Leistungen und psychiatrischen Störungen entstehen unter Mitwirkung von Sprache und Gedächtnis. Es wäre deshalb von Bedeutung für die Psychiatrie, wenn die Neurophysiologie über Mechanismen des Gedächtnisses einiges aussagen könnte.

Seitdem der Psychologe EBBINGHAUS 1885 messende Untersuchungen über Gedächtnis und Vergessen mitgeteilt hat [E 1], sind Lernen und Gedächtnisleistungen ein Arbeitsfeld der Psychologie und Verhaltensforschung geworden. Obwohl viel experimentiert wurde und neue Hypothesen und Lerntheorien entstanden, erzielte die Gedächtnispsychologie seit EBBINGHAUS zunächst nur geringe Fortschritte. Neue Wege wiesen die Reiz-Reaktionsformeln des frühen amerikanischen Behaviorismus am Ende des 19. Jahrhunderts mit den Assoziationsexperimenten THORNDIKES [T 5]. Doch brachte erst die originelle Methode PAWLOWS mit Verwendung der Speichelreflexe einen experimentellen Schlüssel zur Lernforschung bei Tieren [P 4–7]. Dennoch hat die Neurophysiologie lange Zeit nur wenig zu den cerebralen *Mechanismen* der Lern- und Gedächtnisvorgänge beitragen können. Lernen und Gedächtnis wurden von PAWLOW und seiner Schule mit den bedingten Reflexen zunächst nur am ganzen Tier erforscht. Damit konnte ein bestimmter Aspekt des tierischen Lernens sehr exakt in experimentellen Verhaltensstudien, aber noch nicht in seinen cerebralen Einzelmechanismen untersucht werden. Erst seit 20 Jahren hat sich die Elektrophysiologie mit bedingten Reflexen und Lernvorgängen befaßt. Zur Zeit wird in verschiedenen Laboratorien intensiv über neurophysiologische Mechanismen des Lernens gearbeitet. In den letzten Jahren haben die Erfolge der biochemischen Chromosomenforschung über die Erbinformation wiederum neue Aspekte chemischer Gedächtnisspeicherung eröffnet. Es entstanden makromolekulare Hypothesen des Gedächtnisses, die allerdings noch auf eine experimentelle Bestätigung warten. Einige neurophysiologische Ergebnisse und mögliche Beziehungen mit psychologischen, kybernetischen, neurologischen Ergebnissen der Lernforschung sollen im folgenden dargestellt werden.

Die ältere Forschung hatte die Lern- und Gedächtnisprobleme sehr allgemein formuliert. Wie HERING [H 33] in seiner Rede von 1870, SEMON in der „Mneme" [S 24] und BLEULER mit seinem „Mnemismus" [B 49] sah man im Gedächtnis eine allgemeine Funktion der organisierten Materie. In der Physiologie gab es bis etwa 1920 mit Ausnahme von PAWLOWS Konditionierungs-Versuchen nur wenig experimentelle Lern- und Gedächtnisstudien bei Tieren. Auch PAWLOW und seine Schüler hatten meistens auf cerebrale Eingriffe und Untersuchungen der Hirnvorgänge verzichtet und sich auf eine Verhaltensanalyse beschränkt. Über die Vorgänge im Gehirn beim Lernen gab es daher nur spekulative Hypothesen, aber keine experimentellen Befunde, bis K. LASHLEY [L 2–4] systematische Labyrinthversuche bei Ratten mit cerebralen Läsionen durchführte. LASHLEY interpretierte seine Ergebnisse vorwiegend negativ: allgemein gegen eine corticale Lokalisationslehre (vgl. S. 903) und speziell gegen eine cerebrale Lokalisation der „Engramme". Doch mußte er entgegen seiner Massenhypothese der Gedächtnisprozesse auch zugeben, daß bestimmte erlernte Funktionen durch umschriebene Hirnläsionen gestört werden und daß eine durch mehrfache

Wiederholung fixierte Verhaltensweise (habit) auch cerebral lokalisiert sein kann [L 2] (vgl. S. 887 u. 903).

Kurzzeitgedächtnis und Langzeitgedächtnis

Die 1890 von dem amerikanischen Psychologen W. JAMES [J 4] vorgeschlagene Zweiteilung eines kurzen "primary memory" vom länger erinnerten "effective memory" paßte zu schon lange bekannten klinischen Beobachtungen über retrograde Amnesie und ist jetzt als Kurzzeit- und Langzeitgedächtnis allgemein bekannt:

1. Das *Kurzzeitgedächtnis* "short term memory" benutzt in den ersten Sekunden einer Handlungsfolge nur frische für die aktuelle Situation verwendbare Informationen und ermöglicht eine Kontinuität von Handlung und Denken.

2. Das *Langzeitgedächtnis* "long term memory" aktiviert durch Erinnerungsselektion ältere Informationen im vor längerer Zeit *deponierten Gedächtnisspeicher*. Diese zwei Gedächtnisarten sind in den beiden letzten Jahrzehnten genauer definiert [J 14] und mit neurophysiologischen und neurochemischen Begründungen gestützt worden. Man kann das Kurzzeitgedächtnis mit dem *Nachbild,* das Langzeitgedächtnis mit dem *Erinnerungsbild* vergleichen. Wie die kurzdauernden Nachbilder durch neuronale Schaltungen, die länger dauernden Blendungsbilder durch photochemische Prozesse erklärt werden, so könnten auch am Kurz- und Langzeitgedächtnis neurophysiologische und neurochemische Vorgänge mit unterschiedlicher Wertigkeit beteiligt sein. Lernvorgänge brauchen wahrscheinlich beides. Die *retrograde Amnesie* nach Hirntraumen, anoxischen Hirnschädigungen, epileptischen Anfällen und Elektroschocktherapie hatte gezeigt, daß vor allem die *kurz vorher erworbenen Gedächtnisinhalte* ausfallen, während ältere Erinnerungen weniger störbar und offenbar besser fixiert sind. Man muß daher annehmen, daß das Kurzzeitgedächtnis labiler ist, und daß ein neuer Prozeß einsetzen muß, bevor die dauerhafte Fixation im Gedächtnis erfolgt.

Kurzzeit-Gedächtnis und Motorik. Das Kurzzeitgedächtnis wird meistens neurophysiologisch als Erregungskreis in Neuronenketten gedeutet, für die HEBB [H 21] u.a. noch unbewiesene Neuronenmodelle vorgeschlagen haben. Dazu kommen offenbar noch kollaterale Hemmungsvorgänge, obwohl beides noch nicht direkt nachgewiesen ist. Doch wurde, seitdem TÖNNIES [T 9] dem Kleinhirn ein „motorisches Kurzgedächtnis" zuschrieb, oft diskutiert, wieweit die Kleinhirnregulationen, die in den ersten Sekunden eine koordinierte Handlung regeln, mit motorischen Übungs- und Trainingsvorgängen koordiniert sind. Mit dem *motorischen Lernen* würden sie auch das Langzeitgedächtnis einschließen. Da die Kleinhirnrinde mit hemmenden Ausgängen der Purkinje-Zellen arbeitet und damit die Motorik moduliert [E 6], sind auch neuronale *Hemmungsvorgänge,* nicht nur Erregungen beteiligt. Ungeklärt bleibt noch, ob man diese sensomotorischen Kurzzeitverschaltungen, die jede Bewegung und Handlung über Kleinhirn, Großhirn und Hirnstammkerne an die jeweilige Umweltsituation anpassen, also Regulationen im weitesten Sinne darstellen, überhaupt als Kurzgedächtnis klassifizieren soll. Wahrscheinlich ist es zweckmäßiger, das Kurzgedächtnis einfach *zeitlich* zu definieren, als die Merkvorgänge, die in den ersten Sekunden ablaufen und dann z.T. fixiert, z.T. vergessen werden.

Langzeitgedächtnisspeicher. Die für Wochen und Jahre im Zentralnervensystem deponierten *Gedächtnisinhalte*, die in der Motorik als *erlernte Handlungen* und Geschicklichkeit manifest werden und in der Wahrnehmung das *Wiedererkennen* ermöglichen, sind in ihren Mechanismen weithin unbekannt. Auch die Hirnlokalisation mit der Beteiligung von corticalen und cerebellaren Systemen oder des limbischen Systems für die emotionale Fixierung, die oft in Blockschemaschaltungen dargestellt wurden [K 42], ist spekulativ. Man muß annehmen, daß fast alle cerebralen Systeme an Gedächtnisprozessen beteiligt sind. Früher stellte man sich das Langzeitgedächtnis als eine dauerhafte Synapsenbahnung vor. Jetzt nimmt man die Mitwirkung neurochemischer Prozesse an. Die seit CAJAL [C 1], von KONORSKI [K 36], TÖNNIES [T 9], ECCLES [E 5] u.a. postulierten dauerhaften Synapsenveränderungen hat noch niemand exakt nachgewiesen. Sie könnten auch die komplexen Muster und Gestaltungen des kognitiven Gedächtnisses nicht erklären. Auch neuere Parallelen mit Computerschaltungen und Immunprozessen sind Spekulationen. Für neurochemische Fixierungsprozesse würde sprechen, daß das Langzeitgedächtnis vor allem durch *chemische Einwirkungen* gestört wird, z.B. durch die Proteinsynthese hemmende Antibiotika wie AGRANOFF [A 11] u.a. nachgewiesen haben (vgl. S. 1046).

Wie der Übergang von den labilen neuronalen Erregungs- und Hemmungsvorgängen des Kurzzeitgedächtnisses zu dem weitgehend konsolidierten Langzeitgedächtnis vor sich geht, ist unbekannt. Wie die meistens angenommenen „Spuren" der neuronalen Bahnung bestehen bleiben sollen, weiß niemand. Vor allem ist ungeklärt, wie die für lange Zeit fixierten Gedächtnisprogramme wieder aktiviert und *abgerufen* werden können, da Vergleiche mit programmierten Rechenmaschinen und ihren Erkennungs- und Gedächtnisleistungen [S 45, 47] nicht einfach auf die Gehirnfunktionen übertragen werden können. So bleibt das Gedächtnis noch das größte Rätsel der Neurophysiologie und Neurochemie. Bisher gibt es nur Lernversuche, experimentell-psychologische Gedächtnis-Untersuchungen und Trainings-Beobachtungen, die aber alle wenig oder nichts über die zentralen Mechanismen aussagen und die neurochemischen Vorgänge offen lassen. Auch neurologische und neurochirurgische Erfahrungen über schwere amnestische Störungen nach Läsionen des limbischen Systems [M 43–45] bringen keine Lösung der neurochemischen und neurophysiologischen Probleme des Langzeitgedächtnisses.

Gedächtnis und bedingte Reaktionen bei Tieren. Lernvorgänge und Gedächtnisleistungen im weiteren Sinne sind bei Tieren, etwa von den Würmern aufwärts, nachgewiesen, in niederen Tierklassen jedoch unsicher. Regenwürmer lernen, bestimmte Wege und ihre Richtungen nach vielfacher Wiederholung auf Futterbelohnung zu finden. Diese Experimente von YERKES [Y 1] mit niederen Tieren sind Vorstufen oder einfache Formen instrumenteller Konditionierung. Lernprozesse, die näher dem menschlichen Gedächtnis liegen, wurden mit PAWLOWS bedingten Reflexen vor allem bei Hunden experimentell untersucht. Ähnliche Konditionierungsversuche sind bei vielen anderen Tierarten, neuerdings vorwiegend bei Katzen und Affen und schließlich auch beim Menschen durchgeführt worden.

Die hirnelektrischen Begleiterscheinungen der Konditionierung wurden am ausgiebigsten im menschlichen EEG, Einzelneuronenbefunde vorwiegend am Affencortex studiert.

Seit PAWLOW ist die *Methode der bedingten Reflexe* die wichtigste neurophysiologische Technik für *experimentelle Lernuntersuchungen*. Nicht nur das, PAWLOWS Methodik der Verbindung mehrerer Reize verschiedener Sinne in zeitlicher Abfolge ist auch geeignet, die *Konvergenz verschiedener Sinnesmodalitäten* und ihre *zeitliche Ordnung* zu untersuchen. Diese allgemeine Bedeutung hat die bedingte Reflexforschung nach Erweiterung von PAWLOWS klassischer Methodik mit der Speichelfistel auch heute noch, mehr als ein halbes Jahrhundert nach PAWLOWS ersten Mitteilungen.

Die bedingte Reflexforschung und PAWLOWS Lehre

Die Physiologie der bedingten Reflexe und des bedingten Verhaltens ist von PAWLOW in seinen Büchern [P 4, 5] und gesammelten Werken [P 7], und von anderen mit eigenen Arbeiten [H 69] und in Übersichten [P 22, W 30] dargestellt worden. Wir besprechen hier nur, was für die Neurophysiologie von Interesse ist.

Bekanntlich nannte PAWLOW alle angeborenen und im ZNS vorgebildeten Reaktionen bis zum Instinktverhalten „unbedingte Reflexe", alle durch Lernen erworbenen Reaktionen „bedingte Reflexe". Wegen dieser sehr weiten Fassung des in der Neurophysiologie enger gebrauchten Reflexbegriffes sprechen wir im folgenden meist von *bedingten oder erlernten Reaktionen*. Die Vorgänge im ZNS bei bedingten Reaktionen und ihre Verhaltensäquivalente werden mangels eines besseren deutschen Ausdruckes als *Konditionierung* bezeichnet, entsprechend dem angelsächsischen „conditioning".

PAWLOW und seine Schüler arbeiteten vorwiegend mit der Methode *bedingter Nahrungsreflexe* an Hunden mit Speichelfistel und intaktem Gehirn (Abb. 5c). PAWLOWS Vorstellungen über die Rolle des Großhirns bei den bedingten Aktionen wurde zunächst ohne Eingriffe am ZNS entwickelt. Die genauere Untersuchung von Dressur- und Lernvorgängen durch cerebrale Reiz- und Ausschaltungsexperimente wurde erst später mit anderen Konditionierungsmethoden (instrumental conditioning) durchgeführt.

Instrumentelle Konditionierung (instrumental and operant conditioning). Beim „klassischen" Bedingungsexperiment PAWLOWS wird eine einfache Reflexreaktion wie die vegetative Speichelsekretion, die normalerweise (unbedingt) nur durch Futtergabe aktiviert wird, nach Lernen durch einen neuen *bedingten* Reiz ausgelöst, der zeitlich mit der Fütterung verbunden war. Für die Nahrungsaufnahme zunächst nicht bedeutsame Sinnesreize (Licht, Klingeln) können nach häufiger Wiederholung *vor* bedeutsamen Ereignissen (Futtergabe) auch ohne dieses Ereignis bestimmte Reflexmechanismen auslösen. Dagegen verwendet die instrumentelle Konditionierung verschiedene Verhaltensweisen, die selbst *aktiv auf die Versuchssituation zurückwirken,* einen *Belohnungseffekt* erreichen *oder eine Strafwirkung* vermeiden. *Das Versuchstier lernt, spezielle Reaktionen für bestimmte Effekte zu verwenden oder andere Aktionen zu verhindern.* Diese Konditionierungsmethoden wurden mehr in der amerikanischen Physiologie verwendet. Auch die Selbstreizungsmethoden (vgl. S. 955) sind eine Art instrumenteller Konditionierung, die allerdings direkt auf das Gehirn zurückwirkt. Bei anderen instrumentellen Konditionierungen kann eine Reaktion und Verhaltensweise auch normalerweise durch ähnliche Umweltbedingungen ausgelöst werden und das Versuchstier lernt die Einstellung auf spezifische Situationen und die Auslösung oder Vermeidung eigener Aktionen. Die instrumentelle Konditionierung hat mehr Beziehung zu komplexen Verhaltensweisen und höheren psychischen Vorgängen als PAWLOWS Speicheldrüsenexperimente.

PAWLOWs Methoden und die analytische Forschung. PAWLOWs bedingte Reflexphysiologie beschränkte sich zunächst auf reine Eingangs-Ausgangs-Vergleiche durch Beobachtung des intakten Organismus: Er verglich ähnlich wie die spinale Reflexphysiologie, aber auf einer höheren Ebene, die Sinnesreize, die in das Nervensystem hineingehen mit den motorischen Reaktionen, die danach wieder herauskommen. Was zwischen Sinnesreiz und Reaktion im Gehirn ablief, wurde indirekt und hypothetisch erschlossen [P 7]. Die Untersuchung der bedingten Reflexe konnte daher keine direkten Aussagen über die eigentliche Hirntätigkeit machen und es blieb offen, welche Hirnstrukturen und cerebralen Mechanismen an den bedingten Reflexen beteiligt waren. Erst neuere hirnelektrische Ableitungen und Ausschaltungsexperimente bei der bedingten Reflextätigkeit haben diese Vorgänge untersucht. Die Elektrophysiologie war bei PAWLOW noch von der bedingten Reflexforschung ausgeschaltet. Nach wenigen vorangehenden EEG-Versuchen von FESSARD [D 38], MOTOKAWA [M 6] u.Mitarb. hat sich seit 1954 auch die EEG-Forschung und die Elektrophysiologie mit den bedingten Reflexen beschäftigt und dabei neue Ergebnisse über die elektrischen Begleiterscheinungen erhalten. Erste Übersichten gaben das Colloquium in Marseille 1956 [F 11], die Arbeiten von GASTAUT u.Mitarb. [G 11, 12] und die Referate des internationalen Neurologen- und EEG-Kongresses in Brüssel 1957 [R 14]. Ein vollständigeres Bild mit ausgedehnten Diskussionen zwischen Amerikanern, Europäern und russischen Autoren brachte das Colloquium in Moskau 1958 [J 12]. Danach wird die ursprüngliche These von PAWLOW [P 7], daß nur die Großhirnrinde das Substrat der bedingten Reflexe sei, auch von der russischen Schule nicht mehr aufrechterhalten. Jetzt wird dem Hirnstamm, insbesondere dem Thalamus und der Reticularis auch eine wichtige Rolle für die bedingten Reaktionen zugewiesen [A 24–27, B 39].

PAWLOWs Lehre von der höchsten Nerventätigkeit. Ausgehend von seinen Hunden mit Speicheldrüsenfisteln hat PAWLOW die bedingten Reflexe und Lernvorgänge durch objektive Methoden in ihren motorischen und sekretorischen Effekten untersucht (Abb. 5c, d). Er hatte die Tendenz, subjektive Beobachtungen psychischer Vorgänge, die keiner objektiven Prüfung zugänglich sind, so weit wie möglich auszuschalten und durch experimentelle Verhaltensstudien zu ersetzen. PAWLOWs Lehre enthält auch syllogistische, terminologisch bedingte Verallgemeinerungen, die durch spätere Forschungen korrigiert wurden. Wenn PAWLOW von der *„höchsten Nerventätigkeit"* spricht, so meint er einerseits das *Verhalten der Tiere* im bedingten Reflexversuch, andererseits aber auch die physiologische *Tätigkeit der Großhirnhemisphären*. Die Bedeutung subcorticaler Mechanismen beim Lernen wurde daher zunächst unterschätzt.

Einprägsame Metapher und Vorstellungen in PAWLOWS Theorien sind: 1. *Ein Bild für die cerebralen Vorgänge der Aufmerksamkeit und des Bewußtseins:* Ein heller Fleck vermehrter Erregbarkeit läuft über die verschiedenen Regionen des Gehirns und hemmt die übrigen Hirnteile. 2. *Die Unterscheidung einer „äußeren" unbedingten Hemmung und einer „inneren" bedingten Hemmung*, wobei die äußere in allen Teilen des Nervensystems und die innere in den Großhirnhemisphären lokalisiert ist. 3. Die *Wechselwirkung von Hemmung und Erregung* als negative und positive Induktion und die *Beziehung von Schlaf und Hemmung:* Der Schlaf wird als eine Hemmung bezeichnet, die in den Großhirnhemisphären entsteht und sich dann in die Tiefe ausbreitet. 4. Ein *System von corticalen Analysatoren* für die bedingten Reaktionen verschiedener Sinnesqualitäten. 5. *Die Konzeption von zwei Signalsystemen des Gehirns.*

Das erste und zweite Signalsystem. Psychiatrisch bedeutungsvoll ist vor allem PAWLOWS *Lehre von den beiden Signalsystemen:* das *erste Signalsystem* haben Mensch und Tier gemeinsam als Wahrnehmung und Vorstellung. Diese Signale können zwar neurophysiologisch und psychologisch nicht immer genau definiert werden, enthalten aber offenbar anschaulich faßbare zentralnervöse Vorgänge von den Sinneswahrnehmungen bis zur anschaulichen Informationsverarbeitung. BERITOFF [B 37–39] spricht hier von cerebral repräsentierten Bildern. Es mag offen bleiben, ob PAWLOW ein anschauliches Denken mit Bildern als Symbolen, das über sein „gegenständliches Denken" im 1. System hinausreichen würde, nicht schon unter die Abstraktionsprozesse rechnen müßte, die er allein auf sprachlicher Ebene anerkennt. Auf dem ersten Signalsystem baut sich dann ein *zweites Signalsystem* auf, die *Sprache,* „die Signale der Signale". In diesem System vollzieht sich alles *abstrahierende und höhere symbolische Denken,* das für den Menschen spezifisch ist. PAWLOW glaubt, daß diese sprachliche Grundlage alle höheren seelischen Prozesse kennzeichnet und daß es zwecklos ist, allgemeine Theorien über subjektive seelische Vorgänge aufzustellen, ohne die Sprache als Grundlage zu berücksichtigen. Auch die höheren psychischen Prozesse werden dennoch von PAWLOW nach dem Reflexprinzip erklärt. Damit werden alle Lernvorgänge im sprachlichen Bereich nach dem Muster des Hundes mit der Speicheldrüsenfistel als bedingte Reflexe aufgefaßt, nur modifiziert für das 2. Signalsystem.

Die eigenen Worte PAWLOWS bezeichnen am besten seine Lehre von den Signalsystemen: „Wenn unsere Empfindungen und Vorstellungen, die sich auf die Außenwelt beziehen, für uns die ersten und dabei konkreten Signale der Wirklichkeit sind, so bildet die Sprache, und in erster Linie speziell die kinästhetischen Reize, die von den Sprachorganen der Hirnrinde übermittelt werden, eine zweite Ordnung von Signalen, die Signale der Signale. Sie stellen selbst eine Abstraktion von der Wirklichkeit dar und gestatten die Verallgemeinerung, die unser übriges, *speziell menschliches, höheres Denken* bildet, das zuerst die allgemeine menschliche Erfahrung und schließlich die Wissenschaft begründet hat, das Instrument der höchsten Orientierung des Menschen sowohl in bezug auf die Umwelt als auch in bezug auf sich selbst" (PAWLOW, Sämtliche Werke, 3/2, S. 466). Danach ist also Sprache und Denken untrennbar und Ausdruck einer einheitlichen Aktivität des 2. Signalsystems.

Es ist bemerkenswert, wie sehr PAWLOW, der mit Tieren ohne Läsionen des ZNS arbeitet, die *Ganzheitsfunktionen* betont und Psychologisches und Physiologisches darin zusammenfaßt.

Allgemeine Physiologie der bedingten Reaktionen

Die bis 1958 fast ohne gegenseitige Verbindung über die Physiologie der bedingten Reaktionen arbeitenden russischen, amerikanischen und französischen Forschergruppen versuchen allmählich, ihre verschiedenen Konzeptionen zu vereinigen und ihre Terminologie anzugleichen, ohne daß dies bisher voll gelungen ist. Nachdem die bedingten Reflexe ein Aufgabenbereich der Elektrophysiologie des Gehirns wurden, konnten die cerebralen Vorgänge zwischen Sinnesorganen und motorischen Reaktionen mit ihren neuronalen Grundlagen auch für andere erlernte Reaktionen genauer erforscht werden. Auf dem Moskauer Symposion 1958 [J 12] entstand wieder ein persönlicher Kontakt zwischen der westlichen, vorwiegend elektrophysiologisch orientierten Neurophysiologie und der russischen „pawlowistisch" bedingten Reflex-Forschung, die sich fast 30 Jahre getrennt entwickelt hatten.

Vorbedingungen der Konditionierung. Voraussetzung für bedingte Reaktionen sind allgemeine zentralnervöse Einstellungen, vor allem Wachzustand, Aufmerksamkeit und Hinwendungsbereitschaft des Versuchstieres für die Reize. Gewisse Vorstadien der eigentlichen bedingten Reflexe hat PAWLOW als allgemeine *Orientierungsreflexe* beschrieben. Sie wurden von anderen Autoren noch genauer differenziert [A 33, K 37, S 36, W 8].

Was in der Pawlowschen Schule *„Orientierungsreflex"* genannt wird, die unbedingte Habacht-Reaktion mit *Zuwendung auf einen neuen Reiz,* die modalitätsunspezifisch und primär generalisiert ist, wird in der westlichen Literatur meist als *arousal,* als unspezifische Aktivierung oder Aufmerksamkeitsreaktion bezeichnet. Dieses arousal ist nicht nur eine Weckreaktion, sondern enthält vor allem auch optisch-vestibuläre Zuwendungsmechanismen neben vegetativ-ergotroper Aktivierung.

KONORSKI [K 36, 37] hat versucht, den bedingten Reflexbogen auf dem Boden neurophysiologisch bekannter Vorgänge der Nervenleitung und synaptischen Übertragung als Bahnung zu erklären und die Rolle des Cortex und Subcortex genauer zu definieren. Nach seiner Annahme [K 37] führt die Ausschaltung corticaler Verbindungen zu einer selektiven Störung der bedingten Abwehrreflexe, ohne die unbedingte Abwehr zu vermindern. Damit erklärt KONORSKI auch Beobachtungen von KLÜVER, BUCY, SCHREINER u. Mitarb. über Veränderung und Enthemmung affektiver Reaktionen nach temporalen Läsionen im limbischen System (vgl. S. 944) und deutet sie als Ausschaltung höher organisierter bedingter Reaktionen oder phylogenetisch junger unbedingter Reflexe.

Cerebrale Mechanismen der Konditionierung

Wie und wo die neuen zeitweiligen Verbindungen, die PAWLOW forderte, im Gehirn geknüpft werden, war lange Zeit hypothetisch. Schon vor den Ergebnissen der modernen Neurophysiologie hatten Exstirpationen verschiedener corticaler Projektionsfelder, der Sehrinde oder der Hörrinde, gezeigt, daß bedingte Reflexe dieser Sinnesqualitäten auch ohne diese Felder erhalten blieben.

Nach wenigen Experimenten in russischen Laboratorien über bedingte Reflexe bei Tieren mit lokalisierten Hirnläsionen ist die spezielle neurophysiologische Untersuchung der cerebralen Mechanismen bedingter Reaktionen erst seit 1955 in Angriff genommen worden: Systematische Reiz- und Ausschaltungsversuche von Schülern PAWLOWS, vor allem der polnischen Gruppe KONORSKIS [B 69, K 37, Z 2], EEG-Untersuchungen von GASTAUT u.Mitarb. [G 10, 11] und Mikroelektrodenableitungen von JASPER [J 11, R 14], MORRELL [M 57–60] und anderen haben uns einiges über die cerebralen Grundlagen und neuronalen Mechanismen bei den bedingten Reflexen gelehrt.

Cerebrale Lokalisation bedingter Reaktionen. Obwohl bei höheren Tieren offenbar die Großhirnrinde wichtigste Struktur für Lernen und bedingte Reflexe ist, ließ sich die alte Konzeption PAWLOWS von der alleinigen Bedeutung des Cortex der Großhirnhemisphären für die Konditionierung nicht mehr aufrechterhalten. Vor allem die elektrophysiologischen Untersuchungen der letzten Jahre zeigten eine Beteiligung des Subcortex und eine wichtige Rolle des limbischen Systems und des unspezifischen reticulo-thalamischen Systems. PAWLOWS Schüler ANOKHIN hat dies besonders betont und von der „spezifischen" Wirkung der F. reticularis auf die Großhirnrinde in verschiedenen Symposien gesprochen [A 24–27]. Er postuliert auch eine spezifische Beeinflussung der Reticularis durch verschiedene biologische Reize wie Schmerz oder Nahrungsaufnahme bei der Entstehung bedingter Reaktionen.

Die modernen Schemata bedingter Reflexmechanismen zeigen alle eine Beteiligung des *Cortex und Subcortex,* wie das elektrophysiologisch begründete Schema von GASTAUT, ROGER und FESSARD (Abb. 42). EEG-Untersuchungen der bedingten Reflexe bei Mensch und Tier haben die cerebralen Schaltungen noch nicht klären können. Untersuchungen der neuronalen Mechanismen, die JASPER u.Mitarb. 1957 begonnen haben [J 11, R 14], zeigen zunächst nur die Kompliziertheit der beteiligten Neuronenmechanismen und die noch unklare Korrelation mit den langsamen EEG-Wellen. Diese Befunde im motorischen Cortex zeigen verschiedenartige neuronale Reaktionen in einer Hirnregion, die nach PAWLOW eher die höheren, unbedingten Reflexe und ihre gemeinsame Endstrecke mit den bedingten Reaktionen koordiniert, aber noch nicht den corticalen Analysator selbst erfaßt.

Zu den Verbindungen zwischen Isocortex, Thalamus und Reticularis kommt noch der *Allocortex* des limbischen Systems und der Hypothalamus als Substrat für *affektive Konditionierung.*

In der Diskussion zu GASTAUT und ROGER im Moskauer Kolloquium [G 12] berichtet BERITASHVILI (BERITOFF) über *cerebrale Grundlagen affektiver Komponenten der bedingten Reflexe* und die verschiedene Beteiligung des Neo- und Paläocortex. Er fand bedingte Reaktionen mit langdauernden affektiven Veränderungen bei Hunden ohne Neocortex. Wenn auch der Paläocortex entfernt wurde, so waren solche bedingte „Affektreaktionen" nicht mehr auslösbar. Er nennt daher sowohl die Pawlowsche wie die Bechterewsche Form der bedingten Abwehrreflexe „emotional reflexes". Diese bedingten affektiven Reaktionen entstehen unter Mitwirkung des limbischen Systems, werden also wahrscheinlich vom *Allocortex* gesteuert.

Korrelationen der allocorticalen Ammonshornrhythmen mit dem bedingten Verhalten wurden von GRASTYAN [G 38, 39, L 30], ADEY [A 2, 3] und ihren

Mitarbeitern sehr ausführlich untersucht. Beziehungen zu PAWLOWS Orientierungsreaktion sind wahrscheinlich.

Bedingte Reflexe, EEG und Triebmechanismen. Da die bedingten Reaktionen seit PAWLOW durch Speichelreflexe, Futterbelohnung und andere Mechanismen des Nahrungstriebes studiert wurden, war eine Verbindung zu Trieb- und Instinktmechanismen und ihrer Formbarkeit anzunehmen. PAWLOW [P 7] hat daher schon von den Affekten als den *„Energiequellen des Cortex"* gesprochen. Doch blieben Lernen und Triebe zunächst ein Feld der Verhaltensforschung am intakten Organismus. Die Beziehungen der Konditionierung zu Affekten und Trieben in ihren corticalen und subcorticalen Mechanismen wurden bis in die letzten Jahre kaum neurophysiologisch untersucht. Erst EEG-Untersuchungen führten weiter. ROUGEUL [R 35] hat 1958 zuerst bei Nahrungskonditionierung von Katzen langsame EEG-Wellen im Cortex bei Hemmungsreizen beschrieben. GASTAUT [G 11], YOSHII [Y 2] u.a. fanden dann bei Menschen und Tieren unregelmäßige langsame Wellen als Zeichen der *Auslöschung* bedingter Reflexe (extinction). Doch zeigte dies noch keine klare Korrelation zu Triebmechanismen. Erst ANOKHIN beschrieb bei Katzen *während des Fressens schnellere und nach Sättigung langsamere EEG-Wellen im Cortex und Hypothalamus* [A 26]. Die Untersuchungen von WYRWICKA [W 35] über Registrierungen mit implantierten Elektroden in ANAND und BROBECKS [A 21, B 65, 66] „feeding center" des Hypothalamus ergaben deutliche *Korrelationen der Hirnpotentiale mit dem bedingten Nahrungstriebverhalten.*

Neue elektrophysiologische Ergebnisse, die bei bedingten Reaktionen erhalten wurden, bringen noch wenig Licht in das dunkle Gebiet der Gedächtnisprozesse. Sie zeigen zunächst nur, wie kompliziert die hirnelektrischen und neuronalen Vorgänge in den verschiedenen beteiligten Hirnregionen sind.

EEG-Befunde. Das EEG bei bedingten Reaktionen wurde schon seit 1936 untersucht, hatte aber über den neuronalen Mechanismus noch nicht viel aussagen können. Man fand zunächst nur die zu erwartende EEG-Abflachung nach den Sinnesreizen, die eine Zuwendung entsprechend der Pawlowschen Orientierungsreaktion auslösen, aber keine spezifischen Befunde. Genauere Untersuchungen wurden von GASTAUT u.Mitarb. [G 10, 11, 12] beim Menschen durchgeführt und zusammenfassend dargestellt.

Nach diesen EEG-Befunden hat GASTAUT ein noch hypothetisches Schema über die Beteiligung der verschiedenen Hirnregionen vorgeschlagen [G 10, 12] (Abb. 42).

Bei den EEG-Untersuchungen zeigten einige Versuchspersonen eine sehr klare Korrelation mit den bedingten und unbedingten Reizen und einseitigen EEG-Veränderungen. Doch ergeben sich zahlreiche individuelle Variationen und andere Versuchspersonen zeigen weniger klare Befunde und vor allem weniger unilaterale EEG-Veränderungen bei bedingten Reaktionen.

Die EEG-Befunde von GASTAUT [G 11] bei bedingten Reflexen am Menschen sind interindividuell offenbar sehr variabel und in typischer Weise nur bei wenigen Versuchspersonen reproduzierbar. Über den neurophysiologischen Mechanismus der hirnelektrischen Veränderungen bei bedingten Reaktionen weiß man

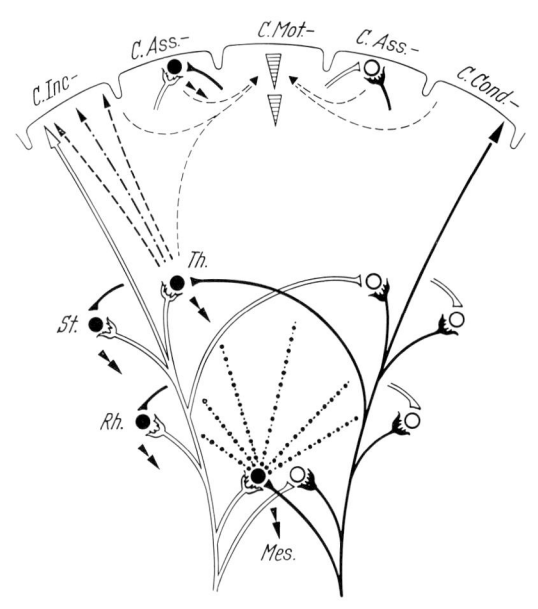

Abb. 42. Hypothetisches Schema subcorticaler und corticaler Neuron-Koordination bei bedingten Reflexen. (Nach GASTAUT und ROGER, 1958)
Die linken hellen Verbindungen sind die Bahnen des *unbedingten* (absolut wirksamen) Reizes. Die dunklen rechten Verbindungen sind die Wege des *bedingten* Reizes. Die Kreise bezeichnen Neurone mit Konvergenz verschiedener Reize, die vor dem Isocortex schon zur Formatio reticularis des Mittelhirns (*Mes*), zum Striatum (*St*) und Rhinencephalon (*Rh*) geleitet werden. Die Rindenfelder des unbedingten Reflexes (*C.Inc*), des bedingten Reflexes (*C.Cond*), der Assoziationsfelder (*C.Ass*) und der motorischen Rinde (*C.Mot*) sind schematisch als koordinierte Regionen angenommen, die auch von den unspezifischen Afferenzen der Reticularis und des Thalamus beeinflußt werden: Die punktierten Linien von den Neuronen der Reticularis sollen eine *unspezifische corticale Aktivierung* andeuten, entsprechend dem „Orientierungsreflex" der russischen Autoren. Die wirksam aktivierten Synapsen sind durch ein Büschel bezeichnet, die nur zur Summation beitragenden durch einen einfachen Endknopf. Die unterbrochenen Linien bilden die *Endkonvergenz zum motorischen Cortex*, der aber nicht allein die bedingte Reaktion steuert. Vielmehr beteiligen sich auch efferente *Neurone subcorticaler Regionen,* deren caudale Projektion jeweils durch schwarze Pfeile angedeutet ist. Sie lösen auch die Aktivierung zusätzlicher vegetativer und affektiver Mechanismen aus, sowohl beim unbedingten wie beim bedingten Reflex

noch wenig. Eine Beziehung zum unspezifischen thalamo-reticulären System ist nach Tierexperimenten wahrscheinlich, aber nicht exakt bewiesen. Das Schema der Abb. 42 von GASTAUT und ROGER ist noch hypothetisch und spekulativ. Vielleicht können die Befunde von WALTER u. Mitarb. [W 10, 11] über elektronegative Potentialverschiebungen bei bedingten Reaktionen und ihre Beziehungen zur sprachlichen Information und Erwartungssituation und ähnliche Potentiale bei erlernten Zielbewegungen (Abb. 11) weiterführen.

WALTERs „Erwartungswelle" bei bedingten Reaktionen. Nach direkten Ableitungen mit intracerebralen Elektroden im Frontalhirn und nach Computer-Auswertung von EEGs der Kopfhaut [W 10, 11] hat W.G. WALTER eine oberflächennegative Potentialänderung vor bedingten Reflexen und bei Erwartungssituationen in unipolaren Ableitungen vom Stirnhirn und Scheitel beim Menschen nachgewiesen (Abb. 43). Er nennt dieses elektronegative Potential „*Erwartungs-*

a

Click — Lichtblitze sollten durch Tastendruck beendet werden, doch beschloß Vp., nur einmal bei 6 Reizen zu reagieren.] 20 μV

1 sec

b

Click — Vp. ist instruiert, daß keine Lichtblitze folgen.

c

Click — Falsche Ankündigung, daß Lichtblitze folgen, die dann ausblieben.

d

Click — Tastendruck nach Zeitschätzung auf 1 sec.

e

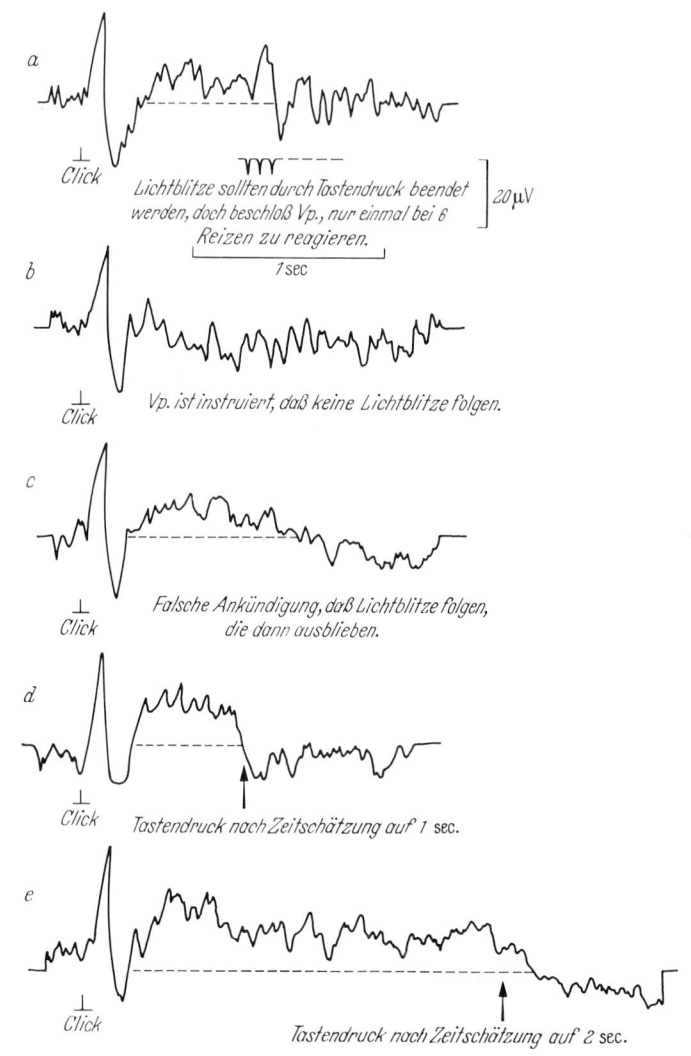

Click — Tastendruck nach Zeitschätzung auf 2 sec.

Abb. 43 a–e. Psychische und verbale Beeinflussung von WALTERS Erwartungswelle bei Kombination von akustischen und Lichtreizen. Nach G. WALTER (1964/65) [W 10]. Die Erwartungswelle im EEG ist eine Vorbereitung der bedingten Reaktion, aber weniger von dieser, als von der psychischen Einstellung abhängig. *a* Verminderte Erwartungswelle nach Knackreiz bei willkürlicher Hemmung der bedingten Reaktion (nur eine Ausführung bei 6 Reizen). *b* Fehlende Erwartungswelle bei Mitteilung, daß keine Lichtblitze folgen. *c* Leichte Erwartungswelle bei Ankündigung folgender Lichtreize, obwohl diese ausbleiben. *d* und *e* Erwartungswelle nach sprachlich gegebenem Auftrag, die Taste nach geschätzter Zeit von 1 oder 2 sec ohne neuen Reiz zu drücken. Ableitungen mit Gleichspannungsverstärker ohne Verzerrung der langsamen Potentiale. Durchschnittskurve von jeweils 6 Reizen mit automatischer Computerauswertung

welle" (expectancy wave) oder später "contingent negative variation" (CNV). Es wurde bei allen Gesunden unter gleichen Bedingungen nachgewiesen, unabhängig vom EEG-Typus und von der Ausprägung der α- oder β-Wellen. Untersucht wurden Kombinationen von optischen und akustischen Reizen in zeitlicher Abfolge [W 10]. Das *oberflächennegative Potential entstand während der Erwartung des zweiten Reizes,* gleichgültig, ob Licht oder Schall erster oder zweiter Reiz war, oder ob die akustischen oder optischen evoked potentials überwogen. Konstant war eine *Beendigung des negativen Potentials und eine oberflächenpositive Schwankung mit der motorischen Reaktion korreliert.*

Abb. 43 zeigt die wesentlichen Befunde. Nach einem kurzen Schallreiz (Click) oder nach Lichtblitzen sieht man im EEG kurzdauernde negative Wellen des evoked potential, die unabhängig von der Konditionierung sind. Nach mehrfacher Wiederholung des unbedingten und bedingten Reizes entsteht zwischen beiden evoked potentials *vor* dem zweiten Reiz in der Erwartungssituation eine negative Potentialverschiebung. Diese endet mit einem positiven Potential, wenn die Versuchsperson durch Tastendruck auftragsgemäß die Lichtblitze unterbricht (Abb. 43d). Die Lokalisation dieser elektronegativen Schwankung ist bei unipolarer Ableitung von der Schädelkonvexität natürlich ungenau. Nach intracerebralen Ableitungen scheint sie vorwiegend in der Frontal- und Parietalregion lokalisiert zu sein [W 9, 10]. Doch ist nach tierexperimentellen Untersuchungen Kornhubers eine multisensorische Konvergenz an corticalen Neuronen auch in verschiedenen occipito-parietalen Rindenfeldern nachgewiesen [J 59].

Beim Menschen hat Kornhuber [K 43] ähnliche Befunde einer negativen Schwankung in der Präcentralregion vor willkürlich eingeleiteten Bewegungen *ohne* Sinnesreize festgestellt (S. 833, Abb. 11 B). Die Potentialverschiebungen sind so klein und langdauernd, daß sie im EEG mit kurzer Zeitkonstante nicht erkennbar sind. Sie müssen mit langer Zeitkonstante oder Gleichspannungsverstärkern registriert werden. Unipolare Ableitungen vom Scheitel zum Ohr sind am geeignetsten.

Psychologisch bemerkenswert ist a) die Korrelation der negativen Welle mit verbalen Informationen und dem Bedeutungscharakter der Erwartungssituation und b) die Beendigung des negativen Potentials mit motorischer Aktion und willkürlichen Handlungen (Abb. 11 u. 43). Die ähnlichen Befunde Walters bei bedingten Reaktionen und Kornhubers bei spontaner Willkürinnervation zeigen, daß es sich nicht um reine Sinnesreaktionen handelt, sondern um *höhere Koordinationen, die mit der Erwartung, der Handlungsvorbereitung und Entschlußfähigkeit zusammenhängen.* Die Beziehungen zu den Bereitschaftspotentialen vor Willkürbewegungen und zu den Zielbewegungspotentialen während sensorisch gesteuerter Handlungen wurde auf S. 833 besprochen und mit Abb. 11 illustriert.

Unklar bleibt, ob die viel größere *oberflächennegative Spannungsverschiebung bei Petit mal-Epilepsie* [J 26] ähnliche Mechanismen betrifft: Beim kleinen epileptischen Anfall ist die oberflächennegative Spannung etwa 10–20mal größer als bei der Erwartungswelle des Gesunden. Ob die negative Gleichspannung beim Petit mal eine extrem pathologische Verstärkung, gewissermaßen eine Karikatur normaler Mechanismen ist, oder eine abnorme Gegenregulation, bleibt offen. Ähnlich wie abnorm synchronisierte Neuronentladungen beim großen epileptischen Anfall zum Bewußtseinsverlust führen, könnten auch beim Petit mal Extremwerte normaler Mechanismen der Bereitschafts- und Erwartungsreaktionen das Bewußtsein ausschalten. Hinweise auf Bereitschaftsmechanismen sind Lehmanns Befunde verkürzter Reaktionszeiten unmittelbar vor dem Bewußtseinsverlust des

Petit mal [L 9]. Gegen eine Bereitschaftsaktivierung im kleinen Anfall selbst spricht das Anfallsverhalten mit Reaktionslosigkeit, Sprachblockierung oder automatischem Fortsetzen von Lokomotionsbewegungen (Laufen, Radfahren) und die Erfahrung, daß während des Anfalls starke Sinnesreize den Patienten wecken und die Krampfpotentiale beenden können [J 26].

Neuronenbefunde im Isocortex bei bedingten Reaktionen. Die bedingten Reaktionen sind mikrophysiologisch bei Affen, Katzen und Ratten an cerebralen Neuronensystemen untersucht worden. Dabei fanden JASPER u.Mitarb. [J 11, R 14] im motorischen Cortex des Affen simultane Hemmung und Erregung verschiedener Neurone ähnlich der reziproken Neuronentätigkeit, die wir im optischen Cortex für Lichtreize beschrieben haben (vgl. Abb. 23). Entsprechend den komplizierteren Verhältnissen mit unbedingten und bedingten Reizreaktionen sind natürlich auch die neuronalen Reaktionen verschieden.

Hypothetische Neuronenschaltungen für den Mechanismus des Orientierungsreflexes und der bedingten Reaktionen [V 12] gibt es viele, aber ihre experimentelle Grundlage ist nicht überzeugend. Meist werden auch Neurone des thalamo-retikulären Systems für die bedingten Reflexschaltungen verwendet. ROITBAK [R 23] spricht von einer antagonistischen und Kontrastfunktion des thalamo-retikulären Systems und seiner Bedeutung für die corticale Hemmung, die Extinktionsphänomene und langsamen Wellen, ANOKHIN [A 27] sogar von einer spezifischen Wirkung der Reticularis auf den Cortex. Entsprechende spezifische Wirkungen haben wir für die optisch-vestibulären Regulationen der Augenbewegungen diskutiert, allerdings für unbedingte Koordinationen. Die Untersuchungen von KORNHUBER und FONSECA [K 44, J 59] über die multisensorische Konvergenz an corticalen Neuronen bringen diese Befunde auch in die Nachbarschaft der bedingten Reaktionen.

Obwohl zahlreiche Neuronenschemata der Gedächtnisfunktionen auf Grund elektrophysiologischer Untersuchungen entworfen wurden, muß man sich darüber klar sein, daß alle diese Neuronenmodelle noch ebenso hypothetisch sind wie die zahlreichen früheren Nervenzellschaltungsbilder der russischen Pawlow-Schule. Die bisherigen Ergebnisse neuronaler Untersuchungen von Konditionierung sind noch nicht so weit fortgeschritten, um die Neuronenmechanismen des Lernens aufzuklären. Trotz aller Bemühungen mit Mikroelektrodenuntersuchungen sind wir noch weit davon entfernt, diese neuronalen Vorgänge in eine klare Ordnung zu bringen. Nach den ersten, 1957 mitgeteilten Ergebnissen [R 14] am motorischen Cortex, hat JASPER [J 12] seine hirnelektrischen Makro- und Mikroableitungen bei bedingten Reaktionen von Affen zusammengefaßt [J 11]. Wie bei den spontanen Hirnpotentialen sind auch bei bedingten Reaktionen keine einfachen Beziehungen der neuronalen Entladungen zu den Makroableitungen des EEG erkennbar. Neuronale Hemmung oder Aktivierung kann sowohl bei α-Blockierung wie bei langsamen Wellen vorkommen. Im sensorischen und motorischen Cortex ist neuronale Aktivierung, in frontalen und parietalen Cortexfeldern neuronale Hemmung häufiger mit EEG-Abflachung verbunden.

Die *neuronale Hemmung* bei bedingten Reizen und Reaktionen entwickelt sich allmählich mit wiederholten Reizen. Bahnung der Neuronentladungen in der Parietalregion und intermittierende Hemmung in zeitlichem Zusammenhang mit dem bedingten Reiz machen es wahrscheinlich, daß die *Parietalregion ein wichtiger Schaltmechanismus für die bedingten Reaktionen* ist. Dies würde auch zu MOUNTCASTLES Korrelation der visuellen Aufmerksamkeit in parietalen Rindenfeldern von Affen [M 73-75] und KORNHUBERs multisensorischer Konvergenz [J 59] in homologen Rindenfeldern der Katze passen.

Allgemeine Physiologie von Lernen und Gedächtnis

Es ist anzunehmen, daß Lernen und Gedächtnis mit irgendwelchen materiellen Begleiterscheinungen in den Neuronensystemen einhergehen, und daß Erinnerungen bestimmte „Spuren" im ZNS zurücklassen müssen. Solche Spuren nennt man seit SEMON [S 25] *Engramme*. Aber niemand hat bis heute eine anatomisch-physiologische oder chemische Spur von Engrammen gefunden, und mit LASHLEY [L 5] ist es üblich geworden, sich über solche Vorstellungen zu mokieren. Noch unbekannter als Engrammschaltungen in Neuronensystemen sind aber chemische „Engramm-Substanzen". Für den Neurophysiologen, der die außerordentliche Kompliziertheit der neuronalen Strukturen kennt, die bereits an einfachen Sinnesvorgängen beteiligt sind, erscheint die Entstehung spezifisch chemischer Substanzen für die Gedächtnisfixierung jedes einzelnen dieser komplexen neuronalen Vorgänge schwer vorstellbar. Noch unverständlicher erscheint ihre Funktion für das Erinnern mit der erneuten Aktivierung komplexer Neuronensysteme. Auch logisch ist nicht zu verstehen, wie chemische Strukturen, die einzelne Gedächtnisvorgänge durch langdauernde molekulare Veränderungen Jahrzehnte relativ konstant bewahren sollen, momentan mit bestimmten Neuronenkonstellationen entstehen und dann in dem dauernden Wechsel der Umweltprozesse und Wahrnehmungsvorgänge jeweils bestimmte Gedächtnisbilder fixieren und wieder reproduzieren sollen. Auch die bis auf wenige Mutationen sehr stabile Genstruktur, die mit der erstaunlichen Konstanz der Arten über Jahrtausende unverändert bleibt, ist nicht einfach mit den labilen und veränderlichen Gedächtnisfunktionen zu vergleichen. Variationen der individuellen Gedächtnisbilder als prinzipiell ähnlich den Varianten des genetischen Artgedächtnisses anzusehen, wäre eine allzu billige Generalisierung. Ein neuester Versuch des Immunologen EDELMAN [E 9], die Selektionsfunktion des Gehirns mit dem modulären Bau [M 74, S 64] des Gehirns und molekulären Prozessen zu erklären und eine Gruppentheorie höherer Hirnfunktionen zu entwickeln, ist noch nicht überzeugend. Bewußtsein und Wachheit wird als Zugang zu modulären Neuronengruppen von etwa 10000 Zellen erklärt, die im Langzeitgedächtnis multimodale und assoziative Muster gespeichert haben. Aber das Hauptproblem, *wie* diese Neuronenmoduls ihre Information speichern, bleibt auch bei EDELMAN ungelöst.

Es bleibt abzuwarten, ob weitere Forschungen makromolekular-chemische Grundlagen des Gedächtnisses feststellen werden. Auch wenn solche gefunden werden sollten, können sie nicht wirksam werden ohne geordnete Systeme von Milliarden von Neuronen, die beim höheren Säuger und Menschen Vorbedingungen für Gedächtnis und Lernfähigkeit sind.

Hypothetische neuronale Gedächtnisgrundlagen. Fast alle neurophysiologischen Lernhypothesen benutzen die *synaptische Bahnung* als Grundlage. Nachdem schon mit den Neuronenschemata der neunziger Jahre ähnliche Vorgänge diskutiert wurden, hat CAJAL 1911 eine Gedächtnisbahnung der Synapsen zuerst klar ausgesprochen [C 1]. ADRIAN [A 8] hat sie 1947 für ebenso unbewiesen wie notwendig erklärt und TÖNNIES [T 9] forderte 1949 eine Art „Punktschweißung" an der erfolgreichen Synapse mit dauernder Verbesserung der synaptischen Übertragung nach häufiger gleichartiger Erregung. Synapsenbahnung wurde auch für die bedingten Reflexe von KONORSKI 1948 angenommen [K 36]. Doch geben diese Hypothesen keine Erklärung für die außerordentlich komplexen Leistungen des Gedächtnisses und der Lernvorgänge. HEBB [H 20] hat zwar versucht, ähnliche einfache neuronale Verbindungen als Grundlage komplexen Verhaltens zu verwenden, aber LASHLEY [L 5] u. a. haben gezeigt, daß alle Schemata neuronaler „Engramme" selbst für die einfachsten Gedächtnisvorgänge ungenügend sind. Noch unerklärbarer durch Synapsenbahnung ist die erstaunliche *zeitliche Ordnung* des Gedächtnisses, durch die wir nicht nur wiedererkennen, sondern das Erkannte auch in zeitliche und höhere Zusammenhänge einordnen können. Solche Gedächtnisordnungen wären nur bei sehr komplizierten, veränderlichen Schaltungen der Neurone möglich, aber nicht durch einfache Bahnung einzelner Synapsen oder gar durch chemisch-molekulare Vorgänge erklärbar (s. S. 1045). Aber auch über langdauernde, einzelne Synapsenbahnungen hat die Neurophysiologie noch keine sehr präzisen Vorstellungen.

Kybernetische Programmierung und Gedächtnis. Die moderne Kybernetik und die seit CRAIK [C 13] oft verwendete Annahme *intracerebraler Modellvorgänge der Außenwelt* haben uns zwar im Verständnis komplexer Schaltungen weitergeführt. Aber sie sind noch weit entfernt von einer Erklärung komplizierter Gedächtnisfunktionen des Gehirns, die auch eine Invariantenbildung von Wahrnehmen und Erkennen einschließt (s. S. 864).

Nachdem es mit einfachen Mitteln und wenigen Elementen gelang, gut funktionierende Modelle für bedingte Reflexe zu bauen (S. 863) erschien es doch zunächst wenig aussichtsvoll, auch die zeitliche Ordnung bedingter Reaktionen zu imitieren. Dies ist jetzt mit komplizierten Rechenmaschinen möglich. Auch die Rechenautomaten und lernenden Maschinen werden für die gedächtnisähnliche Fixierung verschiedener komplexer Reizvorgänge erst nach einer Vorausprogrammierung fähig. Diese *Programmierung* wird für die Maschinen wiederum durch menschliche Gedächtnis- und Kombinationsleistungen ermöglicht. Schon einfache Gehirne von Tieren steuern auf angeborener Grundlage mit Instinktvorgängen äußerst verwickelte, zeitlich geordnete Verhaltensweisen und erlernen nach wenigen einfachen Reizen auch komplizierte Reaktionsweisen. Solche erlernten komplexen Reaktionen sind nicht nur Resultate von Gedächtnis und Übung. Sie setzen sich vielmehr bei genauerer Betrachtung meist aus *angeborenen Teilprozessen* zusammen, die das Nervensystem bereits ohne Lernvorgänge durch seine *geordnete Struktur mit bestimmten Neuronenverbindungen* potentiell in sich trägt. Die neuronale Ordnung des Gehirns, die große Zahl ihrer Elemente und Verbindungen, ihre Muster und „Gestalten" sind zweifellos *Vorbedingungen der Gedächtnisleistungen*. Aber die cerebrale Strukturordnung als solche bringt uns noch keine physiologische Erklärung der Gedächtnisfunktion und des Lernens.

Resonanzhypothese des Gedächtnisses. Gegen die Bahnungshypothesen des Gedächtnisses sind oft Einwände erhoben worden. LASHLEY [L 2–4] hat eine Art Resonanzvorgang in den komplizierten Neuronnetzen des Cortex angenommen. Er bestreitet vor allem eine feste Lokalisation in bestimmten Zentren, muß aber andererseits die Unentbehrlichkeit der primären Sinneszentren zugeben. Nach Exstirpation der corticalen Sehzentren konnte das bereits vor dem Lernversuch geblendete Tier die erlernten Labyrinthwege nicht mehr finden [L 2].

Unbekannte Gedächtniskorrelate. Die Physiologie der *Gedächtnisspeicherung* und *Erinnerungsaktivierung,* englisch kurz „storage" und „retrieval" genannt, bleibt rätselhaft. Wie das Gehirn seine wunderbaren Gedächtnisleistungen vollbringt, wissen wir nicht. Nicht einmal für das Kurzzeit- und Langzeitgedächtnis sind unterschiedliche cerebrale Korrelate nachgewiesen. Alle Gedächtnishypothesen sind auch heute noch Hirnmythologie. Man glaubt zwar allgemein, daß dem Kurzzeitgedächtnis nur eine Fortdauer neuronaler Entladungsmuster in cerebralen Erregungskreisen entspricht und das Langzeitgedächtnis durch dauerhafte „molekularbiologische" Veränderungen in komplexen synaptischen Gehirnstrukturen zustande kommt, aber beides ist noch nicht exakt bewiesen. Während man in den fünfziger Jahren dem reticulären System eine Rolle für die Lernaktivierung zuschrieb, betonen neuere Übersichten von KORNHUBER [K 42a] und ECCLES [E 5b] mehr die Zusammenarbeit des *limbischen Systems* und seiner Erregungskreise mit dem Neocortex für die Motivation und Konsolidierung der Gedächtnisleistungen. Aber auch solche Blockschemata [K 42a] erklären nicht die Gedächtnisfunktion, und die postulierten neuronalen Erregungskreise [E 5b] zeigen nicht mehr als die bekannten anatomischen Verbindungen zwischen limbischem System, medialem Thalamus und den isocorticalen Rindenfeldern. Neue Versuche von ANDERSEN [A 21a], längerdauernde Potentialveränderungen im Ammonshorn nach oft wiederholter Reizung als Grundlage des Lernvorgangs nachzuweisen, können noch keine Allgemeingültigkeit beanspruchen. ECCLES postuliert entsprechend seiner dualistischen Auffassung [P 32, E 6] für das kognitive Gedächtnis und die Erinnerung eine Zusammenarbeit zwischen dem „bewußten Selbst" und dem Großhirn, und für das motorische Lernen eine Koordination mit dem Kleinhirn. Aber da ECCLES' „Selbst" (Welt 2) wie die Seele der alten Religionen und Philosophien nicht mit dem Gehirn identifiziert werden kann, bleiben diese allgemeinen Formulierungen für die Neurophysiologie unbefriedigend.

Neuere Publikationen [B 60a, J 14] über die Physiologie der Gedächtnisvorgänge geben uns leider auch keine klare Vorstellung für die zentralnervösen Mechanismen des Lernens oder der Speicherung und Reaktivierung von Gedächtnisinhalten. JOHN [J 14] trennt bei seinen Flackerlichtreizen und evozierten Potentialen echtes Lernen von einer Pseudokonditionierung mit „sensitisation" und „assimilation" von Hirnrhythmen. KANDEL gibt eine Übersicht über Lernvorgänge von einzelnen Neuronen bei der Meeresschnecke Aplysia [K 1], kann aber aus diesem Neuronenmodell eines wirbellosen Tieres nicht die Gedächtnisleistungen des Menschen ableiten. Die modernen Konzepte der modulären Ordnung der Gehirnfunktionen [E 9, P 32, M 74, S 64] führen uns leider nicht viel weiter als daß sie die Zahl der kombinationsfähigen Einheiten für die Gedächtnisordnung von 10 Milliarden Nervenzellen auf *1–2 Millionen Moduleinheiten* des Gehirns verringern. Wir können weder das Kurzzeitgedächtnis noch die tägliche klinische Erfahrung der retrograden Amnesie erklären. So muß die Neurophysiologie trotz vieler Bemühungen der letzten Jahrzehnte für das Gedächtnis ihr *ignoramus* bekennen, ohne für die Zukunft ein ignorabimus zu behaupten.

Gedächtnis und cerebrale Disposition. Wechselwirkung von Lernen, Instinkten, Affekten und Reflexen

Angeborenes Instinktverhalten und erworbenes Gedächtnis, Triebe und Reflexe, affektive und erfahrungsgesteuerte Reaktionen wirken eng zusammen. Hier gibt es kein „entweder-oder", sondern nur ein „sowohl-als-auch". Dies gilt sowohl für seelisches Erleben und beobachtbares Verhalten beim Menschen, wie auch für somatisch-biologische Vorgänge bei Tieren. Alter und vorangehende Erfahrung verändern biologische und psychologische Vorgänge. Im Gegensatz zur rein physikalisch-chemischen Welt, in der ein Vorgang meistens beliebig reproduzierbar bleibt (Ausnahmen in der organischen und Kolloidchemie können hier unberücksichtigt bleiben), wird die exakte Wiederholbarkeit im biologischen Bereich durch den Lernprozeß selbst und durch die Individualentwicklung eingeschränkt. Organismen werden durch Altersentwicklung und Erfahrung mit Lern- und Gedächtnisvorgängen im weitesten Sinne verändert. So bewirken die gleichen Reize eben durch die Konditionierung nach Wiederholungen verschiedene Effekte. Andererseits wirken auch erste Reize schon vor dem Lernen verschieden bei verschiedenen Individuen. Da dies sowohl am Menschen wie am Tier nachgewiesen ist, berücksichtigte PAWLOW die Temperamente seiner Hunde und bewertete sie als cerebrale Dispositionen.

Bei PAWLOWS Versuchen ist zu beachten, daß die Antriebe des Lernens und der bedingten Reflexe wie bei den meisten Dressurexperimenten aus dem Nahrungstrieb kommen, daß also zur *Motivation der bedingten Reaktionen ein unbedingter angeborener Triebmechanismus gehört* (S. 1032).

Für die cerebrale Wechselwirkung von Trieb, Affekt und Lernen ist folgende Beobachtung BERITASHVILLS (BERITOFF [B 39]) interessant: Er fand bei Katzen und Hunden ohne Neocortex sehr rasch nach wenigen Reizen auftretende typische bedingte Nahrungs- und Abwehrreflexe als emotionale Reaktionen, solange der Paläocortex erhalten ist. Bei Tieren ohne Neo- und Paläocortex waren nur noch allgemeine ungeordnete Affektentladungen, aber keine typischen bedingten emotionalen Reaktionen mehr auslösbar.

Auch auf psychologischer Ebene wird das Lernen durch die verschiedensten Antriebe und Motivationen und durch spezielle Interessen gesteuert. Die „Interessen" sind großenteils *erworben, d.h.* im weiteren Sinne auch erlernt, so daß man innerhalb der Lernmechanismen selbst positive Rückkoppelungsvorgänge der Lernbereitschaft annehmen darf. Die Neurophysiologie solcher feed-back-Mechanismen ist noch nicht bekannt. Man kann annehmen, daß die elektrophysiologischen Vorgänge im Cortex Beziehungen zu der Erwartungswelle WALTERS und dem Bereitschaftspotential KORNHUBERS haben (vgl. S. 833 u. 1034).

Angeborene und erlernte Funktionen. Für die *anatomische* Struktur des Gehirns ist die *genetische Determination* entscheidend, ebenso wie für angeborene Reflexe und Triebe. Diese sind offenbar durch chromosomale Strukturen bestimmt oder, wie man heute gerne sagt, durch Gen-Informationen. Dieses „Erbgedächtnis" wird durch ein lernend erworbenes Individualgedächtnis ergänzt. Bei differenzierten *physiologischen und psychischen Leistungen* der Säuger und des Menschen spielen *erworbene Informations-Verbindungen, Lernfähigkeit und Gedächtnis* für das Individuum eine wichtigere Rolle als die Erbinformation. Die angeborene Ordnung der Strukturen und ihre vorgebildeten Verbindungswege mit der Anlage von Instinkt- und Triebmechanismen sind jeweils *Voraussetzungen* für die Lernfähigkeit und für erworbene bedingte Reaktionen. Erfahrung und Lernen schaffen dann durch Gedächtnismechanismen eine *neue Ordnung*. Ethologen formulieren es so, daß *in die angeborenen Auslösermechanismen der Instinkte hineingelernt* wird. Das Erlernen spezieller Funktionen und Verhaltensweisen ist damit auch von angeborenen *Anlagen und körperlichen Vorbedingungen* abhängig, nicht nur von der allgemeinen Lernfähigkeit des Tieres oder Individuums.

Ein Mensch lernt sprechen, ein Affe nicht. Ein Affe lernt das Baum-zu-Baum-Springen, ein Mensch nicht. Ein anderes Beispiel ist die *Erziehung zur Sauberkeit bei verschiedenen Tierarten*. Katzen und Hunde, die als Raubtiere eine instinktive Tendenz haben, ihre Exkremente an bestimmten Stellen abzusetzen und zu verscharren, sind leicht zur Sauberkeit zu bringen. Affen, obwohl sie eine bessere Lernfähigkeit und ein größeres Repertoire von Verhaltensregulationen haben, sind viel schwieriger oder nie zu einer solchen Sauberkeit zu erziehen, *weil die angeborene instinktive Vorbedingung fehlt*. Offenbar fehlen auch die anatomisch-physiologischen Strukturverbindungen, die das Erlernen ermöglichen, nach dem Sauberkeit für die baumbewohnenden Affen biologisch unwichtig und ohne Selektionswert war.

„Prägung" als einmalig fixierter Lernvorgang mit Instinktverhalten. Die von LORENZ beschriebene *„Prägung"* bei Vögeln ist ein einmaliges kurzdauerndes Lernen, das nur während einer kritischen „sensiblen" Periode des 1. Lebenstages möglich ist und dann eine bleibende Folgereaktion für das geprägte Objekt auslöst. Nach der ethologischen Terminologie handelt es sich um den *Einbau von Erfahrungen in angeborenes Instinktverhalten*: In eine Lücke des angeborenen Auslösemechanismus wird ein neues geprägtes „Bild" eingefügt. Dieses „Bild" erhält der natürlich ausgebrütete Vogel im allgemeinen von der Mutter, während es bei künstlicher Bebrütung von den verschiedensten bewegten Objekten geliefert werden kann [L 36, 38, H 42]. Während der sensiblen Periode läßt sich die Prägung auf beliebige andere Lebewesen und auch auf tote Attrappen durchführen, je nachdem, was der ausgeschlüpfte Vogel zuerst sieht. Deshalb sind Prägungsvorgänge für experimentelle Untersuchungen von Instinkt- und Triebverhalten besonders geeignet und bilden das beste Beispiel für eine *Wechselwirkung von angeborenem und erlerntem Verhalten*. LORENZ und andere Verhaltensforscher haben *echte Prägung nur bei Vögeln, aber nicht bei Säugern und anderen Tieren festgestellt*. Die bekannte „Liebe auf den ersten Blick" ist zwar ein anschauliches und didaktisch brauchbares Bild für den Prägungsvorgang, aber bedeutet nicht mehr als eine Metapher, die weder entsprechende Vorgänge bei Mensch und Vogel wahrscheinlich macht, noch etwas über ähnliche cerebrale Mechanismen aussagt. Nicht jede rasche, emotional gefärbte und dann festgehaltene Fixierung an andere Lebewesen ist mit der Prägung gleichzusetzen.

Affektive Beeinflussung von Gedächtnisvorgängen. Emotional erleichtertes Lernen, Fixierung, Blockierung, oder bessere Erinnerung von affektiv gefärbten Erlebnissen werden alltäglich beobachtet. Doch sind die neurophysiologischen Mechanismen solcher Bahnungen unbekannt. Nach Experimenten und EEG-Untersuchungen bei bedingten Reaktionen wird vermutet, daß die *affektive Bahnung* durch die limbischen und thalamo-reticulären Systeme auf den Isocortex wirkt. Diese selektive Bahnung der Erinnerung ist, wie bei anderen Auswahlvorgängen des Bewußtseins und Lernens, offenbar *mit affektiver Blockierung anderer Gedächtnisinhalte verbunden* oder kann auch in eine Blockierung für dieselben affektbetonten Inhalte umschlagen. Eine ähnliche Blockierung ist wahrscheinlich Grundlage der *Verdrängung* und vielleicht auch der affektiven Sprachhemmung beim Stottern. Klinische Beobachtungen sprechen dafür, daß bei schweren Korsakow-Syndromen und bei senilen und präsenilen Merkfähigkeitsstörungen gewisse emotional gebahnte Gedächtnisvorgänge besser erhalten bleiben. Ob dies auf verschiedenen neurophysiologischen Mechanismen der emotionalen Gedächtnisprozesse oder einfach auf einer stärkeren Bahnung und Fixierung beruht, ist unbekannt: eine unterschiedliche Beteiligung verschiedener Hirnteile ist wahrscheinlich. Auf emotionaler Fixierung und Blockierung komplexer Gedächtnisinhalte beruht vielleicht auch das unveränderliche Festhalten an gewissen politischen und religiösen Überzeugungen bei Gesunden und die unkorrigierbare *Wahnfixierung* bei paranoiden Psychosen. Der cerebrale Mechanismus solcher unbeeinflußbarer Fixierungen bestimmter Ideen und Ideologien ist beim Menschen noch weniger neurophysiologisch erklärbar als die feste Fügung von Prägungsvorgängen bei jungen Vögeln.

Wahrscheinlich handelt es sich beim affektiven Gedächtnis auch um *hirnlokalisatorisch verschiedene Lernvorgänge*. Bereits klinisch-hirnpathologische Beobachtungen an Kranken mit vorwiegend isocorticalen Hirnatrophien und erhaltenem Allocortex, die schwere amnestische Störungen mit besserem affektiven Gedächtnis haben, weisen darauf hin, daß allocorticale Regionen mit dem affektiven Gedächtnis enger verbunden sein können als der Isocortex. Noch beweisender erscheinen experimentelle Untersuchungen bei Affen von PRIBRAM und WEISKRANTZ [P 36] über schwere Störungen der bedingten emotionalen Reaktionen nach frontobasalen und cingulären Läsionen oder Ammonshornschädigungen sowie Erhaltenbleiben des emotionalen Lernens nach ausgedehnten parietalen, occipitalen und temporalen Isocortexverletzungen. Vgl. PLOOG in diesem Band (S. 379).

Zusammenwirken von menschlicher Hirnentwicklung und Lernen. Ein vielbeachteter Unterschied von Mensch und Tier ist die Unreife des menschlichen Kleinkindes und die Parallele von Hirnentwicklung und Lernvorgängen. *Viele spezifisch menschlichen Eigenschaften wie aufrechter Gang, Sprache und soziale Verhaltensweisen werden erst mit der Hirnentwicklung lernend erworben*. Bei Tieren sind Bewegung, Lautäußerungen und soziale Verhaltensweisen dagegen früher entwickelt, stärker durch Triebe und Instinkte fixiert und werden weniger durch Lernen modifiziert, wie die Kaspar-Hauser-Versuche gezeigt haben. Stärkere Plastizität cerebraler Entwicklungsvorgänge mit Umweltveränderung des menschlichen Verhaltens und größere Bedeutung von Lernen und bedingten Reaktionen beim Menschen sind aber nur quantitative, keine prinzipiellen Unterschiede gegenüber den höheren Tieren. Ohne die artspezifischen cerebralen Anlagen für Gangkoordination oder Sprache können diese Leistungen auch nicht erlernt werden.

Grenzen des Lernens. Die erstaunliche Lernfähigkeit des Gehirns, die durch Steuerung bedingter und erworbener Verhaltensweisen die Reaktionen des Organismus auf äußere Reize verändert, findet ihre Grenzen in angeborenen strukturellen und physiologisch vorgebildeten Mechanismen: Ein Huhn kann nicht schwimmen lernen, ein Affe lernt nicht sprechen, ein Schwachsinniger begreift keine Logik. Solche Begrenzungen gelten auch für bestimmte Varianten des Affekt- und Trieblebens und ihre Beherrschung durch bewußte und erlernte Regulationen: Ein Affektlabiler lernt nicht oder nur sehr unvollkommen, seine Gefühlsausbrüche zu beherrschen. Ein Stimmungslabiler bleibt seinen Verstimmungen ausgeliefert, obwohl er damit oft die unangenehmsten bedingten Erfahrungen gemacht hat und gerne gelernt hätte, sie zu vermeiden. Noch deutlicher werden diese Grenzen der Konditionierung und Erziehung bei neurotischen und psychotischen Störungen. Zwar hat die aktive Arbeitstherapie gezeigt, wie sehr auch Geisteskranke und alte psychotische Defektzustände einer Umwelteinwirkung zugänglich sind. Doch wird kein Psychiater nach guten arbeitstherapeutischen Erfolgen glauben, daß Psychosen durch Beschäftigungstherapie heilen. Man sollte erwarten, daß auch für bedingte Reaktionen und Lerntheorien enthusiasmierte Psychologen und Psychotherapeuten die Grenzen des erlernten Verhaltens beachten und die Beeinflußbarkeit des Menschen und seines Verhaltens nicht überschätzen.

Lerntheorien und Psychiatrie. Neuere Studien über die Psychologie der Lernvorgänge treffen sich mit physiologischen Untersuchungen über die bedingten Reaktionen. Bedingte Reaktionen, Gewöhnung und Lernen im weitesten Sinne, werden daher im zunehmenden Maße auch für die Erklärung neurotischer Mechanismen angewandt. Ein Sammelwerk von EYSENCK [E 30] bespricht auch praktisch-psychiatrische Anwendungen für Verhaltenstherapien der Neurosen und versucht, die in psychoanalytischer Dogmatik erstarrte Psychotherapie wieder flott zu machen und mit der Neurophysiologie zu korrelieren.

Tierexperiment und menschliche Beobachtung überschneiden und ergänzen sich auf diesem Gebiet. Der Begriff einer "conditioned emotional reaction", der in der späteren tierexperimentellen Forschung eine so große Rolle spielt, stammt von WATSONS und RAYNERS [W 13] Untersuchungen an Kleinkindern 1920. Die vielzitierten Konzeptionen von HULL [H 92] sind vorwiegend hypothetisch. Er unterscheidet *Leistung* (performance) und *Gewöhnung* (habit) als reizbedingte Antworten des Organismus. Gewöhnung wird aufgefaßt als langdauernde reizbedingte Veränderung im ZNS, die das Lernen ermöglicht, etwa im Sinne neu erworbener Verbindungen der bedingten Reflexforschung. HULL versucht die Lernvorgänge auch mit der Triebpsychologie zu vereinigen, indem er die alte hedonistische Motivationslehre von Lust und Unlust verwendet. Er unterscheidet ferner eine *reaktive Hemmung* und eine *bedingte Hemmung*.

Nachdem weder die Psychophysiologie noch die hirnelektrische und neuronale Erforschung der bedingten Reflexe ein klares Bild der Lernmechanismen geben, müssen zwei allgemeine Gedächtniskonzeptionen kurz erwähnt werden, über die heute viel gesprochen und geschrieben wird: *1. die physikalischen* Gedächtnismodelle der *Kybernetik* und *2.* die *chemisch-molekularen* Gedächtnishypothesen, die aus der biochemischen *Genetik* abgeleitet wurden.

Physikalische Modelle des Gedächtnisses und Kybernetik

Die lernenden Maschinen der modernen Nachrichtentechnik haben uns zahlreiche physikalische Modelle von Gedächtnisvorgängen gebracht. Leider war der Gewinn, den die Neurophysiologie daraus für den Mechanismus der Lernvorgänge ziehen konnte, bisher nur gering. Ob STEINBUCHS Lernmatrizen (s. S. 864) oder einfachere technische Modelle für bedingte Reflexe [G 31, W 7] (s. S. 863) oder für sensomotorische Funktionen [R 5] verwendet wurden, immer war die Schaltung dieser Apparate sehr verschieden von den wirklichen Neuronenschaltungen des Gehirns.

Lernende Maschinen und Kybernetik des Gedächtnisses. Seitdem man lernende Maschinen bauen kann, erwartet die physiologische Erforschung der Lernfunktionen von der Technik manche Anregungen. Doch gelten hier die gleichen Einschränkungen, die allgemein die physiologische Brauchbarkeit technischer Modelle des Nervensystems begrenzen (vgl. S. 875). Besonders leistungsfähige maschinelle Lösungen der Nachrichtentechnik, wie die Lernmatrizen STEINBUCHS sind nicht als Modelle des Nervensystems entworfen, sondern als Apparate für bestimmte *praktische Zwecke* erfunden worden. Parallelen mit der biologischen Kybernetik wurden erst nachträglich von STEINBUCH weiter ausgeführt [S 47]. So interessant und technisch elegant diese Lernmatrizen sind, so wenig sagen sie uns über die physiologischen Vorgänge beim Lernen des Organismus. Die Leistungen dieser Maschinen ersparen dem Neurophysiologen nicht die mühsamen und geduldigen Experimente zur Erforschung der cerebralen Vorgänge beim Lernen und bei den bedingten Reflexen.

Vielleicht sind manche dieser Modellversuche für die Neurophysiologie sogar mehr hinderlich als nützlich, weil sie auf *falsche Wege* führen, die für die Technik zwar gangbar sind, aber die der Organismus nie eingeschlagen hat. So haben auch die verschiedenen Apparate zur Imitierung bedingter Reflexe, die schon vor vielen Jahren z. T. mit sehr einfachen Mitteln gebaut werden konnten [G 31, W 7], die Neurophysiologie der bedingten Reflexvorgänge noch nicht gefördert. Man muß klar aussprechen, daß wir über die *elementarphysiologischen Grundlagen des Lernens im Gehirn noch nichts Exaktes wissen, und daß die kybernetischen Modelle darüber nichts aussagen.* Auch die Millionenzahl der Neurone des Gehirns erschwert durch ihre der Technik fremde Größenordnung eine Korrelation mit den lernenden Maschinen. Solche komplexen hirnähnlichen Modelle wären nicht nur nach anatomischen Daten, sondern auch nach elektrophysiologischen Ergebnissen aufzustellen. Ein neuronales Lernmodell würde neue Schaltbilder erfordern, die der Neurophysiologe noch nicht liefern kann. Die bei bedingten Reaktionen registrierten Neuronentladungen geben auch bei Berücksichtigung der Massenableitungen des EEG mit seinen langsamen Wellen noch keine brauchbare Grundlage für ein neuronales Gedächtnismodell. Selbst wenn es gelänge, die Ableitungstechnik und Aufzeichnung so wesentlich zu verbessern, daß Hunderte und Tausende cerebraler Neuronentladungen simultan registriert werden könnten, würde uns dies noch nicht viel nützen.

Die Analyse komplizierter multipler Neuronenschaltungen würde derart große Anforderungen an die Auswertungsmethoden stellen, daß es fraglich erscheint, ob sich ein solch riesiger Aufwand von Apparaturen und Rechenmaschinen mit seinen enormen Kosten lohnt und ob sie unsere Erkenntnis der Gedächtnismechanismen wesentlich fördert. Ein echtes kybernetisches Hirnmodell neuronaler Gedächtnisschaltungen bleibt daher vorläufig utopisch, obwohl es schon zahlreiche einfachere lernende Maschinen mit leistungsfähigem Gedächtnis gibt.

Speicherung und Auswertung von Informationen durch Lernmatrizen. Unter den zahlreichen lernenden Maschinen wurden STEINBUCHS *Lernmatrizen* bereits im Kybernetik-Kapitel besprochen. STEINBUCHS neueste Konstruktion ist der *„autonome Lernmatrixdipol"* (*ALD*). Anwendungen dieser ALD-Schaltungen mit Beziehungen zu den bedingten Reaktionen sind in der 3. Auflage von STEINBUCHS „Automat und Mensch" dargestellt. Diese Lernmatrizen können sowohl mit starrem inneren Modell der Außenwelt wie mit anpassungsfähigen inneren Außenweltmodellen gebaut und verwendet werden. Psychologisch interessant ist die Auswertung durch „Spielen" des Modells in verschiedenen Außenweltsituationen, die unterschiedliche Reaktionen und *Bewertungen* ermöglichen. Diese ALD-Strukturen können wesentliche Details von unwesentlichen unterscheiden, „gute" und „schlechte" Reaktionen auswählen. Die Apparate suchen durch „Bewertungsschaltungen" nach der besten Reaktion, die jeweils der Außenwelt oder dem inneren Außenweltmodell, das die Maschine selbst hat, adäquat sind.

Bereits für einfache neurobiologische Vorgänge können von der Technik zahlreiche verschiedene Modelle gebaut werden, deren Mechanismen den biologischen Vorgängen völlig fremd sind. Man wird daher von komplexen technischen Modellen für Lern- und Gedächtnisfunktionen vorläufig keinen Aufschluß über die cerebralen Gedächtnisvorgänge erwarten können, solange die physiologischen Grundlagen der biologischen Gedächtnisspeicherung noch unbekannt sind.

Chemisch-makromolekulare Gedächtnishypothesen

Gedächtnis ist zweifellos Informationsspeicherung, aber nicht jedes Speichern von Informationen ist auch Gedächtnis. Wenn ein Lift mehrere Meldungen über die Haltestationen aufbewahrt und richtig ausführt, so mag der Techniker das „Gedächtnis" nennen. Der Neurophysiologe weiß, daß Gedächtnisleistungen der Organismen damit nicht vergleichbar sind. Entsprechende Vergleiche mit der Gedächtnisinformation stammen aus der Genetik.

Unter dem Einfluß der Kybernetik ist der Informationsbegriff heute sehr weit ausgedehnt worden. Die Erfolge der experimentellen und chemischen Genetik mit der Struktur der Nucleinsäuren in Viren und Bakterien haben dazu geführt, biochemische Substanzen als „genetische Information" oder „genetische Code" zu bezeichnen. Da die chemische Genstruktur offenbar geeignet ist, innerhalb des Organismus gleiche Strukturen zu reproduzieren und die Information darüber von Generation zu Generation weiterzugeben, glauben viele an ein *chemisch-molekulares Gedächtnis*. Dabei werden Erfahrungen über das angeborene *„genetische Artengedächtnis"* auf das Gedächtnis im engeren Sinne, die über Sinnesorgane aufgenommenen, cerebral gesteuerten, *erworbenen* Informationsspeicherungen, übertragen, obwohl ähnliche chemische Mechanismen nicht erwiesen sind. Schon vor dieser molekularen Genetik hatte H. FOERSTER 1948 die physikalisch-chemische Variabilität der Eiweiß-Strukturen mit der Variabilität der Gedächtnisvorgänge verglichen [F 17]. Es fehlt aber bis heute jeder Nachweis solcher Korrelationen der makromolekularen Chemie. Im Gegensatz zu den experimentell fundierten Ergebnissen der biochemischen Genetik mit ihren *Desoxyribonucleinsäure-(DNS-) und Ribonucleinsäure-(RNS-)Verbindungen* sind alle neueren chemisch-molekularen Hypothesen für das erworbene Gedächtnis des Gehirns noch Spekulation ohne experimentelle oder substantielle Grundlagen. *Chemisch ausgelöste Gedächtnisstörungen* von FLEXNER und AGRANOFF [F 14, A 11] sprechen für eine *Beziehung zwischen Eiweißsynthese und mnestischen Fixierungsprozessen im Gehirn*: Das Streptomycin-ähnliche Puromycin, das eine spezifische und reversible Hemmung der Eiweißsynthese hervorruft, blockiert für beschränkte Zeit bei intracerebraler Applikation die Gedächtnisretention. Sowohl bei Mäusen [F 14] wie bei Fischen [A 11] ist dies durch Lernversuche experimentell nachgewiesen. AGRANOFF hat bestimmte kritische Zeiten für die mnestische Fixierung von 30 min nach dem Lernexperiment festgestellt und damit bei Fischen die Puromycinwirkung auch zeitlich weiter präzisiert. Die Puromycineffekte wurden mit ähnlichen Wirkungen des Elektrokrampfes verglichen [A 11], der noch dreifach längere Zeiten nach den Lernversuchen mnestisch blockieren kann.

Beim Menschen sind bisher noch keine spezifisch-chemisch ausgelösten Gedächtnisstörungen bekannt, außer dem Korsakow-Syndrom nach B_1-Avitaminose und schweren Vergiftungen mit symptomatischen Psychosen und folgenden amnestischen Syndromen. Traumatische retrograde Amnesien und die amnestischen Störungen nach Elektrokrampf wären eher als physikalische Blockierung der Gedächtnisfixierung zu erklären. Ob die kurzdauernden Amnesiesyndrome unbekannter Ätiologie, die ADAMS [A 1] und andere beschrieben haben, als vasculäre oder Stoffwechselstörung zu deuten sind, ist noch ungeklärt.

Makromolekulare Gedächtniscodierung. F.O. SCHMITTS Vorstellungen über die makromolekulare Neurologie der Gedächtnisfunktionen gehen aus von genetischen und immunologischen Erfahrungen: Die makromolekularen Grundlagen der Gen-Information und ihrer Reproduktion in verschiedenen Körperzellen und die immunologische Reproduktion von Antikörpern im lebenden Organismus sollen Modelle für die Lern- und Gedächtnisleistungen des Gehirns sein. SCHMITT glaubt, daß ähnliche große Moleküle oder Verbände kleiner Moleküle in den Neuronen eine Gedächtniscodierung, Aufbewahrung und Wiederaktivierung von Gedächtnisvorgängen machen können. Da auch die komplexe Hirnentwicklung durch genetische DNS-RNS-Eiweißsysteme geregelt wird, hält SCHMITT es für möglich, daß auch eine *makromolekulare Schaltung an den Synapsen der Neurone* beim Gedächtnisvorgang stattfindet. Wie diese allerdings in den vielen Millionen von Neuronen, die für differenzierte Gedächtnisvorgänge offenbar notwendig sind, koordiniert werden, darüber kann die makromolekulare Hypothese nichts aussagen.

EIGEN [E 13] hat im Anschluß an SCHMITT die Parallele mit Antigen-Antikörperreaktionen weiter ausgeführt. Diese werden als eine Art biologischen Lernvorgangs im Körper aufgefaßt. Die neurochemische Gedächtnistheorie führt in zahlreiche ungelöste Grundprobleme der Biologie und der aktuellen Forschung über die RNS- und DNS-Synthese und den genetischen Code des „Erbgedächtnisses". Deshalb wurde von SCHMITT ein eigenes „Neurosciences-Research-Program" aufgestellt, in dem alte allgemeine Probleme über den Einfluß von Erbanlage, Umwelt und Erziehung zusammen mit modernen biochemischen Ergebnissen diskutiert werden.

Gedächtnisstörungen und Hirnlokalisation

Cerebrale Korrelate von Merkfähigkeitsstörungen beim Menschen. Alle hirnelektrischen Untersuchungen beim Menschen ergaben bei amnestischen Zuständen *Verlangsamungen der EEG-Rhythmen*. Sowohl beim Gesunden während der Schlafamnesie wie bei Kranken mit Korsakow-Syndromen ist diese EEG-Verlangsamung nachweisbar. Bei traumatischen Psychosen findet sich eine gute Korrelation dieser EEG-Allgemeinveränderung mit amnestischen und Bewußtseinsstörungen. Auch toxisch und avitaminotisch bedingte Amnesien des Wernicke-Korsakow-Syndroms zeigen ähnliche EEG-Veränderungen, z.T. mit Herdbefunden, die nach B_1-Therapie rasch reversibel sind.

Solche offenbar flüchtigen Herdstörungen können beim Wernicke-Syndrom wie bei manchen traumatischen Psychosen isolierte EEG-Befunde ohne klinisches Korrelat bleiben, oder mit aphasischen Störungen verbunden sein. Diese *vorübergehenden Herdstörungen* zeigen die Problematik der Korrelation amnestischer Syndrome mit anatomischen Befunden, um die man sich lange bemüht hat. Bei der früher meist tödlich verlaufenden Wernickeschen Encephalopathie sind die anatomischen Herdbefunde im Hirnstamm am stärksten ausgeprägt, so daß GAMPER die Läsion des Corpus mamillare beim amnestischen Syndrom in den Vordergrund stellte [G 5a, 6].

Bei Korsakow-Syndromen des Menschen sind anatomisch vorwiegend Läsionen im *Zwischenhirn* (C. mamillare, Thalamus) und *Riechhirn* (Ammonshorn und Fornix bilateral) beschrieben, ferner im temporalen Neocortex. Doch waren die diencephalen und rhinencephalen Herde nicht streng lokalisiert und nicht auf das limbische System und seine Verbindungen beschränkt.

Amnestische Syndrome, lokalisierte Hirnläsionen und Hirnreizungen beim Menschen. Nachdem GAMPER [G 5a] das amnestische Syndrom durch Läsionen des *Corpus mamillare* und seiner Verbindungen mit Ammonshorn und Thalamus erklären wollte, konzentrierte sich die Amnesieforschung in den letzten Jahren auf den *Thalamus* und das *limbische System* [K 42]. ADAMS u.Mitarb. [A 1] haben die Herdlokalisationen bei Wernicke-Encephalopathie zusammengestellt und fanden schwere Ausfälle im *dorsomedialen Thalamus*, wenn ein Korsakow-Syndrom bestanden hatte. Wernicke-Fälle ohne schwere Merkstörungen hatten dagegen nur geringe oder keine Läsionen dorsalmedialer Thalamuskerne oder des Pulvinar, obwohl die Corpora mamillaria erhebliche Ausfälle zeigten. Beim Menschen beschrieben PENFIELD und MILNER [P 15, M 43–45] und andere schwere Merkstörungen nach *doppelseitigen Ammonshornexstirpationen* und *Fornixläsionen* (vgl. HASSLER in Bd. I/1A der ersten Auflage).

Nachdem bei der *temporalen Epilepsie* mit ihren amnestischen Dämmerattakken und Dämmerzuständen Krampfentladungen im limbischen System (Ammonshorn und Mandelkern) gefunden wurden, lag es nahe, bei stereotaktischen Eingriffen Hirnreizungen und Amnesieprüfungen zu verbinden. *Ammonshorn- und Fornixreizungen* mit implantierten Elektroden beim Menschen erzeugen amnestische Zustände, die nach UMBACH [U 3] und BRAZIER [B 60] der temporalen Epilepsie entsprechen. Die wichtigsten neurophysiologischen Befunde über elektrische Auslösung von amnestischen Zuständen mit retrograder Amnesie sind von BICKFORD bisher nur unvollständig in der Diskussion zu BRAZIER mitgeteilt worden: Er fand bei bipolarer Reizung (20/s und 3 V) in 3 Fällen mit implantierten Elektroden im mittleren Schläfenlappen nur bei bestimmten Elektrodenpositionen im Temporalmark *amnestische Ausfälle, die bei längerer Reizung zunehmend retrograd bis zu 2 Std oder sogar bis zu Wochen rückläufig verlängert werden konnten* (BICKFORD nach [B 60]). Es handelte sich um Patienten mit Epilepsie.

Da die neuropathologischen Befunde meistens nicht mit hirnelektrischen Untersuchungen verbunden waren und bei den intracerebralen Reizungen anatomische Kontrollen fehlten oder epileptische Hirnveränderungen vorlagen, sind alle diese Ergebnisse beim Menschen noch nicht für eine neurophysiologische Erklärung der amnestischen Syndrome zu verwenden. Sie geben nur einige Hinweise, an welchen Hirnregionen physiologische Untersuchungen anzusetzen wären.

Temporaler Neocortex und Gedächtnis. Das Sprachgedächtnis ist nach Aphasieerfahrungen vorwiegend in isocorticalen Feldern des Schläfenlappens lokalisiert. Eine ähnliche Lokalisation gilt vielleicht auch für nicht-sprachliche Erinnerungen: PENFIELD hat bei seinen corticalen Reizversuchen an Epileptikern bestimmte Erinnerungsbilder mit mehreren Sinnesmodalitäten vorwiegend temporal auslösen können [P 9-12]. Er folgerte daraus und aus klinischen Erfahrungen, daß dem Schläfenlappen mit seinen diencephalen Verbindungen eine besondere Rolle für das Gedächtnis zukommt. Allerdings sind diese Reizergebnisse bisher nur bei Epileptikern, ähnlich einer provozierten Aura, gefunden worden, fehlen aber am nicht-epileptischen Gehirn. ORBACH, MILNER und RASMUSSEN [O 10] zeigten bei Affenversuchen mit doppelseitigen Ammonshornläsionen und Schädigungen anderer Allo- und Isocortexteile des Schläfenlappens, daß Störungen der Merkfähigkeit, die bei KLÜVER und BUCYS Experimenten [K 25] weniger betont wurden, vorwiegend durch *allocorticale* Läsionen entstehen, unabhängig vom temporalen Isocortex.

Nach Cortexreizungen bei Epileptikern, die bestimmte Erinnerungen auslösten, hat PENFIELD angenommen, die isocorticale Rinde des Schläfenlappens sei ein *Gedächtnisspeicher,* eine "storehouse of remembered experience" (Lagerhaus der Erinnerung). Da einseitige Temporallappen-Exstirpation die durch den Reiz ausgelösten Erinnerungen nicht zum Verschwinden bringt, sollen diese Gedächtnisspuren *doppelseitig* im Schläfenlappen vertreten sein und aus dem Subcortex aktiviert werden. Die aktivierenden Subcorticalstrukturen, die vorwiegend im medialen Zwischenhirn liegen sollen, werden als *centrencephales System* zusammengefaßt [P 10, 13]. Für die Doppelseitigkeit der Gedächtnismechanismen sprechen neurochirurgische Erfahrungen, daß Gedächtnisstörungen bei bilateralen Schläfenlappen-Exstirpationen wesentlich stärker sind als bei einseitigen [P 15]. Auch der einzige Fall von sicherem Klüver-Bucy-Syndrom beim Menschen, den TERZIAN und DALLE ORE [T 1 a] beschrieben haben, ein mit bilateraler, temporaler Lobotomie operierter Epileptiker, hatte schwerste Störungen des Altgedächtnisses und der Merkfähigkeit. Soweit dies zu untersuchen war, schienen auch frühkindliche Erinnerungen, wie das Wiedererkennen der eigenen Mutter, ausgefallen zu sein.

Fehlende Synthese der Lernforschung. Überblickt man die vielen Experimente über Lernen und Gedächtnis, so wird klar, daß alles im Fluß ist. Noch mehr als in anderen aktuellen Gebieten kommen zahlreiche Anregungen aus verschiedenen Forschungsrichtungen zusammen, ohne daß bisher eine brauchbare Synthese gelungen wäre.

Alle Bemühungen der Neurophysiologen, der Kybernetiker und Biochemiker haben bis heute noch zu keiner brauchbaren Erklärung von Lernen und Gedächtnis geführt. Wie vor 70 Jahren, als PAWLOWS Experimente begannen, bleiben auch heute noch die Gedächtnisvorgänge das größte Rätsel der Hirnfunktionen. Aber niemand kann wissen, wie weit künftige neue Entdeckungen noch führen werden.

Zusammenfassung

Umweltadäquates Verhalten, Erziehung, Sprache und Bildung beruhen auf Lernprozessen und Gedächtnisfunktionen, so daß die Physiologie des Lernens und der Informationsspeicherung auch von psychiatrischem Interesse ist. Seit EBBINGHAUS wurden Gedächtnis, Merkfähigkeit und Vergessen quantitativ psychophysisch untersucht. Dann ermöglichte PAWLOWS Methode der bedingten Reflexe eine tierexperimentelle Untersuchung von Lernvorgängen. PAWLOW unterschied ein „erstes Signalsystem", das Menschen und Tiere für Wahrnehmungen und Vorstellungen gemeinsam haben, von einem „zweiten Signalsystem", das der Sprache und dem abstrahierenden Denken beim Menschen entspricht. Neurophysiologische Korrelate der Konditionierung sind nur unvollkommen mit EEG-Befunden erforscht. Vor bedingten Reaktionen des Menschen erscheint WALTERS „*Erwartungswelle*" oder "contingent negative variation" (CNV) als bilaterale negative corticale Potentialverschiebung der Parietofrontalregionen zwischen dem ersten bedingten Warnreiz und dem zweiten imperativen Reiz. Die Größe der Erwartungswelle wächst mit Motivation, Intention und Erwartungsspannung, ähnlich dem Bereitschaftspotential KORNHUBERS.

Die neurophysiologischen Mechanismen und cerebralen Grundlagen von Lernen und Gedächtnis sind noch ungeklärt. Ob das Kurzzeitgedächtnis wiederholten Erregungskreisen in Neuronenketten entspricht, und das Langzeitgedächtnis eine molekularbiologische Speicherung ist, die komplexe neuronale Erregungsmuster evozieren kann, bleibt offen. Auch die neurochemischen Bedingungen des Kurzzeit- und Langzeitgedächtnisses, der Gedächtnis-Konsolidierung und Reaktivierung sind noch unbekannt, und lernende Maschinen haben nur noch keine kybernetische Erklärung der Programmierung cerebraler Gedächtnisvorgänge geliefert. Amnestische Syndrome können nach bilateralen Läsionen des limbischen Systems und des Zwischenhirns auftreten und sind in der Regel mit Verlangsamung des EEG-Grundrhythmus korreliert, besonders deutlich bei traumatischen Psychosen. Doch kann man aus langsamen EEG-Wellen nicht umgekehrt auf Merkfähigkeitsminderung schließen.

XIII. Grundlagen des Elektrencephalogramms (EEG)

> "The mind is a something with such manifold variety, such fleeting changes, such countless nuances, such wealth of combinations, such heights and depths of mood, such sweeps of passion, such vistas of imagination, that the bald submission of some electrical potentials recognizable in nerve-centres as correlative to all these may seem to the special student of mind almost derisory."
>
> CH. SHERRINGTON: Man on his nature, 1946.

BERGERS Entdeckung des Elektrencephalogramms (EEG) beim Menschen, die ihm – nach älteren Vorversuchen bei Tieren – 1924 bis 1929 gelang, hat eine neue Epoche der Neurophysiologie eingeleitet. Erst diese elektrische Registrierung der Hirnströme von der Kopfhaut oder der Hirnsubstanz ermöglichte eine *direkte* Untersuchung normaler und pathologischer Hirntätigkeit beim Menschen und ihre klinische Anwendung. Bis dahin konnte man nur indirekt aus dem Verhalten des Organismus, aus peripheren Leistungen, Reflex- oder Testuntersuchungen und aus der Introspektion auf zentrale Hirnfunktionen und ihre Störungen schließen.

Der praktischen und theoretischen Bedeutung des EEG für die Diagnostik organischer Hirnkrankheiten in der Neurologie entspricht noch nicht eine ähnlich erfolgreiche hirnelektrische Forschung in der Psychiatrie. Psychiatrisch-diagnostisch brauchbare Veränderungen des EEG beschränken sich vorwiegend auf die Epilepsie, auf hirnorganische Erkrankungen und Psychosen sowie auf Korrelationen mit der psychiatrischen Schocktherapie. Schon BERGER hat die begrenzte Anwendung des EEG auf gewisse organisch-cerebrale Störungen gesehen. Er mußte seine ersten Hoffnungen aufgeben, daß die elektrischen Hirnströme eine Psychophysiologie begründen, zur Lösung des Leib-Seele-Problems beitragen und die Frage „psychischer Energie" beantworten könnten oder daß sie die Erforschung der endogenen Psychosen erleichtern würden. Auch Physiologen wie SHERRINGTON behandelten Beziehungen zwischen psychischen und hirnelektrischen Phänomenen mit größter Skepsis [S 33].

Für die Psychiatrie sind bisher nur folgende Korrelationen von EEG und psychischen Phänomenen genügend sichergestellt und von praktischer Bedeutung: 1. *Beziehungen zwischen EEG und normalen Bewußtseinsänderungen,* die bei Gesunden im Schlaf- und Wachzustand auftreten, und die in Kapitel X und XI dargestellt wurden, 2. *EEG-Veränderungen bei pathologischen Bewußtseinsstörungen,* insbesondere bei *Epilepsien* mit epileptischen Psychosen und Dämmerzuständen, 3. *EEG-Veränderungen bei organischen Psychosen mit amnestischen Syndromen,* 4. *EEG-Veränderungen bei psychiatrischen Somatotherapien.* Die Allgemeinveränderungen des EEG mit Verlangsamung des Grundrhythmus zeigen bei traumatischen Psychosen und nach Elektroschockbehandlung oft gute Korrelationen zum Verlauf amnestischer Syndrome.

Die Technik, Methodik, Diagnostik und Auswertung des EEG sind hier nicht zu behandeln. Ich verweise auf den Beitrag KÜNKELS in diesem Band.

Formen des menschlichen EEG

Die Ordnung der EEG-Wellen. Die für die praktische Diagnostik wichtigsten Formen des EEG zeigt Abb. 44. Beim gesunden Erwachsenen sind im Wachzustand mit geschlossenen Augen, den Standardbedingungen der EEG-Ableitung, meistens nur α- und β-Wellen erkennbar, obwohl das EEG im Schlaf verschiedene schnelle und langsame Wellen enthält (Abb. 39). Langsamere Wellen und abnorme EEG-Formen sind unter Standard-Ableitungsbedingungen Zeichen veränderter Hirnfunktionen, die verschiedene Ursachen haben können. Einige dieser normalen und pathologischen Bedingungen für EEG-Verlangsamung und Beschleunigung sind mit dem Spektrum der EEG-Wellen in Abb. 45 schematisch dargestellt.

Seit BERGER [B 24–27] ist die Bezeichnung der verschiedenen EEG-Wellen mit griechischen Buchstaben üblich. Man unterscheidet nach ihrer Frequenz:
Alpha-Wellen (α): 8 bis 13/s,
Beta-Wellen (β): 14 bis 30/s,
Theta- oder Zwischenwellen (ϑ): 4 bis 7/s,
Delta-Wellen (δ): 1 bis 3,5 s.

Nach ihrer pathologischen Form und Größe bezeichnet man als *Krampfpotentiale* abnorme konvulsive Wellen, die verschiedene charakteristische Formen zeigen und vor allem bei Epilepsie vorkommen.

Die α- und β-Wellen bilden das EEG des gesunden wachen Erwachsenen, die langsameren Zwischen- und δ-Wellen erscheinen erst in der Ermüdung oder

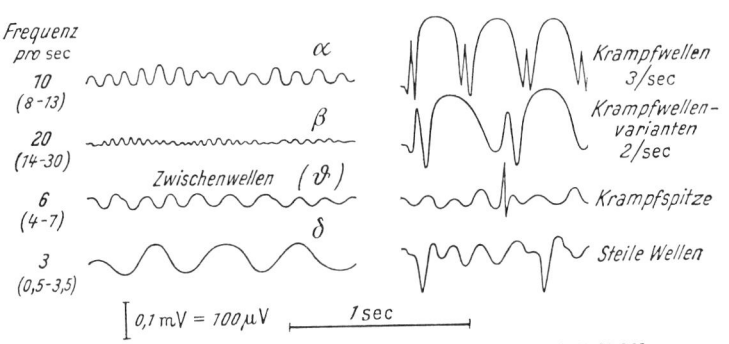

Abb. 44. Hauptformen des EEG. Nach JUNG (1950/53) [J 32]

Links die verschiedenen Wellenarten, die bei Gesunden im Wach- und Schlafzustand vorkommen können. Im Wachzustand sind normalerweise nur α- und β-Wellen erkennbar. Deutliche langsame δ-Wellen finden sich nur bei Kindern und im Schlaf. Wenn sie beim Erwachsenen im Wach-EEG vorkommen, sind sie meistens Zeichen einer Hirnerkrankung, Zwischenwellen von 4–7 sec können gelegentlich auch beim gesunden Erwachsenen in der Ermüdung beobachtet werden.
Rechts die Krampfpotentiale, die vor allem bei Epilepsie vorkommen. Krampfwellen von 3/sec (spike and wave, petit mal) mit Abfolge von raschen und langsamen Abläufen mit großer Amplitude bis 1 mV sind charakteristisch für genuine Epilepsie im jüngeren Alter mit kleinen Anfällen und für Pyknolepsie. Krampfwellenvarianten von 2/sec (petit mal variant) finden sich vor allem bei residualer Epilepsie. Einzelne Krampfspitzen (spikes) kommen über epileptischen Foci vor allem bei symptomatischer Epilepsie vor. Steile Wellen (sharp waves) finden sich sowohl bei genuiner wie bei symptomatischer Epilepsie, besonders temporal. Sie sind ebenso wie die paroxysmale Dysrhythmie charakteristisch für Dämmerattacken (psychomotorische Anfälle)

im Schlaf. Bei kleinen Kindern und Hirnkranken sind solche langsamere Wellen auch ohne Schlaf oft im EEG erkennbar, bei der Epilepsie werden z.T. auch im Anfallsintervall charakteristische Krampfpotentiale im EEG registriert. Beim wachen, entspannten Erwachsenen mit geschlossenen Augen überwiegt eine ziemlich regelmäßige α-Wellentätigkeit von 8 bis 12/s, vor allem über der Occipitalregion. Bei Augenöffnen oder Anspannung der Aufmerksamkeit vermindern sich die α-Wellen (α-Blockierung). Ein gutes Schema der normalen und pathologischen EEG-Potentiale findet man bei GIBBS [G 20]. Eine vereinfachte Übersicht zeigt Abb. 44.

Neben den seit BERGER, GIBBS und WALTER klassifizierten Wellenformen mit den genannten Bezeichnungen ist immer auch die Grundfrequenz der Hauptwellen zu beachten, die Hinweise auf eine allgemeine Hirnveränderung gibt.

Frequenzspektrum und Verlangsamung der EEG-Wellen. Als allgemeine Regel kann man mit wenigen Ausnahmen annehmen, daß eine *Verlangsamung der EEG-Wellen mit einer verminderten Hirntätigkeit einhergeht.* Eine Beschleunigung mit überwiegend schnellen Wellen bedeutet oft eine Aktivierung der Hirnfunktionen entsprechend BERGERS „aktivem EEG". Meistens zeigen pathologische Hirnprozesse eine Verlangsamung der EEG-Wellen, dagegen nur selten, wie bei Krampfentladungen und anderen Reizerscheinungen, eine Beschleunigung. Diese Regeln gelten nur cum grano salis. Bei pharmakologischen Einwirkungen besonders nach Barbituraten, findet man eine biphasische EEG-Veränderung, bei kleinen Dosen zunächst Beschleunigung, dann bei größeren Dosen Verlangsamung (Abb. 45 unten rechts). Ähnliches gilt für das Excitationsstadium der Narkose.

Korrelationen von EEG-Befunden, Hirntätigkeit und Verhalten sind nur in beschränktem Maße möglich und bleiben meist grobe statistische Hinweise,

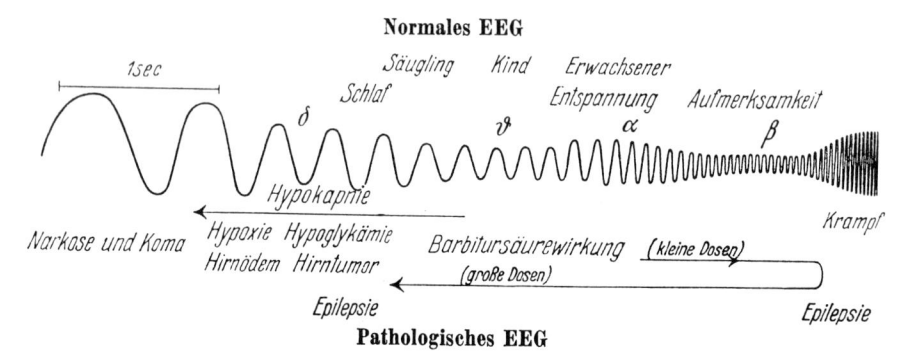

Abb. 45. Frequenzband der Hirnrhythmen. Nach JUNG (1953) [J 32]
Vereinfachtes Schema der Beziehung verschiedener Zustände des normalen und pathologischen EEG zum Frequenzspektrum des Grundrhythmus. *Oben* sind verschiedene Altersstufen und Verhaltensweisen mit der Grundfrequenz des EEG korreliert. *Unten* werden verschiedene Formen des pathologischen EEG mit ihren meist langsameren Grundrhythmen bezeichnet. Fast immer findet sich bei krankhaften Hirnveränderungen eine *Verlangsamung*. Vermehrte schnelle Hirnrhythmen sieht man fast nur bei Epilepsie und unter kleinen Barbituratdosen, bevor große Dosen tiefen Schlaf und Koma erzeugen. Langsame Wellen haben meist größere Amplituden als schnelle Wellen. Nur der normale α-Rhythmus zeigt große Wellen von 10/sec. Die Amplituden des EEG variieren bei gleichen Zuständen stärker als die jeweiligen Frequenzen

die zahlreiche Ausnahmen und individuelle Variationen haben. Dies wurde schon mit den verschiedenen EEG-Formen bei Bewußtseinsänderungen und in den Schlafstadien besprochen. Eine Übersicht über einige Beziehungen schneller und langsamer EEG-Wellen bei verschiedenen Frequenzen des Grundrhythmus im *EEG-Spektrum* zeigt Abb. 45. Dieses Frequenzband gibt nur allgemeine Hinweise auf Veränderungen des normalen und pathologischen EEG, erlaubt aber keine speziellen Aussagen über die physikalisch-chemischen oder physiologischen Charakteristika der einzelnen „Spektralbereiche" von EEG-Wellen. Man weiß zwar, bei welchen Funktionsänderungen und Störungen des Gehirns im EEG vorwiegend α-Wellen, β-Wellen oder δ-Wellen auftreten, aber wie diese Wellen physiologisch zustande kommen und welche Hirnstoffwechselumstellungen die Verlangsamung oder Beschleunigung begleiten, ist weiterhin unbekannt.

Das EEG als Indicator cerebraler Störungen

Da wir noch nicht wissen, wie die EEG-Wellen entstehen und welche Strukturen für sie notwendig sind, kann man das EEG noch nicht zur Erklärung bestimmter Hirnvorgänge verwenden. Dennoch geben EEG-Veränderungen Hinweise auf *Störungen cerebraler Funktionsordnungen*. Dies ist besonders eindrucksvoll bei den Epilepsien, deren EEG-Befunde gut mit verschiedenen Anfallsformen korrelieren, während morphologische Befunde keine befriedigende Erklärung geben. Als ein solcher *Indicator für cerebrale Funktionsstörungen und ihre Lokalisation* ist die EEG-Untersuchung für die neuropsychiatrische Klinik von praktisch-klinischer Bedeutung, obwohl die theoretisch-physiologische Grundlage vorläufig ungewiß bleibt.

Das EEG als cerebrales „Nebengeräusch". Die geringen Korrelationen des EEG mit bestimmten cerebralen Funktionen und die Brauchbarkeit hirnelektrischer Befunde für die Erkennung von Hirnerkrankungen werden vielleicht durch folgenden *Vergleich* verständlicher: Um anschaulich zu machen, wie wenig das EEG über spezielle Hirnvorgänge aussagen kann, habe ich die Hirnwellen mit dem *rhythmischen Geräusch einer Maschine* verglichen: *Das EEG bedeutet für die Hirnfunktion nicht mehr als das Nebengeräusch einer arbeitenden Maschine.* Die Hirnrhythmen des EEG entsprächen dann etwa dem regelmäßigen Takt eines laufenden Motors oder dem Dampfausstoß einer Lokomotive. Solche Geräusche sagen wenig über Funktion und Bau dieser Maschinen, aber wer ihre Arbeitsweise kennt, kann aus der Art und Gleichmäßigkeit des Geräusches und aus Nebengeräuschen schließen, ob die Maschine eine Störung oder einen Defekt hat. Wenn solche abnormen Nebengeräusche von bestimmten Orten des Motors kommen, so kann man den *Ort der Störung*, aber meist nicht ihre Art bestimmen. Dies ist das Lokalisationsprinzip auch in der EEG-Diagnostik: aus dem Ort bestimmter abnormer EEG-Wellen schließen wir auf die Lokalisation von Erkrankungen, deren Natur sehr verschieden sein kann. Bei *generalisierten* abnormen EEG-Wellen nehmen wir an, daß *allgemeine Funktionsstörungen* des Gehirns vorliegen. Diese sind oft metabolische Störungen oder hypoxisch-vasculäre Veränderungen. So wird ein verändertes EEG als Indicator für eine abnorme Hirntätigkeit verwendet, wie ein Störgeräusch einer Maschine deren Reparaturbedürftigkeit anzeigt. Doch wäre derjenige ein schlechter Maschinist, der Reparaturen einer Maschine nur nach Geräuschveränderungen ohne

Kontrolle ihrer Einzelleistungen machen wollte oder der behaupten wollte, eine Maschine mit normalem Motorgeräusch sei auch normal leistungsfähig. Wie ein normales Motorengeräusch nicht beweist, daß die Maschinenfunktionen und Leistungen gut und effektiv sind, so läßt auch ein normales EEG nicht erkennen, ob das betreffende Gehirn intakt ist und mit normaler Wirksamkeit arbeitet. Es gibt bessere und genauere Kriterien für eine Maschinenleistung, wie es neben der EEG-Registrierung viele andere Untersuchungsmethoden des Gehirns gibt. Nur bestimmte cerebrale Funktionsstörungen zeigen sich in einem pathologischen EEG. Dies sind – außer den Herdveränderungen bei groborganischen Hirnerkrankungen, Tumoren, Gefäßläsionen usw. – vor allem *Stoffwechselveränderungen und epileptische Störungen*.

In den letzten Jahren ist es zunehmend wahrscheinlicher geworden, daß nicht nur Allgemeinveränderungen, sondern auch Herdbefunde des EEG durch lokale metabolische und Durchblutungsveränderungen bedingt sind. Für den Herdbefund großer, langsamer Wellen, den sogenannten δ-Focus, haben schon WALTERS erste Untersuchungen 1936 gezeigt, daß sie nicht den Hirntumor, sondern das umgebende *Hirnödem* anzeigen [W 5]. Dies hat sich später oft bestätigt und ist auf Abb. 46 schematisch dargestellt. Schon früher wurde auf die prinzipiell andersartige Lokalisationsbedeutung von EEG-Befunden bei Tumoren hingewiesen [J 32]: *Das EEG zeigt nicht anatomische Hirnveränderungen, sondern Aktivitätsstörungen des Hirngewebes,* im Gegensatz zu anderen diagnostischen Methoden, wie Arteriographie, Pneumencephalographie und Computertomographie mit ihren klaren Lokalbefunden. Dies soll nicht ausschließen, daß EEG-Veränderungen auch mit feinen Störungen submikroskopischer Art einhergehen können, wie sie nach epileptischen Krämpfen elektronenmikroskopisch gefunden wurden. Korrelationen mit lokalen Durchblutungsmessungen durch INGVARS Methode [I 2, 3] versprechen später weitere Aufklärung der Beziehungen des EEG mit Durchblutung und Gewebsstoffwechsel.

Die Begrenzung auf die somatische Forschung weist dem EEG für die eigentliche Psychiatrie der endogenen Psychosen vorläufig eine negative Rolle zu.

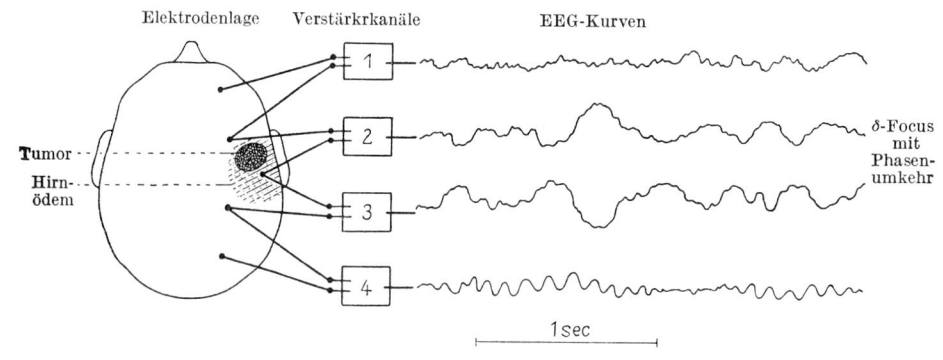

Abb. 46. EEG-Herdbefund mit δ-Focus über dem Hirnödem bei einem kleinen Temporaltumor. Nach JUNG (1953) [J 32]. Die unregelmäßigen langsamen Wellen gehen aus von der gemeinsamen Elektrode des 2. und 3. Verstärkerkanals, so daß in diesen beiden Registrierungen eine Phasenumkehr der langsamen δ-Wellen entsteht. Dieser δ-Focus entsteht nicht im Tumor selbst, sondern durch *Stoffwechselveränderungen des ödematösen Hirngewebes in der Umgebung des Tumors*

Hirnelektrische Untersuchungen dienen mehr dem *Ausschluß* organisch-cerebraler Erkrankungen als der positiven psychiatrischen Diagnose der Psychosen. Bei der psychiatrischen Schockbehandlung gibt das EEG zwar wichtige Hinweise auf vorübergehende therapiebedingte Hirnfunktionsstörungen, aber diese haben wenig Beziehung zu der psychotischen Grunderkrankung. Die EEG-Veränderungen bei der Insulin-, Cardiazol- oder Elektroschocktherapie sind daher nur theoretisch interessant und haben nur geringe praktische und keine diagnostische Bedeutung. Das gleiche gilt für die EEG-Veränderungen durch Psychopharmaka, obwohl Korrelationen der EEG-Befunde zur Prognose neuerdings diskutiert worden sind [H 25]. Erst die weitere Entwicklung wird zeigen, ob hirnelektrische Untersuchungen zusammen mit der Neurochemie noch positivere Ergebnisse für die endogenen Psychosen bringen werden.

Zusammenfassung

Das *Elektrencephalogramm (EEG)*, die Registrierung der in der Großhirnrinde entstehenden elektrischen Hirnströme von der Kopfhaut, kann Veränderungen der normalen und pathologischen Hirntätigkeit anzeigen. Das EEG des Menschen beschränkt sich auf globale elektrische Korrelate synchronisierter Nervenzelltätigkeit, aber kann nicht Einzelneuronentladungen erfassen. EEG-Veränderungen findet man auch bei Stoffwechselstörungen und Durchblutungsminderungen des Gehirns, doch sind die Aussagen über die Lokalisation und die Korrelation mit bestimmten cerebralen Funktionen begrenzt. Man kann das EEG mit dem rhythmischen Geräusch einer arbeitenden Maschine vergleichen, deren Veränderung zwar Tätigkeit oder Störung des Betriebes anzeigt, aber nicht die Leistung der Maschine und nicht die Ursache von Betriebsstörungen erkennen läßt. Für die *Psychiatrie* sind vier Beziehungen von EEG und psychischen Phänomenen von Bedeutung: 1) EEG-Veränderungen bei normalen Bewußtseinsregulationen im Schlaf- und Wachzustand. 2) EEG-Veränderungen bei pathologischen Bewußtseinsstörungen, insbesondere bei Epilepsie. 3) EEG-Veränderungen bei organischen Psychosen. 4) EEG-Veränderungen bei psychiatrischen Somatotherapien.

XIV. Schluß

> "The student of the mind, for instance the practical psychiatrist at the mental hospital, must find the physiology of the brain still remote and vague for his desiderata on his subject ... He may have hoped from it some knowledge which would serve to found the norm from which psycho-pathology could take its points of departure in this direction or in that."
> "The mental is not examinable as a form of energy. That in brief is the gap which parts psychiatry and physiology."
> CH. SHERRINGTON: Man on his nature, 1946.

Die Neurophysiologie hat vor allem durch die hirnelektrische Forschung in drei Jahrzehnten zahlreiche neue Einsichten in die Gehirnfunktionen gebracht, die vor 50 Jahren noch niemand für möglich gehalten hätte. Objektive EEG-Registrierungen cerebraler Begleiterscheinungen des Schlaf- und Wachverhaltens und verschiedener pathologischer Bewußtseinsstörungen bei der Epilepsie und den organischen Psychosen sind auch klinisch bedeutsame Fortschritte. Für die Psychiatrie bedeuten sie allerdings nur Teilaspekte. Die Neurophysiologie hat in der psychiatrischen Forschung zunächst nur begrenzte Möglichkeiten. Vielleicht wird die Neurochemie mit neuen Methoden in den nächsten Jahrzehnten noch weiter in das Gebiet pathologischer Störungen hineinführen, als es die Neurophysiologie vermag. Wahrscheinlich liegt die Bedeutung neurophysiologischer Methoden mit ihrer exakten fortlaufenden Registrierung mehr in der Aufklärung *normaler* Hirnfunktionen als in der Erforschung psychischer Störungen. Denn außer den organischen und epileptischen Psychosen kennen wir noch keine neurophysiologischen Korrelate anderer seelischer Erkrankungen.

Die klinisch-empirische Anwendung der Neurophysiologie in der Psychiatrie ist beschränkt. Das EEG kann dem Kliniker bisher nur auf wenigen Gebieten in der diagnostischen Routinearbeit helfen. Differenziertere Methoden der experimentellen Forschung können lediglich cerebrale Teilmechanismen psychischer Vorgänge aufzeigen. Ohne klinische Synthese und Anwendung bleiben neurophysiologische Einzelmethoden für die psychiatrische Praxis unfruchtbar. Dennoch sind ihre Ergebnisse oft von theoretischer Bedeutung für die Hirnphysiologie und damit auch für die psychiatrische Grundlagenforschung.

Neurophysiologische und psychiatrische Forschung

Eine Schlußbetrachtung soll nicht zusammenfassend wiederholen, was schon mehrfach gesagt wurde, doch seien einige allgemeine Folgerungen nochmals erwähnt.

Experimentelle und klinische Neurophysiologie. Überlegen wir uns, was die Neurophysiologie für die Psychiatrie leisten kann, so ergeben sich zwei Gruppen von theoretischen und praktischen Forschungsergebnissen. *1. Experimentelle Beiträge zur Grundlagenforschung cerebraler Mechanismen:* a) Hirnphysiologische Korrelationen mit Affekten und Triebvorgängen, mit Wachen und Schlafen. b) Objektive Untersuchungen über Sinneswahrnehmungen und ihre Störungen im Gehirn. c) Experimentelle Grundlagen zur Hirnlokalisation und Hirnpathologie durch cerebrale Reizung, Ausschaltung und Hirnpotentialableitung. *2. Praktisch-klinische Leistungen zur Diagnose und Therapie:* a) Hirnelektrische Registrierungen als diagnostische Hilfsmittel zur Erkennung organischer Störungen und Psychosen bei epileptischen und anderen Hirnerkrankungen. b) Ergänzungen der psychiatrischen Diagnostik durch objektive Darstellung somatischer Begleitsymptome psychischer Störungen. c) Untersuchungen neuropharmakologischer und anderer therapeutischer Wirkungsmechanismen mit objektiver Kontrolle cerebraler Veränderungen bei somatischen Behandlungen in der Psychiatrie.

Wechselwirkung von Physiologie und Psychiatrie. *Neurophysiologie und Psychiatrie können voneinander lernen.* Subjektive und objektive Beobachtung müssen sich in beiden Fächern ergänzen. Der *Neurophysiologe* kann vom Psychiater anschaulich-synthetisches Denken und intuitives Erfassen auf der Grundlage subjektiver Erfahrung kennenlernen und damit seine selektive analytische Detailforschung von Einzelmechanismen durch Auswertung von introspektiven und Verhaltensaspekten erweitern. Der *Psychiater* kann vom Neurophysiologen exakte naturwissenschaftliche Methodik, experimentelles analytisches Vorgehen, objektive Registrierungen und quantifizierende Auswertungen erlernen. Im 19. Jahrhundert wurde neben der objektiven Erfassung von Einzelvorgängen seit FECHNER die Messung psychischer Funktionen durch die experimentelle Psychologie zu stark betont. Solche Quantifizierungen wurden damals in der Sinnesphysiologie nur mit subjektiven Methoden der Psychophysik durchgeführt, da die objektiven Registrierungen von Sinnesvorgängen wenig entwickelt waren. Die heftige Reaktion der phänomenologischen Forschung gegen die messende Experimentalpsychologie hat eine Mißachtung experimentell-quantitativer Methoden in der Psychiatrie erzeugt, die lange nachwirkte. Die Testpsychologie und ihre klinische Anwendung hat diese Situation nicht verbessern können. Erst durch naturwissenschaftliche Verfahren der Physiologie, Biochemie, Serologie und zum Teil auch der Anatomie haben messende Methoden in der Neuropsychiatrie wieder praktische Bedeutung erlangt.

Positive Ergebnisse der Neurophysiologie sind objektive Registrierungen von einzelnen Nerven- und Hirnstrukturen und experimentelle Entscheidungen mit streng begrenzter Anwendung. Ihre Resultate und Gesetze bleiben gültig, auch wenn ihre Deutung sich mit Hypothesen und neuen Ergebnissen wandelt. Die wissenschaftlichen Ergebnisse der Psychiatrie sind noch wandelbarer, noch abhängiger vom Zeitgeist und weniger klar begrenzt. Die Psychiatrie will sich nicht mehr, wie vor 50 Jahren auf Geisteskrankheiten und Neurosen beschränken und dringt ein in die verschiedensten Gebiete menschlichen Seelenlebens und menschlichen Verhaltens mit ihrem komplizierten sozialen Gefüge. Die Psychiatrie bezahlt ihr ausgedehntes Interesse für alle menschlichen Fragen mit einer verminderten Exaktheit. Ihre klinische und Laboratoriumsforschung ergab zwar einige naturwissenschaftliche Ergebnisse von dauernder Gültigkeit. Aber nach ihrer Breitenentwicklung und Ausdehnung in viele Grenzgebiete der Sozial- und Geisteswissenschaften kann man bezweifeln, ob eine solche Psychiatrie noch zur Medizin und Naturwissenschaft gehört. Nur soweit die Psychiatrie auch Korrelationen zur Psychologie, Physiologe und Neurologie behandelt, kann sie von neurophysiologischen Experimenten und Ergebnissen Anregung erhalten.

Die Hoffnung scheint begründet, daß systematische Anwendungen naturwissenschaftlicher Methoden mit experimentell oder statistisch nachprüfbaren und korrigierbaren Ergebnissen und Erklärungen die auf Einzelanalysen und Beschreibungen gerichtete psychopathologische Psychiatrie erfolgreich ergänzen werden. Eine solche naturwissenschaftliche Psychiatrie bleibt noch eine Aufgabe der Zukunft. Einige Ansätze für diese Forschungsaufgabe sind vielleicht in den Ergebnissen der modernen Neurophysiologie erkennbar.

Methodische Unterschiede und Quantifizierung. Neurophysiologie und Psychiatrie unterscheiden sich nicht nur in ihren praktischen Zielen, sondern auch in ihren *Methoden,* die auf verschiedener Ebene Funktionen und Leistungen des Gehirns untersuchen. Eine durchgehende Beziehung ist daher nicht zu erwarten. Der *Neurophysiologe* arbeitet vorwiegend mit experimentell prüfbaren, normalen Leistungen und künstlich gesetzten Funktionsstörungen bei Tieren oder mit objektiven Registrierungen beim Menschen und bevorzugt quantifizierbare

Methoden. Den *Psychiater* beschäftigen mehr abnorme Verhaltensweisen und deren subjektive psychische Korrelate bei kranken Menschen, wobei quantitative Methoden oft vernachlässigt werden. Allgemeine Gesetzmäßigkeiten interessieren mehr den Physiologen, individuelle Besonderheiten mehr den Psychiater. Die Sinnesphysiologie überbrückt diese Unterschiede durch Vergleich objektiver physiologischer Registrierungen bei Tieren und subjektiver psychophysischer Beobachtungen beim Menschen zur Erklärung der Sinnestätigkeit. Ähnliche Funktionsgesetze und Strukturen, die das menschliche Gehirn mit dem der höheren Säugetiere gemeinsam hat, ermöglichen experimentelle Hirnuntersuchungen bei Tieren und Parallelen zwischen tierischem und menschlichem Verhalten. *Daher bildet die Verhaltensforschung eine Brücke zwischen Physiologie und Psychologie.*

Individuelle Variationen ähnlicher Funktionen bei verschiedenen Konstitutionen und Rassen, die uns in Psychologie und Psychiatrie begegnen, sind geringer als Unterschiede zwischen verschiedenen Tierarten, mit denen die zoologische Verhaltensforschung rechnen muß. Wenn die Ethologie trotz dieser Speciesdifferenzen gültige Verhaltensregeln findet, so ermutigt dies zu vergleichenden Untersuchungen bei Tieren und Menschen. Gänse und Hühner sind zweifellos sehr verschiedene Tierspecies, aber beide sind Vögel, die bestimmte Merkmale und Hirnstrukturen gemeinsam haben. Affen und Menschen sind ebenfalls verschiedene Arten, doch zeigen sie in Hirnstrukturen und Verhalten gemeinsame Züge und gleichartige Trieb- und Affektmechanismen, so daß man vergleichbare Experimente planen kann. Neurophysiologie und Verhaltensforschung können die Psychiatrie anregen, einige *quantifizierbare* psychische Vorgänge, die in der Naturwissenschaft am wichtigsten sind, mehr zu beachten. Damit kann auch die Psychiatrie, wie andere medizinische Fächer, zum Teil naturwissenschaftlich begründet werden.

Ein Wort EINSTEINS über das Verhältnis von Mathematik und Erfahrungswissenschaft [E 14] wäre auch auf Beziehungen von Physiologie und Psychiatrie anzuwenden: Wie Aussagen der „exakten" Mathematik über die Wirklichkeit nur sehr begrenzt möglich sind, und wie sichere Ergebnisse der Geometrie wenig mit der empirischen Wirklichkeit zu tun haben, so verhält sich auch physiologische Grundlagenforschung zur klinischen Psychiatrie. Ergebnisse neurophysiologischer Experimente können sehr wenig zu klinisch-psychiatrischen Fragen beitragen und wenn solche Aussagen versucht werden, so sind sie mit der empirischen Wirklichkeit schwer zu vereinen. Praktisch brauchbare Resultate ergeben neurophysiologische Methoden nur für begrenzte Fragestellungen der klinischen Empirie. Solche Fragen beantwortet nicht die experimentelle Forschung, sondern die *klinische Neurophysiologie,* z.B. durch EEG-Befunde bei Epilepsien und organischen Psychosen oder der psychiatrischen Somatotherapie.

Neurophysiologie und Psychosen. Bisher gibt es nur wenige Ansätze für allgemeine neurophysiologische Erklärungen psychotischer Phänomene. Vorläufig sind es nicht mehr als hypothetische Parallelen zu hirnelektrischen und Verhaltensbefunden, die zunächst für *organische Psychosen und epileptische Geistesstörungen* brauchbar sind, vielleicht auch für gewisse akute schizophrene Episoden.

Ein weiterer, zu biochemischen und Stoffwechseluntersuchungen führender Ansatz ergab sich aus neuropharmakologischen Erfahrungen. Die starken EEG-

Veränderungen, die bei Einwirkung der modernen Psychopharmaka und nach Entziehung von Barbituraten gefunden wurden, und ähnliche EEG-Befunde bei Epilepsien verschiedener Ursache ermöglichen eine neurophysiologische Deutung der *Entziehungspsychosen* als epilepsieähnliche Hirnveränderungen durch Pharmakaentzug. Es bleibt abzuwarten, ob die Mechanismen dieser cerebralen Störungen durch Veränderungen des Hirnstoffwechsels erklärt werden können.

Physiologische und psychologische *Parallelen von Einschlafdenken, Traum und Psychosen* haben alte Gedanken der Psychiater des 19. Jahrhunderts wieder mit modernen Ergebnissen und Methoden erneuert und durch hirnelektrische Untersuchungen über Schlaf, Schlafmangel und Schlafstörungen bei neurologisch-psychiatrischen Erkrankungen präzisiert. Das Traumstadium des Schlafes gibt durch die verschiedenen Hirnpotentiale im Ammonshorn und Isocortex Hinweise auf Wechselwirkungen von reticulären, limbischen und neocorticalen Funktionen.

Polygraphische Untersuchungen über das Traumstadium beim Menschen lassen Beziehungen zu FREUDS Hypothesen über Triebwirkungen im Traum erkennen (vgl. S. 1013).

Psychoanalytische Sinn- und Kausalzusammenhänge. Trotz der oft erwähnten mechanistisch-materialistischen Grundhaltung der *Psychoanalyse* FREUDS und ihrer Libidomechanik versucht sie doch, im Seelischen wie im Unbewußten einen *Sinn* zu sehen. Diese im Grunde deterministisch-teleologische Tendenz, die oft zu einer Sinngebung des Sinnlosen führt, trennt die Psychoanalyse von rein naturwissenschaftlich-biologischer Forschung. Die Psychoanalyse verwendet mit zielgerichtetem teleologischem Denken psychische Begriffe auch dann, wenn im Unbewußten das eigentlich Psychische verlassen wird. Andererseits verfährt die Freudsche Psychoanalyse auch naturwissenschaftlich, wenn Ursachen neurotischer Störungen in der Vergangenheit gesucht und zeitlich-kausal begründet werden, ohne nach einem etwaigen Zweck der Neurose und ihrer Zukunftsbedeutung zu fragen. Es ist daher verständlich, daß neuere psychoanalytische Autoren versuchen, naturwissenschaftliche Ergebnisse der zoologischen Verhaltens- und Instinktforschung und der modernen Neurophysiologie mit der Psychoanalyse zu vereinigen.

Es ist leicht einzusehen, daß im Psychischen nicht alles sinnvoll ist, wie im biologischen Bereich nicht alles zweckmäßig und in der Physik nicht alles mechanisch sein kann. Erst im gesetzmäßigen Aufbau dieser verschiedenen Schichten, von denen die unteren jeweils die höheren tragen und ermöglichen, und in ihrer Wechselwirkung wird eine Begrenzung verschiedener Prinzipien und Methoden einsichtig.

Doppelwege klinisch-psychiatrischer Untersuchung. Es ist weniger ein Dilemma als eine synthetische Funktion der Psychiatrie, daß sie mit Introspektion und Verhaltensanalyse doppelte Wege subjektiver und objektiver Methoden benutzt. Praktisch wird beides mit sprachlicher *Exploration und Verhaltensbeobachtung* in der Klinik gemeinsam verwendet. Daher sind beide Methoden schwer trennbar. Praktisch-klinische Verbindung mit experimentellen Untersuchungen zeigt die Psychopharmakologie [E 15, 16]. Zwischen sprachlich deskriptiver und experimenteller Analyse versucht die Psychiatrie eine Koexistenz psychischer und somatischer Methoden. Mehr als andere medizinische Fächer reicht sie in verschiedene Schichten der realen Welt und der wissenschaftlichen Methoden (Abb. 1). Daher kann die Psychiatrie von physikalischen und chemischen Untersuchungen bis zur psychologischen und sozialen Kommunikation empirische und gedankliche Synthesen vielseitiger Art unternehmen. Damit vermag sie naturwissenschaftliche und geisteswissenschaftliche Methoden zu vereinen.

Ärztliche Tätigkeit ist in der Psychiatrie wie in der übrigen Medizin eine Verbindung von persönlichem Kontakt mit sachlicher wissenschaftlicher Diagnostik. Wer seinen Patienten wirksam helfen will, kann nicht auf objektive diagnostische Methoden verzichten, auch wenn sie dem Kranken unangenehm sind. Wer nicht reine Psychotherapie ohne Rücksicht auf organische Befunde betreiben will, ist jeweils auf *Kompromisse zwischen streng naturwissenschaftlichen Methoden und ärztlich-menschlichem Verstehen* angewiesen. Auch wenn psychologisches Verstehen und Motivationsklärungen im Vordergrund stehen, bleiben für den Psychiater biologisch-physiologische Analysen des Verhaltens und der Hirnfunktionen mit kausalen Methoden unentbehrlich. Für diese liefert die moderne Neurophysiologie einige Grundlagen, deren mögliche psychiatrische Beziehungen dargestellt werden sollten.

Spezialisierung und Kontaktaufnahme verschiedener Forschungsrichtungen. Die Beziehungen von Neurophysiologie und Psychiatrie entsprechen der allgemeinen Wissenschaftsentwicklung der letzten Jahrzehnte mit ihrer starken Breitenausdehnung und Spezialisierung des Forschungsbetriebs. Dies führte zu einem wissenschaftlichen *Kontaktverlust zwischen den einzelnen Fächern*. Mit dem Überangebot an Publikationen wurde die Forschungsinformation nicht besser, sondern eher schlechter, da das Nebeneinander verschiedener Methoden und Richtungen eine Synthese und einen Informationsaustausch erschwerte. Anregungen aus einem Fachgebiet, die für ein anderes von großem Interesse wären, wurden oft erst nach Jahrzehnten von diesem zweiten Fach aufgegriffen.

Beispiele für *späte Verbindungen zwischen Neurophysiologie und Psychiatrie* findet man genug, wenn man die Forschung des letzten halben Jahrhunderts betrachtet. Nur das EEG wurde ziemlich früh klinisch verwertet, da es von einem Neuropsychiater entdeckt wurde, doch blieb die diagnostische Anwendung auf organische Hirnkrankheiten im Vordergrund. Obwohl das EEG seit 1935 eine objektive Registrierung cerebraler Schlafvorgänge erlaubt, ist die klinische Anwendung für Schlafstörungen erst 2–3 Jahrzehnte später begonnen worden. Wiederum haben klinische Anregungen oft erst sehr spät die Neurophysiologie erreicht. Es hat 40–60 Jahre gedauert, bis FREUDS Traumkonzeption als unbewußte Triebregelung mit neurophysiologischen Untersuchungen über Schlaf und Traum in Verbindung zu bringen war. Die polygraphische Registrierung der Traumstadien, ihrer hirnelektrischen und sexuellen Begleiterscheinungen begann erst in den letzten Jahren (S. 997 u. 1010). So darf es nicht verwundern, daß auch umgekehrt viele Anregungen, welche die Neurophysiologie in den letzten 20 Jahren brachte, noch weit von ihrer psychiatrischen Anwendung entfernt sind. Manches, was heute als experimentelle und rein theoretische Laboratoriumsarbeit erscheint, wird vielleicht morgen von praktisch-klinischer Bedeutung sein. Vorläufig kann die Neurophysiologie der Psychiatrie nur einige ihrer Ergebnisse anbieten. Ihre Anwendung und Weiterentwicklung ist Aufgabe des somatisch interessierten Psychiaters.

Die innere Ordnung des großen Wissensstoffes, der sich in den letzten Jahrzehnten angehäuft hat, braucht Synthesen und Hinweise auf größere Zusammenhänge mit psychologischer Integration vor der praktisch-psychiatrischen Anwendung. Es handelt sich um Grundlagenforschung, die eine klinische Anwendung noch finden muß. Ansätze zu dieser praktischen Verwertung wurden an verschiedenen Stellen erwähnt, müssen aber noch mit neuen Konzeptionen gemeinsam von Klinikern, Physiologen und Verhaltensforschern erarbeitet werden. Erst dann wird eine Synthese verschiedener Forschungsergebnisse möglich sein, die eine naturwissenschaftliche Psychiatrie begründen kann.

Begrenzung naturwissenschaftlicher Forschung in der Psychiatrie

Grenzen neurophysiologischer und anderer somatischer Methoden für den Psychiater. Überblickt man die Leistungen naturwissenschaftlich-somatischer Forschung in der Psychiatrie, so sind viele psychiatrische Krankheitsbilder, mit Ausnahme der endogenen Psychosen und der psychopathisch-neurotischen Störungen allein durch cerebrale Befunde klar definiert worden. Die Ergebnisse der somatischen Forschungsrichtung zeigten, daß die *verschiedenen Forschungsmethoden nur für bestimmte Krankheitsgruppen adäquat waren*. Auch die klinische Neurophysiologie hat ein begrenztes, ihr adäquates Anwendungsbebiet in der Psychiatrie. Man sollte daher außer diesen Teilaspekten nicht zu viel von ihr erwarten.

Die einzelnen somatischen Forschungsrichtungen hatten ihre ersten Erfolge auf verschiedenen Gebieten. Die *Neuropathologie* klärte die senilen und präsenilen Hirnkrankheiten und ermöglichte damit auch eine klinisch-diagnostische Ordnung. Die *Serologie* fand zusammen mit der *Neuropathologie* spezifische Charakteristika der progressiven Paralyse und Neurolues und machte sie objektiv diagnostizierbar. Die *Neuroradiologie* lokalisierte Hirntumoren und Hirnabscesse und ließ das Ausmaß hirnatrophischer Prozesse erkennen. Die *Neurophysiologie* hat die cerebralen Veränderungen der Epilepsie und der organischen Psychosen objektiv registriert. Die epileptischen Hirnveränderungen waren vor 50 Jahren noch ebenso unbekannt wie uns jetzt Hirnfunktionsstörungen der endogenen Psychosen als Rätsel erscheinen. Wenn wir heute wie vordem BERGER im EEG noch keine charakteristischen hirnelektrischen Veränderungen bei schizophrenen und depressiven Psychosen finden, so kann man nur folgern, daß das EEG keine adäquate Methode für solche endogenen Prozesse ist. In diesem Versagen steht die Neurophysiologie nicht allein, denn für die schizophrenen und manisch-depressiven Psychosen gibt es außer der psychopathologischen Diagnostik bisher auch keine andere adäquate objektiv-somatische Erkennungsmethode. Wo sie einmal gefunden wird, läßt sich noch nicht sagen. Jedenfalls ist nicht wahrscheinlich, daß neurophysiologische Methoden viel dazu beitragen würden. Wieweit Biochemie und Neuropharmakologie kommen werden, bleibt abzuwarten. Zunächst sind nur seltene genetische Stoffwechselanomalien untersucht, die zusammen mit erbbiologischen Methoden wenige psychiatrische Anwendungen brachten. Die *Erbbiologie* hat die Erbmodi zahlreicher neurologischer Erkrankungen und bestimmte genetische Chromosomenaberrationen wie beim Mongolismus geklärt. Außer dem Hinweis, daß die endogenen Psychosen genetische Grundlagen haben, hat sie nichts zur Nosologie beigetragen und keine definierten Erbmodi der Schizophrenien und Zyklothymien feststellen können. Es ist unwahrscheinlich, daß den großen psychotischen Krankheitsgruppen einheitliche erbbiologische Biotypen entsprechen, wenn schon seltene neurologische Krankheiten verschiedene Typen des Erbgangs haben. Noch weniger kann die psychopathologische oder gar die philosophisch-existentialistische Betrachtung des psychotischen Erlebens diagnostische oder ätiologische Klärungen bringen. Alle Forschungsrichtungen und Methoden beleuchten nur *Teilaspekte* psychiatrischer Krankheitsbilder. Wenn man sich darüber klar ist, daß dies für sämtliche Forschungsmethoden gilt, so wird man die Beschränktheit neurophysiologischer Einsichten in der Psychiatrie nicht für einen Mangel halten, sondern für eine Notwendigkeit wissenschaftlicher Erkenntnis und ihrer methodischen Begrenzung. Der vorangehende Beitrag konnte auch nur Teilaspekte der Neurophysiologie besprechen, die nach ihrem Interesse für die psychologisch-psychiatrische Grundlagenforschung ausgewählt wurden.

Hier ist nicht der Ort, Wert und Grenzen induktiver empirischer und experimenteller Forschung in Neurophysiologie und Psychiatrie zu bestimmen. Es sei nur erwähnt, daß neben empirischen Einzelbeobachtungen mit ihrer klinischen Synthese und neben geplanten Experimenten der Neurophysiologie in den letzten Jahren zunehmend auch *logische Deduktion und mathematische Begründung mit statistischen Korrelationsmethoden und kybernetischen Modellen* Einfluß gewonnen haben. Mathematische Methoden wurden früher in der Klinik nur wenig verwendet, und die logische Auswertung beschränkte sich auf sprachlich-verbales Gebiet. Obwohl in der Physiologie mathematische und statistische Methoden immer zur Auswertung experimenteller Ergebnisse dienten, galt deduktive Forschung oft nur wenig. Die logische Anwendung kybernetischer und mathematisch berechenbarer Modelle führen damit wieder auf alte Postulate naturwissenschaftlicher Forschung zurück, die LIEBIG vor 100 Jahren in seiner Kritik BACONS vertreten hat: Er betonte schon damals für die Naturwissenschaften den Wert logischer und mathematischer Deduktion gegenüber rein experimentellen, induktiven Methoden [L 23]. Dies entspricht POPPERS [P 31] Prinzipien in der modernen Forschung.

Verhaltensregelung, Lernen und Schichtordnung. Die Triebphysiologie und die Sinnesphysiologie liefern uns neurophysiologische *Modelle für höhere Verhaltensregulationen*. Obwohl durch Lernvorgänge beeinflußt, sind sie stärker an vorgebildete Neuronenschaltungen gebunden. Lernen und Gedächtnisfunktionen sind in ihren speziellen neurophysiologischen Mechanismen noch zu wenig untersucht, um daraus kybernetische Modelle zu entwickeln. Erworbene Ordnungen der psychischen Leistungen und des Verhaltens sind fließender, plastischer und vielfältiger als angeborene Verhaltensweisen auf niederer Ebene, die von einfachen Reflexen bis zum Instinktverhalten reichen. Das angeborene Instinktverhalten gibt Hinweise für *Grenzen des Lernens* und der Plastizität des Nervensystems. Diese Plastizität findet ihre Grenzen in vorgebildeten Strukturen und Verbindungen des Nervensystems, die in einer relativ starren genetischen Anlage bestimmt werden. Die plastischen Funktionen der Lern- und Gedächtnisphänomene mit ihren größeren Freiheitsgraden bilden eine höhere Schicht über den angeborenen

Funktionsstrukturen des Reflex- und Instinktverhaltens. In diesen *Schichtordnungen* des Nervensystems findet man Korrelationen mit NICOLAI HARTMANNS Schichtdependenzen [H 11, 12]. Diese wurden daher ausführlicher dargestellt, nachdem sie bisher in der Physiologie und Psychologie nur wenig verwendet wurden, obwohl CLAUDE BERNARD schon vor 100 Jahren ähnliche Gesetzmäßigkeiten in seiner allgemeinen Physiologie [B 41] erwähnt hat.

Wie überall in der Wissenschaft ergänzen sich auch in der Psychiatrie gedankliche Durchdringung und empirische experimentelle Forschung. Eine rein spekulativ-philosophische Haltung, die von den Ergebnissen der Naturwissenschaften nichts wissen will, versperrt den Weg für eine echte Synthese von Theorie und Experiment. Sie verhindert eine wissenschaftliche Koordination, die heute im Zeitalter der Spezialisierung mehr denn je notwendig ist.

Eine spekulative Psychiatrie, die sich mit verbalen Konstruktionen begnügt, ist ein kranker Zweig am Baume der Wissenschaft. Ein solcher Zweig verdorrt ohne den lebendigen Zustrom aus der Empirie und der somatischen Grundlagenforschung. Andererseits braucht auch die experimentelle Forschung gedankliche Anregungen aus anderen Gebieten, wenn sie nicht zum sterilen Spezialistentum werden will.

Eine Spekulation, die sich mit hochmütiger Ablehnung experimenteller Untersuchungen paart, ist ebenso wenig lebendige Wissenschaft, wie geschäftige Empirie, die nicht die Mühe des Gedankens auf sich nimmt. Um nochmals KANT zu variieren, konnte man sagen: Empirische experimentelle Forschung ohne geistige und gedankliche Schulung ist *blind,* spekulative philosophische Haltung ohne naturwissenschaftliche Anschauung und Ergänzung ist *leer.*

Diagnostisches Primat somatischer Methoden in der Psychiatrie. Daß rein spekulative Methoden in der Naturwissenschaft nicht weiterführen, ist seit KANT auch von der Philosophie anerkannt. In der Psychiatrie entstehen dennoch immer wieder Bestrebungen, die naturwissenschaftlichen Ergebnisse der Hirnforschung zu ignorieren. Vertreter dieser Tendenz nennen das „Überwindung des naturwissenschaftlichen Denkens". Manche „reinen" Psychiater und Psychotherapeuten gehen in der Ablehnung somatischer Methoden so weit, daß sie auf die körperliche Untersuchung der Patienten verzichten.

Wer heute noch glaubt, biologische und pathologische Hirnveränderungen beim Menschen oder Gesetzmäßigkeiten psychischer Funktionen und psychiatrischer Erkrankungen durch philosophische Meditation oder seelische Einfühlung erfassen zu können, den lehrt die klinische Erfahrung bald die enge Grenze des Verstehens und das *Primat der körperlichen Störungen.* Für deren Diagnose verwendet auch der klinische Psychiater oder Psychopathologe mit Nutzen somatische Laboratoriumsmethoden, obwohl die psychiatrische Diagnostik für endogene Psychosen und Neurosen auch heute noch auf psychopathologischen Daten beruht. Diese werden aber *empirisch* und nicht spekulativ festgestellt. Dasselbe gilt für die klinische Psychologie, die zunehmend experimentelle und statistische Methoden verwendet.

Auf dem festen Grund täglicher klinischer Erfahrung mit Hirn- und Geisteskrankheiten werden alle spekulativen Bestrebungen der Psychiatrie an die Notwendigkeit erinnert, körperliche und cerebrale Vorgänge zu untersuchen. Wer eine Psychotherapie beginnt, ohne eine körperliche Störung ausgeschlossen zu haben, mag vielleicht einen ebenso großen diagnostischen Fehler machen, wie ein Arzt, der psychische und „psychosomatische" Störungen als körperliche Krankheiten verkennt. Doch ist die verkannte Diagnose einer körperlichen Krankheit für den Patienten meistens folgenschwerer als die Verkennung einer Neurose. Die als somatische Störung verkannte und behandelte Neurose kostet den Kranken oder die Kasse nur Geld, die als psychogen verkannte Körperkrankheit kann dem Patienten das Leben kosten. Wer dies im psychotherapeutischen Eifer nicht einsieht, dem ist nicht zu helfen. Weder neurophysiologische noch neurochemische Befunde werden ihn überzeugen. Ohne sorgfältige körperliche Untersuchung und Anwendung der notwendigsten Hilfsmethoden des Laboratoriums wird der einseitige Psychotherapeut, der somatische Untersuchung ablehnt, eine Paralyse oder einen Hirntumor psychotherapieren, bis es für eine somatische Behandlung zu spät ist. Oder wenn er internistische Kontrollen für unnötig hält, kann er einem Patienten mit Magencarcinom einreden, daß sein Erbrechen Symptom eines Ehekonfliktes sei, bis sich inoperable Metastasen entwickelt haben. Der Psychotherapeut wird zwar einwenden, daß umgekehrt viele Neurosen fälschlicherweise somatisch behandelt und als körperliche Krankheiten diagnostiziert werden. Aber er muß zugeben, daß dies meistens für Leben und Gesundheit des Patienten weniger schwere Folgen hat und daß viele Neurosen auch ohne Psychotherapie heilen.

Fehlen systematischer Theorien in Neurophysiologie und Psychiatrie. Die Neurophysiologie hat bisher nur klare theoretische Vorstellungen über die Funktion der neuronalen Elemente entwickelt, durch HODGKIN u. HUXLEY für die Nervenfaser [H 73], durch ECCLES für die Nervenzelle [E 2] und ihre Synapsen [E 5]. Doch fehlt eine allgemeine Systemtheorie für koordinative Hirnfunktionen und die Regulationen des Verhaltens. Die *Neuronenlehre* ist zwar eine Grundlage der Neurophysiologie, hat aber nicht die gleiche Exaktheit wie die Quantentheorie in der Physik oder die Atomtheorie in der Chemie. Erst recht fehlen uns allgemeine Konzeptionen, die wie Relativitätstheorie oder Feldtheorien der Physik eine exakte Erfassung von Massenvorgängen im ZNS erlauben. *Dieses Fehlen allgemeiner Theorien betrifft in gleicher Weise Physiologie, Psychologie und Psychiatrie.* Wir haben keine allgemeine Psychiatrie, die mit einer allgemeinen theoretischen Physik oder physikalischen Chemie verglichen werden könnte, oder die durch eine allgemeine Biologie begründet wäre. Die Gestaltpsychologie hat nicht, wie sie zunächst ankündigte, eine entsprechende theoretische Basis der Psychologie geschaffen. Auch die Informationstheorie brachte, entgegen optimistischen Erwartungen einiger Kybernetiker, bisher noch keine gültige theoretische Grundlage der Neurophysiologie und experimentellen Psychologie.

Alle bisherigen Ordnungen sind auch in der Biologie unvollständig und begrenzt. Es bleibt abzuwarten, ob die Informations- und Kommunikationsforschung zu einer kybernetischen Theorie des Organismus führen kann und ob die molekularbiologische Cytologie über die Zell- und Neuronenlehren des vorigen Jahrhunderts hinaus eine cellularbiologische Grundkonzeption entwickeln wird. Heute scheint der *Begriff der Information* eine ähnliche allgemeine Bedeutung in der modernen Naturwissenschaft zu gewinnen, wie im 19. Jahrhundert das Energieprinzip in der Physik oder die Descendenztheorie in der Biologie. Aber auch damals gelang es nicht, aus solchen allgemeinen Konzeptionen eine theoretische Biologie aufzubauen oder mit dem Lokalisationsprinzip in der Hirnforschung und der Assoziationslehre in der Psychologie eine allgemeine Theorie der Hirnfunktionen zu schaffen.

Die heutige Situation der biologisch-physiologischen Forschung im psychologisch-psychiatrischen Gebiet kann vielleicht durch einen *geschichtlichen Vergleich* klargemacht werden. Die biologisch und physiologisch orientierte Psychologie und Psychiatrie hat bis jetzt nur eine *vorläufige Ordnung, aber noch kein theoretisches Gerüst und keine synthetische Konzeption*. Sie kann sich nicht auf allgemeine Prinzipien wie die Physik im 19. Jahrhundert auf das Energieprinzip oder im 20. auf die Atomtheorie stützen. In ihrem Entwicklungsstand *entspricht die Neurophysiologie und Biopsychologie heute etwa der organischen Chemie und Biochemie um 1850*, bevor KEKULÉS und COUPERS Strukturformeln und Bindungsvalenzen eine systematische Darstellung ermöglichten. In der Mitte des 19. Jahrhunderts gab es in der Chemie bereits ein großes spezielles Wissen mit vielen grob empirisch untersuchten Tatsachen und erste Ordnungen mit wenigen Grundkonzeptionen. Die Mengenanalysen mit ihren Bruttoformeln der verschiedenen Stoffe waren annähernd bekannt, die Katalyse war durch MITSCHERLICH und BERZELIUS beschrieben. Grundlegende Untersuchungen von LIEBIG über die organischen Substanzen ließen schon praktische Anwendungen in der Agrikultur und Farbchemie erkennen. Dennoch fehlten klare Theorien der allgemeinen Chemie, und es gab keine praktisch brauchbaren Strukturformeln, die den Molekülaufbau mit den verschiedenen Reaktionen und Valenzen der Einzelelemente klar darstellen ließen. Es fehlte das periodische System der Elemente, dessen Erklärung durch die Atomstruktur erst mehr als ein halbes Jahrhundert später verstanden werden konnte. Ein ähnlicher *Theoriemangel* wie damals in der Chemie besteht heute in der Biologie und Neurobiologie. Der Neurophysiologie und ihren psychologisch-psychiatrischen Entsprechungen fehlen klare Ordnungsprinzipien, die eine Synthese der zahlreichen experimentellen Befunde ermöglichen würden. Gäbe es eine solche Ordnung, so wäre auch eine bessere Quantifizierung neurophysiologischer Befunde möglich, und ihre praktische Anwendung würde zu einer allgemeinen Psychophysiologie und allgemeinen Psychiatrie führen können.

Spezialforschung und Synthese. Sinn dieser Ausführungen war es, einige physiologische und biologische Grundlagen solcher Hirnfunktionen darzustellen, die für psychiatrische Störungen von Bedeutung sein können. Es sollte gezeigt werden, daß allgemeine Ergebnisse und Detailforschung der Neurophysiologie mehr brauchbare Befunde für höhere Hirnleistungen, Verhalten und seelische Funktionen liefern, als von vielen Psychologen und Psychiatern angenommen wird. Diese Anwendungen ergeben sich vorwiegend dann, wenn die allgemeinen *Zusammenhänge* aus der großen Masse von Spezialuntersuchungen herausgearbeitet werden. Solche Zusammenhänge biologisch-physiologischer Funktionen mit psychischen Leistungen sind durch *Verbindungen zwischen verschiedenen Fachgebieten* zu suchen, die Anregungen zu parallelen Untersuchungen ähnlicher Phänomene mit verschiedenen Methoden geben. Solche Verbindungen sind zum Teil noch gedanklich und hypothetisch. Die Korrelationen zwischen Physiologie, Biokybernetik, Verhaltensforschung und Psychologie, die im Vorangehenden betont wurden, bedürfen noch einer gründlichen Bearbeitung.

Gemeinsame Bemühungen von psychologischer und physiologischer Seite in der Sinnesphysiologie, der Schlaf-Wachforschung und in experimentellen Untersuchungen des Triebverhaltens und Lernens haben bereits vielversprechende Ansätze gebracht. Ihre klinischen Anwendungen sind zum Teil noch hypothetisch, aber es besteht begründete Hoffnung, daß manche dieser Ergebnisse auch für die Psychiatrie fruchtbar werden.

Mancher wird fragen, was haben solche allgemeinen Ergebnisse der Neurophysiologie mit der psychiatrischen Klinik zu tun? Entfernt sich die zunehmend spezialisierte neurophysiologische Forschung nicht immer weiter von der klinischen Praxis? Sind manche allgemeine Konzeptionen, die als Fragestellungen und Ordnungsprinzipien dienten, nicht heute überholt? Ist es vielleicht besser, genügsam im Detail zu forschen und zu warten, ob sich daraus praktische und klinisch brauchbare Resultate ergeben, und sollen wir allgemeine Konzeptionen den Philosophen überlassen? Die Antwort kann nur sein: *Reine Spezialforschung führt zur Isolierung und erst die gegenseitige Anregung und Wechselwirkung von Theorie und Praxis, von Laboratorium und Klinik, von einem Fach zum anderen, bedeutet lebendige Forschung.*

Weder fleißig gewonnene Detail-Kenntnisse, noch voreilige mechanistische Erklärungen noch ad hoc konstruierte oder freie Spekulationen bringen allein wissenschaftlichen Gewinn. Aber *Spezialuntersuchungen, biologische Grundlagenforschung, Klinik und theoretisches Denken ergänzen sich*. In der Hirnforschung wie in der Psychiatrie müssen die verschiedenen Aspekte und Schichten der seelischen, vitalen und physikalisch-chemischen Prozesse zwar *methodisch getrennt, aber im Funktionsaufbau gemeinsam erforscht werden*. Innere und äußere Aspekte menschlicher Hirnfunktionen und ihre Funktionsstörungen werden zugänglich durch Introspektion, sprachliche Kommunikation und naturwissenschaftliche Forschungsmethoden. Es wäre verfehlt, aus methodischer Bedenklichkeit auf jede Beziehungssetzung zu verzichten. Nur wer *beide* Seiten des Menschen, seine psychischen und körperlich-cerebralen Funktionen sehen lernt, gewinnt genügende Tiefe in der psychiatrischen Erkenntnis. Innere psychologische und äußere physiologische Aspekte zusammen ermöglichen gewissermaßen räumliches Erkennen in einer neuen 3. Dimension, wie HERING es für die objektive und subjektive Sinnesphysiologie dargestellt hat [H 32, 34]. Wenn auch die Korrelationen der Psychiatrie und Neurophysiologie bis jetzt noch nicht zu einer solchen gemeinsamen Betrachtung ausreichen, so gibt es heute doch viel engere Beziehungen als vor 50 Jahren, vor der Entdeckung des menschlichen EEG durch BERGER. Der Einwand, neurophysiologische Hirnforschung würde dazu führen, die geistigen und sozialen Bedingungen des menschlichen Lebens und der psychischen Störungen zu übersehen, ist falsch. Ein neurophysiologisch erfahrener Forscher kennt die Begrenzungen experimenteller Methoden und die Schwäche seiner Hypothesenbildungen gut genug. Er wird sie daher nicht überwerten oder zu sehr verallgemeinern. Psychiatrische Betrachtung kann weder auf den Zusammenhang geistiger, sozialer und kultureller Werte verzichten, deren Zerstörung oder Verzerrung der Psychiater so oft erleben muß, noch darf die Psychiatrie somatisch-biologische Ergebnisse der Hirnphysiologie und Naturwissenschaft unbeachtet lassen.

Zusammenfassung

Neurophysiologie und Psychiatrie ergänzen sich. Beide können voneinander lernen: der Neurophysiologe vom Psychiater anschaulich-synthetisches Denken und intuitives Erfassen, der Psychiater vom Neurophysiologen exakte Methodik, objektive Registrierung und Quantifizierung. Durch methodologische Begrenzungen bringt die Neurophysiologie für die Psychiatrie nur *Teilaspekte*. Theoretische Grundlagen liefert die experimentelle Erforschung der Hirnmechanismen. Praktisch-klinische Korrelate zur Diagnose und Therapie bringen z.B. EEG-Befunde bei Epilepsien, bei organischen und psycho-pharmakologischen Hirnveränderungen. Die Verhaltensforschung bildet eine Brücke zwischen Psychiatrie und Physiologie. Auch der Psychiater braucht neben der sprachlichen Exploration Verhaltensbeobachtungen und objektive cerebrale Untersuchungsbefunde.

Obwohl naturwissenschaftliche Methoden nicht zum Wesen des Psychischen vordringen, hat die biologisch-somatische Forschungsrichtung eine wichtige Kontrollfunktion. Die Grenzen somatischer Forschung in der Psychiatrie liegen in der begrenzten Anwendung verschiedener Forschungsmethoden, die nur für einzelne Krankheitsgruppen brauchbare Befunde liefern und erst in der *klinischen Synthese* verwertbar sind. In der Neurophysiologie, Psychologie und Psychiatrie fehlen noch systematische Theorien, die der Quantentheorie in der Physik oder der Atomtheorie in der Chemie vergleichbar wären. Spezialuntersuchungen, biologische Grundlagenforschung, klinische und theoretische Forschung ergänzen sich ebenso wie Induktion und Deduktion bei empirischen und logisch-mathematischen Methoden. Kompromisse zwischen streng naturwissenschaftlicher Methodik und verstehendem ärztlich-menschlichem Umgang sind für die Psychiatrie notwendig. In Hirnforschung und Psychiatrie müssen seelische, vitale und physikalisch-chemische Prozesse *methodisch getrennt,* aber in ihrer *Funktionsordnung gemeinsam* erforscht werden.

Für die Überlassung von Abbildungen, Hinweise und Kritik danke ich vor allem: Lord ADRIAN †, Prof. BAUMGARTNER, Zürich, Dr. CALLIERI, Rom, Prof. CASPERS, Münster, Prof. DELGADO, New Haven, Prof. DELL †, Dr. DEMENT, Palo Alto, Prof. ECCLES, Contra, Dr. EHRET, Singen, Dr. EVARTS, Bethesda, Dr. FISHER, New York, Prof. GASTAUT, Marseille, Prof. HASSENSTEIN, Freiburg, Prof. W.R. HESS †, Prof. v. HOLST †, Prof. HUBEL, Boston, Prof. JASPER, Montreal, Prof. JOUVET, Lyon, Prof. O. KOEHLER †, Dr. KUHLO, Wiesbaden, Prof. KORNHUBER, Ulm, Prof. KÜPFMÜLLER †, Prof. LORENZ, Seewiesen, Prof. OHLMEYER, Tübingen, Prof. OLDS †, Prof. PENFIELD †, Prof. ROEDER, Medford, Prof. SHELDON, Eugene, Prof. STEINBUCH, Karlsruhe, Prof. SZENTAGOTHAI, Budapest, Dr. W.G. WALTER †.

Für Hilfe bei Manuskript und Korrektur der ersten Auflage 1967 danke ich Frau FURTWÄNGLER† und Frau HABERSTROH, bei der zweiten Auflage Frau RÖMMELT, Frl. SCHETTER, Frau BRETSCHNEIDER und Frl. SCHRAMM, für die Zeichnungen Herrn Univ.-Zeichner DETTELBACHER †.

Literatur

Der 1967 erschienene Beitrag wurde gekürzt, überarbeitet und ergänzt. Das Literaturverzeichnis wurde in dieser 2. Auflage nur durch wenige Arbeiten bis 1978 erweitert. Die moderne Massenproduktion wissenschaftlicher Literatur macht es zunehmend unmöglich, das Wesentliche auszuwählen. Bevorzugt genannt sind nicht nur neuere Befunde und Zusammenfassungen, sondern auch wichtige Erstbeschreibungen „klassischer" Entdeckungen und älterer Autoren.

Die numerierte Ordnung mit entsprechenden Literaturhinweisen im Text ist nach Buchstaben eingeteilt. Bei *jedem Buchstaben beginnen neue Nummern,* die wie folgt im Text zitiert werden: A 1, B 18 usw.

A

1. Adams, R.D., Collins, G.H., Victor, M.: Troubles de la mémoire et de l'apprentissage chez l'homme; leurs relations avec des lésions des lobes temporaux et du diencéphale (observations anatomo-cliniques). In: Physiologie de l'hippocampe, pp. 273–295. Paris: Centre National de la Recherche Scientifique 1962
2. Adey, W.R.: Studies of hippocampal electrical activity during approach learning. In (A. Fessard et al., eds.): Brain mechanisms and learning, pp. 577–588. Springfield (Ill.): C.C. Thomas 1961
3. Adey, W.R., Dunlop, C.W., Hendrix, C.E.: Hippocampal slow waves: distribution and phase relationships in the course of approach learning. A.M.A. Arch. Neurol. **3**, 74–90 (1960)
4. Adrian, E.D.: The basis of sensation. The action of the sense organs. London: Christophers 1928
5. Adrian, E.D.: Die Untersuchung der Sinnesorgane mit Hilfe elektrophysiologischer Methoden. Ergebn. Physiol. **26**, 501–530 (1928)
6. Adrian, E.D.: The messages in sensory nerve fibres and their interpretation. Proc. R. Soc. Lond. [Biol.] **109**, 1–18 (1931)
7. Adrian, E.D.: Afferent discharges to the cerebral cortex from peripheral sense organs. J. Physiol. (Lond.) **100**, 159–191 (1941)
8. Adrian, E.D.: The physical background of perception. Oxford: Clarendon Press 1947
8a. Adrian, E.D., Bronk, D.W.: The discharge of impulses in motor nerve fibres. Part II. The frequency of discharge in reflex and voluntary contractions. J. Physiol. (Lond.) **67**, 119 (1929)
9. Adrian, E.D., Matthews, B.H.C.: The Berger rhythm. Potential changes from the occipital lobes in man. Brain **57**, 356–385 (1934)
10. Adrian, E.D., Zotterman, Y.: The impulses produced by sensory nerve-endings. Part 2. The response of a single end-organ. J. Physiol. (Lond.) **61**, 151–171 (1926)
11. Agranoff, B.W., Klinger, P.D.: Puromycin effect on memory fixation in the goldfish. Science **146**, 952–953 (1964)
12. Ahlenstiel, H.: Vision und Traum. Betrachtungen über Darstellungsformen in Trugbildern. Stuttgart: Ferd. Enke 1962
13. Ahrens, R.: Störungen von Sukzessivgestalten und Zeiterleben bei Aphasie. In: Zeit in nervenärztl. Sicht. S. 100–103 (Hrsg.: G. Schaltenbrand). Stuttgart: Ferd. Enke 1963
14. Akert, K.: The anatomical substrate of sleep. In: Progress in brain research, Vol. **19**, pp. 9–19. Amsterdam, London, New York: Elsevier Publ. Comp. 1965
14a. Akert, K., Andersson, B.: Experimenteller Beitrag zur Physiologie des Nucleus caudatus. Acta Physiol. Scand. **22**, 281–298 (1951)
15. Akert, K., Gruesen, R.A., Woolsey, C.N., Meyer, D.R.: Klüver-Bucy-syndrome in monkeys with neocortical ablations of temporal lobe. Brain **84**, 480–498 (1961)
16. Akert, K., Hess, W.R.: Über die neurobiologischen Grundlagen akuter affektiver Erregungszustände. Schweiz. Med. Wochenschr. **92**, 1524–1530 (1962)
17. Akimoto, H., Creutzfeldt, O.: Reaktionen von Neuronen des optischen Cortex nach elektrischer Reizung unspezifischer Thalamuskerne. Arch. Psychiatr. Nervenkr. **196**, 494–519 (1957/58)
18. Albe-Fessard, D., Rocha-Miranda, C., Oswaldo-Cruz, E.: Activités évoquées dans le noyeau caudé du chat en résponse à des types divers d'afférences. II. Etude microphysiologique. Electroencephalogr. Clin. Neurophysiol. **12**, 649–661 (1960)
19. Allport, F.H.: Theories of perception and the concept of structure. London, New York: John Wiley & Sons 1955
20. Allport, G.W.: Bemerkungen zum gegenwärtigen Stand der Motivationstheorie in USA. Psychol. Beitr. **1**, 11–29 (1953)

21. Anand, B.K., Dua, S., Singh, B.: Electrical activity of the hypothalamic feeding centres' under the effect of changes in blood chemistry. Electroenceph. Clin. Neurophysiol. **13**, 54–59 (1961)
21a. Andersen, P., Bland, B.H., Dudar, J.D.: Organization of the hippocampal output. Exp. Brain Res. **17**, 152–168 (1973)
22. Anderson, O.D., Liddell, H.S.: Observations on experimental neuroses in sheep. Arch. Neurol. (Chic.) **34**, 330 (1935)
23. Andersson, B., Jewell, P.A., Larsson, S.: An appraisal of the effects of diencephalic stimulation of conscious animals in terms of normal behaviour. In: Ciba Foundation Symposium on the Neurological Basis of Behaviour. **1958**, 76–85
24. Anokhin, P.K.: A new conception of the physiological architecture of conditioned reflex. In (J.F. Delafresnaye, ed.): Brain mechanisms and learning, pp. 189–229. Oxford: Blackwell Scientific Publications 1961
25. Anokhin, P.K.: The multiple ascending influences of the subcortical centers on the cerebral cortex. In (M.A.B. Brazier, ed.): Brain and Behavior, pp. 139–170. Washington: A.I.B.S. 1961
26. Anokhin, P.K.: Electroencephalographic analysis of cortico-subcortical relations in positive and negative conditioned reactions. Ann. N.Y. Acad. Sci. **92**, 899–938 (1961)
27. Anokhin, P.K.: New data on the specific character of ascending activations. Prog. Brain Res. **1**, 325–339 (1963)
28. Arduini, A.: Enduring potential changes evoked in the cerebral cortex by stimulation of brain stem reticular formation and thalamus. In: Henry Ford Hospital International Symp. Reticular Formation of the Brain, pp. 333–351 (eds. Jasper, H.H. et al.). Boston: Little, Brown 1958
28a. Arduini, A.: The tonic discharge of the retina and its central effects. Prog. Brain Res. **1**, 184–206 (1963)
29. Aschoff, J.: Exogene und endogene Komponente der 24-Stunden-Periodik bei Tier und Mensch. Naturwissenschaften **42**, 569–575 (1955)
30. Aschoff, J., Wever, R.: Spontanperiodik des Menschen bei Ausschluß aller Zeitgeber. Naturwissenschaften **49**, 337–342 (1962)
31. Aserinsky, E., Kleitman, N.: Regularly occurring periods of eye motility, and concomitant phenomena during sleep. Science **118**, 273–274 (1953)
32. Aserinsky, E., Kleitman, N.: Two types of ocular motility occurring in sleep. J. Appl. Physiol. **8**, 1–10 (1955)
33. Asratian, E.A.: Compensatory adaptations, reflex activity and the brain. Oxford, London, Edinburgh, New York, Paris, Frankfurt: Pergamon Press 1965
34. Ashby, W. Ross: Design for a brain. The origin of adaptive behaviour. 2. ed. London: Chapman & Hall 1960
35. Assal, G., Hecaen, H.: Neuropsychologie. In (K.P. Kisker, J.E. Meyer, C. Müller, E. Strömgren, Hrsg.): Psych. der Gegenwart. Bd. I/1, S. 211–256. Berlin, Heidelberg, New York: Springer 1979
36. Auchincloss, J.H., Jr., Cook, E., Renzetti, A.D.: Polycythemia of unknown cause with alveolar hypoventilation. J. Clin. Invest. **34**, 1537–1545 (1955)
37. Auersperg, A.: Vorläufige und rückläufige Bestimmung in der Physiogenese. Jahrbuch für Psychologie, Psychotherapie und Medizinische Anthropologie **8**, 223–262 (1960)
38. Avenarius, R.: Philosophie als Denken der Welt gemäß dem Prinzip des kleinsten Kraftmaßes. Prolegomena zu einer Kritik der reinen Erfahrung. 2. Aufl. Berlin: S. Guttentag 1903.

B

1. Baldwin, M.: Electrical stimulation of the mesial temporal region. In (E.R. Ramey, D.S. O'Doherty, eds.): Electrical studies on the unanaesthetized brain, pp. 159–176. New York: P.B. Hoeber Inc. 1960
2. Barahona Fernandes, H.J. de: Nicolai Hartmann und die Psychopathologie. In (H. Kranz, Hrsg.): Psychopathologie heute, S. 6–10. Stuttgart: Thieme 1962
3. Bard, P.: A diencephalic mechanism for the expression of rage with special references to the sympathetic nervous system. Am. Physiol. **84**, 490–515 (1928)
4. Bard, P.: On emotional expression after decortication with some remarks on certain theoretical views. I. u. II. Psychol. Rev. **41**, 309–329, 424–449 (1943)
5. Bard, P.: The hypothalamus and sexual behavior. Res. Publ. Assoc. Nerv. Ment. Dis. **20**, 551–579 (1940)

6. Bard, P., Mountcastle, V.B.: Some forebrain mechanisms involved in expression of rage with special reference to suppression of angry behavior. Res. Publ. Assoc. Res. Nerv. Ment. Dis. **27**, 362–404 (1948)
7. Barlow, H.B.: Possible principles underlying the transformations of sensory messages. In (W.A. Rosenblith, ed.): Sensory communication, pp. 217–234. New York, London: The M.I.T. Press, J. Wiley & Sons, 1961
8. Barlow, H.B.: Three points about lateral inhibition. In (W.A. Rosenblith, ed.): Sensory communication, pp. 782–786. New York, London: The M.I.T. Press, J. Wiley 1961
8a. Barlow, H.B.: The information capacity of nervous transmission. Kybernetik **2**, 1 (1963–1965)
8b. Barlow, H.B., Fitzhugh, R., Kuffler, S.W.: Change of organisation in the receptive fields of the cat's retina during dark adaptation. J. Physiol. (Lond.) **137**, 338–354 (1957)
9. Bates, J.A.V.: Electrical activity of the cortex accompanying movement. J. Physiol. (Lond.) **113**, 240–257 (1951)
10. Batini, C., Moruzzi, G., Palestini, M., Rossi, G.F., Zanchetti, A.: Effects of complete pontine transections on the sleep-wakefulness rhythm: the midpontine pretrigeminal preparation. Arch. Ital. Biol. **97**, 1–12 (1959)
11. Battig, K., Rosvold, H.E., Mishkin, M.: Comparison of the effects of frontal and caudate lesions on delayed response and alternation in monkeys. J. Comp. Physiol. Psychol. **53**, 400–404 (1960)
12. Battig, K., Rosvold, H.E., Mishkin, M.: Comparison of the effects of frontal and caudate lesions on discrimination learning in monkeys. J. Comp. Physiol. Psychol. **55**, 458–463 (1962)
13. Baumgartner, G.: Indirekte Größenbestimmung der rezeptiven Felder der Retina beim Menschen mittels der Hermannschen Gittertäuschung. Pfluegers Arch. **272**, 21 (1960)
14. Baumgartner, G.: Kontrastlichteffekte an retinalen Ganglienzellen: Ableitungen vom Tractus opticus der Katze. In (R. Jung u. H.H. Kornhuber, Hrsg.): Neurophysiologie und Psychophysik des visuellen Systems, S. 45–55. Berlin-Göttingen-Heidelberg: Springer 1961
15. Baumgartner, G.: Die Reaktionen der Neurone des zentralen visuellen Systems der Katze im simultanen Helligkeitskontrast. In (R. Jung u. H.H. Kornhuber, Hrsg.): Neurophysiologie und Psychophysik des visuellen Systems, S. 296–313. Berlin-Göttingen-Heidelberg: Springer 1961
16. Baumgartner, G.: Der Informationswert der on-Zentrum- und off-Zentrum-Neurone des visuellen Systems beim Hell-Dunkel-Sehen und die informative Bedeutung von Aktivierung und Hemmung. In (R. Jung u. H.H. Kornhuber, Hrsg.): Neurophysiologie und Psychophysik des visuellen Systems. Symposion Freiburg, S. 377–379. Berlin-Göttingen-Heidelberg: Springer 1961
17. Baumgartner, G., Creutzfeldt, O., Jung, R.: Microphysiology of cortical neurones in acute anoxia and in retinal ischemia. In (H. Gastaut and J.St. Meyer, eds.): Cerebral anoxia and the electroencephalogram, pp. 5–34. Springfield, Ill.: C. Thomas 1961
18. Baust, W. (Hrsg.): Ermüdung, Schlaf und Traum. Stuttgart: Wissensch. Verlagsg. 1970
18a. Beach, F.A.: Hormones and behavior. 2. ed. New York: Cooper Square Publishers 1961
19. Bechterew, W. v.: Objektive Psychologie oder Psychoreflexologie. Die Lehre von den Associationsreflexen. Leipzig: Teubner 1913
20. Bell, Ch.: The Anatomy and Philosophy of Expression (1. ed. 1806) 3. ed. London: Murray 1844
20a. Bender, H.: Experimentelle Visionen (mit Beschreibung eines neuen Schallaufnahmeverfahrens). Charakter u. Erziehung, XVI. Kongr. d. dtsch. Ges. Psychol., Bayreuth, 261–269 (1938)
21. Berger, H.: Über die körperlichen Äußerungen psychischer Zustände. Weitere experimentelle Beiträge zur Lehre von der Blutzirkulation in der Schädelhöhle des Menschen. I u. II. Jena: Fischer 1904, 1907
22. Berger, H.: Untersuchungen über die Temperatur des Gehirns. Jena: Fischer 1910
23. Berger, H.: Psychophysiologie in 12 Vorlesungen. Jena: Fischer 1921
24. Berger, H.: Über das Elektrenkephalogramm des Menschen. 1. Mitteilung. Arch. Psychiatr. Nervenkr. **87**, 527–570 (1929)
25. Berger, H.: Über das Elektrenkephalogramm des Menschen. 2. Mitteilung. J. Psychol. Neurol. (Lpz.) **40**, 160–179 (1930)
26. Berger, H.: Über das Elektrenkephalogramm des Menschen. 3. Mitteilung. Arch. Psychiatr. Nervenkr. **94**, 16–60 (1931)
27. Berger, H.: Über das Elektrenkephalogramm des Menschen. 6. Mitteilung. Arch. Psychiatr. Nervenkr. **99**, 555–574 (1933)

28. Berger, H.: Physiologische Begleiterscheinungen psychischer Vorgänge. In: Handb. der Neurologie, Bd. 2, Experim. Physiologie, S. 492–526 (Bumke-Foerster, Hrsg.). Berlin: Springer 1937
29. Berger, H.: Das Elektrenkephalogramm des Menschen. 9. Mitteilung. Arch. Psychiatr. Nervenkr. **102**, 538–557 (1938)
30. Berger, H.: Das Elektrenkephalogramm des Menschen. Nova Acta Leopoldina, N.F. **6**, Nr. 38 (1938)
31. Berger, R.J., Olley, P., Oswald, I.: The EEG, eye movements and dreams of the blind. Q. J. Exp. Psychol. **14**, 183–186 (1962)
32. Berger, R.J., Oswald, I.: Effects of sleep deprivation on behavior, subsequent sleep and dreaming. Electroencephalogr. Clin. Neurophysiol. **14**, 294–297 (1962)
33. Bergson, H.: Matière et Mémoire. Essai sur la relation du corps à l'esprit, 46. ed. Paris: Presses Universitaires de France 1946
34. Beringer, K.: Der Meskalinrausch. Seine Geschichte und seine Erscheinungsweise. Monogr. Neur. **49**. Berlin: Springer 1927
35. Beringer, K.: Über Störungen des Antriebs bei einem von der unteren Falxkante ausgehenden doppelseitigen Meningeom. Z. ges. Neurol. Psychiat. **171**, 451–474 (1940)
36. Beringer, K.: Rhythmischer Wechsel von Enthemmtheit und Gehemmtheit als diencephale Antriebsstörung. Nervenarzt **15**, 225–239 (1942)
37. Beritoff, J.S.: Karakteristica i proischoschdenie proiswolnich dwischenii u. wisschich poswonotschnich schiwotnich. J. wisschei nervoi dejatelnosti **12**, 193–201 (1962). [The charact. and origin of voluntary movements in higher vertebrates. J. high. nerve activity **12**, 193–201 (1962)]
38. Beritoff, J.S.: Spatial orientation of man and animals. In: XXII. Int. Congr. Physiol. Sci., Leiden, I, Part I, 1962; Intern. Congr. Ser., No. **47**, 3–4 (1962)
39. Beritoff, J.S. (Beritashvili): Neural mechanisms of higher vertebrate behavior (engl. Übers.). Boston: Little, Brown & Co. 1965
40. Berlucchi, G., Moruzzi, G., Salvi, G., Strata, P.: Pupil behavior and ocular movements during synchronized and desynchronized sleep. Arch. Ital. Biol. **102**, 230–244 (1964)
41. Bernard, C.: Leçons sur les phénomènes de la vie commune aux animaux et aux végétaux. (Cours de physiologie générale du muséum d'histoire naturelle), I/II. Paris: J.-B. Baillière et fils 1878/79
42. Bertalanffy, L. v.: Theoretische Biologie. Bd. 1: Allgemeine Theorie, Physikochemie, Aufbau und Entwicklung des Organismus. Berlin: Gebr. Borntraeger 1932
43. Bickford, R.G., Dodge jr., H.W., Uihlein, A.: Electrographic and behavioral effects related to depth stimulation in human patients. In: Electrical studies on the unanesthetized brain (eds. E.R. Ramey and D.S. O'Doherty), Symposion, pp. 248–261. New York: Paul B. Hoeber Inc., Medical Division of Harper & Brothers 1960
44. Binswanger, L.: Über das Verhalten des psycho-galvanischen Phänomens beim Assoziationsexperiment. Leipzig: Barth 1910
44a. Birkmayer, W., Frühmann, E., Strotzka, H.: Motorische Schablonen im Erwachen nach dem Elektroschock. Arch. Psychiatr. Nervenkr. **193**, 513–525 (1955)
45. Bishop, P.O.: Neurophysiology of binocular single vision and stereopsis. In: (R. Jung, edit): Handbook of sensory physiology, Vol. VII/3 A, pp. 255–305. Berlin, Heidelberg, New York: Springer 1973
46. Bizzi, E., Pompeiano, O., Somogyi, I.: Spontaneous activity of single vestibular neurons of unrestrained cats during sleep and wakefulness. Arch. Ital. Biol. **102**, 308–330 (1964)
47. Blake, H., Gerard, R.W.: Brain potentials during sleep. Am. J. Physiol. **119**, 692–703 (1937)
48. Blake, H., Gerard, R.W., Kleitman, N.: Factors influencing brain potentials during sleep. J. Neurophysiol. **2**, 48–60 (1949)
48a. Blakemore, C.: Binocular depth perception and the optic chiasm. Vision Res. **10**, 43–47 (1970)
49. Bleuler, E.: Mechanismus Vitalismus Mnemismus, Berlin: Springer 1931
50. Bogacz, J., Vanzulli, A., Garcia-Austt, E.: Evoked responses in man. IV. Effects of habituation, distraction and conditioning upon auditory evoked responses. Acta Neurol. Lat.-Am. **8**, 244–252 (1962)
51. Bonhoeffer, K.: Die Entwickelung der Anschauungen von der Großhirnfunktion in den letzten 50 Jahren. Dtsch. Med. Wochenschr. **50**, 1708–1710 (1924)
52. Bonvallet, M., Dell, P., Hiebel, C.: Tonus sympathique et activité électrique corticale. Electroencephalogr. Clin. Neurophysiol. **6**, 119–144 (1954)

53. Borg, G., Diamant, L., Zotterman, Y.: The relation between neural and perceptual intensity: A comparative study on the neural and psychophysical response to taste stimuli. J. Physiol. (Lond.) **192**, 13–20 (1967)
54. Boring, E.G.: Sensation and perception in the history of experimental psychology. New York: Appleton-Century Crofts, Inc. 1942
54a. Boutroux, E.: De la contingence des lois de la nature. (1. Aufl. 1874.) Paris: F. Alcan 1898
54b. Boutroux, E.: De l'idée de loi naturelle dans la science et la philosophie contemporaines. Paris: Lecéne, Oudin et Cie., F. Alcan 1895
55. Brady, J.V.: Animal experimental evaluation of drug effects upon behavior. Res. Publ. Assoc. Nerv. Ment. Dis. **37**, 104–125 (1959)
56. Brady, J.V.: Temporal and emotional effects related to intracranial electrical self-stimulation. In: Electrical studies on the unanesthetized brain (eds. R.R. Ramey, and D.S. O'Doherty), Symposion, pp. 52–77. New York: Paul B. Hoeber Inc., Medical Division of Harper & Brothers 1960
57. Brady, J.V., Schreiner, L., Geller, I., Kling, A.: Subcortical mechanisms in emotional behavior: the effect of rhinencephalic injury upon the acquisition and retention of a conditioned avoidance response in cats. J. Comp. Physiol. Psychol. **47**, 179–186 (1954)
58. Brain, R., The neurology of language. Brain **84**, 145–166 (1961)
59. Brazier, M.A.B.: The action of anesthetics on the nervous system with special reference to the brain stem. In (eds. A. Adrian, F. Bremer, H. Jasper and J.F. Delafresnaye): Brain mechanisms and consciousness, pp. 163–199. Oxford: Blackwell 1954
60. Brazier, M.A.B.: Stimulation of the hippocampus in man using implanted electrodes. In (M.A.B. Brazier, ed.): Brain function, **II**, RNA and brain function memory and learning, pp. 299–310. Berkeley and Los Angeles: University of California Press 1964
60a. Brazier, M.A.B. (ed.): Brain mechanisms in memory and learning: From the single neuron to man (International Brain Res. Organization Monograph Series, Vol. 4). New York: Raven Press 1978
61. Bremer, F.: Cerveau-isolé et physiologie du sommeil. C.R. Soc. Biol. (Paris) **118**, 1235–1242 (1935)
62. Bremer, F.: Nouvelles recherches sur le mécanisme du sommeil. C.R. Soc. Biol. (Paris) **122**, 460–464 (1936)
63. Bremer, F.: Some problems in neurophysiology. University of London: The Athlone Press 1953
64. Bremer, F.: The neurophysiological problem of sleep. In: Brain mechanisms and consciousness, pp. 137–162. Adrian, E.D. et al. Oxford: Blackwell 1954
65. Brobeck, J.R.: Regulation of feeding and drinking. In (J. Field, H.W. Magoun, and V.E. Hall, eds.): Handbook of physiology, Section 1: Neurophysiology, Vol. 2, pp. 1197–1206. Washington: American Physiological Society 1960
66. Brooks, B., Jung, R.: Neuronal physiology of the visual cortex. In: Handbook of sensory physiology, Vol. VII/3B (R. Jung, ed.), pp. 325–440. Berlin Heidelberg New York: Springer 1973
67. Bruesch, S.R., Arey, L.B.: The number of myelinated and unmyelinated fibers in the optic nerve of vertebrates. J. Comp. Neurol. **77**, 631–635 (1942)
68. Brun, R.: Allgemeine Neurosenlehre. Biologie, Psychoanalyse and Psychohygiene leib-seelischer Störungen, 3. Aufl. Basel: Benno Schwabe & Co. 1954
68a. Bruner, J.S.: Neural mechanisms in perception. Psychol. Rev. **64**, 340–358 (1957)
69. Brutkowski, S., Mempel, E.: Disinhibition of inhibitory conditioned responses following selective brain lesions in dogs. Science **134**, 2040–2041 (1961)
70. Bühler, K.: Tatsachen und Probleme zu einer Psychologie der Denkvorgänge I–III: I. Über Gedanken. Arch. ges. Psychol. **9**, 207–365 (1907); II. Über Gedankenzusammenhänge. Arch. ges. Psychol. **12**, 1–23 (1908); III. Über Gedankenerinnerungen. Arch. ges. Psychol. **12**, 24–92 (1908)
71. Bülow, K.: Respiration and wakefulness in man. Acta Physiol. Scand. **59**, Suppl. 209 (1963)
72. Burdach, K.F.: Die Physiologie als Erfahrungswissenschaft, Bd. 1–3, III, S. 460–461. Leipzig: Leopold Voß 1835–1838
73. Bureš, J., Burešová, O.: The use of Leao's spreading depression in the study of interhemispheric transfer of memory traces. J. Comp. Physiol. Psychol. **53** (1960)
74. Burešová, O., Bureš, J.: Interhemispheric synthesis of memory traces. J. Comp. Physiol. Psychol. **59**, 211–214 (1965)

75. Burwell, C.S., Robin, E.D., Whaley, R.D., Bickelman, A.G.: Extreme obesity associated with alveolar hypoventilation. A Pickwickian Syndrome. Am. J. Med. **21**, 811–818 (1956)
76. Buser, P.A., Rougeul-Buser, A. (Hrsg.): Cerebral correlates of conscious experience. Amsterdam, New York, Oxford: North-Holland Publishing Company 1978
77. Buytendijk, F.J.J.: Wesen und Sinn des Spiels. Das Spielen des Menschen und der Tiere als Erscheinungsform der Lebenstriebe. Berlin: Kurt Wolff-Verlag, Der neue Geist-Verlag 1933
78. Buytendijk, F.J.J.: Mensch und Tier. Ein Beitrag zur vergleichenden Psychologie. Berlin. Rowohlt 1958

C

1. Cajal, S.R. y: Histologie du système nerveux de l'homme et des vertébrés, T. 1, 2. Paris: Maloine 1909–1911. Neudruck: Madrid: Instituto Ramon y Cajal 1955
2. Cannon, W.B.: Bodily changes in pain, hunger, fear and rage. New York: Appleton-Century Crofts 1929
3. Cannon, W.B.: The wisdom of the body. London: Kegan Paul 1932
4. Caspers, H.: Changes of cortical d.c. potentials in the sleep wakefulness cycle. In (G.E.W. Wolstenholme, and M. O'Connor, eds.): The nature of sleep. CIBA-Foundation Symposion 237–259. London: J.C.A. Churchill 1961
5. Caspers, H., Schulze, H.: Die Veränderungen der corticalen Gleichspannung während der natürlichen Schlaf-Wach-Perioden beim freibeweglichen Tier. Pfluegers Arch. **270**, 103–120 (1959)
6. Caveness, W.F.: Atlas of electroencephalography in the developing monkey Macaca Mulatta. Reading, Mass., Palo Alto, London: Addison-Wesley Publishing Company 1962
6a. Cherry, C. (ed.): Information theory. Symposion, London 1960. London: Butterworths 1961
7. Cigánek, L.: Die elektroencephalographische Lichtreizantwort der menschlichen Hirnrinde. Bratislava: Akademie d. Wissenschaften 1961
8. Clemente, C.D., Sterman, M.B.: Cortical recruitment and sleep patterns in acute restrained and chronic behaving cats. Electroencephalogr. Clin. Neurophysiol. **14**, 420 (1962)
9. Conrad, K.: Über den Begriff der Vorgestalt und seine Bedeutung für die Hirnpathologie. Nervenarzt **18**, 289–293 (1947)
10. Conrad, K.: Über differentiale und integrale Gestaltfunktion und den Begriff der Protopathie. Nervenarzt **19**, 315–323 (1948)
11. Conrad, K.: Die symptomatischen Psychosen. In (H.W. Gruhle, R. Jung, W. Mayer-Gross u. M. Müller): Psychiatrie der Gegenwart. Forschung und Praxis. Bd. II. Berlin, Göttingen, Heidelberg: Springer 1960
12. Craig, W.: Appetites and aversions as constituents of instincts. Biol. Bull. **34**, 91–107 (1918)
13. Craik, K.J.W.: The nature of explanation. Cambridge: Univ. Press 1943
14. Creed, R.S., Denny-Brown, D., Eccles, J.C., Liddell, E.G.T., Sherrington, C.S.: Reflex activity of the spinal cord. Oxford: Clarendon Press 1932
14a. Cremerius, J., Jung, R.: Über die Veränderungen des Elektrencephalogramms nach Elektroschockbehandlung. Nervenarzt **18**, 193–205 (1947)
15. Creutzfeldt, O., Akimoto, H.: Konvergenz und gegenseitige Beeinflussung von Impulsen aus der Retina und den unspezifischen Thalamuskernen an einzelnen Neuronen des optischen Cortex. Arch. Psychiatr. Nervenkr. **196**, 520–538 (1958)
16. Creutzfeldt, O., Jung, R.: Neuronal discharge in the cat's motor cortex during sleep and arousal. In (G.E.N. Wolstenholme, and M. O'Connor, eds.): The nature of sleep. CIBA-Foundation Symposion, pp. 131–170. London: J. & A. Churchill Ltd. 1961
17. Creutzfeldt, O., Kasamatsu, A., Vaz-Ferreira, A.: Aktivitäts-Änderungen einzelner corticaler Neurone im akuten Sauerstoffmangel. Pfluegers Arch. **263**, 647–667 (1957)
18. Creutzfeldt, O.D., Nothdurft, H.C.: Representation of complex visual stimuli in the brain. Naturwissenschaften **65**, 307–318 (1978)
19. Critchley, M.: Periodic hypersomnia and megaphagia in adolescent males. Brain **85**, 627–656 (1962)
20. Curtiss, S.: Genie: A psycholinguistic study of a Modern-day "Wild Child", p. 288. New York: Academic Press 1977 [138, 139, 140, 141]
21. Curtiss, S., Fromkin, V., Krashen, S., Rigler, D., Rigler, M.: The linguistic development of Genie. Language **50**, 528–554 (1974) [139]

D

1. Darwin, C.: The descent of man and selection in relation to sex. London: John Murray 1871
2. Darwin, C.: The expression of the emotions in man and animals. London: John Murray 1872
3. Dashiell, J.F.: The role of vision in spatial orientation by the white rat. J. Comp. Physiol. Psychol. **52**, 522–526 (1959)
4. Davis, H., Davis, P.A., Loomis, A.L., Harvey, E.N., Hobart, G.: Changes in human brain potentials during the onset of sleep. Science **86**, 448–450 (1937)
5. Davis, H., Davis, P.A., Loomis, A.L., Harvey, E.N., Hobart, G.: Human brain potentials during the onset of sleep. J. Neurophysiol. **1**, 24–38 (1938)
6. Davis, H., Davis, P.A., Loomis, A.L., Harvey, E.N., Hobart, G.: Electrical reactions of the human brain to auditory stimulation during sleep. J. Neurophysiol. **2**, 500–514 (1939)
7. Dawson, G.D.: Cerebral responses to electrical stimulation of peripheral nerve in man. J. Neurol. Neurosurg. Psychiatry N.S. **10**, 134–140 (1947)
8. Dawson, G.D.: Autocorrelation and automatic integration. Electroencephalogr. Clin. Neurophysiol. Suppl. **4**, 26–37 (1953)
9. Dawson, G.D., Scott, J.W.: The recording of nerve action potentials through skin in man. J. Neurol. Neurosurg. Psychiatry **12**, 259–267 (1949)
10. Deecke, L., Scheid, P., Kornhuber, H.H.: Distribution of readiness potential, pre-motion positivity, and motor potential of the human cerebral cortex preceding voluntary finger movements. Exp. Brain Res. **7**, 158–168 (1969)
11. Delafresnaye, J.F. (ed.): Brain mechanisms and consciousness. Symposium. Oxford: Blackwell 1954
12. Delgado, J.M.R.: Effect of brain stimulation on trask-free situations. In (R. Hernándes-Péon, eds.): The physiological basis of mental activity. Electroencephalogr. Clin. Neurophysiol. Suppl. **24**, 260–280 (1963)
13. Delgado, J.M.R.: Cerebral heterostimulation in a monkey colony. Science **141**, 161–163 (1963)
14. Delgado, J.M.R.: Free behavior and brain stimulation. Int. Rev. Neurobiol. **6**, 349–449 (1964)
15. Delgado, J.M.R., Hamlin, H.: Spontaneous and evoked electrical seizures in animals and in humans. In: Electrical studies on the unanesthetized brain (eds. E.R. Ramey, and D.S. O'Doherty), Symposion, pp. 133–158. New York: Paul B. Hoeber Inc., Medical Division of Harper & Brothers 1960
16. Dell, P.: Some basic mechanisms of the translation of bodily needs into behaviour. In (Wolstenholme, G.E.W., and C.M. O'Connor, eds.): Ciba Foundation Symposium on the Neurological Basis of Behavior, pp. 187–201. London: I.A. Churchill 1958
17. Dell, P.: Reticular homeostasis and cortical reactivity. In (G. Moruzzi, A. Fessard, and H.H. Jasper, eds.): Progress in brain research, Vol. I, Brain mechanisms, intern. Colloquium, Pisa, 1961, 82–114. Amsterdam, London, New York: Elsevier Publishing Company 1963
18. Dell, P., Bonvallet, M., Hugelin, A.: Tonus sympathique adrénaline et contrôle réticulaire de la motricité spinale. Electroencephalogr. Clin. Neurophysiol. **6**, 599–618 (1954)
19. Dell, P., Bonvallet, M., Hugelin, A.: Mechanisms of reticular deactivation. In (G.E.W. Wolstenholme and M. O'Connor, eds.): The nature of sleep. London: J. & A. Churchill 1961
20. Dembrowski, J.: Psychologie der Affen. 2. Aufl. Berlin: Akademie-Verlag 1956
21. Dement, W.: The occurrence of low voltage, fast, electroencephalogram patterns during behavioral sleep in the cat. Electroencephalogr. Clin. Neurophysiol. **10**, 291–296 (1958)
22. Dement, W.: The effect of dream deprivation. The need for a certain amount of dreaming each night is suggested by recent experiments. Science **131**, 1705–1707 (1960)
23. Dement, W.: Eye movements during sleep. In (M.B. Bender, ed.): The oculomotor system. Symposion New York, Chapt. 17, 366–416. New York, Evanston, London: Hoeber Medical Division, Harper & Row Publ. 1964
24. Dement, W., Kleitman, N.: The relation of eye movements during sleep to dream activity; an objective method for the study of dreaming. J. Exp. Psychol. **53**, 339–346 (1957)
25. Dement, W., Kleitman, N.: Cyclic variations in EEG during sleep and their relation to eye movements, body motility and dreaming. Electroencephalogr. Clin. Neurophysiol. **9**, 673–690 (1957)

26. Dempsey, E.W., Morison, R.S.: The electrical activity of a thalamocortical relay system. Am. J. Physiol. **138**, 283–296 (1942)
27. Dempsey, E.W., Morison, R.S.: The production of rhythmically recurrent cortical potential after localized thalamic stimulation. Am. J. Physiol. **135**, 293–300 (1942)
28. Denny-Brown, D.: The cerebral control of movement. Liverpool: Liverpool University Press 1966
29. Dichgans, J., Bizzi, E., Morasso, P., Tagliasco, V.: Mechanisms underlying recovery of eye-head coordination following bilateral labyrinthectomy in monkeys. Exp. Brain Res. **18**, 548–562 (1973)
30. Dichgans, J., Brandt, Th.: Visual-vestibular interaction. Effects on self-motion perception and postural control. In: Handbook of Sensory Physiology (R. Held, H. Leibowitz and H.L. Teuber, eds.), Vol. VIII. Berlin, Heidelberg, New York: Springer 1978
31. Dichgans, J., Jung, R.: Attention, eye movements and motion detection: Facilitation and selection in optokinetic nystagmus and railway nystagmus. In (Evans C.R., Mulholland, T.B., eds.): Attention in neurophysiology, pp. 348–375. London: Butterworth 1969
32. Doty, R.W.: The role of subcortical structures in conditioned reflexes. Ann. N.Y. Acad. Sci. **92**, 939–945 (1961)
33. Doty, R.W.: Conditioned reflexes elicited by electrical stimulation of the brain in macaques. J. Neurophysiol. **28**, 623–640 (1965)
34. Doty, R.W., Rutledge, L.T.: "Generalization" between cortically and peripherally applied stimuli eliciting conditioned reflexes. J. Neurophysiol. **22**, 428–435 (1959)
35. Drachman, D.B., Gumnit, R.J.: Periodic alteration of consciousness in the "Pickwickian" syndrome. Arch. Neurol. (Chic.) **6**, 471–477 (1962)
36. Dreyfus-Brisac, C., Fischgold, H.: Veille, sommeil, réactivité sensorielle chez le prématuré, le nouveau-né et le nourisson. Electroencephalogr. Clin. Neurophysiol. Suppl. **6**, 418–440 (1957)
37. Duensing, F., Schaefer, K.-P.: Die Aktivität einzelner Neurone der Formatio reticularis des nicht gefesselten Kaninchens bei Kopfwendungen und vestibulären Reizen. Arch. Psychiatr. Nervenkr. **200**, 97–122 (1960)
38. Durup, G., Fessard, A.: L'électroencéphalogramme de l'homme. Observations psycho-physiologique relatives à l'action des stimuli visuels et auditifs. Ann. psychol. **36**, 1–35 (1936)
39. Dusser de Barenne, J.G., McCulloch, W.S.: The direct functional interrelation of sensory cortex and optic thalamus. J. Neurophysiol. **1**, 176–186 (1938)

E

1. Ebbinghaus, H.: Über das Gedächtnis: Untersuchungen zur experimentellen Psychologie. Leipzig: Duncker u. Humblot 1885
2. Eccles, J.C.: The physiology of nerve cells. Baltimore: Johns Hopkins Press; Oxford: University Press 1957
3. Eccles, J.C.: The physiology of imagination. Sci. Am. **199**, 135–146 (1958)
4. Eccles, J.C.: The mechanism of synaptic transmission. Ergebn. Physiol. **51**, 299–430 (1961)
5. Eccles, J.C.: The physiology of synapses. Berlin, Göttingen, Heidelberg: Springer 1964
5a. Eccles, J.C.: The understanding of the brain. McGraw-Hill Book Co. New York etc. 1973
5b. Eccles, J.C.: An instruction-selection hypothesis of cerebral learning. In: Cerebral correlates of conscious experience (P.A. Buser and A. Rougeul-Buser, eds.), pp. 155–175. Amsterdam, New York, Oxford: North-Holland Publishing Comp. 1978
5c. Eccles, J.C.: Hirn und Bewusstsein. In: Mannheimer Forum 77/78. Mannheim: Boehringer 1978
5d. Eccles, J.C.: The human mystery. The Gifford Lectures University of Edinburgh 1977–1978. Heidelberg, New York: Springer International 1979
6. Eccles, J.C., Ito, I., Szentagothai, J.: The cerebellum as a neuronal machine. Berlin, Heidelberg, New York: Springer 1967
7. Economo, C. v.: Die Encephalitis lethargica. Jb. Psychiat. Neurol. **38**, 1–79 (1917)
8. Economo, C. v.: Schlaftheorie, Ergebn. Physiol. **28**, 312–339 (1929)
9. Edelman, G.M.: Group degenerate selection and phasic reentrant signaling: A theory of higher brain function. In: The mindful brain by M. Edelman, V.B. Mountcastle, and O. Schmitt, pp. 51–100. Cambridge, Mass.: M.I.T. Press 1978

10. Ehrenberg, R.: Theoretische Biologie. Berlin: Julius Springer 1923
11. Ehret, R., Schneider, E.: Photogene Epilepsie mit suchtartiger Selbstauslösung kleiner Anfälle und wiederholten Sexualdelikten. Arch. Psychiatr. Nervenkr. **202**, 75–94 (1961)
12. Eichler, W.: Über die Ableitung der Aktionspotentiale vom menschlichen Nerven in situ. Z. Biol. **98**, 182–214 (1937)
13. Eigen, M.: Chemical means of information, storage and readout in biological systems. Neurosci. Res. Program Bull. **2**, 11–22 (1964)
14. Einstein, A.: Geometrie und Erfahrung. In: Mein Weltbild (Hrsg. C. Seelig). Neue Auflage, S. 156–166. Zürich, Stuttgart, Wien: Europa-Verlag 1953
15. Elkes, J.: Schizophrenic disorder in relation to levels of neural organization: the need for some conceptual points of reference. In (J. Folch-Pi, ed.): Chemical pathology of the nervous system, pp. 648–665. Oxford: Pergamon Press 1961
16. Elkes, J.: Subjective and objective observation in psychiatry. Harvey Lect. Ser. **57**, 63–92 (1963)
17. Endres, G., Frey, W. v.: Über Schlaftiefe und Schlafmenge. Z. Biol. **90**, 70–80 (1930)
18. Engström, H.: Electron micrographic studies of the receptor cells of the organ of corti. In (G.L. Rasmussen, and W. Windle, eds.): Neural mechanisms of the auditory and vestibular systems. Springfield: C.C. Thomas 1961
19. Euler, C. v.: Excitatory and inhibitory mechanisms in hippocampus. In (Tower, D.B., and J.P. Schade, ed.): Structure and function of the cerebral cortex, pp. 272–277. Amsterdam: Elsevier 1960
20. Euler, C. v., Green, J.D., Ricci, G.: The role of hippocampal dendrites in evoked responses and afterdischarges. Acta Physiol. Scand. **42**, 87–111 (1958)
21. Euler, C. v., Green, J.D.: Activity in single hippocampal pyramids. Acta Physiol. Scand. **48**, 95–109 (1960)
22. Evarts, E.V.: Effects of sleep and waking on activity of single units in the unrestrained cat. In (G.E.W. Wolstenholme, and M. O'Connor, eds.): The nature of sleep. CIBA-Foundation Symposion, 171–187. London: J. & A. Churchill Ltd. 1961
22a. Evarts, E.V.: A neurophysiological theory of hallucinations. In (L.J. West, ed.): Hallucinations, pp. 1–14. New York, London: Grune & Stratton 1962
23. Evarts, E.V.: Temporal patterns of discharge of pyramidal tract neurons during sleep and waking in the monkey. J. Neurophysiol. **27**, 152–171 (1964)
24. Evarts, E.V.: Representation of movements and muscles by pyramidal tract neurons of the precental motor cortex. In: M.D. Yahr and D.P. Purpura (eds.): Neurophysiological basis of normal and abnormal motor activity, pp. 215–253. Hewlett, New York: Raven Press 1967
25. Evarts, E.V.: Relation of pyramidal tract activity to force exerted during voluntary movements. J. Neurophysiol. **31**, 14–27 (1968)
26. Evarts, E.V.: Activity of thalamic and cortical neurons in relation to learned movement in the monkey. Int. J. Neurol. **8**, 321–326 (1971)
27. Evarts, E.V., Tanji, J.: Gating of motor cortex reflexes by prior instruction. Brain Res. **71**, 479–494 (1974)
28. Exner, S.: Ueber Sensomobilität. Pfluegers Arch. **48**, 592–613 (1891)
29. Exner, S.: Entwurf zu einer physiologischen Erklärung der psychischen Erscheinungen. 1. Theil. Leipzig, Wien: Franz Deuticke 1894
30. Eysenck, H.J.: Behaviour therapy and the neuroses. Readings in modern methods of treatment derived from learning theory. Oxford, London, New York, Paris: Pergamon Press 1960

F

1. Fabre, J.H.: Souvenirs entomologiques. Vol. 1–10 (1879–1910) 2. ed. def. et ill. Paris: Delgrave 1914–1924
2. Fahrenberg, J.: Psychophysiologie. In (K.P. Kisker, J.E. Meyer, C. Müller, and E. Strömgren, Hrsg.): Psychiatrie der Gegenwart, Bd. I/1, S. 91–210. Berlin, Heidelberg, New York: Springer 1979
3. Fangel, Chr., Kaada, B.R.: Behavior "attention" and fear induced by cortical stimulation in the cat. Electroencephalogr. Clin. Neurophysiol. **12**, 575–588 (1960)

4. Fechner, G.T.: Elemente der Psychophysik, Teil 1 u. 2. Leipzig: Breitkopf und Härtel 1860
5. Fernandez de Molina, A., Hunsperger, R.W.: Central representation of affective reactions in forebrain and brain stem: electrical stimulation of amygdala, stria terminalis and adjacent structures. J. Physiol. (Lond.) **145**, 251–265 (1959)
6. Fernandez de Molina, A., Hunsperger, R.W.: Organization of the subcortical system governing defence and flight reactions in the cat. J. Physiol. (Lond.) **160**, 200–213 (1962)
7. Ferrier, D.: The functions of the brain. London: Smith, Elder & Co. 1876
8. Finke, J., Schulte, W.: Schlafstörungen. Ursachen und Behandlung. Stuttgart: Thieme 1970
9. Fischgold, H.: La conscience et ses modifications systèmes de references en EEG clinique. Ier Congr. Internat. des Scienc. Neurol., Bruxelles, 1957. Vol. Rapp. **2**, 181–206 (1957)
10. Fischgold, H. (ed.): Le sommeil de nuit normal et pathologique. Etudes électroencéphalographiques. Paris: Masson & Cie. 1965
11. Fischgold, H., Gastaut, H. (edit.): Conditionnement et réactivité en électroencéphalographie. Electroencephalogr. Clin. Neurophysiol. Suppl. **6** (1957)
12. Fischgold, H., Schwartz, B.A.: A clinical electroencephalographic and polygraphic study of sleep in the human adult. In (G.E.W. Wolstenholme, and M. O'Connor, eds.): The nature of sleep. CIBA-Foundation Symposion. 209–236. London: J.A. Churchill 1961
12a. Fisher, C.: Psychoanalytic implications of recent research on sleep and dreaming. J. Am. Psychonal. Ass. 13 **2**, 197–303 (1965)
13. Fisher, C.H., Gross, J., Zuch, J.: Cycle of penile erection synchronous with dreaming (REM), sleep. Arch. gen. Psychiat. **12**, 29–45 (1965)
14. Flexner, J.B., Flexner, L.B., Stellar, E.: Memory in mice as affected by intracerebral puromycin. Science **141**, 57–59 (1963)
15. Flourens, P.: Recherches expérimentales sur les propriétés et les fonctions du système nerveux dans les animaux vertèbrés. Paris: Baillière 1842
16. Flynn, W.R.: Visual hallucinations in sensory deprivation. Psychiat. Quart. **36**, 1–10 (1962)
17. Foerster, H.: Das Gedächtnis. Wien: F. Deuticke 1948
17a. Foerster, H. v., Zopf, G.W., jr. (eds.): Principles of selforganization. Symposion. Oxford, London, New York, Paris: Pergamon Press 1962
18. Foerster, O.: Motorische Felder und Bahnen. Sensible corticale Felder. In (O. Bumke, u. O. Foerster, Hrsg.): Handbuch der Neurologie, Bd. VI, S. 1–448. Berlin: Springer 1936
19. Foerster, O., Gagel: Ein Fall von Ependymcyste des III. Ventrikels. Ein Beitrag zur Frage der Beziehungen psychischer Störungen zum Hirnstamm. Z. ges. Neurol. Psychiat. **149**, 312–344 (1934)
20. Foerster, O., Penfield, W.: Der Narbenzug am Gehirn bei traumatischer Epilepsie in seiner Bedeutung für die therapeutische Bekämpfung derselben. Z. ges. Neurol. Psychiat. **125**, 475–572 (1930)
21. Fontana, F.: Dei moti dell'iride. Lucca: Jacopo Giusti 1765
22. Forel, A.: Das Sinnesleben der Insekten. Eine Sammlung von experimentellen und kritischen Studien über Insektenpsychologie. München: Bergmann 1910
23. Frankl, V.E.: Theorie und Therapie der Neurosen. Wien: Urban & Schwarzenberg 1956
24. Freeman, W.J.: An ergometer for measuring work from cats as an index for drive. J. Appl. Physiol. **14**, 1071–1072 (1959)
25. Freeman, W.J.: Comparison of thresholds for behavioral and electrical responses to cortical electrical stimulation in cats. Exp. Neurol. **6**, 315–331 (1962)
26. Freeman, W.J.: Correlation of goal-directed work with sensory cortical excitability. In (J. Wortis, ed.): Recent advances in biological psychiatry, Vol. 7, Chapt. 24, pp. 243–250. New York: Plenum Press 1964
27. Freud, A.: Das Ich und die Abwehrmechanismen. Wien: Intern. Psychoanalyt. Verlag 1936
28. Freud, S.: Entwurf einer Psychologie. (1895). In: S. Freud: Aus den Anfängen der Psychoanalyse. Briefe an Wilhelm Fliess. Abhandlungen und Notizen aus den Jahren 1887–1902. S. 297–384. Frankfurt a.M.: S. Fischer 1962
29. Freud, S.: Die Traumdeutung. Leipzig u. Wien: Franz Deuticke 1900
30. Freud, S.: Gesammelte Werke. Bd. 1–18. London: Imago Publ. 1940
31. Frisch, K. v.: Tanzsprache und Orientierung der Bienen. Berlin, Göttingen, Heidelberg: Springer 1965

31a. Frisch, K.v.: Tiere als Baumeister. Berlin, Frankfurt, Wien: Ullstein 1974
32. Fritsch, G., Hitzig, E.: Über die elektrische Erregbarkeit des Großhirns. Arch. Anat. Physiol. wiss. Med. **37**, 300–332 (1870)
33. Frolov, V.P.: Pavlov and his school. Oxford: University Press 1937
34. Fulton, J.F.: Frontal lobotomy and affective behavior. A neurophysiological analysis. New York: W.W. Norton Co. 1951

G

1. Gänshirt, H., Dransfeld, L., Zylka, W.: Das Hirnpotentialbild und der Erholungsrückstand am Warmblütergehirn nach kompletter Ischämie. Arch. Psychiatr. Nervenkr. **189**, 109–125 (1952)
2. Galambos, R., Morgan, C.T.: The neural basis of learning. In (J. Field, H.W. Magoun, V.E. Hall, eds.): Handbook of physiology, Section 1: Neurophysiology, Vol. 3, pp. 1471–1499. Washington, D.C.: American Physiological Society 1960
3. Galton, F.: Inquiries into human faculty and its development. London: MacMillan 1883
4. Gamper, E.: Bau und Leistungen eines menschlichen Mittelhirnwesens (Arhinencephalie mit Encephalocele). Z. ges. Neurol. Psychiat. **102**, 154–235 (1926)
5. Gamper, E.: Bau und Leistungen eines menschlichen Mittelhirnwesens (Arhinencephalie mit Encephalocele), zugleich ein Beitrag zur Teratologie und Fasersystematik. II. klinischer Teil. Z. ges. Neurol. Psychiat. **104**, 49–120 (1926)
5a. Gamper, E.: Zur Frage der Polioencephalitis haemorrhagica der chronischen Alkoholiker. Anatomische Befunde beim alkaholischen Korsakow und ihre Beziehungen zum klinischen Bild. Dtsch. Z. Nervenheilk. **102**, 122–129 (1928)
6. Gamper, E.: Schlaf, Delirium tremens, Korsakowsches Syndrom. Arch. Psychiatr. Nervenkr. **86**, 294–301 (1929)
7. Gantt, W.H.: Physiological bases of psychiatry. Springfield, Ill.: Charles C. Thomas 1958
8. Gardner, R.A., Gardner, B.T.: Teaching sign language to a chimpanzee. Science **165**, 664–672 (1969)
9. Gassel, M.M., Marchiafava, P.L., Pompeiano, O.: Tonic and phasic inhibition of spinal reflexes during deep, desynchronized sleep in unrestained cats. Arch. Ital. Biol. **102**, 471–499 (1964)
10. Gastaut, H.: Some aspects of the neurophysiological basis of conditioned reflexes and behavior. In (G.E.W. Wolstenholme, and C.M. O'Connor, eds.): Neurological basis of behavior (Ciba Foundation Symposion). Boston: Little, Brown & Co. 1958
10a. Gastaut, H., Collomb, H.: Etude de comportement sexuel chez les épileptiques psychomoteurs. Ann. Medicopsychol. **112**, 657–696 (1954)
11. Gastaut, H.A., Jus, C., Morrell, F., Storm van Leeuwen, W., Dongier, S., Naquet, R., Regis, H., Roger, A., Bekkering, D., Kamp, A., Werre, J.: Étude topographique des réactions électroencéphalographiques conditionnées chez l'homme. Electroencephalogr. Clin. Neurophysiol. **9**, 1–34 (1957)
12. Gastaut, H., Roger, A.: Les mécanismes de l'àctivité nerveuse supérieure envisagés au niveau des grandes structures fonctionelles du cerveau. Electroencephalogr. Clin. Neurophysiol. Suppl. **13**, 13–38 (1960)
12a. Gastaut, H., Roger, J., Ouahchi, S., Timsit, M., Broughton, R.: An electroclinical study of generalized epileptic seizures of tonic expression. Epilepsia **4**, 15–44 (1963)
13. Gaupp, R.: Über den Diabetes insipidus. Z. ges. Neurol. Psychiat. **171**, 514–546 (1941)
14. Gazzaniga, M.S.: The bisected brain. New York: Appleton-Century-Crofts 1970
15. Gehlen, A.: Der Mensch. Berlin: Junker u. Dünnhaupt 1940
15a. Gerard, R.W., Duyff, J.W. (eds.): Information processing in the nervous system, Vol. III. Proc. Internat. Union Physiol. Sci., 22. International Congress Leiden, 1962. Amsterdam, New York, London, Internat. Congr. Ser. No. 49, Excerpta Medica Foundation, 1962
16. Gerardy, W., Herberg, D., Kuhn, H.M.: Vergleichende Untersuchungen der Lungenfunktion und des Elektroencephalogramms bei zwei Patienten mit Pickwickian-Syndrom. Z. klin. Med. **156**, 362–380 (1960)
17. Geschwind, N.: Disconnexion syndromes in animals and man. Part I, Part II. Brain **88**, 237–294, 585–644 (1965)
18. Geschwind, N.: The anatomical basis of hemispheric differentiation. In: Hemisphere function in the human brain. Dimond, S.J., Beaumont, J.G. (eds.), pp. 7–24. New York: John Wiley and Sons 1974 [90]

19. Giaquinto, S., Pompeiano, O., Somogyi, I.: Descending inhibitory influences on spinal reflexes during natural sleep. Arch. Ital. Biol. **102**, 282–307 (1964)
20. Gibbs, F.A.: Electrencephalogramm und Klinik. Der gegenwärtige Stand der klinischen Electrencephalographie. Arch. Psychiatr. Nervenkr. **183**, 2–11 (1949)
21. Gibbs, F.A., Davis, H., Lennox, W.G.: The electroencephalogram in epilepsy and in conditions of impaired consciousness. Arch. Neurol. Psychiat. (Chic.) **34**, 1133–1148 (1935)
22. Gibbs, F.A, Gibbs, E.L.: Atlas of electroencephalography, 2. ed., I: Methodology and controls. Cambridge: Addison-Wesley Press Inc. 1950
23. Gibbs, F.A., Gibbs, E.L.: Atlas of electroencephalography, 2. ed., II. Epilepsy. Cambridge: Addison-Wesley Press, Inc. 1952
24. Gibbs, F.A., Gibbs, E.L.: Fourteen and six per second positive spikes. Electroencephalogr. Clin. Neurophysiol. **15**, 553–558 (1963)
25. Gibbs, F.A., Gibbs, E.L., Lennox, W.G.: Effect on the electroencephalogram of certain drugs which influence nervous activity. Arch. Intern. Med. **60**, 154–166 (1937)
26. Gibbs, F.A., Gibbs, E.L., Lennox, W.G.: The likeness of the cortical dysrhythmias of schizophrenia and psychomotor epilepsy. Am. J. Psychiatry **95**, 255–269 (1938)
27. Gibson, J.G.: The perception of the visual world. Boston: Houghton Mifflin Comp. Cambridge: The Riverside Press 1950
28. Gibson, J.G.: The survival value of sensory perception. In (E.E. Bernard, and M.R. Kare, eds.): Biological prototypes and synthetic systems, Vol. 1 (Symposium), 230–232. New York: Plenum Press 1962
29. Goldstein, K.: Die Lokalisation in der Großhirnrinde. Nach den Erfahrungen am kranken Menschen. In: Bethe-Bergmanns Handbuch der normalen und pathologischen Physiologie, Bd. 10, S. 600–842. Berlin: Springer 1927
30. Goltz, F.: Der Hund ohne Großhirn. Pfluegers Arch. **51**, 570–614 (1892)
31. Gozzano, M., Fontana, A., Folicaldi, G.: Modello elettronico di riflesso condizionato (con presentazione di un nuovo apparecchio). Riv. Neurol. **21**, 440–443 (1951)
32. Granit, R.: Sensory mechanisms of the retina. London: Oxford University Press 1947
33. Granit, R.: Receptors and sensory perception. New Haven: Yale University Press 1955
34. Granit, R.: The purposive brain. Cambridge/Mass., London: The M.I.T. Press 1977
35. Granit, R., Phillips, C.G.: Excitatory and inhibitory processes acting upon individual purkinje cells of the cerebellum in cats. J. Physiol. (Lond.) **133**, 520–547 (1956)
36. Grastyán, E.: The hippocampus and higher nervous activity. In (M.A.B. Brazier, ed.): The central nervous system and behavior. Transactions of the 2. Conference, Febr. 22–25, 1959, Princeton, N.J., pp. 119–205. New York: Josiah Macy jr. Foundation; Washington: The National Science Foundation 1959
37. Grastyán, E., Karmos, G.: A study of a possible "dreaming" mechanism in the cat. Acta Physiol. Acad. Sci. Hung. **20**, Fasc. 1, 41–50 (1961)
38. Grastyán, E., Lissák, K., Madarász, I., Donhoffer, H.: Hippocampal electrical activity during the development of conditioned reflexes. Electroencephalogr. Clin. Neurophysiol. **11**, 409–430 (1959)
39. Grastyán, E., Lissák, K., Szabó, J., Vereby, G.: Über die funktionelle Bedeutung des Hippocampus. In (I. Beritashvili, ed.): Problems of the modern physiology of the nervous and muscle systems, pp. 67–80. Tbilisi (Tiflis), Georgian S.S.R.: Academy of Sciences 1956
40. Green, J.D., Clemente, C.D., Groot, J. de: Rhinencephalic lesions and behavior in cats. An analysis of the Klüver-Bucy-syndrome with particular reference to normal and abnormal sexual behavior. J. Comp. Neurol. **108**, 505–545 (1957)
41. Green, J.D., Machne, X.: Unit activity of rabbit hippocampus. Am. J. Physiol. **181**, 219–224 (1955)
42. Griesinger, W.: Die Pathologie und Therapie der psychischen Krankheiten für Ärzte und Studierende. 2. Aufl. Stuttgart: 1861
43. Grünewald-Zuberbier, E., Grünewald, G.: Goal-directed movement potentials of human cerebral cortex. Exp. Brain Res. **33**, 135–138 (1978)
44. Grünewald-Zuberbier, E., Grünewald, G., Jung, R.: Slow potentials of the human precental and parietal cortex during goal-directed movements (Zielbewegungspotentiale). J. Physiol. (London) **284**, 181–182 P (1978)
45. Grünthal, E.: Über das klinische Bild nach umschriebenem beiderseitigem Ausfall der

Ammonshornrinde, ein Beitrag zur Kenntnis der Funktion des Ammonshornes. Mschr. Psychiat. Neurol. **113**, 1–16 (1947)
46. Grünthal, E.: Über phantastische Gesichtserscheinungen bei langdauerndem Augenschluß. Psychiat. et Neurol. (Basel) **133**, 193–206 (1957)
47. Grüsser, O.-J., Hellner, K.A., Grüsser-Cornehls, U.: Die Informationsübertragung im afferenten visuellen System. Kybernetik **1**, 175–198 (1962)
48. Grüttner, R., Bonkálo, A.: Über Ermüdung und Schlaf auf Grund hirnbioelektrischer Untersuchungen. Arch. Psychiatr. Nervenkr. **111**, 652–665 (1940)

H

1. Hagbarth, K.E., Fex, J.: Centrifugal influences on single unit activity in spinal sensory paths. J. Neurophysiol. **22**, 321–338 (1959)
2. Harlow, H.F., Woolsey, C.N.: Biological and biochemical bases of behavior. Madison: University of Wisconsin Press 1958
3. Harlow, H.F., Akert, K., Schiltz, K.: The effects of bilateral prefrontal lesions on learned behavior of neonatal, infant and preadolescent monkeys. In (J.M. Warren, and K. Akert, eds.): The frontal granular cortex and behavior, Chapter 7, pp. 126–148. New York: McGraw Hill 1964
4. Hartline, H.K.: The response of single optic nerve fibres of the vertebrate eye to illumination of the retina. Am. J. Physiol. **121**, 400–415 (1938)
5. Hartline, H.K.: The receptive fields of optic nerve fibres. Am. J. Psychol. **130**, 690–699 (1940)
6. Hartline, H.K.: Inhibition of activity of visual receptors by illuminating nearby retinal areas in the limulus eye. Fed. Proc. **8**, 69 (1949)
7. Hartmann, E.L. (ed.): Sleep and dreaming. Intern. Psychiatr. Series Vol. 7. Boston: Little Brown 1970
8. Hartmann, M.: Philosophie der Naturwissenschaften. Berlin: J. Springer 1937
9. Hartmann, M.: Allgemeine Biologie. Eine Einführung in die Lehre vom Leben. Jena: Gustav Fischer 1947
10. Hartmann, N.: Philosophische Grundlagen der Biologie. Göttingen: Vandenhoeck u. Ruprecht 1912
11. Hartmann, N.: Der Aufbau der realen Welt. Grundriß der allgemeinen Kategorienlehre. Berlin: W. de Gruyter 1940
12. Hartmann, N.: Neue Wege der Ontologie. 2. Aufl. Stuttgart: W. Kohlhammer 1946
13. Hartmann, N.: Philosophie der Natur; Abriß der speziellen Kategorienlehre. Berlin: W. de Gruyter 1950
14. Hartmann, N.: Teleologisches Denken. Berlin: W. de Gruyter 1951
15. Hassenstein, B.: Die bisherige Rolle der Kybernetik in der biologischen Forschung. Naturwiss. Rundschau **13**, 349–355, 373–382, 419–424 (1960)
15a. Hassenstein, B.: Verhaltensbiologie des Kindes. München: Piper Verlag 1973
16. Hassler, R.: Über die Rinden- und Stammhirnanteile des menschlichen Thalamus. Psychiatr. Neurol. Med. Psychol. (Leipz.) **1**, 181–187 (1949)
17. Hassler, R., Riechert, T.: Wirkungen der Reizungen und Koagulationen in den Stammganglien bei stereotaktischen Hirnoperationen. Nervenarzt **32**, 97–109 (1961)
18. Head, H.: The conception of nervous and mental energy II. Vigilance: a physiological state of the nervous system. Br. J. Psychol. **14**, 126–147 (1923)
19. Head, H.: Aphasia and kindred disorders of speech. Vol. I and II. Cambridge: University Press 1926
20. Hebb, D.O.: The organization of behavior. A neurophysiological theory. New York: J. Wiley; London: Chapman & Hall 1949
21. Hebb, D.O.: A textbook of psychology. Philadelphia: W.B. Saunders Co. 1958
22. Hécaen, H.: Clinical symptomatology in right and left hemispheric lesions. In (V.B. Mountcastle, ed.): Interhemispheric relations and cerebral dominance, pp. 215–243. Baltimore: John Hopkins Press 1962
22a. Hediger, H.: Tierpsychologie im Zoo und im Zirkus. Basel: Reinhardt 1961
23. Heidegger, M.: Sein und Zeit, 1. Hälfte. Jahrb. Philos.-phänomenol. Forschung **8**, 1–438 (1927)

24. Heimann, H.: Psychopathologie. In (K.P. Kisker, J.E. Meyer, C. Müller, und E. Strömgren, Hrsg.): Psychiatrie der Gegenwart. Bd. I/1, S. 1–42. Berlin, Heidelberg, New York: Springer 1979
25. Helmchen, H.: Über zentralnervöse Dekompensation bei psychiatrischer Pharmakotherapie als Beitrag zur experimentellen Psychiatrie. Fortschr. Neurol. Psychiatr. **31**, 160–175 (1963)
26. Helmchen, H., Künkel, H.: Pneumencephalographische und elektroencephalographische Untersuchungen bei Phenothiazin-Behandelten. 2. Mitt.: Paroxysmale Dysrhythmie. Med. exp. **5**, 412–418 (1961)
27. Helmholtz, H. v.: Handbuch der physiologischen Optik. 2. Aufl. Hamburg u. Leipzig: G. Voss 1896
28. Helmholtz, H. v.: Vorträge und Reden, 4. Aufl. Braunschweig: Vieweg u. Sohn 1896
29. Hensel, H., Boman, K.A.: Afferente Impulse im menschlichen Hautnerven. Naturwissenschaften **22**, 634–635 (1959)
30. Hensel, H., Boman, K.A.: Afferent impulses in cutaneous sensory nerves in human subjects. J. Neurophysiol. **23**, 564–578 (1960)
31. Herder, J.G.: Ideen zur Philosophie der Geschichte der Menschheit. Bd. I. Riga, Leipzig: J.F. Hartknoch 1785
31a. Hering, E.: Der Raumsinn und die Bewegungen des Auges. In: Hermanns Handbuch der Physiologie, Bd. 3, I, S. 343–601. Leipzig: F.C.W. Vogel 1879
32. Hering, E.: Grundzüge der Lehre vom Lichtsinn. Berlin: Springer 1920
33. Hering, E.: Über das Gedächtnis als eine allgemeine Funktion der organisierten Materie, 1870. In: Fünf Reden von E. Hering. Leipzig: Engelmann 1921
34. Hering, E.: Wissenschaftliche Abhandlungen. Leipzig: G. Thieme 1931
35. Hermann, L.: Eine Erscheinung des simultanen Contrastes. Pflügers Arch. **3**, 13–15 (1870)
36. Hernández-Peón, R.: Neurophysiological correlates of habituation and other manifestations of plastic inhibition. In: Electroencephalogr. Clin. Neurophysiol. Suppl. **13**, 101–114 (1960)
37. Hernández-Peón, R., Donoso, M.: Influence of attention and suggestion upon subcortical evoked electric activity in the human brain. 1. Internat. Congress of Neurological Sciences, Brussels, 1957, AIII, EEG, Clinical Neurophysiology and Epilepsy, pp. 385–396. New York, Paris: Pergamon Press 1959
38. Hernández-Peón, R., Scherrer, H., Jouvet, M.: Modification of electric activity in cochlear nucleus during "attention" in unanesthetized cats. Science **123**, 331–332 (1956)
39. Heron, W.: Cognitive and physiological effects of perceptual isolation. In (P. Solomon, P.E. Kubzansky, P.H. Leiderman, J.H. Mendelson, R. Trumbull, D. Wexler): Sensory deprivation. A Symposium, pp. 6–33. Cambridge/Mass.: Harvard University Press 1961
40. Heron, W., Bexton, W.H., Hebb, D.O.: Cognitive effects of a decreased variation to the sensory environment. Am. Psychologist **8**, 366 (1953)
41. Herrick, C.J.: Neurological foundations of animal behavior. 2. ed. New York, London: Hafner Publ. Comp. 1962
42. Hess, E.H.: The relationship between imprinting and motivation. In (M.R. Jones, ed.): Nebraska symposium on motivation, 1959, pp. 44–77. Lincoln: University Nebraska Press 1959
43. Hess, E.H., Polt, J.M.: Pupil size as related to interest value of visual stimuli. Science **132**, 349–350 (1960)
44. Hess, R.: Elektrencephalographische Beobachtungen beim kataplektischen Anfall. Arch. Psychiatr. Nervenkr. **183**, 132–141 (1949)
45. Hess, R.: Sleep and sleep disturbances in the electroencephalogram. Progr. Brain Res. **18**, 127–139 (1965)
46. Hess, R., Akert, K., Koella, W.: Les potentiels bioelectriques du cortex et du thalamus et leur altération par stimulation du centre hypnique chez le chat. Rev. neurol. **83**, 537–544 (1950)
47. Hess, R., Koella, W., Akert, K.: Cortical and subcortical recordings in natural and artificially induced sleep in cats. Electroencephalogr. Clin. Neurophysiol. **5**, 75–90 (1953)
48. Hess, W.R.: Über die Wechselbeziehungen zwischen psychischen und vegetativen Funktionen. Zürich, Leipzig, Berlin: O. Füssli 1925
49. Hess, W.R.: Hirnreizversuche über den Mechanismus des Schlafes. Arch. Psychiatr. Nervenkr. **86**, 287–292 (1929)
50. Hess, W.R.: Lokalisatorische Ergebnisse der Hirnreizversuche mit Schlafeffekt. Arch. Psychiatr. Nervenkr. **88**, 813–816 (1929)

51. Hess, W.R.: Die Methodik der lokalisierten Reizung und Ausschaltung subcorticaler Hirnabschnitte. Leipzig: Thieme 1932
52. Hess, W.R.: Der Schlaf. Klin. Wochenschr. **12**, 129–134 (1933)
53. Hess, W.R.: Plastizitätslehre und Lokalisationsfrage. Verh. Dtsch. Ges. Inn. Med. **46**, 212–216 (1934)
54. Hess, W.R.: Kritisches zum Zentrenbegriff. Probl. Biol. et Med. **1935**, 43–49
55. Hess, W.R.: Das Zwischenhirn und die Regulation von Kreislauf und Atmung. Leipzig: G. Thieme 1938
56. Hess, W.R.: Die Motorik als Organisationsproblem. Biol. Zbl. **61**, 545–572 (1941)
57. Hess, W.R.: Teleokinetisches und ereismatisches Kräftesystem in der Biomotorik. Helv. Physiol. Pharmacol. Acta **1**, C 62–C 63 (1943)
58. Hess, W.R.: Induzierte Störungen der optischen Wahrnehmung. Nervenarzt **16**, 57–66 (1943)
59. Hess, W.R.: Das Schlafsyndrom als Folge dienzephaler Reizung. Helv. Physiol. Pharmacol. Acta **2**, 305–344 (1944)
60. Hess, W.R.: Die funktionelle Organisation des vegetativen Nervensystems. Basel: B. Schwabe 1948
61. Hess, W.R.: Das Zwischenhirn. Syndrome, Lokalisationen, Funktionen. Basel: B. Schwabe 1949
62. Hess, W.R.: The diencephalic sleep centre. In: Brain mechanisms and consciousness, p. 117 (ed. E.D. Adrian et al.). Oxford: Blackwell 1954
63. Hess, W.R.: Hypothalamus und Thalamus, Experimental-Dokumente. Stuttgart: Thieme 1956
64. Hess, W.R.: Die Formatio reticularis des Hirnstammes im verhaltenspsychologischen Aspekt. Arch. Psychiatr. Nervenkr. **196**, 329–336 (1957)
65. Hess, W.R.: Psychologie in biologischer Sicht. Stuttgart: Thieme 1962. 2. Aufl. 1968 (Stuttg.)
66. Hess, W.R.: Cerebrale Organisation somatomotorischer Leistungen: I. Physikalische Vorbemerkungen und Analyse konkreter Beispiele. Arch. Psychiatr. Nervenkr. **207**, 33–44 (1965)
67. Hess, W.R., Brügger, M.: Das subcorticale Zentrum der affektiven Abwehrreaktion. Helv. Physiol. Pharmacol. Acta **1**, 33–52 (1943)
68. Hess, W.R., Meyer, A.E.: Triebhafte Fellreinigung der Katze als Symptom diencephaler Reizung. Helv. Physiol. Pharmacol. Acta **14**, 397–410 (1956)
69. Hilgard, E.R., Marquis, D.G.: Conditioning and learning. New York: Appleton-Century 1954
70. Hill, D., Pond, D.A.: Reflections on one hundred capital cases submitted to electroencephalography. J. Ment. Sci. **98**, 23–44 (1952)
71. Hitzig, E.: Untersuchungen über das Gehirn. Berlin: Aug. Hirschwald 1874
72. Hoche, A.: Das träumende Ich, 1. Aufl. Jena: Fischer 1927
73. Hodgkin, A.L., Huxley, A.F.: A quantitative description of membrane current and its application to conduction and excitation in nerve. J. Physiol. (Lond.) **117**, 500–544 (1952)
74. Hoffmann, P.: Die Eigenreflexe (Sehnenreflexe) menschlicher Muskeln. Berlin: Springer 1922
75. Hoffmann, P.: Die physiologischen Eigenschaften der Eigenreflexe. Ergebn. Physiol. **36**, 15–108 (1934)
76. Hoffmann, P.: Die Beziehungen des Willens und der einfachsten Reflexformen zueinander. Arch. Psychiatr. Nervenkr. **185**, 736–742 (1950)
77. Holmgren, F.: Method att objectivera effecten av ljusintryck pa retina. Upsala Läk.-Fören. Förh. **1**, 177–191 (1865–1866)
78. Holst, E. v.: Quantitative Messung von Stimmungen im Verhalten der Fische. Symp. Soc. Exp. Biol. **4**, 143–172 (1950)
79. Holst, E. v.: Zentralnervensystem und Peripherie in ihrem gegenseitigen Verhältnis. Klin. Wochenschr. **29**, 97–105 (1951)
80. Holst, E. v.: Die Auslösung von Stimmungen bei Wirbeltieren durch „punktförmige" elektrische Erregung des Stammhirns. Naturwissenschaften **44**, 549–551 (1957)
81. Holst, E. v.: Zur „Psycho"-Physiologie des Hühnerstammhirns. In (J.D. Achelis u. H. v. Ditfurth): Befinden und Verhalten. „Starnberger Gespräche", S. 55–67. Stuttgart: Georg Thieme 1961
82. Holst, E. v., Mittelstaedt, H.: Das Reafferenzprinzip. Naturwissenschaften **37**, 464–476 (1950)
83. Holst, E. v., Saint Paul, U. v.: Das Mischen von Trieben (Instinktbewegungen) durch mehrfache Stammhirnreizungen beim Huhn. Naturwissenschaften **45**, 579 (1958)

84. Holst, E. v., Saint Paul, U. v.: Vom Wirkungsgefüge der Triebe. Naturwissenschaften **47**, 409–422 (1960)
85. Holzer, H.: Intrazelluläre Regulation des Stoffwechsels, Naturwissenschaften **50**, 260–270 (1963)
86. Hubel, D.H.: Single unit activity in striate cortex of unrestrained cats. J. Physiol. (Lond.) **147**, 226–238 (1959)
87. Hubel, D.H., Wiesel, T.N.: Receptive fields, binocular interaction and functional architecture in the cat's visual cortex. J. Physiol. (Lond.) **160**, 106–154 (1962)
88. Hubel, D.H., Wiesel, T.N.: Receptive fields and functional architecture in two nonstriate visual areas (18 and 19) of the cat. J. Neurophysiol. **28**, 229–289 (1965)
88a. Hubel, D.H., Wiesel, T.N.: Cells sensitive to binocular depth in area 18 of the macaque monkey cortex. Nature (Lond.) **225**, 41–42 (1970)
89. Hugelin, A., Bonvallet, M.: Etude expérimentale des interrelations réticulo-corticales. Proposition d'une théorie de l'asservisement réticulaire a un système diffus cortical. J. Physiol. (Paris) **49**, 1201–1223 (1957)
90. Hugelin, A., Bonvallet, M.: Tonus cortical et controle de la facilitation motrice d'origine réticulaire. J. Physiol. (Paris) **49**, 1171–1200 (1957)
91. Hugger, H.: Zur objektiven Auswertung des Elektrencephalogramms unter besonderer Berücksichtigung der gleitenden Koordination. Pfluegers Arch. **224**, 309–336 (1941)
92. Hull, C.L.: Principles of behavior. New York: Appleton-Century 1943
93. Hunsperger, R.W.: Affektreaktionen auf elektrische Reizung im Hirnstamm der Katze. Helv. Physiol. Pharmacol. Acta **14**, 70–92 (1956)
94. Hunsperger, R.W.: Les représentations centrales des réactions affectives dans le cerveau antérieur et dans le tronc cérèbral. Neuro-chirurgie **5**, 207–233 (1959)
95. Hunsperger, R.W., Brown, J.L., Rosvold, H.E.: Combined stimulation of two hypothalamic areas mediating threatattack and escape behaviour in the cat (22. Internat. Congress of Physiological Sciences). Excerpta med. (Amst.) International Congress Series Nr. **48**, Nr. 1093 (1962)
96. Hurvich, L.M., Jameson, D.: An opponent-process theory of color vision. J. Psychol. Rev. **64**, 384–404 (1957)
97. Huttenlocher, P.R.: Evoked and spontaneous activity in single units of medial brain stem during natural sleep and waking. J. Neurophysiol. **24**, 451–468 (1961)
98. Huxley, J.S.: The courtship habits of the great crested grebe (Podiceps cristatus) with an addition to the theory of sexual selection. Proc. zool. Soc. Lond. **1914**, 491–562

I

1. Iggo, A. (ed.): Somato-sensory system. Handbook of sensory physiology, Vol. II. Berlin, Heidelberg, New York: Springer 1973
2. Ingvar, D.H.: Extraneuronal influences upon the electrical activity of isolated cortex following stimulation of the reticular activating system. Acta Physiol. Scand. **33**, 169–193 (1955)
3. Ingvar, D.H., Söderberg, U.: Correlation of blood flow and EEG. Electroencephalogr. Clin. Neurophysiol. **8**, 699 (1956)
4. Ito, M., Yoshida, M., Obata, K., Kawai, N., Udo, M.: Inhibitory control of intracerebellar nuclei by the Purkinje cell axons. Exp. Brain Res. **10**, 69–80 (1970)

J

1. Jackson, J.H.: Selected writings of John Hughlings Jackson, Vol. 1–2. New York: Basic Books, Inc. 1958
2. Jacob, H.: Der Erlebniswandel bei Späterblindeten (Zur Psychopathologie der optischen Wahrnehmung). Hamburg: H.H. Nölke 1949
3. Jacobson, A., Kales, A., Lehmann, D., Hoedemaker, F.S.: Muscle tonus in human subjects during sleep and dreaming. Exp. Neurol. **10**, 418–424 (1964)
3a. Jacobson, A., Lehmann, D., Kales, A., Wenner, W.H.: Somnambule Handlungen im Schlaf mit langsamen EEG-Wellen. Arch. Psychiatr. Nervenkr. **207**, 141–150 (1965)
4. James, W.: Principles of psychology. New York: H. Holt 1890
5. Janet, P.: L'automatisme psychologique. 2. édit. Paris: Alcan 1894
6. Janzen, R., Kornmüller, A.E.: Hirnbioelektrische Erscheinungen bei Änderungen der Bewußtseinslage. Dtsch. Z. Nervenheilk. **149**, 74–92 (1939)

7. Janzen, R., Behnsen, G.: Beitrag zur Pathophysiologie des Anfallsgeschehens insbesondere des kataplektischen Anfalls beim Narkolepsiesyndrom: Klinische und hirnelektrische Untersuchung. Arch. Psychiatr. Nervenkr. **111**, 178–189 (1940)
8. Jasper, H.: Unspecific thalamocortical relations. In: Handbook of physiology, Section 1: Neurophysiology (eds.: J. Field, H.W. Magoun and V.E. Hall), Vol. 2, pp. 1307–1321. Washington: American Physiological Society 1960
9. Jasper, H.H.: Functional properties of the thalamic reticular system. In (J.F. Delafresnaye, ed.): Brain mechanisms and consciousness, Symposium, pp. 374–401. Oxford: Blackwell Scientific Publications 1954
10. Jasper, H.H., Droogleever-Fortuyn, J.: Experimental studies on the functional anatomy of petit mal epilepsy. Proc. Ass. Res. Nerv. Ment. Dis. **26**, 272–298 (1946)
11. Jasper, H., Ricci, G., Doane, B.: Microelectrode analysis of cortical cell discharge during avoidance conditioning in the monkey. In (H. Jasper, and G.D. Smirnov, eds.): The Moscow Colloquium on Electroencephalography of higher nervous activity. Electroencephalogr. Clin. Neurophysiol. Suppl. **13**, 137–155 (1960)
12. Jasper, H.H., Smirnov, G.D. (ed.): The Moscow Colloquium on Electroencephalography of higher nervous activity. Moskow, Okt. 1958. Electroencephalogr. Clin. Neurophysiol. Suppl. **13**, 1960
13. Jaspers, K.: Allgemeine Psychopathologie. Berlin: Springer 1913, 6. Aufl. 1953
14. John, E.R.: Mechanisms of memory. New York, London: Academic Press 1967
15. Jouvet, M.: Telencephalic and rhombencephalic sleep in the cat. In (G.E. W. Wolstenholme, and M. O'Connor, eds.): The nature of sleep, pp. 188–208. London: J. & A. Churchill Ltd. 1961
16. Jouvet, M.: Recherches sur les structures nerveuses et les mecanismes responsables des differentes phases du sommeil physiologique. Arch. Ital. Biol. **100**, 125–206 (1962)
17. Jouvet, M.: Paradoxical sleep – A study of its nature and mechanisms. In (K. Akert, C. Bally, and J.P. Schadé, eds.): Progr. Brain Res. **18**: Sleep mechanisms, 20–62. Amsterdam, London, New York: Elsevier Publ. Comp. 1965
18. Jouvet, M. (ed.): Aspects anatomofonctionels de la physiologie du sommeil. Coll. internat. CNRS Nr. 127 Centre national de la recherche scientifique Paris 1965
19. Jouvet, M.: The role of monoamines and acetylcholine containing neurons in the regulation of the sleep-waking cycle. Ergebn. Physiol. **64**, 166–307 (1972)
20. Jouvet, M., Pellin, B., Mounier, D.: Etude polygraphique des differentes phases du sommeil au cours des troubles de conscience chroniques (coma prolongés). Rev. neurol. **105**, 181–186 (1961)
21. Jovanović, U.J.: Der Schlaf. Neurophysiologische Aspekte. München: J.A. Barth 1969
22. Jovanović, U.J.: Sexuelle Reaktionen und Schlafperiodik bei Menschen. Stuttgart: F. Enke 1972
23. Judd, D.B.: Basic correlates of the visual stimulus. In (S.S. Stevens, ed.): Handbook of experimental psychology, pp. 811–867. New York, London: J. Wiley, Chapman & Hall 1951
24. Jung, C.G.: Über die Energetik der Seele. Zürich, Leipzig, Stuttgart: Rascher & Cie. 1928
25. Jung, R.: Ein Apparat zur mehrfachen Registrierung von Tätigkeit und Funktionen des animalen und vegetativen Nervensystems (Elektrencephalogramm, Elektrokardiogramm, Muskelaktionsströme, Augenbewegungen, galvanischer Hautreflex, Plethysmogramm, Liquordruck und Atmung). Z. Neurol. **165**, 374–397 (1939)
26. Jung, R.: Über vegetative Reaktionen und Hemmungswirkung von Sinnesreizen im kleinen epileptischen Anfall. Nervenarzt **12**, 169–185 (1939)
27. Jung, R.: Das Elektrencephalogramm und seine klinische Anwendung. I. u. II. Nervenarzt **12**, 559–591 (1939); **14**, 57–70, 104–117 (1941)
28. Jung, R.: Gedanken zur psychiatrischen Schockbehandlung. In (H. Kranz, Hrsg.): Arbeiten zur Psychiatrie, Neurologie und ihren Grenzgebieten, Festschrift Kurt Schneider, S. 99–120. Heidelberg: Scherer 1947
29. Jung, R.: Neurophysiologische Grundlagen der Hirnpathologie. Nervenarzt **19**, 521–524 (1948)
30. Jung, R.: Zur Klinik und Pathogenese der Depression. Zbl. ges. Neurol. Psychiat. **119**, 163 (1952)
31. Jung, R.: Allgemeine Neurophysiologie. Die Tätigkeit des Nervensystems. In (G. v. Bergmann, W. Frey, H. Schwiegk, Hrsg.): Handbuch der inneren Medizin, 4. Aufl., Bd. V/1, Neurologie I, S. 1–181. Berlin, Göttingen, Heidelberg: Springer 1953

32. Jung, R.: Das Elektrencephalogramm (EEG). In (G. v. Bergmann, W. Frey, H. Schwiegk, Hrsg.): Handbuch der inneren Medizin, 4. Aufl., Bd. V/1, Neurologie I, S. 1216–1325. Berlin, Göttingen, Heidelberg: Springer 1953
33. Jung, R.: Nystagmographie. Zur Physiologie und Pathologie des optisch-vestibulären Systems beim Menschen. In (G. v. Bergmann, W. Frey u. H. Schwiegk, Hrsg.): Handbuch der inneren Medizin, 4. Aufl., Bd. V/1, S. 1325–1379. Berlin, Göttingen, Heidelberg: Springer 1953
34. Jung, R.: Neuronal discharge. Electroencephalogr. Clin. Neurophysiol. Suppl. **4**, 57–71 (1953)
35. Jung, R.: Hirnelektrische Befunde bei Kreislaufstörungen und Hypoxieschäden des Gehirns. Verh. Dtsch. Ges. Kreislaufforsch. **19**, 170–196 (1953)
36. Jung, R.: Correlation of bioelectrical and autonomic phenomena with alterations of consciousness and arousal in man. In: Brain mechanisms and consciousness, Symposion (ed. Delafresnaye, Adrian, F. Bremer, and H.H. Jasper), pp. 310–344. Oxford: Blackwell Publ. 1954
37. Jung, R.: Tierexperimentelle Grundlagen und EEG-Untersuchungen bei Bewußtseinsveränderungen des Menschen ohne neurologische Erkrankungen. 1er Congr. Internat. des Scienc. Neurol., Bruxelles, 1957. Vol. Rapp. **2**, 148–179 (1957)
38. Jung, R.: Neuropharmakologie: Zentrale Wirkungsmechanismen chemischer Substanzen und ihre neurophysiologischen Grundlagen. Klin. Wochenschr. **36**, 1153–1167 (1958)
39. Jung, R.: Korrelationen von Neuronentätigkeit und Sehen. In (Jung, R., u. H. Kornhuber, Hrsg.): Neurophysiologie und Psychophysik des visuellen Systems, S. 410–434. Berlin, Göttingen, Heidelberg: Springer 1961
40. Jung, R.: Zusammenfassung. In: Proc. 22. Internat. Congr. Leiden, 1962: Lectures and Symposia **2**, 518–525 (Symposium XI: Optic and vestibula factors in motor coordination). Amsterdam, London, New York: Excerpta med. 1962
41. Jung, R.: Der Schlaf. In: Physiologie und Physiopathologie des vegetativen Nervensystems, Bd. 2, S. 650–684. Stuttgart: Hippokrates Verl. 1963
42. Jung, R.: Neuronale Grundlagen des Hell-Dunkelsehens und der Farbwahrnehmung. Ber. Dtsch. Ophthalmol. Ges. **66**, 69–111 (1964)
43. Jung, R.: Physiologie und Pathophysiologie des Schlafes. Verh. Dtsch. Ges. Inn. Med. **71**, 788–797 (1965)
44. Jung, R.: Kontrastsehen, Konturbetonung und Künstlerzeichnung. Stud. Gen. **24**, 1536–1565 (1971)
45. Jung, R.: Visual perception and neurophysiology. In: (R. Jung, ed.): Handbook of sensory physiology, Vol. VII/3 A, p. 1–152. Berlin, Heidelberg, New York: Springer 1973
46. Jung, R.: Neuropsychologie und Neurophysiologie des Kontur- und Formsehens in Zeichnung und Malerei. In: Psychopathologie musischer Gestaltungen (H.H. Wieck, Hrsg.), S. 29–88. Stuttgart, New York: F.K. Schattauer 1974
47. Jung, R.: Einführung in die Bewegungsphysiologie. In (Gauer, Kramer, Jung, Hrsg.), Physiologie des Menschen: Sensomotorik. Bd. 14, S. 1–97. München, Berlin, Wien: Urban & Schwarzenberg 1976
48. Jung, R.: Über Zeichnungen linkshändiger Künstler von Leonardo bis Klee: Linkshändermerkmale als Zuschreibungskriterien. In: Semper Attentus. Beiträge für Heinz Götze. S. 190–217. Berlin, Heidelberg, New York: Springer 1977
49. Jung, R.: Einführung in die Sehphysiologie. In (Gauer, Kramer, Jung, Hrsg.): Physiologie des Menschen: Sehen. Bd. 13, S. 1–140. München, Wien, Baltimore: Urban & Schwarzenberg 1978
50. Jung, R.: Translokation corticaler Migränephosphene bei Augenbewegungen und vestibularen Reizen. Neuropsychologia **17**, 173–185 (1979)
51. Jung, R.: Sensory Research in Historical Perspective: Some Philosophical Foundations of Perception. In: Handbook of sensory physiology. Sensory processes (ed. I. Darian-Smith). Washington: Amer. Physiol. Soc. 1980
52. Jung, R., Baumgarten, R. v., Baumgartner, G.: Mikroableitungen von einzelnen Neuronen im optischen Cortex der Katze. Die lichtaktivierten B-Neurone. Arch. Psychiatr. Nervenkr. **189**, 521–539 (1952)
53. Jung, R., Baumgartner, G.: Neuronenphysiologie der visuellen und paravisuellen Rindenfelder. 8. Int. Congr. Neurol. Wien Proc. **3**, 47–57 (1965)
54. Jung, R., Carmichael, E.A.: Über vasomotorische Reaktionen und Wärmeregulation im katatonen Stupor. Arch. Psychiatr. Nervenkr. **107**, 300–338 (1937)

55. Jung, R., Creutzfeldt, O., Grüsser, O.J.: Die Mikrophysiologie kortikaler Neurone und ihre Bedeutung für die Sinnes- und Hirnfunktionen. Dtsch. med. Wochenschr. **26**, 1050–1059 (1957)
56. Jung, R., Dietz, V.: Verzögerter Start der Willkürbewegung bei Pyramidenläsionen des Menschen. Arch. Psychiatr. Nervenkr. **221**, 87–109 (1975)
57. Jung, R., Dietz, V.: Übung und Seitendominanz der menschlichen Willkürmotorik: Zur Programmierung der Stoß- und Wurfbewegung im Rechts-Linksvergleich. Arch. Psychiatr. Nervenkr. **222**, 87–116 (1976)
58. Jung, R., Hassler, R.: The extrapyramidal motor system. In: Handbook of physiology, Section 1: Neurophysiology, Vol. 2, pp. 863–927 (eds.: J. Field, H.W. Magoun, and V.E. Hall). Washington: American Physiological Society 1960
59. Jung, R., Kornhuber, H.H., Da Fonseca, J.S.: Multisensory convergence cortical neurons. Neuronal effects of visual, acoustic and vestibular stimuli in the superior convolutions of the cat's cortex. In: Brain mechanisms (G. Moruzzi, A. Fessard, and H.H. Jasper, eds.). Progress in brain research, Vol. 1, pp. 207–240. Amsterdam: Elsevier 1963
60. Jung, R., Kornmüller, A.E.: Eine Methodik der Ableitung lokalisierter Potentialschwankungen aus subcorticalen Hirngebieten. Arch. Psychiatr. Nervenkr. **109**, 1–30 (1939)
61. Jung, R., Kuhlo, W.: Neurophysiological studies of abnormal night sleep and the Pickwickian syndrome. Sleep mechanisms. Progr. Brain Res. **18**, 140–159 (1965)
61a. Jung, R., Spillmann, L.: Receptive-field estimation and perceptual integration in human vision. In: Young, F.A., D.B. Lindlsey (eds.): Early Experience and Visual Information Processing in Perceptual and Reading Disorders, pp. 181–197. Nat. Acad. Sci., Washington, D.C. 1970
62. Jung, R., Tönnies, J.F.: Hirnelektrische Untersuchungen über Entstehung und Erhaltung von Krampfentladungen: Die Vorgänge am Reizort und die Bremsfähigkeit des Gehirns. Arch. Psychiatr. Nervenkr. **185**, 701–735 (1950)

K

1. Kandel, E.R.: Cellular basis of behavior. An introduction to behavioral neurobiology. San Francisco: W.H. Freeman 1976
2. Kandel, E.R., Spencer, W.A.: Hippocampal neuron responses to selective activation of recurrent collaterals of hippocampofugal axons. Exp. Neurol. **4**, 149–161 (1961)
3. Kandel, E.R., Spencer, W.A.: Excitation and inhibition of single pyramidal cells during hippocampal seizure. Exp. Neurol. **4**, 163–179 (1961)
4. Kant, I.: Critik der reinen Vernunft. 2. Aufl. (1. ed. Riga 1781). Riga: J.F. Hartknoch 1787
5. Kant, I.: Kritik der Urtheilskraft. Berlin u. Libau: Lagarde u. Friederich 1790
6. Kasamatsu, A.: Studies on the loss of consciousness induced by inhalation of nitrogen gas. Psychiatr. Neurol. Jpn. **54**, 575–606 (1952)
7. Kasamatsu, A.: An experimental study of consciousness disturbance with some thoughts on the nature of consciousness. Psychiatr. Neurol. Jpn. **54**, 744–755 (1953)
8. Katsuki, Y., Sumi, T., Uchiyama, H., Watanabe, T.: Electric responses of auditory neurons in cat to sound stimulation. J. Neurophysiol. **21**, 569–588 (1958)
9. Kawamura, H., Sawyer, C.H.: D-C potential changes in rabbit brain during slow-wave and paradoxical sleep. Am. J. Physiol. **207**, 1379–1386 (1964)
10. Kawamura, S.: The process of sub-cultural propagation among Japanese macaques. In: C.H. Southwick (ed.) Primate Social Behavior, p. 82–90. Toronto: van Norstrand 1963.
11. Keidel, W.D.: Grenzen der Übertragbarkeit der Regelungslehre auf biologische Probleme. Naturwissenschaften **48**, 264–276 (1961)
12. Keller, H.: Die Geschichte meines Lebens. 60. Aufl. Stuttgart: Robert Lutz 1925
13. Kendel, K., Beck, U., Kruschea-Dubois, H.: Die chronisch-neurasthenische Schlafstörung. Arch. Psychiatr. Nervenkr. **216**, 201–218 (1972)
14. Kety, S.S.: Blood flow and metabolism of the human brain in health and disease. Trans. Stud. Coll. Physicians Phila. **18**, 103–108 (1950)
15. Kinsey, A.C., Pomeroy, W.B., Martin, C.E.: Sexual behavior in the human male. Philadelphia, London: W.B. Saunders Comp. 1948
16. Kleine, W.: Periodische Schlafsucht. Mschr. Psychiat. Neurol. **57**, 285–320 (1925)
17. Kleist, K.: Gehirnpathologie vornehmlich aufgrund der Kriegserfahrungen. Leipzig: J.A. Barth 1934

18. Kleist, K.: Bericht über die Gehirnpathologie in ihrer Bedeutung für Neurologie und Psychiatrie. Z. ges. Neurol. Psychiat. **158**, 159–193 (1937)
19. Kleitman, N.: Nature of dreaming. In (G.E.W. Wolstenholme, and M. O'Connor, eds.): The nature of sleep. CIBA-Foundation Symposion, pp. 349–374. London: J. & A. Churchill 1961
20. Kleitman, N.: Sleep and wakefulness, 1939. Revised edit.: Chicago, London: University of Chicago Press 1963
21. Kleitman, N., Engelmann, Th.G.: Sleep characteristics of infants. J. Appl. Physiol. **6**, 269–282 (1953)
22. Kleitman, N., Kleitman, H.: The sleep-wakefulness pattern in the arctic. Sci. Month. **76**, 349–356 (1953)
23. Klüver, H.: Mechanisms of hallucinations. In: Studies in personality, pp. 175–207, Chapt. 10. USA: McGraw-Hill Book Company 1942
24. Klüver, H.: Behavior mechanisms in monkeys. 2. ed. Chicago: University Press of Chicago 1957
25. Klüver, H., Bucy, P.C.: Preliminary analysis of functions of the temporal lobes in monkeys. Arch. Neurol. Psychiat. (Chic.) **42**, 979–1000 (1939)
26. Koehler, O.: Vom unbenannten Denken. Verh. dtsch. zool. Ges. **1952**, 99–108 (1952)
27. Koehler, O.: Tierische Vorstufen menschlicher Sprache. 1. Arbeitstagg. über zentrale Regulation d. Funktionen des Organismus. Leipzig, Berlin: VEB Verlag Volk u. Gesundheit 1955
28. Koehler, O.: Die Beziehung Mensch-Tier. Verh. Schweiz. naturforsch. Ges. **1960**, 44–47 (1960)
29. Köhler, W.: Intelligenzprüfungen an Anthropoiden. I. Abhandl. kgl. preuß. Akad. Wiss. 1917, physik.-math. Kl. Nr. 1, 1–223. Berlin: Akademie u. G. Reimer 1917
30. Köhler, W.: The mentality of apes. London: Kegan Paul, Trench, Trubner & Co. 1927
31. Köhler, W.: Ein altes Scheinproblem. Naturwissenschaften **17**, 395–401 (1929)
32. Köhler, W.: Gestaltpsychology today. Am. Psychologist **14**, 727–734 (1959)
33. Koella, W.P.: Sleep: Its nature and physiological organization. Springfield, Ill.: C.C. Thomas 1967
34. Koella, W.P., Levin, P. (eds.): Sleep. Physiology, Biochemistry, Psychology, Pharmacology, Clinical Implications. Proc. I. Europ. Congr. Sleep Res. Basel: S. Karger 1973
35. Kohnstamm, O., Quensel, F.: Centrum receptorium der Formatio reticularis und gekreuzt aufsteigende Bahn. Dtsch. Z. Nervenheilk. **35**, 182–188 (1908)
35a. Kohts, N.: A contribution to the problem of "Labour Processes" of monkeys. Moskau: Izdanje gozudarstwennowo darwinowskowo musei 1928
35b. Kohts, N.: Infant ape and human child (instincts, emotions, play, habits). Moscou 1935, 2 vols., 596 pages
36. Konorski, J.: Conditioned reflexes and neuron organization. Cambridge: Univ. Press 1948
37. Konorski, J.: The cortical "representation" of unconditioned reflexes. Electroencephalogr. Clin. Neurophysiol. Suppl. **13**, 81–89 (1960)
38. Kornhuber, H.H.: Zur Situationsabhängigkeit von Bedürfnissen und Neurosen nach Erfahrung in Gefangenenlagern. In (H. Kranz, Hrsg.): Psychopathologie heute. Prof. Dr. Kurt Schneider zum 75. Geburtstag gewidmet, S. 252–257. Stuttgart: Georg Thieme 1962
39. Kornhuber, H.H.: Optisch-vestibuläre und somatisch-vestibuläre Integration an Neuronen der Großhirnrinde: Ein Beitrag zur multimodalen Koordination der Sinnesafferenzen. Freiburg: Habilitationsschrift 1962
40. Kornhuber, H.H.: Zur Funktion der Lust. Antrittsvorlesung 1963, persönl. Mitteilung
41. Kornhuber, H.H.: Motor functions of cerebellum and basal ganglia: the cerebellocortical saccadic (ballistic) clock, the cerebellonuclear hold regulator, and the basal ganglia ramp (voluntary speed smooth movement generator). Kybernetik **8**, 157–161 (1971)
42. Kornhuber, H.H.: Neural control of input into long term memory: limbic system and amnestic syndrome in man. In: Memory and transfer of information. Zippel, H.P. (ed.), pp. 1–22. New York: Plenum Press 1973
42a. Kornhuber, H.H.: A reconsideration of the brain-mind problem. In: Cerebral correlates of conscious experience (P.A. Buser and A. Rougeul-Buser, ed.). 6, pp. 319–334. Amsterdam, New York, Oxford: North-Holland Publishing Comp. 1978
43. Kornhuber, H.H., Deecke, L.: Hirnpotentialänderungen bei Willkürbewegungen und passiven Bewegungen des Menschen: Bereitschaftspotential und reafferente Potentiale. Pfluegers Arch. **284**, 1–17 (1965)

44. Kornhuber, H.H., Fonseca, J.S. da: Optovestibular integration in the cat's cortex: a study of sensory convergence on cortical neurons. In (M.B. Bender, ed.): The oculomotor system, pp. 239–279. New York, Evanston, London: Hoeber Medical Division, Harper & Row, Publ. 1964
45. Kornmüller, A.E., Palme, F., Strughold, H.: Über Veränderungen der Gehirnaktionsströme im akuten Sauerstoffmangel, Luftfahrtmed. **5**, 161–183 (1941)
46. Kraepelin, E.: Psychologische Arbeiten, Bd. 1–9. Leipzig: W. Engelmann 1896–1927
47. Kraines, S.H.: Mental depressions and their treatment. New York: MacMillan Company 1957
48. Kretschmer, E.: Körperbau und Charakter. Untersuchungen zum Konstitutions-Problem zur Lehre von den Temperamenten. Berlin: Springer 1942
49. Kretschmer, E.: Der Begriff der motorischen Schablonen und ihre Rolle in normalen und pathologischen Lebensvorgängen. Arch. Psychiatr. Nervenkr. **190**, 1–3 (1953)
50. Kries, J. v.: Normale und anomale Farbensysteme. Die Theorien des Licht- und Farbensinns. Zusätze zu v. Helmholtz Hdb. der physiol. Optik, 3. Aufl. II, S. 333–378. Hamburg, Leipzig: L. Voss 1911
51. Kries, J. v.: Allgemeine Sinnesphysiologie. Leipzig: F.C.W. Vogel 1923
52. Kries, J. v.: Immanuel Kant und seine Bedeutung für die Naturforschung der Gegenwart. Berlin: J. Springer 1924
53. Kubie, L.S.: The neurotic process as the focus of physiological and psychoanalytic research. J. Ment. Sci. **104**, 518–536 (1958)
54. Kubie, L.S.: The relation of the conditioned reflex to preconscious functions. Trans. Am. Neurol. Ass. **84**, 187–188 (1959)
55. Kühn, H.: Über das Verhältnis der vitalen zu den höheren Persönlichkeitsschichten bei den psychopathischen Formen. Arch. Psychiatr. Nervenkr. **116**, 229–262 (1943)
56. Külpe, O.: Über die Objektivierung und Subjektivierung von Sinneseindrücken. Wundt's philos. Stud. **19**, 508–556 (1902)
57. Küpfmüller, K.: Nachrichtenverarbeitung im Menschen. In (K. Steinbuch, Hrsg.): Taschenbuch der Nachrichtenverarbeitung, S. 1481–1502, Berlin, Göttingen, Heidelberg: Springer 1962
58. Küpfmüller, K.: Grundlagen der Informationstheorie und der Kybernetik. In (Gauer, Kramer, Jung, Hrsg.): Physiologie des Menschen, Bd. 10. Allgemeine Neurophysiologie, S. 195–231. München, Berlin, Wien: Urban & Schwarzenberg 1971
59. Küppers, E.: Der Grundplan des Nervensystems und die Lokalisation des Psychischen. Z. ees. Neurol. Psychiat. **75**, 11–46 (1922)
60. Küppers, E.: Die Grundbegriffe der Psychophysiologie. Schweiz. Arch. Neurol. Neurochir. Psychiatr. **85**, 284–309 (1960)
61. Kuffler, S.: Discharge patterns and functional organization of mammalian retina. J. Neurophysiol. **16**, 37–68 (1953)
62. Kuhlo, W.: Neurophysiologische und klinische Untersuchungen beim Pickwick-Syndrom. Arch. Psychiat. Nervenkr. **211**, 170–192 (1968)
63. Kuhlo, W., Lehmann, D.: Das Einschlaferleben und seine neurophysiologischen Korrelate. Arch. Psychiatr. Nervenkr. **205**, 687–716 (1964)
64. Kummer, H.: Soziales Verhalten einer Mantelpaviangruppe. Beiheft z. Schweiz. Z. Psychol. Bern, Stuttgart: Hans Huber 1957

L

1. Lange, J.: Grundsätzliche Erörterungen zu Kleists hirnpathologischen Lehren. Z. ges. Neurol. Psychiat. **158**, 247–251 (1937)
2. Lashley, K.S.: Brain mechanisms and intelligence. Chicago: Univ. of Chicago Press 1929
3. Lashley, K.S.: Mass action in cerebral function. Science **73**, 245–254 (1931)
4. Lashley, K.S.: Experimental analysis of instinctive behaviour. Psychol. Rev. **45**, 445–471 (1938)
5. Lashley, K.S.: Dynamic process in perception. In (J.F. Delafresnaye, ed.): Brain mechanisms and consciousness, Symposium, pp. 422–469. Oxford: Blackwell Scientific Publications 1954
6. Legendre, R., Piéron, H.: Recherches sur le besoin de sommeil consécutif à une veille prolongée. Z. Allg. Physiol. **14**, 235–262 (1913)
7. Lehmann, A.: Die physischen Äquivalente der Bewußtseinserscheinungen. Leipzig: O.R. Reisland 1901

8. Lehmann, A.: Grundzüge der Psychophysiologie. Leipzig: O.R. Reisland 1912
9. Lehmann, H.J.: Präparoxysmale Weckreaktion bei pyknoleptischen Absencen. Arch. Psychiatr. Nervenkr. **204**, 417–426 (1963)
10. Lehrman, D.S.: A critique of Konrad Lorenz's theory of instinctive behavior. Q. Rev. Biol. **28**, 337–363 (1953)
11. Leibniz, (G.W.): Explication de l'aritmétique binaire, qui se sert des seuls cáractères 0 et 1. ... In: Histoire de l'Academie Royale des Sciences. Anneé 1703, pp. 85–89. Paris: Jean Boudot 1705
12. Lemere, F.: The significance of individual differences in the Berger rhythm. Brain **59**, 366–375 (1936)
13. Lennox, W.G., Gibbs, F.A., Gibbs, E.L.: Effect on the electroencephalogram of drugs and conditions which influence seizures. Arch. Neurol. Psychiat. (Chic.) **36**, 1236–1245 (1936)
14. Leonhard, K.: Die Bedeutung optisch-räumlicher Vorstellungen für das elementare Rechnen. Z. ges. Neurol. Psychiat. **164**, 321–351 (1939)
15. Levin, M.: Periodic somnolence and morbid hunger: A new syndrome. Brain **59**, 494–504 (1936)
15a. Lewin, K.: Vorsatz, Wille und Bedürfnis. Mit Vorbemerkungen über die psychischen Kräfte und die Struktur der Seele. Berlin: Springer 1926
16. Lewin, K.: Der Richtungsbegriff in der Psychologie: der spezielle und allgemeine hodologische Raum. Psychol. Forsch. **19**, 249–299 (1934)
17. Lewin, K.: A dynamic theory of personality. New York, London: McGraw-Hill 1936
18. Lewin, K.: Principles of topological psychology. New York: McGraw-Hill 1936
19. Lewis, H.E.: Sleep patterns on polar expeditions. In (G.E.W. Wolstenholme, and M. O'Connor, eds.): The nature of sleep. CIBA-Foundation Symposion, 322–328. London: J. & A. Churchill 1961
20. Liberson, W.T., Akert, K.: Hippocampal seizure states in guinea pig. Electroencephalogr. Clin. Neurophysiol. (Can.) **7**, 211 (1955)
21. Libet, B., Alberts, W.W., Wright, E.W., Delattre, L.D., Levin, G., Feinstein, B.: Production of threshold levels of conscious sensation by electrical stimulation of human somatosensory cortex. J. Neurophysiol. **27**, 546–578 (1964)
22. Liddell, H.S.: Conditioned reflex methods and experimental neurosis. In: Hunt, J. McV. (ed.). Personality and behavior disorders. New York: Ronald 1944
23. Liebig, J. v.: Über Bacon und die Methode der Naturforschung. 1863. Induction und Deduction, 1865. In: Reden und Abhandlungen, S. 220–254, 296–309. Leipzig und Heidelberg 1874
24. Lilly, J.C.: Learning motivated by subcortical stimulation. The Start and the Stop patterns of behavior. In: Reticular Formation of the Brain. Intern. Symposium (Henry-Ford-Hospital, Detroit), pp. 705–727. Boston, Mass.: Little, Brown & Comp. 1958
25. Lilly, J.C., Miller, A.M.: Operant conditioning of the bottlenose dolphin with electrical stimulation of the brain. J. Comp. Physiol. Psychol. **55**, 73–79 (1962)
26. Lindauer, M.: Orientierung der Tiere in Raum und Zeit. Rev. Physiol. Biochem. Pharmacol. **85**, 1–62 (1979)
27. Lindsley, D.B.: Attention, consciousness, sleep and wakefulness. In (J. Field, H.W. Magoun, and V.E. Hall, eds.): Handbook of physiology, Section 1: Neurophysiology, Vol. 3, pp. 1553–1593. Washington, D.C.: Amer. Physiol. Soc. 1960
28. Lindsley, D.B., Bowden, J.W., Magoun, H.W.: Effect upon the EEG of acute injury to the brain stem activating system. Electroencephalogr. Clin. Neurophysiol. **1**, 475–486 (1949)
29. Lindsley, D.B., Schreiner, L.H., Knowles, W.B., Magoun, H.W.: Behavioral and EEG changes following chronic brain stem lesions in the cat. Electroencephalogr. Clin. Neurophysiol. **2**, 483–498 (1950)
29a. Lissák, K., Endröczi, E.: Die neuroendokrine Steuerung der Adaptationstätigkeit. Budapest: Verlag der ungarischen Akademie der Wissenschaften 1960
30. Lissák, K., Grastyan, E., Csanaky, A., Kéresi, F., Vereby, Gy.: A study of hippocampal function in the waking and sleeping animal with chronically implanted electrodes. Acta Physiol. Pharmacol. Neerl. **6**, 451–459 (1957)
31. Litt, Th.: Mensch und Welt. Grundlinien einer Philosophie. München: I. & S. Federmann 1948

32. Loeb, J.: Forced movements, tropisms and animal conduct. Philadelphia, London: J.B. Lippincott Comp. 1918
33. Loomis, A.L., Harvey, E.N., Hobart, G.: Electrical potentials of the human brain. J. Exp. Psychol. **19**, 249–279 (1936)
34. Loomis, A.L., Harvey, E.N., Hobart, G.A.: Cerebral states during sleep as studied by human brain potentials. J. Exp. Psychol. **21**, 127–144 (1937)
35. Loomis, A.L., Harvey, E.N., Hobart, G.A., III: Distribution of disturbance-patterns in the human electroencephalogram, with special reference to sleep. J. Neurophysiol. **1**, 413–430 (1938)
36. Lorenz, K.: Der Kumpan in der Umwelt des Vogels. J. Ornithol. **83**, 137–213 (1935)
37. Lorenz, K.: Über die Bildung des Instinktbegriffes. Naturwissenschaften **25**, 289–300, 307–318, 324–331 (1937)
38. Lorenz, K.: Die angeborenen Formen möglicher Erfahrung. Z. Tierpsychol. **5**, 235–409 (1943)
39. Lorenz, K.: The comparative method in studying innate behavior patterns. Symp. Soc. Exp. Biol. **4**. New York: Academic Press 1950
40. Lorenz, K.: Die Entwicklung der vergleichenden Verhaltensforschung in den letzten 12 Jahren. Zool. Anz. Suppl. **17**, 36–58 (1953)
41. Lorenz, K.: Methods of approach to the problems of behavior. Harvey Lect. **54**, 60–103 (1958/59)
42. Lorenz, K.: Das sogenannte Böse. Zur Naturgeschichte der Aggression. Wien: Borotha-Schoeler 1963
43. Lotze, R.H.: Medicinische Psychologie (Physiologie der Seele). Leipzig: Weidmann'sche Buchhandlung 1852
44. Lynch, J.C., Mountcastle, V.B., Talbot, W.H., Yin, T.C.T.: Parietal lobe mechanisms for directed visual attention. J. Neurophysiol. **40**, 362–389 (1977)

M

1. Mach, E.: Über die Wirkung der räumlichen Verteilung des Lichtreizes auf die Netzhaut. 1. Sitzber. Akad. Wiss. Wien, math.-nat. Classe, **52/2**, 303–322 (1865)
2. Mach, E.: Die Analyse der Empfindungen und das Verhältnis des Physischen zum Psychischen. 2. Aufl. Jena: Gustav Fischer 1900
3. MacKay, D.M.: Towards an information-flow model of human behaviour. Br. J. Psychol. **47**, 30–43 (1965)
4. MacKay, D.M.: The science of communication. – A bridge between disciplines. Inaug.-Lect. Keele, University of North Staffordshire 1961
5. MacKay, D.M.: Psychophysics of perceived intensity: A theoretical basis for Fechner's and Steven's laws. Science **139**, 1213–1216 (1963)
6. MacKay, D.M.: Perception and brain function. In: (Schmitt, F.O., et al., eds.): The neurosciences, second study programme, pp. 303–316. New York: Rockefeller University Press 1970
7. MacKay, D.M.: Visual stability and voluntary eye movements. In: Handbook of sensory, VII/3 Physiology, pp. 307–331. Edit. R. Jung. Berlin, Heidelberg, New York: Springer 1973
8. MacKay, D.M., McCulloch, W.S.: The limiting information capacity of a neuronal link. Bull. math. Biophys. **14**, 127–135 (1952)
8a. MacLean, P.D.: Some psychiatric implications of physiological studies on fronto-temporal portion of limbic system (visceral brain). Electroencephalogr. Clin. Neurophysiol. **4**, 407–418 (1952)
9. MacLean, P.D. Some psychiatric implications of physiological studies on frontotemporal portion of limbic system (visceral brain). J. Neurosurg. **11**, 29–44 (1954)
10. MacLean, P.D.: The limbic system ("visceral brain") in relation to central gray and reticulum of the brain stem. Evidence of interdependence in emotional processes. Psychosom. Med. **17**, 355–366 (1955)
11. MacLean, P.D.: Chemical and electrical stimulation of hippocampus in unrestrained animals. Part II: Behavioral findings. Arch. Neurol. Psychiat. (Chic.) **78**, 128–142 (1957)
12. MacLean, P.D.: The limbic system with respect to self-preservation and the preservation of the species. J. Nerv. Ment. Dis. **127**, 1–11 (1958)
13. MacLean, P.D.: Contrasting functions of limbic and neocortical system of the brain and their relevance to psycho-physiological aspects of medicine. Am. J. Med. **25**, 611–626 (1958)

14. MacLean, P.D.: Psychosomatics. In (eds. J. Field, H.W. Magoun, V.E. Hall): Handbook of physiology, Section 1: Neurophysiology, Vol. 3, pp. 1723–1744. Washington, D.C.: American Physiological Society 1960
15. MacLean, P.D., Ploog, D.W.: Cerebral representation of penile erection. J. Neurophysiol. **25**, 29–55 (1962)
16. Magnes, J., Moruzzi, G., Pompeiano, O.: Electroencephalogram-synchronizing structures in the lower brain stem. In (G.E.W. Wolstenholme and M. O'Connor, ed.): The nature of sleep, pp. 57–85. London: Churchill 1961
17. Magnus, R.: Körperstellung. Berlin: J. Springer 1924
18. Magoun, H.W.: The ascending reticular system and wakefulness. In (eds. E. Adrian, F. Bremer, H. Jasper, and consciousness, pp. 1–20. Oxford: Blackwell 1954
19. Magoun, H.S.: The waking brain. 2. Aufl. Springfield, Ill.: Charles Thomas; Oxford: Blackwell Scientific Publications Ltd. 1963
20. Magoun, H.W., Rhines, R.: Spasticity: The stretch reflex and extrapyramidal systems. Springfield: Thomas 1947
21. Mahl, G.F., Rothenberg, A., Delgado, J.M.R., Hamlin, H.: Psychological responses in the human to intracerebral electrical stimulation. Psychosom. Med. **26**, 337–368 (1964)
22. Mangold, R., Sokoloff, L., Conner, E., Kleinerman, J., Therman, P.O., Kety, S.S.: The effects of sleep and lack of sleep on the cerebral circulation and metabolism of normal young men. J. Clin. Invest. **34**, 1092–1100 (1955)
22a. Marey, E.-J.: La machine animale. Locomotion terrestre et aérienne. Paris: Germer Baillière 1873
22b. Marey, E.-J.: Le mouvement. Paris: G. Masson 1894
23. Martin, J.P.: Fits of laughter (Sham mirth) in organic cerebral disease. Brain **73**, 453–464 (1950)
24. Masserman, J.H.: Behavior and neurosis. Chicago: University of Chicago Press 1943
25. Masserman, J.H.: Principles of dynamic psychiatry. Philadelphia: W.B. Saunders 1946
26. Masserman, J.H.: Biological Psychiatry. New York: Grune & Stratton 1959
27. Maury, A.: De certains faits observés dans les rêves et dans l'état intermédiaire entre le sommeil et la veille. Ann. méd. psychol. **3**, 157–163 (1857)
28. Maury, L.F.A.: Le sommeil et les rêves. Étude psychologiques sur ces phénomènes. 3. Aufl. Paris: Didier 1865
29. Mayer-Gross, W.: Einschlafdenken und Symptome der Bewußtseinsstörung. Zbl. ges. Neurol. Psychiat. **44**, 552 (1926)
30. Mayer-Gross, W.: Zur Struktur des Einschlaferlebens. Zbl. ges. Neurol. Psychiat. **51**, 246 (1929)
31. Mayer-Gross, W., Stein, J.: Allgemeine Symptomatologie. Pathologie der Wahrnehmung. In (O. Bumke, Hrsg.): Handbuch der Geisteskrankheiten. Allgemeiner Teil I, S. 351–507. Berlin: Springer 1928
32. McCulloch, W.S.: Physiological processes underlying psychoneuroses. Proc. R. Soc. Med. **42**, 71–84 (1949)
33. McCulloch, W.S.: Finality and form. Springfield, Ill.: Ch.C. Thomas 1952
34. McCulloch, W.S., Duchane, E.M., Gesteland, R.C., Lettvin, J.Y., Pitts, W.H., Wall, P.D.: Neurophysiology. A. Stable, reliable and flexible nets of unreliable formal neurons. (A revised and expanded version of "Three of von Neumanns's Biological Questions".) Quart. Prog. Rep. Oct. **15**, 118–129 (1957)
35. McCulloch, W.S., Pfeiffer, J.: Of digital computers called brains. Sci. Monthly **69**, 368–376 (1949)
36. McCulloch, W.S., Pitts, W.: The statistical organization of nervous activity. J. Am. stat. Ass. **4**, 91–99 (1948)
37. McDougal, W.: An outline of abnormal psychology. London: Methuen & Co. Deutsche Übersetzung: Psychopathologie funktioneller Störungen. Leipzig: Joh. Ambr. Barth 1931
37a. Melvill Jones, G., Watt, D.G.D.: Observations on the control of stepping and hopping movements in man. J. Physiol. (Lond.) **219**, 709–727 (1971)
37b. Melvill Jones, G., Watt, D.G.D.: Muscular control of landing from unexpected falls in man. J. Physiol. (Lond.) **219**, 729–737 (1971)
38. Metzger, W.: Gesetze des Sehens. Frankfurt (Main): W. Kramer & Co. 1936.

39. Metzger, W.: Aporien der Psychophysik. In (R. Jung, u. H. Kornhuber, Hrsg.): Neurophysiologie und Psychophysik des visuellen Systems, Symposion, S. 435–444. Berlin, Göttingen, Heidelberg: Springer 1961
39a. Meyer, A.: Epilepsy, Neuropathology. London: E. Arnold Ltd. 1958
40. Meyer, J.E.: Der Bewußtseinszustand bei optischen Sinnestäuschungen. Arch. Psychiatr. Nervenkr. **189**, 477–502 (1952)
41. Meyer-Eppler, W.: Grundlagen und Anwendungen der Informationstheorie. In (W. Meyer-Eppler, Hrsg.): Kommunikation und Kybernetik in Einzeldarstellungen), Bd. I. Berlin, Göttingen, Heidelberg: Springer 1959
42. Miller, V.G.: Learnable drives and rewards. In (S.S. Stevens, ed.): Handbook of experimental psychology. New York: Wiley 1951
43. Milner, B.: Amnesia following operation on the temporal lobes. In: Amnesia, ed. by C.W.M. Whitty and O.L. Zangwill, pp. 109–133. London: Butterworths 1966
44. Milner, B.: Memory and the medial temporal regions of the brain. In: Biology of memory, ed. by K.H. Pribram and D.E. Broadbent, pp. 29–50. New York, London: Academic Press 1970
45. Milner, B.: Disorders of learning and memory after temporal-lobe lesions in man. Clin. Neurosurgery **19**, 421–446 (1972)
46. Milner, P.M.: Note on a possible correspondence between the scotomas of migraine and spreading depression of Leao. Electroencephalogr. Clin. Neurophysiol. **10**, 705–707 (1958)
47. Mishkin, M., Pribram, K.H.: Analysis of the effects of frontal lesions in monkeys: I. Variations of delayed alterations. II. Variations of delayed response. J. Comp. Physiol. Psychol. **48**, 492–495 (1955); **49**, 36–40 (1956)
48. Mittelstaedt, H.: Die Regelungstheorie als methodisches Werkzeug der Verhaltensanalyse. Naturwissenschaften **48**, 246–254 (1961)
49. Mittelstaedt, H.: Bikomponenten-Theorie der Orientierung. Erg. Biol. **26**, 253–258 (1963)
50. Monakow, C. von: Die Lokalisation im Großhirn und der Abbau der Funktion durch kortikale Herde. Wiesbaden: Bergmann 1914
51. Monakow, C. v., Mourgue, R.: Biologische Einführung in das Studium der Neurologie und Psychopathologie. Stuttgart, Leipzig: Hippocrates 1930
52. Monnier, M.: Mesure de la durée d'un processus d'integration corticale: temps d'intégration opto-motrice chez l'homme. Helv. Physiol. Pharmacol. Acta **7**, C 52–53 (1949)
53. Monnier, M.: Moderating brain stem systems inducing synchronization of the neocortex and sleep. Electroencephalogr. Clin. Neurophysiol. **14**, 426 (1962)
54. Moreau, J.: Du Hachisch et de l'aliénation mentale. Études psychologiques. Paris: Fortin, Masson 1845
55. Morgan, C.T., Stellar, E.: Physiological psychology (Revised ed.). New York: McGraw-Hill 1950
56. Morison, R.S., Dempsey, E.W.: A study of thalamocortical relations. Am. J. Physiol. **135**, 281–292 (1942)
57. Morrell, F.: Microelectrode and steady potential studies suggesting a dendritic locus of closure. In (H.H. Jasper, and G.D. Smirnov, eds.): The Moscow Colloquium on electroencephalography of higher nervous activity. Electroencephalogr. Clin. Neurophysiol. **13**, 65–79 (1960)
58. Morrell, F.: Microelectrode studies in chronic epileptic foci. In: Symposion on basic mechanisms of the epileptic discharge. Ann. Meet. of the Amer. Electroencephalographic Society, Cape Cod, 1960. Epilepsia **2**, 81–88 (1961)
59. Morrell, F.: Electrophysiological contributions to the neural basis of learning. Physiol. Rev. **41**, 443–494 (1961)
60. Morrell, F.: Lasting changes in synaptic organization produced by continuous neuronal bombardement. In (J.F. Delafresnaye, ed.): Brain mechanisms and learning, pp. 375–392. Oxford: Blackwell Scientific Publications 1961
61. Morris, G.O., Williams, H.L., Lubin, A.: Misperception and disorientation during sleep deprivation. Arch. Psychiatr. (Chic.) **2**, 247–254 (1960)
61a. Moruzzi, G.: Problems in cerebellar physiology. Springfield, Ill.: Ch.C. Thomas 1950
62. Moruzzi, G.: The physiological properties of the brain stem reticular system. In (eds. E. Adrian, F. Bremer, H. Jasper, and J.F. Delafresnaye): Brain mechanisms and consciousness, pp. 21–53. Oxford: Blackwell 1954

63. Moruzzi, G.: The functional significance of the ascending reticular system. Arch. Ital. Biol. **96**, 17–28 (1958)
64. Moruzzi, G.: Active processes in the brain stem during sleep. Harvey Lect. **58**, 233–297 (1963)
65. Moruzzi, G.: The sleep-waking cycle. Ergebn. Physiol. **64**, 1–165 (1972)
66. Moruzzi, G., Magoun, H.W.: Brain stem reticular formation and activation of the EEG. Electroencephalogr. Clin. Neurophysiol. **1**, 455–473 (1949)
67. Mosowitch, A., Tallaferro, A.: Studies on EEG and sex function orgasm. Dis. Nerv. Syst. **15**, 218–222 (1954)
68. Mosso, A.: Die Furcht. Leipzig: S. Hirzel 1889
68a. Mosso, A.: Die Ermüdung. Leipzig: S. Hirzel 1892
69. Motokawa, K.: Electroencephalograms of man in the generalization and differentiation of conditioned reflexes. Tohoku J. Exp. Med. **50**, 225–234 (1949)
70. Mountcastle, V.B.: Modality and topographic properties of single neurons of cat's somatic sensory cortex. J. Neurophysiol. **20**, 408–434 (1957)
71. Mountcastle, V.B.: Some functional properties of the somatic afferent system. In (W.A. Rosenblith, ed.): Sensory communication, p. 403. New York, London: M.I.T. Press, John Wiley & Sons 1961
72. Mountcastle, V.B. (edit.): Interhemispheric relations and cerebral dominance. Baltimore: Johns Hopkins Press 1962
73. Mountcastle, V.B.: Some neural mechanisms for directed attention. In: Buser [B 76], pp. 37–51 (1978)
74. Mountcastle, V.B.: An organizing principle for cerebral function: The unit module and the distributed system. In: The mindful brain, edit. by M. Edelman, V.B. Mountcastle, and O. Schmitt, pp. 7–50. Cambridge, Mass.: M.I.T. Press 1978
75. Mountcastle, V.B., Lynch, J.C., Georgopopolous, A., Sakata, H., Acuna, C.: Posterior parietal association cortex of the monkey: Command functions for operation within extrapersonal space. J. Neurophysiol. **38**, 871–908 (1975)
76. Mountcastle, V.B., Powell, T.P.S.: Neural mechanisms subserving cutaneous sensibility, with special reference to the role of afferent inhibition in sensory perception and discrimination. Bull. Johns Hopk. Hosp. **105**, 201–232 (1959)
77. Müller, G.E.: Die Gesichtspunkte und die Tatsachen der psychophysischen Methodik. Ergebn. Physiol. **2, II**, 267–516 (1903)
78. Müller, G.E.: Zur Analyse der Gedächtnistätigkeit und des Vorstellungsverlaufes. 3. Bände, Z. Psychol. Ergänzungsbände. Leipzig: J.A. Barth 1911–1917
79. Müller, G.E.: Über das Aubertsche Phänomen. Z. Sinnesphysiol. **49**, 109–246 (1916)
80. Müller, G.E.: Darstellung und Erklärung der verschiedenen Typen der Farbenblindheit. Göttingen: Vandenhoeck und Ruprecht 1924
81. Müller, J.: Über die phantastischen Gesichtserscheinungen. Coblenz: Jacob Hölscher 1826
82. Müller, J.: Zur vergleichenden Physiologie des Gesichtssinnes des Menschen und der Thiere, nebst einem Versuch über die Bewegungen der Augen und über den menschlichen Blick. Leipzig: Knobloch 1826
83. Müller-Limmroth, W.: Elektrophysiologie des Gesichtssinns. Berlin, Göttingen, Heidelberg: Springer 1959
84. Mullan, S., Penfield, W.: Illusions of comparative interpretation and emotion. Arch. Neurol. Psychiat. (Chic.) **81**, 269–284 (1959)
85. Muses, C.A., McCulloch, W.S. (eds.): Aspect of the theory of artificial intelligence. New York: Plenum Press 1963
86. Myers, R.E.: Interocular transfer of pattern discrimination in cats following section of crossed optic fibers. J. Comp. Physiol. Psychol. **48**, 470–473 (1955)
87. Myers, R.E.: Function of corpus callosum in interocular transfer. Brain **79**, 358–363 (1956)
88. Myers, R.E.: Interhemispheric communication through corpus callosum: Limitations under conditions of conflict. J. Comp. Physiol. Psychol. **52**, 6–9 (1959)
89. Myers, R.E.: Localization of function in the corpus callosum. Arch. Neurol. (Chic.) **1**, 74–77 (1959)
90. Myers, R.E.: Transmission of visual information within and between the hemispheres: a behavioral study. In (V.B. Mountcastle, ed.): Interhemispheric relations and cerebral dominance, pp. 51–73. Baltimore: Johns Hopkins 1962

91. Myers, R.E.: Discussion. In (V.B. Mountcastle, ed.): Interhemispheric relations and cerebral dominance, pp. 117–129. Baltimore: Johns Hopkins 1962
92. Myers, R.E., Sperry, R.W.: Interhemispheric communication through the corpus callosum: Mnemonic carryover between the hemispheres. Arch. Neurol. Psychiat. (Chic.) **80**, 298–303 (1958)

N

1. Neumann, J.v.: Die Rechenmaschine und das Gehirn. München: Oldenbourg 1960

O

1. Ohlmeyer, P., Brilmayer, H.: Periodische Vorgänge im Schlaf. II. Mitteilung. Pfluegers Arch. **249**, 50–55 (1947)
2. Ohlmeyer, P., Brilmayer, H., Hülstrung, H.: Periodische Vorgänge im Schlaf. Pfluegers Arch. **248**, 559–560 (1944)
3. Olds, J.: Pleasure centers in the brain. Sci. Am. **195**, 105–114 (1956)
4. Olds, J.: Selective effects of drives and drugs on "reward" systems of the brain. In (Wolstenholme, G.E.W., and Cecilia M. O'Connor, ed.): Neurological basis of behavior. London: J. & A. Churchill Ltd. 1958
5. Olds, J.: Self-stimulation of the brain. Its use to study local effects of hunger, sex and drugs. Science **127**, 315–324 (1958)
6. Olds, J.: Hypothalamic substrates of reward. Physiol. Rev. **42**, 554–604 (1962)
7. Olds, J.: Mechanisms of instrumental conditioning. In (R. Hernández-Peón, eds.): The physiological basis of mental activity, Symposion in Mexico City, 1961. Electroencephalogr. Clin. Neurophysiol. **24**, 219–234 (1963)
8. Olds, J., Milner, P.: Positive reinforcement produced by electrical stimulation of the septal area and other regions of the rat brain. J. Comp. Physiol. Psychol. **47**, 419–427 (1954)
9. Oppelt, W.: Der Automat – das Denkmodell des Ingenieurs für menschliches Verhalten. Elektrotechn. Z. **99**, 105–108, 152–155, 206–210 (1979)
10. Orbach, J., Milner, B., Rasmussen, T.: Learning and retention in monkeys after amygdala-hippocampus resection. Arch. Neurol. (Chic.) **3**, 230–251 (1960)
11. Ostow, M.: A psychoanalytic contribution to the study of brain function. II. The temporal lobes. III. Synthesis. Psychoanal. Quart. **24**, 383 (1955)
12. Oswald, I.: Sleeping and waking. Physiology and psychology. Amsterdam, New York: Elsevier Publishing Comp. 1962
13. Oswald, I.: Some psychophysiological features of human sleep. In (K. Akert, C. Bally, and J.P. Schadé, eds.): Progress in brain research, Vol. 18, Sleep mechanisms, pp. 160–169. Amsterdam, London, New York: Elsevier 1965
14. Oswald, I., Berger, R.J., Jaramillo, R.A., Keddie, K.M.G., Olley, P.C., Plunkett, G.B.: Melancholia and barbiturates: a controlled EEG body and eye-movement study of sleep. Brit. J. Psychiat. **109**, 66–78 (1963)

P

1. Papez, J.W.: A proposed mechanism of emotion. Arch. Neurol. Psychiat. (Chic.) **38**, 725–743 (1937)
2. Parmeggiani, P.L.: Schlafverhalten bei elektrischer Reizung von Hippocampus und Corpus mammillare der nichtnarkotisierten freibeweglichen Katze. Helv. Physiol. Pharmacol. Acta **17**, C34 (1959)
3. Parmeggiani, P.L.: Reizeffekte aus Hippocampus und Corpus mammillare der Katze. Helv. Physiol. Pharmacol. Acta **18**, 523–536 (1960)
4. Passouant, P.: Influence de l'âge sur l'organisation du sommeil de nuit et la période de sommeil avec mouvements oculaires. J. Psychol. norm. path. **1964**, 257–279 (1964)
5. Pawlow, I.P.: Die höchste Nerventätigkeit (das Verhalten) von Tieren. München: J.F. Bergmann 1926
6. Pavlov, I.P.: Lectures on conditioned reflexes. Trans. by W.H. Gantt. New York: International Publ. Co. 1928
7. Pawlow, I.P.: Sämtliche Werke, I–VI. Berlin: Akademie-Verlag 1954

8. Penfield, W.: The cerebral cortex in man. I. The cerebral cortex in consciousness. Arch. Neurol. Psychiat. (Chic.) **40**, 417–442 (1938)
9. Penfield, W.: Memory mechanisms. Arch. Neurol. Psychiat. (Chic.) **67**, 178–191 (1952)
10. Penfield, W.: Studies of the cerebral cortex of man. A review and an interpretation. In (J.F. Delafresnaye, ed.): Brain mechanism and consciousness, Symposium, pp. 283–309. Oxford: Blackwell Scientific Publications 1954
11. Penfield, W.: Mechanisms of voluntary movement. Brain **77**, 1–17 (1954)
12. Penfield, W.: The role of the temporal cortex in certain psychical phenomena. J. Ment. Sci. **101**, 451–465 (1955)
13. Penfield, W.: The rôle of the temporal cortex in recall of past experience and interpretation of the present. In (Wolstenholme, G.E.W., and Cecilia M. O'Connor, ed.): Neurological basis of behavior. London: J. & A. Churchill Ltd. 1958
14. Penfield, W., Jasper, H.: Epilepsy and the functional anatomy of the human brain. Boston: Little Brown 1954
15. Penfield, W., Milner, B.: Memory deficit produced by bilateral lesions in the hippocampal zone. Arch. Neurol. Psychiat. (Chic.) **79**, 475–497 (1958)
16. Penfield, W., Perot, P.: The brain's record of auditory and visual experience. Brain **86**, 595–696 (1963)
17. Penfield, W., Rasmussen, T.: The cerebral cortex of man. New York: The Macmillan Comp. 1950
18. Penfield, W., Roberts, L.: Speech and brain-mechanisms. Princetown, New Jersey: Princetown Univerity Press 1959
19. Peterson, F., Jung, C.G.: Psycho-physical investigations with the galvanometer and pneumograph in normal and insane individuals. Brain **30**, 153–218 (1907)
20. Petsche, H., Stumpf, Ch.: Topographic and toposcopic study of origin and spread of the regular synchronized arousal pattern in the rabbit. Electroencephalogr. Clin. Neurophysiol. **12**, 589–600 (1960)
20a. Pettigrew, J.D., Nikara, T., Bishop, P.O.: Binocular interaction on single units in cat striate cortex. – Simultaneous stimulation by single moving slit with receptive fields in correspondence. Exp. Brain Res. **6**, 391–410 (1968)
21. Phillips, C.G.: Intracellular records from Betz cells in the cat. Quart. J. Exp. Physiol. **41**, 58–69 (1956)
22. Pickenhain, L.: Grundriß der Physiologie der höheren Nerventätigkeit. Berlin: VEB Verlag Volk und Gesundheit 1959
23. Plateau, J.A.F.: Sur la mesure des sensations physiques, et sur la loi qui lie l'intensité de ces sensations à l'intensité de la cause excitante. Bull. Acad. Roy. Scie. Lett. etc. de Belgique (Bruxelles) **33**, 376–385 (1872)
24. Ploog, D.: Über den Einfluß des Schlafes auf das Gedächtnis. Nervenarzt **28**, 277–278 (1957)
25. Ploog, D.W., McLean, P.D.: On functions of the mamillary bodies in the Squirrel monkey. Exp. Neurol. **7**, 76–85 (1963)
26. Poeck, K., Risso, M., Pilleri, G.: Beitrag zur Pathophysiologie und klinischen Systematik des pathologischen Lachens und Weinens. Arch. Psychiatr. Nervenkr. **204**, 181–198 (1963)
27. Pötzl, O.: Experimentell erregte Traumbilder in ihren Beziehungen zum indirekten Sehen. I. Z. ges. Neurol. Psychiat. **37**, 278–349 (1917)
28. Poggio, G.F., Fischer, B.: Binocular interaction and depth sensivity in striate and prestriate cortex of behaving Rhesus monkey. J. Neurophysiol. **40**, 1392–1405 (1977)
29. Pompeiano, O., Swett, J.W.: EEG synchronisation and behavioral manifestations of sleep induced by cutaneous nerve stimulation in normal cats. Arch. Ital. Biol. **100**, 311–342 (1962)
30. Pompeiano, O., Swett, J.E.: Identification of cutaneous and muscular afferent fibers producing EEG synchronization on arousal in normal cats. Arch. Ital. Biol. **100**, 343–380 (1962)
31. Popper, K.R.: Objective knowledge: an evolutionary approach. Oxford: Clarendon Press 1972
32. Popper, K.R., Eccles, J.C.: The self and its brain. Berlin, New York, London: Springer 1977
33. Postman, C.: Perception, motivation and behavior. J. Pers. **22**, 17 (1953)
34. Prast, J.W., Noell, W.K.: Indication of earlier stages of human hypoxia by electroencephalometric means. J. Aviat. Med. **19**, 426–434 (1948)
35. Prechtl, H.F.R.: Neurophysiologische Mechanismen des formstarren Verhaltens. Behaviour **9**, 243–319 (1956)

36. Pribram, K.H., Weiskrantz, L.: A comparison of the effects of medial and lateral cerebral resection on conditioned avoidance behavior in monkeys. J. Comp. Physiol. Psychol. **50**, 74–80 (1957)
37. Purpura, D.P., Cohen, B.: Intracellular recording from thalamic neurons during recruiting responses. J. Neurophysiol. **25**, 621–635 (1962)

Q

1. Quastler, H.: Information theory in biology. Urbana: Univ. of Illinois Press 1958

R

1. Rademaker, G.G.J.: Das Stehen. Statische Reaktionen, Gleichgewichtsreaktionen und Muskeltonus unter besonderer Berücksichtigung ihres Verhaltens bei kleinhirnlosen Tieren. Monogr. Neurol. **59**. Berlin: Springer 1931
2. Radermecker, J.: Leucoencephalite subaigue sclérosante avec lésions des ganglions rachidiens et des nerfs. Rev. neurol. **81**, 1009–1017 (1949)
3. Raehlmann, E., Witkowski, L.: Über atypische Augenbewegungen. Arch. Anat. Physiol. (Physiol. Abt.), 454–471 (1874)
4. Ramey, E.R., O'Doherty, D.S.: Electrical studies on the unanesthetized brain. Symposion. New York: Paul B. Hoeber Inc., Medical Division of Harper & Brothers 1960
5. Ranke, O.F. (Hrsg. W.D. Keidel): Physiologie des Zentralnervensystems vom Standpunkt der Regelungslehre. Berlin: Urban & Schwarzenberg 1960
6. Razran, G.: Raphael's "idealess" behavior. J. Comp. Physiol. Psychol. **54**, 366–367 (1961)
7. Rechtschaffen, A., Wolpert, E.A., Dement, W.C., Mitchell, S.A., Fisher, C.: Nocturnal sleep of narcoleptics. Electroencephalogr. Clin. Neurophysiol. **15**, 599–609 (1963)
8. Reichardt, M.: Theoretisches über die Psyche. J. Psychol. Neurol. **24**, 168–184 (1919)
9. Reichardt, M.: Hirnstamm und Psychiatrie. Mschr. Psychiat. Neurol. **68**, 470–506 (1928)
10. Reichardt, W.: Umwandlung und Verarbeitung von Informationen im Zentralnervensystem und in Automaten. Dtsch. Med. Wochenschr. **85**, 1017–1019 (1960)
11. Reichardt, W., McGinitie, G.: Zur Theorie der lateralen Inhibition. Kybernetik **1**, 155–165 (1962)
11a. Reiss, R.F. (ed.): Neural theory and modeling (Proc. 1962 Ojai Symposium). Stanford, Calif.: Stanford University Press 1964
12. Renqvist-Reenpää, Y.: Allgemeine Sinnesphysiologie. Stellung und Bedeutung des sinnesphysiologischen Versuches im Bereich der Observation, des exakten Experimentes und der Begriffsbildung. Wien: Springer 1936
13. Rey, W. van, Wissfeld, E.: Registrierung von Schlaftiefe und Schlafrhythmus mit einem EEG-Intervallanalysator bei Gesunden und schlafgestörten Depressiven. Zbl. Neurol. Psychiat. **176**, 205 (1962)
14. Ricci, G., Doane, B., Jasper, H.: Microelectrode studies of conditioning: technique and preliminary results. Ier Congres International des Sciences Neurologiques, Bruxelles, 21–28 juillet 1957
15. Richards, W.: The fortification illusion of migraine. Sci. Am. **224**, 89–96 (1971)
16. Richter, C.P.: Biological clocks in medicine and psychiatry: shock-phase hypothesis. Proc. Natl. Acad. Sci. U.S.A. **46**, 1506–1530 (1960)
17. Riechert, T.: Die stereotaktischen Hirnoperationen in ihrer Anwendung bei den Hyperkinesen (mit Ausnahme des Parkinsonismus), bei Schmerzzuständen und einigen weiteren Indikationen (Einführen von radioaktiven Isotopen usw.). Ier Congr. Internat. Neurochir., Bruxelles, Vol. Rapports, 121–160 (1957)
18. Riechert, T., Wolff, M.: Über ein neues Zielgerät zur intrakraniellen elektrischen Ableitung und Ausschaltung. Arch. Psychiatr. Nervenkr. **186**, 225–230 (1951)
19. Rodin, E.A., Luby, E.D., Gottlieb, J.S.: The electroencephalogram during prolonged experimental sleep deprivation. Electroencephalogr. Clin. Neurophysiol. **14**, 544–551 (1962)
20. Roeder, K.D.: Summary, VII. Internationaler Ethologenkongreß. Z. Tierpsychol. **18**, 491–494 (1961)
21. Rohracher, H.: Einführung in die Psychologie, 2. Aufl. Wien: Urban & Schwarzenberg 1947

22. Rohracher, H.: Psychologische Regelprobleme. Z. Exp. Angew. Psychol. **6**, 95–108 (1959)
22a. Rohracher, H.: Permanente rhythmische Mikrobewegungen des Warmblüter-Organismus („Mikrovibration"). Naturwissenschaften **49**, 145–150 (1962)
23. Roitbak, A.I.: Electrical phenomena in the cerebral cortex during the extinction of orientation and conditioned reflexes. Electroencephalogr. Clin. Neurophysiol. Suppl. **13**, 91–100 (1960)
24. Rosenblatt, F.: Principles of neurodynamics. Washington, D.C.: Spartan Books 1962
25. Rosenblith, W.A. (ed.): Sensory communication. Symposium. New York, London: The M.I.T. Press, John Wiley & Sons 1961
26. Rosenkötter, L., Wende, S.: EEG-Befunde beim Kleine-Levin-Syndrom. Mschr. Psychiat. Neurol. **130**, 107–122 (1955)
27. Rossi, G.F.: Sleep inducing mechanisms in the brain stem. Electroencephalogr. Clin. Neurophysiol. Suppl. **24**, 113–131 (1963)
28. Rossi, G.F., Zanchetti, A.: The brain stem reticular formation. Anatomy and physiology. Arch. Ital. Biol. **95**, 199–435 (1957)
29. Rosvold, H.E., Delgado, J.M.R.: The effect on delayed-alternation test performance of stimulating or destroying electrically structures within the frontal lobes of the monkeys brain. J. Comp. Physiol. Psychol. **49**, 365–372 (1956)
30. Rosvold, E.H., Mishkin, M., Szwarcbart, M.K.: Effects of subcortical lesions in monkeys on visual discrimination and single alternation performance. J. Compl. Physiol. Psychol. **51**, 437–444 (1958)
31. Rosvold, H.E., Mishkin, M.: Non-sensory effects of frontal lesions on discrimination learning and performance. In (J.F. Delafresnaye, ed.): Brain mechanisms and learning, pp. 555–576. Oxford: Blackwell 1961
32. Roth, G. (Hrsg.): Kritik der Verhaltensforschung. Konrad Lorenz und seine Schule. München: C.H. Beck 1974
33. Rothacker, E.: Die Schichten der Persönlichkeit, 2. Aufl. Leipzig: Barth 1941
34. Rothschild, F.S.: Symbolik des Hirnbaus. Berlin: S. Karger 1935
35. Rougeul, A.: Observations électroencéphalographiques du conditionnement instrumental alimentaire chez le chat. J. Physiol. (Paris) **40**, 494–496 (1958)
36. Rowland, V.: Electrographic responses in sleeping conditioned animals. In (G.E.W. Wolstenholme, and M. O'Connor, eds.): The nature of sleep. CIBA-Foundation Symposion, 284–306. London: J. & A. Churchill 1961

S

1. Sawyer, C.H.: Reproductive behavior. In (J. Field, H.W. Magoun, and E.V. Hall, eds.): Handbook of physiology, Section I, Neurophysiology, Vol. 2, pp. 1225–1240. Washington: American Physiological Society 1960
2. Sawyer, C.H., Kawakami, M.: Characteristics of behavioral and electroencephalographic afterreactions to copulation and vaginal stimulation in the female rabbit. Endocrinology **65**, 622–630 (1959)
3. Sawyer, C.H., Kawakami, M.: Interactions between the central nervous system and hormones influencing ovulation. In (C.E. Villee, ed.): Control of ovulation, pp. 79–97. Oxford, New York, London, Paris: Pergamon Press 1961
4. Schenkel, R.: Ausdrucksstudien an Wölfen. Behaviour **1**, 81–130 (1947)
5. Schilder, P.: Über Gedankenentwicklung. Z. ges. Neur. Psychiat. **59**, 250–263 (1920)
6. Schjelderup-Ebbe, T.: Beiträge zur Sozialpsychologie des Haushuhnes. Z. Psychol. **88**, 225–252 (1922)
7. Schlag, J.: L'activité spontanée des cellules du système nerveux central. Bruxelles: Editions Arscia S.A. 1959
8. Schlesinger, B.: Higher cerebral functions and their clinical disorders. The organic basis of psychology and psychiatry. New York: Grune & Stratton Inc. 1962
9. Schneider, C.: Psychologie der Schizophrenen. Leipzig: Thieme 1930
10. Schneider, J.: Activités rapides de type particulier et troubles du comportement. Electroencephalogr. Clin. Neurophysiol. Suppl. **6**, 271–281 (1957)
11. Schneider, J., Thomalske, G.: Betrachtungen über den Narkosemechanismus unter besonderer Berücksichtigung des Hirnstammes. Zentralbl. Neurochir. **16**, 185–202 (1956)

12. Schneider, K.: Probleme der klinischen Psychiatrie. Leipzig: Thieme 1932
13. Schneider, K.: Pathopsychologie der Gefühle und Triebe. Leipzig: Thieme 1936
14. Schneider, K.: Nicolai Hartmann zum Gedächtnis. Nervenarzt **22**, 111 (1951)
15. Schneider, K.: Klinische Psychopathologie. 5. Aufl. Stuttgart: Georg Thieme 1959
15a. Schoenfeld, W.N.: An experimental approach to anxiety, escape, and avoidance behavior. In (Hoch, P.H., and J. Zubin, eds.): Anxiety. New York: Grune & Stratton 1950
16. Schreiner, L., Kling, A.: Behavioral changes following rhinencephalic injury in cat. J. Neurophysiol. **16**, 643–659 (1953)
17. Schrödinger, E.: Mind and matter. Cambridge: University Press 1958
18. Schultz, I.H.: Das autogene Training. Leipzig: G. Thieme 1932
19. Schwartz, B.A., Guilbaud, G., Fischgold, H.: Études électroencéphalographiques sur le sommeil de nuit. I. L'"insomnie" chronique. Presse méd. **71**, 1474–1476 (1963)
19a. Schwartz, B.A., Guilbaud, G., Fischgold, H.: Single and multiple spikes in the night sleep of epileptics. Electroencephalogr. Clin. Neurophysiol. **16**, 56–67 (1964)
20. Sears, T.A.: Actionpotentials evoked in digital nerves by stimulation of mechanoreceptors in the human finger. J. Physiol. (Lond.) **148**, 30P–31P (1959)
21. Selbach, C. u. H.: Zur Pathogenese des epileptischen Anfalls. Fortschr. Neur. **18**, 367–401 (1950)
22. Selbach, H.: Zur Regelkreis-Dynamik psychischer Funktionen. In: Dialektik und Dynamik der Person (R. Heiss-Festschrift), 11–35. Köln: Kiepenheuer u. Witsch 1963
22a. Selz, O.: Zur Psychologie des produktiven Denkens und Irrtums. Bonn: 1922
23. Sem-Jacobsen, C.W., Torkildsen, A.: Depth recording and electrical stimulation in the human brain. In: Electrical studies on the unanesthetized brain (eds. E.R. Ramey, and D.S. O'Doherty), Symposion, pp. 275–290. New York: Paul B. Hoeber Inc., Medical Division of Harper & Brothers 1960
24. Semon, R.: Die Mneme als erhaltendes Prinzip im Wechsel des organischen Geschehens. 2. Aufl. Leipzig: W. Engelmann 1908
25. Setschenow, I.M.: Ausgewählte physiologische und psychologsiche Werke (russ.) Moskau: Medgin 1947
26. Shannon, C.E.: Presentation of a maze solving machine. Transact. of the 8th cybernetical conference, New York, p. 173 (1952)
27. Shannon, C.E.: Computers and automata. Proc. Inst. Rad. Eng. **42**, 1234 (1953)
28. Shannon, C.E.: A chess-playing machine. Wld. Math. **4**, 2124–2133 (1956)
29. Shannon, C.E., Weaver, W.: The mathematical theory of communication. Urbana, Ill.: Univ. of Illinois Press 1949
29a. Sharpless, S., Jasper, H.: Habituation of the arousal reaction. Brain **79**, 655–680 (1956)
30. Sheldon, W.H.: The varieties of human physique. New York, London: Harper & Brothers 1940
31. Sheldon, W.H.: The varieties of temperament. A psychology of constitutional differences. New York, London: Harper & Brothers 1942
32. Sherrington, C.S.: The integrative action of the nervous system. New Haven: Yale University Press; London: Constable 1906
33. Sherrington, C.S.: Man on his nature. Edinburgh, The Gifford Lectures, 1937–38. New York: Macmillan; Cambridge: University Press 1941, 1946
34. Shimazono, Y., Horie, T., Yanagisawa, Y., Hori, N., Chikazawa, S., Shozuka, K.: The correlation of the rhythmic waves of the hippocampus with the behaviors of dogs. Neurol. Med. Chir. (Tokyo) **2**, 82–88 (1960)
35. Skinner, B.F.: The behavior of organisms: An experimental analysis. New York: Appleton Century-Crofts 1938
35a. Snider, R.S., Stowell, A.: Receiving areas of the tactile, auditory and visual systems in the cerebellum. J. Neurophysiol. **7**, 331–357 (1944)
36. Sokolov, Y.: Perception and the conditioned reflex. Oxford, London, New York, Paris: Pergamon Press 1963
36a. Solomon, Ph., Kubszansky, Ph., Leiderman, P.H., Mendelson, J.H., Trumbull, R., Wexler, D. (edit.): Sensory deprivation. Cambridge/Mass.: Harvard University Press 1961
37. Sommer, J.: Periphere Bahnung von Muskeleigenreflexen als Wesen des Jendrassik'schen Phänomens. Dtsch. Z. Nervenheilk. **150**, 249–262 (1940)

38. Spalding, I.M.K., Zangwill, O.L.: Disturbance of number-form in a case of brain injury. J. Neurol. Neurosurg. Psychiat. **13**, 24–29 (1950)
39. Sperry, R.W.: Physiological plasticity and brain circuit theory. In (H.F. Harlow, and C.N. Woolsey, ed.): Biological and biochemical bases of behavior, pp. 401–424. Madison: University of Wisconsin Press 1958
40. Sperry, R.W.: Some general aspects of interhemispheric integration. In (V.B. Mountcastle, ed.): Interhemispheric relations and cerebral dominance, pp. 43–49. Baltimore: Johns Hopkins Press 1962
41. Sperry, R.W.: Lateral specialization in the surgically separated hemispheres, pp. 5–19. In: F.O. Schmitt and F.G. Worden (eds.), The neurosciences, third study program. Cambridge, Mass.: The M.I.T. Press 1974
42. Sperry, R.W., Stamm, J.S., Miner, N.M.: Relearning tests for interocular transfer following division of optic chiasma and corpus callosum in cats. J. Comp. Physiol. Psychol. **49**, 529–533 (1956)
43. Spiegel, E.A., Wycis, H.T.: Thalamic recordings in man with special reference to seizure discharges. Electroencephalogr. Clin. Neurophysiol. **2**, 23–29 (1950)
43a. Spillmann, L.: Foveal perceptive fields in the human visual system measured with simultaneous contrast in grids and bars. Pfluegers Arch. **326**, 281–299 (1971)
44. Stein, L.: Effects and interactions of imipramine, chlorpromazine, reserpine and amphetamine on self-stimulation: possible neurophysiological basis of depression. In (J. Wortis, ed.): Recent advances in biological psychiatry, Vol. IV, Proc. 16. Ann. Convention, 9.–11.6.1961, Chapter 27, 288–309. New York: Plenum Press 1962
45. Steinbuch, K.: Die Lernmatrix. Kybernetik **1**, 36–45 (1961)
46. Steinbuch, K. (Hrsg.): Taschenbuch der Nachrichtenverarbeitung. Berlin, Göttingen, Heidelberg: Springer 1962
47. Steinbuch, K.: Automat und Mensch. Über menschliche und maschinelle Intelligenz, 3. Aufl. Berlin, Göttingen, Heidelberg: Springer 1965
48. Steinbuch, K., Frank, H.: Nichtdigitale Lernmatrizen als Perzeptoren. Kybernetik **1**, 117–124 (1961)
49. Steinbuch, K., Kazmierczak, H.: Grundlagen und Anwendungen der automatischen Zeichenerkennung. In: Jahrbuch des elektrischen Fernmeldewesens 1960/61 (Hrsg. K. Herz), S. 314–381. Bad Windsheim: Georg Heidecker 1962
50. Steiniger, F.: Beiträge zur Soziologie und sonstigen Biologie der Wanderratte. Z. Tierpsychol. **7**, 356–379 (1950)
50a. Steinmann, H.W.: Verhaltensänderungen und bioelektrische Erscheinungen bei Mandelkernreizung der Katze. Dtsch. Z. Nervenheilk. **184**, 316–322 (1963)
51. Stellar, E.: Drive and motivation. In (eds.: J. Field, H.W. Magoun, V.E. Hall): Handbook of physiology, Section 1: Neurophysiology, Vol. 3, pp. 1501–1527. Washington, D.C.: American Physiological Society 1960
52. Stevens, S.S.: The psychophysics of sensory function. In (W.A. Rosenblith, ed.): Sensory communication, pp. 1–33. New York, London: John Wiley & Sons 1961
53. Stratton, G.M.: Eye movements and the aisthesis of visual form. Philos. Studien (Wundt) **20**, 336–359 (1902)
54. Straus, E.: Vom Sinn der Sinne. 2. Aufl. Berlin, Göttingen, Heidelberg: Springer 1956
55. Strauss, H.: Das Zusammenschrecken. Experimentell-kinematographische Studie zur Physiologie und Pathophysiologie der Reaktivbewegungen. J. Psychol. Neurol. (Lpz.) **39**, 111–231 (1929)
56. Stumpf, C.: Zur Einteilung der Wissenschaften. Abh. Preuß. Akad. d. Wissensch. Phil. Klasse 1–93, Berlin 1906
57. Svaetichin, G.: Spectral response curves from single cones. Acta Physiol. Scand. **39**, Suppl. 134, 17–46 (1956)
58. Svaetichin, G.: Receptor mechanisms for flicker and fusion. Acta Physiol. Scand. **39**, Suppl. 134, 47–54 (1956)
59. Svaetichin, G.: Component analysis of action potentials from single neurons. Exp. Cell Res. Suppl. **5**, 234–326 (1958)
60. Svaetichin, G., Laufer, M., Mitarai, G., Fatehchand, R., Vallecalle, E., Villegas, J.: Glial control of neuronal networks and receptors. In (R. Jung u. H. Kornhuber): Neurophysiologie und Psychophysik des visuellen Systems, Symposion, S. 445–456. Berlin, Göttingen, Heidelberg: Springer 1961

61. Svaetichin, G., MacNichol, E.F.: Retinal mechanisms for chromatic and achromatic vision. Ann. N.Y. Acad. Sci. **74**, 385–404 (1958)
62. Svaetichin, G., Negishi, K., Fatehchand, R.: Cellular mechanisms of a Young-Hering visual system. In (A.V.S. de Reuck, and J. Knight, eds.): Colour vision. Physiology and experimental psychology. CIBA-Found.-Symposion, 178–207. London: J. & A. Churchill 1965
63. Szentágothai, J.: The 'module-concept' in cerebral cortex architecture. Brain Res. **95**, 475–496 (1975)
64. Szentágothai, J.: Der moduläre Bau nervöser Zentralorgane und dessen funktionelle Bedeutung. Ergebn. exp. Med. **25**, 61–78 (1978)
65. Szentágothai, J., Flerkó, B., Mess, B., Halász, B.: Hypothalamic control of the anterior pituitary. An experimental-morphological study. Budapest: Akademiai Kiadò, Hungarian Academy of Sciences 1962

T

1. Teilhard de Chardin, P.: Le phénomène humain. Paris: Ed. du Seuil 1959
1a. Terzian, H., Dalle Ore, G.: Syndrome of Klüver and Bucy. Reproduced in man by bilateral removal of the temporal lobes. Neurology **5**, 373–380 (1955)
2. Teuber, H.-L.: Perception. In (J. Field, H.W. Magoun, and E. v. Hall, eds.): Handbook of physiology, Section 1, Neurophysiology. Vol. 3, pp. 1595–1688. Washington: American Physiological Society 1960
2a. Teuber, H.-L.: Summation. In (M.A.B. Brazier, ed.): Brain and behavior, I, Proceedings of the First Conference 1961, 393–420. Washington: American Institute of Biological Sciences 1961
3. Thach, W.T.: Cerebellar output: Properties synthesis and uses. Brain Res. **40**, 89–97 (1972)
3a. Thiele, R.: Zur Kenntnis der psychischen Residuärzustände nach Encephalitis epidemica bei Kindern und Jugendlichen, insbesondere der weiteren Entwicklung dieser Fälle. Berlin: S. Karger 1926
4. Thiele, R.: Zur gegenwärtigen Situation in der Gehirnpathologie. Z. ges. Neurol. Psychiat. **158**, 251–257 (1937)
5. Thorndike, E.L.: Animal intelligence: an experimental study of the associative processes in animals. Psychol. Monogr. **2**, No. 8, 1898
6. Thorpe, W.H.: Learning and instinct in animals. Cambridge/Mass.: Harvard University Press; London: Methuen and Co., Ltd. 1956
7. Thorpe, W.H.: Experimental studies of animal behavior. Introduction. In (W.H. Thorpe and O.L. Zangwill): Current problems in animal behavior, Part II, pp. 87–101. Cambridge: University Press 1961
8. Tinbergen, N.: Instinktlehre. Vergleichende Erforschung angeborenen Verhaltens. Berlin, Hamburg: Paul Parey 1952
9. Tönnies, J.F.: Die Erregungssteuerung im Zentralnervensystem. Erregungsfokus der Synapse und Rückmeldung als Funktionsprinzipien. Arch. Psychiatr. Nervenkr. **182**, 478–535 (1949)
10. Tönnies, J.F.: Automatische EEG-Intervall-Spektrumanalyse zur Langzeitdarstellung der Schlaf-Periodik und Narkose. Arch. Psychiatr. Nervenkr. **212**, 423–445 (1969)
11. Tönnies, J.F., Jung, R.: Über rasch wiederholte Entladungen der Motoneurone und die Hemmungsphase des Beugereflexes. Pfluegers Arch. **250**, 667–693 (1948)
11a. Trendelenburg, W.: Die natürlichen Grundlagen der Kunst des Streichinstrumentenspiels. Berlin: J. Springer 1925
12. Tschermak, A.: Der exakte Subjektivismus in der neueren Sinnesphysiologie. Pfluegers Arch. **188**, 1–20 (1921)
13. Tyler, D.B.: Psychological changes during experimental sleep deprivation. Dis. Nerv. Syst. **16**, 293 (1955)
14. Tyler, D.B., Goodman, J., Rothman, T.: The effect of experimental insomnia on the rate of potential changes in the brain. Am. J. Physiol. **149**, 185–193 (1947)

U

1. Uexküll, J. v.: Theoretische Biologie. 2. Aufl. Berlin: Springer 1928
2. Uhthoff, W.: Beiträge zu den Gesichtstäuschungen (Halluzinationen, Illusionen etc.) bei Erkrankungen des Sehorgans. Mschr. Psychiat. Neurol. **5**, 241–264, 370–379 (1899)

3. Umbach, W.: Vegetative Reaktionen bei elektrischer Reizung und Ausschaltung in subcorticalen Hirnstrukturen des Menschen. Acta Neuroveg. (Wien) **23**, 225–245 (1961)
4. Urban, H.: Zur Physiologie der Occipitalregion des Menschen. Z. ges. Neurol. Psychiat. **158**, 257–261 (1937)

V

1. De Valois, R.L.: Color vision mechanisms in the monkey. J. Gen. Physiol. **43**, 115–128 (1960)
2. De Valois, R.L., Jacobs, G.H., Jones, A.E.: Responses of single cells in primate red-green color vision system. Optik **20**, 87–98 (1963)
3. De Valois, R.L., Jones, A.E.: Single cell analysis of the organization of the primate color-vision system. In (R. Jung u. H. Kornhuber, Hrsg.): Neurophysiologie und Psychophysik des visuellen Systems, Symposion Freiburg, S. 178–191. Berlin, Göttingen, Heidelberg: Springer 1961
4. De Valois, R.L., Smith, C.J., Kitai, S.T.: Electrical responses of primate visual system: I. Different layers of macaque lateral geniculate nucleus. J. Comp. Physiol. Psychol. **51**, 662–668 (1958)
5. De Valois, R.L., Smith, C.J., Kitai, S.T.: Electrical responses of primate visual system. II. Recordings from single on-cells of macaque lateral geniculate nucleus. J. Comp. Physiol. Psychol. **52**, 635–641 (1959)
6. Verworn, M.: Kausale und konditionale Weltanschauung. 2. Aufl. Jena: Gustav Fischer 1918
7. Verzeano, M., Negishi, K.: Neuronal activity in cortical and thalamic networks. A study with multiple microelectrodes. J. Gen. Physiol. **43**, 177–195 (1960)
8. Verzeano, M., Negishi, K.: Neuronal activity in wakefulness and in sleep. In (G.E.W. Wolstenholme, and M. O'Connor, eds.): The nature of sleep. CIBA-Foundation Symposion, 108–130. London: J. & A. Churchill Ltd. 1961
9. Vetter, K., Böker, W.: Zur Funktion des K-Komplexes im Schlaf-Elektrencephalogramm. Nervenarzt **33**, 390–394 (1962)
10. Vogt, C. u. O.: Allgemeine Ergebnisse unserer Hirnforschung I–IV. J. Psychol. Neurol. (Lpz.) **25**, Erg.heft 1, 279–462 (1919)
11. Vogt, O.: Psychologie, Neurophysiologie und Neuroanatomie. J. Psychol. Neurol. (Lpz.) **1**, 1–3 (1902/03)
12. Voronin, L.G., Sokolov, E.N.: Certifical mechanisms of the orienting reflex and its relation to the conditioned reflex. Electroencephalogr. Clin. Neurophysiol. Suppl. **13**, 335–346 (1960)

W

1. Wachholder, K.: Willkürliche Haltung und Bewegung. Berlin: Springer 1928 und Ergebn. Physiol. **26**, 568–775 (1928)
2. Wadd Technical Report: Bionics Symposium. Living prototypes – the key to new technology. Ohio: Wright-Patterson Air Force Base 1961
3. Wagner, R.: Über die Zusammenarbeit des Antagonisten bei der Willkürbewegung. I., II. Z. Biol. **83**, 59–93, 120–144 (1925)
4. Wagner, R.: Probleme und Beispiele biologischer Regelung. Stuttgart: Thieme 1954
5. Walter, W.G.: The electro-encephalogram in cases of cerebral tumour. Prov. roy. Scc. Med. **30**, 579–598 (1937)
6. Walter, W.G.: A machine that learns. Sci. Am. **185**, 60–63 (1951)
7. Walter, W.G.: The living brain. London: Duckworth; New York: Norton 1953
8. Walter, W.G.: A statistical approach to the theory of conditioning. Electroencephalogr. Clin. Neurophysiol. Suppl. **13**, 377–391 (1960)
9. Walter, W.G.: Specific and non-specific cerebral responses and autonomic mechanisms in human subjects during conditioning. Progr. Brain Res. **1**, 395–403 (1963)
10. Walter, W.G.: Slow potential waves in the human brain associated with expectancy, attention and decision. Arch. Psychiatr. Nervenkr. **206**, 309–322 (1964)
11. Walter, W.G., Cooper, R., Aldridge, V.J., McCallum, W.C., Winter, A.L.: Contingent negative variation: an electric sign of sensorimotor association and expectancy in the human brain. Nature **203**, 380–384 (1964)
12. Watson, J.B.: Behaviorism. New York: Norton 1925
13. Watson, J.B., Rayner, R.: Conditioned emotional reaction. J. Exp. Psychol. **3**, 1–4 (1920)

14. Weber, E.H.: Der Tastsinn und das Gemeingefühl. In: R. Wagner's Handwörterbuch der Physiologie. Bd. 3, II. S. 481–588. Braunschweig: F. Vieweg 1846
15. Weber, W.C., Jung, R.: Über die epileptische Aura. Z. ges. Neurol. Psychiat. **170**, 211–265 (1940)
16. Weidel, W.: Kybernetik und psychophysisches Grundproblem. Kybernetik **1**, 165–170 (1962)
17. Weigl, E., Kreindler, A.: Beiträge zur Auffassung gewisser aphasischer Störungen als Blockierungserscheinungen. Temporäre Deblockierung sprachmotorischer Reaktionen durch Wortlesen bei motorischer Aphasie. Arch. Psychiatr. Nervenkr. **200**, 306–323 (1960)
18. Weizsäcker, V. v.: Der Gestaltkreis. Theorie der Einheit von Wahrnehmen und Bewegen, 3. Aufl. Stuttgart: Georg Thieme 1947
19. Werner, G.: Die neurophysiologischen Grundlagen der Wirkung von Transquillisatoren. Klin. Wochenschr. **1958**, 404–408 (1958)
20. Wernicke, C.: Grundriß der Psychiatrie in klinischen Vorlesungen. Leipzig: G. Thieme 1906
21. Whitlock, D.G., Arduini, A., Moruzzi, G.: Microelectrode analysis of pyramidal system during transition from sleep to wakefulness. J. Neurophysiol. **16**, 414–429 (1953)
22. Wiener, N.: Cybernetics, or control and communication in the animal and the machine. New York: John Wiley & Sons, Inc. 1948
23. Wiener, N.: Some moral and technical consequences of automation. Science **131**, 1355–1358 (1960)
24. Wiener, N.: Über Informationstheorie. Naturwissenschaften **48**, 174–176 (1961)
24a. Wiener, N., Schade, J.P. (eds.): Progress in brain research, Vol. II, Nerve, brain and memory models. Amsterdam, London, New York: Elsevier Publishing Company 1963
24b. Wiesel, T.N., Hubel, D.H.: Single cell responses in striate cortex of kittens deprived of vision in one eye. J. Neurophysiol. **26**, 1003–1017 (1963)
25. Wieser, St.: Das Schreckverhalten des Menschen. Beiheft z. Schweiz. Z. Psychol. Anwendg., Nr. 42. Bern, Stuttgart: Hans Huber 1961
26. Wieser, St., Domanowsky, K.: Zur Ontogenese und Pathologie des Schreckverhaltens. Arch. Psychiat. Nervenkr. **198**, 267–273 (1958/59)
27. Winterstein, H.: Schlaf und Traum. Berlin: Springer 1932
28. Winterstein, H.: Grundbegriffe der allgemeinen Nervenphysiologie. In: Bumke-Foersters Handbuch der Neurologie, Bd. 2, S. 69–87. Berlin: Springer 1937
29. Wöhlisch, E.: Schlaf und Erholung als Probleme der Energetik und Gefäßversorgung des Gehirns. Klin. Wochenschr. **34**, 720–729 (1956)
30. Wolff, H.-G.: Die bedingte Reaktion. In: Handbuch der Neurologie, Bd. 2, Allgemeine Neurologie II, Experimentelle Physiologie, S. 320–358. Berlin: Springer 1937
31. Wolstenholme, G.E.W., O'Connor, M. (ed.): The nature of sleep. CIBA-Foundation Symposium. London: J. & A. Churchill Ltd. 1961
31a. Woodbury, D.M.: Relation between the adrenal cortex and the central nervous system. Pharmacol. Rev. **10**, 275–357 (1958)
32. Woolsey, C.N.: Patterns of localization in sensory and motor areas of the cerebral cortex. In (S. Cobb): The biology of mental health and disease, pp. 193–206. New York: P. Hoeber 1952
33. Wundt, W.: Grundzüge der physiologischen Psychologie. 5., völlig umgearbeitete Aufl., 3 Bände. Leipzig: W. Engelmann 1902–03
34. Wundt, W.: Grundrisse der Psychologie. 10. Aufl. Leipzig: Engelmann 1911
34a. Wycis, H.T., Lee, A.J., Spiegel, E.A.: Simultaneous records of thalamic and cortical (scalp) potentials in schizophrenics and epileptics. Confin. Neurol. (Basel) **9**, 264–272 (1949)
35. Wyrwicka, W.: Electrical activity of the hypothalamus during alimentary conditioning. Electroencephalogr. Clin. Neurophysiol. **17**, 164–176 (1964)

Y

1. Yerkes, R.M.: The intelligence of earthworms. J. Anim. Behavior **2**, 332–352 (1912)
2. Yoshii, N., Matsumoto, J., Ogura, H., Shimokochi, M., Yamaguchi, Y., Yamasaki, H.: Conditioned reflex and electroencephalography. Electroencephalogr. Clin. Neurophysiol. **13**, 199–208 (1960)

Z

1. Zeigarnik, B.: Über das Behalten erledigter und unerledigter Handlungen. Psychol. Forsch. **9**, 1–85 (1927)
2. Zernicki, B., Santibanez-H., G.: The effects of ablations of "alimentary area" of the cerebral cortex on salivary conditioned and unconditioned reflexes in dogs. Acta Biol. exp. (Warszawa) **21**, 163–176 (1961)
3. Zillig, G.: Über ein Phänomen beim Schreiben mit der linken Hand. Nervenarzt **12**, 512–515 (1939)
4. Zotterman, Y.: Studies in the peripheral nervous mechanism of pain. Acta Med. Scand. **80**, 1–64 (1933)
5. Zotterman, Y.: Touch, pain and tickling: an electrophysiological investigation on cutaneous sensory nerves. J. Physiol. (Lond.) **95**, 1–28 (1939)
6. Zutt, J.: Über die polare Struktur des Bewußtseins. Durch psychiatrische Erfahrungen mit Pervitin angeregte Gedanken. Nervenarzt **16**, 145–162 (1943)

Namenverzeichnis – Author Index

Die *kursiven* Seitenzahlen beziehen sich auf die Literatur. Die in eckigen Klammern stehenden Zahlen bedeuten die Nummern der betreffenden Literaturzitate des Beitrages R. JUNG, S. 1068–1103.
– Page numbers in *italics* refer to the bibliography. The numbers in square brackets indicate the respective references in R. JUNG's contribution, pp. 1068–1103.

Abdel-Latif, A.A., Abood, L.G. 13, *55*
Abele, G., s. Caspers, H. 164, *183*
Abeleen, J.H.F. v. 547, *602*
Åberg, A. 290, *302*
Abood, L.G. 12, *55*
Aboot, L.G., s. Abdel-Latif, A.A. 13, *55*
Abraham, G.E., Maroulis, G.B., Buster, J.E., Chang, R.J., Marshall, J.R. 678, *692*
Abrahams, M.J., Whitlock, F.A. 730, *745*
Abrams, R. 320, *341*
Abrams, R., Taylor, M.A., Gaztanaga, P. 586, *602*
Abrams, R., s. Taylor, M. 580, 581, *616*
Abrams, R., s. Volavka, J. 322, *349*
Abramson, A.S., s. Lisker, L. 440, 441, *533*
Achilles, I., s. Dahme, B. 552, *604*
Ackenheil, M., Hippius, H., Matussek, N. 72, 98, *99*
Ackenheil, M., Hoffmann, G., Markianos, E., Nyström, I., Raese, J. 72, *98*
Ackenheil, M., s. Loosen, P. 72, *104*
Ackenheil, M., s. Matussek, N. 72, 73, 84, 85, *104, 105*
Ackenheil, M., s. Zander, K.J. 92, *109*
Acuna, C., s. Mountcastle, V.B. [M 75] 898, 929, 1037, *1093*
Adametz, J., O'Leary, J.L. 473, *523*

Adams, A., s. Foulds, G.A. 684, *695*
Adams, A., s. Heath, E.S. 333, *345*
Adams, H.B., Cooper, G.D., Carrera, R.N. 741, *745*
Adams, H.B., Robertson, M.H., Cooper, G.D. 741, 742, *745*
Adams, H.B., s. Cooper, G.D. 740, *747*
Adams, R.D., Collins, G.H., Victor, M. [A 1] 1046, 1047, *1068*
Adelman, G., s. Schmitt, F.O. 460, *541*
Adelson, E., Fraiberg, S. 722, *745*
Adelson, E., s. Smith, M.A. 722, *750*
Adelstein, A.M., Downham, D.Y., Stein, Z., Susser, M.W. 661, 663, *692*
Adey, W.R. [A 2] 977, 1031, *1068*
Adey, W.R., Dunlop, C.W., Hendrix, C.E. [A 3] 1031, *1068*
Adey, W.R., Kado, R.T., Walter, D.O. 131, *182*
Adey, W.R., Tokizane, T. 453, *523*
Adrian, E.D. [A 4–8] 843, 851, 882, 907, 908, 909, 910, 936, 1038, *1068*
Adrian, E.D., Bronk, D.W. [A 8a] 850, *1068*
Adrian, E.D., Matthews, B.H.C. [A 9] 804, 805, 976, 982 *1068*
Adrian, E.D., Zotterman, Y. [A 10] 908, 909, *1068*

Änggård, E., s. Jönsson, L.-E. 230, *238*
Affleck, J., s. Forrest, A. 553, *606*
Affleck, J.W., s. Fotherby, K. 69, *102*
Aganati, L., s. Fuxe, K. 34, 58, 110, *112*
Aghajanian, G.K., Bunney, B.S. 211, 215, 220, *234*
Aghajanian, G.K., Bunney, G.S. 211, *234*
Aghajanian, G.K., Foote, W.E., Sheard, M.H. 229, *234*
Aghajanian, G.K., s. Bunney, B.S. 211, 215, *236*
Aghajanian, G.K., s. Nybäck, H.V. 225, *240*
Agid, Y., s. Javoy, F. 219, *238*
Agranoff, B.W. 51, *55*
Agranoff, B.W., Klinger, P.D. [A 11] 1026, 1046, *1068*
Agulnik, P.L., Dimascio, A., Moore, P. 272, *302*
Ahlenius, S., Brown, R., Engel, J., Lundborg, P. 220, 232, 233, *234*
Ahlenius, S., Carlsson, A., Engel, J. *234*
Ahlenius, S., Carlsson, A., Engel, J., Svensson, T., Södersten, P. *234*
Ahlenius, S., Engel, J. 211, 215, 218, 220, 230, *234*
Ahlenius, S., s. Berggren, U. 228, *235*
Ahlestiel, H. [A 12] 931, *1068*
Ahrens, D., s. Zerssen, D. von 675, 677, *705*

Ahrens, R. 411, 415, *523*, [A 13], *1068*
Ainsworth, M.D. 717, 744, *745*
Aird, R.B. 340, *341*
Ajuriaguerra, J. de, s. Talairach, J. 356, *378*
Akert, K. [A 14] 988, *1068*
Akert, K., Andersson, B. [A 14a] 989, *1068*
Akert, K., Gruesen, R.A., Woolsey, C.N., Meyer, D.R. [A 15] 944 *1068*
Akert, K., Hess, W.R. [A 16] 943, *1068*
Akert, K., s. Harlow, H.F. [H 3] 890, *1080*
Akert, K., s. Hess, R. [H 46, 47] 938, *1081*
Akert, K., s. Liberson, W.T. [L 20] *1089*
Akil, H., s. Watson, S.J. 96, *108*, 112, *113*
Akimoto, H., Creutzfeldt, O. [A 17] 936, *1068*
Akimoto, H., s. Creutzfeldt, O. [C 15] 936, *1073*
Akisal, H.S., McKinney, W.T. 501, *523*
Akiskal, H.S., Djenderedjian, A.H., Rosenthal, R.H., Khani, M.K. 582, *602*
Akiskal, H.S., McKinney, T.M. 583, *602*
Alanen, Y.O., Rekola, J., Stewen, A., Tuovinen, M., Takala, K., Rutanen, E. 566, *603*
Alanen, Y., s. Rimon, R. 93, *107*
Alarcón, R. de, Carney, M.W.P. 257, *302*
Albe-Fessard, D. Rocha-Miranda, C., Oswaldo-Cruz, E. [A 18] 842, *1068*
Albeaux-Fernet, M., Bohler, C.C.S.-S., Karpas, A.E. 663, *692*
Albert, H., s. Moccetti, T. 287, *310*
Alberts, W.W., s. Libet, B. [L 21] 886, *1089*
Aldridge, V.J., s. Walter, W.G. 152, *196*, [W 11] 1033, *1101*
Alexander, M., s. Robinson, B.W. 539

Alfredsson, G., s. Sedvall, G. 217, 220, 225, *241*
Alhava, E., s. Idänpään-Heikkilä, J. 291, *308*
Ali, S.I., s. Pandey, G.N. 91, 92, *105*
Allahyari, H., Deisenhammer, E., Weiser, G. 164, *182*
Allen, J.K., s. Nelson, J.F. 26, *61*
Allen, J.L., s. Blackburn, H.L. 253, *304*
Allen, M.G., s. Pollin, W. 555, 556, *613*
Allen, R.P., s. Safer, D.J. 290, *312*
Allen, W.S., Otterbein, E.C., Varma, R., Varma, R.S., Wardi, A.H. 23, *55*
Alleon, A.M., s. Schnetzler, J.P. 289, *312*
Allport, F.H. [A 19] *1068*
Allport, G.W. [A 20] 930, *1068*
Allweis, C., Magnes, J. 7, 8, *55*
Almgren, O., Carlsson, A., Engel, J. 207, *234*
Altherr, P., s. Schmidtke, A. 742, *750*
Altman, J. 47, *55*
Altman, N., s. Sachar, E.J. 77, 78, *107*, 325, 338, *348*
Altmann, S.A. 384, *523*
Altshuler, K.Z., s. Rainer, J.D. 722, *750*
Åmark, C. 599, *603*
Ambrose, J.A. 410, *523*
Amdisen, A., s. Baastrup, P.C. 270, *303*
Amdisen, A., s. Schou, M. 294, *312*
American Psychiatric Association (APA) 316, 333, *341*
Amin, M., s. Simpson, G.M. 297, *313*
Amsler, H.A. 291, *302*
Anagnoste, B., s. Goldstein, M. 216, *238*
Anand, B.K., Dua, S., Singh, B. [A 21] 939, 1032, *1068*
Ananth, J. 294, *302*
Ananth, J., Ban, T.A., Lehmann, H.E., Bennett, J. 94, *99*
Ananth, J., Luchins, D. 267, *302*

Ananth, J.V., Beszterczey, A. 291, *302*
Ananth, J.V., Valles, J.V., Whitelaw, J.P. 291, *302*
Anastasi, A. 673, *692*
Andén, N.-E. 211, 212, 213, 214, 219, *234*
Andén, N.-E., Butcher, S.G., Corrodi, H., Fuxe, K., Ungerstedt, U. 211, 212, *235*
Andén, N.-E., Carlsson, A., Häggendal, J. 15, 55, 201, *235*
Andén, N.-E., Corrodi, H., Fuxe, K. 212, 229, 231, *235*
Andén, N.-E., Dahlström, A., Fuxe, K., Larsson, K. 201, *234*
Andén, N.-E., Roos, B.-E., Werdinius, B. 212, *234*
Andén, N.-E., Stock, G. 213, 220, *234*
Andén, N.-E., Strömbom, U., Svensson, T.H. 75, *99*, 201, *235*
Andén, N.-E., s. Jackson, D.M. 211, *238*
Andersen, A.E., s. Bunney, W.E. Jr. 339, *343*
Andersen, M., s. Eliasen, P. 287, *305*
Andersen, P., Bland, B.H., Dudar, J.D. [A 21a] 1039, *1068*
Andersen, R. 373, *374*
Andersen, T., Astrup, C., Forsdal, A. 587, *603*
Anderson, E.W. 736, *745*
Anderson, O.D., Liddell, A.S. [A 22] 810, 811, *1068*
Anderson, s. Hollister, L.E. 72, *103*
Anderson, V.E., s. Reed, S.C. 553, *613*
Andersson, B., Jewell, P.A., Larsson, S. [A 23] 939, *1069*
Andersson, B., s. Akert, K. [A 14a] 989, *1068*
Ando, K., s. Shagass, C. 175, *194*
Andresen, B., s. Kempe, P. 739, *748*
Andrew, R.J. 384, 406, 412, 426, *523*
Andrews, G., Harris, M.,

Garside, R., Kay, D. 638, *692*

Andrews, P., Hall, J.N., Snaith, R.P. 253, *302*

Andy, O.J., Jurko, M.F. 371, 372, *375*

Angel, C., Roberts, A.J. 340, *341*

Angelergues, R., s. Hecaen, H. 475, 476, *529*

Angeletti, P.U., s. Levi-Montalcini, R. 10, *60*

Angrist, B., Gershon, S. 91, *99*

Angrist, B., Gershon, S., Sathananthan, G., Walker, R.W., Lopez-Ramos, B., Mandel, L.R., Vandenheuvel, W.J.A. 95, *99*

Angrist, B., Sathananthan, G., Gershon, S. 91, *99*

Angrist, B., Sathananthan, G., Wilk, S., Gershon, S. 91, *99*

Angrist, B., Thompson, H., Shopsin, B., Gershon, S. 92, *99*

Angrist, B.M., s. Rotrosen, J. 91, *107*

Angrist, B., s. Sathananthan, G. 91, *107*

Angst, J. 244, 245, 261, 270, 298, *302*, 577, 578, 579, 581, 585, *603*, 642, 649, 661, 684, 686, *692*

Angst, J., Baastrup, P., Grof, P., Hippius, H., Poeldinger, W., Varga, E., Weis, P., Wyss, F. 641, *692*

Angst, J., Baastrup, C., Grof, P., Hippius, H., Poeldinger, W., Weis, P. 642, *692*

Angst, J., Dinkelkamp, T. 244, *302*

Angst, J., Felder, W., Frey, R., Stassen, H.H. 580, *603*

Angst, J., Frey, R. 264, *302*

Angst, J., Perris, C. 578, *603*, 661, *692*

Angst, J., Theobald, W. 262, *302*

Angst, J., Woggon, B. 257, *302*

Angst, J., s. Hucker, H. 257, *308*

Angst, J., s. Kline, N.S. 244, *309*

Angst, J., s. Marussek, N. *105*

Angst, J., s. Woggon, B. 256, 257, *314*

Annell, A.L. 590, *603*

Anokhin, P.K. [A 24–27] 761, 1031, 1032, 1036, *1069*

Anonym 292, 298, *302, 303*

Ansell, G.B., Hawthorne, J.N. 19, *55*

Ansell, G.B., Richter, D. 50, *55*

Anthony, E.J. 569, *603*

Aperia, B., Rönnberg, E., Wetterberg, L. 316, *341*

Aposhian, D., s. Simantov, R. 40, *63*

Appel, S.H., Day, E.D., Mikkey, D.D. 10, 11, 13, 14, *55*

A practising psychiatrist 327, *341*

Aprison, M.H., Takahashi, R., Tachiki, K. 110, *112*

Arbib, M.A. 447, *523*

Arbib, M.A., s. Szentagothai, J. 447, *542*

Archer, J., s. Lloyd, B. 647, *699*

Ardö, A., s. Ingvar, D.H. 162, *188*

Arduini, A. [A 28, 28a] 935, 1004, *1069*

Arduini, A., s. Whitlock, D.G. [W 21] 1005, *1102*

Arey, L.B. s. Bruesch, S.R. [B 67] 878, 913, *1072*

Arfel, G. 159, *182*

Arfel, G., Walter, S. 159, *182*

Arfwidsson, L., Arn, L., Beskow, J., D'Elia, G., Laurell, B., Ottosson, J.-O., Perris, C., Persson, G., Wistedt, B. 332, *342*

Arganian, M. 644, 648, 650, *692*

Arianova, L., s. Jonchev, V. 289, *308*

Arieti, S. *603*, 684, *692*

Arimura, A., s. Hökfelt, T. 15, 40, *58*, 200, *238*

Armington, J.C., Tepas, D.J., Kropfl, W.H., Hengst, D.W.H. 147, *182*

Armocide, C.C., s. Buffa, P. 287, *304*

Armstrong, B., Stevens, N., Doll, R. 292, *303*

Armstrong, G., s. Templer, D.J. 327, *348*

Arneson, G.A., Ourso, R. 335, 341, *342*

Arnl, L., s. Arfwidsson, L. 332, *342*

Arnold, E., s. Diebold, K. 566, *605*, 649, *694*

Arnold, O.H. 570, *603*

Aronoff, M.D., s. Greenspan, K. 72, *103*

Åsberg, M. 69, 70, *99*

Åsberg, M., Bertilsson, L., Tuck, D., Cronholm, B., Sjöqvist, F. 69, *99*

Åsberg, M., Cronholm, B., Sjöqvist, F., Tuck, D. 246, *303*

Åsberg, M., Thoren, P., Träskman, L., Bertilsson, L., Ringberger, V. 69, 70, *99*, 325, 339, *342*

Åsberg, M., s. Bertilsson, L. 225, *235*

Åsberg, M., s. Träskman, L. 109, 110, *113*

Aschoff, J. [A 29] *1069*

Aschoff, J., Wever, R. [A 30] *1069*

Aserinsky, E., Kleitman, N. [A 31, 32] 991, 996, 1008, 1019, *1069*

Ashby, W., Ross [A 34] 853, 863, *1069*

Ashby, W.R. 453, *523*

Ashcroft, G.W., Crawford, T.B.B., Eccleston, D., Sharman, D.F., MacDougall, E.J., Stanton, J.B., Binns, J.K. 69, *99*, 339, *342*

Ashcroft, G.W., Dow, R.C., Yates, C.M., Pullar, J.A. 70, *99*

Ashcroft, G.W., Eccleston, D., Murray, L.G., Glen, A.J., Crawford, T.B.B., Pullar, J.A., Shields, P.J., Walter, D.S., Blackburn, J.M., Chonnechan, J., Lonergan, M. 87, *99*

Ashcroft, G.W., s. Fotherby, K. 69, *102*

Ashcroft, G.W., s. Hitchcock, E. 373, *376*

Asnis, G. 339, *342*

Asper, H., s. Bürki, H.R. 214, *236*
Asratian, E.A. [A 33] 1030, *1069*
Assal, G., Hecaen, H. [A 35] 780, 896, 897, *1069*
Assal, J.P., s. Froesch, E.R. 627, *695*
Ast, M., Rosenberg, S., Metzig, E. 682, *692*
Ast, M., s. Metzig, E. 682, *699*
Astrup, C., Fossum, A., Holmboe, R. 685, *692*
Astrup, C., s. Andersen, T. 587, *603*
Astrup, C., s. Bharnar, E. 587, *603*
Astrup, J., s. Bolwig, T.G. 323, *342*
Atack, C.V., s. Carlsson, A. 204, *236*
Atack, C., s. Kehr, W. 215, *239*
Athen, D., s. Loosen, P. 72, *104*
Athen, D., s. Matussek, N. 72, 85, *104*
Atkinson, M.W., s. Kay, D.W.K. 553, 565, *609*
Atkinson, M.W., s. Stephens, D.A. 553, 558, 564, 565, *616*
Atlas, D., s. Magoun, H.W. 471, *534*
Attewell, P.A., s. Judd, L.L. 687, *697*
Aubert, C. 289, *303*
Auchincloss, J.H., Jr., Cook, E., Renzetti, A.D. [A 36] 1016, *1069*
Auersperg, A. [A 37] 777, *1069*
Austin, L., s. Wellington, B.S. 20, *64*
Autilio-Gambetti, L.A., s. Gambetti, P. 50, *58*
Avenarius, R. [A 38] 774, *1069*
Avery, D., Winokur, G. 330, *342*
Axelrod, J. 35, *55*
Axelrod, J., Whitby, L.G., Hertting, G. 223, *235*
Axelrod, J., s. Glowinski, J. 223, *238*
Axelrod, J., s. Hertting, G. 223, *238*

Axelsson, R., s. Nyberg, G. 217, *240*
Axelsson, T. 218, *235*
Ayd, F.J. Jr. 246, 263, 275, 294, 297, 298, *303*
Aylward, M., Maddock, J. 71, *99*
Azima, H., Cramer, F.J. 740, 745, *746*

Baarfüsser, B., s. Schilkrut, R. 83, *107*
Baastrup, C., s. Angst, J. 642, *692*
Baastrup, C., s. Randrup, A. 75, *106*
Baastrup, P., s. Angst, J. 641, *692*
Baastrup, P.C. 687, *692*
Baastrup, P.C., Poulsen, J.C., Schou, M., Amdisen, A. 270, *303*
Baastrup, P.C., s. Kirk, L. 272, *309*
Baastrup, P.C., s. Kragh-Sörensen, P. 330, *346*
Baastrup, P.C., s. Schou, M. 272, *312*
Bach-Mortensen, N., s. Vendsborg, P.B. 290, *313*
Bachelard, H.S., s. McIlwain, H. 9, *61*
Bachhawat, B.K., s. Balasubramanian, K.A. 24, *55*
Backmund, H., s. Poeppel, E. 448, *539*
Badier, M., s. Gastaut, H. 166, *186*
Baer, L., s. Greenspan, K. 72, *103*
Bäumler, H., Wernecke, K.-D., Michel, J. 140, *182*
Baeyer, W. von 635, 638, *692*
Bagley, C.R., s. Davison, K. 551, 564, *605*
Baig, S., s. Volavka, J. 96, *108*
Bailey, H.R., Dowling, J.L., Swanton, C.H., Davies, E. 357, *375*
Bailey, J., s. Braithwaite, R.A. 246, *304*
Bailey, J., s. Coppen, A. 270, *305*
Bailey, J., s. Kellett, J.M. 272, *309*

Bailey, J., s. Merry, J. 271, *310*
Bailey, P., s. Schaltenbrand, G. 357, *377*
Bakay, L. 16, *55*
Baker, A.A., Game, J.A., Thorpe, J.G. 333, *342*
Baker, H.F., s. Joseph, M.H. *59*
Baker, J.M.H., Johnstone, E.C., Crow, T.J. 92, *99*
Baker, M., s. Murphy, D.L. 74, 96, *105*
Baker, M., s. Winokur, G. 580, 582, 600, *617*
Baker, S.W., s. Ehrhardt, A.A. 647, 648, 678, 690, *695*
Bakkestrøm, E., s. Witkin, H.A. 677, *704*
Bakwin, H. 603, 713, 714, *746*
Balasubramanian, K.A., Bachhawat, B.K. 24, *55*
Balasubramaniam, V., Kanaka, T.S. 369, 370, 373, *375*
Balasubramaniam, V., Kanaka, T.S., Ramanujam, P.B. 361, *375*
Balázs, R., Cocks, W.A. 50, *55*
Balázs, R., Cremer, J.E. 8, 47, *55*
Balázs, R., Lewis, P.D., Patel, A.J. 48, *55*
Balázs, R., Machiyama, Y., Hammond, B.J., Julian, T., Richter, D. 36, 37, *55*
Balázs, R., Patel, A.J., Lewis, P.D. 48, 49, *55*
Balázs, R., Patel, A.J., Richter, D. 47, *55*
Balázs, R., s. Patel, A.J. 36, 49, *61*, *62*
Baldessarini, R.J. 338, *342*
Baldessarini, R.J., s. Granacher, R.P. 299, *306*
Baldessarini, R.J., s. Jacobson, G. 297, *308*
Baldock, G.R., Walter, W.G. 134, *182*
Baldwin, M. [B 1] 886, *1069*
Ballantine, H.T. Jr., Cassidy, W.L., Brodeur, J., Giriunas, I. 361, *375*
Ballantine, H.T. Jr., Cassidy, W.L., Flanagan, N.B., Marino, R. Jr. 361, *375*

Balldin, J., Modigh, K., Walinder, J., Wallin, L., Lindstedt, G. 84, 89, *99*
Ballin, J.C. 287, *303*
Balthasar, K. 163, *182*
Balthazar, E.E., Stevens, H.A. 672, *692*
Bamburg, J.R., s. Pardee, J.D. 20, *61*
Ban, T.A., Lehmann, H.E. 94, *99*
Ban, T.A., s. Ananth, J. 94, *99*
Ban, T.A., s. Nestoros, I.N. 94, *105*
Bandura, A., Walters, R.H. 644, 645, *692*
Banerjee, S.P., Kung, L.S., Riggi, S.J., Chanda, S.K. 88, *99*
Bangham, A.D., s. Ochoa, E.L.M. 26, *61*
Banki, C.M. 69, *99*
Banks, P. 39, *55*
Barahona Fernandes, H.J. de [B 2] 775, *1069*
Barbeau, A., s. Huxtable, R.J. 27, *59*, 199, *238*
Barbeau, S., s. Botez, M.I. 474, *524*
Barbizet, J. 326, 341, *342*
Barchas, J.D., Ciaranello, R.D., Dominic, J.A., Deguchi, T., Orenberg, E.K., Renson, J., Kessler, S. 550, 571, *603*
Barchas, J.D., s. Berger, P.A. 229, *235*
Barchas, J.D., s. Watson, S.J. 96, *108*
Barchas, J., s. Wyatt, R.J. 93, *109*
Barclay, G.L., s. Kline, N.S. 94, 97, *104*
Barley, J., s. Westley, B.R. 26, *64*
Bard, P. [B 3–5] 937, 938, 943, 961, *1069*
Bard, P., Mountcastle, V.B. [B 6] 943, 961, *1069*
Barlow, H.B. [B 7, 8, 8a] 853, 856, 925, 926, *1070*
Barlow, H.B., Fitzhugh, R., Kuffler, S.W. [B 8b] *1070*
Barnett, C., Leiderman, P., Grobstein, R., Klaus, M. 721, 726, *746*

Baron, M., Gershon, E.S., Rudy, V., Jonas, W.Z., Buchsbaum, M. 271, *303*
Baron, M., Stern, M. 566, *603*
Baron, M., s. Gershon, E.S. 578, 579, *607*
Barondes, S.H. 48, *55*
Barondes, S.H., Dutton, G.R. 20, *55*
Barratt, E.S., s. Powell, G.F. 733, *749*
Barrera, S.E., s. Kalinowsky, L.B. 320, *345*
Barron, K., s. Daniels, J.C. 158, *184*
Bartholini, G. *235*
Bartholini, G., Stadler, H. 199, 231, *235*
Bartholini, G., Stadler, H., Gadea-Ciria, M., Lloyd, K.G. 212, 213, 216, *235*
Bartholini, G., Stadler, H., Lloyd, K. 213, 219, *235*
Bartholini, G., s. Stadler, H. 30, *63*, 219, *241*
Bartholomew, A.A. 256, *303*
Bartlett, S.F., Lagercrantz, H., Smith, A.D. 21, 22, *56*
Barton, J.L. 330, *342*
Barton, J.L., Mehta, S., Snaith, R.P. 322, *342*
Baruk, H., Pécheny, J. 287, *303*
Bass, N.H., s. Hess, H.H. 18, *58*
Baštecký, J., Gregová, L. 293, *303*
Bates, J.A.V. [B 9] 831, *1070*
Bateson, P.P.G., Klopfer, P.H. 380, *523*
Batini, C., Moruzzi, G., Palestini, M., Rossi, G.F., Zanchetti, A. [B 10] 989, *1070*
Battig, K., Rosvold, H.E., Mishkin, M. [B 11, 12] 831, *1070*
Bauer, H., Girke, W., Kanowski, S., Krebs, F.A., Müller-Oerlingshausen, B. 272, 298, *303*
Bauer, J. 622, *692*
Baumann, P., Maitre, L. 88, *99*
Baumann, P., Schmocker, M., Reyero, F., Heimann, H. 71, *99*

Baumgart, H.H., s. Meier-Ewert, K. 291, *310*
Baumgarten, R. von, s. Jung, R. [J 52] 766, 844, 908, *1085*
Baumgartner, G. [B 13–16] 912, 913, 915, 918, 922, 924, 925, 989, *1070*
Baumgartner, G., Creutzfeldt, O., Jung, R. [B 17] 922, 982, *1070*
Baumgartner, G., s. Jung, R. [J 52, 53] 766, 844, 908, 926, *1085*
Baust, W. [B 18] 988, *1070*
Baxter, C.F., s. Twomey, S.L. 20, *63*
Bay, E. 475, 476, *523*
Bazett, H.C., Penfield, W.G. 476, *523*
Beach, F.A. [B 18a] 966, *1070*
Beach, F.A., Hebb, D.O., Morgan, C.T., Nissen, H.W. 448, *523*
Beach, F.A., s. Ford, C.S. 622, *695*
Beard, A.W., s. Slater, E. 335, *348*
Beard, W., s. Slater, E. 170, *194*
Beaton, L.E., s. Kelly, A.H. 473, *531*
Beatty, J., McDevitt, C.A. 434, *523*
Bech, P., Vendsborg, P.B., Rafaelsen, O.J. 686, *693*
Bech, P., s. Vendsborg, P.B. 272, 290, *313*
Bechterew, Pavlov 352
Bechterew, W. v. [B 19] 790, *1070*
Beck, A.T., s. Morris, J.B. 271, *311*
Beck, E., s. Meyer, A. 356, *376*
Beck, E.C., s. Lewis, E.G. 161, *190*
Beck, U., s. Kendel, K. [K 13] 1014, *1086*
Becka, D.R., s. Struve, F.A. 172, *195*
Becker, D. 180, *182*
Becker, J. 583, *603*
Becker, P.E. 546, 549, 591, 593, 602, *603*, 681, *693*

Becker, P.E., Schepank, H., Heigl-Evers, A. 592, *603*
Becker, W., s. Deecke, L. 153, *184*
Beckmann, H. 72, *99*
Beckmann, H., Frische, M., Rüther, E., Zimmer, R. 94, *100*
Beckmann, H., Goodwin, F.K. 72, 73, *99*, *100*
Beckmann, H., Strauss, M.A., Ludolph, E. 75, *100*
Beckmann, H., s. Loosen, P. 72, *104*
Beckmann, H., s. Matussek, N. 72, 85, *104*
Beecher, M.D., s. Sinnott, J.M. 443, 444, *541*
Beek, H.H., Bork, I.I. von, Herngreen, H., Most van Spijk, D. van der 171, *182*
Beerstecher, D.M., s. Hurst, L.A. 176, *188*
Beerstecher, D.M., s. Mundy-Castle, A.C. 162, *192*
Behnsen, G., s. Janzen, R. [J 7] 1015, *1084*
Beichl, L. 594, *603*
Bekkering, D., s. Gastaut, H.A. [G 11] 1028, 1031, 1032, *1078*
Belfer, M.L., s. Shader, R.I. 293, *313*
Belizon, N., s. Gershon, E.S. 579, *607*
Bell, B., s. Mednick, S.A. 546, 553, 567, 568, 575, *611*
Bell, D.S. 91, *100*
Bell, R.Q. 720, 721, *746*
Bellabarba, U., Hippius, H., Kanowski, S. 297, *303*
Belluzzi, J.D., s. Wise, C.D. 74, 93, *109*
Bellugi, K., Klima, E.S. 515, *523*
Bellugi, U., s. Klima, E.S. 516, *532*
Belmaker, R., Pollin, W., Wyatt, R.J., Cohen, S. 557, *603*
Belmaker, R., s. Murphy, D.L. *105*
Belmaker, R., s. Wyatt, R.J. 570, *617*
Belmaker, R.H., Ebstein, R., Rimon, R., Wyatt, R.J.,

Murphy, D.L. 570, 583, *603*
Belmaker, R.H., s. Biedermann, J. 92, *100*
Ben-David, M., Danon, A., Sulman, F.G. 292, *303*
Benda, C.E. 469, *523*
Bender, H. [B 20] 931, 948, *1070*
Bender, H.-J., s. Heinrich, K. 297, *307*
Bender, L. 588, 589, *603*
Benington, F., s. Corbett, L. 95, *101*
Benkert, O., Gluba, H., Matussek, N. 74, *100*
Benkert, O., Hippius, H. *100*, 244, *303*
Benkert, O., Renz, A., Marano, C., Matussek, N. 71, 74, *100*
Benkert, O., Renz, A., Matussek, N. *100*
Benkert, O., s. Crombach, G. 71, *101*
Benkert, O., s. Laakmann, G. 82, *104*
Benkert, O., s. Loosen, P. 72, *104*
Benkert, O., s. Matussek, N. 72, 74, 85, *104*, *105*
Benkert, O., s. Strian, F. 92, *108*
Bennet, G. 736, *746*
Bennett, E.L., Diamond, M.C., Krech, D., Rosenzweig, M.R. 49, *56*
Bennett, J., s. Ananth, J. 94, *99*
Benson, D.F. 475, 476, *524*
Bente, D. 171, *182*
Bentinck, C., s. Cleveland, S.E. 741, *747*
Benuck, M., s. Marks, N. 23, *60*
Beppu, H., s. Fujita, K. 93, *102*
Beresford, H.R., Posner, J.B., Plum, F. 322, *342*
Berg, J.M. 632, *693*
Bergamasco, B., s. Bergamini, L. 155, *182*
Bergamasco, B., s. Bergmann, L. *183*
Bergamini, L., Bergamasco, B., Mombelli, A.M., Mutani, R. 155, *182*

Bergamini, L., s. Chatrian, G.E. 121, *183*
Berger, H. 124, 132, 133, 134, 147, 154, 155, 163, 182, *182*, 594, *603*, [B 21–30] 762, 763, 765, 783, 784, 789, 948, 970, 976, 977, 978, 982, 983, 998, 999, 1051, *1070, 1071*
Berger, P.A., Glen, R.E., Barchas, J.D. 229, *235*
Berger, P.A., s. Davis, K.L. 220, *237*
Berger, P.A., s. Watson, S.J. 96, *108*
Berger, R.J., Olley, P., Oswald, I. [B 31] 1011, *1071*
Berger, R.J., Oswald, I. [B 32] 993, 1003, *1071*
Berger, R.J., s. Oswald, I. [O 14] 1015, *1094*
Berggren, U., Tallstedt, L., Ahlenius, S., Engel, J. 228, *235*
Berglund, K., s. Spehr, W. 158, 161, *194*
Bergman, S., s. Nowakowski, H. 677, *700*
Bergman, W. 334, *342*
Bergmann, L., Bergamasco, B. *183*
Bergson, H. [B 33] 1023, *1071*
Beringer, K. [B 34–36] 932, 943, 961 *1071*
Beritoff, J.S. [B 37–39] 1029, 1040, *1071*
Berl, S. 47, *56*
Berl, S., Puszkin, S., Nicklas, W. 20, *56*
Berlucchi, G., Moruzzi, G., Salvi, G., Strata, P. [B 40] 995, 1011, *1071*
Berlyne, N., Strachan, M. 323, 326, *342*
Bernabei, A., s. Kukopulos, A. 330, *346*
Bernard, C. [B 41] 765, 1063, *1071*
Bernasconi, S., s. Samanin, R. 225, *240*
Bernstein, P., s. Papousek, H. 503, *537*
Berrettini, W.H., Vogel, W.H., Clouse, R. 570, *603*
Berson, S., s. Yalow, R. 39, *64*
Bertalanffy, L. von 621, *693*, [B 42] 774, *1071*

Bertelsen, A., Harvald, B., Hauge, M. 578, 579, *603*
Bertelsen, A., s. Leff, J.P. 661, *698*
Berthold, A., s. Crombach, G. 71, *101*
Bertilsson, L., Åsberg, M., Thorén, P. 225, *235*
Bertilsson, L., s. Åsberg, M. 69, 70, *99*, 325, 339, *342*
Bertilsson, L., s. Träskman, L. 109, 110, *113*
Beskow, J., Gottfries, C.G., Roos, B.E., Winblad, B. 67, 68, *100*
Beskow, J., s. Arfwidsson, L. 332, *342*
Besser, G.M. 39, 42, *56*
Besser, G.M., s. Rees, L. 85, *107*
Bessuges, J.M., Ourgaud, J.J. 288, *303*
Beszterczey, A., s. Ananth, J.V. 291, *302*
Bettecken, F., s. Majewski, F. 601, *610*, 673, 674, *699*
Betti, O., s. Schvarcz, J.R. 369, *377*
Beumont, P.J.V., Corker, C.S., Friesen, H.G., Kolakowska, T., Mandelbrote, B.M., Marshall, J., Murray, M.A.F., Wiles, D.H. 293, *303*
Beumont, P.J.V., Gelder, M.G., Friesen, H.G., Harris, G.W., MacKinnon, P.C.B., Mandelbrote, B.M., Wiles, D.H. 293, *304*
Beumont, P.J.V., Harris, G.W., Carr, P.J., Friesen, H.G., Kolakowska, T., MacKinnon, P.C.B., Mandelbrote, B.M., Wiles, D. 292, *303*
Bexton, W.H., s. Heron, W. [H 40] 932, *1081*
Bhargava, K.P., s. Tangri, K.K. 25, *63*
Bharucha, A.D., Elliott, K.A.C. 50, *56*
Bianchi, S., s. Ladinsky, H. 219, *239*
Biase, D.V., Zuckerman, M. *746*
Bickel, H., Kaiser-Grubel, S. 631, 637, *693*

Bickelman, A.G., s. Burwell, C.S. [B 75] 1016, *1073*
Bickford, R.G., Dodge, H.W. Jr., Uihlein, A. [B 43] 886, *1071*
Bickford, R.G., Jacobson, J.L., Langworthy, D. 117, *183*
Biedermann, J., Rimon, R., Ebstein, R., Belmaker, R.H., Davidson, J.T. 92, *100*
Bielski, R.J., Friedel, R.O. 245, *304*, 331, *342*
Bierens de Haan, 800
Bierich, J.R., Majewski, F., Michaelis, R., Tillner, I. 673, 674, 675, *693*
Bierich, J.R., s. Majewski, F. 601, *610*, 673, 674, *699*
Biermann, G., Biermann, R. 714, 718, *746*
Biermann, R., s. Biermann, G. 714, 718, *746*
Bigelow, L.B., Nasrallah, H., Carman, J., Gillin, J.C., Wyatt, R.J. 94, *100*
Bigger, J.T. Jr., s. Kantor, S.J. 287, *309*
Bille, M., s. Weeke, A. 649, 661, *704*
Bilý, J., Hametová, M., Hanus, H., Poláčková, J. 290, *304*
Bilý, J., s. Zapletálek, M. 256, *314*
Bilz, R. 400, 401, *524*
Bineik, E., Bornscheuer, B. 287, *304*
Bingley, T., Leksell, L., Meyerson, B.A., Rylander, G. 364, *375*
Binns, J.K., s. Ashcroft, G.W. 69, *99*, 339, *342*
Binswanger, L. [B 44] 930, *1071*
Bird, E.D., Iversen, L.L. 54, *56*
Bird, E.G., s. Denber, H.C.B. 253, *305*
Bird, R., s. Saldanha, V.F. 293, *312*
Bird, R.L., s. Seager, C.P. 332, *348*
Birdwhistell, R.L. 410, *524*
Birkmayer, W., Frühmann,

E., Strotzka, H., [B 44a] *1071*
Birkmayer, W., Hornykiewicz, O. 74, *100*
Birkmayer, W., Lindauer, W. 71, *100*
Birkmayer, W., Neumayer, E. 91, *100*
Birkmayer, W., Riederer, R. 67, 68, *100*
Birnbaum, D., Karmeli, F. 290, *304*
Birtchnell, J. 730, *746*
Bischof, N. 502, *524*
Bishop, M.P., s. Gallant, D.M. 94, *102*
Bishop, P.O. [B 45] 918, 920, 950, *1071*
Bishop, P.O., s. Pettigrew, J.D. [P 20a] 918, *1095*
Bishop, W., s. McCann, S.M. 220, *239*
Biswas, B., Carlsson, A. 220, 231, *235*
Bizzi, E., Pompeiano, O., Somogyi, I. [B 46] 1005, *1071*
Bizzi, E., s. Dichgans, J. [D 29] 826, *1075*
Bjarnar, E., Reppesgaard, H., Astrup, C. 587, *603*
Bjerkenstedt, L., s. Sedvall, G. 217, 220, 225, *241*
Björklund, A., Lindvall, O. 215, *235*
Blachly, P.H., Denney, D.D. 318, *342*
Blachly, P.H., Gowing, D. 320, 324, *342*
Blackard, W.G., Heidingsfelder, S.A. 81, *100*
Blackburn, H.L., Allen, J.L. 253, *304*
Blackburn, J.M., s. Ashcroft, G.W. 87, *99*
Blacker, K.H., s. Meadow, A. 253, *310*
Blaesig, J., s. Herz, A. 485, *529*
Blair, J.H., Simpson, G.M. 293, *304*
Blake, H., Gerard, R.W. [B 47] 1002, *1071*
Blake, H., Gerard, R.W., Kleitman, N. [B 48] 993, *1071*
Blakemore, C. [B 48a] 918, *1071*

Blanco, I., s. Palacios, J.M. 37, *61*
Bland, B.H., s. Andersen, P. [A 21 a] 1039, *1068*
Blankenburg, W. 673, 685, *693*
Blanksma, L.A., s. Zeller, E.A. 223, *242*
Blazek, R., s. Shaw, D.M. 110, *113*
Blessed, G., s. Perry, E.K. 67, *106*
Bleuler, E. [B 49] 961, 1024, *1071*
Bleuler, M. 551, 553, 561, 564, 566, 567, 576, 586, *603*, *604*, 642, 648, 673, 683, *693*
Blitz, J., s. Ploog, D. 384, 461, 489, *538*
Blix 908
Blizzard, R.M., s. Powell, G.F. 733, *749*
Block, J. 571, *604*
Blomquist, C., s. Cronholm, B. 327, *343*
Bloom, F.E. 32, *56*
Bloom, F.E., s. Iversen, L.L. 36, 37, *59*
Bloom, K. 518, *524*
Blumenbach, J.F. 710, *746*
Blurton Jones, N. 413, 502, *524*
Bobitt, R., s. Jensen, G.D. 489, *531*
Bobrov, A.V., s. Roitbak, A.I. 16, *62*
Bochnik, N., s. Demisch, L. 96, *101*
Bock, E., Hamberger, A. 10, 21, 22, *56*
Bock, M.H., s. Moore, M.T. 295, *311*
Böcker, F. 660, *693*
Boehncke, H., Gerhard, J. 684, *693*
Böker, W., s. Vetter, K. [V 9] 1002, *1101*
Bogacz, J., Vanzulli, A., Garcia-Austt, E. [B 50] 824, *1071*
Bohler, C.C.S.-S., s. Albeaux-Fernet, M. 663, *692*
Bojanovsky, J., Tölle, R. 287, 288, 289, *304*
Bollinelli, R., s. Planques, I. 162, *193*
Bolwig, T.G., Astrup, J., Christoffersen, G.R.J. 323, *342*
Bolwig, T.G., Hertz, M.M., Holm-Jensen, J. 323, 340, *342*
Bolwig, T.G., Hertz, M.M., Paulson, O.B., Spotoft, H., Rafaelson, O.J. 323, 340, *342*
Bolwig, T.G., Hertz, M.M., Westergaard, E. 324, *342*
Bolwig, T.G., s. Brodersen, P. 322, *342*
Boman, K.A., s. Hensel, H. [H 29, 30] 911, *1081*
Bond, E.D. 328, *342*
Bond, E.D., Morris, H.H. 328, *342*
Bond, P.A., Jenner, F.A., Sampson, G.A. 72, *100*
Bonhoeffer, K. [B 51] 905, 943, *1071*
Bone, A.H., s. Sabri, M.T. 50, *62*
Bonetti, U., Johannson, F., Knorring, L. von, Perris, C., Strandman, E. 686, *693*
Bonkálo, A., s. Grüttner, R. [G 48] 856, 993, 1003, *1080*
Bonkowski, L., Dryden, W.F. 28, *56*
Bonsall, R.W., s. Michael, R.P. 461, *536*
Bonvallet, M., Dell, P., Hiebel, C. [B 52] 979, *1071*
Bonvallet, M., s. Dell, P. [D 18, 19] 978, 979, *1074*
Bonvallet, M., s. Hugelin, A. [H 89, 90] 951, 978, *1083*
Borg, G., Diamant, L., Zotterman, Y. [B 53] 911, *1072*
Borge, G., s. Buchsbaum, M. 176, *183*
Boring, E.G. [B 54] 907, 1059, *1072*
Bork, I.I. von, s. Beek, H.H. 171, *812*
Borkowski, W., s. Holt, W.L. Jr. 320, *345*
Borlone, M., s. Lille, F. 159, *190*
Bornscheuer, B., s. Bineik, E. 287, *304*
Borteyru, J.-P., s. Lemoine, P. 673, *698*

Bos, E.R.H., s. Praag, H.M. van 227, *240*
Bosch, G. 587, *604*
Boss, B., s. Vale, W. 40, *64*
Bosse, K., s. Mueller, D. 455, *536*
Bossio, V., s. Pringle, M.L.K. 731, *750*
The Boston Collaborative Drug surveillance Program Research Group, s. Heinonen, O.P. 292, *307*
Bosworth, D.M. 223, *235*
Botez, M.I., Barbeau, S. 474, *524*
Botter, P.A., s. Verhoeven, W.M.A. 97, *108*
Boué, A., s. Boué, J.G. 649, *693*
Boué, J.G., Boué, A. 649, *693*
Bourgeois, M. 293, *304*
Bourne, H.R., Bunney, W.E., Colburn, R.W., Davis, J.M., Shaw, D.M., Coppen, A.J. 68, *100*
Bourne, R.C., s. Joseph, M.H. *59*
Boutroux, E. [B 54a, 54b] 765, *1072*
Bouvet, D., s. Javoy, F. 219, *238*
Bow, J., s. Corter, C. 720, *747*
Bowden, D., Winter, P., Ploog, D. 432, *524*
Bowden, J.W., s. Lindsley, D.B. [L 28] 983, *1089*
Bowers, C., s. Davis, H. 151, 152, *184*
Bowers, M.B. 93, *100*
Bowers, M.B., Henninger, G.R., Gerbode, F.A. 69, *100*
Bowers, M.B. Jr., Rozitis, A. 221, *235*
Bowers, M., s. Sweeny, D. 72, 73, *108*
Bowlby, J. 496, 497, 500, 502, *524*, 715, 717, 718, 725, 728, 744, 746
Bowne, G., s. Robinson, B.W. *539*
Boyd, W.D., s. Wilson, R.G. 292, *314*
Boyns, A.R., s. Wilson, R.G. 292, *314*

Bozza-Marrubini, M.L. 156, *183*
Brace, G.L. 667, *693*
Bradley, P., Fink, M. 180, *183*
Bradley, P.B. 28, *56*
Brady, J.V. [B 55, 56] 817, 955, *1072*
Brady, J.V., Schreiner, L., Geller, I., Kling, A. [B 57] *1072*
Braen, B.B., s. Ross, J.R. 722, *750*
Braestrup, C., s. Squires, R.F. 231, *241*
Bräutigam, W. 685, *693*
Brain, R. 475, 476, *524*, [B 58] 894, *1072*
Braithwaite, R.A., Gouling, R., Théanu, G., Bailey, J., Coppen, A. 246, *304*
Branchey, M.H., s. Simpson, G.M. 220, *241, 313*
Brandt, H.A., Metts, J.C., Kendrick, J.F., Fuster, B., Carney, A. 162, *183*
Brandt, Th., s. Dichgans, J. [D 30] 847, 928, *1075*
Brandt, W. 721, *746*
Brasel, J.A. 733, *746*
Brasel, J.A., s. Powell, G.F. 733, *749*
Bray, D. 9, *56*
Brazeau, W., s. Vale, W. 40, *64*
Brazier, M.A.B. 117, *183*, [B 59, 60, 60a] 982, 1039, 1048, *1072*
Brazier, M.A.B., Cobb, W.A., Fischgold, H., Gastaut, H., Gloor, P., Hess, R., Jasper, H., Loeb, C., Magnus, O., Pampiglione, G., Rémond, A., Storm van Leeuwen, W., Walter, W.G. 121, *183*
Breese, G.R., s. Schanberg, S.M. 72, *107*
Bremer, F. 126, *183*, [B 61–64] 950, 979, 983, 995, *1072*
Brennemann, J. 714, *746*
Brickner, R.M. 353, *375*, 474, *524*
Bridges, C.I., s. Marini, J.L. 271, *310*
Bridges, P.K. 670, *693*

Bridges, P.K., Goktepe, E.O. 367, *375*
Brierly, J.B., s. Meldrum, B.S. 324, *346*
Briggs, D.S., s. Brown, K.G.E. 288, *304*
Brill, H., s. Fieve, R.R. 546, *606*
Brill, N.D., Crumpton, E., Eiduson, S., Grayson, H.M., Hellman, I.I., Richards, R.A. 333, *342*
Brilmayer, H., s. Ohlmeyer, P. [O 1, 2] 996, 997, *1094*
Brinkmann, R., s. Poeppel, E. *539*
Brobeck, J.R. [B 65] 939, 1032, *1072*
Broca, P. 454, 475, *524*
Brockington, I., Crow, T.J., Johnstone, E.C., Owen, F. 570, *604*
Brodersen, P., Paulson, O.B., Bolwig, T.G., Rogon, Z.E., Rafaelsen, O.J., Lassen, N.A. 322, *342*
Brodeur, J., s. Ballantine, H.T. Jr. 361, *375*
Brodie, H.K.H., s. Goodwin, F.K. 74, *103*, 223, 229, 230, *238*
Bronfenbrenner, U. 726, 743, *746*
Bronk, D.W., s. Adrian, E.D. [A 8a] 850, *1068*
Brooks, B., Jung, R. [B 66] 918, 1032, *1072*
Brooks, G.W., s. Ravaris, C.L. 253, *312*
Brooks, H., s. McKenna, G. 317, *346*
Brooks, M., s. Pitts, F.N. 730, *749*
Brostoff, S.W., Karkhanis, Y.D., Carlo, D.J., Reuter, W., Eylar, E.H. 23, *56*
Broughton, R., s. Gastaut, H. [G 12a] *1078*
Broussot, T., s. Margat, M.-P. 292, *310*
Broverman, D.M., s. Klaiber, E.L. 663, *698*
Brown, A.C., s. Shepherd, M. 649, *702*
Brown, A.M., Stafford, R.E., Vandenberg, S.G. 691, *693*

Brown, D.G., Hullin, R.P., Roberts, J.M. 340, *342*
Brown, F. 730, *746*
Brown, G.M. 733, *746*
Brown, G.M., Seggie, J.A., Chambers, H.W., Ettigi, R.G. 81, *100*
Brown, G.M., s. Ettigi, P.G. 338, *344*
Brown, G.M., s. Lal, S. 85, *104*
Brown, J.L., s. Hunsperger, R.W. [H 95] 940, *1083*
Brown, K.G.E., McMichen, H.U.S., Briggs, D.S. 288, *304*
Brown, M., s. Vale, W. 40, *64*
Brown, M.H. 359, *375*
Brown, M.H., Lighthill, J.A. 361, *375*
Brown, R., s. Ahlenius, S. 220, 232, 233, *234*
Brown, R.A. 435, 507, 512, 515, 516, *524*
Brown, S., s. Charalampous, K.D. 93, *101*
Brown, S.L., s. Freedman, D.A. 711, 731, *747*
Brown, W.T. 295, *304*
Bruce, M., s. Hinde, R.A. 407, 496, 500, *530*
Brückel, K.W. 635, *693*
Brügger, M., s. Hess, W.R. [H 67] 937, 943, *1082*
Bruesch, S.R., Arey, L.B. [B 67] 878, 913, *1072*
Brun, R. [B 68] *1072*
Bruner, J.S. 503, *524*, [B 68a] 930, *1072*
Brunngraber, E.G. 23, *56*
Brunswick, D., s. Maany, I. 84, *104*
Brush, R., s. Rosanoff, A.J. 555, 597, 598, *613*
Brutkowski, S., Mempel, E. [B 69] 1031, *1072*
Bruun, R.D., s. Shapiro, A.K. 638, *702*
Bruun, T., s. Partanen, J.K. 599, *612*
Buchanan, E., s. Suedfeld, P. 735, 742, *751*
Bucher, V.M., s. Hunsperger, R.A. 471, *530*
Buchsbaum, M. 150, 175, *183*

Buchsbaum, M., Coursey, R.D., Murphy, D.L. 96, 100, 571, 604
Buchsbaum, M., Goodwin, F., Murphy, D., Borge, G. 176, 183
Buchsbaum, M., s. Baron, M. 271, 303
Buchsbaum, M., s. Murphy, D.L. 681, 700
Buchsbaum, M.A., Pfefferbaum, A. 175, 183
Buchsbaum, M.S., Coursey, R.D., Murphy, D.L. 681, 693
Buchsbaum, M.S., Haier, R.J., Murphy, D.L. 681, 693
Buchsbaum, M.S., s. Davis, G.C. 112, 112
Buchsbaum, M.S., s. Stoddard, F.J. 72, 108
Buck, A.R., s. Carter, C.O. 602, 604
Buck, C., Hobbs, G.E., Simpson, H., Wanklin, J.M. 577, 604
Bucy, P.C., s. Kluever, H. 453, 532, [K 25] 944, 961, 1048, 1087
Buehler, C., Hetzer, H. 415, 416, 417, 524
Bühler, K. [B 70] 789, 971, 1072
Bülow, K. [B 71] 994, 1072
Bürger, M. 634, 693
Bürki, H.R., Ruch, W., Asper, H. 214, 236
Buettner-Janusch, J. 384, 524
Buffa, P., Lacal, C.F., LoGullo, O., Pedretti, A., Armocide, C.C. 287, 304
Bullock, R.J. 298, 304
Bullock, T.H. 434, 442, 524
Bullowa, M. 503, 524
Bullowa, M., Jones, L.G., Duckert, A.R. 521, 524
Bundesminister für Jugend, Familie und Gesundheit 649, 650, 693
Bunge, R.P. 9, 10, 56
Bunney, B.S., Aghajanian, G.K. 215, 236
Bunney, B.S., Walters, J.R., Roth, R.H., Aghajanian, G.K. 211, 236
Bunney, B.S., s. Aghajanian, G.K. 211, 215, 220, 234

Bunney, G.S., s. Aghajanian, G.K. 211, 234
Bunney, W.E., Davis, J.M. 67, 100
Bunney, W.E., Goodwin, F.K., Murphy, D. 74, 101
Bunney, W.E., Murphy, D. 87, 100
Bunney, W.E., Post, R.M. 87, 100
Bunney, W.E. Jr., Post, R.M., Andersen, A.E., Kopanda, R.T. 339, 343
Bunney, W.E., s. Bourne, H.R. 68, 100
Bunney, W.E. Jr., s. Davis, G.C. 112, 112
Bunney, W.E., s. Gershon, E.S. 577, 607, 664, 696
Bunney, W.E., s. Goodwin, F.K. 74, 103, 223, 229, 230, 238
Bunney, W.E., s. Murphy, D.L. 74, 96, 105
Bunney, W.E. Jr., s. Post, R.M. 70, 75, 106
Bunney, W.E., s. Stoddard, F.J. 72, 108
Burbaeva, G.S., s. Vartanian, M.E. 681, 703
Burch 570
Burch, N.R., Nettleton, W.I., Sweeney, J., Edwards, R.J. 134, 183
Burckhardt, G. 351, 352, 375
Burdach, K.F. [B 72] 990, 994, 1072
Burden, J., s. Jones, M.T. 76, 103
Burdick, J.A., Sugerman, A.A., Goldstein, L. 136, 137, 173, 174, 183
Bureš, J., Burešová, O. [B 73] 1072
Bureš, J., s. Burešová, O. [B 74] 1073
Burešová, O., Bureš, J. [B 74] 1073
Burešová, O., s. Bureš, J. [B 73] 1072
Burg, W. van den, s. Praag, H.M. van 227, 240
Burgdorf, I., s. Desmond, M.M. 294, 305
Burgus, R., s. Vale, W. 40, 64
Burkard, W.P., s. Zeller, E.A. 223, 242

Burks, J.B., s. Rubinstein, M. 705
Burks, J.S., Walker, J.E., Rumack, B.H., Ott, J.E. 299, 304
Burlingham, D. 722, 746
Burlingham, D., Freund, A. 721, 746
Burnett, G.B., Little, S.R.C.J., Graham, N., Forrest, A.D. 253, 304
Burns, B.H., s. Coppen, A. 270, 305
Burns, D., s. Mendels, J. 74, 105
Burnstock, G. 27, 56
Burrows, G.D., s. Vohra, J. 287, 288, 313
Burrus, G., s. Morris, D.P. 567, 611
Burt, C.G., s. Hordern, A. 331, 345
Burt, D.R., Larrabee, M.G. 51, 56
Burt, D.R., s. Creese, I. 216, 217, 237
Burt, D.R., s. Snyder, S.H. 216, 217, 241
Burwell, C.S., Robin, E.D., Whaley, R.D., Bickelman, A.G. [B 75] 1016, 1073
Buser, P. 125, 183
Buser, P.A., Rougeul-Buser, A. [B 76] 1073
Busfield, B.L., Schneller, P., Capra, D. 287, 304
Buss, A.H. 684, 688, 693
Buss, A.H., Plomin, R. 669, 693
Busse, G., s. Kubicki, S. 157, 189
Buster, J.E., s. Abraham, G.E. 678, 692
Butcher, R.W., s. Robison, G.A. 26, 30, 62
Butcher, S.G., s. Andén, N.-E. 211, 212, 235
Butler, P.W.P., s. Rees, L. 85, 107
Butler, R.A. 744, 746
Buytendijk, F.J.J. [B 77, 78] 802, 808, 1073

Cabrol, G., s. Lambert, P.A. 287, 309
Cadaldo, M., s. Mendlewicz, J. 580, 583, 611

Cade, J.F. 574, *604*
Cade, R., s. Wagemaker, H. 97, *108*
Cadilhac, J., Ribstein, M. 160, *183*
Cadilhac, J., Ribstein, M., Jean, R. 160, *183*
Cadilhac, J.G., s. Liberson, W.T. 323, 326, *346*
Cadoret, R.J. 565, 577, 579, *604*
Cadoret, R.J., Cunningham, L., Loftus, R., Edwards, J. 596, *604*
Cadoret, R.J., Gath, A. 596, 600, *604*
Cadoret, R.J., s. Fowler, R.C. 558, *606*
Cadoret, R., s. Hill, S. 600, *608*
Cadoret, R.J., s. McCabe, M. 564, *611*
Cadoret, R.J., s. Tsuang, M. 564, *616*
Cadoret, R.J., s. Winokur, G. 580, 582, 600, *617*
Caine, T.M., s. Foulds, G.A. 684, *695*
Cairns, V.M., s. Hitchcook, E. 373, *376*
Cajal, S.R. y [C 1] 1026, 1037, 1038, *1073*
Caliari, B., s. Kukopulos, A. 330, *346*
Callaway, E., Jones, R.T., Layne, R.S. 175, *183*
Callaway, E., s. Jones, R.T. 175, *188*
Calne, D.B., s. Claveria, L.E. 298, *304*
Cammer, L. 586, *604*
Camp, B.W., s. Sterritt, G.M., 722, *751*
Campbell, M., Shapiro, T. 244, *304*
Campbell, M.A., s. Elston, R.C. 562, *605*
Campiche, J. 287, *304*
Camps, F.E., s. Shaw, D.M. 68, *107*
Canal, O., s. Kline, N.S. 271, *309*
Canessa, O.M., s. Lunt, G.G. 51, *60*
Caniglia, A., s. Miani, N. 21, 24, *61*
Cannon, H.E., s. Potkin, S.G. 96, *106*

Cannon, W.B. [C 2, 3] 762, 858, 863, 937, 939, *1073*
Canter, S. s. Claridge, G. 691, *694*
Cantwell, D.P. 596, *604*
Caplan, M.G. 730, *746*
Caplan, M.G., Douglas, V.J. 730, *746*
Capra, D., s. Busfield, B.L. 287, *304*
Capranica, R.R. 469, 514, *524*
Cardon, P.V., s. Pollin, W. 94, *106*
Carendente, F., s. Halberg, F. *187*
Carlisle, S., s. Ström-Olsen, R. 366, 367, *378*
Carlo, D.J., s. Brostoff, S.W. 23, *56*
Carlsson, 260
Carlsson, A. 14, 28, *56*, 198, 201, 205, 208, 210, 212, 219, 226, 229, 230, *236*, 339, *343*
Carlsson, A., Corrodi, H., Fuxe, K., Hökfelt, T. 223, *236*
Carlsson, A., Davis, J.N., Kehr, W., Lindqvist, M., Atack, C.V. 204, *236*
Carlsson, A., Engel, J., Strömbom, U., Svensson, T.H., Waldeck, B. 232, *236*
Carlsson, A., Engel, J., Svensson, T.H. 232, *236*
Carlsson, A., Lindqvist, M. 211, 212, 213, 226, 227, 232, *236*
Carlsson, A., s. Ahlenius, S. *234*
Carlsson, A., s. Almgren, O. 207, *234*
Carlsson, A., s. Andén, N.-E. 15, *55*, 201, *235*
Carlsson, A., s. Biswas, B. 220, 231, *235*
Carlsson, A., s. Cott, J. 220, *237*
Carlsson, A., s. Engel, J. 201, 232, *237*
Carlsson, A., s. Garcia-Sevilla, J.A. 200, *238*
Carlsson, A., s. Kehr, W. 215, *239*
Carlsson, A., s. Magnusson, T. 200, *239*

Carlsson, A., s. Öhman, R. 217, 218, 220, 221, *240*
Carlsson, A., s. Wålinder, J. 218, 225, 227, *242*
Carman, J., s. Bigelow, L.B. 94, *100*
Carman, J.S. 297, *304*
Carman, J.S., s. Post, R.M. 75, *106*
Carman, J.S., s. Stoddard, F.J. 72, *108*
Carmichael, E.A., s. Jung, R. [J 54] 948, *1085*
Carnaps, 910
Carney, A., s. Brandt, H.A. 162, *183*
Carney, M.W.P., Roth, M., Garside, R.F. 330, 331, *343*
Carney, M.W.P., Sheffield, B.F. 256, 257, *304*, 330, *343*
Carney, M.W.P., s. Alarcón, R. de 257, *302*
Carney, R., s. Horn, J.M. 560, *608*
Carpenter, C.R. 384, 489, *524*
Carpenter, W.T., s. Murphy, D.L. *105*
Carr, P.J., s. Beumont, P.J.V. 292, *303*
Carrera, R.N., s. Adams, H.B. 741, *745*
Carroll, B.J. 74, 77, 78, 81, *101*, 111, 112
Carroll, B.J., Curtis, G.C., Mendels, J. 338, *343*
Carroll, B.J., Curtis, G., Mendels, J., Sugerman, A. *101*
Carroll, B.J., Mendels, J. 77, 78, *101*
Carroll, B.J., Mowbray, R.M., Davies, B.M. 74, *101*
Carroll, B.J., s. Mendels, J. 84, *105*
Carter, C.O., Roberts, F.J.A., Evans, K.A., Buck, A.R. 602, *604*
Casey, D.E., Denney, D. 298, *304*
Casirola, G., s. Venezian, E.C. 292, *313*
Casler, L. 719, 723, 732, *745*, *746*
Caspar, R.C., Davis, J.M.,

Pandey, G.N., Garver, D.L., Dekirmenjian, H. 81, 84, 91, *101*
Caspari, E., s. Ehrman, L. 547, 605
Caspers, H. [C 4] 1003, *1073*
Caspers, H., Abele, G. 164, *183*
Caspers, H., Schulze, H. [C 5] 1003, *1073*
Casseday, H.J., s. Neff, W.D. 478, *536*
Cassidy, W.L., s. Ballantine, H.T. Jr. 361, *375*
Castell, R., Krohn, H., Ploog, D. 387, 388, *525*
Catell, s. Eysenck, 593
Caton, R. 147, *183*
Caul, W.F., s. Miller, R.E. 410, *536*
Cavalli-Sforza, L.L., s. Kidd, K.K. 550, 562, *609*
Caveness, W.F. [C 6] 804, 1002, *1073*
Cebiroglu, R., Sümer, E., Polvan, Ö. 590, *604*
Cervós-Navarro, J., s. Matakas, F. 323, *346*
Chabourne, M., s. Planques, I. 162, *193*
Chain, F., s. Lhermitte, F. 479, *533*
Chambers, H.W., s. Brown, G.M. 81, *100*
Chan-Wang, M., s. Seeman, P. 216, 217, *241*
Chance, M.R.A. 402, *525*
Chance, M.R.A., Jolly, C.J. 384, 494, *525*
Chanda, S.K., s. Banerjee, S.P. 88, *99*
Chandra, O., s. Schilkrut, R. 83, *107*
Chang, D., s. Magnusson, T. 200, *239*
Chang, M.M., Leeman, S.E., Niall, H.D. 39, *56*
Chang, M.M., s. Tregear, G.W. 39, *63*
Chang, P.T., s. Singer, K. 679, *702*
Chang, R.J., s. Abraham, G.E. 678, *692*
Chang-Wang, M., s. Seeman, P. 216, 217, *241*
Changeux, J.-P., Kasai, M., Lee, C.Y. 25, *56*

Chanley, J.D., s. Rosenblatt, S. 340, *347*
Chapin, H.D. 714, *746*
Chapman, C.J., s. James, N. 581, 583, *609*
Chapurt, R., s. Ross, J.R. 722, *750*
Charalampous, K.D., Brown, S. 93, *101*
Charlesworth, W.R., Kreutzer, W.R. 411, 414, 417, *525*
Charlesworth, W.R., s. Kreutzer, M.A. 417, *532*
Charriot, G., Resche-Rigon, P. *304*
Chase, G.A., s. Leonard, C.O. 602, *610*
Chase, P.M., s. Squire, L.R. 327, 328, *348*
Chase, T.N., s. Roberts, E. 199, *240*
Chatrian, G.E., Bergamini, L., Dondey, M., Klass, D.W., Lennox-Buchthal, M., Petersen, I. 121, *183*
Chaudhry, Z.A., s. Hussain, M.Z. 291, *308*
Chaulaic, J.L., s. Lambert, P.A. 287, *309*
Chau Wong, M., s. Seeman, P. 571, *614*
Cheadle, J., s. Morgan, R. 253, *311*
Checkley, S.A. 78, 80, *101*
Checkley, S.A., Crammer, J.L. 78, 80, 83, 85, *101*
Chedru, F., s. Lhermitte, F. 479, *533*
Chen, C.H., s. Man, P.L. 287, *310*
Chen, J., s. Kelly, D. 363, 365, *376*
Cheney, D.L., s. Trabucchi, M. 219, *242*
Cherry, C. [C 6a] 855, *1073*
Chesher, G.B. 232, *236*
Chesler, D., s. Kennel, J.H. 726, *748*
Chess, S., s. Thomas, A. 684, *703*
Chethick, M.S.W., s. Smith, M.A. 722, *750*
Chetwynd, J., Hartnett, O. 644, *693*
Chevalier-Skolnikoff, S. 403, 404, 446, *525*

Cheyney, D.L., s. Guidotti, A. 8, *58*
Chiba, Y., s. Halberg, F. *187*
Chien, C.-P., s. Kazamatsuri, H. 298, *309*
Chikazawa, S., s. Shimazono, Y. [S 34] 977, 1019, *1098*
Child, B., s. Leonard, C.O. 602, *610*
Child, J.P., s. Kiloh, L.G. 329, *345*
Childers, R.T. 333, 334, *343*
Chilton, B. 683, *693*
Chomsky, N. 512, *525*, *693*
Chonnechan, J., s. Ashcroft, G.W. 87, *99*
Chow, M., Souney, P. 299, *304*
Chown, B., s. Fouts, R.S. 509, *527*
Christian, S.T., s. Corbett, L. 95, *101*
Christian, W. 117, 167, *183*
Christian, W., s. Lanzinger-Rossnagel, G. 161, *190*
Christiansen, J., Squires, R.F. 216, *237*
Christiansen, K.O. 597, 598, *604*
Christiansen, K.O., s. Witkin, H.A. 677, *704*
Christmann, U., s. Matakas, F. 323, *346*
Christodoulides, H., s. Frangos, E. 297, 298, *306*
Christoffersen, G.R.J., s. Bolwig, T.G. 323, *342*
Ciaranello, R.D., s. Barchas, J.D. 550, 571, *603*
Cigánek, L. 148, 150, *183*, [C 7] 911, *1073*
Ciocco, A. 665, *693*
Ciompi, L., Müller, C. 642, *694*
Ciompi, L., s. Müller, C. 638, 641, 642, *700*
Claeys, M.M., s. Muscettola, G. 110, *113*
Claghorn, J.L., s. Desmond, M.M. 294, *305*
Clancy, H., McBride, G. 722, *746*, *747*
Clancy, J., s. Miller, D.H. 333, *347*
Clancy, J., s. Morrison, J. 586, *611*

Clancy, J., s. Winokur, G. 553, 564, *617*
Clancy, K., Gove, W. 651, *694*
Clanon, T.L., s. Tupin, J.P. 217, *313*
Clare, A. 316, *343*
Claridge, G., Canter, S., Hume, W.I. 691, *694*
Clark, D.L., s. Jones, B.C. 496, *531*
Clarke, B. 690, *694*
Claveria, L.E., Teychenne, P.F., Calne, D.B., Haskayne, L., Petrie, A., Lodge-Patch, I.C. 298, *304*
Clayton, F., s. Wilcox, B. 417, *543*
Clayton, P.L., s. Guze, S.B. 582, *607*
Clemens, J.A., s. Schaar, C.J. 220, *240*
Clement-Cormier, Y.C., Kebabian, J.W., Petzold, G.L., Greengard, P. 216, 217, *237*
Clement-Cormier, Y.C., s. Kebabian, J.W. 30, *59*
Clemente, C.D., Sterman, M.B. [C 8] *1073*
Clemente, C.D. s. Green, J.D. [G 40] 978, *1079*
Cleveland, S.E., Reitman, E.E., Bentinck, C. 741, *747*
Cloninger, C.R., Reich, T., Guze, S.B. 594, 595, *604*, 639, *694*
Cloninger, C.R., s. Reich, T. 550, 561, 600, *613*
Closs, C., s. Kempe, P. 739, *748*
Clouet, D.H., Richter, D. 49, *56*
Clouse, R., s. Berrettini, W.H. 570, *603*
Clyde, D., s. Fink, M. 172, *186*
Cobb, W.A., Duijn, H. van 133, *183*
Cobb, W.A., s. Brazier, M.A.B. 121, *183*
Coceani, F. 19, 32, 38, *56*
Cochran, E., Robins, E., Gorte, S. 67, 68, *101*
Cocks, W.A., s. Balázs, R. 50, *55*

Cohen, B., s. Purpura, D.P. [P 37] *1096*
Cohen, D.J., Dibble, E., Grawe, J.M., Pollin, W. 549, *604*
Cohen, E.L., s. Wurtman, R.J. 71, *109*
Cohen, J. 153, 175, *183*
Cohen, L., s. Smith, D.B.D. 151, *194*
Cohen, L.D., s. Cooper, G.D. 740, *747*
Cohen, M., s. Gershon, E.S. 579, *607*
Cohen, M., s. Leach, B.E. 96, *104*
Cohen, N.H., s. Cohen, W.J. 274, *305*
Cohen, R. 175, *183*
Cohen, S., s. Belmaker, R. 557, *603*
Cohen, S., s. Wyatt, R.J. 570, *617*
Cohen, W.J., Cohen, N.H. 274, *305*
Cohn, C.K., s. Dunner, D.L. 93, *102*, 580, 582, *605*
Cohn, P., Gaitonde, M.K., Richter, D. 49, *56*
Cohn, P., s. Richter, D. 15, *62*
Colburn, R.W., s. Bourne, H.R. 68, *100*
Cole, E.N., s. Wilson, R.G. 292, *314*
Cole, J.O., s. Kazamatsuri, H. 298, *309*
Cole, J.O., s. Klett, C.J. 257, *309*
Cole, J.O., s. Kline, N.S. 94, 97, *104*
Cole, J.O., s. Orlov, P. 257, *311*
Cole, J.O., s. Schildkraut, J.J. 72, *107*
Coleman, R.W., Provence, S. 722, *747*
Collins, G.H. s. Adams, R.D. [A 1] 1046, 1047, *1068*
Collins, M.L., s. Suomi, S.J. 496, *542*
Collins, N. 726, *747*
Collomb, H. s. Gastaut, H. [G 10a] 1018, *1078*
Colony, H.S., Willis, S.E. 171, 172, *184*

Comenius, J.A. 710, *747*
Comer, N.L., Madow, L., Dixon, J.J. 736, *747*
Condon, W.S., Sander, L.W. 517, *525*
Connecticut Lobotomy Committee 375
Conner, E., s. Mangold, R. [M 22] 1007, *1091*
Conrad, K. 475, *525*, 626, 666, 667, 671, *694*, [C 9–11] 789, 901, 988, 1018, 1019, *1073*
Consoli, S., s. Hecaen, H. 476, *529*
Consolo, S., s. Ladinsky, H. 219, *239*
Cook, E., s. Auchincloss, J.H., Jr. [A 36] 1016, *1069*
Cooper, B., s. Shepherd, M. 649, *702*
Cooper, F.S., s. Liberman, A.M. 438, 480, *533*
Cooper, G.D., Adams, H.B., Cohen, L.D. 740, *747*
Cooper, G.D., Adams, H.B., Dickinson, J.R., York, M.W. 742, *747*
Cooper, G.D., s. Adams, H.B. 741, 742, *745*
Cooper, R., Osselton, J.W., Shaw, J.C. 118, 140, *184*
Cooper, R., s. Walter, W.G. 152, *196*, [W 11] 1033, *1101*
Cooper, T.B., Simpson, G.M 274, *305*
Cooper, T.B., s. Kline, N.S. 97, *104*, 271, *309*
Cooper, T.B., s. Wren, J.C. 271, *314*
Cooper, W.E. 442, *525*
Cooper, W.E., s. Eimas, P.D. 442, *527*
Coppen, A. 67, *101*, 339, 340, *343*
Coppen, A., Eccleston, E.G., Peet, M. 71, *101*
Coppen, A., Ghose, K. 110, 111, *112*
Coppen, A., Noguera, R., Bailey, J., Burns, B.H., Swani, M.S., Hare, E.H., Gardner, R., Maggs, R. 270, *305*
Coppen, A., Prange, A.J., Whybrow, P.C., Noguera, R. 69, *101*

Coppen, A., Rama Rao, V.A., Ruthven, C.R.J., Goodwin, B.L., Sandler, M. 72, *101*
Coppen, A., Shaw, D.M., Farrell, J.P. 74, *101*
Coppen, A., Shaw, D.M., Herzberg, B., Maggs, R. 74, *101*
Coppen, A., s. Braithwaite, R.A. 246, *304*
Coppen, A., s. Julian, T. *697*
Coppen, A., s. Merry, J. 271, *310*
Coppen, A.J., 672, *694*
Coppen, A.J., s. Bourne, H.R. 68, *100*
Coppen, A.J., s. Kellett, J.M. 272, *309*
Corbett, L., Christian, S.T., Morin, R.D., Benington, F., Smythies, J.R. 95, *101*
Corbit, J.D., s. Eimas, P.D. 442, *527*
Cording, C., s. Emrich, H.M. 96, *102*
Corker, C.S., s. Beumont, P.J.V. 293, *303*
Corkin, S.H., s. Teuber, H.-L. 359, 362, *378*
Corletto, F., Gentilomo, A., Rosadini, G., Rossi, G., Zattoni, J. 159, *184*
Cornblatt, B., s. Erlenmeyer-Kimling, L. 566, *606*
Cornblatt, B., s. Rutschmann, J. 566, *614*
Cornelissen, G., s. Halberg, F. *187*
Cornu, F. 244, *305*
Corredor, H., s. Talairach, J. 357, *378*
Corrodi, H., Fuxe, K. 225, *327*
Corrodi, H., Hanson, L.C.F. 218, *237*
Corrodi, H., s. Andén, N.-E. 211, 212, 229, 231, *235*
Corrodi, H., s. Carlsson, A. 223, *236*
Corsini, G.U. 89, *101*
Corter, C., Bow, J. 720, *747*
Costa, E., Gessa, G.L., Sandler, M. 201, 202, 231, *237*
Costa, E., Guidotti, A., Mao, C.C. 231, *237*

Costa, E., Trabucchi, M. 97, *101*
Costa, E., s. Trabucchi, M. 219, *242*
Costa, E., s. Zivkovic, B. 213, *242*
Costa, J.L., s. Murphy, D.L. 681, *700*
Costa, L.D., s. Vaughan, H.G. 154, *195*
Costain, D.W., s. Grahame-Smith, D.G. 339, *344*
Cotman, C.W. 13, *56*
Cott, J., Carlsson, A., Engel, J., Lindqvist, M. 220, *237*
Count, E.W. 380, *525*, 625, 633, *694*
Coursey, R.D., s. Buchsbaum, M. 96, *100*, 571, *604*, 681, *693*
Cowburn, D.A., s. Karlin, A. 25, *59*
Cowie, V.A., s. Slater, E. 546, 553, *615*
Coyle, J.T., Snyder, S.H. 31, *56*
Craig, W. [C 12] 801, *1073*
Craik, K.J.W. [C 13] 848, 867, 929, 969, 1038, *1073*
Cramer, F.J., s. Azima, H. 740, 745, *746*
Crammer, J.L., s. Checkley, S.A. 78, 80, 83, 85, *101*
Cramon, D. von, s. Poeppel, E. 448, *539*
Cramon, E., s. Poeppel, E. *539*
Cranach, M. von 380, 402, 446, *525*
Cranach, M. von, Vine, J. 402, *525*
Crawford, R., Forrest, A. 258, *305*
Crawford, T.B.B., s. Ashcroft, G.W. 69, 87, *99*, 339, *342*
Creed, R.S., Denny-Brown, D., Eccles, J.C., Liddell, E.G.T., Sherrington, C.S. [C 14] 822, *1073*
Creese, I., Burt, D.R., Snyder, S.H. 216, 217, *237*
Creese, I., s. Snyder, S.H. 216, 217, *241*
Cremer, J.E., s. Balázs, R. 8, 47, *55*
Cremerius, J., Jung, R. 163, *184*, [C 14a] 1018, *1073*

Creutzfeldt, O., Akimoto, H. [C 15] 936, *1073*
Creutzfeldt, O., Jung, R. [C 16] 1004, *1073*
Creutzfeldt, O., Kasamatsu, A., Vaz-Ferreira, A. [C 17] 982, *1073*
Creutzfeldt, O.D., Nothdurft, H.C. [C 18] 920, *1073*
Creutzfeldt, O. s. Akimoto, H. [A 17] 936, *1068*
Creutzfeldt, O. s. Baumgartner, G. [B 17] 922, 982, *1070*
Creutzfeldt, O., s. Jung, R. [J 55] 982, 1005, *1086*
Creutzfeldt, O., s. Weinmann, H. 150, *196*
Crews, F.T., Smith, C.B. 88, *101*
Criscuoli, P.M. 289, *305*
Crisp, A.H., Kalucy, R.S., Lacey, J.H., Harding, B. 651, *694*
Critchley, M. 736, *747*, [C 19] 1017, *1073*
Crombach, G., Berthold, A., Benkert, O., Matussek, N. 71, *101*
Cronholm, B., Blomquist, C. 327, *343*
Cronholm, B., Ottosson, J.-O. 318, 320, 325, 326, 328, *343*
Cronholm, B., Ottosson, J.-O., Schalling, D. 326, *343*
Cronholm, B., s. Åsberg, M. 69, 99, 246, *303*
Cronholm, B., s. Molander, L. 327, *343*
Cronholm, B., s. Träskman, L. 109, 110, *113*
Crook, J.H., s. Michael, R.P. 381, *536*
Cross, A.J., Crow, T.J., Longden, A., Owen, F., Poulter, M., Riley, G.J. 112, *112*
Cross, A.J., s. Owen, F. 91, *105*
Cross, L.A., s. Offord, D.R. 567, *612*
Crow, T.J., s. Baker, J.M.H. 92, *99*
Crow, T.J., s. Brockington, I. 570, *604*

Crow, T.J., s. Cross, A.J. 112, *112*
Crow, T.J., s. Owen, F. 91, *105*
Crowe, R., s. Morrison, J. 586, *611*
Crowe, R., s. Winokur, G. 553, 564, *617*
Crowe, R.R. 598, *604*
Crowe, R.R., s. Winokur, G. 639, *704*
Crowell, J., s. Van Harreveld, A. 16, *64*
Crumpton, E., s. Brill, N.D. 333, *342*
Cruz, F.F. de la, s. Koch, R. 673, *698*
Cruz, F. de la, s. Lubs, H.A. 601, *610*
Csanaky, A., s. Lisák, K. [L 30] 1031, *1089*
Cuculic, Z., s. Simpson, G.M. 330, 331, *348*
Cumming, E., s. Miller, D.H. 333, *347*
Cunningham, L., s. Cadoret, R.J. 596, *604*
Cunningham, M.R., s. Rosenblatt, P.C. 647, 648, *701*
Curnow, R.N., Smith, C. 562, *604*
Currah, J., s. Kolvin, I. 596, *610*
Curran, D.J., Nagaswami, S., Mohan, K.J. 298, *305*
Curran, J.P. 298, *305*
Curtis, D.R., Game, C.J.A., Lodge, D. 37, *56*
Curtis, D.R., Johnston, G.A.R. 36, *56*
Curtis, D.R., Watkins, J.C. 25, *56*
Curtis, G., s. Carroll, B.J. *101*
Curtis, G.C., Zuckerman, M.A. 735, *747*
Curtis, G.C., s. Carroll, B.J. 338, *343*
Curtis, J., s. Hellmann, L. 77, *103*
Curtiss, S. 523, 525, [C 20] 896, 897, *1073*
Curtiss, S., Fromkin, V., Krashen, S., Rigler, D., Rigler, M. [C 21] 896, 897, *1073*
Curtius, F. 622, 625, 627, 691, *694*

Cutler, R.W.P., s. Korobkin, R.K. 46, *59*
Czernik, A. 78, 79, 81, 82, 86, *101*
Czerny, A. 714, *747*

Dackis, C., s. Sullivan, J. 681, *702*
Da Fonseca, J.S., s. Jung, R. [J 59] 880, 1035, 1036, 1037, *1086*
Dahl, V. 587, 588, 590, *604*
Dahlström, A., Fuxe, K. 15, *57*
Dahlström, A., s. Andén, N.-E. 201, *234*
Dahlström, A., s. Jackson, D.M. 211, *238*
Dahme, B., Achilles, I., Flemming, B., Götze, P., Haag, A., Huse-Klein-Stoll, G., Meffert, J., Polonius, J., Rosewald, G., Speidel, H. 552, *604*
Dahme, B., s. Huse-Kleinstoll, G. 552, *608*
Dalen, J., s. McKenna, G. 317, *346*
Dalén, P. 562, 572, 573, *605*
Dalgard, O.S., Kringlen, E. 596, 597, *605*
Dalle Ore, G., s. Terzian, H. [T 1a] 944, 1049, *1100*
Dalton, R., s. Fleminger, J.J. 682, *695*
Daly, R., s. Sato, S. 298, *312*
D'Andrade, R.G. 648, *694*
Daniel, P.M., Love, E.R., Moorhouse, S.R., Pratt, O.E. 51, *57*
Daniels, J.C., Shokroverty, S., Barron, K. 158, *184*
Danon, A., s. Ben-David, M. 292, *303*
Da Prada, M., Pletscher, A. 212, *237*
Darrusio, J., s. Planques, I. 162, *193*
Darwin, C. 389, 401, 406, 410, 413, 414, 417, 418, 420, 423, 513, *525* [D 1, 2] 803, 808, 947, 948, 965, *1074*
Das, K., s. Ulett, G. *195*
Dashiell, J.F. [D 3] 782, 903, *1074*

Dauner, I., s. Remschmidt, H. 590, *613*
Davenport, R.K., Rogers, M.R., Rumbaugh, D.M. 501, *525*
David, A.R., s. Mandel, P. 12, *60*
David, G.B. 15, *57*
David, M., s. Talairach, J. 356, 357, *378*
Davidson, E.M., s. Goldberg, S.C. 664, *696*
Davidson, J.T., s. Biedermann, J. 92, *100*
Davies, B.M., s. Carroll, B.J. 74, *101*
Davies, E., s. Bailey, H.R. 357, *375*
Davies, R.K., Detre, T.P., Egger, M.D., Tucker, G.J., Wyman, R.J. 318, *343*
Davis, D., s. Ulett, G. *195*
Davis, G.C., Buchsbaum, M.S., Bunney, W.E. Jr. 112, *112*
Davis, H. 147, *184*
Davis, H., Davis, P.A., Loomis, A.L., Harvey, E.N., Hobart., G. [D 4–6] 999, 1002, 1007, 1008, 1009, *1074*
Davis, H., Yoshie, N. 151, *184*
Davis, H., Zerlin, S., Bowers, C., Spoor, A. 151, 152, *184*
Davis, H., s. Davis, P.A. 155, 171, 172, *184*
Davis, H. s. Gibbs, F.A. [G 21] 763, 982, 983, 998, *1079*
Davis, J.M. 75, *101*
Davis, J.M., Janowsky, D.S. 91, *101*
Davis, J.M., s. Bourne, H.R. 68, *100*
Davis, J.M., s. Bunney, W.E. 67, *100*
Davis, J.M., s. Caspar, R.C. 81, 84, 91, *101*
Davis, J.M., s. Dorus, E. 583, *605*
Davis, J.M., s. Fann, W.E. 297, *305*
Davis, J.M., s. Garver, D.L. 338, *344*
Davis, J.M., s. Klein, D.F. 221, *239*

Davis, J.M., s. McKinney, W.T. 500, *535*
Davis, J.M., s. Pandey, G.N. 91, 92, *105*
Davis, J.M., s. Smith, R.C. 92, *108*, 221, *241*
Davis, J.N., Lefkowitz, R.J. 26, 30, *57*
Davis, J.N., s. Carlsson, A. 204, *236*
Davis, K., s. Shopsin, B. 72, *107*
Davis, K.L., Hollister, L.E., Berger, P.A. 220, *237*
Davis, K.L., s. Hollister, L.E. 72, *103*
Davis, K.L., s. Kendler, K.S. 85, *103*
Davis, L.G., s. Volavka, J. 112, *113*
Davis, P.A. 171, 176, *184*
Davis, P.A., Davis, H. 155, 171, 172, *184*
Davis, P.A. s. Davis, H. [D 4–6] 999, 1002, 1007, 1008, 1009, *1074*
Davis, R.T., 384, 505, *525*
Davis, S., s. Itil, T.M. 173, 174, 177, *188*
Davison, A.N. 19, *57*
Davison, A.N., s. Sabri, M.T. 50, *62*
Davison, A.N., s. Spohn, M. 11, *63*
Davison, K. 601, *605*
Davison, K., Bagley, C.R. 551, 564, *605*
Dawson, G.D. 147, 148, 152, *184*, [D 7, 8] 882, 911, *1074*
Dawson, G.D., Scott, J.W. [D 9] 910, 911, *1074*
Dawson, R.M.C. 19, *57*
Dawson, R.M.C., Richter, D. 51, *57*
Dawson, R.M.C., s. Richter, D. 53, *62*
Dawson, R.M.C., s. Wood, J.G. 23, 24, *64*
Day, E.D., s. Appel, S.H. 10, 11, 13, 14, *55*
Dearden, R., s. Stacey, M. 729, *750*
DeBauche, B.A., s. Gershon, E.S. 577, *607*
Debus, G. 247, *305*
Debus, G., s. Janke, W. 247, *308*

Deck, J.H.N., s. Farley, I.J. 93, *102*
Deck, J.H.N., s. Lloyd, K.G. 68, *104*
Deckard, B.S., s. Jarvik, L.F. 577, *609*
Deecke, L., Becker, W., Grözinger, B., Scheid, P., Kornhuber, H. 153, *184*
Deecke, L., Scheid, P., Kornhuber, H.H, [D 10] 832, 834, *1074*
Deecke, L., s. Kornhuber, H.H. 153, *189* [K 43] 789, 831, 832, 833, 834, 848, 882, 1002, 1035, *1087*
Deegener, G. 682, *694*
DeFries, J.C., s. McClearn, G.E. 547, *611*
Degkwitz, R. 244, *305*
Degkwitz, R., Helmchen, H., Kockott, G., Mombour, W. 649, 653, *694*
Deguchi, T., s. Barchas, J.D. 550, 571, *603*
Deisenhammer, E., s. Allahyari, H. 164, *182*
Dekirmenjian, H., s. Caspar, R.C. 81, 84, 91, *101*
Dekirmenjian, H., s. Garver, D.L. 81, 82, 83, *102*, 338, *344*
Dekirmenjian, H., s. Jones, F.D. 72, *103*
Dekirmenjian, H., s. Maas, J.W. 72, *104*
De Kloet, R., s. McEwen, B.S. 26, *60*
Delachaux, A., s. Müller, C. 638, 641, 642, *700*
Delafresnaye, J.F. [D 11] 882, *1074*
Delattre, L.D., s. Libet, B. [L 21] 886, *1089*
Delbrück, H. 680, *694*
Delay, J., Deniker, O. 209, *237*
Deleon-Jones, F., s. Garver, D.L. 81, 82, 83, *102*
Delgado, J.M.R. 482, 486, *525*, [D 12–14] 819, 820, 942, *1074*
Delgado, J.M.R., Hamlin, H. [D 15] 886, *1074*
Delgado, J.M.R., Mir, D. 482, *526*
Delgado, J.M.R., Obrador,

S., Martin-Rodriguez, J.G. 359, *375*
Delgado, J.M.R., s. Mahl, G.F. [M 21] 887, *1091*
Delgado, J.M.R., s. Rosvold, H.E. [R 29] *1097*
D'Elia, G. 318, 321, 327, 337, *343*
D'Elia, G., Fredriksen, S.-O. 316, 336, *343*
D'Elia, G., Laurell, B., Perris, C. 176, *184*
D'Elia, G., Lehmann, J., Raotma, H. 332, 341, *344*
D'Elia, G., Lorentzson, S., Raotma, H., Widepalm, K. 318, 341, *343*, 344
D'Elia, G., Perris, C. 594, *605*
D'Elia, G., Raotma, H. 319, 337, *343*
D'Elia, G., s. Arfwidsson, L. 332, *342*
Delizio, R., s. Suomi, S.J. 500, *542*
Dell, P. [D 16, 17] 838, 951, 978, 979, *1074*
Dell, P., Bonvallet, M., Hugelin, A. [D 18, 19] 978, 979, *1074*
Dell, P. s. Bonvallet, M. [B 52] 979, *1071*
Delse, F., Marsh, G., Thompson, L. 153, *184*
Dembrowski, J. [D 20] *1074*
Dement, W. [D 21–23] 991, 999, 1008, 1010, 1012, *1074*
Dement, W., Kleitman, N. [D 24, 25] 991, 992, 996, 998, 999, 1009, 1010, 1011, *1074*
Dement, W.C., s. Rechtschaffen, A. [R 7] 999, 1009, 1016, *1096*
DeMet, E.M., s. Halaris, A.E. 110, 111, *112*
Deming, W., s. Erlenmeyer-Kimling, L. *606*
Demisch, K. 677, *694*
Demisch, L., Mühlen, H. v.d., Bochnik, N., Seiler, N. 96, *101*
Dempsey, E.W., Morison, R.S. [D 26, 27] 977, *1075*
Dempsey, E.W., s. Morison, R.S. 125, *192*, [M 56] 762, 977, *1092*

Dempsey, G.M., Dunner, D.L., Fieve, R.R., Farkas, T., Wong, J. 290, *305*
Denber, H.C.B., Bird, E.G. 253, *305*
Dencker, S.J., Malm, V., Roos, B.E., Werdenius, B. 69, *102*
Denef, C.J., s. Mc.Ewen, B.S. 465, 466, *535*
Dengler, H.J., Spiegel, H.E., Titus, E.O. 223, *237*
Deniker, O., s. Delay, J. 209, *237*
Dennehy, C.M. 730, *747*
Denney, D., s. Casey, D.E. 298, *304*
Denney, D., s. Heston, L.L. 560, *608*
Denney, D.D., s. Blachly, P.H. 318, *342*
Dennis, M.G., s. Dennis, W. 410, *526*
Dennis, W., Dennis, M.G. 410, *526*
Dennis, W., s. Sayegh, Y. 732, *750*
Denniston, R.H., s. MacLean, P.D. 464, *534*
Denny-Brown, D. [D 28] 829, *1075*
Denny-Brown, D. s. Creed, R.S. [C 14] 822, *1073*
De Potter, W.P., De Schaepdryver, H., Moerman, E., Smith, A.D. 50, *57*
De Robertis, E., Fiszer De Plazas, S. 13, 25, *57*
De Robertis, E., s. Lunt, G.G. 51, *60*
Descartes, R. 791, 821, 906
De Schaepdryver, H., s. De Potter, W.P. 50, *57*
Desmedt, J. 147, *184*
Desmond, M.M., Rudolph, A.J., Hill, R.M., Claghorn, J.L., Dreessen, P.R. Burgdorf, I. 294, *305*
Desmond, M.M., s. Hill, R.M. 294, *307*
Detre, T.P., s. Davies, R.K. 318, *343*
Detre, T.P., s. Kupfer, D.J. 580, *610*
Dev, P., s. Schmitt, F.O. 5, *63*

Devarakonda, R., s. Hess, H.H. 18, *58*
DeVore, I. 384, 494, *526*
DeWied, D. 485, *526*
Diakow, C., s. Pfaff, D. 466, 467, *537*
Diakow, C., s. Pfaff, D.W. 466, 467, 468, *538*
Diamant, L. s. Borg, G. [B 53] 911, *1072*
Diamond, I.T., s. Neff, W.D. 478, *536*
Diamond, L.S., Marks, J.D. 253, *305*
Diamond, M.C., s. Bennett, E.L. 49, *56*
Dibbern, H., s. Wiedemann, H.-R. 627, 673, 674, *704*
Dibble, E., s. Cohen, D.J. 549, *604*
Dicara, L.V. 453, *526*
Dichgans, J., Bizzi, E., Morasso, P., Tagliasco, V. [D 29] 826, *1075*
Dichgans, J., Brandt, Th. [D 30] 847, 928, *1075*
Dichgans, J., Jung, R. [D 31] 782, 847, 860, *1075*
Dick, P. 257, 258, *305*
Dickinson, J.R., s. Cooper, G.D. 742, *747*
Diebold, K. 551, 576, *605*, 681, *694*
Diebold, K., Arnold, E., Pfaff, W. 566, *605*, 649, *694*
Dieckmann, G., Hassler, R., 370, 371, *375*, 455, 457, *526*
Dieckmann, G., s. Hassler, R. 372, *375*
Diener, E., s. Sarason, I.G. 691, *701*
Dieterle, D., s. Nedopil, N. 97, *105*
Dietrich, H. 684, *694*
Dietsch, G. 133, 134, *184*
Dietz, V., s. Jung, R. [J 56, 57] 777, 822, 835, 836, 840, 848, *1086*
Digiacomo, J., s. Mendels, J. 263, *310*
Dilling, H., Weyerer, S. 651, 652, 660, 661, *694*
Dillon, W.S., s. Eisenberg, J.F. 381, *527*
Dimascio, A., s. Agulnik, P.L., 272, *302*

Dimascio, A., s. Orlov, P. 257, *311*
Dimascio, A., s. Shader, R.I. 292, 293, *312*
DiMascio, A., s. Sovner, R. 664, *702*
Dingell, J.V., s. Stawarz, R.J. 213, *241*
Dingell, J.V., s. Vetulani, J. 88, *108*
Dinkelkamp, T., s. Angst, J. 244, *302*
Dittmar, F., s. Doerr, P. 672, 683, *694*
Dittmer, T., s. Loosen, P. 72, *104*
Dittmer, T., s. Matussek, N. 72, 85, *104*
Dittrich, A. 247, *305*
Dixon, J.J., s. Comer, N.L. 736, *747*
Dixon, W.J., s. May, P.R.A. 333, *346*
Djenderedjian, A.H., s. Akiskal, H.S. 582, *602*
Doane, B., s. Jasper, H. [J 11] 880, 929, 1031, 1036, *1084*
Doane, B., s. Ricci, G. [R 14] 817, 1028, 1031, 1036, *1096*
Dodge, H.W. Jr. s. Bickford, R.G. [B 43] 886, *1071*
Dodinval, P. 602, *605*
Doehl, J. 506, 513, *526*
Doehl, J., Podolczak, D. 506, *526*
Dörhöfer, G., s. Faigle, J.W. 292, *305*
Doering, W. 676, 677, *694*
Doerr, P., Kockott, G., Vogt, H.J., Pirke, K.M., Dittmar, F. 672, 683, *694*
Doerr, P., Pirke, K.M., Kockott, G., Dittmar, F. 672, 683, *694*
Dohrenwend, B.S., s. Dohrenwend, B.P. 649, 651, 661, *694*
Dohrenwend, B.P., Dohrenwend, B.S. 649, 651, 661, *694*
Dolan, A.B., s. Matheny, A.P. 549, *610*
Dolce, G., Künkel, H. 133, *184*

Doll, R., s. Armstrong, B. 292, *303*
Dols, L.C.W., s. Praag, H.M. van 227, *240*
Domanowsky, K., s. Wieser, S. [W 26] 950, *1102*
Domek, C.J., s. Suomi, S.J. 498, *542*
Dominic, J.A., s. Barchas, J.D. 550, 571, *603*
Donchin, E. 152, *184*
Donchin, E., Lindsley, D.B. 147, 153, 175, *184*
Donchin, E., s. Smith, D.B.D. 151, *194*
Dondey, M., s. Chatrian, G.E. 121, *183*
Doner, S.M., s. Hill, S. 600, *608*
Dongier, M. 175, *184*
Dongier, M., Dubrowsky, B., Garcia-Rill, E. 175, *184*
Dongier, S. 170, 171, 175, *184*
Dongier, S. s. Gastaut, H.A. [G 11] 1028, 1031, 1032, *1078*
Donhoffer, H. s. Grastyan, E. [G 38] 1031, *1079*
Donnelly, C.H., s. Wyatt, R.J. 570, *617*
Donoso, A.P., s. McCann, S.M. 220, *239*
Donoso, M., s. Hernández-Peón, R. [H 37] 824, *1081*
Dore, J. 516, *526*
Dornbusch, R., Williams, M. 318, 327, *344*
Dornbush, R., s. Volavka, J. 322, *349*
Dorus, E., Pandey, G.N., Davis, J.M. 583, *605*
Dorus, E., Pandey, G.N., Frazer, A. Mendels, J. 583, *605*
Dorzab, J., s. Winokur, G. 580, 582, 600, *617*
Doteuchi, M., s. Guidotti, A. 8, *58*
Doty, R.W. [D 32, 33] 884, *1075*
Doty, R.W., Rutleg de, L.T. [D 34] 884, *1075*
Douglas, J.W.B. 732, 733, *747*

Douglas, J.W.B., Turner, R.K. 733, *747*
Douglas, V.J., s. Caplan, M.G. 730, *746*
Dow, R.C., s. Ashcroft, G.W. 70, *99*
Dow, R.S., Ulett, G., Raaf, J. 163, *185*
Dowdall, M.J., s. Whittaker, V.P. 13, 28, *64*
Dowling, J.E., s. Poeppel, E. 479, *539*
Dowling, J.L., s. Bailey, H.R. 357, *375*
Downham, D.Y., s. Adelstein, A.M. 661, 663, *692*
Doyle, L.N. 263, *305*
Drachman, D.B., Gumnit, R.J. [D 35] 1016, *1075*
Dransfeld, L. s. Gänshirt, H. [G 1] 982, *1078*
Draper, G. 626, 648, *694*
Dreessen, P.R., s. Desmond, M.M. 294, *305*
Dreifuss, J.J., s. Gloor, P. 458, *528*
Dreyer, R. 168, *185*
Dreyfus-Brisac, C., Fischgold, H. [D 36] 1002, *1075*
Dreyfuss, F.E., s. Penry, J.K. 166, *192*
Driollet, R., s. Schvarcz, J.R. 369, *377*
Drohocki, Z. 134, 135, 146, 173, *185*
Droogleever-Fortuyn, J., s. Jasper, H.H. [J 10] 978, *1084*
Droz, B. 14, *57*
Druschky, K.F. 664, 681, *694*
Druschky, K.F., s. Flügel, K.A. 160, *186*
Dryden, W.F., s. Bonkowski, L. 28, *56*
Dua, S. s. Anand, B.K. [A 21] 939, 1032, *1068*
Dua, S., s. MacLean, P.D. 464, *534*
Dubcovich, M.L., Langer, S.Z. 28, *57*
Dubois, E.L., Tallman, E., Wonka, R.A. 292, *305*
Dubois-Reymond, 908
Dubrowsky, B., s. Dongier, M. 175, *184*
Ducame, B., s. Lhermitte, F. 479, *533*

Duchane, E.M., s. McCulloch, W.S. [M 34] 853, 857, *1091*
Duckert, A.R., s. Bullowa, M. 521, *524*
Dudar, J.D. s. Andersen, P. [A 21a] 1039, *1068*
Dudley, W.H.C. Jr., Williams, J.G. 335, *344*
Duecker, G., s. Rensch, B. 506, *539*
Duensing, F. 162, *185*
Duensing, F., Schaefer, K.-P. [D 37] 823, *1075*
Duffy, T.E., s. Plum, F. 322, *347*
Duijn, H. van, s. Cobb, W.A. 133, *183*
Dumermuth, G. 117, 119, 125, 127, 160, 161, *185*
Dumermuth, G., Flühler, H. 134, *185*
Dunham, H.W. 574, *605*
Dunham, H.W., s. Faris, R.E.L. 574, *606*
Dunlon, P.T., s. Meadow, A. 253, *310*
Dunlop, C.W. s. Adey, W.R. [A 3] 1031, *1068*
Dunn, A., Giuditta, A., Wilson, J.E., Glassman, E. 341, *344*
Dunne, D., s. Valentine, M. 318, *348*
Dunner, D.L., Cohn, C.K., Gershon, E.S., Goodwin, F.K. 580, 582, *605*
Dunner, D.L., Cohn C.K., Weinsilboum, R.M., Wyatt, R.J. 93, *102*
Dunner, D.L., Fieve, R.R. 580, 581, *605*
Dunner, D.L., s. Dempsey, G.M. 290, *305*
Dunner, D.L., s. Gershon, E.S. 577, *607*
Dupont, A., s. Weeke, A. 649, 661, *704*
Durell, J., s. Greenspan, K. 72, *103*
Durfee, H., Wolf, K. 715, *747*
Durup, G., Fessard, A. [D 38] 1028, *1075*
Dusser, de Barenne, J.G., McCulloch, W.S. [D 39] 883, *1075*

Dustman, R.E., s. Lewis, E.G. 161, *190*
Dutton, G.R., s. Barondes, S.H. 20, *55*
Du Vignaud, V. 41, *57*
Duyff, J.W. s. Gerard, R.W. [G 15a] 855, *1078*
Dyke, J. van, Rosenthal, D., Rasmussen, P.V. 568, *605*
Dynes, J.B. 295, *305*

Easser, B.R., s. Lesser, S.R. 722, *749*
Eastman, R.F., Mason, W.A. 500, *526*
Eaves, L., Eysenck, H. 593, *605*
Ebara, T., s. Watanabe, S. 272, *314*
Ebbinghaus, H. [E 1] 1024, *1075*
Eberhardt, N.L., Valeana, T., Timiras, P.S. 26, *57*
Ebert, M., Kopin, J.J. 72, *102*
Ebstein, R., s. Belmaker, R.H. 570, 583, *603*
Ebstein, R., s. Biedermann, J. 92, *100*
Ebstein, R., s. Hökfelt, T. 200, *238*
Eccles, J. 155, *185*
Eccles, J.C. [E 2–5, 5a, 5b, 5c, 5d] 781, 791, 792, 793, 794, 795, 824, 844, 845, 904, 1026, 1039, 1064, *1075*
Eccles, J.C., Ito, I., Szentagothai, J. [E 6] 814, 843, 891, 897, 1039, *1075*
Eccles, J.C. s. Creed, R.S. [C 14] 822, *1073*
Eccles, J.C., s. Popper, K.R. [P 32] 779, 791, 792, 793, 794, 902, 904, 1039, *1095*
Eccleston, D., s. Ashcroft, G.W. 69, 87, *99*, 339, *342*
Eccleston, D., s. Moir, A.T.B. 71, *105*
Eccleston, E.G., s. Coppen, A. 71, *101*
Eccleston, E.G., s. Shaw, D.M. 68, *107*
Economo, C.v. [E 7, 8] 762, 977, 988, *1075*
Edelman, G.M. [E 9] 1037, 1039, *1075*

Edelstein, E.L., s. Isac, M. 288, *308*
Edén, S., Modigh, K. 325, *344*
Eden, S., Modigh, S. 88, 89, *102*
Edström, A., Mattsson, H. 5, *57*
Edwards, J., s. Cadoret, R.J. 596, *604*
Edwards, J.H. 561, *605*
Edwards, R.J., s. Burch, N.R. 134, *183*
Edwards, R.J., s. Lester, B.K. 173, *190*
Eerdewegh, M. van, s. Gershon, E.S. 577, *607*
Effendie, S., s. Hökfelt, T. 200, *238*
Efron, D.H., s. Usdin, E. 244, 255, 259, 265, 279, 282, 296, *313*
Egger, M.D., s. Davies, R.K. 318, *343*
Eggers, C. 588, 590, *605*, 632, 641, *695*
Eggers, H., Wagner, K.-D., Wigger, M. 632, *695*
Eggert-Hansen, C., s. Kragh-Sörensen, P. 330, *346*
Ehara, A., s. Kondo, S. 384, *532*
Ehrenberg, R. [E 10] 774, *1076*
Ehret, R., Schneider, E. [E 11] 958, 959, 960, *1076*
Ehrhardt, A.A., Baker, S.W. 647, 648, 678, 690, *695*
Ehrhardt, A.A., s. Money, J. 631, 643, 644, 645, 647, 648, 678, 683, 690, *700*
Ehringer, H., Hornykiewicz, O. 74, *102*
Ehrlich, Y.H., s. Volavka, J. 112, *113*
Ehrman, L., Omenn, G.S., Caspari, E. 547, *605*
Eiband, H.W. 687, 688, 689, *695*
Eibl-Eibesfeldt, I. 390, 395, 401, 402, 408, 410, 411, 414, 417, 418, 421, 425, 488, *526*, 633, *695*
Eibl-Eibesfeldt, I., Wickler, W. 395, *526*
Eibl-Eibesfeldt, I., s. Kurth, G. 381, *532*

Eichberg, J., Hauser, G., Karnovsky, M.L. 19, *57*
Eichler, W. [E 12] 774, 910, 911, *1076*
Eiduson, S., s. Brill, N.D. 333, *342*
Eiff, A.W. von 619, *695*
Eigen, M. [E 13] 1046, *1076*
Eimas, P.D. 437, 442, *526*
Eimas, P.D., Cooper, W.E., Corbit, J.D. 442, *527*
Eimas, P.D., Signeland, E.R., Jusczyk, P., Vigorito, J. 437, 440, 441, 442, *526*
Eimas, P.D., s. Miller, J.L. 442, *536*
Einstein, A. [E 14] 1058, *1076*
Eiseman, J.S., s. Siegel, G.J. 43, *63*
Eisenberg, H.M., s. Lorenzo, A.V. 324, *346*
Eisenberg, J.F., Dillon, W.S. 381, *527*
Ekman, P. 417, 418, 419, 421, 422, *527*
Ekman, P., Friesen, W.V. 413, 419, 420, 421, 438, *527*
Ekman, P., Friesen, W.V., Ellsworth, P. *527*
Elde, R., Hökfelt, T., Johannsson, O., Terenius, L. 26, 40. *57*
Elde, R., s. Hökfelt, T. 15, 40, *58*
Eleftheriou, B.E. 453, 455, *527*
Eleftheriou, B.E., Scott, J.P. 455, *527*
Eliasen, P., Andersen, M. 287, *305*
Elie, R., Morin, L., Tetreault, L. 289, *305*
Elkes, J. [E 15, 16] 783, 863, 966, *1076*
Elkes, J., s. Kety, S.S. 3, *59*
Ellgring, J.H. 402, *527*
Ellingson, R.J. 150, 171, *185*
Elliott, K.A.C., Heller, L.H. 10, *57*
Elliott, K.A.C., Page, I.K., Quastel, J.H. 3, *57*
Elliott, K.A.C., s. Bharucha, A.D. 50, *56*
Ellis, A. 690, *695*
Ellman, S., s. Hellmann, L. 77, *103*

Ellsworth, P., s. Ekman, P. 527
Elmer, E., Gregg, G. 727, 747
Elsässer, G. 586, 589, *605*, 680, *695*
Elston, R.C., Campbell, M.A. 562, *605*
Elston, R.C., s. Tanna, V.L. 582, *616*
Emerson, P.E., s. Schaffer, H.R. 719, 732, *750*
Emrich, H.M., Cording, C., Piree, S., Kölling, A., Möller, H.-J., Zerssen, D. von, Herz, A. 96, *102*
Emrich, H.M., Cording, C., Piree, A., Zerssen, D. von, Herz, A. 96, *102*
Emrich, H.M., Höllt, V., Kissling, W., Fischler, M., Laspe, H., Heinemann, H., Zerssen, D. von, Herz, A. 112, *112*
Emrich, H., s. Hippius, H. 97, *103*
Enders, P., s. Schenck, G.K. 96, *107*
Endler, N.S. 620, *695*
Endo, J., s. Endo, M. 81, *102*
Endo, M. 81, *102*
Endo, M., Endo, J., Nishikubo, M., Yamaguchi, T., Hatotani, N. 81, *102*
Endres, G., Frey, W.v. [E 17] 1014, *1076*
Endröczi, E., s. Lisák, K. [L 29 a] *1089*
Eneroth, P., s. Sedvall, G. 217, 220, 225, *241*
Engel, G.L., Romano, J. 160, *185*
Engel, G.L., Rosenbaum, M. 179, *185*
Engel, G.L., s. Romano, J. *193*
Engel, J., Carlsson, A. 201, 232, *237*
Engel, J., Liljequist, S. 232, *237*
Engel, J., Liljequist, S., Johannesen, K. 221, *237*
Engel, J., Lundborg, P. 233, *237*
Engel, J., s. Ahlenius, S. 211, 215, 218, 220, 230, 232, 233, *234*

Engel, J., s. Almgren, O. 207, *234*
Engel, J., s. Berggren, U. 228, *235*
Engel, J., s. Carlsson, A. 232, *236*
Engel, J., s. Cott, J. 220, *237*
Engel, J., s. Lundborg, P. 221, *239*
Engel, J., s. Öhman, R. 217, 218, 220, 221, *240*
Engel, R. 150, *185*
Engel, R., Halberg, F., Gurly, R. 131, *185*
Engelmann, T.G., s. Kleitman, N. [K 21] 992, *1087*
Engelmeier, H.-M., s. Schenck, G.K. 96, *107*
Engle, R.P. Jr., s. McKenna, G. 317, *346*
Engström, H. [E 18] 824, *1076*
Enterline, J.D., s. Langsley, D.G. 333, *346*
Erdelyi, E., s. Wyatt, R.J. 93, *109*
Ericksen, S., s. Pandey, G.N. 91, 92, *105*
Erickson, G., s. Forrest, F.M. 289, *306*
Erickson, M.T., s. Horn, J.M. 560, *608*
Eriksson, K. 600, *605*
Erlemeyer-Kimling, L. 552, 553, 554, 567, 568, 589, *605*, *606*
Erlenmeyer-Kimling, L., Cornblatt, B., Fleiss, J. 566, *606*
Erlenmeyer-Kimling, L., Nicol, S., Rainer, J., Deming, W. *606*
Erlenmeyer-Kimling, L., Paradowski, W. 577, *606*
Erlenmeyer-Kimling, L., Rainer, J.D., Kallman, F.J. 577, *606*
Erlenmeyer-Kimling, L., s. Rutschmann, J. 566, *614*
Ernst, C., s. Ernst, K. 565, *606*
Ernst, K. 632, 642, 659, *695*
Ernst, K., Ernst, C. 565, *606*
Ernst, K., Kind, H., Rotach-Fuchs, M. 659, *695*
Ervin, F.R., s. Mark, H. 455, *534*

Ervin, F.R., s. Mark, V.H. 372, *376*
Ervin, F., s. Stevens, J.R. 486, *542*
Erwin, T., Maple, T., Mitchel, G., Willott, T. 496, *527*
Escourolle, R., s. Lhermitte, F. 479, *533*
Esquirol, J.E.D. 686, *695*
Essen-Möller, E. 555, 556, 557, 562, 565, 566, 572, 587, *606*
Esser, A.H., s. Kline, N.S. 94, 97, *104*
Essig, C.F., Fraser, H.F. 164, *185*
Essman, W.B. 341, *344*
Essman, W.B., Nakajima, S. 51, *57*
Estess, F., s. Renaud, H. 576, *613*
Ètevenon, P. 133, *185*
Ettigi, P.G., Brown, G.M. 338, *344*
Ettigi, R.G., s. Brown, G.M. 81, *100*
Euler, C.V. [E 19] 977, *1076*
Euler, C.v., Green, J.D. [E 21] 977, *1076*
Euler, C.v., Green, J.D., Ricci, G. [E 20] 977, *1076*
Evans, J.P.M., Grahame-Smith, D.G., Green, A.R., Tordoff, A.F.C. 88, *102*, 325, 339, *344*
Evans, K.A., s. Carter, C.O. 602, *604*
Evarts, E.V. [E 22-26] 833, 844, 847, 935, 936, 1004, 1005, *1076*
Evarts, E.V., Tanji, J. [E 27] 833, 844, *1076*
Evarts, E.V., s. Kety, S.S. *189*
Everett, G.M., Toman, J.E.P. 66, *102*
Everitt, B.J., s. Fuxe, K. 34, *58*
Ewert, J.P. 484, *527*
Ewert, T., s. Schenck, G.K. 96, *107*
Exner, J.E. Jr., Murillo, L.G. 319, 333, *344*
Exner, S. [E 28, 29] 784, 785, 786, 795, 824, 974, *1076*
Eylar, E.H. 22, *57*

Eylar, E.H., s. Brostoff, S.W. 23, 56
Eymer, K.P., s. Kollmannsberger, A. 161, 189
Eysenck, Catell, 593
Eysenck, H., s. Eaves, L. 593, 605
Eysenck, H.J. 626, 670, 671, 678, 688, 695, [E 30] 1043, 1076
Eysenck, H.J., Eysenck, S.B.G. 594, 606
Eysenck, S.B.G., s. Eysenck, H.J. 594, 606

Fabre, J.H. [F 1] 812, 1076
Fahn, S. 298, 305
Fahrenberg, J. 667, 669, 695, [F 2] 780, 783, 1076
Fahy, T., s. Kay, D.W.K. 332, 345
Faigle, J.W., Dörhöfer, G. 292, 305
Fairbanks, L.A., s. McGuire, M.T. 380, 535
Falconer, D.S. 550, 606
Fang, V.S., s. Meltzer, H.Y. 221, 239
Fangel, Chr., Kaada, B.R. [F 3] 1076
Fann, W.E., Davis, J.M., Wilson, I.C. 297, 305
Fann, W.E., Sullivan, J.L. III, Miller, R.D., McKenzie, G.M. 298, 305
Fantz, R.L. 744, 747
Faris, R.E.L., Dunham, H.W. 574, 606
Farkas, T., s. Dempsey, G.M. 290, 305
Farley, I.J., Price, K.S., MacCullough, E., Deck, J.H.N., Hordynski, W., Hornykiewicz, O. 93, 102
Farley, I.J., s. Lee, T. 112, 112
Farley, I.J., s. Lloyd, K.G. 68, 104
Farley, J.D. 561, 606
Farnebo, L.-O., Hamberger, B. 216, 237
Farr, D., s. Wolpert, A. 287, 314
Farrell, J.P., s. Coppen, A. 74, 101
Fatchchand, R., s. Svaetichin, G. [S 60, 62] 787, 913, 1099
Faure, J. 160, 185
Fawcett, C.P., s. McCann, S.M. 220, 239
Fawcett, J.A., s. Jones, F.D. 72, 103
Fawcett, J.A., s. Maas, J.W. 72, 104
Fechner, G.T. [F 4] 761, 781, 782, 787, 868, 870, 907, 908, 913, 1077
Feder, H.H., Wade, G.N. 465, 527
Fedio, P., Ommaya, A.K. 359, 375
Feer, H., s. Thölen, H. 97, 108
Feinstein, B., s. Libet, B. [L 21] 886, 1089
Feldberg, W., Gupta, K.P. 38, 57
Feldberg, W., Vogt, M. 17, 57
Felder, W. 585, 606
Felder, W., s. Angst, J. 580, 603
Feldstein, S., s. Siegman, A.W. 446, 541
Feldstein, S., s. Volavka, J. 322, 349
Felger, H.L. 219, 237
Fenasse, R., Mazet, M., Serment, H. 292, 305
Fenichel, O. 684, 688, 689, 695
Ferber, A., s. Kendon, A. 398, 399, 531
Ferber, G., s. Gutjahr, L. 126, 167, 187
Ferguson, C.A. 520, 527
Ferguson, C.A., Slobin, D.I. 521, 527
Ferillo, F., Rivano, C., Rosadini G., Rossi, G.F., Turelka, C. 155, 185
Fernald, A. 520, 527
Fernandez de Molina, A., Hunsperger, R.W. 458, 527, [F 5, 6] 940, 943, 944, 1077
Fernstrom, J. 71, 102
Fernstrom, J., Wurtman, R.J. 71, 102
Fernstrom, J.D., s. Wurtman, R.J. 71, 109
Ferrier, D. [F 7] 882, 1077
Fessard, A. 126, 185
Fessard, A., Lelord, G. 175, 185
Fessard, A. s. Durup, G. [D 38] 1028, 1075
Feuerbach, A.J.P. von 710, 747
Feuerlein, W. 622, 629, 641, 653, 662, 695
Feuerlein, W., Heyse, H. 680, 695
Fewtrell, C.M.S. 26, 57
Fex, J., s. Hagbarth, K.E. [H 1] 824, 1080
Field, P.M., s. Raisman, G. 466, 539
Fieve, R.R., Rosenthal, D., Brill, H. 546, 606
Fieve, R.R., s. Dempsey, G.M. 290, 305
Fieve, R.R., s. Dunner, D.L. 580, 581, 605
Fieve, R.R., s. Mendlewicz, J. 580, 583, 611
Finance, F., s. Singer, L. 292, 313
Finch, C.E., s. Nelson, J.F. 26, 61
Fink, M. 138, 146, 179, 180, 181, 185, 334, 341, 344
Fink, M., Itil, T.M., Clyde, D. 172, 186
Fink, M., Itil, T.M., Shapiro, D. 179, 186
Fink, M., Kahn, R.L. 164, 186
Fink, M., s. Bradley, P. 180, 183
Fink, M., s. Volavka, J. 322, 349
Finke, J., Schulte, W. [F 8] 1015, 1077
Finkelstein, J., s. Sachar, E.J. 81, 107
Finkelstein, M., s. Silver, H.K. 733, 750
Finner, R.W. 321, 344
Fischbach, R. 290, 305
Fischer, B., s. Poggio, G.F. [P 28] 920, 1095
Fischer, E. 75, 102, 574, 575, 588, 606
Fischer, M. 554, 557, 576, 606
Fischer, M., Harvald, M., Hauge, M. 555, 606
Fischer, M., s. Hauge, M. 574, 608

Fischer, M., s. Leff, J.P. 661, 698
Fischer, S., s. Laska, E.M. 292, 309
Fischgold, H. [F 9, 10] 969, 988, 1077
Fischgold, H., Gastaut, H. 155, 186, [F 11] 969, 1028, 1077
Fischgold, H., Mathis, P. 155, 156, 186
Fischgold, H., Schwartz, B.A. [F 12] 948, 969, 993, 999, 1009, 1077
Fischgold, H., s. Brazier, M.A.B. 121, 183
Fischgold, H. s. Dreyfus-Brisac, C. [D 36] 1002, 1075
Fischgold, H., s. Schwartz, B.A. [S 19, 19a] 1014, 1098
Fischhoff, J., s. Whitten, C.F. 733, 751
Fischler, M., s. Emrich, H.M. 112, 112
Fish, B. 575, 588, 589, 606
Fishbein, L.L. 328, 344
Fisher, C. [F 12a] 1019, 1077
Fisher, C., s. Rechtschaffen, A. [R 7] 999, 1009, 1016, 1096
Fisher, C.H. [F 13] 996, 997, 1077
Fisher, G.H., s. Magnusson, T. 200, 239
Fister, W.P., s. Kennard, M.A. 172, 189
Fiszer De Plazas, S., s. De Robertis, E. 13, 25, 57
Fitzhugh, R. s. Barlow, H.B. [B 8b] 1070
Fjalland, B., s. Möller-Nielsen, I. 221, 240
Flanagan, N.B., s. Ballantine, H.T. Jr. 361, 375
Flätten, O. 316, 344
Fleischhauer, J. 296, 305
Fleiss, J., s. Erlenmeyer-Kimling, L. 566, 606
Fleiss, J.L., s. Mendlewicz, J. 581, 611, 664, 699
Flemenbaum, A. 271, 288, 305, 306
Fleminger, J.J., Dalton, R., Standage, K.F. 682, 695
Flemming, B., s. Dahme, B. 552, 604

Flemming, B., s. Huse-Kleinstoll, G. 552, 608
Flerkó, R., s. Szentagothai, J. [S 65] 860, 861, 939, 1100
Flexner, J.B., Flexner, L.B., Stellar, E. [F 14] 1046, 1077
Flexner, L.B. 48, 52, 57
Flexner, L.B. s. Flexner, J.B. [F 14] 1046, 1077
Fliege, K., s. Zerssen, D. von 687, 704
Flint, B. 732, 747
Floru, L. 272, 280, 295, 306
Floru, L., Floru, L., Tegeler, J. 295, 306
Floru, L., s. Floru, L. 295, 306
Floru, L., s. Haase, H.J. 253, 307
Flourens, P. [F 15] 882, 1077
Flower, R.J., Vane, J.R. 38, 57
Floyd, A., s. Gershon, S. 93, 103
Floyd, A. Jr., s. Gershon, S. 218, 238
Flügel, K.A. 160, 164, 186
Flügel, K.A., Druschky, K.F. 160, 186
Flühler, H., s. Dumermuth, G. 134, 185
Flynn, W.R. [F 16] 934, 1077
Foerster, H. [F 17] 1046, 1077
Foerster, H.v., Zopf, G.W.Jr. [F 17a] 1077
Foerster, O. [F 18] 883, 884, 1077
Foerster, O., Gagel, O. 486, 527, [F 19] 942, 1077
Foerster, O., Penfield, W. [F 20] 884, 934, 1077
Fog, R., s. Randrup, A. 75, 106
Folch-Pi, J. 3, 18, 22, 57
Folch-Pi, J., Lees, M., Sloane-Stanley, G.H. 18, 22, 58
Folch-Pi, J., Stoffyn, P. 19, 22, 57
Foley, J.M., s. Vernon, D.T.A. 729, 751
Folicaldi, G. s. Gozzano, M. [G 31] 863, 1044, 1079
Folkers, J. 714, 747

Folkers, K., s. Magnusson, T. 200, 239
Folstein, M., Folstein, S., McHugh, P.R. 330, 334, 344
Folstein, S., Rutter, M. 589, 606
Folstein, S., s. Folstein, M. 330, 334, 344
Foltz, E.L., White, L.E. 359, 375
Fonseca, J.S., s. Kornhuber, H.H. [K 44] 1036, 1088
Fontana, A. s. Gozzano, M. [G 31] 863, 1044, 1079
Fontana, F. [F 21] 995, 1077
Foote, W., s. Stevens, J. 94, 108
Foote, W.E., s. Aghajanian, G.K. 229, 234
Ford, C.S., Beach, F.A. 622, 695
Forel, A. [F 22] 812, 1077
Forrest, A., Affleck, J. 553, 606
Forrest, A., s. Crawford, R. 258, 305
Forrest, A.D., s. Burnett, G.B. 253, 304
Forrest, A.D., s. Fotherby, K. 69, 102
Forrest, A.D., s. Smith, C. 562, 615
Forrest, A.P.M., s. Wilson, R.G. 292, 314
Forrest, F.M., Snow, H.L. 289, 306
Forrest, F.M., Snow, H.L., Erickson, G., Geiter, C.W., Laxson, G.O. 289, 306
Forsdal, A., s. Andersen, T. 587, 603
Forsman, A. 237
Forsman, A., Öhman, R. 217, 237
Forsman, A., Mårtensson, E., Nyberg, G., Öhman, R. 217, 237
Forssman, H. 337, 344
Fossum, A., s. Astrup, C. 685, 692
Fosvig, L., s. Krogh, H.J. 164, 189
Fotherby, K., Ashcroft, G.W., Affleck, J.W., Forrest, A.D. 69, 102

Fothergrill, L.A., s. Hughes, J. 40, *58*
Foulds, G.A., Caine, T.M., Adams, A., Owen, A. 684, *695*
Fouts, R.S. 507, *527*
Fouts, R.S., Chown, B., Goodin, L. 509, *527*
Fowler, R.C., Tsuang, M.T., Cadoret, R.J., Monelly, E. 558, *606*
Fowler, R.C., s. McCabe, M. 564, *611*
Fowler, R.C., s. Tsuang, M. 564, *616*
Fowler, W. 731, *747*
Fox, M.W. 634, *695*
Fraiberg, S. 722, *747*
Fraiberg, S., s. Adelson, E. 722, *745*
Frances, H., Puech, A., Simon, P. 89, *102*
Frances, H., s. Jouvent, R. 89, *103*
Francis, A., s. Blazek, R. 71
Frangos, E., Christodoulides, H. 297, *298, 306*
Frank, H., s. Steinbuch, K. [S 48] 853, 857, 865, 872, 975, 976, *1099*
Frankl, V.E. [F 23] *1077*
Franks, V., s. Gomberg, E.S. 705
Frantz, A.G., Zimmerman, E.A. 42, *58*
Fraser, H., s. Hökfelt, T. 200, *238*
Fraser, H.F., s. Essig, C.F. 164, *185*
Fraser, H.F., s. Wikler, A. 164, *196*
Frazer, A., Mendels, J. 88, *102*
Frazer, A., s. Dorus, E. 583, *605*
Frazer, A., s. Maany, I. 84, *104*
Frazer, A., s. Mendels, J. 74, 84, *105*
Frederiksen, P.K. 94, *102*, 220, *237*
Fredriksen, S.-O., s. D'Elia, G. 316, 336, *343*
Freedman, D.A. 711, 725, 731, *747*
Freedman, D.A., Brown, S.L. 711, 731, *747*

Freedman, D.G. 410, 415, 502, *527*, 549, *606*, 722, *747*
Freedman, L.S., s. Shopsin, B. 93, *107*
Freeman, W., Watts, J. 354
Freeman, W.J. [F 24–26] 950, *1077*
Frei, D., s. Jones, B.C. 396, *531*
Fremming, K.H., s. Møller, S.E. 71, *105*
Freud, A. [F 27] 940, *1077*
Freud, A., s. Burlingham, D. 721, *746*
Freud, S. 198, *237,238*, 401, 496, *527, 528*, 671, 682, 683, *695*, [F 28–30] 784, 785, 791, 795, 831, 940, 962, 964, 999, 1013, 1018, *1077*
Freud, W. 714, *747*
Freund, K., s. Kolářský, A. 683, 690, *698*
Frey 908
Frey, H.H., s. Kilian, M. 202, *239*
Frey, R. 578, *607*, 686, 687, *695*
Frey, R., s. Angst, J. 264, *302*, 580, *603*
Frey, W.v. s. Endres, G. [E 17] 1014, *1076*
Friedel, R.O., s. Bielski, R.J. 245, *304*, 331, *342*
Friedenberg, P., s. Meier-Ewert, K. 291, *310*
Friedhoff, A.J. 95, *102*
Friedhoff, A.J., Winkle, E. 95, *102*
Friedman, E., s. Shopsin, B.S. 227, *241*
Friedman, R.C., Richart, R.M., Van de Wiele, R.L. 465, *528*
Friesen, H.G., s. Beumont, P.J.V. 292, 293, *303, 304*
Friesen, W.V., s. Ekman, P. 413, 419, 420, 421, 438, *527*
Frisch, K.v. [F 31, 31a] 803, 928, 965, *1077, 1078*
Frische, M., s. Beckmann, H. 94, *100*
Fritsch, G., Hitzig, E. [F 32] 883, 889, *1078*
Fritsch, W. 685, *695*
Froesch, E.R., Assal, J.P. 627, *695*
Frohman, C.E. 96, *102*

Frolov, V.P. [F 33] *1078*
Fromkin, V. s. Curtiss, S. [C 21] 896, 897, *1073*
Frommer, E.A., s. Mendelson, W.B. 590, *611*
Frost, I., s. Lancaster, N. 337, *346*
Frühmann, E. s. Birkmayer, W. [B 44a] *1071*
Fruhstorfer, H., Soveri, P., Järvilehto, T. 152, *186*
Fry, D.B. 438, *528*
Fünfgeld, E.W. 162, *186*
Fuhrmann, W., Vogel. F. 602, *607*, 632, *696*
Fujita, K., Ito, T., Maruta, K., Teradaira, R., Beppu, H., Nakagami, Y., Nagatsu, T., Kato, T. 93, *102*
Fukuda, T., s. Mitsuda, H. 553, *611*
Fulker, D.W. 550, *607*
Fuller, J.L., s. Scott, J.P. 488, *540*
Fulton, Jacobsen, 353
Fulton, J.F. 353, 355, *375*, [F 34] 880, *1078*
Funkenstein, H.H., s. Winter, P. 481, *544*
Furst, S., s. Lajtha, A. 49, *60*
Fushukima, D.K., s. Hellmannn, L. 77, *103*
Fuster, B., s. Brandt, H.A. 162, *183*
Fuxe, K., Everitt, B.J., Agnati, L., Jonsson, G. 34, *58*
Fuxe, K., Ögren, S.-O., Aganati, L., Gustafsson, J.K., Jonsson, G. 110, *112*
Fuxe, K., Sjöqvist, F. 202, *238*
Fuxe, K., s. Andén, N.-E. 201, 211, 212, 229, 231, *234, 235*
Fuxe, K., s. Carlsson, A. 223, *236*
Fuxe, K., s. Corrodi, H. 225, *237*
Fuxe, K., s. Dahlström, A. 15, *57*
Fuxe, K., s. Hökfelt, T. 200, *238*
Fyrö, B., s. Sedvall, G. 217, 220, 225, *241*

Gabriel, E., s. Schuster, P. *312*

Gadea-Ciria, M., s. Bartholini, G. 212, 213, 216, *235*
Gadea-Ciria, M., s. Stadler, H. 30, *63*, 219, *241*
Gänshirt, H., Dransfeld, L., Zylka, W. [G 1] 982, *1078*
Gagel, O., s. Foerster, O. 486, *527*, [F 19] 943
Gaillard, A., s. Lumineau, J.P. 289, *310*
Gaind, R., s. Hirsch, S.R. 256, *307*
Gaitonde, M.K. 22, *58*
Gaitonde, M.K., Richter, D. 49, *58*
Gaitonde, M.K., s. Cohn, P. 49, *56*
Gaitonde, M.K., s. Richter, D. 15, *62*
Galambos, R., Morgan, C.T. [G 2] 761, *1078*
Galambos, R., s. Worden, F.G. 433, 479, *544*
Gallaher, T.F., s. Hellmann, L. 77, *103*
Gallant, D.M., Bishop, M.P., Steele, C.A. 94, *102*
Gallup, G.G. Jr. 381, 506, *528*
Galton, F. [G 3] 931, 935, *1078*
Gambetti, P., Autilio-Gambetti, L.A., Gonatas, N.K., Shafer, B. 50, *58*
Gambill, J.M., Wilson, I.C. 333, *344*
Game, C.J.A., s. Curtis, D.R. 37, *56*
Game, J.A., s. Baker, A.A. 333, *342*
Gamkrelidze, S.A., Putkoradze-Gamkrelidze, N.A. 257, *306*
Gamper, E. [G 4–6] 761, 812, 961, 1047, *1078*
Gancarczyk, E., s. Maj, J. 110, *113*
Ganglberger, J.A., s. Hassler, R. 475, *529*
Gantt, W.H. [G 7] 810, 811, *1078*
Garai, J.E., Scheinfeld, A. 647, *696*
Garattini, S., s. Samanin, R. 225, *240*
Garcia, J. 324, *344*
Garcia-Austt, E. s. Bogacz, J. [B 50] 824, *1071*

Garcia-Rill, E., s. Dongier, M. 175, *184*
Garcia Sainz, M., s. Halberg, F. *187*
Garcia-Sevilla, J.A., Magnusson, T., Carlsson, A. 200, *238*
Gardner, B.T., Gardner, R.A. 509, 516, *528*
Gardner, B.T., s. Gardner, R.A. 507, 509, 515, *528*, [G 8] 893, *1078*
Gardner, L.J. 733, *747*
Gardner, L.J., s. Patton, R.G. 722, 733, *749*
Gardner, R., s. Coppen, A. 270, *305*
Gardner, R., s. Saldanha, V.F. 293, *312*
Gardner, R.A., Gardner, B.T. 507, 509, 515, *528*, [G 8] 893, *1078*
Gardner, R.A., s. Gardner, B.T. 509, 516, *528*
Gardos, G. 252, *306*
Garmezy, N. 171, *186*, 567, *607*
Garner, R.L. 504, *528*
Garraud, M.J., s. Lumineau, J.P. 289, *310*
Garrod, A.E. 3, *58*
Garsche, R. 163, *186*
Garside, R., s. Andrews, G. 638, *692*
Garside, R.F., s. Carney, M.W.P. 330, 331, *343*
Garside, R.F., s. Kay, D.W.K. 332, *345*, 553, 565, *609*
Garside, R.F. III, s. Kolvin, I. 588, 589, *610*
Garside, R.F., s. Kolvin, I. 596, *610*
Garside, R.F., s. Stephens, D.A. 553, 558, 564, 565, *616*
Garver, D.L., Pandey, G.N., Dekirmenjian, H., Davis, J.M. 338, *344*
Garver, D.L., Pandey, G.N., Dekirmenjian, H., Deleon-Jones, F. 81, 82, 83, *102*
Garver, D.L., s. Caspar, R.C. 81, 84, 91, *101*
Garver, D., s. Maas, J.W. 72, *104*

Garver, D.L., s. Pandey, G.N. 91, 92, *105*
Gáspar, M., Poeldinger, W. *306*
Gassel, M.M., Marchiafava, P.L., Pompeiano, O. [G 9] 995, *1078*
Gastaut, H. 155, 158, 167, 172, *186*, [G 10] 1031, 1032, *1078*
Gastaut, H., Collomb, H. [G 10a] 1018, *1078*
Gastaut, H., Naquet, R., Vigourox, R., Roger, A., Badier, M. 166, *186*
Gastaut, H., Roger, A. [G 12] 1028, 1031, 1032, 1033, *1078*
Gastaut, H., Roger, J., Lob, H. 168, *186*
Gastaut, H., Roger, J., Ouahchi, S., Timsit, M., Broughton, R. [G 12a] *1078*
Gastaut, H., Roger, J., Roger, A. 168, *186*
Gastaut, H., Tassinari, C.A. 126, 166, 168, *186*
Gastaut, H., s. Brazier, M.A.B. 121, *183*
Gastaut, H., s. Fischgold, H. 155, *186*, [F 11] 969, 1028, *1077*
Gastaut, H.A., Jus, C., Morrell, F., Storm van Leeuwen, W., Dongier, S., Naquet, R., Regis, H., Roger, A., Bekkering, D., Kamp, A., Werre, J. [G 11] 1028, 1031, 1032, *1078*
Gath, A., s. Cadoret, R.J. 596, 600, *604*
Gaupp, R. [G 13] 939, *1078*
Gay, M.J., Tonge, W.L. 730, *747*
Gaztanaga, P. s. Abrams, R. 586, *602*
Gazzaniga, M.S. [G 14] 890, *1078*
Gehlen, A. 503, 512, 514, *528*, [G 15] 803, *1078*
Geiger, A. 7, *58*
Geiter, C.W., s. Forrest, F.M. 289, *306*
Gelder, M.G., s. Beumont, P.J.V. 293, *304*
Gelder, M.G., s. Kolakowska, T. 292, *309*

Geller, I. s. Brady, J.V. [B 57] *1072*
Gentilomo, A., s. Corletto, F. 159, *184*
George, S., s. Graham, P. 720, *747*
Georgopopolus, A., s. Mountcastle, V.B. [M 75] 898, 929, 1037, *1093*
Gerard, R.W., Duyff, J.W. [G 15a] 855, *1078*
Gerard, R.W. s. Blake, H. [B 47, 48] 993, 1002, *1071*
Gerardy, W., Herberg, D., Kuhn H.M. [G 16] 1016, *1078*
Gerbode, F.A., s. Bowers, M.B. 69, *100*
Gerhard, J., s. Boehncke, H. 684, *693*
Gerhardt, D. 551, *607*
Gerlach, J. 252, *306*
Gerlach, J., Reisby, N., Randrup, A. 298, *306*
Gerlach, J., Thorsen, K. 298, *306*
Gerlach, J., Thorsen, K., Munkvad, I. 271, 298, *306*
Gerlach, J., s. Randrup, A. 75, *106*
Gerlach, J.L., s. McEwen, B.S. 465, 466, *535*
Gerner, R.H., s. Post, R.M. 75, *106*
Gershon, E.S., Baron, M., Leckman, J.F. 578, *607*
Gershon, E.S., Bunney, W.E. 664, *696*
Gershon, E.S., Bunney, W.E., Leckman, J.F., Eerdewegh, M. van, DeBauche, B.A. 577, *607*
Gershon, E.S., Dunner, D.L., Goodwin, F.K. 577, *607*
Gershon, E.S., Jonas, W.Z. 583, *607*
Gershon, E.S., Mark, A., Cohen, M., Belizon, N., Baron, M., Knobe, K.E. 597, *607*
Gershon, E.S., s. Baron, M. 271, *303*
Gershon, E.S., s. Dunner, D.L. 580, 582, *605*
Gershon, S., Heikimian, L.J., Floyd, A. Jr., Hollister, L.E. 93, *103*, 218, *238*

Gershon, S., s. Angrist, B. 91, 92, 95, *99*
Gershon, S., s. Leckmann, J.F. 96, *104*
Gershon, S., s. Rotrosen, J. 91, *107*
Gershon, S., s. Shopsin. B. 272, *313*, 578, *615*
Gershon, S., s. Shopsin, B.S. 93, *107*, 227, *241*
Gershon, S., s. Suslak, L. 578, *616*
Gershon, S., s. Wilk, S. 70, *108*
Gerstein, A., s. Lajtha, A. 49, *60*
Gerstenbrand, F. 158, *186*
Geschwind, N. [G 17, 18] 892, 901, *1078*
Geschwind, N., Lewitzky, W. 682, *696*
Gessa, G.L., s. Costa, E. 201, 202, 231, *237*
Gessa, G.L., s. Gessa, R. 298, *306*
Gessa, R., Tagliamonte, A., Gessa, G.L. 298, *306*
Gesteland, R.C., s. McCulloch, W.S. [M 34] 853, 857, *1091*
Gewirtz, J., s. Rheingold, H.L. 435, 518, *539*, 732, *750*
Gewirtz, J.L. 498, *528*, 708, *747*
Geyer, N., s. Lorenzoni, E. 164, *191*
Ghezzi, D., s. Ladinsky, H. 219, *239*
Ghose, K., s. Coppen, A. 110, 111, *112*
Giannitrapani, D. 174, 178, *186*
Giannitrapani, D., Kayton, L. 174, 178, *186*
Giaquinto, S., Pompeiano, O., Somogyi, I. [G 19] 995, *1079*
Gibbons, J.L. 77, *103*, 340, *344*
Gibbs, E.L., s. Gibbs, F.A. 118, 127, 160, 167, 172, 176, *186*, *187* [G 22–24, 25, 26] 908, 913, 983, 998, 1002, 1017, *1079*
Gibbs, E.L., s. Lennox, W.G. [L 13] 985, *1089*

Gibbs, F.A. 167, 172, *186*, [G 20] 1052, *1079*
Gibbs, F.A., Davis, H., Lennox, W.G. [G 21] 763, 982, 983, 998, *1079*
Gibbs, F.A., Gibbs, E.L. 118, 127, 172, 176, *186*, [G 22–24] 998, 1002, 1017, *1079*
Gibbs, F.A., Gibbs, E.L., Lennox, W.G. 167, *187*, [G 25, 26) 908, 913, 983, *1079*
Gibbs, F.A., Williams, D., Gibbs, E.L. 160, *187*
Gibbs, F.A., s. Lennox, W.G. [L 13] 985, *1089*
Gibson, J.G. [G 27, 28] 929, *1079*
Gibson, P.H., s. Perry, E.K. 67, *106*
Giles, D.E., s. Mai, F.M. 83, *104*
Gill, T.V., s. Rumbaugh, D.M. 512, 515, *540*
Giller, D.R., s. Shader, R.I. 293, *313*
Gilligan, B.S., Wodak, J., Veale, J.L., Munro, O.R. 298, *306*
Gillin, J.C., s. Bigelow, L.B. 94, *100*
Gillin, J.C., s. Post, R.M. 75, *106*
Gillin, J.C., s. Stoddard, F.J. 72, *108*
Gillin, J.C., s. Wyatt, R.J. 75, *109*
Gilman, A., s. Goodman, L.S. 204, *238*
Gindilis, V.M., s. Vartanian, M.A. 570, *617*
Giriunas, I., s. Ballantine, H.T. Jr. 361, *375*
Girke, W., s. Bauer, H. 272, 298, *303*
Giuditta, A., s. Dunn, A. 341, *344*
Gjessing, R. 3, *58*
Glaserfeld, B.C. von, s. Rumbaugh, D.M. 512, *540*
Glasersfeld, E.C. von, Pisani, P.P. 512, *528*
Glasersfeld, E. von, s. Rumbaugh, D.M. 512, *540*
Glassman, A.H., Kantor, S.J., Shostak, M. 331, *344*

Glassman, A.H., s. Kantor, S.J. 287, *309*
Glassmann, A.H., s. Perel, J.M. *311*
Glassman, E., s. Dunn, A. 341, *344*
Glatzel, J. 687, *696*
Glen, A.J., s. Ashcroft, G.W. 87, *99*
Glen, R.E., s. Berger, P.A. 229, *235*
Glithero, E., s. Slater, E. 170, *194*
Gloor, P., Murphy, J.T., Dreifuss, J.J. 458, *528*
Gloor, P., s. Brazier, M.A.B. 121, *183*
Gloor, P., s. Gotman, J. 134, *187*
Glowinski, J., Axelrod, J. 223, *238*
Glowinski, J., s. Javoy, F. 219, *238*
Gluba, H., s. Benkert, O. 74, *100*
Glueck, E., s. Glueck, S. 639, 671, *696*
Glueck, S., Glueck, E. 639, 671, *696*
Gmür, M., s. Matussek, N. *105*
Go, R.C.P., s. Tanna, V.L. 582, *616*
Godtfredsen, K., s. Paikin, H. 558, *612*
Götze, P., s. Dahme, B. 552, *604*
Götze, W., s. Vogel, F. 119, *195*
Goetzl, U., Green, R., Whybrow, P., Jackson, R. 581, 583, *607*
Goff, W.R., s. Heninger, G. 150, *187*
Goktepe, E.O., s. Bridges, P.K. 367, *375*
Goldberg, D. 632, *696*
Goldberg, E.M., Morrison, S.L. 573, *607*
Goldberg, H.L., Nathan, L. 263, *306*
Goldberg, S.C., Schooler, N.R., Davidson, E.M., Kayce, M.M. 664, *696*
Goldfarb, W. 716, 724, *747*
Goldfarb, W., s. Meyers, D. 588, *611*

Goldfarb, W., s. Taft, L. 575, *616*
Goldfield, M.D., s. Schou, M. 289, 294, *312*
Goldfield, M.D., s. Weinstein, M.R. 271, *314*
Goldfoot, D.A. 461, *528*
Goldfoot, D.A., s. Goy, R.W. 465, *528*
Goldman, D. 298, *306*
Goldschneider, 908
Goldstein, K. [G 29] 789, 824, 901 *1079*
Goldstein, L. 134, 135, 136, 137, 173, *187*
Goldstein, L., Sugerman, A.A., Stolberg, H., Murphree, H.B., Pfeiffer, C.C. 172, 173, *187*
Goldstein, L., s. Burdick, J.A. 136, 137, 173, 174, *183*
Goldstein, L., s. Sugerman, A.A. 173, *195*
Goldstein, L.A., Sugerman, A.A. 173, *187*
Goldstein, M., Anagnoste, B., Shirron, C. 216, *238*
Goldstein, M., s. Hökfelt, T. 200, *238*
Goldstein, M., s. Shopsin, B. 93, *107*
Goldstein, M., s. Shopsin, B.S. 227, *241*
Goldstein, S., s. Winsberg, B.G. 287, *314*
Goltz, F. [G 30] 937, 938, 943, *1079*
Gomberg, E.S., Franks, V. 705
Gonatas, N.K., s. Gambetti, P. 50, *58*
Good, W.W., Sterling, M., Holtzman, W.H. 253, *306*
Goodall, J. 381, 398, 506, *528*
Goodall, J.L. van 648, *696*
Goodall, McC. 33, *58*
Goodenough, D.R., s. Witkin, H.A. 677, *704*
Goodin, L., s. Fouts, R.S. 509, *527*
Goodman, J., s. Tyler, D.B. [T 14] 1003, *1100*
Goodman, L.S., Gilman, A. 204, *238*

Goodman, R., s. Simantov, R. 40, *63*
Goodwin, B.L., s. Coppen, A. 72, *101*
Goodwin, D., s. Hill, S. 600, *608*
Goodwin, D., s. Schuckit, M. 600, *614*
Goodwin, D.W., Schulsinger, F., Hermansen, L., Guze, S.B., Winokur, G. 599, *607*
Goodwin, D.W., Schulsinger, F., Møller, N., Hermansen, L., Winokur, G., Guze, S.B. 599, *607*
Goodwin, F., s. Buchsbaum, M. 176, *183*
Goodwin, F.K., Murphy, D.L., Brodie, H.K.H., Bunney, W.E. 74, *103*, 223, 229, 230, *238*
Goodwin, F.K., Post, R.M. 68, 69, 70, *103*
Goodwin, F.K., s. Beckmann, H. 72, 73, *99*, *100*
Goodwin, F.K., s. Bunney, W.E. 74, *101*
Goodwin, F.K., s. Dunner, D.L. 580, 582, *605*
Goodwin, F.K., s. Gershon, E.S. 577, *607*
Goodwin, F.K., s. Murphy, D.L. 74, 96, *105*
Goodwin, F.K., s. Muscettola, G. 110, *113*
Goodwin, F.K., s. Post, R.M. 325, 339, *347*
Goray, A., s. Wojdyslawska, I. 287, *314*
Gordon, B.N., s. Jensen, G.D. 489, *531*
Gordon, E.K., s. Greenspan, K. 72, *103*
Gordon, E.K., s. Post, R.M. 70, *106*
Gordon, W.F., s. Hordern, A. 331, *345*
Gorszcyk, A., s. Maj. J. 110, *113*
Gosling, C., s. Rees, L. 85, *107*
Gotlieb-Jensen, K., s. Hauge, M. 574, *608*
Gotman, J., Gloor, P. 134, *187*
Gottesman, I.I. 591, *607*

Gottesman, I.I., Shields, J. 553, 554, 555, 556, 558, 561, 562, 563, 565, 575, *607*
Gottesman, I.I., s. Hanson, D.R. 553, 568, 569, 575, 588, 589, *608*, 638, 641, *696*
Gottesman, I.I., s. Shields, J. 555, 561, 564, 565, 575, *615*
Gottfries, C.G., s. Beskow, J. 67, 68, *100*
Gottlieb, 96
Gottlieb, J.S., Huston, P.E. 333, *344*
Gottlieb, J.S., s. Rodin, E.A. [R 19] 1003, *1096*
Gottwald, P., s. Ploog, D. 423, 487, *538*
Gouling, R., s. Braithwaite, R.A. 246, *304*
Gove, W., s. Clancy, K. 651, *694*
Gove, W.R., Tudor, J.F. 651, *696*
Gowing, D., s. Blachly, P.H. 320, 324, *342*
Goy, R.W., Goldfoot, D.A. 465, *528*
Gozzano, M., Fontana, A., Folicaldi, G. [G 31] 863, 1044, *1079*
Gradijan, J., s. Lifshitz, K. 173, 174, 177, 178, *190*
Graham, C.W., s. Woods, H.F. 7, *64*
Graham, N., s. Burnett, G.B. 253, *304*
Graham, P., George, S. 720, *747*
Grahame-Smith, D.G., Green, A.R., Costain, D.W. 339, *344*
Grahame-Smith, D.G., s. Evans, J.P.M. 88, *102*, 325, 339, *344*
Grahame-Smith, D.G., s. Green, A.R. 88, 95, *103*, 325, 339, *344*
Grahame-Smith, D.G., s. Woods, H.F. 7, *64*
Granacher, R.P., Baldessarini, R.J. 299, *306*
Granit, R. [G 32–34] 774, 856, 875, 908, 913, 915, *1079*
Granit, R., Phillips, C.G. [G 35] *1079*

Grant, B.R., Waller, R.H. 246, *306*
Grantham, E.G. 356, *375*
Granstýan, E. [G 36] 977, 1019, *1079*
Grastýan, E., Karmos, G. [G 37] 977, *1079*
Granstýan, E., Lissák, K., Madarász, I., Donhoffer, H. [G 38] 1031, *1079*
Grastýan, E., Lissák, K., Szabó, J., Vereby, G. [G 39] 1031, *1079*
Grastýan, E., s. Lisák, K. [L 30] 1031, *1089*
Grau, M., s. Palacios, J.M. 37, *61*
Grawe, J.M., s. Cohen, D.J. 549, *604*
Gray, E.G. 14, *58*
Grayson, H.M., s. Brill, N.D. 333, *342*
Green, A.R., Grahame-Smith, D.G. 88, 95, *103*
Green, A.R., Heal, D.J., Grahame-Smith, D.G. 325, 339, *344*
Green, A.R., Kelly, P.H. 88, *103*
Green, A.R., s. Evans, J.P.M. 88, *102*, 325, 339, *344*
Green, A.R., s. Grahame-Smith, D.G. 339, *344*
Green, A.R., s. Woods, H.F. 7, *64*
Green, J., s. Roth, M. 322, 338, *347*
Green, J.D., Clemente, C.D., Groot, J. de [G 40] 978, *1079*
Green, J.D., Machne, X. [G 41] 977, *1079*
Green, J.D. s. Euler, C. v. [E 20] 977, *1076*
Green, M., s. Horn, J.M. 560, *608*
Green, R., s. Goetzl, U. 581, 583, *607*
Green, R.L., s. Hein, P.L. 172, *187*
Green, S. 434, 470, *528*
Greenblatt, D.J., Koch-Weser, J. 287, *306*
Greenblatt, M., Grosser, G.H., Wechsler, H. 329, *345*

Greenblatt, M., Healy, M.M., Jones, G.A. 171, 176, *187*
Greenfield, S.A., Smith, A.D. 45, *58*
Greengard, P. 30, 32, *58*, 207, 216, *328*
Greengard, P., s. Clement-Cormier, Y.C. 216, 217, *237*
Greengard, P., s. Kebabian, J.W. 30, *59*, 216, *239*
Greengard, P., s. Ueda, T. 30, *63*
Greenspan, K., Schildkraut, J.J., Gordon, E.K., Baer, L., Aronoff, M.D., Durell, J. 72, *103*
Greenup, J., s. Kelly, D. 363, 365, *376*
Greger, J., s. Waldmann, K.-D. 272, 298, *314*
Gregg, G., s. Elmer, E. 727, *747*
Gregová, L., s. Baštecký, J. 293, *303*
Greil, W., s. Matussek, N. 75, *105*
Greiner, A.C. 289, *306*
Grewaal, D.S., s. McGeer, P.L. 219, *239*
Grézes-Rueff, C., s. Planques, I. 162, *193*
Griesinger, W. [G 42] 755, 756, 1018, *1079*
Griffiths, A.B., s. Munro, A. 730, *749*
Griffiths, K., s. Wilson, R.G. 292, *314*
Grinspoon, L., s. Meltzer, H. 94, *105*
Grobstein, R., s. Barnett, C. 721, 726, *746*
Grobstein, R., s. Korner, A.F. 732, *748*
Gröschel, W., s. Waldmann, K.-D. 272, 298, *314*
Grözinger, B., s. Deecke, L. 153, *184*
Grof, P., s. Angst, J. 641, 642, *692*
Groot, J. de, s. Green, J.D. [G 40] 978, *1079*
Gross, G., s. Huber, G. 574, *608*, 630, 685, 689, *697*
Gross, G.W. 14, 20, *58*
Gross, J., Kempe, P., Reimer, C. 736, *748*

Gross, J., Šváb. L. 742, *747*
Gross, J., s. Kempe, P. 740, *748*
Gross, J., s. Šváb, L. 740, *751*
Gross, M., Hitchman, I.L., Reeves, W.P., Lawrence, J., Newell, P.C. 253, *306*
Grosse, F.-R., s. Wiedemann, H.-R. 627, 673, 674, *704*
Grosser, G.H., s. Greenblatt, M. 329, *345*
Grote, S., s. Cochran, E. 67, 68, *101*
Groupe, A., s. Tupin, J.P. 271, *313*
Groves, P.M., Wilson, C.J., Young, S.J., Rebec, G.V. 215, *238*
Gruen, P.H., s. Sachar, E.J. 77, 78, *107*, 325, 338, *348*
Grünberger, J., s. Hofmann, G. 298, *307*
Grünewald, G., s. Grünewald-Zuberbier, E. [G 43, 44] 789, 833, 834, *1079*
Grünewald-Zuberbier, E., Grünewald, G., [G 43] 789, *1079*
Grünewald-Zuberbier, E., Grünewald, G., Jung, R. [G 43, 44] 789, 833, 834, *1079*
Grünthal, E. [G 45, 46] 934, 944, *1080*
Gruesen, R.A., s. Akert, K. [A 15] 944, *1068*
Grüsser, O.J., Hellner, K.A., Grüsser-Cornehls, U. [G 47] 856, *1080*
Grüsser, O.J., s. Jung, R. [J 55] 982, 1005, *1086*
Grüsser-Cornehls, U., s. Grüsser, O.-J. [G 47] 856, *1080*
Grüttner, R., Bonkálo, A. [G 48] 856, 993, 1003, *1080*
Gruhle 775
Grumiller, I., s. Katschnig, H. 649, *697*
Grynbaum, A., s. Marks, N. 23, *60*
Gudeman, J.E., s. Schildkraut, J.J. 72, *107*
Guidotti, A. 231, *238*
Guidotti, A., Cheyney, D.L., Trabucci, M., Doteuchi, M., Wang, C., Hawkins, R.A. 8, *58*
Guidotti, A., s. Costa, E. 231, *237*
Guidotti, A., s. Zivkovic, B. 213, *242*
Guilbaud, F., s. Schwartz, B.A. [S 19, 19a] 1014, *1098*
Guilford, J.P. 667, 669, 670, *696*
Guillemin, R. 41, *58*
Guillemin, R., s. Vale, W. 40, *64*
Guin, T., s. Wilson, I.C. 332, *349*
Gumnit, R.J., s. Drachman, D.B. [D 35] 1016, *1075*
Gunn, D.R. 289, *307*
Gunne, L.M., Lindström, L., Terenius, J. 96, *103*
Gunne, L.-M., s. Jönsson, L.-E. 230, *238*
Gunne, L.-M., s. Lindström, L.H. 112, *112*
Gupta, K.P., s. Feldberg, W. 38, *57*
Gurland, H.J., s. Hippius, H. 97, *103*
Gurland, H.-J., s. Nedopil, N. 97, *105*
Gurly, R., s. Engel, R. 131, *185*
Guroff, G. 30, 32, *58*
Gustafsson, J.K., s. Fuxe, K. 110, *112*
Guterman, B., s. Lennox, M.A. 163, *190*
Gutjahr, L., Künkel, H. 132, *187*
Gutjahr, L., Machleidt, W., Ferber, G. 126, 167, *187*
Guyda, H., s. Lal, S. 85, *104*
Guze, S.B., Woodruff, R.A., Clayton, P.L. 582, *607*
Guze, S.B., s. Cloninger, C.R. 594, 595, *604*, 639, *694*
Guze, S.B., s. Goodwin, D.W. 599, *607*
Guze, S.B., s. Reich, T. 550, 561, 600, *613*
Gyermek, L., s. Sigg, E.B. 223, *241*
Gynther, M.D., s. Smith, K. 334, *348*

Haag, A., s. Dahme, B. 552, *604*
Haag, A., s. Huse-Kleinstoll, G. 552, *608*
Haase, H.-J. 307, 684, 687, *696*, 739, *748*
Haase, H.J., Floru, L., Knaack, M. 253, *307*
Haberlandt, W. 594, *607*
Hacker, M., s. Lieberman, D.M. 172, *190*
Häfner, H. 573, *607*
Häggendal, J., s. Andén, N.-E. 15, *55*, 201, *235*
Hänryd, C., s. Sedvall. G. 217, 220, 225, *241*
Hafner, R.J., s. Kelly, D. 363, 365, *376*
Hagbarth, K.E., Fex, J. [H 1] 824, *1080*
Hagnell, O. 587, *607*, 649, 660, *696*
Hagnell, O., Öjesjö, L. 587, *607*
Haier, R.J., s. Buchsbaum, M.S. 681, *693*
Halaris, A.E., DeMet, E.M. 110, 111, *112*
Halász, B., s. Szentagothai, J. [S 65] 860, 861, 939, *1100*
Halbach, A., s. Matussek, P. 661, *699*
Halberg, F. 131, *187*
Halberg, F., Carendente, F., Cornelissen, G., Katinas, G.S. *187*
Halberg, F., Katinas, G.S., Chiba, Y., Garcia Sainz, M., Kováts, T.G., Künkel, H., Montalbetti, N., Reinberg, A., Scharf, R., Simpson, H. *187*
Halberg, F., s. Engel, R. 131, *185*
Hall, J.N., s. Andrews, P. 253, *302*
Hall, K.R.L. 392, *528*
Halldórsson, S., s. Holmes, L.B. 673, *697*
Hallgren, B. 596, *607*, 638, *696*
Hallgren, B., Sjögren, T. 586, *607*
Halliday, A.M. 148, 152, *187*
Halliday, A.M., McDonald, W.I. 148, *187*

Halliday, A.M., Wakefield, G.S. 152, *187*
Halmy, K. 292, *307*
Halperin, S., s. Menzel, E.W. 505, *535*
Hamberger, A., s. Bock, E. 10, 21, 22, *56*
Hamberger, B., s. Farnebo, L.-O. 216, *237*
Hambert, G. 677, *696*
Hametová, M., s. Bilý, J. 290, *304*
Hamilton, J.R., s. Wilson, R.G. 292, *314*
Hamilton, W.J., s. Marler, P. 428, *535*
Hamlin, H., s. Delgado, J.M.R. [D 15] 886, *1074*
Hamlin, H., s. Mahl, G.F. [M 21] 887, *1091*
Hammerschlag, R., s. Roberts, E. 37, *62*
Hammerstein, J., Meckies, J., Leo-Rossberg, I., Moltz, L., Zielske, F. 678, *696*
Hammond, B.J., s. Balázs, R. 36, 37, *55*
Hampers, C.L., s. Merrill, J.P. 158, *192*
Hampson, J.G., s. Money, J. 690, *700*
Hampson, J.L., s. Money, J. 690, *700*
Handley, P., s. Winter, P. 432, *544*
Handy, L.M., s. Rosanoff, A.J. 555, 597, 598, *613*
Hanhart, E. 594, *607*
Hansen, E., s. Seay, B. 496, *541*
Hanson, D.R., Gottesman, I.I. 588, 589, *608*, 638, 641, *696*
Hanson, D.R., Gottesman, I.I., Heston, L.L. 553, 568, 575, *608*
Hanson, D.R., Gottesman, I.I., Meehl, P.E. 568, 569, *608*
Hanson, L.C.F., s. Corrodi, H. 218, *237*
Hansson, H.-A., Hydén, H., Rönnbäck, L. 21, *58*
Hanus, H., s. Bilý, J. 290, *304*
Harbauer, H. 630, 635, 637, 673, 689, *696*

Hård, G., s. Holmberg, G. 320, *345*
Harder, A., Modestin, J., Steiner, H. 289, *307*
Harding, B., s. Crisp, A.H. 651, *694*
Hare, E.H. 573, 574, *608*
Hare, E.H., Price, J.S. 572, *608*
Hare, E.H., Price, J.S., Slater, E. 572, 573, 574, *608*
Hare, R.D., Schalling, D. 594, *608*
Hare, E.H., s. Coppen, A. 270, *305*
Hare, E.H., s. Price, J.S. 572, *613*
Hare, E.H., s. Spicer, C.C. 582, *615*
Harlow, H., Harlow, M.K. 407, *528*
Harlow, H.F. 407, 492, 493, 496, 501, *528*
Harlow, H.F., Akert, K., Schiltz, K. [H 3] 890, *1080*
Harlow, H.F., Harlow, K. 381, 407, *528*
Harlow, H.F., Harlow, M.K. 407, 489, 493, 496, 498, *528*, 725, 726, 743, *748*
Harlow, H.F., Suomi, S.J. 500, *529*
Harlow, H.F., Zimmermann, R.R. 490, *529*
Harlow, H.F., s. McKinney, W.T. 500, *535*
Harlow, H.F., s. Schrier, A.M. 384, 505, *541*
Harlow, H.F., s. Seay, B. 496, *541*
Harlow, H.F., s. Suomi, S.J. 496, 498, 500, *542*, 725, *751*
Hartline, H.K. [H 4, 5, 6] 908, 910, 913, 915, *1080*
Harlow, K., s. Harlow, H.F. 381, 407, *528*
Harlow, K.E., Woolsey, C.N. [H 2] 824, *1080*
Harlow, M.K., s. Harlow, H. 407, *528*
Harlow, M.K., s. Harlow, H.F. 407, 489, 493, 496, 498, *528*, 725, 726, 743, *748*
Harnad, S.R., Steklis, H.D., Lancaster, J. 503, 508, *529*
Harnad, S.R., s. Steklis, H.D. 513, *542*

Harner, R., Katz, R.I. 157, *187*
Harner, R., Naquet, R. 155, *187*
Harousseau, H., s. Lemoine, P. 673, *698*
Harrer, G. 267, *307*
Harrington, J.A., s. Imlah, N.W. 332, *345*
Harriot, Resche-Rigon 256
Harris, G.W., s. Beumont, P.J.V. 292, 293, *303*, *304*
Harris, M., s. Andrews, G. 638, *692*
Hartelius, H. 323, *345*
Hartley, C., s. Reed, S.C. 553, *613*
Hartmann, E. 93, *103*
Hartmann, E., Keller-Teschke, M. 93, *103*
Hartmann, E., s. Maurus, M. 482, 483, *535*
Hartmann, E.L. [H 7] 988, *1080*
Hartmann, M. [H 8, 9] 771, 774, *1080*
Hartmann, N. [H 10, 11, 12, 13, 14] 764, 765, 767, 768, 770, 771, 772, 773, 774, 775, 776, 777, 778, 779, 793, 795, 846, 847, 848 887, 962, 1063, *1080*
Hartmann, W., s. Waldmann, K.-D. 272, 298, *314*
Hartmann-Wiesner, E., s. Maurus, M. 393, 394, 483, *535*
Hartnett, O., s. Chetwynd, J. 644, *693*
Hartz, S.C., Heinomen, O.P., Shapiro, S., Siskind, V., Slone, D. 294, *307*
Harvald, B., s. Bertelsen, A. 578, 579, *603*
Harvald, B., s. Hauge, M. 574, *608*
Harvald, M., s. Fischer, M. 555, *606*
Harvey, C.A., Milton, A.S. 19, 38, *58*
Harvey, E.N., s. Davis, H. [D 4–6] 999, 1002, 1007, 1008, 1009, *1074*
Harvey, E.N., s. Loomis, A.L. [L 33, 34, 35] 992, 998, 999, 1000, 1009, *1090*

Haskayne, L., s. Claveria, L.E. 298, *304*
Haskell, M.R., Yablonsky, L. 651, *696*
Hassenstein, B. 620, *696*, [H 15, 15a] 806, 853, 854, 855, *1080*
Hassler, R. 451, 457, 475, 486, *529*, [H 16] 884, *1080*
Hassler, R., Dieckmann, G. 372, *375*
Hassler, R., Riechert, T. [H 17] 882, 884, 945, 961, *1080*
Hassler, R., Riechert, T., Mundinger, F., Umbach, W., Ganglberger, J.A. 475, *529*
Hassler, R., s. Dieckmann, G. 370, 371, *375*, 455, 457, *526*
Hassler, R., s. Jung, R. [J 58] 824, 825, 828, 845, *1086*
Hatashita, Y. 286, *307*
Hatotani, N., s. Endo, M. 81, *102*
Hauge, M., Harvald, B., Fischer, M., Gotlieb-Jensen, K., Juel-Nielsen, N., Raebild, I., Shapiro, R., Videbech, T. 574, *608*
Hauge, M., s. Bertelsen, A. 578, 579, *603*
Hauge, M., s. Fischer, M. 555, *606*
Hauge, T., s. Lundervold, A. 156, 157, *191*
Hauser, G., s. Eichberg, J. 19, *57*
Havard, C.W.H., s. Saldanha, V.F. 293, *312*
Hawkins, R.A., s. Guidotti, A. 8, *58*
Hawkins, R.A., s. Veech, R.L. 8, *64*
Hawthorne, J.N., s. Ansell, G.B. 19, *55*
Hayashi, S. 598, *608*
Hayes, C. 507, *529*
Hayes, K.J. 319, *345*
Hays, P. 682, *696*
Head, H. 478, *529*, [H 18, 19] 784, *1080*
Heal, D.J., s. Green, A.R. 325, 339, *344*
Healy, M.M., s. Greenblatt, M. 171, 176, *187*

Heath, E.S., Adams, A., Wakeling, P.L.G. 333, *345*
Heath, R.G. 370, *375*, 681, *696*
Heath, R.G., s. Leach, B.E. 96, *104*
Hebb, D.O. 734, 744, *748*, [20, 21] 790, 932, 1025, 1038, *1080*
Hebb, D.O., s. Beach, F.A. 448, *523*
Hebb, D.O., s. Heron, W. [H 40] 923, *1081*
Hécaen, H. [H 22] 898, *1080*
Hecaen, H., Angelergues, R. 475, 476, *529*
Hecaen, H., Consoli, S. 476, *529*
Hecaen, H., s. Assal, G. [A 35] 780, 896, 897, *1069*
Hecaen, H., s. Talairach, J. 356, *378*
Hecht Orzack, M., Kornetsky, C. 566, *608*
Hediger, H. [H 22a] 949, *1080*
Hedley-Whyte, E.T., s. Lorenzo, A.V. 324, *346*
Heiberg, A., Lingjaerde, O. 289, *307*
Heidegger, M. [H 23] 765, 791, 809, *1080*
Heidingsfelder, S.A., s. Blakkard, W.G. 81, *100*
Heigl-Evers, A., s. Becker, P.E. 592, *603*
Heikimian, L.J., s. Gershon, S. 218, *238*
Heimann, H. 246, *307*, 413, *529*, [H 24] 780, *1081*
Heimann, H., s. Baumann, P. 71, *99*
Hein, P.L., Green, R.L., Wilson, W.P. 172, *187*
Heinemann, H., s. Emrich, H.M. 112, *112*
Heinonen, O.P., Shapiro, S., Laurain, A.R., and The Boston Collaborative Drug surveillance Program Research Group 292, *307*
Heinonen, O.P., Shapiro, S., Tuominen, L., Turunen, M.I. 292, *307*
Heinomen, O.P., s. Hartz, S.C. 294, *307*

Heinrich, K. 95, *103*, 244, 260, *307*
Heinrich, K., Wegener, I., Bender, H.-J. 297, *307*
Heinrich, K., s. Kranz, H. 380, *532*
Heinroth 487
Heinze, G., s. Langer, G. 83, 84, *104*
Heinze, H.J., Künkel, H. 143, 180, *187*
Heiser, J.F., Wilbert, D.E. 299, *307*
Hekimian, L.J., s. Gershon, S. 93, *103*
Held, R. 448, *529*, 721, *748*
Held, R., s. Poeppel, E. 479, *539*
Helgason, T. 642, 649, 659, 660, 661, *696*
Hellbrügge, T. 713, 718, *748*
Heller, L.H., s. Elliott, K.A.C. 10, *57*
Hellman, I.I., s. Brill, N.D. 333, *342*
Hellmann, L., Nakada, F., Curtis, J., Weitzman, E.D., Kream, J., Roffwarg, H., Ellman, S., Fushukima, D.K., Gallaher, T.F. 77, *103*
Hellmann, L., s. Sachar, E.J. 81, *107*
Hellner, K.A., s. Grüsser, O.-J. [G 47] 856, *1080*
Helmchen, H. 165, 171, 176, 177, *187*, 297, *307*, [H 25] 1055, *1081*
Helmchen, H., Kanowski, S., Künkel, H. 128, *187*
Helmchen, H., Künkel, H. 172, *187*, [H 26] *1081*
Helmchen, H., Künkel, H., Oberhoffer, G., Penin, H. 127, *187*
Helmchen, H., Künkel, H., Selbach, H. 149, *187*
Helmchen, H., s. Degkwitz, R. 649, 653, *694*
Helmchen, H., s. Penin, H. 124, 127, *192*
Helmholtz, H. von [H 27, 28] 765, 782, 878, 906, 907, 913, 914, 915, *1081*
Helzer, J.E. 580, *608*
Helzer, J.E., Winokur, G. 580, *608*

Henatsch, H.-D. 449, 451, 452, *519*
Hendrix, C.E., s. Adey, W.R. [A 3] 1031, *1068*
Hendryx, J., s. Kolodny, R.C. 683, *698*
Hengst, D.W.H., s. Armington, J.C. 147, *182*
Heninger, G., McDonald, R.D., Goff, W.R., Sollberger, A. 150, *187*
Henn, F.A. 92, *103*
Henning, M. 202, *238*
Henninger, G.R., s. Bowers, M.B. 69, *100*
Henninger, G.R., s. Mueller, P.S. 81, *105*
Heninger, G.R., s. Pickar, D. 72, *106*
Heninger, G., s. Sweeny, D. 72, 73, *108*
Henry, C.E., s. Obrist, W.D. 162, *192*
Henry, J.L. 40, *58*
Henry, J.P., Stephens, P.M. 619, *696*
Hensel, H., Boman, K.A. [H 29, 30] 911, *1081*
Herbart 786
Herberg, D., s. Gerardy, W. [G 16] 1016, *1078*
Herdemerten, S., s. Schenck, G.K. 96, *107*
Herder, J.G. 512, *529*, [H 31] 804, *1081*
Hering, E. [H 31a, 32, 33, 34] 907, 908, 910, 912, 913, 914, 915, 929, 972, 973, 1022, 1023, 1024, 1066, *1081*
Hermann, L. [H 35] 908, 922, 924, *1081*
Hermansen, L., s. Goodwin, D.W. 599, *607*
Hernandez, A.G. 50, *58*
Hernández-Peón, R. [H 36] 824, *1081*
Hernández-Peón, R., Donoso, M. [H 37] 824, *1081*
Hernández-Peón, R., Scherrer, H., Jouvet, M. [H 38] 824, *1081*
Herner, T. 356, 363, *376*
Herngreen, H., s. Beek, H.H. 171, *182*
Herodet, 395
Heron, W. [H 39] 932, *1081*

Heron, W., Bexton, W.H., Hebb, D.O. [H 40] 932, *1081*
Herrick, C.J. 454, *529*, [H 41] 977, *1081*
Herron, E.W., s. Holtzman, W.H. 363, *376*
Hersher, L., Moore, A., Richmond, J. 726, *748*
Hershon, H.I., Kennedy, P.F., McGuire, R.J. 297, *307*
Hertrich, O. 289, *307*
Hertting, G., Axelrod, J., Kopin, J.J., Whitby, L.G. 223, *238*
Hertting, G., s. Axelrod, J. 223, *235*
Hertz, M.M., s. Bolwig, T.G. 323, 324, 340, *342*
Herz, A., Blaesig, J. 485, *529*
Herz, A., s. Emrich, H.M. 96, *102*, 112, *112*
Herzberg, B., s. Coppen, A. 74, *101*
Herzka, H.S. 410, 413, *529*
Hess, E.H. 408, 487, *529*, 621, *696*, [H 42] 940, 1041, *1081*
Hess, E.H., Polt, J.M. [H 43] 930, 948, *1081*
Hess, H.H., Bass, N.H., Thalheimer, C., Devarakonda, R. 18, *58*
Hess, R. 160, 172, *188*, [H 44, 45] 938, 1015, *1081*
Hess, R., Akert, K., Koella, W. [H 46] 938, *1081*
Hess, R., Koella, W., Akert, K. [H 47] 938, *1081*
Hess, R., s. Brazier, M.A.B. 121, *183*
Hess, W.R. [H 48–66] 758, 762, 774; 783, 784, 817, 818, 823, 824, 825, 827, 828, 829, 838, 841, 858, 859, 882, 883, 900, 903, 937, 938, 939, 950, 977, 978, 979, 988, 989, 990, 995, *1081*
Hess, W.R., Brügger, M. [H 67] 937, 943, *1082*
Hess, W.R., Meyer, A.E. [H 68] 940, *1082*
Hess, W.R. s. Akert, K. [A 16] 943, *1068*
Heston, L.L. 557, 559, 561, 564, *608*
Heston, L.L., Denney, D. 560, *608*

Heston, L.L., Shields, J. 639, 683, *697*
Heston, L.L., s. Hanson, D.R. 553, 568, 575, *608*
Heston, L.L., s. Shields, J. 561, 564, *615*
Hetzer, H., s. Buehler, C. 415, 416, 417, *524*
Hewes, G.W. *529*
Hewes, H. 513, *529*
Hewland, H.R., s. Shaw, D.M. 70, 71, *107*
Hewland, R., s. Blazek, R. 71
Heyde, G., s. Weinmann, H. 150, *196*
Heyse, H., s. Feuerlein, W. 680, *695*
Hickerson, G., s. Langsley, D.G. 333, *346*
Hicks, R.E. 514, *529*
Hiebel, C. s. Bonvallet, M. [B 52] 979, *1071*
Higgins, J. 557, *608*
Higgins, J., s. Mednick, S.A. 546, 553, 567, 568, 575, *611*
Hilbert, 910
Hildemann, W.H. 634, *697*
Hilgard, E.R., Marquis, D.G. [H 69] 1027, *1082*
Hill, D. 171, 172, *188*
Hill, D., Pond, D.A. [H 70] *1082*
Hill, H., s. Stawarz, R.J. 213, *241*
Hill, O.W. 730, *748*
Hill, O.W., Price, J.S. 730, *748*
Hill, R.M., Desmond, M.M., Kay, J.L. 294, *307*
Hill, R.M., s. Desmond, M.M. 294, *305*
Hill, S., Goodwin, D., Cadoret, R., Osterland, K., Doner, S.M. 600, *608*
Hillebrand, G., s. Nedopil, N. 97, *105*
Hillhause, E., s. Jones, M.T. 76, *103*
Hilton, S.M., Zbrozyna, A.W. 458, *529*
Himmelhoch, J.M., s. Kupfer, D.J. 580, *610*
Himwich, H.E. 52, *58*
Hinde, R., s. Rowell, T.E. 432, *540*
Hinde, R.A. 380, 402, 423, 425, 434, 489, 493, 502, *529*

Hinde, R.A., McGinnis, L. 500, *529*
Hinde, R.A., Spencer-Booth, Y. 500, *529*
Hinde, R.A., Spencer-Booth, Y., Bruce, M. 407, 496, 500, *530*
Hinde, R.A., White, L.E. 489, *530*
Hinde, R.A., s. Rowell, T.E.S. 426, 427, 428, 431, *540*
Hines, M. 476, *530*
Hines, O., s. Kiley, J. 161, *189*
Hippius, H., Lange, J. 297, *307*
Hippius, H., Logemann, G. 297, *307*
Hippius, H., Malin, J.-P. 287, *307*
Hippius, H., Matussek, N., Nedopil, N., Strauss, A., Zerssen, G.D. von, Emrich, H., Kolff, W.J., Gurland, H.J. 97, *103*
Hippius, H., s. Ackenheil, M. 72, 98, *99*
Hippius, H., s. Angst, J. 641, 642, *692*
Hippius, H., s. Bellabarba, U. 297, *303*
Hippius, H., s. Benkert, O. 100, 244, *303*
Hippius, H., s. Kalinowsky, L.B. 333, 335, 336, *345*
Hippius, H., s. Loosen, P. 72, *104*
Hippius, H., s. Matussek, N. 72, 84, 85, *104, 105*
Hirsch, S.R., Gaind, R., Rohde, P.D., Stevens, B.C., Wing, J.K. 256, *307*
Hirschhorn, K., s. Witkin, H.A. 677, *704*
Hiscoe, H.B., s. Weiss, P. 50, *64*
Hitchcook, E., Ashcroft, G.W., Cairns, V.M., Murray, L.G. 373, *376*
Hitchman, I.L., s. Gross, M. 253, *306*
Hitzig, E. [H 71] 879, 882, 883, *1082*
Hitzig, E. s. Fritsch, G. [F 32] 883, 889, *1078*

Hjorth, B., s. Spehr, W. 158, 161, *194*
Hoagland, H., Malamud, W., Kaufman, I.C., Pincus, G. 179, *188*
Hobart, G., s. Davis, H. [D 4–6] 999, 1002, 1007, 1008, 1009, *1074*
Hobart, G., s. Loomis, A.L. [L 33] 992, 998, 999, 1000, *1090*
Hobart, G.A., s. Loomis, A.L. [L 34, 35] 998, 999, 1000, 1002, 1009, *1090*
Hobbs, G.E., s. Buck, C. 577, *604*
Hoche, A. [H 72] 935, 1014, *1082*
Hockett, C.F. 512, *530*
Hockman, C.H. 453, *530*
Hodemaker, F.S., s. Jacobson, A. [J 3] 995, *1083*
Hodgkin, A.L., Huxley, A.F. [H 73] 872, 1064, *1082*
Hökfelt, T., Elde, R., Johansson, O., Luft, R., Nilsson, G., Arimura, A. 15, 40, *58*
Hökfelt, T., Johansson, O., Fuxe, K., Löfström, A., Goldstein, M., Park, D., Ebstein, R., Fraser, H., Jeffcoate, S., Effendie, S., Luft, R., Arimura, A. 200, *238*
Hökfelt, T., s. Carlsson, A. 223, *236*
Hökfelt, T., s. Elde, R. 26, 40, *57*
Höllt, V., s. Emrich, H.M. 112, *112*
Hoenig, J., s. Lieberman, D.M. 172, *190*
Hoffer, A., Osmond, H. 94, *103*
Hoffer, A., s. Huxley, J. 577, *608*
Hoffer, A., s. Pollin, W. 555, 556, *613*
Hoffer, B., s. Ungerstedt, U. 221, *242*
Hoffmann, E., Meiers, H.G., Hubbes, A. 678, *697*
Hoffmann, G., s. Ackenheil, M. 72, *98*
Hoffmann, P. [H 74, 75, 76] 822, 824, 830, 835, 860, *1082*

Hofmann, G. 686, *697*
Hofmann, G., Grünberger, J., König, P., Presslich, O., Wolf, R. 298, *307*
Holden, J.M.C., Holden, U.P. 290, *308*
Holden, U.P., s. Holden, J.M.C. 290, *308*
Hole, G., s. Wirz-Justice, A. 71, *108*
Holinger, P.C., Klawans, H.L. 299, *308*
Holinka, C.F., s. Nelson, J.F. 26, *61*
Hollingshead, A.B., Redlich, F.C. 573, *608*
Hollister, L.E., Davis, K.L., Overall, J.E., Anderson, T. 72, *103*
Hollister, L.E., Davis, K.L. 220, *237*
Hollister, L.E., s. Gershon, S. 93, *103*, 218, *238*
Hollstein, H. 288, *308*
Holm-Jensen, J., s. Bolwig, T.G. 323, 340, *342*
Holmberg, G. 317, 320, 321, *345*
Holmberg, G., Hård, G., Ramqvist, N. 320, *345*
Holmberg, G., Thesleff, S. 317, *345*
Holmboe, R., s. Astrup, C. 685, *692*
Holmdahl, M. Jr. 317, *345*
Holmes, L.B., Moser, H.W., Halldórsson, S., Mack, C., Pant, S.S., Matzilewich, B. 673, *697*
Holmgren, F. [H 77] 915, *1082*
Holst, E. von [H 78–81] 819, 823, 853, 856, 859, 860, 876, 889, 929, 935, 939, 941, 950, *1082*
Holst, E. von, Mittelstaedt, H. 451, *530*, [H 82] 853, 856, 859, *1082*
Holst, E. von, Saint Paul, U. von [H 83, 84] 795, 883, 935, 939, 940, 941, 950, 966, *1082, 1083*
Holt, N.F., s. Hordern, A. 331, *345*
Holt, W.L. Jr., Borkowski, W. 320, *345*
Holtzman, W.H., Thorpe,

J.S., Swartz, J.D., Herron, E.W. 363, *376*
Holtzman, W.H., s. Good, W.W. 253, *306*
Holzer, C.E., s. Warheit, G.J. 649, 651, *704*
Holzer, H. [H 85] 860, *1083*
Honigfeld, G., Howard, A. 266, *308*
Honkavaara, S. 416, *530*
Hooff, J.A.R.A.M. van 404, 405, 412, 413, *530*
Hopes, H., s. Lehmann, E. 247, *309*
Hopf, S. 395, 432, 490, 493, 495, *530*
Hopf, S., s. Latta, J. 386, *533*
Hopf, S., s. Ploog, D. 394, 395, 406, 431, 432, 490, 493, *538*
Hoppe, E., s. Vestergaard, P. 69, 70, *108*
Hopwood, N.J., s. Powell, G.F. 733, *749*
Hordern, A., Burt, C.G., Gordon, W.F., Holt, N.F. 331, *345*
Hordern, A., Holt, N.F., Burt, C.G. Gordon, W.F. 331, *345*
Hordynski, W., s. Farley, I.J. 93, *102*
Hori, N., s. Shimazono, Y. [S 34] 977, 1019, *1098*
Horie, T., s. Shimazono, Y. [S 34] 977, 1019, *1098*
Horn, A.S., s. Miller, R.J. 216, *240*
Horn, J.M., Green, M., Carney, R., Erickson, M.T. 560, *608*
Hornung, F., s. Ulett, G. *195*
Hornykiewicz, O., s. Birkmayer, W. 74, *100*
Hornykiewicz, O., s. Ehringer, H. 74, *102*
Hornykiewicz, O., s. Farley, I.J. 93, *102*
Hornykiewicz, O., s. Lee, T. 112, *112*
Hornykiewicz, O., s. Lloyd, K.G. 68, *104*
Horrocks, L.A., s. Toews, A.D. 11, 14, *63*
Horwitz, W.A., s. Kalinowsky, L.B. 320, *345*

Howard, A., s. Honigfeld, G. 266, *308*
Howard, A., s. Rifkin, A. 257, 272, *312*
Howlett, D.R., Jenner, F.A. 72, *103*
Howley, P.H., s. Kirkpatrick, J.B. 14, *59*
Howse, D.C., s. Plum, F. 322, *347*
Hrubec, Z., s. Pollin, W. 555, 556, *613*
Hsu, D.S., s. Lorenzo, A.V. 324, *346*
Hsu, G.L.K., s. Singer, K. 679, *702*
Huang, C.Y., s. Silva, L. de 298, *313*
Hubach, H. 163, 164, *188*
Hubach, H., s. Schneider, E. 163, *193*
Hubbard, B., s. Judd, L.L. 687, *697*
Hubbard, J.I., s. Musick, J. 50, *61*
Hubbes, A., s. Hoffmann, E. 678, *697*
Hubel, D.H. [H 86] 1004, *1083*
Hubel, D.H., Wiesel, T.N. [H 87, 88, 88a] 880, 902, 918, 920, 921, 926, *1083*
Hubel, D.H., s. Wiesel, T.N. [W 24b] 921, *1102*
Huber, G. 622, 639, 661, 685, 689, *697*
Huber, G., Gross, G., Schüttler, R. 574, *608*, 630, 685, 689, *697*
Huber, G., Penin, H. 170, 171, 177, *188*
Hucker, H., Woggon, B., Angst, J. 257, *308*
Hucker, H., s. Woggon, B. 257, *314*
Hueckstedt, B. 416, 424, *530*
Hülstrung, H., s. Ohlmeyer, P. [O 2] 996, 997, *1094*
Huey, L.Y., s. Judd, L.L. 687, *697*
Hugelin, A., Bonvallet, M. [H 89, 90] 951, 978, *1083*
Hugelin, A., s. Dell, P. [D 18, 19] 978, 979, *1074*
Hugger, H. [H 91] 889, *1083*
Hughes, C.C., s. Leighton, A.H. 662, *698*

Hughes, J., Smith, T.W., Kosterlitz, H.W., Fothergrill, L.A., Morgan, B.A., Morris, H.R. 40, *58*
Hughes, J., s. Kosterlitz, H.W. 41, *59*
Hughes, J.T., s. Woods, H.F. 7, *64*
Hull, C.L. [H 92] 790, 1043, *1083*
Hull, R.C., Marshall, J.A. 263, *308*
Hullin, R.P., s. Brown, D.G. 340, *342*
Hulten, K. van, s. Lopes da Silva, F.H. 134, *191*
Humboldt, W. von 512, *530*
Hume, W.I., s. Claridge, G. 691, *694*
Humphrey, J.H., White, R.B. 628, 681, 697
Humphrey, N.R., Weiskrantz, L. 448, *530*
Hunger, H., Leopold, D. 691, *697*
Hunsperger, R.A., Bucher, V.M. 471, *530*
Hunsperger, R.W. [H 93, 94] 819, 940, 941, 942, 943, 944, *1083*
Hunsperger, R.W., Brown, J.L., Rosvold, H.E. [H 95] 940, *1083*
Hunsperger, R.W., s. Fernandez de Molina, A. 458, *527*, [F 5, 6] 940, 943, 944, *1077*
Hupfer, K., Juergens, U., Ploog, D. 479, 480, *530*
Hupfer, K., s. Ploog, D. 394, 430, *538*
Hurst, L.A., Mundy-Castle, A.C., Beerstecher, D.M. 176, *188*
Hurst, L.A., s. Mundy-Castle, A.C. 162, *192*
Hurvich, L.M., Jameson, D. [H 96] 912, 913, *1083*
Huse-Kleinstoll, G., Dahme, B., Flemming, B., Haag, A., Meffert, J., Polonius, M.L., Rosewald, G., Speidel, H. 552, *608*
Huse-Kleinstoll, G., s. Dahme, B. 552, *604*
Hussain, M.Z., Khan, A.G., Chaudhry, Z.A. 291, *308*
Husserl 791

Huston, P.E., Locher, L.M. 328, *345*
Huston, P.E., s. Gottlieb, J.S. 333, *344*
Huszka, L., s. Lovett-Doust, J.W. 295, *310*
Hutchings, B., Mednick, S.A. 598, *608*
Hutchings, B., s. Mednick, S.A. 594, 599, *611*
Hutchinson, J.B. 465, *530*
Hutt, C. 644, 649, 650, *697*
Huttenlocher, P.R. [H 97] 1004, 1005, *1083*
Huttunen, M., s. Niskanen, P. 71, *105*
Huxley, A.F., s. Hodgkin, A.L. [H 73] 872, 1064, *1082*
Huxley, J., Mayr, E., Osmond, H., Hoffer, A. 577, *608*
Huxley, J.S. 384, *530*, [H 98] 802, 947, *1083*
Huxtable, R., Barbeau, A. 199, *238*
Huxtable, R.J., Barbeau, A. 27, *59*
Hvidberg, E.F., s. Kragh-Sörensen, P. 330, *346*
Hyams, L., s. Kirkpatrick, J.B. 14, *59*
Hydén, H., s. Hansson, H.-A. 21, *58*
Hydén, H., Lange, P. 14, 15, *59*
Hyttel, J. 212, 214, *238*

Idänpään-Heikkilä, J., Alhava, E., Olkinuora, M., Palva, I. 291, *308*
Iggo, A. [I 1] 908, 1054, *1083*
Igert, C., Lairy, G.C. 172, *188*
Ignatov, S.A., s. Vartanian, M.E. 681, *703*
Iguchi, K., s. Watanabe, S. 272, *314*
Ikard, F., s. Suedfeld, P. 735, 737, 741, *751*
Ikuta, K., s. Okada, T. 93, *105*
Imbach, P., s. Moccetti, T. 287, *310*
Imlah, N.W., Murphy, K.P. 256, *308*
Imlah, N.W., Ryan, E., Harrington, J.A. 332, *345*

Immelmann, K. 444, *530*
Immich, H. 292, *308*
Impastato, D.J., Karliner, W. 337, *345*
Ingalls, R.P. 637, 673, 689, *697*
Ingersoll, E.H., s. Magoun, H.W. 471, *534*
Inglis, J. 319, *345*
Ingvar, D.H. [I 2] 978, 1054, *1083*
Ingvar, D.H., Lassen, N.A. 6, 7, 53, *59*
Ingvar, D.H., Sjölund, B., Ardö, A. 162, *188*
Ingvar, D.H., Söderberg, U. [I 3] 1007, *1083*
Ingvarsson, C.G. 74, *103*
Inouye, E. 555, *608*
Invernizzi, R., s. Venezian, E.C. 292, *313*
Ippoliti, G., s. Venezian, E.C. 292, *313*
Iqbal, Z., s. Sharma, N.C. 48, *63*
Isaac, W. 744, *748*
Isaacson, R.L. 453, 460, *530*
Isac, M., Stern, S., Edelstein, E.L. 288, *308*
Isbell, H., s. Wikler, A. 164, *196*
Ishino, H., s. Watanabe, S. 271, *314*
Itani, J. 431, *530*
Itard, J., s. Malson, L. 522, *534*, 710, *749*
Itil, T.M. 138, 140, 172, 179, 180, 181, *188*
Itil, T.M., Saletu, B., Davis, S. 173, 174, 177, *188*
Itil, T.M., s. Fink, M. 172, *186*
Itil, T.M., s. Saletu, B. 175, *193*
Ito, I., s. Eccles, J.C. [E 6] 814, 843, 891, 897, 1039, *1075*
Ito, M., Yoshida, M., Obata, K., Kawai, N., Udo, M. [I 4] *1083*
Ito, T., s. Fujita, K. 93, *102*
Ivanitsky, A.M., Natalevich, E.S. 569, *608*
Iversen, L.L. 34, *59*
Iversen, L.L., Bloom, F.E. 36, 37, *59*

Iversen, L.L., Iversen, S.D., Snyder, S.H. 38, *59*
Iversen, L.L., Otsuka, M. 199, *238*
Iversen, L.L., Rogawski, M.A., Miller, R.J. 216, *238*
Iversen, L.L., s. Bird, E.D. 54, *56*
Iversen, L.L., s. Miller, R.J. 216, *240*
Iversen, S.D., s. Iversen, L.L. 38, *59*
Ives, J.O., s. Nies, A. 264, *311*
Ives, J.O., s. Weaver, L.A. Jr. 318, *349*
Izard, C.E. 418, 420, 522, *530*
Izard, C.E., s. Tomkin, S.S. 423, *542*

Jacklin, C.N., s. Maccoby, E.E. 647, *699*
Jackson, C.W. 740, *748*
Jackson, D.M., Andén, N.-E., Dahlström, A. 211, *238*
Jackson, J.H. 448, 449, 451, 478, *530*, [J 1] 771, 879, 884, 888, 897, 898, 902, 906, 968, *1083*
Jackson, R., s. Goetzl, U. 581, 583, *607*
Jacob, H. 134, *188*, [J 2] 934, 935, *1083*
Jacob, H.J. 740, *748*
Jacobitz, K., s. Penin, H. 124, 127, *192*
Jacobs, G.H., s. Valois, R.L. de [V 2] 913, *1101*
Jacobsen, s. Fulton, 353
Jacobsen, B., s. Kety, S.S. 553, 559, 566, *609*
Jacobsen, B., s. Paikin, H. 558, *612*
Jacobsen, B., s. Rimmer, J. 577, *613*
Jacobsen, B., s. Schulsinger, F. 568, *614*
Jacobsen, N., s. Phillips, J.E. 566, *612*
Jacobson, A., Kales, A., Lehmann, D., Hodemaker, F.S. [J 3] 995, *1083*
Jacobson, A., Lehmann, D., Kales, A., Wenner, W.H. [J 3a] 1017, *1083*
Jacobson, G., Baldessarini, R.J., Manschreck, T. 297, *308*

Jacobson, J.L., s. Bickford, R.G. 117, *183*
Jacquet, Y.F., Lajtha, A. 26, 59
Jääskeläinen, J., s. Niskanen, P. 71, *105*
Jaenig, W. 455, 457, 458, *530*
Järvilehto, T., s. Fruhstorfer, H. 152, *186*
Jaffry, N.F., s. Sharma, N.C. 48, *63*
Jakobson, R. 436, *530*
James, J., s. Marjerrison, G. 164, *191*
James, J.H., s. Reich, T. 561, *613*
James, N., Chapman, C.J. 581, 583, *609*
James, W. [J 4] 843, 972, 1021, 1025, *1083*
Jameson, D., s. Hurvich, L.M. [H 96] 912, 913, *1083*
Janet, P. 688, 697 [J 5] 771, 931, *1083*
Janis, I.L. 327, *345*
Janke, W. 247, *308*
Janke, W., Debus, G. 247, *308*
Janowsky, D.S., s. Davis, J.M. 91, *101*
Janowsky, D.S., s. Judd, L.L. 687, *697*
Janz, D. 166, 168, *188*, 335, *345*
Janz, H.W. 641, 660, *697*
Janzarik, W. 380, *530*, 739, *748*
Janzen, R., Behnsen, G. [J 7] 1015, *1084*
Janzen, R., Kornmüller, A.E. [J 6] 985, *1083*
Japanisches Gesundheitsministerium, Abt. f. seelische Gesundheit 649, 651, *697*
Jaramillo, R.A., s. Oswald, I. [O 14] 1015, *1094*
Jarvik, L.F., Deckard, B.S. 577, *609*
Jarvik, L.F., s. Sperber, M.A. 546, 601, *615*
Jarvik, M.E. 210, *238*
Jasper, H. [J 8] 811, 894, 950, 973, *1084*
Jasper, H., Ricci, G., Doane, B., [J 11] 880, 929, 1031, 1036, *1084*

Jasper, H., s. Brazier, M.A.B. 121, *183*
Jasper, H., s. Penfield, W. [P 14] 883, 884, *1095*
Jasper, H., s. Ricci, G. [R 14] 817, 1028, 1031, 1036, *1096*
Jasper, H., s. Sharpless, S. [S 29a] *1098*
Jasper, H.H. [J 9] 811, 973, *1084*
Jasper, H.H., Droogleever-Fortuyn, J. [J 10] 978, *1084*
Jasper, H.H., Koyama, I. 37, 59
Jasper, H.H., Smirnov, G.D. [J 12] 1028, 1030, 1036, *1084*
Jasper, H.H., s. Penfield, W. 126, *192*
Jaspers, K. 685, 688, 697, [J 13] 761, 762, 771, 780, 790, 931, 972, 973, *1084*
Jatzkewitz, H. 571, *609*
Javoy, F., Agid, Y., Bouvet, D., Glowinski, J. 219, *238*
Jean, R., s. Cadilhac, J. 160, *183*
Jeffcoate, S., s. Hökfelt, T. 200, *238*
Jeffrey, P.L., s. Wellington, B.S. 20, *64*
Jellinger, 54
Jellinger, K., Seitelberger, F. 158, *188*
Jenkins, R.B., s. Lebensohn, Z.M. 228, *239*, 339, *346*
Jenner, F.A., s. Bond, P.A. 72, *100*
Jenner, F.A., s. Howlett, D.R. 72, *103*
Jenner, M.R., s. Mai, F.M. 83, *104*
Jenney, E.H., s. Sugerman, A.A. 173, *195*
Jennings, H.S. 447, *531*
Jensen, G.D., Bobitt, R., Gordon, B.N. 489, *531*
Jensen, G.D., Tolman, C.W. 500, *531*
Jensen, J., s. Sørensen, R. 293, 299, *313*
Jensen, K., s. Krogh, H.J. 164, *189*
Jerauld, R., s. Kennel, J.H. 726, *748*

Jerauld, R., s. Klaus, M.H. 726, *748*
Jessell, T., s. Kanazawa, I. 40, 59
Jewell, P.A., s. Andersson, B. [A 23] 939, *1069*
Jimerson, D.C., s. Post, R.M. 75, *106*
Jönsson, L.-E., Gunne, L.-M., Änggård, E. 230, *238*
Johannesen, K., s. Engel, J. 221, *237*
Johannson, F., s. Bonetti, U. 686, *693*
Johansson, H., s. Persson, S.-Å. 229, *240*
Johansson, O., s. Elde, R. 26, 40, *57*
Johansson, O., s. Hökfelt, T. 15, 40, *58*, 200, *238*
John, E.R. [J 14] 1025, 1039, *1084*
Johnson, A.J., s. Shaw, D.M. 70, 71, *107*
Johnson, A.L., s. Patel, A.J. 36, *62*
Johnson, A.L., s. Shaw, D.M. 110, *113*
Johnson, D.A.W., Malik, N.A. 256, *308*
Johnson, F.N. 270, *308*
Johnson, M., s. Sila, B. 172, *194*
Johnson, M., s. Ulett, G. *195*
Johnson, M.W., s. Ulett, G.A. 179, *195*
Johnson, N.A., s. Reed, S.C. 553, *613*
Johnston, G.A.R., s. Curtis, D.R. 36, *56*
Johnstone, E.C. 264, *308*
Johnstone, E.C., s. Baker, J.M.H. 92, *99*
Johnstone, E.C., s. Brockingtone, I. 570, *604*
Jolly, A. 384, 488, 493, *531*
Jolly, C.J., s. Chance, M.R.A. 384, 494, *525*
Jonas, W.Z., s. Baron, M. 271, *303*
Jonas, W.Z., s. Gershon, E.S. 583, *607*
Jonason, J. 205, *238*
Jonchev, V., Arianova, L. 289, *308*
Jonchev, V., Mitkov, V. 298, *308*

Jones, A. 737, *748*
Jones, A.E., s. Valois, R.L. de [V 2, 3] 913, *1101*
Jones, B.C., Clark, D.L. 496, *531*
Jones, F.D., Maas, J.W., Dekirmenjian, H., Fawcett, J.A. 72, *103*
Jones, G.A., s. Greenblatt, M. 171, 176, *187*
Jones, I.H. 401, *531*
Jones, I.H., Frei, D. 396, *531*
Jones, K.L., Smith, D.W., Ulleland, C.N., Pythkowicz Streissguth, A. 673, *697*
Jones, L.G., s. Bullowa, M. 521, *524*
Jones, M.T., Hillhause, E., Burden, J. 76, *103*
Jones, R.T., Callaway, E. 175, *188*
Jones, R.T., s. Callaway, E. 175, *183*
Jonkman, E.J. 150, *188*
Jonsson, E., Nilsson, T. 599, *609*
Jonsson, G., s. Fuxe, K. 34, *58*, 110, *112*
Joseph, M.H., Owen, F., Baker, H.F., Bourne, R.C. *59*
Jotkowitz, M.W. 332, *345*
Jouvent, R., Lecrubier, Y., Puech, A.-J., Frances, H., Simon, P., Wildlocher, D. 89, *103*
Jouvet, M. [J 15–19] 763, 980, 981, 988, 989, 990, 995, 1006, 1007, 1011, 1016, 1020, *1084*
Jouvet, M., Pellin, B., Mounier, D. [J 20] 989, *1084*
Jouvet, M., s. Hernández-Peón, R. [H 38] 824, *1081*
Jovanović, U.J. [J 21, 22] 988, 997, *1084*
Judd, D.B. [J 23] 914, *1084*
Judd, L.L., Hubbard, B., Janowsky, D.S., Huey, L.Y., Attewell, P.A. 687, *697*
Juel-Nielsen, N. 581, *609*
Juel-Nielsen, N., Videbech, T. 594, *609*
Juel-Nielsen, N., s. Hauge, M. 574, *608*
Juel-Nielsen, N., s. Weeke, A. 649, 661, *704*

Juergens, U. 437, 452, 471, 473, 476, 483, *531*
Juergens, U., Mueller-Preuss, P. 474, *531*
Juergens, U., Ploog, D. 425, 436, 437, 471, 473, 477, 478, 513, *531*
Juergens, U., s. Hupfer, K. 479, 480, *530*
Juergens, U., s. Mueller-Preuss, P. 474, *536*
Juergens, U., s. Ploog, D. 394, 430, *538*
Julian, T., Metcalfe, M., Coppen, A. *697*
Julian, T., s. Balázs, R. 36, 37, *55*
Jung, C.G. 688, *697*, [J 24] 784, 791, 930, *1084*
Jung, C.G., s. Peterson, F. [P 19] 930, *1095*
Jung, E.G., Schwarz-Speck, M., Kormany, G. 292, *308*
Jung, G. 119, 167, 170, 171, 172, 178, *188*
Jung, R. 116, 119, 163, *188*, *189*, 450, 452, 483, *531*, 633, *697*, [J 25–51], 763, 766, 770, 780, 789, 822, 825, 826, 844, 846, 862, 868, 880, 881, 888, 891, 893, 898, 899, 900, 905, 908, 910, 911, 912, 913, 915, 917, 920, 928, 934, 935, 948, 970, 971, 973, 977, 979, 982, 984, 985, 988, 994, 999, 1000, 1015, 1035, 1036, 1051, 1052, 1054, *1084*, *1085*
Jung, R., Baumgartner, G. [J 53] 926, *1085*
Jung, R., Baumgarten, R. von, Baumgartner, G. [J 52] 766, 844, 908, *1085*
Jung, R., Carmichael, E.A., [J 54] 948, *1085*
Jung, R., Creutzfeld, O., Grüsser, O.J. [J 55] 982, 1005, *1086*
Jung, R., Dietz, V. [J 56, 57] 777, 822, 835, 836, 840, 848, *1086*
Jung, R., Hassler, R. [J 58] 824, 825, 828, 845, *1086*
Jung, R., Kornhuber, H.H., Da Fonseca, J.S. [J 59] 880, 1035, 1036, 1037, *1086*

Jung, R., Kornmüller, A.E. [J 60] 977, *1086*
Jung, R., Kuhlo, W. [J 61] 1016, *1086*
Jung, R., Spillman, L. [J 61a] 922, *1086*
Jung, R., Tönnies, J.F. 126, *189*, [J 62] 862, 887, *1086*
Jung, R., s. Baumgartner, G. [B 17] 922, 982, *1070*
Jung, R., s. Brooks, B. [B 66] 918, 1032, *1072*
Jung, R., s. Cremerius, J. 163, *184*, [C 14a] 1018, *1073*
Jung, R., s. Creutzfeldt, O. [C 16] 1004, 1005, *1073*
Jung, R., s. Dichgans, J. [D 31] 782, 847, 860, *1075*
Jung, R., s. Grünewald-Zuberbier, E. [G 43, 44] 789, 833, 834, *1079*
Jung, R., s. Tönnies, J.F. [T 11] 858, *1100*
Jung, R., s. Weber, W.C. [W 15] 766, 960, 970, 971, 972, 985, *1102*
Jungkunz, G., Kuss, H.J. 110, *112*
Jurko, M.F., s. Andy, O.J. 371, 372, *375*
Jus, A., Pineau, R., Lachance, R., Pelchat, G., Jus, K., Pires, P., Villeneuve, R. 297, *308*
Jus, C., s. Gastaut, H.A. [G 11] 1028, 1031, 1032, *1078*
Jus, K., s. Jus, A. 297, *308*
Jusczyk, P., s. Eimas, P.D. 437, 440, 441, 442, *526*
Juul-Jensen, P., s. Strömgren, L.S. 164, *195*, 319, *348*

Kaada, B.R., s. Fangel, Chr. [F 3] *1076*
Kablitz, C., s. Spehr, W. 158, 161, *194*
Kacher, H. 399, 491
Kado, R.T., s. Adey, W.R. 131, *182*
Kaelbing, R., s. Litvak, R. 291, *310*
Källén, B., s. Kullander, S. 293, *309*
Käufer, C., s. Penin, H. 155, *192*

Kagan, G., Klein, R.E. 711, 712, 731, 732, *748*
Kahn, R.L., s. Fink, M. 164, *186*
Kaij, L. 599, *609*
Kaij, L., s. McNeil, T.F. 575, *611*
Kaila, E. 415, *531*
Kaira, P.S., s. McCann, S.M. 220, *239*
Kaiser-Grubel, S., s. Bickel, H. 631, 637, *693*
Kajii, T. 649, *697*
Kales, A., s. Jacobson, A. [J 3, 3a] 995, 1017, *1083*
Kalinowsky, L.B., Barrera, S.E., Horwitz, W.A. 320, *345*
Kalinowsky, L.B., Hippius, H. 333, 335, 336, *345*
Kallmann, F.J. 555, 557, 561, 564, *609*
Kallmann, F.J., Roth, B. 588, *609*
Kallmann, F.J., s. Erlenmeyer-Kimling, L. 577, *606*
Kalton, G., s. Shepherd, M. 649, *702*
Kalucy, R.S., s. Crisp, A.H. 651, *694*
Kamberi, I.A., Thorn, N.A. 199, 200, *238*
Kammen, D. von 94, *103*, *112*
Kammen, D.P. van, Murphy, D.L. 271, *308*
Kammen, D.P. van, s. Plantey, F. 94, *106*
Kamp, A., s. Gastaut, H.A. [G 11] 1028, 1031, 1032, *1078*
Kamp, A., s. Storm van Leeuwen, W. 147, *195*
Kamp, A., s. Van der Tweel, L.H. 148, *195*
Kanaka, T.S., s. Balasubramaniam, V. 361, 369, 370, 373, *375*
Kanarek, K.S., Thompson, P.D., Levin, S.E. 299, *308*
Kanazawa, I., Jessell, T. 40, *59*
Kancuká, V., s. Uhlíř, F. 253, *313*
Kandel, E.R. [K 1] 1039, *1086*
Kandel, E.R., Spencer, W.A. [K 2, 3] *1086*

Kane, J., Rifkin, A., Quitkin, F., Klein, D.F. 246, *308*
Kanfer, F.H., Phillips, J.S. 629, 633, *697*
Kanig, K. 563, *609*
Kanner, L. 588, 589, *609*
Kanowski, S., s. Bauer, H. 272, 298, *303*
Kanowski, S., s. Bellabarba, U. 297, *303*
Kanowski, S., s. Helmchen, H. 128, *187*
Kanowski, S., s. Penin, H. 124, 127, *192*
Kant, I. [K 4, 5] 760, 765, 766, 767, 768, 773, 778, 779, 807, 821, 906, 907, 965, *1086*
Kantor, S.J., Bigger, J.T. Jr., Glassman, A.H., Macken, D.L., Perel, J.M. 287, *309*
Kantor, S.J., s. Glassman, A.H. 331, *344*
Kantor, S.J., s. Perel, J.M. *311*
Kapetanakis, S., s. Lazos, G. 292, *309*
Kaplan, A.R. 553, 563, *609*
Karkhanis, Y.D., s. Brostoff, S.W. 23, *56*
Karlin, A., Cowburn, D.A. 25, *59*
Karliner, W., s. Impastato, D.J. 337, *345*
Karlsson, J.L. 557, 561, 562, *609*
Karmeli, F., s. Birnbaum, D. 290, *304*
Karmos, G., s. Grastýan, E. [G 37] 977, *1079*
Karnovsky, M.L., s. Eichberg, J. 19, *57*
Karobath, M., s. Schuster, P. *312*
Karpas, A.E., s. Albeaux-Fernet, M. 663, *692*
Karten, H.J., s. Nauta, W.J.H. 449, *536*
Kasai, M., s. Changeux, J.-P. 25, *56*
Kasamatsu, A. [K 6, 7] 765, 982, 983, *1086*
Kasamatsu, A., s. Creutzfeldt, O. [C 17] 982, *1073*
Kasparian, G., s. Orlov, P. 257, *311*

Kasriel, J., s. Lader, M. 691, *698*
Katinas, G.S., s. Halberg, F. *187*
Kato, T., s. Fujita, K. 93, *102*
Kato, T., s. Okada, T. 93, *105*
Katschnig, H., Grumiller, I., Strobl, R. 649, *697*
Katschnig, H., Steinert, H. 651, *697*
Katschnig, H., Strotzka, H. 660, *697*
Katsuki, Y., Sumi, T., Uchiyama, H., Watanabe, T. [K 8] 908, *1086*
Katz, R.I., s. Harner, R. 157, *187*
Katzman, R. 16, 45, *59*, 705
Kaufman, I.C. 496, 502, *531*
Kaufman, I.C., Rosenblum, L.A. 407, 489, 497, 502, *531*
Kaufman, I.C., s. Hoagland, H. 179, *188*
Kaufman, I.C., s. Rosenblum, L.A. 489, *540*
Kaufman, M.R., s. Rosenblatt, S. 340, *347*
Kawai, M., s. Kondo, S. 384, *532*
Kawai, N., s. Ito, M. [I 4] *1083*
Kawakami, M., s. Sawyer, C.H. [S 2, 3] 862, 940, *1097*
Kawakita, H. 20, 21, *59*
Kawamura, H., Sawyer, C.H. [K 9] *1086*
Kay, D., s. Andrews, G. 638, *692*
Kay, D.W.K. 585, 596, *609*
Kay, D.W.K., Fahy, T., Garside, R.F. 332, *345*
Kay, D.W.K., Roth, M., Atkinson, M.W., Stephens, D.A., Garside, R.F. 553, 565, *609*
Kay, D.W.K., s. Roth, M. 322, 338, *347*
Kay, D.W.K., s. Stephens, D.A. 553, 558, 564, 565, *616*
Kay, J.L., s. Hill, R.M. 294, *307*
Kay, L. *609*
Kayce, M.M., s. Goldberg, S.C. 664, *696*

Kayton, L., s. Giannitrapani, D. 174, 178, *186*
Kazamatsuri, H., Chien, C.-P., Cole, J.O. 298, *309*
Kazmierczak, H., s. Steinbuch, K. [S 49] 853, *1099*
Kebabian, J.W., Clement-Cormier, Y.C., Petzold, G.L., Greengard, P. 30, *59*
Kebabian, J.W., Greengard, P. 216, *239*
Kebabian, J.W., s. Clement-Cormier, Y.C. 216, 217, *237*
Keddie, K.M.G., s. Oswald, I. [O 14] 1015, *1094*
Keddie, K.M.G., s. Valentine, M. 318, *348*
Kehr, W., Carlsson, A., Lindqvist, M. 215, *239*
Kehr, W., Carlsson, A., Lindqvist, M., Magnusson, T., Atack, C. 215, *239*
Kehr, W., Speckenbach, W. 229, *239*
Kehr, W., s. Carlsson, A. 204, *236*
Kehrer, H.E. 637, 690, *697*
Keidel, W.D. [K 10, 11] 877, 908, *1086*
Keidel, W.D., Spreng, M. 151, *189*
Keiner, M., s. Pfaff, D. 466, 467, *537*
Kellaway, P., Petersen, I. 133, *189*
Keller, H. 517, *705*, [K 12] 831, *1086*
Keller-Teschke, M., s. Hartmann, E. 93, *103*
Kellerup, P., s. Krogh, H.J. 164, *189*
Kellett, J.M., Metcalfe, M., Bailey, J., Coppen, A.J. 272, *309*
Kellner, R., s. Simpson, G.M. 330, 331, *348*
Kellogg, L.A., s. Kellogg, W.N. 506, *531*
Kellogg, W.N. 506, *531*
Kellogg, W.N., Kellogg, L.A. 506, *531*
Kelly, A.H., Beaton, L.E., Magoun, H.W. 473, *531*
Kelly, D., Mitchell-Heggs, N. 359, *376*
Kelly, D., Richardson, A., Mitchell-Heggs, N., Greenup, J., Chen, J., Hafner, R.J. 363, 365, *376*
Kelly, D., s. Mitchell-Heggs, N. 363, 365, *376*
Kelly, D., s. Richardson, A.E. 365, *377*
Kelly, D.B., Morell, J.I., Pfaff, D.W. 470, *531*
Kelly, P.H., s. Green, A.R. 88, *103*
Kempe, P. 736, *748*
Kempe, P., Closs, C., Andresen, B., Stemmler, G. 739, *748*
Kempe, P., Reimer, C. 736, *748*
Kempe, P., Schönberger, J., Gross, J. 740, *748*
Kempe, P., s. Gross, J. 736, *748*
Kendel, K., Beck, U., Kruschke-Dubois, H. [K 13] 1014, *1086*
Kendell, R., s. Lader, M. 691, *698*
Kendler, K.S., Davis, K.L. 85, *103*
Kendon, A., Ferber, A. 398, 399, *531*
Kendrick, J.F., s. Brandt, H.A. 162, *183*
Kennard, M.A., Rabinovitch, M.S., Fister, W.P. 172, *189*
Kennard, M.A., Schwartzman, A.G. 172, *189*
Kennedy, A.C., Linton, A.L., Luice, R.G., Renfrew, S. 160, *189*
Kennedy, C., Sokoloff, L. 52, *59*
Kennedy, P.F. 574, *609*
Kennedy, P.F., s. Hershon, H.I. 297, *307*
Kennel, J.H., Jerauld, R., Wolfe, H., Chesler, D., Kreger, N.C., McAlpine, W., Steffa, M., Klaus, M.H. 726, *748*
Kennel, J.H., s. Klaus, M.H. 519, *532*, 720, 721, 726, *748*
Keogh, R.P., s. Marjerrison, G. 173, *191*
Kéresi, F., s. Lisák, K. [L 30] 1031, *1089*
Kessler, S. 562, *609*
Kessler, S., s. Barchas, J.D. 550, 571, *603*

Kety, S., s. Paikin, H. 558, *612*
Kety, S., s. Rosenthal, D. 561, *614*
Kety, S.A., Schmidt, C.F. 6, *59*
Kety, S.S. 6, *59*, 339, 345, [K 14] 1007, *1086*
Kety, S.S., Elkes, J. 3, *59*
Kety, S.S., Evarts, E.V., Williams, H.L. *189*
Kety, S.S., Rosenthal, D., Wender, P.H., Schulsinger, F. 557, 559, 560, 561, 566, *609*
Kety, S.S., Rosenthal, D., Wender, P.H., Schulsinger, F., Jacobsen, B. 553, 559, 566, *609*
Kety, S.S., s. Mangold, R. [M 22] 1007, *1091*
Kety, S.S., s. Pollin, W. 94, *106*
Kety, S.S., s. Rosenthal, D. 553, 558, *614*
Kety, S.S., s. Wender, P.H. 559, 560, *617*
Khan, A.G., s. Hussain, M.Z. 291, *308*
Khan, M.A., s. Krogh, H.J. 164, *189*
Khani, M.K., s. Akiskal, H.S. 582, *602*
Kidd, K.K., Cavalli-Sforza, L.L. 550, 562, *609*
Kidd, K.K., Weissman, M.M. 664, *698*
Kidd, K.K., s. Matthysse, S.W. 562, *611*
Kielholz, P. 86, 97, *103*, 260, *309*, 684, *698*
Kiley, J., Hines, O. 161, *189*
Kiley, J.E. 158, *189*
Kiley, J.E., Woodruff, M.W., Pratt, K.L. 161, *189*
Kilian, M., Frey, H.H. 202, *239*
Kiloh, L.G., Child, J.P., Latner, G. 329, *345*
Kim, L.I., s. Tupin, J.P. 271, *313*
Kimbrough, J.C. 289, *309*
Kimura, B. 649, 661, *698*
Kind, H., s. Ernst, K. 659, *695*
King, J.E., King, P.A. 490, *532*

King, J.S., s. Toews, A.D. 11, 14, *63*
King, P.A., s. King, J.E. 490, *532*
King, P.D. 333, *345*
King, T.L., s. Sara, V.R. 49, *62*
Kinkelin, M. 684, *698*
Kinsey, A.C., Pomeroy, W.B., Martin, C.E. [K 15] 799, 940, *1086*
Kirk, L., Baastrup, P.C., Schou, M. 272, *309*
Kirk, L., s. Møller, S.E. 71, *105*
Kirk, L., s. Schou, M. 272, *312*
Kirkland, R.J.A., s. Whittaker, V.P. 13, 14, *64*
Kirkpatrick, J.B., Hyams, L., Thomas, V.L., Howley, P.H. 14, *59*
Kirman, B.H. 681, *698*
Kirstein, L., Ottosson, J.-O. 321, *346*
Kissling, W., s. Emrich, H.M. 112, *112*
Kitai, S.T., s. Valois, R.L. de [V 4, 5] 913, *1101*
Kitchen, J.H., s. Ruf, K.B. 43, *62*
Kjellberg, B., s. Randrup, A. 75, *106*
Klackenberg, G. 732, *748*
Klages, W., s. Panse, F. 91, *106*
Klaiber, E.L., Broverman, D.M., Vogel, W., Kobayashi, Y. 663, *698*
Klass, D.W., s. Chatrian, G.E. 121, *183*
Klaus, M., s. Barnett, C. 721, 726, *746*
Klaus, M.H., Jerauld, R., Kreger, N., McAlpine, W., Steffa, M., Kennel, J. 726, *748*
Klaus, M.H., Kennel, J. 519, *532*, 720, 721, 726, *748*
Klaus, M.H., s. Kennel, J.H. 726, *748*
Klawans, H.L. Jr., Rubovits, R. 297, 298, *309*
Klawans, H.L., s. Holinger, P.C. 299, *308*
Klee, A. 158, *189*
Klein, A., s. Tamir, H. 26, *63*

Klein, D.F. 78, *103*, 332, *346*
Klein, D.F., Davis, J.M. 221, *239*
Klein, D.F., s. Kane, J. 246, *308*
Klein, D.F., s. Rifkin, A. 257, 272, 292, *312*
Klein, D.F., s. Struve, F.A. 172, *195*
Klein, R.E., s. Kagan, G. 711, 712, 731, 732, *748*
Klein, R.E., s. Lasky, R.E. 440, *533*
Kleine, W. [K 16] 1017, *1086*
Kleinerman, J., s. Mangold, R. [M 22] 1007, *1091*
Kleist, K. 454, *532*, [K 17, 18] 762, 882, 901, 902, 904, 905, 906, 943, 944, 977, 992, *1086*
Kleitman, H., s. Kleitman, N. [K 22] 988, *1087*
Kleitman, N. [K 19, 20] 991, 998, 999, 1008, 1009, 1011, *1087*
Kleitman, N., Engelmann, T.G. [K 21] 992, *1087*
Kleitman, N., Kleitman, H. [K 22] 988, 992, *1087*
Kleitman, N., s. Aserinsky, E. [A 31, 32] 991, 996, 1008, 1019, *1069*
Kleitman, N., s. Blake, H. [B 48] 993, *1071*
Kleitman, N., s. Dement, W. [D 24, 25] 991, 992, 996, 998, 999, 1009, 1010, 1011, *1074*
Klempel, K. 71, 89, *103*, *104*
Klepel, H., s. Rabending, G. 167, *193*
Klerman, G.L., s. Paykel, E.S. 688, *701*
Klett, C.J., Cole, J.O. 257, *309*
Klett, C.J., s. Prien, R.F. 253, *312*
Kley, I.B., s. Pearson, J.S. 567, *612*
Klima, E.S., Bellugi, U. 516, *532*
Klima, E.S., s. Bellugi, K. 515, *523*
Kline, N.S., Angst, J. 244, *309*
Kline, N.S., Barclay, G.L., Cole, J.O., Esser, A.H.,

Lehmann, H., Wittenborn, J.R., 94, 97, *104*
Kline, N.S., Lehmann, H.E., Li, C.H., Cooper, T.B. 97, *104*
Kline, N.S., Mason, B.T., Winick, L. 296, *309*
Kline, N.S., Wren, J.C., Cooper, T.B., Varga, E., Canal, O. 271, *309*
Kline, N.S., s. Loomer, H.P. 223, *239*
Kline, N.S., s. Shopsin, B. 267, *313*
Kline, N.S., s. Singh, M.M. 290, *313*
Kline, N.S., s. Wren, J.C. 271, *314*
Klineberg, O. 410, *532*
Kling, A., s. Brady, J.V. [B 57] *1072*
Kling, A., s. Schreiner, L. [S 16] 961, *1098*
Kling, A., s. Serban, G. 446, *541*
Klinger, P.D., s. Agranoff, B.W. [A 11] 1026, 1046, *1068*
Kloos, G., s. Mueller, D. 455, *536*
Klopfer, P.H., s. Bateson, P.P.G. 380, *523*
Klorman, R., Strauss, J., Kokes, R. 567, *609*
Klorman, R., s. Kokes, R. 567, *610*
Klorman, R., s. Strauss, J. 567, *616*
Klüver, H. 453, 505, 506, *532*, [K 23, 24] 803, 806, 932, 1012, *1087*
Klüver, H., Bucy, P.C. 453, *532*, [K 25] 944, 961, 1048, *1087*
Kluge, H., s. Waldmann, K.-D. 272, 298, *314*
Knaack, M., s. Haase, H.J. 253, *307*
Knapp, S., Mandell, A.J. 228, *239*
Knight, A., s. Westley, B.R. 26, *64*
Knight, D.R., s. Sutherland, E.M. 337, *348*
Knight, G. 356, 357, 366, 367, *376*
Knight, G.C. 366, *376*

Knobe, K.E., s. Gershon, E.S. 579, *607*
Knoers, A.M.P., s. Mönks, F.J. 635, 641, *699*
Knorring, L. von, s. Bonetti, U. 686, *693*
Knott, J.R., s. McCallum, W.C. 147, 153, *191*
Knowles, W.B., s. Lindsley, D.B. [L 29] 983, *1089*
Knussmann, R. 642, *698*
Kobayashi, J., s. Mitsuda, H. 565, *611*
Kobayashi, Y., s. Klaiber, E.L. 663, *698*
Koch, G. 602, *609*
Koch, G., Neuhäuser, G. 675, *698*
Koch, R., Cruz, F.F. de la 673, *698*
Koch-Weser, J., s. Greenblatt, D.J. 287, *306*
Kockott, G., Nusselt, L. 682, 690, *698*
Kockott, G., s. Degkwitz, R. 649, 653, *694*
Kockott, G., s. Doerr, P. 672, 683, *694*
Kockott, G., s. Nusselt, L. 682, 690, *700*
Köhler, G.-H. 170, *189*
Köhler, K.H., s. Schenck, G.K. 96, *107*
Koehler, O. 410, 435, *532*, 710, *748*, [K 26, 27, 28] 803, 807, *1087*
Köhler, W. 406, 407, 411, 506, 513, *532*, [K 29, 30, 31, 32] 789, 803, 806, 870, 913, *1087*
Koella, W.P. [K 33] 988, *1087*
Koella, W.P., Levin, P. [K 34] 988, *1087*
Koella, W., s. Hess, R. [H 46, 47] 938, *1081*
Koelle, G.B. 15, 27, 28, *59*
Koeller, D.-M., s. Zerssen, D. von 548, *618*, 680, *704*, *705*
Kölling, A., s. Emrich, H.M. 96, *102*
Koenig, A., s. Mueller, D. 455, *536*
König, L. 295, *309*
Koenig, O. 395, *532*
König, P., s. Hofmann, G. 298, *307*

Köttgen, U. 711, *748*
Kohn, M. 573, *610*
Kohnstamm, O., Quensel, F. [K 35] 979, 982, *1087*
Kohts, N. [K 35a, 35b] 807, *1087*
Kokes, R., Strauss, J., Klorman, R. 567, *610*
Kokes, R., s. Klorman, R. 567, *609*
Kokes, R., s. Strauss, J. 567, *616*
Kolakowska, T., Wiles, D.H., McNeilly, A.S., Gelder, M.G. 292, *309*
Kolakowska, T., s. Beumont, P.J.V. 292, 293, *303*
Kolárský, A., Freund, K., Machek, J., Polák, O. 683, 690, *698*
Kolff, W.J., s. Hippius, H. 97, *103*
Kollmannsberger, A., Kugler, J., Eymer, K.P. 161, *189*
Kolodny, R.C., Masters, W.H., Hendryx, J., Toro, G. 683, *698*
Koluchová, J. 712, 731, *748*
Kolvin, I., Ounsted, C., Richardson, L., Garside, R.F. III 588, 589, *610*
Kolvin, I., Taunch, T., Currah, J., Garside, R.F., Nolan, J., Shaw, W.B. 596, *610*
Kolyaskina, G.I., s. Vartanian, M.E. 681, *703*
Kommerell, B., s. Lanzinger-Rossnagel, G. 161, *190*
Kondo, S., Kawai, M., Ehara, A. 384, *532*
Konishi, S., s. Otsuka, M. 200, *240*
Konorski, J. [K 36, 37] 1026, 1030, 1031, 1038, *1087*
Konorski, J., Kozniewska, H., Stepien, L., Subczynski, J. 474, 475, *532*
Kooi, K.A., Tipton, A.C., Marshall, R.E. 151, *189*
Kooij, M., s. Kortlandt, A. 513, *532*
Kopanda, R.T., s. Bunney, W.E. Jr. 339, *343*
Kopin, J.J., s. Ebert, M. 72, *102*

Kopin, J.J., s. Hertting, G. 223, *238*
Kopun, M., Propping, P. *610*
Korenyi, C., Lowenstein, B. 293, *309*
Korf, J., s. Praag, H.M. van 69, 93, *106*, 109
Kormany, G., s. Jung, E.G. 292, *308*
Korner, A.F., Grobstein, R. 732, *748*
Kornetsky, C., s. Hecht Orzack, M. 566, *608*
Kornhuber, H.H. 451, *532*, [K 38–42a] 777, 805, 832, 851, 901, 904, 958, 1004, 1026, 1039, *1087*
Kornhuber, H.H., Deecke, L. 153, *189*, [K 43] 789, 831, 832, 833, 834, 848, 882, 1035, *1087*
Kornhuber, H.H., Fonseca, J.S. [K 44] 1036, *1088*
Kornhuber, H.H., s. Deecke, L. 153, *184*, [D 10] 832, 834, *1074*
Kornhuber, H.H., s. Jung, R. [J 59] 880, 1035, 1036, 1037, *1086*
Kornmüller, A.E., Palme, F., Strughold, H. [K 45] 969, 977, 983, *1088*
Kornmüller, A.E., s. Janzen, R. [J 6] 985, *1083*
Kornmüller, A.E., s. Jung, R. [J 60] 977, *1086*
Korobkin, R.K., Cutler, R.W.P. 46, *59*
Korsgaard, S. 298, *309*
Kortlandt, A. 381, *532*
Kortlandt, A., Kooij, M. 513, *532*
Koslow, S.H. 95, *104*
Kosterlitz, H.W., Hughes, J. 41, *59*
Kosterlitz, H.W., s. Hughes, J. 40, *58*
Kotin, J., s. Murphy, D.L. 74, 96, *105*
Kotin, J., s. Post, R.M. 73, *106*
Kováts, T.G., s. Halberg, F. *187*
Kow, L.-M., s. Pfaff, D.W. 466, 467, 468, *538*
Koyama, I., s. Jasper, H.H. 37, *59*

Kozakova, M. 291, *309*
Kozniewska, H., s. Konorski, J. 474, 475, *532*
Krämer, W., s. Prüll, G. 162, *193*
Kraepelin, E. 198, *239*, 380, *532*, 567, 684, 686, *698*, [K 46] 783, *1088*
Kragh-Sörensen, P., Eggert-Hansen, C., Baastrup, P.C., Hvidberg, E.F. 330, *346*
Kraines, S.H. [K 47] *1088*
Král, J., s. Marhold, J. 274, *310*
Kramer, E. 436, *532*
Kramer, M., Taube, C.A. 649, 651, *698*
Kramp, P.L., s. Rafaelsen, O.L. 681, *701*
Kranz, H. 596, 597, *610*
Kranz, H., Heinrich, K. 380, *532*
Krashen, S., s. Curtiss, S. [C 21] 896, 897, *1073*
Krashen, S.D., s. Metzig, E. 682, *699*
Kraus, A. 684, *698*
Krause, A.E., s. Marjerrison, G. 173, *191*
Krauss, W. 688, *698*
Kream, J., s. Hellmann, L. 77, *103*
Krebs, F.A., s. Bauer, H. 272, 298, *303*
Krebs, H.A., s. Page, M.A. 52, *61*
Krech, D., s. Bennett, E.L. 49, *56*
Kreger, N.C., s. Kennel, J.H. 726, *748*
Kreger, N., s. Klaus, M.H. 726, *748*
Kreindler, A., s. Weigl, E. [W 17] *1102*
Kretschmer, E. 158, *189*, 626, 627, 665, 666, 680, 685, 688, *698*, [K 48, 49] 812, 950, 951, *1088*
Kretschmer, W. 666, 673, *698*
Kreutzberg, G.W., s. Schubert, P. 5, *63*
Kreutzer, M.A., Charlesworth, W.R. 417, *532*
Kreutzer, W.R., s. Charlesworth, W.R. 411, 414, 417, *525*
Kries, J. von [K 50, 51, 52] 765, 782, 906, 910, 913, 914, *1088*
Kringlen, E. 555, 561, *610*
Kringlen, E., s. Dalgard, O.S. 596, 597, *605*
Kripke, D.F. 131, *189*
Krishnamoorti, S.R., s. Shagass, C. 150, *194*
Kristensson, K. 45, *60*
Kriszat, G., s. Uexküll, J. von 447, *543*
Krnjević, K. 30, 36, *60*
Krogh, H.J., Khan, M.A., Fosvig, L., Jensen, K., Kellerup, P. 164, *189*
Krohn, H., s. Castell, R. 387, 388, *525*
Kroll, P.D., s. Port, F.K. 97, *106*
Kropfl, W.H., s. Armington, J.C. 147, *182*
Krüger, E., s. Müller, D. 292, *311*
Krulich, L., s. McCann, S.M. 220, *239*
Kruschke-Dubois, H., s. Kendel, K. [K 13] 1014, *1086*
Kubicki, S. 157, *189*
Kubicki, S., Rieger, H., Busse, G. 157, *189*
Kubie, L.S. [K 53, 54] 807, 973, *1088*
Kubszansky, P., s. Solomon, P. [S 36a] 933, *1098*
Kubzansky, E., Leiderman, P.H. 742, *748*
Kuefferle, B., s. Schuster, P. *312*
Kuehlmorgen, B., s. Maurus, M. 393, 394, 482, 483, *535*
Kühn, H. [K 55] 810, *1088*
Külpe, O. [K 56] 789, 929, *1088*
Künkel, H. 125, 131, 133, 134, 142, 146, 171, 173, 177, *189*, *190*
Künkel, H., Luba, A., Niethardt, P. 139, 143, 146, 180, *190*
Künkel, H., Machleidt, W., Niethardt, P. 131, 132, *190*
Künkel, H., s. Dolce, G. 133, *184*
Künkel, H., s. Gutjahr, L. 132, *187*
Künkel, H., s. Halberg, F. *187*
Künkel, H., s. Heinze, H.J. 143, 180, *187*
Künkel, H., s. Helmchen, H. 127, 128, 149, 172, *187*, [H 26] *1081*
Künkel, H., s. Penin, H. 124, 127, *192*
Küpfmüller, K. [K 57, 58] 852, 853, 856, 871, 976, *1088*
Küppers, E. [K 59, 60] 762, 904, *1088*
Kuffler, S. [K 61] 765, 915, *1088*
Kuffler, S.W., s. Barlow, H.B. [B 8b] *1070*
Kugler, J. 117, 150, *190*, 631, 682, *698*
Kugler, J., s. Kollmannsberger, A. 161, *189*
Kuhar, M.J., Pert, C.B., Snyder, S.H. 485, *532*
Kuhar, M.J., s. Pert, C.B. 40, *62*
Kuhlo, W., Lehmann, D. [K 62, 63] 991, 996, 1008, 1009, *1088*
Kuhlo, W., s. Jung, R. [J 61] 1016, *1086*
Kuhn, H.M., s. Gerardy, W. [G 16] 1016, *1078*
Kuhn, R. 223, *239*, 260, 261, *309*
Kukka, E.-K., Vilkki, J., Laitinen, L. 359, *376*
Kukopulos, A., Reginaldi, D., Tondo, L., Bernabei, A., Caliari, B. 330, *346*
Kulhanek, F., s. Pieschl, D. 251, *311*
Kullander, S., Källén, B. 293, *309*
Kullberg, G. 359, 363, 364, *376*
Kummer, H. 389, 390, 405, 494, *532*, [K 64] 810, *1088*
Kung, L.S., s. Banerjee, S.P. 88, *99*
Kunz, E., s. Simpson, G.M. 297, *313*
Kunz-Bartholini, E., s. Simpson, G.M. 290, *313*
Kupfer, D.J., Pickar, D., Himmelhoch, J.M., Detre, T.P. 580, *610*
Kuplic, J.B., s. Munoz, R.A. 299, *311*

Kurland, L.T., s. O'Fallon, W.M., 292, *311*
Kurth, G., Eibl-Eibesfeldt, I. 381, *532*
Kurtin, S.B. 292, *309*
Kurtin, S.B., s. Rifkin, A. 292, *312*
Kurtz, D., s. Rohmer, F. 160, *193*
Kuschinsky, G., Lüllmann, H. 283, *309*
Kuss, H.J., s. Jungkunz, G. 110, *112*
Kuypers, H.G.J.M. 476, *532, 533*
Kvasina, T., s. Talairach, J. 357, *378*

Laakmann, G. 82, *104*
Laakmann, G., Benkert, O. 82, *104*
Labarba, R.C., s. White, J.L. 723, *751*
LaBarre, W. 410, *533*
Labarthe, D.R., s. O'Fallon, W.M. 292, *311*
LaBrie, R.A., s. Schildkraut, J.J. 72, *107*
Labhardt, F. 551, 586, *610*
Lacal, C.F., s. Buffa, P. 287, *304*
Lacey, J.H., s. Crisp, A.H. 651, *694*
Lachance, R., s. Jus, A. 297, *308*
Lachman, M., s. Marhold, J. 274, *310*
Lader, M., Kendell, R., Kasriel, J. 691, *698*
Lader, M., Sartorius, N. 688, *698*
Ladinsky, H., Consolo, S., Bianchi, S., Samanin, R., Ghezzi, D. 219, *239*
Ladygina-Kohts, N.N. 406, 507, *533*
Lagercrantz, H. 31, 32, *60*
Lagercrantz, H., s. Bartlett, S.F. 21, 22, *56*
Lai, D., s. Margolis, R.K. 23, *60*
Lairy, G.C. 171, *190*
Lairy, G.C., s. Igert, C. 172, *188*
Laitinen, L., Toivakka, E., Vilkki, J. 363, *376*

Laitinen, L., s. Kukka, E.-K. 359, *376*
Laitinen, L.V. 367, 368, 373, *376*
Laitinen, L.V., Vilkki, J. 361, 368, *376*
Lajtha, A. 3, 9, 10, 19, *60*
Lajtha, A., Furst, S., Gerstein, A., Waelsch, H. 49, *60*
Lajtha, A., Latzkovits, L., Toth, J. 49, *60*
Lajtha, A., Shershen, H. 50, *60*
Lajtha, A., s. Jacquet, Y.F. 26, *59*
Lal, S., Tolis, G., Martin, J.B., Brown, G.M., Guyda, H. 85, *104*
Lal, S., s. Schlatter, E.K.E. 232, *241*
Lambert, P.A., Chaulaic, J.L., Cabrol, G. 287, *309*
Lambo, T.A., s. Leighton, A.H. 662, *698*
Lamborn, K.R., s. Nies, A. 264, *311*
Lancaster, J., s. Harnad, S.R. 503, 508, *529*
Lancaster, N., Steinert, R., Frost, I. 337, *346*
Landis, D.H., s. Maas, J.W. 72, *104*
Landolt, H. 170, *190*, 335, *346*
Lang, E.M. 400, *533*
Lange, J. 597, *610*, [L 1] 902, *1088*
Lange, J., s. Hippius, H. 297, *307*
Lange, P., s. Hydén, H. 14, 15, *59*
Langer, G., Heinze, G., Reim, B., Matussek, N. 83, 84, *104*
Langer, S.Z. 88, *104*
Langer, S.Z., s. Dubcovich, M.L. 28, *57*
Langfeldt, G. 586, *610*
Langley, G.E., s. Robin, A.A. 331, *347*
Langmeier, L., Matějček, Z. 709, 710, 711, 718, 743, *749*
Lángová, J., s. Šváb, L. 740, *751*
Langsley, D.G., Enterline, J.D., Hickerson, G. 333, *346*

Langworthy, D., s. Bickford, R.G. 117, *183*
Lanzinger-Rossnagel, G., Christian, W., Kommerell, B. 161, *190*
Lapin, I.P., Oxenkrug, G.F. 67, *104*, 339, *346*
Larin, F., s. Wurtman, R.J. 71, *109*
Larrabee, M.G., s. Burt, D.R. 51, *56*
Larson, C., s. Sutton, D. 474, 475, *542*
Larson, C.A., Nyman, G.E. 577, *610*
Larsson, K., s. Andén, N.-E. 201, *234*
Larsson, M., s. Öhman, R. 217, 218, 220, 221, *240*
Larsson, S., s. Andersson, B. [A 23] 939, *1069*
Lasher, R.S. 9, *60*
Lashley, K.S. [L 2–5] 903, 904, 906, 1024, 1025, 1037, 1038, 1039, *1088*
Laska, E.M., Siegel, C., Meisner, M., Fischer, S., Wanderling, J. 292, *309*
Lasky, R.E., Syrdal-Lasky, A., Klein, R.E. 440, *533*
Laspe, H., s. Emrich, H.M. 112, *112*
Lassen, N.A., s. Brodersen, P. 322, *342*
Lassen, N.A., s. Ingvar, D.H. 6, 7, 53, *59*
Latham, K.R., s. Nelson, J.F. 26, *61*
Latner, G., s. Kiloh, L.G. 329, *345*
Latta, J., Hopf, S., Ploog, D. 386, *533*
Latta, J., s. Winter, P. 426, 429, 490, *544*
Latzkovits, L., s. Lajtha, A. 49, *60*
Lauener, H., s. Stille, G. von 212, *241*
Laufer, M., s. Svaetichin, G. [S 60] 787, *1099*
Laurain, A.R., s. Heinonen, O.P. 292, *307*
Laurell, B. 317, 320, 321, 322, *346*
Laurell, B., s. Arfwidsson, L. 332, *342*

Laurell, B., s. D'Elia, G. 176, *184*
Lauter, H. 649, *698*
Lawick-Goodall, J. van 392, 404, 490, 494, 506, 508, *533*
Lawrence, J., s. Gross, M. 253, *306*
Lawson, A.A.H., s. Matthew, H. 299, *310*
Laxson, G.O., s. Forrest, F.M. 289, *306*
Layne, R.S., s. Callaway, E. 175, *183*
Lazanas, J.C., s. Zeller, E.A. 223, *242*
Lazarus, L., s. Sara, V.R. 49, *62*
Lazos, G., Kapetanakis, S., Photiades, H. 292, *309*
Leach, B.E., Cohen, M., Heath, R.G., Martens, S. 96, *104*
Lebensohn, Z.M., Jenkins, R.B. 228, *239*, 339, *346*
Lechner, H., s. Lorenzoni, E. 164, *191*
Leckmann, J.F., Gershon, S., Nichols, A.S., Murphy, D.L. 96, *104*
Leckman, J.F., s. Gershon, E.S. 577, 578, *607*
Lecours, A.-R., s. Yakovlev, P.L. 48, *64*
Lecours, H.R., Lhermitte, F. 475, 476, *533*
Lecrubier, Y., s. Jouvent, R. 89, *103*
Lee, A.J., s. Spiegel, E.A. 356, *378*
Lee, A.J., s. Wyeis, H.T. [W 34a] *1102*
Lee, C.Y., s. Changeux, J.-P. 25, *56*
Lee, J.H., s. Simpson, G.M. *313*, 330, 331, *348*
Lee, T., Seeman, P., Toutellotte, W.W., Farley, I.J., Hornykiewicz, O. 112, *112*
Lee, T., s. Seeman, P. 216, 217, *241*
Leeman, S.E., s. Chang, M.M. 39, *56*
Leeman, S.E., s. Powell, D. 200, *240*
Leeman, S.E., s. Tregear, G.W. 39, *63*

Lees, M., s. Folch-Pi, J. 18, 22, *58*
Leff, J.P., Fischer, M., Bertelsen, A. 661, *698*
Lefkowitz, R.J., s. Davis, J.N. 26, 30, *57*
Legendre, R., Piéron, H. [L 6] 993, *1088*
Le Gras, A.M. 549, *610*
Lehmann, A. [L 7, 8] *1088, 1089*
Lehmann, D., s. Jacobson, A. [J 3, 3a] 995, 1017, *1083*
Lehmann, D., s. Kuhlo, W. [K 62, 63] 991, 996, 1008, 1009, *1088*
Lehmann, E., Hopes, H. 247, *309*
Lehmann, H.E. 248, *309*
Lehmann, H.E., s. Ananth, J. 94, *99*
Lehmann, H.E., s. Ban, T.A. 94, *99*
Lehmann, H.E., s. Kline, N.S. 94, 97, *104*
Lehmann, H.E., s. Nestoros, I.N. 94, *105*
Lehmann, H.J. [L 9] 1036, *1089*
Lehmann, J. 227, *239*
Lehmann, J., s. D'Elia, G. 332, 341, *344*
Lehmeyer, J.E., s. MacLeod, R.M. 220, *239*
Lehr, U. 621, *698*, 720, 721, *749*
Lehrman, D.S. [L 10] 760, *1089*
Leiber, B., s. Majewski, F. 601, *610*, 673, 674, *699*
Leibniz, G.W. [L 11] 851, 852, 906, *1089*
Leiderman, P., s. Barnett, C. 721, 726, *746*
Leiderman, P.H., s. Kubzansky, E. 742, *748*
Leiderman, P.H., s. Solomon, P. [S 36a] 933, *1098*
Leighton, A.H., Lambo, T.A., Hughes, C.C., Leighton, D.C., Murphy, J.M., Macklin, D.B. 662, *698*
Leighton, D.C., s. Leighton, A.H. 662, *698*
Leksell, L. 356, 357, 363, *376*

Leksell, L., s. Bingley, T. 364, *375*
Lelord, G., s. Fessard, A. 175, *185*
Lemere, F. 171, *190*, [L 12] 954, *1089*
Lemoine, P., Harousseau, H., Borteyru, J.-P., Menuet, J.-C. 673, *698*
Lempp, R. 637, 650, *699*
Lenneberg, E.H. 435, 512, 521, 522, *533*, 624, *699*
Lenneberg, E.H., Rebelsky, F.G., Nichols, I.A. 521, *533*
Lennox, M.A., Ruch, T.C., Guterman, B. 163, *190*
Lennox, W.G., Gibbs, F.A., Gibbs, E.L. [L 13] 985, *1089*
Lennox, W.G., s. Gibbs, F.A. 167, *187*, [G 21, 25, 26] 763, 908, 913, 982, 983, 998, *1079*
Lennox-Buchthal, M., s. Chatrian, G.E. 121, *183*
Lenz, W. 596, *610*, 664, *699*, 705
Leo-Rossberg, I., s. Hammerstein, J. 678, *696*
Leonard, C.O., Chase, G.A., Child, B. 602, *610*
Leonhard, K. 413, *533*, 563, 586, *610*, 684, *699*, 710, 749, [L 14] 931, *1089*
Leopold, D., s. Hunger, H. 691, *697*
Lérique, A., s. Lille, F. 159, *190*
Lessa, W.A., s. Tucker, W.B. 624, 665, *703*
Lesser, S.R., Easser, B.R. 722, *749*
Lester, B.K., Edwards, R.J. 173, *190*
Letterer, E. 628, *699*
Lettvin, J.Y., s. McCulloch, W.S. [M 34] 853, 857, *1091*
Levi, G., Raiteri, M. 36, *60*
Levi-Montalcini, R., Angeletti, P.U. 10, *60*
Levin, G., s. Libet, B. [L 21] 886, *1089*
Levin, M. [L 15] 1017, *1089*
Levin, P., s. Koella, W.P. [K 34] 988, *1087*

Levin, S.E., s. Kanarek, K.S. 299, *308*
Levine, J., s. Prien, R.F. 253, *312*
Levine, L. 21, *60*
Levita, E., s. Riklan, M. 478, *539*
Levy, H.B. 298, *310*
Lewandowska, A., s. Maj, J. 110, *113*
Lewin, K. [L 15a–18] 824, 831, 832, *1089*
Lewis, C., s. Pfaff, D. 466, 467, *537*
Lewis, E.G., Dustman, R.E., Beck, E.C. 161, *190*
Lewis, H.E. [L 19] 992, *1089*
Lewis, J.K., McKinney, W.T. Jr. 500, *533*
Lewis, P.D., s. Balázs, R. 48, 49, *55*
Lewitzky, W., s. Geschwind, N. 682, *696*
Leyhausen, P. 402, 407, 423, *533*
Leyton, A.S.F., Sherrington, C.S. 476, *533*
Lhermitte, F., Chain, F., Escourolle, R., Ducarne, B., Pillon, B., Chedru, F. 479, *533*
Lhermitte, F., s. Lecours, H.R. 475, 476, *533*
Li, C.H., s. Kline, N.S. 97, *104*
Liberman, A.M., Cooper, F.S., Shankweiler, D.P., Studdert-Kennedy, M. 438, 480, *533*
Liberman, A.M., Pisoni, D.B. 439, 440, 480, *533*
Liberson, W.T. 172, *190*, 318, *346*
Liberson, W.T., Akert, K. [L 20] *1089*
Liberson, W.T., Cadilhac, J.G. 323, 326, *346*
Libet, B., Alberts, W.W., Wright, E.W., Delattre, L.D., Levin, G., Feinstein, B. [L 21] 886, *1089*
Lichtlen, P., s. Moccetti, T. 287, *310*
Lichtheim, L. 477, *533*
Liddell, A.S., s. Anderson, O.D. [A 22] 810, 811, *1068*

Liddell, E.G.T., s. Creed, R.S. [C 14] 822, *1073*
Liddell, H.S. [L 22] 810, 811, *1089*
Lieberman, D.M., Hoenig, J., Hacker, M. 172, *190*
Liebig, J. von [L 23] 1062, *1089*
Liepman, M.C., Marker, K.R. 673, *699*
Lifshitz, K. 174, 175, *190*
Lifshitz, K., Gradijan, J. 173, 174, 177, 178, *190*
Lighthill, J.A., s. Brown, M.H. 361, *375*
Lilienfeld, A.M., s. Pasamanick, B. 575, *612*
Liljequist, S., s. Engel, J. 221, 232, *237*
Lille, F., Borlone, M., Lérique, A., Scherrer, J., Thieffry, S. 159, *190*
Lilly, J.C. [L 24] 932, 933, 955, 957, *1089*
Lilly, J.C., Miller, A.M. [L 25] 955, 957, *1089*
Lima, A. 353
Limber, J. 508, *533*
Lind, J., Vuorenkoski, V., Rosberg, G., Partanan, T.J., Wasz-Hoeckert, O. 413, *533*
Lind, J., s. Wasz-Hoeckert, O. 413, 434, 435, *543*
Lindauer, M. [L 26] 928, *1089*
Lindauer, W., s. Birkmayer, W. 71, *100*
Lindegård, B., Nyman, G.E. 671, *699*
Lindelius, R. 553, 577, *610*
Lindeman, R.C., s. Sutton, D. 474, 475, *542*
Lindinger, H. 571, *610*
Lindqvist, M., s. Carlsson, A. 204, 211, 212, 213, 226, 227, 232, *236*
Lindqvist, M., s. Cott, J. 220, *237*
Lindqvist, M., s. Kehr, W. 215, *239*
Lindsley, D.B. 155, *190*, 744, 749, [L 27] 950, *1089*
Lindsley, D.B., Bowden, J.W., Magoun, H.W. [L 28] 983, *1089*

Lindsley, D.B., Schreiner, L.H., Knowles, W.B., Magoun, H.W. [L 29] 983, *1089*
Lindsley, D.B., s. Donchin, E. 147, 153, 175, *184*
Lindstedt, G., s. Balldin, J. 84, 89, *99*
Lindström, L.H., Widerlöv, E., Gunne, L.-M., Wahlström, A., Terenius, L. 112, *112*
Lindström, L., s. Gunne, L.M. 96, *103*
Lindström, L., s. Terenius, L. 96, *108*, 112
Lindvall, O., s. Björklund, A. 215, *235*
Lindzey, G., s. Loehlin, J.C. 664, *699*
Ling, N., s. Vale, W. 40, *64*
Lingjaerde, O., s. Heiberg, A. 289, *307*
Linné, K. von 710, *749*
Linnoila, M., s. Viukari, M. 298, *313*
Linton, A.L., s. Kennedy, A.C. 160, *189*
Linton, E.A., Perkins, M.N., Whitehead, S.A. 38, *60*
Lipman, B.S., s. Sterritt, G.M. 722, *751*
Lipsitt, L.P., s. Siqueland, E.R. 503, *541*
Lisák, K., Endröczi, E. [L 29a] *1089*
Lisák, K., Grastyan, E., Csanaky, A., Kéresi, F., Vereby, G. [L 30] 1031, *1089*
Lisák, K., s. Grastyan, E. [G 38, 39] 1031, *1079*
Lisker, L., Abramson, A.S. 440, 441, *533*
Litt, T. [L 31] 772, *1089*
Little, S.R.C.J., s. Burnett, G.B. 253, *304*
Litvak, R., Kaelbing, R. 291, *310*
Livett, B.G., s. Wellington, B.S. 20, *64*
Ljungberg, L. 595, *610*
Ljungberg, T., s. Ungerstedt, U. 221, *242*
Lloyd, B., Archer, J. 647, *699*
Lloyd, K., s. Bartholini, G. 213, 219, *235*

Lloyd, K.B., s. Stadler, H. 219, *241*

Lloyd, K.G., Farley, I.J., Deck, J.H.N., Hornykiewicz, O. 68, *104*

Lloyd, K.G., s. Bartholini, G. 212, 213, 216, *235*

Lloyd, K.G., s. Stadler, H. 30, *63*

Lob, H., s. Gastaut, H. 168, *186*

Lob, H., s. Roger, J. 168, *193*

Locher, L.M., s. Huston, P.E. 328, *345*

Locke, 906

Lockyer, L.A., s. Rutter, M. 589, *614*

Lodemann, E., s. Schenck, G.K. 96, *107*

Lodge, D., s. Curtis, D.R. 37, *56*

Lodge-Patch, I.C., s. Claveria, L.E. 298, *304*

Loeb, C. 157, *190*

Loeb, C., Meyer, J.C. 158, *191*

Loeb, C., s. Brazier, M.A.B. 121, *183*

Loeb, J. [L 32] 841, *1090*

Loeffel, R.G., s. Ulett, G.A. 134, *195*

Löfström, A., s. Hökfelt, T. 200, *238*

Loehlin, J.C., Lindzey, G., Spuhler, J.N. 664, *699*

Loehlin, J.C., Nichols, R.C. 549, *610*

Loehlin, J.C., s. Plomin, R. 549, *612*

Løken, A.C., s. Lundervold, A. 156, 157, *191*

Löser, H., s. Majewski, F. 601, *610*, 673, 674, *699*

Loftus, R., s. Cadoret, R.J. 596, *604*

Logemann, G., s. Hippius, H. 297, *307*

Logothetis, J. 161, *191*

LoGullo, O., s. Buffa, P. 287, *304*

Loizos, C. 406, *534*

Lommen, J.G., s. Lopes da Silva, F.H. 134, *191*

Lonergan, M., s. Ashcroft, G.W. 87, *99*

Longden, A., s. Cross, A.J. 112, *112*

Longden, A., s. Owen, F. 91, *105*

Loomer, H.P., Saunders, J.C., Kline, N.S. 223, *239*

Loomis, A.L., Harvey, E.N., Hobart, G. [L 33] 992, 998, 999, *1090*

Loomis, A.L., Harvey, E.N., Hobart, G.A. [L 34, 35] 998, 999, 1000, 1002, 1009, *1090*

Loomis, A.L., s. Davis, H. [D 4-6] 999, 1002, 1007, 1008, 1009, *1074*

Loosen, P., Ackenheil, M., Athen, D., Beckmann, H., Benkert, O., Dittmer, T., Hippius, H., Matussek, N., Rüther, E., Scheller, M. 72, *104*

Loosen, P., s. Matussek, N. 72, 85, *104*

Lopes da Silva, F.H., Hulten, K. van, Lommen, J.G., Storm van Leeuwen, W., Vellen, C.W.M. van, Vliegenthart, W. 134, *191*

Lopes da Silva, F.H., Rotterdam, A. van 148, *191*

Lopes da Silva, F.A., s. Storm van Leeuwen, W. 147, *195*

Lopez-Ramos, B., s. Angrist, B. 95, *99*

Loranger, A.W. 581, *610*

Lorentzson, S., s. D'Elia, G. 318, 341, *343*, *344*

Lorenz, K. 383, 384, 386, 398, 402, 407, 408, 410, 412, 416, 418, 423, 424, 432, 459, 487, *534*, 633, 699, *705*, [L 36-42] 760, 800, 801, 802, 810, 947, 948, 949, 950, 967, 974, 1041, *1090*

Lorenzo, A.V., Hedley-Whyte, E.T., Eisenberg, H.M., Hsu, D.S. 324, *346*

Lorenzoni, E., Lechner, H., Geyer, N., Manowarda, K., Mauser, H. 164, *191*

Lotze, R.H. [L 43] 783, 924, *1090*

Love, E.R., s. Daniel, P.M. 51, *57*

Lovett Doust, J.W., Raschka, L.B. 323, *346*

Lovett-Doust, J.W., Huszka, L. 295, *310*

Løvtrup-Rein, H., McEwen, B.S. 12, *60*

Low, M.D. 147, 153, 154, *191*

Lowenstein, B., s. Korenyi, C. 293, *309*

Lowrey, L.G. 714, *749*

Lowry, O.H. 14, 15, *60*

Lozovsky, D.V., s. Vartanian, M.E. 681, *703*

Lu, K.-H., s. Meites, J. 220, *239*

Luba, A., s. Künkel, H. 139, 143, 146, 180, *190*

Lubin, A., s. Morris, G.O. [M 61] 1003, *1092*

Lubs, H.A., Cruz, F. de la 601, *610*

Luby, E.D., s. Rodin, E.A. [R 19] 1003, *1096*

Luce, R.A., Rothschild, D. 162, *191*

Luchins, D., s. Ananth, J. 267, *302*

Ludolph, E., s. Beckmann, H. 75, *100*

Lüllmann, H., Lüllmann-Rauch, R., Wassermann, O. 295, *310*

Lüllmann, H., s. Kuschinsky, G. 283, *309*

Lüllmann-Rauch, R., s. Lüllmann, H. 295, *310*

Luft, R., s. Hökfelt, T. 15, 40, 58, 200, *238*

Lugaresi, E., Pazzaglia, P. 166, *191*

Lugaresi, E., Pazzaglia, P., Tassinari, C.A. 168, *191*

Luice, R.G., s. Kennedy, A.C. 160, *189*

Lukačiková, E., s. Uhlíř, F. 253, *313*

Lumineau, J.P., Garraud, M.J., Gaillard, A. 289, *310*

Lumsden, C.E., Pomerat, C.M. 4, *60*

Lundborg, P., Engel, J. 221, *239*

Lundborg, P., s. Ahlenius, S. 220, 232, 233, *234*

Lundborg, P., s. Engel, J. 233, *237*

Lundervold, A. *191*
Lundervold, A., Hauge, T., Löken, A.C. 156, 157, *191*
Lundsteen, C., s. Witkin, H.A. 677, *704*
Lunt, G.G., Canessa, O.M., De Robertis, E. 51, *60*
Luria, A.R. 475, *534*
Lutz, E.G. 253, *310*
Luxenburger, H. 553, 554, 555, *610*
Lynch, J.C., s. Mountcastle, V.B. [M 75] 898, 929, 1037, *1093*
Lynch, J.C., Mountcastle, V.B., Talbot, W.H., Yin, T.C.T. [L 44] 825, 898, *1090*

Maany, I., Mendels, J., Frazer, A., Brunswick, D. 84, *104*
Maas, J.W. 75, *104*
Maas, J.W., Dekirmenjian, H., Garver, D., Redmond, D.E., Landis, D.H. 72, *104*
Maas, J.W., Fawcett, J.A., Dekirmenjian, H. 72, *104*
Maas, J.W., Landis, D.H. 72, *104*
Maas, J.W., s. Jones, F.D. 72, *103*
Maas, J.W., s. Pickar, D. 72, *106*
Maas, J., s. Sweeny, D. 72, 73, *108*
Maccario, M. 158, *191*
Maccoby, E.E., Jacklin, C.N. 647, *699*
MacCullough, E., s. Farley, I.J. 93, *102*
MacDougall, E.J., s. Ashcroft, G.W. 69, *99*, 339, *342*
Machek, J., s. Kolářský, A. 683, 690, *698*
Mach, E. [M 1, 2] 914, *1090*
MacCallum, W.C., s. Walter, W.G. [W 11] 1033, *1101*
Machiyama, Y., s. Balázs. R. 36, 37, *55*
Machleidt, W. 131, *191*
Machleidt, W., s. Gutjahr, L. 126, 167, *187*
Machleidt, W., s. Künkel, H. 131, 132, *190*

Machne, X., s. Green, J.D. [G 41] *1079*
Mack, C., s. Holmes, L.B. 673, *697*
MacKay, D.M. 448, 453, *534*, [M 3–7] 853, 860, 929, 1028, *1090*
MacKay, D.M., McCulloch, W.S. [M 8] 857, *1090*
Macken, D.L., s. Kantor, S.J. 287, *309*
MacKinnon, P.C.B., s. Beumont, P.J.V. 292, 293, 303, *304*
Macklin, D.B., s. Leighton, A.H. 662, *698*
MacLean, P.D. 395, 398, 445, 454, 459, 460, 461, *534*, [M 8a–14] 791, 904, 944, 945, 960, *1090*, *1091*
MacLean, P.D., Denniston, R.H., Dua, S. 464, *534*
MacLean, P.D., Dua, S., Denniston, R.H. 464, *534*
MacLean, P.D., Ploog, D.W. 461, 463, 464, *534*, [M 15] 939, 960, *1091*
MacLean, P.D., s. Ploog, D. 386, 464, *538*
MacLeod, R.M., Lehmeyer, J.E. 220, *239*
MacMahon, J.F., Walter, W.G. 171, *191*
MacNichol, E.F., s. Svaetichin, G. [S 61] 787, *1100*
MacSweeny, D., s. Blazek, R. 71
MacSweeny, D.A., s. Shaw, D.M. 70, 71, *107*
Madarász, I., s. Grastyán, E. [G 38] 1031, *1079*
Maddock, J., s. Aylward, M. 71, *99*
Madow, L., s. Comer, N.L. 736, *747*
Madsen, A., s. Vaernet, K. 367, *378*
Maeno, H., s. Ueda, T. 30, *63*
Maggs, R., Turton, E. 176, *191*
Maggs, R., s. Coppen, A. 74, *101*, 270, *305*
Magnes, J., Moruzzi, G., Pompeiano, O. 125, *191*, [M 16] 989, *1091*

Magnes, J., s. Allweis, C. 7, 8, *55*
Magnus, O., s. Brazier, M.A.B. 121, *183*
Magnus, R. [M 17] 823, *1091*
Magnusson, T., Carlsson, A., Fisher, G.H., Chang, D., Folkers, K. 200, *239*
Magnusson, T., s. Garcia-Sevilla, J.A. 200, *238*
Magnusson, T., s. Kehr, W. 215, *239*
Magoun, H.S. [M 19] 882, 904, 950, 977, 978, 979, 984, *1091*
Magoun, H.W. [M 18] 838, *1091*
Magoun, H.W., Atlas, D., Ingersoll, E.H., Ranson, S.W. 471, *534*
Magoun, H.W., Rhines, R. [M 20] 989, *1091*
Magoun, H.W., s. Kelly, A.H. 473, *531*
Magoun, H.W., s. Lindsley, D.B. [L 28, 29] 983, *1089*
Magoun, H.W., s. Moruzzi, G. [M 66] 762, 904, 977, 995, *1093*
Mahl, G.F., Rothenberg, A., Delgado, J.M.R., Hamlin, H. [M 21] 887, *1091*
Mahler, M. 588, *610*
Mai, F.M., Jenner, M.R., Shaw, B.F., Giles, D.E. 83, *104*
Maier, W.J., s. Schechter, M.D. 741, *750*
Maitre, L., s. Baumann, P. 88, *99*
Maj, J., Gancarczyk, E., Gorszcyk, A., Rantow, A. 110, *113*
Maj, J., Lewandowska, A., Rantow, A. 110, *113*
Majewski, F., Bierich, J.R., Löser, H., Michaelis, R., Leiber, B., Bettecken, F. 601, *610*, 673, 674, *699*
Majewski, F., s. Bierich, J.R. 673, 674, 675, *693*
Majo, E.A., s. Wyatt, R.J. 75, *109*
Malamud, W., s. Hoagland, H. 179, *188*

Malhotra, S.K., s. Van Harreveld, A. 16, *64*
Malik, N.A., s. Johnson, D.A.W. 256, *308*
Malin, J.P., Rosenberg, L. 287, *310*
Malin, J.P., s. Hippius, H. 287, *307*
Mallya, A., s. Volavka, J. 96, *108*
Malm, V., s. Dencker, S.J. 69, *102*
Malpern, F.S., s. Rotrosen, J. 91, *107*
Malson, L., Itard, J., Mannoni, O. 522, *534*, 710, *749*
Malzberg, B. 574, *610*
Man, P.L., Chen, C.H. 287, *310*
Mandel, L.R., s. Angrist, B. 95, *99*
Mandel, P., David, A.R., Pete, N. 12, *60*
Mandelbrote, B.M., s. Beumont, P.J.V. 293, *303, 304*
Mandell, A.J., s. Knapp, S. 228, *239*
Mandels, J., s. Dorus, E. 583, *605*
Mangold, R., Sokoloff, L., Conner, E., Kleinerman, J., Therman, P.O., Kety, S.S. [M 22] 1007, *1091*
Manley, J.A., Mueller-Preuss, P. 481, *534*
Mannon, O., s. Malson, L. 710, *749*
Mannoni, O., s. Malson, L. 522, *534*
Manowarda, K., s. Lorenzoni, E. 164, *191*
Manschreck, T., s. Jacobson, G. 297, *308*
Mao, C.C., s. Costa, E. 231, *237*
Maple, T., s. Erwin, T. 496, *527*
Marangos, P.J., s. Pickel, V.M. 21, *62*
Marano, C., s. Benkert, O. 71, *100*
Marchiafava, P.L., s. Gassel, M.M. [G 9] 995, *1078*
Marcotte, D.B., s. Miller, W.C. Jr. 263, *310*

Marcus, E.M., s. Watson, C.S. 167, *196*
Marey, E.-J. [M 22a, 22b] 835, 846, *1091*
Margat, M.-P., Broussot, T. 292, *310*
Margolis, R.K., Preti, C., Lai, D., Margolis, R.U. 23, *60*
Margolis, R.U., s. Margolis, R.K. 23, *60*
Marhold, J., Zimanová, J., Lachman, M., Král, J., Vojtěchovský, B. 274, *310*
Marini, G., s. Venezian, E.C. 292, *313*
Marini, J.L., Sheard, M.H., Bridges, C.I., Wagner, E. Jr. 271, *310*
Marino, R. Jr., s. Ballantine, H.T. Jr. 361, *375*
Marjerrison, G., James, J., Reichert, H. 164, *191*
Marjerrison, G., Krause, A.E., Keogh, R.P. 173, *191*
Mark, A., s. Gershon, E.S. 579, *607*
Mark, H., Ervin, F.R. 455, *534*
Mark, V.H., Sweet, W.H., Ervin, F.R. 372, *376*
Mark, V.H., s. Stevens, J.R. 486, *542*
Markanen, M., s. Partanen, J.K. 599, *612*
Marker, K.R., s. Liepman, M.C. 673, *699*
Markert, F. 687, *699*
Markey, S.P., s. Muscettola, G. 110, *113*
Markianos, E.S., Nyström, I., Reichel, H., Matussek, N. 93, *104*
Markianos, E., s. Ackenheil, M. 72, *98*
Markland, C., s. Merrill, D.C. 289, *310*
Marks, J. 267, *310*
Marks, J.D., s. Diamond, L.S. 253, *305*
Marks, M., s. Spiegel, E.A. 356, *378*
Marks, N., Grynbaum, A., Benuck, M. 23, *60*
Marks, N., Stern, F. 39, *60*
Marler, P. 425, 426, 431, 433, 444, *534, 535*

Marler, P., Hamilton, W.J. 428, *535*
Marocchino, R., Savio, P.A. 289, *310*
Maroulis, G.B., s. Abraham, G.E. 678, *692*
Marquis, D.G., s. Hilgard, E.R. [H 69] 1027, *1082*
Marsh, G., s. Delse, F. 153, *184*
Marshall, E., Stirling, G.S., Tait, A.C., Todrick, A. 223, *239*
Marshall, J., s. Beumont, P.J.V. 293, *303*
Marshall, J., s. Weiskrantz, L. 448, *543*
Marshall, J.A., s. Hull, R.C. 263, *308*
Marshall, J.R., s. Abraham, G.E. 678, *692*
Marshall, R.E., s. Kooi, K.A. 151, *189*
Martens, S., s. Leach, B.E. 96, *104*
Mårtensson, E., s. Forsman, A. 217, *237*
Martensson, E., s. Nyberg, G. 217, *240*
Martin, C.E., s. Kinsey, A.C. [K 15] 799, 940, *1086*
Martin, G.I., Zaug, P.J. 287, *310*
Martin, J.B., s. Lal, S. 85, *104*
Martin, J.P. [M 23] 961, *1091*
Martin, R. 622, 625, *699*
Martin, W., s. Meyer, G. 362, *376*
Martin-Rodriguez, J.G., s. Delgado, J.M.R. 359, *375*
Martin-Rodriguez, J.G., s. Sweet, W.H. 455, *542*
Martinius, J.W., Papousek, H. 503, *535*
Maruta, K., s. Fujita, K. 93, *102*
Maslowski, J. 94, *104*
Mason, B.T., s. Kline, N.S. 296, *309*
Mason, W.A. 381, 407, 493, 496, 500, *535*
Mason, W.A., s. Eastman, R.F. 500, *526*
Masserman, J.H. [M 24, 25, 26] 810, 811, 962, *1091*

Massini, M.-A., s. Thölen, H. 97, *108*
Masters, W.H., s. Kolodny, R.C. 683, *698*
Mastrogiovanni, P.D. 287, *310*
Matakas, F., Cervós-Navarro, J., Roggendorf, W., Christmann, U., Sasaki, S. 323, *346*
Matejcek, M., Schenk, G.K. 133, *191*
Matějček, Z. 731, *749*
Matějček, Z., s. Langmeier, L. 709, 710, 711, 718, 743, *749*
Matheny, A.P., Wilson, R.S., Dolan, A.B. 549, *610*
Mathias, J., s. Scanlon, W.G. 164, *193*
Mathis, P., s. Fischgold, H. 155, 156, *186*
Matiar-Vahar, H., s. Penin, H. 163, *192*
Matousek, M., s. Volavka, J. 172, *195*
Matsumoto, J., s. Yoshii, N. [Y 2] 1032, *1102*
Matthew, H., Lawson, A.A.H. 299, *310*
Matthews, B.H.C., s. Adrian, E.D. [A 9] 804, 805, 976, 982, *1068*
Matthysse, S.W., Kidd, K.K. 562, *611*
Mattingly, I.G. 443, *535*
Mattsson, H., s. Edström, A. 5, *57*
Matus, A., Mughal, S.M. 21, *60*
Matussek, N. 54, 67, *104*
Matussek, N., Ackenheil, M., Athen, D., Beckmann, H., Benkert, O., Dittmer, T., Hippius, H., Loosen, P., Rüther, E., Scheller, M. 72, 85, *104*
Matussek, N., Ackenheil, M., Hippius, H., Schröder, H.-T., Schultes, H., Wasileski, B. 84, *105*
Matussek, N., Angst, J., Benkert, O., Gmür, M., Papousek, M., Rüther, E., Woggon, B. *105*
Matussek, N., Benkert, O., Schneider, K., Otten, H., Pohlmeier, H. 74, *105*
Matussek, N., Greil, W. 75, *105*
Matussek, N., Pohlmeier, H., Rüther, E. 74, *105*
Matussek, N., Römisch, P., Ackenheil, M. 73, *105*
Matussek, N., s. Ackenheil, M. 72, 98, *99*
Matussek, N., s. Benkert, O. 71, 74, *100*
Matussek, N., s. Crombach, G. 71, *101*
Matussek, N., s. Hippius, H. 97, *103*
Matussek, N., s. Langer, G. 83, 84, *104*
Matussek, N., s. Loosen, P. 72, *104*
Matussek, N., s. Markianos, E.S. 93, *104*
Matussek, N., s. Pohlmeier, H. 74, *106*
Matussek, N., s. Schilkrut, R. 83, *107*
Matussek, P. 684, *699*
Matussek, P., Halbach, A., Troeger, U. 661, *699*
Matz, D., s. Schenck, G.K. 96, *107*
Matzilewich, B., s. Holmes, L.B. 673, *697*
Maurus, M., Hartmann, E., Kuehlmorgen, B. 482, 483, *535*
Maurus, M., Kuehlmorgen, B., Hartmann, E. 483, *535*
Maurus, M., Kuehlmorgen, B., Hartmann-Wiesner, E., Pruscha, H. 393, 394, 483, *535*
Maurus, M., Mitra, J., Ploog, D. 465, *535*
Maurus, M., Ploog, D. 393, 483, *535*
Maurus, M., Pruscha, H. 393, 483, *535*
Maurus, M., s. Pruscha, H. 393, 447, 482, *539*
Maury, A. [M 27] 1008, 1014, *1091*
Maury, L.F.A. [M 28] 1008, 1014, 1018, *1091*
Mauser, H., s. Lorenzoni, E. 164, *191*
Maxwell, J., s. Slater, E. 583, *615*
Maxwell, R.D.H. 318, *346*
May, P.R.A. 333, *346*
May, P.R.A., Tuma, A.H., Dixon, W.J. 333, *346*
May, P.R.A., Tuma, A.H., Yale, C., Potepan, P., Dixon, W.J. 333, *346*
May, V. 256, 288, *310*
Mayanagi, Y., s. Sano, K. 369, *377*
Mayer, W., s. Talmage-Riggs, G. 432, *542*
Mayer-Gross, W. [M 29, 30, 31] 932, 1018, *1091*
Mayer-Gross, W., Slater, E., Roth, M. 622, 635, 641, 642, 649, 661, 666, 684, *699*
Mayo, R. 649, *699*
Mayr, E. 384, *535*
Mayr, E., s. Huxley, J. 577, *608*
Mazer, M. 651, 652, *699*
Mazet, M., s. Fenasse, R. 292, *305*
McAdam, D.W. 153, *191*
McAlpine, W., s. Kennel, J.H. 726, *748*
McAlpine, W., s. Klaus, M.H. 726, *748*
McBride, G., s. Clancy, H. 722, 746, *747*
McBride, W.J., Tassel, J. van 13, *60*
McCabe, M. 585, *611*
McCabe, M., Fowler, R.C., Cadoret, R.J., Winokur, G. 564, *611*
McCabe, M.S. 333, *346*
McCallum, W., Knott, J.R. *191*
McCallum, W.C. 175, *191*
McCallum, W.C., Knott, J.R. 147, 153, *191*
McCallum, W.C., Walter, W.G. 175, *191*
McCallum, W.C., s. Walter, W.G. 152, *196*
McCann, S.M., Kaira, P.S., Donoso, A.P., Bishop, W., Schneider, H.P.G., Fawcett, C.P., Krulich, L. 220, *239*
McCarter, R., s. Tomkin, S.S. 423, *542*
McCarthy, P.S., Walker, R.J., Woodruff, G.N. 40, *60*

McClearn, G.E., DeFries, J.C. 547, *611*
McClure, D.J., s. Papeschi, R. 69, *106*
McClure, J.N. Jr., s. Woodruff, R.A. Jr. 317, *349*
McConaghy, N. 566, *611*
McCulloch, W.S. [M 32, 33] 853, 856, 857, 862, *1091*
McCulloch, W.S., Duchane, E.M., Gesteland, R.C., Lettvin, J.Y., Pitts, W.H., Wall, P.D. [M 34] 853, 857, *1091*
McCulloch, W.S., Pfeiffer, J. [M 35] 856, 857, 858, 859, 862, *1091*
McCulloch, W.S., Pitts, W. [M 36] *1091*
McCulloch, W.S., s. Dusser de Barenne, J.G. [D 39] 883, *1075*
McCulloch, W.S., s. MacKay, D.M. [M 8] 857, *1090*
McCulloch, W.S., s. Muses, C.A. [M 85] 855, *1093*
McCulloch, W.S., s. Pitts, W. 178, *193*
McCurdy, L., s. Miller, W.C. Jr. 263, *310*
McDevitt, C.A., s. Beatty, J. 434, *523*
McDonald, R.D., s. Heninger, G. 150, *187*
McDonald, R.K., s. Mueller, P.S. 81, *105*
McDonald, W.I., s. Halliday, A.M. 148, *187*
McDougal, W. [M 37] 931, *1091*
McElhaney, M., s. Meyer, G. 362, *376*
McEwen, B.S., Denef, C.J., Gerlach, J.L., Plapinger, L. 465, 466, *535*
McEwen, B.S., De Kloet, R., Wallach, G. 26, *60*
McEwen, B.S., s. Løvtrup-Rein, H. 12, *60*
McGeer, P.L., Grewaal, D.S., McGeer, E.G. 219, *239*
McGeer, E.G., s. McGeer, P.L. 219, *239*
McGillivray, B. 134, *191*
McGinitie, G., s. Reichardt, W. [R 11] 853, 865, *1096*

McGinnis, L., s. Hinde, R.A. 500, *529*
McGraw, C.P., s. Meyer, G. 362, *376*
McGregor, D., s. Moore, B.W. 20, *61*
McGrew, W.C. 417, *535*
McGuire, M.T., Fairbanks, L.A. 380, *535*
McGuire, R.J., s. Hershon, H.I. 297, *307*
McHugh, P.R., s. Folstein, M. 330, 334, *344*
McIlwain, H. 38, 46, *61*
McIlwain, H., Bachelard, H.S. 9, *61*
McKenna, G., Engle, R.P. Jr., Brooks, H., Dalen, J. 317, *346*
McKenzie, G.M., s. Fann, W.E. 298, *305*
McKinney, T.M., s. Akiskal, H.S. 583, *602*
McKinney, W.T., Suomi, S.J., Harlow, H.F. 500, *535*
McKinney, W.T., Young, L.D., Suomi, S.J., Davis, J.M. 500, *535*
McKinney, W.T., s. Akisal, H.S. 501, *523*
McKinney, W.T. Jr., s. Lewis, J.K. 500, *533*
McKinney, W.T., s. Suomi, S.J. 725, *751*
McLean, P.D., s. Ploog, D.W. [P 25] 810, *1095*
McLellan, D.L. 298, *310*
McLeod, M., s. McLeod, W.R. 69, *105*
McLeod, W.R., McLeod, M. 69, *105*
McMichen, H.U.S., s. Brown, K.G.E. 288, *304*
McNeil, T.F., Kaij, L. 575, *611*
McNeill, D. 434, 521, *535*
McNeilly, A.S., s. Kolakowska, T. 292, *309*
Meadow, A., Dunlon, P.T., Blacker, K.H. 253, *310*
Meadow, K.P., s. Schlesinger, H.S. 515, *540*
Meckies, J., s. Hammerstein, J. 678, *696*
Medical Record 355, *376*
Medical Research Council 325, 329, 331, 339, *346*

Medical Research Council Brain Metabolism Unit 325, 329, 331, 339, *346*
Mednick, B., s. Mednick, S.A. 567, 575, *611*
Mednick, S.A. 567, 575, *611*
Mednick, S.A., Hutchings, B. 594, 599, *611*
Mednick, S.A., Mura, E., Schulsinger, F., Mednick, B. 567, 575, *611*
Mednick, S.A., Schulsinger, F., Higgins, J., Bell, B. 546, 553, 567, 568, 575, *611*
Mednick, S.A., Wild, C. 566, *611*
Mednick, S.A., s. Hutchings, B. 598, *608*
Mednick, S.A., s. Witkin, H.A. 677, *704*
Meehl, P.E., s. Hanson, D.R. 568, 569, *608*
Meek, J., Werdinius, B. 225, *239*
Meffert, J., s. Dahme, B. 552, *604*
Meffert, J., s. Huse-Kleinstoll, G. 552, *608*
Mehta, S., s. Barton, J.L. 322, *342*
Meier, E., s. Moccetti, T. 287, *310*
Meier-Ewert, K., Baumgart, H.H., Friedenberg, P. 291, *310*
Meierhofer, M. 718, 731, *749*
Meiers, H.G., s. Hoffmann, E. 678, *697*
Meisner, M., s. Laska, E.M. 292, *309*
Meites, J., Lu, K.-H., Wuttke, W., Welsch, C.W., Nagasawa, H., Quadri, S.K. 220, *239*
Meldrum, B.S., Brierly, J.B. 324, *346*
Meldrum, B.S., Vigouroux, R.A., Brierly, J.B. 324, *346*
Melica, A.M., s. Smeraldi, E. 581, *615*
Mellick, R.S., s. Smith, J.S. 335, *348*
Mellström, B., s. Träskman, L. 109, 110, *113*
Melnechuk, T., s. Ploog, D. 393, 503, 508, 511, *538*

Melnechuk, T., s. Schmitt, F.O. 460, *541*
Meltzer, H., Shader, R., Grinspoon, L. 94, *105*
Meltzer, H.Y., Fang, V.S. 221, *239*
Meltzer, H.Y., Stahl, M. 219, 220, 221, 223, *239*
Melvill Jones, G., Watt, D.G.D. [M 37a, 37b] 830, *1091*
Mempel, E., s. Brutkowski, S. [B 69] 1031, *1072*
Mende, W., Ploeger, A. 736, *749*
Mendels, J. 330, 331, *346*
Mendels, J., Digiacomo, J. 263, *310*
Mendels, J., Frazer, A., Carroll, B.J. 84, *105*
Mendels, J., Stinnett, J.L., Burns, D., Frazer, A. 74, *105*
Mendels, J., s. Carroll, B.J. 77, 78, *101*, 338, *343*
Mendels, J., s. Frazer, A. 88, *102*
Mendels, J., s. Maany, I. 84, *104*
Mendelson, J.H., s. Solomon, P. [S 36a] 933, *1098*
Mendelson, M. 687, *699*
Mendelson, W.B., Reid, M.A., Frommer, E.A. 590, *611*
Mendlewicz, J., Fieve, R.R., Rainer, J.D., Cadaldo, M. 580, 583, *611*
Mendlewicz, J., Fieve, R.R., Stallone, F. 583, *611*
Mendlewicz, J., Fleiss, J.L. 581, *611*, 664, *699*
Mendlewicz, J., Rainer, J.D. 578, 579, *611*
Mendlewicz, J., s. Shopsin, B. 578, *615*
Mendlewicz, J., s. Suslak, L. 578, *616*
Mengod, G., s. Palacios, J.M. 37, *61*
Mensokova, Z. 163, *192*
Mentzos, S. 661, *699*
Menuet, J.-C., s. Lemoine, P. 673, *698*
Menzel, E.W. 505, 506, *535*
Menzel, E.W., Halperin, S. 505, *535*

Menzi, R., s. Wirz-Justice, A. 71, *108*
Merkel, C. 621, *699*
Merkenschlager, F., Saller, K. 523, *535*
Merrill, D.C., Markland, C. 289, *310*
Merrill, J.P., Hampers, C.L. 158, *192*
Merry, J., Reynolds, C.M., Bailey, J., Coppen, A. 271, *310*
Merz, F. *705*
Mess, B., s. Szentagothai, J. [S 65] 860, 861, 939, *1100*
Metcalfe, M. *699*
Metcalfe, M., s. Julian, T. *697*
Metcalfe, M., s. Kellett, J.M. 272, *309*
Metrakos, J.D., s. Metrakos, K.O. 167, *192*
Metrakos, K.O., Metrakos, J.D. 167, *192*
Metts, J.C., s. Brandt, H.A. 162, *183*
Metzger, W. [M 38, 39] 781, 790, 870, 913, *1091*
Metzig, E., Rosenberg, S., Ast, M., Krashen, S.D. 682, *699*
Metzig, E., s. Ast, M. 682, *692*
Meyendorf, R. 551, 552, *611*
Meyer, A. [M 39a] 830, *1092*
Meyer, A., Beck, E. 356, *376*
Meyer, A.-E. 678, *699*
Meyer, A.-E., Zerssen, D. von 678, *699*
Meyer, A.E., s. Hess, W.R. [H 68] 940, *1082*
Meyer, A.-E., s. Rieber, I. *539*
Meyer, A.-E., s. Zerssen, D. von 675, 677, *705*
Meyer, D.R., s. Akert, K. [A 15] 944, *1068*
Meyer, G., McElhaney, M., Martin, W., McGraw, C.P. 362, *376*
Meyer, J., s. Pitts, F.N. 730, *749*
Meyer, J.C., s. Loeb, C. 158, *191*
Meyer, J.E. 749, [M 40] 970, 972, 986, *1092*
Meyer-Eppler, W. [M 41] 853, *1092*

Meyer-Mickeleit, R.W. 163, 164, *192*
Meyers, D., Goldfarb, W. 588, *611*
Meyers, F.H., Solomon, P. 244, *310*
Meyerson, B.A., s. Bingley, T. 364, *375*
Miani, N., Caniglia, A., Panetta, V. 21, 24, *61*
Michael, C.M., Morris, D.P., Soroker, E. 567, *611*
Michael, R.P. 465, *536*
Michael, R.P., Bonsall, R.W., Zumpe, D. 461, *536*
Michael, R.P., Crook, J.H. 381, *536*
Michaelis, R., s. Bierich, J.R. 673, 674, 675, *693*
Michaelis, R., s. Majewski, F. 601, *610*, 673, 674, *699*
Michaelson, I.A., s. Whittaker, V.P. 13, 14, *64*
Michalakeas, A.C., s. Shaw, D.M. 110, *113*
Michel, J., s. Bäumler, H. 140, *182*
Micheler, E., s. Strian, F. 92, *108*
Mickey, D.D., s. Appel, S.H. 10, 11, 13, 14, *55*
Mieler, W., s. Pelz, L. 620, 674, *701*
Milazzo-Sayre, L. 649, 651, *699*
Miles, C.C., s. Terman, L.M. 647, *703*
Miles, L.W. 515, 516, *536*
Miller, A.M., s. Lilly, J.C. [L 25] 955, 957, *1089*
Miller, D.H., Clancy, J., Cumming, E. 333, *347*
Miller, H., s. Murphy, D.L. 74, 96, *105*
Miller, J.L., Eimas, P.D. 442, *536*
Miller, P.L., s. Squire, L.R. 326, *348*
Miller, R.D., s. Fann, W.E. 298, *305*
Miller, R.E. 410, *536*
Miller, R.E., Caul, W.F., Mirsky, I.A. 410, *536*
Miller, R.J., Horn, A.S., Iversen, L.L. 216, *240*
Miller, R.J., s. Iversen, L.L. 216, *238*

Miller, V.G. [M 42] 963, *1092*
Miller, W.C. Jr., Marcotte, D.B., McCurdy, L. 263, *310*
Mills, M.J., s. Watson, S.J. 96, *108*
Milner, B. [M 43, 44, 45] 1026, *1092*
Milner, B., s. Orbach, J. [O 10] 944, 1048, *1094*
Milner, B., s. Penfield, W. [P 15] 883, 884, 1047, *1095*
Milner, P., s. Olds, J. [O 8] 954, 955, *1094*
Milner, P., s. Olds, J. 483, *537*
Milner, P.M. [M 46] 934, *1092*
Milton, A.S., Wendlandt, S. 38, *61*
Milton, A.S., s. Harvey, C.A. 19, 38, *58*
Minard, F.N., Richter, D. 50, *61*
Minde, K. *536*
Miner, N.M., s. Sperry, R.W. [S 42] 890, 891, *1099*
Mir, D., s. Delgado, J.M.R. 482, *526*
Mirdal, G.M., Rosenthal, D., Wender, P.H., Schulsinger, F. 575, *611*
Mirsky, I.A., s. Miller, R.E. 410, *536*
Mishkin, M., Pribram, K.H. [M 47] *1092*
Mishkin, M., s. Battig, K. [B 11, 12] 831, *1070*
Mishkin, M., s. Rosvold, H.E. [R 30, 31] *1097*
Misra, N., s. Tangri, K.K. 25, *63*
Mitarai, G., s. Svaetichin, G. [S 60] 787, *1099*
Mitchel, G., s. Erwin, T. 496, *527*
Mitchell, A.B.S. 290, *310*
Mitchell, S.A., s. Rechtschaffen, A. [R 7] 999, 1009, 1016, *1096*
Mitchell-Heggs, N., Kelly, D., Richardson, A.E. 363, 365, *376*
Mitchell-Heggs, N., s. Kelly, D. 359, *376*

Mitchell-Heggs, N., s. Richardson, A.E. 365, *377*
Mitkov, V., s. Jonchev, V. 298, *308*
Mitra, J., s. Maurus, M. 465, *535*
Mitsuda, H. 562, 585, *611*
Mitsuda, H., Fukuda, T. 553, *611*
Mitsuda, H., Sakai, T., Kobayashi, J. 565, *611*
Mittelstaedt, H. [M 48, 49] 827, 853, 875, *1092*
Mittelstaedt, H., s. Holst, E. von 451, *530*, [H 82] 853, 856, 859, *1082*
Mlejnkova, M., s. Rysanek, K. 291, *312*
Mobley, P.L., s. Sulser, F. 88, *108*
Moccetti, T., Lichtlen, P., Albert, H., Meier, E., Imbach, P. 287, *310*
Modestin, J. 288, *311*
Modestin, J., s. Harder, A. 289, *307*
Modigh, K. 88, 89, *105*, 201, 228, *240*, 325, 339, *347*
Modigh, K., Svensson, T.H. 202, *240*
Modigh, K., s. Balldin, J. 84, 89, *99*
Modigh, S., s. Eden, S. 88, 89, *102*, 325, *344*
Möller, H.-J. 244, *311*
Möller, H.-J., s. Emrich, H.M. 96, *102*
Møller, N., s. Goodwin, D.W. 599, *607*
Møller, S.E., Kirk, L., Fremming, K.H. 71, *105*
Möller-Nielsen, I., Fjalland, B., Pedersen, V., Nymark, M. 221, *240*
Mönks, F.J., Knoers, A.M.P., Staay, F.J. van der 635, 641, *699*
Moerman, E., s. De Potter, W.P. 50, *57*
Moffitt, A.R. 437, *536*
Mogenson, G.J. 446, *536*
Mohan, K.J., s. Curran, D.J. 298, *305*
Moir, A.T.B., Eccleston, D. 71, *105*
Molander, L., s. Cronholm, B. 327, *343*

Molander, L., s. Randrup, A. 75, *106*
Moltz, L., s. Hammerstein, J. 678, *696*
Mombelli, A.M., s. Bergamini, L. 155, *182*
Mombour, W., s. Degkwitz, R. 649, 653, *694*
Monakow, C. von [M 50] 897, *1092*
Monakow, C. von, Mourgue, R. [M 51] 800, 896, *1092*
Monelly, E., s. Fowler, R.C. 558, *606*
Monelly, E., s. Tsuang, M. 564, *616*
Money, J. 643, 645, 648, 683, 699, 733, *749*
Money, J., Ehrhardt, A.A. 631, 643, 644, 645, 647, 648, 678, 683, 690, *700*
Money, J., Hampson, J.G., Hampson, J.L. 690, *700*
Moniz, E. 352, 353, *377*
Monnier, M. [M 52, 53] 911, 989, *1092*
Monnier, M., s. Talairach, J. 356, *378*
Montalbetti, N., s. Halberg, F. *187*
Moody, D.B., s. Sinnott, J.M. 443, 444, *541*
Moody, J.P., s. Peet, M. 71, *106*
Moody, J.P., s. Worrall, E.P. 271, *314*
Moore, A., s. Hersher, L. 726, *748*
Moore, B.W. 13, 21, 25, *61*
Moore, B.W., McGregor, D. 20, *61*
Moore, K.L. 643, *700*
Moore, M.T., Bock, M.H. 295, *311*
Moore, P., s. Agulnik, P.L. 272, *302*
Moorhouse, S.R., s. Daniel, P.M. 51, *57*
Morais, T.M. de, Pereira-Reis, M.J., Simao-Bines, J., et al. 256, *311*
Morasso, P., s. Dichgans, J. [D 29] 826, *1075*
Morath, M. 435, *536*
Moraczewski, A.S. 602, *611*
Moreau, J. [M 54] 1018, *1092*

Morell, J.I., s. Kelly, D.B. 470, *531*
Morell, P. 23, *61*
Morgan, B.A., s. Hughes, J. 40, *58*
Morgan, C.T., Stellar, E. [M 55] 858, *1092*
Morgan, C.T., s. Beach, F.A. 448, *523*
Morgan, C.T., s. Galambos, R. [G 2] 761, *1078*
Morgan, L.G. 11, 13, 14, *61*
Morgan, R., Cheadle, J. 253, *311*
Morin, L., s. Elie, R. 289, *305*
Morin, R.D., s. Corbett, L. 95, *101*
Morison, R.S., Dempsey, E.W. 125, *192*, [M 56] 762, 977, *1092*
Morison, R.S., s. Dempsey, E.W. [D 26, 27] 977, *1075*
Moriya, A., s. Uryu, K. 172, *195*
Morrell, F. [M 57–60] 1031, *1092*
Morrell, F., s. Gastaut, H.A. [G 11] 1028, 1031, 1032, *1078*
Morris, C.A., s. Reich, T. 561, *613*
Morris, D. 384, *536*
Morris, D.P., Soroker, E., Burrus, G. 567, *611*
Morris, D.P., s. Michael, C.M. 567, *611*
Morris, G.O., Williams, H.L., Lubin, A. [M 61] 1003, *1092*
Morris, H.H., s. Bond, E.D. 328, *342*
Morris, H.R., s. Hughes, J. 40, *58*
Morris, J.B., Beck, A.T. 271, *311*
Morrison, J., Clancy, J., Crowe, R. 586, *611*
Morrison, J., s. Stewart, M. 596, *616*
Morrison, J., s. Winokur, G. 553, 564, *617*
Morrison, S.L., s. Goldberg, E.M. 573, *607*
Morse, P.A. 437, *536*
Morse, P.A., Snowdon, C.T. 443, 444, *536*

Moruzzi, G. [M 61 a–65] 844, 845, 977, 979, 988, 989, 990, *1092, 1093*
Moruzzi, G., Magoun, H.W. [M 66] 762, 904, 977, 995, *1093*
Moruzzi, G., s. Batini, C. [B 10] 989, *1070*
Moruzzi, G., s. Berlucchi, G. [B 40] 995, 1011, *1071*
Moruzzi, G., s. Magnes, J. 125, *191*, [M 16] 989, *1091*
Moruzzi, G., s. Whitlock, D.G. [W 21] 1005, *1102*
Moser, H.W., s. Holmes, L.B. 673, *697*
Mosowitch, A., Tallaferro, A. [M 67] 940, *1093*
Mosso, A. [M 68, 68 a] 948, *1093*
Most van Spijk, D. van der, s. Beek, H.H. 171, *182*
Mostafapour, S., s. Wurtman, R.J. 71, *109*
Motokawa, K. [M 69] *1093*
Motulsky, A.G., s. Omenn, G.S. 681, *700*
Mounier, D., s. Jouvet, M. [J 20] 989, *1084*
Mountcastle, V.B. [M 70–74] 825, 844, 893, 898, 902, 904, 908, 1037, 1079, *1093*
Mountcastle, V.B., Lynch, J.C., Georgopopolus, A., Sakata, H., Acuna, C. [M 75] 898, 929, 1037, *1093*
Mountcastle, V.B., Powell, T.P.S. [M 76] 844, *1093*
Mountcastle, V.B., s. Bard, P. [B 6] 943, 961, *1069*
Mountcastle, V.B., s. Lynch, J.C. [L 44] 825, 898, *1090*
Mourgue, R., s. Monakow, C. von [M 51] 800, 896, *1092*
Mowbray, R.M., s. Carroll, B.J. 74, *101*
Mowrer, M., s. Sila, B. 172, *194*
Moynihan, M. 426, *536*
Mühlen, H. v.d., s. Demisch, L. 96, *101*
Müller, C., Ciompi, L., Delachaux, A., Rabinowicz, T., Villa, J.L. 638, 641, 642, *700*
Müller, C., s. Ciompi, L. 642, *694*

Müller, D., Krüger, E. 292, *311*
Mueller, D., Orthner, H., Roeder, F., Koenig, A., Bosse, K., Kloos, G. 455, *536*
Mueller, D., Roeder, F., Orthner, H. 370, *377*
Mueller, D., s. Roeder, F. 370, *377*
Müller, G.E. [M 77–80] 781, 782, 786, 787, 870, 931, *1093*
Müller, J. [M 81, 82] 907, 908, 934, 1008, 1016, *1093*
Mueller, P.S., Henninger, G.R., McDonald, R.K. 81, *105*
Mueller, P.S., Vergne, P.M. de la 290, *311*
Müller-Limmroth, W. [M 83] 910, *1093*
Müller-Oerlinghausen, B., s. Bauer, H. 272, 298, *303*
Mueller-Preuss, P., Juergens, U. 474, *536*
Mueller-Preuss, P., s. Juergens, U. 474, *531*
Mueller-Preuss, P., s. Manley, J.A. 481, *534*
Mughal, S.M., s. Matus, A. 21, *60*
Mulder, J., s. Sørensen, R. 293, 299, *313*
Mullan, S., Penfield, W. [M 84] 886, *1093*
Mullaney, J., s. Reich, T. 550, *613*
Muller, H.J. 54, *61*
Mundinger, F., s. Hassler, R. 475, *529*
Mundy-Castle, A.C., Hurst, L.A., Beerstecher, D.M., Prinsloo, T. 162, *192*
Mundy-Castle, A.C., s. Hurst, L.A. 176, *188*
Munkvad, I., s. Gerlach, J. 271, 298, *306*
Munkvad, I., s. Randrup, A. 75, *106*
Munoz, R.A., Kuplic, J.B. 299, *311*
Munro, A. 730, *749*
Munro, A., Griffiths, A.B. 730, *749*
Munro, O.R., s. Gilligan, B.S. 298, *306*

Mura, E., s. Mednick, S.A. 567, 575, *611*
Murillo, L.G., s. Exner, J.E. Jr. 319, 333, *344*
Murken, J.-D. 674, 675, *700*
Murphree, H.B., s. Goldstein, L. 172, 173, *187*
Murphree, H.B., s. Sugerman, A.A. 173, *195*
Murphy, D.L. 81, 96, *105*
Murphy, D.L., Baker, M., Goodwin, F.K., Miller, H., Kotin, J., Bunney, W.E. 74, 96, *105*
Murphy, D.L., Belmaker, R., Carpenter, W.T., Wyatt, R.T. *105*
Murphy, D.L., Weiss, R. 570, *612*
Murphy, D.L., Wright, C., Buchsbaum, M., Nichols, A., Costa, J.L., Wyatt, R.J. 681, *700*
Murphy, D.L., s. Belmaker, R.H. 570, 583, *603*
Murphy, D.L., s. Buchsbaum, M. 96, *100*, 176, *183*, 571, *604*, 681, *693*
Murphy, D., s. Bunney, W.E. 74, 87, *100*, *101*
Murphy, D.L., s. Goodwin, F.K. 74, *103*, 223, 229, 230, *238*
Murphy, D.L., s. Kammen, D.P. van 271, *308*
Murphy, D.L., s. Leckmann, J.F. 96, *104*
Murphy, D.L., s. Potkin, S.G. 96, *106*
Murphy, D.L., s. Wyatt, R.J. 570, *617*
Murphy, J.M., s. Leighton, A.H. 662, *698*
Murphy, J.T., s. Gloor, P. 458, *528*
Murphy, K.P., s. Imlah, N.W. 256, *308*
Murphy, M.R., Schneider, G.E. 461, *536*
Murray, L.G., s. Ashcroft, G.W. 87, *99*
Murray, L.G., s. Hitchcook, E. 373, *376*
Murray, M.A.F., s. Beumont, P.J.V. 293, *303*
Murray, M.R. 10, *61*
Muscettola, G., Goodwin, F.K., Potter, W.Z., Claeys, M.M., Markey, S.P. 110, *113*
Muses, C.A., McCulloch, W.S. [M 85] 855, *1093*
Musick, J., Hubbard, J.I. 50, *61*
Mutani, R., s. Bergamini, L. 155, *182*
Myers, R.E. [M 86–91] 890, 892, *1093*, *1094*
Myers, R.E., Sperry, R.W. [M 92] 882, 890, 892, *1094*
Myrtek, M. 667, 669, *700*

Nadel, A.M., Wilson, W.P. 160, *192*
Nádvornik, P., Šramka, M., Patoprstá, G. 370, 371, *377*
Naef, H. 926
Nagahato, M., s. Narabayashi, H. 372, *377*
Nagao, T., s. Narabayashi, H. 372, *377*
Nagasawa, H., s. Meites, J. 220, *239*
Nagaswami, S., s. Curran, D.J. 298, *305*
Nagatsu, T., s. Fujita, K. 93, *102*
Nagatsu, T., s. Okada, T. 93, *105*
Nagy, A., s. Wålinder, J. 218, 227, *242*
Nakada, F., s. Hellmann, L. 77, *103*
Nakajima, S., s. Essman, W.B. 51, *57*
Nakashima, Y., s. Watanabe, S. 272, *314*
Nakazima, S. 521, *536*
Napier, J.R., Napier, P.N. 390, *536*
Napier, P.N., s. Napier, J.R. 390, *536*
Naquet, R., s. Gastaut, H. 166, *186*
Naquet, R., s. Gastaut, H.A. [G 11] 1028, 1031, 1032, *1078*
Naquet, R., s. Harner, R. 155, *187*
Narabayashi, H. 372, *377*
Narabayashi, H., Nagao, T., Saito, Y., Yoshida, M., Nagahato, M. 372, *377*
Narabayashi, H., Shima, F. 372, *377*
Narabayashi, H., s. Uchimura, Y. 356, *378*
Nash, J. 721, 728, *749*
Nasrallah, H., s. Bigelow, L.B. 94, *100*
Natalevich, E.S., s. Ivanitsky, A.M. 569, *608*
Nathan, L., s. Goldberg, H.L. 263, *306*
Nauta, W.J.H. 365, *377*
Nauta, W.J.H., Karten, H.J. 449, *536*
Nauta, W.J.H., s. Valenstein, E.S. 462, *543*
Nay, L.B. 681, *700*
Naylor, G.J., s. Peet, M. 71, *106*
Naylor, G.J., s. Worrall, E.P. 271, *314*
Návornik, P., Pogády, J., Šramka, M. 372, *377*
Neckers, L.M., s. Träskman, L. 109, 110, *113*
Nedopil, M., Dieterle, D., Hillebrand, G., Gurland, H.-J. 97, *105*
Nedopil, N., s. Hippius, H. 97, *103*
Neff, W.D., Diamond, I.T., Casseday, H.J. 478, *536*
Negishi, K., s. Svaetichin, G. [S 62] 787, *1100*
Negishi, K., s. Verzeano, M. [V 7, 8] 1004, 1005, *1101*
Negri, F., s. Smeraldi, E. 581, *615*
Neilson, M., s. Parker, G. 572, 573, *612*
Nelson, C., s. Sweeny, D. 72, 73, *108*
Nelson, J.F., Holinka, C.F., Latham, K.R., Allen, J.K., Finch, C.E. 26, *61*
Nelson, P., Peacock, J. 9, *61*
Nerenz, K. 299, *311*
Ness, M.L. 722, *749*
Nestoros, I.N., Ban, T.A., Lehmann, H.E. 94, *105*
Netter, P. 672, *700*
Nettleton, W.I., s. Burch, N.R. 134, *183*
Neuhäuser, G., s. Koch, G. 675, *698*
Neumann, F. 642, 643, *700*
Neumann, I. von *1094*

Neumayer, E., s. Birkmayer, W. 91, *100*
Newell, P.C., s. Gross, M. 253, *306*
Newman, J.D. 481, *576*
Newman, J.D., Symmes, D. 433, 481, *536*
Newman, J.D., Wollberg, Z. 481, *537*
Newman, J.D., s. Ploog, D. 394, 430, *538*
Newman, J.D., s. Wollberg, Z. 481, *544*
Newport, E.L. 520, *537*
Newton, 908
Newton, M.P., s. Tooth, G.C. 355, *378*
Newton, R.W. 299, *311*
Niall, H.D., s. Chang, M.M. 39, *56*
Niall, H.D., s. Powell, D. 200, *240*
Niall, H.D., s. Tregear, G.W. 39, *63*
Nichols, A., s. Murphy, D.L. 681, *700*
Nichols, A.S., s. Leckmann, J.F. 96, *104*
Nichols, I.A., s. Lenneberg, E.H. 521, *533*
Nichols, R.C., s. Loehlin, J.C. 549, *610*
Nicklas, W., s. Berl, S. 20, *56*
Nicol, S., s. Erlenmeyer-Kimling, L. *606*
Nicolai, J. 444, *537*
Nicolaou, N., s. Vestergaard, P. 69, 70, *108*
Niedermeyer, E. 162, *192*
Nielsen, J. 587, *612*, 620, 664, 674, 677, *700*
Nies, A., Robinson, D.S., Lamborn, K.R., Ravaris, C.L., Ives, J.O. 264, *311*
Nies, A., s. Weaver, L.A. Jr. 318, *349*
Niethardt, P., s. Künkel, H. 131, 132, 139, 143, 146, 180, *190*
Nikara, T., s. Pettigrew, J.D. [P 20a] 918, *1095*
Nilsson, G., s. Hökfelt, T. 15, 40, *58*
Nilsson, I.M., s. Öhman, R. 217, 218, 220, 221, *240*

Nilsson, T., s. Jonsson, E. 599, *609*
Nishikubo, M., s. Endo, M. 81, *102*
Niskanen, P., Huttunen, M., Tamminen, T., Jääskeläinen, J. 71, *105*
Nissen, G. 590, *612*, 635, 637, 638, 639, 640, 650, *700*
Nissen, H.W., s. Beach, F.A. 448, *523*
Noble, C.E., s. Osborne, R.T. *705*
Noell, W.K., s. Prast, J.W. [P 34] 969, 983, *1095*
Noguera, R., s. Coppen, A. 69, *101*, 270, *305*
Nolan, J., s. Kolvin, I. 596, *610*
Norton, J.C., s. Stark, L.H. 175, *194*
Norton, W.T. 11, 12, 16, 23, *61*
Norton, W.T., Poduslo, S.E. 10, 12, *61*
Nothdurft, H.C., s. Creutzfeldt, O.D. [C 18] 920, *1073*
Nottebohm, F. 444, 508, 514, *537*
Novak, E.N. 291, *311*
Novak, M.A., s. Suomi, S.J. 500, *542*
Nowakowski, H., Zerssen, D. von, Bergman, S., Reitalu, J. 677, *700*
Nugent, A., s. Tupin, J.P. 271, *313*
Nusselt, L., Kockott, G. 682, 690, *700*
Nusselt, L., s. Kockott, G. 682, 690, *698*
Nybäck, H. 225, *240*
Nybäck, H., Sedvall, G. 212, *240*
Nybäck, H.V., Walters, J.R., Aghajanian, G.K., Roth, R.H. 225, *240*
Nybäck, G., s. Sedvall, G. 212, *241*
Nyberg, G., Axelsson, R., Martensson, E. 217, *240*
Nyberg, G., s. Forsman, A. 217, *237*
Nyman, G.E., s. Larson, C.A. 577, *610*

Nyman, G.E., s. Lindegård, B. 671, *699*
Nymark, M., s. Möller-Nielsen, I. 221, *240*
Nyström, I., s. Ackenheil, M. 72, *98*
Nyström, I., s. Markianos, E.S. 93, *104*
Nyström, S. 330, 332, *347*

Obata, K., s. Ito, M. [I 4] *1083*
Oberhoffer, G., s. Helmchen, H. 127, *187*
Obrador, S., s. Delgado, J.M.R. 359, *375*
Obrador, S., s. Sweet, W.H. 455, *542*
Obrist, W.D. 162, *192*
Obrist, W.D., Henry, C.E. 162, *192*
Ochoa, E.L.M., Bangham, A.D. 26, *61*
Ochs, S. 14, 20, *61*
O'Connor, M., s. Wolstenholme, G.E.W. [W 31] 988, *1102*
Ødegaard, Ø. 561, 566, 572, 574, 586, *612*
O'Doherty, D.S., s. Ramey, E.R. [R 4] 886, *1096*
Ögren, S.-O., s. Fuxe, K. 110, *112*
Öhlin, H., s. Wadstein, J. 232, *242*
Öhman, R., Larsson, M., Nilsson, I.M. Engel, J., Carlsson, A. 217, 218, 220, 221, *240*
Öhman, R., s. Forsman, A. 217, *237*
Öjesjö, L., s. Hagnell, O. 587, *607*
Oerter, R. 503, *537*
Oesch, F., Otten, U., Thoenen, H. 31, *61*
O'Fallon, W.M., Labarthe, D.R., Kurland, L.T. 292, *311*
Offir, C., s. Tavris, C. 647, *703*
Offord, D.R., Cross, L.A. 567, *612*
Ogura, H., s. Yoshii, N. [Y 2] 1032, *1102*
Ohlmeyer, P., Brilmayer, H. [O 1] 996, *1094*

Ohlmeyer, P., Brilmayer, H., Hülstrung, H. [O 2] 996, 997, *1094*
Ohno, S. *705*
Okada, T., Shinoda, T., Kato, T., Ikuta, K., Nagatsu, T. 93, *105*
Okada, Y. 219, *240*
O'Keefe, R., Sharman, D.F., Vogt, M. 212, *240*
Okun, L.M. 9, *61*
Oldendorf, W.H. 44, *61*
Oldendorf, W.H., s. Pardridge, W.M. 45, *61*
Olds, J. 483, 484, 485, *537* [O 3–7] 955, 956, 958, 959, 960, 966, *1094*
Olds, J., Milner, P. 483, *537*, [O 8] 954, 955, *1094*
O'Leary, J.L., s. Adametz, J. 473, *523*
Oliver, J.E., s. Sutherland, E.M. 337, *348*
Olkinuora, M., s. Idänpään-Heikkilä, J. 291, *308*
Olley, P. s. Berger, R.J. [B 31] 1011, *1071*
Olley, P.C., s. Oswald, I. [O 14] 1015, *1094*
Olsen, T. 590, *612*
Olson, G.W., Peterson, D.B. 253, *311*
Omenn, G.S. 680, 681, *700*
Omenn, G.S., Motulsky, A.G. 681, *700*
Omenn, G.S., s. Ehrman, L. 547, *605*
Ommaya, A.K., s. Fedio, P. 359, *375*
Oppelt, W. [O 9] 853, 871, *1094*
Oppenheim, G. 289, *311*
Orbach, J., Milner, B., Rasmussen, T. [O 10] 944, 1048, *1094*
Orenberg, E.K., s. Barchas, J.D. 550, 571, *603*
Orley, J., Wing, J.K. 662, *700*
Orlov, P., Kasparian, G., Dimascio, A., Cole, J.O. 257, *311*
Orsulak, P.J., s. Schildkreut, J.J. 72, *107*
Orthner, H., s. Mueller, D. 370, *377*, 455, *536*

Orthner, H., s. Roeder, F. 370, *377*
Osborne, R.T., Noble, C.E., Weyl, N. *705*
Oscarsson, O. 450, *537*
Osmond, H., Smythies, J. 94, *105*
Osmond, H., s. Hoffer, A. 94, *103*
Osmond, H., s. Huxley, J. 577, *608*
Osofsky, J.D. 720, *749*
Osselton, J.W., s. Cooper, R. 118, 140, *184*
Osswald, M., s. Schilkrut, R. 83, *107*
Osterland, K., s. Hill, S. 600, *608*
Ostow, M. [O 11] 791, *1094*
Oswald, I. [O 12, 13] 988, 1019, *1094*
Oswald, I., Berger, R.J., Jaramillo, R.A., Keddie, K.M.G., Olley, P.C., Plunkett, G.B. [O 14] 1015, *1094*
Oswald, I., s. Berger, R.J. [B 31, 32] 993, 1003, 1011, *1071*
Oswaldo-Cruz, E., s. Albe-Fessard, D. [A 18] 842, *1068*
Otsuka, M., Konishi, S., Takahaski, T. 200, *240*
Otsuka, M., s. Iversen, L.L. 199, *238*
Otsuki, S., s. Watanabe, S. 271, 272, *314*
Ott, J.E., s. Burks, J.S. 299, *304*
Otten, H., s. Matussek, N. 74, *105*
Otten, U., s. Oesch, F. 31, *61*
Otterbein, E.C., s. Allen, W.S. 23, *55*
Ottosson, J.-O. 318, 320, 321, 322, 326, 337, 338, 339, *347*
Ottosson, J.-O., Rendahl, I. 336, *347*
Ottosson, J.-O., s. Arfwidsson, L. 332, *342*
Ottosson, J.-O., s. Cronholm, B. 318, 320, 325, 326, 328, *343*

Ottosson, J.-O., s. Kirstein, L. 321, *346*
Ouahchi, S., s. Gastaut, H. [G 12a] *1078*
Ounsted, C., Taylor, D.C. 643, *700*
Ounsted, C., s. Kolvin, I. 588, 589, *610*
Ourgaud, J.J., s. Bessuges, J.M. 288, *303*
Ourso, R., s. Arneson, G.A. 335, 341, *342*
Overall, J.E., s. Hollister, L.E. 72, *103*
Overton, D.A., s. Shagass, C. 175, *194*
Overzier, C. 625, 648, 690, *700*
Owen, A., s. Foulds, G.A. 684, *695*
Owen, D.R., s. Witkin, H.A. 677, *704*
Owen, F., Cross, A.J., Crow, T.J., Longden, A., Poulter, M., Riley, G.J. 91, *105*
Owen, F., s. Brockington, I. 570, *604*
Owen, F., s. Cross, A.J. 112, *112*
Owen, F., s. Joseph, M.H. *59*
Owen, O.E., s. Patel, M.S. 51, *62*
Oxenkrug, G.F., s. Lapin, I.P. 67, *104*, 339, *346*

Paananen, R., s. Weaver, L. 318, *349*
Pach, J., s. Schenck, G.K. 96, *107*
Pacha, W.L., s. Zeller, E.A. 223, *242*
Pacheco, P., s. Stevens, J.R. 486, *542*
Page, I.K., s. Elliott, K.A.C. 3, *57*
Page, L.H. 3, *61*
Page, M.A., Krebs, H.A., Williamson, D.H. 52, *61*
Pagni, C.A. 152, *192*
Paikin, H., Jacobsen, B., Schulsinger, F., Godtfredsen, K., Rosenthal, D., Wender, P., Kety, S. 558, *612*
Pal, S.B. 672, 683, *700*

Palacios, J.M., Mengod, G., Picatoste, F., Grau, M., Blanco, I. 37, *61*
Palestini, M., s. Batini, C. [B 10] 989, *1070*
Palme, F., s. Kornmüller, A.E. [K 45] 969, 977, 983, *1088*
Palmer, B., s. Todd, G.A. 521, *542*
Palva, I., s. Idänpään-Heikkilä, J. 291, *308*
Pampiglione, G., s. Brazier, M.A.B. 121, *183*
Pandey, G.N., Garver, D.L., Tamminga, C., Ericksen, S., Ali, S.I., Davis, J.M. 91, 92, *105*
Pandey, G.N., s. Caspar, R.C. 81, 84, 91, *101*
Pandey, G.N., s. Dorus, E. 583, *605*
Pandey, G.N., s. Garver, D.L. 81, 82, 83, *102*, 338, *344*
Panetta, V., s. Miani, N. 21, 24, *61*
Panse, F., Klages, W. 91, *106*
Pant, S.S., s. Holmes, L.B. 673, *697*
Papeschi, R., McClure, D.J. 69, *106*
Papez, J.W. 355, 365, *377*, 453, 454, *537*, [P 1] 904, 944, *1094*
Papoušek, H. 435, 503, 519, *537*, 720, *749*
Papoušek, H., Bernstein, P. 503, *537*
Papoušek, H., Papoušek, M. 498, 499, 503, 518, 519, 520, *537*, 572, *612*
Papoušek, H., s. Martinius, J.W. 503, *535*
Papoušek, M., s. Matussek, N. *105*
Papoušek, M., s. Papoušek, H. 498, 499, 503, 518, 519, 520, *537*, 572, *612*
Paradowski, W., s. Erlenmeyer-Kimling, L. 577, *606*
Pardee, J.D., Bamburg, J.R. 20, *61*
Pardridge, W.M., Oldendorf, W.H. 45, *61*
Pare, C.M.B. 74, *106*

Pare, C.M.B., Yeung, D.P.H., Price, K., Stacey, R.S. 68, *106*
Park, D., s. Hökfelt, T. 200, *238*
Parker, G., Neilson, M. 572, 573, *612*
Parker, N. 549, *612*
Parmeggiani, P.L. [P 2, 3] 989, *1094*
Parnell, R.W. 667, 671, *700*
Partanen, J.K., Bruun, T., Markanen, M. 599, *612*
Partanan, T.J., s. Lind, J. 413, *533*
Partanan, T., s. Wasz-Hoekkert, O. 413, 434, 435, *543*
Pasamanick, B., Rogers, M., Lilienfeld, A.M. 575, *612*
Passouant, P. [P 4] 858, 881, 1024, 1027, *1094*
Patel, A.J., Balázs, R. 49, *61*
Patel, A.J., Johnson, A.L., Balázs, R. 36, *62*
Patel, A.J., s. Balázs, R. 47, 49, *55*
Patel, M.S., Owen, O.E. 51, *62*
Paterson, D.G. 669, 671, *700*
Patoprstá, G., s. Nádvornik, P. 370, 371, *377*
Patterson, M.M., s. Thompson, R.F. 147, 153, *195*
Patton, R.G., Gardner, L.J. 722, 733, *749*
Pauget, J.D. 289, *311*
Paulson, G.W. 335, *347*
Paulson, O.B., s. Bolwig, T.G. 323, 340, *342*
Paulson, O.B., s. Brodersen, P. 322, *342*
Pavlov 353
Pavlov, s. Bechterew 352
Pawlik, K. 667, 669, *700*
Pawlow, I.P. [P 5–7] 759, 790, 803, 806, 807, 810, 811, 814, 815, 817, 839, 841, 858, 882, 907, 929, 939, 962, 963, 972, 973, 974, 990, 1024, 1027, 1028, 1029, 1032, *1094*
Paykel, E.S., Klerman, G.L., Prusoff, B.A. 688, *701*
Pazzaglia, P., s. Lugaresi, E. 166, 168, *191*
Peacock, J., s. Nelson, P. 9, *61*

Pearson, J.S., Kley, I.B. 567, *612*
Pécheny, J., s. Baruk, H. 287, *303*
Pechstein, J., Siebenmorgen, E., Weitsch, D. 718, 731, *749*
Pedersen, V., s. Möller-Nielsen, I. 221, *240*
Pedretti, A., s. Buffa, P. 287, *304*
Peet, M., Moody, J.P., Worrall, E.P., Walker, P., Naylor, G.J. 71, *106*
Peet, M., s. Coppen, A. 71, *101*
Peiper, A. 434, *537*, 710, *749*
Pelchat, G., s. Jus, A. 297, *308*
Pellin, B., s. Jouvet, M. [J 20] 989, *1084*
Pelz, L., Mieler, W. 620, 674, *701*
Penfield, W. [P 8–13] 784, 880, 883, 884, 904, 906, 978, 1048, *1095*
Penfield, W., Jasper, H.H. 126, 192, [P 14] 883, 884, *1095*
Penfield, W., Milner, B. [P 15] 883, 884, 1047, *1095*
Penfield, W., Perot, P. [P 16] 883, 884, 885, 934, *1095*
Penfield, W., Rasmussen, T. 451, *537* [P 17] 784, 843, 882, 883, 884, 885, 886, 894, 934, 935, *1095*
Penfield, W., Roberts, L. 475, 476, *537*, [P 18] 894, *1095*
Penfield, W., Welch, K. 474, *537*
Penfield, W.G., s. Bazett, H.C. 476, *523*
Penfield, W., s. Foerster, O. [F 20] 884, 934, *1077*
Penfield, W., s. Mullan, S. [M 84] 886, *1093*
Penin, H. 158, 160, 161, 165, 177, *192*
Penin, H., Helmchen, H., Jacobitz, K., Kanowski, S., Künkel, H., Zenker, K. 124, 127, *192*
Penin, H., Käufer, C. 155, *192*

Penin, H., Matiar-Vahar, H. 163, *192*
Penin, H., Schaefer, C.H. 163, *192*
Penin, H., Zeh, W. 160, *192*
Penin, H., s. Helmchen, H. 127, *187*
Penin, H., s. Huber, G. 170, 171, 177, *188*
Pénot, B. 590, *612*
Penry, J.K., Dreyfuss, F.E. 166, *192*
Pereira-Reis, M.J., s. Morais, T.M. 256, *311*
Perel, J.M. 246, 263, *311*
Perel, J.M., Shostak, M., Gann, E., Kantor, S.J., Glassmann, A.H. 311
Perel, J.M., s. Kantor, S.J. 287, *309*
Perel, J.M., s. Winsberg, B.G. 287, *314*
Perez-Cruet, J., s. Volavka, J. 96, *108*
Perez-Reyes, M. 78, *106*
Perkins, M.N., s. Linton, E.A. 38, *60*
Perot, P., s. Penfield, W. [P 16] 883, 884, 885, 934, *1095*
Perrin, G.M. 336, *347*
Perris, C. 335, *347*, 578, 579, 580, 583, 585, *612*, 649, 661, 686, *701*
Perris, C., s. Angst, J. 578, *603*, 661, *692*
Perris, C., s. Arfwidsson, L. 332, *342*
Perris, C., s. Bonetti, U. 686, *693*
Perris, C., s. D'Elia, G. 176, *184*, 594, *605*
Perris, H., Strandman, E. 687, *701*
Perry, E.K., Gibson, P.H., Blessed, G., Perry, R.T., Tomlinson, B.E. 67, *106*
Perry, R.T., s. Perry, E.K. 67, *106*
Persson, G., s. Arfwidsson, L. 332, *342*
Persson, S.-Å., Johansson, H. 229, *240*
Persson, T., Roos, B.E. 93, *106*
Pert, C.B., Kuhar, M.J., Snyder, S.H. 40, *62*

Pert, C.B., s. Kuhar, M.J. 485, *532*
Pescor, F.T., s. Wikler, A. 164, *196*
Pete, N., s. Mandel, P. 12, *60*
Peters, H., s. Sato, S. 298, *312*
Petersen, I., s. Chatrian, G.E. 121, *183*
Petersen, I., s. Kellaway, P. 133, *189*
Peterson, D.B., s. Olson, G.W. 253, *311*
Peterson, F., Jung, C.G. [P 19] 930, *1095*
Peto, R., s. Saxén, E.A. 292, *312*
Petrie, A., s. Claveria, L.E. 298, *304*
Petsche, H., Stumpf, C. [P 20] 918, 977, *1095*
Pettigrew, J.D., Nikara, T., Bishop, P.O. [P 20a] 918, *1095*
Pettit, M.G., s. Whitten, C.F. 733, *751*
Petzold, G.L., s. Clement-Cormier, Y.C. 216, 217, *237*
Petzold, G.L., s. Kebabian, J.W. 30, *59*
Pfaff, D., Lewis, C., Diakow, C., Keiner, M. 466, 467, *537*
Pfaff, D.W., Diakow, C., Zigmond, R.E., Kow, L.-M. 466, 467, 468, *538*
Pfaff, D.W., s. Kelly, D.B. 470, *531*
Pfaff, W., s. Diebold, K. 566, *605*, 649, *694*
Pfanzagl, J. 658, *701*
Pfefferbaum, A., s. Buchsbaum, M.A. 175, *183*
Pfeiffer, C.C., s. Goldstein, L. 172, 173, *187*
Pfeiffer, C.C., s. Sugerman, A.A. 173, *195*
Pfeiffer, J., s. McCulloch, W.S. [M 35] 856, 857, 858, 859, 862, *1091*
Pflanz, M. 629, *701*
Philip, J., s. Witkin, H.A. 677, *704*
Philipp, M. 97, *106*

Phillips, C.G. [P 21] 844, *1095*
Phillips, C.G., s. Granit, R. [G 35] *1079*
Phillips, J.E., Jacobsen, N., Turner, W.J. 566, *612*
Phillips, J.S., s. Kanfer, F.H. 629, 633, *697*
Phillips, V.P., s. Reed, S.C. 553, *613*
Photiades, H., s. Lazos, G. 292, *309*
Piaget, J. 503, *538*
Picatoste, F., s. Palacios, J.M. 37, *61*
Pichot, P. 246, *311*, 591, *612*
Pickar, D., Sweeny, D.R., Maas, J.W., Heninger, G.R. 72, *106*
Pickar, D., s. Kupfer, D.J. 580, *610*
Pickel, V.M., Reis, D.J., Marangos, P.J., Zomely-Neurath, C. 21, *62*
Pickenhain, L. [P 22] 1027, *1095*
Piergies, A., s. Pieschl, D. 251, *311*
Piéron, H., s. Legendre, R. [L 6] 993, *1088*
Pieschl, D. 287, *311*
Pieschl, D., Kulhanek, F., Piergies, A. 251, *311*
Pijnenburg, A.J.J., Woodruff, G.N., Rossum, J.M. van 211, *240*
Pill, R., s. Stacey, M. 729, *750*
Pilleri, G., s. Pock, D.W. [P 26] 961, *1095*
Pillon, B., s. Lhermitte, F. 479, *533*
Pincus, G., s. Hoagland, H. 179, *188*
Pineau, R., s. Jus, A. 297, *308*
Pippard, J. 365, *377*
Piree, S., s. Emrich, H.M. 96, *102*
Pires, P., s. Jus, A. 297, *308*
Pirke, K.M., s. Doerr, P. 672, 683, *694*
Pisani, P.P., s. Glasersfeld, E.C. von 512, *528*
Pisani, P., s. Rumbaugh, D.M. 512, *540*
Pisciotta, A.V. 291, *311*

Pisoni, D.B., s. Liberman, A.M. 439, 440, 480, *533*
Pitts, F.N., Meyer, J., Brooks, M., Winokur, G. 730, *749*
Pitts, F.N., s. Winokur, G. 600, *617*
Pitts, F.N. Jr., s. Woodruff, R.A., Jr. 317, *349*
Pitts, W., McCulloch, W.S. 178, *193*
Pitts, W., s. McCulloch, W.S. [M 36] *1091*
Pitts, W.H., s. McCulloch, W.S. [M 34] 853, 857, *1091*
Planansky, K. 564, *612*
Planques, I., Grézes-Rueff, C., Bollinelli, R., Darrusio, J., Chabourne, M. 162, *193*
Plantey, F., Kammen, D.P. van 94, *106*
Plapinger, L., s. McEwen, B.S. 465, 466, *535*
Plateau, J.A.F. [P 23] 908, *1095*
Platt, D. 634, *701*
Plesset, J., s. Rosanoff, A.J. 555, 597, 598, *613*
Pletscher, A., s. Da Prada, M. 212, *237*
Ploeger, A. 736, *749*
Ploeger, A., s. Mende, W. 736, *749*
Plog, U., s. Spehr, W. 158, 161, *194*
Plomin, R., Willerman, L., Loehlin, J.C. 549, *612*
Plomin, R., s. Buss, A.H. 669, *693*
Ploog, D. 380, 385, 393, 395, 400, 402, 407, 408, 410, 411, 421, 423, 425, 432, 443, 452, 453, 460, 478, 479, 483, 484, 487, 489, 490, 491, 513, *538*, 547, 548, 565, *612*, *613*, 624, 625, 633, *701* [P 24] 759, 797, 808, 811, 813, 939, 940, 1020, *1095*
Ploog, D., Blitz, J., Ploog, F. 384, 461, 489, *538*
Ploog, D., Gottwald, P. 423, 487, *538*
Ploog, D., Hopf, S., Winter, P. 394, 395, 406, 431, 432, 490, 493, *538*
Ploog, D., Hupfer, K., Juergens, U., Newman, J.D. 394, 430, *538*
Ploog, D., MacLean, P.D. 386, 464, *538*
Ploog, D., Melnechuk, T. 393, 503, 508, 511, *538*
Ploog, D., s. Bowden, D. 432, *524*
Ploog, D., s. Castell, R. 387, 388, *525*
Ploog, D., s. Hupfer, K. 479, 480, *530*
Ploog, D., s. Juergens, U. 425, 436, 437, 471, 473, 477, 478, 513, *531*
Ploog, D., s. Latta, J. 386, *533*
Ploog, D., s. MacLean, P.D. 461, 463, 464, *534*
Ploog, D., s. Maurus, M. 393, 465, 483, *535*
Ploog, F., s. Ploog, D. 384, 461, 489, *538*
Ploog, D., s. Talmage-Riggs, G. 432, *542*
Ploog, D., s. Winter, P. 426, 429, 432, 490, *544*
Ploog, D.W., McLean, P.D. [P 25] 810, *1095*
Ploog, D.W., s. MacLean, P.D. [M 15] 939, 960, *1091*
Plum, F., Howse, D.C., Duffy, T.E. 322, *347*
Plum, F., Posner, J.B. 155, 158, *193*
Plum, F., Posner, J.P., Troy, B. 322, *347*
Plum, F., s. Beresford, H.R. 322, *342*
Plum, F., s. Posner, J.B. 322, *347*
Plum, F., s. Raichle, M.E. 5, *62*
Plum, F., s. Wasterlain, C.G. 336, *349*
Plunkett, G.B., s. Oswald, I. [O 14] 1015, *1094*
Pock, K., Risso, M., Pilleri, G. [P 26] 961, *1095*
Podolczak, D., s. Doehl, J. 506, *526*
Poduslo, S.E., s. Norton, W.T. 10, 12, *61*
Pöldinger, W. 244, 280, *311*
Pöldinger, W., Schmidlin, W. 244, *312*
Poeldinger, W., s. Angst, J. 641, 642, *692*
Poeldinger, W., s. Gáspar, M. *306*
Poeppel, E., Brinkmann, R., Cramon, E., Singer, W. *539*
Poeppel, E., Cramon, D. von, Backmund, H. 448, *539*
Poeppel, E., Held, R., Dowling, J.E. 479, *539*
Pötzl, O. [P 27] 894, 1011, *1095*
Pogády, J., s. Návornik, P. 372, *377*
Poggio, G.F., Fischer, B. [P 28] 920, *1095*
Pohlmeier, H., Schön, I., Matussek, N. 74, *106*
Pohlmeier, H., s. Matussek, N. 74, *105*
Poirier, F.E. 488, *539*
Poláčková, J., s. Bilý, J. 290, *304*
Polák, O., s. Kolárský, A. 683, 690, *698*
Polednak, A.P. 666, *701*
Pollack, M., Woerner, M.G. 575, *613*
Pollin, W. 570, *613*
Pollin, W., Allen, M.G., Hoffer, A., Stabenau, J.R. Hrubec, Z. 555, 556, *613*
Pollin, W., Cardon, P.V., Kety, S.S. 94, *106*
Pollin, W., Stabenau, J.R. 570, 575, *613*
Pollin, W., s. Belmaker, R. 557, *603*
Pollin, W., s. Cohen, D.J. 549, *604*
Pollin, W., s. Stabenau, J.R. 685, 691, *702*
Pollin, W., s. Wyatt, R.J. 570, *617*
Pollitt, J. 663, *701*
Pollitt, J.D. 332, *347*
Polonius, J., s. Dahme, B. 552, *604*
Polonius, M.L., s. Huse-Kleinstoll, G. 552, *608*
Polt, J.M., s. Hess, E.H. [H 43] 930, 948, *1081*
Polvan, Ö., s. Cebiroglu, R. 590, *604*
Pomeroy, W.B., s. Kinsey, A.C. 799, 940, *1086*

Pompeiano, O., Swett, J.W. [P 29, 30] 989, *1095*
Pompeiano, O., s. Bizzi, E. [B 46] 1005, *1071*
Pompeiano, O., s. Gassel, M.M. [G 9] 995, *1078*
Pompeiano, O., s. Giaquinto, S. [G 19] 995, *1079*
Pompeiano, O., s. Magnes, J. 125, *191*, [M 16] 989, *1091*
Ponerat, C.M., s. Lumsden, C.E. 4, *60*
Pond, D.A., s. Hill, D. [H 70] *1082*
Pooter, W.Z., s. Muscettola, G. 110, *113*
Popper, K.R. [P 31] 779, 791, 792, 795, 804, 821, 1062, *1095*
Popper, K.R., Eccles, J.C. [P 32] 779, 791, 792, 793, 794, 902, 904, 1039, *1095*
Port, F.K., Kroll, P.D., Swartz, R.D. 97, *106*
Posner, J.B., Plum, F., Van Poznak, A. 322, *347*
Posner, J.B., s. Beresford, H.R. 322, *342*
Posner, J.B., s. Plum, F. 155, 158, *193*, 322, *347*
Posner, J.B., s. Raichle, M.E. 5, *62*
Post, F. 586, *613*
Post, R.M., Gerner, R.H., Carman, J.S., Gillin, J.C., Jimerson, D.C., Goodwin, F.K., Bunney, W.E. Jr. 75, *106*
Post, R.M., Goodwin, F.K. 325, 339, *347*
Post, R.M., Gordon, E.K., Goodwin, F.K., Bunney, W.E. Jr. 70, *106*
Post, R.M., Kotin, J., Goodwin, F.K. 73, *106*
Post, R.M., s. Bunney, W.E. 87, *100*
Post, R.M., s. Bunney, W.E. Jr. 339, *343*
Post, R.M., s. Goodwin, F.K. 68, 69, 70, *103*
Post, R.M., s. Stoddard, F.J. 72, *108*
Postman, C. [P 33] 930, *1095*
Potepan, P., s. May, P.R.A. 333, *346*

Potkin, S.G., Cannon, H.E., Murphy, D.L., Wyatt, R.J. 96, *106*
Potts, J.T., s. Powell, D. 200, *240*
Potts, J.T., s. Tregear, G.W. 39, *63*
Poulsen, J.C., s. Baastrup, P.C. 270, *303*
Poulter, M., s. Cross, A.J. 112, *112*
Poulter, M., s. Owen, F. 91, *105*
Powell, D., Leeman, S.E., Tregear, G.W., Niall, H.D., Potts, J.T. 200, *240*
Powell, G.F., Brasel, J.A., Raiti, S., Blizzard, R.M. 733, *749*
Powell, G.F., Hopwood, N.J., Barratt, E.S. 733, *749*
Powell, T.P.S., s. Mountcastle, V.B. [M 76] 844, *1093*
Praag, H.M. van 67, 68, 69, *106*, 109, *113*, 227, *240*
Praag, H.M. van, Burg, W. van den, Bos, E.R.H., Dols, L.C.W. 227, *240*
Praag, H.M. van, Korf, J. 69, 93, *106*, 109
Praag, H.M. van, s. Verhoeven, W.M.A. 97, *108*
Praag, H.M. van, s. Wied, D. de 97, *108*
Prader, A. 625, 643, *701*
Prange, A.J., s. Coppen, A. 69, *101*
Prast, J.W., Noell, W.K. [P 34] 969, 983, *1095*
Pratt, K.L., s. Kiley, J.E. 161, *189*
Pratt, O.E., s. Daniel, P.M. 51, *57*
Pray, B.J., s. Thornton, W.E. 272, *313*
Prechtl, H.F.R. [P 35] 950, *1095*
Preiningerová, O., s. Zapletálek, M. 256, *314*
Premack, A.J. 509, 510, 511, 512, 516, *539*
Premack, A.J., Premack, D. *539*
Premack, D. 381, 512, 516, *539*
Premack, D., s. Premack, A.J. *539*

Presslich, O., s. Hofmann, G. 298, *307*
Presthus, J., s. Ziegler, D.K. 160, *196*
Preston, E., Schönbaum, E. 32, 33, 34, *62*
Preti, C., s. Margolis, R.K. 23, *60*
Pribram, K.H., Weiskrantz, L. [P 36] 1042, *1096*
Pribram, K.H., s. Mishkin, M. [M 47] *1092*
Price, J.S., Hare, E.H. 572, *613*
Price, J.S., s. Hare, E.H. 572, 573, 574, *608*
Price, J.S., s. Hill, O.W. 730, *748*
Price, J.S., s. Slater, E. 583, *615*
Price, K.S., s. Farley, I.J. 93, *102*
Price, K., s. Pare, C.M.B. 68, *106*
Prien, R.F., Klett, C.J. 253, *312*
Prien, S.F., Levine, J., Switalski, R.W. 253, *312*
Pringle, M.L.K., Bossio, V. 731, *750*
Prinsloo, T., s. Mundy-Castle, A.C. 162, *192*
Pritchard, M. 258, *312*
Pro, J.D., Wells, C.E. 164, *193*
Prokop, O., s. Witkowski, R. 602, *617*
Propping, P. 600, *613*
Propping, P., s. Kopun, M. *610*
Provence, S., s. Coleman, R.W. 722, *747*
Prüll, G., Krämer, W., Rompel, K. 162, *193*
Pruscha, H., Maurus, M. 393, 447, 482, *539*
Pruscha, H., s. Maurus, M. 393, 394, 483, *535*
Prusoff, B.A., s. Paykel, E.S. 688, *701*
Puech, A., s. Frances, H. 89, *102*
Puech, A.-J., s. Jouvent, R. 89, *103*
Pühringer, W., s. Wirz-Justice, A. 71, *108*

Pullar, J.A., s. Ashcroft, G.W. 70, 87, *99*
Purkinje 907, 913
Purpura, D.P., Cohen, B. [P 37] *1096*
Puszkin, S., s. Berl, S. 20, *56*
Putkoradze-Gamkrelidze, N.A., s. Gamkrelidze, S.A. 257, *306*
Puusepp, L. 352, *377*
Pythkowicz Streissguth, A., s. Jones, K.L. 673, *697*

Quadri, S.K., s. Maites, J. 220, *239*
Quandt, J., Sommer, H. 324, *347*
Quarles, R.H. 24, *62*
Quarton, G.C., s. Schmitt, F.O. 460, *541*
Quastel, J.H. 9, *62*
Quastel, J.H., s. Elliott, K.A.C. 3, *57*
Quastler, H. [Q 1] 858, 877, *1096*
Quensel, F., s. Kohnstamm, O. 979, 982, *1087*
Quitkin, F., s. Kane, J. 246, *308*
Quitkin, F., s. Rifkin, A. 257, 272, 292, *312*

Raaf, J., s. Dow, R.S. 163, *185*
Rabending, G., Klepel, H. 167, *193*
Rabinovitch, M.S., s. Kennard, M.A. 172, *189*
Rabinowicz, T., s. Müller, C. 638, 641, 642, *700*
Racagni, G., s. Trabucchi, M. 219, *242*
Rademaker, G.G.J. [R 1] 817, 823, *1096*
Radermecker, J. 132, 157, 163, *193*, [R 2] *1096*
Raebild, I., s. Hauge, M. 574, *608*
Raeburn, S., s. Twomey, S.L. 20, *63*
Raehlmann, E., Witkowski, L. [R 3] 996, *1096*
Raese, J., s. Ackenheil, M. 72, *98*
Rafaelsen, O.J., Kramp, P.L., Shapiro, R.W. 681, *701*
Rafaelsen, O.J., s. Bech, P. 686, *693*
Rafaelsen, O.J., s. Bolwig, T.G. 323, 340, *342*
Rafaelsen, O.J., s. Brodersen, P. 322, 342
Rafaelsen, O.J., s. Vendsborg, P.B. 272, 290, 293, *313*
Rafaelsen, O.J., s. Vestergaard, P. 69, 70, *108*
Raichle, M.E., Posner, J.B., Plum, F. 5, *62*
Rainer, J., s. Erlenmeyer-Kimling, L. 577, *606*
Rainer, J.D., Altshuler, K.Z. 722, *750*
Rainer, J.D., s. Erlenmeyer-Kimling, L. 577, *606*
Rainer, J.D., s. Mendlewicz, J. 578, 579, 580, 583, *611*
Raisman, G., Field, P.M. 466, *539*
Raiteri, M., s. Levi, G. 36, *60*
Raiti, S., s. Powell, G.F. 733, *749*
Rakkolainen, V., s. Rimon, R. 93, *107*
Rall, T.W., s. Sattin, A. 38, *62*
Ramanujam, P.B., s. Balasubramaniam, V. 361, *375*
Rama Rao, V.A., s. Coppen, A. 72, *101*
Ramey, C.T., s. Watson, J.S. 503, *543*
Ramey, E.R., O'Doherty, D.S. [R 4] 886, *1096*
Ramqvist, N., s. Holmberg, G. 320, *345*
Randrup, A., Baastrup, C. 75, *106*
Randrup, A., Munkvad, I., Fog, R., Gerlach, J., Molander, L., Kjellberg, B., Scheel-Krüger, J. 75, *106*
Randrup, A., s. Gerlach, J. 298, *306*
Ranke, O.F. [R 5] 1044, *1096*
Ranson, S.W., s. Magoun, H.W. 471, *534*
Rantow, A., s. Maj, J. 110, *113*
Raotma, H., s. D'Elia, G. 318, 319, 332, 337, *343*, *344*
Rapoport, S.I. 45, *62*

Rapport, M.M., s. Tamir, H. 26, *63*
Raschka, L.B., s. Lovett Doust, J.W. 323, *346*
Rasmussen, T., s. Orbach, J. [O 10] 944, 1048, *1094*
Rasmussen, T., s. Penfield, W. 451, *537* [P 17] 784, 843, 882, 883, 884, 885, 886, 894, 934, 935, *1095*
Rasnussen, P.V., s. Dyke, J. van 568, *605*
Rassin, D.K. 14, *62*
Rauber, A. 710, *750*
Ravaris, C.L., Weaver, L.A., Brooks, G.W. 253, *312*
Ravaris, C.L., s. Nies, A. 264, *311*
Ravaris, C., s. Weaver, L. 318, *349*
Raylor, M.A., s. Abrams, R. 586, *602*
Rayner, R., s. Watson, J.B. [W 13] 1043, *1101*
Razran, G. [R 6] 807, *1096*
Rebec, G.V., s. Groves, P.M. 215, *238*
Rebelsky, F.G., s. Lenneberg, E.H. 521, *533*
Rechtschaffen, A., Wolpert, E.A., Dement, W.C., Mitchell, S.A., Fisher, C. [R 7] 999, 1009, 1016, *1096*
Redlich, F.C., s. Hollingshead, A.B. 573, *608*
Redmond, D.E., s. Maas, J.W. 72, *104*
Ree, J.M. van, Terenius, L. 97, *106*
Ree, J.M. van, s. Verhoeven, W.M.A. 97, *108*
Ree, J.M. van, s. Wied, D. de 97, *108*
Reece, J.C., s. Wilson, J.C. 556, *617*
Reed, S.C. 601, *613*
Reed, S.C., Hartley, C., Anderson, V.E., Phillips, V.P., Johnson, N.A. 553, *613*
Rees, L. 622, 665, 671, 679, *701*
Rees, L., Butler, P.W.P., Gosling, C., Besser, G.M. 85, *107*
Reeves, W.P., s. Gross, M. 253, *306*
Regan, D. 147, 153, 154, *193*

Reginaldi, D., s. Kukopulos, A. 330, *346*
Regis, H., s. Gastaut, H.A. [G 11] 1028, 1031, 1032, *1078*
Reich, T., Cloninger, C.R., Guze, S.B. 550, 561, 600, *613*
Reich, T., James, J.H., Morris, C.A. 561, *613*
Reich, T., Winokur, G., Mullaney, J. 550, *613*
Reich, T., s. Cloninger, C.R. 584, 595, *604*, 639, *694*
Reich, T., s. Winokur, G. 582, 600, *617*
Reich, T., s. Woodruff, R.A. Jr. 689, *704*
Reichardt, M. [R 8, 9] 762, 882, 904, 977, *1096*
Reichardt, W. [R 10] 853, *1096*
Reichardt, W., McGinitie, G. [R 11] 853, 865, *1096*
Reichel, H., s. Markianos, E.S. 93, *104*
Reichert 366
Reichert, H., s. Marjerrison, G. 164, *191*
Reid, M.A., s. Mendelson, W.B. 590, *611*
Reim, B., s. Langer, G. 83, 84, *104*
Reimer, C., s. Gross, J. 736, *748*
Reimer, C., s. Kempe, P. 736, *748*
Reinberg, A., s. Halberg, F. *187*
Reis, D.J., s. Pickel, V.M. 21, *62*
Reisby, N. 553, *613*
Reisby, N., s. Gerlach, J. 298, *306*
Reisner, H. 572, *613*
Reiss, E. 686, *701*
Reiss, R.F. [R 11 a] 855, *1096*
Reitalu, J. 677, *701*
Reitalu, J., s. Nowakowski, H. 677, *700*
Reiter, P.J. 97, *107*
Reitman, E.E., s. Cleveland, S.E. 741, *747*
Rekola, J., s. Alanen, Y.O. 566, *603*

Rémond, A. 133, *193*
Rémond, A., s. Brazier, M.A.B. 121, *183*
Remschmidt, H., Dauner, I. 590, *613*
Renaud, H., Estess, F. 576, *613*
Rendahl, I., s. Ottosson, J.-O. 336, *347*
Renfrew, S., s. Kennedy, A.C. 160, *189*
Renqvist-Reenpää, Y. [R 12] 910, *1096*
Rensch, B. 398, 513, *539*
Rensch, B., Duecker, G. 506, *539*
Renson, J., s. Barchas, J.D. 550, 571, *603*
Renz, A., s. Benkert, O. 71, 74, *100*
Renzetti, A.D., s. Auchincloss, J.H., Jr. [A 36] 1016, *1069*
Reppesgaard, H., s. Bjarnar, E. 587, *603*
Resche-Rigon, P., s. Charriot, G. *304*
Resche-Rigon, s. Harriot 256
Research Committee The Royal College of Psychiatrists 374, *377*
Reuter, W., s. Brostoff, S.W. 23, *56*
Revuelta, A., s. Zivkovic, B. 213, *242*
Rey, E.-R., s. Zerssen, D. von 680, *704* 705
Rey, W. van, Wissfeld, E. [R 13] 1015, *1096*
Rey-Bellet, J. 161, *193*
Reyero, F., s. Baumann, P. 71, *99*
Reynolds, C.M., s. Merry, J. 271, *310*
Reynolds, F., s. Reynolds, V. 426, 427, *539*
Reynolds, V., Reynolds, F. 426, 427, *539*
Rheingold, H.L. 410, *539*, 718, 732, *750*
Rheingold, H.L., Gewirtz, J., Ross, H. 435, 518, *539*, 732, *750*
Rhines, R., s. Magoun, H.W. [M 20] 989, *1091*
Ribstein, M., s. Cadilhac, J. 160, *183*

Ricci, G., Doane, B., Jasper, H. [R 14] 817, 1028, 1031, 1036, *1096*
Ricci, G., s. Euler, C. v. [E 20, 21] 977, *1076*
Ricci, G., s. Jasper, H. [J 11] 880, 929, 1031, 1036, *1084*
Richards, M.P.M. 502, *539*
Richards, R.A., s. Brill, N.D. 333, *342*
Richards, W. [R 15] 934, *1096*
Richardson, A., s. Kelly, D. 363, 365, *376*
Richardson, A.E., Kelly, D., Mitchell-Heggs, N. 365, *377*
Richardson, A.E., s. Mitchell-Heggs, N. 363, 365, *376*
Richardson, L., s. Kolvin, I. 588, 589, *610*
Richart, R.M., s. Friedman, R.C. 465, *528*
Richmond, J., s. Hersher, L. 726, *748*
Richter, C.P. [R 16] *1096*
Richter, D. 3, 50, 52, 53, 54, *62*
Richter, D., Dawson, R.M.C. 53, *62*
Richter, D., Gaitonde, M.K., Cohn, P. 15, *62*
Richter, D., s. Ansell, G.B. 50, *55*
Richter, D., s. Balázs, R. 36, 37, 47, *55*
Richter, D., s. Clouet, D.H. 49, *56*
Richter, D., s. Cohn, P. 49, *56*
Richter, D., s. Dawson, R.M.C. 51, *57*
Richter, D., s. Gaitonde M.K. 49, *58*
Richter, D., s. Minard, F.N. 50, *61*
Richter, K. 119, *193*
Ridges, A.P. 94, 95, 96, *107*
Rieber, I., Meyer, A.-E., Schmidt, G., Schorsch, E., Sigusch, V. *539*
Riechert, T. [R 17] 882, *1096*
Riechert, T., Wolff, M. 356, *377* [R 18] 882, *1096*
Riechert, T., s. Hassler, R. 475, *529*, [H 17] 882, 884, 945, 961, *1080*

Rieder, R.P., s. Rosenthal, D. 561, *614*
Riederer, P. 67, *107*
Riederer, R., s. Birkmayer, W. 67, 68, *100*
Riegel, K.F. 641, *701*
Rieger, H., s. Kubicki, S. 157, *189*
Ries, W. 684, *701*
Rifkin, A., Kurtin, S.B., Quitkin, F., Klein, D.F. 292, *312*
Rifkin, A., Quitkin, F., Howard, A., Klein, D.F. 257, 272, *312*
Rifkin, A., Quitkin, F., Klein, D.F. 272, *312*
Rifkin, A., s. Kane, J. 246, *308*
Riggi, S.J., s. Banerjee, S.P. 88, *99*
Rigler, D., s. Curtiss, S. [C 21] 896, 897, *1073*
Rigler, M., s. Curtiss, S. [C 21] 896, 897, *1073*
Riklan, M., Levita, E. 478, *539*
Riley, G., s. Blazek, R. 71
Riley, G.J., s. Cross, A.J. 112, *112*
Riley, G.J., s. Owen, F. 91, *105*
Riley, G.J., s. Shaw, D.M. 110, *113*
Rimmer, J., Jacobsen, B. 577, *613*
Rimmer, J., s. Winokur, G. 582, 600, *617*
Rimon, R., Roos, B.E., Rakkolainen, V., Alanen, Y. 93, *107*
Rimon, R., s. Belmaker, R.H. 570, 583, *603*
Rimon, R., s. Biedermann, J. 92, *100*
Ringberger, V., s. Åsberg, M. 69, 70, 99, 325, 339, *342*
Ringel, E. 594, *613*
Rios, E., s. Schvarcz, J.R. 369, *377*
Risso, M., s. Pock, K. [P 26] 961, *1095*
Ritter, W., s. Vaughan, H.G. 151, 154, *195*
Rivano, C., s. Ferillo, F. 155, *185*

Rivier, C., s. Vale, W. 40, *64*
Rivier, J., s. Vale, W. 40, *64*
Roberts, A.H. 335, *347*
Roberts, A.J., s. Angel, C. 340, *341*
Roberts, E. 94, *107*
Roberts, E., Chase, T.N., Tower, D.B. 199, *240*
Roberts, E., Hammerschlag, R. 37, *62*
Roberts, F.J.A., s. Carter, C.O. 602, *604*
Roberts, J.A., Walker, M. 178, *193*
Roberts, J.M., s. Brown, D.G. 340, *342*
Roberts, L., s. Penfield, W. 475, 476, *537*, [P 18] 894, *1095*
Roberts, P.J. 25, *62*
Robertson, J. *750*
Robertson, J., Robertson, J. 725, 728, *750*
Robertson, J., s. Robertson, J. 725, 728, *750*
Robertson, M.H., s. Adams, H.B. 741, 742, *745*
Robin, A.A., Langley, G.E. 331, *347*
Robin, E.D., s. Burwell, C.S. [B 75] 1016, *1073*
Robins, E. 638, 639, *701*
Robins, E., s. Cochran, E. 67, 68, *101*
Robins, L.N. 639, 651, *701*
Robins, L.N., s. Woodruff, R.A. Jr. 689, *704*
Robinson, B.W. 471, 478, 482, *539*
Robinson, B.W., Alexander, M., Bowne, G. *539*
Robinson, D., s. Stacey, M. 729, *750*
Robinson, D.S., s. Nies, A. 264, *311*
Robinson, R.J. *539*
Robinson, S.E., s. Stawarz, R.J. 213, *241*
Robison, G.A., Butcher, R.W., Sutherland, E.W. 26, 30, *62*
Rocha-Miranda, C., s. Albe-Fessard, D. [A 18] 842, *1068*
Rodin, E.A., Luby, E.D., Gottlieb, J.S. [R 19] 1003, *1096*

Roeder, F. 370, *377*
Roeder, F., Mueller, D. 370, *377*
Roeder, F., Orthner, H., Mueller, D., 370, *377*
Roeder, F., s. Mueller, D. 370, *377*, 455, *536*
Roeder, K.D. [R 20] 797, 798, 819, *1096*
Roeder-Kutsch, T., Scholz-Wölfing, J. 551, *613*
Römisch, P., s. Matussek, N. 73, *105*
Rönnbäck, L., s. Hansson, H.-A. 21, *58*
Rönnberg, E., s. Aperia, B. 316, *341*
Roffwarg, H., s. Hellmann, L. 77, *103*
Roffwarg, H.P., s. Sachar, E.J. 77, 78, *107*, 325, 338, *348*
Rogawski, M.A., s. Iversen, L.L. 216, *238*
Roger, A., s. Gastaut, H. 166, 168, *186*, [G 12] 1028, 1031, 1032, 1033, *1078*
Roger, A., s. Gastaut, H.A. [G 11] 1028, 1031, 1032, *1078*
Roger, J., Lob, H., Tassinari, C.A. 168, *193*
Roger, J., s. Gastaut, H. 168, *186*, [G 12a] *1078*
Rogers, M., s. Pasamanick, B. 575, *612*
Rogers, M.R., s. Davenport, R.K. 501, *525*
Roggendorf, W., s. Matakas, F. 323, *346*
Roglev, M., s. Raschev, T. 586, *616*
Rogon, Z.E., s. Brodersen, P. 322, *342*
Rohde, P.D., s. Hirsch, S.R. 256, *307*
Rohde, W.A., s. Schildkraut, J.J. 72, *107*
Rohden, F. von 680, *701*
Rohmer, F., Wackenheim, A., Kurtz, D. 160, *193*
Rohmer, F., s. Thiébaut, F. 160, *195*
Rohracher, H. [R 21, 22, 22a] 784, 867, *1096*, *1997*
Roitbak, A.I. [R 23] 1036, *1097*

Roitbak, A.I., Bobrov, A.V. 16, *62*
Rolls, E.T., s. Wauquier, A. 483, 484, 485, *543*
Romano, J., Engel, G.L. *193*
Romano, J., s. Engel, G.L. 160, *185*
Romney, D. 566, *613*
Rompel, K., s. Prüll, G. 162, *193*
Roos, B.E., Sjöström, R. 69, *107*
Roos, B.-E., s. Andén, N.-E. 212, *234*
Roos, B.E., s. Beskow, J. 67, 68, *100*
Roos, B.E., s. Dencker, S.J. 69, *102*
Roos, B.E., s. Persson, T. 93, *106*
Roos, B.E., s. Rimon, R. 93, *107*
Roos, B.-E., s. Sjöström, R. 339, *348*
Roos, B.-E., s. Wålinder, J. 218, 225, 227, *242*
Rosadini, G., s. Corletto, F. 159, *184*
Rosadini, G., s. Ferillo, F. 155, *185*
Rosanoff, A.J., Handy, L.M., Plesset, J., Brush, R. 555, 597, 598, *613*
Rosberg, G., s. Lind, J. 413, *533*
Rose, J.T. 330, *347*
Rose, S.P.R. 10, *62*
Rosenbaum, M., s. Engel, G.L. 179, *185*
Rosenberg, L., s. Malin, J.P. 287, *310*
Rosenberg, S., s. Ast, M. 682, *692*
Rosenberg, S., s. Metzig, E. 682, *699*
Rosenblatt, F. [R 24] 855, *1097*
Rosenblatt, P.C., Cunningham, M.R. 647, 648, *701*
Rosenblatt, S., Chanley, J.D., Sobotka, H., Kaufman, M.R. 340, *347*
Rosenblith, W.A. [R 25] 853, 857, 908, *1097*
Rosenblum, L.A. 384, 489, *539*

Rosenblum, L.A., Kaufman, I.C. 489, *540*
Rosenblum, L.A., s. Kaufman, I.C. 407, 489, 497, 502, *531*
Rosenkötter, L., Wende, S. [R 26] 1017, *1097*
Rosenthal, D. 546, 547, 553, 556, 558, 559, 590, *613*, *614*, 691, *701*
Rosenthal, D., Kety, S.S. 553, 558, *614*
Rosenthal, D., Wender, P.H., Kety, S., Schulsinger, F., Welner, J., Rieder, R.P. 561, *614*
Rosenthal, D., s. Dyke, J. van 568, *605*
Rosenthal, D., s. Fieve, R.R. 546, *606*
Rosenthal, D., s. Kety, S.S. 553, 557, 559, 560, 561, 566, *609*
Rosenthal, D., s. Mirdal, G.M. 575, *611*
Rosenthal, D., s. Paikin, H. 558, *612*
Rosenthal, D., s. Wender, P.H. 559, 560, *617*
Rosenthal, R.H., s. Akiskal, H.S. 582, *602*
Rosenzweig, M.R., s. Bennett, E.L. 49, *56*
Rosewald, G., s. Dahme, B. 552, *604*
Rosewald, G., s. Huse-Kleinstoll, G. 552, *608*
Ross, H., s. Rheingold, H.L. 435, 518, *539*, 732, *750*
Ross, J.R., Braen, B.B., Chapurt, R. 722, *750*
Rossi, A.M. 734, *750*
Rossi, A.M., s. Corletto, F. 159, *184*
Rossi, G.F. [R 27] 989, *1097*
Rossi, G.F., Zanchetti, A. [R 28] 979, *1097*
Rossi, G.F., s. Batini, C. [B 10] 989, *1070*
Rossi, G.F., s. Ferillo, F. 155, *185*
Rossiter, R.J. 20, *62*
Rossum, J.M. van, s. Pijnenburg, A.J.J. 211, *240*
Rosvold, H.E., Delgado, J.M.R. [R 29] *1097*

Rosvold, H.E., Mishkin, M. [R 31] *1097*
Rosvold, H.E., Mishkin, M., Szwarebart, M.K. [R 30] *1097*
Rosvold, H.E., s. Battig, K. [B 11, 12] 831, *1070*
Rosvold, H.E., s. Hunsperger R.W. [H 95] 940, *1083*
Rotach-Fuchs, M., s. Ernst, K. 659, *695*
Roth, B., s. Kallmann, F.J. 588, *609*
Roth, G. [R 32] 760, *1097*
Roth, M. 193, 322, 338, *347*
Roth, M., Kay, D.W.K., Shaw, J., Green, J. 322, 338, *347*
Roth, M., s. Carney, M.W.P. 330, 331, *343*
Roth, M., s. Kay, D.W.K. 553, 565, *609*
Roth, M., s. Mayer-Gross, W. 622, 635, 641, 642, 649, 661, 666, 684, *699*
Roth, M., s. Stephens, D.A. 553, 558, 564, 565, *616*
Roth, R.H., s. Bunney, B.S. 211, *236*
Roth, R.H., s. Nybäck, H.V. 225, *240*
Roth, R.H., s. Walters, J.R. 215, *242*
Rothacker, E. [R 33] 771, *1097*
Rothenberg, A., s. Mahl, G.F. [M 21] 887, *1091*
Rothman, T., s. Tyler, D.B. [T 14] 1003, *1100*
Rothschild, B. 721, *750*
Rothschild, D., s. Luce, R.A. 162, *191*
Rothschild, F.S. [R 34] 791, *1097*
Rothstein, C. 253, *312*
Rotrosen, J., Angrist, B.M., Gershon, S. Sachar, E.J., Malpern, F.S. 91, *107*
Rotterdam, A. van, s. Lopes da Silva, F.H. 148, *191*
Roubicek, J., s. Volavka, J. 172, *195*
Rougeul, A. [R 35] 1032, *1097*
Rougeul-Buser, A., s. Buser, P.A. [B 76] *1073*

Rowell, T.E. 390, 427, 428, *540*
Rowell, T.E.S., Hinde, R.A. 426, 427, 428, 431, *540*
Rowell, T.E., Hinde, R., Spencer-Booth, Y. 432, *540*
Rowland, V. [R 36] 1004, *1097*
Rozitis, A., s. Bowers, M.B. Jr. 221, *235*
Rubens, A.B. 474, *540*
Rubenstein, J. 721, *750*
Rubin, D.B., s. Witkin, H.A. 677, *704*
Rubin, T., s. Swerdloff, R.S. 645, *702*
Rubinstein, M., Burks, J.B. *705*
Rubovits, R., s. Klawans, H.L. Jr. 297, 298, *309*
Ruch, T.C., s. Lennox, M.A. 163, *190*
Ruch, W., s. Bürki, H.R. 214, *236*
Rudolph, A.J., s. Desmond, M.M. 294, *305*
Rudy, V., s. Baron, M. 271, *303*
Rüdin, E. 553, 561, *614*
Rümke 565
Rüther, E., s. Beckmann, H. 94, *100*
Rüther, E., s. Loosen, P. 72, *104*
Rüther, E., s. Matussek, N. 72, 74, 85, *104, 105*
Rüther, E., s. Schilkrut, R. 83, *107*
Ruf, K.B., Kitchen, J.H., Wilkinson, H. 43, *62*
Ruff, C.F., s. Templer, D.J. 327, *348*
Ruh, D., s. Singer, L. 292, *313*
Rumack, B.H., s. Burks, J.S. 299, *304*
Rumbaugh, D.M. 512, *540*
Rumbaugh, D.M., Gill, T.V. 512, 515, *540*
Rumbaugh, D.M., Gill, T.V., Glaserfeld, B.C. von 512, *540*
Rumbaugh, D.M., Gill, T.V., Glaserfeld, E. von, Warner, H., Pisani, P. 512, *540*

Rumbaugh, D.M., s. Davenport, R.K. 501, *525*
Rush, S., s. Weaver, L. 318, 319, 324, *349*
Russell, G.F.M. 340, *347*
Rutanen, E., s. Alanen, Y.O. 566, *603*
Ruthven, C.R.J., s. Coppen, A. 72, *101*
Rutledge, L.T., s. Doty, R.W. [D 34] 884, *1075*
Rutschmann, J., Cornblatt, B., Erlenmeyer-Kimling, L. 566, *614*
Rutter, M. 588, 589, *614*, 650, *701*, 717, 723, 724, 729, 730, 731, 732, 733, 743, *750*
Rutter, M., Lockyer, L.A. 589, *614*
Rutter, M., Schopler, E. *705*
Rutter, M., s. Folstein, S. 589, *606*
Ryan, E., s. Imlah, N.W. 332, *345*
Rylander, G. 356, *377*
Rylander, G., s. Bingley, T. 364, *375*
Rysanek, K., Spankova, H., Mlejnkova, M. 291, *312*

Sabri, M.T., Bone, A.H., Davison, A.N. 50, *62*
Sachar, E.J., Finkelstein, J., Hellmann, L. 81, *107*
Sachar, E.J., Roffwarg, H.P., Gruen, P.H., Altmann, N., Sassin, J. 77, 78, *107*, 325, 338, *348*
Sachar, E.J., s. Rotrosen, J. 91, *107*
Sachs, H. 39, 41, *62*
Sackett, G.P. 407, 408, 409, *540*
Sacksteder, J., s. Strauss, J. 567, *616*
Safer, D.J., Allen, R.P. 290, *312*
Saint Paul, U. von, s. Holst, E. von [H 83, 84] 795, 883, 935, 939, 940, 941, 950, 966, *1082, 1083*
Saito, Y., s. Narabayashi, H. 372, *377*
Sakai, T., s. Mitsuda, H. 565, *611*

Sakata, H., s. Mountcastle, V.B. [M 75] 898, 929, 1037, *1093*
Salaman, D.F., s. Westley, B.R. 26, *64*
Saldanha, V.F., Havard, C.W.H., Bird, R., Gardner, R. 293, *312*
Saletu, B., Itil, T.M., Saletu, M. 175, *193*
Saletu, B., s. Itil, T.M. 173, 174, 177, *188*
Saletu, M., s. Saletu, B. 175, *193*
Salim, T., s. Simpson, G.M. 290, *313*
Saller, K., s. Merkenschlager, F. 523, *535*
Salvi, G., s. Berlucchi, G. [B 40] 995, 1011, *1071*
Salzen, E.A. 408, *540*
Samanin, R., Bernasconi, S., Garattini, S. 225, *240*
Samanin, R., s. Ladinsky, H. 219, *239*
Samaroff, A.J. 503, *540*
Sameroff, A.J. 572, *614*
Sampson, G.A., s. Bond, P.A. 72, *100*
Samuelsson, B. 18, *62*
Sandberg, S. 650, 673, *701*
Sander, 789
Sander, L. 487, *540*
Sander, L.W. 487, *540*
Sander, L.W., s. Condon, W.S. 517, *525*
Sanders, M.D., s. Weiskrantz, L. 448, *543*
Sandifer, M.G., s. Wilson, I.C. 332, *349*
Sandler, M., s. Coppen, A. 72, *101*
Sandler, M., s. Costa, E. 201, 202, 231, *237*
Sankar, S. 589, *614*
Sano, K. 369, *377*
Sano, K., Sekino, H., Mayanagi, Y. 369, *377*
Sano, L. 74, *107*
Santibanez, H.-G., s. Zernikki, B. [Z 2] 1031, *1103*
Sara, V.R., King, T.L., Stuart, M.C., Lazarus, L. 49, *62*
Sarason, I.G., Smith, R.E., Diener, E. 691, *701*

Sartorius, H., s. Spehr, W. 158, 161, *194*
Sartorius, N., s. Lader, M. 688, *698*
Sasaki, S., s. Matakas, F. 323, *346*
Sassin, J., s. Sachar, E.J. 77, 78, *107*, 325, 338, *348*
Sathananthan, G., Angrist, B. 91, *107*
Sathananthan, G., s. Angrist, B. 91, 95, *99*
Sathananthan, G., s. Shopsin, B. 72, *107*
Sato, S., Daly, R., Peters, H. 298, *312*
Sattin, A., Rall, T.W., Zanella, J. 38, *62*
Saunders, J.C., s. Loomer, H.P. 223, *239*
Savio, P.A., s. Marocchino, R. 289, *310*
Sawyer, C.H. [S 1] *1097*
Sawyer, C.H., Kawakami, M. [S 2] [S 3] 862, *1097*
Sawyer, C.H., s. Kawamura, H. [K 9] *1086*
Saxén, E.A., Peto, R. 292, *312*
Sayegh, Y., Dennis, W. 732, *750*
Scanlon, W.G., Mathias, J. 164, *193*
Scarr, S. 549, *614*
Schaar, C.J., Clemens, J.A. 220, *240*
Schachmatowa, E. 564, *614*
Schade, J.P., s. Wiener, N. [W 24a] 855, *1102*
Schaefer, C.H., s. Penin, H. 163, *192*
Schaefer, K.-P., s. Duensing, F. [D 37] 823, *1075*
Schaffer, H.R. 502, *540*, 732, *750*
Schaffer, H.R., Emerson, P.E. 719, 732, *750*
Schaller, G.B. 407, 490, *540*
Schaller, S., s. Schmidtke, A. 742, *750*
Schalling, D. 671, *701*
Schalling, D., s. Cronholm, B. 326, *343*
Schalling, D., s. Hare, R.D. 594, *608*
Schaltenbrand, G. 475, *540*

Schaltenbrand, G., Bailey, P. 357, *377*
Schanberg, S.M., Schildkraut, J.J., Breese, G.R. 72, *107*
Scharf, R., s. Halberg, F. *187*
Scharfetter, C. *312*, 573, *614*
Schatzberg, A.F., s. Schildkraut, J.J. 72, *107*
Schechter, M.D., Shurley, J.T., Toussieng, P.W., Maier, W.J. 741, *750*
Scheel-Krüger, J. 199, 230, 231, *240*, *241*
Scheel-Krüger, J., s. Randrup, A. 75, *106*
Scheid, P., s. Deecke, L. 153, *184*, [D 10] 832, 834, *1074*
Scheinfeld, A., s. Garai, J.E. 647, *696*
Scheller, M., s. Loosen, P. 72, *104*
Scheller, M., s. Matussek, N. 72, 85, *104*
Schenck, G.K., Enders, P., Engelmeier, H.-M., Ewert, T., Herdemerten, S., Köhler, K.-H., Lodemann, E., Matz, D., Pach, J. 96, *107*
Schenk, G.K. 133, *193*
Schenk, G.K., s. Matejcek, M. 133, *191*
Schenk-Danzinger, L. 638, 689, *701*
Schenkel, R. 402, *540*, [S 4] 810, *1097*
Schepank, H. 581, 592, 593, *614*
Schepank, H., s. Becker, P.E. 592, *603*
Scherrer, H., s. Hernández-Peón, R. [H 38] 824, *1081*
Scherrer, J., s. Lille, F. 159, *190*
Schiele, B.C., Schneider, R.A. 333, *348*
Schilder, P. 721, *750*, [S 5] 971, *1097*
Schildkraut, J.J. 67, 72, *107*, 339, *348*
Schildkraut, J.J., Orsulak, P.J., LaBrie, R.A., Schatzberg, A.F., Gudeman, J.E., Cole, J.O., Rohde, W.A. 72, *107*

Schildkraut, J.J., Orsulak, P.J., Schatzberg, A.F., Gudeman, J.E., Cole, J.O., Rohde, W.A., LaBrie, R.A. 72, *107*
Schildkraut, J.J., s. Greenspan, K. 72, *103*
Schildkraut, J.J., s. Schanberg, S.M. 72, *107*
Schilkrut, R., Chandra, O., Osswald, M., Rüther, E., Baarfüsser, B., Matussek, N. 83, *107*
Schiltz, K., s. Harlow, H.F. [H 3] 890, *1080*
Schjelderup-Ebbe, T. [S 6] *1097*
Schlag, J. [S 7] 1005, *1097*
Schlatter, E.K.E., Lal, S. 232, *241*
Schlegel, W.S. 626, *701*
Schleidt, W. 423, *540*
Schlesinger, B. [S 8] 901, 902, 906, *1097*
Schlesinger, H.S., Meadow, K.P. 515, *540*
Schlesser, M.A., Winokur, G., Sherman, B.M. 111, *113*
Schmalohr, E. 710, 718, *750*
Schmidlin, W., s. Pöldinger, W. 244, *312*
Schmidt, C.F., s. Kety, S.A. 6, *59*
Schmidt, G., s. Rieber, I. *539*
Schmidt, P. 257, *312*
Schmidt, R.S. 470, 476, *541*
Schmidt-Kolmer, E. 712, *750*
Schmidtke, A., Schaller, S., Altherr, P. 742, *750*
Schmitt, F.O., Dev, P., Smith, B.H. 5, *63*
Schmitt, F.O., Quarton, G.C., Melnechuk, T., Adelman, G. 460, *541*
Schmitt, F.O., Worden, F.G. 451, *541*
Schmitz, W. 590, *614*
Schmocker, M., s. Baumann, P. 71, *99*
Schneider, C. [S 9] 1018, 1019, *1097*
Schneider, E., Hubach, H. 163, *193*
Schneider, E., s. Ehret, R. [E 11] 958, 959, 960, *1076*
Schneider, G.E. *541*

Schneider, G.E., s. Murphy, M.R. 461, *536*
Schneider, H. 371, *377*, 448, 488, *541*
Schneider, H.P.G., s. McCann, S.M. 220, *239*
Schneider, J. [S 10] 982, *1097*
Schneider, J., Thomalske, G. [S 11] 982, 983, *1097*
Schneider, K. 334, *348*, 591, *614*, [S 12–15] 762, 766, 770, 771, 775, 780, 937, *1098*
Schneider, K., s. Matussek, N. 74, *105*
Schneider, R.A., s. Schiele, B.C. 333, *348*
Schneller, P., s. Busfield, B.L. 287, *304*
Schnetzler, J.P., Alleon, A.M. 289, *312*
Schön, I., s. Pohlmeier, H. 74, *106*
Schönbaum, E., s., Preston, E. 32, 33, 34, *62*
Schönberger, J., s. Kempe, P. 740, *748*
Schoenfeld, W.N. [S 15a] *1098*
Scholz-Wölfing, J., s. Roeder-Kutsch, T. 551, *613*
Schooler, N.R., s. Goldberg, S.C. 664, *696*
Schopler, E., s. Rutter, M. 705
Schorer, C.E. 263, *312*
Schorsch, E., s. Rieber, I. *539*
Schott, A. 649, 661, 662, *702*
Schott, D. 430, 470, *541*
Schott, D., s. Winter, P. 432, *544*
Schou, M. 270, 271, *312*
Schou, M., Amdisen, A. 294, *312*
Schou, M., Amdisen, A., Steenstrup, O.R. 294, *312*
Schou, M., Baastrup, P.C., Kirk, L. 272, *312*
Schou, M., Goldfield, M.D., Weinstein, M.R., Villeneuve, A. 289, 294, *312*
Schou, M., s. Baastrup, P.C. 270, *303*
Schou, M., s. Kirk, L. 272, *309*
Schou, M., s. Sørensen, R. 293, 299, *313*

Schreiber, K. *705*
Schreiner, L., Kling, A. [S 16] 961, *1098*
Schreiner, L., s. Brady, J.V. [B 57] *1072*
Schreiner, L.H., s. Lindsley, D.B. [L 29] 983, *1089*
Schrier, A.M., Harlow, H.F., Stollnitz, F. 384, 505, *541*
Schröder, H.-T., Matussek, N. 84, *105*
Schrödinger, E. [S 17] 908, *1098*
Schubert, P., Kreutzberg, G.W. 5, *63*
Schuckit, M., Goodwin, D., Winokur, G. 600, *614*
Schüttler, R., s. Huber, G. 574, *608*, 630, 685, 689, *697*
Schulman, J.L., s. Vernon, D.T.A. 729, *751*
Schulsinger, F. 568, 594, *614*
Schulsinger, F., Jacobsen, B. 568, *614*
Schulsinger, F., s. Goodwin, D.W. 599, *607*
Schulsinger, F., s. Kety, S.S. 553, 557, 559, 560, 561, 566, *609*
Schulsinger, F., s. Mednick, S.A. 546, 553, 567, 568, 575, *611*
Schulsinger, F., s. Mirdal, G.M. 575, *611*
Schulsinger, F., s. Paikin, H. 558, *612*
Schulsinger, F., s. Rosenthal, D. 561, *614*
Schulsinger, F., s. Wender, P.H. 559, 560, *617*
Schulsinger, F., s. Witkin, H.A. 677, *704*
Schulsinger, H. *614*
Schulte, W. 560, *614*
Schulte, W., Tölle, R. 641, *702*
Schulte, W., s. Finke, J. [F 8] 1015, *1077*
Schultes, H., s. Matussek, N. 84, *105*
Schultz, D.P. 744, *750*
Schultz-Hencke, H. 720, *750*
Schulz, B. 584, 589, *614*
Schulz, B., s. Wittermans, W. 586, *617*
Schulz, I.H. [S 18] 971, *1098*

Schulze, H., s. Carspers, H. [C 5] 1003, *1073*
Schuster, P., Gabriel, E., Kuefferle, B., Karobath, M. *312*
Schvarcz, J.R., Driollet, R., Rios, E., Betti, O. 369, *377*
Schwab, J.J., Schwab, M.E. 649, *702*
Schwab, J.J., s. Warheit, G.J. 649, 651, *704*
Schwab, M.E., s. Schwab, J.J. 649, *702*
Schwartz, B.A., Guilbaud, F., Fischgold, H. [S 19, 19a] 1014, *1098*
Schwartz, B.A., s. Fischgold, H. [F 12] 948, 969, 993, 999, 1009, *1077*
Schwartz, M., s. Shagass, C. 150, 175, *194*
Schwartz, M.A., s. Wyatt, R.J. 93, *109*
Schwartz, T.Z., s. Wyatt, R.J. 93, *109*
Schwartzman, A.G., s. Kennard, M.A. 172, *189*
Schwarz-Speck, M., s. Jung, E.G. 292, *308*
Schweitzer, D. 132, *193*
Schwidetzky, I. 621, 622, 626, 642, 669, 672, *702*
Scott, J.P. 622, *702*
Scott, J.P. 381, 488, 489, *540*
Scott, J.P., Fuller, J.L. 488, *540*
Scott, J.P., s. Eleftheriou, B.E. 455, *527*
Scott, J.W., s. Dawson, G.D. [D 9] 910, 911, *1074*
Scoville, W.B. 356, 357, *378*
Seager, C.P., Bird, R.L. 332, *348*
Sears, T.A. [S 20] 911, *1098*
Seay, B., Hansen, E., Harlow, H.F. 496, *541*
Sebeok, T.A. 384, 503, *541*
Sedvall, G., Alfredsson, G., Bjerkenstedt, L., Eneroth, P., Fyrö, B., Hänryd, C., Swahn, C.-G., Wiesel, F.-A., Wode-Helgodt, B. 217, 220, 225, *241*
Sedvall, G., Nybäck, G. 212, *241*
Sedvall, G., s. Nybäck, H. 212, *240*

Seeman, P., Chau Wong, M., Tedesco, J., Wong, K. 571, *614*
Seeman, P., Lee, T. 216, 217, *241*
Seeman, P., Lee, T., Chan-Wang. M., Wong, K. 216, *241*
Seeman, P., Staiman, A., Lee, T., Chang-Wang, M. 217, *241*
Seeman, P., s. Lee, T. 112, *112*
Seggie, J.A., s. Brown, G.M. 81, *100*
Seiler, N., s. Demisch, L. 96, *101*
Seitelberger, F., s. Jellinger, K. 158, *188*
Sekino, H., s. Sano, K. 369, *377*
Selbach, C., Selbach, H. [S 21] 867, *1098*
Selbach, H. [S 22] 862, *1098*
Selbach, H., s. Helmchen, H. 149, *187*
Selbach, H., s. Selbach, C. [S 21] 867, *1098*
Seltzer, C.C. 671, *702*
Selz, O. [S 22a] 789, *1098*
Sem-Jacobsen, C.W., Styri, O.B. 486, *541*
Sem-Jacobsen, C.W., Torkildsen, A. 486, *541*, [S 23] 887, 955, 958, *1098*
Sem-Jacobsen, C.W., s. Van der Tweel, L.H. 148, *195*
Semon, R. [S 24] 1024, *1098*
Serban, G., Kling, A. 446, *541*
Serment, H., s. Fenasse, R. 292, *305*
Sethy, V.H., Woert, M.H. van 219, *241*
Setschenow, I.M. [S 25] 1037, *1098*
Settler, P., s. Stawarz, R.J. 213, *241*
Shader, R., s. Meltzer, H. 94, *105*
Shader, R.I. 293, 294, *312*
Shader, R.I., Belfer, M.L., Dimascio, A. 293, *313*
Shader, R.I., Dimascio, A. 292, *312*
Shader, R.I., Giller, D.R., Dimascio, A. 293, *313*

Shafer, B., s. Gambetti, P. 50, *58*
Shagass, C. 171, 172, 174, 175, 178, *193*, *194*
Shagass, C., Ando, K. 175, *194*
Shagass, C., Schwartz, M. 175, *194*
Shagass, C., Schwartz, M., Krishnamoorti, S.R. 150, *194*
Shagass, C., Soskis, D.A., Straumanis, J.J., Overton, D.A. 175, *194*
Shagass, C., s. Soskis, D.A. 175, *194*
Shankweiler, D.P., s. Liberman, A.M. 438, 480, *533*
Shannon, C.E. [S 26–28] 852, 853, 858, 877, *1098*
Shannon, C.E., Weaver, W. [S 29] 852, 853, *1098*
Shapiro, A.K., Shapiro, E.S., Bruun, R.D., Sweet, R.D. 638, *702*
Shapiro, D., s. Fink, M. 179, *186*
Shapiro, E.S., s. Shapiro, A.K. 638, *702*
Shapiro, R., s. Hauge, M. 574, *608*
Shapiro, R.W. 581, 592, 593, *614*
Shapiro, R.W., s. Rafaelsen, O.J. 681, *701*
Shapiro, S., s. Hartz, S.C. 294, *307*
Shapiro, S., s. Heinonen, O.P. 292, *307*
Shapiro, T., s. Campbell, M. 244, *304*
Sharma, N.C., Shastri, N., Iqbal, Z., Jaffry, N.F., Talwar, G.P. 48, *63*
Sharma, N.C., Talwar, G.P. 21, *63*
Sharman, D.F., s. Ashcroft, G.W. 69, *99*, 339, *342*
Sharman, D.F., s. O'Keefe, R. 212, *240*
Sharpless, S., Jasper, H. [S 29a] *1098*
Sharrard, G.A.W. 151, *194*
Shashoua, V.E. 51, *63*
Shastri, N., s. Sharma, N.C. 48, *63*

Shaw, B.F., s. Mai, F.M. 83, *104*
Shaw, D.M., Camps, F.E., Eccleston, E.G. 68, *107*
Shaw, D.M., Johnson, A.J., Tidmarsh, S.F., MacSweeny, D.A., Hewland, H.R., Woolcock, N.E. 70, 71, *107*
Shaw, D.M., Riley, G.J., Michalakeas, A.C., Tidmarsh, S.F., Blazek, R., Johnson, A.L. 110, *113*
Shaw, D.M., s. Bourne, H.R. 68, *100*
Shaw, D.M., s. Coppen, A. 74, *101*
Shaw, J., s. Roth, M. 322, 338, *347*
Shaw, J.C. 174, *194*
Shaw, J.C., s. Cooper, R. 118, 140, *184*
Shaw, W.B., s. Kolvin, I. 596, *610*
Sheard, M.H. 271, *313*
Sheard, M.H., s. Aghajanian, G.K. 229, *234*
Sheard, M.H., s. Marini, J.L. 271, *310*
Sheffield, B.F., s. Carney, M.W.P. 256, 257, *304*, 330, *343*
Sheldon, W.H. 626, 627, 665, 666, 671, *702*, [S 30, 31] 952, 953, *1098*
Shepherd, M., Cooper, B., Brown, A.C., Kalton, G. 649, *702*
Sherman, B.M., s. Schlesser, M.A. 111, *113*
Sherrington, C.S. [S 32, 33] 762, 822, 835, 845, 909, 914, 1050, *1098*
Sherrington, C.S., s. Creed, R.S. [C 14] 822, *1073*
Sherrington, C.S., s. Leyton, A.S.F. 476, *533*
Shershen, H., s. Lajtha, A. 50, *60*
Shields, J. 549, 553, 555, 569, 575, 578, 591, 592, 593, 595, 596, 598, 599, *614*, *615*
Shields, J., Gottesman, I.I. 565, 575, *615*
Shields, J., Gottesman, I.I., Slater, E. 555, *615*

Shields, J., Heston, L.L., Gottesman, I.I. 561, 564, *615*
Shields, J., Slater, E. 581, 592, 593, *615*
Shields, J., s. Gottesman, I.I. 553, 554, 555, 556, 558, 561, 562, 563, 565, 575, *607*
Shields, J., s. Heston, L.L. 639, 683, *697*
Shields, J., s. Slater, E. 594, *615*
Shields, P.J., s. Ashcroft, G.W. 87, *99*
Shilcock, G.M., s. Walter, D.S. 72, *108*
Shima, F., s. Narabayashi, H. 372, *377*
Shimazono, Y., Horie, T., Yanagisawa, Y., Hori, N., Chikazawa, S., Shozuka, K. [S 34] 977, 1019, *1098*
Shimkunas, A.M., s. Smith, K. 334, *348*
Shimokochi, M., s. Yoshii, N. [Y 2] 1032, *1102*
Shinoda, T., s. Okada, T. 93, *105*
Shipton, H.W. 134, *194*
Shirron, C., s. Goldstein, M. 216, *238*
Shiwastava, R.K., s. Simpson, G.M. 220, *241*
Shokroverty, S., s. Daniels, J.C. 158, *184*
Shopsin, B., Freedman, L.S., Goldstein, M., Gershon, S. 93, *107*
Shopsin, B., Gershon, S. 272, *313*
Shopsin, B.S., Gershon, S., Goldstein, M., Friedman, E., Wilk, S. 227, *241*
Shopsin, B., Kline, N.S. 267, *313*
Shopsin, B., Mendlewicz, J., Suslak, L., Silbey, E., Gershon, S. 578, *615*
Shopsin, B., Wilk, S., Sathananthan, G., Gershon, S., Davis, K. 72, *107*
Shopsin, B., s. Angrist, B. 92, *99*
Shopsin, B., s. Suslak, L. 578, *616*
Shopsin, B., s. Wilk, S. 70, *108*
Shore, P.A. 223, *241*

Shostak, M., s. Glassman, A.H. 331, *344*
Shostak, M., s. Perel, J.M. *311*
Shozuka, K., s. Shimazono, Y. [S 34] 977, 1019, *1098*
Shurley, J.T., s. Schechter, M.D. 741, *750*
Sidman, R.L. 48, *63*
Siebenmorgen, E., s. Pechstein, J. 718, 731, *749*
Siegel, C., s. Laska, E.M. 292, *309*
Siegel, G.J., Eiseman, J.S. 43, *63*
Siegman, A.W., Feldstein, S. 446, *541*
Sigg, E.B. 223, *241*
Sigg, E.B., Soffer, L., Gyermek, L. 223, *241*
Siggins, G., s. Ungerstedt, U. 221, *242*
Signeland, E.R., s. Eimas, P.D. 437, 440, 441, 442, *526*
Sigusch, V., s. Rieber, I. *539*
Sila, B., Mowrer, M., Ulett, G., Johnson, M. 172, *194*
Silbey, E., s. Shopsin, B. 578, *615*
Silbey, E., s. Suslak, L. 578, *616*
Silva, L. de, Huang, C.Y. 298, *313*
Silver, H.K., Finkelstein, M. 733, *750*
Silverman, C. 649, 661, *702*
Silverman, D. 155, 157, 158, *194*
Silverstone, T. 75, *107*, *108*
Simantov, R., Goodman, R., Aposhian, D., Snyder, S.H. 40, *63*
Simantov, R., s. Snyder, S.H. 41, *63*
Simao-Bines, J., s. Morais, T.M. 256, *311*
Simon, O. 117, *194*
Simon, P., s. Frances, H. 89, *102*
Simon, P., s. Jouvent, R. 89, *103*
Simonds, P.E. 493, 496, *541*
Simons, E.L. 382, 384, *541*
Simpson, G.M., Amin, M., Kunz, E. 297, *313*

Simpson, G.M., Amin, M., Kunz-Bartholini, E., Salim, T., Watts, T.P.S. 290, *313*
Simpson, G.M., Branchey, M.H., Lee, J.H., Voitashevsky, A., Zoubok, B. *313*
Simpson, G.M., Branchey, M.H., Shiwastava, R.K. 220, *241*
Simpson, G.M., Lee, J.H., Cuculic, Z., Kellner, R. 330, 331, *348*
Simpson, G.M., Varga, E. 298, *313*
Simpson, G.M., s. Blair, J.H. 293, *304*
Simpson, G.M., s. Cooper, T.B. 274, *305*
Simpson, H., s. Buck, C. 577, *604*
Simpson, H., s. Halberg, F. *187*
Simpson, J., s. Zellweger, H. 677, *704*
Singer, K., Chang, P.T., Hsu, G.L.K. 679, *702*
Singer, L., Finance, F., Ruh, D. 292, *313*
Singer, W., s. Poeppel, E. *539*
Singh, B., s. Anand, B.K. [A 21] 1032, *1068*
Singh, M.M., Vergel de Dios, L., Kline, N.S. 290, *313*
Sinnott, J.M., Beecher, M.D., Moody, D.B., Stebbins, W.C. 443, 444, *541*
Sipowicz, R.R., s. Vernon, D.T.A. 729, *751*
Siqueland, E.R., Lipsitt, L.P. 503, *541*
Siskind, V., s. Hartz, S.C. 294, *307*
Siuchninska, H., s. Wojdyslawska, I. 287, *314*
Siwers, B. 225, *241*
Sjögren, T., s. Hallgren, B. 586, *607*
Sjölund, B., s. Ingvar, D.H. 162, *188*
Sjöqvist, F., s. Åsberg, M. 69, *99*, 246, *303*
Sjöqvist, F., s. Fuxe, K. 202, *238*
Sjöqvist, F., s. Träskman, L. 109, 110, *113*
Sjöquist, O. 356

Sjöström, R., s. Roos, B.E. 69, *107*, 339, *348*
Skinner, B.F. [S 35] 790, *1098*
Skogstad, W. 601, *615*
Skott, A., s. Wålinder, J. 218, 225, *242*
Slater, E. 555, 561, 586, 593, 595, *615*
Slater, E., Beard, A.W. 335, *348*
Slater, E., Beard, W., Glithero, E. 170, *194*
Slater, E., Cowie, V.A. 546, 553, *615*
Slater, E., Maxwell, J., Price, J.S. 583, *615*
Slater, E., Shields, J. 594, *615*
Slater, E., Slater, P. 689, *702*
Slater, E., Tsuang, M.T. 561, *615*
Slater, E., s. Hare, E.H. 572, 573, 574, *608*
Slater, E., s. Mayer-Gross, W. 622, 635, 641, 642, 649, 661, 666, 684, *699*
Slater, E., s. Shields, J. 555, 581, 592, 593, *615*
Slater, E., s. Spicer, C.C. 582, *615*
Slater, P., s. Slater, E. 689, *702*
Slater, P.C., s. Squire, L.R. 327, *348*
Sloane-Stanley, G.H., s. Folch-Pi, J. 18, 22, *58*
Slobin, D.I., s. Ferguson, C.A. 521, *527*
Slone, D., s. Hartz, S.C. 294, *307*
Small, J.G. 322, *348*
Small, J.G., Small, I.F. 171, 172, 175, 176, *194*
Small, I.F., s. Small, J.G. 171, 172, 175, 176, *194*
Smeraldi, E., Negri, F., Melica, A.M. 581, *615*
Smirnov, G.D., s. Jasper, H.H. [J 12] 1028, 1030, 1036, *1084*
Smith, A.D., s. Bartlett, S.F. 21, 22, *56*
Smith, A.D., s. De Potter, W.P. 50, *57*
Smith, A.D., s. Greenfield, S.A. 45, *58*

Smith, B.H., s. Schmitt, F.O. 5, *63*
Smith, C. 562, *615*
Smith, C., Forrest, A.D. 562, *615*
Smith, C., s. Curnow, R.N. 562, *604*
Smith, C.A., s. Suedfeld, P. 735, 742, *751*
Smith, C.B., s. Crews, F.T. 88, *101*
Smith, C.J., s. Valois, R.L. de [V 4, 5] 913, *1101*
Smith, D.B.D., Donchin, E., Cohen, L., Star, A. 151, *194*
Smith, D.B., s. Tupin, J.P. 271, *313*
Smith, D.W., s. Jones, K.L. 673, *697*
Smith, J.S., Mellick, R.S. 335, *348*
Smith, K., Surphlis, W.R.P., Gynther, M.D., Shimkunas, A.M. 334, *348*
Smith, M.A., Chethick, M.S.W., Adelson, E. 722, *750*
Smith, R.C., Davis, J.M. 221, *241*
Smith, R.C., Tamminga, C., Davis, J.M. 92, *108*
Smith, R.E., s. Sarason, I.G. 691, *701*
Smith, T.W., s. Hughes, J. 40, *58*
Smith, W.K. 356, *378*
Smitt, J.W., Wegener, C.F. 319, *348*
Smythies, J.R. 453, 454, *541*
Smythies, R.J. 94, 95, *108*
Smythies, J.R., s. Corbett, L. 95, *101*
Smythies, J., s. Osmond, H. 94, *105*
Snaith, R.P., s. Andrews, P. 253, *302*
Snaith, R.P., s. Barton, J.L. 322, *342*
Snider, R.S., Stowell, A. [S 35a] 845, *1098*
Snow, C.E. 520, *541*
Snow, H.L., s. Forrest, F.M. 289, *306*
Snowdon, C.T., s. Morse, P.A. 443, 444, *536*

Snyder, S.H. 28, 31, 32, 34, 36, 37, 40, *63*
Snyder, S.H., Burt, D.R., Creese, I. 216, 217, *241*
Snyder, S.H., Simantov, R. 41, *63*
Snyder, S.H., s. Coyle, J.T. 31, *56*
Snyder, S.H., s. Creese, I. 216, 217, *237*
Snyder, S.H., s. Iversen, L.L. 38, *59*
Snyder, S.H., s. Kuhar, M.J. 485, *532*
Snyder, S.H., s. Pert, C.B. 40, *62*
Snyder, S.H., s. Simantov, R. 40, *63*
Snyder, S., s. Usdin, E. 202, 205, 208, *242*
Snyder, S.H., s. Usdin, E. 31, *64*
Snyder, S.H., s. Young, A.B. 25, *64*
Sobotka, H., s. Rosenblatt, S. 340, *347*
Söderberg, U., s. Ingvar, D.H. [I 3] 1007, *1083*
Södersten, P., s. Ahlenius, S. *234*
Sørensen, R., Jensen, J., Mulder, J., Schou, M. 293, 299, *313*
Soffer, L., s. Sigg, E.B. 223, *241*
Sokoloff, L. 53, *63*
Sokoloff, L., s. Kennedy, C. 52, *59*
Sokoloff, L., s. Mangold, R. [M 22] 1007, *1091*
Sokolov, E.N., s. Voronin, L.G. [V 12] 1036, *1101*
Sokolov, Y. [S 36] 1030, *1098*
Sollberger, A., s. Heninger, G. 150, *187*
Solms, H. 641, 653, 662, *702*
Solomon, K., Vickers, R. 273, *313*
Solomon, P. 739, *751*
Solomon, P., Kubszansky, P., Leiderman, P.H., Mendelson, J.H., Trumbull, R., Wexler, D. [S 36a] 933, *1098*
Solomon, P., s. Meyers, F.H. 244, *310*

Somerfeld-Ziskind, E., s. Ziskind, E. 328, *349*
Sommer, H., s. Quandt, J. 324, *347*
Sommer, J. [S 37] 875, *1098*
Sommer, R. 512, *541*
Somogyi, I., s. Bizzi, E. [B 46] 1005, *1071*
Somogyi, I., s. Giaquinto, S. [G 19] 995, *1079*
Sorensen, T., s. Vestergaard, P. 69, 70, *108*
Soroker, E., s. Michael, C.M. 567, *611*
Soroker, E., s. Morris, D.P. 567, *611*
Soskis, D.A., Shagass, C. 175, *194*
Soskis, D.A., s. Shagass, C. 175, *194*
Souney, P., s. Chow, M. 299, *304*
Sourkes, T.L., s. Young, S.N. 227, 228, *242*
Soveri, P., s. Fruhstorfer, H. 152, *186*
Sovner, R., DiMascio, A. 664, *702*
Spalding, I.M.K., Zangwill, O.L. [S 38] *1099*
Spankova, H., s. Rysanek, K. 291, *312*
Spatz, H. 464, *541*
Speckenbach, W., s. Kehr, W. 229, *239*
Spehlmann, R. 148, *194*
Spehr, W., Sartorius, H., Berglund, K., Hjorth, B., Kablitz, C., Plog, U., Wiedemann, P.H., Zapf, K. 158, 161, *194*
Speidel, H., s. Dahme, B. 552, *604*
Speidel, H., s. Huse-Kleinstoll, G. 552, *608*
Spencer, H. 449, *541*
Spencer, W.A., s. Kandel, E.R. [K 2] [K 3] *1086*
Spencer-Booth, Y., s. Hinde, R.A. 407, 496, 500, *529, 530*
Spencer-Booth, Y., s. Rowell, T.E. 432, *540*
Sperber, M.A., Jarvik, L.F. 546, 601, *615*
Sperry, R.W. [S 39–41] 882, 890, 891, 892, *1099*

Sperry, R.W., Stamm, J.S., Miner, N.M. [S 42] 890, 891, *1099*
Sperry, R.W., s. Myers, R.E. [M 92] 882, 890, 892, *1094*
Spicer, C.C., Hare, E.H., Slater, E. 582, *615*
Spiegel, E.A., Wyeis, H.T. [S 43] 882, 924, *1099*
Spiegel, E.A., Wycis, H.T., Marks, M., Lee, A.J. 356, *378*
Spiegel, E.A., s. Wyeis, H.T. [W 34a] *1102*
Spiegel, H.E., s. Dengler, H.J. 223, *237*
Spiel, W. 588, 590, *615*
Spillmann, L. [S 43a] 923, 924, 925, *1099*
Spillman, L., s. Jung, R. [J 61a] 922, *1086*
Spitz, R.A. 416, 496, *541*, 715, 716, 720, 723, 728, *750*
Spitz, R.A., Wolf, K.M. 410, 415, *541*
Spohn, M., Davison, A.N. 11, *63*
Spoor, A., s. Davis, H. 151, 152, *184*
Spotoft, H., s. Bolwig, T.G. 323, 340, *342*
Spreng, M., s. Keidel, W.D. 151, *189*
Spuhler, J.N., s. Loehlin, J.C. 664, *699*
Spunda, C. 162, *194*
Squire, L.R., Chase, P.M. 327, 328, *348*
Squire, L.R., Miller, P.L. 326, *348*
Squire, L.R., Slater, P.C. 327, *348*
Squire, L.R., Slater, P.C., Chase, P.M. 327, *348*
Squires, R.F., Braestrup, C. 231, *241*
Squires, R.F., s. Christiansen, J. 216, *237*
Šramka, M., s. Návornik, P. 370, 371, 372, *377*
Sroufe, L.A., Waters, E. 411, *541*
Stabenau, J.R. 589, *615*
Stabenau, J.R., Pollin, W. 685, 691, *702*
Stabenau, J.R., s. Pollin, W. 555, 556, 570, 575, *613*

Stacey, M., Dearden, R., Pill, R., Robinson, D. 729, *750*
Stacey, R.S., s. Pare, C.M.B. 68, *106*
Stadler, H., Lloyd, K.G., Gadea-Ciria, M., Bartholini, G. 30, *63*, 219, *241*
Stadler, H., s. Bartholini, G. 199, 212, 213, 216, 219, 231, *235*
Stafford, R.E., s. Brown, A.M. 691, *693*
Stahl, M., s. Meltzer, H.Y. 219, 220, 221, 223, *239*
Staiman, A., s. Seeman, P. 217, *241*
Stallone, F., s. Mendlewicz, J. 583, *611*
Stamm, J.S., s. Sperry, R.W. [S 42] 890, 891, *1099*
Standage, K.F., s. Fleminger, J.J. 682, *695*
Stanfield, C.N., s. Sullivan, J. 681, *702*
Stanton, J.B., s. Ashcroft, G.W. 69, *99*, 339, *342*
Star, A., s. Smith, D.B.D. 151, *194*
Stark, L.H., Norton, J.C. 175, *194*
Startsev, V.G. 446, *541*
Stassen, H.H., s. Angst, J. 580, *603*
Staub, H., s. Thölen, H. 97, *108*
Stawarz, R.J., Hill, H., Robinson, S.E., Settler, P., Dingell, J.V., Sulser, F. 213, *241*
Stawarz, R.J., s. Vetulani, J. 88, *108*
Stay, F.J. van der, s. Mönks, F.J. 635, 641, *699*
Stebbins, W.C. 505, *541*
Stebbins, W.C., s. Sinnott, J.M. 443, 444, *541*
Steele, C.A., s. Gallant, D.M. 94, *102*
Steenstrup, O.R., s. Schou, M. 294, *312*
Steffa, M., s. Kennel, J.H. 726, *748*
Steffa, M., s. Klaus, M.H. 726, *748*
Stein, L. 232, *241*, [S 44] *1099*

Stein, L., Wise, C.D. 30, 63, 93, *108*
Stein, L., s. Wise, C.D. 74, 93, *109*
Stein, Z., s. Adelstein, A.M. 661, 663, *692*
Stein, Z.A., Susser, M. 732, *750, 751*
Steinbrecher, W. *702*
Steinbuch, K. [S 45–47] 853, 855, 863, 864, 867, 868, 871, 876, 1026, 1044, *1099*
Steinbuch, K., Frank, H. [S 48] 853, 857, 865, 872, 975, 976, *1099*
Steinbuch, K., Kazmierczak, H. [S 49] 853, *1099*
Steinemann, P. 400
Steiner, H., s. Harder, A. 289, *307*
Steiner, J.E. 413, 424, *541*
Steinert, E. 714, *751*
Steinert, H., s. Katschnig, H. 651, *697*
Steinert, R., s. Lancaster, N. 337, *346*
Steinhausen, H.-C., Wefers, D. 673, *702*
Steiniger, F. [S 50] 810, *1099*
Steinmann, H.W. [S 50a] *1099*
Steklis, H.D., Harnad, S.R. 513, *542*
Steklis, H.D., s. Harnad, S.R. 503, 508, *529*
Stellar, E. [S 51] *1099*
Stellar, E., s. Flexner, J.B. [F 14] 1046, *1077*
Stellar, E., s. Morgan, C.T. [M 55] 858, *1092*
Stemmler, G., s. Kempe, P. 739, *748*
Stenberg, P., s. Wadstein, J. 232, *242*
Stengel, E. 660, *702*
Stenstedt, A. 581, *616*
Stephens, D.A., Atkinson, M.W., Kay, D.W.K., Roth, M., Garside, R.F. 553, 558, 564, 565, *616*
Stephens, D.A., s. Kay, D.W.K. 553, 565, *609*
Stephens, P.M., s. Henry, J.P. 619, *696*
Stepien, L., s. Konorski, J. 474, 475, *532*

Sterling, M., s. Good, W.W. 253, *306*
Sterman, M.B., s. Clemente, C.D. [C 8] 989, *1073*
Stern, D.N. 502, 508, 519, *542*
Stern, F., s. Marks, N. 39, *60*
Stern, M., s. Baron, M. 566, *603*
Stern, S., s. Isac, M. 288, *308*
Sternberg, M. 132, *194*
Sternberg, P. 132, *194*
Sterritt, G.M., Camp, B.W., Lipman, B.S. 722, *751*
Stevens, B. 577, *616*
Stevens, B.C., s. Hirsch, S.R. 256, *307*
Stevens, H.A., s. Balthazar, E.E. 672, *692*
Stevens, J., Wilson, K., Foote, W. 94, *108*
Stevens, J.R. 167, *194*
Stevens, J.R., Mark, V.H., Ervin, F., Pacheco, P., Suematsu, K. 486, *542*
Stevens, N., s. Armstrong, B. 292, *303*
Stevens, S.S. [S 52] 782, 908, 936, *1099*
Stewart, J. 744, *751*
Stewart, M., Morrison, J. 596, *616*
Stewen, A., s. Alanen, Y.O. 566, *603*
Stille, G. von, Lauener, H. 212, *241*
Stinnett, J.L., s. Mendels, J. 74, *105*
Stirling, G.S., s. Marshall, E. 223, *239*
Stock, G., s. Andén, N.-E. 213, 220, *234*
Stocking, M., s. Witkin, H.A. 677, *704*
Stoddard, F.J., Post, R.M., Gillin, J.C., Buchsbaum, M.S., Carman, J.S., Bunney, W.E. 72, *108*
Stoff, D.M., s. Wyatt, R.J. 75, *109*
Stoffyn, P., s. Folch-Pi, J. 19, 22, *57*
Stokoe, W.C. 513, 515, *542*
Stolberg, H., s. Goldstein, L. 172, 173, *187*

Stollnitz, F., s. Schrier, A.M. 384, 505, *541*
Stolz, L.M. 727, *751*
Storm van Leeuwen, W. 151, *194*
Storm van Leeuwen, W., Lopes da Silva, F.A., Kamp, A. 147, *195*
Storm van Leeuwen, W., s. Brazier, M.A.B. 121, *183*
Storm van Leeuwen, W., s. Gastaut, H.A. [G 11] 1028, 1031, 1032, *1078*
Storm van Leeuwen, W., s. Lopes da Silva, F.H. 134, *191*
Storm van Leeuwen, W., s. Van der Tweel, L.H. 148, *195*
Stowell, A., s. Snider, R.S. [S 35a] 845, *1098*
Strachan, M., s. Berlyne, N. 323, 326, *342*
Strandman, E. 687, *702*
Strandman, E., s. Bonetti, U. 686, *693*
Strandman, E., s. Perris, H. 687, *701*
Strata, P., s. Berlucchi, G. [B 40] 995, 1011, *1071*
Stratton, G.M. [S 53] 787, *1099*
Straumanis, J.J., s. Shagass, C. 175, *194*
Straus, E. [S 54] *1099*
Strauss, A., s. Hippius, H. 97, *103*
Strauss, H. [S 55] 950, *1099*
Strauss, J., Klorman, R., Kokes, R., Sacksteder, J. 567, *616*
Strauss, J., s. Klorman, R. 567, *609*
Strauss, J., s. Kokes, R. 567, *610*
Strauss, M.A., s. Beckmann, H. 75, *100*
Strian, F., Micheler, E., Benkert, O. 92, *108*
Stricker, E., s. Thölen, H. 97, *108*
Strobl, R., s. Katschnig, H. 649, *697*
Strömberg, U., Svensson, T.H., Waldeck, B. 230, *241*

Strömberg, U., s. Svensson, T. 230, *242*
Strömbom, U. 75, 90, *108*, 215, *241*
Strömbom, U., s. Anden, N.-E. 75, *99*, 201, *235*
Strömbom, U., s. Carlsson, A. 232, *236*
Strömgren, E. 545, 546, 584, 587, 590, 591, 594, 598, *616*, 649, *702*
Strömgren, E., s. Welner, J. *617*
Strömgren, L.S. 316, 318, 319, 326, 331, 333, 337, *348*
Strömgren, L.S., Juul-Jensen, P. 164, *195*, 319, *348*
Ström-Olsen, R., Carlisle, S. 366, 367, *378*
Strotzka, H., s. Birkmayer, W. [B 44a] *1071*
Strotzka, H., s. Katschnig, H. 660, *697*
Strughold, H., s. Kornmüller, A.E. [K 45] 969, 977, 983, *1088*
Struhsaker, T.T. 426, 427, 432, *542*
Strunk, P. 638, *702*
Struve, F.A., Becka, D.R., Klein, D.F. 172, *195*
Stuart, M.C., s. Sara, V.R. 49, *62*
Studdert-Kennedy, M. 438, *542*
Studdert-Kennedy, M., s. Liberman, A.M. 438, *533*
Stumpf, C. [S 56] 777, *1099*
Stumpf, C., s. Petsche, H. [P 20] 918, *1095*
Stumpfe, K.D. 710, *751*
Stumpfl, F. 597, *616*
Styri, O.B., s. Sem-Jacobsen, C.W. 486, *541*
Subczynski, J., s. Konorski, J. 474, 475, *532*
Suedfeld, P. 735, 737, 740, 741, 744, *751*
Suedfeld, P., Buchanan, E. 735, 742, *751*
Suedfeld, P., Ikard, F. 735, 737, 741, *751*
Suedfeld, P., Smith, C.A. 735, 742, *751*
Suedfeld, P., Vernon, J. 735, 741, *751*

Suematsu, K., s. Stevens, J.R. 486, *542*
Sümer, E., s. Cebiroglu, R. 590, *604*
Sugerman, A.A., Goldstein, L., Murphree, H.B., Pfeiffer, C.C., Jenney, E.H. 173, *195*
Sugerman, A.A., s. Burdick, J.A. 136, 137, 173, 174, *183*
Sugerman, A., s. Carroll, B.J. *101*
Sugerman, A.A., s. Goldstein, L.A. 172, 173, *187*
Suhl, M., s. Wilk, S. 70, *108*
Sullivan, J., Stanfield, C.N., Dackis, C. 681, *702*
Sullivan, J.L. III, s. Fann, W.E. 298, *305*
Sulman, F.G., s. Ben-David, M. 292, *303*
Sulser, F., Vetulani, J., Mobley, P.L. 88, *108*
Sulser, F., s. Stawarz, R.J. 213, *241*
Sulser, F., s. Vetulani, J. 88, *108*
Sumi, T., s. Katsuki, Y. [K 8] 908, *1086*
Sunier, A., s. Verhoeven, W.M.A. 97, *108*
Suomi, S.J., Collins, M.L., Harlow, H.F. 496, *542*
Suomi, S.J., Delizio, R., Harlow, H.F. 500, *542*
Suomi, S.J., Harlow, H.F. 498, 500, *542*
Suomi, S.J., Harlow, H.F., Domek, C.J. 498, *542*
Suomi, S.J., Harlow, H.F., McKinney, W.T. 725, *751*
Suomi, S.J., Harlow, H.F., Novak, M.A. 500, *542*
Suomi, S.J., s. Harlow, H.F. 500, *529*
Suomi, S.J., s. McKinney, W.T. 500, *535*
Surphlis, W.R.P., s. Smith, K. 334, *348*
Suslak, L., Shopsin, B., Silbey, E., Mendlewicz, J., Gershon, S. 578, *616*
Suslak, L., s. Shopsin, B. 578, *615*
Susser, M., s. Stein, Z.A. 732, *750*, *751*

Susser, M.W., s. Adelstein, A.M. 661, 663, *692*
Sutherland, E.M., Oliver, J.E., Knight, D.R. 337, *348*
Sutherland, E.W., s. Robison, G.A. 26, 30, *62*
Sutton, D., Larson, C., Lindeman, R.C. 474, 475, *542*
Suzuki, K. 18, 19, *63*
Šváb, L., Gross, J., Lángová, J. 740, *751*
Šváb, L., s. Gross, J. 742, *747*
Svaetichin, G. [S 57, 58, 59] 787, 913, *1099*
Svaetichin, G., Laufer, M., Mitarai, G., Fatchchand, R., Villegas, J. [S 60] 787, *1099*
Svaetichin, G., MacNichol, E.F. [S 61] 787, *1100*
Svaetichin, G., Negishi, K., Fatchchand, R. [S 62] 787, 913, *1100*
Svensson, T. 230, *241*, *242*
Svensson, T., Strömberg, U. 230, *242*
Svensson, T., s. Ahlenius, S. *234*
Svensson, T.H. 88, *108*
Svensson, T.H., s. Anden, N.-E. 75, *99*, 201, *235*
Svensson, T.H., s. Carlsson, A. 232, *236*
Svensson, T.H., s. Modigh, K. 202, *240*
Svensson, T.H., s. Strömberg, U. 230, *242*
Swahn, C.-G., s. Sedvall, G. 217, 220, 225, *241*
Swani, M.S., s. Coppen, A. 270, *305*
Swanton, C.H., s. Bailey, H.R. 357, *375*
Swartz, J.D., s. Holtzman, W.H. 363, *376*
Swartz, R.D., s. Port, F.K. 97, *106*
Sweeney, D.R., Maas, J.W., Heninger, G.R. *108*
Sweeney, J., s. Burch, N.R. 134, *183*
Sweeny, D., Nelson, C., Bowers, M., Maas, J., Heninger, G. 72, 73, *108*

Sweeny, D.R., s. Pickar, D. 72, *106*
Sweet, R.D., s. Shapiro, A.K. 638, *702*
Sweet, W.H., Obrador, S., Martin-Rodriguez, J.G. 455, *542*
Sweet, W.H., s. Mark, V.H. 372, *376*
Swerdloff, R.S., Rubin, T. 645, *702*
Swett, J.W., s. Pompeiano, O. [P 29] [P 30] 989, *1095*
Switalski, R.W., s. Prien, R.F. 253, *312*
Symmes, D., s. Newman, J.D. 433, 481, *536*
Syndulko, K. 598, *616*
Syrdal-Lasky, A., s. Lasky, R.E. 440, *533*
Szabó, J., s. Grastyán, E. [G 39] 1031, *1079*
Szabó, Z. 619, *702*
Szentágothai, J. [S 63, 64] 860, 902, 913, 1037, 1039, *1100*
Szentágothai, J., Arbib, M.A. 447, *542*
Szentágothai, J., Flerkó, B., Mess, B., Halász, B. [S 65] 860, 861, 939, *1100*
Szentágothai, J., s. Eccles, J.C. [E 6] 814, 843, 891, 897, 1039, *1075*
Szwarebart, M.K., s. Rosvold, E.H. [R 30] *1097*

Tachiki, K., s. Aprison, M.H. 110, *112*
Taft, L., Goldfarb, W. 575, *616*
Tagliamonte, A., s. Gessa, R. 298, *306*
Tagliasco, V., s. Dichgans, J. [D 29] 826, *1075*
Taguchi, K., s. Watanabe, S. 272, *314*
Tait, A.C., s. Marshall, E. 223, *239*
Takahashi, R., s. Aprison, M.H. 110, *112*
Takahaski, T., s. Otsuka, M. 200, *240*
Takala, K., s. Alanen, Y.O. 566, *603*

Talairach, J., David, M., Tournoux, P., Corredor, H., Kvasina, T. 357, *378*
Talairach, J., Hecaen, H., David, M., Monnier, M., Ajuriaguerra, J. de 356, *378*
Talbot, W.H., s. Lynch, J.C. [L 44] 825, 898, *1090*
Tallaferro, A., s. Mosowitch, A. [M 67] 940, *1093*
Tallman, E., s. Dubois, E.L. 292, *305*
Tallstedt, L., s. Berggren, U. 228, *235*
Talmage-Riggs, G., Winter, P., Ploog, D., Mayer, W. 432, *542*
Talwar, G.P., s. Sharma, N.C. 21, 48, *63*
Tamir, H., Klein, A., Rapport, M.M. 26, *63*
Tamminen, T., s. Niskanen, P. 71, *105*
Tamminga, C., s. Pandey, G.N. 91, 92, *105*
Tamminga, C., s. Smith, R.C. 92, *108*
Tandler, J. 622, *702*
Tanghe, A., Vereecken, J.L.T.M. 256, *313*
Tangri, K.K., Misra, N., Bhargava, K.P. 25, *63*
Tanji, J., s. Evarts, E.V. [E 27] 833, 844, *1076*
Tanna, V.L., Winokur, G., Elston, R.C., Go, R.C.P. 582, *616*
Tanna, V.L., s. Winokur, G. 581, *617*
Tanner, J.M. 622, 642, 644, 645, 668, *703*
Taschev, T. 649, 661, *703*
Taschev, T., Roglev, M. 586, *616*
Tassel, J. van, s. McBride, W.J. 13, *60*
Tassinari, C.A., s. Gastaut, H. 126, 166, 168, *186*
Tassinari, C.A., s. Lugaresi, E. 168, *191*
Tassinari, C.A., s. Roger, J. 168, *193*
Tatetsu, S. 601, *616*
Taube, C.A., s. Kramer, M. 649, 651, *698*
Taunch, T., s. Kolvin, I. 596, *610*

Tavris, C., Offir, C. 647, *703*
Taylor, D.C., s. Ounsted, C. 643, *700*
Taylor, M., Abrams, R. 580, 581, *616*
Tecce, J.J. 153, *195*
Tedesco, J., s. Seeman, P. 571, *614*
Tegeler, J., s. Floru, L. 295, *306*
Teilhard de Chardin, P. [T 1] 777, *1100*
Teleki, G. 381, *542*
Tellenbach, H. 335, *348*, 684, 687, *703*
Tellenbach, R. 684, 685, 687, *703*
Templer, D.J., Ruff, C.F., Armstrong, G. 327, *348*
Tepas, D.J., s. Armington, J.C. 147, *182*
Teradaira, R., s. Fujita, K. 93, *102*
Terenius, J., s. Gunne, L.M. 96, *103*
Terenius, L., Wahlström, A., Lindström, L., Widerlöv, E. 96, *108*, 112
Terenius, L., s. Elde, R. 26, 40, *57*
Terenius, L., s. Lindström, L.H. 112, *112*
Terenius, L., s. Ree, J.M. van 97, *106*
Terman, L.M., Miles, C.C. 647, *703*
Terzian, H., Dalle Ore, G. [T 1a] 944, 1049, *1100*
Tetreault, L., s. Elie, R. 289, *305*
Teuber, H.L. 451, *542*, [T 2, 2a] 878, 913, *1100*
Teuber, H.-L., Corkin, S.H., Twitchell, T.E. 359, 362, *378*
Teychenne, P.F., s. Claveria, L.E. 298, *304*
Thach, W.T. [T 3] 840, 845, 905, 965, *1100*
Thalheimer, C., s. Hess, H.H. 18, *58*
Théanu, G., s. Braithwaite, R.A. 246, *304*
Theile, U. 601, *616*, 650, *703*
Theobald, W., s. Angst, J. 262, *302*

Therman, P.O., s. Mangold, R. [M 22] 1007, *1091*
Thesleff, S., s. Holmberg, G. 317, *345*
Thiébaut, F., Rohmer, F., Wackenheim, A. 160, *195*
Thieffry, S., s. Lille, F. 159, *190*
Thiele, R. [T 3a, 4] 902, *1100*
Thölen, H., Stricker, E., Feer, H., Massini, M.-A., Staub, H. 97, *108*
Thoenen, H., s. Oesch, F. 31, *61*
Thomae, H. 622, 635, *703*
Thomä, H. 639, 651, *703*
Thomalske, G., s. Schneider, J. [S 11] 982, 983, *1097*
Thomas, A., Chess, S. 684, *703*
Thomas, D.L.L. 329, *348*
Thomas, P.J., s. Westley, B.R. 26, *64*
Thomas, V.L., s. Kirkpatrick, J.B. 14, *59*
Thompson, H., s. Angrist, B. 92, *99*
Thompson, J. 414, *542*
Thompson, L., s. Delse, F. 153, *184*
Thompson, P.D., s. Kanarek, K.S. 299, *308*
Thompson, R.F., Patterson, M.M. 147, 153, *195*
Thompson, W.R. 635, 690, *703*, 719, *751*
Thoren, P., s. Åsberg, M. 69, 70, *99*, 325, 339, *342*
Thorén, P., s. Bertilsson, L. 225, *235*
Thoren, P., s. Träskman, L. 109, 110, *113*
Thorn, N.A., s. Kamberi, I.A. 199, 200, *238*
Thorndike, E.L. [T 5] 790, 1024, *1100*
Thornton, W.E., Pray, B.J. 272, *313*
Thorpe, J.G., s. Baker, A.A. 333, *342*
Thorpe, J.S., s. Holtzman, W.H. 363, *376*
Thorpe, W.H. 425, *542*, [T 6, 7] *1100*
Thorsen, K., s. Gerlach, J. 271, 298, *306*
Thudichum, J.W.L. 63

Tidmarsch, S., s. Blazek, R. 71
Tidmarsh, S.F., s. Shaw, D.M. 70, 71, *107*, 110, *113*
Tienari, P. 555, 557, *616*, 685, *703*
Tillner, I., s. Bierich, J.R. 673, 674, 675, *693*
Timiras, P.E. 644, *703*
Timiras, P.S., s. Eberhardt, N.L. 26, *57*
Timsit, M., s. Gastaut, H. [G 12a] *1078*
Timsit-Berthier, M. 175, *195*
Tinbergen, N. 383, 384, 407, 410, 423, 459, 461, 466, *542* [T 8] 760, 799, 800, 802, *1100*
Tinklenberg, J.R., s. Wyatt, R.J. 75, *109*
Tipton, A.C., s. Kooi, K.A. 151, *189*
Titus, E.O., s. Dengler, H.J. 223, *237*
Todd, G.A., Palmer, B. 521, *542*
Todrick, A., s. Marshall, E. 223, *239*
Tölle, R. 287, 288, *313*, 639, 642, *703*
Tölle, R., s. Bojanovsky, J. 287, 288, 289, *304*
Tölle, R., s. Schulte, W. 641, *702*
Tönnies, F., s. Jung, R. 126, *189*
Tönnies, J.F. [T 9, 10] 858, 859, 887, 983, 1025, 1026, 1038, *1100*
Tönnies, J.F., Jung, R. [T 11] 858, *1100*
Tönnies, J.F., s. Jung, R. [J 62] 862, 887, *1086*
Toews, A.D., Horrocks, L.A., King, J.S. 11, 14, *63*
Toivakka, E., s. Laitinen, L. 363, *376*
Tokizane, T., s. Adey, W.R. 453, *523*
Tolis, G., s. Lal, S. 85, *104*
Tolman, C.W., s. Jensen, G.D. 500, *531*
Toman, J.E.P., s. Everett, G.M. 66, *102*
Tomkin, S.S. 418, 423, *542*
Tomkin, S.S., Izard, C.E. 423, *542*

Tomkin, S.S., McCarter, R. 423, *542*
Tomlinson, B.E., s. Perry, E.K. 67, *106*
Tonge, W.L., s. Gay, M.J. 730, *747*
Tondo, L., s. Kukopulos, A. 330, *346*
Tooth, G.C., Newton, M.P. 355, *378*
Tordoff, A.F.C., s. Evans, J.P.M. 88, *102*, 325, 339, *344*
Torkildsen, A., s. Sem-Jacobsen, C.W. 486, *541* [S 23] 887, 955, 958, *1098*
Toro, G., s. Kolodny, R.C. 683, *698*
Torrey, E.F. 575, *616*
Toth, J., s. Lajtha, A. 49, *60*
Tournoux, P., s. Talairach, J. 357, *378*
Toussieng, P.W., s. Schechter, M.D. 741, *750*
Toutellotte, W.W., s. Lee, T. 112, *112*
Towbin, A. 551, *616*
Tower, D.B. 446, *542*
Tower, D.B., s. Roberts, E. 199, *240*
Trabucchi, M., Cheney, D.L., Racagni, G., Costa, E. 219, *242*
Trabucchi, M., s. Costa, E. 97, *101*
Trabucci, M., s. Guidotti, A. 8, *58*
Träskman, L., Asberg, M., Bertilsson, L., Cronholm, B., Mellström, B., Neckers, L.M., Sjöqvist, F., Thoren, P., Tybring, G. 109, 110, *113*
Träskman, L., s. Åsberg, M. 325, 339, *342*
Tregear, G.W., Niall, H.D., Potts, J.T., Leeman, S.E., Chang, M.M. 39, *63*
Tregear, G.W., s. Powell, D. 200, *240*
Trendelenburg, W. [T 11a] 829, *1100*
Troeger, U., s. Matussek, P. 661, *699*
Trojan, F. 436, *542*
Trostorff, S. von 563, *616*

Troy, B., s. Plum, F. 322, 347
Trumbull, R., s. Solomon, P. [S 36a] 933, 1098
Tschermak, A. [T 12] 908, 1100
Tsuang, M. 561, 616
Tsuang, M., Fowler, R.C., Cadoret, R.J., Monelly, E. 564, 616
Tsuang, M.T., s. Fowler, R.C. 558, 606
Tsuang, M.T., s. Slater, E. 561, 615
Tuck, D., s. Åsberg, M. 69, 99, 246, 303
Tucker, G.J., s. Davies, R.K. 318, 343
Tucker, W.B., Lessa, W.A. 624, 665, 703
Tudor, J.F., s. Gove, W.R. 651, 696
Tuma, A.H., s. May, P.R.A. 333, 346
Tuominen, L., s. Heinonen, O.P. 292, 307
Tuovinen, M., s. Alanen, Y.O. 566, 603
Tupin, J.P., Smith, D.B., Clanon, T.L., Kim, L.I., Nugent, A., Groupe, A. 271, 313
Turelka, C., s. Ferillo, F. 155, 185
Turner, R.K., s. Douglas, J.W.B. 733, 747
Turner, W.J., s. Phillips, J.E. 566, 612
Turton, E., s. Maggs, R. 176, 191
Turunen, M.I., s. Heinonen, O.P. 292, 307
Twitchell, T.E., s. Teuber, H.-L. 359, 362, 378
Twomey, S.L., Raeburn, S., Baxter, C.F. 20, 63
Tybring, G., s. Träskman, L. 109, 110, 113
Tyler, D.B. [T 13] 1003, 1100
Tyler, D.B., Goodman, J., Rothman, T. [T 14] 1003, 1100

Uchimura, Y., Narabayashi, H. 356, 378
Uchiyama, H., s. Katsuki, Y. [K 8] 908, 1086

Uchtenhagen, A. 661, 703
Udo, M., s. Ito, M. [I 4] 1083
Ueda, T., Maeno, H., Greengard, P. 30, 63
Uexküll, J. von 447, 542, 703 [U 1] 774, 802, 809, 848, 1100
Uexküll, J. von, Kriszat, G. 447, 543
Uhlíř, F., Kancucká, V., Lukačiková, E. 253, 313
Uhthoff, W. [U 2] 934, 1100
Uihlein, A. s. Bickford, R.G. [B 43] 886, 1071
Ujvary, Z. 396, 543
Ulett, G., Das, K., Hornung, F., Davis, D., Johnson, M. 195
Ulett, G.A., Johnson, M.W. 179, 195
Ulett, G.A., Loeffel, R.G. 134, 195
Ulett, G., s. Dow, R.S. 163, 185
Ulett, G., s. Sila, B. 172, 194
Ulleland, C.N., s. Jones, K.L. 673, 697
Umbach, W. [U 3] 1048, 1101
Umbach, W., s. Hassler, R. 475, 529
Undeutsch, U. 673, 703
Ungerstedt, U. 200, 212, 242
Ungerstedt, U., Ljungberg, T., Hoffer, B., Siggins, G. 221, 242
Ungerstedt, U., s. Andén, N.-E. 211, 212, 235
Urban, H. [U 4] 934, 1101
Uryu, K., Moriya, A. 172, 195
Usdin, E. 112, 113
Usdin, E., Efron, D.H. 244, 255, 259, 265, 279, 282, 296, 313
Usdin, E., Snyder, S. 31, 64, 202, 205, 208, 242

Vaernet, K., Madsen, A. 367, 378
Vale, W., Brazeau, W., Rivier, C., Brown, M., Boss, B., Rivier, J., Burgus, R., Ling, N., Guillemin, R. 40, 64
Valeana, T., s. Eberhardt, N.L. 26, 57

Valenstein, E.S. 354, 378, 484, 486, 543
Valenstein, E.S., Nauta, W.J.H. 462, 543
Valentine, M., Keddie, K.M.G., Dunne, D. 318, 348
Vallane, E., s. Wasz-Hoekkert, O. 413, 434, 435, 543
Valles, J.V., s. Ananth, J.V. 291, 302
Valois, R.L. de [V 1] 913, 1101
Valois, R.L. de, Jacobs, G.H., Jones, A.E. [V 2] 913, 1101
Valois, R.L. de, Jones, A.E. [V 3] 913, 1101
Valois, R.L. de, Smith, C.J., Kitai, S.T. [V 4, 5] 913, 1101
Vandenberg, S.G. 547, 616
Vandenberg, S.G., s. Brown, A.M. 691, 693
Vandenheuvel, W.J.A., s. Angrist, B. 95, 99
Van der Tweel, L.H. 147, 148, 195
Van der Tweel, L.H., Sem-Jacobsen, C.W., Kamp, A., Storm van Leeuwen, W., Veringa, F.T.H. 148, 195
Van de Wiele, R.L., s. Friedman, R.C. 465, 528
Van Harreveld, A., Crowell, J., Malhotra, S.K. 16, 64
Van Poznak, A., s. Posner, J.B. 322, 347
Vane, J.R., s. Flower, R.J. 38, 57
Vanzulli, A., s. Bogacz, J. [B 50] 824, 1071
Varga, E., s. Angst, J. 641, 692
Varga, E., s. Kline, N.S. 271, 309
Varga, E., s. Simpson, G.M. 298, 313
Varma, R., s. Allen, W.S. 23, 55
Varma, R.S., s. Allen, W.S. 23, 55
Varon, S. 10, 64
Vartanian, M.A., Gindilis, V.M. 570, 617

Vartanian, M.E., Kolyaskina, G.I., Lozovsky, D.V., Burbaeva, G.S., Ignatov, S.A. 681, *703*
Vatsuro 807
Vaughan, H.G., Costa, L.D., Ritter, W. 154, *195*
Vaughan, H.G., Ritter, W. 151, *195*
Vaz-Ferreira, A. s. Creutzfeldt, O. [C 17] *1073*
Veale, J.L., s. Gilligan, B.S. 298, *306*
Veech, R.L., Hawkins, R.A. 8, *64*
Velde, E. van de, s. Waes, A. van 294, *314*
Vellen, C.W.M. van, s. Lopes da Silva, F.H. 134, *191*
Vendsborg, P.B., Bach-Mortensen, N., Rafaelsen, O.J. 290, *313*
Vendsborg, P.B., Bech, P., Rafaelsen, O.J. 272, 290, *313*
Vendsborg, P.B., Rafaelsen, O.J. 293, *313*
Vendsborg, P.B., s. Bech, P. 686, *693*
Venezian, E.C., Casirola, G., Marini, G., Ippoliti, G., Invernizzi, R. 292, *313*
Verbruegge, L.M. 651, *703*
Vereby, G., s. Grastyan, E. [G 39] 1031, *1079*
Vereby, G., s. Lisák, K. [L 30] 1031, *1089*
Vereecken, J.L.T.M., s. Tanghe, A. 256, *313*
Vergel de Dios, L., s. Singh, M.M. 290, *313*
Verghese, A. 666, *703*
Vergne, P.M. de la, s. Mueller, P.S. 290, *311*
Verhoeven, W.M.A., Praag, H.M. van, Botter, P.A., Sunier, A., Ree, J.M. van Wied, D. de 97, *108*
Verhoeven, W.H., s. Wied, D. de 97, *108*
Veringa, F.T.H., s. Van der Tweel, L.H. 148, *195*
Vernon, D.T.A., Foley, J.M., Sipowicz, R.R., Schulman, J.L. 729, *751*
Vernon, J., s. Suedfeld, P. 735, 741, *751*

Vernon, J.T., s. Wilson, I.C. 332, *349*
Verschuer, O. von 691, *703*
Verworn, M. [V 6] 776, *1101*
Verzeano, M., Negishi, K. [V 7, 8] 1004, 1005, *1101*
Vessey, M.P. 649, *703*
Vestergaard, P., Sorensen, T., Hoppe, E., Rafaelsen, O.J., Yates, C.M., Nicolaou, N. 69, 70, *108*
Vetter, K., Böker, W. [V 9] 1002, *1101*
Vetulani, J., Stawarz, R.J., Dingell, J.V., Sulser, F. 88, *108*
Vetulani, J., s. Sulser, F. 88, *108*
Vickers, R., s. Solomon, K. 273, *313*
Victor, M. s. Adams, R.D. [A 1] 1046, 1047, *1068*
Videbech, T. 684, *703*
Videbech, T., s. Hauge, M. 574, *608*
Videbech, T., s. Juel-Nielsen, N. 594, *609*
Videbech, T., s. Weeke, A. 649, 661, *704*
Viets, H.R. 353, *378*
Vigersky, R.A. 639, *703*
Vigorito, J., s. Eimas, P.D. 437, 440, 441, 442, *526*
Vigourox, R., s. Gastaut, H. 166, *186*
Vigouroux, R.A., s. Meldrum, B.S. 324, *346*
Vilkki, J. 363, 369, *378*
Vilkki, J., s. Kukka, E.-K. 359, *376*
Vilkki, J., s. Laitinen, L. 361, 363, 368, *376*
Villa, J.L., s. Müller, C. 638, 641, 642, *700*
Villegas, J., s. Svaetichin, G. [S 60] 787, *1099*
Villeneuve, A., s. Schou, M. 289, 294, *312*
Villeneuve, R., s. Jus, A. 297, *308*
Vine, J., s. Cranach, M. von 402, *525*
Viukari, M., Linnoila, M. 298, *313*
Vliegenthart, W., s. Lopes da Silva, F.H. 134, *191*
Vogel, F. 119, *195*, 600, *617*

Vogel, F., Götze, W. 119, *195*
Vogel, F., s. Fuhrmann, W. 602, *607*, 632, *696*
Vogel, W., s. Klaiber, E.L. 663, *698*
Vogel, W.H., S. Berrettini 570, *603*
Vogl, G. 685, *703*
Vogt, C., Vogt, O. [V 10] 880, 883, 902, *1101*
Vogt, H.J., s. Doerr, P. 672, 683, *694*
Vogt, M. 33, *64*, 338, *348*
Vogt, M., s. Feldberg, W. 17, *57*
Vogt, M., s. O'Keefe, R. 212, *240*
Vogt, O. [V 11] *1101*
Vogt, O., s. Vogt, C. [V 10] 880, 883, 902, *1101*
Vohra, J., Burrows, G.D. 287, 288, *313*
Voitashevsky, A., s. Simpson, G.M. *313*
Vojtěchovský, B., s. Marhold, J. 274, *310*
Volavka, J., Davis, L.G., Ehrlich, Y.H. 112, *113*
Volavka, J., Feldstein, S., Abrams, R., Dornbush, R., Fink, M. 322, *349*
Volavka, J., Mallya, A., Baig, S., Perez-Cruet, J. 96, *108*
Volavka, J., Matousek, M., Roubicek, J. 172, *195*
Voronin, L.G., Sokolov, E.N. [V 12] 1036, *1101*
Vulpe, M. 292, *314*
Vuorenkoski, V., s. Lind, J. 413, *533*
Vuorenkoski, V., s. Wasz-Hoeckert, O. 413, 434, 435, *543*

Wachholder, K. [W 1] 822, 835, *1101*
Wackenheim, A., s. Rohmer, F. 160, *193*
Wackenheim, A., s. Thiébaut, F. 160, *195*
Wadd Technical Report [W 2] 855, *1101*
Wade, G.N., s. Feder, H.H. 465, *527*
Wadstein, J., Öhlin, H., Stenberg, P. 232, *242*

Waelsch, H. 3, *64*
Waelsch, H., s. Lajtha, A. 49, *60*
Waes, A. van, Velde, E. van de 294, *314*
Wagemaker, H., Cade, R. 97, *108*
Wagner, E. Jr., s. Marini, J.L. 271, *310*
Wagner, J.M. 710, *751*
Wagner, K.-D., s. Eggers, H. 632, *695*
Wagner, R. [W 3, 4] 853, 858, *1101*
Wahlström, A., s. Terenius, L. 96, *108*, *112*
Wahlström, A., s. Lindström, L.H. 112, *112*
Wakefield, G.S., s. Halliday, A.M. 152, *187*
Wakeling, P.L.G., s. Heath, E.S. 333, *345*
Walcher, W. 583, *617*
Waldeck, B. 207, *242*
Waldeck, B., s. Carlsson, A. 232, *236*
Waldeck, B., s. Strömberg, U. 230, *241*
Waldmann, K.-D., Greger, J., Kluge, H., Gröschel, W., Zahlten, W., Hartmann, W. 272, 298, *314*
Walford, R.L. 634, *703*
Wålinder, J. 680, *703*
Wålinder, J., Carlsson, A. 218, *242*
Wålinder, J., Skott, A., Carlsson, A., Roos, B.-E. 225, *242*
Wålinder, J., Skott, A., Nagy, A., Carlsson, A., Roos, B.E. 218, 227, *242*
Wålinder, J., s. Balldin, J. 84, 89, *99*
Walker, J.E., s. Burks, J.S. 299, *304*
Walker, M., s. Roberts, J.A. 178, *193*
Walker, P., s. Peet, M. 71, *106*
Walker, R.J., s. McCarthy, P.S. 40, *60*
Walker, R.W., s. Angrist, B. 95, *99*
Wall, P.D., s. McCulloch, W.S. [M 34] 853, 857, *1091*

Wallace, P.W., Westmoreland, B.F. 161, *195*
Wallach, G., s. McEwen, B.S. 26, *60*
Waller, R.H., s. Grant, B.R. 246, *306*
Wallin, L., s. Balldin, J. 84, 89, *99*
Walter, D.O. 134, 146, *195*
Walter, D.O., s. Adey, W.R. 131, *182*
Walter, D.S., Shilcock, G.M. 72, *108*
Walter, D.S., s. Ashcroft, G.W. 87, *99*
Walter, H. 634, 643, 649, *704*
Walter, P.L. *195*
Walter, P.L., s. Wineburgh, M. *196*
Walter, S., s. Arfel, G. 159, *182*
Walter, W.G. 147, 178, *196*, [W 5–10] 777, 789, 832, 833, 834, 848, 853, 863, 864, 865, 882, 999, 1002, 1004, 1030, 1033, 1034, 1035, 1044, 1054, *1101*
Walter, W.G., Cooper, R., Aldridge, V.J., McCallum, W.C., Winter, A.L. 152, *196* [W 11] 1033, *1101*
Walter, W.G., s. Baldock, G.R. 134, *182*
Walter, W.G., s. Brazier, M.A.B. 121, *183*
Walter, W.G., s. MacMahon, J.F. 171, *191*
Walter, W.G., s. McCallum, W.C. 175, *191*
Walters, J.R., Roth, R.H. 215, 227, *242*
Walters, J.R., s. Bunney, B.S. 211, *236*
Walters, J.R., s. Nybäck, H.V. 225, *240*
Walters, R.H., s. Bandura, A. 644, 645, *692*
Wanderling, J., s. Laska, E.M. 292, *309*
Wang, C., s. Guidotti, A. 8, *58*
Wanklin, J.M., s. Buck, C. 577, *604*
Warburg, O. 9, *64*
Ward, A.A. 126, *196*
Ward, A.A. Jr. 356, *378*

Wardi, A.H., s. Allen, W.S. 23, *55*
Warheit, G.J., Holzer, C.E., Schwab, J.J. 649, 651, *704*
Warner, H. 292, *314*
Warner, H., s. Rumbaugh, D.M. 512, *540*
Warrington, E.K., s. Weiskrantz, L. 448, *543*
Washburn, R.W. 410, 414, *543*
Wasilewski, B., s. Matussek, N. 84, *105*
Wassermann, O., s. Lüllmann, H. 295, *310*
Wasterlain, C.G., Plum, F. 336, *349*
Wasz-Hoeckert, O., Lind, J., Vuorenkoski, V., Partanan, T., Vallane, E. 413, 434, 435, *543*
Wasz-Hoeckert, O., s. Lind, J. 413, *533*
Watanabe, S., Ishino, H., Otsuki, S. 271, *314*
Watanabe, S., Taguchi, K., Nakashima, Y., Ebara, T., Iguchi, K., Otsuki, S. 272, *314*
Watanabe, T., s. Katsuki, Y. [K 8] 908, *1086*
Waters, E., s. Sroufe, L.A. 411, *541*
Waters, R.S., Wilson, W.A. 443, 444, *543*
Watkins, J.C., s. Curtis, D.R. 25, *56*
Watson, C.S., Marcus, E.M. 167, *196*
Watson, J.B. [W 12] 790, *1101*
Watson, J.B., Rayner, R. [W 13] 1043, *1101*
Watson, J.S. 503, *543*
Watson, J.S., Ramey, C.T. 503, *543*
Watson, S.J., Akil, H. 112, *113*
Watson, S.J., Berger, P.A., Akil, H., Mills, M.J., Barchas, J.D. 96, *108*
Watt, D.G.D., s. Melvill Jones, G. [M 37a, 37b] 830, *1091*
Watts, J., s. Freeman, W. 354

Watts, T.P.S., s. Simpson, G.M. 290, *313*
Wauquier, A., Rolls, E.T. 483, 484, 485, *543*
Weaver, L., Ravaris, C., Rush, S., Paananen, R. 318, *349*
Weaver, L., Williams, R., Rush, S. 319, 324, *349*
Weaver, L.A. Jr., Ives, J.O., Williams, R., Nies, A. 318, *349*
Weaver, L.A., s. Ravaris, C.L. 253, *312*
Weaver, W., s. Shannon, C.E. [S 29] 852, 853, *1098*
Weber, E.H. [W 14] 908, *1102*
Weber, W.C., Jung, R. [W 15] 766, 960, 970, 971, 972, 985, *1102*
Wechsler, H., s. Greenblatt, M. 329, *345*
Weeke, A., Bille, M., Videbech, T., Dupont, A., Juel-Nielsen, N. 649, 661, *704*
Wefers, D., s. Steinhausen, H.-C. 673, *702*
Wegener, C.F., s. Smitt, J.W. 319, *348*
Wegener, I., s. Heinrich, K. 297, *307*
Weidel, W. [W 16] 868, 870, *1102*
Weigl, E., Kreindler, A. [W 17] *1102*
Weil-Malherbe, H. 580, *617*
Weinmann, H., Creutzfeldt, O., Heyde, G. 150, *196*
Weinschenk, C. 596, *617*, 689, *704*
Weinsilboum, R.M., s. Dunner, D.L. 93, *102*
Weinstein, M.R., Goldfield, M.D. 271, *314*
Weinstein, M.R., s. Schou, M. 289, 294, *312*
Weis, P., s. Angst, J. 641, 642, *692*
Weisberg, P. 518, *543*
Weiser, G., s. Allahyari, H. 164, *182*
Weiskrantz, L., Warrington, E.K., Sanders, M.D., Marshall, J. 448, *543*
Weiskrantz, L., s. Humphrey, N.R. 448, *530*

Weiskrantz, L., s. Pribram, K.H. [P 36] 1042, *1096*
Weiss, P., Hiscoe, H.B. 50, *64*
Weiss, R., s. Murphy, D.L. 570, *612*
Weissman, M.M., s. Kidd, K.K. 664, *698*
Weitsch, D., s. Pechstein, J. 718, 731, *749*
Weitzman, E.D., s. Hellmann, L. 77, *103*
Weizäcker, V. von [W 18] 777, 824, 901, *1102*
Welch, K., s. Penfield, W. 474, *537*
Wellington, B.S., Livett, B.G., Jeffrey, P.L., Austin, L. 20, *64*
Wells, C.E., s. Pro, J.D. 164, *193*
Wells, D.A. 333, 334, *349*
Welner, J., Strömgren, E. *617*
Welner, J., s. Rosenthal, D. 561, *614*
Welner, J., s. Wender, P.H. 559, 560, *617*
Welsch, C.W., s. Meites, J. 220, *239*
Wende, S., s. Rosenkötter, L. [R 26] 1017, *1097*
Wender, P.H., Rosenthal, D., Kety, S.S. 560, *617*
Wender, P.H., Rosenthal, D., Kety, S.S., Schulsinger, F., Welner, J. 559, 560, *617*
Wender, P.H., s. Kety, S.S. 553, 557, 559, 560, 561, 566, *609*
Wender, P.H., s. Mirdal, G.M. 575, *611*
Wender, P., s. Paikin, H. 558, *612*
Wender, P.H., s. Rosenthal, D. 561, *614*
Wendkos, M.H. 287, *314*
Wendlandt, S., s. Milton, A.S. 38, *61*
Wenner, W.H., s. Jacobson, A. [J 3a] 1017, *1083*
Werdenius, B., s. Dencker, S.J. 69, *102*
Werdinius, B., s. Andén, N.-E. 212, *234*
Werdinius, B., s. Meek, J. 225, *239*

Wernecke, K.-D., s. Bäumler, H. 140, *182*
Werner, G. [W 19] *1102*
Wernicke, C. 475, 478, *543*, [W 20] 884, 905, *1102*
Werre, J., s. Gastaut, H.A. [G 11] 1028, 1031, 1032, *1078*
Wertheimer 789
Westergaard, E., s. Bolwig, T.G. 324, *342*
Westley, B.R., Thomas, P.J., Salaman, D.F., Knight, A., Barley, J. 26, *64*
Westmoreland, B.F., s. Wallace, P.W. 161, *195*
Weston, J. 727, *751*
Wetterberg, L., s. Aperia, B. 316, *341*
Wever, R., s. Aschoff, J. [A 30] *1069*
Wever, R.A. 621, *704*
Wexler, D., s. Solomon, P. [S 36a] 933, *1098*
Weyerer, S., s. Dilling, H. 651, 652, 660, 661, *694*
Weyl, N., s. Osborne, R.T. *705*
Whaley, R.D., s. Burwell, C.S. [B 75] 1016, *1073*
Wheeler, L.R. 672, 679, *704*
Whitby, L.G., s. Axelrod, J. 223, *235*
Whitby, L.G., s. Hertting, G. 223, *238*
White, B.L. 732, *751*
White, J.L., Labarba, R.C. 723, *751*
White, L.E., s. Foltz, E.L. 359, *375*
White, L.E., s. Hinde, R.A. 489, *530*
White, N.F. 380, *543*
White, R.B., s. Humphrey, J.H. 628, 681, *697*
Whitehead, S.A., s. Linton, E.A. 38, *60*
Whitelaw, J.P., s. Ananth, J.V. 291, *302*
Whitlock, D.G., Arduini, A., Moruzzi, G. [W 21] 1005, *1102*
Whitlock, F.A., s. Abrahams, M.J. 730, *745*
Whitman 801
Whittaker, V.P., Dowdall, M.J. 13, 28, *64*

Whittaker, V.P., Michaelson, I.A., Kirkland, R.J.A. 13, 14, *64*
Whitten, C.F., Pettit, M.G., Fischhoff, J. 733, *751*
Whybrow, P., s. Goetzl, U. 581, 583, *607*
Whybrow, P.C., s. Coppen, A. 69, *101*
Wickler, W. 387, 390, 391, 392, 395, 396, 397, *543*
Wickler, W., s. Eibl-Eibesfeldt, I. 395, *526*
Widdowson, E.M. 733, *751*
Widepalm, K., s. D'Elia, G. 318, 341, *343, 344*
Widerlöv, E., s. Lindström, L.H. 112, *112*
Widerlöv, E., s. Terenius, L. 96, *108*, 112
Wied, D. de, Ree, J.M. van, Verhoeven, W.H., Praag, H.M. 97, *108*
Wied, D. de, s. Verhoeven, W.M.A. 97, *108*
Wiedemann, H.-R., Grosse, F.-R., Dibbern, H. 627, 673, 674, *704*
Wiedemann, P.H., s. Spehr, W. 158, 161, *194*
Wiener, N. [W 22–24] 852, 853, 856, 859, 875, *1102*
Wiener, N., Schade, J.P. [W 24a] 855, *1102*
Wiesel, F.-A., s. Sedvall, G. 217, 220, 225, *241*
Wiesel, T.N., Hubel, D.H. [W 24b] 921, *1102*
Wiesel, T.N., s. Hubel, D.H., [H 88, 88a] 880, 902, 918, 920, 921, 926, *1083*
Wieser, S. [W 25] 950, *1102*
Wieser, S., Domanowsky, K. [W 26] 950, *1102*
Wigger, M., s. Eggers, H. 632, *695*
Wikler, A., Fraser, H.F., Isbell, H., Pescor, F.T. 164, *196*
Wikler, A., Pescor, F.T., Fraser, H.F., Isbell, H. 164, *196*
Wilbert, D.E., s. Heiser, J.F. 299, *307*
Wilcox, B., Clayton, F. 417, *543*

Wild, C., s. Mednick, S.A. 566, *611*
Wildlocher, D., s. Jouvent, R. 89, *103*
Wiles, D., s. Beumont, P.J.V. 292, 293, *303, 304*
Wiles, D.H., s. Beumont, P.J.V. 293, *303*
Wiles, D.H., s. Kolakowska, T. 292, *309*
Wilk, S., Shopsin, B., Gershon, S., Suhl, M. 70, *108*
Wilk, S., s. Angrist, B. 91, *99*
Wilk, S., s. Shopsin, B. 72, *107*
Wilk, S., s. Shopsin, B.S. 227, *241*
Wilkinson, H., s. Ruf, K.B. 43, *62*
Willerman, L. *705*
Willerman, L., s. Plomin, R. 549, *612*
Willi, J. 560, *617*
Williams, C. 722, *751*
Williams, D., s. Gibbs, F.A. 160, *187*
Williams, H.L., s. Kety, S.S. *189*
Williams, H.L., s. Morris, G.O. [M 61] 1003, *1092*
Williams, J.G., s. Dudley, W.H.C. Jr. 335, *344*
Williams, M., s. Dornbusch, R. 318, 327, *344*
Williams, R., s. Weaver, L. 319, 324, *349*
Williams, R., s. Weaver, L.A. Jr. 318, *349*
Williamson, D.H., s. Page, M.A. 52, *61*
Willis, S.E., s. Colony, H.S. 171, 172, *184*
Willott, T., s. Erwin, T. 496, *527*
Wilson, C.J., s. Groves, P.M. 215, *238*
Wilson, E.O. 383, 470, *543*
Wilson, I.C., Vernon, J.T., Guin, T., Sandifer, M.G. 332, *349*
Wilson, I.C., s. Fann, W.E. 297, *305*
Wilson, I.C., s. Gambill, J.M. 333, *344*
Wilson, J.C., Reece, J.C. 556, *617*

Wilson, J.D. 642, 643, *704*
Wilson, J.E., s. Dunn, A. 341, *344*
Wilson, J.J. 744, *751*
Wilson, K., s. Stevens, J. 94, *108*
Wilson, N.J., s. Wilson, W.P. 176, *196*
Wilson, R.G., Hamilton, J.R., Boyd, W.D., Forrest, A.P.M., Cole, E.N., Boyns, A.R. Griffiths, K. 292, *314*
Wilson, R.S., s. Matheny, A.P. 549, *610*
Wilson, W.A., s. Waters, R.S. 443, 444, *543*
Wilson, W.P. *196*
Wilson, W.P., Wilson, N.J. 176, *196*
Wilson, W.P., s. Hein, P.L. 172, *187*
Wilson, W.P., s. Nadel, A.M. 160, *192*
Winblad, B., s. Beskow, J. 67, 68, *100*
Wineburgh, M., Walter, P.L. *196*
Wing, J.K., s. Hirsch, S.R. 256, *307*
Wing, J.K., s. Orley, J. 662, *700*
Winick, L., s. Kline, N.S. 296, *309*
Winkle, E., s. Friedhoff, A.J. 95, *102*
Winkler, H. 32, *64*
Winokur, G. 578, *617*, 661, *704*
Winokur, G., Cadoret, R.J., Dorzab, J., Baker, M. 580, 582, 600, *617*
Winokur, G., Crowe, R.R. 639, *704*
Winokur, G., Morrison, J., Clancy, J., Crowe, R. 553, 564, *617*
Winokur, G., Reich, T., Rimmer, J., Pitts, F.N. 600, *617*
Winokur, G., Rimmer, J., Reich, T. 582, 600, *617*
Winokur, G., Tanna, V.L. 581, *617*
Winokur, G., s. Avery, D. 330, *342*

Winokur, G., s. Goodwin, D.W. 599, *607*
Winokur, G., s. Helzer, J.E. 580, *608*
Winokur, G., s. McCabe, M. 564, *611*
Winokur, G., s. Pitts, F.N. 730, *749*
Winokur, G., s. Reich, T. 550, *613*
Winokur, G., s. Schlesser, M.A. 111, *113*
Winokur, G., s. Schuckit, M. 600, *614*
Winokur, G., s. Tanna, V.L. 582, *616*
Winokur, G., s. Woodruff, R.A. Jr. 689, *704*
Winsberg, B.G., Goldstein, S., Yepes, L.E., Perel, J.M. 287, *314*
Winter, A.L., s. Walter, W.G. 152, *196*, [W 11] 1033, *1101*
Winter, E. 680, *704*
Winter, P. 430, 432, *543*
Winter, P., Funkenstein, H.H. 481, *544*
Winter, P., Handley, P., Ploog, D., Schott, D. 432, *544*
Winter, P., Ploog, D., Latta, J. 426, 429, 490, *544*
Winter, P., s. Bowden, D. 432, *524*
Winter, P., s. Ploog, D. 394, 395, 406, 431, 432, 490, 493, *538*
Winter, P., s. Talmage-Riggs, G. 432, *542*
Winterstein, H. [W 27, 28] 900, 987, 991, *1102*
Wirz-Justice, A. 74, *108*
Wirz-Justice, A., Pühringer, W., Hole, G., Menzi, R. 71, *108*
Wise, C.D., Belluzzi, J.D., Stein, L. 74, 93, *109*
Wise, C.D., Stein, L. 93, *109*
Wise, C.D., s. Stein, L. 30, *63*, 93, *108*
Wissfeld, E., s. Rey, W. van [R 13] 1015, *1096*
Wistedt, B., s. Arfwidsson, L. 332, *342*

Witkin, H.A., Mednick, S.A., Schulsiner, F., Bakkestrøm, E., Christiansen, K.O., Goodenough, D.R., Hirschhorn, K., Lundsteen, C., Owen, D.R., Philip, J., Rubin, D.B., Stocking, M. 677, *704*
Witkowski, L., s. Raehlmann, E. [R 3] 996, *1096*
Witkowski, R., Prokop, O. 602, *617*
Wittenborn, J.R. 94, *109*
Wittenborn, J.R., s. Kline, N.S. 94, 97, *104*
Wittermans, W., Schulz, B. 586, *617*
Wodak, J., s. Gilligan, B.S. 298, *306*
Wode-Helgodt, B., s. Sedvall, G. 217, 220, 225, *241*
Wöhlisch, E. [W 29] 1007, *1102*
Woerner, M.G., s. Pollack, M. 575, *613*
Woert, M.H. van, s. Sethy, V.H. 219, *241*
Woggon, B. 246, 256, *314*
Woggon, B., Angst, J. 256, 257, *314*
Woggon, B., Hucker, H., Angst, J. 257, *314*
Woggon, B., s. Angst, J. 257, *302*
Woggon, B., s. Hucker, H. 257, *308*
Woggon, B., s. Matussek, N. *105*
Wojdyslawska, I., Siuchninska, H., Goraj, A. 287, *314*
Wolf, K., s. Durfee, H. 715, *747*
Wolf, K.M., s. Spitz, R.A. 410, 415, *541*
Wolf, M., s. Zerssen, D. von 687, *704*
Wolf, P. 168, 169, *196*
Wolf, R., s. Hofmann, G. 298, *307*
Wolfe, H., s. Kennel, J.H. 726, *748*
Wolff, H.-G. [W 30] 903, 1027, *1102*
Wolff, M., s. Riechert, T. 356, *377*, [R 18] 882, *1096*

Wolff, P.H. 410, 411, 413, 434, 435, 496, 503, *544*, 664, *704*
Wolfgram, F. 22, *64*
Wolkind, S. 731, *751*
Wollberg, Z., Newman, J.D. 481, *544*
Wollberg, Z., s. Newman, J.D. 481, *537*
Wolpert, A., Farr, D. 287, *314*
Wolpert, E.A., s. Rechtschaffen, A. [R 7] 999, 1009, 1016, *1096*
Wolstenholme, G.E.W., O'Connor, M. [W 31] 988, *1102*
Wong, J., s. Dempsey, G.M. 290, *305*
Wong, K., s. Seeman, P. 216, *241*, 571, *614*
Wonka, R.A., s. Dubois, E.L. 292, *305*
Wood, J.G., Dawson, R.M.C. 23, 24, *64*
Woodbury, D.M. [W 31a] *1102*
Woodbury, J.W. 22, *64*
Woodruff, G.N., s. McCarthy, P.S. 40, *60*
Woodruff, G.N., see Pijnenburg, A.J.J. 211, *240*
Woodruff, M.W., s. Kiley, J.E. 161, *189*
Woodruff, R.A. Jr., Pitts, F.N. Jr., McClure, J.N. Jr. 317, *349*
Woodruff, R.A. Jr., Robins, L.N., Winokur, G., Reich, T. 689, *704*
Woodruff, R.A., s. Guze, S.B. 582, *607*
Woods, H.F., Graham, C.W., Green, A.R., Youdin, M.B.H., Grahame-Smith, D.G., Hughes, J.T. 7, *64*
Woolcock, N.E., s. Shaw, D.M. 70, 71, *107*
Woolsey, C.N. [W 32] 882, *1102*
Woolsey, C.N., s. Akert, K. [A 15] 944, *1068*
Woolsey, C.N., s. Harlow, H.F. [H 2] 824, *1080*
Worden, F.G., Galambos, R. 433, 479, *544*

Worden, F.G., s. Schmitt, F.O. 451, *541*
Worrall, E.P., Moody, J.P., Naylor, G.J. 271, *314*
Worrall, E.P., s. Peet, M. 71, *106*
Wren, J.C., Kline, N.S., Cooper, T.B. et al. 271, *314*
Wren, J.C., s. Kline, N.S. 271, *309*
Wright, C., s. Murphy, D.L. 681, *700*
Wright, E.W., s. Libet, B. [L 21] 886, *1089*
Wulff, M.H. 164, *196*
Wundt, W. [W 33, 34] 776, 778, 782, 783, 786, 787, 789, 914, 937, 965, 971, 974, 976, *1102*
Wurtman, R.J. 71, *109*
Wurtman, R.J., Cohen, E.L., Fernstrom, J.D. 71, *109*
Wurtman, R.J., Larin, F., Mostafapour, S., Fernstrom, J.D. 71, *109*
Wurtman, R.J., s. Fernstrom, J. 71, *102*
Wuttke, W., s. Meites, J. 220, *239*
Wyatt, R.J., Gillin, J.C., Stoff, D.M., Majo, E.A., Tinklenberg, J.R. 75, *109*
Wyatt, R.J., Murphy, D.L., Belmaker, R., Cohen, S., Donnelly, C.H., Pollin, W. 570, *617*
Wyatt, R.J., Schwartz, T.Z., Schwartz, M.A., Erdelyi, E., Barchas, J. 93, *109*
Wyatt, R.J., s. Belmaker, R. 557, *603*
Wyatt, R.J., s. Balmaker, R.H. 570, 583, *603*
Wyatt, R.J., s. Bigelow, L.B. 94, *100*
Wyatt, R.J., s. Dunner, D.L. 93, *102*
Wyatt, R.J., s. Murphy, D.L. 681, *700*
Wyatt, R.J., s. Potkin, S.G. 96, *106*
Wyatt, R.T., s. Murphy, D.L. *105*
Wycis, H.T., s. Spiegel, E.A. 356, *378*
Wyeis, H.T., Lee, A.J., Spiegel, E.A. [W 34a] *1102*

Wyeis, H.T., s. Spiegel, E.A. [S 43] 882, 924, *1099*
Wyman, R.J., s. Davies, R.K. 318, *343*
Wyrwicka, W. [W 35] 1032, *1102*
Wyss, F., s. Angst, J. 641, *692*

Yablonsky, L., s. Haskell, M.R. 651, *696*
Yakovlev, P.L., Lecours, A.-R. 48, *64*
Yale, C., s. May, P.R.A. 333, *346*
Yalow, R. Berson, S. 39, *64*
Yamaguchi, T., s. Endo, M. 81, *102*
Yamaguchi, Y., s. Yoshii, N. [Y 2] 1032, *1102*
Yamsaki, H., s. Yoshii, N. [Y 2] 1032, *1102*
Yanagisawa, Y., s. Shimazono, Y. [S 34] 977, 1019, *1098*
Yarrow, L.J. 719, 720, 732, *752*
Yates, C.M., s. Ashcroft, G.W. 70, *99*
Yates, C.M., s. Vestergaard, P. 69, 70, *108*
Yepes, L.E., s. Winsberg, B.G. 287, *314*
Yerkes, A., s. Yerkes, R.M. 406, *544*
Yerkes, R.M. [Y 1] 1026, *1102*
Yerkes, R.M., Yerkes, A. 406, *544*
Yeung, D.P.H., s. Pare, C.M.B. 68, *106*
Yin, T.C.T., s. Lynch, J.C. [L 44] 825, 898, *1090*
York, M.W., s. Cooper, G.D. 742, *747*
Yoshida, M., s. Ito, M. [I 4] *1083*
Yoshida, M., s. Narabayashi, H. 372, *377*
Yoshie, N., s. Davis, H. 151, *184*
Yoshii, N., Matsumoto, J., Ogura, H., Shimokochi, M., Yamaguchi, Y., Yamasaki, H. [Y 2] 1032, *1102*
Yoshimasu, S. 597, *617*

Youdin, M.B.H., s. Woods, H.F. 7, *64*
Young 907, 913, 914
Young, A.B., Snyder, S.H. 25, *64*
Young, J.Z. 448, 453, *544*
Young, L.D., s. McKinney, W.T. 500, *535*
Young, S.J., s. Groves, P.M. 215, *238*
Young, S.N., Sourkes, T.L. 227, 228, *242*

Zahlten, W., s. Waldmann, K.-D. 272, 298, *314*
Zahn, T.P. 568, *617*
Zanchetti, A., s. Batini, C. [B 10] 989, *1070*
Zanchetti, A., s. Rossi, G.F. [R 28] 979, *1097*
Zander, K.J., Ackenheil, M., Zimmer, G. 92, *109*
Zanella, J., s. Sattin, A. 38, *62*
Zangwill, O.L., s. Spalding, I.M.K. [S 38] *1099*
Zapf, K., s. Spehr, W. 158, 161, *194*
Zapletálek, M., Preiningerová, O., Bilý, J. 256, *314*
Zattoni, J., s. Corletto, F. 159, *184*
Zaug, P.J., s. Martin, G.I. 287, *310*
Zbrozyna, A.W., s. Hilton, S.M. 458, *529*
Zeh, W. 124, *196*
Zeh, W., s. Penin, H. 160, *192*
Zeigarnik, B. [Z 1] 832, *1103*
Zeller, E.A., Blanksma, L.A., Burkard, W.P., Pacha, W.L., Lazanas, J.C. 223, *242*
Zellweger, H., Simpson, J. 677, *704*
Zenker, K., s. Penin, H. 124, 127, *192*
Zerbin-Rüdin, E. 54, 547, 548, 551, 553, 577, 578, 579, 595, 596, 599, 602, *617*, *618*
Zerlin, S., s. Davis, H. 151, 152, *184*
Zernicki, B., Santibanez, H.-G. [Z 2] 1031, *1103*

Zerssen, D. von 280, *314*, 576, *618*, 619, 620, 622, 623, 624, 625, 626, 627, 628, 636, 648, 665, 666, 667, 668, 669, 670, 671, 672, 676, 680, 684, 686, 687, 688, *704*
Zerssen, D. von, Fliege, K., Wolf, M. 687, *704*
Zerssen, D. von, Koeller, D.M., Rey, E.-R. 680, *704*, *705*
Zerssen, D. von, Meyer, A.-E., Ahrens, D. 675, 677, *705*
Zerssen, D. von, s. Emrich, H.M. 96, *102*, 112, *112*
Zerssen, G.D. von, s. Hippius, H. 97, *103*
Zerssen, D. von, Koeller, D.-M. 548, *618*
Zerssen, D. von, s. Meyer, A.-E. 678, *699*
Zerssen, D. von, s. Nowakowski, H. 677, *700*
Zetterström, R. 46, *64*

Ziegler, D.K., Presthus, J. 160, *196*
Zielske, F., s. Hammerstein, J. 678, *696*
Zigmond, R.E., s. Pfaff, D.W. 466, 467, 468, *538*
Zillig, G. [Z 3] 892, *1103*
Zimanová, J., s. Marhold, J. 274, *310*
Zimmer, G., s. Zander, K.J. 92, *109*
Zimmer, R., s. Beckmann, H. 94, *100*
Zimmerman, E.A., s. Frantz, A.G. 42, *58*
Zimmermann, R.R., s. Harlow, H.F. 490, *529*
Zingg, R.M. 710, *752*
Ziskind, E., Somerfeld-Ziskind, E., Ziskind, L. 328, *349*
Ziskind, L., s. Ziskind, E. 328, *349*
Zivkovic, B., Guidotti, A., Revuelta, A., Costa, E. 213, *242*

Zomely-Neurath, C., s. Pickel, V.M. 21, *62*
Zopf, G.W. Jr., s. Foerster, H. [F 17a] *1077*
Zotterman, Y. [Z 4, 5] 910, *1103*
Zotterman, Y., s. Adrian, E.D. [A 10] 908, 909, *1068*
Zotterman, Y., s. Borg, G. [B 53] 911, *1072*
Zoubok, B., s. Simpson, G.M. *313*
Zubek, J.P. 738, *752*
Zuckerman, M. 738, 743, 744, *752*
Zuckerman, M., s. Biase, D.V. 746
Zuckerman, M.A., s. Curtis, G.C. 735, *747*
Zuckerman, S. 384, *544*
Züblin, W. 677, *705*
Zumpe, D., s. Michael, R.P. 461, *536*
Zutt, J. [Z 6] 986, *1103*
Zylka, W., s. Gänshirt, H. [G 1] 982, *1078*

Sachverzeichnis – Subject Index

Acetylcholin 28, 199, 219, 980
Adoptionsstudien 549
adrenaline (epinephrine) 32
α-adrenergic blockade 212
Affekt 1040
Affektausdruck 948
– von Angst und Wut 949
Affekte und Triebe 763
– –, Neurophysiologie der 937
affektive Bahnung und Blockierung der Sprach- und Denkleistungen 963
affektive Beeinflussung von Gedächtnisvorgängen 1042
affektive Perseveration 963
affektive Psychosen, Genetik 577f.
– –, prämorbide Besonderheiten 686
Affektivität 902
–, Störungen der 501
– und Kommunikation 445, 452, 496
Affektleere der kybernetischen Maschine 871
Affekt- und Antriebsstörungen nach Hirnläsionen 961
Affekt- und Triebleben 774
Affektvorgänge 786
Aggression, arteigene 947
–, ,,intraspezifische'' 810
Aggressionshemmung bei Tier und Mensch 947
Aggressionstrieb 940, 945
aggressiveness 367
Agnosie 897
Akathisie 257
Aktivierungs-System, unspezifisches des Hirnstamms 763
alcohol, ethyl 232
Alexie 901
Alkohol-Embryopathie 674
Alkoholismus, Erbschäden 600
–, Stoffwechselfaktoren 600
Altersconstitution 625, 634f.
amantedine 230
amino acids γ-aminobutyric acid (GABA) 35
Amnesie, retrograde 1025
Amnesierung des Schlaferlebens 1020
AMP, cyclic 207
Amphetamin 91, 206, 228, 229

Amphetamine, Vergiftungen 301
Amygdala 460
Amygdala-Hypothalamus-Beziehungen 458
amygdalotomy 372
anaklitische Depression (nach R. Spitz) 496, 715, 728
– –, Stufen 716
,,angeborener Auslösemechanismus'', AAM 423
Angriff und Flucht 940
Angst 765, 766
Anlage und Umwelt 760
Anorexia nervosa 639, 651
Antidepressiva 67, 205, 223
–, Applikation 263
–, Behandlungsdauer 264
–, Dauermedikation 264
–, Dosierung 263
–, Indikationen 262
–, intravenöse Infusionsbehandlung 263
–, Klassifikation 260
–, klinische Wirkung 260
–, Kontraindikationen 262
–, Nebenwirkungen 263
– (Thymoleptika), tri- und tetrazyklische 259ff.
–, trizyklische und tetrazyklische Kombination mit MAO-Hemmer 262
–, trizyklische Vergiftungen 299
–, Wirkungseintritt 261
Antidepressivabehandlung, Wirkungslatenz 261
antipsychotic action 213
Antipsychotika 248ff.
Antipsychotika (= s. Neuroleptika) 248
Antizipation 847
Antrieb 951, 973
–, neurophysiologische Grundlagen 950
anxiety 367
Anxiolytika (Tranquilizer) 231, 275ff.
–, Entzugssyndrom 277
–, Indikationen 276
–, klinische Wirkung 275
–, Kontraindikationen 277
–, Nebenwirkungen 277
–, Suchtpotential 277
Aphasie 897

Aphasie, EEG-Befunde bei 894
aphasische Sprachhemmung 885
apomorphine 206, 209
Appetenzverhalten 801
Apraxie 897
Artikulation 436
Assoziationsapparat beim Menschen 761
Aufmerksamkeit 968, 976
–, kybernetisches Schema der Selektion von 975
–, visuelle 898
Augenbewegungen im Nachtschlaf 1011
– – Schlaf 995
Augengruß 421
Auslösermechanismus, angeborener 801
Autismus, frühkindlicher 588
–, –, Schizophreniebelastung 589
–, infantiler 637
„autogenes Training" 971
„Autonomie des Seelischen" 772
autoreceptor, dopaminergic 215

Balken-Funktion 890
Barbiturate, Enzyminduktion 283
–, Vergiftungen 283, 300
Barbituratsucht, Entziehungssymptome 284
Behaviorismus 790
Benzodiazepine, Diphenylhydantoinspiegel 277
–, REM-Schlaf 277
–, Vergiftungen 300
Beratung, genetische 601
Bereitschaftspotential 154
Betablocker 278ff.
–, Indikationen 279, 280
–, Klassifikation 278
–, Nebenwirkungen 280
Bewegungsentwurf 830
Bewußtsein 968, 1028
–, Maschinen 870
–, selektive Funktion 971
Bewußtseinsfrage 867
Bewußtseinsselektion 972
Bewußtseinsstörungen bei Hypoxie und Narkose 981
– – Kranken, Neurophysiologie pathologischer 983
– und hirnelektrische Befunde 985
biogene Amine 67
Biologie, Zwischenstellung der, zwischen Anorganischem und Psychischem 773
–, theoretische 774
Blickkontakt 841
blood-brain barrier 44, 45
brain, energy requirement of the 52

–, frontolimbic 352
–, incorporation of labelled metabolites 7
– lipids, extraction of 17
– –, composition of 18
– mammalian, vivo 4
–, metabolic compartments 8
– metabolism, glucose 52
– metabolism vivo 6
– monoamines 233
–, perfusion techniques 7
–, tissue culture 9ff.
–, tissue slice techniques 8
– water content 16
Bromismus 284
Butyrophenone 91

capsulotomy 363
–, anterior 374
catecholamine synthesis 202, 203
cell nuclei 12
cerebral blood flow 6
Charakterstruktur, prämorbide, Zusammenhänge mit Varianten der allgemeinen Intelligenz 689
– von Neurotikern 688
Charakterstrukturen, Varianten prämorbider, Zusammenhang psychischer Störungen 684
cholinerge Neuronensysteme des Hirnstamms 980
'chromaffin granules' 32
Chromosomenstörung 546, 601
cingulotomy 359, 374
cingulum 356
Clozapin 91, 213
Clozapinbehandlung, Agranulozytose 251
CNV „contingent negative variation" 152
–, Geschlechtsunterschiede 153
–, Methodik 152
–, topographische Verteilung 153
convulsive therapy (CT) 316f.
– –, anesthesiologic principles 317
– –, antidepressive effect 319
– –, cerebral hypoxia 323
– –, electric stimulation 318
– –, – – and psychosyndrome 318
– –, – –, unilateral application 318
– –, pharmacologic 317
corpus callosum 356, 890
Corpus mamillare 761
cortex, ablations of the orbitofrontal 353
–, orbitofrontal 357
Cortexreizungen 884
Cortisolsekretion bei endogen depressiven Patienten 78
–, Regulation 76

–, zirkadianer Rhythmus 77
cryothermia 359
CSF, protein concentration in newborn infants 45
CT, principle of 316

Dämmerzustand 929
Delirien 285
–, Medikation 286
–, Ursachen 285
Delir und Traum 1018
Denken 902, 1029
– beim Menschen 809
–, unbenanntes 807
Depotneuroleptika 255ff.
–, Behandlungsdauer 258
–, Indikationen 256
–, Nebenwirkungen 257
– parenterale Applikation 252
–, Rehospitalisationsquote 256
–, Wirkungsprofil 256
depression 362, 364, 366, 367, 374
– in Parkinsonian patients 227
–, involutional 366
–, neuroendocrinologic research 325
Depression 964, 1018
–, Amindefizit 73
–, Amphetamin 83
–, anaklitische 496
–, Auslöser 583
–, Autopsieuntersuchungen 67
–, Bedeutung der, Adoleszenz 730
–, Blutuntersuchungen 70
–, cholinerges System 75
–, endogene Rezeptorhypothese 89
–, Erbgang 583
–, Hypothalamus-Hypophysen-STH-System 84
–, jugendliche und kindliche 590
–, Katecholamin-Hypothese 67
–, Liquoruntersuchungen 68
–, post- bzw. eine präsynaptische 87
–, Rezeptor-Hypothese der endogenen 86
–, Serotonin 67
–, Urinuntersuchungen 71
–, Transmittersysteme 75
depressiv endogene Cortisolsekretion 79
– – reduzierte α-adrenerge Rezeptorempfindlichkeit 86
– neurotisch-reaktive Cortisolsekretion 79
depressive Schlafstörung 1015
depressives Syndrom 500
– – bei Affen 501
Deprivation 707, 708
– bei Affen- und Menschenkindern 496

– im Kindesalter, „akutes Verlassenheitssyndrom"/„despair-Syndrom" 728–730
– – –, antisoziales Verhalten und Delinquenz 726, 732
– – –, „begleitende Untersuchungstechnik" (R. Spitz) 723
– – –, gefühlsarme Psychopathie ("Affectionless Psychopathy", "Affectionless Character") 731
– – –, geschichtliche Aspekte 709f.
– – –, Langzeitwirkungen, retrospektive Folgestudie 723, 724, 725
– – –, Retardierungssyndrom 731, 732
–, paternale 728
–, sensorische 735
–, spezifische Kurzzeitwirkungen 735
–, Theorien 744
–, therapeutische Einsatzmöglichkeiten 740–742
Deprivationsbedingungen in Säuglings- und Kleinkinderheimen 712
–, Simulation von klinischen 738
Deprivationsexperimente 735
–, Beeinträchtigungen der kognitiven Leistungen 736
–, Körperschemaveränderungen 736
–, kollektive Halluzinationen 736
–, Pseudohalluzinationen 735
–, „Reizhunger" 737
Deprivationsforschung, Deprivation, partielle 734
Deprivationswirkungen, Entstehung 714
developing brain, lipid metabolism 51
Dexamethason-Hemmtest 77
Dissozialität 639
Dominanz des Sehsystems 913
Dominanzsignale 401
dopa 230
Dopamin 67, 980
Dopamin-Hypothese 91
Dopaminrezeptorempfindlichkeit 91, 111
Dopamine 28, 201, 208
–, inhibitory action on neurons 30
–, synthesis and metabolism 29
–, ways of metabolizing 30
dopamine binding and release 216
– neurons 208
– pathway 200
– receptors 210
dopamine-receptor blockade 211
– – –, pharmacokinetic aspects of 217
dopamine, striatal vs limbic 212
dopamine-sensitive adenylate cyclase, effect on 216
dopamine, the possible role of in psychosis 222
dopaminergic autoreceptors, the possible role of 215

dopaminergic receptor 207, 208
dopaminergic synapse 206
Down-Syndrom 469
Drogen 487
Drogensuchten, Entstehung 601
drug addiction 361
Dysarthrie 474, 475
Dyskinesien 257
dysleptische Krisen 286
Dysmelie-Syndrom 680
Dyslexie 596
„Dysrhythmie" 121

ECT (electroconvulsive therapy), amine hypothesis 338
– and electroencephalography 321
and pernicious catatonia 334
–, anterograde amnesia 326
–, antidepressive effect and the delta activity 322
–, – therapy 328
–, British study difference between ECT and imipramine 329
–, cardiovascular effects 336
–, combination with drugs in treatment of depression 332
–, complications 335
–, contraindications 336
–, electrolyte hypothesis 340
– in bromide poisoning 335
– in delirious states 335
–, indications 330
–, influence of age 336
– in mania 333
– in organic brain disease 335
– in psychoses associated with epilepsy 335
– in schizophrenic disorders 333, 334
–, involvement of hypothalamus 338
–, memory disturbance and depression 325
–, modifications minimizing side effect 328
–, monoaminergic activity and neurohormonal activity 324
–, permanent damage 323
–, permeability hypothesis 340
–, retrograde amnesia 327
–, systemic effects 320
EEG (Elektrenzephalogramm) 762, 763, 970, 1032
–, aktives 976
–, akute intermittierende Porphyrie 161
–, Allgemeinveränderung 120
– bei Absencen 166
– bei akuten Hypoxidosen 162, 982
– bei akuter Alkoholintoxikation 164
– bei chronischen zerebralen Gefäßprozessen 162

– bei chronischen zerebralen Hypoxidosen 162
– bei Enzephalitiden und Meningitiden 162, 163
– bei Medikamentenentzugssyndromen 164
– bei Neurolues 163
– bei psychomotorischen Anfällen 166
– bei synkopaler Bewußtseinsstörung 984
–, „burst-suppression"-Aktivität 121
–, Chronobiologie 131
– der verschiedenen Schlafstadien 1000
–, Dysrhythmie, gruppierte 124
–, Endokrinopathien 161
–, genetisch bedingte Stoffwechselstörungen 161
–, Grundaktivität 118
–, Grundlagen 1050
–, Hauptformen des 1051
–, hepatische Enzephalopathie 158
–, Herdstörung 123
–, Hyperglykämie 160
–, hypersynchrone Aktivität 124
–, Hypoglykämie 160
–, hypoglykämisches Koma 158
– Koma, Periodizität 157
–, „Parenrhythmie" 124
–, psychiatrische Bedeutung des 116, 763
–, Rhythmisierung, gruppierte abnorme 124
– und Komatiefe 155
– und Neuronenentladungen bei Narkose 982, 983
– unter Medikamentenwirkung 180
–, Urämie, „Dysäquilibrium-Syndrom" 160
–, urämische Bewußtseinsstörungen 157
–, Vitamin-B_{12}-Mangelsyndrome 161
EEG-Befunde, apallisches Syndrom 158
– – bei Komaformen 155f.
– –, Psychoseverlauf 170
EEG-Beobachtungen bei epileptischen Psychosen 170
EEG, depth, recording 357
EEG-Analyse 133f.
– –, Amplituden-Integration 134
– –, Daten- und Informationsreduktion 146
– –, Leistungs- oder Power-Spektrum 142
– –, period analysis 138
– –, Spektral-Analyse 140
– –, Varianzspektrum 141
EEG-Grundaktivitäten, Altersabhängigkeit 129
– –, geschlechtsabhängige Häufigkeitsunterschiede 128
EEG-Veränderungen 763, 1047
– bei Hirntraumen und posttraumatischen Psychosen 163
EEG-Wellen 1051
–, Frequenzspektrum der 1052

Sachverzeichnis – Subject Index

Ehekonflikt 770
Eidetik 931
electrocoagulation 359
Elektrokrampfbehandlung 228, 316f., 500
Elektrophysiologie des Schlafes 998
Emotion 418, 436
emotionale Bedeutung von Gesichtsausdrücken 420
emotionale Vorgänge, Substrate 944
emotionales Verhalten, zerebrale Korrelate 452
Emotionen, angeborene und erworbene Auslöser 423
encephalins 40
Endhandlung, trieblösende 801
endocrine aspects of neuroleptic action 220
β-Endorphin 112
energetische Konzeptionen 784
Enthemmung 900
Entwicklungsdiagnostik an institutionalisierten Kindern (Untersuchung), (R. Spitz) 715
Enuresis 596, 732
Epilepsie 763
epilepsy 372
epileptische Anfallssucht 958
epileptische Krampfentladung 862
epileptische Störungen 763
Erbanlage 548
Erbfaktoren, Chromosomenaberrationen 546
–, molekulare Ebene 546
–, phänotypische Ebene 546
Erbkoordination 423
Erfahrung und Lernen 760
Erkenntnistheorie, Kants 765
Erlebnisreaktionen und echte Psychosen, Trennung von 770
Erregungszustände 285
– der Nerven und Nervenzentren 786
–, Grundkrankheiten 285
–, Medikation 285
Erwartungswelle, Walters 1034
Ethologie 381, 759, 763, 797
– und Psychiatrie 811
evozierte Potentiale 147
– –, akustische, inter- und intraindividuelle Variabilität 151
– –, akustische, Intervalldauer 151
– –, akustische Reize 148
– –, elektrische Reizung 148
– – im Koma 158
– –, somatosensorisch, Nachweis 152
– –, visuelle, Altersabhängigkeit 150
– –, visuelle Reizung 147
Exhibitionismus 396
Existenzphilosophie 771
–, Heideggers 765
exogene Psychosen 551

experimental allergic encephalitis (EAE) 22
experimentelle Psychologie 786, 788
extrapyramidal effects 213
extrapyramidale Störungssymptome 839
extrapyramidales System 839
„extrauterine Mutter-Kind-Symbiose" 720

Farbenlehre 914
Felder, rezeptive 923
–, – und perzeptive 922
Finalnexus 777
– und Kausalnexus 775
Fluchttrieb 946
Formatio reticularis 950, 977, 994
„Freiheit" des menschlichen Wollens 775
frontal lobes 353
– –, lesions of the 352
–, ventromedial 356

GABA 219
– γ-aminobutyric acid 199
Ganzheitsprinzip 905
Gedächtnis 1021, 1023, 1024
–, physikalische Modelle 1044
–, temporaler Neocortex 1048
– und bedingte Reaktionen bei Tieren 1026
– und Lernen 760
– und zerebrale Disposition 1040
Gedächtnisgrundlagen, hypothetische neuronale 1037
Gedächtnishypothesen, chemisch-makromolekulare 1045
Gedächtnisleistungen, menschliche 761
Gedächtnisstörungen und Hirnlokalisation 1047
Gehirn 794
–, „dreieiniges" 459
– und Bewußtsein 791, 793
Geist, des Leibgebundenheit 772
–, Herrschaft des über die Materie 775
Geisteswissenschaften 777
Genitalpräsentieren 396
Genetik, Depressionen 582
–, Manie 580
–, prospektive Längsschnittuntersuchungen 550
Geschlechtskonstitution 642f.
–, Entwicklungsstufen der 643
Geschlechtsunterschiede in Morbidität und Mortalität 649–664
– – – – –, ätiopathogenetische Interpretation 662
– – – – –, Feldstudie 653
–, psychische 647
Geschlechtsverteilung psychiatrischer Erkrankungen im Erwachsenenalter 651f.

Gesichtsausdruck 414
Gestaltpsychologie 789, 790
glutamic acid 37
glycine 37
glycoproteins 23
Grenzphänomene, Gefühle und Triebe als biologisch seelische 774
Großhirn 761
Großhirn-Hemisphären 890
–, hirnelektrische Koordination beider 889
Großhirnrinde, Entwicklung der 761
Gruppenkonstitution 625
Gyrus cinguli 474

Habitusvariationen, physiologische und biochemische Variablen 669
hallucination 367
Halluzinationen bei Gesunden nach sensorischer Isolierung 932
– bei Kranken ohne Psychose, optische 933
– bei längerer Augenverdunkelung und Blindheit, optische 934
–, experimentelle 932
–, Grundlagen der 935
–, hypnagoge 1008
–, optische 930
–, Sprache 886
haloperidol 206, 213, 217
Handlung 845
–, Zweckrichtung des Wollens und der 778
Handlungen, Konzepte willensgesteuerter Ziele 846
Handlungsbereitschaft 831
Hemisphärendifferenz 884
– und Dominanz 891
5-HIES 68, 69
5-HIES-Konzentration im Liquor 69
„High-Risk-Kinder" 550
Hirnableitungen mit implantierten Elektroden 763
Hirnevolution und Kommunikationsprozesse 444
Hirnkonzeption, SCHLESINGERS 902
Hirnlokalisation von Affekten und Trieben 943
Hirnpathologie 879
–, klinische 889
– und Neurophysiologie, KLEISTS 902
hirnpathologische Störungssyndrome 897
Hirnphysiologie 784
– und Psychologie 783
Hirnreizungen bei Menschen, stereotaktische 886, 884
Hirnrinde und Hirnstamm 763
Hirnveränderungen, organische 763
Hirsutismus der Frau 677

histamine 37
histochemistry 15
Homosexualität, pädophile 370
Hormonregulation 860
Hospitalismus 716
Hunger und Durst 939
5-Hydroxytryptamine (Serotonin), melatonin 34
5-hydroxytryptophan 202
hyperaktive Kinder 596
Hypnotika (=Schlafmittel) 231, 280ff.
–, Durchschlafmittel 281
–, Einschlafmittel 281
–, Indikationen 281
–, Klassifikation 280
–, Kontraindikationen 283
–, Nebenwirkungen 283
hypothalamic regulatory, factors 41
– – –, actions of 42
hypothalamotomy, posteromedial 369
–, ventromedial 370
Hypothalamus 455, 860
Hypothalamus-Hypophysen-Nebennierenrinden-System 76, 111
Hypothalamus-Hypophysen-Wachstumshormon(=STH)-System 81
Hysterie 595

Information, helldunkel 916
–, Spezifizierung und Integration 865
Informationstheorie 857
Instinkt 800, 965, 1040
– und Lernen 760
– - und Triebverhalten, menschliches 760
Instinktbewegung 800
– des Lächelns 411
Instinkthandlungen 812
–, Schlaf als triebhafte 990
Instinktmechanismen 951
Instinktvorgänge, angeborene 824
Intelligenz ohne Sprache 806
Interaktion, kindliche Entwicklung in der 720
Introspektion 789
Invarianz der Wahrnehmung 864

Kataplexie 1015
Kategorienlehre 778
– und Schichtprinzip 767
Kausalbeziehung und Zweckmäßigkeit in Physiologie und Psychologie 779
Kausalnexus 777
Kinderpsychiatrie, geschlechtsspezifische Verteilung des Krankenguts 658
Kleinhirn 845
Klinefelter-Syndrom 675

Körperbau, Beziehung zu Intelligenz 671
–, Faktorenanalysen von Tests zur Erfassung intellektueller Leistungen 669
Koma, Klassifikation 156
Kommunikation bei Tieren, sprachlose Ausdrucks 807
– des Säuglings, phono-audio-visuelle 517
–, sprachliche oder nicht-sprachliche 756
– und Gestimmtheit 486
Kommunikationsforschung, biologische 853
Kommunikationsprozeß, Hirnstrukturen und -funktionen im 444
Kommunikationsprozesse 383
kommunikative Gesten 398
kommunikatives Vermögen der Schimpansen 504
Kondition 619f.
Konditionierung 1027
–, zerebrale Mechanismen 1030
Konstitution 619f.
–, abnorme Varianten 672
–, – – chromosomale Aberrationen 674
–, – – erbliche Form 674
–, – – exogen bedingte 674
–, rassische 626, 664
Konstitutionsanomalien 627
–, psychische im Säuglingsalter 635
Konstitutionsentwicklung, Stufen 636
Konstitutionspathologie 627–630
–, Konsequenzen für die praktisch-klinische Arbeit 630–632
Konstitutionstypen 953
Konstitutionstypologien 625
Krankheitsdisposition 628
Kriminalitätskonkordanzen 597
–, Adoptionsstudie 598
Kultur 804
Kulturwelt 794
Kurzzeitgedächtnis 1025
Kybernetik 759, 852, 1044
–, Bio 879
–, Grenzen technisch-mathematischer 876
–, Vorteile, Nachteile und Grenzen der 872
kybernetische Blockschemata 853
kybernetische Modelle der Gehirnfunktionen 863
kybernetische Programmierung und Gedächtnis 1038
kybernetische Theorien über Bewußtsein 975

Langzeitgedächtnis 1025
Laute, Erkennen der 433, 478
Lautgebung, zerebrale Repräsentation 472
„Leerlauf" 801
Legasthenie 638

Leib-Seele-Problem 867
Leib-Seele-Theorien 792
Lernbehinderte 637
Lernen 760, 1040, 1062
–, Grenzen 1043
– und Gedächtnis, Physiologie von 1037
Lernfähigkeit 760
Lernmatrizen 1045
Lernphysiologie 763
Lernpsychologie 790
Lern- und Verhaltensforschung 760
leukotomy, limbic 364
limbisches System 213, 230, 453, 460, 466, 904, 1047
– –, Anatomie 454
– – des Rhinenzephalons 943
– –, Schema 456
Lithium 228, 270ff.
–, Applikation und Dosierung 273
–, Behandlungsdauer 275
–, Blutspiegelkontrolle 273
–, Indikationen 270
–, klinische Wirkung 270
–, Kombination mit anderen Psychopharmaka 274
–, Kontraindikationen 271
–, renaler Diabetes insipidus 293
–, Schilddrüsenfunktion 293
–, Schwangerschaft 294
–, Vergiftungen 272, 300
–, Wirkungseintritt 270
Lithium-Baby-Register 271
Lithiumpräparate, Nebenwirkungen 271–273
Lithiumresorption, erbliche Unterschiede 583
Lithiumvergiftung 272
lobotomy 355
–, frontal 354
Lokalisations- und Ganzheitslehren 904
LSD-25 229
LTCL (Lithium Toxicity Checklist) 272
luteinizing hormone release factor (LRF) 43
lysergic acid diethylamide 228

manic-depressive illness 374
Manie 943, 964
MAO-Aktivität, Vulnerabilität psychopathologische Auffälligkeiten 96
MAO-Hemmer, Indikationen 266
–, Interaktionsmöglichkeiten, pharmakologische 266
–, klinische Wirkung 264
–, Kontraindikationen 266
–, Nahrungsmittel, Tyramingehalt 266
–, Nebenwirkungen 267

MAO-Hemmer und trizyklische Antidepressiva 267
–, Vergiftungen 299
maprotiline 225
„maternale Deprivation" (nach BOWLBY) 717
maturation of the brain, protein metabolism 49 ff.
Meditation 971
melanocyte-stimulating hormone 42
membrane proteins 21
memory hypotheses 50
mental illness, allergic response 54
– –, biochemical mechanisms 54
– –, metabolic abnormality 54
mental retardation, 'inborn errors' of metabolism 54
Merkfähigkeit und Emotionalität 761
Merkfähigkeitsstörungen, zerebrale Korrelate 1047
mescaline 228
mesoloviotomy 367, 374
metabolic compartmentation 46
metabolism of growth 47
α-methyltyrosine, neuroleptic properties of 218
MHPG 68
– -Ausscheidung im Urin 72, 73, 82
–, Liquor 70
– -Sulfatmengen im Urin schizophrener Patienten 92
microsomal fraction 14
microtubules 14
Milieu, soziales 809
Mimik 415, 421
mimische Ausdrucksformen 405
mimische Signale 403, 410
mitochondria 12
monoamine-degrading enzymes 204
monoamine oxidase inhibitors 224
monoamine precursors as antidepressant agents 226
monoamine re-uptake, inhibitors of 224
monoaminerge Neuronensysteme des Hirnstamms 980
monoaminergic neurons, activity of 208
monoaminergic pathways 200
– –, functional aspects of the 200
monoaminergic receptors 208
Monoaminoxydase, Hauptabbauenzym für Katecholamine für Serotonin 95
Monoaminooxydasehemmer (=MAO-Hemmer) 264 f.
Motivation 929
Motorik 824
–, Analyse der 822
–, Blick 825
–, extrapyramidale 822

–, Programmierung der 839
–, Psycho 823
–, Rechts- und Linkshändigkeit 842
–, Stütz 827
–, Trieb und Lernen 836
–, Willkür 822
–, Ziel 827
motorisches Lernen 840
motorisches Potential 154
Mutismus, akinetischer 474
Mutter-Kind-Beziehung, Einflüsse früher Trennung 726
Mutter-Kind-Dyade 489
Mutter-Kind-Kontakt 806
myelin 11

NA-Rezeptorüberempfindlichkeit 92
–, Urinanalysen 72
Narkolepsie 1015
Naturphilosophien 773
Natur- und Lebensvorgänge, Totalität der Bedingungen von 778
Naturwissenschaft 777
Neglektsyndrome 898
Nervenaktionspotentiale 781
Nervensystem, Forschung am 798
–, Plastizität 1062
–, Schichtenaufbau 887
–, technische Modelle 851
Nervenzellen der Sehrinde 918
neural modulators 38
neurochemistry, development 2
neuroleptic action 210
neuroleptic agents 209, 222
neuroleptics, acute vs long-term effects of 220
–, effect of 213
– on developing brain, effects of 221
– on noncate-cholaminergic systems, effects of 219
Neuroleptika (=s. Antipsychotika, =s. Depotneuroleptika) 248 ff.
–, Absetzstudien 253
–, Agranulozytose 291
–, Behandlungsdauer 253
–, Indikationsstellung 249
–, klinische Wirkung 249
–, kurzwirkende parenterale Applikation 251
–, Kontraindikationen 250
–, Nebenwirkungen 250
„neuroleptische Schwelle" 253
Neuronensysteme des Hirnstamms 981
Neuronentätigkeit im Schlaf 1004
– und Sehen 915
Neuronentheorie 784
Neuron-Koordination bei bedingten Reflexen 1033
Neuropharmakologie 762

Neurophysiologie 755–797, 889
– der Schlafstörungen 1013
– des Sehens 913
– in der Lokalisationsforschung, Methoden der 882
–, Psychiatrie und Philosophie 764, 765, 778
– und Hirnlokalisation 880
neurophysiologische Analyse komplexer motorischer Leistungen 835
neurophysiologische Grundlagen der Hirnlokalisation 879
– – von Lernen 1023
neurophysiologische Untersuchungen über Weckeffekte 976
Neuropsychiatrie 762
Neuropsychologie, klinische 780
neuroreceptor proteins 24
– –, Acetylcholine receptors 25
– –, amino acid receptors 24
– –, Catecholamine receptors 25
– –, L-Glutamic acid 24
Neurosen bei Tieren, experimentelle 811
–, Disposition 593
–, Konfliktsituationen der 770
–, psychische und physiologische Mechanismen der 962
–, spezifisch-menschliche und vital-tierische Anteile bei 813
–, Zwillingsuntersuchung 592
neurosis, anxiety 361, 364
–, obsessional 366
neurostenin 20
"neuroticism score" 593
neurotransmitters 26 ff.
–, chemical transmission 26
nomifensine 226
– (Norepinephrine) 31, 67, 201, 980
Noradrenalindefizit-Hypothese 83
Noradrenalin- und Serotoninsystem 66
noradrenerge Neuronensysteme 1006
noradrenergic pathway 200
Nortriptylin 69
Nucleus amygdalae 455

obsessional 364
obsessive ruminations 367
Östrogene 466
Oligophrenie 637
Ontogenese der Laute 431
opiate receptors 26
Orientierungsleistungen 928
oxytocin 41

pain 362, 374
Parenrhythmie 165

Parietalregion 898
Parkinsonsyndrom 230, 257
Pavor nocturnus 1017
Partialkonstitution, immunologische 681
–, physiologische 681
–, psychische 623, 682 f.
–, somatische 623
–, – und psychische Normabweichungen 679–682
peptide neuroeffectors 39 ff.
– –, metabolism 39
Periodizität, endogene 621
Petit mal-Status und EEG 167
„pharmakogene Depression" 257
Phenothiazine 91
–, Vergiftungen 300
Philosophie 765
phobias 367
Phonationsbalmen 477
Phonemformen 436
Phonemisieren, Wege vom Vokalisieren zum 522
Phonetik 438
Physiologie 758, 780
– von Bewußtsein und Schlaf 763
physiologische Erklärung psychologischer Phänomene 781, 784
physiologische und psychologische Verfahren und Deutungen 779
Pickwick-Syndrom 994, 1016
Porphyrie, intermittierende 681
postparoxysmale Dämmerzustände 167
Potentialveränderungen, kortikale 154
Prägung 408, 1041
Präsentieren, Variationen 389
Primaten, Stammbaum der 382
Privation 708
Progesteron 466
prostaglandins 18, 38
proteins 20 ff.
–, brain-specific soluble 21
–, myelin basic 22
proteolipids 22
Prozesse, evolutive 621
–, involutive 621
Psychiatrie 759, 762, 764, 765, 796
–, Begrenzung naturwissenschaftlicher Forschung in der 1061
–, Lerntheorien 1043
–, organische Grundlagen der 902
– und Neurophysiologie 763, 1056
– – – im Schichtenaufbau 768
psychiatrische Notfallsituationen 284 ff.
„psychische Energie" 784
psychische Erscheinungen, Erklärbarkeit der 786

psychische Kausalität 788
„psychische Kraft" 783
– – und „psychische Energie" 784
Psychoanalyse 791
Psychologie 795, 797
–, Begrenztheit der experimentellen 788
–, experimentelle 786
– im biologischen Aspekt 783
–, physiologische 783
– und Neurophysiologie 779
psychomorphologische Korrelationsstudien 667
Psychomotorik 841
Psychoneurose 591
Psychopathie 361, 591, 594, 639
Psychopharmaka, Akathisie 297
–, Amenorrhoe 292
–, Arzneimittelexantheme 292
–, Delirien 299
–, endokrinologische Nebenwirkungen 292
–, gastrointestinale Nebenwirkungen 289
–, Gewichtszunahme 290
–, hämatologische Nebenwirkungen 291
–, Hautpigmentationen 292
–, Hepatotoxizität 290
–, kardiovaskuläre Nebenwirkungen 286–288
–, manische Syndrome 298
–, Mortalität 295
–, Nebenwirkungen 286ff.
–, organische Verwirrungszustände 299
–, Parkinsonsyndrome 295
–, persistierende Dyskinesien 297
–, pharmakogene Depressionen 298
–, Pigmentablagerungen in den Augen 289
–, sexuelle Störungen 293
–, teratogene Wirkungen 293, 294
–, Tremor 295
–, vegetative Nebenwirkungen 288
Psychopharmakaprüfung 247
Psychopharmaka-Vergiftungen, Therapie 301
Psychopharmakologie 783
Psychophysik 780, 781, 910
– des Sehens 906
Psychophysiologie 782, 783, 785
– des Sehens 913
Psychosen 763, 769, 813
–, affektive 964
–, atypische 582f.
– eineiiger Zwillinge 556
–, endogene 445, 641, 763, 769
–, – im Kindesalter 587f.
–, epileptische 1050
– –, exogene 551
–, Felduntersuchungen, „Lundby-Projekt" 587
–, Hirnmechanismen von 763
–, Neurophysiologie 1058
–, schizophrene 256

–, Schlaf und Traum 1018
–, uni- und bipolare Beziehungen 579
psychosis, manic-depressive 361
psychosomatische Beeinflussung, Grenzen der 769
Psychostimulantien, Amphetamine (Weckamine) und Nicht-Amphetamine 268f.
–, Behandlungsdauer 269
–, Indikationen 268
–, klinische Wirkung 268
–, Kontraindikationen 269
–, Nebenwirkungen 269
–, Suchtgefahr 268
–, Wirkungseintritt 268
psychosurgery 351, 357
Psychosyndrom, frühkindliches exogenes 637
psychotisch-affektive Störung 930
psychotische Bewußtseinsänderungen 986
psychotomimetic agents 228

Reafferenzprinzip 856, 858
Reaktionen im Plethysmogramm, vasomotorische 782
Reaktionsfähigkeit im Schlaf 993
receptor activation 206
receptor proteins for glucocorticoids 26
– – , oestrogen 26
receptor systems for androgens 26
– – – oestrogens 26
Rechenmaschinen, digitale und analoge 855
Reflex 1040
Reflexforschung 763
–, bedingte 1027, 1032
–, PAWLOWs bedingte 759
Regelkreis 854
Regelmechanismus 854
Regelprozesse bei psychischen Vorgängen 867
Regeltechnik, Schwierigkeiten biologischer Anwendungen der 875
Regelung 853
–, biologische 858
Regulation, neuro-endokrine 861
Reiz-Empfindung 782
Reiz und Reizeffekte in der neurophysiologischen Sinnesforschung 909
– und Sinneserregung 782
REM-Schlaf 990
reserpine 206, 210
Resonanzhypothese des Gedächtnisses 1038
Retinaperipherie, Felder in der 925
retikuläres Hirnstammsystem 979
retikulo-thalamische Hirnstammsysteme, Funktionen der „unspezifischen" 977
Rezeptorempfindlichkeit 88
Rezeptor-Hypothese 110
Rhinencephalon 761

Risikofaktoren 629
Ritualisierung 802
„Rooming-in-Konzept" 714, 726
Rückkoppelung im Triebleben 951
–, positive 862
– von triebähnlichen Mechanismen, positive 955

„S-100" protein 21
Schicht, biologische 774
–, psychische 768, 778
–, seelische 774
Schichtenaufbau 769
Schichten des Anorganischen, Organischen und Psychischen 767
–, physikalisch-chemische und biologische 778
–, psychisch-sozial-kulturelle 778
Schichtenprinzip 771, 793
Schichtstruktur der realen Welt 767, 778
Schizoid 564, 565
schizophrene Eltern, Erkrankungsrisiko der Kinder 554
schizophrene Informationsverarbeitung 863
schizophrene Störungen 1019
Schizophrene, Prozeßaktivität, Auftreten von Parenrhythmie 177
–, schizoide Charakterstruktur von 685
schizophrenia 361, 366, 369
–, mimicking paranoid 228
schizophrenic 364
– anxiety 374
– origin, anxiety, tension and fears of 368
Schizophrenie 90, 111, 554–557, 558, 559, 573, 574
–, Adoptionsstudien 557f., 559
–, "Crossfostering Study" 559
–, Diagnosenschema 558
–, EEG 171
–, EEG-Analyse 172
– eine Störung der Adrenalinbildung 94
–, Endorphine 96
–, Erbgangshypothesen 561
–, evozierte und ereignisbezogene Potentiale 175
–, familiäre Transmission 572
–, Familienuntersuchungen 553
–, genetische Aspekte 552f.
–, Gipfel der Erstmanifestation 641
–, Hämodialyse 97
–, Heterogenie 562
–, High-Risk-Kinder 568–569
–, immunbiologische Theorien 570
–, Katecholaminstoffwechsel 93
–, kindliche 588, 589
–, Lerntheorie, MEDNICK 567–568
–, Methionineffekt 95

–, neurochemische Befunde 570
–, perinatale Faktoren 575
–, prospektive Studien 567
–, psychosoziale Ursachen 573
–, Schwellen-Modelle 562
–, Segregationsanalyse 562
–, „Spektrumfälle" 558
–, symptomatologische Beziehungen zu den Neurosen 565
–, Umwelttheorie 571
–, Zwillingsuntersuchungen 554
Schlaf 969, 987, 1029
–, Bewußtseinskontinuität 1021
–, Biochemie und Stoffwechsel 1006
–, Biologie 990
–, Körpermotorik 995
–, periodische Erektionen 996
–, periodischer Ablauf der Nacht 991
–, periphere Funktionsänderungen 994
–, Tonusverlust und Areflexie 995
– und Atmung 994
– und Gedächtnis 1019
– und Hirnstoffwechsel 1007
Schlafauslösung, Tierversuche über 989
Schlafdauer 991
Schlaf-EEG bei Gesunden 988
Schlafentzug 993
– und EEG 1002
Schlafentzugstherapie 72
Schlafmittel (=s. Hypnotika) 280
Schlafregelung, Hirnlokalisation der 989
Schlafregulation, zerebrale 1005
Schlafstadien, neurophysiologische und psychologische Korrelationen in Wach- und 1009
Schlafstadium, „paradoxes" 1010
Schlafstörungen, Ursachen 281
Schlaf-Syndrome, pathologische 1013
–, somnambule 1017
Schlafwandeln 1017
Schlafzustand, das Einschlafstadium als Übergang von Wach- und 1007
Schmerzreize, Unlustreaktionen 785
Schocktherapie 770, 771
sedatives 231
Sehen, hell-dunkel 917
–, neuronales Kontur-, Form- und Tiefen 920
–, räumliches 918
Selbstbeobachtung 788, 789
Selbstmordhäufung, familiäre 594
Selbstreizung bei Affen, Delphinen und Menschen 957
– des Gehirns 954
– und sexuelle Triebhandlungen 958
Selbstschilderung und Verhaltensbeobachtung 789
Selektion als Funktionen von Aufmerksamkeit 974

Selektion der Willensentscheidung und Triebe 965
Semantik 509
Sensomotorik 821
–, antizipierende Koordination in der 824, 825
– und zerebrale Somatotopik 883
sensomotorisches Lernen 838
sensorische Aphasie 478
Septum 460
serotonerge Neuronensysteme 1006
Serotonin 67, 980
Sexualkonstitution, abnorme Varianten 674
Sexualverhalten 466, 760
sexuelle Deviationen 639
Signale, aggressionshemmende 390
– bei Affen, vokale 425
–, mimische 402
–, phonetische 443
–, ritualisierte 388
–, soziogenitale 392
–, zerebrale Erzeugung 446
Signalerkennung beim Menschen 410, 434
Signalfunktion im Kontext des Verhaltens 393
Sinnesbereich, akustischer 781
Sinnesfunktionen, Erforschung der 763
Sinnesinformationen 781
Sinnesmeldungen 794
Sinnesphysiologie 765, 780, 784, 789, 906
–, objektive 782, 907
–, subjektive 781, 907
Sinnesreize, Verhaltensreaktionen nach 781
somato-psychische Störungen 769
somatostatin 40
somatotopische Repräsentation 451
soziale Ordnungen im Tierreich 809
soziale Signale 383
soziogenitales Signal, Imponieren des Totenkopfaffen 385
Sozialisation, Störungen der 496
Sozialisationsprozesse 487
Sozialverhalten, Psychobiologie 407
Soziobiologie der Primaten 379
soziogenitale Signale der Affen 384
– – des Menschen 395
sozio-sexuelles Verhalten, zerebrale Repräsentation 461
Spektrum, bipolar-zyklothymes 582
Sprache 425, 469, 503, 803, 804, 809, 842, 1029
– als semantische Funktion 896
–, Cortexreizung 884
–, Gesten 507
–, Linksdominanz der 892
– oder Vokalsprache, Gesten 513
–, Zeichensprache und 515
Sprachdeprivation 896
Sprachentwicklung, Theorie der 435

Sprachfunktion in der Hirnrinde des Menschen 475
„Sprachzentren" 842
Sprechstörungen 474, 475
Status psychomotorischer Anfälle und EEG 168
Stereotypien 493
steroid hormones 26
Steuerung 853
STH 86
stimulation, electrical 368
Stottern 596
Striatum 213, 230
Stupor 286
subcellular fractionation 11 ff.
subkortikale Mechanismen 761
substance P 39
Sucht, Adoptionsstudie 599, 600
–, Befunde 599
–, elektrischer Selbstreiz 960
–, genetische 599
–, Zwillingsbefunde 599
Suchtverhalten bei Menschen 958
Suizid 594
surface-active detergents, homogenization of neural tissues 22
synaptic membranes 13
synaptic vesicles 14
synaptosomes 13
synkopale Ohnmachten 984
Syntax 509

Tatsachenwissenschaft und Gesetzeswissenschaft 777
Temporallappenläsion 944
Temporalregion 886
Testosteron 466
„thalamoretikuläres System" 904
thalamotomy 371
Thalamus 889, 943, 979
Thalamuskern 460
Thalamusreizversuche 762
theory, autoreceptor 209
Tranquilizer, s. Anxiolytika 231, 275 ff.
Transmethylierungs-Hypothese 94
transmitter 207
Träume als affektive Abreaktionen 1012
Träumen, Psychophysiologie 1010
Traum 987
Traumentzug 1012
Traumstadien, zyklischer Ablauf des Schlafes mit 992, 1008
tricyclic antidepressant 224
Triebe 800, 838, 848, 937, 946, 951, 965, 1040
–, soziale Mitteilung 948
– und Instinkte, Übersprung 946
– und Lernen 963
Triebanlage und Erfahrung 760

Triebbeherrschung 805
Triebinterpretation bei Gesunden und Kranken 961
Triebkonstitution 682–684
Triebmechanismen, sexuelle 939
Triebphysiologie 945
–, allgemeine Beziehungen zur 956
–, psychiatrische Anwendung 961
Triebregulation und Verhalten 952
Triebreizung, soziale Folgen zerebraler 942
Triebstruktur und Konstitution 951
Triebunterdrückung in der sozialen Gemeinschaft 964
Triebverhalten 950
–, menschliches 760
Triebvorgänge, Wechselwirkung verschiedener 941
Tryptophan 71, 226
Tubulin 20
Typensysteme von KRETSCHMER 665
„Typus manicus" 686
„Typus melancholicus" 687
Tyrosin 71

„Übersprung" 802
Umwelt bei Tier und Mensch 808
Unterschiedsschwelle, Methode der 782

Vasopressin 41
Vater-Kind-Beziehung, Einflüsse früher Trennung 727
Verdrängung 1042
Verhalten 201, 969
–, angeborenes 760
–, Ausdrucks 808
–, Blick 402
–, Imponier 396
–, Mutter-Kind 489
–, neurophysiologische Grundlagen des 818, 821
–, Prinzipien der neuralen Organisation 447
– und Erleben, Korrelationen zwischen 764
Verhaltensbeobachtung und Introspektion 814
Verhaltensbiologie 381
Verhaltensdispositionen und psychische Geschlechtsunterschiede 644
Verhaltensforschung 811
– bei Tier und Mensch 799
– und Kybernetik 759
– und psychiatrische Beobachtungen beim Menschen 813
Verhaltensgenetik 547
Verhaltensregelung 1062
Verhaltensstörungen 497
–, kindliche, Familienuntersuchungen 595, 596

Verhaltenstraditionen bei Affen 810
visueller Grenzkontrast 925
visuelle Strukturen, Reizung und Ausschaltung 933
vokales Repertoire des Totenkopfaffen 429
Vokalisation 469
Vokalisationen von Rhesusaffen 428

Wahn 930
Wahrnehmung 845, 908, 929
–, Auswahlkriterien der 929
–, Cortexreizung 885
–, Objekt- und der Orts 448
–, Raum- und Bewegungs 928
Wahrnehmungsbereitschaft, K-Komplex und 1002
Wahrnehmungsprozeß 975
Wechselwirkung, somato-psychische und psycho-somatische 769
Werkzeuggebrauch und Selbsterkennung 506
Werkzeugherstellung 803
Wille 838, 848, 973
Willensbegriff 787
Willkürinnervation 1035
„Würzburger Schule" 789

Zeitparadox der Zweckdetermination 777
Zentrenlehre 900
zerebral auslösbare Bewegung mit Signalcharakter 482
zerebrale Auslösung von Affekten und Trieben 938
zerebrale Bereitschaftspotentiale 832
zerebrale Lokalisation bedingter Reaktionen 1031
zerebrale Repräsentation audio-vokalen Verhaltens 468
zerebrale Selbstreizung 483
zerebrale Systeme der Motorik 843
Zerebralisation und psychische Störanfälligkeit des Menschen 633
Ziel- und Zweckvorgänge 777
Zivilisation und Normabweichung des Verhaltens 634
zoologische Verhaltensforschung 759, 796
Zweckhandlung, Endeffekt einer 776
–, Heterogonie der 777
Zweck- und Zielbegriff 778
Zweck- und Zielbehandlung 776
Zwergwuchs („deprivation dwarfism") 733
Zwillingsforschung 548
„zykloide Psychosen" 585
Zyklothymie 109
–, biochemische Ergebnisse 66
–, neuroendokrinologische Ergebnisse 75